Mechanism-of-Action Illustrations (cont.)

P9-DGV-045

Drugs with illustrated mechanisms of action	Drugs with similar mechanisms of action
isosorbide dinitrate, isosorbide mononitrate	nitroglycerin
lanthanum carbonate	sevelamer hydrochloride
linezolid	none
memantine hydrochloride	none
milrinone lactate	none
nateglinide	repaglinide
olmesartan medoxomil	irbesartan, losartan potassium, valsartan
omeprazole	esomeprazole magnesium, lansoprazole, pantoprazole sodium, rabeprazole sodium
palonosetron hydrochloride	alosetron, dolasetron, granisetron, ondansetron
spironolactone	none
teriparatide	none

Discover the NDH App!

START YOUR FREE 30-DAY TRIAL TODAY!

Experience the convenience of having the trusted drug reference app with you everywhere you go. Designed for today's nurses, you'll love having this app for your classes, clinicals, and throughout your nursing career!

Download the **NDH app** to check out these features:

- Easy navigation
- Improved search
- Personalized note-taking & bookmarking
- Relevant news feed tailored to you
- Top trending drug searches in real-time
- Useful calculators for hard-to-remember formulas
- More to come!

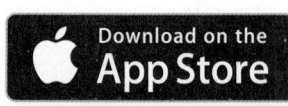

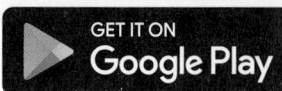

ATTENTION NURSING STUDENTS!

Visit **https://go.jblearning.com/NDHapp** to learn how you can **SAVE 25%** on your annual subscription.

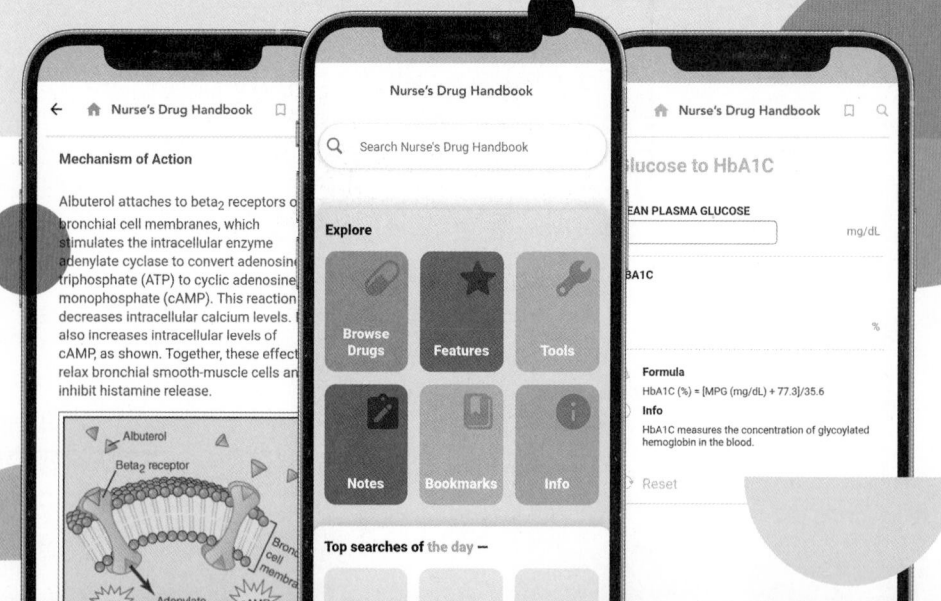

NDH

NURSE'S DRUG HANDBOOK

2023

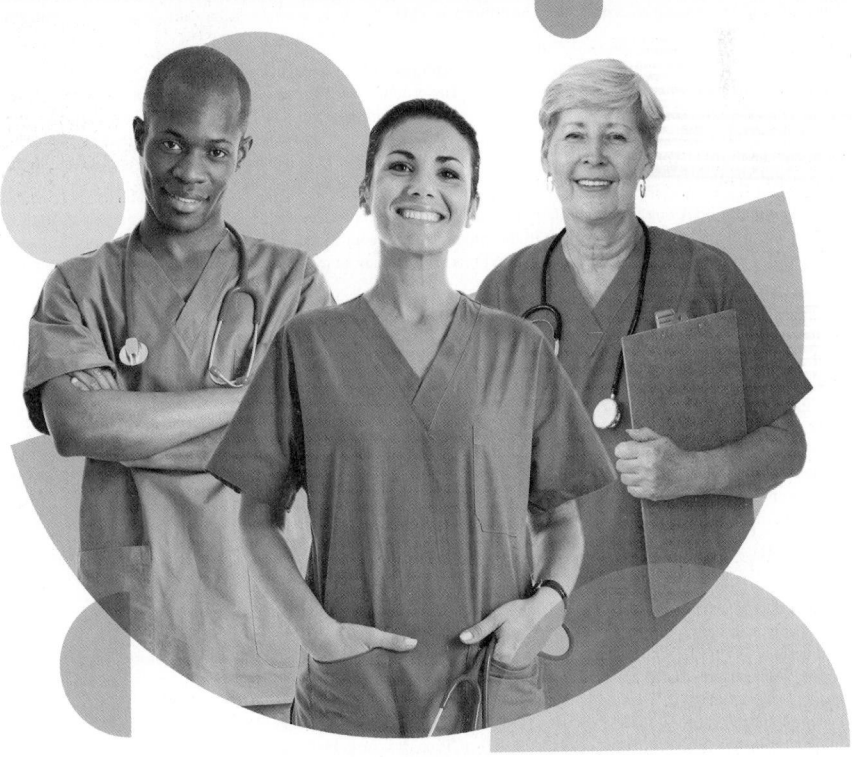

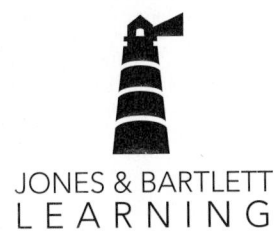

JONES & BARTLETT
LEARNING

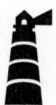

World Headquarters
Jones & Bartlett Learning
25 Mall Road
Burlington, MA 01803
978-443-5000
info@jblearning.com
www.jblearning.com

Jones & Bartlett Learning books and products are available through most bookstores and online booksellers. To contact Jones & Bartlett Learning directly, call 800-832-0034, fax 978-443-8000, or visit our website, www.jblearning.com.

Substantial discounts on bulk quantities of Jones & Bartlett Learning publications are available to corporations, professional associations, and other qualified organizations. For details and specific discount information, contact the special sales department at Jones & Bartlett Learning via the above contact information or send an email to specialsales@jblearning.com.

Copyright © 2023 by Jones & Bartlett Learning, LLC, an Ascend Learning Company

All rights reserved. No part of the material protected by this copyright may be reproduced or utilized in any form, electronic or mechanical, including photocopying, recording, or by any information storage and retrieval system, without written permission from the copyright owner.

The content, statements, views, and opinions herein are the sole expression of the respective authors and not that of Jones & Bartlett Learning, LLC. Reference herein to any specific commercial product, process, or service by trade name, trademark, manufacturer, or otherwise does not constitute or imply its endorsement or recommendation by Jones & Bartlett Learning, LLC and such reference shall not be used for advertising or product endorsement purposes. All trademarks displayed are the trademarks of the parties noted herein. *2023 Nurse's Drug Handbook, Twenty-Third Edition* is an independent publication and has not been authorized, sponsored, or otherwise approved by the owners of the trademarks or service marks referenced in this product.

There may be images in this book that feature models; these models do not necessarily endorse, represent, or participate in the activities represented in the images. Any screenshots in this product are for educational and instructive purposes only. Any individuals and scenarios featured in the case studies throughout this product may be real or fictitious but are used for instructional purposes only.

The authors, editor, and publisher have made every effort to provide accurate information. However, they are not responsible for errors, omissions, or for any outcomes related to the use of the contents of this book and take no responsibility for the use of the products and procedures described. Treatments and side effects described in this book may not be applicable to all people; likewise, some people may require a dose or experience a side effect that is not described herein. Drugs and medical devices are discussed that may have limited availability controlled by the Food and Drug Administration (FDA) for use only in a research study or clinical trial. Research, clinical practice, and government regulations often change the accepted standard in this field. When consideration is being given to use of any drug in the clinical setting, the healthcare provider or reader is responsible for determining FDA status of the drug, reading the package insert, and reviewing prescribing information for the most up-to-date recommendations on dose, precautions, and contraindications, and determining the appropriate usage for the product. This is especially important in the case of drugs that are new or seldom used.

ISBN: 978-1-284-27410-3

Production Credits
Vice President, Product Management: Marisa R. Urbano
Vice President, Content Strategy and Implementation: Christine Emerton
Director, Product Management: Matthew Kane
Product Manager: Joanna Gallant
Director, Content Management: Donna Gridley
Manager, Content Strategy: Carolyn Pershouse
Content Strategist: Christina Freitas
Content Strategist: Paula-Yuan Gregory
Content Coordinator: Samantha Gillespie
Director, Project Management and Content Services: Karen Scott
Manager, Program Management: Kristen Rogers
Project Manager: Belinda Thresher
Senior Digital Project Specialist: Angela Dooley
Director, Marketing: Andrea DeFronzo

Senior Product Marketing Manager: Lindsay White
Content Services Manager: Colleen Lamy
Vice President, Manufacturing and Inventory Control: Therese Connell
Product Fulfillment Manager: Wendy Kilborn
Composition: S4Carlisle Publishing Services
Project Management: S4Carlisle Publishing Services
Cover Design: Timothy Dziewit
Senior Media Development Editor: Troy Liston
Rights & Permissions Manager: John Rusk
Rights Specialist: James Fortney
Cover Image (Title Page, Part Opener, Chapter Opener): © Michaeljung/Shutterstock; © Minerva Studio/Shutterstock; © FabrikaSimf/Shutterstock
Printing and Binding: Mercury Printing

6048

Printed in the United States of America
26 25 24 23   10 9 8 7 6 5 4 3 2

Contents

Reviewers and Clinical Consultants

Reviewers

Peter J. Ambrose, PharmD
Clinical Professor
Los Angeles–Orange County Area Clerkships
University of California
San Francisco, California

Michael C. Barros, PharmD, BCPS, CACP
Clinical Assistant Professor of Pharmacy
  Practice
Temple University School of Pharmacy
Clinical Pharmacist, Heart Failure/Transplant
Temple University Hospital
Philadelphia, Pennsylvania

Edward M. Bednarczyk, PharmD
Clinical Assistant Professor
Pharmacy Practice and Nuclear Medicine
State University of New York at Buffalo
Buffalo, New York

Cristina E. Bello, PharmD
Assistant Professor of Pharmacy Practice
College of Pharmacy
Nova Southeastern University
Fort Lauderdale, Florida

Scott M. Bonnema, PharmD
Consultant Pharmacist
Emissary Pharmacy and Infusion
Casper, Wyoming

Felesia R. Bowen, RN, MS, PNP-C
Clinical Nurse Specialist
Children's Hospital at Robert Wood Johnson
  University Hospital
New Brunswick, New Jersey

Cynthia Burman, PharmD
Clinical Assistant Professor
School of Pharmacy
Temple University
Philadelphia, Pennsylvania

Marlene Ciranowicz, RN, BSN, MSN
Independent Consultant
Binghamton, New York

Jason M. Cota, PharmD, MS, BCPS
Assistant Professor
Department of Pharmacy Practice
University of the Incarnate Word
Feik School of Pharmacy
Infectious Diseases
Clinical Pharmacist
Brooke Army Medical Center
San Antonio, Texas

Kimberly A. Couch, PharmD
Clinical Pharmacy Specialist, Infectious
  Diseases
Department of Pharmacy
Christiana Care Health System
Newark, Delaware

Brenda S. Frymoyer, RN, MSN
Clinical Nurse Specialist
Berks Cardiologists, Inc.
Reading, Pennsylvania

Jason Gallagher, PharmD, BCPS
Associate Professor
Clinical Specialist, Infectious Diseases
Director, Infectious Diseases Pharmacotherapy
  Residency
Temple University
Philadelphia, Pennsylvania

Kimberly A. Galt, PharmD, FASHP
Associate Professor of Pharmacy Practice
Director
Drug Information Services
Co-Director
Center for Practice Improvement and Out-
  comes Research
Creighton University
Omaha, Nebraska

John Gatto, RPh
Clinical Pharmacist
Eckerd Pharmacy
Owego, New York

Deborah L. Green, RN, MSN
Director
Medical Telemetry-CHF Program
Moses H. Cone Health System
Greensboro, North Carolina

Ronald L. Greenberg, PharmD, CPS
Clinical Pharmacy Coordinator
Fairview Ridges Hospital
Burnsville, Minnesota

Jan K. Hastings, PharmD
Assistant Professor
College of Pharmacy
University of Arkansas for Medical Science
Little Rock, Arkansas

Maria Heaney, PharmD
Infectious Diseases Clinical Pharmacist
St. Joseph's University Medical Center
Paterson, New Jersey

Michael D. Hogue, PharmD
Assistant Professor of Pharmacy Practice
McWhorter School of Pharmacy
Samford University
Clinical Coordinator
Walgreens Drug Store
Birmingham, Alabama

Kimberly A. Hunter, PharmD
Assistant Professor of Pharmacy Practice
Albany College of Pharmacy
Albany, New York

William A. Kehoe, Jr., PharmD, CPS, FCCP
Professor of Clinical Pharmacy and Psychology
School of Pharmacy and Health Sciences
University of the Pacific
Stockton, California

Julienne K. Kirk, PharmD, CPS, CDE
Assistant Professor
Department of Family Medicine
School of Medicine
Wake Forest University
Winston-Salem, North Carolina

Peter G. Koval, PharmD, BCPS
Clinical Pharmacist
Moses H. Cone Family Practice
Greensboro, North Carolina

Lisa M. Krupa, RN-C, CEN, FNP
Nurse Practitioner
Medical Specialists
Munster, Indiana

Amista A. Lone, PharmD
Clinical Assistant Professor
College of Pharmacy
University of Arizona
Tucson, Arizona

Jennifer L. Lutz, PharmD
Pharmacy Resident
Samuel S. Stratton Veterans Affairs Medical
  Center
Albany, New York

T. Donald Marsh, PharmD, FASCP, ASHP
Director
Department of Pharmacotherapy
Mountain Area Health Education Center
Asheville, North Carolina

Patrick McDonnell, PharmD
Assistant Professor of Clinical Pharmacy
School of Pharmacy
Temple University
Philadelphia, Pennsylvania

Kenyetta N. Nesbitt, PharmD
Assistant Professor
Wayne State University
Detroit, Michigan

Catherine M. Oliphant, PharmD
Assistant Professor of Pharmacy Practice
School of Pharmacy
University of Wyoming
Laramie, Wyoming

Vinita B. Pai, PharmD
Assistant Professor of Clinical Pharmacy
College of Pharmacy
Ohio State University
Columbus, Ohio

David J. Quan, PharmD
Clinical Pharmacist
University of California, San Francisco
San Francisco, California

Brenda M. Reap-Thompson, RN, MSN
Assistant Clinical Professor
Drexel University
Philadelphia, Pennsylvania

Nancy Jex Sabin, RN, MSN, APRN
Clinical Assistant Professor
University of San Diego
San Diego, California

Elizabeth Sloand, PhD, RN, PNP-BC
Assistant Professor
School of Nursing
Johns Hopkins University
Baltimore, Maryland

Craig Williams, PharmD
Clinical Specialist
Wishard Memorial Hospital
Assistant Professor of Clinical Pharmacy
School of Pharmacy
Purdue University
Indianapolis, Indiana

Clinical Consultants

Madeline Albanese, RN, MSN
Nurse Educator
Hospital of the University of Pennsylvania
Philadelphia, Pennsylvania

Sheree M. Fitzgerald, RN-C, MSN, CNA
Program Coordinator
Ancora Psychiatric Hospital
Hammonton, New Jersey

Maryann Foley, RN, BSN
Independent Consultant
Flourtown, Pennsylvania

Grace Hukushi, RN, BSN, LNC
Critical Care Nurse
Nursing Enterprises, Inc.
Brick, New Jersey

Sammie Justesen, RN, BSN
Independent Nurse Consultant
Providence, Utah

Catherine T. Kelly, RN, PhD, CCRN, CEN, ANP
Faculty
School of Nursing
Mount Saint Mary College
Newburgh, New York

Sharon Kumm, RN, MN, CCRN
Assistant Professor
School of Nursing
University of Kansas
Kansas City, Kansas

Leanne McQuade, RN, BSN, CEN
Staff Nurse
Emergency Department
Doylestown Hospital
Case Manager
CAB Medical Consultant
Doylestown, Pennsylvania

Pamela S. Ronning, RN, MPA
Program Coordinator
Kirkhof College of Nursing
Grand Valley State University
Allendale, Michigan

Maureen Ryan, RN, CS, MSN, FNP
Assistant Professor
Grand Valley State University
Allendale, Michigan
Nurse Practitioner
Emergency Department
St. Mary's Hospital
Grand Rapids, Michigan

Julie M. Smith, RN, BA
Staff Nurse
Radiology-Heart Station
Rancocas Hospital
Willingboro, New Jersey

Aaron J. Strehlow, RN, PhD, FNP
Administrator and Director of Clinical Services
UCLA School of Nursing
Health Center at the Rescue Mission
Los Angeles, California

Maria Wilson, RN, MSN, CCRN
Staff Nurse
Emergency Department
Chestnut Hill Hospital
Philadelphia, Pennsylvania

How to Use This Book

The *Nurse's Drug Handbook* gives you what today's nurses and nursing students need: accurate, concise, and reliable drug facts. This book emphasizes the vital information you need to know before, during, and after drug administration. The information is presented in an easy-to-understand language and organized alphabetically, so you can find what you need quickly.

What's Special

In addition to the drug information you expect to find in each entry (see "Drug Entries" for details), the *Nurse's Drug Handbook* boasts these special features:

- **The design** makes it easy to find the most need-to-know drug information, such as indications, dosages, dosage adjustments, and warnings.
- **Introductory material** reviews essential general information you need to know to administer drugs safely and effectively, including an overview of pharmacology and the principles of drug administration. In addition, the five steps of the nursing process are explained and related specifically to drug therapy.
- **Highly useful illustrations** throughout the text help you visualize selected mechanisms of action by showing how drugs work at the cellular, tissue, and organ levels. In addition, the inside front cover features a table listing all the drugs whose mechanisms of action are illustrated, as well as other drugs with the same mechanisms of action.
- **No-nonsense writing style** speaks in everyday language and uses the terms and abbreviations you typically encounter in your practice and your studies.
- **Up-to-date drug information** includes the latest FDA-approved drugs, new and revised indications, latest drug administration instructions, new warnings, new drug interactions, newly reported adverse reactions, latest childbearing considerations, and changes in the nursing considerations and patient teachings to reflect new information.

- **Dosage adjustment,** headlined in color, alerts you to expected dosage changes for a patient with a specific condition or disorder, such as advanced age or renal impairment or concurrent drug therapy that may require an increase or decrease because of a potential interaction.
- **Warning,** displayed in color, calls attention to important facts that you need to know before, during, and after drug administration. For example, in the beclomethasone entry, this feature informs you that when gradually switching patient from oral corticosteroid to inhaled beclomethasone, you should watch for signs of life-threatening adrenal insufficiency, such as fatigue, hypotension, lassitude, nausea, vomiting, and weakness during the transition period and when exposed to infection, surgery, trauma, or other stressors.
- **Easy-to-use tables** showing route, onset, peak, and duration (see page xi for more details), and other tables in the appendices provide a time-saving way to track and check information. The appendices give you an overview of the most important facts and nursing considerations for important drug groups, including insulin preparations and oral allergen extracts, selected antihistamines, ophthalmics, topical drugs, antivirals, antineoplastic drugs, interferons, and antihypertensive combination drugs, as well as selected obstetrical drugs and vitamins. You'll also find information on less commonly used drugs and handy instructions for calculating drug dosages and I.V. flow rates.

Drug Entries

The *Nurse's Drug Handbook* clearly and concisely presents all the vital facts on the drugs that you'll typically administer. To help you find the information you need quickly, drug entries are organized alphabetically by generic drug name—from abacavir sulfate to zonisamide. For ease of use, every drug entry follows a consistent format.

GENERIC AND TRADE NAMES

First, each entry identifies the drug's main generic name, as well as alternate generic names. (For drugs prescribed by trade name, you can quickly check the comprehensive index, which refers you to the appropriate generic name and page.)

Next, the entry lists the most common U.S. trade names for each drug. It also includes common trade names available only in Canada, marked (CAN).

CLASS AND SCHEDULE

Each entry lists the drug's pharmacologic and therapeutic classes. With this information, you can compare drugs in the same pharmacologic class but in different therapeutic classes, and vice versa.

Where appropriate, the entry also includes the drug's controlled substance schedule. (For details, see *Controlled substance schedules*, page xi.)

INDICATIONS AND DOSAGES

This section lists FDA-approved therapeutic indications. For each indication, you'll find the applicable drug form or route, age group (adults, adolescents, or children), and dosage (which includes amount per dose, timing, and duration, when known and appropriate).

Drug Administration

This section provides you with what you need to know on how to safely administer the drug. The section clearly lists instructions for each route of administration that is possible and includes P.O., I.V., I.M., subcutaneous, inhaled, intranasal, or topical. The section under I.V. ends with a list of incompatibilities as indicated by the manufacturer.

ROUTE, ONSET, PEAK, DURATION, AND HALF-LIFE

Quick-reference tables show the drug's onset, peak, and duration (when known) for each administration route. The onset of action is the time a drug takes to be absorbed, reach a therapeutic blood level, and elicit an initial therapeutic response. The peak therapeutic effect occurs when a drug reaches its highest blood concentration and the greatest amount of drug reaches the site of action to produce the maximum therapeutic response. The duration of action is the amount of time the drug remains at a blood level that produces a therapeutic response. The drug's half-life (when known) determines the time it takes for half of the drug to be eliminated from the body.

Controlled substance schedules

The Controlled Substances Act of 1970 mandated that certain prescription drugs be categorized in schedules based on their potential for abuse. The greater their potential for abuse, the greater the restrictions on their prescription. The controlled substance schedules range from I to V, signifying highest to lowest abuse potential.

I High potential for abuse

No accepted medical use exists for schedule I drugs, which include heroin and lysergic acid diethylamide (LSD).

II High potential for abuse

Use may lead to severe physical or psychological dependence. Prescriptions must be written in ink or typewritten and must be signed by the prescriber. Oral prescriptions must be confirmed in writing within 72 hours and may be given only in a genuine emergency. No renewals are permitted.

III Some potential for abuse

Use may lead to low-to-moderate physical dependence or high psychological dependence. Prescriptions may be oral or written. Up to five renewals are permitted within 6 months.

IV Low potential for abuse

Use may lead to limited physical or psychological dependence. Prescriptions may be oral or written. Up to five renewals are allowed within 6 months.

V Subject to state and local regulation

Abuse potential is low; a prescription may not be required.

MECHANISM OF ACTION

This section concisely describes how a drug achieves its therapeutic effects at cellular, tissue, and organ levels, as appropriate. Illustrations of selected mechanisms of action lend exceptional clarity to sometimes complex processes.

CONTRAINDICATIONS

An alphabetical list details the conditions and disorders that preclude administration of the drug.

INTERACTIONS

This section includes drugs, foods, and activities (such as alcohol use and smoking) that can cause important, problematic, or life-threatening interactions with the topic drug. For each interacting drug, food, or activity, you'll learn the effects of the interaction.

ADVERSE REACTIONS

Organized by body system, this section lists common, serious, and life-threatening adverse reactions. Life-threatening adverse reactions are bolded for easy identification.

CHILDBEARING CONSIDERATIONS

After June 30, 2015, new prescription drugs submitted to the FDA for approval will no longer be allowed to use the lettering system to categorize drugs based on their potential to cause fetal harm such as A, B, C, D, or X. Instead, a new, more comprehensive text is being required in the packaging label to explain the risks. Prescription drugs currently using the lettering system to identify potential for a drug to cause fetal harm will be gradually phased into the new labeling requirement. Labeling of over-the-counter drugs will remain unchanged and is not affected by the FDA mandated change.

The Childbearing Consideration section provides information using the new guidelines. This section is subdivided into four categories consisting of pregnancy risks, labor and delivery risks, and lactation risks, if present, to the fetus or newborn and the fourth category indicating any reproductive risks the drug may pose.

Federal guidelines for drug disposal

Give patients these important instructions for properly disposing of their unwanted prescription drugs:

- Consider mixing discarded prescription drugs with a substance like coffee grounds or used cat litter and putting them in impermeable, nondescript containers, such as empty cans or sealable bags.
- Flush prescription drugs down the toilet only if the label or accompanying patient information specifically tells you to do so.
- See if your community has a pharmaceutical take-back program that allows citizens to bring unused drugs to a central location for proper disposal.

NURSING CONSIDERATIONS

Warnings, general precautions, and key information that you must know before, during, and after drug administration are detailed in this section. Examples include cautions certain populations require and types of monitoring needed.

Patient-teaching information is also included here. You'll find important guidelines for patients, such as how and when to take each prescribed drug, how to spot and manage adverse reactions, which cautions to observe, when to call the prescriber, and more. To save your time, however, this section doesn't repeat basic patient-teaching points. (For a summary of those, see *Teaching your patient about drug therapy*, page xiii, and *Federal guidelines for drug disposal*, page xii.)

In short, the *Nurse's Drug Handbook* is designed expressly to give you more of what you need. It puts vital drug information at your fingertips and helps you always stay current in this critical part of your practice or studies.

Teaching your patient about drug therapy

Your teaching about drug therapy will vary with your patient's needs and your practice setting. To guide your teaching, each drug entry provides key information that you must teach your patient about that drug. For all patients, however, you also should:

- Teach the generic and trade name for each prescribed drug that they'll take after discharge—even if they took the drug before admission.
- Clearly explain why each drug was prescribed, how it works, and what it's supposed to do. To help your patient understand the drug's therapeutic effects, relate its action to their disorder or condition.
- Review the drug form, dosage, and route with the patient. Tell them whether the drug is a tablet, suppository, spray, aerosol, or other form, and explain how to take it correctly. Also, tell them how often to take the drug and for what length of time. Emphasize that they should take the drug exactly as prescribed.
- Describe the drug's appearance, and explain that scored tablets can be broken in half for safe, accurate dosing. Warn the patient not to break unscored tablets, because doing so may alter the drug dosage. If your patient has trouble swallowing capsules, tell them to inquire if the capsule can be opened and sprinkled on food or mixed in a beverage; some can and some cannot. If the capsule should not be opened, have patient ask about being switched to a liquid form, if available. Also, warn them not to crush or chew enteric-coated, extended-release, sustained-release, or similar drug forms.
- Teach the patient about common adverse reactions that may occur. Advise them to notify the prescriber at once if a dangerous adverse reaction, such as syncope, occurs.
- Warn them not to suddenly stop taking a drug if they're bothered by unpleasant adverse reactions, such as nausea or mild itching. Instead, encourage them to discuss the reactions with their prescriber,

who may adjust the dosage or substitute a drug that causes fewer adverse reactions.
- Tell patient that if a drug is known to cause adverse reactions (such as dizziness and drowsiness) that can impair the patient's ability to perform activities that require alertness, help them develop a dosing schedule that minimizes these adverse reactions.
- Inform the patient which adverse reactions resolve with time.
- Teach the patient how to store the drug properly. Let them know if the drug is sensitive to light or temperature and how to protect it from these elements.
- Instruct the patient to store the drug in its original container, if possible, with the drug's name and dosage clearly printed on the label.
- Inform the patient which devices to use— and which to avoid—for drug storage or administration. For example, warn them not to take liquid cyclosporine with a plastic cup or utensils.
- Teach the patient what to do if they miss a dose. Generally, they should take a once-daily drug as soon as they remember—provided it is not close to the end of the 24 hours when the next dose is due. Warn them never to double the dose to make up for a missed dose. If they have questions or concerns about missed doses, tell them to contact their prescriber.
- Provide information specific to the prescribed drug. For example, if a patient takes a diuretic to manage heart failure, instruct them to weigh themselves daily at the same time of day, using the same scale, and wearing the same amount of clothing. Or, if the patient takes digoxin or an antihypertensive drug, teach them how to measure their pulse and blood pressure and how to record the measurements. Then instruct

them to bring the diary to their regular appointments so the prescriber can monitor their response to the drug.
- Advise the patient to refill prescriptions promptly, unless they no longer need the drug. Also instruct them to discard expired drugs because they may become ineffective or even dangerous over time.
- Warn the patient to keep all drugs out of the reach of children at all times.

Foreword

Safe, effective drug therapy is one of your most important responsibilities. Not infrequently, a patient's life will depend on your ability to give drugs accurately and safely. In addition, you must keep up with the latest drug information, including newly approved drugs and recently reported life-threatening adverse reactions, as well as those drugs withdrawn from the market after widespread use.

Despite all the drug information available, medication errors remain one of the greatest threats to patients' well-being and a leading cause of lawsuits against nurses, physicians, and hospitals.

Your Responsibilities in Drug Therapy

Your basic responsibilities in drug therapy include the following:

- Administer the right drug in the right dose by the right route at the right time to the right patient using the right preparation and administration.
- Know the therapeutic use, dosage, interactions, adverse reactions, and warnings of each administered drug.
- Be aware of newly approved drugs that may be prescribed.
- Know about changes to existing drugs, such as new indications and dosages and recently discovered adverse reactions and interactions.
- Concentrate fully when preparing and administering drugs.
- Respond promptly and appropriately to serious or life-threatening adverse reactions, interactions, and complications.
- Instruct each patient about the drug, how it's administered, which effects it causes or may cause, and which reactions to watch for and report.

Several factors may reduce your ability to meet these basic responsibilities—and contribute to medication errors. First, hospitals and other healthcare facilities have budget constraints that may result in elimination of professional nursing positions or the hiring of less qualified technicians to fill them. This forces the remaining nurses to care for more patients. Second, many hospital patients are older and more acutely ill, and they typically receive more complex drug therapy. Together, these factors place greater demands on you—increasing your stress level, reducing the time you have to concentrate on drug administration, and increasing your risk of making medication errors or overlooking serious adverse reactions or interactions.

The same factors reduce your time and energy for learning the latest drug facts—which you need to have at your command. You must have this information at your fingertips because your next patient may need a recently approved drug or a complex and unfamiliar drug regimen.

How can you balance your limited time with your need to know the latest developments?

Meeting Your Needs

Nurses and students need a reliable, accurate, easy-to-use, quick-reference drug book. They need a book clearly written by and for nurses that has been reviewed by experts in nursing and pharmacology. You hold such a book in your hands: the *Nurse's Drug Handbook,* with features that are always current.

The content of the *Nurse's Drug Handbook* was developed, written, and edited by experienced practicing nurses. Expert consultants, reviewers, and advisors—both nurses and pharmacists—help ensure the accuracy and reliability of the information covered in each entry and help target that information to your needs. What's more, every drug fact is checked against the most prominent drug references today, including information approved by the FDA. In addition, to help you quickly access much-needed information, the book is organized alphabetically by generic drug name, follows a consistent format, and is concise.

To ensure that you're always current, the *Nurse's Drug Handbook* is updated every year. This newest edition contains:

- Important new drug entries in the main part of the book and in the appendices.
- New drug facts on hundreds of existing entries, including updated information on new indications and dosages, new guidelines for preparing and administering the drug, new interactions, new adverse reactions, new childbearing considerations, and new nursing considerations.
- Hundreds of patient-teaching guidelines and suggestions.

And as always, you'll find the same color-coded, highly readable type that reduces eyestrain as you speed to the information you need.

Getting More from Your Drug Reference Handbook

Whether you currently work in or are preparing to work in acute care, home care, long-term care, or another healthcare setting, you'll want your own copy of the *Nurse's Drug Handbook*. That's because this book can help you:

- Reduce your risk of medication errors because you'll have easy access to accurate, reliable drug information that's relevant to your practice.
- Stay current on the most up-to-date drug developments of the year.
- Improve your drug administration skills and patient care before, during, and after drug therapy.
- Quickly detect and manage serious or life-threatening adverse reactions and

complications or prevent them from occurring.

- Save time because you won't have to sift through volumes of information to find what you need, search for a book that's up-to-date, or look through several drug handbooks to get enough information.
- Increase your confidence about drug administration and enhance your professional interactions with other healthcare team members.
- Ensure the delivery of safe, effective care.
- Improve the depth and quality of your patient teaching.

Reaping the Rewards

Your patients deserve the best and safest care possible—and you deserve to have the tools to deliver that care. Whether you're a student or an experienced clinician, the *Nurse's Drug Handbook* will help you provide safe, effective drug therapy because of its practical, easy-to-understand, accurate, and reliable information on virtually all the drugs you're likely to administer.

This handbook has aided thousands of nurses in their patient care. Take it with you to the clinical setting, share it with your peers, and use it to enhance your present and future position in the nursing profession.

Kathleen Dracup, RN, FNP, DNSc, FAAN
Dean and Professor
School of Nursing
University of California, San Francisco
San Francisco, California

Overview of Pharmacology

Understanding the basics of pharmacology is an essential nursing responsibility. Pharmacology is the science that deals with the physical and chemical properties, and biochemical and physiologic effects, of drugs. It includes the areas of pharmacokinetics, pharmacodynamics, pharmacotherapeutics, pharmacognosy, and toxicodynamics.

The *Nurse's Drug Handbook* deals primarily with pharmacokinetics, pharmacodynamics, and pharmacotherapeutics—the information you need to administer safe and effective drug therapy (discussed as follows). Pharmacognosy is the branch of pharmacology that deals with the biological, biochemical, and economic features of naturally occurring drugs. Toxicodynamics is the study of the harmful effects that excessive amounts of a drug produce in the body; in a drug overdose or drug poisoning, large drug doses may saturate or overwhelm normal mechanisms that control absorption, distribution, metabolism, and excretion.

Drug Nomenclature

Most drugs are known by several names—chemical, generic, trade, and official—each of which serves a specific function. (See *How drugs are named*.) However, multiple drug names can also contribute to medication errors. You may find a familiar drug packaged with an unfamiliar name if your institution changes suppliers or if a familiar drug is newly approved in a different dose or for a new indication.

How drugs are named

A drug's chemical, generic, trade, and official names are determined at different phases of the drug development process and serve different functions. For example, the various names of the commonly prescribed anticonvulsant divalproex sodium are:

- Chemical name: pentanoic acid, 2-propyl-, sodium salt (2:1), or ($C_{16}H_{31}O_4Na$)
- Generic name: divalproex sodium
- Trade name: Depakote
- Official name: divalproex sodium delayed-release tablets, USP

A drug's chemical name describes its atomic and molecular structure. The chemical name of divalproex sodium—pentanoic acid, 2-propyl-, sodium salt (2:1), or $C_{16}H_{31}O_4Na$ (pronounced valproate semisodium)—indicates that the drug is a combination of two valproic acid compounds with a sodium molecule attached to only one side.

Once a drug successfully completes several clinical trials, it receives a generic name, also known as the nonproprietary name. The generic name is usually derived from, but shorter than, the chemical name. The United States Adopted Names Council is responsible for selecting generic names, which are intended for unrestricted public use.

Before submitting the drug for FDA approval, the manufacturer creates and registers a trade name (or brand name) when the drug appears ready to be marketed. Trade names are copyrighted and followed by the symbol ® to indicate that they're registered and that their use is restricted to the drug manufacturer. Once the original patent on a drug has expired, any manufacturer may produce the drug under its own trade name.

A drug's official name is the name under which it's listed in the United States Pharmacopoeia (USP) and the National Formulary (NF).

Drug Classification

Drugs can be classified in various ways. Most pharmacology textbooks group drugs by their functional classification, such as psychotherapeutics, which is based on common characteristics. Drugs can also be classified according to their therapeutic use, such as antipanic or antiobsessional drugs. Drugs within a certain therapeutic class may be further divided into subgroups based on their mechanisms of action. For example, the therapeutic class antineoplastics can be further classified as alkylating agents, antibiotic antineoplastics, antimetabolites, antimitotics, biological response modifiers, antineoplastic enzymes, and hormonal antineoplastics.

Pharmacokinetics

Pharmacokinetics is the study of a drug's actions—or fate—as it passes through the body during absorption, distribution, metabolism, and excretion.

ABSORPTION

Before a drug can begin working, it must be transformed from its pharmaceutical dosage form to a biologically available (bioavailable) substance that can pass through various biological cell membranes to reach its site of action. This process is known as absorption. A drug's absorption rate depends on its route of administration, its circulation through the tissue into which it's administered, and its solubility—that is, whether it's more water soluble (*hydrophilic*) or fat soluble (*lipophilic*).

Although drugs may penetrate cellular membranes either actively or passively, most drugs do so by *passive diffusion*, moving inertly from an area of higher concentration to an area of lower concentration. Passive diffusion may occur through water or fat. Passive diffusion through water—*aqueous diffusion*—occurs within large water-filled compartments, such as interstitial spaces, and across epithelial membrane tight junctions and pores in the epithelial lining of blood vessels. Aqueous diffusion is driven by concentration gradients. Drug molecules that are bound to large plasma proteins, such as albumin, are too large to pass through aqueous pores in this way. Passive diffusion through fat—*lipid diffusion*—plays an important role in drug metabolism because of the large number of lipid barriers that separate the aqueous compartments of the body. The tendency of a drug to move through lipid layers between aqueous compartments often depends on the pH of the medium—that is, the ability of the water-soluble or fat-soluble drug to form weak acid or weak base.

Drugs with molecules that are too large to readily diffuse may rely on active *diffusion*, in which special carriers on molecules, including peptides, amino acids, and glucose, transport the drug through the membranes. However, some molecules with selective membrane carriers can expel foreign drug molecules; this is why many drugs can't cross the blood–brain barrier.

Drug absorption begins at the administration route. The three main administration route categories are enteral, parenteral, and transcutaneous. Depending on its nature or chemical makeup, a drug may be better absorbed from one site than from another.

Enteral Administration

Enteral administration consists of the oral, nasogastric, and rectal routes.

Oral: Drugs administered orally are absorbed in the GI tract and then proceed by the hepatic portal vein to the liver and into the systemic circulation. Although generally considered the preferred route, oral drug administration has a number of disadvantages:

- The oral route doesn't always yield sufficiently high blood concentrations to be effective.
- Bioavailability may be less than optimal because of incomplete absorption and first-pass elimination (the part of metabolism that occurs during transit through the liver before the drug reaches the general circulation).
- Drug absorption may be incomplete if the drug is degraded by digestive enzymes or the acidic pH in the stomach or if it's excreted from the liver into the bile.
- Food in the GI tract, gastric emptying time, and intestinal motility may also impede drug absorption.

Nasogastric: Drugs administered through a nasogastric tube enter the stomach directly and are absorbed in the GI tract.

Rectal: Rectal drugs and suppositories also enter the GI tract directly after being inserted in the rectum and absorbed through the rectal mucosa. After being absorbed into the lower GI tract, rectal drugs enter the circulation through the inferior vena cava, bypassing the liver and thus avoiding first-pass metabolism. Suppositories, however, tend to travel upward into the rectum, where veins, such as the superior hemorrhoidal vein, lead to the liver. As a result, drug absorption by this route is often unreliable and difficult to predict.

Parenteral Administration

Parenteral routes may be used whenever enteral routes are contraindicated, inadequate, or unavailable. These routes include intramuscular (I.M.), intravenous (I.V.), subcutaneous, and intradermal administration. Drug absorption is much faster and more predictable after parenteral administration than after enteral administration.

I.M.: Drugs administered by the I.M. route are injected deep into the muscle, where they're absorbed relatively quickly. The rate of drug absorption depends on the vascularity of the injection site, the physiochemical properties of the drug, and the solution in which the drug is contained.

I.V.: I.V. drug administration involves injecting or infusing the drug directly into the blood circulation, allowing for rapid distribution throughout the body. This route usually provides the greatest bioavailability.

Subcutaneous: Drugs administered by the subcutaneous route are injected into the connective tissue just below the skin and are absorbed by simple diffusion from the injection site. The factors that affect I.M. absorption also affect subcutaneous absorption. Absorption by the subcutaneous route may be slower than by the I.M. route.

Intradermal: Drugs administered intradermally, such as purified protein derivative (PPD), are injected into the dermis, from which they diffuse slowly into the local microcapillary system.

Transcutaneous Administration

Transcutaneous drug administration allows drug absorption through the skin or soft-tissue surface. Drugs may be inhaled, inserted sublingually, applied topically, or administered to the eyes, ears, nose, or vagina.

Inhalation: Inhaled drugs may be given as a powder and aerosolized or mixed in solution and nebulized directly into the respiratory tract, where they're absorbed through the alveoli. Inhaled drugs are usually absorbed quickly because of the abundant blood flow in the lungs, though some inhaled drugs have low systemic absorption.

Sublingual: Sublingual drug administration involves placing a tablet, troche, or lozenge under the tongue. The drug is absorbed across the epithelial lining of the mouth, usually quickly. This route avoids first-pass metabolism.

Topical: Topical drugs—creams, ointments, lotions, and patches—are placed on the skin and then cross the epidermis into the capillary circulation. They may also be absorbed through sweat glands, hair follicles, and other skin structures. Absorption by the skin is enhanced if the drug is in a solution.

Ophthalmic: Ophthalmic drugs include solutions and ointments that are instilled or applied directly to the cornea or conjunctiva as well as small, elliptical disks that are placed directly on the eyeball behind the lower eyelid. The movements of the eyeball promote distribution of these drugs over the surface of the eye. Although ophthalmic drugs produce a local effect on the conjunctiva or anterior chamber, some preparations may be absorbed systemically and therefore produce systemic effects.

Otic: Drops administered into the external auditory canal, otic drugs are used to treat infection or inflammation and to soften and remove ear wax. Otic solutions exert a local effect and may result in minimal systemic absorption with no adverse effects.

Nasal: Nasal solutions and suspensions are applied directly to the nasal mucosa by instillation or inhalation to produce local effects, such as vasoconstriction to reduce nasal congestion. Some nasal solutions, such as mometasone furoate monohydrate, are administered by this route specifically to produce systemic effects.

Vaginal: Vaginal drugs include creams, suppositories, and troches that are inserted into the vagina, sometimes using a special applicator. These drugs are administered locally to treat such conditions as bacterial and fungal infections.

DISTRIBUTION

Distribution is the process by which a drug is transported by the circulating fluids to various sites, including its sites of action. To ensure maximum therapeutic effectiveness, the drug must permeate all membranes that separate it from its intended site of action. Drug distribution is influenced by blood flow, tissue availability, and protein binding. Drugs that cannot distribute to the tissues in which they are needed are not effective.

METABOLISM

Drug metabolism is the enzymatic conversion of a drug's structure into substrate molecules or polar compounds that are either less active or inactive and are readily excreted. Drugs can also be synthesized to larger molecules. Metabolism may also convert a drug to a more toxic compound. Because the primary site of drug metabolism is the liver, children, the elderly, and patients with impaired hepatic function are at risk for altered therapeutic effects.

Biotransformation is the process of changing a drug into its active metabolite. Compounds that require metabolic biotransformation for activation are known as *prodrugs*. During phase I of biotransformation, the parent drug is converted into an inactive or partially active metabolite. Much of the original drug may be eliminated during this phase. During phase II, the inactive or partially active metabolite binds with available substrates, such as acetic acid, glucuronic acid, sulfuric acid, or water, to form its active metabolite. When biotransformation leads to synthesis, larger molecules are produced to create a pharmacologic effect.

EXCRETION

The body eliminates drugs by both metabolism and excretion. Drug metabolites—and, in some cases, the active drug itself—are eventually excreted from the body, usually through bile, feces, and urine. The primary organ for drug elimination is the kidney. Impaired renal function may alter drug elimination, thereby altering the drug's therapeutic effect. Other excretion routes include evaporation through the skin, exhalation from the lungs, and secretion into saliva and breast milk.

A drug's elimination half-life is the amount of time required for half of the drug to be eliminated from the body. The half-life roughly correlates with the drug's duration of action and is based on normal renal and hepatic function. Typically, the longer the half-life, the less often the drug has to be given and the longer it remains in the body.

Pharmacodynamics

Pharmacodynamics is the study of the biochemical and physiologic effects of drugs and their mechanisms of action. A drug's actions may be structurally specific or nonspecific. Structurally specific drugs combine with cell receptors, such as proteins or glycoproteins, to enhance or inhibit cellular enzyme actions. Drug receptors are the cellular components affected at the site of action. Many drugs form chemical bonds with drug receptors, but a drug can bond with a receptor only if it has a similar shape—much the same way that a key fits into a lock. When a drug combines with a receptor, channels are either opened or closed and cellular biochemical messengers, such as cyclic adenosine monophosphate or calcium ions, are activated. Once activated, cellular functions can be turned either on or off by these messengers.

Structurally nonspecific drugs, such as biological response modifiers, don't combine with cell receptors; rather, they produce changes within the cell membrane or interior.

The mechanisms by which drugs interact with the body are not always known. Drugs may work by physical action (such as the protective effects of a topical ointment) or chemical reaction (such as an antacid's effect on the gastric mucosa), or by modifying the metabolic activity of invading pathogens (such as an antibiotic) or replacing a missing biochemical substance (such as insulin).

AGONISTS

Agonists are drugs that interact with a receptor to stimulate a response. They alter cell physiology by binding to plasma membranes or intracellular structures. *Partial agonists* can't achieve maximal effects even though they may occupy all available receptor sites on a cell. *Strong agonists* can cause maximal effects while occupying only a small number of receptor sites on a cell. *Weak agonists* must occupy many more receptor sites than strong agonists to produce the same effect.

ANTAGONISTS

Antagonists are drugs that attach to a receptor but don't stimulate a response; instead, they inhibit or block responses that would normally be caused by agonists. *Competitive antagonists* bind to receptor sites that are also compatible with an agonist, thus preventing the agonist from binding to the site. *Noncompetitive antagonists* bind to receptor sites that aren't occupied by an agonist; this changes the receptor site so that it's no longer recognized by the agonist. *Irreversible antagonists* work in much the same way that noncompetitive ones do, except that they permanently bind with the receptor.

Antagonism plays an important role in drug interactions. When two agonists that cause opposite therapeutic effects, such as a vasodilator and a vasoconstrictor, are combined, the effects cancel each other out. When two antagonists, such as morphine and naloxone, are combined, both drugs may become inactive.

Pharmacotherapeutics

Pharmacotherapeutics is the study of how drugs are used to prevent or treat disease. Understanding why a drug is prescribed for a certain disease can assist you in prioritizing drug administration with other patient care activities. Knowing a drug's desired and unwanted effects may help you uncover problems not readily apparent from the admitting diagnosis. This information may also help you prevent such problems as adverse reactions and drug interactions.

A drug's *desired effect* is the intended or expected clinical response to the drug. This is the response you start to evaluate as soon as a drug is given. Dosage adjustments and the continuation of therapy often depend on your accurate evaluation and documentation of the patient's response.

An *adverse reaction* is any noxious and unintended response to a drug that occurs at therapeutic doses used for prophylaxis, diagnosis, or therapy. Adverse reactions associated with excessive amounts of a drug are considered drug overdoses. Be prepared to follow your institution's policy for reporting adverse drug reactions.

An *idiosyncratic response* is a genetically determined abnormal or excessive response to a drug that occurs in a particular patient. The unusual response may indicate that the drug has saturated or overwhelmed mechanisms that normally control absorption, distribution, metabolism, or excretion, thus altering the expected response. You may be unsure whether a reaction is adverse or idiosyncratic. Once you report the reaction, the pharmacist usually determines the appropriate course of action.

An *allergic reaction* is an adverse response that results from previous exposure to the same drug or to one that's chemically similar to it. The patient's immune system reacts to the drug as if it were a foreign invader and may produce a mild hypersensitivity reaction, characterized by localized dermatitis or photosensitivity. Allergic reactions should be reported to the prescriber immediately as some reactions may become serious or even life-threatening, requiring the drug to be discontinued. Follow-up care may include giving drugs, including antihistamines and corticosteroids, to counteract the allergic response.

An *anaphylactic reaction* involves an immediate hypersensitivity response characterized by urticaria, pruritus, and angioedema. Left untreated, an anaphylactic reaction can lead to systemic involvement, resulting in shock. It's often associated with life-threatening hypotension and respiratory distress. Be prepared to assist with emergency life-support measures, especially if the reaction occurs in response to I.V. drugs, which have the fastest rate of absorption.

A *drug interaction* occurs when one drug alters the pharmacokinetics of another drug—for example, when two or more drugs are given concurrently. Such concurrent administration can increase or decrease the therapeutic or adverse effects of either drug. Some drug interactions are beneficial. For example, when taken with penicillin, probenecid decreases the excretion rate of penicillin, resulting in higher blood levels of penicillin. Drug interactions also may occur when a drug's metabolism is altered, often owing to the induction of or competition for metabolizing enzymes. For example, H_2-receptor agonists, which reduce secretion of the enzyme gastrin, may alter the breakdown of enteric coatings on other drugs. Drug interactions due to carrier protein competition typically occur when a drug inhibits the kidneys' ability to reduce excretion of other drugs. For example, probenecid is completely reabsorbed by the renal tubules and is metabolized very slowly. It competes with the same carrier protein as sulfonamides for active tubular secretion and so decreases the renal excretion of sulfonamides. This particular competition can lead to an increased risk of sulfonamide toxicity.

Special Considerations

Although every drug has a usual dosage range, certain factors—such as a patient's age, weight, culture and ethnicity, gender, pregnancy status, and renal and hepatic function—may contribute to the need for dosage adjustments. When you encounter special considerations such as these, be prepared to reassess the prescribed dosage to make sure that it's safe and effective for your patient.

CULTURE AND ETHNICITY

Certain drugs are more effective or more likely to produce adverse effects in particular ethnic groups or races. For example, Asian patients being treated for hyperlipidemia with rosuvastatin require a smaller dose to decrease the risk of adverse reactions while African Americans have an increased risk of developing angioedema with angiotensin-converting enzyme (ACE) inhibitors. A patient's religious or cultural background also may call for special consideration. For example, a drug made from porcine products may be unacceptable to a Jewish or Muslim patient.

ELDERLY PATIENTS

Because aging produces certain changes in body composition and organ function, elderly patients present unique therapeutic and dosing problems that require special attention. For example, the weight of the liver, the number of functioning hepatic cells, and hepatic blood flow all decrease as a person ages, resulting in slower drug metabolism. Renal function may also decrease with aging. These processes can lead to the accumulation of active drugs and metabolites as well as increased sensitivity to the effects of some drugs in elderly patients. Because they're also more likely to have multiple chronic illnesses, many elderly patients take multiple prescription drugs each day, thus increasing the risk of drug interactions.

CHILDREN

Because their bodily functions aren't fully developed, children—particularly those under age 12—may metabolize drugs differently than adults. In infants, immature renal and hepatic functions delay metabolism and excretion of drugs. As a result, pediatric drug dosages are very different from adult dosages.

The FDA has provided drug manufacturers with guidelines that define pediatric age categories. Unless the manufacturer provides a specific age range, use these categories as a guide when administering drugs:

- neonates—birth up to age 1 month
- infants—ages 1 month to 2 years
- children—ages 2 to 12
- adolescents—ages 12 to 16

CHILDBEARING CONSIDERATIONS

The many physiologic changes that take place in the body during the childbearing process may affect a drug's pharmacokinetics and alter its effectiveness. Additionally, exposure to drugs may pose risks for the developing fetus. Before administering a drug to a pregnant patient, be sure to check the new more comprehensive text for drugs and intervene appropriately.

Principles of Drug Administration

Because there are thousands of drugs and hundreds of facts about each one, taking responsibility for drug administration can seem overwhelming. One way that you can enhance your understanding of the principles of drug administration is to *associate, ask,* and *predict* during the critical thinking process. For example, associate each drug with general information you may already know about the drug or drug class. *Ask* yourself why a drug is administered by a certain route and why it's given multiple times throughout the day rather than only once. Learn to *predict* a drug's actions, uses, adverse effects, and possible drug interactions based on your knowledge of the drug's mechanism of action. As you apply these principles to drug administration, you'll begin to intuitively know which facts you need to make rational clinical decisions.

Prescriptions for patients in hospitals and other institutions typically are written by a physician, physician assistant, or nurse practitioner on a form called the *physician's order sheet* or they're directly input into a computerized system with an electronic signature. Drugs are prescribed based not only on their specific mechanisms of action but also on the patient's profile, which commonly includes age, ethnicity, gender, pregnancy status, smoking and drinking habits, and use of other drugs.

"Rights" of Drug Administration

Always keep in mind the following "rights" of drug administration: the right drug, right time, right dose, right patient, right route, and right preparation and administration.

RIGHT DRUG

Many drugs have similar spellings, different concentrations, and several generic forms. Before administering any drug, compare the exact spelling and concentration of the prescribed drug that appears on the label with the information contained in the medication administration record or drug profile. Regardless of which drug distribution system your facility uses, you should read the drug label and compare it to the medication administration record at least three times:

- before removing the drug from the dispensing unit or unit dose cart
- before preparing or measuring the prescribed dose
- before opening a unit dose package (just before administering the drug to the patient).

RIGHT TIME

Various factors can affect the time that a drug is administered, such as the timing of meals and other drugs, scheduled diagnostic tests, standardized times used by the institution, and factors that may alter the consistency of blood levels and drug absorption. Before administering any p.r.n. drug, check the patient's chart to ensure that no one else has already administered it and that the specified time interval has passed. Also, document administration of a p.r.n. drug immediately.

RIGHT DOSE

Whenever you're dispensing an unfamiliar drug or are in doubt about a dosage, check the prescribed dose against the range specified in a reliable reference. Be sure to consider any reasons for a dosage adjustment that may apply to your particular patient. Also, make sure you're familiar with the standard abbreviations your institution uses for writing prescriptions.

RIGHT PATIENT

Always compare the name of the patient on the medication record with the name on the patient's identification bracelet. When using a unit dose system, compare the name on the drug profile with that on the identification bracelet.

RIGHT ROUTE

Each drug prescription should specify the administration route. If the administration route is missing from the prescription, consult the prescriber before giving the drug. Never substitute one route for another unless you obtain a prescription for the change.

RIGHT PREPARATION AND ADMINISTRATION

For drugs that have to be mixed, poured, or measured, be sure to maintain aseptic technique. Follow any specific directions included by the manufacturer regarding diluent type and amount and the use of filters, if needed. Clearly label any drug that you've reconstituted with the patient's name, the strength or dose, the date and time that you prepared the drug, the amount and type of diluent that you used, the expiration date, and your initials.

Administration Routes

Drugs may be administered by a variety of routes and dosage forms. A particular route may be chosen for convenience or to maximize drug concentration at the site of action, to minimize drug absorption elsewhere, to prolong drug absorption, or to avoid first-pass metabolism.

Different dosage forms of the same drug may have different drug absorption rates, times of onset, and durations of action. For example, nitroglycerin is a coronary vasodilator that may be administered by the I.V., sublingual, oral, or buccal route, or as a topical ointment or disk. The I.V., sublingual, and buccal forms of nitroglycerin provide a rapid onset of action, whereas the oral, ointment, and disk forms have a slower onset and a prolonged duration of action.

Drug administration routes include the enteral, parenteral, and transcutaneous routes.

ENTERAL

The enteral route consists of oral, nasogastric, and rectal administration. Drugs administered enterally enter the blood circulation by way of the GI tract. This route is considered the most natural and convenient route as well as the safest. As a result, most drugs are taken enterally, usually to provide systemic effects.

Oral

- *Tablets:* Tablets, the most commonly used dosage form, come in a variety of colors, sizes, and shapes. Some tablets are specially coated for various purposes. Enteric coatings permit safe passage of a tablet through the stomach, where some drugs may be degraded or may produce unwanted effects, to the environment of the intestine. Some coatings protect the drug from the destructive influences of moisture, light, or air during storage; some coatings actually contain the drug, such as procainamide; still others conceal a bad taste. Coatings are also used to ensure appropriate drug release and absorption. Some tablets shouldn't be crushed or broken because doing so may alter drug release.
- *Capsules:* Capsules are solid dosage forms in which the drug and other ingredients are enclosed in a hard or soft shell of varying size and shape. Drugs typically are released faster from capsules than from tablets.
- *Solutions:* Drugs administered in solution are absorbed more rapidly than many of those administered in solid form; however, they don't always produce predictable drug levels in the blood. Some drugs in solution should be administered with meals or snacks to minimize their irritating effect on the gastric mucosa.
- *Suspensions:* Suspensions are preparations consisting of finely divided drugs in a suitable vehicle, usually water. Suspensions should be shaken before administration to ensure the uniformity of the preparation and administration of the proper dosage.

Nasogastric

Drugs administered through a nasogastric or gastrostomy tube enter the stomach directly, bypassing the mouth and esophagus. They're usually administered in liquid form because an intact tablet or capsule could cause an obstruction in a gastric tube. Sometimes a tablet may be crushed or a capsule opened for nasogastric administration; however, doing so will affect the drug's release. You may need to consult a pharmacist to determine which tablets can be crushed or capsules opened.

Rectal

Some enteral drugs are administered rectally—as suppositories, solutions, or ointments—to provide either local or systemic effects. When inserted into the rectum, suppositories soften, melt, or dissolve, releasing the drug contained inside them. The rectal route may be preferred for drugs that are destroyed or inactivated by the gastric or intestinal environment or that irritate the stomach. It also may be indicated when the oral route is contraindicated because of vomiting or difficulty swallowing. The drawbacks of rectal administration include inconvenience, noncompliance, and incomplete or irregular drug absorption.

PARENTERAL

In parenteral drug administration, a drug enters the circulatory system through an injection rather than through GI absorption. This administration route is chosen when rapid drug action is desired; when the patient is uncooperative, unconscious, or unable to accept medication by the oral route; or when a drug is ineffective by other routes. Drugs may be injected into the joints, spinal column, arteries, veins, and muscles. However, the most common parenteral routes are the intramuscular (I.M.), intravenous (I.V.), subcutaneous (SubQ), and intradermal (I.D.) routes. Drugs administered parenterally may be mixed in either a solution or a suspension; those mixed in a solution typically act more rapidly than those mixed in a suspension. Parenteral administration has several disadvantages: The drug can't be removed or the dosage reduced once it has been injected, and injections typically are more expensive to administer than other dosage forms because they require strict sterility.

Intramuscular

I.M. injections are administered deep into the anterolateral aspect of the thigh (vastus lateralis), the dorsogluteal muscle (gluteus maximus), the upper arm (deltoid), or the ventrogluteal muscle (gluteus medius). I.M. injections typically provide sustained drug action. This route is commonly chosen for drugs that irritate the subcutaneous tissue. The drug should be injected as far as possible from major nerves and blood vessels.

Intravenous

In I.V. drug administration, an aqueous solution is injected directly into the vein—typically of the forearm. Drugs may be administered as a single, small-volume injection or as a slow, large-volume infusion. Because drugs injected I.V. don't encounter absorption barriers, this route produces the most rapid drug action, making it vital

in emergency situations. Except for I.V. fat emulsions used as nutritional supplements, oleaginous preparations aren't usually administered by this route because of the risk of fat embolism.

Subcutaneous

The subcutaneous route may be used to inject small volumes of medication, usually 1 ml or less. Subcutaneous injections typically are given below the skin in the abdominal area, lateral area of the anterior thigh, posterior surface of the upper arm, or lateral lumbar area. Injection sites should be rotated to minimize tissue irritation if the patient receives frequent subcutaneous injections—as, for example, in a patient who takes insulin.

Intradermal

Common sites for intradermal injection are the arm and the back. Because only about 0.1 ml may be administered intradermally, this route is rarely used except in diagnostic and test procedures, such as screening for allergic reactions.

TRANSCUTANEOUS

In transcutaneous administration, a drug crosses the skin layers from either the outside (dermal) or the inside (mucocutaneous). This route includes sublingual, inhalation, ophthalmic, otic, nasal, topical, and vaginal administration.

Sublingual

In sublingual administration, tablets are placed under the tongue and allowed to dissolve. Nitroglycerin is commonly administered by this route, which allows rapid drug absorption and action. The sublingual route also avoids first-pass metabolism.

Inhalation

Some drugs may be inhaled orally or nasally to produce a local effect on the respiratory tract or a systemic effect. Although drugs given by inhalation avoid first-pass hepatic metabolism, the lungs can also serve as an area of first-pass metabolism by providing respiratory conversion to more water-soluble compounds.

Ophthalmic

Ophthalmic solutions and ointments are applied directly to the cornea or conjunctiva for enhanced local penetration and decreased systemic absorption. Ophthalmic solutions pose a greater risk of drug loss through the nasolacrimal duct into the nasopharynx than ophthalmic ointments do.

Otic

Otic solutions are instilled directly into the external auditory canal for local penetration and decreased systemic absorption. These drugs, which include anesthetics, antibiotics, and anti-inflammatory drugs, usually require occlusion of the ear canal with cotton after instillation.

Nasal

Nasal solutions and suspensions are applied directly to the nasal mucosa for enhanced local penetration and decreased systemic absorption. These drugs are usually used to reduce the inflammation typically associated with seasonal or perennial rhinitis but may also be used for other purposes such as to elicit a systemic response.

Topical

Topical drugs—including creams, ointments, lotions, and pastes—are applied directly to the skin. Transdermal delivery systems, usually in the form of an adhesive patch or a disk, are among the latest developments in topical drug administration. Because they provide slow drug release, these systems are typically used to avoid first-pass metabolism and ensure prolonged duration of action.

Vaginal

Vaginal troches, suppositories, and creams are inserted into the vagina for slow, localized absorption. Body pH that differs from blood pH causes drug trapping or reabsorption, which delays drug excretion through the renal tubules. Vaginal secretions are alkaline, with a pH of 3.4 to 4.2, whereas blood has a pH of 7.35 to 7.45.

Drug Therapy and the Nursing Process

A systematic approach to nursing care, the nursing process helps guide you as you develop, implement, and evaluate your care and ensures that you'll deliver safe, consistent, and effective drug therapy to your patients. The nursing process consists of five steps, including assessment, nursing diagnosis, planning, implementation, and evaluation. Even though documentation is not a step in the nursing process, you're legally and professionally responsible for documenting all aspects of your care before, during, and after drug administration.

Assessment

The first step in the nursing process, assessment involves gathering information that's essential to guide your patient's drug therapy. This information includes the patient's drug history, present drug use, allergies, medical history, and physical examination findings. Assessment is an ongoing process that serves as a baseline against which to compare any changes in your patient's condition; it's also the basis for developing and individualizing your patient's plan of care.

DRUG HISTORY

The patient's drug history is critical in your planning of drug-related care. Ask about his previous use of over-the-counter and prescription drugs, as well as herbal remedies. For each drug, determine:

- the reason the patient took it
- the prescribed dosage
- the administration route
- the frequency of administration
- the duration of the drug therapy
- any adverse reactions the patient may have experienced and how he handled them.

Also determine if the patient has a history of drug abuse or addiction. Depending on his physical and emotional state, you may need to obtain the drug history from other sources, such as family members, friends, other caregivers, and the medical record.

PRESENT DRUG USE

Ask about the patient's current use of over-the-counter and prescription drugs, as well as herbal remedies. As you did in the drug history, find out the specific details for each drug (dosage, route, frequency, and reason for taking). Also ask the patient if he thinks the drug has been effective and when he took the last dose.

If the patient uses herbal remedies, similarly explore the use of these products, because herbs may interact with certain drugs. Also ask about the patient's use of recreational drugs, such as alcohol and tobacco, as well as illegal drugs, such as heroin. If the patient acknowledges use of these drugs, be alert for possible drug interactions. This information also may provide you with insight about the patient's response—or lack of response—to his current drug treatment plan.

Try to find out if the patient has any other problems that might affect his compliance with the drug treatment plan, and intervene appropriately. For instance, a patient who is unemployed and has no health insurance may fail to fill a needed prescription. In such a case, contact an appropriate individual in your facility who may be able to help the patient obtain financial assistance.

Be sure to ask the patient if his drug treatment plan requires special monitoring or follow-up laboratory tests. For example, patients who take antihypertensives need to have their blood pressure checked routinely, and those who take warfarin must have their prothrombin time tested regularly. Other patients must undergo periodic blood tests to assess their hepatic and renal function. Determine whether the patient has complied with this part of his treatment plan, and ask him if he knows the results of the latest monitoring or laboratory tests.

ALLERGIES

Find out if the patient is allergic to any drugs or foods. If he has an allergy, explore it further by determining the type of drug or food that triggers a reaction, the first time he experienced a reaction, the characteristics of the reaction, and other related information. Keep in mind that some patients consider annoying symptoms, such as indigestion, an allergic reaction. However, be sure to document a true allergy according to your facility's policy to ensure that the patient doesn't receive that drug or any related drug that may cause a similar reaction. Also, document allergies to foods because they may lead to drug interactions or adverse drug reactions. For example, sulfite is a food additive as well as a drug additive, so a patient with a known allergy to sulfite-containing foods is likely to react to sulfite-containing drugs.

MEDICAL HISTORY

While reviewing your patient's medical history, determine if he has any acute or chronic conditions that may interfere with his drug therapy. Certain disorders involving major body systems, such as the cardiovascular, GI, hepatic, and renal systems, may affect a drug's absorption, transport, metabolism, or excretion and interfere with its action; they also may increase the incidence of adverse reactions and lead to toxicity. For each disorder identified, try to determine when the condition was diagnosed, what drugs were prescribed, and who prescribed them. This information can help you determine whether the patient is receiving incompatible drugs and whether more than one prescriber is managing his drug therapy.

Ask a female patient if she is or may be pregnant or if she is breastfeeding. Many drugs are safe to use during pregnancy, but others may harm the fetus. Also, some drugs are distributed into breast milk. If your patient is or might be pregnant, check the FDA's recommendation for the prescribed drug and notify the prescriber if the drug may pose a risk to the fetus. If the patient is breastfeeding, find out if the drug is distributed in breast milk and intervene appropriately.

PHYSICAL EXAMINATION FINDINGS

As part of the physical examination, note the patient's age and weight. Be aware that age determines the dosage of certain drugs, such as sedatives and hypnotics, whereas weight determines the dosage of others, including some I.V. antibiotics and antivirals. As you perform the physical examination, note any abnormal findings that may point to body organ or system dysfunction. For example, if you detect liver enlargement and ascites, the patient may have impaired hepatic function, which can affect the metabolism of a drug he's taking and lead to harmful adverse or toxic effects. Also note whether a body organ or system appears to be responding to drug treatment. For example, if a patient has been taking an antibiotic to treat chronic bronchitis, thoroughly evaluate his respiratory status to measure his progress. Be sure to assess the patient for possible adverse reactions to the drugs he's taking.

Assess the patient's neurologic function to make sure that he can understand his drug regimen and carry out required tasks, such as performing a fingerstick to obtain blood for glucose measurement. If the patient can't understand essential drug information, you'll need to identify a family member or another person who is willing to become involved in the teaching process.

Nursing Diagnosis

Based on information derived from the assessment and physical examination findings, the nursing diagnoses are statements of actual or potential problems that a nurse is licensed to treat or manage alone or in collaboration with other members of the healthcare team. They're worded according to guidelines established by NANDA International.

One of the most common nursing diagnoses related to drug therapy is *knowledge deficit*, which indicates that the patient doesn't have sufficient understanding of his drug regimen. However, adverse reactions are the basis for most nursing diagnoses related to drug administration. For example, a patient receiving an opioid analgesic might have a nursing diagnosis of *constipation* related to decreased intestinal motility or *ineffective breathing* pattern related to respiratory depression. A patient receiving long-term, high-dose corticosteroids may have a risk for *impaired skin integrity* related to cortisone acetate or *self-concept disturbance* related to physical changes from prednisone therapy. Many antiarrhythmics cause orthostatic hypotension and thus may place an elderly patient at *high risk for injury* related to possible syncope. Broad-spectrum antibiotics, especially penicillin, may lead to the overgrowth of *Clostridium difficile*, a bacterium that is normally present in the intestine. This overgrowth in turn may lead to pseudomembranous colitis, characterized by abdominal pain and severe diarrhea. The nursing diagnoses in such a case might include *potential for infection* related to bacterial overgrowth, *alteration in comfort* related to abdominal pain, and *fluid balance deficit* related to diarrhea.

Planning

During the planning phase, you'll establish expected outcomes—or goals—for the patient and then develop specific nursing interventions to achieve them. Expected outcomes are observable or measurable goals that should occur as a result of nursing interventions and sometimes in conjunction with medical interventions. Developed in collaboration with the patient, the outcomes should be realistic and objective and should clearly communicate the direction of the plan of care to other nurses. They should be written as behaviors or responses for the patient, not the nurse, to achieve and should include a time frame for measuring the patient's progress. An example of a typical expected outcome is, *The patient will accurately demonstrate self-administration of insulin before discharge.* Based on each outcome statement you establish, you'd then develop appropriate nursing interventions, which might include drug administration techniques, patient teaching, monitoring of vital signs, calculation of drug dosages based on weight, and recording of intake and output.

Implementation

As you implement the nursing interventions, be sure to stringently follow the classic rule of drug administration: administer the right dose of the right drug by the right route to the right patient at the right time. Also, keep in mind that you have a legal and professional responsibility to follow institutional policy regarding standing orders, prescription renewal, and the use of nursing judgment. During the implementation phase, you'll also begin to evaluate the patient's expected outcomes and nursing interventions and make necessary changes to the plan of care.

Evaluation

Evaluation is an ongoing process rather than a single step in the nursing process. During this phase, you evaluate each expected outcome to determine whether or not it has been achieved and whether the original plan of care is working or should be modified. In evaluating a patient's drug treatment plan, you should determine whether or not the drug is controlling the signs and symptoms for which it was prescribed. You also should evaluate the patient for psychological or physiologic responses to the drug, especially adverse reactions. This constant monitoring allows you to make appropriate and timely suggestions for changes to the plan of care, such as dosage adjustments or changes in delivery routes, until each expected outcome has been achieved.

Documentation

You're responsible for documenting all your actions related to the patient's drug therapy, from the assessment phase to evaluation. Each time you administer a drug, document the drug name, dose, time given, and your evaluation of its effect. When you administer drugs that require additional nursing judgment, such as those prescribed on an as-needed basis, document the rationale for administering the drug and follow-up assessment or interventions for each dose administered.

If you decide to withhold a prescribed drug based on your nursing judgment, document your action and the rationale for it, and notify the prescriber of your action in a timely manner. Whenever you notify a prescriber about a significant finding related to drug therapy, such as an adverse reaction, document the date and time, the person you contacted, what you discussed, and how you intervened.

abacavir sulfate
Ziagen

Class and Category
Pharmacologic class: Nucleoside reverse transcriptase inhibitor (NRTI)
Therapeutic class: Antiretroviral

Indications and Dosages
✱ *As adjunct to treat human immunodeficiency virus (HIV)-1 infection*

ORAL SOLUTION, TABLETS
Adults. 600 mg once daily or 300 mg twice daily.
Children, infants 3 months of age and over. 16 mg/kg once daily or 8 mg/kg twice daily. *Maximum:* 600 mg daily.
±**DOSAGE ADJUSTMENT** For patients with mild hepatic impairment, dosage reduced to 200 mg twice daily and only oral solution used to ensure accurate dosage.

Drug Administration
P.O.
- Ensure all patients have been screened for HLA-B*5701 allele before therapy begins.
- Be aware that a scored tablet is available for pediatric patients weighing 14 kg or more, provided the child can swallow tablets.
- Abacavir is given in combination with other antiretroviral agents.

Route	Onset	Peak	Duration
P.O.	Unknown	07–1.7 hr	Unknown

Half-life: 1.5 hr

Mechanism of Action
Blocks an HIV enzyme called reverse transcriptase, which is responsible for starting or increasing the speed of a chemical reaction. By blocking this enzyme, HIV is prevented from multiplying.

Contraindications
Hypersensitivity to abacavir or its components, moderate or severe hepatic impairment, presence of HLA-B*5701 allele

Interactions
DRUGS
methadone: Possibly increased methadone clearance
riociguat: Increased riociguat exposure, increasing risk of riociguat adverse reactions

Adverse Reactions
CNS: Anxiety, chills, depression, dizziness, fatigue, fever, headache, lethargy, malaise, migraines, paresthesia, sleep disorders
CV: Edema, elevated triglyceride levels, **hypotension, MI**
EENT: Conjunctivitis, ENT infections, mouth ulcerations, pharyngitis
ENDO: Cushingoid appearance, fat redistribution, hyperglycemia
GI: Abdominal pain, diarrhea, elevated liver enzymes, gastritis, hyperamylasemia, **liver failure,** nausea, **pancreatitis, severe hepatomegaly with steatosis,** vomiting
GU: Renal dysfunction, **renal failure**
HEME: Anemia, **neutropenia, leukopenia, thrombocytopenia**
MS: Achiness, arthralgia, elevated CPK levels, musculoskeletal pain, myalgia, myolysis
RESP: Adult respiratory distress syndrome, bronchitis, cough, dyspnea, pneumonia, **respiratory failure,** viral respiratory infections
SKIN: Erythema multiforme, rash, **Stevens–Johnson syndrome, toxic epidermal necrolysis**
Other: Anaphylaxis, lactic acidosis, lymphadenopathy, **multiorgan failure,** nonspecific pain

Childbearing Considerations
PREGNANCY
- Pregnancy exposure registry: 1-800-258-4263.
- It is not known if drug can cause fetal harm although it does cross the placental barrier.
- Use with caution only if benefit to mother outweighs potential risk to fetus.

LACTATION
- Drug is present in breast milk.
- The Centers for Disease Control and Prevention recommends that HIV-1-infected mothers not breastfeed to avoid risking postnatal transmission of HIV-1 infection in HIV-negative infants or developing viral resistance in HIV-positive

infants. They also do not recommend breastfeeding because of potential drug-induced adverse reactions in the infant.

Nursing Considerations

- Know that carriers of the HLA-B*5701 allele are at greater risk of developing serious and sometimes fatal hypersensitivity reactions to abacavir.
- Know that a past medical history of an allergic reaction to abacavir, including any abacavir-containing product, is a contraindication for the use of abacavir therapy.
- Use caution when administering abacavir to patients with known risk factors for liver disease.
- Use cautiously in patients with coronary artery disease, because an increase in myocardial infarctions has occurred within 6 months of initiating abacavir therapy.

! **WARNING** Monitor patient closely for any hypersensitivity reaction. If present, notify prescriber immediately and expect drug to be discontinued, especially if a hypersensitivity reaction cannot be ruled out. Obesity, prolonged nucleoside exposure, and being a woman have been identified as risk factors. Know that a hypersensitivity reaction to abacavir usually presents with at least two of the following signs or symptoms: constitutional symptoms (achiness, fatigue, generalized malaise), fever, GI symptoms (abdominal pain, diarrhea, nausea, vomiting), rash, or respiratory symptoms (cough, dyspnea, pharyngitis). Other signs and symptoms that may be present include arthralgia, edema, headache, lethargy, myalgia, myolysis, and paresthesia. Know that adult respiratory distress syndrome, anaphylaxis, hypotension, renal failure, and respiratory failure have also occurred in association with an abacavir-induced hypersensitivity reaction and death has occurred.

- Monitor patient's liver enzymes periodically, as ordered, and monitor patient for any signs and symptoms of lactic acidosis or liver dysfunction such as severe hepatomegaly with steatosis, which may become life-threatening. Be aware that incidence is higher in women and in the presence of obesity. If present, notify prescriber, and expect abacavir therapy to be discontinued even in the absence of marked transaminase elevations.
- Be aware that immune reconstitution syndrome has occurred in patients treated with combination antiretroviral therapy, including abacavir. The inflammatory response predisposes susceptible patients to opportunistic infections such as cytomegalovirus infection, *Mycobacterium avium* infection, *Pneumocystis jiroveci* pneumonia, or tuberculosis. Autoimmune disorders such as Graves' disease, Guillain–Barré syndrome, or polymyositis have also occurred. Report sudden or unusual adverse reactions to prescriber.
- Observe patient for redistribution of body fat, including breast enlargement, central obesity, development of buffalo hump, facial wasting, and peripheral wasting, which may produce a cushingoid-type appearance.

PATIENT TEACHING

- Instruct patient/parents/caregiver to administer drug exactly as prescribed. If a dose is missed, have patient take it as soon as it is remembered. Stress importance of not doubling the next dose or taking more than the prescribed dose.

! **WARNING** Review the warning card and medication guide with patient/parents/caregiver on how to recognize a hypersensitivity reaction. Stress importance of stopping abacavir at the first sign of a hypersensitivity reaction and notifying prescriber.

- Instruct patient/parents/caregiver on the signs and symptoms of lactic acidosis and liver dysfunction. Advise patient to stop taking abacavir if present and notify prescriber.
- Advise patient/parents/caregiver to inform prescriber of any signs or symptoms of an infection, as well as any unusual, persistent severe, or unusual adverse reactions.
- Instruct a mother not to breastfeed while she is receiving abacavir therapy.
- Warn patient that fat distribution may occur with abacavir therapy.
- Tell women of childbearing age to report a known or suspected pregnancy. Provide patient with information on pregnancy exposure registry, if pregnancy occurs.

abaloparatide
Tymlos

Class and Category
Pharmacologic class: Parathyroid hormone analogue
Therapeutic class: Antiosteoporotic

Indications and Dosages
* *To treat postmenopausal women with osteoporosis who are at high risk for fracture, such as a history of multiple risk factors for fracture, have already sustained an osteoporotic fracture, or who have failed or are intolerant to other available osteoporosis therapy*

SUBCUTANEOUS INJECTION
Adult postmenopausal women. 80 mcg once daily.

Drug Administration
SUBCUTANEOUS
- Solution should be clear and colorless. If not, discard the solution.
- Administer into the periumbilical region of abdomen, rotating site every day. Never give intramuscularly or intravenously.
- Give first several doses with patient sitting or lying down, in case orthostatic hypotension occurs.
- Give at about the same time every day.

Route	Onset	Peak	Duration
SubQ	Unknown	0.51 hr	Unknown

Half-life: 1.7 hr

Mechanism of Action
Acts as an agonist at the PTH1 receptor, which activates the cAMP signaling pathway in target cells to increase bone mineral density and content. This in turn increases bone strength at vertebral and/or nonvertebral sites.

Contraindications
Hypersensitivity to abaloparatide or its components

Interactions
DRUGS
None

Adverse Reactions
CNS: Asthenia, dizziness, fatigue, headache, insomnia, lethargy, malaise, vertigo
CV: Orthostatic hypotension, palpitations, tachycardia
GI: Abdominal distention or pain (upper), constipation, diarrhea, nausea, vomiting
GU: Hypercalciuria, urolithiasis
MS: Bone, back, extremity, and joint pain; muscle spasms of back and leg
RESP: Dyspnea
SKIN: Pruritus, rash, urticaria
Other: Anaphylaxis, anti-abaloparatide antibodies, elevated uric acid levels, hypercalcemia, injection-site reactions (bruising, hemorrhage, pain, pruritus, rash, redness, severe edema)

Childbearing Considerations
PREGNANCY
- Drug is not indicated for use in females of reproductive potential.
- No human data with drug use in pregnant women are available.

LACTATION
- Drug is not indicated for use in females that would be breastfeeding.
- There is no information on drug being present in breast milk, effects on the breastfed infant, or the effects on milk production.

Nursing Considerations
- Know that abaloparatide and parathyroid hormone analogues such as teriparatide should not be given for more than 2 years cumulatively during patient's lifetime because of the potential risk of osteosarcoma.
- Be aware that abaloparatide should not be given to patients at increased risk for osteosarcoma. These risks include bone metastases or skeletal malignancies, hereditary disorders predisposing to osteosarcoma, metabolic bone diseases other than osteoporosis (including Paget's disease of the bone), open epiphyses, or prior external beam or implant radiation therapy involving the skeleton.
- Know that abaloparatide should not be given to women with preexisting hypercalcemia or who have an underlying hypercalcemic disorder, such as primary hyperparathyroidism, because of the risk of exacerbating hypercalcemia.

- Monitor patient for orthostatic hypotension for at least 4 hours after each dose.
- Monitor patient's serum calcium levels, as ordered, because drug may increase calcium levels, causing hypercalcemia, hypercalciuria, and urolithiasis. If preexisting hypercalciuria or urolithiasis is suspected, expect to measure the patient's urinary calcium excretion, as ordered.
- Ensure that patient is receiving supplemental calcium and vitamin D if dietary intake is inadequate.

PATIENT TEACHING

- Inform patient that abaloparatide should not be given more than 2 years cumulatively in patient's lifetime because of a potential risk for osteosarcoma. Tell patient to immediately report persistent localized pain or occurrence of a new soft-tissue mass that is tender to touch.
- Instruct patient or caregiver how to administer a subcutaneous injection using the abaloparatide pen and how to properly dispose of the needle and pen.
- Emphasize the importance of not sharing the drug or needles with others. Also tell patient not to transfer the contents of the pen to a syringe.
- Tell patient the pen must be discarded after 30 days of use, even if it still contains unused solution.
- Advise patient to change positions slowly for at least 4 hours after abaloparatide has been given and to watch for a drop in her blood pressure with position changes. Symptoms to be alert for include dizziness, nausea, or a rapid heart rate. If present, tell patient to lie down or sit until symptoms pass.
- Instruct patient to report signs and symptoms of high calcium levels such as constipation, lethargy, muscle weakness, nausea, or vomiting. Inform patient that she will need to have her calcium level checked routinely.
- Review dietary sources of calcium and vitamin D. Inform patient that calcium and vitamin D supplementation will be needed if dietary intake is insufficient.
- Review allergic reactions with patient and stress importance of seeking immediate medical attention if signs of anaphylaxis, dyspnea, or hives occur.

abatacept
Orencia

Class and Category

Pharmacologic class: Selective costimulation modulator
Therapeutic class: Antiarthritic (psoriatic, rheumatic)

Indications and Dosages

✱ *To treat moderate to severe active rheumatoid arthritis as monotherapy or concomitantly with disease-modifying antirheumatic drugs (DMARDs) other than Janus kinase (JAK) inhibitors or biologic disease-modifying antirheumatic drugs (bDMARDs) such as tumor necrosis factor (TNF) antagonists; to treat active psoriatic arthritis*

I.V. INFUSION

Adults weighing more than 100 kg (220 lb). *Initial:* 1,000 mg, repeated at 2 and 4 wk after the first infusion and every 4 wk thereafter.
Adults weighing 60 to 100 kg (132 to 220 lb). *Initial:* 750 mg, repeated at 2 and 4 wk after the first infusion and every 4 wk thereafter.
Adults weighing less than 60 kg (132 lb). *Initial:* 500 mg, repeated at 2 and 4 wk after the first infusion and every 4 wk thereafter.

SUBCUTANEOUS INJECTION

Adults. Following a single I.V. loading dose per body weight categories listed above for treatment of rheumatoid arthritis, 125 mg given within a day after the loading dose, followed by 125 mg once/wk.
125 mg once/wk for treatment of rheumatoid arthritis when I.V. loading dose is not used or to treat psoriatic arthritis.

±**DOSAGE ADJUSTMENT** For patient transitioning from I.V. therapy to subcutaneous injection, first subcutaneous dose should be administered instead of the next scheduled I.V. dose.

✱ *To treat moderate to severe active polyarticular juvenile idiopathic arthritis as monotherapy or concomitantly with methotrexate*

I.V. INFUSION

Children ages 6 to 17 weighing more than 100 kg (220 lb). *Initial:* 1,000 mg, repeated at 2 and 4 wk after the first infusion and every 4 wk thereafter.

Children ages 6 to 17 weighing 75 to 100 kg (165 to 220 lb). *Initial:* 750 mg, repeated at 2 and 4 wk after the first infusion and every 4 wk thereafter.

Children ages 6 to 17 weighing less than 75 kg (165 lb). *Initial:* 10 mg/kg, repeated at 2 and 4 wk after the first infusion and every 4 wk thereafter.

SUBCUTANEOUS INJECTION

Children age 2 and over weighing 50 kg (110 lb) or more. 125 mg once/wk.

Children age 2 and over weighing 25 kg (55 lb) to less than 50 kg (110 lb). 87.5 mg once/wk.

Children age 2 and over weighing 10 kg (22 lb) to less than 25 kg (55 lb). 50 mg once/wk.

＊ *To prevent acute graft versus host disease (aGVHD), in combination with a calcineurin inhibitor and methotrexate in patients undergoing hematopoietic stem cell transplantation (HSCT) from a matched or one allele-mismatched unrelated donor*

I.V. INFUSION

Adults and children age 6 and over. 10 mg/kg on the day before transplantation (day 1), followed by 10 mg/kg on days 5, 14, and 28 after transplantation.

Children age 2 to less than 6 years. 15 mg/kg on the day before transplantation (day 1), followed by 12 mg/kg on days 5, 14, and 28 after transplantation.

☰ Drug Administration

I.V.

- Prepare I.V. injection by reconstituting each vial with 10 ml of Sterile Water for Injection, directing the stream of Sterile Water to the inside glass wall of vial to minimize foaming. Use only the silicone-free disposable syringe with an 18- to 21-gauge needle provided with each vial, because a siliconized syringe may cause translucent particles to form in solution. If the drug is accidently reconstituted with a siliconized syringe, the solution should be discarded. If the provided silicone-free disposable syringe is contaminated or dropped, a new silicone-free disposable syringe should be used. If needed, call 1-800-ORENCIA to obtain new silicone-free syringes.
- After injecting Sterile Water into vial, gently swirl vial until contents are completely dissolved. The solution should appear clear and colorless to pale yellow. To minimize foaming, don't shake and don't prolong or use vigorous agitation. Vent the vial with a needle to dissipate any foam that may be present.
- Dilute further the reconstituted solution with 0.9% Sodium Chloride Injection to achieve a final solution volume of 100 ml. To do so, first withdraw a volume equal to the volume of the reconstituted drug solution required for patient dose from a 100-ml infusion bag or bottle. Then slowly add the reconstituted solution into the infusion bag or bottle using the same silicone-free disposable syringe provided with each vial. Mix gently. Do not shake the bag or bottle.
- Give I.V. dose after dilution over 30 minutes (60 minutes for prevention of aGVHD) using an infusion set and a sterile, nonpyrogenic, low protein-binding filter with a pore size of 0.2 to 1.2 μm. Drug infusion must be completed within 24 hours of reconstitution.
- Be aware that once fully diluted, I.V. solution may be kept for 24 hours at room temperature or refrigerated. If reconstituted solution isn't used within 24 hours, discard.
- *Incompatibilities:* Other drugs in the same intravenous line concurrently

SUBCUTANEOUS

- Administer subcutaneous injection using only the supplied single-dose prefilled glass syringe or the prefilled 125-mg/ml ClickJect autoinjector. Solution should appear clear to slightly opalescent and colorless to pale yellow.
- Know that the prefilled syringe or autoinjector is never to be used for intravenous infusion.
- Rotate sites and never give in areas where the skin is bruised, hard, red, or tender.

Route	Onset	Peak	Duration
I.V./SubQ	Unknown	Unknown	Unknown

Half-life: 13.1 days

☰ Mechanism of Action

Inhibits T-cell activation by binding to CD80 and CD86 to block interaction with CD28. CD28 is part of the costimulatory signal needed for full activation of T cells.

Activated T cells have been implicated in the pathogenesis of rheumatoid arthritis. With decreased proliferation of T cells, inflammation and other evidence of rheumatoid arthritis decrease.

Contraindications

Hypersensitivity to abatacept or its components

Interactions

DRUGS

live-virus vaccines: Possibly decreased response to vaccine, and risk of infection with live virus
tumor necrosis factor antagonists: Increased risk of serious infection

Adverse Reactions

CNS: Dizziness, fever, headache
CV: Hypertension, hypotension
EENT: Epistaxis, nasopharyngitis, rhinitis, sinusitis
GI: Abdominal pain, diarrhea, diverticulitis, dyspepsia, nausea
GU: Acute pyelonephritis, UTI
HEME: Anemia, **decreased CD4 lymphocyte count**
MS: Back or limb pain
RESP: Bronchitis, COPD worsening, cough, dyspnea, **hypoxia,** pneumonia, upper respiratory tract infection, wheezing
SKIN: Cellulitis, flushing, pruritus, rash, urticaria
Other: Anaphylaxis, antibody formation against abatacept, **cytomegalovirus (CMV) infection or reactivation,** Epstein–Barr virus (EBV) reactivation, herpes simplex, herpes zoster infection, flu-like symptoms, **hypermagnesemia, immunosuppression,** malignancies, serious infections such as sepsis, varicella infection

Childbearing Considerations

PREGNANCY

- Pregnancy exposure registry: 1-877-311-8972.
- It is not known if drug can cause fetal harm, including reaction to a live vaccine administered to the infant after exposure in utero.
- Use with caution only if benefit to mother outweighs potential risk to fetus.

LACTATION

- It is not known if drug is present in breast milk.

- Patient should check with prescriber before breastfeeding.

Nursing Considerations

- Screen patient for latent tuberculosis with a tuberculin skin test before starting abatacept. If test is positive, expect to provide treatment, as ordered, before starting abatacept. Also screen patient for hepatitis B. If present, expect abatacept to be withdrawn, because antirheumatic therapies such as abatacept may reactivate hepatitis B. For patient receiving drug to prevent aGVHD, expect patient to be prescribed antiviral prophylactic treatment for Epstein–Barr virus reactivation and to continue it for 6 months following HSCT. Be aware that patient may also receive prophylactic antivirals for cytomegalovirus (CMV) infection/reactivation during treatment and for 6 months following HSCT.
- Review patient's immunization record, and make sure all immunizations are current before therapy starts. Know that while nonlive vaccines may be administered during abatacept therapy, live vaccines should not be given during therapy and for 3 months after drug is discontinued.
- Use cautiously in patients with a history of recurrent infections, underlying conditions that may predispose them to infection, or existing chronic, latent, or localized infection. They have an increased risk of infection with abatacept therapy.
- Use cautiously in patients with COPD and monitor respiratory status closely because abatacept may worsen COPD and increase the risk of adverse respiratory reactions.
- Know that tumor necrosis factor antagonists shouldn't be given with abatacept because of an increased risk of serious infection.
- Watch patient closely for infusion-related reactions that may occur within 1 hour of the start of the infusion. Adverse reactions to be alert for include dizziness, headache, and hypertension. Less commonly a patient may experience cough, dyspnea, flushing, hypersensitivity, hypotension, nausea, pruritus, rash, and wheezing. Notify prescriber if present, but know that most patients need not discontinue abatacept because of these events unless severe.

- Monitor patient closely, after giving drug subcutaneously, for evidence of hypersensitivity reaction such as dyspnea, pruritus, rash, urticaria, or wheezing after administering abatacept. If present, notify prescriber, and provide emergency care, as ordered.
- Monitor patient closely for evidence of infection or malignancy because abatacept inhibits T-cell activation, increasing the risk of both.

PATIENT TEACHING

- Instruct patient receiving abatacept subcutaneously on how to administer the drug. Inform patient that injection sites should be rotated and should never be administered in an area where the skin is tender, bruised, red, or hard.
- Instruct patient self-administering abatacept subcutaneously to use a puncture-resistant container for disposal of needles and syringes. Have patient check with her community guidelines for correct way to dispose of a sharps container and stress the importance of not recycling the sharps container.
- Instruct patient not to receive immunizations with live vaccines during abatacept therapy and for 3 months afterward.
- Advise patient to tell prescriber of all medications being taken, including over-the-counter drugs and other biologic drugs.
- Emphasize need to report any evidence of infection or hypersensitivity to prescriber.
- Alert patient that abatacept may increase the risk of malignancy.
- Warn patient to avoid crowds and people with infections.
- Inform women to report known or suspected pregnancy. Encourage patient to register with the pregnancy exposure registry.

acamprosate calcium

⬛ Class and Category

Pharmacologic class: Amino acid neurotransmitter analogue
Therapeutic class: Alcohol deterrent

⬛ Indications and Dosages

✳ *To maintain abstinence from alcohol for alcohol-dependent patients who are abstinent at the start of treatment*

D.R. TABLETS

Adults. 666 mg three times daily.

±**DOSAGE ADJUSTMENT** For patients with moderate renal impairment (creatinine clearance of 30 to 50 ml/min), initial dosage reduced to 333 mg three times daily.

⬛ Drug Administration

P.O.

- Have patient swallow tablets whole and do not break, crush, or split tablets.

Route	Onset	Peak	Duration
P.O.	Unknown	3–8 hr	Unknown

Half-life: 20–33 hr

⬛ Contraindications

Hypersensitivity to acamprosate or its components, severe renal impairment (creatinine clearance 30 ml/min or less)

⬛ Interactions

DRUGS

None reported

⬛ Adverse Reactions

CNS: Abnormal thinking, amnesia, anxiety, asthenia, chills, depression, dizziness, headache, insomnia, paresthesia, somnolence, **suicidal ideation,** syncope, tremor
CV: Chest pain, hypertension, palpitations, peripheral edema, vasodilation
EENT: Abnormal vision, dry mouth, pharyngitis, rhinitis, taste perversion
GI: Abdominal pain, anorexia, constipation, diarrhea, flatulence, increased appetite, indigestion, nausea, vomiting
GU: **Acute renal failure,** decreased libido, impotence
HEME: **Leukopenia,** lymphocytosis, **thrombocytopenia**
MS: Arthralgia, back pain, myalgia
RESP: Bronchitis, cough, dyspnea
SKIN: Diaphoresis, pruritus, rash
Other: Flu-like symptoms, infection, weight gain

⬛ Childbearing Considerations

PREGNANCY

- It is not known if drug causes fetal harm but animal studies suggest it may.

▤ Mechanism of Action

Chronic alcoholism may alter the balance between excitation and inhibition in neurons in the brain; acamprosate restores it.

When the neurotransmitter gamma-aminobutyric acid (GABA) binds to its receptors in the CNS, it opens the chloride ion channel and releases chloride (Cl^-) into the cell (below left), thereby reducing neuronal excitability by inhibiting depolarization. By interacting with GABA receptor sites, acamprosate prevents GABA from binding (below right).

When glutamate binds to its receptors, it closes the chloride ion channel, increasing neuronal excitability by promoting depolarization (below left). This imbalance fosters a craving for alcohol. By interacting with glutamate receptor sites, acamprosate prevents glutamate from binding (below right).

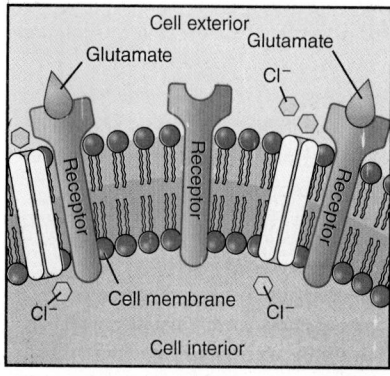

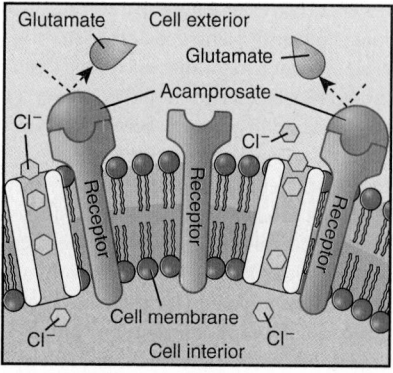

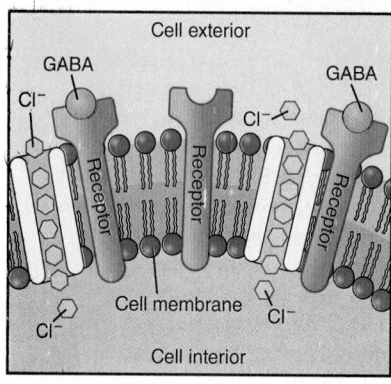

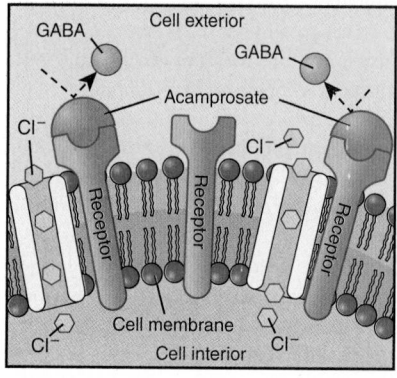

- Use with caution only if benefit to mother outweighs potential risk to fetus.

LACTATION

- It is not known if drug is present in breast milk.
- Patient should check with prescriber before breastfeeding.

▤ Nursing Considerations

- Know that acamprosate should start as soon as possible after patient has undergone alcohol withdrawal and achieved abstinence.

- Continue to give acamprosate even during periods of alcohol relapse, as ordered.

PATIENT TEACHING

- Instruct patient to take acamprosate exactly as prescribed, even if a relapse occurs, and to seek help for a relapse.
- Tell patient to take tablet whole and not to chew, crush, or split it.
- Warn patient that acamprosate won't reduce symptoms of alcohol withdrawal if relapse occurs followed by cessation.
- Urge caregivers to monitor patient for evidence of depression (lack of appetite or

interest in life, fatigue, excessive sleeping, difficulty concentrating) or suicidal tendencies because a small number of patients taking acamprosate have attempted suicide.

- Advise patient to use caution when performing hazardous activities until adverse CNS effects of drug are known.
- Tell female patient to notify prescriber if she is or intends to become pregnant while taking acamprosate; the drug may have to be stopped because fetal risks are unknown.

acetaminophen
(paracetamol)

Oral or rectal: Abenol (CAN), Acephen, Actamin Maximum Strength, Actimol Children's (CAN), Actimol infant (CAN), Altenol, Aminofen, Apra, Atasol (CAN), Cetafen, Children's Mapap, Children's Nortemp, Children's Tylenol Meltaways, Dolono, Febrol, Feverall, Genapap, Genebs, Junior Tylenol Meltaways, Mapap, Pediaphen (CAN), Pyrecot, Pyrigesic, Redutemp, Silapap, Tylenol, Tylenol 8-hr Arthritis Pain Caplets, Tylenol Extra Strength Caplets; *Parenteral:* Ofirmev

Class and Category

Pharmacologic class: Nonsalicylate, para-aminophenol derivative
Therapeutic class: Antipyretic, nonopioid analgesic

Indications and Dosages

* *To relieve mild to moderate pain; to relieve fever*

REGULAR STRENGTH (325 MG): CAPLETS, CAPSULES, CHEWABLE TABLETS, ELIXIR, GELCAPS, LIQUID SOLUTION, SPRINKLES, SUSPENSION, TABLETS

Adults and children 12 yr and over. 640 or 650 mg every 4 to 6 hr, as needed. *Maximum:* 3,250 mg (5 doses) in 24 hr.

EXTRA STRENGTH (500 MG) CAPLETS OR TABLETS

Adults. 1,000 mg every 6 hr, as needed. *Maximum:* 3,000 mg in 24 hr.

8-HR (650 MG) CAPLETS

Adults. 1,300 mg every 8 hr. *Maximum:* 3,900 mg in 24 hr.

CHEWABLE TABLETS, DISINTEGRATING TABLETS, ORAL SUSPENSION, SYRUP

Children age 12 and over weighing 43.5 kg (96 lb) or more. 640 mg every 4 hr, as needed. *Maximum:* 3,200 mg (5 doses) in 24 hr.
Children age 11 weighing 32.6 kg (72 lb) to 43 kg (95 lb). 480 mg every 4 hr, as needed. *Maximum:* 2,400 mg (5 doses) in 24 hr.
Children age 9 to 10 weighing 27 kg (60 lb) to 32 kg (71 lb). 400 mg every 4 hr, as needed. *Maximum:* 2,000 mg (5 doses) in 24 hr.
Children age 6 to 8 weighing 21.5 kg (48 lb) to 26.5 kg (59 lb). 320 mg every 4 hr, as needed. *Maximum:* 1,600 mg (5 doses) in 24 hr.
Children age 4 to 5 weighing 16 kg (35 lb) to 21 kg (47 lb). 240 mg every 4 hr, as needed. *Maximum:* 1,200 mg (5 doses) in 24 hr.
Children age 2 to 3 weighing 10.9 kg (24 lb) to 15.9 kg (35 lb). 160 mg every 4 hr, as needed. *Maximum:* 800 mg (5 doses in 24 hr).

ORAL SUSPENSION, SYRUP

Children age 12 to 23 months weighing 8 to 10.9 kg (17.6 to 24 lb). 120 mg every 4 hr, as needed.
Infants age 4 to 11 months weighing 5 to 8 kg (11 to 17.6 lb). 80 mg every 4 hr, as needed.
Infants 3 months or less weighing 2.7 to 5 kg (6 to 11 lb). 40 mg every 4 hr, as needed.

SUPPOSITORIES

Adults and adolescents. 650 mg every 4 to 6 hr, as needed. *Maximum:* 3,900 mg in 24 hr.
Children ages 6 to 12. 325 mg every 4 to 6 hr, as needed. *Maximum:* 1,625 mg in 24 hr.
Children ages 3 to 6. 120 mg every 4 to 6 hr, as needed. *Maximum:* 600 mg in 24 hr.
Children ages 1 to 3. 80 mg every 4 to 6 hr, as needed. *Maximum:* 400 mg in 24 hr.
Children ages 6 to 11 months. 80 mg every 6 hr, as needed. *Maximum:* 320 mg in 24 hr.

* *To relieve mild to moderate pain; to manage moderate to severe pain with adjunctive opioid analgesics*

I.V. INFUSION (OFIRMEV)

Adults and adolescents age 13 and over weighing 50 kg (110 lb) or more. 650 mg every 4 hr, as needed, or 1,000 mg every 6 hr, as needed. *Maximum:* 1,000 mg as a single dose, a minimum dosing interval of 4 hr, and a maximum dosage of 4,000 mg in 24 hr.

Adults and children age 2 and over weighing less than 50 kg (110 lb). 12.5 mg/kg every 4 hr, as needed, or 15 mg/kg every 6 hr, as needed. *Maximum:* 15 mg/kg (up to 750 mg) in a single dose, a minimum dosing interval of 4 hr, and a maximum dose of 75 mg/kg (up to 3,750 mg) in 24 hr.

✳ *To reduce fever*

I.V. INFUSION (OFIRMEV)

Adults and adolescents age 13 and over weighing 50 kg (110 lb) or more. 650 mg every 4 hr, as needed, or 1,000 mg every 6 hr, as needed. *Maximum:* 1,000 mg as a single dose, a minimum dosing interval of 4 hr, and a maximum dosage of 4,000 mg in 24 hr.

Adults and children age 2 and over weighing less than 50 kg (110 lb). 12.5 mg/kg every 4 hr, as needed, or 15 mg/kg every 6 hr, as needed. *Maximum:* 15 mg/kg (up to 750 mg) in a single dose, a minimum dosing interval of 4 hr, and a maximum dose of 75 mg/kg (up to 3,750 mg) in 24 hr.

Infants 29 days to 2 years. 15 mg/kg every 6 hr, as needed. *Maximum:* 60 mg/kg/day with minimum dosing interval of 6 hr.

Premature neonates at least 32 weeks gestational age and up to 28 days. 12.5 mg/kg every 6 hr, as needed. *Maximum:* 50 mg/kg/day with minimum dosing interval of 6 hr.

± **DOSAGE ADJUSTMENT** For patient with severe renal impairment (creatinine clearance 30 ml/min or less), dosing interval increased and total daily dosage reduced. For patient with mild to moderate hepatic impairment, total daily dosage reduced.

☰ Drug Administration

P.O.

- Extended-release forms should be swallowed whole. Do not crush or split extended-release forms and make sure patient does not chew these forms.
- Shake liquid forms well before measuring dose. Use liquid form for children and adults who have difficulty swallowing. Use a calibrated device to measure dosage.
- Place disintegrating tablets on patient's tongue and allow to dissolve in mouth or tablets can be chewed before swallowing. Tablets may be given with or without water after swallowing.
- Be aware that Pediaphen is a concentrated form of acetaminophen containing 80 mg/0.8 ml (standard liquid forms contain 32 mg/ml). Make sure to use correct concentration and dosage of liquid acetaminophen because serious adverse reactions can result from confusing concentrated form with regular liquid form.

I.V.

- Do not confuse a dose in milligrams with a dose in milliliters when preparing and administering I.V. acetaminophen. Also, make sure the dose is based on the patient's weight and infusion pumps are properly programmed.
- Solution should be clear and container and seals intact before using. Do not use plastic container in series connection.
- Be aware that patients weighing 50 kg (110 lb) or more and requiring 1,000-mg doses of parenteral acetaminophen (Ofirmev) can have the dose administered by inserting a vented intravenous set through the septum of the 100-ml vial. Further dilution is not required.
- For doses less than 1,000 mg, the dose must be withdrawn from the vial and placed into a separate container prior to administration to prevent inadvertent overdose.
- Administer over 15 minutes.
- Place small-volume pediatric doses up to 60 ml in a syringe and administer over 15 minutes using a syringe pump.
- Use parenteral drug within 6 hours once vacuum seal of glass vial has been penetrated or contents transferred to another container.
- *Incompatibilities:* Diazepam and chlorpromazine are physically incompatible; don't mix acetaminophen with other drugs.

P.R.

- If suppository is too soft to administer, either run it under cold water while still in wrapper or refrigerate it for at least 15 minutes.
- Do not take wrapper off until ready to administer.
- Store suppositories under 26.6°C (80°F).

Route	Onset	Peak	Duration
P.O.	30–45 min	30–60 min	4–6 hr
I.V.	15–30 min	15–20 min	4–6 hr
P.R.	1 hr	1.5–3 hr	6+ hr

Half-life: 2–5 hr (neonates: 4–10 hr)

Mechanism of Action

Inhibits the enzyme cyclooxygenase, blocking prostaglandin production and interfering with pain impulse generation in the peripheral nervous system. Acetaminophen also acts directly on temperature-regulating center in the hypothalamus by inhibiting synthesis of prostaglandin E_2.

Contraindications

Hypersensitivity to acetaminophen or its components, severe hepatic impairment, severe active liver disease

Interactions

DRUGS

anticholinergics: Decreased onset of acetaminophen action

barbiturates, carbamazepine, hydantoins, isoniazid, rifampin, sulfinpyrazone: Decreased therapeutic effects and increased hepatotoxic effects of acetaminophen

dasatinib, imatinib: Possibly increased risk of hepatotoxicity

lamotrigine: Possibly decreased therapeutic effects of these drugs

oral contraceptives: Decreased effectiveness of acetaminophen

probenecid: Possibly increased therapeutic effects of acetaminophen

propranolol: Possibly increased action of acetaminophen

warfarin: Possibly increased international normalized ratio

zidovudine: Possibly decreased zidovudine effects

ACTIVITIES

alcohol use: Increased risk of hepatotoxicity

Adverse Reactions

CNS: Agitation, anxiety, fatigue, fever, headache, insomnia

CV: Hypotension, hypertension, peripheral edema

EENT: Stridor (parenteral form)

ENDO: Hypoglycemic coma

GI: Abdominal pain, constipation, diarrhea, **hepatotoxicity,** jaundice, nausea, vomiting

GU: Oliguria (parenteral form)

HEME: Hemolytic anemia (with long-term use), leukopenia, **neutropenia,** pancytopenia, **thrombocytopenia**

MS: Muscle spasm (parenteral form)

RESP: Parenteral form: **atelectasis,** dyspnea, plural effusion, **pulmonary edema,** wheezing

SKIN: Acute generalized exanthematous pustulosis, blisters, pruritus, rash, reddening, **Stevens–Johnson syndrome, toxic epidermal necrolysis,** urticaria

Other: Anaphylaxis, angioedema, hypersensitivity reactions; for parenteral form: hypoalbuminemia, **hypokalemia, hypomagnesemia, hypophosphatemia,** injection-site pain

Childbearing Considerations

PREGNANCY

- Use of drug at any time during pregnancy may increase risk of attention deficit hyperactivity disorder (ADHD) after birth.
- Use with caution only if benefit to mother outweighs potential risk to fetus.

LACTATION

- Drug may be present in breast milk.
- Patient should check with prescriber before breastfeeding.

REPRODUCTION

- Drug may reduce fertility in females and males.

Nursing Considerations

- Use acetaminophen cautiously in patients with hepatic impairment or active hepatic disease, alcoholism, chronic malnutrition, severe hypovolemia, or severe renal impairment.
- Know that before and during long-term therapy including parenteral therapy, liver function test results, including AST, ALT, bilirubin, and creatinine levels, as ordered must be monitored because acetaminophen may cause hepatotoxicity. Ensure that the daily dose of acetaminophen from all sources does not exceed maximum daily limits.
- Monitor renal function in patient on long-term therapy. Keep in mind that blood or albumin in urine may indicate nephritis; decreased urine output may indicate renal failure; and dark brown urine may indicate presence of the metabolite phenacetin.
- Monitor the end of a parenteral infusion to prevent possibility of air embolism.
- Calculate total daily intake of acetaminophen including other products that may contain acetaminophen so maximum daily dosage is not exceeded.

PATIENT TEACHING

- Tell patient that tablets may be crushed or swallowed whole but that extended-release forms should not be broken, chewed, crushed, or split.

- Instruct patient to read manufacturer's label and follow dosage guidelines precisely. Explain that infants' and children's acetaminophen liquid aren't equal in drug concentration and aren't interchangeable. Tell them to use only the measuring device that comes with the bottle to help ensure accurate dosage.
- Caution patient not to exceed recommended dosage or take other drugs containing acetaminophen at the same time because of risk of liver damage. Advise him to contact prescriber before taking other prescription or OTC products because they may contain acetaminophen.
- Teach patient to recognize signs of hepatotoxicity, such as bleeding, easy bruising, and malaise, which commonly occurs with chronic overdose.

! **WARNING** Caution patient that serious skin reactions, although rare, may occur even with first-time use and any time acetaminophen is used, even if no skin reactions occurred with a previous use of drug. Tell patient that if a skin rash, redness, or blisters occur, he should stop using drug and seek emergency treatment immediately.

acetazolamide

acetazolamide sodium

Class and Category

Pharmacologic class: Carbonic anhydrase inhibitor
Therapeutic class: Anticonvulsant, antiglaucoma, diuretic

Indications and Dosages

∗ *As adjunct to treat chronic simple (open-angle) glaucoma*

E.R. CAPSULES

Adults. 500 mg twice daily.

I.V. INJECTION, TABLETS

Adults. 250 to 1,000 mg daily (divided for doses exceeding 250 mg).

∗ *As short-term therapy to treat secondary glaucoma; to treat acute angle-closure glaucoma preoperatively when delay of surgery is needed in order to lower intraocular pressure*

I.V. INJECTION, TABLETS

Adults. 250 mg twice daily or every 4 hr; or 500 mg initially, followed by 125 to 250 mg every 4 hr for severe acute glaucoma. Oral therapy usually started after initial I.V. dose.

∗ *To treat edema caused by congestive heart failure*

I.V. INJECTION, TABLETS

Adults. *Initial:* 250 to 375 mg or 5 mg/kg daily in morning. *Maintenance:* 250 to 375 mg or 5 mg/kg on alternate days or for 2 days followed by a drug-free day.

∗ *To treat drug-induced edema*

I.V. INJECTION, TABLETS

Adults. 250 to 375 mg once daily for 1 to 2 days alternating with a day of rest.

∗ *To treat seizures, including generalized tonic–clonic, absence, and mixed seizures, and myoclonic jerk patterns*

I.V. INJECTION, TABLETS

Adults. 8 to 30 mg/kg daily in divided doses. *Optimal:* 375 to 1,000 mg daily. When used with other anticonvulsants, initially, 250 mg daily, increased as needed to optimal dosage.

∗ *To prevent or relieve symptoms of acute mountain sickness*

E.R. CAPSULES, TABLETS

Adults. 500 to 1,000 mg daily in divided doses, given 24 to 48 hr before ascent and continued for 48 hr or longer while at high altitude, as needed, to control symptoms.

Drug Administration

P.O.

- Administer tablets with a full glass of water. Extended-release capsules should be swallowed whole with a full glass of water.
- Store at controlled room temperature: 20–25°C (68–77°F).

I.V.

- Reconstitute each 500-mg vial with at least 5 ml Sterile Water for Injection.
- Administer by direct I.V. bolus.
- Use within 12 hours because drug has no preservative unless refrigerated (use within 3 days).
- *Incompatibilities:* Multivitamins

Route	Onset	Peak	Duration
P.O.	1–1.5 hr	2–4 hr	8–12 hr
P.O. (E.R.)	2 hr	3–6 hr	18–24 hr
I.V.	2–10 min	15 min	4–5 hr

Half-life: 4–5.8 hr

Mechanism of Action

Inhibits the enzyme carbonic anhydrase, which normally appears in the eyes' ciliary processes, brain's choroid plexus, and kidneys' proximal tubule cells. In the eyes, enzyme inhibition decreases aqueous humor secretion, which lowers intraocular pressure. In the brain, inhibition may delay abnormal, intermittent, and excessive discharge from neurons that cause seizures. In the kidneys, it increases bicarbonate excretion, which carries out water, potassium, and sodium, thus inducing diuresis and metabolic acidosis. This acidosis counteracts respiratory alkalosis and reduces symptoms of mountain sickness, including headache, dizziness, nausea, and dyspnea.

Contraindications

Chronic noncongestive closed-angle glaucoma; cirrhosis; hyperchloremic acidosis; hypersensitivity to acetazolamide, sulfonamides, other sulfonamide derivatives, or their components; hypokalemia; hyponatremia; severe hepatic, renal, or adrenocortical impairment; suprarenal gland failure

Interactions

DRUGS

amphetamines, phenobarbital, procainamide, quinidine: Decreased excretion and possibly toxicity of these drugs
corticosteroids: Increased risk of hypokalemia
cyclosporine: Increased cyclosporine level, possibly nephrotoxicity or neurotoxicity
diflunisal: Possibly significantly decreased intraocular pressure
lithium: Increased excretion and decreased effectiveness of lithium
primidone: Decreased serum and urine primidone levels
salicylates: Increased risk of salicylate toxicity

Adverse Reactions

CNS: Ataxia, confusion, depression, disorientation, dizziness, drowsiness, fatigue, fever, flaccid paralysis, headache, lassitude, malaise, nervousness, paresthesia, **seizures**, tremor, weakness
EENT: Altered taste, tinnitus, transient myopia
GI: Anorexia, constipation, diarrhea, **hepatic dysfunction**, **melena**, nausea, vomiting
GU: Crystalluria, decreased libido, glycosuria, hematuria, impotence, **nephrotoxicity**, phosphaturia, polyuria, renal calculi, renal colic, urinary frequency
HEME: **Agranulocytosis**, **hemolytic anemia**, **leukopenia**, **pancytopenia**, **thrombocytopenia**, **thrombocytopenic purpura**
SKIN: Photosensitivity, pruritus, rash, **Stevens–Johnson syndrome**, urticaria
Other: **Acidosis**, hyperuricemia, **hypokalemia**, weight loss

Childbearing Considerations

PREGNANCY

- It is not known if drug causes fetal harm although animal studies suggest it might.
- Use with caution only if benefit to mother outweighs potential risk to fetus.

LACTATION

- Drug may be present in breast milk.
- A decision should be made to discontinue breastfeeding or the drug to avoid potential serious adverse reactions in the breastfed infant.

Nursing Considerations

- Use acetazolamide cautiously in patients with calcium-based renal calculi, diabetes mellitus, gout, or respiratory impairment.
- Know that acetazolamide may increase risk of hepatic encephalopathy in patients with hepatic cirrhosis.
- Monitor blood tests during acetazolamide therapy to detect electrolyte imbalances.
- Monitor fluid intake and output every 8 hours and body weight daily to detect excessive fluid and weight loss.

PATIENT TEACHING

- Advise patient to take tablets with a full glass of water. If patient is prescribed extended-release capsules, tell patient to swallow capsule whole with a full glass of water.
- Advise patient to avoid hazardous activities if dizziness or drowsiness occurs.
- Instruct patient who takes high doses of salicylates to notify prescriber immediately

about evidence of salicylate toxicity, such as anorexia, tachypnea, and lethargy.
- Tell patient if she plans to mountain climb, urge her to descend mountain gradually and to seek immediate medical care if symptoms of mountain sickness occur.

acetohydroxamic acid
Lithostat

Class and Category
Pharmacologic class: Urease inhibitor
Therapeutic class: Antagonist to bacterial enzyme urease

Indications and Dosages
* *As an adjunct to antimicrobial therapy to treat chronic UTI caused by urea-splitting bacteria*

TABLETS
Adults. *Initial:* 12 mg/kg daily in divided doses every 6 to 8 hr. *Usual:* 250 mg three or four times daily for a total of 10 to 15 mg/kg daily. *Maximum:* 1,500 mg daily.
Children. *Initial:* 10 mg/kg daily in divided doses, increased or decreased as tolerated and needed.
±**DOSAGE ADJUSTMENT** For a patient with a creatinine clearance level above 1.8 mg/dl, dosage interval increased to every 12 hours and maximum daily dosage decreased to 1 g.

Drug Administration
P.O.
- Give drug at same time each day.
- Administer when stomach is empty.

Route	Onset	Peak	Duration
P.O.	Unknown	0.25–1 hr	Unknown

Half-life: 5–10 hr

Mechanism of Action
Inhibits urease, the enzyme that catalyzes urea's hydrolysis to carbon dioxide and ammonia in urine infected with urea-splitting bacteria. This action reduces the urine ammonia level and pH, enhancing antimicrobial drug effectiveness.

Contraindications
Contributing disorder that's treatable by surgery or appropriate antimicrobial therapy, hypersensitivity to acetohydroxamic acid or its components, inadequate renal function (serum creatinine level above 2.5 mg/dl or creatinine clearance below 20 ml/min), risk of pregnancy, UTI caused by nonurease-producing organisms, UTI that could be controlled by appropriate antimicrobial therapy

Interactions
DRUGS
iron: Decreased intestinal absorption of iron, decreased effects of iron and acetohydroxamic acid

ACTIVITIES
alcohol use: Increased risk of severe rash 30 to 45 minutes after drinking alcohol

Adverse Reactions
CNS: Anxiety, depression, fever, headache, lack of coordination, malaise, nervousness, slurred speech, tiredness, tremor
CV: **Deep venous thrombosis,** palpitations, superficial phlebitis
EENT: Pharyngitis, sudden change in vision
GI: Anorexia, nausea, vomiting
HEME: **Hemolytic anemia,** reticulocytosis, **unusual bleeding**
RESP: Dyspnea, **pulmonary emboli**
SKIN: Ecchymosis, hair loss, nonpruritic macular rash

Childbearing Considerations
PREGNANCY
- Drug may cause serious fetal harm.
- Drug is contraindicated in a pregnant woman as well as any childbearing woman who is not using a reliable method of contraception.

LACTATION
- It is not known if drug is present in breast milk.
- A decision should be made to discontinue breastfeeding or the drug to avoid potential serious adverse reactions in the breastfed infant.

REPRODUCTION
- Advise women of childbearing age to use a reliable method of contraception throughout drug therapy.

Nursing Considerations
- Use acetohydroxamic acid cautiously in patients with anemia or chronic renal

disease and those who've had phlebitis or thrombophlebitis.

- Be aware that risk of adverse psychomotor effects increases if patient drinks alcohol or takes drugs that affect alertness and reflexes, such as analgesics, antihistamines, narcotics, sedatives, and tranquilizers.

! **WARNING** Be aware that acetohydroxamic acid chelates with dietary iron. If patient has iron deficiency anemia, expect to administer I.M. iron as needed during acetohydroxamic acid therapy.

- Monitor follow-up laboratory tests to check hepatic and renal function and urine pH, as ordered.

PATIENT TEACHING

- Instruct patient to take drug at same time each day, as prescribed.
- Advise patient to take drug on an empty stomach.
- Tell patient to take a missed dose up to 2 hours after scheduled time. If more than 2 hours have passed, he should wait for next scheduled dose and shouldn't double that dose.
- Warn patient not to take drug with alcohol or iron and to consult prescriber before taking it with any other drug.
- Instruct patient to avoid hazardous activities during therapy.

acetylcysteine
Acetadote, Acetylcysteine 10% or 20%, Cetylev, Parvolex (CAN)

Class and Category
Pharmacologic class: L-cysteine derivative
Therapeutic class: Antidote (for acetaminophen overdose), mucolytic

Indications and Dosages
* *To liquefy abnormal, thickened, or viscid mucus secretions in chronic pulmonary disorders (including bronchiectasis, bronchitis, cystic fibrosis, and emphysema) and in pneumonia, pulmonary complications of cardiovascular or thoracic surgery, and tracheostomy care*

SOLUTION BY DIRECT INSTILLATION INTO TRACHEOSTOMY (ACETYLCYSTEINE)
Adults and children. 1 to 2 ml of 10% or 20% solution instilled every 1 to 4 hr, as needed.

SOLUTION BY INHALATION (ACETYLCYSTEINE)
Adults and children. 1 to 10 ml of 20% solution or 2 to 20 ml of 10% solution nebulized through face mask, mouthpiece, or tracheostomy every 2 to 6 hr. *Usual:* 3 to 5 ml of 20% solution or 6 to 10 ml of 10% solution three or four times daily.
* *To treat acetaminophen overdose*

EFFERVESCENT TABLETS FOR ORAL SOLUTION (CETYLEV), ACETYLCYSTEINE
Adults and children. *Loading dose:* 140 mg/kg. *Maintenance:* 70 mg/kg 4 hr after loading dose and then every 4 hr for a total of 17 doses.

I.V. INFUSION (ACETADOTE)
Adults and children weighing 41 kg (90.2 lb) or more. 150 mg/kg in 200 ml of diluent infused over 60 min, followed by 50 mg/kg in 500 ml of diluent infused over 4 hr, followed by 100 mg/kg in 1,000 ml of diluent infused over 16 hr.
Adults and children weighing 21 kg (46.2 lb) to 41 kg (90.2 lb) 150 mg/kg in 100 ml of diluent infused over 60 min, followed by 50 mg/kg in 250 ml of diluent infused over 4 hr, followed by 100 mg/kg in 500 ml of diluent infused over 16 hr.
Children weighing 5 kg (11 lb) to 20 kg (44 lb). 150 mg/kg in 3 ml/kg of diluent infused over 60 min, followed by 50 mg/kg in 7 ml/kg of diluent infused over 4 hr, followed by 100 mg/kg in 14 ml/kg of diluent infused over 16 hr.

Drug Administration
P.O.
- Follow guidelines when treating acetaminophen overdose with Cetylev. For example, dissolve appropriate number of 2.5-g and/or 500-mg effervescent tablets in water (for patients weighing 19 kg or less, dissolve in 100 ml of water; for patients weighing 20 to 60 kg, dissolve in 150 ml of water; and, for patients weighing 60 kg or more, dissolve in 300 ml of water). Once tablets are dissolved, administer oral solution immediately.
- Repeat dose as prescribed if patient vomits loading dose or any maintenance dose within 1 hour of administration.
- Solution may be administered by nasogastric tube or Miller-Abbott tube, if needed.

I.V.

- Dilute parenteral solution (Acetadote) with 5% Dextrose in Water, 0.45% Sodium Chloride Injection, or Sterile Water for Injection following manufacturer guidelines because dilution is based on dosage. Acetadote may turn from colorless to slight pink or purple once the stopper is punctured, but color change has no effect on product quality.
- Treating acetaminophen overdose with intravenous therapy may require adjusting total administered volume, as ordered, for patients weighing less than 40 kg (88 lb) and for those who need fluid restriction, to avoid fluid overload and possibly fatal hyponatremia or seizures.
- Infuse (150 mg/kg) dose over 60 minutes; second dose (50 mg/kg) over 4 hours; and third dose (100 mg/kg) over 16 hours.
- Diluted solution can be stored for 24 hours at room temperature.
- Discard unused drug.
- *Incompatibilities:* None listed by manufacturer

INHALATION

- It may be necessary to dilute 20% inhalation or instillation solution with normal saline solution or Sterile Water when acetylcysteine is used to liquefy secretions. The 10% solution may be used undiluted.
- Use nebulizers made of aluminum, glass, plastic, or stainless steel. Don't give acetylcysteine with nebulization equipment if drug can contact copper, iron, or rubber.
- Be aware hand bulbs are not recommended to administer drug, because output is too small and in some cases the particle size is too large.
- Have patient wash his face and rinse his mouth at the end of each nebulization treatment because nebulization causes sticky residue on face and in mouth.
- *Incompatibilities for direct instillation or nebulization:* All antibiotics, chymotrypsin, hydrogen peroxide, iodized oil, trypsin

Route	Onset	Peak	Duration
P.O.	Unknown	1–3.5 hr	Unknown
I.V.	Unknown	30–60 min	Unknown
Inhalation	5–10 min	1–2 hr	Unknown

Half-life: 5.6 hr

≣ Mechanism of Action

Decreases viscosity of pulmonary secretions by breaking disulfide links that bind glycoproteins in mucus. Reduces liver damage from acetaminophen overdose. Usually, acetaminophen's toxic metabolites bind with glutathione in the liver, which detoxifies them. When acetaminophen overdose depletes glutathione stores, toxic metabolites bind with protein in liver cells, killing them. Acetylcysteine maintains or restores levels of glutathione or acts as its substitute, which reduces liver damage from acetaminophen overdose.

≣ Contraindications

Hypersensitivity to acetylcysteine or its components, no contraindications when used as antidote

≣ Interactions

DRUGS

activated charcoal: Possibly adsorption and decreased effectiveness of oral acetylcysteine
nitroglycerin: Increased effects of nitroglycerin and possibly significant headache and hypotension

≣ Adverse Reactions

CNS: Chills, dizziness, drowsiness, fever, headache
CV: Edema, hypertension, **hypotension**, tachycardia
EENT: Rhinorrhea, stomatitis, **stridor**, tooth damage
GI: Anorexia, constipation, **hepatotoxicity**, nausea, vomiting
RESP: **Bronchospasm**, chest tightness, cough, **hemoptysis**, **respiratory distress**, shortness of breath, wheezing
SKIN: Clammy skin, erythema, facial flushing, pruritus, rash, urticaria
Other: **Anaphylaxis**, **angioedema**

≣ Childbearing Considerations

PREGNANCY

- It is not known if drug can cause fetal harm.
- Use with caution only if benefit to mother outweighs potential risk to fetus.

LACTATION

- It is not known if drug is present in breast milk.
- Patient should check with prescriber before breastfeeding. Breastfeeding women may

consider pumping and discarding their milk for 30 hours after drug administration.

Nursing Considerations

- Know that acetylcysteine should be used cautiously in patients with asthma or a history of bronchospasm because drug may adversely affect respiratory function.
- Keep in mind that acetylcysteine is most effective if given within 24 hours of acetaminophen ingestion. For specific instructions, contact a regional poison center at 1-800-222-1222 or a special health professional assistance hotline at 1-800-525-6115.
- Be aware that suicidal patient may not provide reliable information about vomiting. Watch such a patient to ensure that he ingests all of prescribed dosage.
- Watch for signs of hepatotoxicity (altered coagulation, easy bruising, and prolonged bleeding time), during treatment for acetaminophen overdose.
- Be aware that acetylcysteine may have a disagreeable odor, which disappears as treatment progresses.
- When drug is given intravenously, acute flushing and erythema of the skin may occur within 30 to 60 minutes of administration and often resolves spontaneously even with continued infusion of drug. However, monitor patient closely for acute hypersensitivity reactions regardless of form of drug administered, such as hypotension, rash, shortness of breath, and wheezing. If present, immediately stop administration of drug, notify prescriber, and provide supportive care according to protocol.
- Assess type, frequency, and characteristics of patient's cough. Particularly note sputum. If cough doesn't clear secretions, prepare to perform mechanical suctioning.
- Monitor patient for tachycardia.

PATIENT TEACHING

- Tell patient receiving acetylcysteine intravenously that facial redness or flushing may occur but usually resolves on its own.
- Instruct patient to notify prescriber immediately about nausea, rash, or vomiting, as well as feeling dizzy or light-headed, shortness of breath, or wheezing.
- Warn patient about acetylcysteine's unpleasant smell; reassure him that it subsides as treatment progresses.

- Urge patient prescribed drug to loosen mucus, to consume 2 to 3 L of fluid daily unless contraindicated by another condition, to decrease mucus viscosity.
- Instruct female patient who is breastfeeding to consider pumping and discarding her milk for 30 hours after acetylcysteine administration.

acitretin
Soriatane

Class and Category

Pharmacologic class: Second-generation retinoid
Therapeutic class: Antipsoriatic

Indications and Dosages

✱ *To treat severe psoriasis*

CAPSULES

Adults. 25 to 50 mg once daily.

Drug Administration

P.O.

- Give with main meal of the day.
- Drug should be kept away from high temperature, humidity, and sunlight.

Route	Onset	Peak	Duration
P.O.	Unknown	2–5 hr	Unknown

Half-life: 49 hr

Mechanism of Action

Binds to several retinoid receptors to regulate gene transcription. Exactly how the action of this second-generation retinoid allows normal growth and development of skin is unknown.

Contraindications

Alcohol consumption; blood donation; breastfeeding; chronic hyperlipidemia; concurrent use of etretinate, methotrexate, or tetracycline; hypersensitivity to acitretin, other retinoids, or their components; pregnancy; severe hepatic or renal impairment

Interactions

DRUGS

methotrexate: Increased risk of hepatitis
oral contraceptives containing only progestin: Possibly decreased effectiveness of oral contraceptive

phenytoin: Possibly decreased protein binding of phenytoin

sulfonylureas: Possibly increased risk of hypoglycemia

tetracyclines: Possibly increased intracranial pressure

vitamin A and other oral retinoids: Increased risk of hypervitaminosis A

ACTIVITIES

alcohol use: Increased risk of adverse reactions and acitretin toxicity

▤ Adverse Reactions

CNS: Aggression, **CVA**, depression, fatigue, headache, hyperesthesia, hypotonia, insomnia, **intracranial hypertension**, paresthesia, peripheral neuropathy, rigors, somnolence, **suicidal ideation**, thirst

CV: Chest pain, decreased high-density lipoproteins, edema, elevated cholesterol or triglyceride levels, **MI**, **thromboembolism**

EENT: Abnormal or blurred vision, blepharitis, conjunctivitis, corneal epithelial abnormality, deafness, decreased night vision, dry eyes or mouth, earache, epistaxis, eye pain, gingival bleeding, gingivitis, increased saliva, photophobia, sinusitis, stomatitis, taste perversion, tinnitus, ulcerative stomatitis

ENDO: Hot flashes, hyperglycemia

GI: Anorexia, abdominal pain, diarrhea, elevated liver enzymes, **hepatitis**, **hepatotoxicity**, nausea, **pancreatitis**

GU: Vulvovaginitis

HEME: **Capillary leak syndrome**, **hemorrhage**, **increased bleeding time**

MS: Arthralgia, arthrosis, back pain, hyperostosis, myalgia, myopathy

SKIN: Abnormal skin or hair texture, alopecia, bullous eruption, cold or clammy skin, dermatitis, diaphoresis, dry or peeling skin, erythematous rash, **exfoliative dermatitis**, erythroderma, flushing, fragility or thinning of skin, loss of eyelashes or eyebrows, photosensitivity, pruritus, purpura, pyogenic granuloma, rash, scaling, seborrhea, skin fissure or ulceration

Other: **Hypervitaminosis A**, increased appetite

▤ Childbearing Considerations

PREGNANCY

- Drug causes fetal harm, especially severe fetal malformations.

- Drug is contraindicated in pregnant women and women of childbearing age who are not using reliable contraception.

- Patient of childbearing age must meet all of the following conditions before drug can be prescribed:
  - 2 negative urine or serum pregnancy tests with a sensitivity of at least 25 mIU/ml; first test done before initial prescription of drug and second test done during the first 5 days of the menstrual cycle immediately preceding the 7 days before drug therapy actually begins.
  - A negative pregnancy test before prescription is refilled monthly.
  - Patient agrees to have a pregnancy test done every 3 months for at least 3 years after drug is discontinued.
  - Patient has selected and is committed to using 2 effective forms of contraception simultaneously, for at least 1 month prior to drug therapy beginning, throughout drug therapy, and for at least 3 years after drug is discontinued.
  - Patient agrees to use at least one contraceptive of a primary form, unless absolute abstinence is the chosen method, patient has undergone a hysterectomy, or is clearly postmenopausal.
  - Patient makes a commitment to undergo counseling about contraception and behaviors associated with an increased risk of pregnancy on a monthly basis and every 3 months for at least 3 years following drug being discontinued.

- Patient agrees to participate in the "Do Your P.A.R.T." (Pregnancy Prevention Actively required During and After Treatment) program.

- Patient understands drug may interfere with the contraceptive effect of microdosed progestin preparations and knows that the microdosed "minipill" is not recommended for use with the drug.

- Patient expresses an understanding that it is not known if there is an interaction between the drug and combined oral contraceptives.

- Patient agrees not to use St. John's wort during drug therapy and for at least 3 years following the discontinuation of the drug because pregnancies have occurred in users of combined hormonal contraceptives and St. John's wort.

- Patient agrees not to donate blood during and for at least 3 years following the completion of drug therapy because women of childbearing potential must not receive blood from patients being treated with drug.

LACTATION

- Drug may be present in breast milk.
- A decision should be made to discontinue breastfeeding or the drug to avoid potential serious adverse reactions in the breastfed infant.

REPRODUCTION

- Pregnancy must be avoided.
- Advise patient to use two reliable contraception forms for at least 1 month before, during drug therapy, and for at least 3 years following drug discontinuation as outlined above.

Nursing Considerations

> ! **WARNING** Don't give acitretin to a pregnant woman, a woman contemplating pregnancy, or a woman who may not use reliable contraception during drug therapy and for at least 3 years afterward, because acitretin causes major fetal abnormalities.

- Make sure patient has had two negative urine or serum pregnancy tests with a sensitivity of at least 25 mIU/ml before receiving acitretin. First test should be obtained when decision is made to use acitretin and second test during first 5 days of the menstrual period just before acitretin therapy starts. For patients with amenorrhea, second test should be done at least 11 days after the last act of unprotected sexual intercourse (which means without using two effective forms of contraception simultaneously).
- Check to make sure female patient of childbearing age has signed the patient agreement and informed consent form before starting acitretin therapy.
- Obtain a lipid profile, as ordered, before acitretin therapy starts and every 1 to 2 weeks for up to 8 weeks or until lipid effects are known. In high-risk patients, such as those with diabetes, obesity, or a history of alcohol abuse and those taking acitretin long term, check lipid profile periodically throughout therapy.
- Monitor liver enzymes, as ordered. If hepatotoxicity is suspected, expect to stop drug and investigate cause.

- Monitor patient closely for capillary leak syndrome demonstrated by localized or generalized edema, weight gain, fever, hypotension, and myalgias. If present, notify prescriber and expect to obtain laboratory studies for evidence of neutrophilia, hypoalbuminemia, and an elevated hematocrit. If confirmed, discontinue acitretin therapy, as ordered.
- Prepare patient for periodic bone radiography if she takes acitretin long term or she develops a skeletal disorder, because ossification abnormalities can occur, especially of the vertebral column, knees, and ankles.
- Monitor patient's eyes for abnormalities throughout therapy. Expect patient to stop drug and have an ophthalmologic examination if eye abnormalities occur.
- Monitor patient for evidence of increased intracranial pressure, such as papilledema, headache, nausea, vomiting, and visual disturbances. If papilledema occurs, stop drug therapy immediately and obtain a neurologic evaluation, as ordered. Patient should never receive a tetracycline while taking acitretin because combined use can increase intracranial pressure.
- Assess patient for suicidal ideation because depression and other psychiatric symptoms, including thoughts of self-harm, may occur with acitretin use. Expect drug to be discontinued if psychiatric symptoms develop.
- Be aware that significantly lower doses of phototherapy are needed during acitretin therapy because drug increases the risk of erythema. If patient develops serious skin reactions, notify prescriber and expect acitretin therapy to be discontinued.

PATIENT TEACHING

> ! **WARNING** Warn women of childbearing age that acitretin causes major fetal abnormalities.

- Inform woman of childbearing age that she must have a pregnancy test before acitretin therapy starts, every month during acitretin therapy, and every 3 months for 3 years after therapy stops.
- Emphasize to woman of childbearing age that she must use two effective forms of contraception simultaneously unless she

has chosen absolute abstinence or has had a hysterectomy. This must begin at least 1 month before acitretin therapy starts and continue throughout therapy and for at least 3 years after therapy ends.

- Caution women taking oral contraceptives that some prescribed and OTC drugs, including herbal supplements such as St. John's wort, may interfere with oral contraceptives. Urge her to tell prescriber about all drugs she takes.
- Alert female patient of childbearing age that any method of birth control can fail, including tubal ligation, and that microdose progestin "minipill" preparations are not recommended to be taken with acitretin. Tell her to seek immediate medical care on how to obtain emergency contraception if sexual intercourse occurs without using two effective forms of contraception simultaneously.
- Caution patient not to consume alcohol or products that contain alcohol during acitretin therapy and for 2 months after therapy ends.
- Inform patient that regular blood tests will be needed to monitor liver function. Tell him to notify prescriber if any of the following develops: nausea and vomiting, loss of appetite, dark urine, or whites of eyes or skin turns yellow.
- Warn patient, male or female of any age, not to donate blood during acitretin therapy and for at least 3 years after it ends.
- Review acitretin medication guide with patient, and answer the patient's questions.
- Inform patient that psoriasis may worsen during initial treatment and that full effects of drug may not be seen for up to 3 months.
- Caution patient to avoid hazardous activities until drug's CNS and ophthalmic effects are known.
- Inform patient that tolerance to contact lenses may decrease during acitretin therapy and for a period of time after treatment ends.
- Advise patient not to take more than the minimum recommended daily allowance of vitamin A during acitretin therapy because of the risk of vitamin A toxicity.
- Caution patient not to use sun lamps and to avoid excessive exposure to sunlight because the effects of UV light are enhanced by retinoids such as acitretin.

- Tell patient to notify prescriber of any new skin changes that become serious or prolonged, as acitretin therapy may have to be discontinued, if present.

acyclovir
Sitavig, Zovirax

acyclovir sodium
Zovirax I.V.

Class and Category
Pharmacologic class: Nucleoside analogue
Therapeutic class: Antiretroviral

Indications and Dosages
* *To treat initial episodes of herpes genitalis*

CAPSULES, ORAL SUSPENSION, TABLETS

Adults. 200 mg every 4 hr, 5 times daily for 10 days.

OINTMENT 5%

Adults. Applied to completely cover all lesions every 3 hr, 6 times daily for 7 days.

* *To treat severe initial episodes of herpes genitalis*

I.V. INFUSION

Adults and adolescents. 5 mg/kg every 8 hr for 5 days.

* *To suppress unusually frequent recurrent episodes of herpes genitalis (6 or more episodes per year)*

CAPSULES, ORAL SUSPENSION, TABLETS

Adults. 200 mg 3 times daily, increased if breakthrough occurs up to 200 mg, 5 times daily. Alternatively, 400 mg twice daily.

* *To treat recurrent episodes of herpes genitalis intermittently*

CAPSULES, ORAL SUSPENSION, TABLETS

Adults. 200 mg every 4 hr, 5 times daily for 5 days.

* *To treat recurrent herpes labialis in immunocompetent patients*

BUCCAL TABLETS (SITAVIG)

Adults. 50 mg as a single dose.

CREAM 5%

Adults and adolescents. Applied 5 times daily for 4 days and initiated as soon as possible following onset of signs and symptoms.

* *To treat non-life-threatening mucocutaneous Herpes simplex virus infections in immunocompromised patients*

OINTMENT 5%

Adults. Applied to completely cover all lesions every 3 hr, 6 times daily for 7 days.

✳ *To treat cutaneous and mucosal herpes simplex (HSV-1 and HSV-2) infections in immunocompromised patients*

I.V. INFUSION

Adults and adolescents. 5 mg/kg every 8 hr for 7 days.

Infants and children 3 months to 12 years. 10 mg/kg every 8 hr for 7 days.

✳ *To treat herpes simplex encephalitis*

I.V. INFUSION

Adults and adolescents. 10 mg/kg every 8 hr for 10 days.

Children 3 months to 12 years. 20 mg/kg every 8 hr for 10 days.

✳ *To treat neonatal herpes simplex virus infections*

I.V. INFUSION

Neonates postmenstrual age of at least 34 weeks. 20 mg/kg every 8 hr for 21 days.

Neonates postmenstrual age of less than 34 weeks. 20 mg/kg every 12 hr for 21 days.

✳ *To treat herpes zoster in immunocompetent patients*

CAPSULES, ORAL SUSPENSION, TABLETS

Adults. 800 mg every 4 hr, 5 times daily for 7 to 10 days with treatment initiated within 72 hr of onset of lesions.

✳ *To treat* Varicella zoster *infections in immunocompetent patients*

CAPSULES, ORAL SUSPENSION, TABLETS

Adults and children weighing over 40 kg (88 lb). 800 mg 4 times daily for 5 days.

Children 2 years and older weighing less than 40 kg (88 kg). 20 mg/kg 4 times daily for 5 days.

✳ *To treat* Varicella zoster *infections in immunocompromised patients*

I.V. INFUSION

Adults and adolescents. 10 mg/kg every 8 hr for 7 days.

Obese adults. 10 mg/kg (based on ideal body weight) every 8 hr for 7 days.

Children. 20 mg/kg every 8 hr for 7 days.

± **DOSAGE ADJUSTMENT** For patients with renal impairment who have genital herpes or *Herpes zoster* infections, oral dosage reduced or dosage interval increased as follows: if dosage is normally 200 mg every 4 hr 5 times daily and creatinine clearance is less than 10 ml/min, dosage interval increased to every 12 hr; if dosage is normally 400 mg every 12 hr and creatinine clearance is less than 10 ml/min, dosage reduced to 200 mg every 12 hr; if dosage is normally 800 mg every 4 hr and creatinine clearance is 10 to 25 ml/min, dosage interval increased to every 8 hr, and if creatinine clearance is less than 10 ml/min, dosage interval increased to every 12 hr. For patients receiving intravenous dosing, dosage reduced or dosage interval increased as follows: if creatinine clearance is 25 to 50 ml/min, dosage interval increased to every 12 hr; if creatinine clearance is 10 to 25 ml/min, dosage interval increased to every 24 hr; if creatinine clearance is 0 to 10 ml/min, dosage is reduced by 50% and dosage interval increased to every 24 hr. For patients receiving hemodialysis, an additional dose is given after each dialysis.

☰ Drug Administration

P.O.

▪ Drug can be given with food if GI upset occurs.

BUCCAL

▪ Apply within 1 hr after onset of symptoms and before the appearance of herpes labialis.

▪ Apply tablet, on same side as the herpes labialis symptoms, to upper gum region just above the incisor tooth using a dry finger covered in a finger cot immediately after taking tablet out of the blister.

▪ Hold in place with slight pressure over the upper lip for 30 seconds to ensure adhesion of tablet so tablet will remain in position as it gradually dissolves during the day.

▪ While either side of the tablet can be applied, the rounded side may be more comfortable for the patient.

▪ Tablet should not be chewed, crushed, sucked on, or swallowed. Food and drink can be taken normally, but chewing gum, touching or pressing the tablet after placement, wearing upper dentures, and brushing teeth should be avoided.

▪ Replace tablet if it does not adhere or falls off within the first 6 hours.

▪ If tablet is swallowed within first 6 hours, have patient drink a glass of water and apply a new tablet.

I.V.

▪ Prepare intravenous infusion by first dissolving the contents of a 10-ml vial containing 500 mg of acyclovir in 10 ml of Sterile Water for Injection or a 20-ml vial containing 1,000 mg of acyclovir in 20 ml of Sterile Water for Injection (do not use Bacteriostatic Water for Injection containing benzyl alcohol or parabens). The result is a concentration of 50 mg acyclovir per milliliter. Shake vial well to ensure that drug has been dissolved.

- Use reconstituted solution within 12 hr. Know that if refrigerated, a precipitate may form but will redissolve at room temperature.
- Remove reconstituted solution from vial and add to any appropriate intravenous solution to deliver concentration needed. Use diluted solution within 24 hr.
- Infuse over 1 hr at a constant rate to reduce risk of renal tubular damage.
- Never administer drug intramuscularly, subcutaneously, or as an I.V. bolus or rapid injection.
- Know that infusion concentrations of about 7 mg/ml or lower are recommended, as higher concentrations may cause inflammation or phlebitis at the injection site if inadvertent extravasation occurs.
- *Incompatibilities:* Blood products, dobutamine, dopamine, morphine sulfate, ondansetron, protein-containing solutions

TOPICAL
- Apply with a rubber glove or finger cot, covering all lesions thoroughly.
- Apply about 1/2-inch ribbon of ointment per 4 square inches of surface area.
- Keep topical product away from eyes.

Route	Onset	Peak	Duration
P.O.	Unknown	1.5–2 hr	Unknown
P.O. (buccal)	Unknown	7 hr	Unknown
I.V.	Immediate	1 hr	Unknown
Topical	Unknown	Unknown	Unknown

Half-life: 2–3 hr

Mechanism of Action
Several actions (inhibition of DNA polymerase, premature termination of DNA synthesis and thymidine kinase specificity) combine to inhibit herpes virus replication.

Contraindications
Hypersensitivity to acyclovir or valacyclovir or any of their components

Interactions
DRUGS
cimetidine, probenecid: Possibly increased acyclovir plasma concentrations
mycophenolate mofetil: Increased plasma concentration of both drugs

Adverse Reactions
CNS: Agitation, asthenia, ataxia, **coma**, confusion, dizziness, **encephalopathy**, fever, hallucinations, headache, malaise, paresthesia, psychotic symptoms, **seizures**, somnolence, tremor
CV: Peripheral edema
EENT: Visual abnormalities
GI: Diarrhea, elevated liver enzymes, gastrointestinal distress, **hepatitis**, hyperbilirubinemia, jaundice, nausea, vomiting
GU: **Acute renal failure**, elevated blood creatinine and blood urea nitrogen, hematuria, **hemolytic uremic syndrome**, renal pain
HEME: Anemia, leukocytosis, **leukopenia**, lymphadenopathy, **neutropenia**, **thrombocytopenia**, **thrombotic thrombocytopenic purpura**
MS: Myalgia
RESP: Dyspnea
SKIN: Alopecia, contact dermatitis (topical), eczema (topical), **erythema multiforme**, photosensitivity, pruritus, rash, **Stevens–Johnson syndrome, toxic epidermal necrolysis**, urticaria
Other: **Anaphylaxis, angioedema,** generalized pain, injection-site reactions (inflammation, phlebitis)

Childbearing Considerations
PREGNANCY
- It is not known if drug can cause fetal harm.
- Use with caution only if benefit to mother outweighs potential risk to fetus.

LACTATION
- Drug is present in breast milk (not known for buccal form).
- Patient should check with prescriber before breastfeeding.

Nursing Considerations
- Know that acyclovir therapy should be initiated as soon as possible after signs and symptoms appear.
- Use caution when administering acyclovir to patients with dehydration or preexisting renal disease or who are receiving other

nephrotoxic drugs, because of increased risk of renal impairment. Also use cautiously in patients with underlying neurologic disorders as well as electrolyte abnormalities, hepatic dysfunction, or significant hypoxia because, although uncommon, encephalopathic changes have occurred with acyclovir administration.

- Ensure that patient receiving acyclovir is adequately hydrated before drug is given, to decrease risk of renal impairment.

! **WARNING** Know that hemolytic uremic syndrome and thrombotic thrombocytopenic purpura have occurred in immunocompromised patients receiving acyclovir therapy and have resulted in death. Report any hematologic or renal dysfunction signs and symptoms to prescriber immediately.

PATIENT TEACHING

- Inform patient that acyclovir does not cure herpes infections but helps to manage the signs and symptoms.
- Tell patient prescribed buccal tablets that it is given as a single dose and should be placed onto the upper gum within 1 hr after the onset of prodromal symptoms and before the appearance of any signs of a cold sore. The tablet should not be chewed, crushed, sucked, or swallowed whole.
- Explain to patient receiving topical form of acyclovir how to apply the cream or ointment ordered, stressing need to completely cover entire lesion area and to apply only to affected areas. Tell patient to use a finger cot or rubber glove to apply to prevent transferring infection to other parts of his body or to other people. Tell patient to start therapy as early as possible following appearance of signs and symptoms. Instruct patient not to apply topical form to the inside of his mouth or nose or to put in his eyes.
- Instruct patient prescribed oral suspension form to use an accurate measuring device when measuring dosage.
- Stress importance of stopping drug therapy and seeking immediate medical attention if any signs and symptoms of an allergic reaction occur.
- Instruct patient to seek medical attention if his symptoms become severe or

he experiences troublesome adverse reactions.
- Tell women of childbearing age to notify prescriber if pregnancy occurs or is suspected.
- Stress importance of maintaining adequate hydration throughout acyclovir therapy to reduce risk of kidney damage.
- Advise patient with genital herpes to avoid contact, including intercourse, when lesions and/or symptoms are present, to avoid infecting partner.
- Instruct patient who requires acyclovir therapy to manage recurrent genital herpes to initiate therapy at the first sign or symptom of an episode.

adalimumab
Humira

adalimumab-adbm
Cyltezo

adalimumab-adaz
Hyrimoz

adalimumab-afzb
Abrilada

adalimumab-atto
Amjevita

adalimumab-bwwd
Hadlima

adalimumab-fkjp
Hulio

☰ Class and Category

Pharmacologic class: Monoclonal antibody
Therapeutic class: Tumor necrosis factor (TNF) blocker

☰ Indications and Dosages

＊ *To reduce signs and symptoms, induce major clinical response, inhibit progression of structural damage, and improve physical function in patients with moderately to severely active rheumatoid arthritis; to reduce signs and symptoms, inhibit progression of structural damage, and improve physical function in patients with psoriatic arthritis; to reduce signs and symptoms in patients with active ankylosing spondylitis*

SUBCUTANEOUS INJECTION (ABRILADA, AMJEVITA, CYLTEZO, HADLIMA, HULIO, HUMIRA, HYRIMOZ)

Adults. 40 mg every other wk.

±**DOSAGE ADJUSTMENT** Dosage may be increased to 40 mg every wk or 80 mg every other wk, as needed, for patients with rheumatoid arthritis not taking methotrexate.

＊ *To reduce signs and symptoms and induce and maintain clinical remission in patients with moderately to severely active Crohn's disease who have had an inadequate response to conventional therapy or who have stopped responding to or have become intolerant of infliximab*

SUBCUTANEOUS INJECTION (ABRILADA, AMJEVITA, CYLTEZO, HADLIMA, HULIO, HUMIRA, HYRIMOZ)

Adults. *Initial:* 160 mg given as four 40-mg injections for 1 day or 80 mg given as two 40-mg injections for 2 consecutive days, followed by 80 mg given as two 40-mg injections on day 15. *Maintenance:* 40 mg every other wk starting on day 29.

＊ *To reduce signs and symptoms and induce and maintain clinical remission in children with moderately to severely active Crohn's disease who have had an inadequate response to conventional therapy or who have had an inadequate response to corticosteroids or immunomodulators such as azathioprine, 6-mercaptopurine, or methotrexate*

SUBCUTANEOUS INJECTION (CYLTEZO, HUMIRA)

Children age 6 and over who weigh 40 kg (88 lb) or more. *Initial:* 160 mg given as four 40-mg injections on day 1 or 80 mg given as two 40-mg injections for 2 consecutive days, followed by 80 mg given as two 40-mg injections on day 15. *Maintenance:* 40 mg every other wk starting on day 29.

Children age 6 and over who weigh less than 40 kg (88 lb) but at least 17 kg (37 lb). *Initial:* 80 mg given as two 40-mg injections on day 1, followed by 40 mg on day 15. *Maintenance:* 20 mg every other wk starting on day 29.

＊ *To reduce signs and symptoms of moderately to severely active polyarticular juvenile idiopathic arthritis*

SUBCUTANEOUS INJECTION (CYLTEZO, HUMIRA)

Children age 2 and over who weigh 30 kg (66 lb) or more. 40 mg every other wk.
Children age 2 and over who weigh less than 30 kg (66 lb) but at least 15 kg (33 lb). 20 mg every other wk.

SUBCUTANEOUS INJECTION (HUMIRA)

Children age 2 and over who weigh less than 15 kg (33 lb) but at least 10 kg (22 lb). 10 mg every other wk.

SUBCUTANEOUS INJECTION (ABRILADA)

Children age 4 and over who weigh 30 kg (66 lb) or more. 40 mg every other wk.
Children age 4 and over who weigh less than 30 kg (66 lb) but at least 15 kg (33 lb). 20 mg every other wk.
Children age 4 and over who weigh less than 15 kg (33 lb) but at least 10 kg (22 lb). 10 mg every other wk.

SUBCUTANEOUS INJECTION (AMJEVITA, HULIO)

Children age 4 and over who weigh 30 kg (66 lb) or more. 40 mg every other wk.
Children age 4 and over who weigh less than 30 kg (66 lb) but at least 15 kg (33 lb). 20 mg every other wk.

SUBCUTANEOUS INJECTION (HADLIMA, HYRIMOZ)

Children age 4 and over who weigh 30 kg (66 lb) or more. 40 mg every other wk.

＊ *To treat moderate to severe chronic plaque psoriasis in patients who are candidates for systemic therapy or phototherapy, and when other systemic therapies are less appropriate*

SUBCUTANEOUS INJECTION (ABRILADA, AMJEVITA, CYLTEZO, HADLIMA, HULIO, HUMIRA, HYRIMOZ)

Adults. *Initial:* 80 mg given as two 40-mg injections on day 1 followed 1 wk later with 40 mg. *Maintenance:* 40 mg every other wk.

To induce and sustain a remission in patients with moderate to severe active ulcerative colitis who have had an inadequate response to immunosuppressants such as azathioprine, corticosteroids, or 6-mercaptopurine

SUBCUTANEOUS INJECTION (ABRILADA, AMJEVITA, CYLTEZO, HADLIMA, HULIO, HUMIRA, HYRIMOZ)

Adults. *Initial:* 160 mg given as four 40-mg injections on day 1 or given as two 40-mg injections on day 1 and repeated on day 2, followed by 80 mg given as two 40-mg injections on day 15 and 40 mg on day 29. *Maintenance:* 40 mg every other wk.

±**DOSAGE ADJUSTMENT** Know that drug should be discontinued if there is no evidence of clinical remission by 8 weeks.

To treat moderate to severe active pediatric ulcerative colitis

SUBCUTANEOUS INJECTION (HUMIRA)

Children age 5 and older weighing 40 kg (88 lb) or more. *Initial:* 160 mg given as four 40-mg injections on day 1 or given as two 40-mg injections on day 1 and repeated on day 2, followed by 80 mg given as two 40-mg injections on days 8 and 15 and 40 mg on day 29. **Maintenance:** 40 mg every wk or 80 mg every other wk.

Children age 5 and older who weigh less than 40 kg (88 lb) but at least 20 kg (44 lb). *Initial:* 80 mg given as two 40-mg injections on day 1 followed by 40 mg on days 8 and 15. *Maintenance:* 20 mg every wk or 40 mg every other wk.

To treat moderate to severe hidradenitis suppurativa

SUBCUTANEOUS INJECTION (HUMIRA)

Adults and adolescents age 12 and over weighing 60 kg (132 lb) or more. *Initial:* 160 mg given as four 40-mg injections on day 1 or two 40-mg injections on day 1 and repeated on day 2, followed by 80 mg given as two 40-mg injections on day 15. *Maintenance:* 40 mg weekly starting on day 29.

Adolescents age 12 and over weighing 30 kg (66 lb) to 60 kg (132 lb). *Initial:* 80 mg given as two 40-mg injections on day 1 followed by 40 mg on day 8. *Maintenance:* 40 mg every other wk starting on day 22 from initial dose.

To treat noninfectious intermediate, posterior, and panuveitis

SUBCUTANEOUS INJECTION (HUMIRA)

Adults. *Initial:* 80 mg given as two 40-mg injections on day 1 followed 1 wk later with 40 mg. *Maintenance:* 40 mg every other wk.

Children age 2 and over weighing 30 kg (66 lb) or more. 40 mg every other wk.

Children age 2 and over weighing less than 30 kg (66 lb) but at least 15 kg (33 lb). 20 mg every other wk.

Children age 2 and over weighing less than 15 kg (33 lb) but at least 10 kg (22 lb). 10 mg every other wk.

Drug Administration

SUBCUTANEOUS

- Know that adalimumab products must be refrigerated but may be left at room temperature with cap or cover on for about 15 to 30 minutes before injecting.
- Inject doses in separate sites in the abdomen or thigh.
- Rotate injection sites and do not give injections into an area where the skin is bruised, hard, red, or tender.
- Activate the protection device on needles of prefilled syringes delivered to institutions by holding the syringe in one hand and, with the other hand, sliding outer protective shield over exposed needle until it locks into place.
- Know that adalimumab may come in a single-use glass vial containing 40 mg (0.8 ml) of adalimumab referred to as an "institutional use vial" because the drug should only be given in a medical institution. Withdraw only one dose when using the "institutional use vial" and administer promptly. Because the vial does not contain preservatives, discard any unused drug.
- Protect drug from light.
- Check product being used to determine if latex may be contained in the pen or prefilled syringe. Do not handle if allergic to latex.

Route	Onset	Peak	Duration
SubQ	Unknown	131–187 hr	Unknown

Half-life: 10–20 days

Mechanism of Action

Binds to tumor necrosis factor (TNF) to block interaction with p55 and p75 cell surface TNF receptors, and lyses surface TNF-expressing cells in the presence of complement. TNF may be a major component of rheumatoid arthritis inflammation and joint destruction. Reduced TNF level in synovial fluid improves signs and symptoms and prevents further structural damage in rheumatoid arthritis. It also causes a decrease in levels of acute phase reactants of inflammation such as C-reactive protein, which may explain why it is useful in alleviating signs and symptoms in other inflammatory disease processes.

Contraindications

Active infection, hypersensitivity to adalimumab or its components

Interactions

DRUGS

abatacept, anakinra, rituximab: Possibly increased risk of serious infection and neutropenia in patients with rheumatoid arthritis
CYP450 substrates with narrow therapeutic index such as cyclosporine, theophylline, warfarin: Possibly altered effectiveness of these drugs
live vaccines: Increased risk of adverse vaccine effects

Adverse Reactions

CNS: Confusion, **CVA**, demyelinating disorders such as **Guillain–Barré syndrome** or multiple sclerosis, fever, headache, **hypertensive encephalopathy**, paresthesia, **subdural hematoma**, syncope, tremor
CV: Arrhythmias, atrial fibrillation, cardiac arrest, chest pain, **congestive heart failure**, coronary artery disease, **deep vein thrombosis**, hypercholesterolemia, hyperlipidemia, hypertension, **MI**, palpitations, **pericardial effusion, pericarditis**, peripheral edema, **systemic vasculitis**, tachycardia
EENT: Cataract, optic neuritis, sinusitis
ENDO: Ketosis, parathyroid disorder
GI: Abdominal pain, cholecystitis, cholelithiasis, diverticulitis, elevated alkaline phosphatase level, elevated liver enzymes, esophagitis, gastroenteritis, **gastrointestinal hemorrhage, hepatic failure or necrosis, hepatitis or reactivation of hepatitis B, large bowel perforation**, nausea, **pancreatitis**, vomiting

GU: Hematuria, paraproteinemia, **pyelonephritis**, UTI
HEME: Agranulocytosis, aplastic anemia, granulocytopenia, leukopenia, lymphocytosis, **pancytopenia**, polycythemia, **thrombocytopenia**
MS: Arthritis (including pyogenic or septic arthritis); back, extremity, pelvic, or thorax pain; bone disorder, fracture, or necrosis; muscle spasms; myasthenia; prosthetic infections; synovitis
RESP: Asthma, bronchitis, **bronchospasm**, decreased pulmonary function, dyspnea, **interstitial lung disease,** pleural effusion, pneumonia, **pulmonary embolism**, tuberculosis (new or reactivation), upper respiratory tract infection
SKIN: Alopecia, cellulitis, cutaneous vasculitis, erysipelas (red skin), **erythema multiforme**, herpes zoster, **lichenoid reaction, melanoma, Merkel cell carcinoma**, new or worsening psoriasis, **nonmelanoma skin cancer**, rash, **Stevens–Johnson syndrome**, urticaria
Other: Anaphylaxis; angioedema; antibody formation against adalimumab; bacterial, mycobacterial, fungal, parasitic, viral, and other opportunistic infections; benign or unspecified cysts or polyps; dehydration; flare-up of disease process; flu-like symptoms; healing abnormalities; injection-site erythema, hemorrhage, itching, pain, or swelling; lupus-like symptoms; **lymphomas and other malignancies such as breast, colon, lung, and prostate**; postsurgical infection; sarcoidosis; **sepsis**

Childbearing Considerations

PREGNANCY

- It is not known if drug can cause fetal harm. However, monoclonal antibodies increasingly cross the placental barrier as pregnancy progresses.
- Infants exposed to drug in utero should have risks and benefits considered before being given live or live-attenuated vaccines.
- Use with caution only if benefit to mother outweighs potential risk to fetus.

LACTATION

- Drug is present in breast milk.
- Patient should check with prescriber before breastfeeding.

≣ Nursing Considerations

- Use adalimumab products cautiously in patients with recurrent infection or increased risk of infection and in patients who live in regions where tuberculosis and certain mycoses, such as *Histoplasma*, are endemic. Be aware that *Legionella* and *Listeria,* two bacterial infections, also have occurred with tumor necrosis factor–alpha blockers such as adalimumab. Monitor patient closely because infections associated with tumor necrosis factor–alpha blocker therapy may involve multiple organ systems and become life-threatening. Be aware that patients over 65 years of age, patients with other diagnoses, and patients taking concomitant immunosuppressants may be at greater risk of infection.

! **WARNING** Assess patient for signs and symptoms of an active infection before beginning adalimumab therapy. If patient has evidence of an active infection when drug is prescribed, therapy shouldn't start until the infection has been treated. Monitor all patients for infection during therapy, especially those receiving concomitant immunosuppressants. If a serious infection develops, drug should be stopped.

- Ensure that children with juvenile idiopathic arthritis are up to date with current immunization guidelines prior to adalimumab therapy being started. However, know that they may receive vaccinations, except for live vaccines, while taking adalimumab, if needed. Be aware that the safety of administering live or live-attenuated vaccines in infants exposed to drug in utero is unknown.
- Use cautiously in a patient with a preexisting or recent onset of a central or peripheral nervous system demyelinating disorder such as Guillain–Barré, multiple sclerosis, or optic neuritis, because, although rare, new onset or exacerbation of demyelinating disorders have occurred with adalimumab therapy. If this occurs, know that drug should be discontinued.
- Make sure patient has a tuberculin skin test before therapy starts. If skin test is positive, treatment of latent tuberculosis will start before adalimumab, as prescribed. Also, ensure that patient previously treated for tuberculosis, including prophylactic treatment, has a tuberculin skin test periodically throughout therapy, as adalimumab products may induce new onset or reactivate tuberculosis. Also monitor patient for signs and symptoms of tuberculosis, as tests for latent tuberculosis infection may be falsely negative while taking adalimumab.
- Review patient's medical and medication history and discuss with prescriber prior to starting an adalimumab product.
- Be aware that adalimumab-adbm is interchangeable with adalimumab.

! **WARNING** Stop adalimumab immediately and tell prescriber if patient has an allergic reaction. Expect to provide supportive care.

- Watch closely for evidence of congestive heart failure (sudden, unexplained weight gain; dyspnea; crackles; anxiety), and notify prescriber if they occur.
- Monitor patient's CBC, as ordered, because adalimumab products may have adverse hematologic effects. Notify prescriber about persistent bleeding, bruising, fever, or pallor.
- Be aware that, although rare, malignancies, especially lymphomas and leukemias, have occurred in patients receiving TNF blockers such as adalimumab products. These malignancies have also occurred in children. Patients with rheumatoid arthritis, especially those with very active disease, and patients with ankylosing spondylitis, Crohn's disease, plaque psoriasis, or psoriatic arthritis are at greatest risk. Monitor patients closely.

PATIENT TEACHING

- Inform patient that the first injection of adalimumab must take place with a healthcare professional present.
- Teach patient or caregiver how to give adalimumab as a subcutaneous injection at home, if applicable. Emphasize importance of injecting the full amount in the syringe to obtain the correct dose.
- Advise patient that the needle cover contains rubber and can cause a latex-induced allergic reaction if touched with bare hands.
- Provide patient or caregiver with a puncture-resistant container for disposal of needles and syringes at home.

- Instruct patient or caregiver to rotate injection sites in the abdomen and thigh and to avoid injecting in any area that's bruised, hard, red, or tender.
- Inform patient that prefilled syringes must be refrigerated (not frozen) but may be left at room temperature for 15 to 30 minutes before injecting to decrease injection discomfort. Keep the cap or cover on while allowing it to reach room temperature. Also keep syringe protected from light and stored in the original container.
- Urge patient to check expiration dates and not to use outdated drug. Also tell patient not to use a prefilled syringe if the liquid is cloudy, discolored, or has flakes or particles in it.
- Review signs and symptoms of an allergic reaction (difficulty breathing, rash, swollen face), and tell patient to seek emergency care immediately if these occur.
- Inform patient that injection-site reactions (such as bruising, itching, rash, redness, and swelling) may occur but are usually mild and transient. Instruct him to apply a towel soaked with cold water on the injection site if it hurts or remains swollen. If reaction does not disappear or seems to worsen, tell patient to call prescriber immediately.
- Inform patient that tuberculosis may occur during adalimumab therapy. Instruct him to report persistent cough, wasting or weight loss, and low-grade fever to prescriber.
- Teach patient how to recognize evidence of infection and bleeding disorders and to tell prescriber if they occur; drug may have to be stopped. Advise patient to avoid people with infections and to have all prescribed laboratory tests.
- Inform patient that the risk of certain kinds of cancer, especially lymphomas, is higher in patients taking adalimumab but still rare. Emphasize the importance of follow-up visits and reporting an unusual or sudden onset of signs or symptoms.
- Caution patient against receiving live-virus vaccines while taking adalimumab because doing so may adversely affect the immune system.
- Inform patient that blood samples may be needed periodically, but especially around week 24 of therapy, to check for autoantibody development. Explain that adalimumab therapy will have to be stopped if it's detected.
- Instruct patient to report lupus-like signs and symptoms that, although rare, may occur during therapy, such as chest pain that doesn't go away, joint pain, a rash on arms or cheeks that is sensitive to the sun, or shortness of breath. Explain that drug may be stopped if these occur.
- Advise patient to inform all healthcare providers about adalimumab use and to inform prescriber about any OTC medications being taken, including herbal remedies and mineral and vitamin supplements.
- Instruct women of childbearing age to notify prescriber immediately if pregnancy is suspected or known, as adalimumab products may affect the immune response of an utero-exposed newborn or infant. Also, emphasize the importance of telling pediatrician if an adalimumab product was taken any time during pregnancy, prior to having infant receive any vaccines.
- Encourage mother wishing to breastfeed infant to discuss with prescriber before doing so.

adefovir dipivoxil
Hepsera

Class and Category
Pharmacologic class: Nucleotide analogue
Therapeutic class: Antiviral

Indications and Dosages
* *To treat chronic hepatitis B in patients with evidence of active viral replication and either evidence of persistent elevations in serum aminotransferases (ALT or AST) or histologically active disease*

TABLETS

Adults and children age 12 and over. 10 mg once daily.

± **DOSAGE ADJUSTMENT** For patients with a creatinine clearance between 30 and 49 ml/min, dosage interval changed to every 48 hr. For patients with a creatinine clearance between 10 and 29 ml/min, dosage interval changed to 72 hr. For patients receiving hemodialysis, dosage interval changed to every 7 days following dialysis.

Drug Administration

P.O.

No special instructions recommended by manufacturer for administration.

Route	Onset	Peak	Duration
P.O.	Unknown	0.5–4 hr	Unknown

Half-life: 7–8 hr

Mechanism of Action

Inhibits hepatitis B virus (HBV) by competing with the natural substrate deoxyadenosine triphosphate and by causing DNA chain termination after its incorporation into viral DNA, which prevents replication.

Contraindications

Hypersensitivity to adefovir dipivoxil or its components

Interactions

DRUGS

drugs that are excreted renally or known to affect renal function, such as *aminoglycosides, cyclosporine, NSAIDs, tacrolimus, and vancomycin:* Possibly increased serum concentrations of adefovir or these drugs or both, increasing risk of adverse reactions

Adverse Reactions

CNS: Asthenia, headache
GI: Abdominal pain, diarrhea, dyspepsia, flatulence, nausea, **pancreatitis, severe acute exacerbations of hepatitis, severe hepatomegaly with steatosis,** vomiting
GU: Abnormal renal function, elevated creatinine level, **Fanconi syndrome, nephrotoxicity, proximal renal tubulopathy, renal failure**
MS: Bone pain, myopathy, osteomalacia
SKIN: Pruritus, rash
Other: HIV resistance, hypophosphatemia, lactic acidosis

Childbearing Considerations

PREGNANCY

- Pregnancy exposure registry: 1-800-258-4263.
- It is not known if drug can cause fetal harm.
- Use with caution only if benefit to mother outweighs potential risk to fetus.

LACTATION

- It is not known if drug is present in breast milk.
- Patient should check with prescriber before breastfeeding.

Nursing Considerations

- Check to be sure HIV antibody testing has been done prior to starting adefovir therapy because treatment with anti-hepatitis B therapies, such as adefovir, may cause an emergence of HIV resistance.
- Use with extreme caution in patients with renal dysfunction. Check to ensure that patient's creatinine clearance is known before adefovir therapy begins and then rechecked periodically throughout therapy, because adefovir may cause a delayed nephrotoxicity that may require dosage interval to be lengthened or drug discontinued. Know that patients at higher risk include those having underlying renal dysfunction and patients taking concomitant nephrotoxic agents such as aminoglycosides, cyclosporine, NSAIDs, tacrolimus, and vancomycin.
- Use caution when administering adefovir to patient with liver dysfunction or known risk factors for liver disease.

! **WARNING** Know that lactic acidosis and severe hepatomegaly with steatosis have occurred with adefovir therapy and death has occurred in some patients. Risk factors include presence of obesity, prolonged nucleoside exposure, and being a woman. However, know that lactic acidosis and severe hepatomegaly with steatosis have also occurred in patients with no known risk factors. Expect drug to be discontinued in any patient who develops clinical or laboratory findings suggestive of lactic acidosis or pronounced hepatotoxicity, even in the absence of marked transaminase elevations.

- Monitor patient throughout treatment for evidence of loss of therapeutic response. Indicators include increasing levels of HBV DNA over time after an initial decline below assay limit, progression of clinical signs or symptoms of hepatic disease and/or worsening of hepatic necroinflammatory findings, or return of persistently elevated ALT levels. These findings may require drug to be discontinued.
- Be aware that immune reconstitution syndrome has occurred in patients treated

with combination antiretroviral therapy, including adefovir. The inflammatory response predisposes susceptible patients to opportunistic infections such as cytomegalovirus infection, *Mycobacterium avium* infection, *Pneumocystis jiroveci* pneumonia, or tuberculosis. Autoimmune disorders such as Graves' disease, Guillain–Barré syndrome, or polymyositis have also occurred. Report sudden or unusual adverse reactions to prescriber.

- Expect patient to be closely monitored for at least several months after adefovir has been discontinued, because exacerbation of hepatitis may occur, some cases of which have been severe.

PATIENT TEACHING

- Instruct patient to take adefovir once daily. If he misses a dose, tell him to take it as soon as he remembers but not to double the next dose or take more than the prescribed dose.
- Advise patient that treatment with adefovir does not reduce the risk of transmission of HBV to others.
- Tell patient to report any new or worsening symptoms to prescriber immediately, because emergence of resistant hepatitis B virus may occur or disease may worsen during treatment.
- Instruct patient with hepatitis B on the importance of testing for HIV before therapy begins and then periodically throughout therapy to avoid development of resistance to HIV treatment.
- Warn patient with hepatitis B that acute severe exacerbations of hepatitis B may occur following discontinuation of adefovir. He should not discontinue drug without prescriber knowledge. Tell patient to report any reappearance of signs and symptoms of hepatitis B.
- Instruct mother not to breastfeed while she is receiving adefovir therapy, as drug is present in human milk.
- Tell women of childbearing age to report a known or suspected pregnancy.

! **WARNING** Alert patient that severe conditions may develop while taking adefovir. Encourage him to stop taking drug and seek medical attention immediately if he experiences any persistent, severe, or unusual symptoms; especially abdominal pain, change

in urine characteristics or urination pattern, loss of appetite, pale stools, muscle pain, or yellowing of the eyes.

adenosine
Adenocard, Adenoscan

Class and Category
Pharmacologic class: Nucleoside
Therapeutic class: Class V antiarrhythmic, diagnostic aid

Indications and Dosages
✱ *To convert paroxysmal supraventricular tachycardia (PSVT) to normal sinus rhythm*

I.V. INJECTION (ADENOCARD)
Adults and children weighing 50 kg (110 lb) or more. *Initial:* 6 mg. If PSVT continues after 1 to 2 min, 12 mg given and repeated in 1 to 2 min, if needed. *Maximum:* 12 mg as a single dose.
Children weighing less than 50 kg. *Initial:* 0.05 to 0.1 mg/kg. If PSVT continues after 1 to 2 min, additional bolus injections are given, incrementally increasing dose by 0.05 to 0.1 mg/kg. Administration continued until PSVT converts to normal sinus rhythm or until patient reaches maximum single dose. *Maximum:* 0.3 mg/kg (12 mg) as a single dose.
✱ *Adjunct to thallium-201 myocardial perfusion scintigraphy in patients unable to exercise adequately during testing*

I.V. INJECTION (ADENOSCAN)
Adults. 140 mcg/kg/min (total infused dose of 0.84 mg/kg).

Drug Administration
I.V.
- Inspect adenosine for crystals before use. If solution isn't clear, discard.
- Give Adenocard by rapid I.V. bolus over 1 to 2 seconds. Slower delivery can cause systemic vasodilation and reflex tachycardia.
- Administer either directly into a central or peripheral vein or, if given into an I.V. line, give as close to patient as possible and follow with a rapid saline flush.
- Don't give single doses of Adenocard more than 12 mg.
- *Incompatibilities:* Other drugs
- Give Adenoscan used as an adjunct to thallium-201 myocardial perfusion

scintigraphy as a continuous peripheral intravenous infusion over 6 minutes. Know that the required dose of thallium-201 should be injected at the midpoint of the Adenoscan infusion. It is compatible with Adenoscan and may be injected directly into the Adenoscan infusion set.

- Store drug at room temperature.
- Discard any unused drug.

Route	Onset	Peak	Duration
I.V.	Immediate	Immediate	Unknown

Half-life: > 10 sec

Mechanism of Action

Slows conduction time through the AV node and can interrupt AV node reentry pathways to restore normal sinus rhythm.

Contraindications

Hypersensitivity to adenosine or its components; second- or third-degree heart block or sick sinus syndrome, except in patients with a functioning artificial pacemaker

Interactions

DRUGS

carbamazepine: Increased degree of heart block
digoxin, verapamil: Possibly increased depressant effect on SA or AV node and increased risk of ventricular fibrillation
dipyridamole: Increased adenosine effects
methylxanthines, such as theophylline: Antagonized adenosine effects

FOODS

caffeine: Antagonized adenosine effects

Adverse Reactions

CNS: Apprehension, CVA, dizziness, headache, heaviness in arms, light-headedness, nervousness, paresthesia, **seizures**
CV: **Atrial fibrillation, bradycardia, cardiac arrest**, chest pain or pressure, **heart block**, hypertension, **hypotension, MI**, palpitations, **prolonged asystole, sinus exit block or pause, sustained ventricular tachycardia**, tachycardia, **torsades de pointes**, transient hypertension, **ventricular fibrillation**
EENT: Blurred vision, metallic taste, **throat tightness**
GI: Nausea, vomiting

MS: Jaw, neck, and back pain
RESP: **Bronchoconstriction, bronchospasm,** dyspnea, hyperventilation, **respiratory arrest**
SKIN: Diaphoresis, erythema, facial flushing, rash
Other: Injection-site reactions including pain, sensitivity reactions

Childbearing Considerations

PREGNANCY

- It is not known if drug can cause fetal harm.
- Use with caution only if benefit to mother outweighs potential risk to fetus.

LACTATION

- It is not known if drug is present in breast milk.
- A decision should be made to discontinue breastfeeding or the drug to avoid potential serious adverse reactions in the breastfed infant.

Nursing Considerations

- Know that Adenoscan should not be given to patients with signs and symptoms of acute myocardial ischemia, as these patients may be at greater risk for serious cardiovascular reactions, including a myocardial infarction during a medical stress test.
- Monitor heart rate and rhythm, blood pressure, and respiratory status often during adenosine therapy.
- Be aware that at the time of conversion to normal sinus rhythm, arrhythmias (such as premature atrial or ventricular contractions, sinus bradycardia, sinus tachycardia, or AV block) may occur for a few seconds, but they don't usually require intervention.

! **WARNING** Stop drug use and notify prescriber immediately if severe respiratory difficulties develop or patient develops other signs of hypersensitivity such as chest discomfort, erythema, flushing, or rash.

PATIENT TEACHING

- Inform patient of increased risk for serious adverse effects. Instruct patient to report chest pain, palpitations, difficulty breathing, or severe headache during adenosine therapy.
- Warn patient that mild, temporary reactions may occur, such as flushing, nausea, and dizziness.

aducanumab-avwa
Aduhelm

Class and Category
Pharmacologic class: Human immunoglobulin gamma 1 monoclonal antibody
Therapeutic class: Anti-dementia

Indications and Dosages
* *To treat Alzheimer's disease in patients with mild cognitive impairment or mild dementia stage of disease*

I.V. INFUSION
Adults. *Initial:* 1 mg/kg every 4 wk for two doses, then 3 mg/kg every 4 wk for two doses, then 6 mg/kg every 4 wk for two doses, followed by 10 mg/kg 4 wk later. *Maintenance:* 10 mg/kg every 4 wk after initial titration.

Drug Administration
I.V.
- Each vial is for single use only. Discard any portion that is unused.
- Calculate the dose, total volume of the drug solution required, and the number of vials needed using the patient's actual body weight. More than one vial may be required to achieve dose required.
- Drug vials come in two different strengths: 170 mg/1.7 ml to yield a 100-mg/ml concentration or 300 mg/3 ml to yield a 100-mg/ml concentration. Select the correct vial(s) for the required volume.
- Drug solution should be clear to opalescent and colorless to yellow. Discard if solution has opaque particles, is discolored, or has other foreign particles.
- Remove flip-off cap, wipe rubber stopper with alcohol, and insert the syringe needle into the vial through the center of the rubber stopper. Withdraw the required volume and add to an infusion bag containing 100 ml of 0.9% Sodium Chloride Injection solution. Do not use other I.V. diluents.
- Gently invert the infusion bag to mix completely. Do not shake.
- Use immediately after dilution, if possible. If not infused immediately, store diluted at room temperature for up to 12 hours or refrigerated up to 3 days. If refrigerated, allow the diluted solution to return to room temperature before administration.
- Infuse using a sterile, low-protein-binding, 0.2- or 0.22-micron in-line filter over 1 hour every 4 weeks and at least 21 days apart.
- Stop infusion immediately at the first sign or symptom of a hypersensitivity reaction.
- When an infusion is missed, expect to resume administration at the same dose as soon as possible.

Route	Onset	Peak	Duration
I.V.	Unknown	Unknown	Unknown

Half-life: 24.8 days

Mechanism of Action
- Reduces amyloid-beta plaques by directly acting against aggregated soluble and insoluble forms of amyloid-beta. Reducing amyloid-beta plaques improves dementia caused by Alzheimer's disease because the accumulation of amyloid-beta plaques in the brain is a known feature of Alzheimer's disease.

Contraindications
Hypersensitivity to aducanumab-avwa or its components

Interactions
None reported by manufacturer

Adverse Reactions
CNS: Altered mental status, amyloid-related imaging abnormalities-edema (ARIA-E), ARIA-H microhemorrhage, ARIA-H siderosis, confusion, delirium, disorientation, dizziness, headache
EENT: Visual changes
GI: Diarrhea, nausea
SKIN: Urticaria
OTHER: Angioedema, antibody formation to aducanumab-avwa

Childbearing Considerations
PREGNANCY
- It is not known if drug can cause fetal harm.
- Use with caution only if benefit to mother outweighs potential risk to fetus.

LACTATION
- It is not known if drug is present in breast milk.
- Patient should check with prescriber before breastfeeding.

Nursing Considerations
- Check that a recent (within 1 year) magnetic resonance imaging (MRI) of the brain has been done prior to treatment being initiated. Know that the MRI should be repeated before the first dose of 10 mg/kg (7th infusion) and again before

the sixth dose of 10 mg/kg (12th infusion). Be aware that if 10 or more new incident microhemorrhages or >2 focal areas of superficial siderosis (radiographic severe ARIA-H) are seen, patient will need a clinical evaluation and a follow-up MRI that demonstrates stabilization such as no increase in size or number of ARIA-H for continued cautious use of drug.

! **WARNING** Monitor patient for signs or symptoms of a hypersensitivity reaction such as angioedema and urticaria. At the first sign discontinue the infusion and notify prescriber. Provide supportive care, as ordered.

PATIENT TEACHING

- Inform patient and caregiver that drug may cause temporary swelling in the brain that usually resolves over time. Tell them some patients are unaware of this. However, tell patient or caregiver to notify prescriber if confusion, dizziness, headache, nausea, or visual changes occur.
- Stress importance of patient compliance with schedule of MRI scans.

! **WARNING** Instruct patient to notify prescriber if hives or swelling, especially of face, tongue, or neck, occurs and to seek immediate medical attention.

albuterol sulfate
(salbutamol sulfate)
AccuNeb, ProAir Digihaler, Proair HFA, ProAir RespiClick, Ventolin HFA, VoSpire ER

⊟ Class and Category
Pharmacologic class: Adrenergic
Therapeutic class: Bronchodilator

⊟ Indications and Dosages
✳ *To prevent exercise-induced bronchospasm*

INHALATION POWDER (PROAIR DIGIHALER, PROAIR RESPICLICK, VENTOLIN HFA)
Adults and children age 4 and over. Two inhalations 15 to 30 min before exercise.

✳ *To prevent or treat bronchospasm in patients with reversible obstructive airway disease*

E.R. TABLETS (VOSPIRE ER)
Adults and children over age 12. *Initial:* 4 or 8 mg every 12 hr. *Maximum:* 32 mg daily in divided doses every 12 hr.
Children ages 6 to 12. *Initial:* 4 mg every 12 hr. *Maximum:* 24 mg daily in divided doses every 12 hr.

SYRUP
Adults and children over age 14. *Initial:* 2 to 4 mg (1 to 2 tsp) three or four times daily. Dosage increased stepwise up to 8 mg four times daily, as needed. *Maximum:* 32 mg daily in divided doses.
Children ages 6 to 14. *Initial:* 2 mg (1 tsp) three or four times daily. Dosage increased stepwise up to maximum dose, as needed. *Maximum:* 24 mg daily in divided doses.
Children ages 2 to 6. *Initial:* 0.1 mg/kg three times daily (not to exceed 2 mg three times daily), increased to 0.2 mg/kg three times daily (not to exceed 4 mg three times daily), as needed. *Maximum:* 12 mg daily in divided doses.

TABLETS
Adults and children over age 12. *Initial:* 2 or 4 mg three or four times daily. Dosage increased stepwise up to 8 mg four times daily, as needed. *Maximum:* 32 mg daily in divided doses.
Children ages 6 to 12. *Initial:* 2 mg three or four times daily. Dosage increased stepwise up to maximum dose, as needed. *Maximum:* 24 mg daily in divided doses.
±**DOSAGE ADJUSTMENT** For elderly patients and patients sensitive to beta-adrenergic stimulation, initial dosage reduced to 2 mg (1 tsp) of syrup three or four times daily or 2 mg of tablets three or four times daily and then slowly increased, if needed, to as much as 8 mg three or four times daily, not exceeding total daily dose of 32 mg in adults and children 12 years and older.

INHALATION SOLUTION (ACCUNEB)
Adults, children age 12 and over and children age 2 to 12 weighing 15 kg (33 lb) or more. 2.5 mg three or four times daily, as needed, by nebulization.
Children ages 2 to 12 weighing 10 kg (22 lb) to less than 15 kg (33 lb). *Initial:* 0.63 mg or 1.25 mg three or four times daily, as needed, by nebulization.

INHALATION POWDER (PROAIR DIGIHALER, PROAIR RESPICLICK)
Adults and children 4 yr and over.
1 inhalation every 4 hr or 2 inhalations every 4 to 6 hr.

Drug Administration

P.O.

- Do not break, crush, or split extended-release tablets or mix with food for administration. E.R. tablets should be swallowed whole.
- Use an accurate measuring device when measuring syrup dosage.

INHALATION

- Use entire contents of a one-unit-dose vial when administering by nebulization. Adjust flow rate to deliver drug solution over 5 to 15 minutes. Do not administer any other drugs in nebulizer. Care for nebulizer following manufacturer instructions.
- Administer pressurized inhalations of albuterol during inspiration, when airways are open wider and aerosol distribution is more effective.
- Advise patient to wait at least 1 minute between inhalations if dosage requires more than one inhalation.
- Shake Proair HFA canister before use and check that a new canister is working by spraying it the appropriate number of times (once to four times based on manufacturer instructions) into the air while looking for a fine mist. However, if using the ProAir Digihaler or ProAir RespiClick device, there is no need to prime and these devices should not be used with a spacer or volume holding chamber.

- Wash mouthpiece with water once a week and let it air-dry if patient is using a Proair HFA device. However, if patient is using a ProAir Digihaler or ProAir RespiClick device, do not wash or put these devices in water. Instead, they should be cleaned by gently wiping the mouthpiece with a dry cloth or tissue, if needed.
- Discard the ProAir Digihaler and ProAir RespiClick devices after 13 months from opening the foil pouch or after the expiration date, whichever comes first. The ProAir RespiClick device should also be discarded before 13 months from opening the foil pouch if the dose counter displays 0.

Route	Onset	Peak	Duration
P.O.	15–30 min	2–3 hr	4–8 hr
P.O. (E.R.)	30 min	2–3 hr	< 12 hr
P.O. (Syrup)	5–15 min	2 hr	< 6 hr
Inhalation (powder)	5–15 min	30 min	4–6 hr
Inhalation (solution)	5–15 min	0.5–2 hr	4–6 hr

Half-life: 3.8–9.3 hr

Contraindications

Hypersensitivity to albuterol or its components

Interactions

DRUGS

beta blockers: Inhibited effects of albuterol
bronchodilators (sympathomimetics), such as theophylline: Possibly adverse CV effects
digoxin: Decreased serum digoxin level

Mechanism of Action

Albuterol attaches to beta$_2$ receptors on bronchial cell membranes, which stimulates the intracellular enzyme adenylate cyclase to convert adenosine triphosphate (ATP) to cyclic adenosine monophosphate (cAMP). This reaction decreases intracellular calcium levels. It also increases intracellular levels of cAMP, as shown. Together, these effects relax bronchial smooth muscle cells and inhibit histamine release.

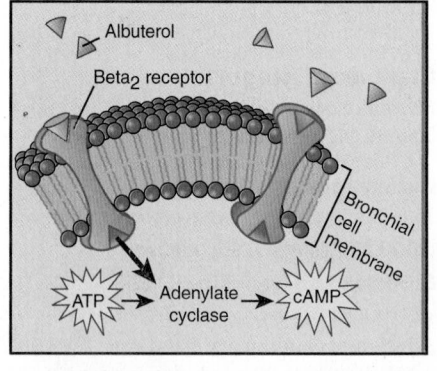

MAO inhibitors, tricyclic antidepressants: Increased vascular effects of albuterol
potassium-lowering drugs: Possibly hypokalemia
potassium-wasting diuretics: Possibly increased hypokalemia

Adverse Reactions

CNS: Anxiety, dizziness, drowsiness, headache, hyperkinesia, insomnia, irritability, nervousness, tremor, vertigo, weakness
CV: Angina, **arrhythmias**, chest pain, hypertension, **hypotension**, palpitations
EENT: Altered taste, dry mouth and throat, ear pain, glossitis, hoarseness, **oropharyngeal edema**, pharyngitis, rhinitis, taste perversion
ENDO: Hyperglycemia
GI: Anorexia, diarrhea, dysphagia, heartburn, nausea, vomiting
GU: UTI
MS: Muscle cramps
RESP: **Bronchospasm**, cough, dyspnea, **paradoxical bronchospasm**, **pulmonary edema**
SKIN: Diaphoresis, flushing, pallor, pruritus, rash, urticaria
Other: **Anaphylaxis**, **angioedema**, **hypokalemia**, infection, **metabolic acidosis**

Childbearing Considerations

PREGNANCY

- Pregnancy exposure registry: 1-877-311-8972 or http://mothertobaby.org/pregnancy studies/.
- It is not known if drug can cause fetal harm.
- Use with caution only if benefit to mother outweighs potential risk to fetus.

LABOR & DELIVERY

- Drug should only be used if benefit to mother during labor clearly outweighs the risk for beta-agonist interference with uterine contractility.
- Drug should not be used for management of preterm labor because serious adverse reactions, including pulmonary edema, have been reported in the mother.

LACTATION

- It is not known if drug is present in breast milk.
- A decision should be made to discontinue breastfeeding or the drug to avoid potential serious adverse reactions in the breastfed infant.

Nursing Considerations

! WARNING Use cautiously in patients with cardiac disorders, diabetes mellitus, digitalis intoxication, hypertension, hyperthyroidism, or history of seizures. Albuterol can worsen these conditions.

- Monitor serum potassium level because albuterol may cause transient hypokalemia.
- Be aware that drug tolerance can develop with prolonged use.

PATIENT TEACHING

- Teach patient how to use inhaler. Tell him if he is prescribed Proair HFA to shake canister before use and to check that a new canister is working by spraying it the appropriate number of times (once to four times based on manufacturer instructions) into the air while looking for a fine mist. However, if patient is prescribed the ProAir Digihaler or ProAir RespiClick device, tell him that they do not require priming and these devices should not be used with a spacer or volume holding chamber.
- Instruct patient to wash mouthpiece with water once a week and let it air-dry if patient is using a Proair HFA device. However, if patient is using a ProAir Digihaler or ProAir RespiClick device, he should not wash or put these devices in water. Instead they should be cleaned by gently wiping the mouthpiece with a dry cloth or tissue, if needed. Tell patient to discard the ProAir Digihaler and ProAir RespiClick devices after 13 months from opening the foil pouch or after the expiration date, whichever comes first. The ProAir RespiClick device should also be discarded before 13 months from opening the foil pouch if the dose counter displays 0.
- Advise patient to wait at least 1 minute between inhalations if dosage requires more than one inhalation.
- Tell patient to check with his prescriber before using other inhaled drugs.
- Warn patient not to exceed prescribed dose or frequency. If doses become less effective, tell patient to contact his prescriber.
- Tell patient to immediately report signs and symptoms of allergic reaction, such as difficulty swallowing, itching, and rash.

alemtuzumab
Lemtrada

Class and Category
Pharmacologic class: Monoclonal antibody
Therapeutic class: Immunomodulator

Indications and Dosages
* *To treat relapsing forms of multiple sclerosis, to include relapsing-remitting disease and active secondary progressive disease in patients who have had an inadequate response to two or more drugs indicated for the treatment of multiple sclerosis*

I.V. INFUSION
Adults. *First treatment course:* 12 mg/day on 5 consecutive days for 60 mg total dose. *Second treatment course:* 12 mg/day on 3 consecutive days for 36 mg total dose administered 12 months after first treatment course. *Subsequent treatment courses:* 12 mg/day on 3 consecutive days, as needed, for 36 mg total dose administered 12 months after last dose of any prior treatment course.

Drug Administration
I.V.
- Premedicate patient with high-dose corticosteroids such as 1,000 mg of methylprednisolone or equivalent, as prescribed, immediately prior to alemtuzumab infusion and for first 3 days of each treatment course to decrease risk of infusion reactions. Antihistamines and/or antipyretics may be prescribed and given prior to infusion.
- Administer antiviral prophylaxis for herpetic viral infections, as prescribed, starting on the first day of each treatment course and continuing for a minimum of 2 months following treatment or until CD4+ lymphocyte count is at least 200 cells per microliter, whichever occurs later.
- Do not freeze or shake vials prior to use. Solution should not be discolored or contain particulate matter.
- Withdraw 1.2 ml from drug vial into a syringe and inject into a 100-ml bag of sterile 0.9% Sodium Chloride, USP or 5% Dextrose in Water, USP. Gently invert bag to mix solution.
- Ensure the sterility of the prepared solution because it contains no antimicrobial preservatives. Also protect it from light. Diluted solution may be stored for up to 8 hours refrigerated or at room temperature.
- Infuse alemtuzumab over 4 hours starting within 8 hours after dilution. Know that duration of infusion may be extended if clinically indicated.
- Do not give drug as a bolus or I.V. push.
- *Incompatibilities:* Other drugs through the same intravenous line

Route	Onset	Peak	Duration
I.V.	Unknown	Unknown	Unknown

Half-life: 2 wk

Mechanism of Action
Possibly binds to CD52, a cell surface antigen present on T and B lymphocytes and on natural killer cells, macrophages, and monocytes. This results in antibody-dependent cellular cytolysis and complement-mediated lysis.

Contraindications
Hypersensitivity to alemtuzumab or its components, presence of active infections or HIV infection

Interactions
DRUGS
antineoplastics, immunosuppressants: Increased risk of immunosuppression
live viral vaccines: Increased risk of infection
myelosuppressive agents: Enhanced myelosuppressive effects

Adverse Reactions
CNS: Anxiety, asthenia, chills, **CVA**, dizziness, fatigue, fever, **Guillain–Barré syndrome**, headache, insomnia, paresthesia, **progressive multifocal leukoencephalopathy, suicidal ideation**
CV: **Cervicocephalic arterial dissection, MI, myocardial ischemia**, peripheral edema, tachycardia, vasculitis
EENT: Epistaxis, nasopharyngitis, oropharyngeal pain, sinusitis, taste distortion
ENDO: Thyroid dysfunction
GI: Abdominal pain, **autoimmune hepatitis**, cholecystitis, diarrhea, dyspepsia, nausea, vomiting
GU: Abnormal uterine bleeding, **antiglomerular basement membrane disease**, hematuria, membranous glomerulonephritis, UTI

HEME: Acquired hemophilia A, **decreased CD4 and CD8 lymphocytes and T-lymphocyte count, hemolytic anemia,** **hemophagocytic lymphohistiocytosis,** **immune thrombocytopenia, lymphopenia,** **neutropenia, pancytopenia, thrombotic** **thrombocytopenic purpura**

MS: Arthralgia; back, extremity, or neck pain; muscle weakness; myalgia

RESP: Cough, dyspnea, **hypersensitivity** **pneumonitis, pneumonitis with fibrosis,** **pulmonary alveolar hemorrhage,** upper respiratory infection

SKIN: Dermatitis, erythema, flushing, pruritus, rash, urticaria

Other: Adult-onset Still's disease (AOSD); alemtuzumab antibody formation; **anaphylaxis;** autoimmune conditions; **bacterial, fungal, herpes, opportunistic,** **or other viral infections** (serious to **life-** **threatening**); flu-like symptoms; **infusion** **reactions** (serious to **life-threatening**); **malignancies; sarcoidosis**

Childbearing Considerations

PREGNANCY

- Pregnancy exposure registry: 1-866-758-2990.
- Drug may cause fetal harm, as placental transfer of antithyroid antibodies to fetus may result in neonatal Graves' disease.
- Use with caution only if benefit to mother outweighs potential risk to fetus.

LACTATION

- It is not known if drug is present in breast milk.
- Patient should check with prescriber before breastfeeding.

REPRODUCTION

- Women of childbearing age should use effective contraceptive measures during drug therapy and for 4 months following that course of treatment.
- Animal studies have shown adverse effects on sperm parameters in males and reduced number of corpora lutea and implantations in females.

Nursing Considerations

- Know that alemtuzumab is only available through a restricted distribution under a Risk Evaluation Mitigation Strategy Program because of the risk of autoimmunity, infusion reactions, and malignancies.

- Complete any necessary immunizations at least 6 weeks prior to treatment, as prescribed. Ensure tuberculosis screening has been done prior to drug therapy.
- Assess patient for signs and symptoms of an infection prior to beginning therapy, and then before each infusion.
- Patients at high risk for hepatitis B or C virus should be screened prior to initiating therapy.
- Expect baseline laboratory tests to be performed prior to alemtuzumab therapy and periodically thereafter as follows: Complete blood count (CBC) with differential prior to and then monthly; serum creatinine levels prior to and then monthly; thyroid function test, such as a thyroid-stimulating hormone level, prior to and then every 3 months; and urinalysis with urine cell counts, including urine protein-to-creatinine ratio, prior to and then monthly. Also expect to check serum transaminase and total bilirubin levels prior to and then periodically and to perform a baseline skin examination followed by yearly exams for melanoma. Expect to continue monitoring these test results for up to 48 months after last dose is infused.

‼ **WARNING** Know that infections frequently occur with alemtuzumab treatment and can become life-threatening. Examples of infections that may occur include serious infections such as appendicitis, gastroenteritis, pneumonia, and tooth infections; Epstein–Barr viral infection; fungal infections; herpes viral infections; human papilloma virus infections; *Listeria monocytogenes* infections; opportunistic infections; and tuberculosis. Know that treatment may be delayed until active infection is under control.

‼ **WARNING** Be aware patients at high risk for hepatitis B or C virus may be at risk of irreversible liver damage caused by a potential virus reactivation.

- Be aware that despite premedicating patient with high-dose corticosteroids as well as antihistamines and/or antipyretics prior to therapy, a serious infusion reaction may still occur. Immediate discontinuation should be considered if a serious infusion reaction occurs.

- Monitor vital signs before infusion and periodically during infusion.

! WARNING Be aware that alemtuzumab may cause serious and life-threatening infusion reactions. These may include anaphylaxis, angioedema, bradycardia, bronchospasm, chest pain, fever, headache, hypertension or hypotension, rash, tachycardia (including atrial fibrillation), or transient neurologic symptoms. Other infusion adverse reactions may include chills, dizziness, dyspepsia, dyspnea, fatigue, insomnia, nausea, pain, pruritus, pulmonary infiltrates, and urticaria. Observe patient during and for at least 2 hours after each infusion. Question patient frequently regarding symptoms they may be experiencing. Be prepared to manage anaphylaxis or serious infusion reactions immediately, if present.

! WARNING Monitor patient for signs and symptoms of neurologic disorders such as Guillain–Barré or progressive multifocal leukoencephalopathy (PML). If any occur, notify prescriber immediately and withhold drug while diagnostic evaluation is ongoing. If confirmed, provide appropriate and supportive care, as prescribed.

! WARNING Know that alemtuzumab causes serious, sometimes fatal, autoimmune conditions such as antiglomerular basement membrane disease and immune thrombocytopenia. Expect to monitor CBC with differential, serum creatinine levels, and urinalysis with urine cell counts at periodic intervals for 48 months after last dose. Also, be aware that adult-onset Still's disease, a rare inflammatory disease, may occur with alemtuzumab therapy. Monitor patient for arthritis (pain, stiffness, and possible swelling of multiple joints), fever (>39°C or 102.2°F lasting more than a week), leukocytosis, and rash with patient having no history or signs and symptoms of infections, malignancies, or other rheumatic conditions. If suspected, notify prescriber and expect drug to be discontinued, if confirmed. In addition, monitor patient for thrombotic thrombocytopenic purpura (fever, microangiopathic hemolytic anemia, neurologic signs and symptoms, renal impairment, and thrombocytopenia). If suspected, notify prescriber immediately and expect drug to be discontinued, if the disorder is confirmed.

- Monitor patient's cardiovascular and pulmonary systems for adverse reactions, such as cervicocephalic arterial dissection involving multiple arteries, MI, and stroke that may occur within 3 days of infusion, with most occurring within 1 day.
- Monitor patient's renal function, as ordered. Notify prescriber immediately of any abnormalities, including hemoptysis (a common lung component), because urgent evaluation and treatment can improve the preservation of renal function. Know that glomerular nephropathies can occur up to 40 months after the last dose of alemtuzumab. Expect patient's urine protein-to-creatinine ratio to be measured if urine dipstick shows 1+ protein or greater.
- Monitor patient for liver dysfunction, because drug can cause significant liver injury, including autoimmune hepatitis. Patients should also be monitored for Graves' disease (hyperthyroidism: palpitations, tachycardia, heat intolerance, frequent bowel movements, eyelid retraction/lag, irritability).
- Be aware that alemtuzumab may cause an increased risk of malignancies, including lymphoproliferative disorders, melanoma, and thyroid cancer. Expect baseline exam and yearly follow-ups to be done.
- Be aware that acquired hemophilia A has occurred in patients taking alemtuzumab. Assess patient frequently for spontaneous subcutaneous hematomas and extensive bruising in addition to epistaxis, gastrointestinal or other types of bleeding, and hematuria. Report findings immediately to prescriber.
- Be aware that alemtuzumab contains the same active ingredient as Campath, which has an orphan designation to treat leukemia. If patient has been previously treated with Campath, monitor patient for additive and long-lasting effects on the immune system.

PATIENT TEACHING

! WARNING Inform patient that alemtuzumab may cause serious to life-threatening infusion reactions requiring patient to stay at infusion center for 2 hours after each infusion. Patient should seek immediate medical attention if a reaction occurs, because reactions can occur for up to 72 hours after infusion.

! WARNING Review signs of an MI or stroke with patient. Instruct patient to seek immediate medical attention if symptoms of stroke occur. Also instruct patient to report any signs and symptoms of infection, as well as other signs and symptoms that are not common to patient, such as chest pain or tightness, cough, hemoptysis, shortness of breath, or wheezing. In addition, review signs and symptoms of adult-onset Still's disease and thrombotic thrombocytopenic purpura and stress importance to immediately notify prescriber if suspected.

- Instruct patients to avoid potential sources of *Listeria monocytogenes,* such as deli meat, dairy products made with unpasteurized milk, poultry, seafood, soft cheeses, or undercooked meat. Review signs and symptoms for *Listeria* infection because the duration of increased risk is unknown. Some cases have been reported up to 8 months after last dose.
- Stress importance of having a yearly skin exam.
- Advise patient to notify prescriber if bleeding, blood in urine, bruising, dark or bloody stools, or nosebleeds occur or painful or swollen joints develop.
- Encourage female patients to have an annual human papilloma virus screening done.

alendronate sodium
Binosto, Fosamax

≣ Class and Category
Pharmacologic class: Bisphosphonate
Therapeutic class: Bone resorption inhibitor

≣ Indications and Dosages
✳ *To prevent postmenopausal osteoporosis*

TABLETS
Adults. 5 mg daily or 35 mg once/wk.
✳ *To treat postmenopausal osteoporosis*

ORAL SOLUTION, TABLETS
Adults. 10 mg (tablet) daily or 70 mg (oral solution or tablet) once/wk.

EFFERVESCENT TABLETS
Adults. 70 mg once/wk.
✳ *To treat Paget's disease of the bone in patients whose alkaline phosphatase level is twice the upper limit of symptomatic and at risk for further complications*

TABLETS
Adults. 40 mg daily for 6 months. Treatment repeated following a 6-month posttreatment evaluation period, if needed, in patients who have failed to normalize their serum alkaline phosphatase levels or have relapsed based on increases in alkaline phosphatase.
✳ *To increase bone mass in men with osteoporosis*

ORAL SOLUTION, TABLETS
Adults. 10 mg (tablet) daily or 70 mg (oral solution or tablet) once/wk.

EFFERVESCENT TABLETS
Adults. 70 mg once/wk.
✳ *To treat glucocorticoid-induced osteoporosis in men and women who receive a daily glucocorticoid dosage of 7.5 mg or greater of prednisone and who have low bone mineral density*

TABLETS
Adults. 5 mg daily.
±**DOSAGE ADJUSTMENT** Dosage for glucocorticoid-induced osteoporosis increased to 10 mg daily for postmenopausal women not receiving estrogen.

≣ Drug Administration
P.O.
- Use only plain water, not flavored or mineral water, that is at room temperature when administering drug.
- Administer after patient awakens and at least 30 minutes before patient eats, drinks, or is given other drugs.
- Administer effervescent form of alendronate by dissolving one tablet in 4 ounces of plain water. Wait at least 5 minutes after effervescence stops and then stir the solution for about 10 seconds before handing to patient to ingest.

- Give tablet form with 6 to 8 ounces of plain water in the morning.
- Give patient at least 2 ounces of plain water following ingestion of oral solution.
- Keep patient in an upright position for 30 minutes after administering drug.

Route	Onset	Peak	Duration
P.O.	Unknown	Unknown	Unknown

Half-life: >10 yr

Mechanism of Action

Reduces activity of cells that cause bone loss, slows rate of bone loss after menopause, and increases amount of bone mass. May act by inhibiting osteoclast activity on newly formed bone resorption surfaces, which reduces the number of sites where bone is remodeled. Bone formation then exceeds bone resorption at these remodeling sites, which gradually increases bone mass. May also inhibit bone dissolution by binding to hydroxyapatite crystals, which are composed of calcium, phosphate, and hydroxide and give bone its rigid structure.

Contraindications

Esophageal abnormalities that delay esophageal emptying, such as achalasia or stricture; hypersensitivity to alendronate or its components; hypocalcemia; inability to stand or sit upright for at least 30 minutes

Interactions

DRUGS

antacids, calcium, iron, multivalent cations: Decreased absorption of alendronate
aspirin: Increased risk of GI distress
levothyroxine: Possibly slight decrease in bioavailability of alendronate

FOODS

any food: Delayed absorption and decreased serum level of alendronate

Adverse Reactions

CNS: Asthenia, dizziness, headache, vertigo
CV: Peripheral edema
EENT: Cholesteatoma of external auditory canal
GI: Abdominal distention and pain, constipation, diarrhea, dysphagia, **esophageal perforation** or ulceration, esophagitis, flatulence, gastritis, gastroesophageal reflux disease, heartburn, indigestion, **melena**, nausea, vomiting
MS: Arthralgia; femoral shaft or subtrochanteric fractures; focal osteomalacia; jaw osteonecrosis; joint swelling; muscle spasms; myalgia; severe bone, joint, and/or muscle pain
RESP: Asthma exacerbation
SKIN: Photosensitivity, pruritus, rash, Stevens–Johnson syndrome, toxic epidermal necrosis
Other: Anaphylaxis, hypocalcemia

Childbearing Considerations

PREGNANCY

- It is not known if drug can cause fetal harm.
- Drug should be discontinued as soon as pregnancy is known.
- Know that there is a theoretical risk of fetal harm, especially skeletal, if a woman becomes pregnant after completing a course of bisphosphonate therapy. Time between cessation of drug therapy to conception, the particular bisphosphonate used, and route of administration causing fetal harm is unknown.

LACTATION

- It is not known if drug is present in breast milk.
- Patient should check with prescriber before breastfeeding.

Nursing Considerations

- Know that alendronate should not be administered to patients who have esophageal disorders, hypocalcemia, or are unable to sit upright or stand for at least 30 minutes.
- Monitor patient's serum calcium level before, during, and after treatment. Expect hypocalcemia to be treated before alendronate therapy begins. If hypocalcemia occurs during therapy, expect prescriber to order a calcium supplement.
- Ensure adequate dietary intake of calcium and vitamin D before, during, and after treatment.
- Be aware that oral osteoporosis drugs such as alendronate may have the potential to increase the risk of esophageal cancer. While studies are underway to determine this potential, assess patient regularly for painful or difficulty swallowing, chest pain, or new or worsening heartburn; notify prescriber if present.

! **WARNING** Monitor patient closely, as alendronate may irritate upper GI mucosa, causing adverse reactions such as esophageal ulceration.

- Monitor patient for jaw pain because alendronate may cause osteonecrosis of the jaw, with risk increasing as therapy duration becomes longer. Patients at increased risk include those who have poor oral hygiene, preexisting dental or periodontal disease, wear ill-fitting dentures, or require an invasive dental procedure. Patients are also at increased risk if they have a cancer diagnosis, concomitant therapy such as chemotherapy or corticosteroid therapy, or other illnesses, such as preexisting dental or periodontal disease, anemia, coagulopathy, or infection.

PATIENT TEACHING

- Advise patient to take alendronate in the morning upon arising with a full glass of plain, room-temperature water, not flavored or mineral water. Explain that drug should be taken at least 30 minutes before eating, drinking, or taking other drugs.
- Instruct patient who is prescribed the effervescent tablet form to dissolve the tablet in 4 ounces of room-temperature water (mineral water or flavored water should not be used). After the effervescence stops, tell patient to wait at least 5 minutes and then stir the solution for about 10 seconds and ingest.
- Tell patient not to chew or suck on tablet, to help reduce esophageal irritation.
- Advise patient taking oral solution form to follow drug with at least 60 ml of room-temperature plain water, not flavored or mineral water.
- Teach patient to remain upright for 30 minutes after taking alendronate and until she has eaten the first food of the day.
- Encourage patient to consume adequate daily amounts of calcium and vitamin D.
- Instruct patient to report to prescriber any new or unusual pain in hip or thigh.
- Tell patient to inform dentist of alendronate therapy prior to dental work and to notify dentist of any signs of infection or delayed healing after an extraction.
- Instruct patient to report any difficulty swallowing or pain when swallowing, chest pain, or new or worsening heartburn to prescriber.
- Inform patient receiving the effervescent tablet form to be aware that each tablet contains 650 mg sodium, which is equivalent to approximately 1,650 mg of salt (sodium chloride) per tablet.
- Warn women of childbearing age to notify prescriber if pregnancy occurs or is suspected.

aliskiren hemifumarate
Rasilez (CAN), Tekturna

⩸ Class and Category
Pharmacologic class: Direct renin inhibitor
Therapeutic class: Antihypertensive

⩸ Indications and Dosages
⁎ *To treat hypertension*

TABLETS
Adults and children age 6 to 17 weighing 50 kg (110 lb) or more. 150 mg once daily, increased to 300 mg once daily, as needed.

⩸ Drug Administration
P.O.
- Avoid giving drug with a high-fat meal, as effectiveness may be reduced.
- Drug should be given at same time every day.

Route	Onset	Peak	Duration
P.O.	Unknown	1–3 hr	Unknown

Half-life: 24 hr

⩸ Mechanism of Action
Inhibits renin secreted by the kidneys in response to decreased blood volume and renal perfusion. Renin cleaves angiotensinogen to form angiotensin I, which is converted to angiotensin II by ACE and non-ACE pathways. Angiotensin II is a powerful vasoconstrictor that induces release of catecholamines from the adrenal medulla and prejunctional nerve endings. It also promotes aldosterone secretion and sodium reabsorption. Together, these actions increase blood pressure. By inhibiting renin release, aliskiren impairs

the renin–angiotensin–aldosterone system. Without the vasoconstrictive effect of angiotensin II, blood pressure decreases.

Contraindications

Children under the age of 2; hypersensitivity to aliskiren or its components, presence of diabetes and concurrent angiotensin-converting enzyme inhibitor (ACEI) or angiotensin receptor blocker (ARB) therapy, pregnancy

Interactions

DRUGS

ACE inhibitors, ARBs: Increased risk of hyperkalemia, hypotension, or renal dysfunction, especially in the elderly and patients who are volume-depleted or already have renal impairment

atorvastatin, cyclosporine, itraconazole, ketoconazole, verapamil: Increased aliskiren blood level

furosemide: Decreased blood furosemide levels

irbesartan: Decreased blood aliskiren level

NSAIDs: Increased risk of decreased renal function and hypotension

P-glycoprotein: Possible alteration in absorption and disposition of aliskiren at Pgp site

potassium-sparing diuretics, potassium supplements: Increased risk of hyperkalemia

FOODS

high-fat food: Decreased aliskiren absorption substantially

Adverse Reactions

CNS: Dizziness, fatigue, headache, **seizures**
CV: Hypotension, peripheral edema
EENT: Nasopharyngitis
GI: Abdominal pain, diarrhea, dyspepsia, elevated liver enzymes, gastroesophageal reflux, **hepatic dysfunction**, nausea, vomiting
GU: Elevated blood creatinine, renal calculi
HEME: Decreased hemoglobin and hematocrit
MS: Back pain
RESP: Increased cough, upper respiratory tract infection
SKIN: Erythema, pruritus, rash, **Stevens–Johnson syndrome, toxic epidermal necrolysis**, urticaria
Other: Anaphylaxis, angioedema, elevated creatine kinase or uric acid level, gout, **hyperkalemia, hyponatremia**

Childbearing Considerations

PREGNANCY

- Drug can cause fetal harm, especially if exposure occurs during the second or third trimester.
- Drug reduces fetal renal function, leading to anuria and renal failure, and increases fetal and neonatal morbidity and death. It can also cause fetal lung hypoplasia, hypotension, and skeletal deformations such as skull hypoplasia.
- Drug is contraindicated in pregnant women and should be discontinued as soon as possible when pregnancy occurs.

LACTATION

- It is not known if drug is present in breast milk.
- Drug is not recommended for use in breastfeeding women, to avoid potential serious adverse reactions including hyperkalemia, hypotension, and renal impairment in the breastfed infant.

Nursing Considerations

- Be aware that aliskiren should not be used in patients with diabetes who are concurrently taking ARBs or ACEIs because of the increased risk of serious adverse effects such as renal dysfunction, hyperkalemia, and hypotension. Also know that aliskiren should not be given to patients with moderate renal impairment (glomerular filtration rate of less than 60 ml/min) who are also receiving ARB or ACEI therapy because renal impairment may worsen.
- Monitor patient's renal function closely, especially in patients receiving drugs such as ARBs, ACEIs, NSAIDs, potassium supplements or potassium-sparing diuretics that affect the renin–angiotensin system. Use aliskiren cautiously in patients whose renal function may depend in part on the activity of this system such as those with renal artery stenosis, severe heart failure, postmyocardial infarction, or who are elderly or experiencing volume depletion because aliskiren therapy increases the risk of renal dysfunction in these patients that could lead to acute renal failure.
- Take measures to correct volume or salt depletion from high-dose diuretic therapy before starting aliskiren, as ordered, to prevent hypotension. If hypotension occurs

during aliskiren therapy, place patient in a supine position and give normal saline solution intravenously, as needed and prescribed.

> ! **WARNING** Watch closely for angioedema of the head or neck. If angioedema occurs, discontinue aliskiren, notify prescriber, and provide supportive therapy until swelling has ceased. If swelling of the tongue, glottis, or larynx is involved, be prepared to give epinephrine solution 1:1,000 (0.3 to 0.5 ml), as prescribed, and provide measures to ensure a patent airway. Be aware that patient shouldn't receive aliskiren again.

- Monitor serum electrolytes, especially potassium levels, as ordered in patients who already are experiencing renal insufficiency or who have diabetes because of increased risk for hyperkalemia in the presence of aliskiren therapy. Also monitor patients who are taking ARBs, ACEIs, or NSAIDs along with aliskiren because of increased risk of hyperkalemia.

PATIENT TEACHING
- Advise patient to avoid high-fat meals while taking aliskiren because fat decreases drug absorption significantly.
- Instruct patient how to monitor blood pressure to determine effectiveness of aliskiren therapy.
- Explain that decreased blood pressure could lead to light-headedness, especially in the first few days of therapy. Advise patient to change positions slowly and, if light-headedness develops, to notify prescriber. Tell patient to stop taking aliskiren and to notify prescriber if she faints.
- Explain that light-headedness and fainting could also result from dehydration caused by inadequate fluid intake, excessive perspiration, diarrhea, or vomiting.
- Instruct patient to avoid using potassium supplements or potassium salt substitutes and to inform all prescribers about her aliskiren and ACE inhibitor or ARD therapy.

> ! **WARNING** Emphasize importance of stopping aliskiren and seeking immediate medical attention if patient has swelling of face, extremities, eyes, lips, or tongue, or if patient has trouble swallowing or breathing.

- Instruct female patient to notify prescriber immediately if she is or could be pregnant because drug will have to be discontinued and another antihypertensive chosen. Also inform mothers that breastfeeding is not recommended while taking aliskiren, as drug can cause high potassium level, kidney impairment, and low blood pressure in a nursing infant.

allopurinol
Purinol (CAN), Zyloprim

allopurinol sodium
Aloprim

Class and Category
Pharmacological class: Xanthine oxidase inhibitor
Therapeutic class: Antigout

Indications and Dosages
✳ *To treat primary gout and hyperuricemia*

TABLETS
Adults. *Initial:* 100 mg daily increased by 100 mg/wk until serum uric acid level is 6 mg/dl or less. Dosages above 300 mg daily given in divided doses. *Maximum:* 800 mg daily.

✳ *To prevent uric acid nephropathy*

TABLETS
Adults. 600 to 800 mg daily for 2 to 3 days, then adjusted to keep serum uric acid level within normal limits.

✳ *To treat secondary hyperuricemia caused by leukemia, lymphoma, and other malignancies such as solid tumors*

TABLETS
Adults. 600 to 800 mg daily for 2 to 3 days, then adjusted to keep serum uric acid level within normal limits.
Children ages 6 to 10. 300 mg daily, adjusted after 48 hr, depending on response to treatment.
Children under age 6. 150 mg daily, adjusted after 48 hr, depending on response to treatment.

I.V. INFUSION
Adults. 200 to 400 mg/m^2 daily as a single infusion or in equally divided doses every 6, 8, or 12 hr beginning 24 to 48 hr before

initiation of chemotherapy. *Maximum:* 600 mg daily.

Children. *Initial:* 200 mg/m^2 daily as a single infusion or in equally divided doses every 6, 8, or 12 hr beginning 24 to 48 hr before initiation of chemotherapy. Dosage then titrated according to uric acid levels.

✳ *To treat recurrent calcium oxalate calculi*

TABLETS

Adults. 200 to 300 mg daily as a single dose or in divided doses, adjusted based on 24-hr urine urate level.

±**DOSAGE ADJUSTMENT** For patient with impaired renal function, dosage adjusted to 200 mg daily if creatinine clearance is 10 to 20 ml/min, 100 mg daily if creatinine clearance is 3 to 10 ml/min, or 100 mg at extended intervals if creatinine clearance falls below 3 ml/min.

Drug Administration

P.O.

- No special instructions recommended by manufacturer for administration.

I.V.

- Administer 24 to 48 hours before chemotherapy, if possible.
- Reconstitute each 30-ml vial with 25 ml of Sterile Water for Injection. Solution should appear clear, almost colorless with no more than a slight opalescence. Further dilute to desired concentration, but no greater than 6 mg/ml, with 0.9% Sodium Chloride Injection or Dextrose 5% Water for Injection.
- Infuse at a rate based on the volume of the infusion solution.
- Diluted solution should be used within 10 hours and stored only at room temperature that does not exceed 25°C (77°F).
- *Incompatibilities:* Amikacin sulfate, amphotericin B, carmustine, cefotaxime sodium, chlorpromazine hydrochloride, cimetidine hydrochloride, clindamycin phosphate, cytarabine, dacarbazine, daunorubicin hydrochloride, diphenhydramine hydrochloride, doxorubicin hydrochloride, doxycycline hyclate, droperidol, floxuridine, gentamicin sulfate, haloperidol lactate, hydroxyzine hydrochloride, idarubicin hydrochloride, imipenem-cilastatin sodium, mechlorethamine hydrochloride, meperidine hydrochloride, metoclopramide hydrochloride, methylprednisolone sodium succinate, minocycline hydrochloride, nalbuphine hydrochloride, netilmicin sulfate, ondansetron hydrochloride, prochlorperazine edisylate, promethazine hydrochloride, sodium bicarbonate, streptozocin, tobramycin sulfate, vinorelbine tartrate

Route	Onset	Peak	Duration
P.O.	Unknown	1.5 hr	1–2 wk
I.V.	Unknown	30 min	Unknown

Half-life: 1–2 hr

☰ Mechanism of Action

Inhibits uric acid production by inhibiting xanthine oxidase, the enzyme that converts hypoxanthine and xanthine to uric acid. Allopurinol is metabolized to oxipurinol, which also inhibits xanthine oxidase.

☰ Contraindications

Hypersensitivity to allopurinol or its components

☰ Interactions

DRUGS

ACE inhibitors: Increased risk of hypersensitivity reactions
amoxicillin, ampicillin: Increased risk of rash
azathioprine, mercaptopurine: Increased plasma levels of these drugs with increased risk of toxicity
chlorpropamide: Increased risk of hypoglycemia in patients with renal insufficiency
cyclophosphamide, other cytotoxic drugs: Enhanced bone marrow suppression
dicumarol: Increased half-life and anticoagulant action of dicumarol
thiazide diuretics: Possibly increased risk of allopurinol toxicity
uricosuric agents: Increased urinary excretion of uric acid

☰ Adverse Reactions

CNS: Chills, drowsiness, fever, headache, neuritis, paresthesia, peripheral neuropathy, somnolence
CV: Vasculitis
EENT: Epistaxis, loss of taste
GI: Abdominal pain, diarrhea, dysphagia, elevated liver enzymes, gastritis,

granulomatous hepatitis, **hepatic necrosis,** hepatomegaly, jaundice, nausea, vomiting
GU: Exacerbated renal calculi, **renal failure**
HEME: Agranulocytosis, **aplastic anemia, bone marrow depression,** eosinophilia, leukocytosis, **leukopenia, thrombocytopenia**
MS: Arthralgia, exacerbation of gout, myopathy
SKIN: Alopecia; ecchymosis; maculopapular, scaly, or **exfoliative rash,** pruritus; urticaria
OTHER: Drug hypersensitivity syndrome (DHA), drug reaction with eosinophilia and systemic symptoms (DRESS)

Childbearing Considerations
PREGNANCY
- It is not known if drug can cause fetal harm.
- Use with caution only if benefit to mother outweighs potential risk to fetus.

LACTATION
- Drug is present in breast milk.
- Patient should check with prescriber before breastfeeding.

Nursing Considerations
- Obtain baseline CBC and uric acid level, as ordered, and review results of renal and liver function tests before and during allopurinol therapy.

! **WARNING** Discontinue allopurinol and notify prescriber immediately at first sign of hypersensitivity reaction, such as rash, which may precede more severe reactions.

- Be aware that the HLA-B*58:01 allele is a genetic marker for severe skin hypersensitivity reactions to allopurinol. The frequency is higher in patients of African, Asian (e.g., Han Chinese, Korean, Thai), and Native Hawaiian/Pacific Islander ancestry. The use of allopurinol is not recommended in patients with this genetic marker. Hypersensitivity reactions may also be increased in patients with renal impairment, especially if patient is receiving a thiazide diuretic.
- Maintain a fluid intake to produce a daily urinary output of 2 L daily. Also, don't give vitamin C because the pH of urine should be kept neutral to slightly alkaline.
- Monitor patient for the development of a skin rash that may occur 1 week or more after allopurinol therapy is initiated. If present, notify prescriber immediately because this could be a sign of DRESS, which may become life-threatening. Expect drug to be discontinued.

PATIENT TEACHING
- Advise patient to take allopurinol after meals and to drink enough water (8 to 10 full glasses) to produce a daily urinary output of at least 2 L.
- Instruct patient to report unusual bleeding or bruising, chills, fever, gout attack, numbness, and tingling.
- Inform patient that acute gout attacks may occur more often early in allopurinol treatment and that results may not be noticeable for 2 weeks or longer.
- Instruct patient not to drive or perform hazardous tasks if drug causes drowsiness.
- Tell patient to notify prescriber immediately if a rash develops and to stop taking drug until the rash is evaluated.

almotriptan malate
Axert

Class and Category
Pharmacologic class: Selective serotonin receptor agonist (5-T_1)
Therapeutic class: Antimigraine drug

Indications and Dosages
∗ *To treat acute migraine in adults with history of migraine and in adolescents with history of migraine usually lasting more than 4 hours when untreated*

TABLETS
Adults and adolescents ages 12 to 17.
Initial: **6.**25 or 12.5 mg as a single dose, repeated in 2 hr as needed. *Maximum:* 25 mg/24 hr or 4 migraine treatments/mo.
±**DOSAGE ADJUSTMENT** For patient with impaired hepatic or renal function or patients receiving potent CYP3A4 inhibitors such as ketoconazole, initial dose reduced to 6.25 mg with maximum daily dose of 12.5 mg.

Drug Administration
P.O.
- Expect to give first dose of almotriptan in a medical facility for patient with risk factors for coronary artery disease (CAD) but no known cardiovascular abnormalities.

- Obtain an ECG immediately after first dose of almotriptan, as ordered, in patient with risk factors for CAD because cardiac ischemia can occur without causing clinical symptoms.
- Repeat dose after 2 hours if patient's migraine continues. Do not administer more than four doses in a 30-day period.

Route	Onset	Peak	Duration
P.O.	Rapid	1–3 hr	Unknown

Half-life: 3–4 hr

Mechanism of Action

May stimulate 5-HT$_1$ receptors on intracranial blood vessels and sensory nerves in trigeminal vascular system. By activating these receptors, almotriptan selectively constricts dilated and inflamed cranial blood vessels and inhibits production of proinflammatory neuropeptides. It also interrupts transmission of pain signals to the brain.

Contraindications

Basilar or hemiplegic migraine, cerebrovascular, or peripheral vascular disease, hypersensitivity to almotriptan or its components, hypertension (uncontrolled), ischemic or vasospastic coronary artery disease (CAD), use within 24 hours of other serotonin receptor agonists or ergotamine-containing or ergot-type drugs

Interactions

DRUGS

ergotamine-containing drugs: Prolonged vasospastic reactions
erythromycin, itraconazole, ketoconazole, MAO inhibitors, ritonavir, verapamil: Possibly increased blood almotriptan level
selective serotonin reuptake inhibitors (such as citalopram, escitalopram, fluoxetine, fluvoxamine, paroxetine, sertraline), serotonin norepinephrine reuptake inhibitors (such as duloxetine, venlafaxine): Increased risk of serotonin syndrome

Adverse Reactions

CNS: Confusion, dizziness, headache, hemiplegia, hypoesthesia, malaise, paresthesia, restlessness, **seizures, serotonin syndrome**, somnolence, syncope, vertigo
CV: Angina pectoris, **coronary artery vasospasm**, hypertension, **ischemia, MI,** palpitations, tachycardia, vasodilation, **ventricular fibrillation, or tachycardia**
EENT: Blepharospasm, dry mouth, oral hypoesthesia, swollen tongue, visual impairment
GI: Abdominal pain or discomfort, colitis, nausea
MS: Arthralgia, extremity coldness or pain, myalgia
SKIN: Cold sweat, diaphoresis, erythema
Other: **Anaphylaxis, angioedema**

Childbearing Considerations

PREGNANCY

- It is not known if drug can cause fetal harm.
- Use with caution only if benefit to mother outweighs potential risk to fetus.

LACTATION

- It is not known if drug is present in breast milk.
- Patient should check with prescriber before breastfeeding.

Nursing Considerations

! **WARNING** Monitor patient with CAD for angina because almotriptan can cause coronary artery vasospasm. Because it may cause peripheral vasospastic reactions, such as ischemic bowel disease, watch for abdominal pain and bloody diarrhea.

- Monitor blood pressure regularly during therapy in patients with hypertension because almotriptan may produce a transient increase in blood pressure.

! **WARNING** Monitor patient for evidence of serotonin syndrome, such as agitation, chills, confusion, diaphoresis, diarrhea, fever, hyperactive reflexes, poor coordination, restlessness, shaking, talking or acting with uncontrolled excitement, tremor, and twitching. In its most severe form, serotonin syndrome can resemble neuroleptic malignant syndrome, which includes autonomic instability with possible fluctuations in vital signs, high fever, mental status changes, and muscle rigidity.

- Monitor patients hypersensitive to sulfonamides for hypersensitivity to almotriptan because cross-sensitivity may occur.

A

PATIENT TEACHING

- Inform patient that almotriptan is used to treat acute migraine and that he shouldn't take it to treat nonmigraine headaches.
- Advise patient to consult prescriber before taking any OTC or prescription drugs.
- Advise patient not to take more than maximum prescribed dosage, as medication overuse can cause migraine-like daily headaches or a marked increase in frequency of migraine attacks requiring detoxification to treat, which could lead to withdrawal symptoms.
- Caution patient that drug may cause adverse CNS reactions, and advise him to avoid hazardous activities until he knows how drug affects him.
- Instruct patient to seek emergency care immediately for signs of hypersensitivity such as breathing difficulties, itching, or a rash; cardiac symptoms (such as heaviness, pain, pressure, or tightness in chest, jaw, neck, or throat); or if multiple new symptoms develop (such as diarrhea, high fever, incoordination, mental changes nausea, vomiting) after taking the drug.
- Advise women of childbearing age to notify prescriber if pregnancy is suspected or occurs. Also advise mothers who wish to breastfeed to discuss with prescriber first.

alogliptin benzoate
Nesina

≡ Class and Category
Pharmacologic class: Dipeptidyl peptidase-4 (DPP-4) inhibitor
Therapeutic class: Oral antidiabetic

≡ Indications and Dosages
∗ *As adjunct to diet and exercise to achieve control of glucose levels in type 2 diabetes mellitus as monotherapy or in conjunction with combination therapy*

TABLETS
Adults. 25 mg once daily.
±**DOSAGE ADJUSTMENT** For patients with moderate renal impairment (creatinine clearance less than 60 ml/min but equal to or greater than 30 ml/min), dosage decreased to 12.5 mg once daily. For patients with severe renal impairment (creatinine clearance less than 30 ml/min but equal to or greater than 15 ml/min) or patients with end-stage renal disease or who are on hemodialysis, dosage decreased to 6.25 mg once daily.

≡ Drug Administration
P.O.
Administer drug at about the same time every day.

Route	Onset	Peak	Duration
P.O.	Unknown	1–2 hr	Unknown

Half-life: 21 hr

≡ Mechanism of Action
Inhibits the dipeptidyl peptidase-4 enzyme to slow inactivation of incretin hormones. These hormones are released by the intestine in response to a meal. When blood glucose level is increased, incretin hormones increase insulin synthesis and release from pancreatic beta cells. One type of incretin hormone, glucagon-like peptide (GLP-1), also lowers glucagon secretion from pancreatic alpha cells, which reduces hepatic glucose production. These combined actions decrease blood glucose level in type 2 diabetes.

≡ Contraindications
Diabetic ketoacidosis; hypersensitivity to alogliptin or its components including anaphylaxis, angioedema, or severe cutaneous adverse reactions; type 1 diabetes

≡ Interactions
DRUGS
insulin, sulfonylureas: Possibly increased risk of hypoglycemia

≡ Adverse Reactions
CNS: Headache
CV: Heart failure
EENT: Nasopharyngitis
ENDO: Hypoglycemia
GI: Acute pancreatitis, constipation, diarrhea, elevated liver enzymes, fulminant hepatic failure, ileus, nausea
MS: Arthralgia (disabling and severe), joint pain (severe), rhabdomyolysis
RESP: Upper respiratory tract infection
SKIN: Bullous pemphigoid, rash, Stevens–Johnson syndrome, urticaria
Other: Anaphylaxis, angioedema, serum sickness

Childbearing Considerations

PREGNANCY

- It is not known if drug can cause fetal harm.
- Use with caution only if benefit to mother outweighs potential risk to fetus.

LACTATION

- It is not known if drug is present in breast milk.
- Patient should check with prescriber before breastfeeding.

Nursing Considerations

- Use alogliptin cautiously in patients with a history of angioedema to another drug in the same class because it is not known if patient will be predisposed to angioedema with alogliptin therapy.
- Determine patient's history for prior history of heart failure and a history of renal impairment, because drug may increase risk for heart failure.
- Assess patient's renal function before starting alogliptin therapy. Know that in moderate to severe renal dysfunction, dosage will have to be reduced.
- Assess patient's liver function before starting alogliptin therapy. If abnormalities are present, monitor patient closely for signs and symptoms of liver dysfunction. If patient develops anorexia, dark urine, fatigue, jaundice, or right upper abdominal discomfort during therapy, notify prescriber and expect liver enzymes to be assessed. If elevated, expect drug to be discontinued.
- Monitor patient for serious hypersensitivity reactions, including severe cutaneous adverse reactions. If present, notify prescriber, expect alogliptin to be discontinued, and provide supportive care, as ordered.
- Check patient's blood glucose level, as ordered, to determine effectiveness of alogliptin therapy.

! **WARNING** Monitor patient for signs and symptoms of acute pancreatitis, such as acute upper abdominal pain, fever, nausea, and vomiting. If suspected, notify prescriber and expect alogliptin to be discontinued, if confirmed.

PATIENT TEACHING

- Emphasize the need to follow an exercise program and a diet control program during alogliptin therapy. Tell patient to take drug at about the same time every day.
- Advise patient to notify prescriber immediately if he has trouble breathing, develops swelling or skin reactions such as hives, rash, or other cutaneous abnormalities.
- Inform patient that periodic blood tests will be done to determine effectiveness of drug.
- Teach patient how to monitor blood glucose level and when to report changes.
- Caution patient that taking other drugs used to decrease blood glucose level may lead to hypoglycemia. Review signs, symptoms, and appropriate treatment.
- Instruct patient to contact prescriber if he develops other illnesses, such as infection, or experiences trauma or surgery, because his diabetes medication may need adjustment.
- Advise patient to carry identification indicating that he has diabetes.
- Instruct patient to stop taking alogliptin and to report persistent severe abdominal pain, possibly radiating to the back, that may or may not be accompanied by vomiting.
- Alert patient that if severe joint pain occurs, he should notify prescriber as alogliptin may have to be discontinued.
- Review signs and symptoms of heart failure with patient and instruct her to notify prescriber immediately if present.

alprazolam

Alprazolam Intensol, Apo-Alpraz (CAN), Xanax, Xanax TS (CAN), Xanax XR

Class, Category, and Schedule

Pharmacologic class: Benzodiazepine
Therapeutic class: Anxiolytic, antipanic
Controlled substance schedule: IV

Indications and Dosages

* *To treat generalized anxiety disorder*

ORAL SOLUTION, ORALLY DISINTEGRATING TABLETS, TABLETS

Adults. *Initial:* 0.25 to 0.5 mg three times daily and increased, as needed, every 3 to 4 days. *Maximum:* 4 mg daily in divided doses.

* *To treat panic disorder*

ORAL SOLUTION, ORALLY
DISINTEGRATING TABLETS, TABLETS

Adults. *Initial:* 0.5 mg three times daily,
increased every 3 to 4 days by no more
than 1 mg daily, based on patient response.
Maximum: 10 mg in equally divided doses
three or four times daily.

E.R. TABLETS

Adults. *Initial:* 0.5 to 1 mg daily, increased every
3 to 4 days by no more than 1 mg daily, based
on patient response. *Usual:* 3 to 6 mg once daily.
Maximum: 10 mg daily as single dose.

± **DOSAGE ADJUSTMENT** For elderly or
debilitated patients or patients with advanced
hepatic disease, initial dosage decreased
to 0.25 mg twice daily or three times daily
(immediate-release form) and increased
gradually, as needed and tolerated; initial
dose of extended-release form kept at 0.5 mg
daily, then gradually increased, as needed.
For patient starting ritonavir therapy, dosage
decreased by 50%, then dosage increased to
target dose after 10 to 14 days (immediate-
release form) or gradually (extended-release
form), as needed.

Drug Administration

P.O.

- Use dry gloved hands to remove orally
disintegrating tablet from bottle just prior to
administration. Have patient immediately
place tablet on top of the tongue to dissolve.
There is no need for patient to drink a liquid
beverage after taking this form of drug.
- Use calibrated dropper provided with
drug to measure dosage of oral solution.
Administer oral solution with either
a beverage or semisolid food such
as applesauce or pudding. Give drug
immediately after mixing.
- Do not break, crush, or split extended-
release tablet.
- Administer extended-release tablets in
morning.
- Dosage should be reduced slowly when
drug is discontinued because of potential
dependency.

Route	Onset	Peak	Duration
P.O.	15–30 min	1.5 hr	6 hr
P.O. (E.R.)	Unknown	1.6 hr	11.3 hr

Half-life: 6.3–26.9 hr

Mechanism of Action

May increase effects of gamma-aminobutyric
acid (GABA) and other inhibitory
neurotransmitters by binding to specific
benzodiazepine receptors in cortical and
limbic areas of the CNS. GABA inhibits
excitatory stimulation, which helps control
emotional behavior. The limbic system
contains many benzodiazepine receptors,
which may help explain drug's antianxiety
effects.

Contraindications

Acute angle-closure glaucoma;
hypersensitivity to alprazolam, its
components, or other benzodiazepines; strong
CYP3A inhibitors (except for ritonavir) such
as itraconazole or ketoconazole

Interactions

DRUGS

*anticonvulsants; antidepressants;
antihistamines; other benzodiazepines, CNS
depressants, psychotropics:* Possibly increased
CNS depressant effects
*CYP3A inducers such as carbamazepine,
phenytoin:* Decreased plasma level of
alprazolam and potential decreased
effectiveness
*CYP3A inhibitors (except for ritonavir)
such as itraconazole, ketoconazole:* Possibly
profound effect on clearance of alprazolam,
causing elevated concentrations of
alprazolam and increased risk of adverse
reactions
digoxin: Possibly increased serum digoxin
level, causing digitalis toxicity
opioids: Increased risk of significant
respiratory depression
ritonavir: Administration for less than
14 days possibly increases alprazolam
exposure

ACTIVITIES

alcohol use: Enhanced adverse CNS effects
of alprazolam; increased risk of significant
sedation and somnolence, especially if
combined with an opioid

Adverse Reactions

CNS: Abnormal involuntary movements,
agitation, akathisia, anxiety, confusion,
cognitive disorder, depersonalization,
depression, derealization, disinhibition,
dizziness, drowsiness, fatigue, hallucinations,

headache, hypomania, insomnia, irritability, lack of coordination, light-headedness, mania, memory loss, muscle twitching, nervousness, paresthesia, rigidity, sedation, **seizures,** speech problems, syncope, talkativeness, tremor, weakness

CV: Chest pain, edema, **hypotension,** nonspecific ECG changes, palpitations, peripheral edema, tachycardia

EENT: Altered salivation or taste, blurred vision, diplopia, dry mouth, nasal congestion, tinnitus

ENDO: Galactorrhea, gynecomastia, hyperprolactinemia

GI: Abdominal discomfort, anorexia, constipation, diarrhea, elevated bilirubin or liver enzymes, **hepatitis, hepatic failure,** jaundice, nausea, vomiting

GU: Altered libido, incontinence, menstrual disorders, urinary hesitancy

MS: Dysarthria, muscle rigidity and spasms

RESP: Apnea, hypoventilation, respiratory depression, upper respiratory tract infection

SKIN: Dermatitis, diaphoresis, photosensitivity, pruritus, rash, **Stevens– Johnson syndrome**

Other: Angioedema, physical and psychological dependence, protracted withdrawal syndrome, weight gain or loss

☰ Childbearing Considerations

PREGNANCY

- Pregnancy exposure registry: 1-866-961- 2388 or https://womensmentalhealth .org/clinical-and-research-programs /pregnancyregistry/other medications/
- Drug can potentially cause fetal harm, especially congenital abnormalities, when taken during the first trimester of pregnancy. During later stages of pregnancy, neonatal respiratory depression, sedation, and withdrawal may occur at birth.
- Drug should not be used during pregnancy.

LABOR & DELIVERY

- Drug has no established use during labor and delivery.

LACTATION

- Drug is present in breast milk.
- A decision should be made to discontinue breastfeeding or the drug to avoid potential adverse reactions in the breastfed infant.

☰ Nursing Considerations

! WARNING Be aware that opioid therapy should only be used concomitantly with alprazolam in patients for whom other treatment options are inadequate. If prescribed together, expect dosing and duration of the opioid to be limited. Monitor patient closely for signs and symptoms of decrease in consciousness, including coma, profound sedation, and significant respiratory depression. Notify prescriber immediately and provide emergency supportive care, as death may occur.

- Be aware that alprazolam therapy can result in significant dependence even with short- term use and dosages less than 4 mg daily. Monitor patient closely. A sudden cessation of therapy can result in acute withdrawal reactions. In certain individuals, withdrawal symptoms may last for weeks to up to more than 12 months. Notify prescriber if physical and psychological dependence is suspected.
- Monitor patient closely if depression occurs because of the potential for episodes of hypomania, mania, and suicidal ideation.

! WARNING Monitor patient with impaired respiratory function closely because severe pulmonary dysfunction may occur. Notify prescriber immediately if apnea, hypoventilation, or respiratory depression occurs and provide supportive care.

PATIENT TEACHING

- Warn against stopping drug abruptly because withdrawal symptoms may occur.
- Instruct patient never to increase prescribed dose because of risk of dependency.
- Tell patient prescribed orally disintegrating tablets to use dry hands to remove tablet from bottle just prior to administration. Then she should immediately place the tablet on top of her tongue to dissolve. Inform patient that drinking a liquid beverage is not necessary after taking this form of alprazolam.

! WARNING Warn patient not to consume alcohol or take an opioid during alprazolam treatment without prescriber knowledge, as severe respiratory depression can occur and may lead to death. Instruct patient to inform all prescribers of alprazolam use, especially if pain medication may be prescribed.

- Advise patient to avoid driving and activities that require alertness until alprazolam's effects are known.
- Instruct female patient of childbearing age to notify prescriber immediately if she becomes or might be pregnant. Drug isn't recommended during pregnancy.

alteplase
(tissue plasminogen activator, recombinant)
Activase, Activase rt-PA (CAN), Cathflo Activase

☰ Class and Category
Pharmacologic class: Tissue plasminogen activator (tPA)
Therapeutic class: Thrombolytic

☰ Indications and Dosages
✳ *To treat acute MI for reduction of mortality and incidence of heart failure*

I.V. INJECTION COMBINED WITH ACCELERATED I.V. INFUSION
Adults weighing more than 67 kg (148 lb). 15-mg bolus given over 1 to 2 min, followed by 50 mg infused over 30 min and then 35 mg infused over next 60 min. *Maximum:* 100 mg.
Adults weighing 67 kg (148 lb) or less. 15-mg bolus given over 1 to 2 min, followed by 0.75 mg/kg (up to 50 mg) infused over 30 min and then 0.5 mg/kg (up to 35 mg) infused over next 60 min. *Maximum:* 100 mg.

I.V. INJECTION COMBINED WITH 3-HOUR I.V. INFUSION
Adults weighing 65 kg (143 lb) or more. 6 to 10 mg by bolus over first 1 to 2 min, then as an infusion, 50 to 54 mg over remainder of first hour, 20 mg over second hour, and 20 mg over third hour. *Maximum:* 100 mg.
Adults weighing less than 65 kg (143 lb). 0.075 mg/kg by bolus over first 1 to 2 min, then as an infusion, 0.675 mg/kg over remainder of first hour, 0.25 mg/kg over second hour, and 0.25 mg/kg over third hour. *Maximum:* 100 mg.

✳ *To treat acute ischemic stroke within 3 hr after onset of stroke symptoms and only after computed tomography or other diagnostic imaging method excludes intracranial hemorrhage.*

I.V. INJECTION COMBINED WITH I.V. INFUSION
Adults. 0.9 mg/kg infused over 60 min, with 10% of total dose given as bolus over first min. *Maximum:* 90 mg.

✳ *To treat acute massive pulmonary embolism*

I.V. INFUSION
Adults. 100 mg infused over 2 hr.

✳ *To restore function of occluded central venous access devices*

I.V. INJECTION (CATHFLO ACTIVASE)
Adults and children weighing 30 kg (66 lb) or more. 2 mg/2 ml instilled into occluded catheter; if unsuccessful, may repeat once after 2 hr.
Adults and children weighing less than 30 kg (66 lb). 110% of the lumen volume (not to exceed 2 mg/2 ml) instilled into occluded catheter; if unsuccessful, may repeat once after 2 hr.

☰ Drug Administration
I.V. (ACTIVASE)
- Know that drug may be given prior to availability of coagulation results in patients without recent use of oral anticoagulants or heparin.
- Do not use drug vial if vacuum is not present.
- Drug may be administered reconstituted at 1 mg/ml or further diluted immediately before administration in an equal volume of 0.9% Sodium Chloride Injection or 5% Dextrose Injection, to yield a concentration of 0.5 mg/ml. Administer in either polyvinyl chloride bags or glass vials.
- Avoid excessive agitation during dilution; mix gently by swirling and/or slow inversion.
- Reconstitute 50-mg vial using an 18-gauge needle and a syringe by adding the contents of the accompanying 50-ml vial of Sterile Water for Injection. Direct the stream into the lyophilized cake in the drug vial.
- Reconstitute 100-mg vial using only preservative-free Sterile Water for Injection (100-ml vial) and the transfer device that comes with the drug. Remove one of the

protective caps from the transfer device and insert the piercing pin vertically into the center of the stopper of the Sterile Water for Injection vial, keeping the vial upright. Holding the drug vial upside down, position it so that the center of the stopper is directly over the exposed pin of the transfer device. Push drug vial down onto the transfer device, ensuring that the piercing pin is inserted through the center of the stopper. Invert the two vials so that the drug vial is on the bottom (upright) and the vial of Sterile Water for Injection is upside down. Allow the entire contents of the vial of Sterile Water for Injection to flow down through the transfer device into the drug vial. Be aware that about 0.5 ml of Sterile Water for Injection will be left in the diluent vial. Remove the transfer device and the empty Sterile Water for Injection vial from the drug vial. Discard both. Mix solution with a gentle swirl. Do not shake. Know that slight foaming may occur; this is normal. Leave solution undisturbed for several minutes to allow any large bubbles to dissipate. Resultant solution should be colorless to pale yellow transparent looking.

- The bolus dose should be prepared by removing the appropriate volume from the vial of the reconstituted (1 mg/ml) drug using a syringe and needle. If a 50-mg vial is used, the syringe should not be primed with air and the needle should be inserted into the drug vial stopper. If the 100-mg drug vial is used, the needle should be inserted away from the puncture mark made by the transfer device. Remove the appropriate volume from a port on the infusion line after the infusion set is primed. Program an infusion pump to deliver the bolus over 1 to 2 minutes.

- After the bolus has been given, follow with the infusion. If using 50-mg vials, administer the infusion using either a polyvinyl chloride bag or glass vial and infusion set. If using 100-mg vials for the infusion, remove any amount of drug in excess of the dose to be given from the drug vial. Insert the spike end of an infusion set through the same puncture site created by the transfer device in the stopper of the vial of the reconstituted drug. Peel the clear plastic hanger from the vial label. Hang the drug vial from the resulting loop. Program the infusion to deliver the infusion at the rate prescribed for the condition being treated.

- Reconstituted solution should be discarded if not used within 8 hours; if further diluted, solution must be used immediately.

- Monitor I.V. infusion site. If extravasation occurs causing ecchymosis or inflammation, stop the infusion and apply local therapy. Move I.V. drug site to another location.

I.V. (CATHFLO ACTIVASE)

- Reconstitute Cathflo Activase to a final concentration of 1 mg/ml immediately before administration.

- Withdraw 2.2 ml of Sterile Water for Injection. Do not use Bacteriostatic Water for Injection. Inject the 2.2 ml of Sterile Water for Injection into the drug vial, directing the diluent stream into the powder. Slight foaming may occur but is not unusual. Leave drug undisturbed for several minutes to allow large bubbles to dissipate.

- Mix by gently swirling contents until completely dissolved, usually within 3 minutes. Do not shake. Solution should be colorless to pale yellow transparent.

- Solution may be stored for up to 8 hours following reconstitution when stored at 2–30°C (36–86°F).

- Withdraw 2 mg/2 ml solution from vial and instill into the occluded catheter. Do not use excessive pressure while instilling drug into catheter, to avoid rupturing the catheter or expelling a clot into the circulation. Wait 30 minutes and check catheter function by attempting to aspirate blood. If still occluded, expect to wait an additional 90 minutes before assessing again. If still occluded, expect to repeat dose.

- Once catheter function is restored, aspirate 4 to 5 ml of blood in patients weighing 10 kg (22 lb) or more or 3 ml in patients weighing less than 10 kg (22 lb) to remove the drug and residual clot, then gently irrigate the catheter with 0.9% Sodium Chloride Injection.

- *Incompatibilities:* Other drugs

Route	Onset	Peak	Duration
I.V.	Unknown	Unknown	Unknown

Half-life: < 5 min

Mechanism of Action

Binds to fibrin in a thrombus and converts trapped plasminogen to plasmin. Plasmin breaks down fibrin, fibrinogen, and other clotting factors, which dissolves the thrombus.

Contraindications

For all indications: Active internal bleeding, arteriovenous malformation or aneurysm, bleeding diathesis, hypersensitivity to alteplase or its components, intracranial neoplasm, severe uncontrolled hypertension
For acute MI and pulmonary embolism only: History of stroke, intracranial or intraspinal surgery or trauma in past 3 months
For acute ischemic stroke only: Recent head trauma, recent intracranial or intraspinal surgery or trauma in past 3 months, recent stroke, seizure activity at onset of stroke, subarachnoid hemorrhage, suspicion or history of intracranial hemorrhage

Interactions

DRUGS

angiotensin-converting enzyme (ACE) inhibitors: Possible increased risk of angioedema
anticoagulants, antiplatelets, vitamin K antagonists: Increased risk of bleeding

Adverse Reactions

CNS: Cerebral edema or herniation, CVA, fever, **seizures**
CV: Arrhythmias (including bradycardia and electromechanical dissociation), cardiac arrest, cardiac tamponade, cardiogenic shock, cholesterol embolism, coronary thrombolysis, heart failure, hypotension, mitral insufficiency, myocardial reinfarction or rupture, pericardial effusion, pericarditis, venous embolism, or thrombosis
EENT: Epistaxis, gingival bleeding, **laryngeal edema**
GI: GI bleeding, nausea, **retroperitoneal bleeding**, vomiting
GU: GU bleeding
HEME: Bleeding that may be severe
RESP: Pleural effusion, **pulmonary edema, pulmonary reembolization**
SKIN: Bleeding at puncture sites, ecchymosis, rash, urticaria
Other: Anaphylaxis, angioedema

Childbearing Considerations

PREGNANCY

- It is not known if drug may cause fetal harm but some evidence suggests the possibility exists.
- Drug should only be used in pregnant women in life-threatening situations if no other safer alternative is available, as pregnancy increases risk of bleeding.

LACTATION

- It is not known if drug is present in breast milk.
- Patient should check with prescriber before breastfeeding, once condition has stabilized, as its effect on the breastfed infant is unknown.

Nursing Considerations

! WARNING Know that treatment for acute ischemic stroke must begin within 3 hours after onset of stroke symptoms and only after computed tomography or other diagnostic imaging method excludes intracranial hemorrhage to avoid complications.

! WARNING Monitor patient closely for hypersensitivity reactions which may be life-threatening (angioedema, laryngeal edema, rash, shock) during alteplase administration and for several hours after infusion is completed. If hypersensitivity occurs, discontinue the alteplase infusion immediately and institute appropriate emergency interventions such as administering antihistamines, epinephrine, or intravenous corticosteroids as prescribed.

! WARNING Know that alteplase can cause internal bleeding that could be severe and sometimes fatal, as well as external bleeding, especially at arterial and venous puncture sites. Avoid intramuscular injections and trauma to patient receiving drug. Discontinue alteplase immediately if serious bleeding occurs. Be aware that the following conditions increases risk: advanced age, especially if patient is currently receiving anticoagulant therapy; acute pericarditis; cerebrovascular disease; diabetic hemorrhagic retinopathy or other hemorrhagic ophthalmic conditions; hemostatic defects including those secondary to severe hepatic or renal disease; hypertension (diastolic above 110 mm/Hg or systolic above 175 mm Hg); pregnancy; recent gastrointestinal or genitourinary bleeding, intracranial hemorrhage, or trauma; septic thrombophlebitis or occluded AV cannula at seriously infected site; significant hepatic dysfunction; or subacute bacterial endocarditis.

- Minimize bleeding from noncompressible sites by avoiding internal jugular and subclavian venous puncture sites.
- Apply pressure at puncture site for at least 30 minutes, followed by a pressure dressing after administering alteplase.
- Assess blood pressure and heart rate and rhythm frequently during and after therapy.

! **WARNING** Monitor continuous ECG for arrhythmias during drug therapy because alteplase therapy may cause arrhythmias from sudden reperfusion of the myocardium.

- Be aware that the use of thrombolytics such as alteplase can increase the risk of thromboembolic events in patients with high risk of left heart thrombus, such as patients with atrial fibrillation or mitral stenosis. Also know that the drug does not adequately treat underlying deep vein thrombosis in patients with a pulmonary embolism. Watch this type of patient closely for reembolization.
- Know that the most common complication of thrombolytic therapy is bleeding and that pregnancy may increase this risk. Monitor pregnant patient closely for evidence of bleeding.

PATIENT TEACHING
- Tell patient to immediately report bleeding, including from the nose or gums.
- Advise patient to limit physical activity during alteplase administration to reduce risk of injury and bleeding.

aluminum carbonate
Basalgel

aluminum hydroxide
Alternagel, Alu-Cap, Alugel (CAN), Alu-Tab, Amphojel, Dialume

≡ Class and Category
Pharmacologic class: Aluminum salt
Therapeutic: Antacid, phosphate binder

≡ Indications and Dosages
✳ *To treat hyperacidity associated with gastric hyperacidity, gastritis, hiatal hernia, peptic esophagitis, and peptic ulcers; to prevent phosphate renal calculus formation*

CAPSULES, SUSPENSION, TABLETS (ALUMINUM CARBONATE)
Adults. 2 capsules or tablets or 10 ml suspension every 2 hr up to 12 times daily, as needed.

CAPSULES, TABLETS (ALUMINUM HYDROXIDE)
Adults. 500 to 1,500 mg in divided doses 3 to 6 times daily.

SUSPENSION
Adults. 5 to 30 ml, as needed.

✳ *To reduce hyperphosphatemia in chronic renal failure*

ORAL SUSPENSION
Adults. 300 mg to 600 mg three times daily.
Children. 50 to 150 mg/kg/day in 4 to 6 divided doses.

≡ Drug Administration
P.O.
- Have patient chew tablets thoroughly before swallowing and then have patient drink a full glass of water.
- Shake suspension well before administering and use a calibrated measuring device to measure dose.
- Administer aluminum hydroxide between meals and at bedtime.
- Don't give aluminum hydroxide within 1 to 2 hours of other oral drugs.

Route	Onset	Peak	Duration
P.O.	20 min	Unknown	20–180 min

Half-life: Unknown

≡ Mechanism of Action
Neutralizes or reduces gastric acidity, increasing stomach and duodenal alkalinity. Protects stomach and duodenum lining by inhibiting pepsin's proteolytic activity. Binds with phosphate ions in intestine to form insoluble aluminum–phosphate compounds, which lower blood phosphate level.

≡ Contraindications
Hypersensitivity to aluminum or its components

≡ Interactions

DRUGS

allopurinol, chloroquine, corticosteroids, diflunisal, digoxin, ethambutol, H₂-receptor blockers, iron, isoniazid, phenothiazines, tetracyclines, thyroid hormones, ticlopidine: Decreased effects of these drugs

benzodiazepines: Increased benzodiazepine effects

≡ Adverse Reactions

CNS: Encephalopathy
GI: Constipation, intestinal obstruction, white-speckled stool
MS: Osteomalacia, osteoporosis
Other: Aluminum intoxication, electrolyte imbalances

≡ Childbearing Considerations

PREGNANCY

- It is not known if drug can cause fetal harm.
- Use with caution only if benefit to mother outweighs potential risk to fetus.

LACTATION

- It is not known if drug is present in breast milk.
- Patient should check with prescriber before breastfeeding.

≡ Nursing Considerations

- Know that two 0.6-g aluminum hydroxide tablets can neutralize 16 mEq of acid.
- Monitor patient's serum levels of sodium, phosphate, and other electrolytes, as appropriate.

PATIENT TEACHING

- Instruct patient to chew tablets thoroughly before swallowing and then to drink a full glass of water.
- Advise patient using suspension form to shake container before use and to use a calibrated device when measuring dose, not a household spoon.
- Warn patient not to take maximum dosage for more than 2 weeks unless prescribed because doing so may cause stomach to secrete excess hydrochloric acid.
- Teach patient to prevent constipation with a high-fiber diet and increased fluid intake (2 to 3 L daily), if appropriate.
- Advise patient to notify prescriber about taking other medications and supplements before taking aluminum because of risk of interactions.
- Advise patient to notify prescriber if symptoms worsen or don't subside.

amantadine hydrochloride

Gocovri, Osmolex ER

A

≡ Class and Category

Pharmacologic class: Dopamine agonist
Therapeutic class: Antidyskinetic, antiviral

≡ Indications and Dosages

✴ *To manage symptoms of Parkinson's disease, including arteriosclerotic Parkinsonism, idiopathic Parkinsonism, and postencephalitic Parkinsonism types; to relieve signs and symptoms of Parkinsonism caused by carbon monoxide poisoning*

CAPSULES, ORAL SOLUTION, TABLETS

Adults who do not have serious medical illnesses or who are not receiving other antiparkinson drugs. 100 mg twice daily and increased, as needed. *Maximum:* 300 mg daily in divided doses.

Adults with serious associated medical illnesses or who are receiving other antiparkinson drugs. 100 mg once daily, increased after 1 to several weeks to 100 mg twice daily, if needed. *Maximum:* 400 mg daily in divided doses.

✴ *To treat drug-induced extrapyramidal reactions*

CAPSULES, ORAL SOLUTION, TABLETS

Adults. *Initial:* 100 mg twice daily and then increased, as needed. *Maximum:* 300 mg daily in divided doses.

✴ *To prevent and treat respiratory tract infection caused by influenza A virus*

CAPSULES, ORAL SOLUTION, TABLETS

Adults up to age 65 and children age 12 and over. *Initial:* 200 mg once daily or 100 mg twice daily and continued for at least 10 days following exposure or, if used in conjunction with inactivated influenza A virus vaccine, until protective antibody responses develop, continued for 2 to 4 wk after vaccine has been given. *Maximum:* 200 mg daily.

Adults age 65 and over. 100 mg daily and continued for at least 10 days following exposure or, if used in conjunction with inactivated influenza A virus vaccine, until protective antibody responses develop, continued for 2 to 4 wk after vaccine has been given.

Children ages 9 to 12. 100 mg twice daily. *Maximum:* 200 mg daily.

Children ages 1 to 9. 4.4 to 8.8 mg/kg daily. *Maximum:* 150 mg/day.

±**DOSAGE ADJUSTMENT** For all indications in adult patient receiving immediate-release form with a creatinine clearance of 30 to 50 ml/min, 200 mg on day 1 and then 100 mg daily. For patient with a creatinine clearance of 15 to 29 ml/min, 200 mg on day 1 and then 100 mg every other day. For patient with creatinine clearance less than 15 ml/min or patient on hemodialysis, 200 mg weekly. For patients with congestive heart failure, orthostatic hypotension, or peripheral edema, dosage may have to be reduced. For patient who develops central nervous system adverse effects or other effects while taking 200-mg daily dose, dosage decreased to 100 mg once daily.

＊ *To treat dyskinesia in patients with Parkinson's disease receiving levodopa-based therapy; as adjunct to patients receiving levodopa/carbidopa for Parkinson's disease and experiencing "off" episodes*

E.R. CAPSULES (GOCOVRI)

Adults. *Initial:* 137 mg once daily. After 1 wk, increased to 274 mg once daily.

±**DOSAGE ADJUSTMENT** (Gocovri) For patient with a creatinine clearance of 30 to 59 ml/min, initial dosage reduced to 68.5 mg once daily at bedtime, with maximum dosage not to exceed 137 mg once daily at bedtime. For patient with a creatinine clearance of 15 to 29 ml/min, dosage reduced to 68.5 mg once daily at bedtime with no increased dosage adjustment.

＊ *To treat Parkinson's disease; to treat drug-induced extrapyramidal reactions*

E.R. TABLETS (OSMOLEX ER)

Adults. *Initial:* 129 mg once daily with dosage increased weekly to 322 mg, as needed. *Maximum:* 322 mg given as a 129-mg and 193-mg tablet in morning.

±**DOSAGE ADJUSTMENT** (Osmolex ER) For patient with a creatinine clearance of 30 to 59 ml/min, dosage titration done every 3 weeks instead of weekly and dosing frequency increased to one dose every 48 hours. For patients with a creatinine clearance of 15 to 29 ml/min, dosage titration interval increased to every 4 weeks instead of weekly, and dosing frequency increased to one dose every 96 hours.

Drug Administration

P.O.

- Treatment to prevent influenza started as soon as possible, preferably within 24 to 48 hr after onset of signs and symptoms and continued for 24 to 48 hr after signs and symptoms disappear.
- Use a calibrated device to measure dosage of oral solution.
- Administer immediate-release capsules and tablets whole. Do not break, crush, or split tablets or open capsules.
- Extended-release capsules and tablets should not be chewed, crushed, or split but swallowed whole.
- E.R. capsules may be opened and contents sprinkled on a teaspoon of soft food, such as applesauce, and then administered immediately. Mixture should be swallowed immediately without chewing and not stored for future use.
- Administer extended-release capsules at bedtime and extended-release tablets in the morning.

Route	Onset	Peak	Duration
P.O.	Unknown	1–4 hr	Unknown
P.O. (E.R.)	Unknown	12 hr	Unknown

Half-life: 10–31 hr

Mechanism of Action

Affects dopamine, a neurotransmitter that is synthesized and released by neurons leading from substantia nigra to basal ganglia and is essential for normal motor function. In Parkinson's disease, progressive degeneration of these neurons reduces intrasynaptic dopamine. Amantadine may cause dopamine to accumulate in the basal ganglia by increasing dopamine release or by blocking dopamine reuptake into the presynaptic neurons of the CNS. Amantadine also may stimulate dopamine receptors or make postsynaptic receptors more sensitive to dopamine. These actions help control alterations in involuntary muscle movements, such as tremors and rigidity, that are associated with Parkinson's disease. Amantadine may inhibit influenza A viral replication by blocking uncoating of virus and release of viral nucleic acid into respiratory epithelial cells. It also may interfere with early replication of viruses that have already penetrated cells.

Contraindications

End-stage renal disease (Gocovri, Osmolex ER only), hypersensitivity to amantadine or its components

Interactions

DRUGS

anticholinergics or other drugs with anticholinergic activity: Possibly increased anticholinergic effects and risk of paralytic ileus

CNS stimulants: Excessive CNS stimulation, possibly causing arrhythmias, insomnia, irritability, nervousness, or seizures

live-virus vaccines: Possibly interference with vaccine effectiveness

quinidine, quinine, trimethoprim-sulfamethoxazole: Increased blood amantadine level

urine acidifying drugs: Increased elimination of amantadine with possible decrease in effectiveness

urine alkaline drugs: Decreased elimination of amantadine with possible increase in adverse reactions

ACTIVITIES

alcohol use: Possibly increased risk of CNS effects such as confusion, dizziness, light-headedness, and orthostatic hypotension

Adverse Reactions

CNS: Agitation, amnesia, anxiety, ataxia, confusion, depression, dizziness, dream abnormalities, drowsiness, euphoria, fatigue, fever, hallucinations, headache, hypokinesia, insomnia, irritability, light-headedness, mental impairment, nervousness, **neuroleptic malignant syndrome**, nightmares, psychiatric behavior, **seizures**, slurred speech, somnolence, **suicidal ideation**, syncope, weakness

CV: **Arrhythmias, cardiac arrest, congestive heart failure**, hypertension, orthostatic hypotension, peripheral edema, tachycardia

EENT: Blurred vision; corneal edema or opacity; dry mouth, nose, or throat; keratitis; light sensitivity; mydriasis; optic nerve palsy

GI: Anorexia, constipation, diarrhea, dysphagia, nausea, vomiting

GU: Decreased libido, dysuria, urinary retention

HEME: **Agranulocytosis, leukopenia, neutropenia**

RESP: **Acute respiratory failure, pulmonary edema**, tachypnea

SKIN: Diaphoresis, eczematoid dermatitis, livedo reticularis (purplish, netlike rash), pruritus, rash

Other: **Anaphylaxis**; intense urges to perform certain activities, such as gambling or sexual acts

Childbearing Considerations

PREGNANCY

- It is not known if drug can cause fetal harm, although some evidence exists that drug may have the potential to cause developmental issues, including cardiovascular, skeletal, and visceral malformations when administered in the first trimester.
- Use with caution only if benefit to mother outweighs potential risk to fetus.

LACTATION

- Drug is present in breast milk.
- Drug may alter breast milk excretion or production.
- Breastfeeding should not be undertaken during immediate-release drug therapy; patient should check with prescriber if taking extended-release form before breastfeeding.

Nursing Considerations

- Be aware that amantadine should not be used as the first drug of choice to prevent or treat influenza A because of high levels of resistance to the drug that have developed over the past several years.
- Monitor patients who have a history of psychiatric illness or substance abuse because amantadine may worsen these conditions. Some patients taking amantadine have attempted suicide or had suicidal ideation.
- Monitor for weight gain and edema because drug may cause redistribution of body fluid.
- Be aware that amantadine may increase seizure activity in patients with a history of seizures.

! **WARNING** Monitor patient for evidence of neuroleptic malignant syndrome during dosage reduction or discontinuation of therapy. These include fever, hypertension or hypotension, involuntary motor activity, mental changes, muscle rigidity, tachycardia, and tachypnea. Be prepared to provide supportive treatment and additional drug therapy, as prescribed.

- Be aware that patients receiving more than 200 mg daily are more likely to experience adverse or toxic reactions.
- Monitor patient for decreased drug effectiveness over time. If therapeutic response declines, expect to increase dosage or discontinue drug temporarily, as ordered.
- Assess patient regularly for skin changes because melanoma risk is higher in those with Parkinson's disease. It isn't clear whether the risk is increased by the disease or by its treatment.

PATIENT TEACHING

- Instruct patient to take amantadine exactly as prescribed and not to stop abruptly.
- Instruct patient to use a calibrated measuring device if using oral solution or to swallow immediate-release tablets and capsules whole and not to break, chew, or crush drug.
- Instruct patient taking Osmolex ER tablets to swallow tablets whole and not to chew, crush, or divide tablets. Advise patient to notify prescriber if drug becomes less effective.
- Instruct patient taking Gocovri ER capsules to swallow capsules whole. However, for patient unable to swallow capsules, the capsules may be opened and contents sprinkled on a teaspoon of soft food, such as applesauce, and then administered immediately. Mixture should be swallowed immediately without chewing and not stored for future use.
- Tell patient to notify prescriber if influenza symptoms don't improve after 2 to 3 days.

! **WARNING** Advise patient or family member to notify prescriber immediately if patient reveals thoughts of suicide.

- Encourage patient to avoid consuming alcohol during amantadine therapy because alcohol may increase the risk of confusion, dizziness, light-headedness, or orthostatic hypotension.
- Advise patient to avoid driving and other activities that require a high level of alertness until he knows how the drug affects him because it may cause blurred vision and mental impairment.
- Advise patient to change positions slowly to minimize effects of orthostatic hypotension.
- Tell patient to use ice chips or sugarless candy or gum to relieve dry mouth.
- Caution patient to resume physical activities gradually as signs and symptoms improve.
- Urge patient to have regular skin examinations by a dermatologist or other qualified health professional.
- Instruct patient to notify prescriber about intense urges, such as for gambling or sex, because dosage may have to be reduced or drug discontinued.

amikacin sulfate
Arikayce

Class and Category
Pharmacologic class: Aminoglycoside
Therapeutic class: Antibiotic

Indications and Dosages

✻ *To treat serious gram-negative bacterial infections (including bone, burns, CNS, joint, intra-abdominal, postoperative infections, respiratory tract, skin and soft tissue; neonatal sepsis; septicemia; and serious, complicated, and recurrent UTI) caused by* Acinetobacter, Enterobacter, Escherichia coli, Klebsiella, Proteus, Providencia, Pseudomonas, and Serratia; *and susceptible strains of staphylococci in patients allergic to other antibiotics, and in mixed staphylococcal/gram-negative infections*

I.V. INFUSION, I.M. INJECTION

Adults and children. 15 mg/kg daily in equal doses at equally spaced intervals (7.5 mg/kg every 12 hr or 5 mg/kg every 8 hr) for 7 to 10 days.

Neonates. *Loading dose:* 10 mg/kg. *Maintenance:* 7.5 mg/kg every 12 hr for 7 to 10 days. *Maximum:* 15 mg/kg daily.

✻ *To treat uncomplicated UTI*

I.V. INFUSION, I.M. INJECTION

Adults. 250 mg twice daily for 7 to 10 days.

±**DOSAGE ADJUSTMENT** For patients with impaired renal function, loading dose of 7.5 mg/kg daily; then maintenance dosage based on creatinine clearance and serum creatinine level and given every 12 hr. For morbidly obese patients, dosage not to exceed 1.5 g daily.

* *To treat refractory* Mycobacterium avium complex (MAC) *lung disease for patients who did not achieve negative sputum cultures after a minimum of 6 consecutive months of a multidrug background regimen therapy*

ORAL INHALATION (ARIKAYCE)
Adults. 590 mg once daily using the Lamira Nebulizer System.

Drug Administration
I.V.
- Prepare amikacin I.V. solution by adding contents of 500-mg vial to 100 or 200 ml of sterile diluent such as 0.9% Sodium Chloride Injection, 5% Dextrose Injection, or other compatible solutions listed in manufacturer guidelines.
- Infuse drug over 30 to 60 minutes for adults and children and 1 to 2 hours for neonates.
- *Incompatibilities:* Other drugs

I.M.
- Give I.M. injection in large muscle mass.

ORAL INHALATION
- Know that Arikayce is for oral inhalation use only and should be at room temperature before administration.
- Administer by nebulization only using the Lamira Nebulizer System. The handset and aerosol head must be cleaned and disinfected before using them for the first time, as well as after every use.
- Administer bronchodilator, if prescribed, before administering amikacin oral inhalation.
- Prior to opening glass vial, shake vial well for at least 10 to 15 seconds until the contents appear uniform and well mixed. Open the vial by flipping up the plastic top of the vial then pulling downward to loosen the metal ring. The metal ring and rubber stopper should be removed carefully. Then pour contents of vial into the medication reservoir of the nebulizer handset.
- Expect the inhalation treatment to take about 14 minutes, although it may take as long as 20 minutes.
- After 7 uses, the aerosol head will have to be replaced.

Route	Onset	Peak	Duration
I.V.	Immediate	30 min	8–12 hr
I.M.	Rapid	1 hr	8–12 hr
Oral inhalation	Unknown	Unknown	Unknown

Half-life: 2 hr (oral inhalation: 5.9–19.5 hr)

Mechanism of Action
Binds to negatively charged sites on bacteria's outer cell membrane, disrupting cell integrity. Also binds to bacterial ribosomal subunits and inhibits protein synthesis. Both actions lead to cell death.

Contraindications
Hypersensitivity to amikacin, other aminoglycosides, or their components

Interactions
DRUGS
general anesthetics: Increased risk of neuromuscular blockade
loop diuretics: Increased risk of ototoxicity
neuromuscular blockers: Possibly increased neuromuscular blockade and prolonged respiratory depression
penicillins: Possibly inactivation of or synergistic effects with amikacin
other nephrotoxic drugs: Increased risk of nephrotoxicity

Adverse Reactions
CNS: Drowsiness, headache, loss of balance, **neuromuscular blockade**, tremor, vertigo
EENT: Hearing loss, ototoxicity, tinnitus
GI: Nausea, vomiting
GU: **Azotemia**, dysuria, **nephrotoxicity**, oliguria or polyuria, proteinuria
MS: **Acute muscle paralysis**; arthralgia; muscle fatigue, spasms, and weakness
RESP: **Apnea**; *Inhalation form:* **bronchospasm**, exacerbation of underlying pulmonary disease, **hemoptysis**, **hypersensitivity pneumonitis**
Other: **Anaphylaxis, angioedema, hyperkalemia, hypersensitivity reactions**

Childbearing Considerations
PREGNANCY
- Drug may cause fetal harm such as total, irreversible, bilateral deafness in pediatric patients exposed in utero.
- Drug should not be given to pregnant women unless no other alternative is available.

LACTATION

- It is not known if drug is present in breast milk.
- A decision should be made to discontinue breastfeeding or the drug to avoid potential adverse reactions in the breastfed infant.

Nursing Considerations

- Expect to obtain results of culture and sensitivity testing before therapy begins.
- Obtain patient's weight prior to treatment for calculation of correct dosage.
- Watch for signs of ototoxicity, such as tinnitus and vertigo, especially during high-dosage or prolonged amikacin therapy.

! **WARNING** Assess renal function before and daily during therapy, as ordered because amikacin may produce nephrotoxic effects. To minimize renal tubule irritation, maintain hydration during therapy.

- Be aware that amikacin may exacerbate muscle weakness in such conditions as myasthenia gravis and Parkinson's disease.
- Measure serum amikacin concentrations as ordered, usually 30 to 90 minutes after injection (for peak concentration) and just before administering next parenteral dose (for trough concentration).

PATIENT TEACHING

- Tell patient that daily laboratory tests are necessary during treatment.
- Instruct patient to report ringing in ears, hearing changes, headache, nausea, vomiting, and changes in urination.
- Instruct patient prescribed oral inhalation amikacin therapy how to administer drug. Tell patient that drug is to be administered by nebulization only using the Lamira Nebulizer System. Advise patient that the handset and aerosol head will have to be cleaned and disinfected before using them for the first time, as well as after each use. Prior to opening glass vial, instruct patient to shake vial well for at least 10 to 15 seconds until the contents appear uniform and well mixed. Then patient should open the vial by flipping up the plastic top of the vial then pulling downward to loosen the metal ring. The metal ring and rubber stopper should be removed carefully. Then tell patient to pour the contents of the vial into the medication reservoir of

the nebulizer handset and then follow manufacturer instructions on use of the nebulizer unit.

- Advise patient that the Lamira aerosol head will have to be replaced with a new one after seven uses.
- Tell patient using oral inhalation form that if he misses a daily dose, he should administer the next dose the next day and not double the dose.

! **WARNING** Alert patient taking drug by oral inhalation to seek immediate medical attention if he experiences breathing difficulty.

amiloride hydrochloride
Midamor (CAN)

Class and Category

Pharmacologic class: Potassium-sparing diuretic
Therapeutic class: Diuretic

Indications and Dosages

＊ *As adjunct to loop or thiazide diuretic therapy in patient with heart failure or hypertension to correct diuretic-induced hypokalemia or to prevent diuretic-induced hypokalemia that increases the risk of arrhythmias or other complications*

TABLETS

Adults. 5 mg daily as single dose; if hypokalemia persists, increased to 10 mg. If hypokalemia continues to persist, increased to 15 mg daily and then 20 mg daily, as needed.

Drug Administration

P.O.

- Administer with food to reduce GI upset.

Route	Onset	Peak	Duration
P.O.	2 hr	3–4 hr	24 hr
Half-life: 6–9 hr			

Mechanism of Action

Inhibits sodium reabsorption in distal convoluted tubules and cortical collecting ducts, causing sodium and water loss and enhancing potassium retention.

Contraindications

Hypersensitivity to amiloride or its components; impaired renal function; serum potassium level above 5.5 mEq/L; therapy with another potassium-sparing diuretic, such as spironolactone or triamterene, or a potassium supplement

Interactions

DRUGS

angiotensin-converting enzyme inhibitors, angiotensin II receptor antagonists, cyclosporine, enalapril, lisinopril, potassium products, spironolactone: Increased risk of hyperkalemia
digoxin: Decreased effectiveness of digoxin
lithium: Reduced renal clearance of lithium and increased risk of lithium toxicity
NSAIDs: Reduced diuretic effect of amiloride

FOODS

high-potassium food: Increased risk of hyperkalemia

Adverse Reactions

CNS: Confusion, depression, dizziness, drowsiness, **encephalopathy**, fatigue, headache, insomnia, nervousness, paresthesia, somnolence, tremor, vertigo
CV: Angina, **arrhythmias**, orthostatic hypotension, palpitations
EENT: Dry mouth, increased intraocular pressure, nasal congestion, tinnitus, vision disturbances
GI: Abdominal pain or fullness, anorexia, appetite changes, constipation, diarrhea, **GI bleeding**, heartburn, indigestion, jaundice, nausea, thirst, vomiting
GU: Bladder spasms, dysuria, impotence, loss of libido, polyuria
HEME: **Aplastic anemia, neutropenia**
MS: Arthralgia, muscle spasms, or weakness
RESP: Cough, dyspnea
SKIN: Alopecia, pruritus, rash
Other: Dehydration, hyperchloremia, **hyperkalemia, hypernatremia, metabolic acidosis**

Childbearing Considerations

PREGNANCY

- It is not known if drug can cause fetal harm.
- Use with caution only if benefit to mother outweighs potential risk to fetus.

LACTATION

- It is not known if drug is present in breast milk.
- A decision should be made to discontinue breastfeeding or the drug to avoid potential adverse reactions in the breastfed infant.

Nursing Considerations

- Monitor renal function test results, fluid intake and output, and weight. Also monitor serum potassium level to detect hyperkalemia.

! WARNING Don't administer amiloride with other potassium-sparing diuretics.

PATIENT TEACHING

- Instruct patient to take drug with food.
- Warn patient to avoid high-potassium food and salt substitutes that contain potassium.
- Advise patient to consult prescriber before taking other drugs, including OTC remedies, especially sympathomimetics.
- Tell patient to report dizziness, trembling, numbness, and muscle weakness or spasms.
- Advise patient to increase fluid and fiber intake to prevent constipation.
- Warn patient to expect reversible hair loss and impotence.

amiodarone hydrochloride
Nexterone, Pacerone

Class and Category

Pharmacologic class: Benzofuran derivative
Therapeutic class: Class III antiarrhythmic

Indications and Dosages

* *To treat life-threatening, recurrent ventricular fibrillation and hemodynamically unstable ventricular tachycardia when these arrhythmias don't respond to other drugs or when patient can't tolerate other drugs*

TABLETS (PACERONE)

Adults. *Loading:* 800 to 1,600 mg daily in divided doses for 1 to 3 wk. Once arrhythmia is controlled or side effects become prominent, dosage reduced to 600 to 800 mg daily in divided doses for 1 mo and then reduced to 400 mg daily if cardiac rhythm is stable. *Maintenance:* 400 mg daily.

* *To treat or prevent life-threatening, recurrent ventricular fibrillation and hemodynamically unstable ventricular tachycardia when these arrhythmias don't respond to other drugs, when patient can't tolerate other drugs, or when oral amiodarone is indicated but patient is unable to take oral medication*

I.V. INFUSION (NEXTERONE)

Adults. *Loading:* 150 mg (15 mg/min) of 150 mg/100 ml solution infused over 10 min followed by 360 mg (1 mg/min) of 360 mg/200 ml solution infused over 6 hr followed by 540 mg (0.5 mg/min) of 360 mg/200 ml solution infused over remaining 18 hr. *Maintenance:* 720 mg (0.5 mg/min) of 360 mg/200 ml solution infused over 24 hr and repeated every 24 hr for up to 2 to 3 wk, as needed. Changed to oral form as soon as possible.

* *To treat breakthrough episodes of ventricular fibrillation or hemodynamically unstable ventricular tachycardia*

I.V. INFUSION (NEXTERONE)

Adults. 150 mg (15 mg/min) of 150 mg/100 ml solution infused over 10 min.

Drug Administration

P.O.

- Administer consistently with regard to meals because food affects absorption.
- Doses should be divided for total daily doses of 1,000 mg or higher, or when gastrointestinal intolerance develops.
- Expect dosage to be reduced if excessive gastrointestinal intolerance occurs.

I.V.

- Know that Nexterone is already premixed and does not require further dilution. Solution should appear clear. Check for minute leaks prior to use by squeezing the bag firmly.
- Use an in-line filter during administration. Also use a central venous catheter whenever possible. A central venous catheter is required when infusion rate exceeds 2 mg/ml because drug may cause peripheral vein phlebitis at higher rates.
- Use only a volumetric infusion pump to administer drug.
- Don't use plastic containers in series connections because this could result in an air embolism.
- Know that after the initial rate, subsequent infusions are given at different rates depending on the dose and sequence given.

- Monitor patient's blood pressure and pulse rate frequently throughout infusion as bradycardia and hypotension may occur and may require infusion rate to be decreased and possibly additional supportive care given, as prescribed. Expect to have a temporary pacemaker available if patient is at risk for bradycardia or AV block.
- Protect from light until ready to use; does not have to be protected from light during administration.
- Drug should be changed to oral form as soon as possible.
- *Incompatibilities:* Aminophylline, amoxicillin sodium-clavulanic acid, ampicillin sodium-sulbactam sodium, argatroban, bivalirudin, cefamandole nafate, cefazolin sodium, ceftazidime, digoxin, furosemide, heparin sodium, imipenem-cilastatin sodium, magnesium sulfate, mezlocillin sodium, micafungin, piperacillin tazobactam sodium, potassium phosphates, sodium bicarbonate, sodium nitroprusside, and sodium phosphates

Route	Onset	Peak	Duration
P.O.	2 days–3 wk	3–7 hr	Weeks–months
I.V.	Hours–3 days	Unknown	Weeks–months

Half-life: 26–107 days (I.V.: 9–36 days)

Mechanism of Action

Acts on cardiac cell membranes, prolonging repolarization and the refractory period and raising ventricular fibrillation threshold. Drug relaxes vascular smooth muscles, mainly in coronary circulation, and improves myocardial blood flow. It relaxes peripheral vascular smooth muscles, decreasing peripheral vascular resistance and myocardial oxygen consumption.

Contraindications

Bradycardia that causes syncope (unless pacemaker present), cardiogenic shock, hypersensitivity to amiodarone or its components, SA node dysfunction, second- and third-degree AV block (unless pacemaker present)

Interactions

DRUGS

anticoagulants: Increased anticoagulant response and possibly serious bleeding

anesthetic agents, azole antifungals, Class I and III antiarrhythmics, fluoroquinolones (selected ones), halogenated inhalation, lithium, loratadine, macrolide antibiotics (selected ones), phenothiazines (selected ones), trazodone, tricyclic antidepressants: Increased risk of prolonged QT interval and life-threatening arrhythmias such as torsades de points

beta blockers, clonidine, digoxin, diltiazem, ivabradine: Potentiate amiodarone effects with increased risk of AV block, bradycardia, and hypotension

calcium channel blockers: Increased serum levels of these drugs and increased risk of AV block, bradycardia, and hypotension

cholestyramine, phenytoin, rifampin: Decreased amiodarone level

cimetidine, protease inhibitors (selected ones): Increased amiodarone level

cyclosporine: Increased cyclosporine level

CYP450 inducers such as St. John's Wort: Reduced exposure of amiodarone

CYP450 inhibitors such as azole antifungals, cimetidine, and selected fluoroquinolone and macrolide antibiotics: Increased exposure of amiodarone

dabigatran, dextromethorphan, phenytoin: Possible increased serum levels of these drugs

dextromethorphan, methotrexate, phenytoin: Increased serum levels of these drugs and increased risk of toxicity

digoxin: Increased serum digoxin level and risk of digitalis toxicity

fentanyl: Increased serum fentanyl level with increased risk of bradycardia, decreased cardiac output, and hypotension

flecainide procainamide, quinidine: Increased serum levels of these drugs

HMG-CoA reductase inhibitors such as atorvastatin, lovastatin, and simvastatin: Increased risk of myopathy and rhabdomyolysis

ledipasvir/sofosbuvir, sofosbuvir/simeprevir: May cause serious symptomatic bradycardia

protease inhibitors: Possibly increased risk of elevated amiodarone levels and toxicity

sofosbuvir: Increased risk of symptomatic bradycardia requiring possible pacemaker insertion

theophylline: Increased serum theophylline level; increased risk of theophylline toxicity

warfarin: Potentiated anticoagulant response with possible serious or fatal bleeding

FOODS

grapefruit juice: Increased amiodarone level

Adverse Reactions

CNS: Abnormal gait, ataxia, confusion, delirium, demyelinating polyneuropathy, disorientation, dizziness, fatigue, fever, hallucinations, headache, insomnia, involuntary motor activity, lack of coordination, malaise, paresthesia, parkinsonian symptoms, peripheral neuropathy, **pseudotumor cerebri**, sleep disturbances, tremor

CV: Arrhythmias (including AV block, bradycardia, electromechanical dissociation, torsades de pointes, and ventricular tachycardia or fibrillation), cardiac arrest, cardiogenic shock, edema, **heart failure, hypotension, QT prolongation,** vasculitis

EENT: Abnormal salivation, abnormal taste and smell, blurred vision, corneal microdeposits, dry eyes or mouth, halo vision, lens opacities, macular degeneration, optic neuritis, optic neuropathy, papilledema, permanent blindness, photophobia, scotoma

ENDO: Hyperthyroidism, hypothyroidism, syndrome of inappropriate ADH secretion, thyroid nodules, **thyroid cancer**

GI: Abdominal pain, anorexia, **cirrhosis,** constipation, diarrhea, elevated bilirubin or liver enzymes, **hepatic failure, hepatitis,** nausea, **pancreatitis,** vomiting

GU: Acute renal failure, decreased libido, epididymitis, impotence, **renal insufficiency**

HEME: Agranulocytosis, aplastic or hemolytic anemia, coagulation abnormalities, neutropenia, pancytopenia, spontaneous bruising, **thrombocytopenia**

MS: Muscle weakness, myopathy, **rhabdomyolysis**

RESP: Acute respiratory distress syndrome in postoperative setting; bronchiolitis obliterans organizing pneumonia; bronchospasm; **eosinophilic pneumonia; infiltrates that lead to** dyspnea, cough, **hemoptysis, hypoxia, pulmonary fibrosis, pulmonary alveolar hemorrhage, pulmonary interstitial pneumonitis;** crackles and wheezing; pleural effusion; pleuritis; pneumonia; pulmonary inflammation, **pulmonary fibrosis; respiratory arrest or failure**

SKIN: Alopecia, bluish gray pigmentation, bullous dermatitis, eczema, **erythema multiforme, exfoliative dermatitis,** flushing, photosensitivity, pruritus, rash, **skin cancer,** solar dermatitis, **Stevens–Johnson syndrome, toxic epidermal necrolysis,** urticaria

Other: Anaphylaxis including shock, angioedema, **drug reaction with eosinophilia and systemic symptoms (DRESS),** lupus-like syndrome

Childbearing Considerations

PREGNANCY

- Drug crosses the placental barrier and has the possibility to cause fetal harm.
- Fetal adverse effects may include arrhythmias such as bradycardia, periodic ventricular extrasystoles, and QT prolongation; growth restriction; neurodevelopmental abnormalities, such as ataxia, delayed motor development, jerk nystagmus, and speech delay with difficulties with written language and math later in childhood; premature birth; and thyroid dysfunction, such as hyperthyroxinemia or hypothyroidism.
- Drug should not be given to pregnant women unless benefit to the mother outweighs potential risk to fetus.

LABOR & DELIVERY

- Newborn should be monitored for signs and symptoms of cardiac arrhythmias and thyroid dysfunction.

LACTATION

- Drug is present in breast milk.
- Breastfeeding is not recommended during drug therapy.

REPRODUCTION

- Drug may reduce female and male fertility, but it is not known if this effect is reversible.
- Women of childbearing age should use effective contraception to avoid pregnancy.

Nursing Considerations

- Check patient's implantable cardiac device (if present), as ordered, at the start of and during amiodarone therapy because drug may affect pacing or defibrillating thresholds.
- Monitor all patients but especially elderly patients closely when conversion to oral amiodarone is made for continued effectiveness.

! **WARNING** Be aware that amiodarone may cause or worsen pulmonary disorders that may develop days to weeks after therapy and progress to respiratory failure or even death. Expect to obtain chest x-ray and pulmonary function tests before therapy starts and then chest x-ray and follow-up exams every 3 to 6 months during therapy.

- Monitor vital signs and oxygen level often during and after giving amiodarone. Keep emergency equipment and drugs nearby.

! **WARNING** Monitor continuous ECG; check for increased PR and QRS intervals, arrhythmias, and heart rate below 60 beats/min because amiodarone may cause sinus arrest or symptomatic bradycardia and new ventricular arrhythmias or worsen existing arrhythmias as well as increasing resistance to cardioversion. Electrolyte imbalance or use of concomitant antiarrhythmics or other interacting drugs may increase the development of these arrhythmias. Expect to correct electrolyte imbalance, as ordered, prior to initiating treatment with amiodarone.

- Monitor serum amiodarone level, which normally ranges from 1.0 to 2.5 mcg/ml.
- Assess thyroid hormone levels; drug inhibits conversion of T_4 to T_3 and may cause drug-induced hyperthyroidism, thyrotoxicosis, and new or worsened arrhythmias. If new signs of thyroid dysfunction or arrhythmias occur, notify prescriber at once.
- Monitor liver enzymes, as ordered. If elevations become persistent and significant, notify prescriber and expect maintenance dosage to be reduced or drug discontinued.
- Be aware that patient should undergo regular ophthalmic examinations including fundoscopy and slit-lamp examination during amiodarone therapy because drug can cause serious visual impairment including permanent blindness.

PATIENT TEACHING

- Instruct patient to take oral drug consistently with regard to meals.
- Explain that patient will need frequent monitoring and laboratory tests during treatment.

- Advise patient to report cough, dark urine, dyspnea, fainting, fatigue, light-headedness, nausea, swollen feet and hands, vomiting, wheezing, yellow sclerae or skin, or a sudden change in quality or rapidity of pulse.
- Instruct patient to report abnormal bleeding or bruising. Also tell patient to report any sign of visual impairment or decreased or increased levels of energy.
- Stress importance of informing all prescribers of amiodarone use, as serious drug interactions may occur.
- Advise patient to avoid corneal refractive laser surgery while taking drug.
- Warn female patient of childbearing age that amiodarone can cause fetal harm. Instruct her to use effective contraceptive measures and report suspected or known pregnancy immediately.
- Advise female patient who has been breastfeeding to discontinue nursing, because drug is excreted in human milk and may cause potential harm.
- Advise patient to avoid drinking grapefruit juice or taking St. John's wort while receiving amiodarone.
- Warn patient that adverse reactions or interactions may persist following the discontinuation of amiodarone. If serious, prescriber should be notified.

amisulpride
Barhemsys

Class and Category
Pharmacologic class: Dopamine-2 receptor antagonist
Therapeutic class: Antiemetic

Indications and Dosages
* *To prevent postoperative nausea and vomiting, either alone or in combination with an antiemetic of a different class*

I.V. INJECTION
Adults. 5 mg at the time of induction of anesthesia.
* *To treat postoperative nausea and vomiting in patients who have received antiemetic prophylaxis with an antiemetic of a different class or who have not received prophylaxis*

I.V. INJECTION
Adults. 10 mg as a single dose.

Drug Administration
I.V.
- Dilution not required.
- Compatible with 0.9% Sodium Chloride Injection, 5% Dextrose Injection, and Water for Injection, or Lactated Ringer's Solution, which may be used to flush I.V. line before and after administration.
- Protect from light.
- Administer within 12 hours of removal of vial from the protective carton.
- Inject over 1 to 2 minutes as a single I.V. injection.
- *Incompatibilities:* None listed by manufacturer

Route	Onset	Peak	Duration
I.V.	Immediate	1–2 min	Unknown

Half-life: 12 hr

Mechanism of Action
Blocks the dopamine-2 receptor sites located in the chemoreceptor trigger zone. Inhibition of these sites prevents stimulation of the vomiting center, which prevents or stops nausea and vomiting.

Contraindications
Hypersensitivity to amisulpride or its components

Interactions
DRUGS
dopamine agonists: Reciprocal antagonism of effects between amisulpride and dopamine agonists, especially with levodopa, which should not be given with amisulpride
drugs prolonging QT interval: Potential additive effects; droperidol should not be administered with amisulpride and other drugs that prolong QT interval and require ECG monitoring

Adverse Reactions
CNS: Chills
CV: **Hypotension**
ENDO: Elevated prolactin levels
GI: Abdominal distention
OTHER: **Hypokalemia**, infusion-site pain

Childbearing Considerations
PREGNANCY
- It is not known if drug can cause fetal harm.

- Use with caution only if benefit to mother outweighs potential risk to fetus.

LACTATION

- Drug is present in breast milk.
- Pumping breast milk and discarding for 48 hours after drug is given will help minimize drug exposure of breastfed infant. However, patient should check with prescriber before breastfeeding.

⌇ Nursing Considerations

- Be aware that amisulpride should not be given to patients with severe renal impairment (eGFR less than 30 ml/min) because it is substantially excreted by the kidneys and may increase risk of adverse reactions. It may be used in patients with mild to moderate renal impairment.
- Know that amisulpride should not be given to patients with congenital long QT syndrome or concurrent administration with droperidol because of risk of QT prolongation.
- Expect to monitor patient's ECG in patients with concurrent therapy of drugs known to prolong QT interval or for patients with conditions known to prolong QT interval. ECG monitoring is also recommended in patients with congestive heart failure, electrolyte abnormalities such as hypokalemia or hypomagnesemia, or in the presence of preexisting arrhythmias/cardiac conduction disorders.

PATIENT TEACHING

- Instruct patient to immediately report a change in heart rate or if he feels faint or light-headed.
- Advise patient to inform anesthesiologist about drugs being taken prior to surgery.

amitriptyline hydrochloride
Elavil (CAN)

⌇ Class and Category
Pharmacologic class: Tricyclic antidepressant
Therapeutic class: Antidepressant

⌇ Indications and Dosages
✳ *To relieve depression, especially when accompanied by anxiety and insomnia*

TABLETS

Adults. *Outpatient:* 75 mg daily in divided doses, increased to 150 mg daily, if needed. Alternatively, 50 to 100 mg at bedtime, increased by 25 to 50 mg, as needed, to 150 mg daily. *Inpatient:* 100 mg daily, gradually increased to 300 mg daily, if needed. *Maintenance:* 40 to 100 mg daily at bedtime.

±**DOSAGE ADJUSTMENT** Dosage reduced to 10 mg three times a day plus 20 mg for adolescent and elderly patients at bedtime.

⌇ Mechanism of Action

Normally, when an impulse reaches adrenergic nerves, the nerves release serotonin and norepinephrine from their storage sites. Most of this is taken back into the nerves and stored by the reuptake mechanism, as shown below on the left.

Amitriptyline blocks serotonin and norepinephrine reuptake by adrenergic nerves. By doing so, it raises serotonin and norepinephrine levels at nerve synapses. This action may elevate mood and reduce depression.

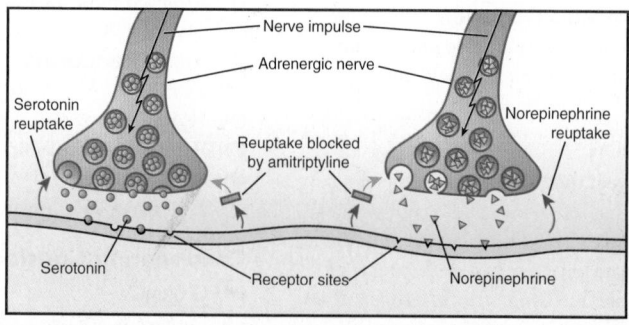

Drug Administration
P.O.
- Increase in dosage made preferably in late afternoon and/or bedtime doses to decrease daytime sedation.

Route	Onset	Peak	Duration
P.O.	7–14 days	2–5 hr	Unknown

Half-life: 13–36 hr

Contraindications
Acute recovery phase after MI, concurrent therapy with cisapride, hypersensitivity to amitriptyline or its components, MAO inhibitor therapy within 14 days

Interactions
DRUGS
anticholinergics, epinephrine, norepinephrine: Increased effects of these drugs
barbiturates: Decreased amitriptyline level
carbamazepine: Decreased serum amitriptyline level and increased serum carbamazepine level, which increases therapeutic and toxic effects of carbamazepine
cimetidine, disulfiram, fluoxetine, fluvoxamine, haloperidol, H₂-receptor antagonists, methylphenidate, oral contraceptives, paroxetine, phenothiazines, sertraline: Increased serum amitriptyline level
cisapride: Possibly prolonged QT interval and increased risk of arrhythmias
clonidine, guanethidine, and other antihypertensives: Decreased antihypertensive effects
dicumarol: Increased anticoagulant effect
levodopa: Decreased levodopa absorption; sympathetic hyperactivity, sinus tachycardia, hypertension, agitation
MAO inhibitors: Possibly seizures and death
thyroid replacement drugs: Arrhythmias and increased antidepressant effects

ACTIVITIES
alcohol use: Enhanced CNS depression
smoking: Decreased amitriptyline effects

Adverse Reactions
CNS: Anxiety, ataxia, **coma**, chills, delusions, disorientation, drowsiness, extrapyramidal reactions, fatigue, fever, headache, insomnia, nightmares, peripheral neuropathy, **suicidal ideation**, tremor

CV: **Arrhythmias (including prolonged AV conduction, heart block**, and tachycardia), **cardiomyopathy**, hypertension, **MI**, nonspecific ECG changes, orthostatic hypotension, palpitations

EENT: Abnormal taste, black tongue, blurred vision, dry mouth, increased salivation, nasal congestion, tinnitus

ENDO: Gynecomastia, hyperglycemia, **hypoglycemia**, increased prolactin level, syndrome of inappropriate ADH secretion

GI: Abdominal cramps, constipation, diarrhea, flatulence, ileus, increased appetite, nausea, vomiting

GU: Impotence, libido changes, menstrual irregularities, testicular swelling, urinary hesitancy, urine retention

HEME: **Agranulocytosis, bone marrow depression**, eosinophilia, **leukopenia, thrombocytopenia**

SKIN: Alopecia, flushing, purpura

Other: Weight gain

Childbearing Considerations
PREGNANCY
- It is not known if drug can cause fetal harm but limited studies suggest it may.
- Know that drug is a tricyclic antidepressant. This type of antidepressant has been known to cause withdrawal symptoms such as agitation and respiratory depression in the neonate when given to the mother during the last trimester of pregnancy. Also, urinary retention in the neonate has been reported when mother has taken drug during pregnancy.
- Use with caution only if benefit to mother outweighs potential risk to fetus.

LACTATION
- Drug is present in breast milk.
- A decision should be made to discontinue breastfeeding or the drug to avoid potential adverse reactions in the breastfed infant.

Nursing Considerations
- Use caution if patient has a history of seizures, urine retention, or angle-closure glaucoma because of amitriptyline's atropine-like effects.

! **WARNING** Don't give an MAO inhibitor within 14 days of amitriptyline because of the risk of seizures and death.

- Closely monitor patient with CV disorder because amitriptyline may cause arrhythmias, such as sinus tachycardia.
- Watch patients closely (especially adolescents and young adults), for suicidal tendencies, particularly when therapy starts and dosage changes. Depression may worsen temporarily during these times.
- Monitor blood pressure for hypotension or hypertension.
- Stay alert for behavior changes, such as hallucinations and decreased interest in personal appearance. Be aware that psychosis may develop in schizophrenic patients, and symptoms may increase in paranoid patients.
- Avoid abrupt withdrawal after long use because nausea, headache, vertigo, and nightmares may occur.

PATIENT TEACHING

- Instruct patient to avoid using alcohol or OTC drugs that contain alcohol during amitriptyline therapy because alcohol enhances CNS depressant effects.
- Urge family or caregiver to watch patient closely for suicidal tendencies, especially when therapy starts or dosage changes and particularly if patient is a teenager or young adult.

amlodipine benzoate
Katerzia

amlodipine besylate
Norvasc

Class and Category
Pharmacologic class: Calcium channel blocker
Therapeutic class: Antianginal, antihypertensive

Indications and Dosages
✳ *To control hypertension*

ORAL SUSPENSION, TABLETS
Adults. *Initial:* 5 mg daily, increased gradually over 10 to 14 days, as needed. *Maximum:* 10 mg daily.
Children age 6 to 17 years. 2.5 to 5 mg once daily. Maximum: 5 mg once daily.

± **DOSAGE ADJUSTMENT** Initially 2.5 mg daily for elderly, fragile, or small patients or patients with impaired hepatic function. Increased gradually over 7 to 14 days based on response.

✳ *To treat chronic stable angina and vasospastic angina (Prinzmetal's or Variant angina); to reduce risk of hospitalization for angina and the risk of coronary revascularization procedure in patients with recently documented coronary artery disease without heart failure or an ejection fraction less than 40%*

ORAL SUSPENSION, TABLETS
Adults. 5 to 10 mg daily.
± **DOSAGE ADJUSTMENT** 2.5 to 5 mg daily for elderly patients and those with impaired hepatic function.

Drug Administration
P.O.
- Shake oral suspension container before measuring dose. Use a calibrated device to measure dosage.
- Administer with food if GI upset occurs.

Route	Onset	Peak	Duration
P.O.	Unknown	6–12 hr	24 hr

Half-life: 30–50 hr

Mechanism of Action
Binds to dihydropyridine and nondihydropyridine cell membrane receptor sites on myocardial and vascular smooth muscle cells and inhibits influx of extracellular calcium ions across slow calcium channels. This decreases intracellular calcium level, inhibiting smooth muscle cell contractions and relaxing coronary and vascular smooth muscles, decreasing peripheral vascular resistance, and reducing systolic and diastolic blood pressure. Decreased peripheral vascular resistance also decreases myocardial workload, oxygen demand, and possibly angina. Also, by inhibiting coronary artery muscle cell contractions and restoring blood flow, drug may relieve Prinzmetal's angina.

Contraindications
Hypersensitivity to amlodipine or its components

Interactions
DRUGS
ACE inhibitors, aliskiren (in patients with diabetes or renal impairment): Increased risk

of hyperkalemia, hypotension, and renal dysfunction

cyclosporine, simvastatin, tacrolimus: Possibly increased blood levels of these drugs

CYP3A4 inhibitors such as diltiazem, ketoconazole, itraconazole, and ritonavir: Possibly increased blood amlodipine level

sildenafil: Possibly excessive hypotension

Adverse Reactions

CNS: Anxiety, dizziness, extrapyramidal disorder, fatigue, headache, lethargy, light-headedness, paresthesia, somnolence, syncope, tremor

CV: **Arrhythmias**, chest pain, **hypotension**, palpitations, peripheral edema

EENT: Dry mouth, gingival hyperplasia, pharyngitis

ENDO: Hot flashes

GI: Abdominal cramps or pain, anorexia, constipation, diarrhea, dysphagia, elevated liver enzymes, esophagitis, flatulence, indigestion, jaundice, nausea, **pancreatitis**, vomiting

GU: Decreased libido, impotence, urinary frequency

MS: Myalgia

RESP: Dyspnea

SKIN: Dermatitis, flushing, rash

Other: Weight loss

Childbearing Considerations

PREGNANCY

- It is not known if drug can cause fetal harm.
- Use with caution only if benefit to mother outweighs potential risk to fetus.

LACTATION

- Drug is present in breast milk.
- Patient should check with prescriber before breastfeeding.

Nursing Considerations

- Use amlodipine cautiously in patients with heart block, heart failure, impaired renal function, hepatic disorder, or severe aortic stenosis.
- Monitor patient with impaired hepatic function closely because amlodipine is extensively metabolized by the liver, and expect to titrate dosage slowly when administering drug to patients with severe hepatic impairment.
- Monitor blood pressure while adjusting dosage, especially in patients with heart

failure or severe aortic stenosis, because symptomatic hypotension may occur.

- Assess patient frequently for chest pain when starting or increasing the dose of amlodipine, because worsening of angina or an acute myocardial infarction can occur, especially in patients with severe obstructive coronary artery disease.

PATIENT TEACHING

- Instruct patient to shake container of oral suspension before measuring dose and to use a calibrated device to measure dosage.
- Suggest taking amlodipine with food to reduce GI upset.
- Tell patient to take missed dose as soon as remembered and next dose in 24 hours.
- Tell patient to immediately notify prescriber of dizziness, arm or leg swelling, difficulty breathing, hives, or rash.
- Advise patient to have blood pressure checked routinely for possible hypotension.
- Tell mothers interested in breastfeeding to discuss with prescriber, because amlodipine is present in human milk.

amoxicillin trihydrate
(amoxycillin)
Amoxil, Apo-Amoxi (CAN), Novamoxin (CAN)

Class and Category
Pharmacologic class: Aminopenicillin
Therapeutic class: Antibiotic

Indications and Dosages
✽ *To treat ear, nose, throat, GU tract, skin, and soft-tissue infections; to treat pharyngitis, tonsillitis, or both secondary to* Streptococcus pyogenes *infection*

CAPSULES, CHEWABLE TABLETS, ORAL SUSPENSION, TABLETS

Adults and children weighing 40 kg (88 lb) or more. 250 mg every 8 hr; for severe infections, 500 mg or 875 mg every 12 hr. Given at least 10 days for pharyngitis and tonsillitis.

Children age 12 wk and over weighing less than 40 kg. 20 mg/kg daily in divided doses every 8 hr; for severe infections, 40 to 45 mg/kg/day in divided doses every 12 hr. Given at least 10 days for pharyngitis and tonsillitis.

Children under age 12 wk. Up to 30 mg/kg/day in divided doses every 12 hr. Given at least 10 days for pharyngitis and tonsillitis.

* *To treat lower respiratory tract infections*

CAPSULES, CHEWABLE TABLETS, ORAL SUSPENSION, TABLETS

Adults and children weighing 40 kg (88 lb) or more. 875 mg every 12 hr or 500 mg every 8 hr.

Children age 12 wk and over weighing less than 40 kg (88 lb). 40 mg/kg in divided doses every 8 hr or 45 mg/kg in divided doses every 12 hr.

Children under age 12 wk. Up to 30 mg/kg daily in divided doses every 12 hr.

* *As adjunct to eradicate* Helicobacter pylori *to reduce risk of duodenal ulcer recurrence*

CAPSULES, CHEWABLE TABLETS, ORAL SUSPENSION, TABLETS

Adults. 1 g every 12 hr with 500 mg of clarithromycin every 12 hr and 30 mg of lansoprazole every 12 hr for 14 days, or 1 g every 8 hr with 30 mg of lansoprazole every 8 hr for 14 days.

±**DOSAGE ADJUSTMENT** For patients with impaired renal function with a glomerular filtration rate less than 30 ml/min, dosage reduced to less than 875 mg; for a glomerular filtration rate of 10 to 30 ml/min dosage reduced to 500 mg or 250 mg every 12 hr; for a glomerular filtration rate less than 10 ml/min dosage reduced to 500 mg or 250 mg and frequency reduced to every 24 hr.

≡ Drug Administration

P.O.

- Shake oral suspension well before each use. Use a calibrated device to measure dosage.
- Administer oral suspension form to children by dropping directly on child's tongue to swallow. If this does not work, mix dose of suspension with formula or cold drink (milk, fruit juice, ginger ale, water) and have child drink it immediately.
- Refrigerate reconstituted suspension. Discard after 14 days.
- Chewable tablets should not be swallowed whole.
- Each 200-mg chewable tablet contains 1.82 mg phenylalanine; each 400-mg chewable tablet contains 3.64 mg phenylalanine. Suspension does not contain phenylalanine.

Route	Onset	Peak	Duration
P.O.	Unknown	1–2 hr	6–8 hr

Half-life: 9–11 hr

≡ Mechanism of Action

Kills bacteria by binding to and inactivating penicillin-binding proteins on the inner bacterial cell wall, weakening the bacterial cell wall and causing lysis.

≡ Contraindications

Hypersensitivity including severe reactions (anaphylaxis or Stevens–Johnson syndrome) to amoxicillin, other beta-lactam antibiotics, or their components

≡ Interactions

DRUGS

allopurinol: Increased risk of rash

chloramphenicol, erythromycins, sulfonamides, tetracyclines: Reduced bactericidal effect of amoxicillin

methotrexate: Increased risk of methotrexate toxicity

oral anticoagulants: Possible prolonged prothrombin time (increased international normalized ratio)

oral contraceptives with estrogen: Possibly reduced effectiveness of contraceptive

probenecid: Increased amoxicillin effects

≡ Adverse Reactions

CNS: Agitation, anxiety, behavior changes, confusion, dizziness, insomnia, reversible hyperactivity, **seizures**

CV: Hypersensitivity vasculitis

EENT: Black, hairy tongue; mucocutaneous candidiasis; tooth discoloration

GI: *Clostridium difficile*–associated diarrhea, diarrhea, elevated liver enzymes, **hemorrhagic or pseudomembranous colitis, hepatic dysfunction,** jaundice, nausea, vomiting

GU: Crystalluria, vaginal mycosis

HEME: **Agranulocytosis,** anemia (including **hemolytic anemia**), eosinophilia, granulocytosis, **leukopenia, thrombocytopenia, thrombocytopenic purpura**

SKIN: **Erythema multiforme,** erythematous maculopapular rash, generalized exanthematous pustulosis, **Stevens–Johnson syndrome, toxic epidermal necrolysis,** urticaria

Other: Allergic reactions, anaphylaxis, serum sickness-like reaction (such as arthralgia, arthritis, fever, myalgia, rash, and urticaria)

Childbearing Considerations

PREGNANCY

- It is not known if drug can cause fetal harm.
- Use with caution only if benefit to mother outweighs potential risk to fetus.

LABOR & DELIVERY

- It is not known if drug given to mother during labor has immediate or delayed adverse effects on the fetus.

LACTATION

- Drug is present in breast milk and may lead to sensitization in infant.
- Patient should check with prescriber before breastfeeding.

Nursing Considerations

- Know that patients with mononucleosis shouldn't receive amoxicillin because this class of drugs may cause an erythematous rash.
- Use drug cautiously in patients with hepatic impairment. Monitor hepatic and renal function and CBC, as ordered, in patients on prolonged therapy. Also use cautiously in breastfeeding and elderly patients.
- Expect to start therapy before culture and sensitivity test results are known.

! **WARNING** Stop amoxicillin immediately and provide emergency care as indicated and ordered if an allergic reaction occurs.

- Monitor patient closely for diarrhea, which may indicate pseudomembranous colitis caused by *Clostridium difficile.* If diarrhea occurs, notify prescriber, expect to withhold amoxicillin, and treat with fluids, electrolytes, protein, and an antibiotic effective against *C. difficile.*
- Monitor patient for superinfection. If it occurs, expect to discontinue drug and provide treatment as ordered.

PATIENT TEACHING

- Tell patient to refrigerate reconstituted suspension and to shake well before each use. Advice patient to use a calibrated measuring device and not a household spoon to ensure accurate dosing.
- Know that when amoxicillin suspension is prescribed for a child, instruct parents

to place it directly on child's tongue to swallow. If this does not work, tell parents to mix dose of suspension with formula or cold drink (milk, fruit juice, ginger ale, water) and have child drink it immediately.
- Tell patient to chew or crush chewable tablets and not to swallow them whole.
- Urge patient to take amoxicillin for full length of time prescribed, even if he feels better.
- Teach patient to report adverse reactions and notify prescriber if infection worsens or doesn't improve after 72 hours.
- Urge patient to tell prescriber about diarrhea that's severe or lasts longer than 3 days. Remind patient that watery or bloody stools can occur 2 or more months after antibiotic therapy and may be serious, requiring prompt treatment.
- Inform patient with diabetes who is using glucose tests based on the Benedict's copper reduction reaction that false-positive reactions may occur when testing for glucose in urine. Advise patient to use glucose tests based on enzymatic glucose oxidase reaction instead.

amphetamine
Dyanavel XR

amphetamine sulfate
Evekeo ODT

dextroamphetamine sulfate
Dexedrine ER, ProCentra, Zenzedi

Class and Category
Pharmacologic class: Phenethylamine
Therapeutic class: CNS stimulant
Controlled substance schedule: II

Indications and Dosages
∗ To treat attention deficit hyperactivity disorder (ADHD)

ORAL SOLUTION (PROCENTRA), TABLETS (ZENZEDI)

Children age 6 and over. *Initial:* 5 mg daily or twice daily. Increased by 5 mg daily at 1-wk intervals until desired response occurs. Rarely, dosage above 40 mg daily is needed.
Children ages 3 to 6. *Initial:* 2.5 mg daily. Increased by 2.5 mg daily at 1-wk intervals until desired response occurs.

ORAL DISINTEGRATING TABLETS (EVEKEO ODT)

Children age 6 and over. *Initial:* 5 mg once daily or twice daily. An additional dose given 4 to 6 hr later, if needed. Increased by 2.5 mg or 5 mg at 1-wk intervals until desired response occurs. Rarely, dosage above 40 mg daily is needed.
Children age 3 to 6. *Initial:* 2.5 mg once daily or twice daily. An additional dose given 4 to 6 hr later, if needed. Increased by 2.5 mg at 1-wk intervals until desired response occurs.

E.R. CAPSULES (DEXEDRINE ER)

Children age 6 and over. *Initial:* 5 mg daily or twice daily. Increased by 5 mg daily at 1-wk intervals until desired response occurs.

E.R. ORAL SUSPENSION (DYANAVEL XR), E.R. TABLETS (DYANAVEL XR)

Children age 6 and over. *Initial:* 2.5 or 5 mg once daily. Increased by 2.5 to 10 mg every 4 to 7 days. *Maximum:* 20 mg daily.

✶ *To treat narcolepsy*

E.R. CAPSULES (DEXEDRINE ER), ORAL SOLUTION (PROCENTRA), TABLETS (ZENZEDI)

Adults. 5 to 60 mg daily in divided doses, depending on response.
Children age 12 and over. *Initial:* 10 mg daily. Increased by 10 mg daily at 1-wk intervals until desired response occurs.
Children ages 6 to 12. *Initial:* 5 mg daily. Increased by 5 mg daily at 1-wk intervals until desired response occurs.

± **DOSAGE ADJUSTMENT** For patient with narcolepsy who develops adverse reactions such as anorexia or insomnia, dosage is reduced.

⊟ Drug Administration

P.O.

- Do not substitute one amphetamine product for another on a milligram-per-milligram basis, because of different amphetamine salt compositions and differing pharmacokinetic profiles. The exception is Dyanavel XR tablets and Dyanavel XR suspension, which may be used interchangeably.
- Administer first dose in the morning. Do not administer the last dose, if more than one daily dose is prescribed, late in evening because insomnia may occur.
- Each 5 ml of oral solution contains 5 mg of dexamphetamine.
- Use a calibrated measuring device for accurate dosing of oral suspension and shake bottle before measuring dose. Wash oral dosing syringe or measuring device after each use.
- Dyanavel XR tablets may be chewed or swallowed whole.
- Administer disintegrating tablets by first carefully removing tablets from package (avoid pushing tablets through the foil) with gloved hand. Tablet should be immediately placed on patient's tongue and allowed to dissolve without chewing or crushing.
- E.R. capsules should be swallowed whole.

Route	Onset	Peak	Duration
P.O.	20–90 min	1–2 hr	3–6 hr
P.O. (E.R.)	Unknown	4–5 hr	Unknown

Half-life: 9–12 hr

⊟ Mechanism of Action

May produce its CNS stimulant effects by facilitating release and blocking reuptake of norepinephrine at adrenergic nerve terminals and by direct stimulation of alpha and beta receptors in the peripheral nervous system. It also releases and blocks reuptake of dopamine in limbic regions of the brain. The drug's main action appears to be in the cerebral cortex and, possibly, the reticular activating system. These actions cause decreased motor restlessness, increased alertness, and diminished drowsiness and fatigue. Its peripheral actions include increased blood pressure and mild bronchodilation and respiratory stimulation.

⊟ Contraindications

Advanced arteriosclerosis, agitation (for narcolepsy treatment), glaucoma, history of drug abuse, hypersensitivity or idiosyncratic reaction to sympathomimetic amines, hyperthyroidism, MAO inhibitor therapy including I.V. methylene blue or linezolid within 14 days, moderate to severe hypertension, symptomatic cardiovascular disease

Interactions
DRUGS
acetazolamide, alkalinizers (such as sodium bicarbonate), some thiazides: Increased blood level and effects of amphetamine
adrenergic blockers: Inhibited adrenergic blockade
antihistamines: Possibly reduced sedation from antihistamine
antihypertensives: Possibly decreased antihypertensive effects
buspirone, CYP206 inhibitors, fentanyl, lithium, MAO inhibitors, selective serotonin reuptake inhibitors, serotonin norepinephrine reuptake inhibitors, St. John's wort, tramadol, tricyclic antidepressants, triptans: Increased risk of serotonin syndrome
chlorpromazine: Inhibited CNS stimulant effects of amphetamine
ethosuximide: Possibly delayed ethosuximide absorption
GI acidifiers (such as ascorbic acid), reserpine: Decreased amphetamine absorption
guanethidine: Decreased antihypertensive effect and decreased amphetamine absorption
haloperidol: Decreased CNS stimulation
lithium carbonate: Possibly decreased anorectic and stimulant effects of amphetamine
MAO inhibitors: Potentiated effects of amphetamine; possibly hypertensive crisis
meperidine: Increased analgesia
methenamine: Increased urine excretion and decreased effects of amphetamine
norepinephrine: Possibly increased adrenergic effect of norepinephrine
phenobarbital, phenytoin: Synergistic anticonvulsant action
propoxyphene: Increased CNS stimulation, potentially fatal seizures
proton pump inhibitors: Possibly decreased effectiveness of amphetamines
tricyclic antidepressants: Possibly enhanced antidepressant effects and decreased effects of amphetamine
urinary acidifiers (such as ammonium chloride and sodium acid phosphate): Increased amphetamine excretion and

decreased amphetamine blood level and effects
veratrum alkaloids: Decreased hypotensive effect

FOODS
acidic fruit juices: Decreased amphetamine absorption

Adverse Reactions
CNS: Aggression, anger, anxiety, depression, dizziness, dyskinesia, dysphoria, euphoria, exacerbation of motor and phonic tics and Tourette's syndrome, excessive talkativeness, hallucinations, headache, insomnia, irritability, overstimulation, paranoia, paresthesia, psychotic episodes, restlessness, **serotonin syndrome**, tremor
CV: Cardiomyopathy, hypertension, MI, palpitations, Raynaud's phenomenon, tachycardia
EENT: Blurred vision, dry mouth, mydriasis, teeth grinding, unpleasant taste
ENDO: Growth suppression in children and teens (long-term use)
GI: Anorexia, constipation, diarrhea
GU: Frequent or prolonged erections, impotence, libido changes
MS: Rhabdomyolysis
SKIN: Alopecia, excessive skin picking, rash, **Stevens–Johnson syndrome, toxic epidermal necrolysis**, urticaria
Other: Anaphylaxis, angioedema, weight loss

Childbearing Considerations
PREGNANCY
- Pregnancy exposure registry: 1-866-961-2388 or https://womensmentalhealth.org/clinical-and-research-programs/pregnancyregistry/othermedictions/.
- Drug may cause fetal harm because amphetamines cause vasoconstriction, which results in decreased placental perfusion.
- Use with caution only if benefit to mother outweighs potential risk to fetus.

LABOR & DELIVERY
- Know that infants born to mothers dependent on amphetamines have an increased risk of premature delivery and low birth weight because amphetamines can cause contractions.
- Monitor infants born to mothers dependent on amphetamines for withdrawal symptoms

such as agitation and significant lassitude as well as feeding difficulties and irritability in the postnatal period.

LACTATION
- Drug is present in breast milk.
- A decision should be made to discontinue breastfeeding or the drug to avoid potential adverse reactions in the breastfed infant.

⬛ Nursing Considerations
- Keep in mind that when symptoms of ADHD occur with acute stress reactions, treatment with amphetamines usually isn't indicated.

> ! **WARNING** Don't give amphetamine during or for up to 14 days after MAO therapy to prevent hypertensive crisis.

- Expect to decrease dosage if patient has bothersome adverse reactions, such as insomnia and anorexia. To minimize insomnia, administer drug earlier in day.
- Be alert for evidence of long-term amphetamine abuse, such as hyperactivity, irritability, marked insomnia, personality changes, and severe dermatoses. If patient suddenly stops drug after long-term, high-dose regimen, watch for extreme fatigue and depression.

> ! **WARNING** Monitor patient closely for evidence of serotonin syndrome, such as agitation, coma, diarrhea, hallucinations, hyperreflexia, hyperthermia, incoordination, labile blood pressure, nausea, tachycardia, and vomiting. Notify prescriber immediately because serotonin syndrome reactions may be life-threatening. Expect to discontinue amphetamine therapy and any other serotonergic agents patient may be taking. Be prepared to provide supportive care.

- Monitor children and teens receiving drug long term for growth suppression or not gaining weight.

PATIENT TEACHING
- Instruct breastfeeding patient to avoid breastfeeding during amphetamine therapy because drug is excreted in breast milk.
- Advise women of childbearing age to notify prescriber if pregnancy occurs.
- Teach patient to take first dose on awakening and subsequent doses as prescribed. Tell him not to take last dose late in evening because insomnia may occur.
- Inform patient or caregiver to use a calibrated measuring device for accurate dose.
- Instruct patient prescribed orally disintegrating tablets how to remove tablets from package and to avoid pushing tablets through the foil. Tablet should be immediately placed on the tongue and allowed to dissolve without chewing or crushing.
- Inform patient or caregiver that if Dyanavel XR tablets are prescribed, the tablets may be chewed or swallowed whole.
- Urge patient to avoid hazardous activities until drug's effects are known.
- Advise patient not to take amphetamine with acidic fruit juice because doing so decreases drug absorption.
- Explain drug's abuse potential, and caution against altering dosage unless prescribed.
- Instruct patient to notify prescriber before taking any new drugs, including over-the-counter preparations.
- Tell patient to report any new or worsening behavior and thought problems; new or worsening bipolar illness; new manic symptoms; or new psychotic symptoms such as believing things that are not true, feeling suspicious, or hearing voices.

amphotericin B

amphotericin B lipid complex
Abelcet

amphotericin B liposomal complex
AmBisome

⬛ Class and Category
Pharmacologic class: Amphoteric polyene
Therapeutic class: Antifungal

Indications and Dosages

* *To treat severe life-threatening fungal infections*

I.V. INFUSION (AMPHOTERICIN B)

Adults and adolescents. *Initial:* 1-mg test dose in 20 ml of D_5W infused over 20 to 30 min; if test dose is tolerated, then 0.25 to 0.3 mg/kg daily, given over 2 to 6 hr. Increased in 5- to 10-mg increments, based on patient tolerance and infection severity, to a final daily dose of 0.5 to 0.7 mg/kg but not to exceed a total daily dose of 1.5 mg/kg. *Usual range:* Up to 1 mg/kg daily or 1.5 mg/kg every other day.

* *To provide empirical therapy for presumed fungal infection in febrile, neutropenic patients*

I.V. INFUSION (AMBISOME)

Adults and children. 3 mg/kg daily.

* *To treat oral candidiasis*

ORAL SUSPENSION (AMPHOTERICIN B)

Adults and children. 1 ml (100 mg) four times daily for 14 days.

* *To treat invasive fungal infections in patients who are refractory to or intolerant of conventional amphotericin B therapy*

I.V. INFUSION (ABELCET)

Adults and children. 5 mg/kg daily.

* *To treat severe aspergillosis, candidiasis, or cryptococcosis refractory to amphotericin B deoxycholate or in patients whose renal impairment or unacceptable toxicity precludes the use of amphotericin B deoxycholate*

I.V. INFUSION (AMBISOME)

Adults and children. 3 to 5 mg/kg daily.

* *To treat visceral leishmaniasis*

I.V. INFUSION (AMBISOME)

Immunocompetent adults and children. 3 mg/kg daily on days 1 through 5 and on days 14 and 21. A repeat course of therapy given, as needed.

Immunocompromised adults and children. 4 mg/kg daily on days 1 through 5 and days 10, 17, 24, 31, and 38.

* *To treat cryptococcal meningitis in patients with HIV*

I.V. INFUSION (AMBISOME)

Adults and children. 6 mg/kg daily.

Drug Administration

P.O.

- Shake well before giving amphotericin B oral suspension.

- Drop suspension on tongue with calibrated dropper. Then tell patient to swish suspension in mouth for as long as possible before swallowing.
- If drug must be swabbed on, use a nonabsorbent swab.
- Give amphotericin B oral suspension between meals to permit prolonged contact with oral lesions.

I.V.

- Expect to give an antihistamine, antipyretic, or corticosteroid, if prescribed, just before infusing amphotericin B to help minimize fever and shaking chills.
- Each product of amphotericin B is not interchangeable on a milligram-per-milligram basis with other amphotericin B products.
- Avoid rapid infusion because arrhythmias, hypokalemia, hypotension, and shock may occur.
- *Incompatibilities for all products:* Other I.V. drugs, saline products

AMPHOTERICIN B

- Reconstitute drug by rapidly directing 10 ml Sterile Water for Injection without a bacteriostatic agent into the lyophilized cake, using a 20 G needle. Shake vial immediately until the colloidal solution is clear.
- Further dilute with 5% Dextrose Injection with a pH above 4.2 to yield a concentration of 0.1 mg/ml of amphotericin B. The pH of each container of Dextrose Injection should be ascertained before use. If the pH is below 4.2, then a buffer should be added before it is used to dilute the concentrated solution of amphotericin B following manufacturer guidelines.
- An in-line membrane filter may be used as long as it is not less than 1.0 micron to ensure passage of the antibiotic dispersion.
- Administer by slow infusion over 2 to 6 hours (depending on the dose).

AMPHOTERICIN B LIPOSOMAL COMPLEX

- An in-line membrane filter may be used if the mean pore diameter is more than 1 micron to prevent significant drug removal, because reconstituted amphotericin B liposomal complex is a colloidal suspension.
- To reconstitute, add 12 ml of Sterile Water for Injection to each drug vial to obtain a concentration of 4 mg/ml. Do

not reconstitute with saline or add saline to reconstituted concentration. The use of any solution other than Sterile Water for Injection, including Bacteriostatic Water, may cause precipitation of drug. Shake drug vial vigorously for 30 seconds to completely disperse the drug. It will form a yellow, translucent suspension.

- The reconstituted drug concentrate may be stored for up to 25 hours at 2–8°C (36–46°F). Do not freeze.
- Withdraw amount needed from drug vial. Attach the 5-micron filter provided to the syringe. Inject the syringe contents through the filter into the appropriate amount of 5% Dextrose Injection (use only one filter per drug vial) to obtain a final concentration of 1 to 2 mg/ml prior to administration. Lower concentrations (0.2 to 0.5 mg/ml) may be used for infants and small children to provide sufficient volume for infusion.
- Administer the diluted solution within 6 hours.
- Flush existing intravenous line with 5% Dextrose in Water before administering drug. If this is not possible, a separate intravenous line must be used.
- Infuse over 2 hours using a controlled infusion device. Time may be reduced to 1 hour in patients in whom drug is well tolerated, or the infusion time may be increased if patient experiences discomfort during infusion.

AMPHOTERICIN B LIPID COMPLEX

- Prepare amphotericin B lipid complex by shaking vial gently until no yellow sediment is seen. Using an 18G needle, withdraw prescribed dose from required number of vials into one or more 20-ml syringes. Replace needle with 5-micron filter needle supplied with each vial.
- Empty syringe contents into a bag of 5% Dextrose in Water so that final concentration is 1 mg/ml. Expect to use a concentration of 2 mg/ml for children and patients with cardiovascular disease. Before infusing, shake bag until contents are mixed thoroughly.
- Do not use an in-line filter.
- Flush an existing I.V. line with 5% Dextrose Injection before infusion or use a separate infusion line for drug administration. Infuse at 2.5 mg/kg/hr.

- If infusion exceeds 2 hours, shake infusion bag every 2 hours.
- The admixed drug in 5% Dextrose Injection may be stored for up to 48 hours at 2–8°C (36–46°F) and an additional 6 hours at room temperature. Do not freeze.

Route	Onset	Peak	Duration
I.V.	Immediate	Unknown	Unknown

Half-life: 24 hr–15 days

Mechanism of Action

Binds to sterols in fungal cell plasma membranes, which changes membrane permeability and allows loss of potassium and small molecules from cells. This action results in fungal cell impairment or death.

Contraindications

Hypersensitivity to amphotericin B or its components

Interactions

DRUGS

antineoplastics: Increased risk of bronchospasm, hypotension, and nephrotoxicity
corticosteroids, corticotropin: Increased risk of hypokalemia and cardiac dysfunction
cyclosporine, nephrotoxic drugs: Increased risk of nephrotoxicity
digitalis glycosides: Possibly hypokalemia and more severe digitalis toxicity
flucytosine: Possibly increased flucytosine toxicity
imidazoles such as clotrimazole, fluconazole, ketoconazole, miconazole: Possibly induced resistance to amphotericin
leukocyte transfusion: Possibly acute pulmonary toxicity
skeletal muscle relaxants: Possibly hypokalemia and increased muscle relaxation

Adverse Reactions

CNS: Fever, headache, shaking chills, tiredness, weakness
CV: Chest pain, **hypotension**, irregular heartbeat
EENT: Difficulty swallowing, pharyngitis
GI: Abdominal pain, anorexia, diarrhea, **hepatic failure**, indigestion, jaundice, nausea, vomiting

GU: Decreased or increased urine output, hemorrhagic cystitis, impaired renal function
HEME: Agranulocytosis, anemia, **leukopenia, thrombocytopenia, unusual bleeding** or bruising
MS: Arthralgia, muscle spasms, myalgia, **rhabdomyolysis**
RESP: Apnea, bronchospasm, cyanosis, dyspnea, **hypoventilation, hypoxia, pulmonary edema**, tachypnea
SKIN: Erythema, flushing, maculopapular rash, pruritus and redness especially around ears, urticaria
Other: Anaphylaxis, angioedema, hypocalcemia, hypokalemia, hypomagnesemia, infusion-site pain, thrombophlebitis

Childbearing Considerations
PREGNANCY
- It is not known if drug can cause fetal harm.
- Use with caution only if benefit to mother outweighs potential risk to fetus.

LACTATION
- It is not known if drug is present in breast milk.
- Breastfeeding should be discontinued during drug therapy.

Nursing Considerations
- Assess I.V. insertion site regularly to detect extravasation of amphotericin B, which may cause severe local irritation. To minimize local thrombophlebitis, plan to add heparin to infusion or expect to administer amphotericin on alternate days, which also may help prevent anorexia. Alternate-day dose shouldn't exceed 1.5 mg/kg.
- Monitor renal function because of the risk of renal impairment. Plan to obtain serum creatinine level every other day while amphotericin B dosage is increasing and then at least twice weekly during therapy. If serum creatinine or BUN level increases significantly, expect to stop amphotericin B until renal function improves. Know that a cumulative dose of more than 4 g may cause irreversible renal dysfunction.
- Expect to monitor CBC and platelet count weekly during therapy to detect adverse hematologic effects. Also monitor serum calcium, magnesium, and potassium levels twice weekly to detect abnormalities.

- Be aware that false elevations of serum phosphate may occur when samples are analyzed using the PHOSm assay.

PATIENT TEACHING
- Instruct patient to shake bottle of oral suspension well before each dose; to drop suspension directly on his tongue using calibrated dropper; and then to swish suspension in his mouth for as long as possible before swallowing. If prescriber orders drug to be swabbed onto oral lesions, tell patient to use nonabsorbent swab. Instruct him to take drug four times a day (between meals and at bedtime).
- Tell patient to notify prescriber if he develops local irritation, if existing symptoms worsen or return, or if new symptoms arise.

ampicillin

ampicillin sodium

ampicillin trihydrate

Class and Category
Pharmacologic class: Aminopenicillin
Therapeutic class: Antibiotic

Indications and Dosages
✳ *To treat GI infections and genitourinary infections (other than gonorrhea) caused by susceptible strains of* Shigella, Salmonella typhi *and other species,* Escherichia coli, Proteus mirabilis, *and enterococci*

CAPSULES, ORAL SUSPENSION
Adults and children weighing more than 20 kg (44 lb). 500 mg every 6 hr.
Children weighing 20 kg (44 lb) or less. 100 mg/kg daily in divided doses every 6 hr.

I.M. INJECTION, I.V. INFUSION, I.V. INJECTION
Adults and children weighing 40 kg (88 lb) or more. 500 mg every 6 hr.
Children weighing less than 40 kg. 50 mg/kg daily in divided doses every 6 to 8 hr.
✳ *To treat uncomplicated gonorrhea caused by susceptible strains of non–penicillinase-producing* Neisseria gonorrhoeae

CAPSULES, ORAL SUSPENSION

Adults and children weighing more than 20 kg (44 lb). 3.5 g as a single dose with 1 g of probenecid.

✴ *To treat respiratory tract infections caused by susceptible strains of non–penicillinase-producing* Haemophilus influenzae, *staphylococci, and streptococci, including* Streptococcus pneumoniae; *to treat soft-tissue infections caused by susceptible strains of staphylococci and streptococci organisms*

CAPSULES, ORAL SUSPENSION

Adults and children weighing more than 20 kg (44 lb). 250 mg every 6 hr.

Children weighing 20 kg (44 lb) or less. 50 mg/kg daily in divided doses every 6 to 8 hr.

I.M. INJECTION, I.V. INFUSION, I.V. INJECTION

Adults and children weighing 40 kg (88 lb) or more. 250 to 500 mg every 6 hr.

Children weighing less than 40 kg. 25 to 50 mg/kg daily in divided doses every 6 to 8 hr.

✴ *To treat septicemia; to treat bacterial meningitis caused by susceptible strains of* Neisseria meningitidis

I.M. INJECTION, I.V. INFUSION, I.V. INJECTION

Adults and children. 150 to 200 mg/kg daily in divided doses every 3 to 4 hr. Dosage may initially be administered I.V. for at least 3 days and then continued I.M.

Neonates greater than 34 weeks gestation and less than or equal to 28 days postnatal. 15 mg/kg daily in divided doses every 8 hr.

Neonates less than or equal to 34 weeks gestation but greater than or equal to 8 days but less than 28 days postnatal. 150 mg/kg daily in divided doses every 12 hr.

Neonates less than or equal to 34 weeks gestation but less than or equal to 7 days postnatal. 100 mg/kg daily in divided doses every 12 hr.

✴ *To treat urethritis in males due to* N. gonorrhoeae

I.M. INJECTION, I.V. INFUSION, I.V. INJECTION

Adult men. Two doses of 500 mg at 8- or 12-hr intervals. May repeat or extend treatment, if needed.

⦚ Drug Administration

P.O.

▪ Give with 8 ounces of water 30 minutes before or 2 hours after meals.

▪ Shake suspension well before each use and keep bottle tightly closed between uses. Use a calibrated device to measure dosage. Discard unused portion after 14 days if refrigerated or 7 days if stored at room temperature.

I.V.

▪ For direct I.V. administration, reconstitute by adding 5 ml of Sterile Water for Injection or Bacteriostatic Water for Injection to 250- or 500-mg vial and administer slowly over 3 to 5 minutes or dilute with 7.4 ml to 1-g vial or 14.8 ml to 2-g vial and administer over 10 to 15 minutes. Do not exceed 100 mg/min. More rapid administration may cause seizures.

▪ Do not reconstitute using Bacteriostatic Water for Injection if giving drug to newborns.

▪ For intermittent infusion, reconstitute solution as outlined above and then dilute with 50 to 100 ml of intravenous solution such as 0.9% Sodium Chloride Injection or Lactated Ringer's Injection (see manufacturer list for other suitable solutions). Maximum concentration should not exceed 30 mg/ml. Infuse over 15 to 30 minutes. Administer within 1 hour after preparation because potency may decrease significantly after this period.

▪ *Incompatibilities:* None listed by manufacturer

I.M.

▪ Reconstitute by adding 1 ml of Sterile Water for Injection or Bacteriostatic Water for Injection to each 250-mg vial, 1.8 ml of diluent to each 500-mg vial, 3.5 ml of diluent to each 1-g vial, or 6.8 ml of diluent to each 2-g vial.

▪ Do not use Bacteriostatic Water for Injection when drug will be given to newborns.

▪ Use within 1 hour after preparation because potency may decrease significantly after this period.

Route	Onset	Peak	Duration
P.O.	Unknown	1–2 hr	6–8 hr
I.V.	Immediate	Unknown	Unknown
I.M.	Unknown	1 hr	Unknown

Half-life: 1–1.8 hr

Mechanism of Action

Inhibits bacterial cell wall synthesis. The rigid, cross-linked cell wall is assembled in several steps. Ampicillin exerts its effects on susceptible bacteria in the final stage of the cross-linking process by binding with and inactivating penicillin-binding proteins (enzymes responsible for linking the cell wall strands). This action causes bacterial cell lysis and death.

Contraindications

Hypersensitivity to ampicillin, other penicillins, or their components; infection caused by penicillinase-producing organism

Interactions

DRUGS

allopurinol: Increased risk of rash, particularly in hyperuricemic patient
aminoglycosides: Possibly inactivated action
bacteriostatic antibiotics such as chloramphenicol, erythromycins, sulfonamides, tetracyclines: Possibly impaired action of ampicillin
live-virus vaccines such as BCG (intravesical) and typhoid: May decrease effectiveness of vaccine
oral anticoagulants: Increased risk of bleeding
oral contraceptives: Possibly reduced contraceptive effectiveness and breakthrough bleeding

Adverse Reactions

CNS: Chills, fatigue, fever, headache, malaise
CV: Chest pain, edema, thrombophlebitis
EENT: Epistaxis, glossitis, **laryngeal stridor**, mucocutaneous candidiasis, stomatitis, **throat tightness**
GI: Abdominal distention, *Clostridium difficile*-**associated diarrhea**, diarrhea, enterocolitis, flatulence, gastritis, nausea, **pseudomembranous colitis**, vomiting
GU: Dysuria, urine retention, vaginal candidiasis
HEME: **Agranulocytosis**, anemia, eosinophilia, **leukopenia**, **thrombocytopenia, thrombocytopenic purpura**
SKIN: **Erythema multiforme**; erythematous, mildly pruritic maculopapular rash or other types of rash; **exfoliative dermatitis**; pruritus; urticaria
Other: **Anaphylaxis, angioedema**, injection-site pain

Childbearing Considerations

PREGNANCY

- It is not known if drug can cause fetal harm.
- Use with caution only if benefit to mother outweighs potential risk to fetus.

LABOR & DELIVERY

- Oral drug is poorly absorbed during labor.
- It is not known if drug has any immediate or delayed adverse effects on the fetus, prolongs the duration of labor, or increases the likelihood that forceps delivery or other obstetrical intervention or resuscitation of the newborn will be needed.

LACTATION

- Drug is present in breast milk.
- Patient should check with prescriber before breastfeeding.

Nursing Considerations

- Avoid giving ampicillin to patients with mononucleosis because of increased risk of rash.
- Expect to give ampicillin for 48 to 72 hours after patient becomes asymptomatic. For streptococcal infection, expect to give ampicillin for at least 10 days after cultures show streptococcal eradication to reduce risk of rheumatic fever or glomerulonephritis.
- Monitor patient closely for anaphylaxis, which may be life-threatening. Patients at greatest risk are those with a history of multiple allergies, hypersensitivity to cephalosporins, or a history of asthma, hay fever, or urticaria.

! **WARNING** Stop drug in an anaphylactic reaction, notify prescriber immediately, and provide immediate treatment with epinephrine, airway management, oxygen, and I.V. corticosteroids, as needed.

- Notify prescriber if patient has evidence of superinfection; expect to stop drug and provide appropriate treatment.
- Closely monitor results of renal and liver function tests and CBCs if long-term or high-dose ampicillin therapy is required.
- Monitor patient closely for diarrhea, which may be pseudomembranous colitis caused by *Clostridium difficile*. If diarrhea occurs, notify prescriber and expect to withhold ampicillin and administer fluids,

electrolytes, protein, and an antibiotic effective against *C. difficile*.

PATIENT TEACHING

- Emphasize the importance of taking the full course of ampicillin exactly as prescribed.
- Tell patient to take oral dose with 8 ounces of water 30 minutes before or 2 hours after meals.
- Instruct patient to shake suspension well before each use, keep bottle tightly closed between uses, and discard unused portion after 14 days if refrigerated or 7 days if stored at room temperature.
- Review signs of allergic reaction; if they occur, tell patient to hold next ampicillin dose and contact prescriber immediately.
- Urge patient to tell prescriber about diarrhea that's severe or lasts longer than 3 days. Remind patient that watery or bloody stools may occur 2 or more months after antibiotic therapy and may be serious, requiring prompt treatment.

angiotensin II
Giapreza

Class and Category
Pharmacologic class: Peptide hormone of the renin–angiotensin–aldosterone system
Therapeutic class: Antihypertensive

Indications and Dosages
＊ *To increase blood pressure in patients with septic or other distributive shock*

I.V. INFUSION

Adults. *Initial:* 20 ng/kg/min continuously then increased in increments of up to 15 ng/kg/min every 5 minutes, as needed, to achieve or maintain target blood pressure. When no longer needed, dosage decreased in increments of up to 15 ng/kg/min every 5 to 15 minutes, with adjustments made based upon blood pressure. *Maximum:* For first 3 hr, dosage should not exceed 80 ng/kg/min; maintenance dosage should not exceed 40 ng/kg/min.

±**DOSAGE ADJUSTMENT** Dosage may be decreased to as low as 1.25 ng/kg/min in patients sensitive to angiotensin II effects.

Drug Administration
I.V.

- Dilute drug in 0.9% Sodium Chloride solution prior to use to achieve a final concentration of 5,000 ng/ml or 10,000 ng/ml.
- To prepare a 5,000 ng/ml solution, use 2.5 mg/ml vial and withdraw 1 ml from vial. Add to 500-ml infusion bag of 0.9% Sodium Chloride. To prepare a 10,000 ng/ml solution, use 2.5 mg/ml vial and withdraw 1 ml from vial. Add to a 250-ml infusion bag of 0.9% Sodium Chloride.
- Administer as a continuous infusion and preferably through a central venous line. Adjust dosage every 5 minutes as needed.
- Know that diluted solution may be stored at room temperature or in refrigerator. Discard unused prepared solution after 24 hours regardless of how it was stored.
- *Incompatibilities:* None listed by manufacturer

Route	Onset	Peak	Duration
I.V.	Within 1 min	5 min	Unknown

Half-life: > 1 min.

Mechanism of Action
Binds to the G-protein-coupled angiotensin II receptor type I on vascular smooth muscle cells, which stimulates myosin and causes smooth muscle contraction. These actions raise blood pressure by increasing aldosterone release and causing vasoconstriction.

Contraindications
Hypersensitivity to angiotensin II components

Interactions
DRUGS

angiotensin-converting enzyme (ACE) inhibitors: Possibly increased response to angiotensin II
angiotensin II receptor blockers (ARBs): Possibly decreased response to angiotensin II

Adverse Reactions
CNS: Delirium
CV: Arterial and venous thrombotic events, deep vein thrombosis, peripheral ischemia, tachycardia
ENDO: Hyperglycemia
HEME: Thrombocytopenia
Other: Acidosis, fungal infection

Childbearing Considerations
PREGNANCY

- It is not known if drug can cause fetal harm.
- Use with caution only if benefit to mother outweighs potential risk to fetus.

LACTATION

- It is not known if drug is present in breast milk.
- Patient should check with prescriber before breastfeeding, once condition has stabilized.

Nursing Considerations

- Take blood pressure every 5 minutes for the first 3 hours and monitor blood pressure every 5 to 15 minutes thereafter, as needed.
- Monitor patient closely for thrombotic events. Take precautions to prevent these events, especially deep venous thromboses.

PATIENT TEACHING

- Instruct patient on angiotensin II use, if patient's condition allows for understanding.
- Tell patient to report any abnormal symptoms, if patient is able to understand.

anidulafungin

Eraxis

Class and Category

Pharmacologic class: Echinocandin
Therapeutic class: Antifungal

Indications and Dosages

✳ *To treat Candidemia and other forms of* Candida *infections (intra-abdominal abscess and peritonitis)*

I.V. INFUSION

Adults. *Initial:* 200 mg on day 1 followed by 100 mg once daily and continued for at least 14 days following last positive culture.
Children and infants 1 month of age and over. *Initial:* 3 mg/kg (not to exceed 200 mg) loading dose on day 1, followed by 1.5 mg/kg (not to exceed 100 mg) once daily thereafter and continued for at least 14 days after the last positive culture.

✳ *To treat esophageal candidiasis*

I.V. INFUSION

Adults. 100 mg on day 1, followed by 50 mg once daily for a minimum of 14 days and continued for at least 7 days following resolution of symptoms.

Drug Administration

I.V.

- Reconstitute each 50-mg vial with 15 ml of Sterile Water for Injection and each 100-mg vial with 30 ml of Sterile Water for Injection to provide a concentration of 3.33 mg/ml.
- Transfer the contents of the reconstituted vial(s) into the appropriately sized I.V. bag or bottle containing either 5% Dextrose Injection or 0.9% Sodium Chloride Injection as follows: 50 ml of infusion volume for 50-mg dose for total volume of 65 ml; 100-ml infusion volume for 100-mg dose for a total volume of 130 ml; and 200-ml infusion volume for 200-mg dose for a total volume of 260 ml.
- If total infusion volume is 65 ml, infuse at least over 45 minutes; if total infusion volume is 130 ml, infuse over at least 90 minutes; if total infusion volume is 260 ml, infuse over at least 180 minutes.
- Infusion rate should not exceed 1.1 mg/min (equivalent to 1.4 ml/min or 84 ml/hour) when reconstituted and diluted.
- Administer with a programmable infusion pump.
- The reconstituted solution can be stored for up to 24 hours and the infusion solution for up to 48 hours if kept at 25°C (77°F).
- Follow adult preparation for children with prescribed doses above 50 mg.

Children with prescribed doses below 50 mg

- Calculate the dose and reconstitute vials according to manufacturer instructions to provide a concentration of 3.33 mg/ml.
- Calculate the volume (ml) of reconstituted drug required as follows: Volume of reconstituted drug (ml) = Dose in mg divided by 3.33 ml.
- Then calculate the total volume of the infusion solution (ml) that contains a final concentration of 0.77 mg/ml as follows: Total volume of infusion solution (ml) = drug dose (mg) divided by 0.77 mg/ml
- Calculate the volume of diluent (5% Dextrose in Water or 0.9% Sodium Chloride) required to prepare the infusion solution as follows: Volume of diluent (ml) = Total volume of final infusion solution (ml) − Volume of reconstituted drug (ml).
- Prepare the infusion solution by transferring the required volumes (ml) of the reconstituted drug and diluent into an infusion syringe or I.V. infusion bag for administration.
- Infusion rate should not exceed 1.1 mg/min (equivalent to 1.4 ml/min or 84 ml/min) when reconstituted and diluted.

- Administer with a programmable syringe or infusion pump.
- *Incompatibilities:* Other intravenous additives, medications, or other solutions other than 5% Dextrose Injection and 0.9% Sodium Chloride Injection

Route	Onset	Peak	Duration
I.V.	Unknown	Unknown	Unknown

Half-life: 40–50 hr

Mechanism of Action

Inhibits glucan synthase, an enzyme present in fungal cells. This results in inhibition of the formation of an essential D-glucan component of the fungal cell wall, thereby eliminating the fungal infection.

Contraindications

Hypersensitivity to anidulafungin, other echinocandins or their components; presence of hereditary fructose intolerance

Interactions

None reported

Adverse Reactions

CNS: Confusion, depression, dizziness, fever, headache, insomnia, rigors, **seizures**
CV: Atrial fibrillation, chest pain, **deep vein thrombosis**, hypertension, **hypotension**, peripheral edema, **QT prolongation**, right bundle branch block, sinus arrhythmia, superficial thrombophlebitis, **ventricular extrasystoles**
EENT: Blurred vision, epistaxis, eye pain, oral candidiasis, visual disturbance
ENDO: Hot flashes, hyperglycemia, **hypoglycemia**
GI: Abdominal pain, cholestasis, constipation, diarrhea, dyspepsia, elevated liver enzymes, **hepatic failure or necrosis, hepatitis**, nausea, vomiting
GU: Elevated blood creatinine levels, UTI
HEME: Anemia, **leukocytosis, prolonged prothrombin time, thrombocytopenia**
MS: Back pain
RESP: Bronchospasm, cough, dyspnea, pleural effusion, pneumonia, **respiratory distress**
SKIN: Diaphoresis, erythema, flushing, pruritus, rash, ulceration, urticaria
Other: Anaphylaxis, angioedema, bacteremia, clostridial infection, dehydration, **hyperkalemia, hypokalemia,**

hypomagnesemia, infusion-related reactions, **multiorgan failure, sepsis**, systemic *Candida* infection in the arm used for infusion

Childbearing Considerations

PREGNANCY

- It is not known if drug can cause fetal harm although animal studies suggest it may.
- Use with caution only if benefit to mother outweighs potential risk to fetus.

LACTATION

- It is not known if drug is present in breast milk.
- Patient should check with prescriber before breastfeeding.

Nursing Considerations

! WARNING Know that patients with hereditary fructose intolerance should not receive anidulafungin because it contains fructose and may precipitate a life-threatening metabolic crisis if patient is exposed.

- Monitor patient's liver function and enzyme levels closely during anidulafungin therapy because significant hepatic dysfunction, hepatitis, or hepatic failure have been reported, although a causal relationship has not been established. If patient begins to complain of fatigue and shows signs of jaundice or his liver enzymes become abnormal, notify prescriber, as drug may be discontinued.

! WARNING Monitor patient closely for hypersensitivity reactions that could lead to anaphylactic reactions, including shock. If present, withhold drug, notify prescriber, and be prepared to provide emergency treatment.

PATIENT TEACHING

- Instruct patient to promptly report any hypersensitivity reaction such as flushing, hives, itching, rash, difficulty breathing, or dizziness.
- Advise patient to comply with blood tests that may be ordered to monitor reaction to anidulafungin.
- Review signs and symptoms of liver dysfunction and advise patient to notify prescriber if present.
- Tell women of childbearing age that anidulafungin may cause fetal harm. If pregnancy is suspected or confirmed, or patient is planning to breastfeed, advise patient to alert prescriber.

antihemophilic factor (recombinant) PEGylated-aucl

Jivi

Class and Category

Pharmacologic class: Coagulation Factor VIII
Therapeutic class: Coagulant

Indications and Dosages

❋ *To treat on-demand and control of bleeding episodes in previously treated patients with hemophilia A*

I.V. INFUSION

Adults and adolescents. *For minor bleeding:* 10 to 20 international units/kg and repeated every 24 to 48 hr until bleeding resolved. *For moderate bleeding:* 15 to 30 international units/kg and repeated every 24 to 48 hr until bleeding resolved. *For major bleeding:* 30 to 50 international units/kg and repeated every 8 to 24 hr until bleeding is resolved.

❋ *To manage perioperative bleeding in previously treated patients with hemophilia A*

I.V. INFUSION

Adults and adolescents. *For minor surgery:* 15 to 30 international units/kg and repeated every 24 hr for at least 1 day and until healing is achieved. *For major surgery:* 40 to 50 international units/kg and repeated every 12 to 24 hr until adequate wound healing is complete, then therapy continued for at least another 7 days to maintain Factor VIII activity of 30% to 60%.

❋ *To reduce frequency of bleeding episodes in previously treated patients with hemophilia A*

I.V. INFUSION

Adults and adolescents. *Initial:* 30 to 40 international units/kg twice weekly with regimen adjusted to 45 to 60 international units/kg every 5 days based on bleeding episodes. Dosing then adjusted to less or more frequent dosing as needed.

Drug Administration

I.V.

- Calculation of the required dose of Factor VIII is based on one international unit of Factor VIII/kilogram ability to increase the plasma Factor VIII level by 2 international units/dl.

- Prepare antihemophilic factor (recombinant) PEGylated-aucl by first warming both the unopened vial and prefilled diluent syringe in your hands to a comfortable temperature (not to exceed 37°C [99°F]).

- Remove the protective cap from vial and cleanse the rubber stopper with a sterile alcohol swab, being careful not to touch the rubber stopper.

- Place vial on a firm, nonskid surface.

- Peel off the paper cover on the vial adapter plastic housing. Do not remove the adapter from the plastic housing. Holding the adapter housing, place it over the product vial and firmly press down. The adapter will snap over the vial cap. Do not remove the adapter housing at this step. Holding the syringe by the barrel, snap the syringe cap off the tip. Do not touch the syringe tip with your hand or any surface. Set the syringe aside.

- Remove and discard the adapter plastic housing. Attach the prefilled syringe to the vial adapter thread by turning clockwise. Remove the clear plastic plunger rod from the carton. Grasp the plunger rod by the top plate. Avoid touching the sides and threads of the plunger rod. Attach the plunger rod by turning it clockwise into the threaded rubber stopper of the prefilled syringe.

- Inject the diluent slowly by pushing down on the plunger rod. Swirl vial gently until all powder on all sides of the vial is dissolved. Do not shake vial. Be sure that all powder is completely dissolved. Do not use if solution contains visible particles or is cloudy.

- Push down on the plunger to push all air back into the vial. Then, while holding the plunger down, turn the vial with syringe upside down (inverted) so the vial is now above the syringe.

- Know that if the dose requires more than one vial, each vial must be reconstituted as described above with the diluent syringe provided. Use a larger plastic syringe (not supplied) to combine the contents of the vials into one syringe.

- Filter the reconstituted product to remove potential particulate matter in the solution. Filtering is achieved by using the vial adapter. Withdraw all the solution through the vial adapter into the syringe by pulling the plunger rod back slowly and smoothly. Tilt the vial to the side and back to make sure all the solution has been drawn toward the large opening in the rubber stopper and into the syringe. Remove as much air as possible before removing the syringe from the vial by slowly and carefully pushing the air back into the vial.

- Detach the syringe with the plunger rod from the vial adapter by turning counterclockwise. Attach the syringe to the infusion set provided.
- Administer the reconstituted drug as soon as possible after preparation. If unable to do so, store at room temperature for no longer than 3 hours.
- Infuse intravenously over 1 to 15 minutes, adapting the rate of administration to patient's response. Do not exceed the maximum infusion rate of 2.5 ml/min.
- *Incompatibilities:* None listed by manufacturer

Route	Onset	Peak	Duration
I.V.	Unknown	Unknown	Unknown

Half-life: 17.9 hr

Mechanism of Action

Temporarily replaces the missing coagulation Factor VIII.

Contraindications

Hypersensitivity to antihemophilic factor (recombinant) PEGylated-aucl or to hamster or mouse proteins, polyethylene glycol, or their components

Interactions

DRUGS

None reported

Adverse Reactions

CNS: Dizziness, fever, headache, insomnia
CV: Chest tightness, hypotension (mild)
EENT: Distorted sense of taste, **throat tightness**
GI: Abdominal pain, nausea, vomiting
RESP: Cough
SKIN: Erythema, **erythema multiforme,** flushing, pruritus, rash
Other: Anaphylaxis, anti-PEG antibody formation, injection-site reactions (pruritus, rash), neutralizing antibodies

Childbearing Considerations

PREGNANCY

- It is not known if drug can cause fetal harm.
- Use with caution only if benefit to mother outweighs potential risk to fetus.

LACTATION

- It is not known if drug is present in breast milk.
- Patient should check with prescriber before breastfeeding.

Nursing Considerations

- Know that dosage and duration of treatment depend on the severity of the Factor VIII deficiency, the location and extent of bleeding, and the patient's clinical condition.
- Be aware that potency assignment for the drug is determined using a chromogenic substrate assay.
- Monitor the Factor VIII activity of the drug in plasma, as ordered, knowing that the activity will be assessed using either a validated chromogenic substrate assay or a validated one-stage clotting assay.
- Monitor patient for hypersensitivity reactions that could progress to anaphylaxis. If any signs or symptoms of an allergic reaction occur, immediately discontinue administration of the drug, notify prescriber, and initiate treatment according to institutional protocol.
- Be aware that neutralizing antibodies may form following the administration of antihemophilic factor (recombinant) PEGylated-aucl. If plasma Factor VIII activity levels are not attained or if bleeding is not controlled as expected with the administered dose, suspect the presence of a neutralizing antibody and notify prescriber. Expect testing for Factor VIII inhibitors and Factor VIII recovery. A low postinfusion Factor VIII level in the absence of detectable Factor VIII inhibitors indicates that the loss of drug effect is likely due to anti-PEG antibodies. In this situation, expect drug to be discontinued and know that patient will need to be switched to a previously effective Factor VIII product.

PATIENT TEACHING

- Instruct patient to report early signs of an allergic reaction such as dizziness, nausea, and tightness of his chest or throat during or after the infusion. If patient is home, stress importance of seeking immediate emergency attention, as the reaction can progress to a life-threatening situation.

- Tell patient to notify prescriber or treatment center if he experiences a lack of response to the drug.
- Advise patient to consult his prescriber prior to traveling.

apixaban
Eliquis

Class and Category
Pharmacologic class: Factor Xa inhibitor
Therapeutic class: Anticoagulant

Indications and Dosages
✻ *To reduce the risk of stroke and systemic embolism in patients with nonvalvular atrial fibrillation*

TABLETS
Adults. 5 mg twice daily.

±**DOSAGE ADJUSTMENT** For patients with at least two of the following characteristics: 80 years or older, body weight of 60 kg (132 lb) or less, or a serum creatinine of 1.5 mg/dl or greater; dosage decreased to 2.5 mg twice daily.

✻ *To prevent deep vein thrombosis following hip or knee replacement surgery*

TABLETS
Adults. 2.5 mg twice daily beginning 12 to 24 hours after surgery and lasting 12 days for knee replacement and 35 days for hip replacement.

✻ *To treat deep vein thrombosis and pulmonary embolism*

TABLETS
Adults. 10 mg twice daily for 7 days followed by 5 mg twice daily.

✻ *To reduce risk of recurrence of deep vein thrombosis and pulmonary embolism*

TABLETS
Adults. 2.5 mg twice daily following 6 months of treatment for deep vein thrombosis or pulmonary embolism.

±**DOSAGE ADJUSTMENT** For patients receiving 5-mg or 10-mg dosage twice daily, dosage reduced by 50% if patient also receiving combined strong dual inhibitors

of cytochrome P450 3A4 (CYP3A4) and P-glycoprotein (P-gp) such as itraconazole, ketoconazole, or ritonavir. For patients receiving 2.5-mg dosage twice daily, coadministration with combined strong CYP3A4 and P-gp inhibitors are avoided.

Drug Administration
P.O.
- Crush tablet and mix with apple juice or water or put in applesauce and administer immediately for patient unable to swallow whole tablets.
- For patient with a nasogastric tube, crush tablet and suspend in 60 ml of 5% Dextrose in Water or plain water and immediately administer through the nasogastric tube.
- Be aware that crushed tablets are stable in apple juice, 5% Dextrose in Water, plain water, or applesauce for up to 4 hours.

Route	Onset	Peak	Duration
P.O.	Rapid	3–4 hr	Unknown

Half-life: 12 hr

Mechanism of Action
Inhibits free and clot-bound factor Xa and prothrombinase activity. Although apixaban has no direct effect on platelet aggregation, it does indirectly inhibit platelet aggregation induced by thrombin. By inhibiting factor Xa, apixaban decreases thrombin generation and thrombus development.

Contraindications
Active pathological bleeding, severe hypersensitivity to apixaban or its components

Interactions
DRUGS
antiplatelets, aspirin, fibrinolytics, heparin NSAIDs (chronic use): Increased risk of bleeding
strong dual inducers of CYP3A4 and P-gp such as carbamazepine, phenytoin, rifampin, St. John's wort: Decreased effectiveness of apixaban
strong dual inhibitors of CYP3A4 and P-gp such as itraconazole, ketoconazole, ritonavir: Increased effects of apixaban

Adverse Reactions
CNS: Hemorrhagic stroke, syncope
CV: Hypotension

EENT: Epistaxis, gingival bleeding, ocular hemorrhage

GI: Elevated bilirubin and liver enzymes, GI bleeding or hemorrhage, fresh bleeding from rectum, hematemesis, melena, rectal hemorrhage

GU: Hematuria, vaginal hemorrhage

HEME: Excessive bleeding, including hemorrhage, hemorrhagic anemia, thrombocytopenia

SKIN: Ecchymosis, petechiae, rash

MS: Muscle hemorrhage

RESP: Hemoptysis

Other: Anaphylaxis, angioedema, elevated alkaline phosphatase, hematomas at injection sites

Childbearing Considerations
PREGNANCY
- It is not known if drug can cause fetal harm but there is the potential for hemorrhage.
- Drug use is not recommended during pregnancy unless no other alternative is available.

LABOR & DELIVERY
- Use with caution only if absolutely necessary and no other alternative is available because there is a potential for hemorrhage. A shorter acting anticoagulant should be considered as delivery approaches.

LACTATION
- It is not known if drug is present in breast milk.
- A decision should be made to discontinue breastfeeding or the drug to avoid potential adverse reactions in the breastfed infant.

REPRODUCTION
- Drug may cause significant abnormal uterine bleeding, possibly requiring surgical intervention. If female patient is of reproductive age, plans for a pregnancy should be made known to the prescriber.

Nursing Considerations
- Know that apixaban should not be given to patients with severe hepatic dysfunction. Drug should also not be given to patient with triple positive antiphospholipid syndrome because drug therapy has been associated with increased rates of recurrent thrombotic events.
- Expect apixaban to be discontinued 48 hours before an invasive procedure or surgery if patient has a moderate or high risk of hemorrhage and 24 hours before an invasive procedure or surgery if patient has a mild risk of hemorrhage.
- Be aware that manufacturer guidelines should be followed when patient is switching from or to other anticoagulants. For example, when patient is switching from warfarin to apixaban therapy, expect warfarin to be discontinued and apixaban started when the international normalized ratio (INR) is below 2. When switching from apixaban to warfarin, expect apixaban to be discontinued and both a parenteral anticoagulant and warfarin given at the time the next dose of apixaban would have been given. Then the parenteral anticoagulant is discontinued when INR reaches an acceptable range. When switching between apixaban and anticoagulants other than warfarin, expect to discontinue the one being taken and begin the other at the next scheduled dose.
- Be aware that if apixaban is discontinued prematurely and adequate alternative anticoagulation is not present, the risk of thrombosis increases.

! **WARNING** Monitor patient closely for bleeding, as apixaban may cause life-threatening bleeding. Expect drug to be discontinued with active pathological hemorrhage and expect to give the antidote, coagulation factor Xa (recombinant), inactivated-zhzo (Andexxa) to reverse effects of anticoagulation. Know that effects of apixaban may persist for at least 24 hours after the last dose, but that activated oral charcoal can reduce the absorption of apixaban, thereby lowering apixaban plasma concentration if given close to last dose of apixaban.

PATIENT TEACHING
- Emphasize the importance of taking apixaban exactly as prescribed.
- Tell patient unable to swallow whole tablets to crush tablet and mix with apple juice or water or mix with applesauce and take immediately.
- Tell patient not to stop taking apixaban without first consulting prescriber. If patient misses a dose, instruct him to take it as soon as possible on the same day and resume

the dosing schedule the next day. Caution patient not to double dose to make up for the missed dose the day before.

- Advise patient to report any unusual bleeding or bruising to the prescriber. Inform patient that it may take longer for her to stop bleeding and to take bleeding precautions, such as avoiding the use of a razor and using a soft-bristle toothbrush.
- Tell patient to alert all prescribers to use of apixaban therapy before any invasive procedure, including dental work, is scheduled.
- Tell women of childbearing age to discuss plans for a possible pregnancy with prescriber. Advise female patient to notify prescriber immediately if pregnancy is suspected or known.

apremilast
Otezla

☰ Class and Category
Pharmacologic class: Phosphodiesterase 4 inhibitor
Therapeutic class: Antirheumatic

☰ Indications and Dosages
✴ *To treat active psoriatic arthritis; to treat moderate to severe plaque psoriasis in patients who are candidates for phototherapy or systemic therapy; to treat oral ulcers associated with Behçet's Disease.*

TABLETS
Adults. *Initial:* 10 mg in a.m. on day 1; 10 mg in a.m. and p.m. on day 2; 10 mg in a.m. and 20 mg in p.m. on day 3; 20 mg in a.m. and p.m. on day 4; 20 mg in a.m. and 30 mg in p.m. on day 5; and 30 mg in a.m. and p.m. on day 6 and thereafter. *Maintenance:* 30 mg in a.m. and p.m.

±**DOSAGE ADJUSTMENT** For patients with severe renal impairment (creatinine clearance less than 30 ml/min), dosage titration decreased to once daily using only the a.m. titration schedule and maintenance dosage kept at 30 mg once daily in a.m.

☰ Drug Administration
P.O.
- Do not have patient chew tablets and do not crush or split tablets. Tablets should be swallowed whole.

Route	Onset	Peak	Duration
P.O.	Unknown	2.5 hr	Unknown

Half-life: 6–9 hr

☰ Mechanism of Action
Inhibits phosphodiesterase 4, which is specific for cyclic adenosine monophosphate (cAMP). This action results in increased intracellular cAMP levels, which are thought to help relieve symptoms of psoriatic arthritis.

☰ Contraindications
Hypersensitivity to apremilast or its components

☰ Interactions
DRUGS
strong CYP450 inducers such as rifampin: Decreased apremilast exposure with loss of effectiveness

☰ Adverse Reactions
CNS: Depression, fatigue, headache, insomnia, migraine, **suicidal ideation**
EENT: Nasopharyngitis
GI: Anorexia, diarrhea, dyspepsia, gastroesophageal reflux disease, nausea, upper abdominal pain, vomiting
MS: Arthralgia, back pain
RESP: Bronchitis, cough, upper respiratory infection
SKIN: Infected hair follicles, rash
Other: **Anaphylaxis, angioedema,** weight loss

☰ Childbearing Considerations
PREGNANCY
- Pregnancy exposure registry: 1-877-311-8972 or https://mothertobaby.org/ongoing-study/otezla/.
- It is not known if drug can cause fetal harm although some studies suggest an increased risk for fetal loss.
- Use with caution only if benefit to mother outweighs potential risk to fetus.

LACTATION
- It is not known if drug is present in breast milk.
- Patient should check with prescriber before breastfeeding.

☰ Nursing Considerations
- Watch patient closely for evidence of depression, especially when apremilast therapy begins, because apremilast therapy may increase risk of depression and possibly lead to suicidal thinking or behavior.

! WARNING Monitor patient for hypersensitivity reactions that could include anaphylaxis and angioedema. If a hypersensitivity reaction occurs, notify prescriber immediately, expect drug to be discontinued, and provide supportive care, as prescribed.

- Monitor patient's weight regularly because apremilast may cause weight loss. Notify prescriber if weight loss occurs that is unexplained or is significant.
- Monitor patients 65 years and older for signs and symptoms of hypotension or dehydration that may occur as a result of severe diarrhea, nausea, or vomiting.

PATIENT TEACHING
- Tell patient to follow titration schedule exactly, as this will help reduce the incidence and severity of gastrointestinal symptoms associated with initial therapy.
- Instruct patient to swallow the tablets whole and not to chew, crush, or split, the tablets.

! WARNING Review allergic reactions with patient and stress importance of notifying prescriber, if present, and seeking emergency medical care, if severe.

- Advise patient to notify prescriber if severe diarrhea, nausea, or vomiting occurs.
- Instruct caregivers to watch patient closely for evidence of suicidal tendencies, especially when therapy starts, and to report concerns to prescriber immediately.
- Instruct patient to weigh themselves regularly and report any significant weight loss.

aprepitant
Cinvanti, Emend

fosaprepitant dimeglumine
Emend for Injection

Class and Category
Pharmacologic class: Substance P/neurokinin 1 (NK1) receptor antagonist
Therapeutic class: Antiemetic

Indications and Dosages
* *As adjunct to prevent acute and delayed nausea and vomiting associated with moderately to highly emetogenic chemotherapy, including high-dose cisplatin*

CAPSULES (EMEND)
Adults and children age 12 and over. 125 mg 1 hr before chemotherapy treatment, followed by 80 mg daily 1 hr before chemotherapy on day 2 and 3, or if no chemotherapy, 80 mg in morning on day 2 and 3.

ORAL SUSPENSION (EMEND)
Adults and children age 12 and over who cannot swallow oral capsules. 125 mg 1 hr before chemotherapy treatment on day 1, followed by 80 mg daily 1 hr before chemotherapy on days 2 and 3, or if no chemotherapy, 80 mg in morning on days 2 and 3.

Children 6 months to less than 12 years. 3 mg/kg (maximum 125 mg) on day 1, followed by 2 mg/kg (maximum 80 mg) 1 hr before chemotherapy on days 2 and 3, or if no chemotherapy, 2 mg/kg (maximum 80 mg) in morning on days 2 and 3.

I.V. INFUSION (EMEND FOR INJECTION)
Adults receiving a single-dose regimen. 150 mg as a single dose infused over 20 to 30 min before chemotherapy.

I.V. INFUSION (CINVANTI)
Adults receiving a single-dose regimen. 130 mg as a single dose infused over 30 min and completed about 30 min prior to chemotherapy on day 1 only.

I.V. INJECTION (CINVANTI)
Adults receiving a single-dose regimen. 130 mg as a single dose administered over 2 minutes and given 30 minutes prior to chemotherapy.

I.V. INFUSION (CINVANTI) FOLLOWED BY CAPSULES (EMEND)
Adults receiving moderately emetogenic cancer chemotherapy as a 3-day regimen. 100 mg as a single dose infused over 30 min about 30 min prior to chemotherapy on day 1, followed by 80 mg of oral aprepitant on days 2 and 3.

I.V. INJECTION (CINVANTI) FOLLOWED BY CAPSULES (EMEND)
Adults receiving moderately emetogenic cancer chemotherapy as a 3-day regimen. 100 mg as a single dose administered over

2 minutes and given 30 minutes before chemotherapy on day 1, followed by 80 mg of oral aprepitant on days 2 and 3.

✳ *To prevent nausea and vomiting associated with moderately to highly emetogenic chemotherapy with single-day pediatric chemotherapy regimens*

I.V. INFUSION (EMEND FOR INJECTION)

Adolescents age 12 to 17. 150 mg as a single dose infused over 30 min and completed about 30 min prior to chemotherapy on day 1 only.

Children age 2 to less than 12. 4 mg/kg (maximum 150 mg) as a single dose infused over 60 min and completed about 30 min prior to chemotherapy on day 1 only.

Children 6 months to less than 2 years weighing at least 6 kg (13.2 lb). 5 mg/kg (maximum 150 mg) as a single dose infused over 60 min and completed about 30 min prior to chemotherapy on day 1 only.

✳ *To prevent nausea and vomiting associated with moderately to highly emetogenic chemotherapy with multi-day pediatric chemotherapy regimens*

I.V. INFUSION (EMEND FOR INJECTION), CAPSULES (EMEND), ORAL SUSPENSION (EMEND)

Adolescents age 12 to 17. 115 mg as a single dose infused over 30 min and completed about 30 min prior to chemotherapy on day 1 followed by 80 mg daily of oral aprepitant on days 2 and 3.

Children age 6 months to less than 12 years weighing at least 6 kg (13.2 lb). 3 mg/kg (maximum 115 mg) as a single dose infused over 60 min and completed about 30 min prior to chemotherapy on day 1, followed by 2 mg/kg (maximum 80 mg) daily of oral aprepitant in suspension form on days 2 and 3.

Drug Administration

- Expect to administer aprepitant with dexamethasone and a 5-HT3 antagonist, such as dolasetron, granisetron, or ondansetron, for maximum antiemetic effects.

P.O.

- Administer 1 hour before chemotherapy.
- Administer capsule form only to children age 12 and over. Suspension form should be administered to children under 12 or to an older patient who cannot swallow capsules.
- Capsules must be swallowed whole.

- Oral suspension will be prepared by a health care provider and put in an oral dispenser after mixing.
- Administer by first taking cap off the dispenser and then placing the dispenser in the patient's mouth along the inner cheek on either the left or right side. Slowly dispense the drug.
- Refrigerate prepared oral suspension until administered.
- May be stored at room temperature for up to 3 hours before use.
- Discard any dose remaining after 72 hours.

I.V.

Cinvanti

- *For 30-minute I.V. infusion:* Reconstitute by filling an infusion bag with 100 ml of 0.9% Sodium Chloride Injection, USP, or 5% Dextrose for Injection, USP. Then withdraw 18 ml for 130-mg dose or 14 ml for 100-mg dose from drug vial and transfer it into the infusion bag.
- Gently invert the bag four or five times. Avoid shaking. Before administration, inspect bag for particulate matter and discoloration.
- Diluted solution is stable at ambient room temperature for up to 6 hours in Sodium Chloride Injection or 12 hours in 5% Dextrose Injection or up to 72 hours if stored under refrigeration with either solution.
- *For 2-minute I.V. push:* Prepare by withdrawing 18 ml for the 130-mg dose or 14 ml for the 100-mg dose from the vial. Do not dilute. Flush infusion line with 0.9% Sodium Chloride for Injection solution before and after administration.

Emend

- Reconstitute by injecting 5 ml 0.9% Sodium Chloride for Injection along vial wall to prevent foaming. Swirl vial gently. Withdraw contents from vial and add to an infusion bag containing 145 ml 0.9% Sodium Chloride Injection. Gently invert the bag two or three times.
- Determine volume to be administered based on dosage prescribed. For adults, the entire prepared infusion bag of 150 ml should be administered. For patients 12 years and older, the volume to be administered is calculated as follows: Volume to administer (ml) = the recommended dose (mg).

In patients 6 months of age to less than 12 years, the volume to be administered is calculated as follows: Volume to administer (ml) = recommended dose (mg/kg) × weight (kg). The dose to be administered should never exceed the maximum dose. If necessary, for volumes less than 150 ml, the calculated volume can be transferred to an appropriate size bag or syringe prior to administration.

- Administer by infusion at the rate given under Indications and Dosages section for the indication and age of patient being treated.
- Reconstituted solution may be stored at room temperature for 24 hours.
- *Incompatibilities for both products:* Any solution containing divalent cations such as calcium and magnesium, including Lactated Ringer's Solution and Hartmann's Solution

Route	Onset	Peak	Duration
P.O.	1 hr	4 hr	24 hr
I.V.	Unknown	>1 hr	Unknown

Half-life: 9–13 hr

Mechanism of Action

Crosses the blood–brain barrier to occupy brain NK1 receptors, which prevents nerve transmission of signals that cause nausea and vomiting.

Contraindications

Concurrent use of pimozide, hypersensitivity to aprepitant or its components

Interactions

DRUGS

carbamazepine, other CYP3A4 inducers, phenytoin, rifampin: Possibly decreased blood aprepitant level
CYP3A4 inhibitors (such as clarithromycin, diltiazem, itraconazole, ketoconazole, nefazodone, nelfinavir, ritonavir, and troleandomycin): Increased blood aprepitant level
CYP3A4 substrates (such as astemizole, benzodiazepines, cisapride, docetaxel, etoposide, imatinib, irinotecan, paclitaxel, pimozide, terfenadine, vinblastine, vincristine, and vinorelbine): Increased level of CYP3A4 substrates, resulting in possibly serious or life-threatening adverse reactions

dexamethasone, methylprednisolone: Increased effects of these drugs and risk of adverse reactions
ifosfamide: Increased risk of neurotoxicity and possibly other serious or life-threatening adverse reactions
oral contraceptives: Possibly decreased effectiveness of hormonal contraceptives
paroxetine: Possibly decreased blood level of both drugs
warfarin: Decreased effectiveness of warfarin and decreased prothrombin time

Adverse Reactions

CNS: Anxiety, asthenia, confusion, depression, dizziness, fatigue, fever, headache, hypoesthesia, hypothermia, insomnia, malaise, peripheral or sensory neuropathy, rigors, somnolence, syncope, tremor
CV: Bradycardia, deep vein thrombosis, edema, hypertension, hypotension, MI, palpitations, peripheral edema, tachycardia, thrombophlebitis at injection site
EENT: Conjunctivitis, dry mouth, increased salivation, mucous membrane alteration, nasal discharge, oral candidiasis, oropharyngeal pain, pharyngitis, stomatitis, taste perversion, tinnitus, vocal disturbance
ENDO: Hot flashes, hyperglycemia
GI: Abdominal pain, anorexia, constipation, diarrhea, dysphagia, elevated liver enzymes, epigastric discomfort, flatulence, gastritis, gastroesophageal reflux, heartburn, hiccups, nausea, obstipation (intractable constipation), vomiting
GU: Dysuria, elevated BUN and serum creatinine levels, hematuria, leukocyturia, proteinuria, renal insufficiency, UTI
HEME: Anemia, febrile neutropenia, hematoma, leukocytosis, leukopenia, neutropenia, thrombocytopenia
MS: Arthralgia, back pain, muscle weakness, musculoskeletal pain, myalgia, pelvic pain
RESP: Cough, dyspnea, hypoxia, non–small-cell lung carcinoma, pneumonitis, pulmonary embolism, respiratory depression or insufficiency, respiratory tract infection
SKIN: Acne, alopecia, diaphoresis, flushing, pruritus, rash, Stevens–Johnson syndrome, toxic epidermal necrolysis, urticaria
Other: Anaphylaxis, anaphylactic shock, angioedema, candidiasis, dehydration,

elevated alkaline phosphatase, herpes simplex, **hypokalemia**, **hyponatremia**, infusion-site pain or induration, **malignant neoplasm**, **septic shock**, weight loss

Childbearing Considerations

PREGNANCY
- It is not known if drug can cause fetal harm.
- Use with caution only if benefit to mother outweighs potential risk to fetus.

LACTATION
- It is not known if drug is present in breast milk.
- Patient should check with prescriber before breastfeeding.

REPRODUCTION
- Drug may reduce hormonal contraceptive effectiveness.
- Patient should be instructed to use an effective alternative or backup nonhormonal contraceptive, such as spermicides or male partners' use of condoms, during therapy and for 1 month following last dose.

Nursing Considerations
- Use caution when giving aprepitant to patients with severe hepatic insufficiency because drug's effects on such patients aren't known.

! WARNING Monitor patient closely for hypersensitivity reactions, which could include anaphylaxis and anaphylactic shock during or soon after *administration* of drug. Symptoms to be alert for include dyspnea, erythema, flushing, hypotension, and syncope. If a hypersensitivity reaction occurs, stop infusion *or injection* if still being given, notify prescriber, expect drug to be discontinued, and be prepared to provide supportive care.

- Be aware that ifosfamide-induced neurotoxicity may occur after aprepitant and ifosfamide have been coadministered.

PATIENT TEACHING
- Instruct patient to take 125-mg dose of oral aprepitant 1 hour before chemotherapy, 80-mg dose in the morning for 2 days after chemotherapy. Tell patient capsule should be swallowed whole and not chewed, crushed, or opened.
- Instruct patient using oral suspension form that drug will be premixed and placed in a

dispenser for use. Tell patient to administer by first taking cap off the dispenser and then placing the dispenser in mouth along the inner cheek on either the left or right side. The patient should then slowly dispense the drug.
- Remind patient to refrigerate the prepared oral suspension until administered and that it can be stored only for up to 3 hours at room temperature before use. Have patient discard suspension if not used after 72 hours.

! WARNING Instruct patient to report an allergic reaction such as difficulty breathing or swallowing, dizziness, fainting, flushing, hives, itching, or rash and seek immediate medical attention.

- Tell female patients taking hormonal contraceptives to use an alternative or backup method of contraception during aprepitant therapy and for 1 month after last dose because drug reduces effectiveness of hormonal contraceptives.
- Tell patient taking chronic warfarin therapy to have clotting status monitored closely especially at 7 to 10 days during each chemotherapy cycle in which the drug is used.
- Caution patient to inform prescriber of any drugs he's taking, including OTC drugs and herbal preparations, because they may interact with aprepitant.

argatroban

Class and Category
Pharmacologic class: Direct thrombin inhibitor
Therapeutic class: Anticoagulant

Indications and Dosages
✴ *To prevent or treat thrombosis in patients with heparin-induced thrombocytopenia (HIT)*

I.V. INFUSION
Adults without hepatic impairment.
2 mcg/kg/min. *Maximum:* 10 mcg/kg/min.
±**DOSAGE ADJUSTMENT** Dosage adjusted as prescribed to maintain patient's APTT at 1.5 to 3 times the initial baseline value, not to exceed 100 sec. Initial dosage reduced to

0.5 mcg/kg/min for patients with moderate or severe hepatic impairment.

＊ *To prevent or treat thrombosis in patients with or at risk for HIT when undergoing percutaneous coronary intervention (PCI)*

I.V. INFUSION, I.V. INJECTION

Adults without hepatic impairment. *Initial:* 350 mcg/kg bolus followed by 25 mcg/kg/min infusion.

±**DOSAGE ADJUSTMENT** Dosage adjusted as prescribed to keep activated clotting time (ACT) at 300 to 450 sec. If ACT is less than 300 sec, additional I.V. bolus dose of 150 mcg/kg given and infusion increased to 30 mcg/kg/min; if ACT exceeds 450 sec, dosage reduced to 15 mcg/kg/min. For dissection, impending abrupt closure, thrombus formation during PCI, or inability to reach or keep ACT above 300 sec, additional bolus doses of 150 mcg/kg may be given and infusion increased to 40 mcg/kg/min.

Drug Administration

I.V.

- 50 mg/ml single-dose vial is ready for use and does not require dilution. The 250 mg/2.5 ml single-dose vial must be diluted 100-fold prior to infusion. Dilute each 2.5-ml vial with 250 ml of room-temperature diluent using 0.9% Sodium Chloride Injection, 5% Dextrose Injection, or Lactated Ringer's Injection to a final concentration of 1 mg/ml. Drug solution should appear clear, colorless to pale yellow.
- Give bolus dose over 3 to 5 minutes.
- For continuous infusion, invert diluent bag repeatedly for 1 minute to mix completely before administering. Initially the solution may appear to have a slight haziness but this rapidly disappears upon mixing. Final solution should be clear.
- Solution is stable at room temperature of 20–25°C (68–77°F) in ambient indoor light for 24 hours. Prepared solution does not require light-resistant measures such as foil protection for I.V. tubing when administering drug. However, drug should not be exposed to direct sunlight.
- *Incompatibilities:* Other I.V. drugs

Route	Onset	Peak	Duration
I.V.	Immediate	1–3 hr	2–4 hr

Half-life: 39–51 min

Mechanism of Action

Exerts its anticoagulant effects by inhibiting thrombin-catalyzed or induced reactions, including fibrin formation, activation of coagulation factors, V, VIII, and XIII; protein C; and platelet aggregation.

Contraindications

Active major bleeding, hypersensitivity to argatroban or its components

Interactions

DRUGS

heparin, oral anticoagulants: Increased risk of bleeding

Adverse Reactions

CNS: **Cerebrovascular bleeding**, fever, headache

CV: **Atrial fibrillation, cardiac arrest, hypotension, unstable angina, ventricular tachycardia**

GI: Abdominal pain, anorexia, diarrhea, elevated liver enzymes, **GI bleeding, melena,** nausea, vomiting

GU: Elevated BUN and serum creatinine levels, hematuria (microscopic), UTI

HEME: **Hemorrhage, hypoprothrombinemia, unusual bleeding or bruising**

RESP: Cough, dyspnea, **hemoptysis,** pneumonia

SKIN: Bleeding at puncture site, rash

Other: **Sepsis**

Childbearing Considerations

PREGNANCY

- Drug may cause fetal harm due to increased risk of bleeding.
- Use with caution only if benefit to mother outweighs potential risk to fetus.

LABOR & DELIVERY

- Use with caution during labor and delivery.
- Use of drug increases risk of bleeding for both the mother and fetus/neonate.

LACTATION

- It is not known if drug is present in breast milk.
- Patient should check with prescriber before breastfeeding.

Nursing Considerations

! WARNING Know that argatroban isn't recommended for PCI patients with significant hepatic disease or AST/ALT levels three times or more the upper limits of normal.

! WARNING Monitor patients with thrombocytopenia or those receiving daily doses of salicylates greater than 6 g for signs and symptoms of bleeding; these patients are at increased risk of bleeding from hypoprothrombinemia.

! WARNING Expect to perform blood coagulation tests before and 2 hours after start of therapy because of the major risk of bleeding associated with argatroban. Be aware that coagulopathy must be ruled out before therapy starts. When giving drug to a patient undergoing PCI, expect to check ACT 5 to 10 minutes after each bolus and each infusion rate change and every 20 to 30 minutes during the PCI.

- Monitor the following patients for signs and symptoms of bleeding which may become severe and occur at any site in the body because they're at increased risk during argatroban therapy: patients who have recently had a large vessel puncture or organ biopsy, lumbar puncture, major bleeding (including intracranial, GI, intraocular, retroperitoneal, or pulmonary bleeding), major surgery (including brain, eye, or spinal cord surgery), spinal anesthesia, or stroke; patients with vascular or organ abnormalities, such as advanced renal disease, dissecting aortic aneurysm, diverticulitis, hemophilia, hepatic disease (especially if associated with a deficiency of vitamin K-dependent clotting factors), infective endocarditis inflammatory bowel disease, or peptic ulcer disease such as severe uncontrolled hypertension; and women with active menstruation. Risk of bleeding, especially hemorrhage, is also increased with concomitant use with other anticoagulants, antiplatelets, and thrombolytics.
- Avoid I.M. injections, whenever possible, in patients receiving argatroban, to decrease the risk of bleeding.
- Be aware that thrombin times may not be helpful for monitoring argatroban activity because the drug affects all thrombin-dependent coagulation tests.

- Monitor pregnant women during labor and delivery for excessive bleeding or unexpected changes in coagulation parameters. Know that exposure to argatroban may increase the risk of bleeding in the fetus and neonate. Monitor closely.
- Expect dosage to be tapered before stopping to prevent the risk of rebound hypercoagulopathy; drug's effects last only a short time once drug is discontinued.

PATIENT TEACHING

- Inform patient that argatroban is a blood thinner that's given in the hospital by infusion into a vein. If he needs long-term anticoagulation, he'll be switched to another drug before discharge.
- Advise patient to report immediately any unusual or unexplained bleeding, such as blood in urine, easy bruising, nosebleeds, tarry stools, and vaginal bleeding.
- Instruct patient to avoid injury while receiving argatroban. For example, suggest that he brush his teeth gently, using a soft-bristled toothbrush, and take special care when flossing.

aripiprazole
Abilify, Abilify Maintena, Abilify Mycite

aripiprazole lauroxil
Aristada, Aristada Initio

☰ Class and Category
Pharmacologic class: Atypical antipsychotic
Therapeutic class: Antipsychotic

☰ Indications and Dosages
∗ *To treat acute schizophrenia; to maintain stability in patients with schizophrenia*

ORAL SOLUTION, ORALLY DISINTEGRATING TABLETS, TABLETS (ABILIFY)

Adults. *Initial:* 10 or 15 mg daily. Increased to 30 mg daily, as needed, with dosage adjustments at 2-wk intervals.
Adolescents. *Initial:* 2 mg daily for 2 days, then increased to 5 mg daily for 2 days, then increased to 10 mg daily. Further increased in 5-mg increments as needed. *Maximum:* 30 mg daily.

I.M. INJECTION (ABILIFY MAINTENA)

Adults. 400 mg monthly (no sooner than 26 days after the previous injection) into the deltoid or gluteal muscle. Dosage reduced to 300 mg monthly if adverse reactions occur.

I.M. INJECTION (ARISTADA), ORAL SOLUTION, ORALLY DISINTEGRATING TABLETS, OR TABLETS

Adults. *Initial:* 441 mg every month in the deltoid muscle if patient is currently taking 10 mg daily of aripiprazole P.O.; 662 mg every month, 882 mg every 6 wk, or 1064 mg every 2 months given in the gluteal muscle if patient is currently taking 15 mg daily of aripiprazole P.O.; or 882 mg each month given in the gluteal muscle if patient is currently taking 20 mg or higher daily doses of aripiprazole P.O. Dosage initiated in one of two ways. *Option 1:* Administer first injection along with one 30-mg oral dose of drug along with one 675-mg injection of Aristada Initio. *Option 2:* Oral drug given for 21 days with first injection.

TABLET (ABILIFY MYCITE)

Adults. *Initial:* 10 or 15 mg daily, with dosage increased no sooner than every 2 wk. *Maximum:* 30 mg daily.

✳ *As adjunct with oral aripiprazole to initiate Aristada treatment for patients with schizophrenia*

I.M. INJECTION (ARISTADA INITIO), ORAL SOLUTION, ORALLY DISINTEGRATING TABLETS, OR TABLETS

Adults. 675 mg as a single dose into the deltoid or gluteal muscle and given at the same time as a 30-mg oral dose of aripiprazole. First dose of Aristada is then administered on the same day or up to 10 days thereafter.

✳ *To reinitiate treatment with Aristada following a missed dose of Aristada in patients with schizophrenia*

I.M. INJECTION (ARISTADA INITIO)

Adults taking 441 mg of Aristada. If time lapse from last dose of Aristada is greater than 6 weeks but 7 weeks or less, 675 mg as a single dose of Aristada Initio given in the deltoid or gluteal muscle.

Adults taking 662 mg or 882 mg of Aristada. If time lapse from last dose of Aristada is greater than 8 wk but 12 wk or less, 675 mg as a single dose of Aristada Initio given into the deltoid or gluteal muscle.

Adults taking 1064 mg of Aristada. If time lapse from last dose of Aristada is greater than 10 wk but 12 weeks or less, 675 mg as a single dose of Aristada Initio into the deltoid or gluteal muscle.

I.M. INJECTION (ARISTADA INITIO) PLUS ORAL SOLUTION, ORALLY DISINTEGRATING TABLETS, OR TABLETS

Adults taking 441 mg of Aristada. If time lapse from last dose of Aristada is greater than 7 wk, 675 mg given into the deltoid or gluteal muscle as a single dose of Aristada Initio plus a single 30-mg oral dose of aripiprazole.

Adults taking 662 mg, 882 mg, or 1064 mg of Aristada. If time lapse from last dose of Aristada is greater than 12 wk, 675 mg as a single dose of Aristada Initio given into the deltoid or gluteal muscle plus a single 30-mg oral dose of aripiprazole.

✳ *To treat acute manic and mixed episodes in bipolar I disorder with or without psychotic features; to maintain stability in patients with bipolar I disorder; as adjunct with lithium or valproate in patients with bipolar I disorder*

ORAL SOLUTION, ORALLY DISINTEGRATING TABLETS, TABLETS (ABILIFY)

Adults. *Initial:* 15 mg daily (10 to 15 mg if lithium or valproate coadministered), increased to 30 mg daily, as needed. *Maintenance:* 15 to 30 mg daily. *Maximum:* 30 mg daily.

Children ages 10 to 17. *Initial:* 2 mg daily, increased after 2 days to 5 mg daily and then after 2 days to 10 mg daily. Increased in 5-mg increments, as needed, at 2-wk intervals. *Maintenance:* Lowest dose possible to maintain remission. *Maximum:* 30 mg daily.

TABLETS (ABILIFY MYCITE)

Adults with acute and mixed episodes of bipolar I disorder. *Initial:* 15 mg once daily. *Maximum:* 30 mg daily.

Adults with bipolar I disorder receiving adjunct treatment with lithium or valproate. *Initial:* 10 to 15 mg once daily. *Maximum:* 30 mg daily.

✳ *To maintain stability with monotherapy treatment of bipolar I disorder*

I.M. INJECTION (ABILIFY MAINTENA)

Adults. 400 mg monthly (no sooner than 26 days after the previous injection) into the deltoid or gluteal muscle. Dosage reduced to 300 mg monthly if adverse reactions occur.

* *As adjunct to treat depression in patients already taking an antidepressant*

ORAL SOLUTION, ORALLY DISINTEGRATING TABLETS, TABLETS (ABILIFY)

Adults. *Initial:* 2 to 5 mg daily, with dosage increased by 5 mg daily at 1-wk intervals, as needed. *Maximum:* 15 mg daily.

TABLETS (ABILIFY MYCITE)

Adults. *Initial:* 2 to 5 mg daily, increased as needed, in increments of up to 5 mg daily no less than once a wk. *Maximum:* 15 mg daily.

* *To treat irritability associated with autistic disorder*

ORAL SOLUTION, ORALLY DISINTEGRATING TABLETS, TABLETS (ABILIFY)

Children ages 6 to 17. *Initial:* 2 mg daily, with dosage increased after 1 wk to 5 mg daily and then after 1 wk to 10 mg daily and then after 1 wk to 15 mg daily, as needed.

* *To treat Tourette's disorder*

ORAL SOLUTION, ORALLY DISINTEGRATING TABLETS, TABLETS (ABILIFY)

Children ages 6 to 18 weighing 50 kg (110 lb) or more. *Initial:* 2 mg daily for 2 days, then 5 mg daily for 5 days, followed by dosage increased to 10 mg daily on day 8. Dosage increased 5 mg daily at weekly intervals, as needed, to control tics. *Maximum:* 20 mg daily.

Children age 6 to 18 weighing less than 50 kg (110 lb). *Initial:* 2 mg daily for 2 days, with dosage increased to 5 mg daily on day 3. Dosage increased to 10 mg/kg daily after at least 1 wk, as needed, to control tics. *Maximum:* 10 mg daily.

* *To treat agitation associated with bipolar mania or schizophrenia*

I.M. INJECTION (ABILIFY)

Adults. 5.25 to 9.75 mg, repeated, as needed, after 2 or more hr. *Maximum:* Cumulative daily doses up to 30 mg with dosing intervals of 2 hr or more.

±**DOSAGE ADJUSTMENT** Aristada Initio administration avoided in patients who are known CYP2D6 poor metabolizers or in patients taking strong CYP2D6 or CYP3A4 inhibitors or strong CYP3A4 inducers because dosage adjustment cannot be made, as product is only available in a single strength. For other aripiprazole products, dosage reductions made for patients who are known CYP2D6 poor metabolizers and patients taking concomitant CYP2D6 inhibitors, CYP3A4 inhibitors, and/or CYP3A4 inducers for more than 14 days. Dosage reduction individualized taking into account current dosage prescribed and type of aripiprazole formulation being used. Dosage of Abilify formulation doubled over 1 to 2 weeks for patients taking strong CYP3A4 inducers such as carbamazepine or rifampin.

Drug Administration

P.O.

- Oral solution may be given on a milligram-per-milligram basis in place of tablets up to 25 mg.
- Abilify Mycite tablets should be swallowed whole. Tablets should not be chewed, crushed, or split because tablet contains a sensor to track patient compliance.
- When ready to administer orally disintegrating tablets, open the blister pack by peeling back the foil carefully. Do not push tablet through the foil because doing so could damage the tablet. Have patient place the tablet on his tongue without breaking it and let it dissolve. If needed, a drink may be given afterward.

I.M.

- Tolerability must be established with oral form for patients who have never taken aripiprazole prior to initiating parenteral therapy.
- Do not confuse the various types of I.M. preparations. They are not interchangeable.

Abilify
- Draw up the required volume of solution into a syringe as follows: 0.7 ml for a 5.25-mg single dose; 1.3 ml for a 9.75-mg dose; and 2 ml for a 15-mg dose.
- Inject slowly and deeply into the muscle mass.
- Do not administer intravenously or subcutaneously.

Abilify Maintena
- After first dose of Abilify Maintena, expect to continue to administer oral aripiprazole (10 to 20 mg) for 14 consecutive days to achieve a therapeutic level during the initiation of the intramuscular injection.

- Abilify Maintena comes in two types of kits: prefilled chamber syringe or single-use vial.
- Reconstitute Abilify Maintena lyophilized powder in prefilled dual-chamber syringe by pushing plunger rod slightly to engage threads. Then rotate plunger rod until the rod stops rotating to release diluent. After plunger rod is at a complete stop, middle stopper will be at the indicator line. Vertically shake the syringe vigorously for 20 seconds until drug is uniformly milky white.
- Reconstitute Abilify Maintena using a single-use vial by using the syringe with the pre-attached needle to withdraw 1.9 ml of Sterile Water for Injection for a 400-mg vial and 1.5 ml of Sterile Water for Injection for a 300-mg vial. Slowly inject the solution into the drug vial. Withdraw air to equalize the pressure, then remove the needle from the vial. Engage the needle safety device by using the one-handed technique. Gently press the sheath against a flat surface until the needle is firmly engaged in the needle protection sheath and discard appropriately. Shake the drug vial vigorously for 30 seconds until the reconstituted suspension appears uniform. It should be opaque and milky white in color. If the injection is not given immediately after reconstitution, keep the vial at room temperature and shake the vial vigorously for at least 60 seconds to resuspend prior to administration. Do not store the reconstituted suspension in a syringe.
- Prepare Abilify Maintena prior to injection after reconstituting from a single-use vial by removing cover from the vial adapter package, but do not remove the vial adapter from the package. Using the vial adapter package to handle the vial adapter, attach the prepackaged BD Luer-Lok syringe to the vial adapter. Use the syringe to remove the vial adapter from the package and discard the vial adapter package. Do not touch the spike tip of the adapter at any time. Determine the recommended volume for injection using the manufacturer chart for size vial being used and dosage prescribed. After wiping top of vial with a sterile alcohol swab, place and hold vial of the reconstituted suspension on a hard surface. Attach the adapter syringe assembly to the vial by holding the outside of the adapter and pushing the adapter's spike firmly through the rubber stopper until the adapter snaps in place. Slowly withdraw the recommended volume from the vial into the syringe. Prior to injection, detach the Luer-Lok syringe containing the recommended volume of reconstituted Abilify Maintena suspension from the vial.

- Once the drug is reconstituted, select the appropriate hypodermic safety needle provided by the manufacturer to use for the injection. When selecting the deltoid site for a nonobese patient, use a 23 G, 1-inch needle; for an obese patient use a 22 G, 1.5-inch needle. When selecting the gluteal site, for a nonobese patient, use a 22 G, 1.5-inch needle; for an obese patient use a 21 G, 2-inch needle.
- Inject Abilify Maintena form slowly, deep into the deltoid or gluteal muscle, and never I.V. or subcutaneously. Do not massage the injection site.
- Use following guide for determining when to administer missed doses of the long-acting formulation, Abilify Maintena:
  - If a second or third dose is missed and it's been more than 4 weeks but less than 5 weeks since the last injection, administer the injection as soon as possible. If more than 5 weeks have elapsed since the last injection, restart concomitant oral aripiprazole, as ordered, for 14 days with the next administered injection.
  - If a fourth or subsequent doses are missed and it's been more than 4 weeks but less than 6 weeks since the last injection, administer the injection as soon as possible. If more than 6 weeks have elapsed since the last injection, restart concomitant oral aripiprazole, as ordered, for 14 days with the next administered injection.

Aristada
- Prepare Aristada for injection by first tapping the syringe at least 10 times and then shaking syringe vigorously for 30 seconds to ensure a uniform suspension. If pen is not used within 15 minutes, shake again for 30 seconds. Select needle length based on injection site and attach to syringe. For administration in the deltoid muscle, use a 21 G, 1-inch or 20 G, 1½-inch needle; for administration in the gluteal

muscle, use a 20 G, 1½-inch or 20 G, 2-inch needle. Prime the syringe to remove air.

- Administer Aristada formulation into the gluteal muscle by I.M. injection only for all dosages except the 441-mg dose, which may also be administered into the deltoid muscle. Inject in a rapid and continuous manner in less than 10 seconds.
- Follow manufacturer guidelines when a dose of Aristada is missed; these are based upon the dosage missed and length of time that has elapsed. However, be aware that Aristada Initio may have to be used to reinitiate treatment with Aristada.

Aristada Initio

- Prepare Aristada Initio for injection in the same manner as Aristada. The kit contains three safety needles (a 2-inch 20-gauge needle with a yellow needle hub, a 1½-inch 20-gauge needle with a yellow needle hub, and a 1-inch 21-gauge needle with a green needle hub). Select the injection needle to use (deltoid administration requires a 20- to 21-gauge needle and gluteal administration requires a 20-gauge needle). Avoid overtightening the needle when attaching to syringe because needle hub may crack.
- Inject in a rapid and continuous manner intramuscularly. Do not inject by any other route.

Route	Onset	Peak	Duration
P.O.	Unknown	3–5 hr	Unknown
I.M.	Unknown	4–7 days	Unknown

Half-life: 75–94 hr

Mechanism of Action

May produce antipsychotic effects through partial agonist and antagonist actions. Aripiprazole acts as a partial agonist at dopamine (especially D_2) receptors and serotonin (especially $5\text{-}HT_{1A}$) receptors. The drug acts as an antagonist at $5\text{-}HT_{2A}$ serotonin receptor sites.

Contraindications

Hypersensitivity to aripiprazole or its components

Interactions

DRUGS

antihypertensives: Possibly enhanced antihypertensive effects

benzodiazepines such as lorazepam: Increased risk of orthostatic hypotension and sedation
strong CYP3A4 inducers such as carbamazepine, rifampin: Possibly increased clearance and decreased blood level of aripiprazole
strong CYP34A inhibitors such as clarithromycin, itraconazole; strong CYP2D6 inhibitors such as fluoxetine, quinidine, paroxetine: Increased exposure of aripiprazole and increased risk of adverse reactions

ACTIVITIES

alcohol use: Increased CNS depression

Adverse Reactions

CNS: Abnormal gait, aggression, agitation, akathisia, anxiety, asthenia, catatonia, cognitive and motor impairment, confusion, CVA (elderly), delusions, depression, dizziness, dream disturbances, dystonia, extrapyramidal reactions, fatigue, fever, hallucinations, headache, homicidal ideation, hostility, insomnia, intracranial hemorrhage, lethargy, light-headedness, mania, nervousness, neuroleptic malignant syndrome, paranoia, Parkinsonism, restlessness, schizophrenic reaction, seizures, sleep walking, somnolence, suicidal ideation, tardive dyskinesia, transient ischemic attack (elderly), tremor

CV: Angina pectoris, arrhythmias, bradycardia, cardiopulmonary arrest, chest pain, circulatory collapse, deep vein thrombosis, dyslipidemia, elevated serum CK levels, heart failure, hyperlipidemia, hypertension, MI, orthostatic hypotension, palpitations, peripheral edema, prolonged QT interval, tachycardia

EENT: Blurred vision, conjunctivitis, diplopia, dry mouth, increased salivation, hiccups, laryngospasm, nasal congestion, nasopharyngitis, oculogyric crisis, oropharyngeal spasm, pharyngitis, photophobia, rhinitis, sinusitis

ENDO: Blood glucose fluctuation, breast pain, gynecomastia, hyperglycemia, diabetes mellitus

GI: Abdominal discomfort, constipation, decreased appetite, diarrhea, difficulty swallowing, GI bleeding, gastroesophageal reflux disease, hepatitis, hiccups, indigestion, jaundice, nausea, vomiting

GU: Decreased or increased libido, erectile dysfunction, menstrual disorders, nocturia, priapism, **renal failure**, urinary incontinence or retention

HEME: **Agranulocytosis**, anemia, **leukopenia**, **neutropenia**, **thrombocytopenia**

MS: Arthralgia, joint stiffness, muscle spasms or weakness, musculoskeletal pain, myalgia, neck and limb rigidity, **rhabdomyolysis**, trismus

RESP: **Apnea**, **aspiration**, **asthma**, cough, dyspnea, pneumonia, **pulmonary edema or embolism**, **respiratory failure**

SKIN: Alopecia, diaphoresis, dry skin, ecchymosis, photosensitivity, pruritus, rash, ulceration, urticaria

Other: **Anaphylaxis**; **angioedema**; dehydration; **drug reaction with eosinophilia and systemic symptoms (DRESS)**; elevated blood creatine phosphokinase (Aristada); flu-like symptoms; **heat stroke**; injection-site induration, pain, redness, swelling (Aristada); **hypokalemia**; **hyponatremia**; intense uncontrollable urges to perform certain activities, such as gambling and sexual acts; weight gain

Childbearing Considerations

PREGNANCY

- Pregnancy exposure registry: 1-866-961-2388 or http://womensmentalhealth.org/clinical-and-research-programs/pregnancyregistry/.
- Drug may cause fetal harm. Neonates exposed to drug during the third trimester of pregnancy are at risk for extrapyramidal and withdrawal symptoms.
- Use with caution only if benefit to mother outweighs potential risk to fetus and no other alternative is available.

LACTATION

- Drug is present in human milk.
- Patient should check with prescriber before breastfeeding.

Nursing Considerations

- Know that aripiprazole shouldn't be used to treat dementia-related psychosis in the elderly because of an increased risk of death.
- Use cautiously in patients with cardiovascular disease, cerebrovascular disease, or conditions that would predispose them to hypotension. Also use cautiously in those with a history of seizures or with conditions that lower the seizure threshold, such as Alzheimer's disease.
- Use cautiously in elderly patients because of increased risk of serious adverse cerebrovascular effects, such as stroke and transient ischemic attack.
- Be aware that Abilify Mycite is a drug-device combination product comprised of aripiprazole tablets embedded with an ingestible event marker (IEM) sensor intended to track drug ingestion. Other ways used to track ingestion of aripiprazole include a Mycite patch, which is a wearable sensor that detects signals from the IEM sensor after ingestion of aripiprazole and transmits data to a smartphone. Alternatively, there is a Mycite app, which is a smartphone application, which is used with a compatible smartphone to display information for the patient and web-based portal for healthcare professionals and caregivers to track compliance.
- Know that most ingestions can be tracked with Abilify Mycite within 30 minutes, but it may take up to 2 hours for the smartphone app and web portal to detect that the tablet has been taken.
- Apply the Abilify Mycite patch to the left side of the body just above the lower edge of the rib cage. Do not place it in areas where the skin is cracked, inflamed, irritated, or scraped or in a location that overlaps the area of the most recently removed patch. Be aware that the patch must be removed before patient undergoes an MRI.
- Monitor patient for difficulty swallowing or excessive somnolence, which could predispose to accidental injury or aspiration. For patients with medical conditions or who are taking medications that could exacerbate CNS effects, complete a fall risk assessment and institute safety measures.

! WARNING Be aware that aripiprazole rarely may cause neuroleptic malignant syndrome, seizures, and tardive dyskinesia. Monitor patient closely throughout therapy, and take safety precautions as needed. Be aware that tardive dyskinesia may resolve, partially or completely, if aripiprazole is discontinued.

- Watch patients closely (especially children, adolescents, and young adults) for suicidal tendencies, particularly when therapy starts and dosage changes, because depression may worsen temporarily during these times.

- Monitor patient's CBC, as ordered, because serious adverse hematologic reactions may occur, such as agranulocytosis, leukopenia, and neutropenia. Assess more often during first few months of therapy if patient has a history of drug-induced leukopenia or neutropenia or a significantly low WBC count. If abnormalities occur during therapy, watch for fever or other signs of infection, notify prescriber and, if severe, expect drug to be stopped.

- Monitor patient's weight, blood glucose level, and lipid levels, as ordered, because atypical antipsychotic drugs such as aripiprazole may cause metabolic changes. If patient is already a diabetic, monitor blood glucose levels more closely.

PATIENT TEACHING

- Instruct patient prescribed orally disintegrating tablets to open the blister pack only when ready to take the tablet. Tell him to peel back the foil carefully and not to push tablet through the foil because doing so could damage the tablet. Tell him to place the tablet on his tongue without breaking it and let it dissolve. If needed, he may take a drink.

- Instruct patient how to use the Abilify Mycite system, which will have to be downloaded and compatibility with patient's smartphone checked. Once downloaded, patient should followed manufacturer instructions. Inform patient that a functioning pod will be needed before using the Maintenance Kit.

- If taking drug orally, tell patient to swallow tablets whole and not to chew, crush, or divide them. Tell patient that most ingestions will be detected within 30 minutes on the app; however, it can take more than 2 hours for the smartphone app and web portal to detect ingestion of Abilify Mycite. In some cases, the ingestion of the tablet may not be detected. If it is not, stress that dose should not be repeated.

- Tell patient using the patch to keep it on when exercising, showering, and swimming. Tell patient the patch will have to be changed at least weekly. Inform patient that the app will prompt patient to change the patch and will direct patient on how

to apply and remove the patch correctly. If skin irritation or a rash develops, the patch should be removed and prescriber notified. Inform patient that if undergoing an MRI, the patch must be removed and a new one applied after the test.

- Advise patient to get up slowly from a lying or sitting position during aripiprazole therapy to minimize orthostatic hypotension.

- Urge patient to avoid alcohol during aripiprazole therapy.

- Instruct patient to avoid hazardous activities until drug's effects are known. Also, alert patient and family of increased risk for falls, especially if patient has other medical conditions or takes medication that may affect the nervous system.

- Urge patient to avoid activities that raise body temperature suddenly, such as strenuous exercise and exposure to extreme heat, and to compensate for situations that cause dehydration, such as vomiting or diarrhea.

- Instruct patient and caregivers to notify prescriber about intense urges, such as for gambling or sex, because dosage may have to be reduced or drug discontinued.

- Instruct patient to inform all prescribers of any drugs he's taking, including OTC drugs, because of risk of interactions.

- Advise female patient of childbearing age to notify prescriber if she intends to become or suspects that she is pregnant during therapy.

- Instruct diabetic patient to monitor blood glucose levels closely, especially if taking the oral solution form because each milliliter of solution contains 400 mg of sucrose and 200 mg of fructose.

- Urge family or caregiver to watch patient closely for suicidal tendencies, especially when therapy starts or dosage changes, and particularly if patient is a child, teenager, or young adult.

armodafinil
Nuvigil

Class and Category
Pharmacologic class: Analeptic modafinil derivative
Therapeutic class: CNS stimulant
Controlled substance schedule: IV

▤ Indications and Dosages

✳ *To treat narcolepsy or as adjunct to standard therapy for excessive daytime sleepiness in obstructive sleep apnea/hypopnea syndrome*

TABLETS

Adults. 150 or 250 mg once daily.

✳ *To improve daytime wakefulness in patients with excessive sleepiness from circadian rhythm disruption (shift-work sleep disorder)*

TABLETS

Adults. 150 mg once daily.

±**DOSAGE ADJUSTMENT** Dosage decreased for patients who are elderly or have severe hepatic impairment.

▤ Drug Administration

P.O.

▪ Administer drug in the morning or 1 hr before start of work shift.
▪ Drug should be given consistently with or without food, as food may delay effect.

Route	Onset	Peak	Duration
P.O.	Unknown	2–6 hr	Unknown

Half-life: 15 hr

▤ Mechanism of Action

May produce CNS stimulant effects by binding to dopamine transporter in the brain and inhibiting dopamine reuptake in limbic regions. These actions increase alertness and reduce drowsiness and fatigue.

▤ Contraindications

Hypersensitivity to armodafinil, modafinil, or their components

▤ Interactions

DRUGS

cyclosporine: Possibly decreased blood cyclosporine level and increased risk of organ transplant rejection
CYP2C19 substrates such as clomipramine, diazepam, omeprazole, and propranolol: Possibly prolonged elimination time and increased blood levels of these drugs
CYP3A4/5 substrates such as midazolam, triazolam: Possibly decreased effectiveness of these drugs
fosphenytoin, mephenytoin, phenytoin: Possibly decreased effectiveness of armodafinil, increased blood phenytoin level, and increased risk of phenytoin toxicity

MAO inhibitors: Increased risk of serious adverse reactions
oral steroidal contraceptives: Possibly decreased effectiveness of oral contraceptive and for one month following discontinuation
warfarin: Possibly decreased warfarin metabolism and increased risk of bleeding

FOODS

all foods: 2- to 4-hr delay for armodafinil to reach peak levels and possibly delayed onset of action
caffeine: Increased CNS stimulation

ACTIVITIES

alcohol use: Possibly adverse CNS effects

▤ Adverse Reactions

CNS: Aggression, agitation, anxiety, attention disturbance, delusions, depression, dizziness, drowsiness, excessive sleepiness, fatigue, fever, hallucinations, headache (including migraine), insomnia, irritability, mania, nervousness, paresthesia, **suicidal ideation**, thirst, tremor
CV: Increased heart rate, palpitations
EENT: Dry mouth, mouth sores
GI: Abdominal pain (upper), anorexia, constipation, diarrhea, dyspepsia, loose stools, nausea, vomiting
GU: Polyuria
RESP: **Bronchospasm**, dyspnea
SKIN: Contact dermatitis, **Stevens–Johnson syndrome, toxic epidermal necrolysis**
Other: **Anaphylaxis, angioedema, drug reaction with eosinophilia and system symptoms (DRESS)**, flu-like illness

▤ Childbearing Considerations

PREGNANCY

▪ Pregnancy exposure registry: 1-866-404-4106.
▪ Limited data suggest drug may cause fetal harm. Intrauterine growth restriction and spontaneous abortion have been reported in association with the drug.
▪ Use with caution only if benefit to mother outweighs potential risk to fetus.

LACTATION

▪ It is not known if drug is present in breast milk.
▪ Patient should check with prescriber before breastfeeding.

REPRODUCTION

▪ The effectiveness of oral hormonal contraceptives can be reduced during drug therapy. Women of childbearing age using this type of contraception should use an additional barrier or alternative nonhormonal type of contraception during drug therapy and for 1 month after drug is discontinued.

Nursing Considerations

- Know that armodafinil shouldn't be given to patients with mitral valve prolapse syndrome or a history of left ventricular hypertrophy because drug may cause ischemic changes.

! **WARNING** Know whether patient has a history of alcoholism, stimulant abuse, or other substance abuse, and ensure compliance with armodafinil therapy. Watch for signs of misuse or abuse, including frequent prescription refill requests, increased frequency of dosing, and drug-seeking behavior. Also watch for evidence of excessive armodafinil use, including agitation, anxiety, diarrhea, nausea, nervousness, palpitations, sleep disturbances, and tremor.

- Know that armodafinil, like other CNS stimulants, may alter mood, perception, thinking, judgment, feelings, and motor skills and may produce signs that patient needs sleep.
- Giving drug to patient with a history of psychosis, emotional instability, or psychological illness with psychotic features may require a baseline behavioral assessment or frequent clinical observation.
- Stop drug at first sign of rash, and notify prescriber. Although rare, rash may indicate a potentially life-threatening event.
- Monitor patient for signs and symptoms of multisystem organ hypersensitivity, such as a fever, hematologic abnormalities, hepatitis, myocarditis, pruritus, rash, or any other serious abnormality because multiorgan hypersensitivity may vary in its presentation. While multisystem organ hypersensitivity has only occurred with modafinil, the possibility that it may occur with armodafinil cannot be ruled out because the two drugs are very closely related. Therefore, if suspected, notify prescriber immediately, expect to

discontinue drug, and provide supportive care, as ordered.
- Watch closely for suicidal tendencies, especially in patients with a psychiatric history.

PATIENT TEACHING

- Inform patient that armodafinil can help, but not cure, narcolepsy and that drug's full effects may not be seen right away.
- Instruct patient to take drug in the morning or 1 hr before start of work shift.
- Advise patient to avoid taking armodafinil within 2 hours of eating because food may delay time to peak drug effect and onset of action. If patient drinks grapefruit juice, encourage him to drink a consistent amount daily.

! **WARNING** Tell patient to stop taking armodafinil immediately and seek emergency medical treatment if he experiences an allergic reaction such as difficulty breathing or swallowing; hives; or swelling of eyes, face, lips, or tongue.

- Inform patient that drug can affect his concentration and ability to function and can hide signs of fatigue. Urge him not to drive or perform activities that require mental alertness until drug's full CNS effects are known.
- Instruct patient to continue previously prescribed treatments such as CPAP and not to stop without consulting prescriber first.
- Tell patient to contact prescriber immediately if she begins to experience psychiatric symptoms such as anxiety, depression, or signs of mania or psychosis.
- Advise patient to avoid alcohol with armodafinil because drug may decrease alertness.
- Encourage a regular sleeping pattern.
- Caution patient to avoid excessive intake of foods, beverages, and OTC drugs that contain caffeine because caffeine may lead to increased CNS stimulation.
- Advise patient to report the presence of blisters, mouth sores, peeling, or rash immediately to prescriber and to stop taking armodafinil. Also encourage patient to report any unusual or persistent signs and symptoms to prescriber.

- Inform woman that armodafinil can decrease effectiveness of certain contraceptives, including birth control pills and implantable hormonal contraceptives. If she uses such contraceptives, urge her to use an alternate birth control method during armodafinil therapy and for up to 1 month after it stops. Tell patient to notify prescriber if pregnancy is suspected or occurs and encourage her to notify the pregnancy exposure registry.
- Instruct patient to notify prescriber before taking any new medication, including over-the-counter preparations.
- Urge family or caregiver to watch patient closely for abnormal behaviors, including suicidal tendencies, especially if patient has a psychiatric history.
- Advise patient to keep follow-up appointments with prescriber so that her progress can be monitored.

asenapine
Secuado

asenapine maleate
Saphris

Class and Category
Pharmacologic class: Dopamine-serotonin antagonist
Therapeutic: Atypical antipsychotic

Indications and Dosages
✷ *To treat schizophrenia*
SUBLINGUAL TABLETS
Adults. *Initial:* 5 mg twice daily, increased to 10 mg twice daily after 1 wk, if needed and tolerated. *Maximum:* 10 mg twice daily.
TRANSDERMAL (SECUADO)
Adults. *Initial:* 3.8 mg/24 hr, increased to 5.7 mg/24 or 7.6/24 hr, if needed and tolerated.
✷ *To treat manic or mixed episodes associated with bipolar I disorder as monotherapy*
SUBLINGUAL TABLETS
Adults. 5 to 10 mg twice daily and then if 5-mg dose is used it may be increased to 10 mg, if needed and tolerated. *Maximum:* 10 mg twice daily.

Children age 10 and over. *Initial:* 2.5 mg twice daily increased after 3 days to 5 mg twice daily and after an additional 3 days to 10 mg twice daily, as needed and tolerated. *Maximum:* 10 mg twice daily.
✷ *To provide maintenance monotherapy in adults in the treatment of bipolar I disorder*
SUBLINGUAL TABLETS
Adults. 5 or 10 mg twice daily, whichever dosage patient was stabilized on. Then dosage decreased, if needed. *Maximum:* 10 mg twice daily.
✷ *As adjunct therapy with lithium or valproate to treat bipolar I disorder*
SUBLINGUAL TABLETS
Adults. *Initial:* 5 mg twice daily, increased to 10 mg twice daily, as needed. *Maximum:* 10 mg twice daily.
±**DOSAGE ADJUSTMENT** Dosage may be decreased to 5 mg twice daily if adverse reactions occur.

Drug Administration
P.O.
- Sublingual tablet should be removed from package only when ready for administration, using dry gloved hands. Firmly press and hold thumb button, and then pull out tablet pack from case. Then peel back the colored tab, being careful not to push tablet through the tab because doing so could damage tablet. Have patient place tablet under the tongue and let it dissolve completely. Slide tablet pack back into case until it clicks.
- Sublingual tablets should not be chewed, crushed, or swallowed.
- Patient should not eat or drink for at least 10 minutes after taking oral asenapine.

TRANSDERMAL
- Each transdermal system is to be worn for 24 hours only and only one transdermal system should be worn at any one time.
- Apply to a clean, dry, and intact skin area on the abdomen, hip, or upper arm or back. The transdermal system should be applied to a different application site each time a new transdermal system is applied.
- Do not cut open the pouch until ready to apply. Do not cut the transdermal system.
- If the transdermal system lifts at the edges, reattach by pressing firmly and smoothing down the edges. However, if it comes off, a new transdermal system should be applied.

- Discard each used transdermal system by folding it so the adhesive side sticks to itself and then discard.

Route	Onset	Peak	Duration
P.O.	Unknown	30–90 min	Unknown

Half-life: 24 hr

Mechanism of Action

May produce antipsychotic effects through antagonist actions at dopamine receptors, especially D_2, and serotonin receptors, especially 5-HT$_{2A}$.

Contraindications

Hypersensitivity to asenapine or its components, severe hepatic impairment

Interactions

DRUGS

antihypertensives, CNS depressants: Possibly enhanced effects

class I A and III antiarrhythmics, gatifloxacin, moxifloxacin, other antipsychotic drugs: Increased risk of prolonged QT interval

paroxetine: Possibly increased paroxetine effect

ACTIVITIES

alcohol use: Possibly enhanced effect

Adverse Reactions

CNS: Agitation, akathisia, anger, anxiety, depression, dizziness, dyskinesia, dystonia, extrapyramidal symptoms, fatigue, fever, gait disturbance, headache, hyperkinesia, insomnia, irritability, mania, masked facies, **neuroleptic malignant syndrome**, Parkinsonism, **seizures**, somnolence, **suicidal ideation**, syncope, tardive dyskinesia, torticollis, tremor

CV: Hyperlipidemia, hypertension, orthostatic hypotension, peripheral edema, **prolonged QT interval**, tachycardia, temporary bundle branch block

EENT: Accommodation disorder; blepharospasm; blurred vision; **choking**; diplopia; dry mouth; nasopharyngitis; nasal congestion; oral hypoesthesia or paresthesia; salivary hypersecretion; sublingual application-site reactions such as blisters, inflammation, oral ulcers, peeling, or sloughing; oropharyngeal pain; swollen tongue; taste perversion; toothache

ENDO: Hyperglycemia, diabetes mellitus, hyperprolactinemia

GI: Abdominal pain, constipation, dyspepsia, dysphagia, elevated liver enzymes, gastroesophageal reflux disease, increased appetite, stomach discomfort, vomiting

GU: Dysmenorrhea, enuresis (children)

HEME: Anemia, **leukopenia**, **neutropenia**, **thrombocytopenia**

MS: Arthralgia, dysarthria, extremity pain, muscle rigidity, myalgia

RESP: Dyspnea

SKIN: Photosensitivity reaction

Other: **Anaphylaxis**, **angioedema**, dehydration, elevated creatine kinase, **hyponatremia**, weight gain

Childbearing Considerations

PREGNANCY

- Pregnancy exposure registry: 1-866-961-2388 or http://womensmentalhealth.org / clinical-and-research-programs/pregnancy registry/.
- Drug may cause fetal harm. Neonates exposed to drug during the third trimester of pregnancy are at risk for extrapyramidal and withdrawal symptoms.
- Use with caution only if benefit to mother outweighs potential risk to fetus.

LACTATION

- It is not known if drug is present in breast milk.
- Patient should check with prescriber before breastfeeding.

Nursing Considerations

- Avoid asenapine in patients with a history of cardiac arrhythmias; conditions that might prolong the QT interval, such as bradycardia, hypokalemia, or hypomagnesemia; or congenital QT interval prolongation because of increased risk of torsades de pointes or sudden death.
- Know that asenapine shouldn't be used for dementia-related psychosis in elderly patients because of an increased risk of death.
- Use cautiously in patients with mild to moderate hepatic impairment.
- Use cautiously in patients with a history of seizures or who have conditions that may lower the seizure threshold, such as Alzheimer's dementia, because drug increases risk of seizures in these patients.

! **WARNING** Monitor patient closely even with the first dose for life-threatening hypersensitivity reactions that may include anaphylaxis and angioedema.

- Monitor elderly patients with psychosis closely for adverse effects because asenapine drug exposure has been found to be higher in these patients than in younger adult patients.
- Monitor patient's blood glucose level, lipid levels and weight, as ordered, because atypical antipsychotic drugs such as asenapine may cause metabolic changes. If patient is already diabetic, monitor blood glucose levels more closely.
- Know that the smallest dose of asenapine and the shortest duration of treatment should be used to minimize the risk of the patient developing tardive dyskinesia, which may become irreversible. If signs and symptoms appear, notify the prescriber, and know that the drug may have to be discontinued.

! **WARNING** Know that asenapine rarely may cause neuroleptic malignant syndrome or tardive dyskinesia. Monitor patient closely throughout therapy, and take safety precautions as needed. Expect to stop drug if any of these adverse effects occur.

- Monitor patient's CBC regularly, as ordered. Notify prescriber of any change because drug may have to be stopped.
- Monitor patient for trouble swallowing or excessive somnolence, which could predispose him to aspiration, choking, or injury.

PATIENT TEACHING

- Tell patient to remove tablet from package only when ready to take it and to use dry hands. Tell him to firmly press and hold thumb button, and then pull out tablet pack from case. Then, he should peel back the colored tab, being careful not to push tablet through the tab because doing so could damage tablet. Instruct patient to place tablet under his tongue and let it dissolve completely. Tell him to then slide tablet pack back into case until it clicks.
- Caution patient not to crush, chew, or swallow the sublingual tablets.
- Advise him not to eat or drink for at least 10 minutes after taking oral asenapine.
- Inform patient that application-site reactions may occur in the sublingual area, which may include blisters, inflammation, oral ulcers, peeling, or sloughing of tissue. Also inform patient that numbness or tingling of his mouth or throat may occur after administration of asenapine, but that it usually resolves within 1 hour.
- Teach patient how to apply the transdermal system if prescribed. Tell patient each transdermal system is to be worn for 24 hours only and only one transdermal system should be worn at any one time. Instruct patient to apply to a clean, dry, and intact skin area on the abdomen, hip, or upper arm or back. The transdermal system should be applied to a different application site each time a new transdermal system is applied. Caution the patient not to cut open the pouch until ready to apply, nor should the patient cut the transdermal system in any way. Tell patient if the transdermal system lifts at the edges to reattach by pressing firmly and smoothing down the edges. However, if it comes off, a new transdermal system should be applied.
- Tell patient using the transdermal system to discard each used transdermal system by folding it so the adhesive side sticks to itself and then discard. Advise patient if burning or irritation occurs, the transdermal system should be removed and a new one applied in a different site. Although patient may shower, inform the patient that it is not known if swimming or taking a bath is safe. Caution patient not to apply external heat sources over the transdermal system.
- Teach patient the signs and symptoms of a serious allergic reaction and to seek immediate emergency treatment if present. Also inform patient of other serious adverse reactions and tell patient to report any persistent, severe, or unusual effects to prescriber immediately, including abnormal movements.
- Urge patient to avoid alcohol while taking asenapine.
- Instruct diabetic patient taking asenapine to monitor blood glucose levels closely because hyperglycemia may occur.

- Advise patient to get up slowly from lying or sitting position during asenapine therapy to minimize orthostatic hypotension.
- Caution patient to avoid hazardous activities until drug's effects are known. Also, alert patient and family of increased risk for falls, especially if patient has other medical conditions or takes medication that may affect the nervous system.
- Urge patient to avoid activities that raise body temperature suddenly, such as strenuous exercise and exposure to extreme heat, and to compensate for situations that cause dehydration, such as vomiting or diarrhea.
- Tell patient that if he has a preexisting low WBC or a history of drug-induced low WBC, he should have his CBC monitored throughout asenapine therapy.
- Inform prescriber of any new medication being prescribed or use of any over-the-counter drugs.
- Advise female patient of childbearing age to notify prescriber if she intends to become or suspects that she is pregnant during therapy, because drug may affect the fetus. Inform her that if she does become pregnant she should contact the pregnancy registry.

aspirin
(acetylsalicylic acid, ASA)
Aspir-81, Aspirin, Aspir-Low, Bayer, Durlaza, Ecotrin, Empirin, Miniprin, Novasen (CAN), St. Joseph Children's, Supasa (CAN), Vazalore, Zorprin

☰ Class and Category
Pharmacologic class: Salicylate
Therapeutic class: NSAID (anti-inflammatory, antiplatelet, antipyretic, nonopioid analgesic)

☰ Indications and Dosages
✳ *To relieve mild pain or fever*
CHEWABLE TABLETS, CONTROLLED-RELEASE TABLETS, ENTERIC-COATED TABLETS, SOLUTION, TABLETS, TIMED-RELEASE TABLETS, SUPPOSITORIES
Adults and adolescents. 325 to 650 mg every 4 hr, as needed; or 500 mg every 3 hr, as needed; or 1,000 mg every 6 hr, as needed. *Maximum:* 4,000 mg daily.

Children ages 2 to 12. 10 to 15 mg/kg/dose every 4 hr, as needed, up to 80 mg/kg daily.
✳ *To relieve mild to moderate pain from inflammation, as in rheumatoid arthritis and osteoarthritis*
CAPSULES (VAZALORE), CHEWABLE TABLETS, CONTROLLED-RELEASE TABLETS, ENTERIC-COATED TABLETS, SOLUTION, TABLETS, TIMED-RELEASE TABLETS, SUPPOSITORIES
Adults and adolescents. 3 g daily in divided doses.
✳ *To treat juvenile rheumatoid arthritis*
CAPSULES (VAZALORE), CHEWABLE TABLETS, CONTROLLED-RELEASE TABLETS, ENTERIC-COATED TABLETS, SOLUTION, TABLETS, TIMED-RELEASE TABLETS, SUPPOSITORIES
Children. 90 to 130 mg/kg daily in divided doses every 6 to 8 hr.
✳ *To reduce the risk of recurrent transient ischemic attacks or ischemic stroke*
CAPSULES (VAZALORE), TABLET
Adults. 50 to 325 mg once daily.
✳ *To reduce the severity of or prevent acute MI*
TABLETS
Adults. *Initial:* 160 to 325 mg as soon as MI is suspected. *Maintenance:* 160 to 325 mg daily for 30 days.
✳ *To treat suspected acute MI*
CAPSULES (VAZALORE)
Adults. 160 mg given as soon as infarction is suspected, then once daily for 30 days postinfarction.
✳ *To reduce risk of MI in patients with previous MI, stable angina, or unstable angina*
CAPSULES (VAZALORE), TABLETS
Adults. 75 to 325 mg daily.
✳ *To reduce the risk of death and MI in patients with chronic coronary artery disease; to reduce risk of death and recurrent stroke in patients who have had an ischemic stroke or transient ischemic attack*
E.R. CAPSULES (DURLAZA)
Adults. 162.5 mg once daily.
✳ *To prepare patient for carotid endarterectomy*
CAPSULES (VAZALORE), TABLETS
Adults. 80 mg once daily to 650 mg twice daily, started presurgery.
✳ *Adjunct therapy with coronary artery bypass graft*

CAPSULES (VAZALORE), TABLETS

Adults. 325 mg daily starting 6 hr after procedure and continued for 1 yr.

✻ *Adjunct treatment for percutaneous transluminal coronary angioplasty*

TABLETS

Adults. 325 mg 2 to 3 hr before procedure, then 160 to 325 mg daily.

✻ *To treat spondyloarthropathies*

CAPSULES (VAZALORE), TABLETS

Adults. Up to 4 g daily in divided doses.

✻ *To treat arthritis and pleurisy of systemic lupus erythematosus (SLE)*

CAPSULES (VAZALORE), TABLETS

Adults. *Initial:* 3 g daily, then dosage adjusted as needed.

⬚ Drug Administration

P.O.

- Administer with food and a full glass of water to reduce adverse gastrointestinal effects.
- Have patient swallow whole enteric-coated or extended-release forms. These forms should not be chewed, crushed, or split.
- Extended-release capsules should be taken with a full glass of water at the same time every day. Capsules should be swallowed whole.
- For suspected MI, patient should chew non-enteric-coated, immediate-release aspirin to speed its anti-blood-clotting properties.
- Use calibrated device to measure dosage when administering solution form.

RECTAL

- Suppositories should be refrigerated until time of administration.

Route	Onset	Peak	Duration
P.O. (chewable)	20 min	20 min	1–4 hr
P.O. (tabs)	5–30 min	25–40 min	1–4 hr
P.O. (buffered)	5–30 min	1–2 hr	1–4 hr
P.O. (E.R.)	5–30 min	1–4 hr	4–6 hr
P.O. (Enteric)	5–30 min	Unknown	1–4 hr
P.O. (Solution)	5–30 min	15–40 min	1–4 hr
P.R.	Unknown	3–4 hr	Unknown

Half-life: 15 min–6 hr

⬚ Mechanism of Action

Blocks the activity of cyclooxygenase, the enzyme needed for prostaglandin synthesis. Prostaglandins, important mediators in the inflammatory response, cause local vasodilation with swelling and pain. With blocking of cyclooxygenase and inhibition of prostaglandins, inflammatory symptoms subside. Pain is also relieved because prostaglandins play a role in pain transmission from the periphery to the spinal cord. Aspirin inhibits platelet aggregation by interfering with production of thromboxane A2, a substance that stimulates platelet aggregation. Aspirin acts on the heat-regulating center in the hypothalamus and causes peripheral vasodilation, diaphoresis, and heat loss.

⬚ Contraindications

Active bleeding or coagulation disorders; breastfeeding (continuous high dose); fever, chickenpox, or flu-like symptoms in children and teens; current or recent GI bleed or ulcers; hypersensitivity to aspirin, aspirin products, other NSAIDs, tartrazine dye, or their components; third trimester of pregnancy

⬚ Interactions

DRUGS

ACE inhibitors: beta blockers: Decreased antihypertensive effect

acetazolamide: Possibly acetazolamide toxicity

ammonium chloride and other urine acidifiers: May increase level of aspirin with possibility of aspirin toxicity

antacids, urine alkalinizers: Decreased aspirin effectiveness

anticoagulants, antiplatelets: Increased risk of bleeding; prolonged bleeding time

corticosteroids: Increased excretion and decreased blood level of aspirin

digoxin: Increased risk of digitalis toxicity

diuretics: Possibly decreased diuretic effectiveness, especially in patients with renal impairment

heparin: Increased risk of bleeding

ibuprofen, naproxen: Possibly reduced cardioprotective and stroke preventive effects of aspirin

methotrexate: Increased blood level and decreased excretion of methotrexate, causing toxicity

other NSAIDs: Possibly decreased blood NSAID level and increased risk of adverse GI effects *oral antidiabetic agents:* Possibly enhanced hypoglycemic effects

selective serotonin reuptake inhibitors (SSRIs): Increased risk of upper gastrointestinal bleeding

uricosuric agents: Decreased uricosuric effect

valproic acid: Possibly increased valproic acid level and incidence of adverse reactions

ACTIVITIES

alcohol use: Increased risk of ulcers

Adverse Reactions

CNS: Confusion, **CNS depression**
EENT: Hearing loss, tinnitus
GI: Diarrhea, **GI bleeding**, heartburn, **hepatotoxicity**, nausea, stomach pain, vomiting
HEME: Decreased blood iron level, **leukopenia, prolonged bleeding time**, shortened life span of RBCs, **thrombocytopenia**
RESP: Bronchospasm
SKIN: Ecchymosis, rash, urticaria
Other: Angioedema, Reye's syndrome, salicylism (CNS depression, confusion, diaphoresis, diarrhea, difficulty hearing, dizziness, headache, hyperventilation, lassitude, tinnitus, and vomiting) with regular use of large doses

Childbearing Considerations

PREGNANCY

- Drug can cause fetal harm especially in the third trimester, as drug may cause premature closure of the ductus arteriosus in the fetus.
- Salicylates have also been associated with altered maternal and neonatal hemostasis mechanisms, decreased birth weight, and perinatal mortality.
- Drug is generally not recommended for use during pregnancy and drug should not be used at 20 weeks gestation or later. Low-dose aspirin (60 to 100 mg daily) may be used sometimes with clotting disorders, recurrent pregnancy loss, or preeclampsia.

LABOR & DELIVERY

- Drug should not be used 1 week before and during labor and delivery because of the potential for bleeding at delivery.

LACTATION

- Drug is present in breast milk.
- A decision should be made to discontinue breastfeeding or the drug to avoid potential adverse reactions in the breastfed infant unless low-dose aspirin is prescribed as an antiplatelet.
- If low-dose aspirin is used, infant should be monitored for bleeding and bruising.

Nursing Considerations

- Be aware that elderly patients and dehydrated febrile children are at higher risk for toxicity.
- Monitor salicylate level in patients receiving long-term therapy. Ask about tinnitus. This reaction usually occurs when blood aspirin level reaches or exceeds maximum dosage for therapeutic effect.
- Expect aspirin therapy to be temporarily halted 5 to 7 days before elective surgery to reduce risk of bleeding.

PATIENT TEACHING

! WARNING Advise parents not to give aspirin to a child or adolescent with chickenpox or flu symptoms because of risk of Reye's syndrome (rare life-threatening reaction). Tell them to consult prescriber for alternative drugs.

- Advise adult patient taking low-dose aspirin not to also take ibuprofen or naproxen because these drugs may reduce the cardioprotective and stroke preventive effects of aspirin.
- Instruct patient to take aspirin with food or after meals because it may cause GI upset if taken on an empty stomach.
- Advise patient prescribed Durlaza to take the capsule with a full glass of water at the same time every day and to swallow the capsule whole.
- Advise patient to avoid alcohol while taking aspirin to decrease risk of ulcers.
- Instruct patient to stop taking aspirin and notify prescriber if any symptoms of stomach or intestinal bleeding occur, such as passage of bloody or tarry stools or if patient is coughing up blood or vomit that looks like coffee grounds.
- Advise patient with tartrazine allergy not to take aspirin.
- Tell patient to consult prescriber before taking aspirin with any prescription drug for blood disorder, diabetes, gout, or arthritis.
- Tell patient not to use aspirin if it has a strong vinegar-like odor.

- Advise pregnant women to check with prescriber before taking aspirin at 20 weeks or later. Likewise, tell breastfeeding mothers breastfeeding is usually not recommended with aspirin use. If low-dose aspirin is prescribed, caution mother to monitor breastfed infant for bleeding and bruising.

atazanavir sulfate
Reyataz

⬓ Class and Category
Pharmacologic class: Protease inhibitor
Therapeutic class: Antiretroviral

⬓ Indications and Dosages
✳ *As adjunct to treat HIV-1 infection*

CAPSULES, ORAL POWDER
Adults who are treatment-experienced or treatment-naïve. 300 mg once daily in combination with ritonavir 100 mg once daily.

Adults who are HIV treatment-naïve and cannot tolerate ritonavir. 400 mg once daily.

Adults who are HIV treatment-naïve and also taking efavirenz, adults who are treatment-experienced and also taking both H2RA and tenofovir DF. 400 mg once daily in combination with ritonavir 100 mg once daily.

Children ages 13 to 18 who weigh at least 40 kg (88 lb) and are HIV treatment-naïve and cannot tolerate ritonavir. 400 mg once daily.

Children ages 6 to 18 who weigh at least 35 kg (77 lb) who are treatment-experienced or treatment-naïve. 300 mg once daily in combination with ritonavir 100 mg once daily.

Children ages 6 to 18 who weigh less than 35 kg (77 lb) but at least 15 kg (33 lb) who are treatment-experienced or treatment-naïve. 200 mg once daily in combination with ritonavir 100 mg once daily.

ORAL POWDER
Children up to age 6 who weigh less than 25 kg (55 lb) but at least 15 kg (33 lb) who are treatment-experienced or treatment-naïve. 250 mg once daily in combination with ritonavir 80 mg once daily.

Infants 3 months of age and over who weigh less than 15 kg (33 lb) but at least 5 kg (11 lb) who are treatment-experienced or treatment-naïve. 200 mg once daily in combination with ritonavir 80 mg once daily.

±**DOSAGE ADJUSTMENT** For HIV treatment-experienced pregnant patients who are in the second or third trimester and also being treated with either H2RA or tenofovir DF, atazanavir dosage increased to 400 mg once daily and given with ritonavir 100 mg once daily. For HIV treatment-naïve adults with mild hepatic impairment, atazanavir dosage increased to 400 mg once daily and given without ritonavir. For HIV treatment-naïve adults with moderate hepatic impairment, atazanavir dosage kept at 300 mg once daily but given without ritonavir. For pediatric patient who weighs 5 kg (11 lb) to less than 10 kg (22 lb) and does not tolerate the 200-mg (4 packets) dose of oral powder and has not previously taken an HIV protease inhibitor, dosage may be decreased to 150 mg (3 packets) with close HIV viral load monitoring.

⬓ Drug Administration

P.O.
- Do not administer atazanavir at the same time as H_2-receptor antagonists or proton pump inhibitors.
- Administer atazanavir with food.
- If patient changes from capsule form to oral powder or vice versa, dosage adjustment may be needed.
- Capsules should be swallowed whole by the patient. Do not open.
- Mix oral powder as follows: Determine number of packets needed and tap each packet to settle powder. Using a clean pair of scissors, cut each packet along the dotted line. Mix with food such as applesauce or yogurt using a minimum of 1 tablespoon of food mixed in a container and then administered to patient. Follow with mixing second tablespoon in container with food and administering the residual mixture.
- For infants, oral powder may be mixed with 30 ml of infant formula, milk, or water if infant can drink from a cup. After administering drug in this way, add 15 ml of liquid to the cup and have child drink the residual mixture. If water was used to mix the drug, the child should immediately be given something to eat.

- For infants less than 6 months old who cannot drink from a cup or eat solid food, mix with 10 ml of infant formula in a medicine cup and give using an oral dosing syringe and administer into either inner cheek of infant. Add an additional 10 ml of formula to cup used to mix drug and formula, draw up residual mixture, and administer to infant.
- Do not use an infant bottle to administer drug, because full dose may not be delivered.
- When drug is mixed with food or liquid, it must be administered within 1 hr of preparation. Mixture may remain at room temperature during this time.
- Administer ritonavir, if prescribed, immediately after atazanavir.
- Oral powder contains 35 mg of phenylalanine, which can be harmful if patient has phenylketonuria. Capsules contain no phenylalanine.

Route	Onset	Peak	Duration
P.O.	Unknown	2–3 hr	Unknown

Half-life: 7–8 hr

☰ Mechanism of Action

Selectively inhibits the virus-specific processing of specific polyproteins in HIV-1-infected cells to prevent formation of mature virions.

☰ Contraindications

Concurrent therapy with alfuzosin, cisapride, dihydroergotamine, elbasvir/grazoprevir, ergonovine, ergotamine, glecaprevir/pibrentasvir, indinavir, irinotecan, lovastatin, lurasidone, methylergonovine, midazolam (oral), nevirapine, pimozide, rifampin, sildenafil (when used for treatment of pulmonary arterial hypertension), simvastatin, St. John's wort, triazolam; hypersensitivity to atazanavir or any of its components

☰ Interactions

DRUGS

amiodarone, atorvastatin, bepridil, buprenorphine, colchicine, diltiazem, ethinyl and norethindrone, felodipine, fluticasone, ketoconazole, itraconazole, immunosuppressants, lidocaine (systemic) lurasidone, midazolam, nicardipine, nifedipine, norbuprenorphine, PDE5 inhibitors

(sildenafil, tadalafil, vardenafil), quetiapine, rifabutin, quinidine, rosuvastatin, salmeterol, trazodone, tricyclic antidepressants, verapamil, voxilaprevir: Increased plasma concentrations of these drugs with possible increased risk of adverse effects that could be serious or life-threatening

antacids, buffered medications, efavirenz, H_2-receptor antagonists, proton pump inhibitors: Decreased plasma concentration of atazanavir, decreasing effectiveness

boceprevir: Decreased plasma concentrations of both atazanavir and ritonavir when administered together, decreasing effectiveness of both drugs

bosentan: Decreased plasma concentration of atazanavir and increased plasma concentration of bosentan

carbamazepine: Decreased plasma concentration of atazanavir and increased plasma concentration of carbamazepine, increasing risk of serious carbamazepine-induced adverse reactions

clarithromycin: Increased plasma concentration of both atazanavir and clarithromycin, increasing risk of QT prolongation

didanosine: Decreased plasma concentration of both atazanavir and didanosine, with decreased effectiveness

ethinyl estradiol and norgestimate: Decreased plasma concentration of ethinyl estradiol and increased plasma concentration of norgestimate, possibly affecting contraceptive effectiveness

lamotrigine: Possibly decreased plasma concentration of lamotrigine, with increased risk of seizure activity

other protease inhibitors such as saquinavir: Possibly increased plasma concentration of protease inhibitor

phenobarbital, phenytoin: Decreased plasma concentration of atazanavir, phenobarbital, and phenytoin, decreasing effectiveness and increasing risk of seizures

ritonavir: Increased plasma concentration of atazanavir and risk of serious adverse reactions

tenofovir disoproxil fumarate: Decreased plasma concentration of atazanavir; increased plasma concentration of tenofovir

voriconazole: Decreased plasma concentrations of both atazanavir and voriconazole in patients with a functional

CYP2C19 allele; decreased plasma concentration of atazanavir and increased plasma concentration of voriconazole in patients without a functional CYP2C19 allele

warfarin: Increased plasma concentration of warfarin, increasing risk of serious or life-threatening bleeding

Adverse Reactions

CNS: Depression, dizziness, fever, headache, insomnia, peripheral nervous system abnormalities

CV: Cardiac conduction abnormalities (second- or third-degree AV block, left bundle branch block), edema, elevated cholesterol and triglyceride levels, peripheral edema, **QT prolongation**

EENT: Nasal congestion (children), oropharyngeal pain (children), rhinorrhea (children), scleral icterus

ENDO: Diabetes mellitus, fat redistribution, hyperglycemia, **hypoglycemia (children)**

GI: Abdominal pain, cholecystitis, cholelithiasis, cholestasis, diarrhea, elevated liver and pancreatic enzymes, **hepatic dysfunction,** hyperbilirubinemia, jaundice, nausea, **pancreatitis,** vomiting

GU: Chronic kidney disease, granulomatous interstitial nephritis, interstitial nephritis, nephrolithiasis

HEME: Decreased hemoglobin or platelet count, **neutropenia**

MS: Arthralgia, elevated creatine kinase, extremity pain (children), myalgia

RESP: Cough (children), wheezing (children)

SKIN: Alopecia, **erythema multiforme,** pruritus, rash, **Stevens–Johnson syndrome, toxic skin eruptions**

Other: Angioedema, drug reaction with eosinophilia and systemic symptoms (DRESS), immune reconstitution syndrome

Childbearing Considerations

PREGNANCY

- Pregnancy exposure registry: 1-800-258-4263.
- It is not known if drug can cause fetal harm.
- Use with caution only if benefit to mother outweighs potential risk to fetus.
- Drug has potential to increase risk for hyperbilirubinemia and lactic acidosis syndrome in mother during pregnancy.

LABOR & DELIVERY

- Drug can cause increased risk of adverse reactions in mother during the first

2 months after delivery because drug exposure could be higher during this time.
- Neonate may develop severe hyperbilirubinemia during the first few days following birth if exposed to drug in utero.

LACTATION

- Drug is present in breast milk.
- The Centers for Disease Control and Prevention recommends that HIV-1 infected mothers not breastfeed to avoid risking postnatal transmission of HIV-1 infection as well as the possibility of potential drug-induced adverse reactions in the infant.

Nursing Considerations

- Be aware that atazanavir is not recommended for HIV treatment-experienced patients with end-stage renal disease managed with hemodialysis. Expect all patients to have renal laboratory testing prior to atazanavir being initiated and periodically throughout drug therapy. Testing should include estimated creatinine clearance, serum creatinine, and urinalysis with microscopic examination. If kidney disease occurs and becomes progressive, expect that atazanavir may be discontinued.
- Expect patients with underlying hepatitis B or C viral infections or marked elevations in transaminases that have occurred before atazanavir treatment to have hepatic function evaluated prior to start of therapy and periodically during treatment, because these patients may experience further transaminase elevations or hepatic decompensation while taking atazanavir.
- Be aware that capsule form, without concomitant ritonavir therapy, is not recommended for the treatment-experienced patient with prior virologic failure.
- Be aware that patients with preexisting conduction system disease should be monitored by ECG.
- Monitor patient closely for the appearance of a rash. Although common and usually not affecting the use of atazanavir, some rashes may become severe and life-threatening. Report all rashes to prescriber and expect drug to be discontinued if rash becomes severe.
- Report signs or symptoms suggestive of cholelithiasis or nephrolithiasis to prescriber, as drug may have to be

temporarily interrupted or discontinued if confirmed.

- Monitor patient's blood glucose level throughout atazanavir therapy, because drug has been associated with new-onset diabetes mellitus and exacerbation of preexisting diabetes mellitus. Treat hyperglycemia as prescribed.
- Be aware that immune reconstitution syndrome has occurred in patients treated with combination antiretroviral therapy, including atazanavir. The inflammatory response predisposes susceptible patients to opportunistic infections such as cytomegalovirus infection, *Mycobacterium avium* infection, *Pneumocystis jiroveci* pneumonia, or tuberculosis. Autoimmune disorders such as Graves' disease, Guillain–Barré syndrome, or polymyositis have also occurred. Report sudden or unusual adverse reactions to prescriber.
- Monitor patients with hemophilia for increased bleeding, because spontaneous skin hemarthrosis and hematomas have occurred in these patients while taking atazanavir. Provide supportive care as prescribed.

PATIENT TEACHING

- Instruct patient to take atazanavir with food.
- Instruct patient prescribed capsule form of atazanavir not to open capsule and to ingest it whole.
- Instruct patient, parent, or caregiver how to mix oral powder form, if prescribed. Tell parent/caregiver of an infant younger than 6 months who cannot drink from a cup or eat solid food to mix with infant formula but to administer it with an oral dosing syringe. The drug should not be delivered using an infant bottle.
- Alert patient, parent, or caregiver using the oral powder form of atazanavir that it contains 35 mg of phenylalanine, which can be harmful if patient has phenylketonuria. The capsule form of drug contains no phenylalanine.
- Tell patient prescribed both atazanavir and ritonavir to take atazanavir first and then immediately take ritonavir.
- Stress importance of maintaining adequate hydration while taking drug because of risk of chronic kidney disease.
- Alert patient that atazanavir may redistribute or cause accumulation of body fat which may include breast enlargement,

a buffalo hump on the back of the neck, central obesity, and wasting appearance of extremities and face.

- Advise patient to report the appearance of a rash to prescriber. Inform patient that severe skin reactions may occur that begin with a rash and caution patient to report any rash immediately to prescriber.
- Advise patient to report dizziness or light-headedness to prescriber because drug may causes changes in how the heart functions. Also tell patient to report any yellowing of the skin or whites of the eyes.
- Stress importance of maintaining adequate hydration throughout therapy, as drug may cause chronic kidney disease.
- Review signs and symptoms of the presence of gallbladder or kidney stones with patient and advise patient to notify prescriber if any such signs and symptoms develop, as drug may have to be temporarily withheld or discontinued.
- Stress importance of informing all prescribers of atazanavir therapy, because drug interacts with many other drugs. Tell patient not to take any over-the-counter medication, including herbals, without consulting prescriber first.
- Tell patient with diabetes mellitus to monitor glucose levels during atazanavir therapy, as adjustments in her diabetes treatment regimen may be needed. Also review signs and symptoms of diabetes mellitus with all patients, because new-onset diabetes mellitus has occurred during atazanavir therapy.
- Instruct patient to report any signs and symptoms of infection or persistent or unusual adverse effects to prescriber.
- Encourage women who become pregnant to register on the pregnancy exposure registry through their prescriber.
- Instruct women not to breastfeed while taking atazanavir, as drug may pass through breast milk to the infant.

atenolol

Tenormin

Class and Category

Pharmacologic class: Beta-adrenergic blocker (beta$_1$ and at high doses beta$_2$)

Therapeutic class: Antianginal,
antihypertensive

Indications and Dosages

* *To treat angina pectoris; to treat hypertension*

TABLETS

Adults. 50 mg daily increased, as needed,
after 1 to 2 wk to 100 mg daily. *Maximum:*
100 mg for treatment of hypertension;
200 mg for treatment of angina pectoris.

* *To treat acute myocardial infarction in
hemodynamically stable patients*

I.V. INJECTION

Adults. 5 mg followed in 10 min by 5 mg.

TABLETS

Adults. *Initial:* 50 mg following last I.V. dose,
then 50 mg 12 hr later. *Maintenance:* 100 mg
once daily or 50 mg twice daily for 6 to 9 days
or until discharge.

±**DOSAGE ADJUSTMENT** Dosage usually not
increased above 50 mg daily P.O. for the
elderly and for patients with a creatinine
clearance of 15 to 35 ml/min. For patients
with creatinine clearance less than
15 ml/min, dosage reduced to 25 mg daily.

Drug Administration

P.O.

- Take patient's apical pulse and blood
pressure before each dose.
- Administer at about the same time each day.
- Do not discontinue abruptly.

I.V.

- Drug should be administered in a coronary
care or similar unit immediately after patient's
hemodynamic condition has stabilized.
- Administer each I.V. injection dose over
5 minutes.
- Protect from light.
- Keep ampules in outer packaging until time
of use.
- Store at controlled room temperature of
20–25°C (68–77°F).
- *Incompatibilities:* None reported by
manufacturer

Route	Onset	Peak	Duration
P.O.	1 hr	2–4 hr	24 hr

Half-life: 6–7 hr

Mechanism of Action

Inhibits stimulation of beta$_1$-receptor sites,
located mainly in the heart, decreasing
cardiac excitability, cardiac output, and
myocardial oxygen demand. Atenolol also
acts to decrease release of renin from the
kidneys, aiding in reducing blood pressure.
At high doses, it inhibits stimulation of beta$_2$
receptors in the lungs, which may cause
bronchoconstriction.

Contraindications

Anesthesia with agents that produce
myocardial depression, cardiogenic shock,
heart block greater than first degree,
hypersensitivity to atenolol, other beta
blockers or their components, overt heart or
uncontrolled failure, hypotension, metabolic
acidosis, pheochromocytoma in the absence
of alpha-blockade, right ventricular failure
secondary to pulmonary hypertension,
severe peripheral arterial disorders, sick sinus
syndrome, sinus bradycardia

Interactions

DRUGS

*amiodarone and class I antiarrhythmics such
as disopyramide:* Additive atenolol effects
with increased risk of asystole, heart failure,
and severe bradycardia
anesthetic agents: Possibly induced
hypotensive state with associated reflex
tachycardia
*calcium channel blockers, such as verapamil
and diltiazem:* Possibly symptomatic
bradycardia and conduction abnormalities
*catecholamine-depleting drugs, such
as guanethidine, reserpine:* Additive
antihypertensive effect
clonidine: Possible rebound hypertension
following discontinuation of clonidine
digoxin, fingolimod: Possible potentiate
bradycardia
dihydropyridines such as nifedipine:
Increased risk of cardiac failure and
hypotension in patients with latent cardiac
insufficiency
NSAIDs: Possible blunting of the
antihypertensive effect of atenolol

Adverse Reactions

CNS: Depression, disorientation, dizziness,
drowsiness, emotional lability, fatigue, fever,
lethargy, light-headedness, short-term
memory loss, vertigo
CV: Arrhythmias, including bradycardia
and heart block; cardiogenic shock;
cold arms and legs; mitral insufficiency;

myocardial reinfarction; orthostatic hypotension; Raynaud's phenomenon
EENT: Dry eyes, **laryngospasm**, pharyngitis
GI: Diarrhea, **ischemic colitis, mesenteric artery thrombosis**, nausea
GU: Renal failure
HEME: Agranulocytosis
MS: Leg pain
RESP: Bronchospasm, dyspnea, **pulmonary emboli, respiratory distress**, wheezing
SKIN: Erythematous rash
Other: Allergic reaction

Childbearing Considerations
PREGNANCY
- Drug crosses placental barrier and can cause fetal harm.
- Use of drug starting in the second trimester has caused a lower birth rate for gestational age of fetus; in the third trimester bradycardia may occur in the fetus.
- Use with caution only if benefit to mother outweighs potential risk to fetus.

LABOR & DELIVERY
- Newborns are at risk for bradycardia and hypoglycemia if exposed to drug in utero.

LACTATION
- Drug is present in breast milk.
- Patient should check with prescriber before breastfeeding because breastfed infant may be at risk for bradycardia and hypoglycemia.

Nursing Considerations
- Use atenolol cautiously in patients with heart failure controlled by digitalis glycosides or diuretics, patients with conduction abnormalities or left ventricular dysfunction who take verapamil or diltiazem, patients with arterial circulatory disorders, and patients with impaired renal function.
- Use atenolol cautiously in diabetic patients because it may mask tachycardia caused by hypoglycemia. Unlike other beta-adrenergic blockers, it doesn't mask other signs of hypoglycemia, cause hypoglycemia, or delay the return of blood glucose to a normal level.
- Monitor patient for heart failure. At first sign of heart failure, expect patient to receive a digitalis glycoside, a diuretic, or both and to be monitored closely. If failure continues, expect to stop atenolol.
- Closely monitor patient with hyperthyroidism because atenolol may

mask some signs of thyrotoxicosis. Abrupt withdrawal of atenolol may precipitate thyrotoxicosis.
- Know that if patient also receives clonidine, expect to stop atenolol several days before gradually withdrawing clonidine. Then expect to restart atenolol therapy several days after clonidine has been discontinued.
- Stop atenolol and notify prescriber if patient develops bradycardia, hypotension, or other serious adverse reaction.
- Be aware that chronic beta blocker therapy such as atenolol is not routinely withheld prior to major surgery because the benefits outweigh the risks associated with its use with general anesthesia and surgical procedures.

PATIENT TEACHING
- Instruct patient to take drug at about the same time daily and not to stop taking atenolol abruptly. Otherwise, angina may worsen, and an MI or arrhythmia may occur.
- Tell him to perform minimal physical activity to prevent chest pain when he is being weaned from atenolol therapy.
- Instruct patient to take a missed dose as soon as possible. However, if it's within 8 hours of the next scheduled dose, tell him to skip the missed dose and return to his regular schedule.
- Explain that atenolol may alter serum glucose level and mask hypoglycemia.
- Inform the patient that he may experience fatigue and reduced tolerance to exercise and that he should notify his prescriber if this interferes with his normal lifestyle.

atogepant
Qulipta

Class and Category
Pharmacologic class: Calcitonin gene-related peptide (CGRP) receptor antagonist
Therapeutic class: Antimigraine drug

Indications and Dosages
⁎ To prevent episodic migraine

TABLETS
Adults. 10 mg, 30 mg, or 60 mg once daily.

±**DOSAGE ADJUSTMENT** For patients with severe renal impairment and end-stage renal disease or who are taking strong CYP3A4 inhibitors, dosage limited to 10 mg once daily. For patients who are taking OATP inhibitors, dosage limited to 10 mg or 30 mg once daily. For patients who are taking strong or moderate CYP3A4 inducers, dosage limited to 30 mg or 60 mg once daily.

Drug Administration

P.O.

- Do not administer drug with grapefruit juice.
- Administer drug after dialysis for patients with end-stage renal disease undergoing intermittent dialysis.

Route	Onset	Peak	Duration
P.O.	Unknown	1–2 hr	Unknown

Half-life: 11 hr

Mechanism of Action

Blocks the CGRP protein from attaching to receptors to prevent migraine headaches.

Contraindications

Hypersensitivity to atogepant or its components

Interactions

DRUGS

CYP3A4 strong or moderate inducers such as carbamazepine, efavirenz, etravirine, phenytoin, rifampin, St. John's wort: Decreased exposure to atogepant with decreased effectiveness

FOODS

grapefruit, grapefruit juice: Increased exposure of atogepant with increased risk of adverse reactions

Adverse Reactions

CNS: Fatigue, somnolence
GI: Anorexia, constipation, elevated liver enzymes, fatigue
OTHER: Weight loss

Childbearing Considerations

PREGNANCY

- It is not known if drug can cause fetal harm.
- Use with caution only if benefit to mother outweighs potential risk to fetus.
- Be aware that women with migraine may be at increased risk of gestational hypertension and preeclampsia during pregnancy.

LACTATION

- It is not known if drug is present in breast milk.
- Patient should check with prescriber before breastfeeding.

Nursing Considerations

- Know that atogepant should not be administered to patients with severe hepatic impairment.
- Be aware that the starting dose for patients age 65 and over should be initiated at the low end of the dosing range because of increased frequency of decreased cardiac, hepatic, and renal function.

PATIENT TEACHING

- Advise patient to report all drug use to prescriber, including over-the-counter medication and herbal products.
- Instruct patient to avoid eating grapefruit or drinking grapefruit juice while taking atogepant.

atomoxetine hydrochloride

Strattera

Class and Category

Pharmacologic class: Selective norepinephrine reuptake inhibitor
Therapeutic class: Anti–ADHD agent

Indications and Dosages

✳ *To treat attention deficit hyperactivity disorder (ADHD)*

CAPSULES

Adults and children weighing more than 70 kg (154 lb). *Initial:* 40 mg daily, increased after at least 3 days to 80 mg daily. After 2 to 4 additional wk, dosage may be increased to 100 mg daily if optimal response hasn't been achieved. *Maximum:* 100 mg daily.
Adults and children weighing 70 kg (154 lb) or less. *Initial:* 0.5 mg/kg daily, increased after at least 3 days to 1.2 mg/kg daily as needed. *Maximum:* 1.4 mg/kg or 100 mg daily, whichever is less.

±**DOSAGE ADJUSTMENT** For patients with moderate (Child-Pugh Class B) hepatic impairment, dosage reduced by 50%. For patients with severe (Child-Pugh Class C) hepatic impairment, dosage reduced by 75%.

For patients weighing more than 70 kg and taking strong CYP2D6 inhibitors (fluoxetine, paroxetine, or quinidine), initial dosage of 40 mg daily increased to 80 mg daily only if symptoms fail to improve after 4 wk. For patients weighing 70 kg or less and taking strong CYP2D6 inhibitors or are CYP2D6 poor metabolizers, initial dosage of 0.5 mg/kg daily increased to 1.2 mg/kg daily only if symptoms fail to improve after 4 wk.

Drug Administration

P.O.

- Administer capsules whole. Do not open capsules for administration.
- If capsule inadvertently opens, immediately wash hands and any surface drug touched.

Route	Onset	Peak	Duration
P.O.	Unknown	1–2 hr	>24 hr

Half-life: 5.2 hr

Mechanism of Action

Selectively inhibits presynaptic norepinephrine transport in the nervous system to increase attention span and produce a calming effect.

Contraindications

Angle-closure glaucoma, hypersensitivity to atomoxetine or its components, pheochromocytoma, severe cardiovascular disorders, use within 14 days of MAO inhibitor therapy

Interactions

DRUGS

albuterol and other beta$_2$ agonists: May potentiate action of albuterol and other beta$_2$ agonists on cardiovascular system
antihypertensives, pressor agents: Possibly increased blood pressure
CYP2D6 inhibitors (such as fluoxetine, paroxetine, and quinidine): Increased blood atomoxetine level
MAO inhibitors: Possibly induced hypertensive crisis

Adverse Reactions

CNS: Aggressiveness, anxiety, chills, crying, CVA, depression, dizziness, early morning awakening, fatigue, headache, hostility, hypoesthesia, insomnia, irritability, jittery feeling, lethargy, mood changes, paresthesia (children and adolescents), peripheral coldness, pyrexia, rigors, sedation, **seizures**, sensory disturbances, sleep disturbance, somnolence, **suicidal ideation**, syncope, tics, tremor, unusual dreams
CV: Chest pain, hypertension, orthostatic hypotension, **MI**, palpitations, **QT interval prolongation**, Raynaud's phenomenon, tachycardia
EENT: Blurred vision, conjunctivitis, dry mouth, ear infection, mydriasis, nasal congestion, nasopharyngitis, pharyngitis, rhinorrhea, sinus congestion
ENDO: Hot flashes
GI: Abdominal pain (upper), anorexia, constipation, diarrhea, dyspepsia, elevated liver enzymes, flatulence, gastroenteritis (viral), indigestion, nausea, **severe hepatic dysfunction**, vomiting
GU: Decreased libido, dysmenorrhea, dysuria, ejaculation disorders, erectile dysfunction, impotence, male pelvic pain, menstrual irregularities, orgasm abnormality, priapism, prostatitis, urinary hesitancy (children and adolescents), urine retention (children and adolescents)
MS: Arthralgia, back pain, myalgia, **rhabdomyolysis**
RESP: Cough, upper respiratory tract infection
SKIN: Alopecia, dermatitis, diaphoresis, hyperhidrosis, pruritus, rash, urticaria
Other: **Anaphylaxis, angioedema**, flu-like symptoms, weight loss

Childbearing Considerations

PREGNANCY

- Pregnancy Exposure Registry: 1-866-961-2388 or https://womensmentalhealth.org/adhd-medications/
- It is not known if drug can cause fetal harm although some animal studies suggest adverse developmental risks may occur.
- Drug is not recommended during pregnancy unless benefit to mother outweighs potential risk to fetus.

LACTATION

- It is not known if drug is present in breast milk.
- Patient should check with prescriber before breastfeeding.

REPRODUCTION

- Women of childbearing age should avoid pregnancy during drug therapy by using an effective contraceptive.

⬚ Nursing Considerations

- Know that patient should be screened for a personal or family history of bipolar disorder, hypomania, or mania before atomoxetine therapy is begun. This is because drug can increase risk for exacerbation of these disorders. In addition, drug may cause manic or psychotic symptoms even in patients without a prior history at normal doses. Monitor patient carefully throughout therapy, and if symptoms such as delusional thinking, hallucinations, or mania occur, notify prescriber and expect drug to be discontinued.
- Use atomoxetine cautiously in patients with cerebrovascular or CV disease (especially hypertension or tachycardia) because drug may increase blood pressure and heart rate. Also use cautiously in those prone to orthostatic hypotension and those with serious structural cardiac abnormalities, cardiomyopathy, serious heart rhythm abnormalities, or other serious cardiac problems because drug may increase risk of sudden death from these conditions.

! **WARNING** Monitor patient closely for evidence of suicidal thinking and behavior as well as for psychotic or manic symptoms such as hallucinations, delusional thinking, or mania because atomoxetine increases the risk of suicidal ideation and the onset of psychotic or manic symptoms. In addition, monitor patients, especially children and adolescents with ADHD, for the appearance or worsening of aggressive behavior or hostility. Notify prescriber if psychiatric adverse reactions are observed during atomoxetine therapy.

- Obtain baseline blood pressure and heart rate before starting therapy. Monitor patient's vital signs after dosage increases and periodically during therapy.
- Monitor patient closely for allergic reactions. If these occur, notify prescriber.
- Monitor child's or adolescent's growth and weight. Expect to interrupt therapy, as prescribed, if patient isn't growing or gaining weight appropriately.
- Monitor patient's liver function studies, as ordered. Notify prescriber immediately if enzyme levels are elevated or patient has evidence of hepatic dysfunction. Expect to stop drug permanently.

PATIENT TEACHING

- Instruct patient to swallow capsule whole and not to chew, crush, or open capsule. If a capsule opens, urge patient to promptly wash his hands and any surface drug touches. If drug gets in his eyes, tell him to flush immediately with water and seek medical care.
- Instruct patient or parent to immediately report to prescriber any adverse reactions to atomoxetine therapy, such as facial swelling, itching, or rash.

! **WARNING** Urge parents to watch their child or adolescent closely for evidence of abnormal thinking or behavior, or increased aggression or hostility. Emphasize need to notify prescriber about unusual changes.

- Urge patient to tell prescriber immediately about dark urine, flu-like symptoms, itchiness, right upper abdominal pain, or yellowing of his skin or eyes. Also tell patient to notify prescriber immediately if he experiences exertional chest pain, unexplained syncope, or other symptoms suggestive of heart disease.
- Caution patient to assume sitting or standing position slowly because of drug's potential effect on blood pressure.
- Urge male patient to seek immediate medical attention for a penile erection that becomes prolonged or painful.
- Advise patient to report urinary hesitancy or urine retention to prescriber.
- Remind patient of the importance of alerting all prescribers to any OTC drugs, dietary supplements, or herbal remedies he's taking.
- Caution patient to avoid hazardous activities until drug's CNS effects are known.
- Reassure patient or parent that drug doesn't cause physical or psychological dependence.
- Instruct patient or parent to monitor weight during therapy.

atorvastatin calcium
Lipitor

⬚ Class and Category
Pharmacologic class: HMG-CoA reductase inhibitor
Therapeutic class: Antihyperlipidemic

Indications and Dosages

* *To control lipid levels as adjunct to diet in primary (heterozygous familial and nonfamilial) hypercholesterolemia and mixed dyslipidemia*

TABLETS

Adults. *Initial:* 10 or 20 mg once daily; then increased according to lipid level. *Maintenance:* 10 to 80 mg once daily.

±**DOSAGE ADJUSTMENT** Initial dose may be increased to 40 mg once daily for patients who need cholesterol level reduced more than 45%.

* *As adjunct to control lipid levels in homozygous familial hypercholesterolemia*

TABLETS

Adults. 10 to 80 mg daily.

* *As adjunct to control lipid levels in pediatric heterozygous familial hypercholesterolemia*

TABLETS

Adolescents and children ages 10 to 17. *Initial:* 10 mg daily, adjusted at intervals of 4 wk or more, as needed. *Maximum:* 20 mg daily.

* *To reduce risk of acute cardiovascular events such as angina, CVA, or MI and to reduce risk for revascularization procedures or hospitalization for congestive heart failure in patients with coronary heart disease (CAD); to reduce risk of angina, CVA, or MI in patients without clinical evidence of CAD but with multiple risk factors for CAD such as age, family history of early CAD, hypertension, low HDL-C, or smoking; to reduce risk of CVA or MI in patients with type 2 diabetes without clinical evidence of CAD but with multiple risk factors for CAD such as albuminuria, hypertension, retinopathy, or smoking*

TABLETS

Adults. 10 to 80 mg once daily.

±**DOSAGE ADJUSTMENT** for all indications For patient with HIV taking lopinavir plus ritonavir, lowest dosage should be used. For patient taking clarithromycin, darunavir plus ritonavir, elbasvir plus grazoprevir, fosamprenavir, fosamprenavir plus ritonavir, itraconazole, letermovir, or saquinavir plus ritonavir, dosage should not exceed 20 mg daily. For patient taking nelfinavir, dosage should not exceed 40 mg daily.

Drug Administration

P.O.

- Give drug at the same time of day to maintain effects.

Route	Onset	Peak	Duration
P.O.	Unknown	1–2 hr	Unknown

Half-life: 14 hr

Mechanism of Action

Reduces plasma cholesterol and lipoprotein levels by inhibiting HMG-CoA reductase and cholesterol synthesis in the liver and by increasing the number of LDL receptors on liver cells to enhance LDL uptake and breakdown.

Contraindications

Active hepatic disease, breastfeeding, hypersensitivity to atorvastatin or its components, pregnancy, unexplained persistent rise in serum transaminase level

Interactions

DRUGS

azole antifungals, colchicine, erythromycin, gemfibrozil, lipid-modifying doses of niacin, other fibrates: Increased risk of myopathy and rhabdomyolysis

cyclosporine, CYP3A4 and/or OATP1B1 strong inhibitors such as clarithromycin, HIV and HCV protease inhibitors including combination drugs, itraconazole, letermovir: Possibly increased plasma concentrations of atorvastatin and adverse reactions such as myopathy and rhabdomyolysis

digoxin: Increased digoxin level and increased risk of toxicity

efavirenz, rifampin, other CYP450 3A4 inducers: Possible decreased plasma atorvastatin level and effectiveness

oral contraceptives such as ethinyl estradiol and norethindrone: Increased hormone levels

FOODS

grapefruit juice: Increased blood atorvastatin level

Adverse Reactions

CNS: Abnormal dreams, amnesia, asthenia, cognitive impairment, depression, dizziness, emotional lability, facial paralysis, fatigue, fever, headache, hyperkinesia, lack of coordination, malaise, paresthesia, peripheral neuropathy, somnolence, syncope, weakness

CV: **Arrhythmias**, orthostatic hypotension, palpitations, phlebitis, vasodilation

EENT: Amblyopia, altered refraction, dry eyes or mouth, epistaxis, eye hemorrhage, gingival hemorrhage, glaucoma, glossitis, hearing loss, lip swelling, loss of taste, pharyngitis, sinusitis, stomatitis, taste perversion, tinnitus

ENDO: Hyperglycemia, **hypoglycemia**

GI: Abdominal or biliary pain, anorexia, colitis, constipation, diarrhea, duodenal or stomach ulcers, dysphagia, elevated liver enzymes, eructation, esophagitis, flatulence, gastroenteritis, **hepatic failure**, **hepatitis**, increased appetite, indigestion, jaundice, melena, **pancreatitis**, **rectal hemorrhage**, vomiting

GU: Abnormal ejaculation; cystitis; decreased libido; dysuria; epididymitis; hematuria; impotence; nephritis; nocturia; renal calculi; urinary frequency, incontinence, or urgency; urine retention; vaginal hemorrhage

HEME: Anemia, **thrombocytopenia**

MS: Arthralgia, back or muscle pain, bursitis, elevated creatine kinase, gout, **immune-mediated necrotizing myopathy**, leg cramps, myalgia, myasthenia gravis, myopathy, myositis, neck rigidity, **rhabdomyolysis**, tendon contracture or rupture, tenosynovitis, torticollis

RESP: Dyspnea, pneumonia

SKIN: Acne, alopecia, contact dermatitis, diaphoresis, dry skin, ecchymosis, eczema, **erythema multiforme**, petechiae, photosensitivity, pruritus, rash, seborrhea, **Stevens–Johnson syndrome**, **toxic epidermal necrolysis**, ulceration, urticaria

Other: **Anaphylaxis**, **angioedema**, flu-like symptoms, infection, lymphadenopathy, weight gain

Childbearing Considerations

PREGNANCY

- Drug may cause fetal harm.
- Drug is contraindicated during pregnancy.

LACTATION

- It is not known if drug is present in breast milk.
- Drug is contraindicated during breastfeeding because of potential for serious adverse reactions in breastfed infant.

REPRODUCTION

- Women of childbearing age should use effective contraception during drug therapy.

Nursing Considerations

- Know that atorvastatin is used in patients with homozygous familial hypercholesterolemia as an adjunct to other lipid-lowering treatments or alone only if other treatments aren't available.
- Know that treatment of heterozygous familial hypercholesterolemia, in children who have failed an adequate trial of diet therapy, may include atorvastatin therapy if their LDL-C is 190 mg/dl or greater, or their LDL-C is 160 mg/dl or greater and they have a positive family history of familial hypercholesterolemia or premature cardiovascular disease in a first- or second-degree relative, or two or more other cardiovascular risk factors are present.
- Be aware that atorvastatin may be used with colestipol or cholestyramine for additive antihyperlipidemic effects.
- Know that atorvastatin should not be used in patients taking cyclosporine, gemfibrozil, tipranavir plus ritonavir, or telaprevir because of high risk for rhabdomyolysis with acute renal failure.
- Use atorvastatin cautiously in patients who consume substantial quantities of alcohol or have a history of liver disease because atorvastatin use increases risk of liver dysfunction.
- Expect liver function tests to be performed before atorvastatin therapy starts and then thereafter as clinically necessary. If clinical symptoms such as hyperbilirubinemia and jaundice occur, notify prescriber and expect atorvastatin therapy to be discontinued until cause of liver dysfunction has been identified. If no cause can be found, expect drug to be discontinued permanently.
- Expect to measure lipid levels 2 to 4 weeks after therapy starts, to adjust dosage as directed, and to repeat periodically until lipid levels are within desired range.
- Monitor diabetic patient's blood glucose levels because atorvastatin therapy can affect blood glucose control.

! **WARNING** Notify prescriber immediately and expect to withhold atorvastatin therapy if patient develops an acute condition suggestive of a myopathy (unexplained muscle pain, tenderness or weakness, especially if accompanied by elevated CPK level, fever, or malaise) or has a risk factor predisposing to the development of renal failure secondary to rhabdomyolysis, such as an acute severe infection; hypotension; major surgery; severe electrolyte, endocrine, or metabolic disorder; or uncontrolled seizures.

PATIENT TEACHING

- Emphasize that atorvastatin is an adjunct to—not a substitute for—a low-cholesterol diet.
- Tell patient to take drug at the same time each day to maintain its effects.
- Instruct patient to take a missed dose as soon as possible. If it's almost time for his next dose, he should skip the missed dose. Tell him not to double the dose.
- Instruct patient to consult prescriber before taking OTC niacin because of increased risk of rhabdomyolysis.
- Advise patient to notify prescriber immediately if he develops unexplained muscle pain, tenderness, or weakness, especially if accompanied by fatigue or fever.
- Reinforce the benefits of therapy, and urge patient to comply if possible.
- Advise patient with diabetes to monitor blood glucose levels closely.
- Inform women of childbearing age to use effective contraception while taking atorvastatin because atorvastatin is contraindicated in pregnancy. Tell female patient to notify prescriber immediately if pregnancy is suspected or known, as drug will have to be discontinued. Also tell mothers that breastfeeding is contraindicated during atorvastatin therapy.

atovaquone
Mepron

≣ Class and Category
Pharmacologic class: Ubiquinone analogue
Therapeutic class: Antiprotozoal

≣ Indications and Dosages
✳ *To prevent* Pneumocystis jiroveci
pneumonia in patients who can't tolerate
trimethoprim-sulfamethoxazole

SUSPENSION

Adults and adolescents. 1,500 mg (10 ml) once daily.

✳ *To treat mild to moderate* P. jiroveci
pneumonia in patients who can't tolerate
trimethoprim-sulfamethoxazole

SUSPENSION

Adults and adolescents. 750 mg (5 ml) twice daily for 21 days. *Maximum:* 1,500 mg/day.

≣ Drug Administration
P.O.

- Administer with meals to enhance absorption.
- Shake bottle gently before opening to measure dose. Use a calibrated device to measure dosage.
- If administering drug from a foil pouch, open pouch by removing tab at perforation and tear at notch. Administer entire contents from pouch directly into the patient's mouth, or it can be poured into a dosing spoon or cup prior to administration. Expect to use the entire contents of 2 pouches for a 10-ml dose.

Route	Onset	Peak	Duration
P.O.	Unknown	Unknown	Unknown

Half-life: 2–4 days

≣ Mechanism of Action
May destroy *P. jiroveci* organisms by inhibiting the enzymes needed to synthesize nucleic acid and adenosine triphosphate.

≣ Contraindications
Hypersensitivity to atovaquone or its components

≣ Interactions
DRUGS

indinavir: Possible loss of efficacy of indinavir
metoclopramide, rifabutin, rifampin,
tetracycline: Possibly decreased blood atovaquone level

≣ Adverse Reactions
CNS: Fever, headache, insomnia
EENT: Rhinitis, **throat tightness**, vortex keratopathy
GI: Abdominal pain, diarrhea, elevated liver enzymes, **hepatic failure**, **hepatitis**, nausea, **pancreatitis**, vomiting
GU: **Acute renal dysfunction**
HEME: Anemia, **thrombocytopenia**
RESP: Bronchospasm, cough, dyspnea
SKIN: Desquamation, **erythema multiforme**, rash, **Stevens–Johnson syndrome**, urticaria

Other: Allergic reaction, angioedema, methemoglobinemia

Childbearing Considerations

PREGNANCY
- It is not known if drug can cause fetal harm.
- Use with caution only if benefit to mother outweighs potential risk to fetus.

LACTATION
- It is not known if drug is present in breast milk.
- Centers for Disease Control and Prevention recommend women infected with HIV-1 not breastfeed their infant to avoid risking postnatal transmission of HIV-1.

Nursing Considerations
- Use atovaquone cautiously in patient with severe hepatic impairment because, although rare, serious adverse reactions affecting liver function may occur.
- Monitor blood test results because atovaquone may decrease serum sodium, hemoglobin levels, and neutrophil count; and may increase AST, ALT, alkaline phosphatase, and serum amylase levels.

PATIENT TEACHING
- Instruct patient to take atovaquone with meals for maximum effectiveness.
- Remind patient to shake the suspension gently before using each time and to use a calibrated device to measure dosage.
- Instruct patient to take a missed dose as soon as possible. If it's almost time for the next dose, tell him to skip the missed dose. Tell him not to double the next dose.
- Tell patient to notify prescriber if his condition doesn't improve in a few days or if he develops signs of an allergic reaction, such as fever or rash.

atropine
AtroPen

atropine sulfate

Class and Category
Pharmacologic class: Anticholinergic
Therapeutic class: Antiarrhythmic, antimuscarinic

Indications and Dosages
* *To treat bradyasystolic cardiac arrest*

I.V. INJECTION (ATROPINE SULFATE)
Adults. 1 mg, repeated every 3 to 5 min, as needed. *Maximum:* 3 mg total dose.

* *To provide temporary blockade of severe or life-threatening muscarinic anticholinesterase effects from muscarinic mushroom or organophosphorus poisoning*

I.V. INJECTION (ATROPINE SULFATE)
Adults. 2 to 3 mg, repeated every 20 to 30 min, as needed, until signs of poisoning are significantly lessened or signs of atropine toxicity occur.

* *To treat exposure to chemical nerve agent or insecticide*

I.M. INJECTION (ATROPINE)
Adults and children weighing over 41 kg (90 lb) with two or more mild symptoms. 2 mg, if severe symptoms develop at any time after injection, two or more 2-mg injections given in rapid succession.

Adults and children weighing over 41 kg (90 lb) who are unconscious or have other severe symptoms. 2 mg given immediately 3 times in rapid succession.

Children weighing 18 to 41 kg (40 to 90 lb) with two or more mild symptoms. 1 mg, if severe symptoms develop at any time after injection, two more 1-mg injections given in rapid succession.

Children weighing 18 to 41 kg (40 to 90 lb) who are unconscious or exhibit any other severe symptoms. 1 mg given immediately 3 times in rapid succession.

Children weighing 7 to 18 kg (15 to 40 lb) with two or more mild symptoms. 0.5 mg. If severe symptoms develop at any time after injection, two more 0.5-mg injections given in rapid succession.

Children weighing 7 to 18 kg (15 to 40 lb) who are unconscious or exhibit any other severe symptoms. 0.5 mg given immediately three times in rapid succession.

Children weighing less than 7 kg (15 lb) with two or more mild symptoms. 0.25 mg. If severe symptoms develop at any time after injection, two more 0.25-mg injections given in rapid succession.

Children weighing less than 7 kg (15 lb) who are unconscious or exhibit any other severe symptoms. 0.25 mg given immediately three times in rapid succession.

⦀ Drug Administration

I.V.

- Administer into a large vein or I.V. tubing over 1 to 2 minutes.
- *Incompatibilities:* Floxacillin as an additive, cimetidine with pentobarbital in same syringe, thiopental with a Y-site, and other drugs such as ampicillin, diazepam, epinephrine, and norepinephrine with atropine solution

I.M.

- AtroPen has no absolute contraindications when used to treat life-threatening nerve gas or insecticide exposure. However, the 2-mg atropine autoinjector should not be used in children weighing 41 kg (90 lb) or less for any indication, as its safety and effectiveness have not been established.
- Can be given through clothing.
- Administer by firmly jabbing tip into midlateral thigh at a 90-degree angle. If patient is thin, pinch the skin before injecting into the site.
- Hold the AtroPen firmly in place for at least 10 seconds to allow the injection to finish. After removing, massage the injection site for several seconds.
- After injection, make sure needle is visible on autoinjector. If not, repeat administration, jabbing more firmly than first time.

Route	Onset	Peak	Duration
I.V.	Immediate	2–4 min	Brief
I.M.	Rapid	3 min	Brief

Half-life: 2–10 hr, and age-dependent

⦀ Mechanism of Action

Inhibits acetylcholine's muscarinic action at the neuroeffector junctions of smooth muscles, cardiac muscles, exocrine glands, SA and AV nodes, and the urinary bladder. In small doses, atropine inhibits salivary and bronchial secretions and diaphoresis. In moderate doses, it increases impulse conduction through the AV node and increases heart rate. In large doses, it decreases GI and urinary tract motility and gastric acid secretion.

⦀ Contraindications

Hypersensitivity to atropine or other belladonna alkaloids or their components

⦀ Interactions

DRUGS

amantadine, anticholinergics, antidyskinetics, glutethimide, meperidine, muscle relaxants, phenothiazines, tricyclic antidepressants and other drugs with anticholinergic properties, including antiarrhythmics (disopyramide, procainamide, quinidine), antihistamines, buclizine: Increased atropine effects

barbiturates: Potentiated effects of barbiturates

ketoconazole: Decreased ketoconazole absorption

levodopa: Decreased plasma levodopa concentration and effectiveness

opioid analgesics: Increased risk of ileus, severe constipation, and urine retention

potassium chloride, especially wax-matrix forms: Possibly GI ulcers

pralidoxime: May potentiate the effect of atropine causing atropinization (dryness of mouth and nose, flushing, mydriasis, and tachycardia)

urinary alkalizers (calcium or magnesium antacids, carbonic anhydrase inhibitors, citrates, sodium bicarbonate): Delayed excretion, increased risk of adverse atropine effects

⦀ Adverse Reactions

CNS: Agitation, amnesia, anxiety, ataxia, Babinski's or Chaddock's reflex, behavioral changes, CNS stimulation (at high doses), **coma,** confusion, decreased concentration, decreased tendon reflexes, delirium, dizziness, drowsiness, EEG abnormalities, excessive thirst, fatigue, fever, hallucinations, headache, **hyperpyrexia,** hyperreflexia, insomnia, lethargy, mania, mental disorders, nervousness, paranoia, restlessness, **seizures,** sensation of intoxication, somnolence, stupor, syncope, vertigo, weakness

CV: Arrhythmias, bradycardia (at low doses), cardiac dilation, chest pain, hypertension, **hypotension, left ventricular failure, MI,** palpitations, tachycardia (at high doses), **weak or impalpable peripheral pulses**

EENT: Acute angle-closure glaucoma, altered taste, blepharitis, blindness, blurred vision, conjunctivitis, cyclophoria, cycloplegia, decreased visual acuity or accommodation, dry eyes or conjunctiva, dry mucous membranes, dry mouth, eye irritation, eyelid crusting, heterophoria, increased intraocular pressure, keratoconjunctivitis, lacrimation, laryngitis, **laryngospasm,** mydriasis, nasal congestion, oral lesions, photophobia, pupils poorly reactive to light, strabismus, tongue chewing

ENDO: Hyperglycemia, **hypoglycemia**

GI: Abdominal distention and pain, bloating, constipation, decreased bowel sounds or food absorption, delayed gastric emptying, dysphagia, heartburn, ileus, nausea, vomiting

GU: Bladder distention, difficulty urinating, elevated BUN, enuresis, impotence, loss of libido, polydipsia, urinary hesitancy, urinary urgency, urine retention

HEME: Anemia, elevated erythrocytes and hemoglobin, leukocytosis

MS: Dysarthria, hypertonia, muscle twitching

RESP: Bradypnea, **exacerbation of chronic lung disease,** dyspnea, **inspiratory stridor, pulmonary edema, respiratory failure, shallow breathing, subcostal recession,** tachypnea

SKIN: Cold skin, decreased or excessive sweating, dermatitis, **exfoliative dermatitis,** flushing, rash, urticaria

Other: **Anaphylaxis,** dehydration, **hypokalemia, hyponatremia,** injection-site pain, sensations of warmth

⬚ Childbearing Considerations

PREGNANCY

- It is not known if drug can cause fetal harm, although it does cross the placental barrier.
- Use with caution only if benefit to mother outweighs potential risk to fetus.

LACTATION

- Drug is present in breast milk.
- Patient should check with prescriber before breastfeeding.

⬚ Nursing Considerations

! WARNING Know that for patient prescribed atropine for suspected nerve gas or insecticide exposure, dosage is determined by severity of symptoms. Mild symptoms include acute onset of stomach cramps, blurred vision, bradycardia, chest tightness, difficulty breathing, excessive unexplained teary eyes or runny nose, increased salivation, miosis, muscle twitching, nausea, tachycardia, unexplained wheezing or coughing, and vomiting. Severe symptoms include confusion or other strange behavior, extreme secretions from airway or lungs, involuntary urination and defecation, seizures, severe difficulty breathing, severe muscle twitching and general weakness, tremors, and unconsciousness.

! WARNING Monitor patient closely for hypersensitivity reactions, including anaphylaxis, after drug is given.

- Be aware that high-dose atropine sulfate should not be used in patients with ulcerative colitis because of risk of toxic megacolon or in patients with hiatal hernia and reflux esophagitis because of risk of esophagitis.
- Caution should be used when atropine is given to patients with known cardiac conduction problems or cardiovascular disease because of its effect on the heart. Caution should also be used when atropine is given to patients with acute glaucoma, partial pyloric stenosis, or significant bladder outflow obstruction.
- Monitor patients with chronic lung disease because atropine may cause thickening of bronchial secretions and formation of dangerous viscid plugs.

! WARNING Assess for symptoms of toxic doses of atropine, such as agitation, confusion, drowsiness, and excitement, which are likely to affect elderly patients even with low doses. If symptoms occur, take safety precautions to prevent injury.

- Monitor elderly patients receiving atropine closely because they are more susceptible to the effects of the drug.
- Assess bowel and bladder elimination. Notify prescriber of constipation, diarrhea, urinary hesitancy, or urine retention.

PATIENT TEACHING

- Teach patient prescribed an AtroPen, because of risk of nerve gas or insecticide exposure, when and how to self-administer the drug. Remind patient that if the AtroPen is used, this is only an initial emergency treatment and they still need to seek additional emergency care.
- Advise patient to notify prescriber if he has constipation, difficulty urinating, or persistent or severe diarrhea.

- Inform patient that atropine may inhibit sweating. Advise patient to avoid excessive exercise or heat exposure, which can lead to heat injury.

avanafil
Stendra

Class and Category
Pharmacologic class: Phosphodiesterase 5 (PDE5) inhibitor
Therapeutic class: Erectile dysfunction

Indications and Dosages
✱ *To treat erectile dysfunction*

TABLETS
Adults. 100 mg before sexual activity as needed. *Maximum:* One dose daily.
±**DOSAGE ADJUSTMENT** Dosage may be increased to 200 mg before sexual activity or decreased to 50 mg before sexual activity, as needed. For patient who is stable on alpha blocker therapy or who is taking a moderate CYP3A4 inhibitor such as amprenavir, aprepitant, diltiazem, erythromycin, fluconazole, fosamprenavir, or verapamil, dosage is limited to 50 mg in 24-hr period.

Drug Administration
P.O.
- 100-mg and 200-mg doses may be taken as early as 15 minutes before sexual activity.
- 50-mg dose may be taken as early as 30 minutes before sexual activity.

Route	Onset	Peak	Duration
P.O.	Rapid	> 30 min	6 hr
Half-life: 3–5 hr			

Mechanism of Action
Enhances the effect of nitric oxide released in the penis through stimulation. Nitric oxide increases cGMP level, relaxes smooth muscle, and increases blood flow to the corpus cavernosum, thus producing an erection.

Contraindications
Concomitant therapy with strong CYP3A4 inhibitors (including atazanavir, clarithromycin, indinavir, itraconazole, ketoconazole, nefazodone, nelfinavir, ritonavir, saquinavir, and telithromycin) or riociguat, hypersensitivity to avanafil or its components, nitrate therapy

Interactions
DRUGS
alpha blockers and other antihypertensives: Increased risk of hypotension
amlodipine, ritonavir: Increased effect of avanafil with possible increased risk of adverse reactions
CYP3A4 inhibitors: Possibly increased plasma levels of avanafil
guanylate cyclase stimulators such as riociguat: Possibly increased risk of hypotension
nitrates: Profound hypotension

ACTIVITIES
alcohol use: Increased risk of orthostatic hypotension

Adverse Reactions
CNS: Depression, dizziness, fatigue, headache, insomnia, somnolence, vertigo
CV: **Abnormal ECG**, angina, **deep vein thrombosis**, hypertension, palpitations, peripheral edema
EENT: Epistaxis, eyelid swelling, hearing or vision loss, nasal or sinus congestion, nasopharyngitis, nonarteritic anterior ischemic optic neuropathy, oropharyngeal pain, sinusitis, tinnitus
ENDO: Hyperglycemia, **hypoglycemia**
GI: Constipation, diarrhea, dyspepsia, elevated liver enzymes, gastric pain, gastritis, gastroesophageal reflux disease, nausea, vomiting
GU: Hematuria, nephrolithiasis, pollakiuria, prolonged erection, urinary tract infection
MS: Arthralgia, back or musculoskeletal pain, muscle spasms, myalgia
RESP: Bronchitis, cough, exertional dyspnea, upper respiratory infection, wheezing
SKIN: Flushing, pruritus, rash
Other: Flu-like symptoms

Childbearing Considerations
PREGNANCY
- Not for use in women.

LACTATION
- Not for use in women.

Nursing Considerations
- Be aware that avanafil should not be used in a patient taking a strong CYP3A4 inhibitor (such as atazanavir, clarithromycin, indinavir, itraconazole, ketoconazole,

nefazodone, nelfinavir, ritonavir, saquinavir, telithromycin) because of increased risk of elevated avanafil levels that could cause serious adverse effects.

- Know that although nitrate therapy is a contraindication to avanafil therapy, in a life-threatening situation, at least 12 hours should elapse after the last dose of avanafil before nitrate administration is given. In this situation, be prepared to hemodynamically monitor the patient and expect hypotension to be treated, if it occurs.

- Use avanafil cautiously in a patient with preexisting cardiovascular disease because of the potential for increased cardiac adverse effects during sexual activity. Patient with left ventricular outflow obstruction or severely impaired autonomic control of blood pressure may be especially sensitive to the vasodilatation effect of avanafil.

- Use avanafil cautiously in the elderly and patients with mild to moderate renal or hepatic dysfunction. The effects of avanafil in the presence of severe renal or hepatic dysfunction are unknown.

- Monitor the patient's vision, especially in patients over age 50; who have diabetes, hypertension, coronary artery disease, or hyperlipidemia; or who smoke, because avanafil rarely may cause nonarteritic anterior ischemic optic neuropathy that may lead to decreased vision or permanent vision loss.

PATIENT TEACHING

- Explain to patient that avanafil should be taken as early as 15 minutes (30 minutes for 50-mg dose) before sexual activity and that sexual stimulation is required for drug to be effective.

- Remind patient that avanafil should not be taken more than once a day.

! **WARNING** Warn patient not to take avanafil if he also takes any form of organic nitrate, either continuously or intermittently or other PDE5 inhibitors, because profound hypotension and death could result.

- Tell patient to stop taking drug and contact prescriber immediately if vision decreases suddenly in one or both eyes, or if he has a sudden loss of hearing, possibly with dizziness and tinnitus.

- Advise patient taking avanafil to seek sexual counseling to enhance the drug's effects.

- Instruct patient to notify prescriber immediately if erection is painful or lasts longer than 4 hours.

- Warn patient that alcohol ingestion may increase risk of low blood pressure, accompanied by dizziness when changing position, increased heart rate, and headache.

avatrombopag
Doptelet

☰ Class and Category

Pharmacologic class: Thrombopoietin receptor agonist
Therapeutic class: Hematopoietic

☰ Indications and Dosages

✳ *To treat thrombocytopenia in patients with chronic liver disease who are scheduled to undergo a procedure*

TABLETS

Adults with a platelet count 40 to less than 50×10^9/L. 40 mg once daily for 5 days starting 10 to 13 days prior to procedure.
Adults with a platelet count less than 40×10^9/L. 60 mg once daily for 5 days starting 10 to 13 days prior to procedure.

✳ *To treat thrombocytopenia in patients with chronic immune thrombocytopenia (ITP) who have had an insufficient response to a previous treatment*

TABLETS

Adults. *Initial:* 20 mg once daily. If platelet count remains less than 50×10^9/L after 2 wk, dosage increased to 40 mg three times a wk and 20 mg on the remaining days of each wk. If platelet count remains less than 50×10^9/L after an additional 2 wk, dosage increased to 40 mg once daily. If platelet count following initial dosage is between 200 and 400×10^9/L after 2 wk, dosage decreased to 20 mg three times a wk. If platelet count remains between 200 and 400×10^9/L after an additional 2 wk, dosage further decreased to 20 mg twice weekly or 40 mg once weekly. *Maximum:* 40 mg once daily. *Discontinuation:* If platelet count does not increase to greater than or equal to 50×10^9/L after 4 wk of dosing at maximum dose, drug discontinued. If platelet count is greater than 400×10^9/L after 2 wk of dosing at 20 mg once weekly, drug is discontinued.

± DOSAGE ADJUSTMENT For patients taking moderate or strong dual CYP2C9 and CYP3A4 inhibitors, initial dosage decreased to 20 mg three times a week. For patients taking moderate or strong dual CYP2C9 and CYP3A4 inducers, initial dosage increased to 40 mg once daily.

Drug Administration

P.O.

- Tablets must be taken with food.
- When used in patients with chronic liver disease scheduled to undergo a procedure, the five-dosage regimen must be completed 5 to 8 days before the procedure.

Route	Onset	Peak	Duration
P.O.	Unknown	5–8 hr	Unknown

Half-life: 19 hr

Mechanism of Action

Stimulates differentiation and proliferation of megakaryocytes from bone marrow progenitor cells to increase platelet production.

Contraindications

Hypersensitivity to avatrombopag or its components

Interactions

DRUGS

moderate or strong dual inducers of CYP2C9 and CYP3A4: Possibly decreased effectiveness of avatrombopag
moderate or strong dual inhibitors of CYP2C9 and CYP3A4: Possibly increased risk of avatrombopag toxicity

Adverse Reactions

CNS: Fatigue, fever, headache
CV: **Arterial/vein thromboembolism,** peripheral edema, **portal vein thrombosis**
EENT: Epistaxis, gingival bleeding, nasopharyngitis
GI: Abdominal pain, nausea
HEME: Anemia
MS: Arthralgia, myalgia
RESP: Upper respiratory tract infection
SKIN: Bruise, petechiae
Other: **Hyponatremia**

Childbearing Considerations

PREGNANCY

- Drug may cause fetal harm based on animal studies.
- Use with caution and only if benefit to mother outweighs potential risk to fetus.

LACTATION

- It is not known if drug is present in breast milk.
- Breastfeeding is not recommended during drug therapy and for 2 weeks after last dose.
- If drug is being given for brief periods, such as prior to an invasive procedure, breastfeeding must be interrupted, with breast milk pumped and discarded during drug therapy and for 2 weeks after last dose of drug.

Nursing Considerations

- Expect to obtain a platelet count prior to starting avatrombopag therapy in patients with chronic liver disease undergoing a procedure and repeated on the day of the procedure to ensure that an adequate increase in platelet count has occurred.
- Be aware that patients with chronic immune thrombocytopenia should be prescribed the lowest dose needed to achieve and maintain a platelet count greater than or equal to 50×10^9 as needed to reduce the risk for bleeding. The drug should not be used to normalize platelet counts.

! **WARNING** Monitor patients for signs and symptoms of thromboembolic events and notify prescriber immediately if present, because avatrombopag increases thrombotic risk.

- Monitor patient's platelet counts weekly in patients with chronic immune thrombocytopenia until a stable platelet count greater than or equal to 50×10^9 has been achieved, and then monthly thereafter. Platelet counts should be checked weekly for at least 4 weeks after drug is discontinued.

PATIENT TEACHING

- Tell patient to take drug with food.
- Instruct patient with chronic liver disease undergoing a procedure to take avatrombopag beginning 10 to 13 days prior to procedure for 5 consecutive days only. Educate patient on the importance of not missing doses. If a dose is missed, instruct patient to take it as soon as it is remembered but not to take two doses at

the same time to make up for a missed dose. The next dose should be taken at the usual time the next day.

! WARNING Review signs and symptoms of thrombotic conditions with patient. If present, stress importance of notifying prescriber and seeking emergency care immediately.

- Instruct patient to notify prescriber if taking any new medication, whether prescribed or over the counter, including herbal substances.
- Tell women of childbearing age to notify prescriber if pregnancy is suspected or confirmed.
- Advise women who are breastfeeding and receiving drug short term for a procedure to pump and discard breast milk during treatment and for 2 weeks following last dose of drug. Inform women wishing to breastfeed during chronic therapy that breastfeeding is not recommended.

azathioprine
Azasan, Imuran

azathioprine sodium
Imuran I.V.

☰ Class and Category

Pharmacologic class: Purine antagonist
Therapeutic class: Immunosuppressant, antirheumatic

☰ Indications and Dosages

✴ *To prevent kidney rejection after homotransplantation*

TABLETS (AZASAN, IMURAN)

Adults and children. *Initial:* 3 to 5 mg/kg daily as a single dose on, or 1 to 3 days before, day of transplantation then decreased according to patient's response and tolerance to 1 to 3 mg/kg daily following surgery. *Maintenance:* 1 to 3 mg/kg daily.

I.V. INFUSION (IMURAN I.V.)

Adults unable to tolerate oral dosage.
Initial: 3 to 5 mg/kg as a single dose on, or 1 to 3 days daily before, day of transplantation, then decreased according to patient's

response and tolerance to 1 to 3 mg/kg daily following surgery until P.O. dose is tolerated (usually 1 to 4 days).

±**DOSAGE ADJUSTMENT** Dosage reduced for patients with oliguria (as from tubular necrosis) after transplantation and in patients with heterozygous deficiency of nucleotide diphosphatase (NUDT15) or thiopurine *S*-methyl transferase (TPMT).

✴ *To reduce signs and symptoms of acute rheumatoid arthritis*

TABLETS (AZASAN, IMURAN)

Adults. *Initial:* 1 mg/kg (50 to 100 mg) daily as a single dose or on a twice-daily schedule for 6 to 8 wk. *Maintenance:* If initial therapy doesn't produce therapeutic effects or no serious adverse effects occur after 6 to 8 wk, dosage increased every 4 wk in 0.5-mg/kg increments up to 2.5 mg/kg/daily.

±**DOSAGE ADJUSTMENT** Dosage reduced to 25% to 33% of usual dosage for patients who also take allopurinol. Dosage reduced for patients with reduced thiopurine *S*-methyl transferase (TPMT) activity.

☰ Drug Administration

P.O.

- Give with meals if GI upset occurs.
- Expect to use lowest possible maintenance dosage for rheumatoid arthritis, reducing it gradually in 0.5-mg/kg (about 25-mg) increments at 4-week intervals, as ordered.
- Know that drug can be stopped abruptly, but its effects may persist for several days.

I.V.

- Follow procedure for proper handling and disposal of this immunosuppressive antimetabolite drug.
- Use restricted to patients who can't tolerate oral form of drug.
- Reconstitute by adding 10 ml of Sterile Water for Injection and swirl until solution is clear.
- Further dilute in 0.9% Sodium Chloride or 5% Dextrose in Water, with final volume dependent on infusion time.
- Infuse over 30 to 60 minutes (most common) but know that it may be infused as short as 5 minutes and as long as 8 hours for the daily dose.
- Drug switched to oral form as soon as patient can tolerate it, which is usually in 1 to 4 days.

- *Incompatibilities:* None reported by manufacturer

Route	Onset	Peak	Duration
P.O./I.V.	Unknown	1–2 hr	Unknown

Half-life: 5 hr

Mechanism of Action

May prevent proliferation and differentiation of activated B and T cells by interfering with purine (protein) and nucleic acid (DNA and RNA) synthesis.

Contraindications

Hypersensitivity to azathioprine or its components, treatment of rheumatoid arthritis in pregnant women

Interactions

DRUGS

ACE inhibitors and drugs that affect bone marrow and cell development in bone marrow, such as trimethoprim-sulfamethoxazole: Possibly severe leukopenia
cyclosporine: Possibly decreased plasma cyclosporine level
ribavirin: Possibly induced severe pancytopenia and possibly increased risk of azathioprine-related myelotoxicity
xanthine oxidase inhibitors such as allopurinol, febuxostat: Increased plasma azathioprine levels possibly leading to azathioprine toxicity
warfarin: Possibly inhibited anticoagulant effect of warfarin

Adverse Reactions

CNS: Fever, malaise, **progressive multifocal leukoencephalopathy**
GI: Abdominal pain, diarrhea, **hepatotoxicity**, nausea, **pancreatitis**, steatorrhea, vomiting
HEME: Immunosuppression (severe), **leukopenia**, macrocytic anemia, **pancytopenia, thrombocytopenia**
MS: Arthralgia, myalgia
SKIN: Acute febrile neutrophilic dermatosis (Sweet's syndrome), alopecia, **cancer**, rash
RESP: **Interstitial pneumonitis**
Other: Infection, **lymphomas and other neoplasms**, negative nitrogen balance

Childbearing Considerations

PREGNANCY

- Drug can cause fetal harm.

- Drug is contraindicated for use during pregnancy for treatment of rheumatoid arthritis.
- Use should be avoided to treat renal homotransplantation during pregnancy, if possible. Drug should not be used to treat rheumatoid arthritis in pregnant women.

LACTATION

- Drug is present in breast milk.
- A decision should be made to discontinue breastfeeding or the drug because of the potential risk for tumor formation in the infant.

REPRODUCTION

- Women of childbearing age should be advised to avoid becoming pregnant during drug therapy.

Nursing Considerations

- Obtain results of baseline laboratory tests, including WBC, RBC, and platelet counts. Expect to monitor results once a week during first month of therapy, twice a month during second and third months, and once a month or more thereafter.
- Know that hematologic reactions typically are dose-related and may occur late in therapy, especially in patients with transplant rejection.

! **WARNING** Expect to reduce dosage or discontinue azathioprine, if WBC count decreases rapidly or remains significantly and consistently low.

! **WARNING** Monitor patient closely for abnormal signs and symptoms suggestive of lymphomas, especially in adolescent and young adult males who have a history of inflammatory bowel disease, in patients who have received a renal transplant, or in patients with rheumatoid arthritis, because the majority of patients who develop a lymphoma fall into one of these categories.

- Monitor liver enzymes, as ordered, for early signs of hepatotoxicity.
- Take action if patient develops thrombocytopenia, such as bleeding precautions, such as avoiding I.M. injections and venipunctures, applying ice to areas of trauma, and checking I.V. infusion sites every 2 hours for bleeding.
- Be aware that patients with low or absent thiopurine *S*-methyl transferase (TPMT)

or nucleotide diphosphatase (NUDT15) levels are at risk for developing severe and life-threatening myelosuppression. Expect patient to be tested for these disorders if significant myelosuppression occurs. If confirmed, expect dosage to be decreased in the presence of heterozygous deficiency and drug discontinued in the presence of homozygous deficiency.

- Monitor patient's prothrombin time if he also receives an oral anticoagulant.
- Be aware that azathioprine therapy increases risk of bacterial, fungal, protozoal, and viral infections. Watch for evidence of infection, such as fever, chills, sore throat, and mouth sores. Expect to administer aggressive antibiotic, antiviral, or other drug therapy and reduce azathioprine dosage.
- Minimize the risk of infection. If patient has severe leukopenia, take neutropenic precautions, such as placing him in a private room and limiting visitors.
- Know that rheumatoid arthritis requires at least 12 weeks of azathioprine therapy. During this time, continue other pain-relief measures, such as physical therapy, rest, and other drugs, such as salicylates and corticosteroids if it causes GI upset.

PATIENT TEACHING

- Advise patient to take oral drug with food or meals to minimize GI upset.

! **WARNING** Teach patient to recognize and report signs of infection, such as sore throat and fever, and to seek medical attention for any abnormal signs and symptoms that might be suggestive of a malignancy.

- Teach patient how to reduce the risk of bleeding and falling.
- Inform women of childbearing age to use effective contraception during drug therapy and not to breastfeed.

azelastine hydrochloride
Astelin, Astepro

☰ Class and Category

Pharmacologic class: H$_1$-receptor antagonist
Therapeutic class: Antihistamine

☰ Indications and Dosages

✳ *To treat symptoms of seasonal allergic rhinitis*

NASAL SPRAY (ASTELIN)

Adults and children age 12 and over. 1 or 2 sprays in each nostril twice daily.
Children age 5 to 11 years. 1 spray in each nostril twice daily.

NASAL SPRAY (ASTEPRO)

Adults and children age 12 and over. 1 or 2 sprays (0.1% or 0.15%) in each nostril twice daily. Alternatively, 0.15% solution may be administered as 2 sprays in each nostril once daily.
Children age 6 to 11 years. 1 spray (0.1% or 0.15%) in each nostril twice daily.
Children age 2 to 5 years: 1 spray (0.1%) in each nostril twice daily.

✳ *To treat symptoms of perennial allergic rhinitis*

NASAL SPRAY (ASTEPRO)

Adults and children age 12 and over. 2 sprays (0.15%) in each nostril twice daily.
Children age 6 to 11. 1 spray (0.1% or 0.15%) in each nostril twice daily.
Children age 6 months to 5 years: 1 spray (0.1%) in each nostril twice daily.

✳ *To treat symptoms of vasomotor rhinitis*

NASAL SPRAY (ASTELIN)

Adults and adolescents 12 years and older. 2 sprays in each nostril twice daily.

☰ Drug Administration

INTRANASAL

- Prime pump before administering for first time by placing thumb on base and the index and middle fingers on shoulder area of bottle and then pressing thumb firmly and quickly against bottle four times (Astelin) or six times (Astepro), or until fine mist appears.
- If spray hasn't been used in more than 3 days, the container will have to be reprimed by pumping two sprays or until fine mist appears.
- Have patient clear nostrils gently, if needed, before using spray.
- Have patient inhale deeply after each spray and then exhale through her mouth and tilt her head back so drug can spread over nasopharynx.
- Wipe tip of spray container with a clean tissue after each use.
- Store bottle upright and keep it tightly closed.

Route	Onset	Peak	Duration
Intranasal	30 min	2–3 hr	12 hr

Half-life: 22–25 hr

≣ Mechanism of Action

Binds nonselectively to central and peripheral H_1 receptors, preventing histamine from reaching its site of action, which reduces or prevents most of histamine's physiologic effects. By blocking histamine at its site of action, azelastine inhibits GI, respiratory, and vascular smooth muscle contraction; decreases capillary permeability, which reduces flares, itching, and wheals; and decreases lacrimal and salivary gland secretions.

≣ Contraindications

Hypersensitivity to azelastine or its components

≣ Interactions

DRUGS

cimetidine: Possibly increased blood azelastine level
CNS depressants: Possibly increased sedative effects and reduced mental alertness

ACTIVITIES

alcohol use: Possibly increased sedative effects and reduced mental alertness

≣ Adverse Reactions

CNS: Dizziness, fatigue, headache, somnolence
CV: **Atrial fibrillation**, palpitations
EENT: Bitter taste, dry mouth, epistaxis, nasal burning, paroxysmal sneezing, pharyngitis, rhinitis
GI: Nausea
Other: Weight gain

≣ Childbearing Considerations

PREGNANCY

- It is not known if drug can cause fetal harm.
- Use with caution only if benefit to mother outweighs potential risk to fetus.

LACTATION

- It is not known if drug is present in breast milk.
- Patient should check with prescriber before breastfeeding.
- Breastfed infants should be monitored for signs of milk rejection.

≣ Nursing Considerations

- Assess for changes in alertness, and take safety precautions, if needed.

PATIENT TEACHING

- Teach patient how to use azelastine nasal spray properly to achieve maximum therapeutic effects.
- Instruct patient to prime pump before using for first time by placing his thumb on base and his index and middle fingers on shoulder area of bottle and then pressing thumb firmly and quickly against bottle four times if using Astelin or six times if using Astepro, or until fine mist appears.
- Tell patient if he hasn't used spray in more than 3 days, he will need to reprime pump with two sprays or until fine mist appears.
- Advise patient to clear nostrils gently, if needed, before using spray.
- Teach patient to inhale deeply after each spray and then exhale through his mouth and tilt his head back so drug can spread over nasopharynx.
- Advise patient to store bottle upright and keep it tightly closed.

! WARNING Emphasize that patient must consult prescriber before taking any OTC drug, such as cough syrup or a cold remedy, because of the risk of extreme CNS depression.

- Inform patient that decreased alertness may occur. Advise him to avoid hazardous activities or those that require alertness, such as driving or operating machinery, until drug's effects are known.
- Inform breastfeeding mothers to monitor infant for milk rejection because drug may cause a bitter taste in breast milk.

azithromycin
Zithromax

azithromycin dihydrate
Zmax

≣ Class and Category

Pharmacologic class: Macrolide
Therapeutic class: Antibiotic

☰ Indications and Dosages

✻ *To treat mild community-acquired pneumonia, pharyngitis, tonsillitis, and uncomplicated skin and soft-tissue infections caused by susceptible bacteria*

ORAL SUSPENSION, TABLETS (ZITHROMAX)

Adults. 500 mg as a single dose on day 1, followed by 250 mg daily on days 2 through 5.

✻ *To treat pediatric community-acquired pneumonia*

ORAL SUSPENSION (ZITHROMAX)

Children age 6 months and over. 10 mg/kg as a single dose (not to exceed 500 mg daily) on day 1, followed by 5 mg/kg (not to exceed 250 mg daily) daily on days 2 through 5.

✻ *To treat pediatric otitis media*

ORAL SUSPENSION (ZITHROMAX)

Children age 6 months and over. 30 mg/kg as a single dose. Alternatively, 10 mg/kg once daily for 3 days, or 10 mg/kg as a single dose on day 1 followed by 5 mg/kg on days 2 through 5.

✻ *To treat pediatric pharyngitis or tonsillitis*

ORAL SUSPENSION (ZITHROMAX)

Children age 2 years and older. 12 mg/kg once daily for 5 days.

✻ *To treat community-acquired pneumonia caused by* Chlamydophila pneumoniae, Haemophilus influenzae, Legionella pneumophila, Moraxella catarrhalis, Mycoplasma pneumoniae, Staphylococcus aureus, *or* Streptococcus pneumoniae *and requiring initial I.V. therapy*

ORAL SUSPENSION, TABLETS, I.V. INFUSION (ZITHROMAX)

Adults. 500 mg I.V. as a single dose daily for at least 2 days, followed by 500 mg P.O. as a single dose daily until patient completes 7 to 10 days of therapy.

✻ *To treat community-acquired pneumonia caused by* C. pneumoniae, H. influenzae, M. pneumoniae, *or* S. pneumoniae

E.R. ORAL SUSPENSION (ZMAX)

Adults and children weighing 34 kg (75 lb) or more. 2 g as a single dose.

Children age 6 months and over weighing less than 34 kg (75 lb). 60 mg/kg as a single dose.

✻ *To treat acute bacterial sinusitis caused by* Haemophilus influenzae, Moraxella catarrhalis, *or* Streptococcus pneumoniae

ORAL SUSPENSION, TABLETS (AZITHROMYCIN)

Adults. 500 mg once daily for 3 days.

Children age 6 months and over. 10 mg/kg once daily for 3 days.

E.R. ORAL SUSPENSION (ZMAX)

Adults and children weighing 34 kg (75 lb) or more. 2 g as a single dose.

Children age 6 months and over weighing less than 34 kg (75 lb). 60 mg/kg as a single dose.

✻ *To treat acute bacterial exacerbations of COPD including chronic bronchitis caused by* H. influenzae, M. catarrhalis, *or* S. pneumoniae

ORAL SUSPENSION, TABLETS (ZITHROMAX)

Adults. 500 mg daily for 3 days, or 500 mg as a single dose on day 1, followed by 250 mg daily on days 2 through 5.

✻ *To treat nongonococcal cervicitis and urethritis caused by* Chlamydia trachomatis

ORAL SUSPENSION, TABLETS (ZITHROMAX)

Adults. 1 g as a one-time dose.

✻ *To treat urethritis or cervicitis caused by* Neisseria gonorrhoeae

ORAL SUSPENSION, TABLETS (ZITHROMAX)

Adults. 2 g as a one-time dose.

✻ *To prevent* Mycobacterium avium *complex (MAC) in patients with advanced HIV infection*

ORAL SUSPENSION, TABLETS (ZITHROMAX)

Adults. 1.2 g once weekly, as indicated.

As adjunct to treat MAC in patients with advanced HIV infection

ORAL SUSPENSION, TABLETS (ZITHROMAX)

Adults. 600 mg daily in combination with ethambutol 15 mg/kg daily.

✻ *To treat pelvic inflammatory disease caused by* Chlamydia trachomatis, Neisseria gonorrhoeae, *or* Mycoplasma hominis *and requiring initial I.V. therapy*

ORAL SUSPENSION, TABLETS, I.V. INFUSION (ZITHROMAX)

Adults. 500 mg I.V. as a single dose daily for 1 to 2 days, followed by 250 mg P.O. as a single dose daily until patient completes 7 days of therapy.

Drug Administration

P.O.

- Administer Zmax on an empty stomach at least 1 hour before or 2 hours following a meal. Zithromax can be administered with or without food.
- Reconstitute oral suspension by adding 60 ml of water to the container. Shake well before administering. Do not refrigerate. Constituted suspension should be consumed within 12 hours. Any suspension remaining after dosing must be discarded.
- For children weighing less than 34 kg (75 lb) and prescribed oral suspension, use a calibrated dosing device to measure dose.

I.V.

- Reconstitute by adding 4.8 ml of Sterile Water for Injection to the 500-mg drug vial and shaking until all the drug is dissolved. Each ml of reconstituted solution contains 100 mg of azithromycin. Solution is stable for 24 hours when stored below 30°C (86°F).
- Use a standard (non-automated) 5-ml syringe to ensure that an accurate amount of 4.8 ml is withdrawn for reconstitution.
- Dilute further to provide a concentration range of 1–2 mg/ml by transferring 5 ml of the reconstituted solution into 0.9% Sodium Chloride Injection, 5% Dextrose in Water, or any of the other solutions recommended by the manufacturer. To achieve a final infusion solution concentration of 1 mg/ml, use 500 ml of diluting solution; to achieve 2 mg/ml, use 250 ml of diluting solution.
- Infuse a 2 mg/ml infusion over 1 hour and a 1 mg/ml infusion over 3 hours. Do not give as a bolus or as an intramuscular injection.
- Diluted drug may be stored at or below room temperature of 30°C (86°F) for 24 hours or for 7 days if refrigerated.
- *Incompatibilities:* Other intravenous additives or drugs

Route	Onset	Peak	Duration
P.O.	Unknown	2.5–4.5 hr	Unknown
I.V.	Unknown	1–2 hr	Unknown

Half-life: 2–3 days

Mechanism of Action

Binds to a ribosomal subunit of susceptible bacteria, blocking peptide translocation and inhibiting RNA-dependent protein synthesis. Drug concentrates in phagocytes, macrophages, and fibroblasts, which release it slowly and may help move it to infection sites.

Contraindications

History of cholestatic jaundice or hepatic dysfunction associated with prior use of azithromycin; hypersensitivity to azithromycin, erythromycin, ketolide antibiotics, other macrolide antibiotics or their components

Interactions

DRUGS

antacids that contain aluminum or magnesium: Possibly decreased peak blood azithromycin level
nelfinavir: Possibly increased blood levels of these drugs
oral anticoagulants such as warfarin: Possibly potentiated effects of oral anticoagulants
other macrolides: Possible adverse effects

FOODS

any food: Altered absorption rate of azithromycin

Adverse Reactions

CNS: Aggressiveness, agitation, anxiety, asthenia, dizziness, fatigue, headache, hyperactivity, malaise, nervousness, paresthesia, **seizures**, somnolence, syncope, vertigo
CV: **Arrhythmias**, chest pain, edema, **hypotension**, palpitations, **prolonged QT interval**, **torsades de pointes**, **ventricular tachycardia**
EENT: Hearing loss, oral candidiasis, perversion or loss of taste or smell, tinnitus, tongue discoloration
ENDO: Hyperglycemia
GI: Abdominal pain, anorexia, cholestatic jaundice, *Clostridioides difficile*–**associated diarrhea,** constipation, diarrhea, dyspepsia, elevated liver enzymes, flatulence, **hepatic necrosis or failure, hepatitis,** nausea, **pancreatitis,** pyloric stenosis, **pseudomembranous colitis,** vomiting
GU: **Acute renal failure,** elevated BUN and serum creatinine levels, nephritis, vaginal candidiasis
HEME: **Leukopenia, neutropenia, thrombocytopenia**

MS: Arthralgia, elevated creatine kinase levels
SKIN: Acute generalized exanthematous pustulosis, **erythema multiforme,** photosensitivity, pruritus, rash, **Stevens–Johnson syndrome, toxic epidermal necrolysis,** urticaria
Other: Allergic reaction, anaphylaxis, angioedema, drug reaction with eosinophilia and systemic symptoms (DRESS), elevated serum phosphorus level, **hyperkalemia,** infusion-site reaction (such as pain and redness), new or worsening myasthenia syndrome, superinfection

Childbearing Considerations
PREGNANCY
- It is not known if drug can cause fetal harm.
- Use with caution only if benefit to mother outweighs potential risk to fetus.

LACTATION
- Drug is present in breast milk.
- Patient should check with prescriber before breastfeeding.
- If breastfeeding occurs, mother should monitor breastfed infant for diarrhea, rash, or vomiting.

Nursing Considerations
- Be aware that azithromycin should not be used in patients with known QT prolongation, bradyarrhythmias, congenital long QT syndrome, uncompensated heart failure, or history of torsades de pointes; patients with ongoing proarrhythmic conditions such as uncorrected hypokalemia or hypomagnesemia, or significant bradycardia; or patients receiving drugs known to prolong the QT interval such as class IA (procainamide, quinidine) or class III (amiodarone, dofetilide, sotalol) antiarrhythmic agents because of increased risk of life-threatening arrhythmias such as torsades de pointes.
- Know that azithromycin should not be used in patients who have undergone donor stem cell transplant for cancer of the blood or lymph nodes because of an increased risk for cancer relapse and possibly death.

! **WARNING** Be aware that azithromycin therapy has been linked to an increased risk for acute cardiovascular death, with the risk being greatest during the first 5 days

of therapy. The risk can occur in patients with or without a history of preexisting cardiovascular disease.

- Monitor elderly patients closely for arrhythmias because they are more susceptible to drug effects on the QT interval.
- Obtain culture and sensitivity test results, if possible, before starting therapy.
- Use azithromycin cautiously in patients with hepatic dysfunction not associated with prior use of azithromycin (drug is metabolized in the liver) or renal dysfunction (effects are unknown in this group).
- Monitor liver enzymes closely in patients with impaired liver function and expect to discontinue drug immediately if signs and symptoms of hepatitis occur.
- Assess patient for bacterial or fungal superinfection, which may occur with prolonged or repeated therapy. If it occurs, expect to give another antibiotic or antifungal.
- Monitor bowel elimination; if needed, obtain stool culture to rule out pseudomembranous colitis. If it occurs, expect to stop azithromycin and give fluid, electrolytes, and antibiotics effective with *Clostridium difficile.*
- Be aware that laboratory abnormalities may occur during azithromycin therapy. If present, alert prescriber, as changes can be reversible.

PATIENT TEACHING
- Tell patient to take Zmax oral suspension 1 hour before or 2 to 3 hours after food. Instruct patient to take Zithromax tablets without regard to food.
- Urge patient to consult prescriber before taking OTC drugs, including antacids. If they're prescribed, tell patient to take azithromycin 1 hour before or 2 to 3 hours after taking antacids. Also advise patient to inform prescriber of all prescriptions and drugs being taken, including over-the-counter and herbal preparations.

! **WARNING** Tell patient to report signs and symptoms of allergic reaction (such as chest tightness, hives, itching, rash, and trouble breathing) immediately.

A

- Warn patient that abdominal pain and loose, watery stools may occur. If diarrhea persists or becomes severe, urge him to contact prescriber and replace fluids.
- Teach patient to watch for and immediately report signs of superinfection, such as white patches in the mouth.

! **WARNING** Inform patient that drug may cause serious heart rhythm changes. Stress importance of seeking immediate emergency help if chest discomfort, dizziness, or feeling faint occurs or heart feels like it's pounding or racing or the heartbeat is irregular.

aztreonam
Azactam, Cayston

Class and Category
Pharmacologic class: Monobactam
Therapeutic class: Antibiotic

Indications and Dosages
✱ *To improve respiratory symptoms in cystic fibrosis patients with* Pseudomonas aeruginosa

INHALATION (CAYSTON)
Adults and children age 7 and over. 75 mg (1 vial) 3 times a day with doses at least 4 hr apart for 28 days (followed by 28 days off of therapy).

✱ *To treat infections of the female reproductive tract; lower respiratory tract, skin, soft tissue, or urinary tract; intra-abdominal infections; septicemia; and surgical abscesses caused by susceptible strains of gram-negative bacteria*

I.V. INFUSION, I.V. OR I.M. INJECTION (AZACTAM)
Adults with a urinary tract infection. 500 mg or 1 g every 8 or 12 hours.
Adults with moderately severe systemic infections. 1 or 2 g given every 8 to 12 hrs.
Adults with severe systemic or life-threatening infections or an infection due to *Pseudomonas aeruginosa.* 2 g every 6 or 8 hrs. *Maximum:* 8 g daily.

I.V. INFUSION OR INJECTION (AZACTAM)
Children ages 9 months and over with mild to moderate infections. 30 mg/kg every 8 hr. *Maximum:* 120 mg/kg daily.
Children ages 9 months and over with moderate to severe infections. 30 mg/kg

every 6 to 8 hr up to 120 mg/kg daily. *Maximum:* 120 mg/kg/daily.
±**DOSAGE ADJUSTMENT** If creatinine clearance is 10 to 30 ml/min, initial dose is 1 to 2 g; then 50% of usual dose at usual interval. If creatinine clearance is less than 10 ml/min, initial dose is 500 mg to 2 g; then 25% of the usual dose every 6, 8, or 12 hr. For hemodialysis patients with serious or life-threatening infections, in addition to the maintenance doses, one-eighth of the initial dose given after each hemodialysis session.

Drug Administration
I.V.
- For bolus injection, reconstitute by injecting 6 to 10 ml of Sterile Water for Injection into drug vial. Immediately shake vial vigorously to mix. After withdrawing prescribed dose, discard unused solution. Reconstituted solution will be colorless to light straw yellow but may turn light pink on standing at room temperature. This doesn't affect drug potency.
- Give I.V. bolus injection directly into I.V. tubing slowly over 3 to 5 minutes after flushing line with a compatible solution, if needed. Once administered, flush I.V. line again, if necessary.
- If drug is to be administered as an I.V. infusion, the 15-ml drug vial should first be reconstituted with at least 3 ml of Sterile Water for Injection for each gram of aztreonam to be administered. Further dilute drug with an I.V. solution such as 0.9% Sodium Chloride, 5% Dextrose in Water, Lactated Ringer's Injection, or any other solution recommended by manufacturer to a final concentration not to exceed 20 mg/ml.
- Administer I.V. infusion over 20 to 60 minutes.
- Flush I.V. tubing with a solution, such as 0.9% Sodium Chloride for Injection, before and after administering I.V. infusion.
- If drug solution is frozen, thaw it, but do not immerse drug in water baths or microwave irradiation to thaw it. After thawing is complete, invert the container to ensure a well-mixed solution. Administer only as an I.V. infusion.
- *Incompatibilities:* Cephradine, metronidazole, or nafcillin sodium; other admixtures

I.M.

- Reconstitute with at least 3 ml of Bacteriostatic Sodium Chloride Injection, 0.9% Sodium Chloride Injection, Sterile Water for Injection, or Sterile Bacteriostatic Water for Injection for each gram of aztreonam to be administered.
- Do not admix with any local anesthetic agent.
- Administer as a deep injection into a large muscle mass (such as the upper outer quadrant of the gluteus maximus or lateral part of the thigh).

INHALATION

- Dilute each vial of inhalation solution with 1 ampule of the diluent that comes with drug. To do so, open the glass drug vial carefully, remove metal ring by pulling the tab, and remove the gray rubber stopper. Twist the tip off the diluent ampule and squeeze the liquid into the glass drug vial. Replace the rubber stopper, then gently swirl the vial until contents have been completely dissolved.
- Administer immediately, using only an Altera Nebulizer System. After placing the diluted drug into the handset of the nebulizer, turn the unit on. Then place the mouthpiece of the handset into the patient's mouth. Have patient breathe normally through his mouth. Expect to administer drug over 2 to 3 minutes.
- Bronchodilators should be given prior to aztreonam inhalation therapy. A short-acting bronchodilator should be used at least 15 minutes before but no sooner than 4 hours prior to aztreonam inhalation therapy, or a long-acting bronchodilator at least 30 minutes before but no longer than 12 hours prior to aztreonam inhalation therapy. If patient is receiving multiple inhaled therapies, administer the bronchodilator first, followed by mucolytics, and last aztreonam.

Route	Onset	Peak	Duration
I.V.	Unknown	Immediate	Unknown
I.M.	Unknown	60 min	Unknown
Inhalation	Unknown	60 min	Unknown

Half-life: 1.5–2 hr

Mechanism of Action

Inhibits bacterial cell wall synthesis in susceptible aerobic gram-negative bacteria. These bacteria assemble rigid, cross-linked cell walls in several steps. Aztreonam affects the final cross-linking step by inactivating penicillin-binding protein 3 (the enzyme that links cell wall strands), which causes cell lysis and death.

Contraindications

Hypersensitivity to aztreonam or its components

Interactions

DRUGS

None reported

Adverse Reactions

CNS: Confusion, dizziness, **encephalopathy,** fever, headache, insomnia, malaise, paresthesia, **seizures,** vertigo

CV: Chest pain, **hypotension,** transient ECG changes

EENT: Altered taste, diplopia, halitosis, mouth ulcers, mucocutaneous candidiasis, nasal congestion, sneezing, tinnitus, tongue numbness

GI: Abdominal cramps, diarrhea, elevated enzymes, **GI bleeding, hepatitis,** jaundice, nausea, **pseudomembranous colitis,** vomiting

GU: Breast tenderness, elevated serum creatinine level, vaginal candidiasis

HEME: Anemia, eosinophilia, leukocytosis, **neutropenia, pancytopenia,** positive Coombs' test, **prolonged PT and APTT, thrombocytopenia,** thrombocytosis

MS: Arthralgia, joint swelling, myalgia

RESP: **Bronchospasm,** dyspnea, wheezing

SKIN: Diaphoresis, **erythema multiforme, exfoliative dermatitis,** flushing, petechiae, pruritus, purpura, rash, **toxic epidermal necrolysis,** urticaria

Other: **Anaphylaxis, angioedema,** injection-site reaction (pain, phlebitis, swelling, or thrombophlebitis)

Childbearing Considerations

PREGNANCY

- It is not known if drug can cause fetal harm although it does cross the placental barrier.
- Cystic fibrosis may increase the risk for preterm delivery.

- Use with caution only if benefit to mother outweighs potential risk to fetus.

LACTATION

- Drug is present in breast milk.
- Breastfeeding should be withheld during drug therapy when Azactam is used. Patient should check with prescriber before breastfeeding when Cayston is used.

Nursing Considerations

- Obtain culture and sensitivity test results, if possible, before starting aztreonam therapy. If patient is acutely ill, expect to begin therapy before results are available.
- Keep in mind that other antimicrobials may be used with aztreonam in seriously ill patients at risk for gram-positive infection.
- Expect to use I.V. route for patients who need single doses over 1 g and those with life-threatening systemic infections, such as septicemia or peritonitis.

! WARNING Monitor patient for a hypersensitivity reaction, which could become life-threatening.

- Assess for signs of bacterial or fungal superinfection, which may occur with prolonged or repeated therapy. If superinfection occurs, treat it as prescribed.
- Monitor bowel elimination; if needed, obtain stool culture to rule out pseudomembranous colitis. If it occurs,

expect to discontinue aztreonam and administer fluid, electrolytes, and antibiotics effective against *Clostridium difficile*.

- Evaluate patient's renal and liver function test results, as ordered, if patient has renal or hepatic impairment.
- Monitor renal function if patient is receiving an aminoglycoside because of the increased risk of nephrotoxicity.

PATIENT TEACHING

- Emphasize the need to take full course of aztreonam exactly as prescribed, even if patient feels better before finishing it.
- Instruct patient how to dilute and administer inhalation form of drug, if ordered.

! WARNING Teach patient to recognize and immediately report signs and symptoms of allergic reactions, such as chest tightness, difficulty breathing, hives, itching, and rash.

- Warn patient that abdominal pain and loose, watery stools may occur 2 months or more after aztreonam therapy stops. If diarrhea persists or becomes severe, urge him to contact prescriber and replace fluids.
- Teach patient to watch for and immediately report signs of superinfection, such as white patches in mouth.

B

baloxavir marboxil
Xofluza

Class and Category
Pharmacologic class: Polymerase acidic endonuclease inhibitor
Therapeutic class: Influenza antiviral

Indications and Dosages
* *To treat acute uncomplicated influenza in patients who have been symptomatic for no more than 48 hours and who are otherwise healthy, or at high risk of developing influenza-related complications; to prevent influenza following contact with an individual who has influenza*

ORAL SUSPENSION, TABLETS
Adults and children 12 years and over weighing at least 80 kg (176 lb). 80 mg as a single dose.
Adults and children 12 years and over weighing 40 kg (88 lb) to less than 80 kg (176 lb). 40 mg as a single dose.

Drug Administration
P.O.
- Do not give drug with antacids, calcium-fortified beverages, dairy products, oral supplements (calcium, iron, magnesium, selenium, or zinc), or polyvalent cation-containing laxatives.
- Tablets should be swallowed whole.
- Oral suspension can be constituted with 20 ml of plain or Sterile Water to a volume of suspension of 40 mg/20 ml (2 mg/ml). Gently swirl the suspension. Do not shake. More than one bottle may be needed for adults and adolescents weighing at least 80 kg.
- Use a calibrated measuring device to ensure correct dosage.
- For enteral administration, flush tube with 1 ml of water, administer the suspension with an enteral syringe, and reflush tube with 1 ml of water after administration.
- Drug does not contain preservatives and must be administered within 10 hours after constitution. During that time it may be stored at room temperature. Discard if not used within 10 hours or if suspension has been stored above 25°C (77°F).

Route	Onset	Peak	Duration
P.O.	Unknown	4 hr	Unknown

Half-life: 79.1 hr

Mechanism of Action
Inhibits the endonuclease activity of the polymerase acidic protein, an influenza virus-specific enzyme required for viral gene transcription. This action prevents the influenza virus from being replicated.

Contraindications
Hypersensitivity to baloxavir marboxil or its components

Interactions
DRUGS
antacids, laxatives, oral supplements, and other polyvalent cation-containing products (e.g., calcium, iron, magnesium, selenium, or zinc): Possibly decreased plasma concentrations of baloxavir which may reduce its effectiveness
live attenuated intranasal influenza vaccine: Possibly decreased effectiveness of vaccination

FOODS
calcium-fortified beverages, dairy products: Possibly decreased effectiveness of baloxavir

Adverse Reactions
CNS: Abnormal behavior, delirium, hallucinations, headache
EENT: Nasopharyngitis, sinusitis
GI: Bloody diarrhea, colitis, diarrhea, nausea, vomiting
RESP: Bronchitis
SKIN: Erythema multiforme, rash, urticaria
Other: Anaphylactic shock, anaphylaxis, angioedema, hypersensitivity reactions

Childbearing Considerations
PREGNANCY
- It is not known if drug can cause fetal harm.
- Use with caution only if benefit to mother outweighs potential risk to fetus.

LACTATION
- It is not known if drug is present in breast milk.
- Patient should check with prescriber before breastfeeding.

⬚ Nursing Considerations

- Be aware that baloxavir is not effective in treating infections other than influenza.
- Know that baloxavir should be administered to patients who have had flu symptoms for no more than 48 hours.
- Do not administer baloxavir with calcium-fortified beverages, dairy products, or drugs that contain cation-containing products such as calcium, iron, magnesium, selenium, or zinc.

> **! WARNING** Monitor patient closely for hypersensitivity reactions that could be life-threatening. Be prepared to provide emergency treatment per institutional protocol.

PATIENT TEACHING

- Inform patient that baloxavir will be administered only once.
- Instruct patient that drug must not be taken with a calcium-fortified beverage or a meal containing dairy products. Also, tell patient to alert prescriber if he is taking any drugs that contain calcium, iron, magnesium, selenium, or zinc, because baloxavir may not be as effective when taken with such drugs.
- Tell patient that an oral suspension is available if he has difficulty swallowing tablets. If oral suspension is needed, explain how to mix the suspension and emphasize importance of discarding suspension after 10 hours. Tell patient to use a calibrated measuring device to ensure accurate dosing, not a household spoon.

> **! WARNING** Warn patient that drug can cause severe allergic reactions. Tell patient to seek immediate medical attention if an allergic reaction occurs.

- Advise patient to check with prescriber before receiving live attenuated influenza vaccines after taking drug.

balsalazide disodium
Colazal, Giazo

⬚ Class and Category

Pharmacologic class: Aminosalicylate
Therapeutic class: Anti-inflammatory

⬚ Indications and Dosages

✳ *To treat mildly to moderately active ulcerative colitis*

CAPSULES (COLAZAL)

Adults. 2.25 g three times daily for up to 8 to 12 wk. *Maximum:* 6.75 g daily for 12 wk.
Children ages 5 to 17. 750 mg or 2.25 g three times daily for up to 8 wk.

TABLETS (GIAZO)

Male adults. 3.3 g twice daily for up to 8 wk.

⬚ Drug Administration

P.O.

- Capsules and tablets should be swallowed whole and not chewed or crushed. However, if patient cannot swallow capsule whole, it can be opened and contents sprinkled on applesauce. Mixture should be swallowed immediately. Patient may chew contents once mixed, if needed. Color variation ranging from orange to yellow of the powder is normal if capsule is opened.
- Capsules and tablets should be given with a full glass of water.

Route	Onset	Peak	Duration
P.O.	10–14 days	1–2 hr	Unknown

Half-life: Unknown

⬚ Mechanism of Action

After it has been metabolized to 5-ASA, balsalazide may reduce inflammation by inhibiting the enzyme cyclooxygenase and decreasing production of arachidonic acid metabolites, which may be increased in patients with inflammatory bowel disease.

Cyclooxygenase is needed to form prostaglandin from arachidonic acid. Prostaglandin mediates inflammatory activity and produces signs and symptoms of inflammation. By inhibiting prostaglandin synthesis, balsalazide may reduce signs and symptoms of inflammation in inflammatory bowel disease.

Balsalazide also interferes with leukotriene synthesis and inhibits the enzyme lipoxygenase. These substances are involved in the inflammatory response.

⬚ Contraindications

Hypersensitivity to balsalazide, salicylates, or their components

≡ Interactions

DRUGS

6-mercaptopurine, azathioprine: Possibly increased risk for blood disorders, bone marrow failure, and associated complications

nephrotoxic drugs such as NSAIDs: Possible increased risk of adverse renal effects

≡ Adverse Reactions

CNS: Fatigue, fever, headache, insomnia
CV: Myocarditis, pericarditis, vasculitis
EENT: Dry mouth, nasopharyngitis, pharyngitis, rhinitis, stomatitis
GI: Abdominal cramps or pain, anorexia, cholestatic jaundice, **cirrhosis,** constipation, diarrhea, dyspepsia, elevated bilirubin or liver enzyme levels, exacerbation of colitis, flatulence, **hepatic failure, hepatotoxicity,** jaundice, **liver necrosis,** nausea, **pancreatitis,** vomiting
GU: Acute and chronic interstitial nephritis, dysmenorrhea, interstitial nephritis, nephrolithiasis, **renal failure,** UTI
MS: Arthralgia, myalgia
RESP: Alveolitis, **asthma exacerbation,** cough, **eosinophilic pneumonia, interstitial pneumonitis,** pleural effusion, pleurisy, pneumonia, respiratory tract infection
SKIN: Acute generalized exanthematous pustulosis, alopecia, dry skin, erythema nodosum, photosensitivity, pruritus, psoriasis, pyoderma gangrenosum, **Stevens–Johnson syndrome (SJS), toxic epidermal necrolysis (TEN),** urticaria
Other: Anaphylaxis, flu-like syndrome, **Kawasaki-like syndrome, mesalamine-induced acute intolerance syndrome**

≡ Childbearing Considerations

PREGNANCY

- It is not known if drug can cause fetal harm.
- Be aware that women with ulcerative colitis who develop an increased disease activity during pregnancy are at risk of developing adverse pregnancy outcomes such as low birth weight or small for gestational age of neonate and preterm delivery.
- Use with caution only if benefit to mother outweighs potential risk to fetus.

LACTATION

- Drug may be present in breast milk in small amounts.

- Patient should check with prescriber before breastfeeding. If breastfeeding is undertaken, infant should be monitored for diarrhea.

≡ Nursing Considerations

- Know that patient's renal function should be assessed prior to starting balsalazide therapy and then periodically during therapy because drug may cause renal impairment that could be serious.

! WARNING Monitor patients who are sensitive to olsalazine or sulfasalazine for possible cross-sensitivity to balsalazide.

- Monitor patients with pyloric stenosis for decreased or delayed drug effects due to prolonged gastric retention of balsalazide capsules.
- Monitor patient for possible exacerbation of colitis symptoms.

! WARNING Monitor patient for mesalamine-induced acute intolerance syndrome (abdominal pain, bloody diarrhea, cramping, fever, headache, and rash). If suspected, notify prescriber and expect drug to be discontinued because, although uncommon, it could become life-threatening.

! WARNING Monitor patients with known liver impairment for hepatic failure as a result of balsalazide being converted to mesalamine.

! WARNING Monitor patient for signs and symptoms of severe cutaneous adverse reactions, which have occurred with the use of mesalamine, the active moiety of balsalazide. These reactions may become life-threatening. If patient develops a rash, blistering lesions, or other skin abnormalities, contact prescriber immediately, and expect drug to be discontinued.

- Ensure that patient is adequately hydrated during therapy because mesalamine (main active moiety of balsalazide) has been associated with nephrolithiasis.
- Be aware that each 1.1-g tablet of balsalazide contains 126 mg of sodium. The daily dose of 6.6 grams/day provides about 756 mg of sodium per day. Monitor patients on a sodium-restricted diet or

B

patients at risk for congestive heart failure for adverse effects.

- Be aware that drug may lead to elevated test results when measuring urinary normetanephrine by liquid chromatography with electrochemical detection.

PATIENT TEACHING

- Inform patient that balsalazide is used to reduce bowel inflammation and pain in ulcerative colitis and to minimize recurring inflammation.
- Instruct patient to swallow capsules whole and not to chew or crush them. However, capsules can be opened and mixed with applesauce if patient is unable to swallow the capsules whole. If mixed, drug should be taken immediately. Contents of capsule can be chewed, if needed. Reassure patient that color variation of the powder inside the capsule may range from orange to yellow but is normal.
- Administer drug with a full glass of water.
- Advise patient to notify prescriber of any other drugs she may be taking, including herbal products, nutritional supplements, and OTC drugs, because they may interact with balsalazide.
- Instruct patient to notify prescriber immediately if colitis symptoms worsen.
- Instruct patient to be compliant with all blood tests ordered while taking balsalazide.

! **WARNING** Review signs and symptoms of allergic reactions, mesalamine-induced acute intolerance syndrome, and severe skin disorders. Advise patient to notify prescriber immediately, if present.

- Review signs and symptoms of liver impairment, especially for patients with known liver disease, and instruct patient to report such effects to prescriber.
- Advise patient to avoid sun exposure, use a broad-spectrum sunscreen, and wear protective clothing when outdoors.
- Alert patients on a sodium-restricted diet or patients at risk of developing congestive heart failure of the sodium content of tablets.
- Inform patient that she can expect some improvement in symptoms in 3 to 21 days but that optimal results may take up to 6 weeks of treatment.

baricitinib
Olumiant

Class and Category
Pharmacologic class: Janus kinase inhibitor
Therapeutic class: Antirheumatic

Indications and Dosages
✱ *To treat moderate to severe active rheumatoid arthritis in patients who have had an inadequate response to one or more tumor necrosis factor (TNF) antagonist therapies*

TABLETS
Adults. 2 mg once daily.

±**DOSAGE ADJUSTMENT** For patients with moderate renal impairment (estimated glomerular filtration rate between 30 and 60 ml/min) or patients taking strong organic anion transporter 3 (OAT3) inhibitors such as probenecid, dosage reduced to 1 mg once daily. For patients who develop an absolute lymphocyte count (ALC) less than 500 cells/mm^3, drug withheld until ALC is 500 cells/mm^3 or greater. For patients who develop an absolute neutrophil count (ANC) less than 1,000 cells/mm^3, drug withheld until ANC is 1,000 cells/mm^3 or greater. For patients who develop a hemoglobin value less than 8 g/dl, drug withheld until hemoglobin is 8 g/dl or greater.

Drug Administration
P.O.
- No specific instructions recommended by manufacturer for administration.

Route	Onset	Peak	Duration
P.O.	Unknown	1 hr	Unknown

Half-life: 12 hr

Mechanism of Action
Janus kinases are intracellular enzymes that influence cellular processes of hematopoiesis and immune cell function. Janus kinase inhibitors interfere with these actions, thereby reducing the signs and symptoms of rheumatoid arthritis, which is thought to be an autoimmune disorder.

Contraindications
Hypersensitivity to baricitinib or its components

Interactions

DRUGS

Strong organic anion transporter 3 inhibitors, such as probenecid: Increased baricitinib exposure, increasing risk of adverse reactions
Live vaccines: Decreased effectiveness of vaccine

Adverse Reactions

CV: Elevated lipid levels, **thrombosis (including arterial and deep vein thrombosis)**
GI: Elevated liver enzymes, **gastrointestinal perforation**, nausea
GU: UTI
HEME: Anemia, **elevated platelet count, lymphopenia, neutropenia**
MS: Elevated creatine phosphokinase (CPK) levels
RESP: Bronchitis, pneumonia, **pulmonary embolus**, upper respiratory infections
SKIN: Acne, **nonmelanoma skin cancers**, rash, urticaria
Other: **Angioedema**; infections such as bacterial, fungal (invasive), mycobacterial, viral, or other opportunistic infections; **lymphomas and other malignancies**

Childbearing Considerations

PREGNANCY

- It is not known if drug can cause fetal harm.
- Use with caution only if benefit to mother outweighs potential risk to fetus.

LACTATION

- It is not known if drug is present in breast milk.
- Breastfeeding should be avoided during drug therapy.

Nursing Considerations

- Be aware that baricitinib should not be used in patients with an ALC less than 500 cells/mm^3, ANC less than 1,000 cells/mm^3, or hemoglobin level less than 8 g/dl.
- Know that baricitinib therapy should also be avoided in patients with an active, serious infection, including localized infections. In addition, drug is not recommended in patients with a glomerular filtration rate less than 30 ml/min or patients who have severe hepatic impairment.
- Be aware that patients who are 50 years or older with at least one cardiovascular risk factor, including being a current or past smoker, may have a higher risk for

sudden cardiovascular death, MI, or stroke because higher rates have occurred with use of another Janus kinase inhibitor. Monitor patient closely for cardiovascular abnormalities and expect drug to be discontinued, if any occurs.

- Test patients for latent tuberculosis, as ordered, prior to initiating baricitinib therapy. If positive, expect patient to receive treatment. Monitor all patients for signs and symptoms of tuberculosis throughout therapy, including patients who were negative for latent tuberculosis infection prior to initiating therapy. Know that tuberculosis therapy also may be prescribed for patients with a history of active or latent tuberculosis in whom an adequate course of treatment cannot be confirmed and for patients with a negative test for latent tuberculosis but who have risk factors for tuberculosis.

- Expect liver enzymes to be determined prior to baricitinib therapy and periodically throughout therapy, because drug can affect liver function. Know that if increases in liver enzymes occur and liver injury is suspected, drug therapy should be stopped until liver dysfunction is ruled out.

! WARNING Monitor patient closely for hypersensitivity reactions such as angioedema, rash, and urticaria. Reactions may become serious. If present, notify prescriber and expect baricitinib to be discontinued. Provide supportive care per institutional protocol.

- Be aware that viral reactivation, including herpes zoster, may occur. If patient develops herpes zoster during therapy with baricitinib, expect drug therapy to be interrupted until the episode has been resolved. Know that patients should be screened for viral hepatitis before initiating therapy with baricitinib.

- Use baricitinib cautiously in patients who may be at increased risk for gastrointestinal perforation or thrombosis, as drug use may increase the risk for these life-threatening disorders.

! WARNING Monitor patient's complete blood count closely, as drug may cause anemia, lymphopenia, or neutropenia. Expect drug to be withheld if patient develops an ALC less than 500 cells/mm^3 until ALC is 500 cells/mm^3 or greater; an ANC less than 1,000 cells/mm^3 until ANC is 1,000 cells/mm^3 or greater; or a hemoglobin value becomes less than 8 g/dl until the hemoglobin level is 8 g/dl or greater.

- Assess patient regularly for signs and symptoms of infection, because serious and sometimes fatal infections due to bacterial, invasive fungal, mycobacterial, viral, or other opportunistic pathogens may occur. Patients at higher risk are those who are taking immunosuppressants such as corticosteroids or methotrexate. Notify prescriber if infection is suspected and expect antibiotic therapy to be prescribed, if confirmed. Know that baricitinib may be temporarily stopped if patient is not responding to antibiotic therapy and not restarted until the infection is under control.
- Be aware that baricitinib increases the risk of cancer. Assess patient regularly, especially for nonmelanoma skin cancers. Also, know that higher rates of lung cancers and lymphomas have occurred with use of another Janus kinase inhibitor.

! **WARNING** Assess patient regularly for thrombosis, including arterial, deep venous thrombosis, and pulmonary embolism, as drug increases risk of thrombus formation, especially in patients who are 50 years or older and have at least one cardiovascular risk factor.

- Monitor patient for new-onset abdominal symptoms, especially patients with a history of diverticulitis, because baricitinib increases the risk for gastrointestinal perforation.
- Monitor patient's lipid profile periodically, as ordered, during baricitinib therapy. Know that a lipid profile should be performed about 12 weeks into baricitinib therapy to determine if management of hyperlipidemia is needed.
- Avoid giving patient live vaccines during baricitinib therapy because drug may reduce effectiveness of the vaccination.

PATIENT TEACHING
- Instruct patient to take baricitinib exactly as prescribed.

! **WARNING** Stress importance of seeking immediate medical attention if an allergic reaction such as hives; rash; or swelling of

lips, tongue, or throat occurs and to stop taking baricitinib.

- Inform patient of her risk for infections. Review signs and symptoms of infection and stress importance of notifying prescriber if an infection is suspected or develops. Also tell patient that herpes zoster may also occur. Because it could become quite serious, it should be reported.
- Tell patient that baricitinib therapy increases the risk of certain cancers. Encourage her to report any unusual, persistent, or severe signs or symptoms to prescriber. Also instruct patient to periodically examine her skin for signs of skin cancer.
- Review signs and symptoms of a blood clot, MI, or stroke with patient and stress importance of seeking immediate medical attention if suspected.
- Alert patient that laboratory abnormalities such as an elevated lipid profile or liver enzymes may occur during baricitinib therapy and may require treatment. Stress importance of complying with ordered laboratory tests.
- Advise mothers not to breastfeed during treatment with baricitinib.
- Instruct patient not to receive vaccinations containing live virus during baricitinib therapy.

beclomethasone dipropionate
QNASL, QVAR Redihaler

beclomethasone dipropionate monohydrate
Beconase AQ

⬛ Class and Category
Pharmacologic class: Corticosteroid
Therapeutic class: Antiasthmatic, anti-inflammatory

⬛ Indications and Dosages
✱ *To maintain treatment of asthma as prophylactic therapy*

ORAL INHALATION AEROSOL (QVAR REDIHALER)

Adults and adolescents who are not on an inhaled corticosteroid. *Initial:* 1 to 2 inhalations (40 to 80 mcg) twice daily, depending on strength used. *Maximum:* 4 to 8 inhalations (up to 320 mcg) twice daily, depending on strength used.

Adults and adolescents switching from another inhaled corticosteroid. *Dependent on strength of previous inhaled corticosteroid and disease severity:* 1 inhalation (40 mcg), 1 or 2 inhalations (80 mcg) depending on dosage strength, 2–4 inhalations (160 mcg) depending on dosage strength, or 4 inhalations (320 mcg) using 80-mcg strength twice daily. *Maximum:* 320 mcg twice daily.

Children ages 4 to 11. 1 inhalation (40 mcg) twice daily, increased after 2 wk to 2 inhalations (80 mcg) twice daily, as needed. *Maximum:* 2 inhalations (80 mcg) twice daily.

✱ *To relieve symptoms of seasonal or perennial allergic and nonallergic (vasomotor) rhinitis; to prevent recurrence of nasal polyps after surgical removal*

NASAL SPRAY (BECONASE AQ)

Adults and children age 12 and older. 1 or 2 inhalations (42 or 84 mcg) in each nostril twice daily for total dose of 168 or 336 mcg daily.

Children ages 6 to 12. *Initial:* 1 spray (42 mcg) in each nostril twice daily, increased to 2 sprays (84 mcg) in each nostril twice daily, as needed. Once control is achieved, dosage decreased to 1 spray (42 mcg) in each nostril twice daily. *Maximum:* 336 mcg (2 sprays in each nostril) daily given in two divided doses 12 hr apart.

✱ *To treat nasal symptoms associated with perennial or seasonal allergic rhinitis*

NASAL SPRAY (QNASI)

Adults and children 12 years and older. 2 inhalations (using 80-mcg strength) in each nostril once daily for a total dose of 320 mcg daily. *Maximum:* 4 inhalations (320 mcg) per day.

Children ages 4 to and including 11. 1 inhalation (using 40-mcg strength) in each nostril once daily for a total dose of 80 mcg daily. *Maximum:* 2 inhalations (80 mcg) per day.

☰ Drug Administration

NASAL SPRAY

- Daily dosages given twice daily should be spaced about 12 hours apart.
- Have patient blow nose and then hand device to patient to hold upright and insert actuator tip into one nostril. Have patient point device slightly away from the nasal septum while holding other nostril closed.
- Have patient hold breath while pressing down completely on the canister to release 1 spray. The patient should hold breath for 5 seconds and then breathe out through the mouth. Then device should be removed from nostril. Steps are repeated for the dose in the other nostril.
- Do not allow patient to blow nose for the next 15 minutes.

±**BECONASE AQ**

- Pump nasal spray 6 times or until a fine mist is seen before using for the first time. If drug has not been used for a week, repeat priming.
- Shake well before using.
- Clean nasal applicator by washing in cold water, dry, and replace cap and safety clip back in position.

±**QNASI**

- Does not have to be primed. Before using a new container, spray counter should read 120.
- Use a clean, dry tissue to clean tip. Do not wash in water.

ORAL INHALATION

±**QVAR REDIHALER**

- Do not use with a spacer or volume holding chamber.
- Does not require priming or shaking before administration.
- Before using a new container, spray counter should read 120.
- Inhaler should be held in an upright position with the mouthpiece positioned down. There is no button to push. The white cap on the inhaler must be closed before each inhalation. Have patient insert mouthpiece into mouth and close lips around it. Have patient inhale deeply to release drug. Then have patient remove inhaler and hold breath for 5 to 10 seconds, then breathe out slowly. If more than one inhalation is required, repeat the same steps.

B

- Have patient rinse mouth with water without swallowing after each dose.
- Clean mouthpiece by gently wiping with a dry cloth or tissue. Never place inhaler in water.

Route	Onset	Peak	Duration
Inhalation	1–2 wk	30 min	Unknown
Intranasal	2 wk	Unknown	Unknown

Half-life: 2.9–4 hr

Mechanism of Action

May decrease number and activity of cells involved in the inflammatory response of allergies, asthma, and rhinitis, such as basophils, eosinophils, lymphocytes, macrophages, mast cells, and neutrophils. Also may inhibit production or secretion of chemical mediators, such as cytokines, eicosanoids, histamine, and leukotrienes. May produce direct smooth-muscle cell relaxation and decrease airway hyperresponsiveness.

Contraindications

Hypersensitivity to beclomethasone or its components, relief of acute bronchospasm or acute asthma, or status asthmaticus (QVAR)

Interactions

DRUGS

None reported

Adverse Reactions

CNS: Aggression, depression, fatigue, fever, headache, insomnia, light-headedness, mania, psychomotor hyperactivity, sleep disorders, **suicidal ideation**
CV: Chest pain, tachycardia
EENT: Blurred vision, burning sensation in nasal passages, cataracts, central serous chorioretinopathy, dry mouth, dysphonia, earache, elevated intraocular pressure, epistaxis, glaucoma, hoarseness, lacrimation, loss of smell and taste, nasal congestion or ulceration, nasal septal perforation, nose and throat dryness and irritation, nose and oral candidiasis (inhaler), pharyngitis, rhinorrhea, sinusitis, sneezing, unpleasant smell and taste
ENDO: Adrenal insufficiency, cushingoid symptoms
GI: Diarrhea, indigestion, nausea, **rectal hemorrhage**
GU: Dysmenorrhea, UTI

MS: Arthralgia, growth suppression in children, reduction in bone mineral density (long-term therapy)
RESP: Bronchitis, **bronchospasm**, chest congestion, cough, **pulmonary infiltrates**, upper respiratory tract infection, wheezing
SKIN: Acne, eczema, pruritus, rash, skin discoloration, urticaria
Other: **Anaphylaxis, angioedema,** flu-like symptoms, impaired wound healing, lymphadenopathy, weight gain

Childbearing Considerations

PREGNANCY

- It is not known if drug can cause fetal harm.
- Use with caution only if benefit to mother outweighs potential risk to fetus.

LACTATION

- Drug may be present in breast milk.
- Patient should check with prescriber before breastfeeding.

Nursing Considerations

- Be aware that beclomethasone should not be used with patients who have experienced recent nasal septal ulcers, nasal surgery, or nasal trauma, because of corticosteroids' adverse effects on wound healing.
- Know that drug should be used with extreme caution but preferably not at all in patients with active or quiescent respiratory tuberculosis or untreated bacterial, parasitic, fungal, or viral infections or in the presence of ocular herpes simplex. Monitor patient closely throughout therapy for signs and symptoms of infection because immunosuppression occurs with corticosteroid therapy.
- Know that if patient also takes an oral corticosteroid, expect to taper dosage slowly (by decreasing daily dosage or taking drug every other day, as ordered) about 1 week after beclomethasone therapy begins.

! **WARNING** Be aware that when gradually switching patient from oral corticosteroid to inhaled beclomethasone, watch for signs of life-threatening adrenal insufficiency, such as fatigue, hypotension, lassitude, nausea, vomiting, and weakness, during transition period and when exposed to infection, surgery, trauma, or other stressor. If signs occur, notify prescriber immediately.

- Expect to resume oral corticosteroid during a stressful period or severe asthma attack.
- Watch for signs of adrenal insufficiency during periods of stress because beclomethasone may be absorbed systemically.
- Be prepared, if patient has acute asthma attack or increased wheezing after receiving beclomethasone, to give a fast-acting bronchodilator, as prescribed. Expect to discontinue beclomethasone.
- Assess for signs of candidiasis, such as thick white coating or plaques on tongue and sides of mouth. Tell patient to rinse mouth with water without swallowing after inhalation; this may help to prevent oral candidiasis. If present, notify prescriber and expect to reduce dose or frequency or to stop beclomethasone. Also anticipate treatment with antifungal drug.
- Assess nasal discharge regularly when patient is prescribed nasal spray. Look for color or consistency changes, which may indicate infection when patient is using beclomethasone nasal spray.
- Monitor the growth of children receiving beclomethasone nasally.
- Monitor patients with a change in vision or a history of blurred vision, cataracts, glaucoma, or intraocular pressure because use of intranasal and inhaled corticosteroids may cause eye abnormalities. If adverse eye symptoms develop, notify prescriber and expect patient to be referred to an ophthalmologist.
- Monitor patient closely for altered thinking such as suicidal thoughts. If present, notify prescriber because drug will have to be discontinued.

PATIENT TEACHING

- Advise patient not to abruptly stop taking beclomethasone because adrenal insufficiency may occur. Urge her to notify prescriber if she develops signs of adrenal insufficiency, such as anorexia, dizziness, dyspnea, fainting, fatigue, fever, hypotension, malaise, or nausea.
- Instruct her, if prescribed Beconase AQ, to prime pump before using nasal spray for first time by placing her thumb on its base, and her index and middle fingers on its shoulder area (the canister should be on top, pointing down), and then pressing her thumb firmly and quickly against the bottle six times into the air away from eyes and face. If nasal spray has not been used for 7 consecutive days, remind patient that container needs to be primed by spraying two times prior to use. Before patient uses nasal inhalation canister for first time, instruct her to shake it and check that it's working properly by spraying it once in the air while looking for fine mist.
- Tell patient prescribed Qnasl or Qvar Redihaler that the container does not have to be primed prior to use.
- Teach patient to inhale deeply after each nasal spray or inhalation, exhaling through mouth and tilting head back to let drug spread over the nasopharynx.
- Teach patient how to properly use oral inhalation aerosol, shaking canister well before using.
- Advise patient prescribed two inhalations to wait a minute between them.
- Tell patient prescribed an inhaled bronchodilator with beclomethasone oral inhalation to use bronchodilator first, wait for 5 minutes, and then use beclomethasone.

! WARNING Warn patient that beclomethasone isn't intended to relieve acute bronchospasm. Urge patient to notify prescriber if asthma symptoms don't respond.

- Advise patient to wear medical identification that states need for supplemental oral corticosteroids during severe asthma attack or stress. Inform patient that prescriber may order high-dose oral corticosteroid therapy.
- Warn patient and caretakers to report any abnormal thinking such as suicidal thoughts immediately to prescriber.

! WARNING Caution patient to avoid exposure to chickenpox and measles because drug may cause immunosuppression. If she's exposed to these disorders, urge her to notify prescriber immediately. Also, review signs and symptoms of infection to report to prescriber and infection control precautions to take.

- Tell patient to report any changes in vision to prescriber.

belimumab
Benlysta

Class and Category

Pharmacologic class: Monoclonal antibody
Therapeutic class: Immunosuppressant

Indications and Dosages

* *To treat active lupus nephritis in patients who are receiving standard therapy*

I.V. INFUSION

Adults. 10 mg/kg at 2-wk intervals for the first 3 doses and at 4-wk intervals thereafter.

SUBCUTANEOUS INJECTION

Adults. *Initial:* 400 mg (given as two 200-mg injections) once/wk for 4 doses, then 200 mg thereafter.

Adults transitioning from intravenous therapy. 200 mg once/wk, with first dose given 1 to 4 wk after the last I.V. dose.

Drug Administration

- Be aware that vials containing belimumab are intended for intravenous use only and autoinjectors and prefilled syringes are intended for subcutaneous use only.

I.V.

- Patient should be premedicated prior to receiving each dose of belimumab to prevent hypersensitivity and infusion reactions, as prescribed.
- Remove vial from refrigerator and allow to stand 10 to 15 minutes prior to reconstitution.
- Reconstitute with 1.5 ml of Sterile Water for Injection, USP for a 120-mg vial and 4.8 ml of Sterile Water for Injection, USP when reconstituting a 400-mg vial. When injecting diluent solution into the vial, direct stream of Sterile Water toward the side of the vial to minimize foaming. Gently swirl vial for 60 seconds every 5 minutes until the powder is dissolved. Do not shake or refrigerate during this process. It typically takes 10 to 15 minutes for powder to dissolve but may take as long as 30 minutes. Once reconstituted, protect from sunlight. When using a mechanical reconstitution device (swirler), do not exceed 500 rpm, and swirl no longer than 30 minutes.

Solution should appear opalescent and colorless to pale yellow without particles. Small air bubbles may be present and are acceptable.

- Use only 0.9% Sodium Chloride Injection, 0.45% Sodium Chloride Injection, or Lactated Ringer's Injection to further dilute the drug to a volume of 250 ml (100 ml for patients who weigh less than or equal to 45 kg [99 lb]). Withdraw amount of solution from the infusion bag or bottle equivalent to the vial contents of reconstituted drug required for patient's dose. Then add the required volume of the reconstituted solution of the drug into the infusion bag or bottle. Gently invert bag or bottle to mix the solution.
- Discard any unused solution left in the vial(s). The solution should be stored in the refrigerator, protected from direct sunlight, if not used immediately.
- Infuse over 1 hour. The total time from reconstitution to completion of infusion should not exceed 8 hours.
- If an infusion reaction occurs, slow the rate of infusion or stop it temporarily, as ordered.
- *Incompatibilities:* Dextrose intravenous solutions; other drugs infused concomitantly in the same I.V. line. Is compatible with polyolefin or polyvinylchloride bags

SUBCUTANEOUS

- First subcutaneous injection should be given under the supervision of a healthcare professional.
- Remove the autoinjector or prefilled syringe from the refrigerator and allow it to sit at room temperature for 30 minutes prior to administering. Do not warm the drug any other way. Solution should appear clear to opalescent and colorless to pale yellow. Discard if product exhibits discoloration or particulate matter or if the autoinjector or prefilled syringe is accidentally dropped on a hard surface.
- Inject into the abdomen or thigh. When administering a 400-mg dose in the same area, administer the two injections at least 5 cm (2 inches) apart. Use a different injection site each week; do not give the injection into areas where the skin is bruised, hard, red, or tender.

Route	Onset	Peak	Duration
I.V.	Unknown	Unknown	Unknown
SubQ	Unknown	2–6 days	Unknown

Half-life: 18–19 days

Mechanism of Action

Blocks the binding of soluble B-cell lymphocyte stimulator protein, a B-cell survival factor, to its receptors on B cells. This action causes cell death, which helps to relieve the signs and symptoms of active, autoantibody-positive, systemic lupus erythematosus.

Contraindications

Hypersensitivity to belimumab or its components

Interactions

DRUGS

Live virus vaccines: Possibly suppressed immune response and increased adverse effects of vaccine

Adverse Reactions

CNS: Anxiety, depression, fatigue, fever, headache, insomnia, migraines, myalgia, **progressive multifocal leukoencephalopathy, suicidal ideation**
CV: **Bradycardia, hypotension**
EENT: Nasopharyngitis, pharyngitis, sinusitis
GI: Diarrhea, nausea
GU: Cystitis, lupus nephritis, UTI
HEME: **Leukopenia**
MS: Extremity pain, myalgia
RESP: Bronchitis, dyspnea, pneumonia, upper respiratory tract infection
SKIN: Cellulitis, nonmelanoma skin cancers, pruritus, rash, urticaria
Other: **Anaphylaxis, angioedema,** antibelimumab antibody formation, flu-like symptoms, infusion reactions, injection-site reactions (erythema, hematoma, induration, pain, pruritus), **malignancies,** serious infections

Childbearing Considerations

PREGNANCY

- Pregnancy exposure registry: 1-877-681-6296.
- Drug may cause fetal harm. Drug actively crosses placental barrier with largest amount transferred in the third trimester, which may affect fetal immune response in utero.
- Use with caution only if the benefit to the mother outweighs the potential risk to the fetus.
- Monitor neonate and infant if drug exposure occurred in utero for B-cell reduction and other immune dysfunction.

LACTATION

- It is not clear if drug is present in breast milk.
- Patient should check with prescriber before breastfeeding.

REPRODUCTION

- Women of childbearing age should avoid pregnancy by using effective contraception during drug therapy and for at least 4 months after final dose of the drug.

Nursing Considerations

- Know that belimumab should not be used to treat patients who are receiving drug therapy to treat a chronic infection. Monitor patient closely for signs and symptoms of infections during belimumab therapy. If present, notify prescriber. If the infection is determined to be new, belimumab therapy may have to be interrupted until infection is resolved.
- Be aware that patients with a history of multiple drug allergies or significant hypersensitivity may be at increased risk for an allergic reaction or an infusion reaction. If an infusion reaction occurs, slow or temporarily stop the infusion, as ordered. If a serious hypersensitivity reaction occurs, discontinue drug immediately and notify prescriber. Know that a nonacute hypersensitivity reaction that may be evident as facial edema, fatigue, headache, myalgia, nausea, and rash may occur up to a week after an infusion.

! **WARNING** Monitor patient for a hypersensitivity reaction following administration of belimumab because hypersensitivity reactions, including anaphylaxis, may occur on the same day of infusion. Notify prescriber immediately if a reaction occurs, because death has occurred with some patients experiencing hypersensitivity reactions. Expect to provide emergency medical treatment as ordered and indicated by severity of reaction.

B

- Monitor African American patients closely during belimumab therapy for decreased effectiveness, because clinical trials have shown the response rate may be lower in these patients.
- Watch for evidence of infection (such as cough, fever, malaise, pain) because patients receiving immunosuppressants such as belimumab are at increased risk for serious infections such as bronchitis, cellulitis, pneumonia, and urinary tract infection. If patient develops an infection, notify prescriber, monitor patient closely, and know that drug therapy may be interrupted until infection is gone.
- Be aware that other biologic therapies, such as B-cell targeted therapies or intravenous cyclophosphamide therapy, are not recommended during belimumab therapy because potential drug interactions are unknown.

PATIENT TEACHING

- Instruct patient who will be self-injecting belimumab, as a subcutaneous injection, how to administer the injection and dispose of needle and syringe after injection.
- Tell patient to remove the autoinjector or prefilled syringe from the refrigerator and allow it to sit at room temperature for 30 minutes prior to administering. Tell patient not to warm the drug in any other way. Have patient inspect the solution. The solution should appear clear to opalescent and colorless to pale yellow. Instruct patient to discard if product exhibits discoloration or particulate matter or if the autoinjector or prefilled syringe is accidentally dropped on a hard surface. Tell patient to use a different injection site each week and not to give the injection into areas where the skin is bruised, hard, red, or tender.
- Advise patient that if a subcutaneous dose is missed, she should administer a dose as soon as she remembers. Then patient can resume dosing on the usual day of administration or start a new weekly schedule from the day that the missed dose was administered. Tell patient not to administer two doses on the same day.
- Instruct patient to report any signs of a hypersensitivity reaction such as difficulty breathing, hives, itching, or a rash to prescriber, and to seek medical attention immediately.

- Caution patient to report new or worsening depression, suicidal thoughts, or other mood changes.
- Tell patient to contact the prescriber if he develops new or worsening neurologic symptoms such as confusion, difficulty talking or walking, dizziness, loss of balance, memory loss, or vision problems.
- Advise patient not to receive any immunization with live vaccines for 30 days before or concurrently with belimumab and to avoid contact with anyone who has an infection.
- Tell female patient of childbearing age to use effective contraception during treatment and for at least 4 months after the final treatment because of potential adverse effects to infants exposed to drug in utero. Advise her to notify prescriber if pregnancy occurs and encourage her to enroll in the belimumab pregnancy registry.
- Encourage patient to report any persistent, severe, or unusual signs and symptoms to prescriber because drug may increase risk for cancer and infections.

bempedoic acid
Nexletol

Class and Category
Pharmacologic class: Adenosine triphosphate-citrate lyase inhibitor
Therapeutic class: Antilipid

Indications and Dosages
* *Adjunct to diet and maximally tolerated statin therapy for the treatment of heterozygous familial hypercholesterolemia or established atherosclerotic cardiovascular disease in patients who require additional lowering of LDL-C*

TABLETS
Adults. 180 mg once daily.

Drug Administration
P.O.
- Give in combination with maximally tolerated statin therapy.

Route	Onset	Peak	Duration
P.O.	Unknown	3.5 hr	Unknown

Half-life: 15–24 hr

Mechanism of Action
Inhibits cholesterol synthesis in the liver.

Contraindications
Hypersensitivity to bempedoic acid or its components

Interactions
DRUGS
pravastatin, simvastatin: Increased blood levels of these drugs with possible increased risk of myopathy

Adverse Reactions
CV: Atrial fibrillation
GI: Abdominal discomfort or pain, diarrhea, elevated liver enzymes
GU: Benign prostatic hyperplasia, elevated blood urea nitrogen and creatinine levels, prostatomegaly
HEME: Anemia, decreased hemoglobin, **elevated platelet count, leukopenia**
MS: Back or extremity pain, elevated creatine kinase, muscle spasms, tendon rupture
RESP: Bronchitis, upper respiratory infection
OTHER: Gout, hyperuricemia

Childbearing Considerations
PREGNANCY
- Pregnancy Exposure Registry: 1-833-377-7633.
- Drug may cause fetal harm based on its mechanism of action.
- Drug should be discontinued during pregnancy.

LACTATION
- It is not known if drug is present in breast milk.
- Drug is not recommended during breastfeeding.

Nursing Considerations
- Be aware that bempedoic acid may increase risk of patient developing gout, because it may increase blood uric acid levels. Monitor patient's serum uric acid levels, if ordered. Report to prescriber any signs or symptoms of hyperuricemia.
- Know that bempedoic acid increases risk of tendon injury or rupture, especially in patients over 60 years of age, patients taking corticosteroid or fluoroquinolone drugs, or patients with a history of previous tendon disorders or who have renal failure. Monitor patient for joint inflammation, pain, or swelling. Alert prescriber if signs or symptoms of tendinitis or tendon rupture occur. Drug may have to be discontinued for tendinitis and immediately discontinued if rupture of a tendon occurs.
- Expect to determine patient's lipid levels within 8 to 12 weeks after starting bempedoic acid therapy to evaluate the effectiveness of the drug.
- Know that pravastatin should not be coadministered in a dose greater than 40 mg and simvastatin should not be coadministered in a dose greater than 20 mg daily.

PATIENT TEACHING
- Advise patient to alert prescriber if taking more than 40 mg of pravastatin or 20 mg of simvastatin before starting bempedoic acid therapy.
- Tell patient that periodic blood studies may be ordered to check effectiveness of drug and monitor for increased uric acid levels.
- Review signs and symptoms of hyperuricemia with patient and tell patient to alert prescriber if present.
- Teach patient the signs and symptoms of tendinitis and tendon rupture. Advise patient to rest at the first sign of either and to immediately contact prescriber.
- Instruct female patients to notify prescriber if pregnancy is suspected or known.

benazepril hydrochloride
Lotensin

Class and Category
Pharmacologic class: Angiotensin-converting enzyme (ACE) inhibitor
Therapeutic class: Antihypertensive

Indications and Dosages
✶ *To control hypertension alone or with a thiazide diuretic*
SUSPENSION, TABLETS
Adults who aren't receiving a diuretic.
Initial: 10 mg daily. *Maintenance:* 20 to 40 mg daily as a single dose or in two equally divided doses.
Adults who are receiving a diuretic.
5 mg daily.
±**DOSAGE ADJUSTMENT** Initial dosage of 5 mg/day for adult patients with impaired

renal function and creatinine clearance less than 30 ml/min; then increased gradually until blood pressure is controlled or dosage reaches maximum of 40 mg daily.

SUSPENSION, TABLETS

Children age 6 and over with glomerular filtration rate of 30 ml/min or higher.
Initial: 0.2 mg/kg daily. *Maximum:* 0.6 mg/kg daily or 40 mg daily.

Drug Administration

P.O.

- Shake suspension before each use. Use calibrated device when measuring dosage.
- Suspension should be refrigerated and can be stored for up to 30 days.

Route	Onset	Peak	Duration
P.O.	1 hr	1–2 hr	24 hr

Half-life: 10–11 hr

Mechanism of Action

May reduce blood pressure by affecting renin–angiotensin–aldosterone system. By inhibiting angiotensin-converting enzyme, benazepril:

- prevents conversion of angiotensin I to angiotensin II, a potent vasoconstrictor that also stimulates aldosterone release
- may inhibit renal and vascular production of angiotensin II
- decreases serum angiotensin II level and increases serum renin activity. This decreases aldosterone secretion, slightly increasing serum potassium level and fluid loss.
- decreases vascular tone and blood pressure
- inhibits aldosterone release, which reduces sodium and water resorption, increases their excretion, and reduces blood pressure

Contraindications

Aliskiren therapy in patients with diabetes; concurrent therapy with a neprilysin inhibitor (e.g., sacubitril) or within 36 hours of switching to or from sacubitril/valsartan combination; history of angioedema; hypersensitivity to benazepril, other ACE inhibitors, or their components

Interactions

DRUGS

aliskiren (in patients with diabetes or renal impairment), angiotensin receptor blockers, *other ACE inhibitors:* Increased risk of hyperkalemia, hypotension, and renal dysfunction
antidiabetics (oral), insulin: Possibly increased risk of hypoglycemia
diuretics: Possibly excessive hypotension
gold salts: Possibly nitritoid reaction including facial flushing, hypotension, nausea, and vomiting
lithium: Increased serum lithium level and risk of lithium toxicity
mTOR inhibitors (everolimus, sirolimus, temsirolimus), neprilysin inhibitors: Increased risk for angioedema
NSAIDs: Possible decreased renal function in patients who are elderly, volume depleted, or have a compromised renal function; may increase antihypertensive effect of benazepril
potassium preparations, potassium-sparing diuretics: Possibly increased serum potassium level

Adverse Reactions

CNS: Anxiety, asthenia, dizziness, drowsiness, fatigue, headache, hypertonia, insomnia, nervousness, paresthesia, sleep disturbance, somnolence, syncope, weakness
CV: Angina, ECG changes, hypotension, orthostatic hypotension, palpitations, peripheral edema
EENT: Sinusitis
ENDO: Hyperglycemia
GI: Abdominal pain, acute liver failure, cholestatic hepatitis, constipation, elevated liver enzymes, gastritis, hepatic necrosis, melena, nausea, pancreatitis, small bowel angioedema, vomiting
GU: Acute renal failure, decreased libido, elevated BUN and serum creatinine levels, frequent urination, impotence, nephrotic syndrome, oliguria, progressive azotemia, proteinuria, renal insufficiency, UTI
HEME: Agranulocytosis, decreased hemoglobin level, hemolytic anemia, leukopenia, neutropenia, thrombocytopenia
MS: Arthralgia, arthritis, myalgia
RESP: ACE cough, asthma, bronchitis, bronchospasm, dyspnea
SKIN: Alopecia, dermatitis, diaphoresis, flushing, pemphigus, photosensitivity, pruritus, rash, Stevens–Johnson syndrome
Other: Anaphylaxis, angioedema, hyperkalemia, hyponatremia

≡ Childbearing Considerations

PREGNANCY

- Drug can cause fetal harm, especially during the second and third trimesters of pregnancy.
- Oligohydramnios that occurs in pregnant women as a result of the drug can cause reduced fetal renal function leading to anuria and renal failure, fetal lung hypoplasia, and skeletal deformations, including skull hypoplasia. In addition, hypotension and death may occur.
- Drug should not be given during pregnancy and drug should be discontinued as soon as possible if pregnancy occurs.

LACTATION

- Drug is present in breast milk.
- Patient should check with prescriber before breastfeeding.

REPRODUCTION

- Women of childbearing age should be advised to avoid pregnancy by using effective contraception during drug therapy.

≡ Nursing Considerations

- Evaluate blood pressure with patient lying down, sitting, and standing before starting benazepril and then regularly, as appropriate, to monitor effectiveness.
- Monitor urine output and BUN and serum creatinine levels, as needed, before therapy and then during therapy, especially in patients with renal artery stenosis, severe heart failure, postmyocardial infarction or in patients who are volume depleted. Also monitor patients closely who are also receiving NSAID or angiotensin receptor blocker therapy because these patients may be at increased risk for developing acute renal failure.

! **WARNING** Monitor patient closely during dialysis because sudden and potentially life-threatening anaphylactoid reactions have occurred in some patients dialyzed with high-flux membranes while receiving an ACE inhibitor like benazepril. If anaphylaxis occurs, institute emergency measures, as ordered, and stop dialysis.

- Monitor liver enzymes regularly, as ordered. Assess patient routinely for signs and symptoms of liver dysfunction, such as jaundice and fatigue. Notify prescriber if patient develops jaundice or exhibits elevated liver enzyme levels, as drug will have to be discontinued.

! **WARNING** Be alert for angioedema, especially after first dose. If it extends to larynx and patient has laryngeal stridor or signs of airway obstruction, prepare to give epinephrine subcutaneously immediately, as prescribed, and discontinue benazepril. Be aware that African-American patients have a higher incidence of angioedema compared to other groups.

- Monitor WBC count periodically to detect neutropenia and agranulocytosis.
- Check serum potassium and other electrolyte levels to detect electrolyte imbalances.
- Take safety precautions, such as having patient change positions slowly and sit on edge of bed before arising, to prevent injury caused by orthostatic hypotension.

PATIENT TEACHING

- Advise patient to shake suspension before each use and to measure dose with a calibrated device, not an ordinary spoon. Tell patient to keep suspension in refrigerator and to discard after 30 days.
- Teach patient how to monitor blood pressure, if appropriate, and how to recognize signs of hypertension and hypotension.

! **WARNING** Urge patient to contact prescriber before using any OTC salt substitutes, which may contain potassium, or potassium supplements. These substances increase the risk of hyperkalemia.

- Explain that a persistent dry cough may develop and may not subside unless benazepril is stopped. If cough becomes bothersome or interferes with sleep or activities, patient should notify prescriber.

! **WARNING** Instruct patient to contact prescriber immediately if she has signs of angioedema, such as swelling of the face, eyes, lips, or tongue.

- Caution patient to avoid sudden position changes and to rise slowly from sitting or lying to minimize orthostatic hypotension.

! **WARNING** Advise patient to stop benazepril and notify prescriber as soon as possible if she experiences syncope.

! **WARNING** Caution women of childbearing age to use reliable contraception and to notify prescriber immediately if pregnancy is suspected. Benazepril may cause fetal harm and should be discontinued.

benralizumab

Fasenra

Class and Category

Pharmacologic class: Monoclonal antibody
Therapeutic class: Antiasthmatic

Indications and Dosages

* As adjunct to treat severe asthma as an add-on maintenance treatment in patients with eosinophilic phenotype

SUBCUTANEOUS INJECTION

Adults and children age 12 and over. 30 mg once every 4 wk for the first 3 doses, then once every 8 wk.

Drug Administration

SUBCUTANEOUS

- Administer drug using the prefilled syringe.
- Prior to administration, warm drug by leaving carton at room temperature for about 30 minutes. Drug should appear clear to opalescent, colorless to slightly yellow, and may contain a few translucent or white to off-white particles. Do not use if solution is cloudy, discolored, or large particles or foreign particulate matter is visible.
- Do not expel any small air bubbles prior to administration.
- Administer into the abdomen, thigh, or upper arm. Inject by pushing plunger all the way until the plunger head is completely between the needle guard activation clip, which is needed to activate the needle guard. After injection, maintain pressure on the plunger head and remove the needle. Release pressure on the plunger head to allow the needle guard to cover the needle.
- Be aware that the single-dose autoinjector pen device is intended for use by the patient or caregiver.

Route	Onset	Peak	Duration
SubQ	Rapid	Unknown	Unknown

Half-life: 15.5 days

Mechanism of Action

Binds to the alpha subunit of the human interleukin-5 receptor, which is expressed on the surface of basophils and eosinophils. Eosinophils play a part in the inflammatory process, which is present in the pathogenesis of asthma. When binding to the interleukin-5 receptor occurs, eosinophils are reduced through an antibody-dependent cell-mediated cytotoxicity to help relieve inflammation found in asthma.

Contraindications

Hypersensitivity to benralizumab or its components

Interactions

DRUGS

None reported

Adverse Reactions

CNS: Fever, headache
EENT: Pharyngitis
SKIN: Rash, urticaria
Other: Anaphylaxis, angioedema, benralizumab antibody formation, injection-site reactions (erythema, pain, papule, pruritus)

Childbearing Considerations

PREGNANCY

- Pregnancy exposure registry: 1-877-311-8972 or mothertobaby.org/Fasenra.
- It is not known if drug can cause fetal harm. Drug actively crosses placental barrier with largest amount transferred in the third trimester.
- Use cautiously only if the benefit to the mother outweighs the potential risk to the fetus.

LACTATION

- It is not clear if drug is present in breast milk.
- Patient should check with prescriber before breastfeeding.

Nursing Considerations

- Expect to treat patients with preexisting parasitic (helminth) infections before benralizumab therapy is begun, because it is not known if the drug will influence a patient's response to treatment for such an infection. If patient develops a parasitic infection while taking benralizumab and does not respond to treatment, expect benralizumab to be discontinued until the infection is resolved.

! **WARNING** Know that benralizumab should never be used to treat acute asthma symptoms, acute bronchospasms, acute exacerbations of asthma, or status asthmaticus.

! **WARNING** Monitor patient closely for hypersensitivity reactions that may occur within hours after benralizumab has been administered. If present, notify prescriber, provide supportive emergency care, and expect drug to be discontinued.

- Expect inhaled or systemic corticosteroids used to treat asthma to be gradually withdrawn, if no longer needed. Corticosteroid therapy should never be withdrawn abruptly.

PATIENT TEACHING
- Teach patient and caregivers how to use the autoinjector (Fasenra Pen), if prescribed, by using the "Instructions for Use" that comes with it. Also teach patient how to administer a subcutaneous injection using the autoinjector. Tell patient to inject the drug either into the abdomen or thigh. A caregiver may also use the upper arm.
- Instruct patient that benralizumab is not effective in treating acute asthma symptoms or acute exacerbations. If asthma remains uncontrolled or worsens after benralizumab therapy is begun, tell patient to notify prescriber or seek emergency medical care.

! **WARNING** Tell patient to report any signs of an allergic reaction such as difficulty breathing, hives, or rash immediately. Remind patient that although an allergic reaction usually occurs within hours after benralizumab is administered, a delayed reaction could occur even days later.

- Emphasize importance of not decreasing any prescribed inhaled or systemic corticosteroid dosage without prescriber knowledge.

benztropine mesylate
Cogentin

B

Class and Category
Pharmacologic class: Anticholinergic
Therapeutic class: Antiparkinsonian, central-acting anticholinergic

Indications and Dosages
＊ *As adjunct, to treat all forms of Parkinson's disease*

I.M. OR I.V. INJECTION
Adults with Parkinson's disease. *Initial:* 0.5 to 1 mg daily, increased gradually in increments of 0.5 mg at 5- or 6-day intervals, as needed. *Maximum:* 6 mg daily.
Adults with idiopathic Parkinson's disease. *Initial:* 0.5 to 1 mg daily. *Maximum:* 4 to 6 mg daily.
Adults with postencephalitic Parkinson's disease. *Initial:* 0.5 mg to 2 mg in one or more divided doses and then increased in increments of 0.5 mg at 5–6 day intervals as needed. *Maximum:* 6 mg daily.
＊ *To control extrapyramidal symptoms (except tardive dyskinesia) caused by phenothiazines and other neuroleptics*

I.M. OR I.V. INJECTION
Adults. 1 to 4 mg once or twice daily.
＊ *To treat acute dystonic reactions*

I.M. INJECTION
Adults. *Initial:* 1 to 2 mg as a single dose.

Drug Administration
I.V.
- Rarely used because I.M. administration is just as effective.
- Manufacturer does not provide specific instructions for administration because there usually is no need to use this route.

I.M.
- Use a filtered needle when drawing drug up from vial.

Route	Onset	Peak	Duration
P.O.	1 hr	7 hr	24 hr
I.V., I.M.	15 min	Unknown	24 hr

Half-life: Unknown

Mechanism of Action

Blocks acetylcholine's action at cholinergic receptor sites. This restores the brain's normal dopamine and acetylcholine balance, which relaxes muscle movement and decreases drooling, rigidity, and tremor. Benztropine also may inhibit dopamine reuptake and storage, which prolongs dopamine's action.

Contraindications

Children younger than age 3, hypersensitivity to benztropine mesylate or its components

Interactions

DRUGS

amantadine, phenothiazines, tricyclic antidepressants: Possibly increased adverse anticholinergic effects
haloperidol: Possibly decreased haloperidol effects and development of tardive dyskinesia

Adverse Reactions

CNS: Agitation, confusion, delirium, delusions, depression, disorientation, dizziness, drowsiness, euphoria, excitement, fever, hallucinations, headache, light-headedness, listlessness, memory loss, nervousness, paranoia, psychosis, weakness
CV: Hypotension, mild bradycardia, orthostatic hypotension, palpitations, tachycardia
EENT: Blurred vision, diplopia, dry mouth, increased intraocular pressure, mydriasis, narrow-angle glaucoma, suppurative parotitis
GI: Constipation, duodenal ulcer, epigastric distress, ileus, nausea, vomiting
GU: Dysuria, urinary hesitancy, urine retention
MS: Muscle spasms, muscle weakness
SKIN: Decreased sweating, dermatoses, flushing, rash, urticaria

Childbearing Considerations

PREGNANCY

- It is not known if drug can cause fetal harm.
- Use with caution only if benefit to mother outweighs potential risk to fetus.

LACTATION

- It is not known if drug is present in breast milk.
- Patient should check with prescriber before breastfeeding as drug may suppress lactation.

Nursing Considerations

- Assess muscle rigidity and tremor at baseline. Then monitor them often for improvement, which indicates drug's effectiveness.

! WARNING Know that when giving drug to patient with drug-induced extrapyramidal reactions, watch for worsening psychiatric symptoms.

- Monitor patient's movements closely. High-dose benztropine therapy may cause weakness and inability to move specific muscle groups. If this occurs, expect to reduce benztropine dosage.
- Know that benztropine therapy should not be abruptly discontinued.

PATIENT TEACHING

- Warn patient that drug has a cumulative effect, increasing risk of adverse reactions and overdose.
- Caution against driving and similar activities until benztropine's effects are known because it may cause blurred vision, dizziness, or drowsiness.

! WARNING Know that because benztropine decreases sweating, urge patient to avoid extremely hot or humid conditions to reduce risk of heatstroke and severe hyperthermia. This is especially important for elderly patients and those who abuse alcohol or have chronic illness or CNS disease.

- Stress need for periodic eye examinations and intraocular pressure measurements because drug may cause narrow-angle glaucoma and increase intraocular pressure.

bethanechol chloride
Duvoid, Urecholine

Class and Category

Pharmacologic class: Cholinergic agonist
Therapeutic class: Urinary tract stimulant

Indications and Dosages

✽ *To treat acute postoperative and postpartum nonobstructive (functional) urine retention; to treat neurogenic atony of bladder with retention*

TABLETS

Adults. 10 to 50 mg three times daily or four times daily. *To determine minimum effective dose:* 5 to 10 mg repeated every hour until response is obtained or maximum of 50 mg is reached.

Drug Administration
P.O.

- Give drug 1 hour before or 2 hours after meals. If taken soon after eating, nausea and vomiting may occur.

Route	Onset	Peak	Duration
P.O.	30 min	60–90 min	1 hr

Half-life: Unknown

Mechanism of Action

Acts directly on muscarinic receptors of the parasympathetic nervous system, increasing detrusor muscle tone in the bladder and allowing contraction strong enough to start voiding. Like natural neurotransmitter acetylcholine, bethanechol stimulates gastric motility, increases gastric tone, and enhances peristalsis.

Contraindications

Acute inflammatory lesions of GI tract, bronchial asthma, coronary artery disease, epilepsy, hypersensitivity to bethanechol or its components, hyperthyroidism, marked vagotonia, mechanical obstruction of GI or GU tract, Parkinson's disease, peptic ulcer disease, peritonitis, pronounced bradycardia or hypotension, questionable integrity of GI or GU mucosa, spastic GI disorders, vasomotor instability

Interactions
DRUGS

cholinergic drugs: Possibly increased effects of bethanechol
ganglionic blockers: Possibly severe hypotension, usually first manifested by severe adverse GI reactions
procainamide, quinidine: Possibly decreased effects of bethanechol

Adverse Reactions

CNS: Headache, malaise
CV: Hypotension with reflex tachycardia, vasomotor response
EENT: Excessive salivation, lacrimation, miosis
GI: Abdominal cramps, colicky pain, diarrhea, eructation, nausea, vomiting
GU: Urinary urgency
RESP: Asthma attack, bronchoconstriction

Childbearing Considerations
PREGNANCY

- It is not known if drug can cause fetal harm.
- Use with caution only if benefit to mother outweighs potential risk to fetus.

LACTATION

- It is not known if drug is present in breast milk.
- A decision should be made to discontinue breastfeeding or the drug to avoid potential serious adverse reactions in the breastfed infant.

Nursing Considerations

- Assess urine elimination before starting bethanechol therapy.

> **! WARNING** Be aware that patient must have functioning urinary sphincter because a sphincter that doesn't relax when bladder contracts can push urine upward into renal pelvis and cause reflux infection.

PATIENT TEACHING

- Advise patient to take bethanechol on an empty stomach 1 hour before or 2 hours after meals to reduce risk of nausea and vomiting.

bezlotoxumab
Zinplava

Class and Category

Pharmacologic class: Monoclonal antibody
Therapeutic class: Clostridium difficile recurrence inhibitor

Indications and Dosages

✳ *To reduce recurrence of Clostridium difficile infection (CDI) in patients who are receiving antibacterial drug treatment for CDI and are at a high risk for CDI recurrence*

I.V. INFUSION

Adults. 10 mg/kg as a single dose.

Drug Administration
I.V.

- Prepare diluted solution immediately after removal of the vial(s) from refrigerator or, if left at room temperature no longer than 24 hours.
- Dilute by withdrawing the required volume from drug vial based on patient's weight in kg and transfer into an intravenous bag containing either 0.9% Sodium Chloride Injection USP or 5% Dextrose Injection

USP with a final concentration ranging from 1 to 10 mg/ml.
- Mix diluted solution by gentle inversion. Do not shake.
- Store diluted solution at room temperature up to 16 hours or under refrigeration for up to 24 hours prior to administration. If refrigerated, allow the intravenous bag to come to room temperature before administering. Do not allow total time following mixture and including duration of infusion to exceed 16 hours if kept at room temperature or 24 hours if refrigerated.
- Using a sterile, nonpyrogenic, low-protein binding 0.2-micron to 5-micron in-line or add-on filter, infuse over 60 minutes.
- May be infused through a central line or peripheral catheter. Do not administer as an intravenous bolus or push.
- *Incompatibilities:* Other drugs infused simultaneously through same infusion line

Route	Onset	Peak	Duration
I.V.	Unknown	Unknown	Unknown

Half-life: 19 days

Mechanism of Action

Binds to *C. difficile* toxin B and neutralizes its effects.

Contraindications

Hypersensitivity to bezlotoxumab or its components

Interactions

DRUGS
None reported

Adverse Reactions

CNS: Dizziness, fatigue, fever, headache
CV: Heart failure, hypertension, ventricular tachyarrhythmia
GI: Nausea
RESP: Dyspnea
Other: Antibezlotoxumab antibodies, infusion-related reactions

Childbearing Considerations

PREGNANCY
- It is not known if drug can cause fetal harm.
- Use with caution only if benefit to mother outweighs potential risk to fetus.

LACTATION
- It is not known if drug is present in breast milk.

- Patient should check with prescriber before breastfeeding.

Nursing Considerations

- Be aware that bezlotoxumab alone is not to be used to treat *C. difficile* infection (CDI), as it is not an antibacterial drug. It should only be used in conjunction with antibacterial drug treatment of CDI.
- Use with extreme caution in patients with a history of congestive heart failure, as drug may exacerbate congestive heart failure and may become severe enough to cause death.
- Monitor patient for adverse reactions, especially infusion reactions that may include dizziness, dyspnea, fatigue, fever, hypertension, and nausea. Know that these reactions usually resolve within 24 hours.

! **WARNING** Monitor patient closely for signs and symptoms of congestive heart failure, especially in patients with a history of the disorder. Notify prescriber immediately if such signs or symptoms are present and expect to provide supportive care.

PATIENT TEACHING

- Remind patient that bezlotoxumab does not take the place of the prescribed antibacterial therapy. Reinforce need to continue taking the antibacterial agent as prescribed.
- Reassure patient that although infusion reactions may occur, they usually resolve within 24 hours and are not usually serious.

! **WARNING** Urge patient to seek immediate medical attention if signs and symptoms of congestive heart failure occur.

bisoprolol fumarate

Class and Category

Pharmacologic class: Beta$_1$-adrenergic blocker
Therapeutic class: Antihypertensive

Indications and Dosages

✱ *To treat hypertension, alone or with other antihypertensives*

TABLETS

Adults. 2.5 to 5 mg daily, increased to 10 to 20 mg daily if blood pressure doesn't respond to lower dosage.

±**DOSAGE ADJUSTMENT** Dosage reduced to 2.5 mg daily initially and then increased gradually for patients with impaired renal function and creatinine clearance less than 40 ml/min; who have impaired hepatic function, as from cirrhosis or hepatitis; or patients who have bronchospastic disease.

Drug Administration

P.O.

- Store at room temperature.
- Keep in tight container to protect from moisture.

Route	Onset	Peak	Duration
P.O.	1–2 hr	2–4 hr	Unknown

Half-life: 9–12 hr

Mechanism of Action

Inhibits stimulation of beta$_1$-receptors primarily in the heart, which decreases cardiac excitability, cardiac output, and myocardial oxygen demand. Bisoprolol also decreases renin release from kidneys, which helps reduce blood pressure.

Contraindications

Cardiogenic shock, hypersensitivity to bisoprolol or its components, overt heart failure, second- or third-degree heart block, sinus bradycardia

Interactions

DRUGS

antiarrhythmics such as disopyramide; calcium channel blockers such as diltiazem, verapamil: Increased risk of conduction delay and decreased heart rate
beta blockers, digoxin: Increased risk of bradycardia
catecholamine-depleting drugs such as guanethidine, reserpine: Increased risk of bradycardia or hypotension
clonidine: Possibly severe hypertension from withdrawal of clonidine or both drugs
rifampin: Possibly increased bisoprolol metabolism with decreased bisoprolol effects

Adverse Reactions

CNS: Anxiety, confusion, depression, dizziness, emotional lability, fatigue, fever, hallucinations, headache, insomnia, malaise, nightmares, paresthesia, sleep disturbances, syncope, tremor, unsteadiness, vertigo

CV: Bradycardia, heart block, and other arrhythmias; chest pain; claudication; edema; heart failure; hypercholesterolemia; hyperlipidemia; hypotension; MI; orthostatic hypotension; palpitations; peripheral vascular insufficiency

EENT: Altered taste, blurred vision, dry mouth, eye pain or pressure, hearing loss, increased salivation, laryngospasm, pharyngitis, rhinitis, sinusitis, tinnitus

GI: Constipation, diarrhea, epigastric pain, gastritis, indigestion, ischemic colitis, mesenteric artery thrombosis, nausea, vomiting

GU: Cystitis, decreased libido, impotence, Peyronie's disease, renal artery thrombosis, renal colic

HEME: Agranulocytosis, eosinophilia, leukopenia, thrombocytopenia, thrombocytopenic purpura

MS: Arthralgia, cold extremities, gout, muscle twitching, neck pain

RESP: Asthma, bronchitis, bronchospasm, cough, dyspnea, respiratory distress, upper respiratory tract infection

SKIN: Alopecia, dermatitis, diaphoresis, eczema, exfoliative dermatitis, flushing, pruritus, psoriasis, rash

Other: Angioedema, hyperkalemia, hyperuricemia, weight gain

Childbearing Considerations

PREGNANCY

- It is not known if drug can cause fetal harm.
- Use with caution only if benefit to mother outweighs potential risk to fetus.

LACTATION

- It is not known if drug is present in breast milk.
- Patient should check with prescriber before breastfeeding.

Nursing Considerations

- Administer bisoprolol cautiously in patients with peripheral vascular disease because reduced cardiac output can cause or worsen arterial insufficiency. Assess patient's arms and legs for changes in color, temperature, and pulses; ask about numbness, tingling, and pain.
- Be aware that chronic beta blocker therapy, such as bisoprolol, is not routinely withheld prior to major surgery because the benefits outweigh the risks associated with its use with general anesthesia and surgical procedures.

- Measure blood pressure with patient lying, sitting, and standing before starting bisoprolol and then every 4 to 8 hours, as appropriate, to evaluate effectiveness.
- Know that if patient has diabetes, patient should be monitored closely for signs of hypoglycemia, which drug may mask.
- Be aware that if patient has hyperthyroidism, she should be watched for tachycardia and hypertension, which may be masked by bisoprolol.

! **WARNING** Keep in mind that abrupt withdrawal of bisoprolol may cause or worsen thyroid storm. During drug withdrawal, monitor patient closely.

- Expect to stop bisoprolol over 1 to 2 weeks to prevent MI, ventricular arrhythmias, and, possibly, death from catecholamine hypersensitivity caused by beta blocker therapy.
- Monitor patient's blood pressure. If systolic blood pressure falls to less than 90 mm Hg, expect to discontinue drug. Prepare for hemodynamic monitoring, if needed.

! **WARNING** Expect to discontinue bisoprolol about 48 hours beforehand if patient is scheduled for surgery with general anesthesia, to reduce risk of excessive myocardial depression during anesthesia.

PATIENT TEACHING

- Teach patient how to monitor her blood pressure, if appropriate, and to recognize signs of hypertension and hypotension.
- Instruct patient to avoid sudden position changes and to rise slowly from a lying or sitting position to minimize the effects of orthostatic hypotension.
- Advise patient to avoid driving and other activities that require mental alertness until bisoprolol's CNS effects are known.
- Instruct patient to contact prescriber before using any OTC product, such as a cold remedy or nasal decongestant.

bivalirudin
Angiomax, Angiomax RTU

Class and Category
Pharmacologic class: Direct thrombin inhibitor
Therapeutic class: Anticoagulant

Indications and Dosages
✳ *To provide anticoagulation in patients undergoing percutaneous coronary intervention (PCI), including patients with heparin-induced thrombocytopenia and heparin-induced thrombocytopenia and thrombosis syndrome*

I.V. INFUSION, I.V. INJECTION
Adults. *Initial:* Immediately before procedure, 0.75-mg/kg bolus; then 1.75 mg/kg/hr infusion for duration of procedure. Five minutes after bolus dose and with continuous infusion running, another 0.3-mg/kg bolus may be given, if needed. After procedure, 1.75 mg/kg/hr may be continued for up to 4 hr for patients with ST segment elevation MI (STEMI).

±**DOSAGE ADJUSTMENT** Infusion dosage reduced to 1 mg/kg/hr for patients with severe renal impairment (glomerular filtration rate less than 30 ml/min) and to 0.25 mg/kg/hr for patients on hemodialysis.

Drug Administration
I.V.
- Expect to give 300 to 325 mg of aspirin P.O. daily with bivalirudin therapy.

ANGIOMAX
- Thaw premixed frozen solution at room temperature or under refrigeration. Do not thaw by bath immersion or in microwave.
- For bolus dose and continuous infusion, reconstitute by adding 5 ml Sterile Water for Injection to 250-mg vial and swirl gently until dissolved. Solution should appear slightly opalescent, colorless to slightly yellow solution.
- Withdraw and discard 5 ml from a 50-ml infusion bag of either 0.9% Sodium Chloride Injection or 5% Dextrose in Water. Then add reconstituted contents of vial to infusion bag to yield 5 mg/ml.
- Use diluted solution to administer bolus dose first and then immediately follow with a continuous infusion at a rate of 1.75 mg/kg/hr. After 5 minutes, administer another reduced bolus, if needed, with continuous infusion running. Administer a reduced rate as indicated above for patients with severe renal impairment or who are on hemodialysis.

- If a low-rate infusion is ordered following initial infusion, dilute reconstituted drug in 500 ml of 0.9% Sodium Chloride Injection or 5% Dextrose in Water to yield a final concentration of 0.5 mg/ml.

ANGIOMAX RTU

- Store in refrigerator. Remove only when ready to administer.
- This form need not be reconstituted or diluted.
- Administer initial bolus followed by the continuous infusion at a rate of 1.75 mg/kg/hr. After 5 minutes another reduced bolus may be given, if needed, with continuous infusion running.
- *Incompatibilities for both products:* Alteplase, amiodarone, amphotericin B, chlorpromazine HCl, diazepam, dobutamine, prochlorperazine edisylate, reteplase, streptokinase, vancomycin HCl

Route	Onset	Peak	Duration
I.V.	Rapid	Immediate	1 hr after end of infusion

Half-life: 25 min

Mechanism of Action

Selectively binds to thrombin, including thrombin trapped in established clots. Without thrombin, fibrinogen can't convert to fibrin, producing an anticoagulation effect.

Contraindications

Active major bleeding, hypersensitivity to bivalirudin or its components

Interactions

DRUGS

glycoprotein IIb/IIIa inhibitors, heparin, thrombolytics, warfarin: Risk of bleeding

Adverse Reactions

CNS: Headache, intracranial hemorrhage
CV: Acute stent thrombosis (patients with ST segment elevation myocardial infarction), cardiac tamponade, hypotension, thrombosis during PCI
EENT: Epistaxis, gingival bleeding
GI: Abdominal cramps, diarrhea, **GI or retroperitoneal bleeding**, nausea, vomiting
GU: Hematuria, vaginal bleeding
HEME: Absence of anticoagulant effect, bleeding events, decreased hemoglobin, increased INR, severe bleeding

MS: Back pain
RESP: Hemoptysis, **hemothorax, pulmonary hemorrhage**
SKIN: Ecchymosis
Other: Anaphylaxis, antibody formation to bivalirudin, injection-site bleeding, hematoma, or pain

Childbearing Considerations

PREGNANCY

- It is not known if drug can cause fetal harm.
- Use with caution only if benefit to mother outweighs potential risk to fetus.

LABOR AND DELIVERY

- Drug should not be used during labor and delivery because of the potential for drug-induced hemorrhage during delivery.

LACTATION

- It is not known if drug is present in breast milk.
- Patient should check with prescriber before breastfeeding.

Nursing Considerations

- Be aware drug should be given with aspirin.

! **WARNING** Monitor blood coagulation tests before and regularly during therapy; bleeding is a major bivalirudin risk. Be aware that drug affects international normalized ratio (INR), so INR may not be useful for determining an appropriate warfarin dose.

! **WARNING** Monitor patient often for bleeding because there's no antidote for bivalirudin. All patients with unexplained drop in blood pressure or hematocrit should be evaluated for bleeding. If life-threatening bleeding occurs, notify prescriber immediately, stop drug, and monitor APTT and other coagulation tests as ordered. Blood transfusions may be needed. Patients with increased bleeding risk include menstruating women; patients with large vessel or lumbar puncture, major surgery (including brain, eye, or spinal cord), major bleeding (including GI, intracranial, intraocular, pulmonary bleeding, or retroperitoneal), organ biopsy, recent stroke, or spinal anesthesia; and patients with organ or vascular abnormalities, such as advanced renal disease, dissecting aortic aneurysm, diverticulitis, hemophilia, hepatic disease (especially from deficient vitamin K–dependent clotting factors), infective endocarditis, inflammatory bowel disease, peptic ulcer disease, or severe uncontrolled hypertension. These patients should be monitored more frequently for bleeding. Patients with unstable angina also may experience major bleeding events such as intracranial bleeding, retroperitoneal bleeding, or a drop in hemoglobin of 3 g/dl or more.

- Know that if patient is receiving gamma brachytherapy, watch closely for evidence of thrombosis (weak or absent pulse, pallor, pain); use of bivalirudin may increase the risk in these patients.
- Avoid I.M. injections of any kind, if possible, to decrease the risk of bleeding.
- Discard any unused portion of drug.

PATIENT TEACHING

- Inform patient that bivalirudin is a blood thinner administered only in the hospital.
- Urge patient to check her skin for bruising or red spots and to immediately report back for stomach pain, dizziness, fainting, trouble breathing, and unusual bleeding (black, tarry stool; blood in urine; coughing blood; heavy menses; nosebleeds). Drug may have to be stopped.
- Encourage patient to reduce the risk of injury while receiving bivalirudin, such as by brushing her teeth gently with a soft-bristled toothbrush.
- Caution patient not to take anti-inflammatories, such as aspirin or aspirin-like products, ibuprofen, ketoprofen, and naproxen, or other blood thinners, such as warfarin, while receiving bivalirudin unless directed.

brexpiprazole
Rexulti

⬛ Class and Category
Pharmacologic class: Atypical antipsychotic
Therapeutic class: Antipsychotic

⬛ Indications and Dosages
✳ *Adjunct treatment of major depressive disorder*

TABLETS
Adults. *Initial:* 0.5 or 1 mg once daily, then increased to 1 or 2 mg once daily after 1 wk. Further increase in 1-mg increments weekly, as needed. *Maximum:* 3 mg once daily.

✳ *To treat schizophrenia*

TABLETS
Adults. *Initial:* 1 mg once daily for 4 days, followed by 2 mg once daily for 3 days, then increased to 4 mg once daily. *Maximum:* 4 mg once daily.

Adolescents. *Initial:* 0.5 mg once daily for 4 days, followed by 1 mg once daily for 3 days, then increased in 1-mg increments weekly, as needed. *Maximum:* 4 mg once daily.

±**DOSAGE ADJUSTMENT** For patients with moderate to severe hepatic impairment or moderate to severe or end-stage renal impairment (creatinine clearance less than 60 ml/min), maximum dosage should not exceed 2 mg once daily for patients with major depressive disorder and 3 mg for patients with schizophrenia. For patient who is a CYP2D6 poor metabolizer or patient is taking strong CYP2D6 or CYP3A4 inhibitors, dosage reduced by 50%. For patient who is a CYP2D6 poor metabolizer who is also taking moderate to strong CYP3A4 inhibitors or patient taking both a moderate to strong CYP2D6 inhibitor and a moderate to strong CYP3A4 inhibitor, dosage reduced by 75%. For patient taking strong CYP3A4 inducers, dosage doubled over 1 to 2 wk.

⬛ Drug Administration
P.O.
- Store at room temperature.

Route	Onset	Peak	Duration
P.O.	Unknown	4 hr	Unknown

Half-life: 91 hr

⬛ Mechanism of Action
May produce antipsychotic effects through partial agonist and antagonist actions. Brexpiprazole acts as a partial agonist at dopamine (especially D_2) receptors and serotonin (especially 5-HT1A) receptors. The drug acts as an antagonist at 5-HT2A serotonin receptor sites.

⬛ Contraindications
Hypersensitivity to brexpiprazole or its components

Interactions

DRUGS

clarithromycin, itraconazole, ketoconazole, and other strong CYP3A4 inhibitors: combination of a strong CYP3A4 inhibitor/strong CYP2D6 inhibitor (itraconazole/quinidine), moderate CYP3A4 inhibitor/strong CYP2D6 inhibitor (fluconazole/paroxetine), strong CYP3A4 inhibitor/moderate CYP2D6 inhibitor (itraconazole/duloxetine), moderate CYP3A4 inhibitor/moderate CYP2D6 inhibitor (fluconazole/duloxetine)

fluoxetine, paroxetine, quinidine, and other strong CYP2D6 inhibitors: Increased brexpiprazole exposure and possibly increased adverse brexpiprazole-related reactions

rifampin, St. John's wort, and other strong CYP3A4 inducers: Decreased brexpiprazole exposure and effectiveness

Adverse Reactions

CNS: Abnormal dreams, akathisia, anxiety, body temperature dysregulation, **CVA**, dizziness, dyskinesia, dystonia, fatigue, headache, impaired cognitive and motor skills, insomnia, **neuroleptic malignant syndrome**, restlessness, **seizures**, somnolence, **suicidal ideation**, syncope, tardive dyskinesia, tremor

CV: Dyslipidemia, orthostatic hypotension

EENT: Blurred vision, dry mouth, excessive salivation, nasopharyngitis

ENDO: Decreased blood cortisol levels, elevated prolactin levels, hyperglycemia

GI: Abdominal pain, constipation, diarrhea, dyspepsia, flatulence, increased appetite, nausea

GU: UTI

HEME: **Agranulocytosis, leukopenia, neutropenia**

MS: Myalgia

SKIN: Hyperhidrosis

Other: Increased blood creatine phosphokinase level, pathological gambling and other compulsive behaviors, weight gain

Childbearing Considerations

PREGNANCY

- Pregnancy exposure registry: 1-866-961-2388 or http://womensmentalhealth.org/clinical-and-research-programs/pregnancyregistry/.

- It is not known if drug can cause fetal harm. However, extrapyramidal and/or withdrawal symptoms have been reported in neonates whose mothers were exposed to antipsychotic drugs during the third trimester of pregnancy.
- Use with caution only if benefit to mother outweighs potential risk to fetus.

LACTATION

- It is not known if drug is present in breast milk.
- Patient should check with prescriber before breastfeeding.

Nursing Considerations

- Be aware that brexpiprazole shouldn't be used to treat dementia-related psychosis in the elderly because of an increased risk of death.
- Use brexpiprazole cautiously in patients with a history of seizures or with conditions that lower the seizure threshold. Also use cautiously in patients at risk for aspiration pneumonia because esophageal dysphagia has been associated with antipsychotic drug use.
- Monitor patient's CBC, as ordered, because serious adverse hematologic reactions, such as agranulocytosis, leukopenia, and neutropenia, may occur with atypical antipsychotic therapy. Assess more often during first few months of therapy if patient has a history of drug-induced leukopenia or neutropenia or a significantly low WBC count. If abnormalities occur during therapy, watch for fever or other signs of infection, notify prescriber and, if severe, expect drug to be stopped.
- Monitor patient for tardive dyskinesia, especially in elderly women. Know that it has the potential to be irreversible and the risk for developing tardive dyskinesia increases the longer brexpiprazole is used and the higher the total cumulative dose. If it occurs, notify prescriber and expect drug to be discontinued, if possible.

! **WARNING** Monitor patient's blood glucose level, lipid levels, and weight, as ordered, because atypical antipsychotic drugs such as brexpiprazole may cause metabolic changes. If patient is already a diabetic, monitor blood glucose levels more closely because hyperglycemia may become extreme, causing hyperosmolar coma, ketoacidosis, or even death. Know that even in patients with no history of diabetes mellitus, hyperglycemia may develop.

! **WARNING** Know that antipsychotic drugs may cause neuroleptic malignant syndrome. Monitor patient closely throughout brexpiprazole therapy. If suspected, notify prescriber immediately, be prepared to provide emergency supportive care, and expect drug to be discontinued.

- Watch patients closely for suicidal tendencies, particularly when therapy starts and dosage changes, because depression may worsen temporarily during these times.

PATIENT TEACHING
- Instruct patient to follow dosage increases exactly as ordered.
- Advise patient to get up slowly from a lying or sitting position during brexpiprazole therapy to minimize a drop in blood pressure.
- Instruct patient to avoid hazardous activities until drug's effects are known. Also, alert patient and family of increased risk for falls, especially if patient has other medical conditions or takes medication that may affect the nervous system.
- Urge patient to avoid activities that raise body temperature suddenly, such as strenuous exercise and exposure to extreme heat, and to compensate for situations that cause dehydration, such as vomiting or diarrhea.
- Advise patient to report any persistent, severe, or unusual signs and symptoms to prescriber, especially abnormal movements.
- Instruct patient to inform all prescribers of any drugs he's taking, including OTC drugs, because of risk of interactions.
- Advise female patient of childbearing age to notify prescriber if she intends to become or suspects that she is pregnant during therapy.
- Instruct patient on the signs and symptoms of an elevated blood glucose level. Tell diabetic patient to monitor blood glucose levels closely. If abnormalities occur, prescriber should be notified.

- Tell family or caregiver to watch patient closely for suicidal tendencies, especially when therapy starts or dosage changes.
- Inform patient and family or caregiver that drug may cause intense urges, particularly for gambling, but may also cause sexual urges, uncontrollable shopping, binge eating, and other impulsive or compulsive behaviors. These behaviors may not be recognized as abnormal by patient. Urge the reporting of such behaviors, as a dosage reduction or discontinuation of the drug may be required to protect patient from these harmful effects.

brivaracetam
Briviact

☰ Class, Category, Schedule
Pharmacologic class: Anticonvulsant
Therapeutic class: Anticonvulsant
Controlled substance schedule: V

☰ Indications and Dosages
✴ *To treat partial-onset seizures*
ORAL SOLUTION, TABLETS
Adults and adolescents age 16 and over.
Initial: 50 mg twice daily followed by dosage reduction to 25 mg twice daily or dosage increase to 100 mg twice daily depending on therapeutic response and patient tolerance.
Children age 4 to 16 weighing 50 kg (110 lb) or more. *Initial:* 25 to 50 mg twice daily followed by dosage adjustment depending on patient tolerance and therapeutic response. Dosage maybe be reduced to 25 mg twice daily if dose started at 50 mg twice daily or dosage increased to 100 mg twice daily, if needed.
Children age 4 to 16 weighing 20 kg (44 lb) to less than 50 kg (110 lb). *Initial:* 0.5 mg/kg to 1 mg/kg twice daily followed by dosage adjustment depending on therapeutic response and patient tolerance. Dosage maybe reduced to 0.5 mg/kg if dose started at 1 mg/kg twice daily or dosage increased to 2 mg/kg twice daily, if needed.
Children age 4 to 16 weighing 11 kg (24.2 lb) to less than 20 kg (44 lb). *Initial:* 0.5 mg/kg to 1.25 mg/kg twice daily followed by dosage adjustment depending on therapeutic response and patient tolerance. Dosage may

be decreased to 0.5 mg/kg if dose started at 1.25 mg/kg twice daily or dosage increased to 2.5 mg/kg twice daily, if needed.

Infants 1 month of age or older and children weighing less than 11 kg (24.2 lb). *Initial:* 0.75 mg/kg to 1.5 mg/kg twice daily followed by dosage adjustment depending on therapeutic response and patient tolerance. Dosage may be decreased to 0.75 mg/kg if dose started at 1.5 mg/kg twice daily or dosage increased to 3 mg/kg twice daily, if needed.

I.V. INJECTION

Adults and adolescents age 16 and over. *Initial:* 50 mg twice daily followed by dosage reduction to 25 mg twice daily or dosage increase to 100 mg twice daily depending on therapeutic response and patient tolerance.

±**DOSAGE ADJUSTMENT** For adult patient and pediatric patient weighing 50 kg (110 lb) or more with hepatic impairment of any severity, initial dosage reduced to 25 mg twice daily, with maximum dosage not to exceed 75 mg twice daily. For pediatric patient with hepatic impairment weighing 11 kg (24.2 lb) to less than 50 kg (110 lb), initial dosage not to exceed 0.5 mg/kg twice daily. For pediatric patient with hepatic impairment weighing 20 kg (44 lb) to less than 50 kg (110 lb), maximum dosage not to exceed 1.5 mg/kg twice daily and for pediatric patient with hepatic impairment weighing 11 kg (24.2 lb) to less than 20 kg (44 lb), maximum dosage not to exceed 2 mg/kg twice daily. For infants and children weighing less than 11 kg (24.2 lb), initial dose not to exceed 0.75 mg/kg twice daily, maximum dosage not to exceed 2.25 mg/kg twice daily. For patient receiving rifampin concurrently, dosage of brivaracetam doubled.

☰ Drug Administration

- Drug can be initiated with either intravenous or oral administration in adults. Intravenous administration is not approved for children under the age of 16.

P.O.

- Tablets should be swallowed whole and given with a beverage. Tablets should not be chewed or crushed.
- Use a calibrated measuring device to measure and deliver the prescribed dose of oral solution.

- Oral solution may be administered without dilution into a gastrostomy or nasogastric tube. Flush tube afterwards.
- Oral solution should be discarded after 5 months of first opening bottle.

I.V.

- Can be administered intravenously without further dilution or mixed with 0.9% Sodium Chloride Injection, 5% Dextrose Injection, or Lactated Ringer's Injection.
- Do not store diluted solution for more than 4 hours at room temperature. It may be stored in polyvinyl chloride bags.
- Administer over 2 to 15 minutes.
- *Incompatibilities:* None listed by manufacturer

Route	Onset	Peak	Duration
P.O.	Unknown	1 hr	Unknown
I.V.	Unknown	Unknown	Unknown

Half-life: 9 hr

☰ Mechanism of Action

Displays a high and selective affinity for synaptic vesicle protein 2A (SV2A) in the brain, which may contribute to the anticonvulsant effect, although the exact mechanism is unknown.

☰ Contraindications

Hypersensitivity to brivaracetam or its components

☰ Interactions

DRUGS

carbamazepine: Possibly increased exposure of carbamazepine that may lead to adverse reactions
phenytoin: Increased plasma concentrations of phenytoin that may lead to adverse reactions
rifampin: Decreased plasma concentrations of brivaracetam significantly interfering with its effectiveness and requiring a dosage increase to compensate

☰ Adverse Reactions

CNS: Abnormal behavior, acute psychosis, adjustment disorder, affect lability, aggression, agitation, altered mood, anger, anxiety, apathy, balance and cerebellar coordination disturbances, belligerence, depression, dizziness, dysgeusia (parenteral form), euphoria (parenteral form), fatigue, feeling drunk (parenteral form), hallucinations, irritability, mood swings, nervousness, paranoia, psychomotor hyperactivity, psychotic behavior or disorder, restlessness, sedation, somnolence, **suicidal ideation**

EENT: Taste disturbance (parenteral form)

GI: Anorexia (children), constipation, nausea, vomiting

HEME: Leukopenia, neutropenia

RESP: Bronchospasm

Other: Angioedema, infusion-site pain (parenteral form)

Childbearing Considerations
PREGNANCY
- Pregnancy exposure registry: 1-888-233-2334 or http://www.aedpregnancyregistry.org/.
- It is not known if drug can cause fetal harm.
- Use with caution only if benefit to mother outweighs potential risk to fetus.

LACTATION
- It is not known if drug is present in breast milk.
- Patient should check with prescriber before breastfeeding.

Nursing Considerations
- Be aware that brivaracetam oral solution may be administered via a gastrostomy or nasogastric tube.

! **WARNING** Monitor patient closely for abnormal behavior or thoughts, because brivaracetam may increase risk of suicidal thoughts or behavior.

! **WARNING** Monitor patient for hypersensitivity reactions, especially angioedema and bronchospasm. If present, notify prescriber, expect brivaracetam to be discontinued, and be prepared to provide supportive care.

- Take safety measures to prevent patient from falling, because brivaracetam may cause dizziness and disturbances in coordination and gait.
- Know that brivaracetam may cause psychiatric adverse reactions. Notify prescriber, if present, and take measures to keep patient calm and safe.
- Be aware that brivaracetam should not be discontinued abruptly, because of increased risk of seizure frequency and the potential for status epilepticus.

PATIENT TEACHING
- Inform patient prescribed tablet form to swallow tablets whole with a beverage. Tell patient tablets should not be chewed or crushed.
- Inform patient prescribed oral solution form to use a calibrated measuring device to measure and deliver the prescribed dose. Remind patient that a household tablespoon or teaspoon is not an adequate measuring device. Tell patient the oral solution need not be diluted. Have patient discard any unused oral solution after 5 months of first opening the bottle.

! **WARNING** Have family or caregiver monitor patient closely for abnormal behavior or thoughts, because drug may increase risk of suicidal thoughts and behavior.

- Advise patient to avoid performing hazardous activities such as driving or operating machinery until central nervous system effects of brivaracetam are known and have abated.
- Remind patient to be careful and use safety precautions when walking or performing physical activities because brivaracetam may cause disturbances in coordination and gait and dizziness.
- Advise patient and family or caregiver that brivaracetam may cause changes in behavior such as aggression, agitation, anger, anxiety, and irritability along with psychotic symptoms. Instruct patient or family/caregiver to report these changes immediately to the prescriber.
- Tell women of childbearing age to notify prescriber if pregnancy is suspected or known. If confirmed, encourage patient to enroll in the pregnancy exposure registry by calling 1-888-233-2334.

brodalumab
Siliq

Class and Category
Pharmacologic class: Monoclonal IgG2 antibody
Therapeutic class: Antipsoriatic

Indications and Dosages

* *To treat moderate to severe plaque psoriasis in patients who are candidates for systemic therapy or phototherapy and have failed to respond or have lost response to other systemic therapies*

SUBCUTANEOUS INJECTION

Adults. *Initial:* 210 mg followed by 210 mg repeated at wk 1 and 2, and then 210 mg every 2 wk.

Drug Administration

SUBCUTANEOUS

- Allow prefilled syringe to reach room temperature before administering, which is about 30 minutes. Do not warm any other way and do not remove the gray needle cap on the prefilled syringe while allowing it to reach room temperature.
- Do not shake the prefilled syringe.
- Solution in the pen should appear clear to slightly opalescent, colorless to slightly yellow, and may have a few translucent to white particles. Do not use if cloudy or discolored or if foreign matter is present.
- Do not use the prefilled syringe if it has been dropped on a hard surface.
- Administer only as a subcutaneous injection into the patient's abdomen, thigh, or upper arm, injecting the full amount in the syringe to provide the correct dosage.
- Do not inject into an area that is affected by psoriasis or is bruised, hard, red, scaly, tender, or thick.
- Store in original carton to protect from light in refrigerator or at room temperature. However, do not place back into refrigerator if stored at room temperature; carton must be discarded after 14 days if stored at room temperature.

Route	Onset	Peak	Duration
SubQ	Unknown	3 days	Unknown

Half-life: Unknown

Mechanism of Action

Binds to human IL-17RA and inhibits its interactions with selective cytokines. This inhibits the release of proinflammatory chemokines and cytokines, which are thought to be part of the pathogenesis of plaque psoriasis.

Contraindications

Crohn's disease, hypersensitivity to brodalumab or its components

Interactions

DRUGS

CYP450 substrates such as cyclosporine or warfarin: Possibly altered effectiveness of these drugs

live vaccines: Failure to produce an adequate immune response

Adverse Reactions

CNS: Headache, fatigue, **suicidal ideation**
EENT: Nasopharyngitis, oropharyngeal pain, pharyngitis
GI: Crohn's disease, diarrhea, nausea
GU: UTI
HEME: **Neutropenia**
MS: Arthralgia, myalgia
RESP: Bronchitis, upper respiratory infections
SKIN: Tinea infections, urticaria
Other: Antibrodalumab antibody formation, flu-like symptoms, injection-site reactions (bruising, erythema, hemorrhage, pain, pruritus)

Childbearing Considerations

PREGNANCY

- It is not known if drug can cause fetal harm. However, human IgG antibodies are known to cross the placental barrier; therefore, drug may be transmitted from the mother to the fetus.
- Use with caution only if benefit to mother outweighs potential risk to fetus.

LACTATION

- It is not known if drug is present in breast milk.
- Patient should check with prescriber before breastfeeding.

Nursing Considerations

- Expect patient to be evaluated for tuberculosis before brodalumab therapy is begun. If present, know that brodalumab should not be initiated until treatment for latent tuberculosis has been given. Monitor all patients for signs and symptoms of tuberculosis during and after brodalumab therapy.
- Use cautiously in patients with a chronic infection or who have a history of recurrent infections, because brodalumab increases

B

the risk of infections, especially fungal infections. If an infection occurs and does not respond to standard therapy for the infection, expect brodalumab to be withheld until the infection is resolved.

> **! WARNING** Know that brodalumab is only available through a restricted program because of its potential to cause suicidal behavior and thoughts. Monitor patient closely and expect drug to be discontinued if suicidal ideation is present.

- Monitor patient for Crohn's disease and know that brodalumab must be discontinued if patient develops this disease while taking the drug.
- Avoid administering live vaccines while patient is receiving brodalumab because vaccines may not be effective.

PATIENT TEACHING

- Instruct patient self-administering brodalumab how to properly administer a subcutaneous injection and sites for administration. Tell patient not to inject the drug in an area that is affected by psoriasis or is bruised, hard, scaly, tender, or thick.
- Tell patient to allow the prefilled syringe to reach room temperature (which takes about 30 minutes) before injecting the drug. Remind patient not to remove the gray needle cap on the syringe while allowing it to reach room temperature and not to shake the syringe. Prior to injection, tell patient to look at solution inside the syringe. It should be clear to slightly opalescent, colorless to slightly yellow. A few translucent to white particles may be present. If solution appears cloudy or discolored or if foreign matter is present, the syringe should be discarded and a replacement obtained. Also tell patient not to use if syringe is dropped onto a hard surface. Tell patient to inject the full amount of solution contained in the prefilled syringe. Advise patient to rotate sites.
- Advise patient to seek medical attention if signs or symptoms of infection occur.
- Tell patient to notify prescriber if persistent or severe bowel problems develop. If Crohn's disease is diagnosed, inform patient that brodalumab therapy must be discontinued.

> **! WARNING** Alert patient or family that drug may produce suicidal behavior or thoughts. If present, suicide precautions should be undertaken, prescriber notified, and drug discontinued.

budesonide

Entocort EC, Ortikos, Pulmicort Flexhaler, Pulmicort Respules, Pulmicort Turbuhaler (CAN), Rhinocort Allergy, Uceris

Class and Category

Pharmacologic class: Corticosteroid
Therapeutic class: Antiasthmatic, anti-inflammatory

Indications and Dosages

* *To manage symptoms of seasonal or perennial allergic rhinitis*

NASAL SPRAY (BUDESONIDE)

Adults and children age 6 and over. 32 mcg in each nostril daily. *Maintenance:* Lowest dosage that controls symptoms.
Maximum: For adults and children age 12 and over: 256 mcg once daily administered as four sprays (32 mcg/spray) per nostril. For children age 6 to less than 12 years of age: 128 mcg once daily administered as two sprays (32 mcg/spray) per nostril.

NASAL SPRAY (RHINOCORT ALLERGY)

Adults and children 12 years of age and older. *Initial:* 64 mcg (2 sprays) in each nostril once daily, reduced to 32 mcg (1 spray) in each nostril once daily when symptoms improve.
Children age 6 to under 12 years. *Initial:* 32 mcg (1 spray) in each nostril once daily, increased to 64 mcg (2 sprays) in each nostril once daily, if needed. Once symptoms are under control, dosage reduced back to 32 mcg (1 spray) in each nostril once daily.

* *To provide maintenance therapy as prophylactic therapy in asthma*

ORAL INHALATION (PULMICORT FLEXHALER)

Adults and adolescents age 18 and over. *Initial:* 180 or 360 mcg twice daily, increased as needed. *Maximum:* 720 mcg twice daily.

Children ages 6 to 17. *Initial:* 180 or 360 mcg twice daily. *Maximum:* 360 mcg twice daily.

NEBULIZED INHALATION (PULMICORT RESPULES)

Children ages 1 to 8 previously on bronchodilators alone. 0.25 mg twice daily. or 0.5 mg daily by jet nebulizer. *Maximum:* 0.5 mg/day.

Children ages 1 to 8 previously on inhaled steroids. 0.25 mg twice daily or 0.5 mg daily inhaled by jet nebulizer. *Maximum:* 1 mg/day.

Children ages 1 to 8 previously on systemic corticosteroids. 0.5 mg twice daily or 1 mg daily inhaled by jet nebulizer. *Maximum:* 1 mg/day.

ORAL INHALATION (PULMICORT TURBUHALER)

Adults and children over 12 years of age upon initiation of inhaled glucocorticoids, during periods of severe asthma, and when oral glucocorticoid dosages are being decreased or discontinued.
Initial: 400 to 2400 mcg daily evenly divided into 2 to 4 times daily. Alternatively, doses of 400 mcg may be given once daily in the morning or evening. *Maintenance:* 200 to 400 mcg twice daily.

Children age 6 to and including 12 years of age upon initiation of inhaled glucocorticoids, during periods of severe asthma, and when oral glucocorticoid dosages are being decreased or discontinued. *Initial:* 100 to 200 mcg twice daily.

✳ *To treat mild to moderate active Crohn's disease involving the ileum, the ascending colon, or both*

DELAYED-RELEASE CAPSULES (ENTOCORT EC), E.R. CAPSULES (ORTIKOS)

Adults. 9 mg daily for up to 8 wk. Course may be repeated for recurring episodes of active disease.
Children age 8 to 17 weighing more than 25 kg (55 lb). 9 mg once daily for 8 wk, followed by 6 mg once daily for 2 wk.

✳ *To maintain clinical remission of mild to moderate Crohn's disease involving the ileum, the ascending colon, or both*

E.R. CAPSULES (ENTOCORT EC), E.R. CAPSULES (ORTIKOS)

Adults. 6 mg daily for up to 3 mo.

± **DOSAGE ADJUSTMENT** *For Entocort EC:* For adult patients with moderate hepatic impairment, dosage reduced to 3 mg once daily for duration of treatment.

✳ *To induce remission in patients with active, mild to moderate ulcerative colitis*

E.R. TABLETS (UCERIS)

Adults. 9 mg daily for up to 8 wk.

✳ *To induce remission in patients with active, mild to moderate distal ulcerative colitis extending up to 40 cm from the anal verge*

RECTAL FOAM (UCERIS)

Adults. 1 metered dose (2 mg) twice daily for 2 wk followed by 1 metered dose (2 mg) once daily for 4 wk.

▤ Drug Administration

P.O.

EXTENDED-RELEASE TABLETS

- Administer in morning.
- Tablets should be swallowed whole with water and not broken, chewed, or crushed.

DELAYED- OR EXTENDED-RELEASE CAPSULES

- Administer in morning.
- Capsules should be swallowed whole and not chewed or split.
- Entocort EC Capsules may be opened and granules sprinkled onto 1 tablespoon of applesauce. Mix the granules with the applesauce and administer entire contents within 30 minutes of mixing. Stress importance of not chewing or crushing the granules.
- After administration either way, have patient drink 8 ounces of water.
- Mixture should not be saved for future use.
- Ortikos brand is not interchangeable with other budesonide products.

NASAL SPRAY

- Prime bottle before first use by pumping the bottle 8 times or until a fine spray comes out. If bottle is not used for 2 days, it will have to be primed again. If bottle is not used for more than 14 days, clean the spray tip and prime it again by releasing two sprays.
- Shake bottle before each use. Have patient blow her nose, tilt her head slightly forward, and insert tip into a nostril, pointing toward inner corner of eye, away from nasal septum. The other nostril should be held closed while patient inhales gently. Then repeat in the other nostril.

B

ORAL INHALER

- Prime oral inhaler before using it for first time by holding canister upright with mouthpiece on top and twisting base of device fully to right and then fully to left until it clicks.
- Load each dose just before use in the same way. Once loaded, do not shake device.
- Do not use with a spacer device.
- Have patient turn head away from device and exhale. Then have her hold device upright, place her lips around mouthpiece, and inhale deeply. Device will discharge a dose. Have her remove her lips from mouthpiece to exhale.
- Have patient rinse mouth with water without swallowing after each dose.
- Keep canister away from heat sources, as its contents are flammable.

NEBULIZED INHALATION

- Use with a compressed-air–driven jet nebulizer only. It must have an adequate air flow and a suitable face mask or nose piece.
- Do not mix other drugs in the nebulizer.
- Have patient rinse mouth with water after each treatment without swallowing the water.
- Discard ampules if not used within 2 weeks of opening the protective aluminum foil envelope. Do not refrigerate or freeze drug.

RECTAL FOAM

- Have patient empty bowels before administering rectal foam. Although product is lubricated, use additional petroleum jelly, if needed.
- Warm the canister in hands while shaking it vigorously for 10 to 15 seconds prior to use.
- Administer in the morning and evening for the first 2 weeks, then once daily in the evening.
- When administering in the evening, do so immediately before bedtime. Patient should not try to empty bowels again until morning.

Route	Onset	Peak	Duration
P.O./D.R.	Unknown	0.5–10 hr	Unknown
P.O./E.R.	Unknown	7.4–19.2 hr	Unknown
Intranasal	10 hr	30 min	Unknown
Oral inhalation	24 hr	10–30 min	Unknown
Nebulization	2–8 days	2 min	Unknown
P.R.	Unknown	Unknown	Unknown

Half-life: 2–3.6 hours

Mechanism of Action

Inhibits inflammatory cells and mediators, possibly by decreasing influx into nasal passages, bronchial walls, or the intestines. As a result, nasal or airway inflammation decreases. Oral inhalation form also inhibits mucus secretion in airways, decreasing the amount and viscosity of sputum.

Contraindications

Hypersensitivity to budesonide or its components, recent septal ulcers or nasal surgery or trauma (nasal spray); status asthmaticus or other acute asthma episodes (oral inhalation)

Interactions

DRUGS

antacids, H2 blockers, proton pump inhibitors (oral Uceris): Dissolution of the coating of oral Uceris may be altered
clarithromycin, erythromycin, itraconazole, ketoconazole, and other strong CYP3A4 inhibitors such as atazanavir, clarithromycin, indinavir, itraconazole, nefazodone, nelfinavir, ritonavir, saquinavir, telithromycin: Possibly increased blood budesonide level

FOODS

grapefruit juice: Possibly increased blood budesonide level

Adverse Reactions

CNS: Amnesia, asthenia, **benign intracranial hypertension**, changes in mood, dizziness, fatigue, fever, headache
CV: Hypertension, peripheral edema
EENT: Bad taste, cataracts, dry mouth, epistaxis, glaucoma, nasal irritation, oral or pharyngeal candidiasis, pharyngitis, rhinitis, sinusitis
ENDO: Adrenal insufficiency, growth suppression in children, hypercorticism
GI: Abdominal pain, diarrhea, dyspepsia, flatulence, indigestion, nausea, **pancreatitis, rectal bleeding**, vomiting
GU: UTI
MS: Arthralgia, back pain, muscle cramps and spasms
RESP: Bronchospasm, increased cough, respiratory tract infection
SKIN: Allergic or contact dermatitis, maculopapular rash, pruritus, purpura, rash, urticaria
Other: Anaphylaxis, angioedema, increased risk of infection

Childbearing Considerations

PREGNANCY

- Drug may cause fetal harm, as it crosses the placental barrier.
- Hypoadrenalism in infants may occur when mothers have received substantial doses of corticosteroids during pregnancy, especially oral forms. Inhaled corticosteroids pose less risk.
- Use with caution only if benefit to mother outweighs potential risk to fetus.

LACTATION

- Drug is present in breast milk following inhalation of the drug. It is unknown if drug is present in breast milk following oral administration.
- Patient should check with prescriber before breastfeeding.

Nursing Considerations

- Use budesonide cautiously if patient has ocular herpes simplex; tubercular infection; or untreated fungal, bacterial, or systemic viral infection.
- Closely monitor a child's growth pattern; budesonide may stunt growth.

! WARNING Assess patient who switches from a systemic corticosteroid to inhaled budesonide for adrenal insufficiency (fatigue, hypotension, lassitude, nausea, vomiting, weakness), which may be life-threatening. Hypothalamic–pituitary–adrenal axis function may take several months to recover after stopping systemic corticosteroids. Stopping budesonide abruptly may cause adrenal insufficiency.

- Monitor patient exposed to chickenpox. Know that he may receive varicella zoster immune globulin or pooled I.V. immunoglobulin. If chickenpox develops, give antiviral as ordered. A patient exposed to measles may need pooled I.M. immunoglobulin.
- Assess patient for effectiveness of budesonide therapy, especially if being weaned from a systemic corticosteroid. If patient has increased asthma or an immunologic condition previously suppressed by systemic corticosteroid— such as arthritis, conjunctivitis, an eosinophilic condition, eczema, or rhinitis—notify prescriber.

- Determine if patient has a milk allergy. Pulmicort Flexhaler contains small amounts of lactose, which may trigger coughing, wheezing, or bronchospasm in a patient with a severe milk-protein allergy.
- Monitor patient for evidence of hypersensitivity. If present, notify prescriber immediately. Expect to stop budesonide and provide emergency supportive care.
- Monitor patients with conditions such as diabetes mellitus, glaucoma or cataracts, hypertension, osteoporosis, or peptic ulcer, as glucocorticosteroid therapy may increase adverse effects. Also monitor patients with a family history of diabetes or glaucoma.

PATIENT TEACHING

- Urge patient taking oral delayed-release or E.R. capsules or E.R. tablets to swallow them whole and not to chew or break them. However, for the patient who cannot swallow an intact capsule, tell her to place one tablespoonful of applesauce into an empty bowl if she is prescribed Entocort EC capsules. Applesauce should not be hot and should be soft enough to swallow without chewing. Then patient should open Entocort EC capsule and carefully empty all the granules inside onto the applesauce. She should mix the granules with the applesauce and consume the entire contents within 30 minutes of mixing followed immediately by drinking an 8-ounce glass of cool water. Stress importance of not chewing or crushing the granules, nor should she save the applesauce and granules for future use. Patient should drink 8 ounces of water after taking oral budesonide.
- Tell patient using nasal spray form to prime bottle before first use by pumping the bottle 8 times or until a fine spray comes out. If bottle is not used for 2 days, it will have to be primed again. If bottle is not used for more than 14 days, patient should clean the spray tip and prime it again by releasing two sprays. Instruct patient to shake bottle before each use. Instruct her to blow her nose, tilt her head slightly forward, and insert tube into a nostril, pointing toward inner corner of eye, away from nasal septum. Tell her to hold the other nostril closed and spray while inhaling gently. Then have her repeat in the other nostril.

B

- Instruct patient to prime oral inhaler before using it for first time by holding canister upright with mouthpiece on top and twisting base of device fully to right and then fully to left until it clicks. Teach her to load each dose just before use in the same way. After loading a dose, caution patient not to shake device or blow into it. Tell patient to turn her head away from device and exhale. Then have her hold device upright, place her lips around mouthpiece, and inhale deeply. Device will discharge a dose. Tell patient to remove her lips from mouthpiece to exhale.
- Instruct patient to empty her bowels before using rectal foam. Although product is lubricated, tell patient she may use petroleum jelly if more lubrication is needed. Tell her to warm the canister in her hands while shaking it vigorously for 10 to 15 seconds prior to use. Inform her that she may apply the rectal foam while standing, lying, or sitting. When applied in the evening, instruct her to do so immediately before bedtime and advise her to try not to empty her bowels again until morning. Warn patient to keep canister away from heat sources, as its contents are flammable.
- Caution patient not to use an oral inhaler with a spacer device.
- Advise patient to rinse her mouth with water after each orally inhaled dose and to spit the water out. Tell her to contact her prescriber if she develops a mouth or throat infection.
- Instruct patient not to use budesonide as a rescue inhaler.
- Tell patient to contact prescriber if symptoms persist or have worsened after 3 weeks. Caution against increasing the dose on her own.
- Inform parents of small children using nebulized Respules that improvement may begin within 2 to 8 days but that full effect may not be evident for 4 to 6 weeks.
- Caution patient to avoid exposure to chickenpox and measles and, if exposed, to contact prescriber immediately.
- Caution against stopping drug abruptly.
- Instruct patient on long-term therapy to have regular eye examinations.

- Urge female patient to notify prescriber if she is or could be pregnant.
- Strongly encourage mothers who wish to breastfeed an infant to discuss breastfeeding with prescriber before doing so.

bumetanide
Bumex

Class and Category
Pharmacologic class: Loop diuretic as sulfonamide derivative
Therapeutic class: Diuretic

Indications and Dosages
❋ *To treat edema caused by heart failure, hepatic disease, and renal disease, including nephrotic syndrome*

TABLETS
Adults. 0.5 to 2 mg daily, increased as needed, with a second or third dose every 4 to 5 hr or 0.5 to 2 mg every other day or daily for 3 or 4 days each week. *Maximum:* 10 mg daily.

I.M. INJECTION, I.V. INFUSION, I.V. INJECTION
Adults. 0.5 to 1 mg daily, increased as needed with a second or third dose every 2 to 3 hr. *Maximum:* 10 mg daily.

Drug Administration
P.O.
- No special instructions for administration given by manufacturer.

I.V.
- Given only if impaired absorption is suspected or oral administration is not practical.
- Dilute for infusion by adding to 250 ml of 0.9% Sodium Chloride Injection or 5% Dextrose in Water Injection. Administer infusion at 0.2 mg/hr to 1 mg/hr.
- Administer undiluted as an injection over 1 to 2 minutes.
- Discard unused solution 24 hours after preparation.
- *Incompatibilities:* None reported by manufacturer

I.M.
- Given only if impaired absorption is suspected or oral administration is not practical.

Route	Onset	Peak	Duration
P.O.	30–60 min	1–2 hr	4–6 hr
I.V.	>5 min	15–30 min	3.5–4 hr
I.M.	30–60 min	30 min	4–5 hr

Half-life: 1–1.5 hr

⋮ Mechanism of Action

Inhibits reabsorption of sodium, chloride, and water in the ascending limb of the loop of Henle, which promotes their excretion and reduces fluid volume.

⋮ Contraindications

Anuria, hepatic coma, hypersensitivity to bumetanide or its components, marked increase in BUN or creatinine levels or development of oliguria if progressive renal disease is present, severe electrolyte depletion

⋮ Interactions

DRUGS

aminoglycosides: Increased risk of ototoxicity
antihypertensives: Increased hypotensive effect
indomethacin: Slowed increase in urine and sodium excretion, inhibited plasma renin activity
lithium: Reduced lithium renal clearance, increased risk of lithium toxicity
nephrotoxic drugs: Potential for adverse renal effects
probenecid: Reduced sodium excretion

⋮ Adverse Reactions

CNS: Dizziness, **encephalopathy**, headache
CV: Hypotension
EENT: Ototoxicity
ENDO: Hyperglycemia
GI: Nausea
GU: Azotemia, elevated serum creatinine level
MS: Muscle spasms
SKIN: Stevens–Johnson syndrome, toxic epidermal necrolysis
Other: Hyperuricemia, **hypocalcemia**, hypochloremia, **hypokalemia, hyponatremia**, hypovolemia

⋮ Childbearing Considerations

PREGNANCY

- It is not known if drug can cause fetal harm.
- Use with caution only if benefit to mother outweighs potential risk to fetus.

LACTATION

- It is not known if drug is present in breast milk.
- Breastfeeding is not recommended during drug therapy.

⋮ Nursing Considerations

! WARNING Know that a patient hypersensitive to sulfonamides may be hypersensitive to bumetanide. Monitor such a patient closely when starting therapy.

- Assess fluid and electrolyte balance closely because bumetanide is a potent diuretic (40 to 60 times more potent than furosemide). Monitor fluid intake and output once every 8 hours, evaluate serum electrolyte levels when ordered, and assess for imbalances.

! WARNING Be aware that high-dose or too-frequent administration can cause profound diuresis and water and electrolyte depletion, especially in elderly patients.

- Monitor serum potassium level regularly to check for hypokalemia, especially if patient takes a digitalis glycoside for heart failure or has aldosteronism, ascites, diarrhea, hepatic cirrhosis, potassium-losing nephropathy, or a history of ventricular arrhythmias.
- Assess for evidence of ototoxicity, such as tinnitus, daily. Rarely, drug may cause ototoxicity, especially with I.V. use, high doses, and increased frequency of dosing in a patient with renal impairment.
- Monitor results of renal function tests during therapy to detect adverse reactions.

PATIENT TEACHING

- Advise patient to avoid hazardous activities until drug's CNS effects are known.
- Stress importance of monitoring fluid intake and output and watching for evidence of electrolyte imbalance, such as dizziness, headache, and muscle spasms.
- Review adverse reactions, and tell patient to report severe or persistent reactions.
- Review potassium-rich foods, and urge patient to include them in her daily diet.
- Urge patient to return for appropriate follow-up care, especially if she's receiving bumetanide for a chronic condition.

B

- Tell diabetic patient to monitor blood glucose level regularly and to notify prescriber about persistent hyperglycemia.
- Advise patient to report any changes in skin that are new, unusual, persistent, or severe.

buprenorphine
Butrans, Sublocade

buprenorphine hydrochloride
Belbuca, Buprenex

☰ Class, Category, and Schedule
Pharmacologic class: Opioid
Therapeutic class: Opioid analgesic
Controlled substance schedule: III

☰ Indications and Dosages
✳ *To control pain severe enough to require opioid treatment and for which alternative treatment options (i.e., nonopioid analgesics or opioid combination products) are inadequate or not tolerated*

I.V. OR I.M. INJECTION (BUPRENEX)
Adults and adolescents. 0.3 mg up to 6 hr intervals, as needed. A second 0.3-mg dose may be given 30 to 60 min after first dose, if needed.
Children 2 to 12 years of age. 2 to 6 mcg/kg every 4 to 6 hr, as needed. *Maximum:* 6 mcg/kg

±**DOSAGE ADJUSTMENT** For adult patients not at high risk for opioid toxicity, I.M. dose increased to 0.6 mg and given as a single dose, if needed, depending on pain severity and patient response. For elderly or debilitated patients and patients who have respiratory disease or also use another CNS depressant, I.V. or I.M. dose kept at minimum dose.

✳ *To control severe chronic pain in patients requiring a continuous, around-the-clock opioid analgesic for an extended period of time for which alternative treatment options are inadequate*

TRANSDERMAL PATCH (BUTRANS)
Opioid-naïve adults. *Initial:* 5 mcg/hr with dosage titrated every 72 hr, as needed, to achieve pain relief with patch changed every 7 days. *Maximum:* 20 mcg/hr.

Adults whose daily dose of oral morphine or equivalent was less than 30 mg. *Initial:* 5 mcg/hr, increased after 72 hr, as needed, to 10 mcg/hr with patch changed every 7 days. *Maximum:* 20 mcg/hr.

Adults whose daily dose of oral morphine or equivalent was between 30 and 80 mg. *Initial:* Current around-the-clock opioid use tapered for up to 7 days to no more than 30 mg of morphine or equivalent per day. Then a 10 mcg/hr patch applied, increased after 72 hr, as needed, to 20 mcg/hr with patch changed every 7 days. *Maximum:* 20 mcg/hr.

BUCCAL FILM (BELBUCA)
Opioid-naïve and opioid-nontolerant adults. *Initial:* 75 mcg once daily or, if tolerated every 12 hr for at least 4 days, then increased to 150 mcg every 12 hr. Dosage further titrated, as needed, in increments of 150 mcg every 12 hr every 4 or more days. *Maximum:* 450 mcg every 12 hr.

Adults already on opioids. *Initial:* 75 mcg once daily or every 12 hr for patients whose daily dose of oral morphine sulfate equivalent (MSE) is less than 30 mg; 150 mcg every 12 hr for patients whose daily dose of oral MSE is between 30 and 89 mg; and 300 mcg every 12 hr for patients whose daily dose of oral MSE is between 90 and 160 mg. Then dosage titrated, as needed, no more than every 4 days in increments of 150 mcg every 12 hr. *Maximum:* 900 mcg every 12 hr.

±**DOSAGE ADJUSTMENT** For patients with oral mucositis or severe hepatic impairment, initial dose and subsequent titrations, dosage decreased by half.

✳ *To treat opioid dependence*

SUBLINGUAL TABLETS (BUPRENORPHINE HYDROCHLORIDE)
Adults. *Induction:* 8 mg daily on day 1 followed by 16 mg daily on day 2. *Maintenance:* 4 to 24 mg daily, with increases or decreases in 2- to 4-mg increments, as needed. *Maximum:* 24 mg daily.

±**DOSAGE ADJUSTMENT** For patients with severe hepatic impairment, initial dose and subsequent titrations, dosage decreased by half.

✳ *To treat moderate to severe opioid use disorder in patients who have initiated treatment with a transmucosal buprenorphine-containing product, followed by dose adjustment for a minimum of 7 days*

SUBCUTANEOUS INJECTION (SUBLOCADE)

Adults. 300 mg monthly for first 2 months followed by maintenance dose. *Maintenance:* 100 mg monthly. Maintenance dose may be increased to 300 mg monthly, if needed.

▤ Drug Administration

P.O.
Buccal film
- Have patient wet the inside of cheek. Have patient place the yellow side of the film against the inside of cheek immediately after removing film from the package. Using clean, dry fingers, it should be held in place for 5 seconds. The film will dissolve, usually within 30 minutes. Patient should not eat or drink until film is dissolved nor should patient try to manipulate film with tongue or fingers while dissolving.
- Dispose of unused film by removing from the foil packages. Dispose of foil packages in the trash.

Sublingual tablets
- Have patient place sublingual tablets under the tongue until dissolved. If more than two tablets per dose is prescribed, all tablets are placed under the tongue at the same time. If they won't fit, two tablets at a time can be placed under the tongue until full dose has been given.
- Sublingual tablets should not be swallowed.

I.V.
- Give I.V. injection slowly over at least 2 minutes.
- Store avoiding excessive heat and prolonged exposure to light.
- *Incompatibilities:* None listed by manufacturer

I.M.
- Administer as a deep intramuscular injection.

SUBCUTANEOUS
- Administer monthly with a minimum of 26 days between doses.
- Remove subcutaneous form from refrigerator at least 15 minutes prior to administration to allow drug to reach room temperature. Then remove the foil pouch and safety needle from the carton. Open pouch and remove the syringe. Check

the solution, which should be colorless to yellow to amber. Attach the safety needle. Do not remove the plastic cover from the needle at this time.
- Choose an injection site on patient's abdomen between the transpyloric and transtubercular planes that has adequate subcutaneous tissue that is free of excessive pigment, lesions, or nodules. Also, do not inject into an area where the skin is bruised, infected, irritated, reddened, or scarred in any way.
- Have patient assume a supine position.
- Clean injection site with an alcohol swab.
- Remove excess air from syringe and administer drug. Use a slow, steady push to inject drug until all of the drug is given. Withdraw the needle, lock the needle guard, and discard the syringe.
- Do not massage or rub injection site.

TRANSDERMAL
- Place patch only on intact skin that is hairless and clean (washed with water only) and dry. If a hairless site is not available, clip, not shave, area prior to application. Do not apply patch to irritated skin.
- Apply patch immediately after its removal from pouch to upper outer arm, upper back, upper chest, or the side of chest. Rotate sites and wait at least a minimum of 21 days before reapplying to the same site.
- If problems with adhesion occur, tape the edges of the patch with first-aid tape. If the patch should fall off during the 7-day interval, dispose of the patch and apply a new one at a different skin site.
- When removing the patch, fold it over on itself and discard.

Route	Onset	Peak	Duration
Buccal film	Unknown	2.5–3 hr	Unknown
Sublingual	Unknown	3–4 hr	Unknown
I.V.	Immediate	2 min	6 hr
I.M.	15 min	1–2 hr	6 hr
SubQ	Unknown	24 hr	Unknown
Transdermal	17 hr	Unknown	7 days

Half-life: Depends on route; up to 60 days

▤ Mechanism of Action
May bind with CNS receptors to alter the perception of and emotional response to pain.

Buprenorphine may act by displacing narcotic agonists from their binding sites and competitively inhibiting their actions.

Contraindications

Acute or severe bronchial asthma in an unmonitored setting or in the absence of resuscitative equipment, hypersensitivity to buprenorphine or its components, known or suspected GI obstruction including paralytic ileus, significant respiratory depression

Interactions

DRUGS

anticholinergic drugs: Increased risk of urinary retention and/or severe constipation that could lead to paralytic ileus

antimigraine agents, cyclobenzaprine; dextromethorphan; dolasetron; granisetron; linezolid; MAO inhibitors; methylene blue; ondansetron; palonosetron; selected psychiatric drugs such as amoxapine, buspirone, lithium, mirtazapine, nefazodone, trazodone, vilazodone; selective serotonin reuptake inhibitors; serotonin-norepinephrine reuptake inhibitors; St. John's wort; tricyclic antidepressants; tryptophan: Increased risk of serotonin syndrome

benzodiazepines, CNS depressants, other opioids, sedating antihistamines, tricyclic antidepressants: Increased risk of significant respiratory depression and other life-threatening adverse effects

CNS depressants, MAO inhibitors: Additive hypotensive and respiratory and CNS depressant effects of these drugs that may be life-threatening

CYP3A4 inducers such as carbamazepine, phenytoin, rifampin: Possibly decreased plasma concentration of buprenorphine

CYP3A4 inhibitors such as azole-antifungals (ketoconazole), macrolide antibiotics (erythromycin), protease inhibitors (ritonavir): Increased plasma concentration of buprenorphine, causing increased or prolonged opioid effects

diuretics: Possibly reduced effectiveness of diuretics

mixed agonist/antagonist and partial agonist opioid analgesics such as butorphanol, nalbuphine, pentazocine: Possibly reduced analgesic effect of buprenorphine and/or precipitate withdrawal symptoms

muscle relaxants: Possibly enhanced neuromuscular blocking action of skeletal muscle relaxants; increased degree of respiratory depression

nonnucleoside reverse transcriptase inhibitors (NNRTIs) such as delavirdine, efavirenz: Significant pharmacokinetic interactions that have potential to affect action of buprenorphine

protease inhibitors such as atazanavir, ritonavir: Increased levels of buprenorphine causing symptoms of opioid excess, including increased sedation

ACTIVITIES

alcohol use: Increased serum buprenorphine levels possibly resulting in fatal overdose owing to CNS and respiratory depression

Adverse Reactions

CNS: **CNS depression**, dizziness, headache, sedation, **seizures**, vertigo

CV: **Bradycardia**, hypertension, **hypotension, QT prolongation**

EENT: Miosis; *Sublingual form:* Burning mouth syndrome, glossitis, mucosal erythema, oral hypoesthesia, stomatitis

ENDO: **Adrenal insufficiency (rare)**

GI: Elevated liver enzymes or serum amylase level, **hepatitis, hepatotoxicity**, jaundice, nausea, spasm of the sphincter of Oddi, vomiting

GU: Androgen deficiency with chronic use, decreased libido, erectile dysfunction, impotency, infertility, lack of menstruation

RESP: **Bronchospasm, hypoventilation, respiratory depression**

SKIN: Diaphoresis, pruritus, rash, urticaria

Other: **Anaphylaxis; angioedema;** application-site inflammation, burns, discharge, and vesicle occurrence; injection site pain, pruritus, redness, and swelling; physical and psychological dependence

Childbearing Considerations

PREGNANCY

- It is not known if drug can cause fetal harm but neonatal opioid withdrawal syndrome may occur in newborn infants of mothers receiving the drug.
- Use with caution only if benefit to mother outweighs potential risk to fetus.

LABOR & DELIVERY

- Mothers who are opioid dependent on buprenorphine maintenance therapy may require additional analgesia during labor.

- Be aware that, as with all opioids, use of the drug prior to delivery may result in respiratory depression in the newborn.

LACTATION

- Drug is present in breast milk.
- Breastfeeding is usually not recommended.
- If breastfeeding occurs, mother should be instructed to monitor infant for breathing difficulties and drowsiness.

REPRODUCTION

- Chronic use of opioids may cause reduced fertility in females of childbearing age and in males.
- It is not known whether these effects on fertility are reversible.

Nursing Considerations

- Evaluate patient's risk for abuse and addiction prior to the start of buprenorphine therapy, as excessive use of drug may lead to abuse, addiction, misuse, overdose, and possibly death. Be prepared to monitor patient's intake throughout therapy. Because of the potential risks associated with buprenorphine therapy, be aware that the FDA now requires a Risk Evaluation and Mitigation Strategy (REMS) for buprenorphine use.
- Know that the transdermal patch should not be used in patients whose prior total daily dose of opioid use is greater than 80 mg of oral morphine equivalents per day because the maximum 20 mcg/hr dosage may not provide adequate analgesia. An alternate analgesic should be considered.
- Be aware that opioids like buprenorphine should not be given to women during pregnancy and labor and while breast-feeding, as the newborn or infant may experience neonatal opioid withdrawal syndrome (NOWS). This syndrome may exhibit as excessive or high-pitched crying, poor feeding, rapid breathing, or trembling.

! **WARNING** Be aware that opioid therapy like buprenorphine should only be used concomitantly with benzodiazepine therapy in patients for whom other treatment options are inadequate. If prescribed together, expect dosing and duration of the opioid to be limited. Monitor patient closely for signs and symptoms of decrease in consciousness, including coma, profound sedation, and significant respiratory depression. Notify prescriber immediately and provide emergency supportive care, as death may occur.

- Use buprenorphine cautiously in patients with adrenal insufficiency, alcohol withdrawal syndrome, acute alcoholism, biliary tract dysfunction, CNS depression, coma, hypothyroidism, kyphoscoliosis, myxedema, prostatic hypertrophy, psychosis, severe hepatic or renal impairment, toxic psychosis, or urethral stricture. Also use cautiously in patients who take a drug that decreases hepatic clearance, are known drug abusers, or have been addicted to opioids.
- Use drug cautiously in patients with head injury, intracranial lesions, or other conditions that could increase CSF pressure. Be particularly cautious when administering drug to patients with chronic obstructive pulmonary disease or cor pulmonale and in patients who have decreased respiratory reserve, hypoxia, hypercapnia, or preexisting respiratory depression.
- Know that to avoid causing withdrawal, drug shouldn't be given for opioid dependence until signs of withdrawal occur.
- Expect to obtain liver function tests prior to initiation of buprenorphine therapy and periodically throughout therapy because drug may cause hepatic dysfunction ranging from transient asymptomatic elevations in liver enzymes to hepatic failure and death. Acute hepatitis may also occur and, in some cases, require the drug to be discontinued, although in other cases even a dosage reduction of buprenorphine may not be needed. Monitor patient closely and report any signs and symptoms of hepatic dysfunction to prescriber.
- Know that an extended-release formulation (Sublocade) given as a subcutaneous injection monthly is available for patients who have initiated treatment with a transmucosal buprenorphine-containing product, followed by dose adjustment, for a minimum of 7 days. If Sublocade is discontinued, monitor patient for several months for signs and symptoms of withdrawal and treat as prescribed.
- Monitor the injection site when administering Sublocade subcutaneously

for injection-site reactions such as pain, redness, and pruritis. However, know that injection-site reactions may also include abscess formation, necrosis, and ulceration that may require antibiotic therapy and surgical removal or debridement. Know that the drug (Sublocade) may be removed from a subcutaneous site surgically under local anesthesia within 14 days of the injection. If removed, monitor patient for signs and symptoms of withdrawal and treat appropriately, as prescribed. Be aware that serious injection-site reactions may be increased with inadvertent intramuscular or intradermal administration. Inject this form of drug only by subcutaneous injection.

- Inspect injection site for local reactions; don't use the same site twice.
- Monitor vital signs and response to drug often, especially after giving first dose and if patient develops a fever. Be aware that drug may cause severe hypotension, including orthostatic hypotension and syncope in ambulatory patients.

! WARNING Monitor patient closely for respiratory depression, especially in cachectic, debilitated, or elderly patients; when initiating and titrating dosages; or when other drugs that depress respiration are given together. Report respiratory depression immediately, because respiratory arrest may occur. Be prepared to provide emergency supportive care.

- Monitor patient with a seizure disorder, as buprenorphine may worsen seizure control.
- Assess elderly patients for signs and symptoms of toxicity or overdose, as these patients may be at increased risk because of decreased cardiac, hepatic, or renal function and the presence of concomitant disease and other drug therapy.

! WARNING Know that many drugs may interact with opioids like buprenorphine to cause serotonin syndrome. Monitor patient closely for signs and symptoms such as agitation, diaphoresis, diarrhea, fever, hallucinations, labile blood pressure, muscle twitching or stiffness, nausea, shakiness, shivering, tachycardia, trouble with coordination, or vomiting. Notify prescriber at once because serotonin syndrome may be

life-threatening. Be prepared to discontinue drug, if possible and ordered, and provide supportive care.

- Monitor patient for adrenal insufficiency. Although rare, this can be life-threatening. Monitor patient for anorexia, dizziness, fatigue, hypotension, nausea, vomiting, or weakness. Notify prescriber if adrenal insufficiency is suspected and expect diagnostic testing to be done to determine if present. If diagnosis is confirmed, expect to administer corticosteroids and wean patient off buprenorphine, if possible.
- Do not discontinue therapy abruptly when buprenorphine therapy is no longer needed. Instead, expect a gradual downward titration of the dose to prevent signs and symptoms of withdrawal.
- Be aware that dosage adjustments of buprenorphine may be required during pregnancy even if patient was stable prior to pregnancy. Monitor pregnant patient closely for signs and symptoms of withdrawal and expect dosage to be adjusted as needed.

PATIENT TEACHING

- Warn patient not to take more drug than prescribed and not to take it longer than absolutely needed, because excessive or prolonged use can lead to abuse, addiction, misuse, overdose, and possibly death.
- Advise patient that if a dose is missed, patient should take it as soon as it is remembered but if it is almost time for the next dose, the missed dose should be skipped and the next dose taken at the regular time. Dose should never be doubled to make up for a missed dose.

! WARNING Warn patient not to consume alcohol or take benzodiazepines or other CNS depressants, including other opioids, during buprenorphine therapy without prescriber knowledge, as severe respiratory depression can occur that may lead to death.

! WARNING Inform patient about potentially fatal additive effects of combining buprenorphine with benzodiazepines or other opioids. Instruct patient to inform all prescribers of buprenorphine use.

- Explain that buprenorphine may be habit forming. Urge patient to notify prescriber if she develops any unusual or persistent symptoms.

- Instruct patient taking sublingual form to place tablets under her tongue until they dissolve. If patient takes more than two tablets per dose, tell her to place all tablets under her tongue at the same time. If they won't fit, tell her to place two at a time under her tongue until full dose has dissolved. Caution against swallowing tablets.

! WARNING Instruct patient not to crush or dissolve tablet form of drug and then inject it, as life-threatening infections, precipitated withdrawal, and other serious health problems could occur.

- Instruct patient prescribed the transdermal patch to place patch only on intact skin that is hairless and clean (washed with water only) and dry. If a hairless site is not available, instruct patient to clip, not shave, area prior to application. Emphasize importance of not applying patch to irritated skin. Inform patient patch must be applied immediately after its removal from pouch and placed on her upper outer arm, upper back, upper chest, or the side of her chest. Instruct patient to rotate sites and not to use same site for at least 21 days. Tell patient patch is to be worn for 7 days and that she should not cut the patch. If problems with adhesion occur, she may tape the edges of the patch with first-aid tape. If the patch should fall off during the 7-day interval, tell her to dispose of the patch and apply a new one at a different skin site. When removing the patch, tell patient to fold it over on itself and flush it down the toilet or seal it in the patch disposal unit provided and dispose of it in the trash.
- Instruct patient prescribed the buccal film form to first use his tongue to wet the inside of his cheek or rinse his mouth with water to wet the area. Then, he should place the yellow side of the film against the inside of his cheek after immediately removing it from the package and using clean, dry fingers, hold it in place for 5 seconds following which the film should be left in place until fully dissolved, usually within 30 minutes. Doing this time he should not manipulate the film with his tongue or

fingers nor should he eat or drink anything until the film has dissolved. Remind patient to dispose of unused film by removing from the foil packages and flush down the toilet. Discard foil packaging in the trash. He should not flush the drug down the toilet in the foil package. Encourage patient to have regular dental examinations because dental problems may occur with this form of drug.

- Tell patient receiving the drug as an extended-release subcutaneous injection that a lump may appear at injection site and last for several weeks. Tell patient not to massage or rub the injection site and to be careful of the placement of any belts or clothing waistbands so as not to irritate the site. If other symptoms develop, instruct patient to have prescriber evaluate injection site.
- Caution patient to keep drug, including patch form, out of the reach of others, especially children, as exposure to even one dose or patch could be fatal.
- Inform patient wearing a buprenorphine patch not to expose it to any external heat source such as heating pads, electric blankets, heat lamps, saunas, heated water beds or hot tubs, as absorption may be affected.
- Warn patient not to stop taking drug abruptly.
- Advise patient to get up slowly from a lying or sitting position to avoid a sudden drop in blood pressure.
- Caution patient to avoid hazardous activities while receiving buprenorphine.
- Instruct patient not to drink alcohol or take CNS depressants or sleep aids without checking with prescriber first.
- Inform patient that long-term use of opioids like buprenorphine may decrease sex hormone levels causing decreased libido, erectile dysfunction, impotence, infertility, or lack of menstruation. Encourage patient to report any such symptoms.
- Advise patient to report any persistent, severe, or unusual signs and symptoms to prescriber.
- Advise patient to keep buprenorphine in a safe place and to protect it from theft because of it being an opioid.
- Advise patient to notify prescriber if she becomes pregnant or is breastfeeding,

as drug may have to be discontinued or dosage altered. Also tell mothers who are taking buprenorphine while breastfeeding to monitor their infant for breathing difficulties and increased drowsiness. If present, tell patient to stop breastfeeding and notify prescriber.

- Caution patient to dispose of expired, unwanted, or unused drug properly. Tell patients to visit the website: www.fda.gov /drugdisposal for instructions. The drug can also be flushed down the toilet after removing foil, if present, if a drug take-back option is not available.

bupropion hydrobromide
Aplenzin

bupropion hydrochloride
Forfivo XL, Wellbutrin, Wellbutrin SR, Wellbutrin XL, Zyban

⋮ Class and Category
Pharmacologic class: Aminoketone
Therapeutic class: Antidepressant, smoking cessation adjunct

⋮ Indications and Dosages
✳ *To treat depression*

E.R. TABLETS (WELLBUTRIN SR)
Adults. *Initial:* 150 mg daily for 3 days; then 150 mg twice daily with at least 8 hr between successive doses and, after several wk, 200 mg twice daily, as needed and tolerated. *Maximum:* 400 mg daily, given as 200 mg twice daily. Single doses should not exceed 200 mg/dose.

E.R. TABLETS (WELLBUTRIN XL)
Adults. *Initial:* 150 mg daily for 4 days; then 300 mg daily.

E.R. TABLETS (APLENZIN)
Adults. *Initial:* 174 mg daily for 4 days. Then, if tolerated well, dosage increased to 348 mg daily.

E.R. TABLETS (FORFIVO XL)
Adults. *Initial:* 300 mg daily of another bupropion product for at least 2 wk before

maintenance with Forfivo XL is begun. *Maintenance:* 450 mg once daily.

TABLETS (WELLBUTRIN)
Adults. *Initial:* 100 mg twice daily, increased after 3 or more days to 100 mg three times daily with at least 6 hr between successive doses, as needed. *Maximum:* 450 mg daily or 150 mg/dose.

✳ *To aid in smoking cessation*

E.R. TABLETS (ZYBAN)
Adults. *Initial:* 150 mg daily for 3 days and then 150 mg twice daily with at least 8 hr between each dose for 7 to 12 wk. *Maximum:* 300 mg daily or 150 mg/dose.

✳ *To prevent seasonal major depressive episodes in patient with seasonal affective disorder*

E.R. TABLETS (WELLBUTRIN XL)
Adults. *Initial:* 150 mg once daily starting in autumn, increased after 1 wk to 300 mg once daily in morning, if tolerated and needed. Decreased to 150 mg once daily 2 wk before stopping in early spring if dosage was 300 mg once daily.

E.R. TABLETS (APLENZIN)
Adults. *Initial:* 174 mg once daily starting in autumn, increased after 1 wk to 348 mg once daily if tolerated and needed. Decreased to 174 mg once daily 2 wk before stopping in early spring if dosage was 348 mg once daily.

±**DOSAGE ADJUSTMENT** For patients with severe hepatic cirrhosis, no more than 75 mg daily of Wellbutrin, 100 mg daily or 150 mg every other day of Wellbutrin SR, 150 mg every other day of Wellbutrin XL or Zyban, and 174 mg every other day of Aplenzin. In renal impairment, dosage or frequency decreased on an individual basis.

⋮ Drug Administration
P.O.
- Use of Zyban for smoking cessation should be started a week or two before patient quits smoking.
- Administer daily doses or first dose of the day in the morning.
- E.R. tablets should be swallowed whole and not cut, crushed, or chewed.
- Adhere to manufacturer instructions on length of time to wait between doses, if applicable.
- Store tablets at room temperature while keeping tablets dry and out of the light.

Route	Onset	Peak	Duration
P.O.	Unknown	2 hr	1–2 days
P.O./E.R.	Unknown	5 hr	1–2 days
P.O./SR	Unknown	3 hr	1–2 days

Half-life: 21 hr

☰ Mechanism of Action

May inhibit dopamine, norepinephrine, and serotonin uptake by neurons, which significantly relieves evidence of depression.

☰ Contraindications

Hypersensitivity to bupropion or its components, seizure disorder or conditions that increase risk of seizures (i.e., abrupt discontinuation of alcohol, antiepileptic drugs, barbiturates, or benzodiazepines); anorexia nervosa or bulimia; use within 14 days of an MAO inhibitor (MAOI), including reversible MAOIs such as linezolid or intravenous methylene blue; use of another form of bupropion concurrently

☰ Interactions

DRUGS

amantadine, levodopa: Increased CNS adverse reactions to bupropion
antidepressants, antipsychotics, concurrent use of other bupropion products, systemic corticosteroids, theophylline: Increased risk of seizures
carbamazepine, phenobarbital, phenytoin: Increased bupropion metabolism resulting in decreased bupropion exposure
CYP2B6 inducers such as efavirenz, lopinavir, ritonavir: Possibly decreased bupropion exposure and subsequent effectiveness
CYP2B6 inhibitors such as clopidogrel, ticlopidine: Possibly increased bupropion exposure and risk of adverse reactions
digoxin: Possibly decreased digoxin levels
drugs metabolized by CYP2D6 such as certain antidepressants (i.e. desipramine, fluoxetine, imipramine, nortriptyline, paroxetine, sertraline, venlafaxine), antipsychotics (i.e. haloperidol, risperidone, thioridazine), beta blockers (i.e. metoprolol), type IC antiarrhythmics (i.e. flecainide, propafenone): Increased blood exposure of these drugs and risk of adverse reactions
MAO inhibitors including reversible MAOIs such as linezolid and intravenous methylene blue: Increased risk of acute bupropion toxicity and serious hypertensive reactions
tamoxifen: Possibly reduced effectiveness of tamoxifen

ACTIVITIES

alcohol use, recreational drug abuse: Possible rare adverse neuropsychiatric events; reduced alcohol tolerance

☰ Adverse Reactions

CNS: Abnormal coordination, abnormal EEG, aggression, agitation, akathisia, akinesia, anxiety, aphasia, asthenia, CNS stimulation, **coma**, confusion, **CVA**, decreased concentration or memory, delirium, delusions, depersonalization, depression, dizziness, dream abnormalities, emotional lability, euphoria, extrapyramidal syndrome, fever, general or migraine headache, hallucinations, **homicidal ideation**, hostility, hyperkinesia, hypertonia, hyperesthesia, insomnia, irritability, mania, nervousness, neuralgia, neuropathy, panic, paranoia, paresthesia, parkinsonism, psychosis and other neuropsychiatric reactions, restlessness, **seizures**, sleep disorder, somnolence, **suicidal ideation**, syncope, tremor, unmasking tardive dyskinesia, vertigo
CV: Arrhythmias, chest pain, **complete AV block**, **extrasystoles**, hypertension, **MI**, orthostatic hypotension, palpitations, phlebitis, tachycardia, vasodilation
EENT: Acute-angle glaucoma, altered taste, amblyopia, blurred vision, dry mouth, gum hemorrhage, hearing loss, increased ocular pressure, increased salivation, mydriasis, pharyngitis, sinusitis, taste perversion, tinnitus
ENDO: Hyperglycemia, **hypoglycemia**, syndrome of inappropriate ADH secretion
GI: Abdominal pain, anorexia, colitis, constipation, diarrhea, dysphagia, esophagitis, flatulence, **GI hemorrhage**, GI ulceration, **hepatic dysfunction**, **hepatitis**, increased appetite, **intestinal perforation**, nausea, **pancreatitis**, vomiting
GU: Abnormal ejaculation, cystitis, decreased or increased libido, dyspareunia, dysuria, incontinence, painful erection, prostate disorder, salpingitis, urinary frequency and urgency, UTI, vaginal hemorrhage, vaginitis
HEME: Anemia, leukocytosis, **leukopenia**, lymphadenopathy, **pancytopenia**, **thrombocytopenia**

MS: Arthralgia; arthritis; muscle rigidity, twitching, and weakness; myalgia; **rhabdomyolysis**
RESP: **Bronchospasm**, cough, dyspnea, pneumonia, **pulmonary embolism**
SKIN: Alopecia, diaphoresis, **erythema multiforme**, **exfoliative dermatitis**, flushing, hirsutism, pruritus, rash, **Stevens–Johnson syndrome**, urticaria
Other: **Anaphylaxis**, **angioedema**, generalized pain, hot flashes, **hyponatremia**, infection, serum sickness–like reaction, weight loss

Childbearing Considerations

PREGNANCY

- Pregnancy exposure registry: 1-844-405-6185 or visit https://womensmentalhealth .org/clinical-and-research-programs /pregnancyregistry/antidepressants/.
- It is not known if drug can cause fetal harm.
- Use with caution only if benefit to mother outweighs potential risk to fetus.

LACTATION

- Drug is present in breast milk.
- Patient should check with prescriber before breastfeeding.

Nursing Considerations

- Know that certain forms of bupropion are not approved for smoking cessation treatment, such as Aplenzin, Forfivo XL, Wellbutrin SR, and Wellbutrin XL.
- Be aware that Forfivo XL should not be used in patients with hepatic or renal impairment because the only dosage available for Forfivo XL is 450 mg once daily, which may be too high a dose for the kidneys or liver to handle.
- Use cautiously in patients with renal impairment (all other brands); drug is excreted by kidneys.
- Know that Forfivo XL should never be used to initiate treatment of depression because the dose is too high. Only after the patient has received other bupropion products first and then requires a 450-mg dose should Forfivo XL be used.
- Assess patient's blood pressure before bupropion therapy begins and monitor periodically during therapy because bupropion may cause hypertension.
- Monitor depressed patients closely for worsened depression and increased suicide

risk, especially when therapy starts or dosage changes.
- Monitor patient taking bupropion to stop smoking for neuropsychiatric symptoms, including suicidal ideation. If present, notify prescriber immediately, begin safety measures, and expect to discontinue drug.

! WARNING Monitor patient for seizures. To reduce seizure risk, allow at least 4 hours (tablets) or 8 hours (E.R. tablets) between doses. Know that maximum dosage should not be exceeded and dosage reduction should be gradual because risk of seizures is dose-related.

- Use seizure precautions, especially in patients who are addicted to cocaine, opioids, or stimulants; have a history of CNS tumors, head trauma, or seizures; have hyponatremia, hypoxia, or severe hepatic cirrhosis; take drugs that lower the seizure threshold; take insulin or an oral antidiabetic; take OTC stimulants or anorectics; or use excessive alcohol, benzodiazepines, hypnotics, or sedatives.
- Know that using transdermal nicotine with bupropion may cause hypertension. Watch closely.

PATIENT TEACHING

- Advise patient to take bupropion for 7 or more days before stopping smoking.
- Tell patient to swallow E.R. tablets whole and not to cut, crush, or chew them.
- Tell patient to take daily dose or first dose of the day in the morning and to store tablets at room temperature while keeping tablets dry and out of the light.
- Emphasize importance of maintaining length of time between dosages of formulation prescribed, if applicable.
- Urge patient to avoid or minimize consuming alcohol and sedatives during therapy and not to stop drug abruptly or exceed dosage prescribed because seizures may occur. Also warn patient not to abruptly stop taking antiseizure drugs or prescribed benzodiazepines or sedatives.

! WARNING Advise patient to seek medical help immediately and stop taking drug if signs of rash, itching, hives, chest pain, shortness of breath, or swelling, especially of face, occurs.

- Urge caregivers to monitor depressed patient closely for worsened depression, especially when therapy starts or dosage changes. Also inform caregiver that drug may cause a variety of neuropsychiatric adverse events that could be serious. If changes in behavior or thought patterns emerge with bupropion use, instruct caregiver to notify prescriber immediately.
- Alert patient that drug may cause mild pupillary dilation, which can lead to an episode of acute-closure glaucoma. Encourage him to have an eye exam to determine if he is susceptible to angle closure.
- Warn patient taking bupropion for smoking cessation by explaining that it may cause serious adverse effects, including suicidal thoughts and behavior. If present, patient should notify prescriber immediately and expect to discontinue drug.
- Alert patient that bupropion therapy may produce a false-positive urine screening test for amphetamines even after drug has been discontinued. Other tests may be required to distinguish bupropion from amphetamines.

buspirone hydrochloride

Class and Category
Pharmacologic class: Azapirone
Therapeutic class: Anxiolytic

Indications and Dosages
* *To manage anxiety*
TABLETS
Adults. *Initial:* 7.5 mg twice daily increased by 5 mg daily at 2- to 3-day intervals until desired response occurs. *Maintenance:* 20 to 30 mg daily (usual therapeutic range) in divided doses. *Maximum:* 60 mg daily.
±**DOSAGE ADJUSTMENT** When used with CYP3A4 inhibitors, dosage reduced.

When used with nefazodone, dosage decreased to 2.5 mg daily. Concomitant therapy with CYP3A4 inducers may require dosage to be increased.

Drug Administration
P.O.
- Administer consistently, either always with or always without food.

Route	Onset	Peak	Duration
P.O.	Slow	40–90 min	Unknown

Half-life: 18 hr

Mechanism of Action
May act as a partial agonist at serotonin 5-hydroxytryptamine$_{1A}$ receptors in the brain, producing antianxiety effects.

Contraindications
Hypersensitivity to buspirone or its components, severe hepatic or renal impairment

Interactions
DRUGS
CYP3A4 inducers, such as certain anticonvulsants (carbamazepine, phenobarbital, phenytoin) and dexamethasone: Possibly increased rate of buspirone metabolism and decreased effectiveness of buspirone
CYP3A4 inhibitors, such as ketoconazole and ritonavir: Possibly inhibited buspirone metabolism and increased blood level of buspirone
diltiazem, erythromycin, itraconazole, nefazodone, nordiazepam, verapamil: Increased blood level and adverse effects of buspirone
haloperidol: Increased haloperidol level
MAO inhibitors: Increased risk of hypertension
rifampin: Decreased blood buspirone level and pharmacodynamic effects
FOODS
any food: Possibly decreased buspirone clearance
grapefruit juice: Increased blood buspirone level

Adverse Reactions
CNS: Akathisia, anger, ataxia, cogwheel rigidity, confusion, decreased concentration, depression, dizziness, dream disturbances,

drowsiness, dyskinesias, dystonia, excitement, extrapyramidal symptoms, fatigue, headache, hostility, insomnia, lack of coordination, light-headedness, mood swings, nervousness, paresthesia, parkinsonism, restless leg syndrome, restlessness, **serotonin syndrome**, transient recall impairment, tremor, weakness
CV: Chest pain, palpitations, tachycardia
EENT: Blurred vision, dry mouth, nasal congestion, pharyngitis, tinnitus, tunnel vision
GI: Abdominal or gastric distress, constipation, diarrhea, nausea, vomiting
GU: Urine retention
MS: Myalgia
SKIN: Diaphoresis, ecchymosis, rash, urticaria
Other: Angioedema

Childbearing Considerations
PREGNANCY
- It is not known if drug can cause fetal harm.
- Use with caution only if benefit to mother outweighs potential risk to fetus.

LACTATION
- It is not known if drug is present in breast milk.
- Drug use during breastfeeding is not recommended.

Nursing Considerations
- Use buspirone cautiously in patients with hepatic or renal impairment.
- Institute safety precautions because of possible adverse CNS reactions.
- Follow closely if patient is being withdrawn from long-term therapy with benzodiazepines or other sedative-hypnotic drugs while starting buspirone, because buspirone won't prevent withdrawal symptoms.

PATIENT TEACHING
- Advise patient to take buspirone consistently, either always with or always without food.
- Caution patient to avoid drinking large amounts of grapefruit juice.
- Inform patient that 1 to 2 weeks of therapy may be needed before she notices drug's antianxiety effect.
- Emphasize the importance of not taking more buspirone than prescribed.
- Advise patient to avoid hazardous activities until drug's CNS effects are known.

butorphanol tartrate

Class, Category, and Schedule
Pharmacologic class: Opioid agonist–antagonist
Therapeutic class: Anesthesia adjunct, opioid analgesic
Controlled substance schedule: IV

Indications and Dosages
* To manage pain severe enough to require an opioid analgesic and for which alternative treatments are inadequate

I.V. INJECTION
Adults. 0.5 to 2 mg (usually 1 mg) every 3 to 4 hr, as needed.

I.M. INJECTION
Adults. 1 to 4 mg (usually 2 mg) every 3 to 4 hr, as needed. *Maximum:* 4 mg/single dose.

NASAL SPRAY
Adults. 1 mg (1 spray) in one nostril. Dose repeated after 60 to 90 min, as needed; two-dose sequence repeated every 3 to 4 hr after the second dose of the sequence, as needed. For severe pain, 2 mg (1 spray in each nostril) every 3 to 4 hr, as needed.
±**DOSAGE ADJUSTMENT** Dose maintained at 1 spray in one nostril for elderly patients and those with impaired hepatic or renal function. Dose repeated after 90 to 120 min, as needed; two-dose sequence repeated every 6 hr or more, as needed.
* As adjunct to provide preoperative anesthesia

I.M. INJECTION
Adults. Individualized. *Usual:* 2 mg 60 to 90 min before surgery.
* Adjunct to balanced anesthesia

I.V. INJECTION
Adults. 2 mg shortly before induction and/or 0.5 to 1 mg in increments during anesthesia, as needed. Increments may be increased up to 0.06 mg/kg, if needed. *Usual range*: 4 mg to 12.5 mg
* To relieve pain during labor

I.M. INJECTION, I.V. INJECTION
Pregnant women at full term in early labor. 1 to 2 mg repeated in 4 hr.
±**DOSAGE ADJUSTMENT** For elderly patients and patients with impaired hepatic or renal function, initial parenteral dose kept at 1 mg followed, if needed, by 1 mg in 90 to 120 min

and dosage interval for subsequent doses increased to at least 6 hr or more.

DRUG ADMINISTRATION

I.V.

- Administer by direct injection.
- Protect from light.
- If skin contact occurs, rinse skin with cool water.
- *Incompatibilities:* None reported by manufacturer

I.M.

- Protect vial from light.
- If skin contact occurs, rinse skin with cool water.

NASAL INHALATION

- Have patient blow nose.
- Pull clear cover from the pump unit and remove protective clip from its neck.
- Prime pump unit by placing the nozzle between first and second fingers with thumb on the bottom of the bottle. Then pump sprayer unit firmly and quickly until a fine spray appears (7 or 8 strokes).
- Insert spray tip about 1 cm (one-third inch) into one nostril, pointing tip toward the back of the nose. Close other nostril with one finger and tilt head slightly forward. Then pump sprayer firmly and quickly by pushing down on the pump unit's finger grips and against the thumb at the bottom of the bottle.
- Have patient sniff gently with mouth closed.
- After spraying, remove pump from nose, have patient tilt head back, and sniff gently for a few more seconds.
- Replace protective clip and clear cover.

Route	Onset	Peak	Duration
I.V.	1–3 min	30–60 min	3–4 hr
I.M.	5–10 min	30–60 min	3–4 hr
Inhalation	15 min	1–2 hr	4–5 hr

Half-life: 4–10 hr

Mechanism of Action

Binds with specific CNS receptors to alter the perception of and emotional response to pain.

Contraindications

Acute or severe bronchial asthma in an unmonitored setting or in the absence of resuscitative equipment; GI obstruction, including paralytic ileus; hypersensitivity to butorphanol or its components (including the preservative benzethonium chloride); significant respiratory depression

Interactions

DRUGS

benzodiazepines, other CNS depressants: Additive CNS depression that can be significant, causing coma, prolonged sedation, or significant respiratory depression
Nasal vasoconstrictors, such as oxymetazoline: Decreased absorption rate and delayed onset of butorphanol
serotonergic drugs: Increased risk of serotonin syndrome

ACTIVITIES

alcohol use: Additive CNS depression that could be significant

Adverse Reactions

CNS: Anxiety, confusion, difficulty making purposeful movements, difficulty speaking, dizziness, euphoria, floating feeling, headache, insomnia (with nasal form), lethargy, nervousness, paresthesia, sensation of heat, somnolence, syncope, tremor, vertigo
CV: Chest pain, **hypotension**, palpitations, tachycardia, vasodilation
EENT: Blurred vision, dry mouth, ear pain, epistaxis, nasal congestion or irritation (with nasal form), pharyngitis, rhinitis, sinus congestion, sinusitis, tinnitus, unpleasant taste
GI: Anorexia, constipation, epigastric pain, nausea, vomiting
RESP: **Apnea**, bronchitis, cough, dyspnea, **respiratory depression**, **shallow breathing**, upper respiratory tract infection
SKIN: Clammy skin, pruritus

Childbearing Considerations

PREGNANCY

- Drug can cause fetal harm such as physical dependence in the neonate and neonatal opioid withdrawal syndrome shortly after birth.
- Use with caution only if benefit to mother outweighs potential risk to fetus.

LABOR & DELIVERY

- Drug may prolong labor.
- Use of drug during pregnancy for prolonged time may cause neonatal opioid withdrawal syndrome in infants, causing respiratory depression and excessive sedation in the neonate shortly after birth.

LACTATION

- Drug may be present in breast milk.
- Patient should check with prescriber before breastfeeding.
- If breastfeeding occurs, mother should be instructed to monitor infant for breathing difficulties and drowsiness.
- Withdrawal symptoms can occur in breastfed infants when mother stops taking drug or breastfeeding stops.

REPRODUCTION

- Women of childbearing age should avoid pregnancy during drug use and report known or suspected pregnancy to prescriber.
- Chronic use of opioids may reduce fertility and it is not known if effects on fertility are reversible.

Nursing Considerations

- Know that butorphanol should be used cautiously, if at all, in patients with depression, suicidal tendency, history of drug abuse, or hepatic or renal dysfunction.
- Use it cautiously, if at all, in patients with head injury because drug can raise CSF pressure. Because it can increase cardiac workload, use with extreme caution in patients with acute MI, ventricular dysfunction, or coronary insufficiency.
- Be aware that butorphanol has a high potential for abuse.
- Monitor patient after first dose of nasal form; hypotension and syncope may occur.
- Take safety precautions because butorphanol causes CNS depression.
- Assess respiratory status closely because drug causes respiratory depression, which could become life-threatening.
- Monitor blood pressure often after giving drug. If severe hypertension develops (rare),

stop drug at once and notify prescriber. If patient isn't narcotic-dependent, expect to administer naloxone to reverse butorphanol's effects.

PATIENT TEACHING

- Emphasize the importance of taking butorphanol exactly as prescribed because it can be addictive. Warn patient not to increase the dose or decrease the dosage interval without consulting prescriber.
- Teach patient how to use nasal form properly by giving these instructions: After blowing nose to clear the nostrils, pull clear cover from the pump unit and remove protective clip from its neck. Prime pump unit by placing the nozzle between first and second fingers with thumb on the bottom of the bottle. Then pump sprayer unit firmly and quickly until a fine spray appears (7 or 8 strokes). Insert spray tip about 1 cm (one-third inch) into one nostril, pointing tip toward the back of the nose. Close other nostril with one finger and tilt head slightly forward. Then pump sprayer firmly and quickly by pushing down on the pump unit's finger grips and against the thumb at the bottom of the bottle. Sniff gently with mouth closed. After spraying, remove pump from nose, tilt head back, and sniff gently for a few more seconds. Then replace protective clip and clear cover.
- Advise patient to avoid hazardous activities until drug's CNS effects are known.
- Tell patient to avoid alcohol and other CNS depressants, including OTC drugs, while taking butorphanol, because of additive adverse CNS reactions.

cabergoline
Dostinex

Class and Category
Pharmacologic class: Dopamine agonist
Therapeutic class: Antihyperprolactinemic

Indications and Dosages
* *To treat idiopathic or pituitary adenoma-induced hyperprolactinemic disorders*

TABLETS
Adults. *Initial:* 0.25 mg twice/wk. Increased by 0.25 mg twice/wk at 4-wk intervals, if needed, up to 1 mg twice/wk.

Drug Administration
P.O.
- Administer with meals to minimize adverse GI effects.

Route	Onset	Peak	Duration
P.O.	Unknown	2–3 hr	>14 days

Half-life: 63–69 hr

Mechanism of Action
Binds with dopamine D_2 receptors to block prolactin synthesis and secretion by the anterior pituitary gland, thereby reducing the serum prolactin level.

Contraindications
History of cardiac valvular, pericardial, pulmonary, or retroperitoneal fibrotic disorders; hypersensitivity to cabergoline, ergot derivatives, or their components; uncontrolled hypertension

Interactions
DRUGS
antihypertensives: Increased risk of hypotension
dopamine antagonists (butyrophenones, metoclopramide, phenothiazines, or thioxanthenes): Decreased cabergoline effectiveness

ACTIVITIES
alcohol use: May increase risk of adverse CNS effects

Adverse Reactions
CNS: Aggression, asthenia, compulsive/impulse control behaviors (hypersexuality, increased libido, pathological gambling), depression, fatigue, headache, nervousness, paresthesia, somnolence, psychotic disorder, vertigo
CV: Orthostatic hypotension, **valvulopathy**
EENT: Dry mouth
ENDO: Breast pain
GI: Abdominal pain, constipation, diarrhea, flatulence, indigestion, nausea, vomiting
GU: Dysmenorrhea, increased libido
RESP: Pulmonary effusion, **pulmonary fibrosis**
SKIN: Alopecia
Other: Extracardiac fibrotic reactions

Childbearing Considerations
PREGNANCY
- It is not known if drug can cause fetal harm. However, dopamine agonists in general should not be used in patients with pregnancy-induced hypertension or postpartum hypertension unless absolutely necessary.
- Use with caution only if benefit to mother outweighs potential risk to fetus.

LACTATION
- It is not known if drug is present in breast milk.
- A decision should be made to discontinue breastfeeding or the drug.

Nursing Considerations
- Ensure that patient has undergone a cardiovascular evaluation, including an echocardiogram, to determine the presence of valvular disease prior to administering cabergoline because the presence of valvular disease is a contraindication to the use of cabergoline therapy.
- Obtain a chest x-ray, an erythrocyte sedimentation rate, and serum creatinine measurement, as ordered, prior to initiating cabergoline therapy and repeat during therapy if the patient develops any signs and symptoms of an extracardiac fibrotic reaction.
- Check serum prolactin level to assess cabergoline's effectiveness before each dose increase.
- Know that if patient has moderate to severe hepatic impairment, monitor closely for adverse reactions because of decreased cabergoline metabolism.

- Expect patient who takes cabergoline long term to undergo periodic reassessment of cardiac status, including echocardiography, because valvulopathy can occur with prolonged cabergoline use.
- Monitor erythrocyte sedimentation rate, as it may increase in a patient with pleural effusion or pleural fibrosis.

! **WARNING** Monitor patient for evidence of overdose, such as hallucinations, light-headedness, nasal congestion, syncope, and tachycardia. If present, prescribe and treat as ordered.

PATIENT TEACHING

- Urge patient to read and follow printed information that explains how to use cabergoline for best therapeutic results.
- Advise patient to take drug with meals to help decrease GI distress.
- Tell patient to take a missed dose as soon as possible within 1 to 2 days. If missed dose isn't remembered until it's time for the next dose, instruct him to double the dose if drug is generally well tolerated and doesn't cause nausea. If drug isn't well tolerated, instruct patient to consult prescriber before taking the missed dose.
- Urge patient to change positions slowly to avoid orthostatic hypotension. Tell him to notify prescriber if it occurs.
- Urge patient to keep regular appointments to monitor drug effectiveness.
- Advise patient that drug therapy will end when serum prolactin level is normal for 6 months. Explain that he'll need periodic monitoring to determine whether therapy should resume.
- Tell female patient of childbearing age to notify prescriber if she is, could be, or plans to become pregnant during therapy; drug may have to be discontinued. Inform breastfeeding mothers that the drug will have to be discontinued when breastfeeding.
- Inform patient that cabergoline may cause compulsive or impulse control behaviors such as hypersexuality, increased libido, and pathological gambling. If present, patient should contact prescriber because a dosage reduction or discontinuation of the drug may be needed. Caution patient to avoid gambling during therapy.

cabotegravir
Vocabria

Class and Category
Pharmacologic class: HIV-1 integrase strand transfer inhibitor (INSTI)
Therapeutic class: Antiviral

Indications and Dosages
* *As adjunct for short-term treatment of HIV-1 infection for patients who are virologically suppressed (HIV-1 RNA less than 50 copies/ml) and on a stable antiretroviral regimen with no history of treatment failure and with no known or suspected resistance to either cabotegravir or rilpivirine; to assess tolerability of cabotegravir prior to administration of the combination drug, cabotegravir and rilpivirine, as an E.R. injectable suspension*

TABLET
Adults. 30 mg (1 tablet) in combination with 25 mg (1 tablet) of rilpivirine once daily for at least 28 days with last oral dose given on the same day injections of the combination drug, cabotegravir and rilpivirine, are started.

As adjunct for short-term treatment of HIV-1 infection for patients who are virologically suppressed (HIV-1 RNA less than 50 copies/ml) and on a stable antiretroviral regimen with no history of treatment failure and with no known or suspected resistance to either cabotegravir or rilpivirine when planned injection dosing with cabotegravir-rilpivirine will be missed for more than 7 days

TABLET
Adults. Initial: 30 mg (1 tablet) in combination with 25 mg (1 tablet) of rilpivirine once daily initiated about 1 month after the last injection dose of the combination drug, cabotegravir and rilpivirine, and continued until the day the injection of the combination drug is restarted. Maximum: Replacement for up to 2 consecutive monthly injections.

Drug Administration
P.O.
- Administer drug at about the same time each day.
- Administer with a meal.

Route	Onset	Peak	Duration
P.O.	Unknown	Unknown	Unknown

Half-life: 40 hr

Mechanism of Action

Binds to the integrase active site and blocks the strand transfer step of retroviral deoxyribonucleic acid (DNA) integration, which is essential for HIV replication.

Contraindications

Concurrent use of anticonvulsants (carbamazepine, oxcarbazepine, phenobarbital, phenytoin), antimycobacterials (rifampin, rifapentine), and the combination drug, cabotegravir and rilpivirine E.R. injectable suspension with rifabutin; hypersensitivity to cabotegravir or its components

Interactions

DRUGS

- *antacids containing polyvalent cations such as aluminum or magnesium hydroxide or calcium carbonate:* Decreased absorption of cabotegravir decreasing effectiveness
- *anticonvulsants such as carbamazepine, oxcarbazepine, phenobarbital, phenytoin:* Decreased cabotegravir plasma concentrations leading to potential for loss of effectiveness and increased risk of development of resistance
- *antimycobacterials such as rifampin, rifapentine:* Decreased cabotegravir plasma concentration decreasing effectiveness

Adverse Reactions

CNS: Abnormal dreams, anxiety, asthenia, depression, headache, insomnia, mood swings, suicidal ideation
GI: Elevated liver enzymes, hepatotoxicity, nausea
MS: Myalgia
Other: Hypersensitivity reaction

Childbearing Considerations

PREGNANCY

- Pregnancy exposure registry: 1-800-258-4263
- Potential increased risk for fetal neural tube defects when administered at the time of conception or in early pregnancy.
- Use with caution only if benefit to mother outweighs potential risk to fetus.

LACTATION

- It is not known if drug is present in breast milk.
- The Centers for Disease Control and Prevention recommends that HIV-1-infected mothers not breastfeed, to avoid risking postnatal transmission of HIV-1 infection to infants. They also do not recommend breastfeeding because of potential drug-induced adverse reactions in the infant.

Nursing Considerations

- Know that patients with underlying liver disease or who have marked elevations in liver enzymes before cabotegravir therapy is initiated may develop worsening of liver function or further increased liver enzymes during cabotegravir therapy. Monitor closely for decreased liver function even in patients without known hepatic disease and expect liver enzymes to be monitored throughout drug therapy.

! **WARNING** Monitor patient closely for hypersensitivity reaction because other integrase inhibitors have caused hypersensitivity reactions. At the first sign of a hypersensitivity reaction (angioedema, blisters, conjunctivitis, difficulty breathing, eosinophilia, facial edema, fatigue, general malaise, hepatitis, joint or muscle aches, oral blisters or lesions), stop administering drug and notify prescriber. Provide supportive care as needed and prescribed.

- Monitor patient for depressive disorders such as depression and mood swings. Report changes to prescriber, as cabotegravir may have to be discontinued.

PATIENT TEACHING

- Advise patient to take cabotegravir with a meal and at about the same time every day.
- Stress importance of not missing a dose of cabotegravir because this can cause resistance to the drug to develop. Patient should take drug as soon as remembered but not to double the dose.

! **WARNING** Instruct patient to notify prescriber immediately if a rash develops. Tell patient to stop drug and seek immediate medical attention if rash is accompanied by any other symptoms.

! WARNING Stress importance of complying with ordered blood tests used to monitor liver function. Tell patient to watch for signs of liver dysfunction such as dark or tea-colored urine, loss of appetite, nausea, pale-colored stools, pain or sensitivity on the right side below the ribs, or yellowing of the skin or whites of the eyes. If present, stress importance of notifying prescriber, as liver function will have to be assessed through laboratory tests and additional treatment may be needed.

- Inform patient and family or caregiver that cabotegravir may affect patient's mood enough to cause depression or even suicidal ideology. If present, patient should be reevaluated to determine if drug should be discontinued.
- Tell patient to keep prescriber informed of all drug use, including prescribed drugs, over-the-counter drugs, and herbal products being taken.
- Advise mothers receiving cabotegravir not to breastfeed their infant.

calcitonin, salmon

Calcimar (CAN), Miacalcin, Miacalcin Nasal

Class and Category

Pharmacologic class: Hormone
Therapeutic class: Antihypercalcemic, anti-osteoporotic

Indications and Dosages

✳ *To treat an early hypercalcemic emergency*

I.M. OR SUBCUTANEOUS INJECTION (MIACALCIN)

Adults. *Initial:* 4 international units/kg every 12 hr. Increased after 1 or 2 days, if needed, to 8 international units/kg every 12 hr and then 8 international units/kg every 6 hr after 2 more days, if needed. *Maximum:* 8 international units/kg every 6 hr.

✳ *To treat postmenopausal osteoporosis in women who are at least 5 years postmenopausal*

I.M. OR SUBCUTANEOUS INJECTION (MIACALCIN)

Adults. *Initial:* 100 international units daily.

NASAL SPRAY (MIACALCIN NASAL)

Adults. 200 international units (1 spray) daily, alternating nostrils.

✳ *To treat symptomatic Paget's disease of the bone*

I.M. OR SUBCUTANEOUS INJECTION (MIACALCIN)

Adults. *Initial:* 100 international units daily.

Drug Administration

- Expect to perform a skin test before giving drug if sensitivity to drug is suspected. Prepare a mixture of 10 international units/ml by withdrawing 0.05 ml from a 200-international unit solution in a tuberculin syringe and filling the syringe to 1 ml with Sodium Chloride for Injection. Mix well, discard 0.9 ml, and inject 0.1 ml intradermally on the inner forearm. Observe the site for 15 minutes after injection. If you detect evidence of sensitivity, such as more than mild erythema or a wheal, notify prescriber.

I.M.

- Route preferred if dose volume exceeds 2 ml with total dose distributed across multiple injection sites. Solution should appear clear and colorless.

SUBCUTANEOUS

- Route can be used if dose volume is less than 2 ml.

NASAL SPRAY

- Store unopened bottles in refrigerator. Once opened, bottle may be stored at room temperature but away from heat and light.
- Before first use, activate nasal pump by holding bottle upright and depressing the two white side arms of the pump toward the bottle. When bottle emits a full spray, pump is activated.
- Have patient gently blow nose first.
- Insert tip of bottle into one nostril while patient holds head upright.
- Depress pump firmly. Patient should not sniff, inhale deeply, or blow nose for a few minutes afterwards.
- Alternate nostrils daily.
- Bottle should be thrown away after 30 doses regardless if anything is still left in bottle.

Route	Onset	Peak	Duration
I.M., SubQ	15 min	4 hr	8–24 hr
Nasal spray	>10 min	31–39 min	Unknown
Half-life: 43–60 min			

Mechanism of Action

Directly inhibits bone resorption. Besides reducing the serum calcium level, this action slows bone metabolism (a major factor in the development of Paget's disease) and calcium loss from the bone (a major factor in the development of osteoporosis).

Contraindications

Hypersensitivity to calcitonin salmon or its components

Interactions

DRUGS

lithium: Possibly decreased lithium level

Adverse Reactions

CNS: Agitation, anxiety, **CVA**, dizziness, fatigue, headache, insomnia, neuralgia, paresthesia, tremor, vertigo
CV: **Bundle branch block**, hypertension, **MI**, palpitations, peripheral edema, tachycardia, thrombophlebitis
EENT: Blurred vision; dry mouth; earache; epistaxis; eye pain; hearing loss; nasal irritation or ulceration (nasal spray), lesions, or redness; pharyngitis; rhinitis; salty taste; sinusitis; taste perversion; tinnitus; vitreous floaters
ENDO: Goiter, hyperthyroidism
GI: Abdominal pain, anorexia, cholelithiasis, diarrhea, epigastric discomfort, flatulence, gastritis, **hepatitis**, increased appetite, nausea, thirst, vomiting
GU: Hematuria, nocturia, polyuria, **pyelonephritis**, renal calculi
HEME: Anemia
MS: Arthralgia, arthrosis, back or musculoskeletal pain, joint stiffness, polymyalgia rheumatica
RESP: Bronchitis, **bronchospasm**, cough, dyspnea, pneumonia, upper respiratory tract infection
SKIN: Alopecia, diaphoresis, eczema, flushing of face or hands, pruritus of earlobes, rash, ulceration, urticaria
Other: Anaphylaxis, **anaphylactic shock**, **angioedema**, antibody formation, feverish sensation, **hypocalcemia**, influenza-like symptoms, injection-site inflammation, lymphadenopathy, **malignancies**, mild tetanic symptoms

Childbearing Considerations

PREGNANCY

▪ It is not known if drug can cause fetal harm.

▪ Use with caution only if benefit to mother outweighs potential risk to fetus.

LACTATION

▪ It is not known if drug is present in breast milk.
▪ Drug is not recommended for women who are breastfeeding or wish to breastfeed, because drug action may interfere with lactation.

Nursing Considerations

! WARNING Monitor all patients for hypersensitivity reactions, which could be severe. Have appropriate equipment and drugs present to treat a hypersensitivity reaction if it occurs. Notify prescriber, expect drug to be discontinued, and provide supportive care, as directed by prescriber.

▪ Monitor serum calcium level, as ordered, if patient receives calcitonin for hypercalcemia. During first several doses, keep parenteral calcium available in case the calcium level is inadvertently overcorrected.
▪ Know that for patient receiving calcitonin for postmenopausal osteoporosis, hypocalcemia, and other mineral metabolism disorders, such as vitamin D deficiency, must be corrected before calcitonin therapy begins. These patients should also be monitored during therapy for signs and symptoms of hypocalcemia such as muscle cramps, twitching, and seizures. Also, expect to give 1.5 g of supplemental calcium carbonate and at least 400 units of vitamin D daily. Plan to provide a balanced diet that includes foods high in calcium and vitamin D.
▪ Periodically examine patient using nasal spray for nasal ulcers. If severe ulceration of the nasal mucosa occurs (ulcers greater than 1.5 mm, ulcers penetrating below the mucosa, or ulcers causing heavy bleeding), notify prescriber and expect nasal spray form to be discontinued. Also, know that nasal spray should be discontinued for smaller or less severe ulcers until healing occurs.
▪ Assess for nausea, especially with the first dose. Nausea tends to decrease or disappear with continued use.
▪ Be aware if patient with Paget's disease relapses after treatment, check for antibody formation, as ordered.

PATIENT TEACHING

- Tell patient to refrigerate injection or unopened nasal spray container.
- Teach patient how to self-administer injections.
- Teach patient how to administer nasal spray, if ordered. Explain how to activate nasal pump by holding bottle upright and depressing two white side arms toward the bottle until a full spray is seen. Tell patient to store activated nasal pump upright at room temperature and to discard it after 30 days.
- Instruct patient to place nozzle firmly into one nostril while holding head upright. Tell her to then depress the pump toward the bottle.
- Remind patient that she doesn't need to reactivate the pump before each dose.
- Instruct patient to report nasal symptoms to prescriber.
- Be aware that if patient has postmenopausal osteoporosis, teach her about dietary needs, including foods rich in calcium and vitamin D.

calcitriol
(1,25-dihydroxy-cholecalciferol)
Rocaltrol

⬚ Class and Category
Pharmacologic class: Vitamin D analogue
Therapeutic class: Antihypocalcemic

⬚ Indications and Dosages
✴ *To treat hypocalcemia in dialysis patients*

CAPSULES, ORAL SOLUTION (ROCALTROL)
Adults. *Initial:* 0.25 mcg daily. Increased by 0.25 mcg daily every 4 to 8 wk, if needed. *Usual:* 0.5 to 1 mcg daily.

I.V. INJECTION (CALCITRIOL)
Adults. *Initial:* 1–2 mcg three times weekly, approximately every other day, increased in increments of 0.5 to 1 mcg at 2- to 4-wk intervals, if needed.

±**DOSAGE ADJUSTMENT** Initial doses for I.V. administration may begin as small as 0.5 mcg and as large as 4 mcg three times a week, if needed. Patients with normal or only slightly reduced serum calcium levels and receiving oral therapy, dosage kept at

0.25 mcg but dosage frequency increased to every other day.

✴ *To treat hypocalcemia in predialysis patients*

CAPSULES, ORAL SOLUTION (ROCALTROL)
Adults and children age 3 and over. *Initial:* 0.25 mcg daily. Increased, if needed, to 0.5 mcg daily.

ORAL SOLUTION
Children up to age 3. *Initial:* 10 to 15 ng/kg daily.

✴ *To treat hypoparathyroidism*

CAPSULES, ORAL SOLUTION (ROCALTROL)
Adults and children age 6 and over. *Initial:* 0.25 mcg daily in the morning. Increased every 2 to 4 wk, if needed. *Usual:* 0.5 to 2 mcg daily.
Children ages 1 to 5. *Usual:* 0.25 to 0.75 mcg daily in the morning.

⬚ Drug Administration
P.O.
- Measure dosage of oral solution using a calibrated device.
- Capsules should be swallowed whole and not chewed, crushed, or opened.

I.V.
- No dilution is needed.
- Administer rapidly as a bolus at the end of hemodialysis.
- *Incompatibilities:* None reported by manufacturer.

Route	Onset	Peak	Duration
P.O.	2.6 hr	3–6 hr	3–5 days
I.V.	Immediate	Unknown	3–5 days

Half-life: 5–8 hr

⬚ Mechanism of Action
Binds to specific receptors on intestinal mucosa to increase calcium absorption from intestine. Drug may also regulate calcium ion transfer from bone to blood and stimulate calcium reabsorption in the distal renal tubules, making more calcium available in the body.

⬚ Contraindications
Hypercalcemia, hypersensitivity to calcitriol or its components, vitamin D toxicity

⬚ Interactions
DRUGS
calcium supplements: Increased risk of hypercalcemia

cholestyramine: Decreased calcitriol absorption
corticosteroids: Possibly inhibits calcium absorption
digitalis glycosides: Possibly arrhythmias
ketoconazole: Decreased calcitriol level
magnesium-containing antacids Hypermagnesemia
mineral oil: Decreased blood calcitriol level (with prolonged use of mineral oil)
phenobarbital, phenytoin: Decreased synthesis and blood level of calcitriol
phosphate-binding agents: Possibly altered phosphate transport in bone, intestine, and kidneys
thiazide diuretics: Hypercalcemia
vitamin D: Additive effects, including possible hypercalcemia

Adverse Reactions
SKIN: Erythema multiforme, lip swelling, pruritus, rash, urticaria
Other: Anaphylaxis

Childbearing Considerations
PREGNANCY
- It is not known if drug can cause fetal harm. However, upon birth, the neonate may exhibit mild signs and symptoms of hypercalcemia for several days.
- Use with caution only if benefit to mother outweighs potential risk to fetus.

LACTATION
- Drug may be present in breast milk.
- Breastfeeding should not be done during drug therapy.

Nursing Considerations
- Check to be sure patient receives enough calcium.
- Monitor patient closely. In high-dose or long-term calcitriol therapy, be alert for vitamin D toxicity. Early evidence includes abdominal or bone pain, constipation, dry mouth, headache, metallic taste, myalgia, nausea, somnolence, vomiting, and weakness. Late evidence includes albuminuria, anorexia, arrhythmias, azotemia, conjunctivitis (calcific), decreased libido, elevated AST and ALT levels, elevated BUN level, vascular calcification, hypercholesterolemia, hypertension, hyperthermia, irritability, mild acidosis, nephrocalcinosis, nocturia, pancreatitis, photophobia, polydipsia, polyuria, pruritus, rhinorrhea, and weight loss.

PATIENT TEACHING
- Warn patient not to take other forms of vitamin D while taking calcitriol.
- Tell patient to swallow whole and not to chew, crush, or open capsules. If oral solution is prescribed, tell patient to use a calibrated device to measure dosage, not a household spoon.
- Instruct patient to take a missed dose as soon as possible.
- Advise patient to notify prescriber immediately about possible toxicity, such as headache, irritability, nausea, photophobia, vomiting, weakness, and weight loss.

calcium acetate
Calphron, Phoslyra

calcium carbonate
Apo-Cal (CAN), Calci-Mix, Calsan (CAN), Liqui-Cal, Liquid Cal-600, Titralac

calcium chloride
Calciject (CAN)

calcium citrate
Cal-C Cap, Cal-Cee, Citracal

calcium gluconate

calcium lactate
Cal-Lac

Class and Category
Pharmacologic class: Calcium salts
Therapeutic class: Antacid, antihypermagnesemic, antihyperphosphatemic, antihypocalcemic, calcium replacement, cardiotonic

Indications and Dosages
✳ *To treat hyperphosphatemia*

CAPSULES, TABLETS (CALCIUM ACETATE)
Adults. *Initial:* 2 capsules or tablets three times daily. Dosage increased every 2 to 3 wk

to reduce serum phosphorus level below 6 mg/dl as long as hypercalcemia doesn't develop. *Usual:* 3 or 4 capsules or tablets three times daily.

ORAL SOLUTION (CALCIUM ACETATE)

Adults. *Initial:* 10 ml three times daily. Dosage increased every 2 to 3 wk to reduce serum phosphorus levels to the target range, as long as hypercalcemia doesn't develop. *Usual:* 15 to 20 ml three times daily.

✳ *To prevent hypocalcemia with oral supplementation*

CAPSULES, ORAL SUSPENSION, TABLETS (CALCIUM CARBONATE); EFFERVESCENT TABLETS, TABLETS (CALCIUM CITRATE); TABLETS (CALCIUM GLUCONATE OR LACTATE)

Adults. 1,000 to 1,200 mg daily RDA elemental calcium.

Pregnant and breastfeeding women. 1,000 to 1,300 mg daily RDA elemental calcium.

Children ages 9 to 18. 1,300 mg daily RDA elemental calcium.

Children ages 4 to 8. 800 mg daily RDA elemental calcium.

Children ages 1 to 4. 500 mg daily RDA elemental calcium.

Children ages 7 to 12 months. 270 mg daily RDA elemental calcium.

Infants up to 6 months. 210 mg daily RDA elemental calcium.

✳ *To provide antacid effects*

CHEWABLE TABLETS, ORAL SUSPENSION, TABLETS (CALCIUM CARBONATE)

Adults and children age 12 and over. 350 to 1,500 mg, as needed.

✳ *To provide emergency treatment for acute symptomatic hypocalcemia*

I.V. INJECTION (10% CALCIUM CHLORIDE)

Adults. 500 to 1,000 mg, repeated as needed, in intervals of 1 to 3 days.

I.V. INFUSION (CALCIUM GLUCONATE)

Adults. *Initial:* 500 to 2,000 mg (5 to 20 ml) not to exceed a rate of 0.5 to 2 ml/min. Dosage increased as needed in intervals of 1 to 3 days. *Usual daily dose, if needed:* 1,000 to 1,500 mg in divided doses as a bolus or continuous infusion initiated at a rate not to exceed 0.5 to 2 ml/min, with adjustments made as needed.

Children age more than 1 month to 17 years. *Initial:* 29–60 mg/kg. *Subsequent doses, if needed:* 29–60 mg/kg every 6 hr as a bolus or continuous infusion initiated at 8 to 13 mg/kg/hr, with adjustments made as needed.

Neonates 1 month or less. *Initial:* 100–200 mg/kg. *Subsequent doses, if needed:* 100 to 200 mg/kg every 6 hr as a bolus or continuous infusion initiated at 17–33 mg/kg/hr, with adjustments made as needed.

✳ *As adjunct to treat magnesium intoxication*

I.V. INFUSION (CALCIUM GLUCONATE)

Adults. 1,000 to 2,000 mg as a one-time dose not to exceed a rate of 0.5 to 2 ml/min. Dosage repeated in severe cases.

✳ *To treat hyperkalemia*

I.V. INFUSION (CALCIUM GLUCONATE)

Adults. 500 to 3,000 mg as a one-time dose not to exceed a rate of 0.5 to 2 ml/min. Dosage repeated in extreme hyperkalemia cardiotoxicity.

✳ *To provide calcium during exchange transfusion*

I.V. INFUSION (CALCIUM GLUCONATE)

Adults. 300 mg with each 100 ml of citrated blood not to exceed a rate of 0.5 to 2 ml/min.

▤ Drug Administration

P.O.

- Administer calcium acetate with meals; calcium carbonate 1 hour after meals and at bedtime.
- Chewable tablets must be chewed thoroughly before swallowing and followed with a glass of water.
- Shake suspension bottle well before each use.
- Use a calibrated device to measure oral solution or suspension dosage.
- Dissolve calcium citrate effervescent tablets in water and have patient drink immediately.
- Avoid administering calcium within 2 hours of other drugs.
- Store oral calcium at room temperature away from heat, moisture, and light. Do not freeze oral solution or suspension.

I.V.

- Administer calcium chloride and calcium gluconate only intravenously, preferably in a central or large, deep vein. Do not administer as an I.M. or subcutaneous injection. Also do not administer in a small hand or foot vein or into a scalp vein in neonates.

- Warm solution to body temperature, if time permits.
- Administer through a small needle into a large vein or through a free-flowing compatible I.V. solution.
- Administer 10% calcium chloride slowly over 5 to 10 minutes, not exceeding 1 ml/min.
- For calcium gluconate bolus administration, dilute in a compatible I.V. solution such as Sodium Chloride Injection or 5% Dextrose Injection to a concentration of 10–50 mg/ml. Solution should appear clear and colorless to slightly yellow. Use immediately. Administer slowly and do not exceed a rate of 200 mg/min in adults and 100 mg/min in pediatric patients, including neonates.
- For calcium gluconate continuous infusion, dilute drug in 0.9% Sodium Chloride Injection or 5% Dextrose Injection to a concentration of 5.8 to 10 mg/ml. For adults, initiate rate at 5.4 to 21.5 mg/kg/hr; for children older than 1 month to 17 years, initiate at 8–13 mg/kg/hr; and for neonates 1 month or less, initiate at 17–33 mg/kg/hr. Rate then adjusted according to serum calcium levels.
- Stop infusion if patient experiences pain or discomfort and notify prescriber.
- Keep patient in a recumbent position for at least 15 minutes after I.V. administration.
- *Incompatibilities:* Calcium chloride, none reported by manufacturer; calcium gluconate-ceftriaxone, I.V. fluids containing bicarbonate or phosphate, minocycline

Route	Onset	Peak	Duration
P.O.	Unknown	Unknown	Unknown
I.V.	Immediate	Immediate	30–120 min

Half-life: Unknown

Mechanism of Action

Increases levels of intracellular and extracellular calcium, which is needed to maintain homeostasis, especially in the nervous and musculoskeletal systems. Also plays a role in normal cardiac and renal function, respiration, coagulation, and cell membrane and capillary permeability. Helps regulate the release and storage of neurotransmitters and hormones. Oral forms also neutralize or buffer stomach acid to relieve discomfort caused by hyperacidity.

Contraindications

Cardiac resuscitation with risk of existing digitalis toxicity or presence of ventricular fibrillation (I.V.), concurrent use of calcium supplements, hypercalcemia, hypersensitivity to calcium salts or their components, hypophosphatemia, renal calculi

Interactions
DRUGS

bisphosphonates (alendronate, etidronate, ibandronate, risedronate): Possibly decreased absorption of bisphosphonates
calcium supplements, magnesium-containing preparations: Increased serum calcium or magnesium level, especially in patients with impaired renal function
digitalis glycosides: Increased risk of arrhythmias
fluoroquinolones: Reduced fluoroquinolone absorption by calcium carbonate
iron salts: Decreased gastric iron absorption
levothyroxine: Decreased absorption of levothyroxine
tetracyclines: Decreased tetracycline absorption and blood level, leading to decreased anti-infective response
thiazide diuretics: Possibly hypercalcemia
verapamil: Reversed verapamil effects
vitamin D (high doses): Excessively increased calcium absorption

FOODS

caffeine, high-fiber food: Possibly decreased calcium absorption

ACTIVITIES

alcohol use (excessive), smoking: Possibly decreased calcium absorption

Adverse Reactions

CNS: Paresthesia (parenteral form)
CV: Hypotension, irregular heartbeat (parenteral form)
GI: Nausea or vomiting (parenteral form)
SKIN: Diaphoresis, flushing, or sensation of warmth (parenteral form)
Other: Aluminum toxicity (calcium gluconate); hypercalcemia; injection-site burning, pain, rash, or redness (parenteral form)

Childbearing Considerations
PREGNANCY

- It is not known if drug can cause fetal harm.
- Be aware that pregnancy may alter dosage needs for mother.

- Use with caution only if benefit to mother outweighs potential risk to fetus.

LACTATION
- Drug is present in breast milk.
- Patient should check with prescriber before breastfeeding. Dosage needs for mother may change if breastfeeding.

Nursing Considerations
- Check intravenous site regularly for infiltration because calcium causes necrosis. If infiltration occurs, stop infusion and tell prescriber immediately.
- Be aware that patients with kidney failure on dialysis may develop hypercalcemia when treated with calcium. Monitor patient closely. Know that these patients should not take calcium supplements, including antacids containing calcium.
- Monitor serum calcium level in all patients, as ordered, and evaluate therapeutic response by assessing for Chvostek's and Trousseau's signs, which shouldn't appear.
- Be aware that calcium chloride injection contains three times as much calcium per milliliter as calcium gluconate injection.
- Monitor patient for aluminum toxicity when receiving calcium gluconate because calcium gluconate contains up to 100 mcg per liter of aluminum, increasing patient's risk for aluminum toxicity.

PATIENT TEACHING
- Urge patient to chew chewable tablets thoroughly before swallowing and to drink a glass of water afterward.
- Tell patient to shake bottle well before each use if suspension form is prescribed.
- Tell patient to dissolve calcium citrate effervescent tablets in water and drink immediately.
- Instruct patient to take calcium carbonate tablets 1 to 2 hours after meals and other forms with meals.
- Advise storing calcium at room temperature away from heat, moisture, and light. Warn against freezing suspension or syrup.
- Urge patient to ask prescriber before taking OTC drugs because of risk of interactions.
- Tell patient to avoid excessive use of tobacco and excessive consumption of alcoholic beverages, caffeine-containing products, and high-fiber foods because these substances may decrease calcium absorption.

- Remind patient to take calcium separate from other prescribed drugs. For example, tell the patient to take fluoroquinolone at least 2 hours before or 6 hours after calcium; if prescribed levothyroxine, to take it at least 4 hours before or after calcium; if prescribed a tetracycline, to take it at least 1 hour before calcium. Advise patient to avoid taking calcium within 2 hours of other oral drugs.

canagliflozin
Invokana

Class and Category
Pharmacologic class: Sodium-glucose co-transporter 2 (SGLT2) inhibitor
Therapeutic class: Antidiabetic

Indications and Dosages
✳ *Adjunct to control blood glucose level in type 2 diabetes mellitus; to reduce the risk of major adverse cardiovascular events such as nonfatal myocardial infarction and nonfatal stroke in patients with type 2 diabetes mellitus and established cardiovascular disease; to reduce the risk of end-stage kidney disease (ESKD), doubling of serum creatinine, cardiovascular death, and hospitalization for heart failure in patients with type 2 diabetes mellitus and diabetic nephropathy with albuminuria greater than 300 mg/day.*

TABLETS
Adults. 100 mg once daily, followed by dosage increase to 300 mg once daily, if needed, and patient has a glomerular filtration rate of 60 ml/min or greater. *Maximum:* 300 mg once daily.

±**DOSAGE ADJUSTMENT** For patients with glomerular filtration rate less than 60 ml/min but at least 30 ml/min, dosage limited to 100 mg once daily. For patients with a glomerular filtration rate less than 30 ml/min, initiation is not recommended but patient with albuminuria greater than 300 mg/day may continue 100 mg once daily to reduce the risk of end-stage kidney disease, doubling of serum creatinine, CV death, and hospitalization for heart failure. For patients receiving an UDP-glucuronosyltransferase (UGT) enzyme inducer such as phenobarbital, phenytoin, rifampin, or ritonavir and have a glomerular filtration rate of 60 ml/min or greater, dosage may be increased to 200 mg once daily if patient is tolerating 100 mg daily or increased to 300 mg once daily if patient is tolerating 200 mg daily. For patients receiving an UGT enzyme inducer as indicated above and the glomerular filtration rate is less than 60 ml/min, dosage increased to 200 mg once daily in patients tolerating 100 mg once daily.

Drug Administration

P.O.

- Administer before first meal of the day.

Route	Onset	Peak	Duration
P.O.	>24 hr	1–2 hr	Unknown
Half-life: 10.6–13.1 hr			

Mechanism of Action

Inhibits sodium-glucose co-transporter 2 (SGLT2) responsible for the majority of the reabsorption of filtered glucose from the tubular lumen in the kidneys. By inhibiting SGLT2, reabsorption of filtered glucose is reduced along with a lowering of the renal threshold for glucose, which increases urinary glucose excretion.

Contraindications

Hypersensitivity to canagliflozin or its components, use of dialysis

Interactions

DRUGS

digoxin: Possibly increased serum digoxin levels and digitalis toxicity
insulin, insulin secretagogues: Possibly increased risk of hypoglycemia
phenobarbital, phenytoin, rifampin, ritonavir: Decreased effectiveness of canagliflozin

Adverse Reactions

CNS: Asthenia, excessive thirst, fatigue, postural dizziness, syncope
CV: Elevation of low-density lipoprotein cholesterol (LDL-C) and non-high-density lipoprotein cholesterol (non-HDL-C), **hypotension**, orthostatic hypotension
ENDO: **Hypoglycemia, ketoacidosis**
EENT: Dry mouth
GI: Abdominal pain, constipation, nausea, **pancreatitis**
GU: **Acute renal failure**, decreased glomerular filtration rate, elevated serum creatinine levels, genital mycotic infections, **necrotizing fasciitis of the perineum (Fournier's gangrene), pyelonephritis,** polyuria, renal impairment, UTIs, vulvovaginal pruritus, **urosepsis**
HEME: Elevated hemoglobin
MS: Bone fracture, decreased bone density, lower-limb amputation
SKIN: Erythema, photosensitivity, pruritus, rash**,** urticaria
Other: **Anaphylaxis, angioedema,** dehydration, **hyperkalemia, hyperphosphatemia, hypermagnesemia**

Childbearing Considerations

PREGNANCY

- Drug may cause fetal harm by adversely affecting kidney function of the fetus.
- Drug is not recommended during the second and third trimester of pregnancy.

LACTATION

- It is not known if drug is present in breast milk.
- Drug should not be given to women who are breastfeeding since kidney maturation in infant continues for 2 years following birth.

Nursing Considerations

- Use drug cautiously in patients with chronic kidney insufficiency, congestive heart failure, decreased blood volume, and in patients taking medications such as angiotensin-converting enzyme inhibitors and angiotensin receptor blockers, diuretics, and NSAIDs because these conditions and treatments may predispose patient to acute kidney injury while receiving canagliflozin. Ensure that kidney function has been assessed prior to start of canagliflozin therapy and then periodically thereafter.
- Know that patients with volume depletion should have the condition corrected before canagliflozin therapy is begun because drug causes intravascular volume contraction. Patients especially at risk for symptomatic hypotension caused by volume depletion include patients with impaired renal function, the elderly, patients taking either diuretics or drugs that interfere with the renin–angiotensin–aldosterone system, or patients with low systolic blood pressure.

- Expect drug to be temporarily discontinued in patients who develop a reduced oral intake, such as in an acute illness or fasting, or who experience excessive fluid losses because of significant heat exposure or gastrointestinal illness, to reduce risk of acute kidney injury.
- Be aware that canagliflozin dosage should only be increased in patients who have at least a glomerular filtration rate of 60 ml/min and need greater glucose control.
- Assess renal function, as ordered prior to starting canagliflozin therapy and then periodically thereafter, because canagliflozin may cause renal impairment, especially in patients with hypovolemia. Expect drug to be discontinued if patient develops acute kidney injury. Also monitor patient for a UTI, because canagliflozin increases risk of UTIs. Report promptly and expect to treat because the UTI can quickly become serious, developing into pyelonephritis and urosepsis.
- Monitor serum potassium levels regularly, as ordered, during canagliflozin therapy in patients with impaired renal function and in patients predisposed to hyperkalemia due to medications or other medical conditions.
- Monitor patient's blood glucose levels to determine effectiveness of canagliflozin therapy. Be aware that canagliflozin can increase urinary glucose excretion, leading to positive urine glucose tests, and should not be used to monitor glucose levels in patients with diabetes mellitus. Assess patient also receiving insulin or insulin secretagogues for hypoglycemia.

! WARNING Monitor patient closely for ketoacidosis that may occur despite the patient having type 2 diabetes and may be present even if a blood glucose level is less than 250 mg/dl. If signs and symptoms occur such as dehydration, fruity odor to breath, malaise, nausea, shortness of breath, and vomiting, notify prescriber and expect drug to be discontinued. Provide supportive care, as ordered.

- Be aware that patients with a history of genital mycotic infections, as well as uncircumcised males, are at greater risk for developing genital mycotic infections.

! WARNING Report immediately signs and symptoms of necrotizing fasciitis of the perineum (Fournier's gangrene), a rare but serious and life-threatening necrotizing infection that has been linked to canagliflozin therapy. Report patient's complaints of erythema, pain or tenderness, or swelling in the genital or perineal area, along with fever or malaise, as treatment requires urgent surgical intervention along with immediate broad-spectrum antibiotic therapy. If confirmed, expect canagliflozin to be discontinued and an alternative treatment for glycemic control prescribed.

- Monitor patient's lipid levels and expect to treat if an elevation occurs.

! WARNING Assess patient for hypersensitivity reactions such as angioedema and generalized urticaria, especially within hours to days after canagliflozin therapy is begun. The hypersensitivity reaction can become severe, causing anaphylaxis. If hypersensitivity to canagliflozin occurs, expect drug to be discontinued and provide supportive care as ordered.

- Institute safety precautions to prevent falls because drug may increase risk of falls leading to bone fracture. The risk of bone fracture may occur as early as 12 weeks after therapy is begun.
- Be aware that canagliflozin has been linked to an increase in foot and leg amputations in patients receiving the drug. Assess patient's feet and legs regularly for any abnormalities and notify prescriber immediately if present. Be aware that patients may be at higher risk of lower-limb amputation if they have had diabetic foot sores or ulcers, have had blocked or narrowed blood vessels (usually in leg), have had damage to the nerves (neuropathy) in the leg, or have a history of amputation, heart disease, or are at risk for heart disease. Know that canagliflozin may be discontinued if abnormalities develop.

PATIENT TEACHING

- Instruct patient to take canagliflozin before the first meal of the day. Tell her that if a dose is missed, she should take it as soon as she remembers unless it is almost time for the next dose. Then patient should skip the missed dose and take her normal dose of canagliflozin at the regular time. She should never double the dose.

- Urge patient not to skip doses or increase dosage without consulting prescriber. However, tell patient to notify prescriber if he is unable to take a normal amount of daily fluids due to illness or fasting or experiences an excessive loss of fluids from excessive perspiration or gastrointestinal illnesses, as drug may have to be temporarily withheld.
- Emphasize importance of reporting signs of hypoglycemia, such as anxiety, confusion, dizziness, excessive sweating, headache, and nausea.
- Tell patient to carry identification indicating that he has diabetes.
- Teach patient how to monitor his blood glucose level. Advise patient with diabetes mellitus not to use urine glucose tests to monitor her glycemic control, as drug will cause a false-positive result. Review signs and symptoms of ketoacidosis with patient and urge her to seek immediate medical attention, if present, even if blood glucose level is less than 250 mg/dl.
- Inform patient that canagliflozin is not a substitute for diet and exercise management.
- Inform patient that drug may increase his risk for bone fractures and to take safety precautions to prevent falls.
- Advise patient to avoid direct sunlight and to wear sunscreen when outdoors.
- Instruct patient to notify prescriber right away if he notices any new pain or tenderness, sores or ulcers, or symptoms of infections in his feet or legs. Tell patient this is very important, because canagliflozin therapy increases the risk of lower-limb amputations.
- Advise patient to seek medical care promptly if pain or tenderness, redness, or swelling of the genitals or the area from the genitals back to the rectum occurs, along with a fever above 38°C (100.4°F) or malaise develops.

candesartan cilexetil
Atacand

≡ Class and Category
Pharmacologic class: Angiotensin receptor blocker
Therapeutic class: Antihypertensive

≡ Indications and Dosages
✳ *To manage, or as adjunct in managing, hypertension*

ORAL SUSPENSION, TABLETS
Adults. *Initial:* 16 mg once daily. *Maintenance:* 8 to 32 mg once daily or 4 to 16 mg twice daily. *Maximum:* 32 mg daily.
Children ages 6 to 17 weighing more than 50 kg (110 lb). *Initial:* 8 to 16 mg daily. *Maintenance:* 4 to 32 mg once daily or 2 to 16 mg twice daily. *Maximum:* 32 mg daily.
Children ages 6 to 17 weighing 50 kg (110 lb) or less. *Initial:* 4 to 8 mg daily. *Maintenance:* 2 to 16 mg once daily or 1 to 8 mg twice daily. *Maximum:* 16 mg daily.

ORAL SUSPENSION
Children ages 1 to 6. *Initial:* 0.20 mg/kg daily. *Maintenance:* 0.05 to 0.4 mg/kg daily or 0.025 to 0.2 mg/kg twice daily. *Maximum:* 0.4 mg/kg daily.
±**DOSAGE ADJUSTMENT** For adult patients with moderate hepatic impairment, initial dosage reduced to 8 mg daily.
✳ *To treat heart failure in patients with an ejection fraction of 40% or less and NYHA class II–IV to reduce the risk of death from cardiovascular causes and reduce hospitalizations for heart failure*

ORAL SUSPENSION, TABLETS
Adults. *Initial:* 4 mg once daily for 2 wk; then doubled every 2 wk as tolerated until reaching target dose of 32 mg once daily.

≡ Drug Administration
P.O.
- Tablets should be swallowed whole.
- Administer oral suspension to patients who cannot swallow tablets.
- Shake suspension well before each dose and use a calibrated device to measure dose.
- Store suspension at room temperature. Use within 30 days of opening bottle or discard. Also discard after 100 days if not opened.

Route	Onset	Peak	Duration
P.O.	2–3 hr	6–8 hr	>24 hr

Half-life: 5–9 hr, dose-dependent

≡ Mechanism of Action
Selectively blocks binding of angiotensin (AT) II to AT_1 receptor sites in many tissues, including adrenal glands and vascular smooth muscle. This inhibits vasoconstrictive

and aldosterone-secreting effects of AT II, which reduces blood pressure.

Contraindications

Concurrent aliskiren therapy in presence of diabetes, hypersensitivity to candesartan or its components

Interactions

DRUGS

aliskiren (in presence of diabetes or renal impairment), angiotensin-converting enzyme inhibitors, angiotensin receptor blockers: Increased risk of hypotension, hyperkalemia, and renal dysfunction
lithium: Increased blood lithium level
NSAIDs: Possible decreased renal function in patients who are elderly, volume-depleted, or have a compromised renal function
potassium-sparing diuretics, potassium supplements, potassium-containing salt substitutes: Possibly increased risk of hyperkalemia

Adverse Reactions

CNS: Dizziness, headache
CV: Hypotension
EENT: Pharyngitis, rhinitis
GI: Elevated liver enzymes, hepatitis, impaired liver function
GU: Elevated BUN and serum creatinine levels
HEME: Agranulocytosis, leukopenia, neutropenia
MS: Back pain, rhabdomyolysis
RESP: Cough, upper respiratory tract infection
SKIN: Pruritus, rash, urticaria
Other: Angioedema, hyperkalemia, hyponatremia

Childbearing Considerations

PREGNANCY

- Drug can cause fetal harm.
- Drug given during the second or third trimester reduces fetal renal function and increases fetal and neonatal morbidity and death. Resulting oligohydramnios can cause fetal lung hypoplasia and skeletal malformations.
- Drug is contraindicated during pregnancy.

LACTATION

- It is not known if drug is present in breast milk.
- Breastfeeding is not recommended during drug therapy.

Nursing Considerations

- Determine if patient has fluid or salt depletion prior to starting candesartan. If patient has known or suspected hypovolemia and/or salt depletion such as may occur with prolonged diuretic therapy, dietary salt restriction, dialysis, diarrhea or vomiting, expect to provide treatment, such as I.V. normal saline solution, as prescribed, to correct it before starting candesartan. Continue to monitor blood pressure throughout candesartan therapy, especially after a dosage increase.
- Monitor patient closely during major surgery and anesthesia because candesartan increases risk of hypotension by blocking renin–angiotensin system.
- Watch for elevated BUN and serum creatinine levels, especially if patient has heart failure or impaired renal function; drug may cause acute renal failure. Report significant or persistent increases immediately.

! **WARNING** Know that if patient receives a diuretic or antihypertensive with candesartan, has heart failure, or is elderly, assess blood pressure often because of added risk of hypotension.

- Monitor patient for hypotension. If patient develops hypotension, expect to stop drug temporarily. Immediately place patient in supine position and prepare to give I.V. normal saline solution, as prescribed. Expect to resume therapy after blood pressure stabilizes.
- Monitor patient for fluid deficit. If patient receives a diuretic, provide hydration, as ordered, to help prevent hypovolemia. Watch for evidence, such as hypotension with dizziness and fainting. If patient has heart failure and develops hypotension, dosage of diuretic, candesartan, or both may be reduced when blood pressure stabilizes and therapy resumes.
- Check CBC for decreases in hemoglobin and hematocrit. If they're significant or persistent, notify prescriber immediately.

PATIENT TEACHING

- Advise patient that full effects of candesartan may not occur for 4 to 5 weeks.
- Instruct patient to swallow tablets whole and not to chew, crush, or divide. Instruct

patient receiving oral suspension to shake bottle well before measuring dose and to use a calibrated dosing device, not a household spoon, for accuracy of dosing. Tell patient to store suspension at room temperature and use within 30 days of opening bottle or discard. Also tell patient to discard bottle after 100 days if not opened.

- Explain importance of lifestyle choices in controlling hypertension.
- Advise female patient of childbearing age to immediately report known or suspected pregnancy. Explain that if she becomes pregnant, candesartan will have to be discontinued as soon as possible and treatment started with another antihypertensive that's safe to use during pregnancy.

cangrelor

Kengreal

Class and Category

Pharmacologic class: P2Y$_{12}$ platelet inhibitor
Therapeutic class: Antiplatelet

Indications and Dosages

* *Adjunct to percutaneous coronary intervention (PCI) to reduce risk of periprocedural myocardial infarction, repeat coronary revascularization and stent thrombosis in patients who have not been treated with a P2Y12 platelet inhibitor and are not being given a glycoprotein IIb/IIIa inhibitor*

I.V. INFUSION, I.V. INJECTION

Adults. 30 mcg/kg I.V. bolus prior to PCI followed immediately by a 4 mcg/kg/min infusion for at least 2 hr or for the duration of PCI, whichever is longer.

Drug Administration

I.V.

- Reconstitute each 50-mg vial by adding 5 ml of Sterile Water for Injection. Swirl gently until all material is dissolved. Avoid vigorous mixing. Allow any foam to settle. Ensure that contents are fully dissolved and the reconstituted material is clear and colorless to pale yellow.
- Dilute reconstituted solution immediately with 0.9% Sodium Chloride Injection or 5% Dextrose Injection. Withdraw the

contents from one reconstituted vial and add to one 250-ml bag of I.V. solution. Mix the bag thoroughly. This will result in a concentration of 200 mcg/ml and last for about 2 hours of infusion. Know that patients weighing 100 kg or more will require a minimum of two bags.

- Diluted cangrelor is stable for 12 hr if diluted in 5% Dextrose Injection and 24 hr if diluted in 0.9% Sodium Chloride Injection and kept at room temperature.
- Administer via a dedicated I.V. line.
- Administer the bolus rapidly in less than 1 minute from the diluted bag via manual I.V. push or pump. Make sure the bolus is completely administered before the start of PCI and then start infusion immediately after administration of the bolus at a rate of 4 mcg/kg/min.
- *Incompatibilities:* None reported by manufacturer

Route	Onset	Peak	Duration
I.V.	2 min	2 min	1 hr after infusion stopped

Half-life: 3–6 min

Mechanism of Action

Blocks ADP-induced platelet activation and aggregation by binding selectively and reversibly to the P2Y$_{12}$ receptor to prevent further signaling and platelet activation.

Contraindications

Hypersensitivity to cangrelor or its components, significant active bleeding

Interactions

DRUGS

thienopyridines such as clopidogrel, prasugrel: Elimination effect of these drugs if given during cangrelor infusion; these drugs should be administered after cangrelor infusion is discontinued

Adverse Reactions

CNS: Intracranial bleeding or hemorrhage
CV: Coronary artery dissection or perforation
EENT: Stridor
GU: Decreased renal function
HEME: Bleeding events
RESP: Bronchospasm, dyspnea
Other: Anaphylaxis including shock, angioedema

☰ Childbearing Considerations
PREGNANCY
- It is not known if drug can cause fetal harm.
- Use with caution only if benefit to mother outweighs potential risk to fetus.

LABOR & DELIVERY
- Drug may increase risk of maternal bleeding and hemorrhage.
- Drug should be discontinued 1 hour prior to labor, delivery, or neuraxial blockade, if possible.

LACTATION
- It is not known if drug is present in breast milk.
- Patient should check with prescriber before breastfeeding.

☰ Nursing Considerations
- Be aware that after cangrelor is discontinued, an oral P2Y$_{12}$ platelet inhibitor should be administered such as clopidogrel 600 mg after discontinuation of cangrelor, prasugrel 60 mg immediately after discontinuation of cangrelor, or ticagrelor 180 mg at any time during cangrelor infusion or immediately after discontinuation.
- Monitor patient closely for bleeding that can range from being minor to severe. Be prepared to treat bleeding events immediately and notify prescriber. Know that once cangrelor is discontinued, there is no antiplatelet effect after an hour.

! **WARNING** Monitor patient closely for allergic reactions following administration. Alert prescriber immediately, if present, and be prepared to discontinue drug and provide supportive emergency care, as ordered.

PATIENT TEACHING
- Tell patient to alert medical staff immediately if difficulty breathing occurs.
- Inform patient that the effects of cangrelor are gone after 1 hour of the drug being discontinued.

captopril

☰ Class and Category
Pharmacologic class: Angiotensin-converting enzyme (ACE) inhibitor

Therapeutic class: Antihypertensive, vasodilator

☰ Indications and Dosages
✻ *To control hypertension*

TABLETS
Adults. *Initial:* 25 mg twice daily or three times daily. Increased to 50 mg twice daily or three times daily after 1 to 2 wk, if needed. If blood pressure isn't well controlled at this dosage after an additional 1–2 wk, diuretic added. If blood pressure is still not controlled, dosage increased to 100 mg twice daily or three times daily and then, if needed, to 150 mg twice daily or three times daily while continuing diuretic. *Maximum:* 450 mg daily.

✻ *To control accelerated or malignant hypertension when temporary discontinuation of current antihypertensive therapy isn't practical or when prompt titration of blood pressure is needed*

TABLETS
Adults. *Initial:* 25 mg twice daily or three times daily while continuing diuretic but discontinuing other current antihypertensive drug. Increased every 24 hr or less, as needed, until satisfactory response is obtained or maximum dosage is reached. *Maximum:* 450 mg daily.

✻ *To treat congestive heart failure*

TABLETS
Adults with normal or low blood pressure, who have been vigorously treated with diuretics. *Initial:* 6.25 mg or 12.5 mg three times daily, increased gradually over several days to 50 mg three times daily. Further increases done in 2-wk intervals, as needed. *Maximum:* 450 mg daily.

Adults. *Initial:* 25 mg three times daily. Increased to 50 mg three times daily, as needed. After 14 days, increased to 100 mg three times daily and then to 150 mg three times daily, if needed. *Maximum:* 450 mg daily.

✻ *To treat left ventricular dysfunction after MI*

TABLETS
Adults. *Initial:* 6.25 mg as single dose starting 3 days after MI and then 12.5 mg three times daily. Increased to 25 mg three times daily over several days and then again to maintenance dosage over next several wk. *Maintenance:* 50 mg three times daily.

✴ *To treat diabetic nephropathy*

TABLETS
Adults. 25 mg three times daily.

±**DOSAGE ADJUSTMENT** For patient with renal impairment, initial dosage reduced and smaller increments utilized for titration.

⬚ Drug Administration

P.O.
- Administer on an empty stomach one hour before meals.

Route	Onset	Peak	Duration
P.O.	>15 min	60–90 min	Unknown
Half-life: 1.7 hr			

⬚ Mechanism of Action
By inhibiting angiotensin-converting enzyme, captopril:
- prevents conversion of angiotensin I to angiotensin II, a potent vasoconstrictor that also stimulates the adrenal cortex to secrete aldosterone. Inhibiting aldosterone increases sodium and water excretion, reducing blood pressure and water retention.
- may inhibit renal and vascular production of angiotensin II.
- decreases serum angiotensin II level and increases renin activity. This decreases aldosterone secretion, slightly increasing serum potassium level and fluid loss.
- decreases vascular tone and blood pressure.

⬚ Contraindications
Combination therapy with a neprilysin inhibitor (e.g., sacubitril) or within 36 hours of switching to or from sacubitril/valsartan; concurrent aliskiren use in patients with diabetes or patients with renal impairment (GFR less than 60 ml/min); hypersensitivity to captopril, other ACE inhibitors, or their components

⬚ Interactions

DRUGS
adrenergic neuron-blocking drugs, beta adrenergic drugs, ganglionic blocking drugs: Possibly increased risk of hypotension
aliskiren in patients with diabetes, other ACE inhibitors, angiotensin receptor blockers: Increased risk of hypotension, hyperkalemia, and renal impairment
antacids: Possibly impaired captopril absorption
capsaicin: Possibly cause or worsening of cough from ACE inhibitor
diuretics; hypotension-producing drugs, such as hydralazine: Additive hypotensive effects
gold: Increased risk of nitritoid reaction, including facial flushing, hypotension, nausea, and vomiting
lithium: Increased risk of lithium toxicity
mTOR (everolimus, sirolimus, temsirolimus), neprilysin inhibitor such as sacubitril: Increased risk for angioedema
nitrates, other vasodilators: Possibly potentiated effects
NSAIDs: Decreased antihypertensive response to captopril; possible decreased renal function in elderly patients or those who are volume-depleted or already have existing impaired renal function
potassium-containing drugs, potassium-sparing diuretics, potassium supplements: Increased risk of hyperkalemia

ACTIVITIES
alcohol use: Additive hypotensive effects

FOOD
moderate to high-potassium-containing foods: Possibly increased risk of hyperkalemia

⬚ Adverse Reactions
CNS: Fever
CV: Chest pain, **hypotension**, orthostatic hypotension, palpitations, tachycardia
EENT: Loss of taste
GU: Dysuria, impotence, **nephrotic syndrome**, nocturia, oliguria, polyuria, proteinuria, urinary frequency
HEME: Eosinophilia
MS: Arthralgia
RESP: Cough
SKIN: Photosensitivity, pruritus, rash
Other: Angioedema, hyperkalemia, hyponatremia, positive ANA titer

⬚ Childbearing Considerations

PREGNANCY
- Drug can cause fetal harm.
- Drug given during the second or third trimester reduces fetal renal function and increases fetal and neonatal morbidity and death. Resulting oligohydramnios can cause fetal lung hypoplasia and skeletal malformations.
- Drug is contraindicated in pregnancy and should not be given to a pregnant woman unless no alternative is available.

LACTATION

- Drug is present in breast milk.
- A decision should be made to discontinue breastfeeding or the drug to avoid potential serious adverse reactions in the breastfed infant.

Nursing Considerations

- Monitor closely patient's blood pressure, especially when therapy starts and dosage increases. Also know that excessive hypotension, although rare, may occur in hypertensive patients when captopril is used in patients with heart failure or those who are undergoing renal dialysis or in patients with salt/volume depletion (such as occurs with vigorous treatment with diuretics). Keep patient supine if hypotension occurs.
- Monitor patient's blood pressure and electrolytes routinely if patient is receiving other drugs that also affect the renin–angiotensin system because hypotension and hyperkalemia may occur.
- Monitor renal function tests for signs of nephrotic syndrome, such as proteinuria and increased BUN and serum creatinine levels. Also watch for such renal evidence as oliguria, polyuria, and urinary frequency or other signs of impaired renal function, especially in patients who are receiving other drugs that also affect the renin–angiotensin system.
- Monitor WBC regularly, as ordered, especially if patient has collagen vascular disease or renal disease.

PATIENT TEACHING

- Instruct patient to take captopril 1 hour before meals.
- Tell patient to rise slowly from sitting or lying to minimize orthostatic hypotension.
- Tell patient to avoid sunlight or wear sunscreen in direct sunlight because photosensitivity may occur.
- Warn patient not to stop taking drug abruptly.
- Urge patient not to use salt substitutes that contain potassium and to consult prescriber before increasing potassium intake, to avoid increasing risk of hyperkalemia.
- Urge patient to tell prescriber about signs and symptoms of infection, such as sore throat or fever.
- Advise female patient of childbearing age to notify prescriber immediately if pregnancy occurs.

carbamazepine

Carbatrol, Epitol, Equetro, Tegretol, Tegretol-XR

Class and Category

Pharmacologic class: Iminostilbene derivative
Therapeutic class: Analgesic, anticonvulsant

Indications and Dosages

* *To treat epilepsy with generalized tonic–clonic seizures, mixed seizure patterns, and partial seizures with complex symptomatology*

E.R. CAPSULES (CARBATROL), E.R. TABLETS (TEGRETOL-XR)

Adults and children age 12 and over. *Initial:* 200 mg twice daily. Increased weekly by up to 200 mg daily, if needed, and given in divided doses twice daily. *Maximum:* 1,600 mg daily in adults, 1,200 mg daily in children age 16 to 18, and 1,000 mg daily in children ages 12 to 15.

Children ages 6 to 12. *Initial:* 100 mg twice daily. Increased weekly by 100 mg daily, if needed, and given in divided doses twice daily. *Maximum:* 1,000 mg daily.

E.R. CAPSULES (EQUETRO)

Adults and children age 12 and over. *Initial:* 200 mg twice daily. Increased weekly by up to 200 mg daily, if needed, and given in divided doses twice daily. *Maximum:* 1,600 mg daily in adults, 1,200 mg daily in children ages 16 to 18, and 1,000 mg daily in children ages 12 to 15.

Children under the age of 12.
Individualized and based on body weight with dosage under 35 mg/kg/24 hr. *Maximum:* 35 mg/kg/24 hr.

ORAL SUSPENSION (TEGRETOL)

Adults and children age 12 and over.
Initial: 100 mg four times daily. Increased weekly by up to 200 mg daily, if needed, given in divided doses three times daily or four times daily. *Maximum:* 1,600 mg daily in adults, 1,200 mg daily in children age 16 and over, and 1,000 mg daily in children ages 12 to 15.

Children ages 6 to 12. *Initial:* 50 mg four times daily. Increased weekly by 100 mg daily, if needed, given in divided doses three times daily or four times daily. *Maximum:* 1,000 mg daily.

Children up to age 6. *Initial:* 10 to 20 mg/kg/day in divided doses four times daily. *Maximum:* 35 mg/kg daily.

TABLETS (TEGRETOL)

Adults and children age 12 and over. *Initial:* **200 mg twice daily.** Increased weekly by up to 200 mg/day, if needed, given in divided doses three times daily or four times daily *Maximum:* 1,600 mg daily in adults, 1,200 mg daily in children age 16 and over, and 1,000 mg daily in children ages 12 to 15.

Children ages 6 to 12. *Initial:* 100 mg twice daily. Increased weekly by up to 100 mg daily, if needed, given in divided doses three times daily or four times daily. *Maximum:* 1,000 mg daily.

Children up to age 6. *Initial:* 10 to 20 mg/kg daily in divided doses twice daily or three times daily. Increased weekly, if needed, divided and given three times daily or four times daily. *Maximum:* 35 mg/kg/day.

✳ *To relieve pain in trigeminal neuralgia*

E.R. TABLETS (TEGRETOL-XR), TABLETS (TEGRETOL)

Adults. *Initial:* 100 mg twice daily. Increased by up to 200 mg daily, if needed, in increments of 100 mg every 12 hr. *Maintenance:* 200 to 1,200 mg daily although usual maintenance dosage is 400 to 800 mg/day. *Maximum:* 1,200 mg daily.

E.R. CAPSULES (CARBATROL, EQUETRO)

Adults. *Day 1:* 200 mg given as one 200-mg capsule. Increased by up to 200 mg/day, if needed, in increments of 100 mg every 12 hr. *Maintenance:* 200 mg to 1,200 mg daily with usual dosage between 400 to 800 mg daily. *Maximum:* 1,200 mg daily.

ORAL SUSPENSION (TEGRETOL)

Adults. 50 mg four times daily. Increased by up to 200 mg daily, if needed, in increments of 50 mg four times daily. *Maintenance:* 400 to 800 mg daily. *Maximum:* 1,200 mg daily.

✳ *To treat acute manic and mixed episodes in bipolar disorder*

E.R. CAPSULES (EQUETRO)

Adults. *Initial:* 200 mg twice daily, increased as needed in 200-mg increments. *Maximum:* 1,600 mg daily.

Drug Administration

P.O.

- Shake oral suspension well before administering and use a calibrated device to measure dosage.
- *Incompatibility: with oral suspension:* Other liquid medications or diluents, especially liquid chlorpromazine or thioridazine (a precipitate may form).
- Administer tablets with food.
- Examine tablets before administration for chips or cracks. If present, discard and obtain new one.
- E.R. capsules or tablets should not be chewed or crushed. In addition, tablets should not be split.
- E.R. capsules may be opened and sprinkled over a teaspoon of soft food such as applesauce for administration if patient has difficulty swallowing. E.R. capsules need not be taken with food.

Route	Onset	Peak	Duration
P.O.	Unknown	4.5 hr	Unknown
P.O./E.R.	Unknown	3–12 hr	Unknown
Oral susp.	Unknown	1.5 hr	Unknown

Half-life: 10–40 hr

Contraindications

Concurrent therapy with boceprevir, delavirdine or other non-nucleoside reverse transcriptase inhibitors, or nefazodone; history of bone marrow depression; hypersensitivity to carbamazepine, tricyclic compounds, or their components; MAO inhibitor therapy within 14 days

Interactions

DRUGS

acetaminophen (long-term use): Increased metabolism, leading to acetaminophen-induced hepatotoxicity or decreased acetaminophen effectiveness

acetazolamide, aprepitant, cimetidine, ciprofloxacin, clarithromycin, danazol, delavirdine or other non-nucleoside reverse transcriptase inhibitors, diltiazem, erythromycin, fluconazole, fluoxetine, fluvoxamine, ibuprofen, isoniazid, itraconazole, ketoconazole, loratadine, macrolides, niacinamide, nicotinamide, olanzapine, omeprazole, oxybutynin, propoxyphene, protease inhibitors, terfenadine, ticlopidine, trazodone, troleandomycin, verapamil, voriconazole: Increased blood carbamazepine level

albendazole, alprazolam, amitriptyline, apixaban, aripiprazole, bupropion, buspirone,

citalopram, clobazam, clonazepam, clozapine, corticosteroids, dabigatran, delavirdine, desipramine, diazepam, dicumarol, doxycycline, edoxaban, ethosuximide, felbamate, felodipine, haloperidol, itraconazole, lamotrigine, levothyroxine, methadone, midazolam, nefazodone, nortriptyline, olanzapine, oral and other hormonal contraceptives, oxcarbazepine, phenytoin, praziquantel, protease inhibitors, quetiapine, risperidone, rivaroxaban, theophylline, topiramate, tramadol, trazodone, triazolam, valproate, warfarin, ziprasidone, zonisamide: Decreased blood levels of these drugs
aminophylline, cisplatin, doxorubicin, felbamate, fosphenytoin, loxapine, phenobarbital, phenytoin, primidone, quetiapine, rifampin, theophylline, valproic acid: Decreased blood carbamazepine level
cyclophosphamide: Possibly increased cyclophosphamide toxicity
furosemide, hydrochlorothiazide: Possibly increased risk of symptomatic hyponatremia
isoniazid: Increased risk of carbamazepine toxicity and isoniazid hepatotoxicity
hormonal contraceptives: Possibly less effectiveness of hormonal contraceptives
lithium: Increased risk of CNS toxicity
MAO inhibitors: Increased risk of serotonin syndrome
nondepolarizing neuromuscular blockers: Possibly reduced duration or decreased effectiveness of neuromuscular blocker
oral anticoagulants (direct acting such as apixaban, dabigatran, edoxaban, rivaroxaban): Increased metabolism and decreased effectiveness of anticoagulant

FOODS
grapefruit juice: Increased blood carbamazepine level

ACTIVITIES
alcohol use: Increased sedative effect

Adverse Reactions

CNS: Chills, confusion, dizziness, drowsiness, fatigue, fever, headache, **suicidal ideation**, syncope, talkativeness, unsteadiness, visual hallucinations
CV: Arrhythmias, including AV block; edema; **heart failure;** hypertension; **hypotension; thromboembolism;** thrombophlebitis; worsened coronary artery disease
EENT: Blurred vision, conjunctivitis, dry mouth, glossitis, **laryngeal edema,** nystagmus, oculomotor disturbances, stomatitis, tinnitus, transient diplopia
ENDO: Syndrome of inappropriate ADH secretion, water intoxication
GI: Abdominal pain, anorexia, constipation, diarrhea, dyspepsia, elevated liver enzymes, **hepatitis,** jaundice, nausea, **pancreatitis,** vanishing bile duct syndrome, vomiting
GU: Acute urine retention, albuminuria, **azotemia,** glycosuria, impotence, oliguria, **renal failure,** urinary frequency
HEME: Acute intermittent porphyria, **agranulocytosis, aplastic anemia, bone marrow depression,** eosinophilia, leukocytosis, **leukopenia, pancytopenia, thrombocytopenia**
MS: Arthralgia, leg cramps, myalgia, osteoporosis
RESP: Pulmonary hypersensitivity (dyspnea, fever, pneumonia, or pneumonitis)
SKIN: Aggravation of disseminated lupus erythematosus, alopecia, altered skin pigmentation, diaphoresis, **erythema multiforme,** erythema nodosum, **exfoliative dermatitis,** nail shedding (onychomadesis), photosensitivity reactions, pruritic and

Mechanism of Action

Normally, sodium moves into a neuronal cell by passing through a gated sodium channel in the cell membrane. Carbamazepine may prevent or halt seizures by closing or blocking sodium channels, as shown here, thus preventing sodium from entering the cell. Keeping sodium out of the cell may slow nerve impulse transmission, thus slowing the rate at which neurons fire.

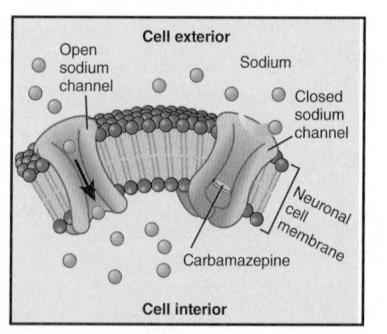

erythematous rash, purpura, **Stevens–Johnson syndrome, toxic epidermal necrolysis**, urticaria
Other: Adenopathy, **anaphylaxis, angioedema, drug reaction with eosinophilia and systemic symptoms (DRESS), multiorgan hypersensitivity or other hypersensitivity, hypocalcemia, hypogammaglobulinemia, hyponatremia,** lymphadenopathy

☰ Childbearing Considerations
PREGNANCY
- Pregnancy exposure registry: 1-888-233-2334 or http://www.aedpregnancyregistry.org/.
- Drug can cause fetal harm including anomalies of various body systems such as cardiovascular malformations, congenital malformations such as spina bifida, and developmental disorders.
- Drug should not be used in pregnancy unless the benefit to the mother outweighs the potential risk to the fetus.
- Be aware that drug should not be discontinued abruptly if used to prevent major seizures in mother because of potential for status epilepticus.
- There is a higher incidence of teratogenic effects associated with the use of anticonvulsants in combination therapy so if therapy must be continued in pregnancy, monotherapy is recommended.

LACTATION
- Drug is present in breast milk.
- A decision should be made to discontinue breastfeeding or the drug to avoid potential serious adverse reactions in the breastfed infant.

☰ Nursing Considerations
- Avoid using carbamazepine in patients with a history of hepatic porphyria because it may prompt an acute attack. Also, be aware that the Tegretol brand suspension contains sorbitol and should not be given to a patient with fructose intolerance.

! **WARNING** Note patient's ancestry. If patient has Asian ancestry, make sure he has been evaluated for the genetic allelic variant HLA-B 1502 before starting carbamazepine therapy. If patient has African-American, Chinese, European, Indian including Native American, Japanese, Korean, Latin American, Taiwanese, or Thai ancestry, make sure he has been evaluated for the genetic allelic variant HLA-A 3101 before starting carbamazepine therapy. Patients positive for HLA-A 3101 or HLA-B 1502 shouldn't take carbamazepine because of the risk of serious, sometimes fatal, dermatologic reactions. The risk is between 5% and 15% in patients with these variants.

- Use carbamazepine cautiously in patients with impaired hepatic function because it's mainly metabolized in the liver. Monitor liver function tests, as directed.

! **WARNING** Be aware that anaphylaxis and angioedema may occur in patients after taking the first or subsequent doses of carbamazepine. Monitor patient closely.

- Monitor patient closely for other adverse reactions because many of them are serious and some can become life-threatening, such as DRESS multiorgan hypersensitivity.
- Periodically monitor blood carbamazepine level, as ordered, to assess for therapeutic and toxic levels; a blood level of 6 to 12 mcg/ml is optimal for anticonvulsant effects.
- Monitor patient's electrolytes, especially sodium level, as ordered. Hyponatremia may occur as an adverse reaction to carbamazepine therapy, especially in the elderly and patients treated with diuretics. Assess patient regularly for signs and symptoms of hyponatremia such as confusion, difficulty concentrating, headache, memory impairment, unsteadiness, and weakness. If present, notify prescriber and expect drug to be discontinued.

! **WARNING** Monitor WBC and platelet counts monthly for first 2 months. Decreased counts may indicate bone marrow depression. Monitor patient closely, especially for agranulocytosis or aplastic anemia.

- Monitor patient closely for evidence of suicidal thinking or behavior, especially when therapy starts or dosage changes.

C

- Withdraw carbamazepine gradually to minimize risk of seizures.
- Monitor renal function in patients who are receiving carbamazepine intravenously, as they may be at greater risk of developing adverse effects on the renal system. Know that intravenous form should not be used in patients with moderate or severe renal impairment.

PATIENT TEACHING
- Tell patient to take carbamazepine with food (except the oral suspension form, which shouldn't be taken with other liquid drugs or diluents and extended-release capsules).
- Inform patient that coating of E.R. tablets isn't absorbed and may appear in stool.
- Advise patient not to crush or chew E.R. capsules or tablets. If he can't swallow capsules whole, have him open them and sprinkle contents on soft food.

! **WARNING** Instruct patient to seek immediate medical care and to stop taking carbamazepine if difficulty in breathing or swallowing occurs or swelling of eyes, face, lips, or tongue develops.

- Urge patient to wear sunscreen and protective clothing to reduce photosensitivity.
- Warn patient about possible blurred vision, dizziness, and unsteadiness.
- Tell patient to report bruising, fever, mouth ulcers, rash, or unusual bleeding or bruising.
- Tell female patient of childbearing age that drug decreases oral contraceptive effectiveness, and urge her to use different contraception. Because drug may cause fetal harm, tell her to notify prescriber about possible pregnancy.
- Instruct caregivers to watch patient closely for evidence of suicidal tendencies, especially when therapy starts or dosage changes, and to report such tendencies to prescriber immediately.
- Advise patient to inform all prescribers of carbamazepine therapy. This is especially important if patient has had a hypersensitivity reaction to carbamazepine because about one-third of such patients will also experience hypersensitivity to oxcarbazepine.

cariprazine hydrochloride
Vraylar

Class and Category
Pharmacologic class: Atypical antipsychotic
Therapeutic class: Antipsychotic

Indications and Dosages
✳ *To treat schizophrenia*

CAPSULES

Adults. *Initial:* 1.5 mg once daily, then increased to 3 mg once daily on day 2, as needed, with further increases in 1.5-mg to 3-mg increments, as needed. *Usual:* 1.5 mg to 6 mg once daily. *Maximum:* 6 mg once daily.

✳ *To treat acute manic or mixed episodes associated with bipolar I disorder*

CAPSULES

Adults. *Initial:* 1.5 mg once daily, then increased to 3 mg once daily on day 2, with further increases in 1.5- to 3-mg increments, as needed. *Usual:* 3 mg to 6 mg once daily. *Maximum:* 6 mg once daily.

✳ *To treat depressive episodes associated with bipolar I disorder*

CAPSULES

Adults. *Initial:* 1.5 mg once daily, increased to 3 mg once daily on day 15, as needed and tolerated. *Maximum:* 3 mg once daily.

±**DOSAGE ADJUSTMENT** For patient initiating cariprazine therapy while already taking a strong CYP3A4 inhibitor, a dose of 1.5 mg given on day 1 and day 3 with no dose on day 2. From day 4 onward, 1.5 mg daily given with possible increase to a maximum dose of 3 mg daily, as needed. For patient prescribed a strong CYP3A4 inhibitor after being on a stable dose of cariprazine, dosage reduced by half; if patient is taking 4.5 mg daily, dosage decreased to 1.5 or 3 mg daily; if patient is taking 1.5 mg, dosing frequency reduced to every other day.

Drug Administration
P.O.
- Capsules should be swallowed whole and not chewed, crushed, or opened.
- Protect 3-mg and 4.5-mg capsules from light to prevent potential color fading.

Route	Onset	Peak	Duration
P.O.	Unknown	3–6 hr	Unknown

Half-life: 2–4 days

Mechanism of Action

May produce antipsychotic effects through partial agonist and antagonist actions. Cariprazine acts as a partial agonist at dopamine (especially D2) receptors and serotonin (especially 5-HT1A) receptors. The drug acts as an antagonist at 5-HT2A serotonin receptor sites.

Contraindications

Hypersensitivity to cariprazine or its components

Interactions

DRUGS

CYP3A4 inducers such as carbamazepine, rifampin: Possibly decreased effectiveness of cariprazine
CYP3A4 strong inhibitors such as itraconazole, ketoconazole: Increased exposure of cariprazine and risks of adverse reactions

Adverse Reactions

CNS: Agitation, akathisia, anxiety, body temperature dysregulation, **CVA**, dystonia, dizziness, extrapyramidal symptoms, fatigue, fever, headache, insomnia, **neuroleptic malignant syndrome**, Parkinsonism, restlessness, **seizures**, somnolence, **suicidal ideation**, syncope, tardive dyskinesia
CV: Hyperlipidemia, hypertension, orthostatic hypotension, tachycardia
EENT: Blurred vision, dry mouth, nasopharyngitis, oropharyngeal pain
ENDO: **Diabetic ketoacidosis**, hyperglycemia **(may be extreme)**, **hyperosmolar coma**
GI: Abdominal pain, anorexia, constipation, diarrhea, dyspepsia, dysphagia, elevated liver enzymes, nausea, vomiting
GU: UTI
HEME: **Agranulocytosis, leukopenia, neutropenia**
MS: Arthralgia, back or extremity pain, elevated creatine phosphokinase, musculoskeletal stiffness, **rhabdomyolysis**
RESP: Cough
SKIN: Rash, **Stevens–Johnson syndrome**
Other: **Hyponatremia**, weight gain

Childbearing Considerations

PREGNANCY

- Pregnancy exposure registry: 1-866-961-2388 or http://womensmentalhealth.org/clinical-and-research-programs/pregnancyregistry/
- It is not known if drug can cause fetal harm. However, neonates exposed to antipsychotic drugs such as cariprazine during the third trimester are at risk for extrapyramidal and/or withdrawal symptoms following delivery.
- Use with caution only if the benefit to the mother outweighs the potential risk to the fetus.

LACTATION

- It is not known if drug is present in breast milk.
- Patient should check with prescriber before breastfeeding.

Nursing Considerations

- Know that cariprazine should not be given to patients with severe hepatic or renal impairment nor to patients receiving a CYP3A4 inducer.
- Be aware that cariprazine should not be used to treat dementia-related psychosis in the elderly because of an increased risk of death.
- Use cautiously in patients with CV disease, cerebrovascular disease, seizure disorders, or conditions that would predispose them to hypotension. Also use cautiously in elderly patients because of increased risk of serious adverse effects such as MI or stroke.
- Monitor patient for difficulty swallowing or excessive somnolence, which could predispose to accidental injury or aspiration.
- Watch patient closely for suicidal tendencies, particularly when therapy starts and with dosage changes.

! **WARNING** Know that atypical antipsychotics such as cariprazine rarely may cause neuroleptic malignant syndrome, seizures, or tardive dyskinesia. Monitor patient closely throughout therapy, and take safety precautions as needed.

- Monitor patient's CBC, as ordered, because serious adverse hematologic reactions may occur, such as agranulocytosis, leukopenia, and neutropenia. Assess more often during first few months of therapy if patient has a history of drug-induced leukopenia or neutropenia or a significantly low WBC count. If abnormalities occur during therapy, watch for fever or other signs of infection, notify prescriber, and, if severe, expect drug to be discontinued.

- Monitor patient's blood glucose level, lipid levels, and weight, as ordered, because atypical antipsychotic drugs such as cariprazine may cause metabolic changes. If patient is already a diabetic, monitor blood glucose levels more closely.

- Assess patient for late-occurring adverse reactions, especially akathisia or extrapyramidal symptoms that may first appear several weeks after cariprazine therapy begins. Also be on the alert for an increase in adverse reactions after each dosage increase. If late-effect adverse reactions occur, notify prescriber, and expect dosage to be reduced or drug discontinued.

PATIENT TEACHING

- Tell patient to swallow capsule whole and not to chew, crush, or open it.
- Advise patient to get up slowly from a lying or sitting position during cariprazine therapy to minimize orthostatic hypotension and syncope.
- Instruct patient to avoid hazardous activities until drug's effects are known. Also, alert patient and family of increased risk for falls, especially if patient has other medical conditions or takes medication that may affect the nervous system.
- Urge patient to avoid activities that raise body temperature suddenly, such as strenuous exercise and exposure to situations that cause dehydration.
- Instruct patient to inform all prescribers of any drugs she's taking, including OTC drugs, because of risk of interactions.
- Advise female patient of childbearing age to notify prescriber if she intends to become or suspects that she is pregnant during therapy.
- Instruct diabetic patient to monitor blood glucose levels closely.
- Urge family or caregiver to watch patient closely for suicidal tendencies, especially when therapy is started and dosage changes are made.

carisoprodol
Soma

Class and Category
Pharmacologic class: Carbamate derivative
Therapeutic class: Skeletal muscle relaxant
Controlled substance schedule: IV

Indications and Dosages
✳ *As adjunct to relieve acute musculoskeletal pain and stiffness*

TABLETS

Adults and adolescents over age 16. 250 to 350 mg three times daily and at bedtime. *Maximum:* 3 weeks duration of therapy.

Drug Administration
P.O.
- Administer with a meal if GI upset occurs.
- Store tablets in a tight container at room temperature away from light and moisture.

Route	Onset	Peak	Duration
P.O.	30 min	1.5–2 hr	4–6 hr

Half-life: 2 hr

Mechanism of Action
Blocks interneuronal activity in descending reticular formation and spinal cord, producing muscle relaxation and sedation.

Contraindications
History of acute, intermittent porphyria; hypersensitivity to carisoprodol, its components, or to meprobamate-related compounds

Interactions
DRUGS
CNS depressants, psychotropic drugs: Additive CNS depression
CYP2C19 inducers such as rifampin or St. John's wort: Decreased carisoprodol level
CYP2C19 inhibitors such as fluvoxamine, omeprazole: Increased blood carisoprodol level

ACTIVITIES
alcohol use: Additive CNS depression

Adverse Reactions
CNS: Agitation, ataxia, depression, dizziness, drowsiness, fever, headache, insomnia, irritability, **seizures**, somnolence, syncope, tremor, vertigo

CV: Orthostatic hypotension, tachycardia
EENT: Diplopia, transient vision loss
GI: Epigastric discomfort, hiccups, nausea, vomiting
HEME: Eosinophilia
SKIN: **Erythema multiforme**, facial flushing, pruritus, rash
Other: Drug dependence or withdrawal

Childbearing Considerations
PREGNANCY
- It is not known if drug can cause fetal harm.
- Use with caution only if benefit to mother outweighs potential risk to fetus.

LACTATION
- Drug is present in breast milk.
- Patient should check with prescriber before breastfeeding.
- Breastfed infant should be monitored for drowsiness.

Nursing Considerations
- Use carisoprodol cautiously in patients with history of drug addiction and in patients taking other CNS depressants, including alcohol.
- Know that carisoprodol therapy should last no longer than 3 weeks.
- Monitor patient closely for hypersensitivity or idiosyncratic reactions. They typically occur before the fourth dose in patients who have no previous carisoprodol exposure.
- Provide rest and other pain-relief measures.
- Expect to taper therapy as prescribed, rather than stopping it abruptly, in order to avoid mild withdrawal symptoms.

PATIENT TEACHING
- Tell patient to take carisoprodol with meals if GI distress occurs.
- Caution patient that drug dependence and withdrawal may occur, especially if therapy lasts a long time or patient changes dosage without consulting prescriber.
- Warn patient about possible dizziness, drowsiness, syncope, and vertigo. Discourage hazardous activities, such as driving, until effects of drug are known.
- Inform patient that abruptly stopping drug can cause headache, insomnia, nausea, and other adverse reactions.
- Instruct patient to avoid alcohol and other CNS depressants while taking drug.

- Explain that saliva, sweat, and urine may appear darker (red, brown, or black). Reassure him that this discoloration is harmless but may stain garments.
- Tell patient to store drug in a tightly capped container at room temperature.
- Tell patient not to store drug in bathroom, near kitchen sink, or in other damp places to protect it from heat and moisture.
- Advise mothers who are breastfeeding while taking carisoprodol to monitor the infant for sedation.

carvedilol
Coreg

carvedilol phosphate
Coreg CR

Class and Category
Pharmacologic class: Nonselective beta blocker and alpha-1 blocker
Therapeutic class: Antihypertensive, heart failure treatment adjunct

Indications and Dosages
✳ *To control hypertension*
TABLETS (COREG)
Adults. 6.25 mg twice daily for 7 to 14 days, if tolerated. Then dosage increased to 12.5 mg twice daily for 7 to 14 days, and then up to 25 mg twice daily, if tolerated and needed. *Maximum:* 50 mg daily.
E.R. CAPSULES (COREG CR)
Adults. *Initial:* 20 mg once daily. After 7 to 14 days, increased to 40 mg once daily. After another 7 to 14 days, increased to 80 mg once daily. *Maximum:* 80 mg once daily.
✳ *As adjunct to treat mild to severe chronic heart failure of ischemic or cardiomyopathic origin*
TABLETS (COREG)
Adults. 3.125 mg twice daily for 2 wk; then increased to 6.25, 12.5, and 25 mg twice daily at successive 2-wk intervals, as tolerated. *Maximum for patients with mild to moderate heart failure:* 50 mg twice daily if patient weighs more than 85 kg (187 lb).
E.R. CAPSULES (COREG CR)
Adults. *Initial:* 10 mg once daily for 2 wk. Then increased to 20 mg once daily, as

needed. Subsequent dosage increased by 20 mg every 2 wk, as needed. *Maximum:* 80 mg once daily.

✳ *To reduce CV mortality after acute phase of MI in patients with left ventricular ejection fraction of 40% or less*

TABLETS (COREG)

Adults. 6.25 mg twice daily for 3 to 10 days, if tolerated. Then dosage increased to 12.5 mg twice daily for 3 to 10 days and up to 25 mg twice daily, if needed and tolerated.

E.R. CAPSULES (COREG CR)

Adults. *Initial:* 10 to 20 mg once daily. After 3 to 10 days, increased to 20 to 40 mg once daily. Increased again as needed every 3 to 10 days until reaching tolerance or target dose of 80 mg once daily. *Maximum:* 80 mg once daily.

±**DOSAGE ADJUSTMENT** For patient with fluid retention or low blood pressure or heart rate, starting dosage may be decreased, titration may be slowed, or both.

≋ Drug Administration

P.O.

- Administer tablets with food.
- Administer E.R. capsules with food in the morning.
- E.R. capsules should be swallowed whole and not chewed or crushed. Capsule may be opened and contents sprinkled on a spoonful of cold applesauce if swallowing a capsule is difficult. Administer immediately. Mixture should not be chewed.

Route	Onset	Peak	Duration
P.O.	30 min	1–2 hr	7–10 hr
P.O./E.R.	30 min	5 hr	24 hr

Half-life: 7–10 hr

≋ Mechanism of Action

Reduces cardiac output and tachycardia, causes vasodilation, and decreases peripheral vascular resistance, which reduces blood pressure and cardiac workload. When given for at least 4 weeks, carvedilol reduces plasma renin activity.

≋ Contraindications

Bronchial asthma or related bronchospastic conditions; cardiogenic shock; decompensated heart failure that requires I.V. inotropics; history of serious hypersensitivity reactions, such as anaphylaxis, angioedema, or Stevens–Johnson syndrome; hypersensitivity to carvedilol or its components; second- or third-degree AV block, severe bradycardia, or sick sinus syndrome unless pacemaker is in place; severe hepatic impairment

≋ Interactions

DRUGS

amiodarone; other CYP2C9 inhibitors, such as fluconazole: Increased risk of bradycardia or heart block

anesthetic agents that depress myocardial function (such as cyclopropane, trichloroethylene): Increased risk of depressed myocardial function

beta blockers, digoxin: Increased risk of bradycardia and hypotension

calcium channel blockers (especially diltiazem and verapamil): Abnormal cardiac conduction

catecholamine-depleting drugs (such as MAO inhibitors, reserpine): Additive effects, increased risk of severe bradycardia and hypotension

cyclosporine, digoxin: Increased blood levels of these drugs

insulin, oral antidiabetics: Increased risk of hypoglycemia

potent CYP2D6 inhibitors such as fluoxetine, paroxetine, propafenone, quinidine: Possibly increased blood carvedilol levels

rifampin: Decreased significantly blood carvedilol level

≋ Adverse Reactions

CNS: Asthenia, **CVA**, depression, dizziness, fatigue, fever, headache, hypesthesia, hypotonia, insomnia, light-headedness, malaise, paresthesia, somnolence, syncope, vertigo

CV: Angina, **AV block**, **bradycardia**, edema, **heart failure**, hyperglycemia, hypertension, hypertriglyceridemia, orthostatic hypotension, palpitations, peripheral vascular disorder

EENT: Blurred vision, dry eyes, periodontitis, pharyngitis, rhinitis

ENDO: Hyperglycemia, **hypoglycemia**

GI: Abdominal pain, diarrhea, elevated liver enzymes, jaundice, **melena**, nausea, vomiting

GU: Albuminuria, hematuria, elevated BUN and creatinine levels, impotence, incontinence, **renal insufficiency**, UTI

HEME: Aplastic anemia, decreased PT, thrombocytopenia, unusual bleeding or bruising
MS: Arthralgia, arthritis, back pain, muscle cramps
RESP: Dyspnea, increased cough, interstitial pneumonitis
SKIN: Erythema multiforme, pruritus, purpura, Stevens–Johnson syndrome, toxic epidermal necrolysis, urticaria
Other: Anaphylaxis, angioedema, gout, hyperkalemia, hyperuricemia, hyponatremia, hypovolemia, viral infection, weight gain or loss

Childbearing Considerations

PREGNANCY

- It is not known if drug can cause fetal harm. However, use of beta blockers during the third trimester of pregnancy may increase the risk of neonatal bradycardia, hypoglycemia, hypotension, and respiratory depression.
- Use with caution only if benefit to mother outweighs potential risk to fetus.

LACTATION

- It is not known if drug is present in breast milk.
- Patient should check with prescriber before breastfeeding.

Nursing Considerations

- Use carvedilol cautiously in patients with peripheral vascular disease because it may aggravate symptoms of arterial insufficiency. In patients with diabetes mellitus it may mask signs of hypoglycemia, such as tachycardia, and may delay recovery.
- Monitor patient's blood glucose level, as ordered, during carvedilol therapy because drug may alter blood glucose level.

! **WARNING** Avoid stopping drug abruptly in patients with hyperthyroidism because thyroid storm may occur, and in patients with angina because it may worsen or MI may occur.

- Know that if patient has heart failure, expect to also give digoxin, a diuretic, and an ACE inhibitor.
- Be aware that chronic beta blocker therapy such as carvedilol is not routinely withheld prior to major surgery because the benefits outweigh the risks associated with its use with general anesthesia and surgical procedures.

PATIENT TEACHING

- Advise patient prescribed tablet form to take drug with food.
- Instruct patient to swallow extended-release capsules whole. If swallowing capsules is difficult, tell patient he may open capsule and sprinkle beads on a spoonful of cold applesauce and then eat the applesauce immediately without chewing. Tell patient to take capsule form in the morning with food.
- Warn patient that drug may cause dizziness, light-headedness, and orthostatic hypotension; advise him to take precautions.
- Tell patient with heart failure to notify prescriber if he gains 5 lb or more in 2 days or if shortness of breath increases, which may signal worsening heart failure.
- Alert patient with diabetes to monitor his glycemic control closely because drug may increase blood glucose level or mask symptoms of hypoglycemia.
- Emphasize the need to seek emergency care if patient develops hives or swelling of the face, lips, tongue, or throat that causes trouble swallowing or breathing.
- Advise patient to notify ophthalmologist of carvedilol therapy because if cataract surgery is required, modifications of the surgical technique may be necessary.
- Tell patient to notify prescriber of all medications taken, including over-the-counter preparations, before using them.
- Tell women of childbearing age to inform prescriber if pregnancy is known or suspected, as safety in pregnancy is unknown. Also, tell mothers wishing to breastfeed to discuss this decision with prescriber before doing so.

caspofungin acetate
Cancidas

Class and Category

Pharmacologic class: Echinocandins
Therapeutic class: Antifungal

Indications and Dosages

✽ *To treat invasive aspergillosis in patients refractory to or intolerant of other therapies;*

to treat candidemia and candidal infections in intra-abdominal abscesses, peritonitis, and pleural space infections

I.V. INFUSION

Adults. *Initial:* 70 mg on day 1, followed by 50 mg once daily for at least 14 days after last positive culture for candidemia and other candidal infections; duration individualized for invasive aspergillosis.

Children ages 3 months to 17 years. *Initial:* 70 mg/m^2 on day 1, followed by 50 mg/m^2 once daily and increased to 70 mg/m^2 once daily, if needed and tolerated. Continued at least 14 days after last positive culture for candidemia and other candidal infections; duration individualized for invasive aspergillosis. *Maximum:* 70 mg once daily for both loading and maintenance doses.

✷ *To treat presumed fungal infections in febrile, neutropenic patients*

I.V. INFUSION

Adults. *Initial:* 70 mg on day 1, followed by 50 mg once daily for at least 14 days and continued for at least 7 days after neutropenia and symptoms have resolved. Increased to 70 mg once daily, as needed. *Maximum:* 70 mg once daily.

Children ages 3 months to 17 years. *Initial:* 70 mg/m^2 on day 1, followed by 50 mg/m^2 once daily for at least 14 days, and continued for at least 7 days after neutropenia and symptoms have resolved. *Maximum:* 70 mg once daily for both loading and maintenance doses.

✷ *To treat esophageal candidiasis*

I.V. INFUSION

Adults. 50 mg once daily for 7 to 14 days after symptoms have resolved.

Children ages 3 months to 17 years. *Initial:* 70 mg/m^2 on day 1, followed by 50 mg/m^2 once daily and increased to 70 mg/m^2, if needed. Continued for 7 to 14 days after symptoms have resolved. *Maximum:* 70 mg once daily for both loading and maintenance doses.

±**DOSAGE ADJUSTMENT** For patients with moderate hepatic insufficiency, dosage reduced to 35 mg daily after initial 70-mg loading dose, if a loading dose is required. For patients receiving carbamazepine, dexamethasone, efavirenz, nevirapine, phenytoin, or rifampin, dosage may be increased to 70 mg once daily for adults and 70 mg/m^2 once daily for children (not to exceed 70 mg daily).

☰ Drug Administration

I.V.

- Reconstitute vial by adding 10.8 ml of 0.9% Sodium Chloride Injection, Sterile Water for Injection, Bacteriostatic Water for Injection with methylparaben and propylparaben, or Bacteriostatic Water for Injection with 0.9% benzyl alcohol to the vial. Mix gently until a clear solution is obtained. Concentration will be 5 mg/ml for a 50-mg vial; 7 mg/ml for a 70-mg vial. A 50-mg vial should be used for children requiring a dose of 50 mg or less (with a concentration of 5 mg/ml) and the 70-mg vial used for a dose greater than 50 mg.
- Store reconstituted solution up to one hour at room temperature prior to further dilution.
- Dilute reconstituted solution by withdrawing prescribed dose from drug vial and adding to 250 ml of 0.9%, 0.45%, or 0.225% Sodium Chloride Injection or Lactated Ringer's Injection. Alternatively, drug can be added to a reduced volume of I.V. solution, not to exceed a final concentration of 0.5 mg/ml. Use within 24 hours if stored at room temperature or within 48 hours if refrigerated.
- Infuse slowly over 1 hour. Never administer as an I.V. bolus.
- *Incompatibilities:* Diluents containing dextrose, other drugs infused at the same time

Route	Onset	Peak	Duration
I.V.	Unknown	Unknown	Unknown

Half-life: 9–11 hr

☰ Contraindications

Hypersensitivity to caspofungin acetate or its components

☰ Interactions

DRUGS

carbamazepine, dexamethasone, efavirenz, nelfinavir, nevirapine, phenytoin, rifampin: Possibly decreased blood caspofungin level
cyclosporine: Transient increases in ALT and AST levels
tacrolimus: Possibly decreased blood tacrolimus level

⦚ Mechanism of Action

Caspofungin acetate interferes with fungal cell membrane synthesis by inhibiting the synthesis of β (1, 3)-D-glucan. A polypeptide, β (1, 3)-D-glucan is the essential component of the fungal cell membrane that makes it rigid and protective. Without it, fungal cells rupture and die. This mechanism of action is most effective against susceptible filamentous fungi, such as *Aspergillus*.

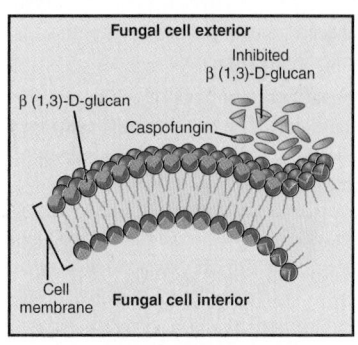

⦚ Adverse Reactions

CNS: Asthenia, anxiety, chills, confusion, depression, dizziness, fatigue, fever, headache, insomnia, paresthesia, **seizures,** somnolence, tremor, warmth sensation

CV: Hypertension, **hypotension,** peripheral edema, phlebitis, tachycardia, thrombophlebitis

EENT: Epistaxis, mucosal inflammation, **stridor**

ENDO: Hyperglycemia

GI: Abdominal distention or pain, anorexia, constipation, diarrhea, dyspepsia, elevated bilirubin or liver enzymes, **hepatic dysfunction or necrosis,** hepatomegaly, hyperbilirubinemia, jaundice, nausea, **pancreatitis,** vomiting

GU: Elevated BUN or serum creatinine level, hematuria, proteinuria, **renal failure or insufficiency,** UTI

HEME: Decreased hemoglobin, hematocrit, and white blood cell count

MS: Arthralgia, back or extremity pain, myalgia

RESP: Adult respiratory distress syndrome, bronchospasm, cough, crackles, dyspnea, **hypoxia,** pleural effusion, pneumonia, **pulmonary edema, respiratory failure,** tachypnea

SKIN: Diaphoresis, erythema, **erythema multiforme,** flushing, petechiae, pruritus, rash, sensation of warmth, skin exfoliation, **Stevens–Johnson syndrome, toxic epidermal necrolysis,** urticaria

Other: Anaphylaxis, angioedema, bacteremia, decreased serum bicarbonate level, elevated alkaline phosphatase, elevated gamma-glutamyltransferase level, **hypercalcemia, hyperkalemia,** **hyperphosphatemia, hypokalemia, hypomagnesemia,** infusion-site reaction, **sepsis, septic shock**

⦚ Childbearing Considerations

PREGNANCY

- Drug may cause fetal harm based on animal studies.
- Use with caution only if benefit to mother outweighs potential risk to fetus.

LACTATION

- It is not known if drug is present in breast milk.
- Patient should check with prescriber before breastfeeding.

⦚ Nursing Considerations

- Use cautiously in patients with a history of allergic skin reactions because caspofungin may cause serious skin reactions such as Stevens–Johnson syndrome and toxic epidermal necrolysis, which can be life-threatening.
- Watch for flushed skin, and assess patient often for unexplained temperature elevation.

! **WARNING** Monitor patient for possible histamine-mediated adverse reactions such as angioedema, bronchospasm, facial swelling, pruritus, rash, or warmth sensation. Report these symptoms immediately and expect caspofungin therapy to be discontinued.

! **WARNING** Assess for airway patency if patient develops excessive facial edema or respiratory stridor. Provide emergency airway management if complete obstruction occurs.

- Monitor patient's liver function test results, as ordered, and report abnormalities.

PATIENT TEACHING

- Urge patient to notify prescriber immediately if he has difficulty talking, swallowing, or breathing during drug administration.

! WARNING Review signs and symptoms of an allergic reaction. If present, tell patient to notify prescriber. Stress importance of seeking immediate medical treatment if reaction is severe.

- Advise women of childbearing age to report suspected or known pregnancy to prescriber, as drug may cause fetal harm.

cefaclor
Ceclor (CAN)

Class and Category
Pharmacologic class: Second-generation cephalosporin
Therapeutic class: Antibiotic

Indications and Dosages
* *To treat otitis media caused by* Haemophilus influenzae, *staphylococci,* Streptococcus pneumoniae, *or* Streptococcus pyogenes; *lower respiratory tract infections, including pneumonia caused by* H. influenzae, S. pneumoniae, *or* S. pyogenes; *pharyngitis and tonsillitis caused by* S. pyogenes; *UTI, including cystitis and pyelonephritis, caused by* Escherichia coli, Klebsiella *species,* Proteus mirabilis, *or coagulase-negative staphylococci and skin and soft-tissue infections caused by* S. pyogenes *or* Staphylococcus aureus

CAPSULES

Adults and adolescents. 250 mg every 8 hr. For severe infections, such as pneumonia, or those caused by less susceptible organisms, 500 mg every 8 hr. *Maximum:* 4 g daily.

CHEWABLE TABLETS, ORAL SUSPENSION

Adults and adolescents. 250 mg every 8 hr. For severe infections, such as pneumonia, or those caused by less susceptible organisms, 500 mg every 8 hr. *Maximum:* 4 g daily.
Children. 20 mg/kg daily in divided doses every 8 hr. For serious infections, otitis media, and infections caused by less susceptible

organisms, 40 mg/kg daily in divided doses every 8 hr. For otitis media and pharyngitis, total daily dosage divided and given every 12 hr, if needed. *Maximum:* 1 g daily.

* *To treat acute bacterial infection in chronic bronchitis or secondary bacterial infection in acute bronchitis caused by* H. influenzae, Moraxella catarrhalis, *or* S. pneumoniae

E.R. TABLETS

Adults and adolescents age 16 and over. 500 mg every 12 hr for 7 days.

* *To treat pharyngitis and tonsillitis caused by* S. pyogenes

E.R. TABLETS

Adults and adolescents age 16 and over. 375 mg every 12 hr for 10 days.

* *To treat uncomplicated skin and soft-tissue infections caused by* S. aureus

E.R. TABLETS

Adults and adolescents age 16 and over. 375 mg every 12 hr for 7 to 10 days.

Drug Administration
P.O.

- Administer drug with food or within 30 minutes of a meal.
- Capsules and E.R. tablets should be swallowed whole. Do not break or crush them.
- Give capsules or E.R. tablets with a full glass of water.
- Patient must chew chewable tablets before swallowing.
- Shake oral suspension well before measuring and use a calibrated measuring device to measure dose.
- Refrigerate oral suspension and discard unused portion after 14 days.

Route	Onset	Peak	Duration
P.O.	Unknown	0.5–1 hr	Unknown
P.O./E.R.	Unknown	1.5–2.5 hr	Unknown

Half-life: Unknown

Mechanism of Action
Interferes with bacterial cell wall synthesis by inhibiting cross-linking of peptidoglycan strands, which stiffen cell membranes. As a result, bacterial cells rupture.

Contraindications
Hypersensitivity to cefaclor, other cephalosporins, or their components

Interactions
DRUGS
aminoglycosides, loop diuretics: Increased risk of nephrotoxicity
antacids: Decreased blood cefaclor level (E.R. tablets)
oral anticoagulants: Increased anticoagulation
probenecid: Increased serum cefaclor levels

Adverse Reactions
CNS: Chills, fever, headache, **seizures**
CV: Edema
EENT: Hearing loss, oral candidiasis
GI: Abdominal cramps, diarrhea, elevated liver enzymes, **hepatic failure**, hepatomegaly, nausea, **pseudomembranous colitis**, vomiting
GU: Elevated BUN level, **nephrotoxicity**, **renal failure**, vaginal candidiasis
HEME: Eosinophilia, **hemolytic anemia**, **hypoprothrombinemia**, **neutropenia**, **thrombocytopenia**, **unusual bleeding**
MS: Arthralgia
RESP: Dyspnea
SKIN: Ecchymosis, erythema, **erythema multiforme**, pruritus, rash, **Stevens–Johnson syndrome**
Other: **Anaphylaxis**, superinfection

Childbearing Considerations
PREGNANCY
- It is not known if drug can cause fetal harm.
- Use with caution only if benefit to mother outweighs potential risk to fetus.

LACTATION
- Drug is present in breast milk.
- Patient should check with prescriber before breastfeeding.

Nursing Considerations
- Use cefaclor cautiously in patients with impaired renal function or a history of GI disease, particularly colitis, and in patients who are hypersensitive to penicillin; about 10% of them have cross-sensitivity.
- Obtain culture and sensitivity test results, if possible and as ordered, before giving drug.
- Monitor BUN and serum creatinine levels for early signs of nephrotoxicity. Also monitor fluid intake and output; decreasing urine output may indicate nephrotoxicity.
- Be aware that an allergic reaction may occur a few days after therapy starts.

- Assess bowel pattern daily; severe diarrhea may indicate pseudomembranous colitis.
- Assess patient for superinfection: cough or sputum changes, diarrhea, drainage, fever, malaise, pain, perineal itching, rash, redness, and swelling.

PATIENT TEACHING
- Instruct patient to complete the prescribed course of therapy, even if he feels better.
- Tell patient to swallow capsules and E.R. tablets whole and not to break, chew, or crush them.
- Advise patient to take drug with food or within 30 minutes of a meal to enhance absorption.
- Instruct patient to take capsules or E.R. tablets with a full glass of water.
- Tell patient to shake oral suspension well before measuring and to use a calibrated measuring device to ensure accurate dose.
- Tell patient to refrigerate oral suspension and to discard unused portion after 14 days.
- Instruct patient to chew chewable tablets before swallowing.
- Instruct patient to report severe diarrhea to prescriber immediately.
- Explain that buttermilk and yogurt protect intestinal flora and decrease diarrhea.
- Urge patient to report evidence of superinfection.

cefazolin sodium
Cefazolin, Cefazolin and Dextrose

Class and Category
Pharmacologic class: First-generation cephalosporin
Therapeutic class: Antibiotic

Indications and Dosages
* *To treat respiratory tract infections caused by* Haemophilus influenzae, Klebsiella *species,* Staphylococcus aureus, Streptococcus pneumoniae, *or group A beta-hemolytic* streptococci; *skin and soft-tissue infections caused by* S. aureus, *group A beta-hemolytic* streptococci, *or other strains of* streptococci; *biliary or urinary tract infections caused by* Escherichia coli, Proteus mirabilis, S. aureus, *or various strains of streptococci; bone and joint infections caused by* S. aureus;

genital infections, such as epididymitis and prostatitis, caused by E. coli, Klebsiella *species,* P. mirabilis, *and some strains of* enterococci; *septicemia caused by* E. coli, Klebsiella *species,* P. mirabilis S. aureus, *and* S. pneumoniae; *and endocarditis caused by* S. aureus *or group A beta-hemolytic* streptococci

I.V. INFUSION, I.V. OR I.M. INJECTION

Adults with a creatinine clearance equal to or greater than 55 ml/min. For mild infections caused by susceptible gram-positive cocci, 250 to 500 mg every 8 hr; for moderate to severe infections, 500 to 1,000 mg every 6 to 8 hr; and for severe life-threatening infections, 1,000 to 1,500 mg every 6 hr. *Maximum:* 12 g daily in divided doses for severe, life-threatening infections. **Children with a creatinine clearance equal to or greater than 70 ml/min.** For mild to moderate infections, 25 to 50 mg/kg daily divided equally and given three times daily or four times daily; for severe infections, 100 mg/kg daily divided equally and given three times daily or four times daily.

✻ *To treat pneumococcal pneumonia*

I.V. INFUSION, I.V. OR I.M. INJECTION

Adults. 500 mg every 12 hr.

✻ *To treat acute uncomplicated UTI caused by* E. coli, Klebsiella *species, or* P. mirabilis, *and some strains of* Enterobacter *and* Enterococcus

I.V. INFUSION, I.V. OR I.M. INJECTION

Adults. 1 g every 12 hr.

✻ *To provide surgical prophylaxis*

I.V. INFUSION, I.V. OR I.M. INJECTION

Adults with a creatinine clearance equal to or greater than 55 ml/min. 1 g 30 to 60 min before surgery; 0.5 to 1 g every 6 to 8 hr for 24 hr after surgery. *For surgeries expected to last 2 hours or longer:* 2 g 30 to 60 min before surgery; 0.5 to 1 g during surgery; and 0.5 to 1 g every 6 to 8 hr for 24 hr after surgery although drug therapy may continue for 3 to 5 days after surgery if the occurrence of an infection may be devastating such as open-heart surgery or prosthetic arthroplasty.

I.V. INFUSION (CEFAZOLIN AND DEXTROSE)

Children age 10 to 17 years with a creatinine clearance equal to or greater than 70 ml/min weighing 50 kg (110 lb) or greater and undergoing a surgical procedure expected to last 2 hours or longer. 2 g 20 to 60 min before surgery; 0.5 to 1 g during surgery; and 0.5 to 1 g for 24 hours every 6 to 8 hours after surgery although drug therapy may continue for 3 to 5 days after surgery if the occurrence of an infection may be devastating, such as in open-heart surgery or prosthetic arthroplasty. **Children age 10 to 17 years with a creatinine clearance equal to or greater than 70 ml/min and weighing less than 50 kg (110 lb).** 1 g 30 to 60 min before surgery and 0.5 to 1 g every 6 to 8 hours for 24 hours after surgery.

±**DOSAGE ADJUSTMENT** After initial loading dose appropriate to infection's severity, dosage interval restricted to at least 8 hr or longer for adults with creatinine clearance of 35 to 54 ml/min; dosage reduced by 50% and given every 12 hr for adults with creatinine clearance of 11 to 34 ml/min; and dosage reduced by 50% and given every 18 to 24 hr for adults with creatinine clearance of 10 ml/min or less. Dosage reduced to 60% and given every 12 hr for children with creatinine clearance of 40 to 70 ml/min; dosage reduced to 25% and given every 12 hr for children with creatinine clearance of 20 to 40 ml/min; and dosage reduced to 10% and given every 24 hr for children with creatinine clearance of 5 to 20 ml/min.

Drug Administration

I.V.

- Only single-dose vials may be given by I.V. infusion or by I.V. or I.M. injection. ADD-Vantage vials and Duplex containers are only administered as an I.V. infusion.

ADD-Vantage vials

- Open diluent container by peeling overwrap at corner and remove solution container. Some opacity of the plastic may be present but this is normal. The opacity will diminish gradually.

- Assemble vial and flexible diluent container by removing the protective covers from the top of the vial and the vial port on the diluent container by swinging the pull ring over the top of the vial and pulling down far enough to start the opening; then pull straight up to remove the cap. To remove the vial port cover, grasp the tab on the pull ring, pulling up to break the three tie strings, then pull back to remove the cover. Screw the vial into the vial port until it will go no further. Label appropriately.

- Squeeze the bottom of the diluent container gently to inflate the portion of the container surrounding the end of the drug vial. With the other hand, push the drug vial down into the container, telescoping the walls of the container. Grasp the inner cap of the vial through the walls of the container. Pull the inner cap from the drug vial, allowing the drug and diluent to mix. Mix thoroughly.
- Prepare to administer by checking for leaks by squeezing container firmly. If present, discard and obtain a new one. Attach administration set. Lift the free end of the hanger loop on the bottom of the vial, breaking the two tie strings. Bend loop outward to lock it in the upright position, then suspend from hanger. Attach administration set.
- Administer drug as an intermittent infusion over 30 minutes.
- Drug is stable for 24 hours after reconstitution.

Single-use regular vials
- Reconstitute with 2 ml of Sterile Water for Injection for 500-mg vial and 2.5 ml of Sterile Water for Injection for 1-g vial. Shake well until dissolved. Solution will appear pale yellow to yellow.
- For direct I.V. injection, further dilute reconstituted solution with at least 5 ml of Sterile Water for Injection. Inject slowly over 3 to 5 minutes through tubing of a flowing compatible I.V. solution.
- For intermittent I.V. infusion, reconstitute 500 to 1,000 mg in 50 to 100 ml of 0.9% Sodium Chloride Injection, 5% Dextrose in Water, or 5% Lactated Ringer's Solution. See manufacturer list for other compatible solutions.
- Administer I.V. infusion over 30 minutes.
- Store reconstituted drug up to 24 hours at room temperature or 10 days refrigerated.

Duplex Container
- Keep container in folded position until activation is intended. Remove from refrigerator and allow to come to room temperature.
- Unlatch side tab and unfold container. Visually inspect diluent chamber. Use only if container and seals are intact.

- Inspect drug powder by peeling foil strip from drug chamber. Protect from light after removal of foil strip. If foil strip is removed but administration is delayed, refold container and latch side tab. Product then must be used within 7 days.
- To reconstitute, unfold container and point the set port in a downward direction. Starting at the hanger tab end, fold the container just below the diluent meniscus, trapping all air above the fold. To activate, squeeze the folded diluent chamber until the seal between the diluent and powder opens, releasing diluent into the drug powder chamber. Agitate the liquid-powder mixture until completely dissolved. Once dissolved, drug must be used within 24 hours if stored at room temperature or 7 days if refrigerated.
- To administer, point the set port in a downward direction. Starting at the hanger tab end, fold the container just below the solution meniscus, trapping all air above the fold. Squeeze the folded container until the seal between the reconstituted drug and set port opens, releasing the solution to set port. Squeeze container firmly to check for minute leaks. Then peel foil cover from the set port and attach administration set.
- Do not use in series connections.
- Do not introduce additives to the container.
- Administer as an infusion over about 30 minutes.
- *Incompatibilities:* None reported by manufacturer

I.M.
- Reconstitute with 2 ml of Sterile Water for Injection for 500-mg vial and 2.5 ml of Sterile Water for Injection for 1-g single-dose vial. Shake well until dissolved. Solution will appear pale yellow to yellow.
- Administer I.M. injection deep into large muscle mass, such as the gluteus maximus.

Route	Onset	Peak	Duration
I.V.	Immediate	Immediate	Unknown
I.M.	Unknown	1–2 hr	Unknown

Half-life: 1.8 hr

≡ Mechanism of Action
Interferes with bacterial cell wall synthesis by inhibiting the final step in the cross-linking of peptidoglycan strands. Peptidoglycan

makes cell membranes rigid and protective. Without it, bacterial cells rupture and die.

Contraindications

Hypersensitivity to cefazolin, other cephalosporins or their components

Interactions

DRUGS

aminoglycosides, loop diuretics: Additive nephrotoxicity
probenecid: Increased and prolonged blood cefazolin level due to renal excretion of cefazolin being inhibited

Adverse Reactions

CNS: Chills, confusion, dizziness, fainting, fever, headache, light-headedness, **seizures, somnolence, tiredness, weakness**
CV: Edema, **hypotension**
EENT: Hearing loss, oral candidiasis
GI: Abdominal cramps, *Clostridioides difficile–associated* **diarrhea,** diarrhea, elevated liver enzymes, **hepatic failure, hepatitis,** hepatomegaly, nausea, **pseudomembranous colitis,** vomiting
GU: Acute tubulointerstitial nephritis, elevated BUN and serum creatinine levels, **nephrotoxicity, renal failure,** vaginal candidiasis
HEME: Eosinophilia, **hemolytic anemia, hypoprothrombinemia, neutropenia, thrombocytopenia, unusual bleeding**
MS: Arthralgia
RESP: Dyspnea
SKIN: Acute generalized exanthematous pustulosis (AGEP), ecchymosis, erythema, **erythema multiforme,** pruritus, rash, **Stevens–Johnson syndrome**
Other: **Anaphylaxis;** injection-site pain, phlebitis, redness, and swelling; serum sickness–like reaction; superinfection

Childbearing Considerations

PREGNANCY

- It is not known if drug can cause fetal harm.
- Use with caution only if benefit to mother outweighs potential risk to fetus.

LACTATION

- Drug is present in breast milk.
- Patient should check with prescriber before breastfeeding.

Nursing Considerations

- Use cefazolin cautiously in patients with impaired renal function or a history of GI disease, particularly colitis. Also use cautiously in patients hypersensitive to penicillin, because cross-sensitivity has occurred in about 10% of such patients.
- Obtain culture and sensitivity test results, if possible and as ordered, before giving drug.
- Monitor I.V. site for irritation, phlebitis, and extravasation.
- Monitor BUN and serum creatinine for early signs of nephrotoxicity. Also monitor fluid intake and output; decreasing urine output may indicate nephrotoxicity.

> **! WARNING** Be aware that an allergic reaction may occur a few days after therapy starts. Monitor patient closely.

- Assess bowel pattern daily; severe diarrhea may indicate *Clostridioides difficile*–associated diarrhea or pseudomembranous colitis.
- Watch for evidence of superinfection: cough, diarrhea, drainage, fever, malaise, pain, perineal itching, rash, redness, swelling.
- Assess for arthralgia, bleeding, ecchymosis, and pharyngitis; they may indicate a blood dyscrasia.
- Institute seizure precautions and monitor patient closely for seizures, especially patients with renal impairment. If seizures occur, manage according to institutional protocol and notify prescriber. Drug may have to be discontinued or dosage adjusted.

PATIENT TEACHING

- Instruct patient to complete the prescribed course of therapy.
- Reassure patient that I.M. injection doesn't typically cause pain.

> **! WARNING** Alert patient to potential for serious allergic reactions. If present, have patient notify prescriber and if severe to seek immediate medical attention.

- Tell patient to report watery, bloody stools to prescriber immediately, even up to 2 months after drug therapy has ended.
- Warn patient of the possibility of seizures. Review seizure precautions and advise patient to notify prescriber if any occur, as drug may have to be discontinued or dosage adjusted.

- Advise diabetic patient who is testing urine for glucose to use an enzymatic glucose oxidase test while taking drug, to avoid false-positive reactions.

cefdinir

▤ Class and Category

Pharmacologic class: Third-generation cephalosporin
Therapeutic class: Antibiotic

▤ Indications and Dosages

✴ *To treat community-acquired pneumonia caused by* Haemophilus influenzae *(including beta-lactamase–producing strains),* H. parainfluenzae *(including beta-lactamase–producing strains),* Moraxella catarrhalis *(including beta-lactamase-producing strains), and* Streptococcus pneumoniae *(penicillin-susceptible strains only); acute exacerbations of chronic bronchitis caused by* H. influenzae *(including beta-lactamase–producing strains),* H. parainfluenzae *(including beta-lactamase–producing strains),* S. pneumoniae *(penicillin-susceptible strains only), and* M. catarrhalis *(including beta-lactamase–producing strains)*

CAPSULES

Adults and adolescents. 300 mg every 12 hr for 10 days for pneumonia and 5–10 days for bronchitis. *Maximum:* 600 mg daily.

✴ *To treat pharyngitis or tonsillitis caused by* Streptococcus pyogenes

CAPSULES

Adults and adolescents. 300 mg every 12 hr for 5 to 10 days or 600 mg every 24 hr for 10 days. *Maximum:* 600 mg daily.

ORAL SUSPENSION

Children ages 6 months to 12 years. 7 mg/kg every 12 hr for 5 to 10 days or 14 mg/kg every 24 hr for 10 days.

✴ *To treat acute maxillary sinusitis caused by* H. influenzae *(including beta-lactamase–producing strains),* S. pneumoniae *(penicillin-susceptible strains only), and* M. catarrhalis *(including beta-lactamase–producing strains)*

CAPSULES

Adults and adolescents. 300 mg every 12 hr or 600 mg every 24 hr for 10 days. *Maximum:* 600 mg daily.

ORAL SUSPENSION

Children ages 6 months to 12 years. 7 mg/kg every 12 hr or 14 mg/kg every 24 hr for 10 days.

✴ *To treat uncomplicated skin and soft-tissue infections caused by* Staphylococcus aureus *(including beta-lactamase–producing strains) and* S. pyogenes

CAPSULES

Adults and adolescents. 300 mg every 12 hr or 600 mg every 24 hr for 10 days. *Maximum:* 600 mg daily.

ORAL SUSPENSION

Children ages 6 months to 12 years. 7 mg/kg every 12 hr for 10 days.

✴ *To treat acute bacterial otitis media caused by* H. influenzae *(including beta-lactamase–producing strains),* S. pneumoniae *(penicillin-susceptible strains only), and* M. catarrhalis *(including beta-lactamase–producing strains)*

ORAL SUSPENSION

Children ages 6 months to 12 years. 7 mg/kg every 12 hr for 5 to 10 days or 14 mg/kg every 24 hr for 10 days.

±**DOSAGE ADJUSTMENT** For adults with creatinine clearance less than 30 ml/min, dosage not to exceed 300 mg daily; for children with creatinine clearance less than 30 ml/min, dosage not to exceed 7 mg/kg (up to 300 mg) daily. For patients undergoing intermittent hemodialysis, dosage is 300 mg or 7 mg/kg every other day, beginning at the end of each hemodialysis session.

▤ Drug Administration

P.O.

- Reconstitute cefdinir powder for oral suspension by tapping bottle to loosen powder, and then dilute with water to 125 mg/5 ml.
- Shake well before each use and use a calibrated device to measure dose.
- Keep suspension bottle tightly closed, and store it at room temperature. Discard any unused portion after 10 days.
- Capsules should be swallowed whole and not chewed, crushed, or opened.
- Give antacids that contain aluminum or magnesium and iron salts at least 2 hours before or after cefdinir.

Route	Onset	Peak	Duration
P.O.	Unknown	2–4 hr	Unknown

Half-life: 1.75 hr

Mechanism of Action

Interferes with bacterial cell wall synthesis by inhibiting the final step in the cross-linking of peptidoglycan strands. Peptidoglycan makes cell membranes rigid and protective. Without it, bacterial cells rupture and die.

Contraindications

Hypersensitivity to cefdinir, other cephalosporins, or their components

Interactions

DRUGS

antacids that contain aluminum or magnesium: Decreased cefdinir absorption if given within 2 hours of antacid
iron salts: Reduced cefdinir absorption if given within 2 hours of iron
probenecid: Increased blood level and prolonged half-life of cefdinir

Adverse Reactions

CNS: Asthenia, dizziness, drowsiness, headache, insomnia, somnolence
EENT: Dry mouth, pharyngitis, rhinitis
GI: Abdominal pain, anorexia, constipation, diarrhea, flatulence, indigestion, nausea, **pseudomembranous colitis**, stool discoloration, vomiting
GU: Leukorrhea, vaginal candidiasis, vaginitis
HEME: Leukopenia
SKIN: Pruritus, rash
Other: Anaphylaxis, serum sickness–like reaction

Childbearing Considerations

PREGNANCY

- It is not known if drug can cause fetal harm.
- Use with caution only if benefit to mother outweighs potential risk to fetus.

LACTATION

- It is not known if drug is present in breast milk.
- Patient should check with prescriber before breastfeeding.

Nursing Considerations

- Monitor patient allergic to penicillin for evidence of hypersensitivity reaction, from a mild rash to fatal anaphylaxis, because cross-sensitivity can occur.
- Monitor patient with a chronic GI condition, such as colitis, for signs and symptoms of a drug-related exacerbation.
- Know that because all cephalosporins have the potential to cause bleeding, monitor elderly patients and patients with a preexisting coagulopathy, including vitamin K deficiency, for elevated PT or APTT.
- Monitor patient closely for diarrhea, which may indicate pseudomembranous colitis caused by *Clostridium difficile*. If diarrhea occurs, notify prescriber and expect to withhold cefdinir and treat with fluids, electrolytes, protein, and an antibiotic effective against *C. difficile*.
- Assess for other evidence of superinfection, including perineal itching; loose, foul-smelling stools; and vaginal drainage.

PATIENT TEACHING

- Advise patient taking cefdinir oral suspension to shake bottle well before use and to use a liquid-measuring device to ensure accurate dose. Tell patient suspension should be discarded after 10 days.
- Instruct patient to swallow capsule form whole and not to chew or crush capsule.
- Instruct patient to complete entire course of therapy, even if he feels better.
- Advise patient to take iron salts and aluminum- or magnesium-containing antacids at least 2 hours before or after taking cefdinir.
- Inform patient with history of colitis that cefdinir may worsen it; urge him to notify prescriber promptly if symptoms develop.
- Inform patient with diabetes mellitus that oral suspension contains 2.86 g of sucrose per teaspoon; advise him to monitor his blood glucose levels as appropriate.
- Teach patient to recognize and report evidence of superinfection, such as perineal itching; loose, foul-smelling stools; and vaginal drainage.
- Inform patient that buttermilk and yogurt can help prevent superinfection and may decrease diarrhea.
- Urge patient to tell prescriber about diarrhea that's severe or lasts longer than 3 days. Remind patient that watery or bloody stools can occur 2 or more months after antibiotic therapy and can be serious, requiring prompt treatment.

cefditoren pivoxil

Class and Category

Pharmacologic class: Third-generation cephalosporin
Therapeutic class: Antibiotic

Indications and Dosages

✷ *To treat mild to moderate acute bacterial exacerbation of chronic bronchitis or community-acquired pneumonia caused by* Haemophilus influenzae *(including beta-lactamase–producing strains),* Haemophilus parainfluenzae *(including beta-lactamase–producing strains),* Streptococcus pneumoniae *(penicillin-susceptible strains), or* Moraxella catarrhalis *(including beta-lactamase–producing strains)*

TABLETS

Adults and children age 12 and over.
400 mg twice daily for 10 days or for 14 days for community-acquired pneumonia.

✷ *To treat mild to moderate pharyngitis and tonsillitis caused by* Streptococcus pyogenes

TABLETS

Adults and children age 12 and over.
200 mg twice daily for 10 days.

✷ *To treat mild to moderate uncomplicated skin and soft-tissue infections caused by* Staphylococcus aureus *(including beta-lactamase–producing strains) or* S. pyogenes

TABLETS

Adults and children age 12 and over.
200 mg twice daily for 10 days.

±**DOSAGE ADJUSTMENT** For patient with a creatinine clearance of 30 to 49 ml/min, maximum dosage reduced to 200 mg twice daily. For patient with a creatinine clearance less than 30 ml/min, maximum dosage reduced to 200 mg daily.

Drug Administration

P.O.

- Administer with meals to enhance absorption.

Route	Onset	Peak	Duration
P.O.	Unknown	1.5–3 hr	Unknown

Half-life: 1.2–2 hr

Mechanism of Action

Interferes with bacterial cell wall synthesis by inhibiting the final step in the cross-linking of peptidoglycan strands. Peptidoglycan makes the cell membrane rigid and protective. Without it, bacterial cells rupture and die. This mechanism of action is most effective against bacteria that divide rapidly, including many gram-positive and gram-negative bacteria. Cefditoren isn't inactivated by beta lactamase produced by some bacteria.

Contraindications

Carnitine deficiency or inborn metabolic disorder that causes it; hypersensitivity to cefditoren, other cephalosporins or their components, or to milk

Interactions

DRUGS

aluminum- and magnesium-containing antacids, H_2-receptor antagonists: Reduced cefditoren absorption
H_2-receptor antagonists such as famotidine: Possibly reduced absorption of cefditoren
probenecid: Increased and prolonged blood cefditoren level

FOODS

any food: Increased cefditoren absorption

Adverse Reactions

CNS: Headache, hyperactivity, hypertonia, **seizures**
GI: Abdominal pain, diarrhea, dyspepsia, **hepatic dysfunction**, nausea, **pseudomembranous colitis**, vomiting
GU: **Acute renal failure, renal dysfunction, toxic nephropathy**
HEME: **Aplastic anemia, hemolytic anemia, hemorrhage, thrombocytopenia**
MS: Arthralgia
RESP: Pneumonia
SKIN: **Erythema multiforme, Stevens–Johnson syndrome, toxic epidermal necrolysis**
Other: Allergic reaction, **anaphylaxis**, carnitine deficiency, drug fever, serum sickness–like reaction, superinfection

Childbearing Considerations

PREGNANCY

- It is not known if drug can cause fetal harm.
- Use with caution only if benefit to mother outweighs potential risk to fetus.

C

- It is not known if drug is present in breast milk.
- Patient should check with prescriber before breastfeeding.

Nursing Considerations

! **WARNING** Be aware that before starting cefditoren therapy, determine if patient is hypersensitive to milk protein because cefditoren contains sodium caseinate, a milk protein. Drug should not be given to patient with this hypersensitivity. Also determine if patient has had a hypersensitivity reaction to cefditoren or other cephalosporins (because drug is contraindicated in these patients) or to penicillin (because cross-sensitivity has occurred in about 10% of such patients).

- Know that cefditoren shouldn't be used for prolonged treatment because of the risk of carnitine deficiency.
- Obtain culture and sensitivity test results before giving cefditoren, if possible and as ordered.
- Assess patient for evidence of *Clostridium difficile* infection and pseudomembranous colitis, such as profuse, watery diarrhea. For mild cases, expect to discontinue cefditoren. For moderate to severe cases, expect to also give fluids and electrolytes, protein supplementation, and an antibacterial drug effective against *C. difficile.*
- Monitor patient for an allergic reaction. If an allergic reaction occurs, expect to discontinue drug, as prescribed. For serious acute hypersensitivity reactions, expect to also give antihistamines, corticosteroids, epinephrine, I.V. fluids, oxygen, and vasopressors, as prescribed.
- Monitor BUN and serum creatinine levels to detect early signs of renal dysfunction. Also monitor fluid intake and output.
- Watch for a decreased PT, as ordered, in at-risk patients, such as those with renal or hepatic impairment, those with a poor nutritional state, and those receiving anticoagulant or prolonged antibiotic therapy. Notify prescriber if a decrease occurs, and give vitamin K as ordered.

PATIENT TEACHING

- Urge patient to complete prescribed course of therapy.

- Instruct patient to take cefditoren with meals to enhance drug absorption.
- Advise patient not to take cefditoren with aluminum- or magnesium-containing antacids or other drugs used to reduce stomach acids because these drugs may interfere with cefditoren absorption.
- Explain that buttermilk and yogurt help maintain normal intestinal flora and can decrease diarrhea during therapy.
- Instruct patient to report severe diarrhea to prescriber immediately.

cefepime hydrochloride
Maxipime

Class and Category
Pharmacologic class: Fourth-generation cephalosporin
Therapeutic class: Antibiotic

Indications and Dosages
✳ *To treat mild to moderate UTI caused by* Escherichia coli, Klebsiella pneumoniae, *or* Proteus mirabilis

I.V. INFUSION, I.M. INJECTION (ONLY FOR UTI CAUSED BY *E. COLI*)
Adults and children age 16 and over. 500 to 1,000 mg every 12 hr for 7 to 10 days.
Children ages 2 months to 16 years weighing up to 40 kg (88 lb). 50 mg/kg/dose every 12 hr for 7 to 10 days. *Maximum:* Not to exceed adult dose.

✳ *To treat severe UTI caused by* E. coli *or* K. pneumoniae, *uncomplicated skin and soft-tissue infections caused by* Staphylococcus aureus *or* Streptococcus pyogenes

I.V. INFUSION
Adults and children age 16 and over. 2 g every 12 hr for 10 days.
Children ages 2 months to 16 years weighing up to 40 kg (88 lb). 50 mg/kg/dose every 12 hr for 10 days. *Maximum:* Not to exceed adult dose.

✳ *To treat moderate to severe pneumonia caused by* Enterobacter *species,* K. pneumoniae, Pseudomonas aeruginosa, *or* Streptococcus pneumoniae

I.V. INFUSION

Adults and children age 16 and over. 2 g every 8 hr if caused by *P. aeruginosa* or 1 to 2 g every 12 hr for other infections for 10 days.

✳ *To treat moderate to severe pneumonia caused by* P. aeruginosa

I.V. INFUSION

Children ages 2 months to 16 years weighing up to 40 kg (88 lb). 50 mg/kg/dose every 8 hr for 10 days. *Maximum:* Not to exceed adult dose.

✳ *To treat febrile neutropenia*

I.V. INFUSION

Adults and children age 16 and over. 2 g every 8 hr for 7 days or until neutropenia resolves.

Children ages 2 months to 16 years weighing up to 40 kg (88 lb). 50 mg/kg/dose every 8 hr for 7 days or until neutropenia resolves. *Maximum:* Not to exceed adult dose.

✳ *To treat complicated intra-abdominal infections (together with metronidazole) caused by* Bacteroides fragilis, E. coli, Enterobacter *species,* K. pneumoniae, P. aeruginosa, *or viridans group streptococci*

I.V. INFUSION

Adults and children age 16 and over. 2 g every 8 to 12 hr for 7 to 10 days.

±**DOSAGE ADJUSTMENT** For adult patient with creatinine clearance between 30 and 60 ml/min, dosing interval increased to every 24 hr if dosing interval had been every 12 hr, and dosing interval increased to every 12 hr if dosing interval had been every 8 hr. For adult patient with creatinine clearance between 11 and 29 ml/min, dosage decreased to 500 mg every 24 hr if dosage had been 1 g every 24 hr; dosage decreased to 1 g every 24 hr if dosage had been 2 g every 12 hr; and dosing interval decreased to 24 hr if dosing interval had been every 8 hr while maintaining a dosage of 2 g. For adult patient with creatinine clearance less than 11 ml/min, dosage decreased to 250 mg every 24 hr if dosage had been 500 mg or 1 g every 12 hr; dosage decreased to 500 mg every 24 hr if dosage had been 2 g every 12 hr; and dosage decreased to 1 g every 24 hr if dosage had been 2 g every 8 hr. For adult patient on continuous abdominal peritoneal dialysis or hemodialysis, dosage interval and dosage

further altered. For pediatric patient, dosage decreased and dosage interval increased in similar proportion as adults.

≣ Drug Administration

I.V.

- For I.V. infusion, reconstitute using manufacturer's guidelines. Reconstitution varies with product used.
- Use only solutions recommended by manufacturer, as type of diluent varies with the product used.
- Use a Y-type administration set but discontinue primary I.V. solution during cefepime infusion.
- Infuse over 30 minutes.
- Reconstituted solution is stable for 24 hours at room temperature or 7 days in refrigerator with selected diluents (see manufacturer guidelines).
- Color of solution may darken while stored but product potency is not affected.
- *Incompatibilities:* Solutions that contain ampicillin in a concentration of more than 40 mg/ml; solutions that contain aminophylline, gentamycin, metronidazole, netilmicin sulfate, tobramycin, or vancomycin

I.M.

- Reconstitute 500-mg vial of drug with 1.3 ml of diluent, such as Sterile Water for Injection (or 1-g vial with 2.4 ml of diluent). See manufacturer guidelines for complete list of appropriate diluents.
- Reconstituted solution is stable for 24 hours at room temperature or 7 days in refrigerator with selected diluents (see manufacturer guidelines).
- Color of solution may darken while stored but product potency is not affected.

Route	Onset	Peak	Duration
I.V.	Unknown	30 min	Unknown
I.M.	Unknown	1–2 hr	Unknown

Half-life: 2–2.3 hr

≣ Mechanism of Action

Interferes with bacterial cell wall synthesis by inhibiting the final step in the cross-linking of peptidoglycan strands. Peptidoglycan makes cell membranes rigid and protective. Without it, bacterial cells rupture and die.

Contraindications

Hypersensitivity to cefepime, other beta-lactam antibiotics, other cephalosporins, penicillins, or their components

Interactions

DRUGS

aminoglycosides: Increased risk of nephrotoxicity and ototoxicity
potent diuretics such as furosemide: Increased risk of nephrotoxicity

Adverse Reactions

CNS: Aphasia, chills, **coma**, confusion, **encephalopathy**, fever, hallucinations, headache, myoclonus, **neurotoxicity**, **nonconvulsive status epilepticus, seizures**, stupor
CV: Edema
EENT: Hearing loss, oral candidiasis
GI: Abdominal cramps, *Clostridioides difficile–associated* diarrhea, diarrhea, elevated liver enzymes, **hepatic failure**, hepatomegaly, nausea, **pseudomembranous colitis**, vomiting
GU: Elevated BUN level, **nephrotoxicity**, **renal failure**, vaginal candidiasis
HEME: **Agranulocytosis, decreased prothrombin activity**, eosinophilia, **hemolytic anemia, hypoprothrombinemia, leukopenia, neutropenia**, positive direct Coombs tests, **thrombocytopenia, unusual bleeding**
MS: Arthralgia
RESP: Dyspnea
SKIN: Ecchymosis, erythema, **erythema multiforme**, pruritus, rash, **Stevens–Johnson syndrome**
Other: **Anaphylaxis**; injection-site pain, redness, and swelling; superinfection

Childbearing Considerations

PREGNANCY

- It is not known if drug can cause fetal harm.
- Use with caution only if benefit to mother outweighs potential risk to fetus.

LACTATION

- Drug is present in breast milk.
- Patient should check with prescriber before breastfeeding.

Nursing Considerations

- Use cefepime cautiously in patients with impaired renal function or a history of GI disease, particularly colitis. Also use cautiously in patients hypersensitive to other cephalosporins, other drugs, or penicillins because cross-sensitivity has occurred.
- Obtain culture and sensitivity test results, if possible and as ordered, before giving drug.

! WARNING Monitor patient closely for hypersensitivity reactions. Be aware that an allergic reaction may occur even up to a few days after therapy starts. Notify prescriber immediately and expect cefepime to be discontinued. Be prepared to administer treatment with corticosteroids, epinephrine, intravenous fluids, intravenous antihistamines, oxygen, pressor amines, and airway management, if reaction is severe.

- Monitor BUN and serum creatinine levels for early signs of nephrotoxicity. Also monitor fluid intake and output; decreasing urine output may indicate nephrotoxicity.
- Assess bowel pattern daily; severe diarrhea may indicate *Clostridioides difficile–* associated diarrhea or pseudomembranous colitis. Be aware that, if present, drug will have to be discontinued and supportive care given, as prescribed.
- Assess for signs of superinfection, such as cough or sputum changes, diarrhea, drainage, fever, malaise, pain, perineal itching, rash, redness, and swelling.
- Be aware that prothrombin time activity may decrease, especially in patients with hepatic or renal impairment, or a poor nutritional state. A protracted course of antimicrobial therapy may also decrease prothrombin activity. Expect to monitor prothrombin time in patients at risk and have exogenous vitamin K ready for administration, if needed.
- Assess for arthralgia, bleeding, ecchymosis, and pharyngitis; they may indicate a blood dyscrasia. Be aware that positive direct Coombs tests may occur with cefepime use. Expect drug to be discontinued and appropriate therapy instituted if patient develops hemolytic anemia.
- Monitor patient for evidence of neurotoxicity such as aphasia, encephalopathy, myoclonus, nonconvulsive status epilepticus, or seizures. Be prepared to provide immediate treatment, as ordered. Be aware that although most cases occurred in patients with renal

impairment who did not receive appropriate dosage adjustment, some did not.

PATIENT TEACHING

- Tell patient to immediately report severe diarrhea to prescriber, even if it occurs as late as 2 or more months after the last dose was taken.
- Instruct patient and caregiver to immediately seek emergency care for any change in mental status, development of seizure activity, difficulty speaking or understanding spoken or written words, or sudden jerking movements. Cefepime should be stopped until patient is evaluated.
- Alert patients with diabetes that cefepime therapy may result in a false-positive reaction for glucose in the urine when using some methods such as Clinitest tablets.

cefiderocol sulfate tosylate
Fetroja

Class and Category

Pharmacologic class: Cephalosporin
Therapeutic class: Antibiotic

Indications and Dosages

✳ *To treat complicated urinary tract infections, including pyelonephritis caused by* Enterobacter cloacae *complex,* Escherichia coli, Klebsiella pneumoniae, Proteus mirabilis, *or* Pseudomonas aeruginosa; *to treat hospital-acquired bacterial pneumonia and ventilator-associated bacterial pneumonia caused by* Acinetobacter baumannii *complex,* Enterobacter cloacae *complex,* Escherichia coli, Klebsiella pneumoniae, Pseudomonas aeruginosa, *or* Serratia marcescens

I.V. INFUSION

Adults with a creatinine clearance between 60 and 119 ml/min. 2 g every 8 hr for 7 to 14 days.

±**DOSAGE ADJUSTMENT** For patients with renal impairment and a creatinine clearance between 30 to 59 ml/min, dosage reduced to 1.5 g every 8 hr; creatinine clearance between 15 to 29 ml/min, dosage reduced to 1 g every 8 hr; and for creatinine clearance of less than 15 ml/min, dosage reduced to 0.75 g every 12 hr. For patients who are

receiving intermittent hemodialysis, dosage reduced to 0.75 g every 12 hr. For patients with a creatinine clearance of 120 ml/min or greater, dosage remains at 2 g but dosage interval decreases to every 6 hr. All dosage adjustments infused over 3 hr. For patient receiving continuous renal replacement therapy (CRRT), dosage is based on the effluent flow rate in CRRT as follows: 4.1 L/hr or greater, dosage is 2 grams every 8 hours; 3.1 to 4 L/hr, dosage is 1.5 grams every 8 hours; 2.1 to 3 L/min, dosage is 2 grams every 12 hours; and 2 L/hr or less, dosage is 1.5 grams every 12 hours.

Drug Administration

I.V.

- Reconstitute powder in drug vial with 10 ml of either 0.9% Sodium Chloride Injection, USP, or 5% Dextrose Injection, USP, and gently shake to dissolve.
- Allow vial to stand until foaming generated on surface has disappeared (typically 2 minutes).
- Final volume of reconstituted solution will be about 11.2 ml/vial.
- Immediately (or up to 1 hour if kept at room temperature) withdraw appropriate volume of reconstituted solution from vial(s) (22.4 ml for a 2-g dose, 16.8 ml for a 1.5-g dose, 11.2 ml for a 1-g dose, and 8.4 ml for a 0.75-g dose) and add to 100-ml infusion bag containing either 0.9% Sodium Chloride Injection, USP, or 5% Dextrose Injection, USP. Solution should be clear and colorless.
- Diluted solution may be stored for up to 6 hours at room temperature or up to 24 hours refrigerated. Must be protected from light.
- Infuse over 3 hours.
- Infusion should be completed within 6 hours after removal from refrigerator.
- *Incompatibilities:* Solution other than 0.9% Sodium Chloride, USP, or 5% Dextrose Injection, USP; other drugs

Route	Onset	Peak	Duration
I.V.	Unknown	Unknown	Unknown

Half-life: 2–3 hr

Mechanism of Action

Interferes with bacterial cell wall synthesis by inhibiting cross-linking of peptidoglycan strands. Peptidoglycan makes the cell membrane rigid and protective. Without it, bacterial cells rupture and die.

Cefiderocol is also a siderophore cephalosporin. It binds with extracellular free ferric iron to form a chelated complex, which then uses bacterial iron transport systems to be delivered across the outer cell membrane of the organism.

Contraindications

Hypersensitivity to cefiderocol, other beta-lactam antibacterials, or their components

Interactions

DRUGS

None reported by manufacturer

Adverse Reactions

CNS: Dysgeusia, fever, headache, insomnia, restlessness, **seizures**

CV: **Atrial fibrillation**, atrial flutter, **bradycardia**, **congestive heart failure**, **fluid overload**, **MI**, peripheral edema

EENT: Dry mouth, oral candidiasis, stomatitis

GI: Abdominal pain, anorexia, cholecystitis, cholelithiasis, cholestasis, **Clostridium difficile colitis**, constipation, diarrhea, elevated liver enzymes, gallbladder pain, nausea, vomiting

GU: Acute interstitial nephritis, candiduria, urine positive for red blood cells, vulvovaginal candidiasis

HEME: **Prolonged activated partial thromboplastin time**, **prolonged prothrombin time**, **increased international normalized ratio (INR)**, **thrombocytopenia**, thrombocytosis

MS: Elevated creatine phosphokinase

RESP: Cough, dyspnea, pleural effusion

SKIN: Pruritis, rash

Other: **Hypersensitivity reactions**, **including anaphylaxis**, **hypocalcemia**, **hypokalemia**; **hypomagnesemia**; infusion-site reactions (erythema, inflammation, pain, phlebitis, pruritis)

Childbearing Considerations

PREGNANCY

- It is not known if drug causes fetal harm.
- Use with caution only if benefit to mother outweighs potential risk to fetus.

LACTATION

- It is not known if drug is present in breast milk.
- Patient should check with prescriber before breastfeeding.

Nursing Considerations

! WARNING Be aware that drug may cause an increase in mortality compared to treatment with other drugs. Monitor patient response closely and alert prescriber, if patient's condition deteriorates.

! WARNING Monitor patient for hypersensitivity reactions that could become severe, especially with the first dose. Patients who have had previous hypersensitivity reactions to other beta-lactams (including cephalosporins) or other allergens may be at higher risk for developing a serious reaction. If present, discontinue drug immediately, notify prescriber, and be prepared to provide emergency supportive care, as prescribed.

- Monitor patients for adverse reactions, especially patients with renal impairment, because drug is substantially excreted by the kidney.
- Put seizure precautions in place because cefiderocol has been implicated in triggering seizures, especially in patients with epilepsy and/or when dosage was not reduced in patients with impaired renal function. Patient should also be monitored for other signs of neurotoxicity, including confusion, tremors, or extra muscle action. Patients should be educated to report any of these signs.
- Be aware that cefiderocol may result in false-positive results in dipstick tests (ketones, occult blood, urine protein), thus requiring alternate clinical laboratory methods of testing to confirm positive tests.
- Assess bowel function daily; severe diarrhea may indicate pseudomembranous colitis caused by *C. difficile*. If diarrhea occurs, notify prescriber and expect to treat with electrolytes, fluids, protein, and an antibiotic effective against *C. difficile*. Cefiderocol may also have to be withheld.
- Monitor urine output hourly. Urine output less than 0.3 mL/kg/h or less than 500 mL/day should be reported to the physician.

! WARNING Monitor patient closely for seizures, especially if patient has a history of epilepsy or has renal impairment, because drug may trigger seizures.

PATIENT TEACHING

> **! WARNING** Urge patient to immediately report any hypersensitivity reactions, such as hives, itching skin, or rash.

- Tell patient that diarrhea is a common problem caused by antibacterial drugs such as cefiderocol. However, if patient develops watery, bloody stools that may occur even up to 2 months after drug therapy has ended, prescriber should be notified immediately.

cefixime

≡ Class and Category

Pharmacologic class: Third-generation cephalosporin
Therapeutic class: Antibiotic

≡ Indications and Dosages

✶ *To treat uncomplicated UTI caused by* Escherichia coli *or* Proteus mirabilis; *pharyngitis and tonsillitis caused by* S. pyogenes; *acute bronchitis and acute exacerbations of chronic bronchitis caused by* H. influenzae *or* Streptococcus pneumoniae

CAPSULES, CHEWABLE TABLETS, ORAL SUSPENSION, TABLETS

Adults and children weighing 45 kg (99 lb) or more. 400 mg once daily or 200 mg every 12 hr.

CHEWABLE TABLETS, ORAL SUSPENSION

Children age 6 months to 12 years weighing less than 45 kg (99 lb). 8 mg/kg once daily or 4 mg/kg every 12 hr.

✶ *To treat otitis media caused by* Haemophilus influenzae, Moraxella catarrhalis, *or* Streptococcus pyogenes

CHEWABLE TABLETS, ORAL SUSPENSION

Adults and children weighing 45 kg (99 lb) and over. 400 mg once daily or 200 mg every 12 hr.

Children age 6 months to 12 years weighing less than 45 kg (99 lb). 8 mg/kg once daily or 4 mg/kg every 12 hr.

✶ *To treat uncomplicated gonorrhea caused by* Neisseria gonorrhoeae

CAPSULES, TABLETS

Adults. 400 mg as a single dose.

±**DOSAGE ADJUSTMENT** Dosage reduced for patients with renal impairment with a creatinine clearance less than 60 ml/min, patients on hemodialysis, and patients on continuous ambulatory peritoneal dialysis.

≡ Drug Administration

P.O.

- Shake oral suspension well before pouring dose and use a calibrated device to obtain an accurate dose.
- Store oral suspension at room temperature or in refrigerator and discard unused portion after 14 days.
- Chewable tablets should be chewed completely and swallowed.
- Chewable tablets contain aspartame, a source of phenylalanine, which can be harmful to patients with phenylketonuria (PKU).
- Tablets shouldn't be substituted for chewable tablets or oral suspension in the treatment of otitis media because these forms produce a higher peak blood level than do tablets when administered at the same dose.

Route	Onset	Peak	Duration
P.O.	Unknown	4 hr	Unknown

Half-life: 3–4 hr

≡ Mechanism of Action

Interferes with bacterial cell wall synthesis by inhibiting the final step in the cross-linking of peptidoglycan strands. Peptidoglycan makes cell membranes rigid and protective. Without it, bacterial cells rupture and die.

≡ Contraindications

Hypersensitivity to cefixime, other cephalosporins, or their components

≡ Interactions

DRUGS

anticoagulants such as warfarin: Increased prothrombin time; increased risk of bleeding
carbamazepine: Increased blood carbamazepine level

≡ Adverse Reactions

CNS: Chills, dizziness, fever, headache, **seizures**
CV: Edema, elevated LDH level
EENT: Hearing loss, oral candidiasis
GI: Abdominal cramps, diarrhea, elevated liver enzymes, **hepatic failure, hepatitis,**

hepatomegaly, hyperbilirubinemia, jaundice, nausea, **pseudomembranous colitis**, vomiting
GU: Elevated BUN or creatinine levels, genital pruritus, **nephrotoxicity, renal failure**, vaginal candidiasis
HEME: Agranulocytosis, eosinophilia, **hemolytic anemia, hypoprothrombinemia, leukopenia, neutropenia, pancytopenia, prolonged prothrombin time, thrombocytopenia, unusual bleeding**
MS: Arthralgia
RESP: Dyspnea
SKIN: Ecchymosis, erythema, **erythema multiforme**, pruritus, rash, **Stevens–Johnson syndrome, toxic epidermal necrolysis,** urticaria
Other: Anaphylaxis, angioedema, drug fever, serum sickness–like reactions, superinfection

Childbearing Considerations
PREGNANCY
- It is not known if drug can cause fetal harm.
- Use with caution only if benefit to mother outweighs potential risk to fetus.

LACTATION
- It is not known if drug is present in breast milk.
- Patient should check with prescriber before breastfeeding.

Nursing Considerations
- Use cefixime cautiously in patients with impaired renal function or a history of GI disease, especially colitis. Also use cautiously in patients hypersensitive to penicillin, because cross-sensitivity has occurred in about 10% of such patients.
- Obtain culture and sensitivity test results, if possible and as ordered, before giving drug.
- Monitor BUN and serum creatinine for early signs of nephrotoxicity. Also monitor fluid intake and output; decreasing urine output may indicate nephrotoxicity.
- Be aware that an allergic reaction may occur a few days after therapy starts.
- Assess bowel pattern daily; severe diarrhea may indicate pseudomembranous colitis.
- Assess for signs of superinfection, such as cough or sputum changes, diarrhea, drainage, fever, malaise, pain, perineal itching, rash, redness, and swelling.
- Assess for arthralgia, bleeding, ecchymosis, and pharyngitis; they may indicate a blood dyscrasia.

PATIENT TEACHING
- Instruct patient to complete the prescribed course of therapy.
- Advise patient to shake oral suspension well before pouring dose and to use a calibrated device to obtain an accurate dose.
- Instruct patient to store oral suspension at room temperature or refrigerate and to discard unused portion after 14 days.
- Alert patient that chewable tablets contain aspartame, a source of phenylalanine, which can be harmful to patients with phenylketonuria (PKU).
- Tell patient to report severe diarrhea to prescriber immediately; this may occur even up to 2 months after cefixime therapy has been discontinued.
- Inform patient that buttermilk and yogurt can help maintain intestinal flora and decrease diarrhea.
- Teach patient to recognize and report signs of superinfection, such as furry tongue, perineal itching, and loose, foul-smelling stools.

cefotaxime sodium

Class and Category
Pharmacologic class: Third-generation cephalosporin
Therapeutic class: Antibiotic

Indications and Dosages
⁎ *To provide perioperative prophylaxis in contaminated or potentially contaminated surgery*
I.V. INFUSION, I.V. OR I.M. INJECTION
Adults and children weighing 50 kg (110 lb) or more. 1 g 30 to 90 min before surgery.
⁎ *To provide perioperative prophylaxis related to cesarean section*
I.V. INFUSION, I.V. OR I.M. INJECTION
Adults. 1 g as soon as cord is clamped, then 1 g every 6 hr for up to two doses.
⁎ *To treat gonococcal urethritis and cervicitis in men and women*
I.M. INJECTION
Adults. 500 mg as a single dose.
⁎ *To treat rectal gonorrhea in women*
I.M. INJECTION
Adults. 500 mg as a single dose.

* *To treat rectal gonorrhea in men*

I.M. INJECTION
Adults. 1 g as a single dose.

* *To treat uncomplicated infections caused by susceptible organisms*

I.V. INFUSION, I.V. OR I.M. INJECTION
Adults and children weighing 50 kg (110 lb) or more. 1 g every 12 hr.
Children ages 1 month to 12 years weighing less than 50 kg. 50 to 180 mg/kg daily in four to six divided doses.
Neonates ages 1 to 4 weeks. 50 mg/kg I.V. every 8 hr.
Neonates age 1 week and under. 50 mg/kg I.V. every 12 hr.

* *To treat moderate to severe infections caused by susceptible organisms*

I.V. INFUSION, I.V. OR I.M. INJECTION
Adults and children weighing 50 kg (110 lb) or more. 1 to 2 g every 8 hr.
Children ages 1 month to 12 years weighing less than 50 kg. 50 to 180 mg/kg daily in four to six divided doses. For more serious infections, including meningitis, the higher dosages are used.
Neonates ages 1 to 4 weeks. 50 mg/kg I.V. every 8 hr.
Neonates age 1 week and younger. 50 mg/kg I.V. every 12 hr.

* *To treat septicemia and other infections that commonly require antibiotics in higher doses than those used to treat moderate to severe infections*

I.V. INFUSION OR INJECTION
Adults and children weighing 50 kg (110 lb) or more. 2 g every 6 to 8 hr. I.V. infusion given over longer than 5 minutes.

* *To treat life-threatening infections caused by susceptible organisms*

I.V. INFUSION OR INJECTION
Adults and children weighing 50 kg (110 lb) or more. 2 g every 4 hr. *Maximum:* 12 g daily.
Children ages 1 month to 12 years weighing less than 50 kg. 50 to 180 mg/kg daily in four to six divided doses.
Neonates ages 1 to 4 weeks. 50 mg/kg every 8 hr.
Neonates age 1 week and younger. 50 mg/kg every 12 hr.

±**DOSAGE ADJUSTMENT** Dosage reduced by 50% for patients with estimated creatinine clearance below 20 ml/min.

Drug Administration

I.V.
- Reconstitute each 0.5-, 1-, or 2-g vial with 10 ml of Sterile Water for Injection. Shake to dissolve. Color should be a very pale yellow to light amber.
- Administer I.V. injection over 3 to 5 minutes through tubing of a free-flowing compatible I.V. solution. Temporarily stop other solutions being given through same I.V. site.
- For I.V. infusion, further dilute in 50 to 100 ml of 0.9% Sodium Chloride Injection or 5% Dextrose Injection.
- Administer I.V. infusion over 15 to 30 minutes.
- *Incompatibilities:* Aminoglycosides

I.M.
- Reconstitute each 500-mg vial with 2 ml Sterile Water for Injection or Bacteriostatic Water for Injection; each 1-g vial with 3 ml diluent; and each 2-g vial with 5 ml diluent. Shake to dissolve. Don't use diluent that contains benzyl alcohol when preparing drug for a neonate.
- Inject deep into a large muscle such as the gluteus maximus or lateral side of thigh. Doses of 2 g may be given, if divided and injected into different sites.
- Discard unused drug after 12 hours if stored at room temperature, 5 days in plastic syringes, or 7 days in original containers, if refrigerated.
- Protect powder and solution from heat and light.

Route	Onset	Peak	Duration
I.V.	Unknown	Unknown	Unknown
I.M.	Unknown	30 min	Unknown

Half-life: 1–1.5 hr

Mechanism of Action
Interferes with bacterial cell wall synthesis by inhibiting cross-linking of peptidoglycan strands. Peptidoglycan makes cell membranes rigid and protective. Without it, bacterial cells rupture and die.

Contraindications
Hypersensitivity to cefotaxime, other cephalosporins, or their components

Interactions

DRUGS
aminoglycosides, loop diuretics, NSAIDs: Increased risk of nephrotoxicity
probenecid: Increased and prolonged blood cefotaxime level

Adverse Reactions
CNS: Chills, fever, headache, **seizures**
CV: Edema
EENT: Hearing loss, oral candidiasis
GI: Abdominal cramps, cholestasis, diarrhea, elevated enzymes, **hepatic failure, hepatitis,** hepatomegaly, jaundice, nausea, **pseudomembranous colitis,** vomiting
GU: Elevated BUN level, **nephrotoxicity, renal failure,** vaginal candidiasis
HEME: Eosinophilia, **hemolytic anemia, hypoprothrombinemia, neutropenia, thrombocytopenia, unusual bleeding**
MS: Arthralgia
RESP: Dyspnea
SKIN: Ecchymosis, erythema, **erythema multiforme,** pruritus, rash, **Stevens–Johnson syndrome, toxic epidermal necrolysis**
Other: **Anaphylaxis;** injection-site pain, redness, and swelling; superinfection

Childbearing Considerations

PREGNANCY
- It is not known if drug can cause fetal harm.
- Use with caution only if benefit to mother outweighs potential risk to fetus.

LACTATION
- Drug is present in breast milk.
- Patient should check with prescriber before breastfeeding.

Nursing Considerations
- Use cefotaxime cautiously in patients with impaired renal function, a history of GI disease (especially colitis), or hypersensitivity to penicillin, because cross-sensitivity has occurred in about 10% of such patients.
- Obtain culture and sensitivity test results, if possible and as ordered, before giving drug.
- Monitor I.V. sites for signs of phlebitis or extravasation. Rotate I.V. sites every 72 hours.
- Monitor BUN and serum creatinine levels and fluid intake and output for signs of nephrotoxicity.
- Be aware that allergic reaction may occur a few days after cefotaxime therapy starts.

- Assess bowel pattern daily; severe diarrhea may indicate pseudomembranous colitis caused by *Clostridium difficile.* If diarrhea occurs, notify prescriber and expect to withhold cefotaxime and treat with fluids, electrolytes, protein, and an antibiotic effective against *C. difficile.*
- Assess patient for arthralgia, bleeding, ecchymosis, and pharyngitis, which may indicate a blood dyscrasia. Monitor bleeding time, CBC, and PT, as ordered.
- Monitor patient closely for superinfection. If evidence appears, notify prescriber and expect to stop drug and provide care.
- Be aware that cephalosporins, such as cefotaxime, may produce a positive direct Coombs test.

PATIENT TEACHING
- Explain that I.M. injection may be painful.
- Instruct patient to report watery, bloody stools to prescriber immediately, even up to 2 months after drug therapy has ended.

cefotetan disodium

Class and Category
Pharmacologic class: Second-generation cephalosporin
Therapeutic class: Antibiotic

Indications and Dosages
✳ *To provide surgical prophylaxis*

I.V. INJECTION
Adults. 1 to 2 g given 30 to 60 min before surgery or, in cesarean section, as soon as cord is clamped.

✳ *To treat lower respiratory tract infections caused by* Escherichia coli, Haemophilus influenzae, Klebsiella *species,* Proteus mirabilis, Serratia marcescens, Staphylococcus aureus, *or* Streptococcus pneumoniae; *gynecologic infections caused by* Bacteroides *species (excluding* B. distasonis, B. ovatus, *or* B. thetaiotaomicron*),* E. coli, Fusobacterium *species, gram-positive anaerobic cocci,* Neisseria gonorrhoeae, P. mirabilis, S. aureus, Staphylococcus epidermidis, *or* Streptococcus *species (excluding enterococci); intra-abdominal infections caused by* Bacteroides *species (excluding* B. distasonis, B. ovatus, *or* B. thetaiotaomicron*),* Clostridium *species (other than* Clostridium difficile*),* E. coli, Klebsiella *species, or* Streptococcus *species (excluding* enterococci*); and bone and joint infections caused by* S. aureus

I.V. INFUSION, I.V. OR I.M. INJECTION

Adults. For mild to moderate infections, 1 g every 12 hr or 2 g I.V. every 24 hr.

I.V. INFUSION OR INJECTION

Adults. For severe infections, 2 g every 12 hr; for life-threatening infections, 3 g every 12 hr.

✳ *To treat UTI caused by* E. coli, Klebsiella *species,* Morganella morganii, P. mirabilis, P. vulgaris, *or* Providencia rettgeri

I.V. INFUSION, I.V. OR I.M. INJECTION

Adults. 0.5 to 2 g every 12 hr or 1 to 2 g every 24 hr.

✳ *To treat skin and soft-tissue infections caused by* E. coli, Klebsiella pneumoniae, Peptostreptococcus *species,* S. aureus, S. epidermidis, Streptococcus pyogenes, *and* Streptococcus *species (excluding enterococci)*

I.V. INFUSION, I.V. OR I.M. INJECTION

Adults. For mild to moderate infections due to *K. pneumoniae,* 1 or 2 g every 12 hr. For mild to moderate infections caused by other organisms, 1 g I.M. or I.V. every 12 hr or 2 g I.V. every 24 hr; for severe infections, 2 g I.V. every 12 hr.

±**DOSAGE ADJUSTMENT** Dosing interval reduced to 24 hr if creatinine clearance is 10 to 30 ml/min or dosage reduced by 50% while maintaining a dosage interval of 12 hours; dosage interval reduced to 48 hr if creatinine clearance is less than 10 ml/min or dosage reduced by 75% while maintaining a dosage interval of 12 hours.

≡ Drug Administration

I.V.

Vials

- Reconstitute each 1-g vial of drug with 10 ml Sterile Water for Injection. For each 2-g vial, use 10 to 20 ml diluent. Shake to dissolve and let stand until clear.
- For direct I.V. injection, give drug slowly over 3 to 5 minutes through tubing of a flowing compatible I.V. solution.
- For I.V. infusion, further dilute solution in 50 to 100 ml 0.9% Sodium Chloride Injection or 5% Dextrose in Water solution. Do not use in series connections.
- For I.V. infusion, infuse over 30 minutes.

Duplex Container

- Keep container in folded position until activation is intended. Remove from

refrigerator and allow to come to room temperature.

- Unlatch side tab and unfold container. Visually inspect diluent chamber. Use only if container and seals are intact.
- Inspect drug powder by peeling foil strip from drug chamber. Protect from light after removal of foil strip. If foil strip is removed but administration is delayed, refold container and latch side tab. Product then must be used within 7 days.
- To reconstitute, unfold container and point the set port in a downward direction. Starting at the hanger tab end, fold the container just below the diluent meniscus, trapping all air above the fold. To activate, squeeze the folded diluent chamber until the seal between the diluent and powder opens, releasing diluent into the drug powder chamber. Agitate the liquid-powder mixture until completely dissolved. Once dissolved, drug must be used within 24 hours if stored at room temperature or 7 days if refrigerated.
- To administer, point the set port in a downward direction. Starting at the hanger tab end, fold the container just below the solution meniscus, trapping all air above the fold. Squeeze the folded container until the seal between the reconstituted drug and set port opens, releasing the solution to set port. Squeeze container firmly to check for minute leaks. Then peel foil cover from the set port and attach administration set.
- Do not use in series connections.
- Do not introduce additives to the container.
- Administer as an infusion over about 30 minutes.

- *Incompatibilities:* Aminoglycosides

I.M.

- Reconstitute each 1-g vial of drug with 2 ml of Sterile or Bacteriostatic Water for Injection, 0.9% Sodium Chloride for Injection, 0.5% Lidocaine Hydrochloride, or 1% Lidocaine Hydrochloride. For a 2-g vial, use 3 ml diluent. Shake to dissolve and let stand until clear.
- Inject deeply into a large muscle mass such as the gluteus maximus.
- Protect reconstituted solution from light, and store for up to 24 hours at

room temperature or 96 hours under refrigeration.

Route	Onset	Peak	Duration
I.V.	Immediate	10 min	Unknown
I.M.	Unknown	1.5–3 hr	Unknown

Half-life: 3–4.6 hr

Mechanism of Action

Interferes with bacterial cell wall synthesis by inhibiting the final step in the cross-linking of peptidoglycan strands. Peptidoglycan makes cell membranes rigid and protective. Without it, bacterial cells rupture and die.

Contraindications

History of cephalosporin-induced hemolytic anemia; hypersensitivity to cefotetan, other cephalosporins, or their components

Interactions

DRUGS

aminoglycosides, loop diuretics: Increased risk of nephrotoxicity
probenecid: Increased and prolonged blood cefotetan level

ACTIVITIES

alcohol use: Disulfiram-like reaction

Adverse Reactions

CNS: Chills, fever, headache, **seizures**
CV: Edema
EENT: Hearing loss, oral candidiasis
GI: Abdominal cramps, diarrhea, elevated liver enzymes, **hepatic failure**, hepatomegaly, nausea, **pseudomembranous colitis**, vomiting
GU: Elevated BUN level, **nephrotoxicity**, **renal failure**, vaginal candidiasis
HEME: Eosinophilia, **hemolytic anemia**, **hypoprothrombinemia**, **neutropenia**, **thrombocytopenia**, **unusual bleeding**
MS: Arthralgia
RESP: Dyspnea
SKIN: Ecchymosis, erythema, **erythema multiforme**, pruritus, rash, **Stevens–Johnson syndrome**
Other: **Anaphylaxis**; injection-site pain, redness, and swelling; superinfection

Childbearing Considerations

PREGNANCY

- It is not known if drug can cause fetal harm.
- Use with caution only if benefit to mother outweighs potential risk to fetus.

LACTATION

- Drug is present in breast milk.
- Patient should check with prescriber before breastfeeding.

Nursing Considerations

- Use cefotetan cautiously in patients with impaired renal function or a history of GI disease, especially colitis. Also use cautiously in patients hypersensitive to penicillin, because cross-sensitivity has occurred in about 10% of such patients.
- Obtain culture and sensitivity test results, if possible and as ordered, before giving drug.
- Be aware that an allergic reaction may occur a few days after therapy starts.
- Monitor BUN and serum creatinine levels and fluid intake and output for signs of nephrotoxicity.
- Monitor patient receiving even short-term cefotetan therapy for signs and symptoms of hemolytic anemia, such as marked pallor and fatigue.
- Monitor ALT, AST, bilirubin, CBC, LD, and serum alkaline phosphatase levels if patient receives long-term therapy.
- Assess patient's bowel pattern daily; severe diarrhea may indicate pseudomembranous colitis.
- Watch for arthralgia, bleeding, ecchymosis, and pharyngitis which may indicate a blood dyscrasia. Monitor PT and bleeding time, as ordered. Be prepared to give vitamin K, if ordered, to treat hypoprothrombinemia.

PATIENT TEACHING

- Explain that I.M. injection may be painful.
- Tell patient to immediately report severe diarrhea to prescriber even up to 2 months after therapy has stopped.
- Urge patient to avoid alcohol during and for at least 3 days after cefotetan therapy.

cefoxitin sodium
Cefoxitin, Cefoxitin and Dextrose

Class and Category

Pharmacologic class: Second-generation cephalosporin
Therapeutic class: Antibiotic

Indications and Dosages

* *To provide surgical prophylaxis in patients undergoing uncontaminated abdominal*

or vaginal hysterectomy or gastrointestinal surgery

I.V. INFUSION OR INJECTION (CEFOXITIN, CEFOXITIN AND DEXTROSE)

Adults. 2 g 30 to 60 min before surgery and then 2 g every 6 hr after first dose for up to 24 hr.

I.V. INFUSION OR INJECTION (CEFOXITIN)

Children age 3 months or over. 30 to 40 mg/kg 30 to 60 min before surgery and every 6 hr after first dose, if needed, for up to 24 hr.

✴ *To provide surgical prophylaxis for cesarean section*

I.V. INFUSION OR INJECTION (CEFOXITIN, CEFOXITIN AND DEXTROSE)

Adults. 2 g as a single dose as soon as cord is clamped; or 2 g as soon as cord is clamped, followed by 2 g 4 and 8 hr after initial dose.

✴ *To treat bone and joint infections caused by* Staphylococcus aureus; *gynecological infections, including endometritis and pelvic cellulitis or inflammatory disease caused by* Bacteroides *species,* Clostridium *species,* E. coli, Neisseria gonorrhoeae, Peptococcus niger, Peptostreptococcus *species, or* Streptococcus agalactiae; *intra-abdominal infections including intra-abdominal abscess and peritonitis caused by* Bacteroides *or* Clostridium *species,* E. coli, *or* Klebsiella *species; lower respiratory infections, including lung abscess and pneumonia caused by* Bacteroides *species,* E. coli, Haemophilus influenzae, Klebsiella *species,* S. aureus, Streptococcus pneumoniae, *and other streptococci (excluding* enterococci); *skin and skin structure infections caused by* Bacteroides *and* Clostridium *species,* Enterococcus faecalis, E. coli, P. niger, Peptostreptococcus *species,* Proteus mirabilis, S. aureus, S. epidermidis, S. pyogenes, *and other streptococci (excluding* enterococci); *septicemia caused by* Bacteroides species, E. coli, Klebsiella *species,* S. aureus *or* S. pneumoniae; *and urinary tract infections caused by* E. coli, Klebsiella *species,* Morganella morganii, P. mirabilis, P. vulgaris, *or* Providencia species

I.V. INFUSION OR INJECTION (CEFOXITIN, CEFOXITIN AND DEXTROSE)

Adults. For uncomplicated infections, 1 g every 6 to 8 hr; for moderate to severe infections, 1 g every 4 hr or 2 g every 6 to 8 hr. For infections that commonly require high-dose antibiotics (such as gas gangrene), 2 g every 4 hr, or 3 g every 6 hr.

I.V. INFUSION OR INJECTION (CEFOXITIN)

Children age 3 months or over. 80 to 160 mg/kg daily in equally divided doses given every 4 to 6 hr (higher dosages used for more severe infections). *Maximum:* 12 g daily.

± **DOSAGE ADJUSTMENT** Dosage reduced to 1 to 2 g every 8 to 12 hr if creatinine clearance is 30 to 50 ml/min; 1 to 2 g every 12 to 24 hr if clearance is 10 to 29 ml/min; 0.5 to 1 g every 12 to 24 hr if clearance is 5 to 9 ml/min; and 0.5 to 1 g every 24 to 48 hr if clearance is less than 5 ml/min.

☰ Drug Administration

I.V.
Vials

- Reconstitute each 1-g vial of drug with 10 ml 0.9% Sodium Chloride Injection, 5% Dextrose Injection, Bacteriostatic Water for Injection, or Sterile Water for Injection. For each 2-g vial, use 10 to 20 ml diluent. Shake to dissolve and let stand until clear.
- For I.V. injection, give drug slowly over 3 to 5 minutes through tubing of a flowing compatible I.V. solution.
- For I.V. infusion, further dilute solution in 50 to 100 ml 0.9% Sodium Chloride Injection, 5% Dextrose Injection, or 0.9% Sodium Chloride Injection and 5% Dextrose Injection.
- Do not use in series connections.
- For I.V. infusion, infuse over 30 minutes while temporarily discontinuing administration of any other solutions at the same site.
- Discard unused drug after 6 hours if stored at room temperature, or after 1 week if refrigerated.
- Be aware that powder or solution may darken during storage, which doesn't reflect altered potency.

Duplex

- Keep container in folded position until activation is intended. Remove from refrigerator and allow to come to room temperature.
- Unlatch side tab and unfold container. Visually inspect diluent chamber. Use only if container and seals are intact.
- Inspect drug powder by peeling foil strip from drug chamber. Protect from light

after removal of foil strip. If foil strip is removed but administration is delayed, refold container and latch side tab. Product then must be used within 7 days.

- To reconstitute, unfold container and point the set port in a downward direction. Starting at the hanger tab end, fold the container just below the diluent meniscus, trapping all air above the fold. To activate, squeeze the folded diluent chamber until the seal between the diluent and powder opens, releasing diluent into the drug powder chamber. Agitate the liquid-powder mixture until completely dissolved. Once dissolved drug must be used within 24 hours if stored at room temperature or 7 days if refrigerated.
- To administer, point the set port in a downward direction. Starting at the hanger tab end, fold the container just below the solution meniscus, trapping all air above the fold. Squeeze the folded container until the seal between the reconstituted drug and set port opens, releasing the solution to set port. Squeeze container firmly to check for minute leaks. Then peel foil cover from the set port and attach administration set.
- Do not use in series connections.
- Do not introduce additives to the container.
- Administer as an infusion over about 30 minutes.
- *Incompatibilities:* Aminoglycosides; Y-site: fenoldopam mesylate, filgrastim, hetastarch in 0.9% Sodium Chloride Injection, pemetrexed disodium, pentamidine isethionate

Route	Onset	Peak	Duration
I.V.	Immediate	>5 min	Unknown

Half-life: 45–60 min.

Mechanism of Action

Interferes with bacterial cell wall synthesis by inhibiting the final step in the cross-linking of peptidoglycan strands. Peptidoglycan makes cell membranes rigid and protective. Without it, bacterial cells rupture and die.

Contraindications

Hypersensitivity to cefoxitin, other cephalosporins, or their components

Interactions

DRUGS

aminoglycosides, loop diuretics: Increased risk of nephrotoxicity

Adverse Reactions

CNS: Chills, fever, headache, **seizures**
CV: Edema
EENT: Hearing loss, oral candidiasis
GI: Abdominal cramps, diarrhea, elevated liver enzymes, **hepatic failure**, hepatomegaly, nausea, **pseudomembranous colitis**, vomiting
GU: Elevated BUN level, **nephrotoxicity**, **renal failure**, vaginal candidiasis
HEME: Eosinophilia, **hemolytic anemia**, **hypoprothrombinemia**, **neutropenia**, **thrombocytopenia**, **unusual bleeding**
MS: Arthralgia
RESP: Dyspnea
SKIN: Ecchymosis, erythema, **erythema multiforme**, flushing, pruritus, rash, **Stevens–Johnson syndrome**, urticaria
Other: **Anaphylaxis**; injection-site pain, redness, and swelling; superinfection

Childbearing Considerations

PREGNANCY

- It is not known if drug can cause fetal harm.
- Use with caution only if benefit to mother outweighs potential risk to fetus.

LACTATION

- Drug is present in breast milk.
- Patient should check with prescriber before breastfeeding.

Nursing Considerations

- Use cefoxitin cautiously in patients hypersensitive to penicillin; cross-sensitivity has occurred in about 10% of such patients.
- Use cautiously in patients with a history of GI disease, particularly colitis, because of an increased risk of pseudomembranous colitis.
- Obtain culture and sensitivity test results, if possible and as ordered, before giving drug.
- Be aware that an allergic reaction may occur a few days after therapy starts.
- Monitor BUN and serum creatinine for early signs of nephrotoxicity. Also monitor fluid intake and output; decreasing urine output may indicate nephrotoxicity.
- Assess patient's bowel pattern daily; severe diarrhea may indicate pseudomembranous colitis.

- Assess for arthralgia, bleeding, ecchymosis, and pharyngitis; they may indicate a blood dyscrasia.

PATIENT TEACHING

- Tell patient to report severe diarrhea to prescriber immediately.
- Instruct patient to complete the course of therapy as prescribed.

cefpodoxime proxetil

☰ Class and Category
Pharmacologic class: Third-generation cephalosporin
Therapeutic class: Antibiotic

☰ Indications and Dosages
❋ *To treat acute community-acquired pneumonia caused by* Haemophilus influenzae *or* Streptococcus pneumoniae

ORAL SUSPENSION, TABLETS
Adults and adolescents. 200 mg every 12 hr for 14 days.

❋ *To treat acute bacterial exacerbation of chronic bronchitis caused by* H. influenzae, Moraxella catarrhalis, *or* S. pneumoniae

ORAL SUSPENSION, TABLETS
Adults and adolescents. 200 mg every 12 hr for 10 days.

❋ *To treat uncomplicated gonorrhea in men and women and rectal gonococcal infections in women caused by* Neisseria gonorrhoeae

ORAL SUSPENSION, TABLETS
Adults. 200 mg as a single dose.

❋ *To treat uncomplicated UTI caused by* Escherichia coli, Klebsiella pneumoniae, Proteus mirabilis, *or* Staphylococcus saprophyticus

ORAL SUSPENSION, TABLETS
Adults and adolescents. 100 mg every 12 hr for 7 days.

❋ *To treat uncomplicated skin and soft-tissue infections caused by* S. aureus or S. pyogenes

ORAL SUSPENSION, TABLETS
Adults and adolescents. 400 mg every 12 hr for 7 to 14 days.

❋ *To treat acute otitis media caused by* H. influenzae, M. catarrhalis, S. pneumoniae, *or* S. pyogenes

ORAL SUSPENSION, TABLETS
Children ages 2 months through 12 years. 5 mg/kg every 12 hr for 5 days. *Maximum:* 200 mg/dose.

❋ *To treat pharyngitis and tonsillitis caused by* S. pyogenes

ORAL SUSPENSION, TABLETS
Adults and adolescents. 100 mg every 12 hr for 5 to 10 days.
Children ages 2 months through 12 years. 5 mg/kg every 12 hr for 5 to 10 days. *Maximum:* 100 mg/dose.

❋ *To treat acute maxillary sinusitis caused by* H. influenzae, M. catarrhalis, *or* S. pneumoniae

ORAL SUSPENSION, TABLETS
Adults and adolescents. 200 mg every 12 hr for 10 days.
Children ages 2 months through 12 years. 5 mg/kg every 12 hr for 10 days. *Maximum:* 200 mg/dose.

±**DOSAGE ADJUSTMENT** Dosing interval increased to 24 hr in patients with creatinine clearance less than 30 ml/min. For patients on hemodialysis, dosage frequency reduced to 3 times a week and given after hemodialysis.

☰ Drug Administration
P.O.

- Administer tablets with food to enhance absorption.
- Oral suspension may contain aspartame, depending on the manufacturer. Check for absence of aspartame before administering to a patient with phenylketonuria.
- Shake oral suspension bottle well before pouring dose and use a calibrated device to ensure accurate doses. It need not be given with food.
- Refrigerate oral suspension and discard after 14 days.

Route	Onset	Peak	Duration
P.O.	Unknown	1 hr	Unknown

Half-life: 2–3 hr

☰ Mechanism of Action
Interferes with bacterial cell wall synthesis by inhibiting the final step in the cross-linking of peptidoglycan strands. Peptidoglycan makes cell membranes rigid and protective. Without it, bacterial cells rupture and die.

☰ Contraindications

Hypersensitivity to cefpodoxime, other cephalosporins, or their components

☰ Interactions

DRUGS

aminoglycosides, loop diuretics: Increased risk of nephrotoxicity
antacids (high doses of aluminum hydroxide or sodium bicarbonate), H₂-receptor antagonists: Reduced bioavailability and blood level of cefpodoxime
probenecid: Possibly increased and prolonged blood cefpodoxime level

☰ Adverse Reactions

CNS: Chills, fever, headache, **seizures**
CV: Edema
EENT: Hearing loss, oral candidiasis
GI: Abdominal cramps, diarrhea, elevated liver enzymes, **hepatic failure**, hepatomegaly, nausea, **pseudomembranous colitis**, vomiting
GU: Elevated BUN level, **nephrotoxicity**, **renal failure**, vaginal candidiasis
HEME: Eosinophilia, **hemolytic anemia**, **hypoprothrombinemia**, **neutropenia**, **thrombocytopenia**, **unusual bleeding**
MS: Arthralgia
RESP: Dyspnea
SKIN: Ecchymosis, erythema, **erythema multiforme**, pruritus, rash, **Stevens–Johnson syndrome**
Other: **Anaphylaxis**, superinfection

☰ Childbearing Considerations

PREGNANCY

- It is not known if drug can cause fetal harm.
- Use with caution only if benefit to mother outweighs potential risk to fetus.

LACTATION

- Drug is present in breast milk.
- A decision should be made to discontinue breastfeeding temporarily during drug therapy or discontinue the drug to avoid potential serious adverse reactions in the breastfed infant.

☰ Nursing Considerations

- Use cefpodoxime cautiously in patients who have impaired renal function or are receiving potent diuretics. Also use drug cautiously in patients hypersensitive to penicillin, because cross-sensitivity has occurred in about 10% of such patients.
- Obtain culture and sensitivity test results, if possible and as ordered, before giving cefpodoxime.
- Assess patient's bowel pattern daily; severe diarrhea may indicate pseudomembranous colitis.
- Be aware that an allergic reaction may occur a few days after therapy starts.

PATIENT TEACHING

- Urge patient to complete the prescribed course of therapy.
- Tell patient to take tablets with food to enhance absorption.
- Tell patient prescribed oral suspension that it does not have to be given with food. However, ensure patient with phenylketonuria checks if product contains aspartame before taking, as some oral suspension products do.
- Instruct patient to shake oral suspension bottle well before pouring dose and to use a calibrated liquid-measuring device to ensure accurate doses.
- Advise patient to refrigerate oral suspension and discard after 14 days.
- Inform patient that buttermilk and yogurt can help maintain intestinal flora and decrease diarrhea.
- Warn patient not to take an antacid within 2 hours before or after taking cefpodoxime.
- Tell patient to report watery, bloody stools to prescriber immediately, even up to 2 months after drug therapy has ended.

cefprozil

☰ Class and Category

Pharmacologic class: Second-generation cephalosporin
Therapeutic class: Antibiotic

☰ Indications and Dosages

✳ *To treat secondary bacterial infections in patients with acute bronchitis and acute bacterial exacerbations of chronic bronchitis caused by* Haemophilus influenzae, Moraxella catarrhalis, *and* Streptococcus pneumoniae

ORAL SUSPENSION, TABLETS

Adults and adolescents. 500 mg every 12 hr for 10 days.

* *To treat uncomplicated skin and soft-tissue infections caused by* Staphylococcus aureus *and* Streptococcus pyogenes

ORAL SUSPENSION, TABLETS

Adults and adolescents. 250 mg every 12 hr or 500 mg every 12 or 24 hr for 10 days.
Children ages 2 to 12. 20 mg/kg every 24 hr for 10 days. *Maximum:* Not to exceed adult dose.

* *To treat pharyngitis and tonsillitis caused by* S. pyogenes

ORAL SUSPENSION, TABLETS

Adults and adolescents. 500 mg every 24 hr for 10 days.
Children ages 2 to 12. 7.5 mg/kg every 12 hr for 10 days. *Maximum:* Not to exceed adult dose.

* *To treat otitis media caused by* H. influenzae, M. catarrhalis, *and* S. pneumoniae

ORAL SUSPENSION, TABLETS

Children ages 6 months to 12 years. 15 mg/kg every 12 hr for 10 days. *Maximum:* Not to exceed adult dose of 500 mg/dose or 1,000 mg/day.

* *To treat acute sinusitis caused by* H. influenzae, M. catarrhalis, *and* S. pneumoniae

ORAL SUSPENSION, TABLETS

Adults and adolescents. 250 to 500 mg every 12 hr for 10 days.
Children ages 6 months to 12 years. 7.5 or 15 mg/kg every 12 hr for 10 days. *Maximum:* Not to exceed adult dose.

±**DOSAGE ADJUSTMENT** Dosage reduced by half and given at usual intervals in patients with creatinine clearance less than 30 ml/min.

Drug Administration

P.O.
- Administer without regard to meals.
- Check oral suspension for the aspartame that is added by some manufacturers. Patients with phenylketonuria should only be given oral suspension without aspartame.
- Shake oral suspension well before pouring and use a calibrated measuring device to ensure accurate doses.
- Tell patient to refrigerate oral suspension and discard after 14 days.

Route	Onset	Peak	Duration
P.O.	Immediate	1.5 hr	Unknown

Half-life: 1.25 hr

Mechanism of Action

Interferes with bacterial cell wall synthesis by inhibiting the final step in the cross-linking of peptidoglycan strands. Peptidoglycan makes the cell membrane rigid and protective. Without it, bacterial cells rupture and die.

Contraindications

Hypersensitivity to cefprozil, other cephalosporins, or their components

Interactions

DRUGS
aminoglycosides, loop diuretics: Increased risk of nephrotoxicity
probenecid: Increased blood cefprozil level

Adverse Reactions

CNS: Chills, fever, headache, **seizures**
CV: Edema
EENT: Hearing loss, oral candidiasis
GI: Abdominal cramps, diarrhea, elevated liver enzymes, **hepatic failure**, hepatomegaly, nausea, **pseudomembranous colitis**, vomiting
GU: Elevated BUN level, **nephrotoxicity, renal failure**, vaginal candidiasis
HEME: Eosinophilia, **hemolytic anemia, hypoprothrombinemia, neutropenia, thrombocytopenia, unusual bleeding**
MS: Arthralgia
RESP: Dyspnea
SKIN: Ecchymosis, erythema, **erythema multiforme**, pruritus, rash, **Stevens–Johnson syndrome**
Other: **Anaphylaxis**, superinfection

Childbearing Considerations

PREGNANCY
- It is not known if drug can cause fetal harm.
- Use with caution only if benefit to mother outweighs potential risk to fetus.

LACTATION
- Drug is present in breast milk.
- Patient should check with prescriber before breastfeeding.

Nursing Considerations

- Use cefprozil cautiously in patients who have impaired renal function or a history of GI disease, especially colitis. Also use drug cautiously in patients who are hypersensitive to penicillin, because cross-sensitivity has occurred in about 10% of such patients.

- Obtain culture and sensitivity test results, if possible and as ordered, before giving drug.
- Monitor BUN and serum creatinine levels to detect early signs of nephrotoxicity. Also monitor fluid intake and output; decreasing urine output may indicate nephrotoxicity.

! **WARNING** Be aware that an allergic reaction may occur a few days after therapy starts. Monitor patient closely, notify prescriber if present, and provide supportive care, as ordered.

- Assess patient's bowel pattern daily; severe diarrhea may indicate pseudomembranous colitis.

PATIENT TEACHING

- Urge patient to complete the prescribed course of therapy.
- Tell patient to refrigerate oral suspension and discard after 14 days.
- Instruct patient to shake oral suspension well before pouring and to use a calibrated measuring device to ensure accurate doses.
- Alert patient with phenylketonuria that oral suspension may contain aspartame, depending on manufacturer.
- Inform patient that an allergic reaction may occur even a few days after therapy begins. Stress importance of notifying prescriber or seeking immediate emergency care, if severe.
- Inform patient that buttermilk and yogurt can help maintain intestinal flora and decrease diarrhea.
- Tell patient to report watery, bloody stools to prescriber immediately, even up to 2 months after drug therapy has ended.

ceftaroline fosamil

Teflaro

☰ Class and Category

Pharmacologic class: Fifth-generation cephalosporin
Therapeutic class: Antibiotic

☰ Indications and Dosages

✳ *To treat acute bacterial skin and skin structure infection caused by* Escherichia coli, Klebsiella oxytoca, K. pneumoniae, Staphylococcus aureus, Streptococcus agalactiae, *or* S. pyogenes

I.V. INFUSION

Adults. 600 mg every 12 hr for 5 to 14 days.
Children ages 2 to 18 years weighing more than 33 kg (72.5 lb). 400 mg every 8 hr or 600 mg every 12 hr for 5 to 14 days.
Children ages 2 to 18 years weighing 33 kg (72.5 lb) or less. 12 mg/kg every 8 hr for 5 to 14 days.
Children 2 months to less than 2 years. 8 mg/kg every 8 hr for 5 to 14 days.
Newborns (gestational age 34 weeks and older and postnatal age 12 days and older) to less than 2 months of age. 6 mg/kg every 8 hours for 5 to 14 days.

✳ *To treat community-acquired bacterial pneumonia caused by* E. coli, Haemophilus influenzae, K. oxytoca, K. pneumoniae, S. aureus, *or* S. pneumoniae

I.V. INFUSION

Adults. 600 mg every 12 hr for 5 to 7 days.
Children ages 2 to 18 years weighing more than 33 kg (72.5 lb). 400 mg every 8 hr or 600 mg every 12 hr for 5 to 14 days.
Children ages 2 to 18 years weighing 33 kg (72.5 lb) or less. 12 mg/kg every 8 hr for 5 to 14 days.
Children 2 months to less than 2 years. 8 mg/kg every 8 hr for 5 to 14 days.
±**DOSAGE ADJUSTMENT** For adult patients with a creatinine clearance above 30 ml/min but no higher than 50 ml/min, dosage reduced to 400 mg every 12 hr; for adult patients with a creatinine clearance above 15 ml/min but no higher than 30 ml/min, dosage reduced to 300 mg every 12 hr; for adult patients with a creatinine clearance of less than 15 ml/min, including those on hemodialysis, dosage reduced to 200 mg every 12 hr. For pediatric patients, dosage adjustment is unknown if creatinine clearance is below 50 ml/min.

☰ Drug Administration

I.V.

- Reconstitute each drug vial with 20 ml of 0.9% Sodium Chloride Injection, 5% Dextrose in Water, Lactated Ringer's Injection, or Sterile Water for Injection. Mix gently to ensure drug is completely dissolved. Color may range from clear to light to dark yellow, depending on the concentration and storage conditions.
- Drug must be diluted after reconstitution with 45% or 0.9% Sodium Chloride

Injection, 2.5% or 5% Dextrose Injection, or Lactated Ringer's Injection. Do not use Sterile Water for Injection for dilution.

- If diluting 600 mg of reconstituted solution in a 50-ml infusion bag for adult administration, withdraw 20 ml of diluent from the infusion bag. Then inject entire content of the drug vial into the bag to provide a total volume of 50 ml. Concentration will be 12 mg/ml.
- If diluting 400 mg of reconstituted solution in a 50-ml infusion bag for adults or pediatric patients weighing more than 33 kg (72.5 lb), withdraw 20 ml of diluent from the infusion bag. Inject entire content of drug vial into the bag to provide a total volume of 50 ml. Concentration will be 8 mg/ml.
- If diluting reconstituted solution for pediatric patients weighing 33 kg (72.5 lb) or less, amount of solution withdrawn from the reconstituted drug vial for dilution in infusion bag will vary according to the age and weight of the child (see manufacturer guidelines). The concentration should not exceed 12 mg/ml.
- Reconstituted drug may also be diluted in 250 ml of recommended solution for adult administration.
- Color of infusion solution varies from clear, light to dark yellow depending on the concentration and storage.
- Infuse diluted solution within 6 hours of mixing if stored at room temperature or within 24 hours if refrigerated.
- For adults and children 2 months of age and older, administer infusion as an I.V. infusion over 5 minutes to 1 hour.
- For infants less than 2 months of age, infuse over 30 to 60 minutes.
- *Incompatibilities:* Aminoglycosides, other drugs

Route	Onset	Peak	Duration
I.V.	Unknown	5 min after infusion	Unknown

Half-life: 2.6 hr

Mechanism of Action

Interferes with bacterial cell wall synthesis by inhibiting the final step in the cross-linking of peptidoglycan strands. Peptidoglycan makes the cell membrane rigid and protective. Without it, bacterial cells rupture and die.

Contraindications

Hypersensitivity to ceftaroline, other cephalosporins, or their components

Drug Reactions

None reported by manufacturer

Adverse Reactions

CNS: Dizziness, **encephalopathy**, fever, headache, **seizures**
CV: **Bradycardia**, palpitations, phlebitis
ENDO: Hyperglycemia
GI: Abdominal pain, *Clostridium difficile*–associated diarrhea, constipation, diarrhea, elevated liver enzymes, **hepatitis**, nausea, vomiting
GU: **Renal failure**
HEME: **Agranulocytosis**, anemia, eosinophilia, **hemolytic anemia**, **leukopenia**, **neutropenia**, **thrombocytopenia**
RESP: **Eosinophilic pneumonia**
SKIN: Pruritus, rash, urticaria
Other: **Anaphylaxis**, direct Coombs test seroconversion, **hyperkalemia**, **hypokalemia**, **hypersensitivity reactions**

Childbearing Considerations

PREGNANCY

- It is not known if drug can cause fetal harm.
- Use with caution only if benefit to mother outweighs potential risk to fetus.

LACTATION

- It is not known if drug is present in breast milk.
- Patient should check with prescriber before breastfeeding.

Nursing Considerations

- Use ceftaroline cautiously in patients hypersensitive to penicillins or carbapenems, because cross-sensitivity may occur.
- Obtain culture and sensitivity results, if possible and as ordered, before giving drug.

! **WARNING** Monitor patient for hypersensitivity to ceftaroline. If present, discontinue ceftaroline, as ordered, and prepare to provide emergency supportive care.

- Assess bowel pattern daily; severe diarrhea may indicate pseudomembranous colitis caused by *C. difficile*. If diarrhea occurs, notify prescriber and expect to withhold drug and treat with electrolytes, fluids, protein, and an antibiotic effective against *C. difficile*.

- Be aware that seroconversion from a negative to a positive direct Coombs test result may occur. If anemia develops during or after ceftaroline therapy, expect a direct Coombs test to be ordered. If drug-induced hemolytic anemia is suspected, expect to discontinue drug and provide supportive care, as indicated.

- Monitor patient closely for adverse neurological reactions such as encephalopathy and seizures, especially in patients with renal impairment. If present, notify prescriber, as drug may have to be discontinued or dosage adjusted.

PATIENT TEACHING

! **WARNING** Urge patient to report hypersensitivity reactions, such as a rash, immediately.

- Instruct patient to report watery, bloody stools to prescriber immediately, even up to 2 months after drug therapy has ended.

- Warn patient that adverse neurological adverse reactions may occur, such as seizures. If any occur, tell patient to notify prescriber immediately, as dosage may have to be changed or drug discontinued.

ceftazidime
Fortaz, Tazicef

⦀ Class and Category
Pharmacologic class: Third-generation cephalosporin
Therapeutic class: Antibiotic

⦀ Indications and Dosages
✳ *To treat UTI caused by* Enterobacter *species,* Escherichia coli, Klebsiella *species,* Proteus mirabilis *and other species such as* indole-positive Proteus, *or* Pseudomonas aeruginosa

I.V. INFUSION, I.V. INJECTION (TAZICEF), I.M. INJECTION
Adults and children age 12 and over. 250 mg every 12 hr. for uncomplicated UTI and 500 mg every 8 to 12 hours for complicated UTI.

I.V. INFUSION, I.V. INJECTION (TAZICEF)
Children age 1 month to 12 years. 30 to 50 mg/kg every 8 hr. *Maximum:* 6 g daily.
Neonates up to 4 weeks. 30 mg/kg every 8 hr.

✳ *To treat uncomplicated pneumonia, caused by* Citrobacter *species,* Enterobacter *species,* Escherichia coli, Haemophilus influenzae, Klebsiella *species,* P. mirabilis, P. aeruginosa *and other* Pseudomonas *species,* Serratia *species,* Staphylococcus pneumoniae, *or* Streptococcus pneumoniae; *mild skin and skin structure infections caused by* Enterobacter *species,* E. coli, Klebsiella *species,* P. mirabilis *and other* Proteus *species including indole-positive* Proteus, Pseudomonas aeruginosa, Serratia *species,* S. aureus, *or* Streptococcus pyogenes (*group A beta-hemolytic streptococci*)

I.V. INFUSION, I.V. INJECTION (TAZICEF), I.M. INJECTION
Adults and children age 12 and over. 0.5 to 1 g every 8 hr.

I.V. INFUSION, I.V. INJECTION (TAZICEF)
Children age 1 month to 12 years. 30 to 50 mg/kg every 8 hr. *Maximum:* 6 g daily.
Neonates up to 4 weeks. 30 mg/kg every 8 hr.

✳ *To treat bone and joint infections caused by* Enterobacter *species,* Klebsiella *species,* P. aeruginosa, *or* S. aureus

I.V. INFUSION, I.V. INJECTION (TAZICEF)
Adults and children age 12 and over. 2 g every 12 hr.
Children age 1 month to 12 years. 30 to 50 mg/kg every 8 hr. *Maximum:* 6 g daily.
Neonates up to 4 weeks. 30 mg/kg every 8 hr.

✳ *To treat serious gynecologic* infections caused by E. coli; *to treat intra-abdominal infections caused by* E. coli, Klebsiella species, *or* S. aureus; *to treat meningitis caused by* H. influenzae *or* Neisseria meningitidis; *and life-threatening infections, such as bacterial septicemia caused by* E. coli, H. influenzae, Klebsiella *species,* P. aeruginosa, Serratia *species,* S. aureus, *or* S. pneumoniae *especially in immunocompromised patients*

I.V. INFUSION, I.V. INJECTION (TAZICEF)
Adults and children age 12 and over. 2 g every 8 hr.
Children age 1 month to 12 years. 30 to 50 mg/kg every 8 hr. *Maximum:* 6 g daily.
Neonates up to 4 weeks. 30 mg/kg every 8 hr.

✳ *To treat pseudomonal lung infection in patients with cystic fibrosis and normal renal function*

I.V. INFUSION, I.V. INJECTION (TAZICEF)
Adults and children 1 month and over. 30 to 50 mg/kg every 8 hr. *Maximum:* 6 g daily.
Neonates from birth to 4 weeks. 30 mg/kg every 12 hr.

± **DOSAGE ADJUSTMENT** Dosage reduced to 1 g every 12 hr if creatinine clearance is 31 to 50 ml/min; to 1 g every 24 hr if 16 to 30 ml/min; to 0.5 g every 24 hr if 6 to 15 ml/min; and to 0.5 g every 48 hr if less than 6 ml/min. For hemodialysis patients, a loading dose of 1 g given followed by 1 g after each session.

Drug Administration

I.V.

- Administration of fractional doses is not recommended.

Vials

- Do not use pharmacy bulk package for I.V. injection.
- Protect ceftazidime powder and reconstituted drug from heat and light; both tend to darken during storage.
- Thaw frozen solution at room temperature, not in water bath or microwave. Do not refreeze.
- Don't use diluents containing benzyl alcohol when administering to neonates.
- All drug vials are under reduced pressure. Carbon dioxide will be released during dissolution, causing positive pressure to develop in the drug vial.
- Consult recommended manufacturer instructions to reconstitute drug, as instructions vary among products.
- Administer I.V. injection (Tazicef) slowly over 3 to 5 minutes through tubing of a flowing compatible I.V. fluid.
- For intermittent infusion, administer over about 30 minutes.
- Avoid using Sodium Bicarbonate Injection as a diluent because drug is least stable in it.
- During administration, temporarily stop other solutions being given at the same I.V. site.
- Rotate I.V. sites every 72 hours.
- Store solution for up to 12 hours at room temperature or 7 days in refrigerator. Thawed solution may be stored for up to 8 hours at room temperature and 4 days if stored in refrigerator.

Duplex

- Keep container in folded position until activation is intended. Remove from refrigerator and allow to come to room temperature.
- Unlatch side tab and unfold container. Visually inspect diluent chamber. Use only if container and seals are intact.
- Inspect drug powder by peeling foil strip from drug chamber. Protect from light after removal of foil strip. If foil strip is removed but administration is delayed, refold container and latch side tab. Product then must be used within 7 days.
- To reconstitute, unfold container and point the set port in a downward direction. Starting at the hanger tab end, fold the container just below the diluent meniscus, trapping all air above the fold. To activate, squeeze the folded diluent chamber until the seal between the diluent and powder opens, releasing diluent into the drug powder chamber. Agitate the liquid-powder mixture until completely dissolved. Once dissolved, drug must be used within 24 hours if stored at room temperature or 7 days if refrigerated.
- To administer, point the set port in a downward direction. Starting at the hanger tab end, fold the container just below the solution meniscus, trapping all air above the fold. Squeeze the folded container until the seal between the reconstituted drug and set port opens, releasing the solution to set port. Squeeze container firmly to check for minute leaks. Then peel foil cover from the set port and attach administration set.
- Do not use in series connections.
- Do not introduce additives to the container.
- Administer as an infusion over about 30 minutes.
- *Incompatibilities:* Aminoglycosides, vancomycin

I.M.

- Reconstitute each gram with 3 ml Sterile Water for Injection, Bacteriostatic Water for Injection, or 0.5% or 1% Lidocaine Hydrochloride Injection.
- Give I.M. injection deep into large muscle mass, such as the gluteus maximus or lateral part of the thigh.

Route	Onset	Peak	Duration
I.V.	Immediate	30 min	Unknown
I.M.	Unknown	1 hr	Unknown

Half-life: 2 hr

Mechanism of Action

Interferes with bacterial cell wall synthesis by inhibiting the cross-linking of peptidoglycan strands. Peptidoglycan makes the cell membrane rigid and protective. Without it, bacterial cells rupture and die.

Contraindications

Hypersensitivity to ceftazidime, other beta-lactam or cephalosporins, penicillins or their components

Interactions

DRUGS

aminoglycosides, loop diuretics: Increased risk of nephrotoxicity
chloramphenicol: Antagonistic effect on ceftazidime
oral combined estrogen–progesterone contraceptives: Decreased effectiveness of oral contraceptive

Adverse Reactions

CNS: Chills, **coma, encephalopathy,** fever, headache, irregular lapses of posture, **nonconvulsive status epilepticus,** myoclonus, neuromuscular excitability, **seizures**
CV: Edema
EENT: Hearing loss, oral candidiasis
GI: Abdominal cramps, *Clostridioides difficile*–associated diarrhea, diarrhea, elevated liver enzymes, **hepatic failure,** hepatomegaly, nausea, **pseudomembranous colitis,** vomiting
GU: Elevated BUN level, **nephrotoxicity, renal failure,** vaginal candidiasis
HEME: Eosinophilia, **hemolytic anemia, hypoprothrombinemia, neutropenia, thrombocytopenia, unusual bleeding**
MS: Arthralgia
RESP: Dyspnea
SKIN: Ecchymosis, erythema, **erythema multiforme,** pruritus, rash, **Stevens–Johnson syndrome**
Other: **Anaphylaxis;** injection-site pain, redness, and swelling; superinfection

Childbearing Considerations

PREGNANCY

- It is not known if drug can cause fetal harm.

- Use with caution only if benefit to mother outweighs potential risk to fetus.

LACTATION

- Drug is present in breast milk.
- Patient should check with prescriber before breastfeeding.

Nursing Considerations

- Use ceftazidime cautiously in patients hypersensitive to penicillin, because cross-sensitivity occurs in about 10% of such patients.
- Use cautiously in patients with a history of GI disease, particularly colitis, because risk of pseudomembranous colitis is increased.
- Use cautiously in patients with renal insufficiency, because high and prolonged serum ceftazidime concentrations can occur from usual dosages. This can lead to asterixis, coma, encephalopathy, myoclonia, neuromuscular excitability, nonconvulsive status epilepticus, and seizures. Ensure that patients with significant renal insufficiency are receiving reduced dosage based on their creatinine clearance.
- Obtain culture and sensitivity test results, if possible and as ordered, before giving drug.

! **WARNING** Monitor patient for allergic reactions a few days after therapy starts. If present, notify prescriber and provide supportive care as ordered.

- Assess patient's bowel pattern daily; severe diarrhea may indicate *Clostridioides difficile*–associated diarrhea or pseudomembranous colitis. If confirmed, drug may have to be discontinued and additional supportive care given, as ordered.
- Monitor ALT, AST, bilirubin, CBC, hematocrit, LD, and serum alkaline phosphatase, levels during long-term therapy.
- Monitor PT, as ordered, in at-risk patients, such as those with hepatic or renal impairment or poor nutritional state and those receiving anticoagulant or prolonged antibiotic therapy. Notify prescriber if PT decreases, and expect to give vitamin K.
- Assess for signs of superinfection, such as cough or sputum changes, diarrhea, drainage, fever, malaise, pain, perineal itching, rash, redness, and swelling.

- Watch for arthralgia, bleeding, ecchymosis, and pharyngitis (possible blood dyscrasia). Monitor PT and bleeding time.

PATIENT TEACHING

- Tell patient to take ceftazidime exactly as prescribed.
- Tell patient to report evidence of blood dyscrasia or superinfection to prescriber immediately.

> **! WARNING** Alert patient that allergic reactions can occur, especially after a few days of drug therapy. Instruct patient to notify prescriber if present and seek immediate medical attention if severe.

- Urge patient to report watery, bloody stools to prescriber immediately, even up to 2 months after drug therapy has ended.
- Review signs and symptoms of types of neurologic adverse reactions that may occur with ceftazidime therapy. If present, urge patient to notify prescriber.
- Urge diabetic patients testing urine for glucose to use an enzymatic glucose oxidase reactor during drug therapy.

ceftriaxone sodium

☰ Class and Category

Pharmacologic class: Third-generation cephalosporin
Therapeutic class: Antibiotic

☰ Indications and Dosages

* *To treat infections such as bacterial septicemia caused by* Escherichia coli, Haemophilus influenzae, Klebsiella pneumoniae, Staphylococcus aureus, *or* Streptococcus pneumoniae; *bone and joint infections caused by* Enterobacter *species,* E. coli, K. pneumoniae, Proteus mirabilis, S. aureus, *or* S. pneumoniae; *intra-abdominal infections caused by* Bacteroides fragilis, Clostridium *species,* E. coli, K. pneumoniae, *or* Peptostreptococcus *species; lower respiratory tract infections caused by* Enterobacter aerogenes, E. coli, H. influenzae, H. parainfluenzae, K. pneumoniae, P. mirabilis, Serratia marcescens, S. aureus, *or* S. pneumoniae; *pelvic inflammatory disease caused by* Neisseria gonorrhoeae; *skin and soft-tissue infections caused by* Acinetobacter

calcoaceticus, B. fragilis, E. cloacae, E. coli, K. pneumoniae, K. oxytoca, Morganella morganii, Peptostreptococcus species, P. mirabilis, Pseudomonas aeruginosa, Serratia marcescens, S. aureus, S. epidermidis, S. pyogenes, *or* Viridans *group streptococci; and urinary tract infections caused by* E. coli, K. pneumoniae, M. morganii, P. mirabilis, *or* P. vulgaris

I.V. INFUSION, I.M. INJECTION

Adults. 1 to 2 g daily or in equally divided doses twice daily for 4 to 14 days, although complicated infections may require longer therapy. Infections caused by *Streptococcus pyogenes* should be continued for at least 10 days.

Children. 50 to 75 mg/kg daily or in equally divided doses every 12 hr. *Maximum:* 2 g daily.

* *To treat meningitis caused by* H. influenzae, Neisseria meningitidis, *or* S. pneumoniae

I.V. INFUSION

Adults. 1 to 2 g daily or in equally divided doses twice daily for 4 to 14 days, although a complicated infection may require longer therapy. *Maximum:* 4 g daily.

Children. *Initial:* 100 mg/kg on first day, then 100 mg/kg daily or in divided doses every 12 hr for 7 to 14 days. *Maximum:* 4 g daily.

* *To treat acute bacterial otitis media caused by* H. influenzae, Moraxella catarrhalis, *or* S. pneumoniae

I.M. INJECTION

Children. 50 mg/kg as a single dose. *Maximum:* 1 g.

* *To treat uncomplicated gonorrhea (cervical/urethral, pharyngeal, or rectal) caused by* Neisseria gonorrhoeae

I.M. INJECTION

Adults. 250 mg as a single dose.

* *To provide surgical prophylaxis*

I.V. INFUSION

Adults. 1 g 30 min to 2 hr before surgery.

☰ Drug Administration

I.V.

ADD-Vantage vials

- Open diluent container by peeling overwrap at corner and remove solution container. Some opacity of the plastic may be present, but this is normal. The opacity will diminish gradually.

- Assemble vial and flexible diluent container by removing the protective covers from the top of the vial and the vial port on the diluent container by swinging the pull ring over the top of the vial and pulling down far enough to start the opening; then pull straight up to remove the cap. To remove the vial port cover, grasp the tab on the pull ring, pulling up to break the three tie strings, then pull back to remove the cover. Screw the vial into the vial port until it will go no further. Label appropriately.
- Squeeze the bottom of the diluent container gently to inflate the portion of the container surrounding the end of the drug vial. With the other hand, push the drug vial down into the container, telescoping the walls of the container. Grasp the inner cap of the vial through the walls of the container. Pull the inner cap from the drug vial, allowing the drug and diluent to mix. Mix thoroughly.
- Prepare to administer by checking for leaks by squeezing container firmly. If present, discard and obtain a new one. Attach administration set. Lift the free end of the hanger loop on the bottom of the vial, breaking the two tie strings. Bend loop outward to lock it in the upright position, then suspend from hanger. Attach administration set.
- Do not use plastic containers in series connections.
- Administer over 30 minutes.

Single-use regular vials
- If using drug vials, reconstitute with an appropriate diluent, such as Sterile Water for Injection, 0.9% Sodium Chloride for Injection, or 5% Dextrose Injection (see manufacturer guidelines for other solutions that can be used) as follows: for 250-mg vial, add 2.4 ml; for 500-mg vial, add 4.8 ml; for 1-g vial, add 9.6 ml; and for 2-g vial, add 19.2 ml to yield 100 mg/ml.
- After reconstitution, further dilute to 50 to 100 ml with diluent indicated above and infuse over 30 minutes (60 minutes for neonates).
- Do not use plastic containers in series connections.
- If administering with a pump, take care to discontinue pumping action before the container runs dry, or an air embolism may result.

- Store drug powder at room temperature and protect from light. After reconstitution, protection from light is not necessary. Check manufacturer guidelines for length of storage based upon concentration and diluent used.

Duplex
- Keep container in folded position until activation is intended. Remove from refrigerator and allow to come to room temperature.
- Unlatch side tab and unfold container. Visually inspect diluent chamber. Use only if container and seals are intact.
- Inspect drug powder by peeling foil strip from drug chamber. Protect from light after removal of foil strip. If foil strip is removed but administration is delayed, refold container and latch side tab. Product then must be used within 7 days.
- To reconstitute, unfold container and point the set port in a downward direction. Starting at the hanger tab end, fold the container just below the diluent meniscus, trapping all air above the fold. To activate, squeeze the folded diluent chamber until the seal between the diluent and powder opens, releasing diluent into the drug powder chamber. Agitate the liquid-powder mixture until completely dissolved. Once dissolved, drug must be used within 24 hours if stored at room temperature or 7 days if refrigerated.
- To administer, point the set port in a downward direction. Starting at the hanger tab end, fold the container just below the solution meniscus, trapping all air above the fold. Squeeze the folded container until the seal between the reconstituted drug and set port opens, releasing the solution to set port. Squeeze container firmly to check for minute leaks. Then peel foil cover from the set port and attach administration set.
- Do not use in series connections.
- Do not introduce additives to the container.
- Administer as an infusion over about 30 minutes.
- *Incompatibilities:* Aminoglycosides; amsacrine; calcium solutions such as Ringer's solution or Hartmann's solution, including parenteral nutrition; fluconazole; vancomycin. For patients

other than neonates, ceftriaxone and calcium-containing solutions may be given sequentially if infusion lines are thoroughly flushed with a compatible fluid between infusions.

I.M.

- Reconstitute with an appropriate diluent, such as Sterile Water for Injection or 0.9% Sodium Chloride for Injection, by adding 1.8 ml to a 500-mg vial to make a concentration of 250 mg/ml and 1 ml to a 500-mg vial to make a 350-mg/ml concentration. Using a 1-gram vial, add 3.6 ml to make a 250-mg/ml concentration and 2.1 ml to make a 350-mg/ml concentration.
- Shake well.
- Inject deep into large muscle mass, such as the gluteus maximus.
- Know that lidocaine can be used instead of Sterile Water for Injection as a diluent to lessen the pain of an I.M. injection (follow manufacturer instructions when doing so). However, it is not without risk.
- Store drug powder at room temperature and protect from light. After reconstitution, protection from light is not necessary. Check manufacturer guidelines for length of storage based upon concentration and diluent used.

Route	Onset	Peak	Duration
I.V.	Immediate	30 min	Unknown
I.M.	Unknown	1.5–4 hr	Unknown

Half-life: 5–9 hr

▤ Mechanism of Action

Interferes with bacterial cell wall synthesis by inhibiting cross-linking of peptidoglycan strands. Peptidoglycan makes the cell membrane rigid and protective. Without it, bacterial cells rupture and die.

▤ Contraindications

Hyperbilirubinemic or premature neonates (up to a postmenstrual age of 41 weeks); hypersensitivity to ceftriaxone, other beta-lactam antibacterials or cephalosporins, penicillins, or their components; intravenous administration of ceftriaxone solutions containing lidocaine; neonates who are 28 days old or less if they're expected to need calcium-containing solutions, including parenteral nutrition.

▤ Interactions

DRUGS

aminoglycosides, loop diuretics: Increased risk of nephrotoxicity

▤ Adverse Reactions

CNS: Chills, fever, headache, hypertonia, reversible hyperactivity, **seizures**
CV: Edema
EENT: Glossitis, hearing loss, stomatitis
GI: Abdominal cramps, cholestasis, *Clostridium difficile*–associated **diarrhea**, diarrhea, elevated liver enzymes, gallbladder dysfunction, **hepatic failure**, **hepatitis**, hepatomegaly, nausea, oral candidiasis, **pancreatitis**, pseudolithiasis, **pseudomembranous colitis**, vomiting
GU: **Acute renal failure**, elevated BUN level, **nephrotoxicity**, oliguria, vaginal candidiasis, ureteric obstruction, urolithiasis
HEME: **Agranulocytosis, aplastic anemia**, eosinophilia, **hemolytic anemia**, **hemorrhage, hypoprothrombinemia**, **leukopenia, neutropenia, thrombocytopenia**
MS: Arthralgia
RESP: **Allergic pneumonitis**, dyspnea
SKIN: Allergic dermatitis, ecchymosis, erythema, **erythema multiforme**, exanthema, pruritus, rash, **Stevens–Johnson syndrome**, **toxic epidermal necrolysis**, urticaria
Other: **Anaphylaxis**; drug fever; injection-site pain, redness, and swelling; serum sickness; superinfection

▤ Childbearing Considerations

PREGNANCY

- It is not known if drug can cause fetal harm.
- Use with caution only if benefit to mother outweighs potential risk to fetus.

LACTATION

- Drug is present in breast milk.
- Patient should check with prescriber before breastfeeding.

▤ Nursing Considerations

! **WARNING** Be aware that calcium-containing products must not be given I.V. within 48 hours of ceftriaxone, including solutions given through a different I.V. line and at a different site, in neonates because a ceftriaxone-calcium salt may precipitate in the lungs and kidneys and could be fatal.

- Use ceftriaxone cautiously in patients who are hypersensitive to penicillins, because cross-sensitivity has occurred in about 1% to 3% of such patients.

! **WARNING** Ask patient if an allergic reaction was ever experienced when given other antibiotics. Patients who have had previous hypersensitivity reactions to carbapenems, other cephalosporins, penicillins, or other drugs may be at high risk for developing a serious reaction that may be fatal. Monitor all patients closely for a hypersensitivity reaction. If present, discontinue ceftriaxone immediately, notify prescriber, and be prepared to provide emergency supportive care, as prescribed.

- Obtain culture and sensitivity results, if possible and as ordered, before giving drug.
- Be aware that local anesthetics such as lidocaine used to lessen the pain of an I.M. injection may cause methemoglobinemia as late as several hours after the injection. Monitor patient closely.
- Monitor BUN and serum creatinine levels to detect early signs of nephrotoxicity. Also monitor fluid intake and output; decreasing urine output may indicate nephrotoxicity. Also be alert for precipitates in the patient's urine, especially children. If any sign of renal dysfunction occurs, notify prescriber, expect ceftriaxone to be discontinued, and provide supportive care, as prescribed.
- Assess ALT, AST, bilirubin, CBC, hematocrit, LD, and serum alkaline phosphatase levels during long-term therapy. If abnormalities occur, notify prescriber. Drug may have to be discontinued.
- Assess bowel pattern daily; severe diarrhea may indicate pseudomembranous colitis caused by *C. difficile*. If diarrhea occurs, notify prescriber and expect to treat with electrolytes, fluids, protein, and an antibiotic effective against *C. difficile*. Ceftriaxone therapy may be withheld also.
- Monitor patient for evidence of gallbladder disease (abdominal pain, nausea, vomiting) because drug may cause ceftriaxone-calcium salt to deposit in the gallbladder, which may mimic gallstones. Expect drug to be discontinued if gallbladder disorders arise.

- Assess for signs of superinfection, such as cough or sputum changes, diarrhea, drainage, fever, malaise, pain, perineal itching, rash, redness, and swelling.
- Assess for arthralgia, bleeding, ecchymosis, and pharyngitis; they may indicate a blood dyscrasia.

PATIENT TEACHING
- Tell patient to report evidence of blood dyscrasia or superinfection to prescriber immediately.
- Urge patient to report watery, bloody stools to prescriber immediately, even up to 2 months after drug therapy has ended.

! **WARNING** Advise patient to report any hypersensitivity reactions, such as a rash, itching skin, or hives, to prescriber immediately and to stop taking the drug.

- Tell patient that if he received drug as an I.M. injection that used lidocaine as the diluent, he should watch for signs and symptoms such as fatigue; headache; light-headedness; skin color change of blue, gray, or pale; rapid heart rate; or shortness of breath. If present, patient should seek immediate medical attention.

cefuroxime axetil

cefuroxime sodium
Zinacef

⧉ Class and Category
Pharmacologic class: Second-generation cephalosporin
Therapeutic class: Antibiotic

⧉ Indications and Dosages
✳ *To treat pharyngitis and tonsillitis caused by* Streptococcus pyogenes

TABLETS
Adults and adolescents. 250 mg every 12 hr for 10 days.

✳ *To treat acute otitis media caused by* Haemophilus influenzae, Moraxella catarrhalis, Streptococcus pneumoniae, *or* S. pyogenes

TABLETS
Children under age 13 who can swallow tablets. 250 mg every 12 hr for 10 days.

* *To treat acute bacterial maxillary sinusitis caused by* H. influenzae *or* S. pneumoniae

TABLETS

Adults, adolescents, and children under age 13 who can swallow tablets. 250 mg every 12 hr for 10 days.

* *To treat acute bacterial exacerbations of chronic bronchitis (mild to moderate) caused by* H. influenzae, Haemophilus parainfluenzae, *or* S. pneumoniae

TABLETS

Adults and adolescents. 250 or 500 mg every 12 hr for 10 days.

* *To treat uncomplicated skin and skin structure infections caused by* Enterobacter *species,* E. coli, Klebsiella *species,* S. aureus, *or* S. pyogenes

TABLETS

Adults and adolescents. 250 or 500 mg every 12 hr for 10 days.

I.V. INFUSION, I.V. OR I.M. INJECTION (ZINACEF)

Adults and adolescents. 750 mg every 8 hr for 5 to 10 days.

* *To treat secondary bacterial infections of acute bronchitis caused by* S. aureus *or* S. pyogenes

TABLETS

Adults and adolescents. 250 or 500 mg every 12 hr for 5 to 10 days.

* *To treat lower respiratory tract infections including pneumonia caused by* E. coli, H. influenzae, Klebsiella *species,* S. aureus, S. pneumoniae, *or* S. pyogenes

I.V. INFUSION, I.V. OR I.M. INJECTION (ZINACEF)

Adults. 750 mg to 1.5 g every 8 hr for 5 to 10 days.

* *To treat early Lyme disease caused by* Borrelia burgdorferi

TABLETS

Adults and adolescents. 500 mg every 12 hr for 20 days.

* *To treat uncomplicated UTI caused by* E. coli *or* Klebsiella pneumoniae

TABLETS

Adults. 250 mg every 12 hr for 7 to 10 days.

I.V. INFUSION, I.V. OR I.M. INJECTION (ZINACEF)

Adults. 750 mg every 8 hr for 5 to 10 days.

* *To treat uncomplicated gonorrhea caused by* Neisseria gonorrhoeae

TABLETS

Adults. 1 g as a single dose.

I.M. INJECTION (ZINACEF)

Adults. 1.5 g as a single dose and given with oral probenecid 1 g.

* *To treat bone and joint infections caused by* S. aureus

I.V. INFUSION, I.V. OR I.M. INJECTION (ZINACEF)

Adults. 1.5 g every 8 hr.

Children over age 3 months. 150 mg/kg daily in divided doses every 8 hr. *Maximum:* Adult dose.

* *To treat bacterial meningitis caused by* H. influenzae, Neisseria meningitidis, S. aureus, *or* S. pneumoniae

I.V. INFUSION, I.V. INJECTION (ZINACEF)

Adults. 1.5 to 3 g every 8 hr.

Children over age 3 months. 200 to 240 mg/kg/daily in divided doses every 6 to 8 hr.

* *To treat moderate infections other than those listed above*

I.V. INFUSION, I.V. OR I.M. INJECTION (ZINACEF)

Adults. 750 mg every 8 hr for 5 to 10 days.

I.V. INFUSION OR INJECTION (ZINACEF)

Children over age 3 months. 50 mg/kg daily in equally divided doses every 6 to 8 hr.

* *To treat severe or complicated infections other than those listed above*

I.V. INFUSION OR INJECTION (ZINACEF)

Adults. 1.5 g every 8 hr.

Children over age 3 months. 100 mg/kg daily in equally divided doses every 6 to 8 hr.

* *To treat life-threatening infections other than those listed above*

I.V. INFUSION OR INJECTION (ZINACEF)

Adults. 1.5 g every 6 hr.

* *To provide perioperative prophylaxis*

I.V. INJECTION (ZINACEF)

Adults. 1.5 g 30 to 60 min before surgery (at induction of anesthesia for open-heart surgery), and then 0.75 g every 8 hr for prolonged procedures (1.5 g every 12 hr for total of 6 g with open-heart surgery).

±**DOSAGE ADJUSTMENT** Parenteral dosage for adults reduced to 0.75 g every 12 hr if creatinine clearance is 10 to 20 ml/min or to 0.75 g every 24 hr if creatinine clearance is less than 10 ml/min. For parenteral dosage for children, frequency expanded to every 12 hr if creatinine clearance is 10 to 20 ml/min or to 24 hr if creatinine clearance is less than 10 ml/min.

▤ Drug Administration

P.O.

- Tablet should be swallowed whole and not chewed, crushed, or split.
- Administer with food.
- Make sure lid on container is put on tightly.

I.V.

Vials

- Reconstitute each 750-mg vial with 8.3 ml of Sterile Water for Injection and each 1.5-gram vial with 16 ml of Sterile Water for Injection.
- For I.V. injection, administer slowly into a vein over 3 to 5 minutes through the tubing system of a free-flowing intravenous solution.
- For intermittent I.V. infusion with a Y-type administration set, temporarily discontinue administration of any other solution at the same site. Dilute reconstituted drug with 100 ml of 0.9% Sodium Chloride Injection or 5% Dextrose Injection and infuse over 15 to 60 minutes.
  - Follow manufacturer instructions for use of TwistVials when used to prepare an intermittent I.V. infusion.
- For continuous I.V. infusion, add reconstituted drug to 0.9% Sodium Chloride Injection or 5% Dextrose Injection (see manufacturer guidelines for other solutions that may be used) to provide a concentration between 1 and 30 mg/ml.
- Store reconstituted or diluted solution for 24 hours at room temperature or 48 hours refrigerated.

Galaxy Plastic Containers

- Follow manufacturer instructions on use of Galaxy plastic containers used for intermittent or continuous infusions.

Duplex

- Keep container in folded position until activation is intended. Remove from refrigerator and allow to come to room temperature.
- Unlatch side tab and unfold container. Visually inspect diluent chamber. Use only if container and seals are intact.
- Inspect drug powder by peeling foil strip from drug chamber. Protect from light after removal of foil strip. If foil strip is removed but administration is delayed, refold container and latch side tab. Product then must be used within 7 days.
- To reconstitute, unfold container and point the set port in a downward direction. Starting at the hanger tab end, fold the container just below the diluent meniscus, trapping all air above the fold. To activate, squeeze the folded diluent chamber until the seal between the diluent and powder opens, releasing diluent into the drug powder chamber. Agitate the liquid-powder mixture until completely dissolved. Once dissolved, drug must be used within 24 hours if stored at room temperature or 7 days if refrigerated.
- To administer, point the set port in a downward direction. Starting at the hanger tab end, fold the container just below the solution meniscus, trapping all air above the fold. Squeeze the folded container until the seal between the reconstituted drug and set port opens, releasing the solution to set port. Squeeze container firmly to check for minute leaks. Then peel foil cover from the set port and attach administration set.
- Do not use in series connections.
- Do not introduce additives to the container.
- For intermittent infusion, administer over 15 to 60 minutes.
- *Incompatibilities:* Aminoglycosides

I.M.

- Reconstitute 750-mg vial with 3 ml of Sterile Water for Injection.
- Inject into a large muscle mass such as the gluteus maximus or the lateral side of the thigh.
- Store reconstituted solution for 24 hours at room temperature or 48 hours refrigerated.

Route	Onset	Peak	Duration
P.O.	Unknown	2–3 hr	Unknown
I.V.	Immediate	2–3 min	Unknown
I.M.	Unknown	15–30 min	Unknown

Half-life: 1–2 hr

▤ Mechanism of Action

Interferes with bacterial cell wall synthesis by inhibiting the final step in the cross-linking of peptidoglycan strands. Peptidoglycan makes the cell membrane rigid and protective. Without it, bacterial cells rupture and die.

Contraindications

Hypersensitivity to cefuroxime, other cephalosporins, or their components

Interactions

DRUGS

aminoglycosides, loop diuretics: Increased risk of nephrotoxicity
antacids, histamine-2 antagonists, proton pump inhibitors: Possibly lower bioavailability of oral cefuroxime
oral combined estrogen–progesterone contraceptives: Decreased effectiveness of oral contraceptive

Adverse Reactions

CNS: Chills, fever, headache, **seizures**
CV: Acute myocardial ischemia with or without MI, edema
EENT: Hearing loss, oral candidiasis
GI: Abdominal cramps, diarrhea, elevated liver enzymes, **hepatic failure**, hepatomegaly, nausea, **pseudomembranous colitis,** vomiting
GU: Elevated BUN level, **nephrotoxicity, renal failure**, vaginal candidiasis
HEME: Eosinophilia, **hemolytic anemia, hypoprothrombinemia, neutropenia, thrombocytopenia, unusual bleeding**
MS: Arthralgia
RESP: Dyspnea
SKIN: Cutaneous vasculitis, ecchymosis, erythema, **erythema multiforme**, pruritus, rash, **Stevens–Johnson syndrome**
Other: Anaphylaxis; angioedema; injection-site edema, pain, and redness; serum sickness–like reaction; superinfection

Childbearing Considerations

PREGNANCY

- It is not known if drug can cause fetal harm.
- Use with caution only if benefit to mother outweighs potential risk to fetus.

LACTATION

- Drug is present in breast milk.
- Patient should check with prescriber before breastfeeding.

Nursing Considerations

- Use cefuroxime cautiously in patients hypersensitive to penicillin, because cross-sensitivity has occurred in about 10% of such patients.

- Obtain culture and sensitivity results, if possible and as ordered, before giving drug.
- Monitor I.V. site for extravasation and phlebitis.
- Monitor BUN and serum creatinine levels and fluid intake and output to detect signs of nephrotoxicity. Monitor patients with renal impairment closely because they may have greater toxic reactions to cefuroxime.

! **WARNING** Monitor patient for allergic reactions that may occur a few days after therapy starts. Patients with a history of some form of allergy, especially to drugs, are at increased risk for an allergic reaction. Be aware that acute myocardial ischemia with or without MI can be part of the allergic reaction.

- Assess bowel pattern daily; severe diarrhea may indicate pseudomembranous colitis. If it's suspected, stop drug, as ordered, and provide treatment as prescribed.
- Assess patient for arthralgia, bleeding, ecchymosis, and pharyngitis, which may indicate a blood dyscrasia.
- Monitor bleeding time and PT, as ordered. Be prepared to administer vitamin K, if ordered, to treat hypothrombinemia.

PATIENT TEACHING

- Inform patient that buttermilk and yogurt help maintain intestinal flora and can decrease diarrhea during therapy.
- Instruct patient to report evidence of blood dyscrasia to prescriber immediately.
- Urge patient to report watery, bloody stools to prescriber immediately, even up to 2 months after drug therapy has ended.

! **WARNING** Alert patient that drug can cause an allergic reaction even up to a few days after drug therapy starts. Stress importance of notifying prescriber, if present, and to seek immediate medical attention if severe.

celecoxib

Celebrex, Elyxyb

Class and Category

Pharmacologic class: NSAID
Therapeutic class: Analgesic, anti-inflammatory, antirheumatic

≡ Indications and Dosages

＊ *To relieve signs and symptoms of osteoarthritis*

CAPSULES

Adults. 200 mg daily or 100 mg twice daily.

＊ *To relieve signs and symptoms of rheumatoid arthritis*

CAPSULES

Adults. 100 to 200 mg twice daily.

＊ *To relieve signs and symptoms of juvenile rheumatoid arthritis*

CAPSULES

Children age 2 and over weighing more than 25 kg (55 lb). 100 mg twice daily.
Children age 2 and over weighing 10 to 25 kg (22 to 55 lb). 50 mg twice daily.

＊ *To relieve pain from ankylosing spondylitis*

CAPSULES

Adults. 200 mg daily or 100 mg twice daily. Dosage increased to 400 mg daily or 200 mg twice daily after 6 weeks, if needed.

＊ *To manage acute pain, to treat primary dysmenorrhea*

CAPSULES

Adults. 400 mg, followed by 200 mg, if needed, on 1st day. On subsequent days, 200 mg twice daily, as needed.

＊ *To treat acute migraine*

ORAL SOLUTION (ELYXYB)

Adults. 120 mg as a single dose. *Maximum:* 120 mg in a 24-hr period.

±**DOSAGE ADJUSTMENT** Daily dosage reduced by 50% for patients with moderate hepatic impairment. For patients who are poor CYP2C9 metabolizers, starting dosage should be half the lowest recommended dose and the maximum dose for the treatment of migraine headaches should not exceed 60 mg in a 24-hour period.

≡ Drug Administration

P.O.

- Capsule may be opened and sprinkled onto a level teaspoon of cool or room-temperature applesauce and given with water, if capsule cannot be swallowed whole. Mixture should not be chewed.
- Drug-and-applesauce mixture may be stored up to 6 hours in refrigerator.
- Use a calibrated device to measure dose of oral solution. The concentration is 120 mg/4.8 ml.
- Store at room temperature.

Route	Onset	Peak	Duration
P.O.	Unknown	3 hr	Unknown

Half-life: 11 hr

≡ Mechanism of Action

Selectively inhibits the enzymatic activity of cyclooxygenase-2 (COX-2), the enzyme needed to convert arachidonic acid to prostaglandin. Prostaglandins are responsible for mediating the inflammatory response and causing local vasodilation, swelling, and pain. Prostaglandins also play a role in peripheral pain transmission to the spinal cord. By inhibiting COX-2 activity and prostaglandin production, this reduces inflammatory symptoms and relieves pain.

≡ Contraindications

Allergic reaction (such as anaphylaxis or angioedema) to aspirin, other NSAIDs, or sulfonamide derivatives or history of aspirin-induced nasal polyps with bronchospasm; hypersensitivity to celecoxib or its components; treatment of pain after coronary artery bypass graft surgery

≡ Interactions

DRUGS

ACE inhibitors, angiotensin II receptor antagonists, beta blockers: Decreased antihypertensive effect of these drugs, increased risk of renal failure in patients who are elderly, have existing renal dysfunction, or are volume-depleted

anticoagulants such as warfarin, antiplatelet drugs such as aspirin and other salicylates, corticosteroids, selective serotonin reuptake inhibitors: Increased risk of GI ulceration and other GI complications, increased risk of bleeding

cyclosporine: Increased risk of cyclosporine-induced nephrotoxicity

CYP2C9 inducers such as rifampin: Possibly decreased effectiveness of celecoxib

CYP2C9 inhibitors such as fluconazole: Possibly increased risk of celecoxib toxicity

CYP2D6 substrates: Possibly enhance the exposure and toxicity of these drugs

digoxin: Increased risk of digitalis toxicity

furosemide, thiazide diuretics: Reduced diuretic effects of these drugs, increased risk of renal failure

lithium: Possibly elevated blood lithium level

methotrexate: Increased risk of methotrexate toxicity (neutropenia, renal dysfunction, thrombocytopenia)
pemetrexed: Increased risk of myelosuppression, GI, and renal toxicity

Adverse Reactions

CNS: Aseptic meningitis, **cerebral hemorrhage, CVA,** depression, dizziness, fever, headache, insomnia, **suicidal ideation,** syncope, transient ischemic attacks, vertigo
CV: **Aortic valve incompetence, bradycardia,** chest pain, **congestive heart failure, deep vein thrombosis,** fluid retention, hypertension, **MI,** palpitations, peripheral edema, tachycardia, **thrombosis, unstable angina,** vasculitis, **ventricular fibrillation, ventricular hypertrophy**
EENT: Conjunctival hemorrhage, deafness, labyrinthitis, nasopharyngitis, pharyngitis, rhinitis, sinusitis, vitreous floaters
ENDO: Hyperglycemia, **hypoglycemia**
GI: Abdominal pain, diarrhea, elevated liver enzymes, **esophageal perforation,** flatulence, **GI bleeding** or ulceration, **hepatic failure,** ileus, indigestion, jaundice, nausea, **pancreatitis, perforation of intestines or stomach,** vomiting
GU: **Acute renal failure,** interstitial nephritis, ovarian cyst, proteinuria, urinary incontinence, UTI
HEME: **Agranulocytosis, aplastic anemia,** decreased hematocrit and hemoglobin, **leukopenia, pancytopenia, prolonged APTT, thrombocytopenia**
MS: Arthralgia, back pain, elevated serum creatine kinase level, epicondylitis, tendon rupture
RESP: **Bronchospasm,** cough, dyspnea, pneumonia, **pulmonary embolism,** upper respiratory tract infection
SKIN: **Erythema multiforme, exfoliative dermatitis,** phototoxicity, rash, **Stevens–Johnson syndrome, toxic epidermal necrolysis,** urticaria
Other: **Anaphylaxis, angioedema, drug reaction with eosinophilia and systemic symptoms (DRESS), hyperkalemia, hypernatremia, hyponatremia, sepsis**

Childbearing Considerations

PREGNANCY

- Drug increases risk of premature closure of the fetal ductus arteriosus if given during the third trimester of pregnancy and fetal renal dysfunction causing oligohydramnios and possibly neonatal renal impairment if given during the second or third trimester of pregnancy.
- Drug is not recommended in pregnant women starting at 20 weeks of gestation.

LACTATION

- Drug may be present in breast milk in low concentrations.
- Patient should check with prescriber before breastfeeding.

REPRODUCTION

- Drug may delay or prevent rupture of ovarian follicles, which may result in infertility that is reversible once drug therapy has been discontinued.
- Drug may have to be withheld in women who are having difficulty conceiving or who are being tested for infertility.

Nursing Considerations

- Know that NSAIDs like celecoxib should be avoided in patients with a recent MI because risk of reinfarction increases with NSAID therapy. If therapy is unavoidable, monitor patient closely for signs of cardiac ischemia.
- Be aware that NSAIDs such as celecoxib should not be given to patients with severe heart failure because risk of heart failure increases with NSAID use. If use is unavoidable, monitor patient for worsening of heart failure.
- Use celecoxib with extreme caution in patients who have a history of GI bleeding or ulcer disease because NSAIDs, such as celecoxib, increase the risk of GI bleeding and ulceration. In these patients, drug should be used for shortest time possible.
- Be aware that serious GI tract ulceration and bleeding, as well as perforation of intestine or stomach, can occur without warning or symptoms. Debilitated or elderly patients are at greatest risk along with patients with a prior history of GI bleeding and/or peptic ulcer disease who used NSAIDs. Other patients who may be at risk include patients with advanced liver disease and/or coagulopathy, patients in poor health, smokers, use of certain drugs (antiplatelets, anticoagulants, oral corticosteroids, selective serotonin reuptake

inhibitors), and use of alcohol. If patient develops GI distress, withhold celecoxib and notify prescriber immediately.

- Use celecoxib cautiously in patients with hypertension, and monitor blood pressure closely throughout therapy, because drug can start or worsen hypertension.
- Use celecoxib cautiously in children with systemic onset juvenile rheumatoid arthritis because serious adverse reactions can occur, including disseminated intravascular coagulation.
- Use celecoxib cautiously in patients known to be poor CYP2C9 metabolizers based on history or experience with other CYP2C9 substrates, such as phenytoin or warfarin. For patients with juvenile rheumatoid arthritis who are also poor CYP2C9 metabolizers, alternative management should be considered.

! **WARNING** Know that use of NSAIDs like celecoxib increases risk of serious cardiovascular thrombotic events, including MI and stroke, which can be life-threatening. These events may occur early in treatment and risk increases with duration of use. Be aware that these events have occurred even in patients who do not have a history or known risk factors for cardiovascular disease. Monitor patient for warning signs such as chest pain, shortness of breath, slurring of speech, or weakness. If any signs and symptoms develop, withhold celecoxib, alert prescriber immediately, and provide supportive care, as prescribed.

! **WARNING** Expect to monitor laboratory results (including WBC) and assess for infection in patient who has bone marrow suppression such as occurs with antineoplastic therapy, because celecoxib's anti-inflammatory and antipyretic actions may mask signs and symptoms, such as fever and pain.

- Monitor patient—especially if elderly or receiving long-term celecoxib therapy— for less common but serious adverse GI reactions, including anorexia, constipation, diverticulitis, dysphagia, esophagitis, gastritis, gastroenteritis, gastroesophageal reflux disease, hemorrhoids, hiatal hernia, melena, stomatitis, and vomiting.

- Monitor liver enzymes because, in rare cases, elevation may progress to severe hepatic reaction, including fatal hepatitis, or hepatic failure or necrosis.
- Monitor BUN and serum creatinine levels in elderly patients; patients taking ACE inhibitors, angiotensin II receptor antagonists, or diuretics; and patients with heart failure, impaired hepatic dysfunction or renal function because drug may cause renal failure.
- Monitor CBC for decreased hemoglobin level and hematocrit because drug may worsen anemia.
- Assess patient's skin regularly for signs of rash or other hypersensitivity reaction because celecoxib is a sulfur drug and may cause serious skin reactions without warning, even in patients with no history of sensitivity to sulfur. Drug may also cause DRESS, often with early symptoms of a fever, lymphadenopathy, and rash that can proceed to severe signs and symptoms. At first sign of reaction, stop drug and notify prescriber.
- Avoid using celecoxib with a nonaspirin NSAID, regardless of the dose, because celecoxib reduces inflammation and fever, which may mask signs of infection.

PATIENT TEACHING

- Instruct patient to swallow celecoxib capsules whole with a full glass of water and with food or milk to prevent stomach upset.
- Inform patient that if capsule can't be swallowed, patient should open capsule and sprinkle contents on a teaspoon of cool or room-temperature applesauce and take with water. Inform patient that the mixture may be stored in refrigerator for up to 6 hours.
- Advise patient prescribed oral solution to use a calibrated device when measuring dose. Warn not to use a regular teaspoon or tablespoon, as accurate dosage may not be obtained.
- Tell patient to take celecoxib exactly as prescribed and not to increase dosage or take drug longer than prescribed because serious adverse reactions can occur.
- Advise patient to notify prescriber if pain continues or is poorly controlled.
- Explain that celecoxib may increase the risk of serious adverse CV events; urge patient to seek immediate medical attention if signs or symptoms arise, such as chest pain,

shortness of breath, slurred speech, and weakness.

- Inform patient that the risk of congestive heart failure increases with NSAID use. Instruct patient to promptly report any evidence of edema, shortness of breath, or unexplained weight gain.
- Tell patient that celecoxib may increase the risk of serious adverse GI reactions. Stress the need to seek immediate medical attention if signs or symptoms develop, such as abdominal or epigastric, black or tarry stools, indigestion, and vomiting blood or material that resembles coffee grounds.
- Alert patient that celecoxib may cause serious skin reactions. Advise immediate medical attention if signs or symptoms develop, such as rash, blisters, fever, itching, or other evidence of hypersensitivity.
- Urge patient to avoid alcohol consumption and smoking during celecoxib therapy because they may increase the risk of adverse GI reactions.
- Inform pregnant women of fetal risks if taking drug. Stress importance of not taking celecoxib if pregnant, especially at 20 weeks or later.
- Advise patient not to take other NSAIDs or salicylates while taking celecoxib. Also advise patient to consult prescriber before taking low-dose aspirin.

cenobamate
Xcopri

Class and Category
Pharmacologic class: Sodium channel antagonist
Therapeutic class: Anticonvulsant
Controlled substance schedule: V

Indications and Dosages
✴ *To treat partial-onset seizures as adjunct or monotherapy*

TABLETS
Adults. *Initial:* 12.5 mg once daily for 2 wk, then titrated as follows: 25 mg once daily for wk 3 and wk 4, 50 mg once daily for wk 5 and wk 6, 100 mg once daily for wk 7 and wk 8, and 150 mg once daily for wk 9 and wk 10. *Maintenance:* 200 mg once daily beginning wk 11. Dosage further increased in increments of 50 mg once daily every

2 wk, based on response and tolerability. *Maximum:* 400 mg once daily.

±**DOSAGE ADJUSTMENT** For patients with mild to moderate hepatic impairment, maximum dosage 200 mg once daily.

Drug Administration
P.O.
- Tablets should be swallowed whole and taken with a liquid.
- Do not have patient chew tablets and do not crush tablets.

Route	Onset	Peak	Duration
P.O.	Unknown	1–4 hr	Unknown

Half-life: 50–60 hr

Mechanism of Action
May reduce repetitive neuronal firing by inhibiting voltage-gated sodium currents. It also is a positive allosteric modulator of the γ-aminobutyric acid (GABA$_A$) ion channel.

Contraindications
Familial short QT interval, hypersensitivity to cenobamate or its components

Interactions
DRUGS
carbamazepine, CYP2B6 substrates, CYP3A substrates, lamotrigine, oral contraceptives: Decreased plasma concentrations of these drugs, decreasing effectiveness
clobazam, CYP2C19 substrates, phenobarbital, phenytoin: Increased plasma concentrations of these drugs, increasing risk of adverse reactions
CNS depressants: Increased risk of neurological adverse reactions, including sedation and somnolence
drugs that shorten QT interval: Potential greater shortening of QT interval

ACTIVITIES
alcohol use: Increased risk of neurological adverse reactions, including sedation and somnolence

Adverse Reactions
CNS: Aphasia, asthenia, ataxia, balance disorder, confusion, dizziness, euphoric mood, fatigue, gait disturbance, irritability, headache, memory impairment, migraine, sedation, somnolence, **suicidal ideation**, tremor, vertigo
CV: Palpitations, **QT shortening**

EENT: Blurred vision, diplopia, dry mouth, nasopharyngitis, nystagmus, pharyngitis, taste distortion

GI: Abdominal pain, anorexia, constipation, diarrhea, dyspepsia, elevated liver enzymes, nausea, vomiting

GU: Dysmenorrhea, pollakiuria, UTI

MS: Back pain, dysarthria, musculoskeletal chest pain

RESP: Dyspnea, hiccups

SKIN: Pruritus, rash

Other: Appendicitis, **drug reaction with eosinophilia and systemic symptoms (DRESS)/multiorgan hypersensitivity, hyperkalemia**, weight loss

Childbearing Considerations

PREGNANCY

- Pregnancy exposure registry: 1-888-233-2334 or visit http://www.aedpregnancyregistry.org.
- It is not known if drug causes fetal harm.
- Use with caution only if benefit to mother outweighs potential risk to fetus.

LACTATION

- It is not known if drug is present in breast milk.
- Patient should check with prescriber before breastfeeding.

REPRODUCTION

- Women of childbearing age taking an oral contraceptive will need to use an additional alternative nonhormonal method during drug therapy.

Nursing Considerations

- Know that cenobamate should not be given to patients with familial short QT syndrome because of risk of synergistic effect on the QT interval that would increase the risk of sudden death and ventricular arrhythmias.
- Use cenobamate cautiously in patients also receiving other medications known to shorten QT intervals, as a synergistic effect could occur.
- Maintain titration schedule, as rapid titration may cause adverse reactions that could be serious.

! **WARNING** Monitor patient for signs and symptoms of **drug reaction with eosinophilia and systemic symptoms (DRESS)**, such as facial swelling, fever, lymphadenopathy, and rash, in addition to other organ system involvement such as hematological abnormalities, hepatitis, myocarditis, myositis, or nephritis. Eosinophilia is often present. Early manifestations such as fever or lymphadenopathy may be present without a rash. Notify prescriber immediately if suspected, as DRESS can be life-threatening. Expect cenobamate to be discontinued.

- Monitor patient for emergence of or worsening depression, suicidal thoughts or behavior, and/or any unusual changes in behavior or mood, because cenobamate increases risk of suicidal behavior and thoughts. Suicidal ideation has occurred as early as 1 week after starting drug therapy and can persist for duration of therapy.
- Discontinuing drug requires a gradual reduction over a period of at least 2 weeks, unless safety concerns require abrupt withdrawal.
- Be aware that patient may develop a tolerance to drug and potentially abuse it. Discuss any concerns with prescriber.

PATIENT TEACHING

- Tell patient to take tablets whole with liquid and not to chew or crush tablets. Let patient know that cenobamate can be taken with or without food.
- Instruct patient to notify prescriber of persistent, severe, or unusual signs and symptoms, especially if a fever or rash, along with other signs or symptoms, is present.
- Urge family or caregiver to monitor patient closely for suicidal tendencies, especially when therapy starts or dosage changes, and report any concerns to prescriber.
- Instruct patient to inform prescriber of all drugs taken, including over-the-counter and herbal preparations.
- Tell patient alcohol should be avoided while taking cenobamate.
- Advise women of childbearing age using oral contraceptives to use additional or an alternative nonhormonal contraceptive during cenobamate therapy. Cenobamate may reduce the efficacy of oral contraceptives.

! **WARNING** Tell patient and family members to seek immediate emergency care if patient becomes unconscious or experiences prolonged palpitations.

- Urge patient to avoid hazardous activities until drug's CNS and visual effects are known.
- Counsel patient not to stop taking cenobamate abruptly, as drug must be gradually discontinued to minimize the potential for increased seizure frequency or other withdrawal effects.
- Warn patient that drug can cause physical and psychological dependence. Stress importance of not altering dosage without consulting prescriber.

cephalexin hydrochloride

cephalexin monohydrate

Keflex

Class and Category

Pharmacologic class: First-generation cephalosporin
Therapeutic class: Antibiotic

Indications and Dosages

✳ *To treat bone infections caused by* Proteus mirabilis *or* Staphylococcus aureus; *genitourinary tract infections caused by* Escherichia coli, Klebsiella pneumoniae, *or* P. mirabilis; *respiratory infections caused by* Streptococcus pneumoniae *or* S. pyogenes; *and skin and skin structure infections caused by* S. aureus *or* S. pyogenes

CAPSULES, ORAL SUSPENSION, TABLETS
Adults and adolescents age 15 and over. 250 mg every 6 hr or 500 mg every 12 hr for 7 to 14 days. *For severe infections:* Up to 4 g daily in 2 to 4 equally divided doses for 7 to 14 days. **Children ages 1 to 15.** 25 to 50 mg/kg daily given in equally divided doses for 7 to 14 days. *For severe infections:* 50 to 100 mg/kg daily given in equally divided doses for 7 to 14 days.

✳ *To treat otitis media caused by* Haemophilus influenzae, Moraxella catarrhalis, S. aureus, S. pneumoniae, *or* S. pyogenes

ORAL SUSPENSION
Children. 75 to 100 mg/kg daily in equally divided doses every 6 hr.

± **DOSAGE ADJUSTMENT** For patients with a creatinine clearance of 30 to 59 ml/min, maximum dosage not to exceed 1 g; for creatinine clearance of 15 to 29 ml/min, dosage reduced to 250 mg every 8 or 12 hr; for creatinine clearance of 5 to 14 ml/min and patient not yet on dialysis, dosage reduced to 250 mg every 24 hr; and for creatinine clearance of 1 to 4 ml/min and patient not yet on dialysis, dosage reduced to 250 mg every 48 or 60 hr.

Drug Administration
P.O.
- Capsules and tablets should be swallowed whole without chewing or crushing.
- Prepare oral suspension as follows: Tap bottle to loosen powder. Then add 71 ml of water to 125 mg/5 ml or 250 mg/5 ml bottle to make a 100-ml suspension or add 140 ml to 125 mg/5 ml or 250 mg/5 ml to make a 200-ml suspension. Add the water in two portions, shaking well after each addition.
- Shake oral suspension well before measuring each dose and use a calibrated device to ensure an accurate dose.
- Store oral suspension in refrigerator. Discard after 14 days.

Route	Onset	Peak	Duration
P.O.	Unknown	1 hr	Unknown

Half-life: 30–75 min

Contraindications
Hypersensitivity to cephalexin, other cephalosporins, or their components

Interactions
DRUGS
metformin: Increased plasma metformin levels and increased risk of adverse reactions
probenecid: Increased and prolonged blood cephalexin level

Adverse Reactions
CNS: Chills, fever, headache, **seizures**
CV: Edema
EENT: Hearing loss, oral candidiasis
GI: Abdominal cramps, diarrhea, elevated liver enzymes, **hepatic failure**, hepatomegaly, nausea, **pseudomembranous colitis**, vomiting
GU: Elevated BUN level, **nephrotoxicity**, **renal failure**, vaginal candidiasis

☰ Mechanism of Action

Like all cephalosporins, cephalexin interferes with bacterial cell wall synthesis by inhibiting the final step in the cross-linking of peptidoglycan strands. Peptidoglycan makes the cell membrane rigid and protective. Without it, bacterial cells rupture and die. This mechanism of action is most effective against bacteria that divide rapidly, including many gram-positive and gram-negative bacteria.

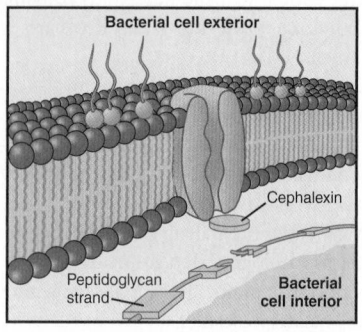

HEME: Eosinophilia, **hemolytic anemia, hypoprothrombinemia, neutropenia, thrombocytopenia, unusual bleeding**
MS: Arthralgia
RESP: Dyspnea
SKIN: Ecchymosis, erythema, **erythema multiforme,** pruritus, rash, **Stevens–Johnson syndrome**
Other: **Anaphylaxis,** superinfection

☰ Childbearing Considerations

PREGNANCY

- It is not known if drug can cause fetal harm.
- Use with caution only if benefit to mother outweighs potential risk to fetus.

LACTATION

- Drug is present in breast milk.
- Patient should check with prescriber before breastfeeding.

☰ Nursing Considerations

- Use cephalexin cautiously in patients hypersensitive to penicillin, because cross-sensitivity occurs in about 10% of them.
- Obtain culture and sensitivity test results, if possible and as ordered, before giving drug.
- Monitor patient's BUN and serum creatinine levels to detect early signs of nephrotoxicity. Also monitor fluid intake and output; decreasing urine output may indicate nephrotoxicity. Expect to monitor a patient who already has renal impairment longer for nephrotoxicity, because drug clearance is slowed.
- Monitor for allergic reactions a few days after therapy starts.
- Assess ALT, AST, bilirubin, CBC, hematocrit, LD, and serum alkaline phosphatase, levels during long-term therapy.
- Assess patient's bowel pattern daily; severe diarrhea may indicate pseudomembranous

colitis caused by *Clostridium difficile.* If diarrhea occurs, notify prescriber and expect to withhold cefotaxime and treat with electrolytes, fluids, protein, and an antibiotic effective against *C. difficile.*
- Assess patient for arthralgia, bleeding, ecchymosis, and pharyngitis; they may indicate a blood dyscrasia.

PATIENT TEACHING

- Advise patient to complete prescribed course of therapy.
- Instruct patient to shake oral suspension well before measuring each dose and to use a calibrated liquid-measuring device to ensure an accurate dose. Suspension should be stored in the refrigerator and discarded after 14 days.
- Tell patient that buttermilk and yogurt can help maintain intestinal flora and decrease diarrhea during therapy.
- Urge patient to report watery, bloody stools to prescriber immediately, even if they occur up to 2 months after cephalexin therapy has ended.

certolizumab pegol
Cimzia

☰ Class and Category

Pharmacologic class: Tumor necrosis factor (TNF) blocker
Therapeutic class: Immunomodulator, disease modifying antirheumatic drug (DMARD)

☰ Indications and Dosages

∗ *To reduce signs and symptoms of Crohn's disease and maintain clinical response in patients with moderately to severely active disease who have had an inadequate response to conventional therapy*

SUBCUTANEOUS INJECTION

Adults. *Initial:* 400 mg (given as two 200-mg injections) and repeated at wk 2 and 4. *Maintenance:* 400 mg (given as two 200-mg injections) every 4 wk if clinical response occurs.

✷ *To treat active ankylosing spondylitis, active psoriatic arthritis, moderate to severe active rheumatoid arthritis or nonradiographic axial spondyloarthritis*

SUBCUTANEOUS INJECTION

Adults. *Initial:* 400 mg (given as two 200-mg injections) and repeated at wk 2 and 4 followed by 200 mg every other week. *Maintenance:* 200 mg every other wk, or 400 mg (given as two 200-mg injections) every 4 wk if clinical response occurs.

✷ *To treat moderate to severe plaque psoriasis in patients who are candidates for phototherapy or systemic therapy*

SUBCUTANEOUS INJECTION

Adults. 400 mg (given as two 200-mg injections) every other wk.

±**DOSAGE ADJUSTMENT** For patient with plaque psoriasis who weighs 90 kg (198 lb) or more, dosage may be changed to 400 mg (given as two 200-mg injections) and repeated at wk 2 and 4, followed by 200 mg every other week.

Drug Administration

SUBCUTANEOUS

- Reconstitute two 200-mg certolizumab vials for each 400-mg dose and one 200-mg vial for a 200-mg dose after drug has reached room temperature.
- Inject 1 ml Sterile Water for Injection into each vial needed, using the 20 G needle provided. Direct the stream at the vial wall rather than directly onto drug.
- Gently swirl vial(s) without shaking for about 1 minute. Continue swirling every 5 minutes as long as undissolved particles are observed, which may take as long as 30 minutes. Solution should be clear to opalescent, colorless to pale yellow. The final reconstituted solution will be 200 mg/ml.
- Do not leave at room temperature, once reconstituted, for more than 2 hours before administration. If administration will be delayed, reconstituted drug can be refrigerated for up to 24 hours. Do not let drug freeze.
- Administer drug only when solution has reached room temperature.
- Using a 20 G needle, withdraw drug from vial using a separate syringe and needle for each vial.
- Switch to a 23 G needle and administer subcutaneously into patient's abdomen (staying at least 2 inches away from navel) or thigh. Do not exceed 200 mg per site and do not inject into skin that is bruised, hard, red, or tender or where there are scars or stretch marks.
- When using the prefilled syringe, know that the needle shield inside the removable cap of the prefilled syringe contains a derivative of natural rubber latex, which may cause allergic reactions if touched by latex-sensitive persons.

Route	Onset	Peak	Duration
SubQ	Unknown	54–171 hr	Unknown

Half-life: 14 days

Mechanism of Action

Binds to human tumor necrosis factor (TNF) alpha, inhibiting it. TNF alpha stimulates production of inflammatory mediators, including interleukin-1, nitric oxide, platelet activating factor, and prostaglandins. TNF alpha level is increased in patients with Crohn's disease and rheumatoid arthritis. Inhibition of TNF alpha causes C-reactive protein level to decline in patients with Crohn's disease, and the disease improves.

Contraindications

Hypersensitivity to certolizumab or its components

Interactions

DRUGS

abatacept, anakinra, natalizumab, rituximab: Possibly increased risk of serious infection and neutropenia

immunosuppressants: Possibly increased risk of infection

live-virus vaccines: Increased risk of adverse vaccine effects

Adverse Reactions

CNS: Anxiety, bipolar disorder, dizziness, fever, headache, malaise, **suicidal ideation**, syncope

CV: Angina, **arrhythmias**, **heart failure**, hypertension, **hypotension**, **MI**, **pericardial effusion**, **pericarditis**, peripheral edema, vasculitis

EENT: Optic neuritis, retinal hemorrhage, uveitis

ENDO: Hot flashes

GI: Abdominal pain, diarrhea, elevated liver enzymes, **hepatitis**, **intestinal obstruction**

GU: Menstrual dysfunction, **nephrotic syndrome**, **pyelonephritis**, **renal failure**, UTI

HEME: Anemia, **leukemia**, **leukopenia**, lymphadenopathy, **pancytopenia**, thrombophilia

MS: Arthralgia, extremity pain

RESP: Cough, dyspnea, pneumonia, upper respiratory infection

SKIN: Allergic dermatitis, alopecia, change of plaque psoriasis into a different psoriasis subtype, **erythema multiforme**, erythema nodosum, lichenoid skin reaction, **melanoma**, **Merkel cell carcinoma**, new or worsening psoriasis, rash, **Stevens–Johnson syndrome**, **toxic epidermal necrolysis**, urticaria

Other: **Anaphylaxis**; **angioedema**; antibody formation to certolizumab; bacterial, invasive fungal, mycobacterial, parasitic, viral or other opportunistic infections including aspergillosis, blastomycosis, candidiasis, coccidioidomycosis, histoplasmosis, legionellosis, listeriosis, pneumocystosis, and tuberculosis; herpes infections; injection-site reactions (bruising, discoloration, pain, redness, swelling); **lymphomas and other malignancies**; lupus-like syndrome; sarcoidosis, serum sickness

Childbearing Considerations

PREGNANCY

- Pregnancy exposure registry: 1-877-311-8972 or http://mothertobaby.org/pregnancy-studies/.
- It is not known if drug can cause fetal harm although it may affect fetal immune responses.
- Use with caution only if benefit to mother outweighs potential risk to fetus.
- Know that the safety of administering live or live-attenuated vaccines in neonates exposed to drug in utero is unknown.

LACTATION

- Drug is present in breast milk.

- Patient should check with prescriber before breastfeeding.

Nursing Considerations

- Be aware that certolizumab should not be initiated in a patient with an active infection, including serious localized infections.
- Use certolizumab cautiously in patients with recurrent or increased risk of infection, patients who live in regions where histoplasmosis and tuberculosis are endemic, and patients with a history of CNS demyelinating disorders because any of these disorders can occur, rarely, during certolizumab therapy. Be aware that a falsely negative antigen and antibody test for histoplasmosis may occur in some patients during certolizumab therapy, even when an active infection is present. Patient should be monitored closely throughout therapy.
- Use cautiously in patients who are chronic carriers of hepatitis B virus because drug may reactivate the virus. Assess patient for evidence of hepatitis B viral infection before starting and periodically throughout certolizumab therapy. If HBV reactivation occurs, notify prescriber, stop drug, and start appropriate therapy, as ordered.
- Make sure patient has a tuberculin skin test before therapy starts. If skin test is positive (induration 5 mm or greater), treatment of latent tuberculosis must start before certolizumab is given, as prescribed. In addition, expect antituberculosis therapy to be given to a patient with a past history of latent or active tuberculosis in whom an adequate course of treatment cannot be confirmed, and for patients with a negative test for latent tuberculosis but having risk factors for tuberculosis infection. Be aware that a falsely negative test for latent tuberculosis may occur during certolizumab therapy, so any signs and symptoms suggestive of tuberculosis should be carefully evaluated.

! **WARNING** Monitor all patients for infection during therapy, especially those who are at higher risk for infection, such as patients receiving immunosuppressants, those who are over 65 years of age, or who have comorbid conditions. If serious infection develops, expect prescriber to stop drug.

! **WARNING** Stop drug immediately and notify prescriber if patient has an allergic reaction. Expect to provide supportive care.

- Monitor patient closely for evidence of congestive heart failure (anxiety; crackles; dyspnea; sudden, unexplained weight gain), and notify prescriber if they occur.
- Monitor patient's CBC, as ordered, because certolizumab may have adverse hematologic effects. Notify prescriber about persistent bleeding, bruising, fever, or pallor.
- Be aware that certolizumab is a TNF inhibitor. Although rare, malignancies (especially lymphomas and leukemias) have been reported in patients receiving these drugs, including children. Patients with rheumatoid arthritis, especially those with very active disease, and patients with disorders that certolizumab treats are at greatest risk. Monitor these patients closely.
- Assess patient's skin regularly, especially for patients who are at risk for skin cancer, as drug may cause melanomas and Merkel cell carcinoma as well as other life-threatening disorders such as Stevens–Johnson syndrome. At the first sign of a rash, notify prescriber.

PATIENT TEACHING

- Instruct patient on how to administer a subcutaneous injection using the prefilled syringe. Tell patient to keep drug in refrigerator until about 30 min before administering to allow it to warm up to room temperature. Caution him not to warm up the drug any other way. Check with patient about a latex allergy because the needle shield inside the removeable cap of the prefilled syringe contains a derivative of natural rubber latex, which may cause allergic reactions if touched by latex-sensitive persons. Tell him to inject the drug either into his abdomen or thigh and to make sure he injects the full amount. Review how to safely discard the needle and syringe after the injection.
- Inform patient that he may receive vaccinations, except for live or live-attenuated vaccines.

! **WARNING** Review signs and symptoms of allergic reaction (rash, swollen face, trouble breathing), and tell patient to seek emergency care immediately if these occur.

- Inform patient that injection-site reactions such as pain or redness may occur and usually are mild and transient. Instruct him to apply a towel soaked in cold water to the site if it hurts. Tell patient to call prescriber if reaction persists or worsens.
- Inform patient that drug may lower the ability of the immune system to fight infections. Tell patient to report any signs and symptoms of infection, including tuberculosis or reactivation of hepatitis B virus infections, that may occur during therapy. Instruct him to report fever, including a low-grade fever, persistent cough, or wasting or weight loss to prescriber.
- Tell patient to report evidence of bleeding disorders and infections to prescriber; drug may have to be stopped. Advise patient to avoid people with infections and to comply with all prescribed tests.
- Inform patient that certain kinds of cancer, especially leukemias and lymphomas, are more likely in patients taking certolizumab but still rare. Emphasize need to keep follow-up visits and to report sudden or unusual signs or symptoms. Also advise patient to have periodic skin examinations, especially if they are at risk for skin cancer.
- Instruct patient to report lupus-like signs and symptoms that, although rare, may occur during therapy, such as chest pain that doesn't go away, joint pain, rash on cheeks or arms that's sensitive to the sun, or shortness of breath. Explain that drug may have to be discontinued if these occur.
- Advise patient to inform all healthcare providers about certolizumab use and to inform prescriber about any herbal remedies, vitamin and mineral supplements, and OTC medications being taken.
- Advise patient to report any signs of new or worsening health issues such as autoimmune disorders, heart disease, or neurological disease, especially bleeding, bruising, or a persistent fever.
- Tell women of childbearing age to notify prescriber if pregnancy occurs or is suspected, because drug's effects on the fetus are unknown. If pregnancy is confirmed, encourage patient to enroll in the pregnancy exposure registry by calling 1-877-311-8972. Also tell mothers wishing to breastfeed their infant to discuss breastfeeding with prescriber before doing so.

cetirizine hydrochloride

Quzyttir, Zyrtec

Class and Category

Pharmacologic class: Histamine-1 (H-1) receptor antagonist
Therapeutic class: Antihistamine

Indications and Dosages

＊ *To treat acute urticaria*

I.V. INJECTION (QUZYTTIR)

Adults and adolescents age 12 and older. 10 mg every 24 hr, as needed.
Children age 6 to 11. 5 or 10 mg, depending on severity, every 24 hr, as needed.
Children 6 months to 5 years with normal hepatic and renal function. 2.5 mg every 24 hr, as needed.

＊ *To treat chronic urticaria, perennial allergic rhinitis, or seasonal allergic rhinitis*

CHEWABLE TABLETS, DISSOLVE TABLETS, SYRUP, TABLETS (ZYRTEC)

Adults and children age 6 and older. 5 or 10 mg once daily.
Children age 2 to 5. 2.5 mg once daily, increased to 5 mg once daily or 2.5 mg every 12 hr, if needed.

SYRUP

Children age 6 to 24 months. 2.5 mg once daily. For children that are between 12 and 24 months, dosage may be increased to 2.5 mg every 12 hr, if needed.

Drug Administration

P.O.

- Chewable tablets should be chewed completely before swallowing.
- Dissolve tablets are meant to be dissolved in mouth but the tablets can be chewed or swallowed. May be taken with or without water.
- Syrup should be measured with a calibrated device to ensure accurate dose.

I.V.

- Withdraw dosage from a single-use vial. Each ml contains 10 mg of cetirizine hydrochloride.
- Administer only as an I.V. injection over 1 to 2 minutes.

- Do not administer to children under the age of 6 years with impaired hepatic or renal function.
- *Incompatibilities:* None listed by manufacturer

Route	Onset	Peak	Duration
P.O.	Unknown	1 hr	Unknown
I.V.	Unknown	Unknown	Unknown

Half-life: 8.3 hr

Mechanism of Action

The antihistaminic activity of cetirizine is mediated via selective inhibition of peripheral H_1-receptors to alleviate urticaria.

Contraindications

Hypersensitivity to cetirizine, hydroxyzine, levocetirizine, or their components

Interactions

DRUGS

CNS depressants: Increased CNS impairment
theophylline: Possibly decreased clearance of cetirizine, increasing plasma cetirizine levels

ACTIVITIES

alcohol use: Increased CNS impairment

Adverse Reactions

CNS: Dizziness, fatigue, feeling hot, headache, insomnia, irritability, paresthesia, presyncope, sedation, somnolence
EENT: Dry mouth, epistaxis, pharyngitis, taste alteration
GI: Abdominal pain, diarrhea, dyspepsia, nausea, vomiting
RESP: Bronchospasm, cough
SKIN: Diaphoresis

Childbearing Considerations

PREGNANCY

- It is not known if drug causes fetal harm.
- Use with caution only if benefit to mother outweighs potential risk to fetus.

LACTATION

- Drug may be present in breast milk.
- Patient should check with prescriber before breastfeeding.

Nursing Considerations

- Institute safety precautions, because drug can cause sedation and somnolence.

PATIENT TEACHING

- Instruct patient on how to take form of drug prescribed: chewable tablets should be chewed completely before swallowing; dissolvable tablets are meant to be dissolved in mouth but the tablets may be chewed or swallowed and may be taken with or without water; and syrup should be measured with a calibrated device, not a household spoon, to ensure accurate dose.

- Instruct patient to avoid hazardous activities until drug's CNS effects are known. Warn her that taking other CNS depressants, including over-the-counter products, increases sedation and somnolence.
- Warn patient not to drink alcohol while receiving cetirizine, because alcohol also increases sedation and somnolence.
- Keep oral drug out of reach of small children.

chlordiazepoxide hydrochloride

≡ Class, Category, and Schedule
Pharmacologic class: Benzodiazepine
Therapeutic class: Anxiolytic
Controlled substance schedule: IV

≡ Indications and Dosages
✷ *To provide short-term management of mild to moderate anxiety*

CAPSULES
Adults. 5 to 10 mg three or four times daily.
Children over age 6. 5 mg two to four times daily, increased, as needed, to 10 mg two or three times daily.

✷ *To provide short-term management of severe anxiety*

CAPSULES
Adults. 20 to 25 mg three or four times daily.

✷ *To provide short-term treatment of acute alcohol withdrawal*

CAPSULES
Adults. *Initial:* 50 to 100 mg. Repeated in 2 to 4 hr followed by individualized dosage if needed to control symptoms. *Maximum:* 300 mg daily.

✷ *To provide perioperative relaxation and reduce apprehension and anxiety*

CAPSULES
Adults. 5 to 10 mg P.O. three or four times daily several days before surgery.

± **DOSAGE ADJUSTMENT** Dosage reduced to 5 mg P.O. two to four times daily, as needed, for elderly or debilitated patients. For patients with a creatinine clearance less than 10 ml/min, dosage reduced by 50%.

≡ Drug Administration
P.O.
- Capsule should be swallowed whole and not chewed, crushed, or opened.
- Administer with water.

I.V.
- Reconstitute 100 mg with 5 ml of preservative-free Sterile Water for Injection or 0.9% Sodium Chloride for Injection. Agitate gently until completely dissolved. Resulting concentration should be 20 mg/ml.
- Never give the reconstituted I.M. preparation I.V. because gas bubbles develop in the solution when the special I.M. diluent supplied by the manufacturer is added.
- Administer immediately but slowly over more than 1 minute.
- *Incompatibilities:* Cefepime if used at a Y-site

I.M.
- Do not give the reconstituted preparation for I.V. use as an I.M. injection because it may cause pain at the injection site.
- Reconstitute only with diluent provided by manufacturer.
- Reconstitute 100 mg by adding the 2 ml of diluent to the drug ampule with gentle pressure to minimize surface bubbles. Gently agitate the ampule until drug is completely dissolved. The concentration should then be 50 mg/ml.
- Administer immediately after preparing.
- Inject slowly and deeply, preferably into the upper outer quadrant of the gluteus muscle.

Route	Onset	Peak	Duration
P.O.	Unknown	0.5–4 hr	Unknown

Half-life: 24–48 hr

≡ Mechanism of Action
May potentiate the effects of gamma-aminobutyric acid (GABA) and other inhibitory neurotransmitters by binding to specific benzodiazepine receptors

in cortical and limbic areas of the CNS. By binding to these receptors, chlordiazepoxide increases GABA's inhibitory effects and blocks cortical and limbic arousal, which helps control emotional behavior. It also helps relieve symptoms of alcohol withdrawal by causing CNS depression.

Contraindications

Hypersensitivity to chlordiazepoxide or its components

Interactions

DRUGS

antacids: Delayed absorption of chlordiazepoxide

cimetidine, disulfiram: Increased blood chlordiazepoxide level

CNS depressants, opioids, other benzodiazepines, sedating antihistamines, tricyclic antidepressants: Increased risk of sedation and somnolence and other CNS effects

digoxin, phenytoin: Increased blood level and risk of toxicity with digoxin and phenytoin

levodopa: Decreased efficacy of levodopa's antiparkinsonian effects

opioids: Increased risk of significant respiratory depression

ACTIVITIES

alcohol use: Increased CNS effects, including severe respiratory depression and significant sedation and somnolence

heavy smoking: Reduced effectiveness of chlordiazepoxide

Adverse Reactions

CNS: Ataxia, confusion, depression, drowsiness, sedation, **suicidal ideation**

CV: ECG changes, hypotension,

GI: Elevated liver enzymes, **hepatic dysfunction**, jaundice

HEME: Agranulocytosis

RESP: Respiratory depression

Other: Injection-site pain, redness, and swelling

Childbearing Considerations

PREGNANCY

- Drug may increase risk of congenital malformations if used during the first trimester of pregnancy and may cause withdrawal symptoms and other adverse reactions in the neonate if given to mothers late in pregnancy.

- Drug is not recommended during pregnancy and should be discontinued if pregnancy occurs.

LACTATION

- It is unknown if drug is present in breast milk.
- A decision should be made to discontinue breastfeeding or the drug to avoid potential serious adverse reactions in the breastfed infant.

Nursing Considerations

- Use chlordiazepoxide cautiously in patients with hepatic or renal impairment or porphyria.

! **WARNING** Be aware that benzodiazepine therapy such as chlordiazepoxide should only be used concomitantly with opioid therapy in patients for whom other treatment options are inadequate. If prescribed together, expect dosing and duration of the opioid to be limited. Monitor patient closely for signs and symptoms of decrease in consciousness, including coma, profound sedation, and significant respiratory depression. Notify prescriber immediately and provide emergency supportive care, as death may occur.

! **WARNING** Be aware that prolonged use of chlordiazepoxide at therapeutic doses can lead to dependence.

- Monitor liver enzymes during therapy.
- Know that if patient is an aggressive, hyperactive child or has a history of psychiatric disorders, watch for paradoxical reactions, such as acute rage excitement, and stimulation, during first 2 weeks of therapy.
- Watch patients closely (especially children, adolescents, and young adults) for suicidal tendencies, particularly when chlordiazepoxide therapy starts and dosage changes.

PATIENT TEACHING

- Warn that drug may cause drowsiness.

! **WARNING** Warn patient not to consume alcohol or take an opioid during chlordiazepoxide therapy without prescriber knowledge, as severe respiratory depression can occur that may lead to death.

! WARNING Inform patient about potentially fatal additive effects of combining a benzodiazepine like chlordiazepoxide with an opioid. Instruct patient to inform all prescribers of chlordiazepoxide use, especially if pain medication may be prescribed.

- Advise patient to avoid other CNS depressants during therapy.
- Warn patient not to take antacids with chlordiazepoxide.
- Urge family or caregiver to watch patient closely for suicidal tendencies, especially when therapy starts or dosage changes and particularly if patient is a child, teenager, or young adult.

chlorothiazide

chlorothiazide sodium

☰ Class and Category
Pharmacologic class: Thiazide diuretic
Therapeutic class: Antihypertensive, diuretic

☰ Indications and Dosages
❋ *To treat hypertension*

ORAL SUSPENSION, TABLETS
Adults. 500 to 1,000 mg (10- to 20-ml ml oral suspension) daily in a single dose or divided doses twice daily. *Maximum:* 2,000 mg daily in divided doses.
Children age 6 months and over. 10 to 20 mg/kg daily in a single dose or divided doses twice daily. *Maximum:* 1,000 mg daily for ages 2 to 12; 375 mg daily for ages 6 months to 2 years.
Children under age 6 months. Up to 30 mg/kg daily in divided doses given twice daily.

❋ *As adjunct therapy to treat edema associated with corticosteroid and estrogen therapy, congestive heart failure, hepatic cirrhosis, and renal dysfunction*

ORAL SUSPENSION, TABLETS
Adults. 500 to 1,000 mg (10- to 20-ml oral suspension) once or twice a day. Administered on an intermittent schedule, if needed, such as alternate days or 3 to 5 days/wk.

Children age 6 months and over. 10 to 20 mg/kg daily in a single dose or divided doses twice daily. *Maximum:* 1,000 mg daily for children ages 2 to 12; 375 mg daily for children ages 6 months to 2 years.
Children under age 6 months. Up to 30 mg/kg daily in divided doses twice daily.

I.V. INFUSION OR INJECTION
Adults. 500 mg to 1 g once or twice daily. *Maximum:* 2,000 mg daily.

☰ Drug Administration
P.O.
- Shake suspension before measuring dose.
- Use calibrated device to measure dose of oral suspension.
- Administer with food or milk if GI upset occurs.
- Administer single daily dose in morning.
- Store oral suspension at room temperature.

I.V.
- Don't give by I.M. or subcutaneous route.
- For I.V. use, reconstitute with at least 18 ml of Sterile Water for Injection. Solution should be clear.
- Administer I.V. injection slowly over at least 5 minutes.
- Dilute further for I.V. infusion with 0.9% Sodium Chloride for Injection or 5% Dextrose Injection (check manufacturer guidelines for other appropriate solutions).
- Administer I.V. infusion over 30 minutes.
- Discard unused solution after 24 hours.
- *Incompatibilities:* Amikacin, chlorpromazine, hydralazine, insulin regular, levorphanol, morphine sulfate, multivitamin additives, norepinephrine bitartrate, polymyxin sulfate, procaine, prochlorperazine, promazine, promethazine, streptomycin, triflupromazine, vancomycin

Route	Onset	Peak	Duration
P.O.	2 hr	4 hr	6–12 hr
I.V.	15 min	30 min	Unknown

Half-life: 45–120 min

☰ Mechanism of Action
May promote chloride, sodium, and water excretion by inhibiting sodium reabsorption in the kidneys' distal tubules. Initially, chlorothiazide may reduce blood pressure by decreasing cardiac output, extracellular

fluid volume, and plasma volume. It also may dilate arteries directly, reducing peripheral vascular resistance. After several weeks, cardiac output, extracellular fluid, and plasma volume return to normal, but peripheral vascular resistance remains decreased.

Contraindications

Hypersensitivity to chlorothiazide, sulfonamides, or their components

Interactions

DRUGS

ACTH, corticosteroids: Intensified electrolyte depletion, especially potassium
angiotensin II antagonist or angiotensin-converting enzyme inhibitor in combination with NSAIDS: Increased risk of renal dysfunction in patients with compromised renal function, especially the elderly or patients who are volume-depleted
barbiturates, narcotics: Possibly increased risk of orthostatic hypotension
cholestyramine, colestipol: Decreased chlorothiazide absorption
insulin, oral hypoglycemics: Possible alteration in blood glucose control
lithium: Increased risk of lithium toxicity
nondepolarizing skeletal muscle relaxants: Possibly increased effects of muscle relaxants
NSAIDs: Possibly reduced diuretic effect of chlorothiazide
other antihypertensives: Increased antihypertensive effect

ACTIVITIES

alcohol: Increased risk of orthostatic hypotension

Adverse Reactions

CNS: Dizziness, headache, paresthesia, restlessness, vertigo, weakness
CV: Orthostatic hypotension
ENDO: Hyperglycemia
GI: Abdominal cramps, anorexia, constipation, diarrhea, gastric irritation, jaundice, nausea, **pancreatitis**, vomiting
GU: Glycosuria, hematuria (I.V. form), impotence, interstitial nephritis, renal dysfunction, **renal failure**
HEME: **Agranulocytosis, aplastic anemia, hemolytic anemia, leukopenia, thrombocytopenia**
MS: Muscle spasms
SKIN: Photosensitivity, purpura, rash, urticaria

Other: **Anaphylactic reactions, hypercalcemia,** hyperuricemia, hypochloremic alkalosis, **hypokalemia, hypomagnesemia, hyponatremia,** hypovolemia

Childbearing Considerations

PREGNANCY

- Drug may cause fetal or neonatal harm such as jaundice, thrombocytopenia, and possibly other adverse reactions as it does cross the placental barrier.
- Use with caution only if benefit to mother outweighs potential risk to fetus.

LACTATION

- It is unknown if drug is present in breast milk.
- A decision should be made to discontinue breastfeeding or the drug to avoid potential serious adverse reactions in the breastfed infant.

Nursing Considerations

- Watch I.V. site closely. If extravasation occurs, stop infusion and tell prescriber at once.
- Weigh patient daily to assess fluid loss and drug effectiveness. If used to treat hypertension, check blood pressure often; antihypertensive effect may not appear for days.
- Assess patient for electrolyte imbalances.
- Monitor renal function closely, especially in elderly patients, because risk of toxicity increases with renal impairment.

PATIENT TEACHING

- Tell patient to take chlorothiazide early in the day to avoid nocturia and to take it with food or milk if GI distress occurs.
- Advise patient taking oral suspension form to shake suspension before use and to use a calibrated device to measure dosage, not a household spoon. Tell patient drug should be stored at room temperature.
- Urge patient to eat a high-potassium diet.
- Instruct patient to rise slowly to minimize effects of orthostatic hypotension.
- Urge patient to weigh himself at least weekly and to notify prescriber if weight rises or falls by 5 lb (2.25 kg) or more in 2 days.
- Tell patient to immediately notify prescriber if he develops cramps, diarrhea, dizziness, drowsiness, excessive thirst,

increased heart rate, nausea, restlessness, sudden joint pain, tiredness, vomiting, or weakness.

- Know that if patient has diabetes mellitus, tell him to check blood glucose level often. Insulin or oral antidiabetic dosage may have to be increased.
- Tell patient to avoid prolonged exposure to sun, use sunscreen, and wear protective clothing.
- Advise patient to consult prescriber or pharmacist before using alcohol and such OTC drugs as those used for appetite control, colds, cough, hay fever, and sinus problems.

chlorpromazine

chlorpromazine hydrochloride

Class and Category

Pharmacologic class: Phenothiazine
Therapeutic class: Antiemetic, antipsychotic, tranquilizer

Indications and Dosages

✳ *To manage symptoms of psychotic disorders or control manic manifestations of manic-depression in outpatient*

TABLETS

Adults. 30 to 75 mg/day divided equally into 2 to 4 doses, increased as needed. *Usual maintenance:* 200 mg/day. *Maximum:* 800 mg/day.

✳ *To control acutely disturbed or manic hospitalized patients*

I.M. INJECTION

Adults. 25 mg. 25 to 50 mg repeated in 1 hr, if needed. Increased gradually over several days up to 400 mg every 4 to 6 hr for severe cases until behavior is controlled. Then, regimen switched to oral form and outpatient dosage.

✳ *To treat severe behavioral problems in children*

SYRUP, TABLETS

Children ages 6 months to 12 years.
0.55 mg/kg every 4 to 6 hr, as needed.

SUPPOSITORIES

Children ages 6 months to 12 years.
1 mg/kg every 6 to 8 hr, as needed.

I.M. INJECTION

Children ages 6 months to 12 years.
0.55 mg/kg every 6 to 8 hr. *Maximum:* 75 mg daily for children ages 5 to 12 years or weighing 23 to 45 kg (50.6 to 99 lb) except in unmanageable cases; 40 mg daily for children up to age 5 or weighing up to 23 kg (50.6 lb).

✳ *To treat nausea and vomiting*

SYRUP, TABLETS

Adults and adolescents. 10 to 25 mg every 4 to 6 hr, as needed.
Children ages 6 months to 12 years.
0.55 mg/kg every 4 to 6 hr, as needed.

I.M. OR I.V. INJECTION

Adults. 25 mg. If no hypotension occurs, 25 to 50 mg every 4 to 6 hr, as needed, until vomiting stops; then drug switched to oral form.
Children age 6 months and over. 0.55 mg/kg every 6 to 8 hr, as needed. *Maximum:* 75 mg daily for children ages 5 to 12 or weighing 23 to 45 kg (50.6 to 99 lb); 40 mg daily for children up to age 5 or weighing up to 23 kg (50.5 lb).

SUPPOSITORIES

Adults and adolescents. 50 to 100 mg every 6 to 8 hr, as needed.
Children ages 6 months to 12 years.
1 mg/kg every 6 to 8 hr, as needed.

✳ *To treat intractable hiccups*

TABLETS

Adults. 25 to 50 mg three times daily or four times daily. If hiccups last longer than 2 to 3 days, route switched to I.M., as prescribed.

I.M. INJECTION

Adults. 25 to 50 mg every 3 to 4 hr, as needed, given only if oral route is ineffective. If symptoms persist, route switched to I.V., as prescribed.

I.V. INFUSION

Adults. 25 to 50 mg.

✳ *To provide preoperative relaxation*

SYRUP, TABLETS

Adults and adolescents. 25 to 50 mg 2 to 3 hr before surgery.
Children ages 6 months to 12 years.
0.55 mg/kg 2 to 3 hr before surgery.

I.M. INJECTION

Adults. 12.5 to 25 mg 1 to 2 hr before surgery.
Children age 6 months and over. 0.55 mg/kg 1 to 2 hr before surgery.

＊ *To provide intraoperative sedation*

I.V. INJECTION

Adults. 25 mg. *Maximum:* 25 mg.
Children age 6 months and over. 1 mg/ml. May repeat regimen in 30 min, if needed. *Maximum:* 0.25 mg/kg

I.M. INJECTION

Adults. 12.5 mg. Repeated in 30 min if needed and no hypotension occurs.
Children age 6 months and over. 0.25 mg/kg. Repeated in 30 min if needed and tolerated.

＊ *To treat acute intermittent porphyria*

TABLETS

Adults and adolescents. 25 to 50 mg three times daily or four times daily.

I.M. INJECTION

Adults. 25 mg three times daily or four times daily until oral route is possible.

＊ *As adjunct to treat tetanus (usually with barbiturates)*

I.V. INJECTION

Adults. 25 to 50 mg every 6 to 8 hr.
Children age 6 months and over. 0.55 mg/kg every 6 to 8 hr. *Maximum:* 75 mg daily for children ages 5 to 12 years or weighing 23 to 45 kg (50.5 lb to 99 lb); 40 mg daily for children up to age 5 years or weighing up to 45 kg (50.6 lb).

I.M. INJECTION

Adults. 25 to 50 mg three times daily or four times daily.
Children age 6 months and over. 0.55 mg/kg every 6 to 8 hr. *Maximum:* 75 mg daily for children ages 5 to 12 or weighing 23 to 45 kg (50.6 to 99 lb); 40 mg daily for children up to age 5 years or weighing up to 23 kg (50.6 lb).

±**DOSAGE ADJUSTMENT** Dosage possibly reduced for patients with hepatic dysfunction. Dosage reduced to one-third to one-half the normal adult dosage for elderly or debilitated patients.

☰ Drug Administration

P.O.

- Capsules should be swallowed whole and not chewed, crushed, or opened.
- Tablets should be swallowed whole and not chewed, crushed, or split.
- Use calibrated device to measure dosage given as a syrup.
- Administer oral form with food or a full glass of milk or water.
- Do not administer an antacid within 2 hours of chlorpromazine administration.

I.V.

- Wear gloves when working with injectable form because parenteral solution may cause contact dermatitis.
- Dilute with 0.9% Sodium Chloride Injection to a concentration of 1 mg/ml. Never administer undiluted.
- For I.V. injection, administer at no more than 0.5 mg/min for children and 1 mg/min for adults.
- For I.V. infusion, further dilute with 500 to 1,000 ml of 0.9% Sodium Chloride Injection and administer slowly with patient supine.
- Have patient lie down for at least 30 minutes after drug is administered.
- *Incompatibilities:* Atropine, thiopental, or other drugs; solutions that don't have a pH of 4 to 5.

I.M.

- Don't inject drug by subcutaneous route because it can cause severe tissue necrosis.
- Give I.M. injection slowly and deep into upper outer quadrant of buttocks in the gluteus maximus.
- Have patient lie down for at least 30 minutes after drug is administered.
- Rotate sites.
- If patient develops irritation, dilute with 0.9% Sodium Chloride or add 2% procaine, as ordered.

P.R.

- If suppository is too soft to administer, keep in wrapper while holding it under cool water or place it in a refrigerator for up to 30 minutes to harden it before removing from the wrapper.

Route	Onset	Peak	Duration
P.O.	0.5–1 hr	Unknown	4–6 hr
P.O./E.R.	0.5–1 hr	Unknown	10–12 hr
I.V./I.M.	>15 min	30 min	Unknown
P.R.	>1 hr	Unknown	3–4 hr
Half-life: 30 hr			

Mechanism of Action

Depresses brain areas that control activity and aggression, including the cerebral cortex, hypothalamus, and limbic system, by an unknown mechanism. Prevents nausea and vomiting by inhibiting or blocking dopamine receptors in the medullary chemoreceptor trigger zone and peripherally by blocking the vagus nerve in the GI tract. May relieve anxiety by indirect reduction in arousal and increased filtering of internal stimuli to the reticular activating system in the brain stem.

Contraindications

Comatose states; hypersensitivity to chlorpromazine, phenothiazines, or their components; use of large amounts of CNS depressants

Interactions
DRUGS

anticonvulsants: Possibly lowered convulsive threshold
CNS depressants such as anesthetics, barbiturates, narcotics: Prolonged and intensified CNS depression
metrizamide: Possibly lowered seizure threshold
oral anticoagulants: Decreased anticoagulation
propranolol: Increased plasma levels of both drugs
thiazide diuretics: Possibly increased orthostatic hypotension

ACTIVITIES

alcohol use: Prolonged and intensified CNS depression

Adverse Reactions

CNS: Drowsiness, extrapyramidal reactions (such as dystonia, fever, motor restlessness, pseudoparkinsonism, and tardive dyskinesia), **neuroleptic malignant syndrome, seizures**
CV: ECG changes, such as nonspecific, usually reversible Q- and T-wave changes; orthostatic hypotension; tachycardia
EENT: Blurred vision, dry mouth, nasal congestion, ocular changes (fine particle deposits in lens and cornea) with long-term therapy
ENDO: Gynecomastia, hyperglycemia, **hypoglycemia**, lactation, moderate breast engorgement
GI: Constipation, ileus, nausea

GU: Amenorrhea, ejaculation disorders, impotence, priapism, urine retention
HEME: Agranulocytosis, aplastic anemia, eosinophilia, **hemolytic anemia, leukopenia, pancytopenia, thrombocytopenic purpura**
SKIN: Exfoliative dermatitis, photosensitivity, tissue necrosis, urticaria

Childbearing Considerations
PREGNANCY

- It is not known if drug can cause fetal harm.
- Extrapyramidal and/or withdrawal symptoms have occurred in neonates exposed to phenothiazines during the third trimester of pregnancy. In addition, prolonged jaundice may also occur in the neonate.
- Drug should not be used in pregnant women or those likely to become pregnant, unless the expected benefit to the mother outweighs the potential risk to the fetus.

LACTATION

- Drug is present in breast milk.
- A decision should be made to discontinue breastfeeding or the drug to avoid potential serious adverse reactions in the breastfed infant.

Nursing Considerations

- Know that chlorpromazine shouldn't be used to treat dementia-related psychosis in the elderly because of an increased risk of death.
- Use chlorpromazine cautiously in patients (especially children) with chronic respiratory disorders (such as severe asthma or emphysema) or acute respiratory tract infections because drug has CNS depressant effect. Also use cautiously in patients with cardiovascular, hepatic, or renal disease because of increased risk of developing arrhythmias, heart failure, and hypotension.
- Use drug cautiously in patients with glaucoma because of its anticholinergic effects. Also use it cautiously in those who are exposed to extreme heat or organophosphate insecticides and those receiving atropine or related drugs.

! **WARNING** Stay alert for possible suppressed cough reflex, which increases the risk of the patient's aspirating vomitus.

- Monitor patient for increased sensitivity to drug's CNS effects if patient has a history of hepatic encephalopathy from cirrhosis.

! WARNING Notify prescriber immediately if neuroleptic malignant syndrome (altered mental status, autonomic instability hyperpyrexia, muscle rigidity) develops, and expect to stop drug and start intensive treatment. Watch for recurrence if patient resumes antipsychotic therapy.

PATIENT TEACHING

- Tell patient not to take drug within 2 hours of an antacid. Advise him to take drug with food or a full glass of milk or water.
- Tell patient using suppository form to chill the suppository, moisten it with cold water, and insert it well into rectum.
- Know that because of possible blurred vision, dizziness, and drowsiness (especially during the first few days of therapy), advise patient to avoid hazardous activities until drug's CNS effects are known.
- Tell patient to avoid alcohol because of possible additive effects and hypotension.
- Advise patient, especially if elderly, to rise slowly from a supine or seated position to avoid dizziness, fainting, and light-headedness.
- Tell patient to inform doctors and dentists that he's taking chlorpromazine before he has dental work, medical tests, or surgery.
- Explain that drug may reduce the body's response to cold and heat; tell patient to avoid temperature extremes, as in a hot tub, sauna, or very cold or hot shower. Remind patient to dress warmly in cold weather.
- Warn patient not to take OTC drugs for an allergy or a cold because they can increase the risk of heatstroke and other unwanted effects.
- Inform patient that drug increases sensitivity to sunlight; tell him to stay out of the sun as much as possible and to protect his skin.
- Suggest fluids, hard candy, or sugarless gum for patient who is experiencing a dry mouth.
- Urge patient to report sudden sore throat or other signs of infection.
- Advise female patient of childbearing age to notify prescriber if she intends to become or suspects that she is pregnant during therapy.

chlorzoxazone
Lorzone

≡ Class and Category
Pharmacologic class: Benzoxazole derivative
Therapeutic class: Skeletal muscle relaxant

≡ Indications and Dosages
✳ *As adjunct to relieve acute discomfort associated with painful musculoskeletal conditions*

TABLETS
Adults. *Initial:* 375 mg to 500 mg three or four times daily, decreased or increased according to response. *Maximum:* 750 mg three or four times daily.

≡ Drug Administration
P.O.
- Crush chlorzoxazone tablets and mix with food or liquid for easier swallowing, if needed.
- If GI upset occurs, administer drug with food or milk.

Route	Onset	Peak	Duration
P.O.	1 hr	1–2 hr	3–6 hr

Half-life: 1 hr

≡ Mechanism of Action
Reduces muscle spasm by inhibiting multisynaptic reflex arcs at the level of the spinal cord and subcortical areas of the brain that are active in producing and maintaining skeletal muscle spasm.

≡ Contraindications
Hypersensitivity to chlorzoxazone or any of its components

≡ Interactions
DRUGS
CNS depressants: Additive CNS depression
ACTIVITIES
alcohol use: Additive CNS depression

≡ Adverse Reactions
CNS: Dizziness, drowsiness, headache, light-headedness, malaise, paradoxical stimulation
GI: Abdominal cramps or pain, constipation, diarrhea, **GI bleeding**, heartburn, **hepatotoxicity**, nausea, vomiting
GU: Urine discoloration

HEME: **Agranulocytosis**, anemia
SKIN: Allergic dermatitis, ecchymosis, petechiae
Other: **Anaphylaxis**, **angioedema**

Childbearing Considerations

PREGNANCY
- It is not known if drug can cause fetal harm.
- Use with caution only if benefit to mother outweighs potential risk to fetus.

LACTATION
- It is not known if drug is present in breast milk.
- Patient should check with prescriber before breastfeeding.

Nursing Considerations
- Assess patients, especially those who have a history of allergies, for evidence of hypersensitivity, such as hives, itching, and rash.

! **WARNING** Monitor patient for signs of hepatotoxicity, including darkened urine, fever, jaundice, and rash. Notify prescriber immediately and expect to discontinue drug if any of these signs or symptoms occur. Monitor patient for abnormal liver function test results, such as elevated ALT, AST, alkaline phosphatase, and bilirubin levels, and expect to discontinue drug, as ordered, if any of these occurs.

- Ensure adequate rest, and provide other pain-relief measures as needed.
- Institute safety measures to prevent falls or injury until drug's full CNS effects are known.

PATIENT TEACHING
- Instruct patient having difficulty swallowing tablet that it may be crushed and mixed with food or liquid for easier swallowing. Also, advise patient that if stomach upset occurs, drug can be taken with food or milk.
- Advise patient to take a missed dose of chlorzoxazone as soon as possible unless it's almost time for the next dose.
- Advise patient to avoid hazardous activities until drug's CNS effects are known.
- Instruct patient to avoid alcohol and other CNS depressants during therapy.
- Inform patient that, in rare instances, urine may turn orange or reddish purple during therapy.

- Advise patient to store drug in a tightly capped container at room temperature.

cholestyramine
Prevalite

Class and Category
Pharmacologic class: Bile acid sequestrant
Therapeutic class: Antihyperlipidemic, antipruritic (cholestasis)

Indications and Dosages
✳ *As adjunct to reduce serum cholesterol level in patients with primary hypercholesterolemia; to reduce LDL cholesterol in patients who also have hypertriglyceridemia when hypertriglyceridemia is not the abnormality of most concern; to relieve pruritus associated with partial biliary obstruction*

ORAL SUSPENSION
Adults. *Initial:* 4 g once or twice daily, increased every 4 wk or more, as needed. *Maintenance:* 8 to 16 g equally divided and given 1 to 6 times a day. *Maximum:* 24 g daily.

Drug Administration

P.O.
- Administer drug at mealtime.
- Never administer the dry powder without mixing it as follows: Place amount of powder needed for dose in any 60 to 180 ml of noncarbonated beverage or water and stir vigorously. After patient drinks mixture, rinse glass with more liquid, and have patient swallow it to make sure full dose is given.
- Drug also may be mixed in thin soups or moist, pulpy fruits, such as applesauce or crushed pineapple.
- Administer other oral drugs 1 hour before or at least 4 hours after cholestyramine to avoid interfering with absorption.

Route	Onset	Peak	Duration
P.O.	24–48 hr	7–21 days	2–4 wk

Half-life: Unknown

Mechanism of Action
Increases bile acid excretion in feces. The resulting decreased bile acid level increases the activity of the enzyme that regulates

C

cholesterol synthesis in the liver. As a result, the liver increases its cholesterol synthesis to produce more bile acids. However, the liver's synthesis of cholesterol typically can't match the amount needed to synthesize bile acids, which reduces the cholesterol level. Also, a decreased cholesterol level causes liver cells to increase their uptake of LDLs, which further reduces the cholesterol level. Cholestyramine may relieve pruritus by decreasing the body's bile acid level. This reduces the amount of excess bile acids that are deposited in the dermis and that typically cause pruritus in patients with cholestasis.

Contraindications

Complete biliary obstruction (when bile isn't secreted into intestine), hypersensitivity to cholestyramine or its components

Interactions

DRUGS

oral drugs such as chenodiol, digitalis glycosides, estrogens, fat-soluble vitamins, folic acid, gemfibrozil, penicillin G (oral), phenobarbital (oral), phenylbutazone, progestins, propranolol (oral), tetracyclines (oral), thiazide diuretics (oral), thyroid hormones, ursodiol, vancomycin (oral), warfarin: Decreased absorption and effects of these drugs

Adverse Reactions

CNS: Dizziness, headache
GI: Bloating, constipation, diarrhea, epigastric pain, eructation, fecal impaction, flatulence, indigestion, nausea, vomiting

Childbearing Considerations

PREGNANCY

- It is not known if drug causes fetal harm.
- Be aware that drug interferes with absorption of fat-soluble vitamins, which may make regular prenatal supplementation inadequate.
- Use with caution only if benefit to mother outweighs potential risk to fetus.

LACTATION

- It is not known if drug is present in breast milk.
- Patient should check with prescriber before breastfeeding.
- Be aware that the possibility of a lack of proper vitamin absorption may affect the breastfed infant.

Nursing Considerations

! WARNING Be aware that long-term use may increase bleeding tendency from hyperprothrombinemia caused by vitamin K deficiency. If this occurs, patient will require treatment with vitamin K_1.

- Monitor for deficiencies of fat-soluble vitamins, such as A and D. If long-term therapy prevents absorption of these vitamins, expect to provide supplementation.

PATIENT TEACHING

- Urge patient to follow a low-cholesterol, low-fat diet and regular exercise program.
- Tell patient to take drug before meals.
- Instruct patient to mix dry powder as follows: Place amount of powder needed for dose in any beverage and stir vigorously. Then, vigorously stir in another 2 to 4 ounces of beverage. After drinking mixture, rinse glass with more liquid, and swallow it to make sure full dose is taken. Patient also may mix drug in thin soups or moist, pulpy fruits, such as applesauce or crushed pineapple.
- Tell patient to drink plenty of fluids and increase bulk in his diet to minimize constipation; remind him to notify prescriber if constipation, nausea, or other adverse GI reactions develop.
- Explain that serum cholesterol level will have to be measured often for first few months of therapy and periodically thereafter.
- Advise patient to take other drugs at least 1 hour before or 4 to 6 hours after cholestyramine to avoid interference with their absorption.
- Tell patient to take a missed dose as soon as he remembers but not to take double or extra doses.

ciclesonide

Alvesco, Omnaris, Zetonna

Class and Category

Pharmacologic class: Corticosteroid
Therapeutic class: Antiasthmatic, anti-inflammatory

Indications and Dosages

✳ *To provide prophylactic maintenance therapy for patients with asthma*

INHALATION AEROSOL (ALVESCO)

Adults and children age 12 and over who received bronchodilator therapy. *Initial:* 80 mcg twice daily. *Maximum:* 160 mcg twice daily.

Adults and children age 12 and over who received inhaled corticosteroid. *Initial:* 80 mcg twice daily, adjusted to lowest effective dose when stabilized. *Maximum:* 320 mg twice daily.

Adults and children age 12 and over who received oral corticosteroid therapy. *Initial and maximum:* 320 mcg twice daily, adjusted to lowest effective dose when stabilized.

✱ *To treat nasal congestion in seasonal allergic rhinitis*

NASAL SPRAY (OMNARIS)

Adults and children age 6 and over. 200 mcg once daily as 2 sprays in each nostril.

NASAL AEROSOL (ZETONNA)

Adults and children age 12 and over. 74 mcg once daily as 1 spray (37 mcg) in each nostril.

✱ *To treat nasal congestion in perennial allergic rhinitis*

NASAL SPRAY (OMNARIS)

Adults and children age 12 and over. 200 mcg once daily as 2 sprays in each nostril.

NASAL AEROSOL (ZETONNA)

Adults and children age 12 and over. 74 mcg once daily as 1 spray (37 mcg) in each nostril.

⬚ Drug Administration

INHALATION

- Use inhalation form only with the actuator supplied with the product.
- Prime Alvesco before first use by actuating the inhaler 3 times; repeat priming if inhaler is not used for more than 10 days.
- Have patient gargle and rinse mouth after each dose to help prevent dry mouth and throat, relieve throat irritation, and prevent oral yeast infection.
- Clean mouthpiece weekly with a clean, dry tissue, both inside and out. Wipe over the front of the small hole where the drug comes out with a dry, folded tissue. Do not wash or put any part of the unit in water or any other liquid.
- When the dose indicator shows a red zone in the window, this indicates a need for

a refill. When the indicator shows zero, discard the inhaler.

INTRANASAL

- Avoid spraying drug directly onto the nasal septum.

Omnaris

- Gently shake nasal spray before each use. On first use, spray eight times into the air, looking for a fine mist. If drug hasn't been used for more than 4 days, it should be primed again with one spray or until a fine mist appears. Discard after 120 actuations following initial priming or after 4 months after bottle is removed from the foil pouch, whichever occurs first.

Zetonna

- Nasal spray should be primed before first use, by actuating three times. If drug hasn't been used for than 10 days, it should be primed again by actuating three times. If canister is dropped and actuator becomes separated, reassemble and test spray once into the air before using. When the Zetonna dose indicator shows a red zone in the window, this indicates a need for a refill. When the indicator shows zero, discard the canister.

Route	Onset	Peak	Duration
Inhalation	>4 wk	1 hr	Unknown
Intranasal	1–2 days	1–5 wk	Unknown

Half-life: Inhalation, 0.7 hr; intranasal, unknown

⬚ Mechanism of Action

Inhibits cells involved in the asthma inflammatory response, such as basophils, eosinophils, lymphocytes, macrophages, mast cells, and neutrophils. Ciclesonide also inhibits production or secretion of chemical mediators, such as cytokines, eicosanoids, histamine, and leukotrienes.

⬚ Contraindications

Hypersensitivity to ciclesonide or its components, primary treatment of status asthmaticus or other acute asthma episodes that require intensive measures (Alvesco)

⬚ Interactions

DRUGS

ketoconazole: Increased exposure time of ciclesonide

Adverse Reactions

CNS: Dizziness, fatigue, headache

EENT: Cataracts, conjunctivitis, dry mouth or throat, dysphonia, epistaxis, glaucoma, hoarseness, nasal congestion or ulceration, nasal septal perforation, nasopharyngitis, oral candidiasis, pharyngolaryngeal pain, sinusitis

ENDO: Adrenal insufficiency, cushingoid symptoms, decreased bone mineral density, hyperglycemia, slower growth in children

GI: Nausea

MS: Arthralgia, back or limb pain, musculoskeletal chest pain

RESP: Bronchospasm, cough, pneumonia, upper respiratory tract infection

SKIN: Urticaria

Other: Angioedema, flu-like symptoms, infections

Childbearing Considerations

PREGNANCY

- It is not known if drug can cause fetal harm although hypoadrenalism may occur in neonates born of mothers receiving corticosteroids during pregnancy.
- Use with caution only if benefit to mother outweighs potential risk to fetus.

LACTATION

- It is not known if drug is present in breast milk.
- Patient should check with prescriber before breastfeeding.

Nursing Considerations

- Know that ciclesonide should not be used in patients with recent nasal septal ulcers, nasal surgery, or nasal trauma until healing has occurred.
- Use cautiously in patients with tuberculosis; bacterial, fungal, parasitic, or viral infection; ocular herpes simplex; or chickenpox or measles, because these conditions may worsen with ciclesonide therapy.
- Also use cautiously in patients with a history of cataracts, glaucoma, or increased intraocular pressure because ciclesonide may increase intraocular pressure or cause cataract formation; and in patients with major risk factors for decreased bone mineral content, such as family history of osteoporosis, prolonged immobilization, or long-term use of drugs that can reduce bone mass, such as anticonvulsants and oral corticosteroids.
- Inspect patient's oral cavity if using inhaler form, or nasal cavity if using nasal spray regularly for abnormalities. If nasal or oral candidiasis occurs, expect to continue ciclesonide therapy, unless severe. If nasal erosion, ulceration, or perforation occurs, notify prescriber and expect nasal spray to be discontinued.
- Be aware that if patient takes a systemic corticosteroid, expect to taper dosage by no more than 2.5 mg/day at weekly intervals, starting 1 week after ciclesonide therapy begins.

! **WARNING** Know that if patient is switched from systemic corticosteroid to ciclesonide, assess for adrenal insufficiency (fatigue, hypotension, lassitude, nausea, vomiting, weakness) early in therapy and whenever patient has infection, stress, surgery, or trauma, or other steroid-depleting conditions or procedures. Notify prescriber immediately if signs or symptoms develop.

- Administer a fast-acting inhaled bronchodilator, as prescribed, if an acute asthma attack occurs. Ciclesonide inhalation is not a bronchodilator and its action takes longer than needed to abort acute asthma symptoms. If bronchospasm occurs immediately after ciclesonide use, expect to stop drug and start another drug regimen.
- Monitor growth in children because ciclesonide may suppress growth.

PATIENT TEACHING

- Urge patient to use ciclesonide regularly, as prescribed, but not for acute bronchospasm. Also tell her never to increase or decrease the dosage without consulting prescriber.
- Advise patient, on first use, to spray three times into the air and away from her eyes (Alvesco, Zetonna) or eight times (Omnaris), looking for a fine mist. Tell patient that if inhaler or spray hasn't been used for more than 4 days (Omnaris) or 10 days (Alvesco, Zetonna), it should be primed again.
- Tell patient to use inhalation form only with the actuator supplied with the product. Explain that when the dose indicator shows a red zone in the window, about 20 inhalations are left, indicating a need for a refill. When the indicator shows zero,

she should discard the inhaler. Advise against relying solely on the dose indicator, especially if inhaler has been dropped, but to keep track of number of inhalations used.

- Instruct patient to use inhaler form according to package instructions. Emphasize need to make sure canister is firmly seated in the plastic mouthpiece adapter before each use and to press inhaler slowly but firmly until it can go no further in the adapter for each spray. Inform patient that she doesn't need to shake inhaler before use. Tell patient to always replace cap on inhaler after use, to keep mouthpiece clean, and to clean mouthpiece once a week with a clean, dry tissue or cloth. Warn patient never to wash inhaler with water.
- Advise patient using nasal spray form to avoid spraying the drug directly onto the nasal septum.
- Instruct patient to gargle and rinse her mouth after each dose of inhaler to help prevent dry mouth and throat, relieve throat irritation, and prevent oral yeast infection.
- Explain that the full effect of drug may not occur for 4 weeks or more.
- Stress importance of notifying prescriber if symptoms continue or worsen.
- Instruct patient to notify prescriber immediately if asthma attacks don't respond to bronchodilators during ciclesonide inhaler use.
- Make patient aware that if she is switching from an oral corticosteroid to inhaled ciclesonide, she should carry medical identification indicating the need for supplemental systemic corticosteroids during a severe asthma attack or stress.
- Caution patient to avoid contact with people who have infections, because drug suppresses the immune system, increasing the risk of infection. Instruct patient to notify prescriber about exposure to chickenpox, measles, or other infections, because additional treatment may be needed.

cilostazol

☰ Class and Category

Pharmacologic class: Phosphodiesterase 3 (PDE 3) inhibitor
Therapeutic class: Antiplatelet

☰ Indications and Dosages

✳ *To reduce symptoms of intermittent claudication*

TABLETS

Adults. 100 mg twice daily.

±**DOSAGE ADJUSTMENT** For patient taking a moderate or strong CYP3A4 inhibitor (diltiazem, erythromycin, itraconazole, ketoconazole) or taking a CYP2C19 inhibitor (fluconazole, omeprazole, ticlopidine), dosage reduced to 50 mg twice daily.

☰ Drug Administration

P.O.

- Administer at least 30 minutes before or 2 hours after breakfast and dinner.
- Don't administer with grapefruit juice.

Route	Onset	Peak	Duration
P.O.	Unknown	Unknown	Unknown

Half-life: 11–13 hr

☰ Mechanism of Action

May inhibit phosphodiesterase, decreasing phosphodiesterase activity and suppressing cyclic adenosine monophosphate (cAMP) degradation. This action increases cAMP in platelets and blood vessels, which inhibits platelet aggregation and causes vasodilation. This in turn relieves symptoms of claudication.

☰ Contraindications

Heart failure, hypersensitivity to cilostazol or its components

☰ Interactions

DRUGS

CYP2C19 inhibitors (e.g., fluconazole, omeprazole, ticlopidine) or CYP3A4 inhibitors (e.g., diltiazem, erythromycin, omeprazole, ticlopidine): Increased plasma cilostazol level

FOODS

grapefruit: Increased risk of adverse reactions
high-fat foods: Faster cilostazol absorption and increased risk of adverse reactions

ACTIVITIES

smoking: Decreased cilostazol effects by about 20%

☰ Adverse Reactions

CNS: Cerebral hemorrhage, dizziness, headache, paresthesia
CV: Angina, chest pain, hypertension, hypotension, left ventricular outflow tract

obstruction (patients with sigmoid-shaped interventricular septum), palpitations, peripheral edema, **prolonged OT interval, supraventricular or ventricular tachycardia, thrombosis, torsades de pointes**
EENT: Pharyngitis, rhinitis
ENDO: Diabetes mellitus, hot flashes, hyperglycemia
GI: Abdominal pain, abnormal stool, diarrhea, elevated liver enzymes, flatulence, **GI hemorrhage, hepatic dysfunction,** indigestion, jaundice, vomiting
GU: Elevated BUN level, hematuria
HEME: **Agranulocytosis, aplastic anemia, bleeding tendency, decreased platelet count, granulocytopenia, leukopenia, pancytopenia, thrombocytopenia**
MS: Back pain, myalgia
RESP: Cough, **interstitial pneumonia, pulmonary hemorrhage**
SKIN: Eruptions, pruritus, rash, **Stevens–Johnson syndrome**
Other: Infection, increased blood uric acid level

Childbearing Considerations
PREGNANCY
- It is not known if drug can cause fetal harm.
- Use with caution only if benefit to mother outweighs potential risk to fetus.

LACTATION
- It is not known if drug is present in breast milk.
- A decision should be made to discontinue breastfeeding or the drug to avoid potential serious adverse reactions in the breastfed infant.

Nursing Considerations
- Monitor patient's vital signs and cardiovascular status closely because cilostazol may cause cardiovascular lesions, which could lead to problems, such as endocardial hemorrhage.
- Be aware that left ventricular outflow tract obstruction has been reported in patients with sigmoid-shaped interventricular septum. Monitor patients for development of new cardiac symptoms, including a systolic murmur, after starting cilostazol.
- Monitor blood glucose level to detect hyperglycemia. Also assess for signs of type 2 diabetes mellitus, such as fatigue, polydipsia, polyphagia, and polyuria.

PATIENT TEACHING
- Instruct patient to take cilostazol on an empty stomach 30 minutes before breakfast and dinner or 2 hours after these meals, because high-fat foods can increase the risk of adverse reactions.
- Warn patent to avoid grapefruit juice during therapy because it can increase the risk of adverse reactions.
- Urge patient not to smoke because it decreases drug's effects.
- Explain that assessment of drug effectiveness is based on ability to walk increased distances. Stress that drug effects won't appear until 2 to 4 weeks after therapy starts and that full effects may take up to 12 weeks.

cimetidine
Tagamet HB

cimetidine hydrochloride

Class and Category
Pharmacologic class: Histamine H_2 antagonist
Therapeutic class: Antiulcer agent

Indications and Dosages
✲ *To treat and prevent recurrence of duodenal ulcer*

ORAL SOLUTION, TABLETS
Adults and adolescents age 16 and over.
Initial: 800 mg (or 1,600 mg if ulcer is greater than 1.0 cm and patient is heavy smoker) once daily. Alternatively, 300 mg four times daily, or 400 mg twice daily for 4 to 6 wk. *Maintenance:* 400 mg once daily.

I.M. INJECTION
Adults. *Initial:* 300 mg every 6 to 8 hr.

I.V. INJECTION, I.V. INTERMITTENT INFUSION
Adults. *Initial:* 300 mg every 6 to 8 hr. Frequency of a 300-mg dose increased as needed. *Maximum:* 2,400 mg daily.

I.V. CONTINUOUS INFUSION
Adults. 37.5 mg/hr. *Maximum:* 900 mg daily.
✲ *To treat active, benign gastric ulcer*

ORAL SOLUTION, TABLETS
Adults and adolescents age 16 and over.
800 mg once daily or 300 mg four times daily for up to 8 wk.

I.M. INJECTION
Adults and adolescents age 16 and over.
300 mg every 6 to 8 hr.

I.V. INJECTION, I.V. INTERMITTENT INFUSION
Adults. *Initial:* 300 mg every 6 to 8 hr. Frequency of a 300-mg dose increased as needed. *Maximum:* 2,400 mg daily.

I.V. CONTINUOUS INFUSION
Adults and adolescents age 16 and over.
Initial: 37.5 mg/hr. *Maximum:* 900 mg daily.

❋ *To manage erosive gastroesophageal reflux disease*

ORAL SOLUTION, TABLETS
Adults. 1,600 mg daily in divided doses (800 mg twice daily or 400 mg four times daily) for up to 12 wk.

❋ *To treat pathological hypersecretory conditions, such as Zollinger–Ellison syndrome*

ORAL SOLUTION, TABLETS
Adults and adolescents age 16 and over.
300 mg four times daily increased in dosage and/or frequency, if needed. *Maximum:* 2,400 mg daily.

I.M. INJECTION
Adults and adolescents age 16 and over.
300 mg every 6 to 8 hr.

I.V. INJECTION, I.V. INTERMITTENT INFUSION
Adults. *Initial:* 300 mg every 6 to 8 hr. Frequency of a 300-mg dose increased as needed. *Maximum:* 2,400 mg daily.

I.V. CONTINUOUS INFUSION
Adults. *Initial:* 37.5 mg/hr. *Maximum:* 900 mg daily.

❋ *To treat heartburn and acid indigestion*

ORAL SOLUTION, TABLETS
Adults and children age 12 and over.
Initial: 200 mg, as needed, up to twice daily. *Maximum:* 400 mg every 24 hr for no more than 2 wk unless prescribed.

❋ *To prevent stress-related upper GI bleeding during hospitalization*

I.V. CONTINUOUS INFUSION
Adults. 37.5 mg/hr for 7 days.

±**DOSAGE ADJUSTMENT** For patient with severe renal impairment, dosage reduced to 300 mg and frequency lengthened to every 12 hr (and increased to every 8 hr with caution, if needed). For patient with both renal and liver impairment, dosage decreased even further. For patient with a creatinine clearance less than 30 ml/min and being treated to prevent stress-related upper GI bleeding during hospitalization, dosage reduced by 50%.

☰ Drug Administration
P.O.
- For treatment other than use as an antacid or for acid indigestion, once-daily doses given at bedtime; twice-daily doses given in morning and at bedtime; four-times-a-day doses given with meals and at bedtime.
- For use as an antacid or for acid indigestion, administer with water at onset of symptoms or up to 30 minutes before eating.
- Use calibrated device when measuring oral solution dosage.
- Do not administer an antacid within 1 hour of administering cimetidine.

I.V.
- Solutions compatible for use to dilute drug include 0.9% Sodium Chloride Injection, 5% Dextrose Injection, Lactated Ringer's, and 5% Sodium Bicarbonate Injection.
- Diluted solutions may be stored for up to 48 hours at room temperature.
- Do not administer rapidly. For I.V. injection, dilute to a total volume of 20 ml. Inject over 5 minutes or more.
- For intermittent infusion, dilute in at least 50 ml I.V. solution. Infuse over 15 to 20 minutes.
- For continuous infusion, dilute 900 mg in 100- to 1,000-ml I.V. solution (volume used individualized). Use a volumetric pump to infuse drug if volume is less than 250 ml. Administer at a rate of 37.5 mg/hr.
- *Incompatibilities:* None listed by manufacturer

I.M.
- Administer undiluted.
- Inform patient the injection may be painful.

Route	Onset	Peak	Duration
P.O.	1 hr	45–90 min	4–5 hr
I.V.	30 min	Immediate	4–5 hr
I.M.	Unknown	15 min	4–5 hr
Half-life: 2 hr			

C

Mechanism of Action

Blocks histamine's action at H_2-receptor sites on stomach's parietal cells. This action reduces gastric fluid volume and acidity. Cimetidine also decreases the amount of gastric acid secreted in response to betazole, caffeine, food, insulin, or pentagastrin.

Contraindications

Hypersensitivity to cimetidine or its components

Interactions

DRUGS

antacids, metoclopramide: Decreased cimetidine absorption
chlordiazepoxide, diazepam, lidocaine, metronidazole, nifedipine, phenytoin, propranolol, quinidine, theophylline, tricyclic antidepressants (certain ones), warfarin: Reduced metabolism and increased blood levels and effects of these drugs, possibly toxicity from these drugs
digoxin, ketoconazole: Altered absorption of these drugs
warfarin: Increased risk of bleeding

FOODS

caffeine: Reduced metabolism and increased blood level and effects of caffeine

ACTIVITIES

alcohol use: Possibly increased blood alcohol level

Adverse Reactions

CNS: Confusion, dizziness, hallucinations, headache, peripheral neuropathy, somnolence
ENDO: Mild gynecomastia if used longer than 1 month
GI: Mild and transient diarrhea
GU: Impotence, transiently elevated serum creatinine level
SKIN: Rash
Other: Pain at I.M. injection site

Childbearing Considerations

PREGNANCY

- It is not known if drug can cause fetal harm.
- Use with caution only if benefit to mother outweighs potential risk to fetus.

LACTATION

- Drug is present in breast milk.
- Breastfeeding is not recommended during drug therapy.

Nursing Considerations

- Be alert for confusion in debilitated or elderly patients who receive cimetidine.

PATIENT TEACHING

- Tell patient to use a liquid-measuring device to ensure accurate dose of solution.
- Advise patient that for treatment (other than used as an antacid or for acid indigestion), once-daily doses given at bedtime; twice-daily doses given in morning and at bedtime; four-times-a-day doses given with meals and at bedtime.
- Instruct patient using drug as an antacid or for acid indigestion to take drug with water at onset of symptoms or up to 30 minutes before eating.
- Advise patient to avoid alcohol while taking cimetidine, to prevent interactions.
- Instruct patient to avoid taking antacids within 1 hour of taking cimetidine.
- Warn patient that cigarette smoking increases gastric acid secretion and can worsen gastric disease.
- Caution patient not to take drug for more than 14 days, unless prescribed.

cinacalcet hydrochloride

Sensipar

Class and Category

Pharmacologic class: Calcimimetic
Therapeutic class: Calcium reducer

Indications and Dosages

* *To treat secondary hyperparathyroidism in patients with chronic renal disease who are on dialysis*

TABLETS

Adults. *Initial:* 30 mg once daily, increased by 30 mg every 2 to 4 wk daily, as needed. *Maximum:* 180 mg daily.

* *To treat hypercalcemia in patients with parathyroid carcinoma; to treat primary hyperparathyroidism in patients who are unable to undergo parathyroidectomy*

TABLETS

Adults. *Initial:* 30 mg twice daily, increased in 2 to 4 wk to 60 mg twice daily, then in 2 to 4 wk to 90 mg twice daily, and then in

2 to 4 wk to 90 mg three times daily or four times daily, as needed to normalize serum calcium level.

Drug Administration

P.O.

- Administer drug with food or shortly after a meal.
- Tablet should be swallowed whole and not chewed, crushed, or split.

Route	Onset	Peak	Duration
P.O.	Unknown	2–6 hr	Unknown

Half-life: 30–40 hr

Mechanism of Action

Increases sensitivity of calcium-sensing receptors on the surface of parathyroid cells to extracellular calcium. This sensitivity directly reduces parathyroid hormone (PTH) level, which in turn decreases serum calcium level.

Contraindications

Hypersensitivity to cinacalcet or its components, hypocalcemia

Interactions

DRUGS

CYP2D6 substrates, such as carvedilol, desipramine, metoprolol; drugs that have a narrow therapeutic index, such as flecainide, tricyclic antidepressants (most): Possibly increased blood level of these drugs
other calcium-lowering drugs including other calcium-sensing receptor agonists: Increased risk of severe hypocalcemia
strong CYP3A4 inhibitors such as itraconazole, ketoconazole: Possibly increased blood cinacalcet level

Adverse Reactions

CNS: Asthenia, dizziness, **seizures**
CV: Arrhythmias, hypertension, **hypotension** (in the presence of impaired cardiac function), **worsening heart failure** (in the presence of impaired cardiac function)
GI: Anorexia, diarrhea, **gastrointestinal bleeding**, nausea, vomiting
MS: Adynamic bone disease, myalgia
SKIN: Rash, urticaria
Other: Acute pseudogout, **allergic reaction, angioedema, hypocalcemia**, noncardiac chest pain

Childbearing Considerations

PREGNANCY

- It is not known if drug can cause fetal harm.
- Use with caution only if benefit to mother outweighs potential risk to fetus.

LACTATION

- It is not known if drug is present in breast milk.
- Patient should check with prescriber before breastfeeding.

Nursing Considerations

- Be aware that cinacalcet is not recommended for use in patients with chronic kidney disease who are not on dialysis, because of an increased risk of hypocalcemia.
- Use cinacalcet cautiously in patients with a history of seizures because reduced blood calcium level may lower seizure threshold. Also use cautiously in patients with hepatic insufficiency because cinacalcet metabolism may be reduced.

! **WARNING** Monitor patient for hypocalcemia exhibited by cramping, myalgia, paresthesia, prolonged QT interval that may cause ventricular arrhythmias, seizures, and tetany. Also monitor patient's blood calcium and phosphorus levels within 1 week after starting therapy or adjusting dosage, and every month or two once maintenance dose is established, as ordered. If hypocalcemia develops, notify prescriber immediately because treatment to raise calcium level will be needed. Treatment may include giving supplemental calcium, starting or increasing dosage of calcium-based phosphate binder or vitamin D sterols, or temporarily withholding cinacalcet.

- Be aware that if patient starts or stops therapy with a strong CYP3A4 inhibitor, such as itraconazole, or ketoconazole, cinacalcet dosage may have to be adjusted.
- Monitor dialysis patient's intact PTH levels 1 to 4 weeks after therapy starts or dose is adjusted and then every 1 to 3 months thereafter, as ordered. Keep in mind that adynamic bone disease may develop if iPTH levels drop below 100 pg/ml. Expect to reduce dosage or discontinue cinacalcet, as ordered, in a patient whose intact PTH level falls below the target range of 150 to 300 pg/ml.

C

- Monitor patient for worsening of common gastrointestinal adverse reactions of nausea and vomiting associated with cinacalcet therapy and for signs and symptoms of GI bleeding and ulcerations. Risk factors include esophagitis, gastritis, severe vomiting, or ulcers. Notify prescriber if such symptoms present, and provide supportive care, as ordered.

PATIENT TEACHING

- Instruct patient to take cinacalcet with food or shortly after a meal.
- Caution patient to take tablet whole and not divide it or crush it.
- Review signs and symptoms of hypocalcemia with patient and urge him to notify prescriber of changes.
- Advise patient to report any symptoms of gastrointestinal bleeding, nausea, or vomiting to prescriber.
- Alert patient with heart failure that cinacalcet may worsen the heart failure, requiring additional monitoring of their condition.
- Inform patient that regular blood tests will be ordered to monitor the safe use of cinacalcet and the importance of actually having the tests done.

ciprofloxacin

Cipro, Cipro I.V., Cipro XR, Otiprio

Class and Category

Pharmacologic class: Fluoroquinolone derivative
Therapeutic class: Antibiotic

Indications and Dosages

❋ *To prevent inhalation anthrax after exposure*

I.V. INFUSION FOLLOWED BY ORAL SUSPENSION, OR TABLETS

Adults. 400 mg I.V. every 12 hr and switched to 500 mg P.O. every 12 hr, as soon as possible, for a total of 60 days.

Children. 10 mg/kg I.V. every 12 hr and switched to 15 mg/kg P.O. every 12 hr, as soon as possible, for a total of 60 days. *Maximum:* 400 mg per dose I.V.; 500 mg per dose P.O.

❋ *To treat acute sinusitis caused by susceptible organisms*

ORAL SUSPENSION, TABLETS

Adults. 500 mg every 12 hr for 10 days.

I.V. INFUSION

Adults. 400 mg every 12 hr for 10 days.

❋ *To treat bone and joint infections caused by susceptible organisms*

ORAL SUSPENSION, TABLETS

Adults. For mild to moderate infections, 500 mg every 12 hr for 4 to 8 wk. For severe or complicated infections, 750 mg every 12 hr for 4 to 8 wk.

I.V. INFUSION

Adults. For mild to moderate infections, 400 mg every 12 hr for 4 to 8 wk. For severe or complicated infections, 400 mg every 8 hr for 4 to 8 wk.

❋ *To treat skin and soft-tissue infections caused by susceptible organisms*

ORAL SUSPENSION, TABLETS

Adults. For mild to moderate infections, 500 mg every 12 hr for 7 to 14 days. For severe or complicated infections, 750 mg every 12 hr for 7 to 14 days.

I.V. INFUSION

Adults. For mild to moderate infections, 400 mg every 12 hr for 7 to 14 days. For severe or complicated infections, 400 mg every 8 hr for 7 to 14 days.

❋ *To treat chronic bacterial prostatitis caused by susceptible organisms*

ORAL SUSPENSION, TABLETS

Adults. 500 mg every 12 hr for 28 days.

I.V. INFUSION

Adults. 400 mg every 12 hr for 28 days.

❋ *To treat infectious diarrhea caused by susceptible organisms*

ORAL SUSPENSION, TABLETS

Adults. 500 mg every 12 hr for 5 to 7 days.

❋ *To treat UTI caused by susceptible organisms*

ORAL SUSPENSION, TABLETS

Adults. For mild to moderate infections, 250 mg every 12 hr for 7 to 14 days. For severe or complicated infections, 500 mg every 12 hr for 7 to 14 days.

I.V. INFUSION

Adults. For mild to moderate infections, 200 mg every 12 hr for 7 to 14 days. For severe or complicated infections, 400 mg every 8 hr for 7 to 14 days.

❋ *To treat complicated UTI and pyelonephritis*

ORAL SUSPENSION, TABLETS

Children from age 1 to 17. *For mild to moderate infections:* 10 mg/kg every 12 hr for

10 to 21 days. *For severe infections*: 20 mg/kg every 12 hr for 10 to 21 days. *Maximum* 750 mg per dose.

I.V. INFUSION

Children age 1 to 17. 6 to 10 mg/kg every 8 hr for 10 to 21 days.

* *To treat acute uncomplicated cystitis*

ORAL SUSPENSION, TABLETS

Adults. 250 mg every 12 hr for 3 days.

E.R. TABLETS

Adults. 500 mg once daily for 3 days.

* *To treat acute uncomplicated pyelonephritis; to treat complicated urinary tract infection*

E.R. TABLETS

Adults. 1,000 mg once daily for 7 to 14 days.

* *To treat or prevent plague, including pneumonic and septicemic plague, due to Yersinia pestis*

ORAL SUSPENSION, TABLETS

Adults. 500 to 750 mg every 12 hr for 14 days.
Children. 15 mg/kg every 8 to 12 hr for 14 days. *Maximum:* 500 mg/dose.

I.V. INFUSION

Adults. 400 mg every 8 to 12 hr for 14 days.
Children. 10 mg/kg every 8 to 12 hr for 10 to 14 days. *Maximum:* 400 mg/dose.

* *To treat lower respiratory tract infections caused by susceptible organisms*

ORAL SUSPENSION, TABLETS

Adults. For mild to moderate infections, 500 mg every 12 hr for 7 to 14 days. For severe or complicated infections, 750 mg every 12 hr for 7 to 14 days.

I.V. INFUSION

Adults. For mild to moderate infections, 400 mg every 12 hr for 7 to 14 days. For severe or complicated infections, 400 mg every 8 hr for 7 to 14 days.

* *To treat nosocomial pneumonia caused by susceptible organisms*

I.V. INFUSION

Adults. 400 mg every 8 hr for 10 to 14 days.

* *To treat complicated intra-abdominal infections caused by susceptible organisms*

ORAL SUSPENSION, TABLETS

Adults. 500 mg every 12 hr for 7 to 14 days.

I.V. INFUSION

Adults. 400 mg every 12 hr for 7 to 14 days.

* *To treat typhoid fever caused by susceptible organisms*

ORAL SUSPENSION, TABLETS

Adults. 500 mg every 12 hr for 10 days.

* *To treat uncomplicated urethral or cervical gonococcal infections caused by N. gonorrhoeae*

ORAL SUSPENSION, TABLETS

Adults. 250 mg as a single dose.

* *To provide empirical therapy in febrile neutropenic patients*

I.V. INFUSION

Adults. 400 mg every 8 hr for 7 to 14 days given concomitantly with piperacillin.

* *To treat acute otitis externa caused by Pseudomonas aeruginosa or Staphylococcus aureus*

OTIC SUSPENSION (OTIPRIO)

Children age 6 months and over. 0.2 ml (12 mg) as a single dose to the external ear canal of each affected ear.

±**DOSAGE ADJUSTMENT** For patients taking oral suspension or tablets, dosage reduced to 250 to 500 mg every 12 hr if creatinine clearance is 30 to 50 ml/min; and to 250 to 500 mg every 18 hr if creatinine clearance is 5 to 29 ml/min. For patient on dialysis, dosage reduced to 250 mg to 500 mg every 24 hr and given after dialysis. For patient with a creatinine clearance of 30 ml/min or less taking E.R. tablets, dosage reduced to 500 mg daily and drug administered after dialysis, if patient is receiving dialysis. For patient receiving drug intravenously and who has a creatinine clearance between 5 to 29 ml/min, dosage reduced to 200 to 400 mg every 18 to 24 hr.

Drug Administration

P.O.

- E.R. and immediate-release tablets aren't interchangeable.
- Tablets are scored and may be split in half to provide correct dosage. Tablets should be swallowed without chewing or crushing.
- E.R. tablets should be swallowed whole and not chewed, crushed, or split.
- Administer with a main meal, preferably the evening meal.
- To mix oral suspension, know that the small bottle contains the microcapsules and the large bottle contains the diluent. Open both bottles and pour the microcapsules completely into the larger bottle of diluent. Do not add water to the suspension.

Remove the top layer of the diluent bottle label to reveal the Cipro Oral Suspension label. Close the large bottle according to the directions on the cap and shake vigorously for about 15 seconds. Write expiration date on bottle label.

- Reconstituted drug may be stored at room temperature for 14 days. Avoid freezing suspension.
- To administer oral suspension, shake bottle vigorously for 15 seconds prior to dose. Use the co-packaged graduated teaspoon provided. Tell patient not to chew the microcapsules in the suspension but to swallow them whole. Give patient water to drink after administration.
- Wash the graduated spoon afterwards with soap and water and dry thoroughly.
- Oral suspension should not be administered through a feeding or nasogastric tube.
- Administer at least 2 hours before or 6 hours after aluminum/magnesium antacids; polymeric phosphate binders (lanthanum carbonate, sevelamer) or sucralfate; didanosine chewable or buffered tablets or pediatric powder for oral solution; other highly buffered drugs; or products containing calcium, iron, or zinc.
- Do not administer drug with dairy products or calcium-fortified juices; however, drug may be given with a meal that contains these products.

I.V.

- Intravenous drug comes in a premixed solution in flexible containers of 200 ml. The solution in the flexible containers need not be diluted.
- Administer infusion over 60 minutes.
- Slowing infusion of a dilute solution into a larger vein will minimize patient discomfort and reduce the risk of venous irritation.
- *Incompatibilities:* Aminophylline, amoxicillin, cefepime, clindamycin, dexamethasone, floxacillin, furosemide, heparin, phenytoin

OTIC SUSPENSION

- During preparation of the suspension, the drug must be kept cold. If solution thickens during preparation, vial should be placed back in refrigeration.
- Shake vial for 5 to 8 seconds to mix well until a visually homogenous suspension is

obtained. Hold vial by the aluminum seal to prevent gelation when shaking vial.

- Using an 18- to 21-gauge needle, withdraw 0.3 ml of the suspension into the 1-ml syringe. Replace the needle with a 20- to 24-gauge, 1.5-inch blunt, flexible catheter.
- Prime the syringe after the administration catheter has been attached by leaving a dose of 0.2 ml in the syringe. Know that the syringes can be kept at room temperature or in the refrigerator prior to administration, but the syringes must be kept on their sides.
- Discard syringes if not administered in 3 hours.

Route	Onset	Peak	Duration
P.O.	Unknown	1–2 hr	Unknown
P.O./E.R.	Unknown	1–4 hr	Unknown
I.V.	Unknown	Unknown	Unknown
Otic	Unknown	Unknown	Unknown

Half-life: 3–5 hr

☰ Mechanism of Action

Inhibits the enzyme DNA gyrase, which is responsible for the unwinding and supercoiling of bacterial DNA before it replicates. By inhibiting this enzyme, ciprofloxacin causes bacterial cells to die.

☰ Contraindications

Concurrent therapy with tizanidine; hypersensitivity to ciprofloxac*in*, other quinolones, or their components

☰ Interactions

DRUGS

antacids, didanosine, iron supplements, multivitamins that contain iron or zinc sucralfate: Decreased ciprofloxacin absorption
caffeine, clozapine, duloxetine, methotrexate, methylxanthines, olanzapine, ropinirole, sildenafil, zolpidem: Increased plasma levels of these drugs and increased risk of serious adverse reactions including toxicity
cyclosporine: Elevated serum creatinine
drugs that prolong QT interval such as class IA or III antiarrhythmics, antipsychotics, macrolides, tricyclic antidepressants: Increased risk of further QT prolongation
NSAIDs (except acetylsalicylic acid): Increased risk of seizures with high doses of ciprofloxacin
oral anticoagulants: Enhanced anticoagulant effects

oral hypoglycemics: Possibly increased risk of hypoglycemia that may be severe (especially with glyburide)

phenytoin: Increased or decreased blood phenytoin level

probenecid: Increased blood ciprofloxacin level and, possibly, toxicity

theophylline: Increased risk of CNS or other serious adverse reactions

tizanidine: Potentiation of hypotensive and sedative effects of tizanidine

FOODS

caffeine: Increased caffeine effects

dairy products: Delayed drug absorption

Adverse Reactions

CNS: Abnormal gait, agitation, anxiety, ataxia, **cerebral thrombosis**, confusion delirium, depersonalization, depression, disorientation, disturbance in attention, dizziness, drowsiness, fever, hallucinations, headache, **increased intracranial pressure including pseudotumor cerebri**, insomnia, irritability, lethargy, light-headedness, malaise, manic reaction, memory impairment, migraine, nervousness, nightmares, paranoia, paresthesia, peripheral neuropathy, phobia, restlessness, **seizures, status epilepticus, suicidal ideation**, syncope, tremor, toxic psychosis, unresponsiveness, weakness

CV: Angina, **aortic aneurysm and dissection, atrial flutter, cardiopulmonary arrest, cardiovascular collapse,** hypertension, **MI**, orthostatic hypotension, palpitations, phlebitis, tachycardia, **torsades de pointes**, vasculitis, **ventricular ectopy**

EENT: Oral candidiasis

ENDO: Hyperglycemia, **hypoglycemia**

GI: Abdominal pain, anorexia, **Clostridioides difficile–associated diarrhea**, constipation, diarrhea, dysphagia, elevated liver enzymes, flatulence, **GI bleeding, hepatic failure or necrosis, hepatitis,** indigestion, **intestinal perforation**, jaundice, nausea, **pancreatitis, pseudomembranous colitis**, vomiting

GU: **Acute renal failure or insufficiency**, crystalluria, hematuria, increased serum creatinine level, interstitial nephritis, **nephrotoxicity**, renal calculi, urine retention, vaginal candidiasis

HEME: **Agranulocytosis, aplastic or hemolytic anemia, bone marrow** **depression, leukopenia**, lymphadenopathy, **pancytopenia, thrombocytopenia**

MS: Arthralgia, myalgia, tendinitis, tendon rupture

RESP: **Allergic pneumonitis, bronchospasm, pulmonary embolism, respiratory arrest**

SKIN: Acute generalized exanthematous pustulosis (AGEP), **erythema multiforme, exfoliative dermatitis**, photosensitivity, rash, **Stevens–Johnson syndrome, toxic epidermal necrolysis**, urticaria

Other: **Acidosis, anaphylaxis, angioedema,** serum sickness–like reaction

Childbearing Considerations

PREGNANCY

- It is not known if drug can cause fetal harm.
- Use with caution only if benefit to mother outweighs potential risk to fetus.

LACTATION

- Drug is present in breast milk.
- A decision should be made to discontinue breastfeeding temporarily during drug therapy or discontinue the drug to avoid potential serious adverse reactions in the breastfed infant except for postexposure with inhalation anthrax. If breastfeeding is temporarily stopped, mother could consider pumping and discarding breast milk during therapy and for an additional 2 days after the last dose.
- If breastfeeding does occur, mother should monitor her breastfed infant for bloody or loose stools and candidiasis (diaper rash, thrush).

Nursing Considerations

- Obtain culture and sensitivity test results, as ordered, before giving ciprofloxacin.
- Know that ciprofloxacin should not be used in a patient with myasthenia gravis as it may exacerbate muscle weakness.
- Know that ciprofloxacin should not be given to patients with a known aortic aneurysm or patients who are at greater risk for aortic aneurysms, unless no alternative antibacterial treatment is available. This is because studies suggest an increased risk of aortic aneurysm and dissection within 2 months following use of fluoroquinolones, especially in the elderly.
- Use drug cautiously in patients with CNS disorders and disorders that may predispose

C

patient to seizures, such as history of epilepsy or conditions that may lower the seizure threshold, such as history of altered brain structure, reduced cerebral blood flow, severe cerebral arteriosclerosis, or stroke. Take seizure precautions. If a seizure occurs, expect ciprofloxacin to be discontinued immediately.

- Use drug cautiously in patients who may be more susceptible to drug's effect on QT interval, such as those taking Class IA or III antiarrhythmics; those with uncorrected hypokalemia or hypomagnesemia; or in the presence of a history of cardiac disease such as heart failure, QT-interval prolongation, or torsades de pointes.

- Be aware that patient should be well hydrated during therapy to help prevent alkaline urine, which may lead to crystalluria and nephrotoxicity.

- Assess patient's hematologic, hepatic, and renal functions periodically, as ordered. Report any abnormalities, including signs and symptoms of dysfunction, to prescriber. For example, severe liver toxicity has occurred with ciprofloxacin use (within 1 to 39 days of therapy) and has been associated more frequently with hypersensitivity reactions. If dysfunction occurs, expect drug to be discontinued and provide supportive care, as ordered and needed.

- Assess patient routinely for signs of rash or other hypersensitivity reactions, even after patient has received multiple doses. Stop drug at first sign of rash, or other sign of hypersensitivity, and notify prescriber immediately. Be prepared to provide supportive emergency care.

- Monitor patient closely for diarrhea, which may reflect *C. difficile*–associated diarrhea. If it occurs, notify prescriber and expect to withhold drug and treat diarrhea.

- Assess patient for evidence of peripheral neuropathy. Notify prescriber and expect to stop drug if patient complains of burning, numbness, pain, tingling, or weakness in extremities or if physical examination reveals deficits in light touch, motor strength, pain, position sense, temperature, or vibratory sensation.

- Monitor patients (especially children, elderly patients, patients receiving corticosteroids,

and patients who have renal failure or who have had a heart, kidney, or lung transplant) for evidence of tendon rupture, such as inflammation, pain, and swelling at the site. Be aware that tendon rupture may occur within the first 48 hours of therapy, throughout therapy, or months after ciprofloxacin therapy. Notify prescriber about suspected tendon rupture, and have patient rest and refrain from exercise until tendon rupture has been ruled out. If present, expect to provide supportive care as ordered.

- Monitor patient closely for changes in behavior or mood that may be caused by ciprofloxacin-induced depression or worsening psychotic reactions potentially resulting in self-injurious behavior, such as suicide. Be aware these reactions may occur even after just one dose. Notify prescriber immediately and expect to discontinue ciprofloxacin therapy, if present, and institute precautions to keep patient safe until adverse effects have disappeared.

- Monitor patient's blood glucose levels, especially diabetic patients, and for signs and symptoms of changes in blood glucose levels. Both symptomatic hyperglycemia and hypoglycemia may occur as a result of ciprofloxacin therapy. If present, alert prescriber and initiate appropriate treatment, as prescribed. Also be aware that severe hypoglycemia has occurred when drug has been administered intravenously. If a hypoglycemic reaction occurs in a patient receiving drug intravenously, discontinue administration immediately and initiate appropriate emergency treatment for hypoglycemia.

PATIENT TEACHING

- Urge patient to complete the prescribed course of therapy, even if he feels better before it's finished.

- Tell patient not to take drug with calcium-fortified juices or dairy products.

- Advise patient to take ciprofloxacin 2 hours before or 6 hours after antacids, iron supplements, or multivitamins that contain iron or zinc. Tell him to shake oral suspension for 15 seconds, not to chew microcapsules, and not to chew, crush, or split E.R. tablets. Immediate-release tablets may be split in half. Advise patient to take drug about the same time every day and if prescribed a twice-daily dose to take first dose in the morning and second dose in the evening about 12 hours apart.

- Encourage patient to drink plenty of fluids during therapy to help prevent crystalluria.
- Urge patient to avoid caffeinated products, because caffeine may accumulate in the body during ciprofloxacin therapy and cause excessive stimulation.
- Stress importance of stopping ciprofloxacin therapy if adverse reactions occur and to contact prescriber for advice on completing treatment with another antibiotic.

! WARNING Instruct patient to seek emergency medical help immediately if sudden back, chest, or stomach pain occurs.

- Caution patient to avoid excessive exposure to sunlight or artificial ultraviolet light because severe sunburn may result. Tell patient to notify prescriber if sunburn develops; drug will have to be stopped.
- Urge patient to avoid hazardous activities until CNS effects of drug are known.
- Advise patient to notify prescriber about changes in limb movement or sensation and about inflammation, pain, or swelling over a joint. Urge patient to rest the affected limb at the first sign of discomfort.
- Tell patient to stop taking drug and to notify prescriber at first sign of rash or other hypersensitivity reaction.
- Urge patient to report bloody, watery stools to prescriber immediately, even up to 2 months after drug therapy has ended.
- Urge caregivers to monitor patient closely for suicidal tendencies if he develops depression or worsening of psychotic behavior and to notify prescriber.
- Warn patient, especially diabetic patient, that ciprofloxacin may alter blood glucose levels. Review signs and symptoms of hyperglycemia and hypoglycemia. Tell patient to report symptomatic changes in blood glucose levels immediately to prescriber and review how to treat hypoglycemia.
- Inform mothers who are breastfeeding to consider pumping and discarding breast milk during treatment and an additional 2 days after the last dose.

citalopram hydrobromide
Celexa

Class and Category
Pharmacologic class: Selective serotonin reuptake inhibitor (SSRI)
Therapeutic class: Antidepressant

Indications and Dosages
✳ *To treat depression*
ORAL SOLUTION, TABLETS
Adults. *Initial:* 20 mg daily. Increased to 40 mg daily, after 1 wk as needed. *Maximum:* 40 mg daily.
±**DOSAGE ADJUSTMENT** Dosage should not exceed 20 mg daily in patients taking concomitant cimetidine or CYP2C19 inhibitors, who are poor CYP2C19 metabolizers, who have hepatic impairment, or who are older than 60 years of age.

Drug Administration
P.O.
- Use calibrated measuring device to measure dose of oral solution.

Route	Onset	Peak	Duration
P.O.	1–2 wk	4 hr	1–2 days
Half-life: 24–48 hr			

Mechanism of Action
Blocks serotonin reuptake by adrenergic nerves, which normally release this neurotransmitter from their storage sites when activated by a nerve impulse. This blocked reuptake increases serotonin levels at nerve synapses, which may elevate mood and reduce depression.

Contraindications
Hypersensitivity to citalopram or its components, pimozide therapy, use within 14 days of MAO inhibitor therapy including I.V. methylene blue or linezolid

Interactions
DRUGS
antidepressants, buspirone, fentanyl, isoniazid, linezolid, lithium, MAO inhibitors, methylene blue, other selective serotonin reuptake inhibitors (escitalopram,

fluoxetine, fluvoxamine, paroxetine, sertraline), pentamidine, selegiline, serotonin norepinephrine reuptake inhibitors (desvenlafaxine, duloxetine, milnacipran, venlafaxine), St. John's wort, tramadol, triptans, tryptophan: Increased risk of life-threatening serotonin syndrome

antipsychotics, Class IA and Class III antiarrhythmics, CYP2C19 inhibitors, gatifloxacin, methadone, moxifloxacin, pimozide: Increased risk of QT prolongation and torsades de pointes

aspirin, NSAIDs, warfarin: Increased risk of bleeding ranging from ecchymoses to life-threatening hemorrhage

carbamazepine: Possibly increased clearance of citalopram

cimetidine: Possibly increased blood citalopram level and increased risk of QT prolongation

clozapine: Substantial increases in plasma clozapine levels

CNS depressants: Possible potentiated CNS effect

diuretics: Possibly increased risk of hyponatremia

ketoconazole: Decreased peak concentrations of ketoconazole

metoprolol, tricyclic antidepressants such as desipramine or imipramine: Possibly increased blood levels of these drugs; possibly life-threatening serotonin syndrome

Adverse Reactions

CNS: Agitation, akathisia, amnesia, anxiety, apathy, asthenia, confusion, CVA, delirium, depression, dizziness, drowsiness, dyskinesia, fatigue, fever, impaired concentration, insomnia, migraine, myoclonus, **neuroleptic malignant syndrome**, paresthesia, **seizures**, **serotonin syndrome**, **suicidal ideation**, tremor

CV: Angina, bundle branch block, chest pain, **heart failure**, MI, orthostatic hypotension, **prolonged QT interval**, tachycardia, **thrombosis**, **ventricular arrhythmias**

EENT: Abnormal accommodation, acute-angle glaucoma, blurred vision, dry mouth, rhinitis, sinusitis, taste perversion

GI: Abdominal pain, anorexia, diarrhea, flatulence, **GI bleeding**, **hepatic necrosis**, indigestion, nausea, **pancreatitis**, vomiting

GU: **Acute renal failure**, amenorrhea, anorgasmia, decreased libido, dysmenorrhea,

ejaculation disorders, impotence, polyuria, priapism

HEME: Abnormal bleeding, **decreased PT**, **hemolytic anemia**, **thrombocytopenia**

MS: Arthralgia, myalgia, **rhabdomyolysis**

RESP: Cough, upper respiratory tract infection

SKIN: Diaphoresis, ecchymosis, **erythema multiforme**, pruritus, rash

Other: **Anaphylaxis**, **angioedema**, **hyponatremia**, weight gain or loss

Childbearing Considerations

PREGNANCY

- Pregnancy exposure registry: 1-844-405-6185 or http://womensmentalhealth.org/research/pregnancyregistry/antidepressants.
- Drug may cause fetal harm if given late in the third trimester evident as early as immediately after birth with neonate exhibiting constant crying and irritability, feeding difficulty, temperature instability, respiratory distress and/or seizures.
- Use with caution only if benefit to mother outweighs potential risk to fetus.

LACTATION

- Drug is present in breast milk.
- Patient should check with prescriber before breastfeeding.
- If breastfeeding occurs, mother should monitor infant for decreased feeding, excessive somnolence, irritability, restlessness, and weight loss.

Nursing Considerations

! **WARNING** Monitor patient for possible serotonin syndrome, when dosage increases and which may include agitation, chills, confusion, diaphoresis, diarrhea, fever, hyperactive reflexes, poor coordination, restlessness, shaking, talking, or acting with uncontrolled excitement, tremor, and twitching. In its most severe form, serotonin syndrome can resemble neuroleptic malignant syndrome, which includes a high fever, muscle rigidity, or autonomic instability with possible changes in vital signs, and mental status changes.

- Be aware that citalopram should not be given to patients with congenital long QT syndrome, bradycardia, hypokalemia or hypomagnesemia, recent acute myocardial infarction, or uncompensated heart failure because of increased risk of prolonged QT interval and torsades de pointes. It should also not be given to patients who are taking other drugs that prolong the QT interval. Expect hypokalemia and hypomagnesemia to be corrected before citalopram therapy is begun.

- Use citalopram cautiously in patients with other cardiac conditions. ECG monitoring may be ordered to monitor the patient's QT interval and detect the development of serious arrhythmias.
- Use citalopram cautiously in patients with hepatic impairment because citalopram clearance is affected and can lead to increased plasma citalopram levels.
- Be aware that effective antidepressant therapy may convert depression into mania in predisposed people. If patient develops symptoms of mania, notify prescriber immediately and expect to discontinue citalopram.
- Assess elderly patients and those taking diuretics for signs suggesting syndrome of inappropriate secretion of antidiuretic hormone, including hyponatremia and increased serum and urine osmolarity.
- Monitor patient closely for suicidal tendencies, especially when therapy starts or dosage changes, because depression may worsen at these times.
- Expect to reduce dosage gradually when drug is no longer needed to avoid serious adverse reactions.

PATIENT TEACHING

- Instruct patient taking oral solution to use a calibrated measuring device, not a household spoon.
- Inform patient that citalopram's full effects may take up to 4 weeks.
- Advise patient not to self-medicate for allergies, colds, or coughs without consulting prescriber because these preparations can increase the risk of adverse reactions.
- Caution patient not to stop citalopram abruptly because doing so may lead to serious adverse reactions.
- Urge caregivers to monitor patient closely for suicidal tendencies, especially when therapy starts or dosage changes.
- Caution against taking OTC aspirin, NSAIDs, or other remedies (including herbal products, such as St. John's wort) while taking citalopram because they may increase the risk of bleeding.
- Advise patient that drug may cause mild pupillary dilation, which may lead to an episode of acute closure glaucoma. Encourage patient to have an eye exam before starting therapy to see if he is at risk.
- Urge patient to report sudden, severe, or unusual adverse reactions promptly to prescriber. Although uncommon, life-threatening adverse effects may occur.
- Alert patient that use of drug may cause symptoms of sexual dysfunction in both females and males. Tell patient to discuss concerns with prescriber.

cladribine
Mavenclad

Class and Category
Pharmacologic class: Purine antimetabolite
Therapeutic class: Antineoplastic

Indications and Dosages
⁕ *To treat relapsing forms of multiple sclerosis (MS), to include relapsing-remitting disease and active secondary progressive disease, in patients who have had an inadequate response to, or are unable to tolerate, an alternate drug indicated for the treatment of MS*

TABLETS

Adults. 3.5 mg/kg divided into 2 yearly treatment courses (1.75 mg/kg/treatment course with each treatment course further divided into two treatment cycles). First course/first cycle is begun at any time, followed by first course/second cycle administered 23 to 27 days after last dose of first course/first cycle. Second course/first cycle administered at least 43 wk after last dose of first course/second cycle. Second course/second cycle administered 23 to 27 days after last dose of second course/first cycle. Administer each cycle dosage divided over 4 to 5 consecutive days with once-daily dose given as one or two 10-mg tablets. Do not administer more than 20 mg once daily. Cycle dosage based on weight as follows: **For adults weighing 110 kg (242 lb) or above.** 100 mg for cycle one and 100 mg for cycle two.

For adults weighing 100 kg (220 lb) to less than 110 kg (242 lb). 100 mg for cycle one and 90 mg for cycle two.

For adults weighing 90 kg (198 lb) to less than 100 kg (220 lb). 90 mg for cycle one and 80 mg for cycle two.

For adults weighing 80 kg (176 lb) to less than 90 kg (198 lb). 80 mg for cycle one and 70 mg for cycle two.

For adults weighing 70 kg (154 lb) to less than 80 kg (176 lb). 70 mg for cycle one and 70 mg for cycle two.

For adults weighing 60 kg (132 lb) to less than 70 kg (154 lb). 60 mg for cycle one and 60 mg for cycle two.

For adults weighing 50 kg (110 lb) to less than 60 kg (132 lb). 50 mg for cycle one and 50 mg for cycle two.

For adults weighing 40 kg (88 lb) to less than 50 kg (110 lb). 40 mg for cycle one and 40 mg for cycle two.

Drug Administration

P.O.

- Drug is a cytotoxic drug and requires special handling and disposal procedures.
- If tablet is left on a surface, or if a broken or fragmented tablet is released from the blister, the area must be thoroughly washed with water.
- Upon removal from blister pack, tablets should immediately be swallowed whole and taken with water.
- Tablets should not be chewed or crushed.
- Avoid prolonged skin contact with tablets.
- Separate doses of drug from other oral drugs by at least 3 hours during the 4- to 5-day treatment cycles.

Route	Onset	Peak	Duration
P.O.	Unknown	0.5–1.5 hr	Unknown

Half-life: 24 hr

Mechanism of Action

May involve cytotoxic effects on B and T lymphocytes through impairment of DNA synthesis, resulting in depletion of lymphocytes.

Contraindications

Active chronic infections such as hepatitis or tuberculosis, breastfeeding (avoid for 10 days following last dose), HIV infection, hypersensitivity to cladribine or its components, current malignancy, patient of reproductive potential who does not plan to use effective contraception during cladribine therapy and for 6 months after last dose in each treatment course, pregnancy

Interactions

DRUGS

antiviral and antiretroviral drugs such as lamivudine, ribavirin, stavudine, zalcitabine, zidovudine: Possible interference with cladribine effectiveness

hepatotoxic drugs: Increased risk of serious adverse reactions because of additive hematological effects

immunomodulatory, immunosuppressive, myelosuppressive drugs: Increased risk of serious adverse reactions because of additive effects on immune system

interferon-beta: Possibly increased lymphopenia risk

potent BCRP CNT, ENT transporter inhibitors such as cilostazol, curcumin, cyclosporine, dilazep, dipyridamole, eltrombopag, nifedipine, reserpine, ritonavir, sulindac: Possible alteration of bioavailability, intracellular distribution, and renal elimination of cladribine

potent BCRP and P-gp transporter inducers: Possible decreased exposure of cladribine, decreasing effectiveness

Adverse Reactions

CNS: Depression, fever, headache, insomnia, **seizures,** vertigo

CV: Cardiac failure, hypertension

EENT: Diplopia, mucous membrane ulceration, oral herpes, **throat swelling**

GI: Activation of latent hepatitis infections, anorexia, elevated bilirubin and liver enzymes, **fulminant hepatitis,** jaundice, nausea

GU: Pyelonephritis

HEME: Anemia, **decreased platelet count, lymphopenia, neutropenia, pancytopenia, thrombocytopenia**

MS: Arthralgia, back pain

RESP: Bronchitis, upper respiratory infection

SKIN: Alopecia, dermatitis, pruritus, rash

Other: Bacterial, fungal, herpes viral, opportunistic, tuberculosis infections; **hypersensitivity reactions; malignancies**

Childbearing Considerations

PREGNANCY

- A negative pregnancy test must be obtained before drug therapy begins.
- Drug causes fetal harm.

- Drug is contraindicated during pregnancy.
- If pregnancy occurs during treatment, drug is discontinued.

LACTATION

- It is not known if drug is present in breast milk.
- Drug is contraindicated in breastfeeding women.

REPRODUCTION

- Female patients and partners of male patients who are of childbearing age must use effective contraception during cladribine therapy and for 6 months after last dose in each treatment course.
- Instruct female patients of childbearing age to immediately report suspected or confirmed pregnancy to prescriber.
- Women using systemically acting hormonal contraceptives need to add a barrier method during cladribine therapy and for at least 4 weeks after last dose in each treatment course, because it is unknown if drug may reduce effectiveness of hormonal contraceptives.

≡ Nursing Considerations

- Know that cladribine is not recommended for patients with clinically isolated syndrome, because drug is deemed unsafe.

! **WARNING** Be aware that cladribine may increase the risk of malignancy and is contraindicated in patients who currently have a malignancy. Expect patient to be screened for cancer before cladribine therapy begins and follow standard cancer screening guidelines during and after drug therapy. Known that as an antineoplastic drug, the intravenous form of drug is used to treat hairy cell leukemia.

- Ensure that all women of childbearing age have had a negative pregnancy test prior to cladribine therapy, because drug can cause fetal harm.
- Obtain a complete blood count, including lymphocyte count, before cladribine therapy begins. Lymphocytes must be within normal limits before initiating first treatment course and at least 800 cells/microliter before initiating second treatment course. Second treatment course may have to be delayed for up to 6 months to allow for recovery of lymphocytes to

at least 800 cells/microliter. However, if recovery takes longer than 6 months, expect drug to be discontinued.

- Assess patient for the presence of infection prior to starting cladribine therapy. This includes evaluating patient for acute infection (cladribine therapy may have to be delayed until infection is under control), excluding presence of hepatitis B and C and HIV infections (screen for hepatitis B and C before first and second treatment courses), tuberculosis screening (before first and second treatment courses), and varicella zoster virus screening (vaccination for patients who are antibody-negative).
- Expect to obtain a baseline (within 3 months) magnetic resonance imaging prior to first treatment course because of risk of progressive multifocal leukoencephalopathy (PML) and assess alkaline phosphatase, total bilirubin, and serum aminotransferase levels prior to starting cladribine therapy.
- Administer all immunizations, as ordered, according to immunization guidelines prior to starting cladribine therapy. Expect to administer live-attenuated or live vaccines at least 4 to 6 weeks prior to starting drug therapy.
- Be aware that following the administration of two treatment courses, drug should not be administered during the next 2 years because of risk of malignancy.
- Expect to administer antiherpes prophylaxis in patients with lymphocyte counts less than 200 cells/microliter, as ordered.
- Ensure that complete blood counts with differential, including lymphocyte count, are performed as follows: before initiating first course, before initiating second course, 2 to 3 months after starting treatment in each treatment course (if lymphocyte count at month 2 is below 200 cells/microliter, expect monthly monitoring until month 6), and periodically thereafter and when clinically indicated.
- Withhold drug after consulting with prescriber if lymphocyte count is below 200 cells/microliter.
- Monitor patient for signs and symptoms of infection throughout drug therapy, especially if lymphocyte count is below 500 cells/microliter. Know that infections occur in about half of patients, with the most serious being herpes zoster and

pyelonephritis. At first sign of infection, notify prescriber, because drug therapy may have to be delayed or interrupted. Institute infection control measures.

- Monitor patient for liver dysfunction such as abdominal pain, anorexia, dark urine, fatigue, jaundice, unexplained nausea, or vomiting. If present, notify prescriber and expect liver enzymes to be obtained. If elevated, expect drug to be interrupted or discontinued.
- Monitor patient for hypersensitivity reactions such as dermatitis and pruritus. Serious reactions can occur involving diplopia, headache, rash, and throat swelling. Stop cladribine immediately and notify prescriber. Provide supportive emergency care according to protocol, as prescribed.
- Monitor patient for heart failure such as edema, irregular or rapid heartbeat, or shortness of breath, because cladribine may induce heart failure.

! WARNING Monitor patient for signs and symptoms of progressive multifocal leukoencephalopathy (PML), such as changes in memory, orientation, or thinking leading to confusion and personality changes, as well as clumsiness of limbs, progressive weakness on one side of the body, and visual disturbances. Although no reports of PML have occurred with cladribine for treating relapsing forms of MS, it is a possibility. At first sign of PML, notify prescriber, expect cladribine to be withheld, and ensure that appropriate diagnostic evaluation is done. Know that MRI findings may reveal problems before clinical signs or symptoms appear.

- Be aware that if patient requires a blood transfusion, irradiation of cellular blood components is recommended, prior to administration, to decrease risk of transfusion-related graft-versus-host disease. Expect a hematologist to be consulted.

PATIENT TEACHING

- Stress importance of taking cladribine exactly as prescribed. If a dose is missed, tell patient not to double next dose or take extra doses. Instead, the patient should take the missed dose on the following day and extend the number of days in that treatment cycle. If two consecutive doses are missed, treatment cycle is extended by 2 days.
- Instruct patient to take tablets with water and swallow them whole without chewing or crushing them. Inform patient that drug may be taken with or without food.
- Instruct patient that once tablet is removed from the blister, tablet must be swallowed immediately. If tablet is left on a surface or if a broken or fragmented tablet is released from the blister, area must be thoroughly washed with water. Patient must have dry hands when handling tablets and hands must be washed thoroughly afterward. Tell patient to avoid contact with skin.
- Tell patient to separate taking cladribine from all other oral drugs by at least 3 hours during the 4- or 5-day treatment cycles.
- Tell patient to notify prescriber immediately if edema, irregular or rapid heartbeat, or shortness of breath occurs.

! WARNING Tell men and women of reproductive potential to use effective contraception during cladribine therapy and for 6 months after the last dose in each treatment course. Stress importance of informing prescriber immediately if pregnancy is suspected or confirmed, as drug must be discontinued.

- Inform women using systemically acting hormonal contraceptives to add a barrier method during cladribine therapy and for at least 4 weeks after the last dose in each treatment course, because it is unknown if drug may reduce effectiveness of hormonal contraceptives. Also tell women breastfeeding is contraindicated during drug therapy.

clarithromycin

Class and Category

Pharmacologic class: Macrolide
Therapeutic class: Antibiotic

Indications and Dosages

* *To treat pharyngitis and tonsillitis caused by Streptococcus pyogenes*

ORAL SUSPENSION, TABLETS

Adults. 250 mg every 12 hr for 10 days.

Children age 6 months and older. 7.5 mg/kg every 12 hr for 10 days.

✶ *To treat acute maxillary sinusitis caused by* Haemophilus influenzae, Moraxella catarrhalis, *or* Streptococcus pneumoniae

ORAL SUSPENSION, TABLETS

Adults. 500 mg every 12 hr for 14 days.
Children age 6 months and older. 7.5 mg/kg every 12 hr for 10 days.

E.R. TABLETS

Adults. 1,000 mg every 24 hr for 14 days.

✶ *To treat acute exacerbations of chronic bronchitis caused by* H. influenzae, H. parainfluenzae, M. catarrhalis, *or* S. pneumoniae

ORAL SUSPENSION, TABLETS

Adults. 250 mg every 12 hr for 7 to 14 days if caused by *M. catarrhalis* or *S. pneumoniae*, 500 mg every 12 hr for 7 to 14 days if caused by *H. influenzae,* or 500 mg every 12 hr for 7 days if caused by *H. parainfluenzae.*

E.R. TABLETS

Adults. 1,000 mg every 24 hr for 7 days.

✶ *To treat uncomplicated skin and soft-tissue infections caused by* Staphylococcus aureus *or* S. pyogenes

ORAL SUSPENSION, TABLETS

Adults. 250 mg every 12 hr for 7 to 14 days.
Children 6 months and older. 7.5 mg/kg every 12 hr for 10 days.

✶ *To treat community-acquired pneumonia caused by* Chlamydia pneumoniae, Mycoplasma pneumoniae, *or* S. pneumoniae

ORAL SUSPENSION, TABLETS

Adults. 250 mg every 12 hr for 7 to 14 days.
Children 6 months and older. 7.5 mg/kg every 12 hr for 10 days.

✶ *To treat community-acquired pneumonia caused by* H. influenzae

ORAL SUSPENSION, TABLETS

Adults. 250 mg every 12 hr for 7 days.

E.R. TABLETS

Adults. 1,000 mg every 24 hr for 7 days.

✶ *To treat community-acquired pneumonia caused by* H. parainfluenzae *or* M. catarrhalis

E.R. TABLETS

Adults. 1,000 mg every 24 hr for 7 days.

✶ *To treat acute otitis media caused by* H. influenzae, M. catarrhalis, *or* S. pneumoniae

ORAL SUSPENSION, TABLETS

Children 6 months and older. 7.5 mg/kg every 12 hr for 10 days.

✶ *To reduce the risk of active duodenal ulcer recurrence caused by* Helicobacter pylori

ORAL SUSPENSION, TABLETS

Adults. 500 mg every 8 hr for 14 days with omeprazole 40 mg daily in the morning for 14 days. Then, omeprazole continued at 20 mg daily in the morning days 15 through 28. Or, 500 mg every 12 hr for 14 days with lansoprazole 30 mg and amoxicillin 1 g every 12 hr for 10 to 14 days. Alternatively, 500 mg every 12 hr with omeprazole 20 mg and amoxicillin 1 g every 12 hr for 10 days.

✶ *To prevent or treat* Mycobacterium avium complex in patients with advanced HIV infection

ORAL SUSPENSION, TABLETS

Adults. 500 mg every 12 hr.
Children. 7.5 mg/kg every 12 hr.

±**DOSAGE ADJUSTMENT** For patient with severe renal impairment (creatinine clearance less than 30 ml/min), dosage reduced by 50%. For patient with moderate renal impairment (creatinine clearance 30 to 60 ml/min) who is also taking atazanavir or ritonavir, dosage reduced by 50%. For patient with severe renal impairment (creatinine clearance less than 30 ml/min) who is also taking atazanavir or ritonavir, dosage reduced by 75%.

Drug Administration

P.O.

- To reconstitute granules to make oral suspension, mix 27 ml of water to make 50 ml of suspension and 55 ml to make 100 ml of suspension. Add half the water to the bottle and shake vigorously, then add remainder of water and shake again.
- Shake oral suspension well before each use and use a calibrated device to measure dose.
- Oral suspension does not have to be taken with food.
- Store oral suspension at room temperature; do not refrigerate.
- Discard after 14 days.
- Administer E.R. tablets with food. E.R. tablets should not be chewed or crushed but must be swallowed whole.
- Immediate-release tablets can be taken with or without food.

Route	Onset	Peak	Duration
P.O.	Unknown	2–3 hr	Unknown
P.O./E.R.	Unknown	5–8 hr	Unknown

Half-life: 3–7 hr

Mechanism of Action

Inhibits RNA-dependent protein synthesis in many types of aerobic, anaerobic, gram-negative, and gram-positive bacteria. By binding with the 50S ribosomal subunit of the bacterial 70S ribosome, clarithromycin causes bacterial cells to die.

Contraindications

Concurrent therapy with cisapride, colchicine (in patients with renal or hepatic impairment), dihydroergotamine, ergotamine, lomitapide, lovastatin, pimozide, or simvastatin; history of cholestatic jaundice or hepatic dysfunction; hypersensitivity to clarithromycin, erythromycin, or any macrolide antibiotic or their components

Interactions

DRUGS

alfentanil, bromocriptine, cilostazol, cyclosporine, methylprednisolone, phenobarbital, St. John's wort, tacrolimus, vinblastine: Possibly increased risk of adverse reactions

alprazolam, midazolam (oral), triazolam: Possibly increased effects of these triazolobenzodiazepines, including increased and/or prolonged sedation

antiarrhythmics such as amiodarone, disopyramide, dofetilide, procainamide, quinidine, sotalol: Increased risk of prolonged QT interval, torsades de pointes, or other life-threatening arrhythmias

atazanavir, ritonavir: Increased clarithromycin levels

calcium channel blockers; Increased risk of acute kidney dysfunction and hypotension, especially in patients 65 years or older

carbamazepine, other drugs metabolized by cytochrome P450 enzyme system, tolterodine: Increased blood levels of these drugs

cisapride, pimozide: Increased risk of cardiac arrhythmias

colchicine: Increased risk of colchicine toxicity

colchicine: Increased risk of life-threatening colchicine toxicity

digoxin: Increased serum digoxin level, increasing risk of toxicity

dihydroergotamine, ergotamine: Risk of acute ergot toxicity

disopyramide: Hypoglycemia, increased risk of torsades de pointes

efavirenz, nevirapine, rifampicin, rifabutin, rifapentine: Decreased concentration of clarithromycin with decreased effectiveness

hexobarbital, phenytoin, valproate: Increased risk of adverse reactions

insulin, oral hypoglycemics such as nateglinide, pioglitazone, repaglinide, rosiglitazone: Increased risk of severe hypoglycemia

itraconazole: Increased plasma concentration of clarithromycin and itraconazole with increased risk of adverse reactions that may become prolonged

lomitapide: Markedly increased transaminases levels

maraviroc: Possibly increased maraviroc exposure, resulting in increased risk of adverse reactions

nifedipine: Potential for hypotension and peripheral edema

omeprazole: Increased clarithromycin concentrations in gastric tissue and mucus

oral anticoagulants: Potentiated anticoagulant effects

quetiapine: Increased quetiapine exposure and related toxicity

rifabutin: Decreased clarithromycin serum levels, increased rifabutin serum levels, increased risk of uveitis

sildenafil, tadalafil, vardenafil: Possibly increased exposure of these phosphodiesterase inhibitors

statins such as atorvastatin, lovastatin, pravastatin, simvastatin: Increased risk of rhabdomyolysis

theophylline: Increased blood theophylline level

tolterodine: Significant increase in tolterodine level in patients with a deficiency in CYP2D6 activity

verapamil: Increased risk of bradyarrhythmias, hypotension, and lactic acidosis

zidovudine: Decreased blood zidovudine level

Adverse Reactions

CNS: Anxiety, confusion, disorientation, dizziness, fatigue, hallucinations, headache, insomnia, mania, nightmares, **seizures,** somnolence, tremor, vertigo

CV: Prolonged QT interval, ventricular arrhythmias

EENT: Altered smell, altered taste, glossitis, hearing loss, oral moniliasis, stomatitis, tinnitus, tongue or tooth discoloration

ENDO: Hypoglycemia
GI: Abdominal pain, anorexia, **cholestatic hepatitis**, diarrhea, elevated liver enzymes, **hepatic dysfunction, hepatitis, hepatotoxicity**, indigestion, jaundice, nausea, **pancreatitis, pseudomembranous colitis**, vomiting
GU: Elevated BUN level
HEME: Increased prothrombin time, leukopenia, neutropenia, thrombocytopenia
MS: Rhabdomyolysis
SKIN: Acute generalized exanthematous pustulosis, Henoch–Schönlein purpura, pruritus, rash, **Stevens–Johnson syndrome, toxic epidermal necrolysis**, urticaria
Other: Anaphylaxis, angioedema, drug reaction with eosinophilia and systemic symptoms (DRESS), new or worsening myasthenia gravis symptoms, superinfection

Childbearing Considerations
PREGNANCY
- It is not known if drug can cause fetal harm.
- Drug should be used with caution during pregnancy only if benefit to mother outweighs potential risk to fetus and if no alternative therapy is available.

LACTATION
- Drug is present in breast milk.
- Patient should check with prescriber before breastfeeding.

Nursing Considerations
- Expect to obtain a specimen for culture and sensitivity tests before giving first dose.
- Know that clarithromycin therapy should be avoided in patients at risk for QT prolongation such as uncorrected hypokalemia or hypomagnesemia or significant bradycardia, and in patients receiving Class IA or Class III antiarrhythmics. Elderly patients are more susceptible to clarithromycin's effect on the QT interval, as well.

! **WARNING** Be aware that use of clarithromycin in patients with coronary artery disease is not recommended because of an increased risk of heart problems or death that may occur even years after exposure to drug.

- Use clarithromycin cautiously in patients with renal impairment. Be aware that patients with severe renal impairment may need decreased dosage.

- Monitor patient closely for acute hypersensitivity reactions such as anaphylaxis and serious skin disorders. If present, expect clarithromycin therapy to be discontinued immediately and appropriate emergency treatment initiated.
- Monitor patient for signs and symptoms of liver dysfunction, especially hepatitis (anorexia, dark urine, jaundice, pruritus, or tender abdomen). Notify prescriber immediately if present, and expect clarithromycin to be discontinued.
- Monitor patients with diabetes who are also receiving insulin or oral hypoglycemics closely for hypoglycemia, which could be severe.
- Be watchful for an elevated INR and prothrombin time in patients who are also taking warfarin, as serious bleeding may occur.
- Assess patient's bowel pattern daily; severe diarrhea may indicate pseudomembranous colitis caused by *Clostridium difficile*. If diarrhea occurs, notify prescriber and expect to withhold clarithromycin and treat with fluids, electrolytes, protein, and an antibiotic effective against *C. difficile*.

PATIENT TEACHING
- Emphasize importance of taking the full course of clarithromycin exactly as prescribed, even after feeling better, because skipped doses or not completing the full course prescribed may hinder drug from eliminating the bacterial infection and increases risk of bacterial resistance.
- Caution patient not to chew or crush E.R. tablets but to swallow them whole.
- Advise patient to take drug with food if he takes E.R. tablets or has GI distress.
- Instruct patient taking suspension form not to refrigerate it. Tell patient to shake suspension before each use and to use a calibrated device to measure dosage, not a household spoon. Suspension should be discarded after 14 days.
- Tell patient to report itching, rash, severe nausea, or any other persistent, severe, or unusual reaction to prescriber immediately.
- Instruct patient not to take OTC or prescription drugs without consulting prescriber of clarithromycin.
- Urge patient to report bloody, watery stools to prescriber immediately, even if they occur 2 months or more after therapy has ended.

C

- Advise patient to report signs and symptoms of liver dysfunction immediately to prescriber.
- Instruct patient not to perform hazardous activities such as driving until effects on the nervous system such as confusion and dizziness are known.
- Instruct patient with diabetes who is also taking insulin or an oral hypoglycemic agent to monitor his blood glucose level closely.

! **WARNING** Advise patient who has coronary artery disease to continue lifestyle modifications and medications for the heart condition, because clarithromycin may be associated with increased risk for worsening heart problems or mortality years after the end of clarithromycin therapy. Review signs and symptoms of heart disease with all patients, because some patients may not know coronary artery disease is present. Emphasize importance of reporting such signs and symptoms to prescriber even if it is years after exposure to clarithromycin.

- Advise women of childbearing age to use contraception throughout clarithromycin therapy, because drug may cause fetal harm.

clindamycin hydrochloride

Cleocin, Dalacin C (CAN)

clindamycin palmitate hydrochloride

Cleocin Pediatric, Dalacin C Flavored Granules (CAN)

clindamycin phosphate

Cleocin, Clindesse 2%, Dalacin C Phosphate (CAN), Evoclin, Xaciato

Class and Category

Pharmacologic class: Lincosamide
Therapeutic class: Antibiotic

Indications and Dosages

* *To treat serious respiratory tract infections caused by anaerobes such as occur with anaerobic pneumonitis, empyema, and lung abscess and those caused by pneumococci, staphylococci, and streptococci; serious skin and soft-tissue infections caused by anaerobes, staphylococci, and streptococci; septicemia caused by anaerobes; intra-abdominal infections caused by anaerobes such as occur with intra-abdominal abscess and peritonitis; infections of the female pelvis and genital tract caused by anaerobes such as occur with endometritis, nongonococcal tubo-ovarian abscess, pelvic cellulitis, and postsurgical vaginal cuff infection*

CAPSULES, ORAL SOLUTION

Adults and adolescents. For serious infections, 150 to 300 mg every 6 hr; for severe infections, 300 to 450 mg every 6 hr. **Children.** For serious infections, 8 to 16 mg/kg daily in equally divided doses three times daily or four times daily; for severe infections, 16 to 20 mg/kg/day in equally divided doses three times daily or four times daily.

I.V. INFUSION, I.M. INJECTION

Adults and adolescents age 16 and over. For serious infections, 600 to 1,200 mg daily in equally divided doses twice daily to four times daily; for severe infections, 1,200 to 2,700 mg daily in equally divided doses twice daily to four times daily; for life-threatening infections, up to 4,800 mg daily in equally divided doses twice daily to four times daily. **Children ages 1 month to 16 years.** 20 to 40 mg/kg daily in equally divided doses three times daily or four times daily, depending on severity of infection. **Neonates less than age 1 month.** 15 to 20 mg/kg daily in equally divided doses three times daily or four times daily, depending on severity of infection. **Neonates with postmenstrual age (PMA) greater than or equal to 32 but less than or equal to 40.** 7 mg/kg every 8 hr. **Neonates with a PMA less than 31.** 5 mg/kg every 8 hr.

* *To treat bone and joint infections caused by Staphylococcus aureus; as adjunct therapy in chronic bone and joint infections*

I.V. INFUSION, I.M. INJECTION

Adults and adolescents age 16 and over. *For serious infections:* 600 to 1,200 mg daily in equally divided doses twice daily to four times daily. *For severe infections:* 1,200 to 2,700 mg daily in equally divided doses twice daily to four times daily. *For life-threatening infections:* 4,800 mg daily in equally divided doses twice daily to four times daily.

✴ *To treat bacterial vaginosis caused by anaerobes,* Corynebacterium, Gardnerella, *or* Haemophilus

VAGINAL CREAM 2%

Nonpregnant females. 100 mg (1 applicatorful) into vagina daily, preferably at bedtime, for 3 to 7 consecutive days.

Pregnant females in second or third trimester. 100 mg (1 applicatorful) into vagina daily, preferably at bedtime, for 7 consecutive days.

VAGINAL CREAM (CLINDESSE 2%)

Nonpregnant females. 5 g (1 applicatorful) into vagina as a single dose.

VAGINAL GEL 2% (XACIATO)

Adult women and adolescent girls. 5 g (1 applicatorful) into vagina as a single dose.

✴ *To treat acne vulgaris*

FOAM (EVOCLIN)

Adults and adolescents. Apply to affected area once daily, using enough to cover the entire affected area(s).

▤ Drug Administration

P.O.

- Capsules should be swallowed whole and not chewed, crushed, or opened. Give with 8 ounces of water.
- Prepare oral solution 100-ml bottles by adding a large portion but not all of 75 ml of water. Shake vigorously and then add remainder of water for a total of 75 mg/5 ml and shake until the solution is uniform.
- Store at room temperature. Do not refrigerate reconstituted solution, as it may thicken and be difficult to pour.
- Use a calibrated measuring device when measuring oral solution dosage and shake container before measuring dose.
- Discard solution after 2 weeks.

I.V.

- Ensure prescriber is aware drug solution contains benzyl alcohol, which can cause Gasping Syndrome in neonates and premature infants, before administering drug solution to these patients. While the therapeutic dose delivers substantially

less than those reported to cause Gasping Syndrome in other products, the minimum amount of benzyl alcohol, which may cause toxicity, is not known. In addition, total daily benzyl alcohol exposure may be increased with other drugs. Premature and low birth weight infants may be more likely to develop toxicity.

- Solutions used for diluting drug include 0.9% Sodium Chloride Injection, 5% Dextrose Injection, or Lactated Ringer's Injection (see manufacturer instructions for complete list).
- The concentration of clindamycin in diluent for infusion should not exceed 18 mg/ml. Infusion rate should not exceed 30 mg/min.
- For intermittent infusion, dilute 300-mg dose with 50 ml and infuse over 10 minutes; 600-mg dose diluted with 50 ml and infused over 20 min; 900-mg dose diluted with 50 to 100 ml and infused over 30 min; and 1,200-mg dose diluted in 100 ml and infused over 40 min.
- Administration of more than 1,200 mg in a single 1-hour infusion is not recommended.
- Alternatively, a rapid I.V. infusion given over 30 minutes for first dose followed by a continuous infusion rate that varies between 0.75 mg/min and 1.25 mg/min, depending on the clindamycin level to be maintained, can be administered, if prescribed.
- Prepare drug to be used in the ADD-Vantage system by reconstituting with 50 ml of 0.9% Sodium Chloride Injection or 5% Dextrose Injection for 300- or 600-mg dose and 100 ml of same solutions for 900-mg dose in the ADD-Vantage diluent container.
- Frozen solutions should be thawed at room temperature before use and not refrozen.
- For premixed drug solution in a plastic container, check for minute leaks prior to use by squeezing bag firmly. Do not add supplementary drugs to solution. Do not use unless solution is clear and seal is intact.
- Do not use plastic containers in series connections which could result in air embolism.
- *Incompatibilities:* allopurinol (Y-site), aminophylline, azithromycin (Y-site), caspofungin acetate (Y-site), ceftriaxone sodium, ciprofloxacin, doxapram hydrochloride (Y-site), filgrastim (Y-site), fluconazole (Y-site), gentamicin sulfate with cefazolin sodium, idarubicin hydrochloride

(Y-site), oritavancin diphosphate (Y-site), tramadol hydrochloride

I.M.

- Single injections greater than 600 mg are not recommended.
- Administer undiluted.

TOPICAL FOAM

- Wash the affected area with mild soap, let it dry fully, and then apply foam to entire affected area.

VAGINAL CREAM

- Follow manufacturer's instructions for administration.

Route	Onset	Peak	Duration
P.O.	Unknown	45–60 min	Unknown
I.V.	Immediate	Immediate	Unknown
I.M.	Unknown	1–3 hr	Unknown
Topical	Unknown	Unknown	Unknown

Half-life: 2–3 hr

Mechanism of Action

Inhibits protein synthesis in susceptible bacteria by binding to the 50S subunits of bacterial ribosomes and preventing peptide bond formation, which causes bacterial cells to die.

Incompatibilities

To prevent physical incompatibility, don't administer with aminophylline, ampicillin, barbiturates, calcium gluconate, magnesium sulfate, or phenytoin.

Contraindications

Hypersensitivity to clindamycin or any of its components

Interactions

DRUGS

CYP3A4 and CYP3A5 inducers: Possibly decreased plasma concentrations of clindamycin decreasing its effectiveness
CYP3A4 and CYP3A5 inhibitors: Possibly increase plasma concentrations of clindamycin with potential for adverse reactions
erythromycin: Possibly blocked access of clindamycin to its site of action
kaolin-pectin antidiarrheals: Decreased absorption of oral clindamycin
neuromuscular blockers: Increased neuromuscular blockade

Adverse Reactions

CNS: Fatigue, headache
CV: Hypotension, thrombophlebitis (after I.V. injection)
EENT: Eye pain (topical), glossitis, metallic or unpleasant taste (with high I.V. doses), stomatitis
GI: Abdominal pain, acute kidney injury, *Clostridioides difficile*–associated diarrhea, diarrhea, elevated liver enzymes, esophagitis, jaundice, nausea, **pseudomembranous colitis,** vomiting
GU: Cervicitis, renal dysfunction, vaginitis, and vulvar irritation (with vaginal form)
HEME: Agranulocytosis, eosinophilia, **leukopenia, neutropenia, thrombocytopenic purpura**
MS: Polyarthritis
SKIN: Acute generalized exanthematous pustulosis, contact dermatitis (topical), **erythema multiforme, exfoliative dermatitis,** irritation, maculopapular rash, pruritus, rash, **Stevens–Johnson syndrome, toxic epidermal necrolysis,** urticaria
Other: Anaphylaxis; angioedema; drug reaction with eosinophilia and systemic symptoms (DRESS); induration, pain, or sterile abscess after injection; superinfection

Childbearing Considerations

PREGNANCY

- It is not known if drug can cause fetal harm.
- Drug should be used with caution during pregnancy, especially during the first trimester, only if benefit to mother outweighs potential risk to fetus.

LACTATION

- Drug is present in breast milk.
- Patient should check with prescriber before breastfeeding.
- An alternative drug should be substituted if breastfeeding occurs. If this is not possible, infant should be monitored for blood in the stool, diarrhea, and candidiasis (thrush, diaper rash).

Nursing Considerations

- Expect to obtain a specimen for culture and sensitivity testing before giving first dose.
- Use clindamycin cautiously in patients who have a history of asthma, GI disease, or significant allergies; in those with hepatic or renal dysfunction; and in atopic or elderly patients. Infants and children should

be monitored closely for organ system dysfunction.

- Check I.V. site often for phlebitis and irritation.
- Be aware that if dermatitis or irritation develops after use of topical foam, notify prescriber, as drug will have to be discontinued.
- Monitor results of CBC, liver enzymes, and platelet counts during prolonged therapy.
- Observe patient for signs and symptoms of superinfection, such as sore mouth and vaginal itching, which may occur 2 to 9 days after therapy begins.
- Assess patient's skin regularly for abnormalities because clindamycin may cause severe skin reactions. If present, notify prescriber, expect drug to be discontinued, and be prepared to administer supportive treatment, as prescribed.
- Assess patient's bowel pattern daily; severe diarrhea may indicate pseudomembranous colitis caused by *C. difficile*. If diarrhea occurs, notify prescriber and expect to withhold clindamycin and treat with fluids, electrolytes, protein, and an antibiotic effective against *C. difficile*.

PATIENT TEACHING

- Tell patient to complete the prescribed course of therapy, even if he feels better before it's finished.
- Instruct patient to take clindamycin capsule with at least 8 ounces of water to prevent esophageal irritation.
- Advise patient to take oral drug with food, if needed, to reduce GI distress.
- Tell patient not to refrigerate reconstituted oral solution because it may become thick and difficult to pour. Patient should discard unused drug after 14 days. Advise patient to shake container before each use and to use a calibrated device to measure dose.
- Tell patient using topical foam to wash affected area with mild soap, let it dry fully, and then apply foam to entire area. Caution against dispensing foam directly onto hands or face because foam will melt when it contacts warm skin. Instead, patient should dispense amount to be used into the cap or onto a cool surface. Tell patient to pick up a small amount with fingertips and gently massage into affected area until foam disappears. If foam feels warm or looks

runny, tell patient to run the can under cold water before dispensing.

- Advise patient using topical foam to avoid contact with eyes, lips, mouth, other mucous membranes or areas of broken skin. If contact occurs, tell patient to rinse area thoroughly with water.
- Instruct patient how to administer vaginal cream. Warn patient not to rely on latex or rubber condoms and diaphragms for 72 hours after vaginal treatment because mineral oil in vaginal cream may weaken these items.
- Explain that having sexual intercourse after using vaginal cream can increase irritation.
- Inform patient that I.M. injection may be painful.
- Tell patient to immediately report an inflamed mouth or vagina, and lesions or rash. Also tell patient to immediately report any skin abnormalities such as rash, pruritus, or urticaria.
- Urge patient to report bloody, watery stools to prescriber immediately, even up to 2 months after drug therapy has ended.
- Advise mothers not to breastfeed because drug does appear in breast milk and cause adverse gastrointestinal effects for infant.

clobazam
Onfi, Sympazan

Class and Category

Pharmacologic class: Benzodiazepine
Therapeutic class: Anticonvulsant
Controlled substance schedule: IV

Indications and Dosages

* *Adjunct treatment of seizures associated with Lennox–Gastaut syndrome*

ORAL DISSOLVING FILM STRIPS, ORAL SUSPENSION, TABLETS

Adults and children age 2 and over weighing more than 30 kg (66 lb). *Initial:* 5 mg twice daily increased to 10 mg twice daily on day 7 and further increased to 20 mg twice daily on day 14. *Maximum:* 40 mg daily. **Adults and children age 2 and over weighing less than or equal to 30 kg (66 lb).** *Initial:* 5 mg once daily increased to 5 mg twice daily on day 7 and further increased to 10 mg twice daily on day 14. *Maximum:* 20 mg daily.

±**DOSAGE ADJUSTMENT** For elderly patients and patients who are CYP2C19 poor metabolizers or those with hepatic dysfunction, initial dose begun at 5 mg once daily regardless of weight and then titrated according to weight, but only to half the dose normally given for weight category. If needed, an additional titration to the maximum dose for the patient's weight may be started on day 21.

Drug Administration

P.O.

- Tablet may be given as a whole tablet or crushed and mixed in applesauce.
- Shake oral suspension container well before every dose.
- Use only the oral dosing syringe provided with the product to measure dosage. Firmly insert adapter into the neck of the bottle before the first use and keep it there. To withdraw the dose, pull back on dosing syringe to dosage amount, insert the dosing syringe into the adapter, invert bottle, slowly push the air from the syringe into the bottle and then slowly pull back the plunger to the prescribed dose. Slowly squirt the suspension into the corner of patient's mouth. Rinse syringe well with warm water.
- Discard oral suspension after 90 days.
- Place dissolving film strip form on top of patient's tongue and allow it to dissolve. Patient should refrain from chewing, spitting, or talking until it is dissolved. Although it can be taken with or without food, it should not be taken with liquids. If more than one film strip is needed, wait until the first film strip is dissolved before placing the second film strip on the tongue.
- Do not stop drug abruptly. Expect to decrease total daily dose by 5 to 10 mg/day on a weekly basis until discontinued, as ordered.

Route	Onset	Peak	Duration
P.O.	Rapid	0.5–4 hr	Unknown

Half-life: 36–82 hr

Mechanism of Action

May possibly involve potentiation of GABAergic neurotransmission, which causes binding at the benzodiazepine site of the GABA$_A$ receptor to stop seizure activity.

Contraindications

Hypersensitivity to clobazam or its components

Interactions

DRUGS

benzodiazepines, opioids: Increased risk of significant respiratory depression
cannabidiol: Increased risk of clobazam-related adverse reactions
CNS depressants, opioids, other benzodiazepines, sedating antihistamines, tricyclic antidepressants: Increased risk of significant change in level of mental status leading to coma, respiratory depression, sedation, and somnolence
fluconazole, fluvoxamine, ticlopidine and other strong inhibitors of CYP2C19 and omeprazole, a moderate inhibitor of CYP2C19 drugs: Increased action of clobazam and adverse effects
CYP2D6 drugs: Possibly altered metabolism of these drugs
midazolam: Decreased effect of midazolam
opioids: Increased risk of significant respiratory depression
oral contraceptives: Possible diminished effectiveness of oral contraceptive

ACTIVITIES

alcohol use: Additive CNS effect including severe respiratory depression and significant sedation and somnolence; increased effect of clobazam

Adverse Reactions

CNS: Aggression, agitation, anxiety, apathy, ataxia, confusion, depression, delirium, delusion, fatigue, hallucination, insomnia, irritability, lethargy, psychomotor hyperactivity, pyrexia, sedation, somnolence, **suicidal ideation**
EENT: Blurred vision, diplopia, drooling
GI: Abdominal distention, change in appetite, constipation, dysphagia, elevated liver enzymes, vomiting
GU: UTI
HEME: Anemia, eosinophilia, **leukopenia, thrombocytopenia**
MS: Dysarthria, muscle spasms
RESP: Bronchitis, cough, pneumonia, **respiratory depression**, upper respiratory infection
SKIN: Rash, **Stevens–Johnson syndrome, toxic epidermal necrolysis**, urticaria

Other: Physical and psychological dependence

Childbearing Considerations
PREGNANCY
- Pregnancy exposure registry: 1-888-233-2334 or http://www.aedpregnancyregistry.org/.
- Drug can cause fetal harm if administered during pregnancy, especially late in pregnancy possibly causing neonatal abstinence syndrome and withdrawal that can occur within hours to weeks after birth and persist for hours to months.
- Drug should be used with caution during pregnancy, especially in third trimester, only if benefit to mother outweighs potential risk to fetus.

LABOR & DELIVERY
- Administration of benzodiazepines such as clobazam immediately prior to or during childbirth can cause floppy infant syndrome (difficulty feeding, hypothermia, hypotonia, respiratory depression), which can last up to 14 days.
- Drug is not recommended during labor and delivery.

LACTATION
- Drug is present in breast milk.
- Patient should check with prescriber before breastfeeding.
- If breastfeeding takes place, advise mother to monitor infant for drowsiness and poor sucking.

Nursing Considerations
- Assess patient before therapy is begun and throughout therapy for patient's risk for abuse, misuse, and addiction such as physical and psychological dependence (strong desire or need to increase dose to maintain drug effects), especially in patients with a history of substance abuse. Alert prescriber, if present.

! **WARNING** Be aware that benzodiazepine therapy like clobazam should only be used concomitantly with opioids in patients for whom other treatment options are inadequate. If prescribed together, expect dosing and duration of the opioid to be limited. Monitor patient closely for signs and symptoms of decrease in consciousness, including coma, profound sedation, and significant respiratory depression. Notify prescriber immediately and provide emergency supportive care, as death may occur.

- Monitor patient closely for skin reactions, especially during the first 8 weeks of therapy or when reintroducing clobazam therapy. If the patient develops a rash, notify prescriber immediately and expect drug to be discontinued, as serious dermatological adverse reactions have occurred with clobazam therapy.
- Monitor patient for suicidal tendencies, particularly when therapy starts and dosage changes.

PATIENT TEACHING
- Advise patient or parents that clobazam prescribed as a tablet may be given as a whole tablet or crushed and mixed in applesauce.
- Instruct patient prescribed oral suspension form to shake container well before every administration. The oral dosing syringe provided with the product should be the only device used to measure dosage. Tell patient to firmly insert adapter into the neck of the bottle before the first use and keep it there. To withdraw the dose, she should pull back on dosing syringe to dosage amount that will be withdrawn from bottle, insert the dosing syringe into the adapter, invert bottle, slowly push the air from the syringe into the bottle and then slowly pull back the plunger to the prescribed dose. After removing the syringe from the bottle adapter, the patient should be told to slowly squirt the suspension into the corner of her mouth. Then she should replace the cap over the adapter until next dose is due and rinse syringe well with warm water.
- Tell patient prescribed the oral dissolving film strip form to place the film on top of the tongue and allow it to dissolve. As the film dissolves, saliva should be swallowed in a normal manner, but tell patient to refrain from chewing, spitting, or talking. Although it can be taken with or without food, it should not be taken with liquids. Remind patient that only one film strip should be taken at a time. If more than one film strip is needed, patient should wait until the first film strip is dissolved before placing the second film strip on the tongue.

- Tell patient not to take more drug or more often, or for a longer time than prescribed. Warn her that physical and psychological dependence can occur and teach her to recognize the signs. Stress importance of not stopping drug abruptly, as withdrawal may occur. Warn her that protracted withdrawal has occurred with symptoms lasting weeks to more than a year.

! **WARNING** Warn patient not to consume alcohol or take an opioid during clobazam therapy without prescriber knowledge, as severe respiratory depression can occur and may lead to death.

! **WARNING** Inform patient about potentially fatal additive effects of combining clobazam with an opioid. Instruct patient to inform all prescribers of clobazam use, especially if an opioid pain medication may be prescribed.

- Warn patient to stop taking drug at the first sign of a rash and to notify prescriber immediately.
- Instruct patient to avoid performing hazardous activities such as driving until the effects of clobazam are known.
- Tell patient not to stop taking clobazam abruptly, as withdrawal symptoms may occur.
- Urge family or caregiver to watch patient closely for suicidal tendencies, especially when therapy starts or dosage changes.
- Inform female patient of childbearing age to discuss clobazam therapy with her prescriber because drug could interfere with the effectiveness of oral contraceptives. Additional nonhormonal forms of contraception should be used during clobazam therapy if pregnancy is not desired.
- Inform women of childbearing age to notify prescriber of pregnancy, as drug may possibly harm the fetus.
- Advise mothers not to breastfeed while taking clobazam, because the drug is found in breast milk. If breastfeeding does occur, tell mothers to monitor the infant for poor sucking and possible sedation. If present, breastfeeding should be discontinued.

clomipramine hydrochloride
Anafranil

≣ Class and Category
Pharmacologic class: Tricyclic antidepressant
Therapeutic class: Antiobsessional agent

≣ Indications and Dosages
✳ *To treat obsessive–compulsive disorder*
CAPSULES
Adults. *Initial:* 25 mg daily. Gradually increased to 100 mg daily in divided doses over 2 wk, then up to 250 mg daily in divided doses over next few weeks, as needed.
Children age 10 and over. *Initial:* 25 mg daily. Gradually increased to the lesser of 3 mg/kg daily or 100 mg daily in divided doses over 2 wk, then up to 3 mg/kg daily or 200 mg daily, whichever is less.

≣ Drug Administration
P.O.
- Capsules should be swallowed whole and not chewed, crushed, or opened.
- Administer with meals.
- After titration is done, total daily dose may be given at bedtime.
- Drug should not be stopped abruptly.

Route	Onset	Peak	Duration
P.O.	1–2 wk	2–6 wk	1–2 days

Half-life: 19–37 hr

≣ Mechanism of Action
May inhibit neuronal reuptake of norepinephrine and serotonin, which may be a factor in normalizing neurotransmission in obsessive–compulsive behavior.

≣ Contraindications
Acute recovery period after MI, hypersensitivity to clomipramine or its components, linezolid or methylene blue (I.V.) administration, use of an MAO inhibitor within 14 days

≣ Interactions
DRUGS
anticholinergics, sympathomimetics: Altered blood levels possibly requiring dosage adjustment of clomipramine
barbiturates, phenytoin: Possibly decreased level and effects of clomipramine; additive

CNS depression; possibly increased barbiturate effect

cimetidine, flecainide, haloperidol, H2-receptor antagonists, methylphenidate, other antidepressants, phenothiazines, propafenone, quinidine, selective serotonin reuptake inhibitors: Possibly increased blood level and adverse effects of clomipramine; possibly altered plasma concentrations of these drugs

clonidine: Antagonized antihypertensive effect of clonidine, possibly causing increased blood pressure and risk of hypertensive crisis

CNS depressants: Increased CNS depression

digoxin, warfarin: Possibly increased blood levels of these drugs and adverse reactions

guanethidine: Antagonized antihypertensive effect of guanethidine

MAO inhibitors: Increased risk of coma, seizures, or death

ACTIVITIES

alcohol use: Increased CNS depression

Adverse Reactions

CNS: Anxiety, confusion, depersonalization, depression, dizziness, drowsiness, emotional lability, fatigue, headache, insomnia, panic reaction, paresthesia, **serotonin syndrome**, somnolence, **suicidal ideation (children and teens)**, syncope, tremor, unusual dreams, yawning

CV: Orthostatic hypotension, palpitations, tachycardia

EENT: Acute-angle glaucoma, blurred vision, dry mouth, epistaxis, pharyngitis, rhinitis, sinusitis, unpleasant taste

ENDO: Syndrome of inappropriate antidiuretic hormone secretion (SIADH)

GI: Abdominal pain, anorexia, constipation, diarrhea, flatulence, increased appetite, indigestion, nausea, vomiting

GU: Dysmenorrhea, ejaculation failure, impotence, urinary hesitancy, urine retention

RESP: **Bronchospasm**

SKIN: Abnormal skin odor, acne, dermatitis, dry skin, photosensitivity, rash, urticaria

Other: Drug reaction with eosinophilia and systemic symptoms (DRESS), hyponatremia, weight gain

Childbearing Considerations

PREGNANCY

- Drug may cause fetal harm if administered up to time of delivery, possibly causing withdrawal symptoms in neonate after birth.

- Use with caution during pregnancy only if benefit to mother outweighs potential risk to fetus.

LACTATION

- Drug is present in breast milk.
- A decision should be made to discontinue breastfeeding or the drug to avoid potential serious adverse reactions in the breastfed infant.

REPRODUCTION

- Male patients may experience sexual dysfunction such as ejaculatory failure and impotence during drug therapy.

Nursing Considerations

! **WARNING** Don't give drug within 14 days of an MAO inhibitor to avoid possible coma, seizures, or possibly death.

! **WARNING** Monitor patient closely for evidence of suicidal ideation; clomipramine increases the risk.

- Monitor patient for hyponatremia such as confusion, difficulty concentrating, headache, unsteadiness, and weakness. More severe reactions may present as coma, hallucinations, seizures, and syncope which can lead to respiratory arrest and death if left untreated. Hyponatremia occurs as a result of SIADH that may be an adverse reaction to clomipramine. Patients at greater risk are the elderly and patients taking diuretics or who are experiencing volume depletion. Notify prescriber immediately if hyponatremia occurs, expect appropriate medical treatment to raise the sodium level, and anticipate that drug will be discontinued.

! **WARNING** Monitor patient closely for evidence of serotonin syndrome, such as agitation, coma, diarrhea, hallucinations, hyperreflexia, hyperthermia, incoordination, labile blood pressure, nausea, tachycardia, or vomiting. Notify prescriber at once because serotonin syndrome may be life-threatening. Be prepared to discontinue drug and provide supportive care.

PATIENT TEACHING

- Instruct patient to swallow capsules whole and not to chew, crush, or open capsules.

- Tell patient to take drug with meals. Inform patient that after titration is done, total daily dose may be taken at bedtime.
- Instruct patient to take a missed dose as soon as he remembers unless it's almost time for the next scheduled dose, in which case he should skip the missed dose. Warn against doubling the next dose.
- Tell patient not to use alcohol, barbiturates, or other CNS depressants; clomipramine increases their effects.

! **WARNING** Urge families to watch patient closely for abnormal thinking or behavior, or increased aggression or hostility. Emphasize the need to notify prescriber if they occur.

- Inform male patients about risk of sexual dysfunction while taking drug.
- Caution patient that drug may cause drowsiness, especially during initial dosage adjustment.
- Warn patient not to stop taking drug abruptly.
- Teach patient how to prevent photosensitivity reactions.
- Tell patient to report difficulty urinating, dizziness, dry mouth, mental changes, or sedation.
- Advise patient that drug may cause mild pupillary dilation, which may lead to an episode of acute-angle glaucoma. Encourage patient to have an eye exam before starting therapy to see if he is at risk.
- Caution patient to avoid hazardous activities until CNS effects of drug are known.
- Warn patient to seek medical attention if he experiences confusion, difficulty concentrating or thinking, feeling unsteady and having headaches, memory problems, or weakness.

clonazepam
Klonopin , Klonopin ODT

Class, Category, and Schedule
Pharmacologic class: Benzodiazepine
Therapeutic class: Anticonvulsant, antipanic
Controlled substance schedule: IV

Indications and Dosages
✴ *As adjunct or to treat Lennox–Gastaut syndrome (petit mal variant) and akinetic and myoclonic seizures*

ORAL DISINTEGRATING TABLETS, TABLETS
Adults and children over age 10 or weighing more than 30 kg (66 lb). *Initial:* 1.5 mg daily in divided doses three times daily. Increased by 0.5 to 1 mg every 3 days, if needed, until seizures are controlled or adverse reactions make further increases undesirable. *Maximum:* 20 mg daily.
Children age 10 or under weighing 30 kg (66 lb) or less. *Initial:* 0.01 to 0.03 mg/kg daily in divided doses twice daily or three times daily. Increased by 0.25 to 0.5 mg every third day up to maintenance dosage unless seizures are controlled or adverse reactions make further increases undesirable. *Maintenance:* 0.1 to 0.2 mg/kg daily, preferably in three equal doses.

✴ *To treat panic disorder*

ORALLY DISINTEGRATING TABLETS, TABLETS
Adults. *Initial:* 0.25 mg twice daily. Increased, if needed, to 1 mg daily after 3 days. If more than 1 mg daily is required, dosage increased in increments of 0.125 to 0.25 mg twice daily every 3 days until panic disorder is controlled or adverse reactions make further increases undesirable. *Maximum:* 4 mg daily.

Drug Administration
P.O.
- To administer a dissolving disintegrating tablet, first peel back the foil on the blister. Do not push tablet through foil. Immediately, and using dry gloved hands, remove tablet and place in patient's mouth or have patient place in mouth. It can be swallowed with or without water.
- Regular tablet should be swallowed whole with water. Tablet should not be broken, chewed, or crushed.
- Drug should not be stopped abruptly. Expect to taper dosage gradually by 0.125 mg twice daily every 3 days, until the drug is completely discontinued.

Route	Onset	Peak	Duration
P.O.	20–40 min	1–4 hr	6–12 hr

Half-life: 17–60 hr

Mechanism of Action
Although unknown, drug is thought to prevent panic and seizures by potentiating the effects of gamma-aminobutyric

acid (GABA), which is an inhibitory neurotransmitter. This action is also thought to suppress the spread of seizure activity caused by seizure-producing foci in the cortex, limbic, and thalamus structures.

Contraindications

Acute–narrow-angle glaucoma; hepatic disease; hypersensitivity to clonazepam, other benzodiazepines, or their components

Interactions

DRUGS

antianxiety drugs, antipsychotics (butyrophenone and thioxanthene classes), barbiturates, CNS depressants, MAO inhibitors, narcotics, nonbarbiturate hypnotics, other benzodiazepines, phenothiazines, sedating antihistamines, tricyclic antidepressants: Increased risk of CNS depression including significant change in mental status possibly leading to coma, respiratory depression, sedation, and somnolence

carbamazepine, lamotrigine, phenobarbital, phenytoin: Possibly decreased plasma clonazepam levels with potential for interference with its effectiveness

fluconazole: Possibly impaired clonazepam metabolism with potential for exaggerated concentrations and effects

opioids: Increased risk of severe respiratory depression

phenytoin: Possibly altered plasma concentrations of phenytoin

ACTIVITIES

alcohol use: Increased CNS depression, including severe respiratory depression and significant sedation and somnolence

Adverse Reactions

CNS: Abnormal dreams, aggression, agitation, amnesia, anxiety, apathy, ataxia, attention disturbance, confusion, depersonalization, depression, dizziness, drowsiness, emotional lability, excessive dreaming, fatigue, hallucinations, headache, hostility, hysteria, insomnia, irritability, memory loss, nervousness, nightmares, organic disinhibition, psychosis, reduced intellectual ability, sedation, sleep disturbances, **suicidal ideation**
CV: Palpitations
EENT: Blurred vision, eyelid spasm, increased salivation, loss of taste, pharyngitis, rhinitis, sinusitis, yawning

GI: Abdominal pain, anorexia, constipation, increased appetite
GU: Altered libido, difficult ejaculation, dysmenorrhea, dysuria, enuresis, impotence, nocturia, urine retention, UTI
HEME: Anemia, eosinophilia, **leukopenia, thrombocytopenia**
MS: Dysarthria, myalgia
RESP: Bronchitis, cough, **respiratory depression**
Other: **Allergic reaction,** physical and psychological dependence

Childbearing Considerations

PREGNANCY

- Pregnancy exposure registry: 1-888-233-2334 or http://www.aedpregnancyregistry.org/.
- Drug can cause fetal harm if administered late in pregnancy, possibly causing neonatal abstinence syndrome or withdrawal that can occur within hours to weeks after birth and persist for hours to months.
- Drug should be used with caution during pregnancy, especially in third trimester, only if benefit to mother outweighs potential risk to fetus.

LABOR & DELIVERY

- Administration of benzodiazepines such as clonazepam immediately prior to or during childbirth can cause floppy infant syndrome (difficulty feeding, hypothermia, hypotonia, respiratory depression), which can last up to 14 days.
- Drug is not recommended during labor and delivery.

LACTATION

- Drug is present in breast milk.
- Patient should check with prescriber before breastfeeding.
- If breastfeeding takes place, advise mother to monitor infant for drowsiness and poor sucking.

Nursing Considerations

- Assess patient before therapy is begun and throughout therapy for patient's risk for abuse, misuse, and addiction such as physical and psychological dependence (strong desire or need to increase dose to maintain drug effects), especially in patients with a history of substance abuse. Alert prescriber, if present.
- Use clonazepam cautiously in patients with mixed seizure disorder (because drug can

increase the risk of generalized tonic–clonic seizures), renal failure, or troublesome secretions (because clonazepam increases salivation) and in elderly patients (because they're more sensitive to drug's CNS effects). Also use cautiously in patients with compromised respiratory function and porphyria.

- Monitor blood drug level, CBC, and liver enzymes during long-term or high-dose therapy, as ordered.
- Monitor patient closely for signs of loss of effectiveness of anticonvulsant activity, especially within the first 3 months of administration. Notify prescriber if noted, because a dosage adjustment may reestablish effectiveness.
- Monitor patient closely for evidence of suicidal thinking or behavior, especially when therapy starts or dosage changes.
- Be aware that paradoxical and psychiatric reactions have occurred with benzodiazepines. Because clonazepam is a benzodiazepine, monitor patient for aggression, agitation, anger, anxiety, hallucinations, irritability, nightmares, and psychoses. Children and elderly patients are at greater risk of developing paradoxical reactions. If noted, notify prescriber and expect drug to be discontinued gradually.

! **WARNING** Be aware that benzodiazepine therapy like clonazepam should only be used concomitantly with opioids in patients for whom other treatment options are inadequate. If prescribed together, expect dosing and duration of the opioid to be limited. Monitor patient closely for signs and symptoms of decrease in consciousness, including coma, profound sedation, and significant respiratory depression. Notify prescriber immediately and provide emergency supportive care, as death may occur.

- Know that although the risk of teratogenicity is inconclusive, administration of benzodiazepines like clonazepam immediately before or during childbirth can cause a syndrome of difficulty feeding, hypothermia, hypotonia, and respiratory depression in the infant after birth. Also know that if mothers have taken clonazepam during the later stages of pregnancy, their infants may develop a dependency on the drug and experience withdrawal after birth.

PATIENT TEACHING

- Tell patient to take drug exactly as prescribed. Explain that stopping abruptly can cause seizures and withdrawal symptoms. Inform patient that in some cases, protracted withdrawal syndromes have occurred lasting weeks to more than a year.
- Instruct patient how to take a dissolving disintegrating tablet by first peeling back the foil on the blister. Caution patient not to push tablet through foil. Immediately, and using dry hands, tell patient to remove tablet and place in mouth. Tell patient the ODT tablet can be swallowed with or without water.
- Tell patient regular tablet should be swallowed whole with water and not broken, chewed, or crushed.
- Urge patient to carry medical identification of his seizure disorder and drug therapy.
- Warn patient about possible drowsiness.
- Instruct patient to report difficulty urinating, palpitations, persistent drowsiness, seizure activity, severe dizziness, and other disruptive adverse reactions.
- Suggest that parents monitor child's performance in school because clonazepam can cause drowsiness or inattentiveness.
- Urge caregivers to watch patient closely for evidence of suicidal tendencies, especially when therapy starts or dosage changes, and to report concerns to prescriber immediately.

! **WARNING** Warn patient not to consume alcohol or take an opioid during clonazepam therapy without prescriber knowledge, as severe respiratory depression can occur and may lead to death.

! **WARNING** Inform patient about potentially fatal additive effects of combining clonazepam with an opioid. Instruct patient to inform all prescribers of clonazepam use, especially if pain medication may be prescribed.

- Warn women of childbearing age who become pregnant while taking clonazepam to notify prescriber of pregnancy.

- Tell patient to let prescriber know about any new drug prescribed by another healthcare provider or before using any new over-the-counter preparations.

clonidine
Catapres-TTS

clonidine hydrochloride
Catapres, Dixarit (CAN), Duraclon, Kapvay

≡ Class and Category
Pharmacologic class: Centrally acting alpha agonist
Therapeutic class: Analgesic, antihypertensive, behavior modifier

≡ Indications and Dosages
✽ *To manage hypertension*

TABLETS
Adults. *Initial:* 0.1 mg twice daily, increased by 0.1 mg/wk to produce desired response. *Maintenance:* 0.2 to 0.6 mg daily in divided doses. *Maximum:* 2.4 mg daily.

TRANSDERMAL PATCH (CATAPRES-TTS)
Adults. *Initial:* 0.1-mg patch applied every 7 days. After 1 to 2 wk, if blood pressure isn't controlled, two 0.1-mg patches or one 0.2-mg patch applied. Dosage adjusted, as needed, every 7 days. *Maximum:* Two 0.3-mg patches worn at same time.

±**DOSAGE ADJUSTMENT** Dosage may be initially reduced for patients with renal failure.

✽ *To treat attention deficit hyperactivity disorder (ADHD) alone or as adjunct therapy with stimulant drugs*

E.R. TABLETS (KAPVAY)
Children age 6 to 17. *Initial:* 0.1 mg at bedtime, increased in increments of 0.1 mg daily at weekly intervals, as needed, with total daily dosage equally divided and given twice a day with equal or higher dose given at bedtime. *Maximum:* 0.4 mg/day.

✽ *As adjunct to relieve severe pain (in cancer patients) that isn't adequately relieved by opioid analgesics alone*

CONTINUOUS EPIDURAL INFUSION (DURACLON)
Adults. *Initial:* 30 mcg/hr. Titrated up or down, if needed, depending on comfort. *Maximum:* 40 mcg/hr.
Children old enough to tolerate epidural infusion. *Initial:* 0.5 mcg/kg/hr. Dosage then adjusted cautiously, as needed.

≡ Drug Administration
P.O.
- Extended-release tablets are not interchangeable with immediate-release tablets.
- E.R. tablets should be swallowed whole and never chewed, crushed, or cut.
- Administer once-a-day E.R. tablets at bedtime. If more than one daily dose is ordered, administer second dose of an equal or higher split at bedtime.
- Dosage should be decreased by 0.1 mg every 3 to 7 days when it is being discontinued.
- When switching patient from oral use to transdermal patch, expect to do the following: On day 1 apply patch and administer 100% of oral dose; day 2 administer 50% of oral dose; day 3 administer 25% of oral dose; and on day 4 discontinue oral dose, as ordered.

TRANSDERMAL
- Apply patch to a nonhairy site of intact skin on chest or upper arm.
- If a transdermal patch loosens during 7-day application period, place adhesive overlay directly over patch to ensure adhesion.
- Rotate transdermal sites.
- Remove patch and place a fresh one on another site if skin irritation, rash, or redness develops at patch site.
- Fold used transdermal patch in half with adhesive sides together and discard it out of the reach of children.

EPIDURAL INFUSION
- Dilute 500-mcg/ml concentrate to 100 mcg/ml with 0.9% Sodium Chloride Injection prior to administration. Drug should not be used with a preservative.
- Administered as a continuous infusion by healthcare professional familiar with epidural techniques and patient management problems associated with this route.
- A controlled-infusion device should be used for administration.

C

- Monitor infusion pump function and inspect the catheter tubing for obstruction or dislodgement to reduce risk of inadvertent abrupt withdrawal of the epidural infusion.

Route	Onset	Peak	Duration
P.O.	30–60 min	1–3 hr	6–10 hr
P.O./E.R.	1–2 wk	7–8 hr	Unknown
Transdermal	2–3 days	2–3 days	7–8 days
Epidural	Unknown	30–60 min	Unknown

Half-life: 12–20 hr

Mechanism of Action

Stimulates peripheral alpha-adrenergic receptors in the CNS to produce transient vasoconstriction and then stimulates central alpha-adrenergic receptors in the brain stem to reduce heart rate, peripheral vascular resistance, and systolic and diastolic blood pressure. Although alpha$_2$ adrenergic receptors in the brain are stimulated, the precise action that calms children with ADHD is unknown. May produce analgesia by preventing transmission of pain signals to the brain at presynaptic and postjunctional alpha$_2$-adrenoreceptors in the spinal cord. With epidural administration, clonidine produces analgesia in body areas innervated by the spinal cord segments in which the drug concentrates.

Contraindications

Anticoagulant therapy (epidural infusion); bleeding diathesis (epidural infusion); hypersensitivity to clonidine or its components, including adhesive used in transdermal patch; injection-site infection (epidural infusion)

Interactions

DRUGS

barbiturates, other CNS depressants: Increased depressant effects of these drugs
beta blockers, calcium channel blockers, digoxin: Additive effects, such as bradycardia and AV block; increased risk of worsened hypertensive response when clonidine is withdrawn (beta blockers only)
diuretics, other antihypertensive drugs: Increased hypotensive effect
epidural local anesthetics: Prolonged effects of epidural local anesthetics when used with epidural clonidine

fluphenazine: Possible development of acute delirium
tricyclic antidepressants: Decreased antihypertensive effect of clonidine

ACTIVITIES

alcohol use: Enhanced CNS depressant effects of alcohol

Adverse Reactions

CNS: Agitation, delusional perception, depression, dizziness, drowsiness, fatigue, hallucinations, headache, malaise, nervousness, paresthesia, sedation, syncope, weakness, tremor
CV: **Arrhythmias, AV block, bradycardia (severe)**, chest pain, **congestive heart failure**, orthostatic hypotension, Raynaud's phenomenon
EENT: Accommodation disorder, blurred vision, burning eyes, decreased lacrimation, dry eyes and mouth, salivary gland pain
GI: Constipation, **hepatitis**, mildly elevated liver enzymes, nausea, vomiting
GU: Decreased libido, erectile dysfunction, nocturia
HEME: Thrombocytopenia
SKIN: Pruritus, rash, urticaria
Other: **Angioedema**, weight gain, withdrawal symptoms

Childbearing Considerations

PREGNANCY

- Pregnancy exposure registry: 1-866-961-2388 or https://womensmentalhealth.org/adhd-medications/.
- It is not known if drug can cause fetal harm.
- Drug (except for epidural clonidine) should be used with caution during pregnancy only if benefit to mother outweighs potential risk to fetus. Epidural clonidine is contraindicated for use in obstetric, postpartum, or perioperative pain management because it may cause hemodynamic instability.

LACTATION

- Drug is present in breast milk.
- Patient should check with prescriber before breastfeeding for oral clonidine but breastfeeding or the drug should be discontinued when epidural clonidine is used.
- If breastfeeding occurs, infant should be monitored for symptoms of bradycardia or hypotension, such as lethargy, poor feeding, rapid breathing, or sedation.

REPRODUCTION

- Drug may impair fertility in females and males according to animal studies.

☰ Nursing Considerations

- Be aware that clonidine should not be used in most patients with severe cardiovascular disease or in those who are not hemodynamically stable because of the potential for severe hypotension.
- Use clonidine cautiously in elderly patients, who may be more sensitive to its hypotensive effect.
- Monitor blood pressure and heart rate often during clonidine therapy because clonidine may worsen AV block and sinus node dysfunction, especially if patient is taking another sympatholytic drug. If severe bradycardia occurs, be prepared to administer I.V. atropine or isoproterenol and assist with insertion of temporary cardiac pacing.
- Expect transdermal clonidine to take 2 to 3 days to lower blood pressure.
- Remove patch before patient has an MRI to avoid possible burns at the patch site.
- Be aware that stopping drug abruptly can elevate serum catecholamine levels and cause such withdrawal symptoms as agitation, confusion headache, nervousness, rebound hypertension, and tremor.
- Monitor patient with AV block and sinus node dysfunction closely if patient is taking sympatholytics concurrently with clonidine because these conditions may worsen, causing severe bradycardia, requiring treatment with I.V. atropine or isoproterenol therapy and temporary cardiac pacing.
- Expect hypertension to return within 48 hours after drug is discontinued.

PATIENT TEACHING

- Advise patient to take drug exactly as prescribed and not to stop abruptly because severe hypertension and withdrawal symptoms may occur.
- Instruct patient to apply transdermal patch to a hairless site of intact skin on chest or upper arm.
- Instruct patient that if a transdermal patch loosens during 7-day application period, he should place adhesive overlay directly over patch to ensure adhesion.
- Tell patient to rotate transdermal sites.

- Instruct patient to remove patch and place a fresh one on another site if skin irritation, rash, or redness develops at patch site.
- Advise patient to fold used transdermal patch in half with adhesive sides together and discard it out of the reach of children.
- Instruct patient to swallow E.R. tablets whole and never chew, crush, or cut the tablets.
- Advise patient to avoid hazardous activities until drug's CNS effects are known. Caution patient that these effects are increased by concomitant use of alcohol, barbiturates, or other sedating drugs.
- Advise men that libido may decrease or erectile dysfunction may occur.
- Instruct patient to report chest pain, dizziness with position changes, excessive drowsiness, rash, urine retention, and vision changes. As needed, tell patient to rise slowly to avoid hypotensive effects.
- Inform patient who wears contact lenses that clonidine may cause dry eyes.
- Advise patient who has a history of syncope or has a condition that predisposes him to syncope such as bradycardia, dehydration, hypotension, or orthostatic hypotension to avoid becoming dehydrated or overheated during therapy.

! WARNING Advise patient to stop taking drug and seek immediate medical attention if an allergic reaction occurs.

clopidogrel bisulfate
Plavix

☰ Class and Category

Pharmacologic class: P2Y$_{12}$ platelet inhibitor
Therapeutic class: Platelet aggregation inhibitor

☰ Indications and Dosages

✳ *To reduce the rate of CVA and MI in patient with established peripheral arterial disease or a history of recent MI or CVA*

TABLETS

Adults. 75 mg once daily.

✳ *To reduce rate of CVA and MI in patients with non-ST-segment elevation acute coronary syndrome (unstable angina/non-ST-elevation myocardial infarction), including patients*

*who are to be managed medically and those
who are to be managed with coronary
revascularization*

TABLETS

Adults. *Loading dose:* 300 mg as a single
dose. *Maintenance:* 75 mg once daily.

Drug Administration

P.O.

- Drug should not be discontinued abruptly.
- Expect drug to be given with aspirin.

Route	Onset	Peak	Duration
P.O.	2 hr	45 min	5 days

Half-life: 6 hr

Mechanism of Action

Binds to adenosine diphosphate (ADP)
receptors on the surface of activated platelets.
This action blocks ADP, which deactivates
nearby glycoprotein IIb/IIIa receptors
and prevents fibrinogen from attaching to
receptors. Without fibrinogen, platelets can't
aggregate and form thrombi.

Contraindications

Active pathological bleeding, including
intracranial hemorrhage and peptic ulcer;
hypersensitivity to clopidogrel or its
components

Interactions

DRUGS

aspirin: Increased risk of bleeding
CYP1C19 inducers (strong) such as rifampin:
Increased plasma clopidogrel level increasing
risk of bleeding
*CYP2C19 inhibitors, such as dexlansoprazole,
esomeprazole, lansoprazole, omeprazole,
pantoprazole:* Decreased plasma clopidogrel
level, decreased platelet inhibition
*NSAIDs, serotonin norepinephrine reuptake
inhibitors (SNRIs), selective serotonin reuptake
inhibitors (SSRIs):* Increased risk of GI
bleeding
opioid agonists: Delayed and reduced
absorption of clopidogrel
repaglinide and other CYP2C8 inhibitors:
Increased repaglinide and other CYP2C8
inhibitors exposure possibly increasing
risk of adverse reactions, especially
hypoglycemia
warfarin: Prolonged bleeding time, increased
risk of bleeding

Adverse Reactions

CNS: Confusion, depression, dizziness,
fatal intracranial bleeding, fatigue, fever,
hallucinations, headache
CV: Chest pain, edema,
hypercholesterolemia, hypertension,
hypotension, vasculitis
EENT: Altered or loss of taste; conjunctival,
ocular, or retinal bleeding; epistaxis; rhinitis;
stomatitis; taste disorders
**ENDO: Insulin autoimmune syndrome,
severe hypoglycemia**
GI: Abdominal pain; **acute liver failure**;
colitis; diarrhea; duodenal, gastric, or peptic
ulcer; elevated liver enzymes; gastritis;
**gastrointestinal and retroperitoneal
hemorrhage**; indigestion; nausea;
noninfectious hepatitis, pancreatitis
GU: Elevated serum creatinine level,
glomerulopathy, UTI
**HEME: Acquired hemophilia A,
agranulocytosis, aplastic anemia,
neutropenia, pancytopenia, prolonged
bleeding time, thrombocytopenic purpura,
thrombotic thrombocytopenic purpura,
unusual bleeding** or bruising
MS: Arthralgia, back pain, musculoskeletal
bleeding, myalgia
RESP: Bronchitis, **bronchospasm**, cough,
dyspnea, **eosinophilic pneumonia,
interstitial pneumonitis, respiratory tract
bleeding**, upper respiratory tract infection
SKIN: Acute generalized exanthematous
pustulosis, bullous dermatitis, eczema,
**erythema multiforme, exfoliative
dermatitis**, lichen planus, pruritus, skin
bleeding, **Stevens–Johnson syndrome, toxic
epidermal necrolysis**, urticaria
**Other: Anaphylaxis, angioedema, drug
reaction with eosinophilia and systemic
symptoms (DRESS)**, flu-like symptoms,
serum sickness

Childbearing Considerations

PREGNANCY

- It is not known if drug can cause fetal harm.
- Drug should be used with caution during
  pregnancy only if benefit to mother
  outweighs potential risk to fetus.

LABOR & DELIVERY

- Drug may cause maternal bleeding and
  hemorrhage if given during labor and
  delivery.

- Know that drug should be temporarily withheld for 5 to 7 days prior to labor, delivery, or use with neuraxial anesthesia, if possible.

LACTATION
- It is not known if drug is present in breast milk.
- Patient should check with prescriber before breastfeeding.

Nursing Considerations
- Avoid clopidogrel in patients who have a genetic variation in CYP2C19 or are receiving CYP2C19 inhibitors. Platelet inhibition may decline, increasing the risk of adverse cardiovascular effects after MI.
- Determine if patient has a history of hypersensitivity that may have included a hematologic reaction to any other thienopyridine drug, such as prasugrel or ticlopidine, because allergic cross-reactivity has been reported.
- Use clopidogrel cautiously in patients with severe hepatic or renal disease, risk of bleeding from surgery or trauma, or conditions that predispose to bleeding (such as peptic ulcer disease or thrombotic thrombocytopenic purpura).

! **WARNING** Be aware that clopidogrel prolongs bleeding time; expect to stop it 5 days before elective surgery.

- Obtain blood cell count, as ordered, whenever signs and symptoms suggest a hematologic problem.
- Monitor patient closely for increased bleeding because concurrent aspirin therapy increases the risk.

PATIENT TEACHING
- Remind patient to adhere to aspirin therapy that has to be taken with clopidogrel therapy.
- Caution patient not to use NSAIDs, including OTC preparations such as proton pump inhibitors, during clopidogrel therapy because of potential for bleeding.
- Caution patient that bleeding may continue longer than usual. Instruct him to report unusual bleeding or bruising.
- Urge patient to inform all other healthcare providers, including dentists, that he takes clopidogrel before having surgery or other

procedures or taking a new drug, because he has an increased risk of bleeding.
- Advise patient to notify prescriber promptly if he experiences extreme skin paleness, fever, neurologic changes, purple skin patches, weakness, or yellowing of his skin or eyes.
- Instruct patient not to discontinue clopidogrel abruptly or without first consulting prescriber.

! **WARNING** Warn patient that drug may cause low blood sugar levels. Review signs and symptoms of hypoglycemia and how to treat. Tell patient to notify prescriber if hypoglycemia occurs because it can cause persistent hypoglycemia, which could become severe.

clozapine
Clozaril, FazaClo, Versacloz

Class and Category
Pharmacologic class: Atypical antipsychotic
Therapeutic class: Atypical antipsychotic

Indications and Dosages
* *To treat severe schizophrenia unresponsive to standard drugs; to reduce risk of recurrent suicidal behavior in schizophrenia or schizoaffective disorders*

ORALLY DISINTEGRATING TABLETS, ORAL SUSPENSION, TABLETS
Adults. *Initial:* 12.5 mg once or twice daily. Increased by 25 to 50 mg daily to 300 to 450 mg daily in divided doses by the end of 2 wk. Subsequently, dosage titration shouldn't exceed 100 mg twice per wk. *Maximum:* 900 mg daily in divided doses.

±**DOSAGE ADJUSTMENT** If patient is receiving a strong CYP1A2 inhibitor such as ciprofloxacin, enoxacin, or fluvoxamine concurrently, dosage decreased by two-thirds and then adjusted according to clinical response. If a patient is receiving a CYP1A2 inducer (tobacco smoking) or CYP3A4 inducers such as carbamazepine, phenytoin, rifampin, or St. John's wort concurrently, clozapine dosage may have to be increased if clinical response is ineffective. If patient has significant renal or hepatic impairment or is a CYP2D6 poor metabolizer, clozapine dosage may be decreased if patient develops significant adverse reactions.

Drug Administration

P.O.

- Administer single daily doses at bedtime. If more than one dose is given daily, the dose may be split unequally so a larger dose is given at bedtime.
- Administer orally disintegrating tablets by peeling foil back to remove tablet (rather than pushing tablet through foil) with dry, gloved hand and then immediately place or have patient place tablet in mouth and let it dissolve before swallowing. No water is needed.
- Shake oral suspension container for 10 seconds before every use. The oral dosing syringe provided with the product should be the only device used to measure dosage. Firmly insert adapter into the neck of the bottle before the first use and keep it there. Then fill the syringe with air equivalent to the dose being withdrawn from the bottle. To withdraw the dose, insert the dosing syringe into the adapter and push air from syringe into the bottle. Then invert bottle and slowly pull back the plunger to the prescribed dose. After removing the syringe from the bottle adapter, slowly squirt the suspension into patient's mouth. Replace the cap over the adapter until next dose is due and rinse syringe well with warm water and dry.

Route	Onset	Peak	Duration
P.O.	15 min	1.5–2.5 hr	4–12 hr

Half-life: 12 hr

Mechanism of Action

May produce antipsychotic effects by interfering with dopamine binding to dopamine—especially D_4—receptors in the limbic region of the brain and by antagonizing adrenergic, cholinergic, histaminic, and serotoninergic receptors.

Contraindications

Absolute neutrophil count (ANC) below 1,500/mm^3 for general population and at least 1,000/mm^3 for patients with Benign Ethnic Neutropenia, hypersensitivity to clozapine or its components

Interactions

DRUGS

antidepressants (selected ones); carbamazepine; class IC antiarrhythmics such as encainide, flecainide, propafenone; phenothiazines: Increased levels of these drugs with possible increased adverse reactions

bupropion, cimetidine, ciprofloxacin, duloxetine, enoxacin, erythromycin, escitalopram, fluoxetine, fluvoxamine, oral contraceptives, paroxetine, quinidine, sertraline, terbinafine: Possibly increased blood clozapine level and increased risk of adverse reactions

carbamazepine, phenytoin, rifampin, St. John's wort: Decreased blood clozapine level with decreased effectiveness

chlorpromazine, class 1a antiarrhythmias such as quinidine or procainamide, class III antiarrhythmias such as amiodarone or sotalol, dolasetron, droperidol, erythromycin, gatifloxacin, halofantrine, iloperidone, levomethadyl, mesoridazine, mefloquine, methadone, moxifloxacin, pentamidine, pimozide, probucol, sparfloxacin, tacrolimus, thioridazine ziprasidone: Possible increased risk of prolonged QT interval

CNS depressants: Increased CNS depression

other anticholinergic drugs: Increased risk for anticholinergic toxicity or severe GI adverse reactions

ACTIVITIES

alcohol use: Increased CNS depression
caffeine: Increased blood clozapine level
smoking: Decreased blood clozapine level

Adverse Reactions

CNS: Agitation, akinesia, anxiety, ataxia, cholinergic rebound adverse reactions postdiscontinuation, confusion, delirium, depression, dizziness, drowsiness, dystonia, EEG abnormality, fatigue, fever, headache, hyperkinesia, hypokinesia, insomnia, lethargy, myoclonic jerks, **neuroleptic malignant syndrome**, nightmares, obsessive–compulsive symptoms, paresthesia, possible cataplexy, restlessness, restless leg syndrome, rigidity, sedation, **seizures**, sleep disturbance including **sleep apnea**, slurred speech, **status epilepticus**, syncope, tardive dyskinesia, tremor, vertigo, weakness

CV: Atrial or ventricular fibrillation, **bradycardia, cardiac arrest, cardiomyopathy,** chest pain, **deep vein thrombosis,** dyslipidemia, **ECG changes,** hypercholesterolemia, hypertension, hypertriglyceridemia, **hypotension,** leukocytoclastic vasculitis, **MI, mitral valve incompetence, myocarditis,** orthostatic hypotension, palpitations, **QT-interval prolongation,** tachycardia, **torsades de pointes,** vasculitis, **ventricular tachycardia**
EENT: Blurred vision, dry mouth, increased nasal congestion, increased salivation, narrow-angle glaucoma, periorbital edema, pharyngitis, salivary gland swelling, tongue numbness or soreness
ENDO: Ketoacidosis, **pseudopheochromocytoma, severe hyperglycemia**
GI: Abdominal discomfort, **acute pancreatitis,** anorexia, cholestasis, colitis, constipation, diarrhea, dysphagia, elevated liver enzymes, heartburn, **hepatic cirrhosis or fibrosis, hepatitis, hepatotoxicity, intestinal ischemia or infarction,** jaundice, **liver failure or injury, megacolon,** nausea, vomiting
GU: Abnormal ejaculation including retrograde; acute interstitial nephritis; nocturnal enuresis; priapism; **renal failure;** urinary frequency, urgency, and incontinence; urine retention
HEME: Agranulocytosis; elevated hemoglobin, hematocrit and erythrocyte sedimentation rate; eosinophilia; **granulocytopenia; leukopenia; neutropenia (may become severe); thrombocytopenia;** thrombocytosis
MS: Back or leg pain, elevated creatine phosphokinase, muscle spasm or weakness, myalgia, myasthenic syndrome, **rhabdomyolysis**
RESP: Aspiration, dyspnea, lower respiratory tract infection, pleural effusion, pneumonia, **pulmonary embolism, respiratory arrest**
SKIN: Erythema multiforme, photosensitivity, pigmentation disorder, pruritus, rash, **Stevens–Johnson syndrome,** urticaria
Other: Angioedema, anticholinergic toxicity, **hypersensitivity reactions,** hyperuricemia, **hyponatremia,** inflammation of serous membranes, **sepsis,** systemic lupus erythematosus, weight gain or loss

⬚ Childbearing Considerations

PREGNANCY

- Pregnancy Exposure Registry: 1-866-961-2388 or http://womensmentalhealth.org/clinical-and-research-programs/pregnancyregistry/.
- It is not known if drug can cause fetal harm. However, neonates exposed to antipsychotic drugs such as clozapine in utero are at risk for extrapyramidal and/or withdrawal symptoms following delivery.
- Drug should be used with caution during pregnancy only if benefit to mother outweighs potential risk to fetus.

LACTATION

- Drug is present in breast milk.
- Patient should check with prescriber before breastfeeding. If breastfeeding occurs, infant should be monitored for excess sedation.

⬚ Nursing Considerations

- Use clozapine cautiously in patients with cardiovascular, hepatic, or renal disease, because they have increased risk of serious or fatal adverse reactions. Also use cautiously in patients with risk factors for a stroke because drug use may increase risk of cerebrovascular adverse events.
- Be aware that clozapine should not be given to elderly patients with dementia-related psychosis.
- Use cautiously in patients with a history of prolonged QT syndrome or who have existing conditions that might prolong the QT interval such as a recent MI, serious cardiac arrhythmia, or uncompensated heart failure. Drug should also be used cautiously in patients with cardiovascular disease or a family history of prolonged QT syndrome because clozapine therapy may increase the QT interval enough to cause life-threatening arrhythmias such as torsades de pointes, especially in patients who are hypokalemic. Know that hypokalemia should be corrected, if present, before clozapine therapy begins and the serum potassium level monitored closely throughout therapy. If QT prolongation occurs, notify prescriber and expect drug to be discontinued if the QT interval exceeds 500 msec.

! WARNING Know that, rarely, clozapine causes severe or life-threatening adverse reactions, such as agranulocytosis, cardiac or respiratory arrest, deep vein thrombosis, myocarditis (especially in first month), neuroleptic malignant syndrome, and severe hyperglycemia with ketoacidosis in nondiabetic patients. It also may cause seizures and tardive dyskinesia. Monitor patient closely. Know that these risks are often dose-related. Expect therapy to begin with a dose as low as 12.5 mg with titration done slowly and divided daily dosing used.

! WARNING Check patient's baseline complete blood count (CBC), including differential before therapy and weekly for first 6 months, as ordered. Know that the baseline absolute neutrophil count (ANC) must be at least 1,500/µl for the general population; and must be at least 1,000/µl for patients with documented Benign Ethnic Neutropenia (BEN) before therapy can begin. If ANC remains equal to or greater than 1,500/µl during the first 6 months, expect to check the patient's ANC to check every 2 weeks for next 6 months, as ordered. If counts remain stable, expect to continue checking every 4 weeks thereafter. Also, know that laboratory monitoring may be reduced for hospice patients with an estimated life expectancy of 6 months or less. Be aware that because of the risk for severe neutropenia, clozapine is only available through a restricted program.

- Be aware that because of the risk of severe neutropenia, clozapine is available only through a restricted program called the Clozapine REMS Program. If patient develops mild neutropenia (1,000 to 1,499/µl), treatment should be expected to continue but ANC monitoring should be increased to three times weekly until level reaches 1,500/µl. If patient develops moderate neutropenia (500 to 999/µl), expect treatment to be interrupted and daily monitoring of the patient's ANC done until the level reaches 1,000/µl, then three-times-a-week monitoring until level reaches 1,500/µl. Expect therapy to be resumed once ANC reaches 1,000/µl. If patient develops severe neutropenia (less than 500/µl), expect drug to be discontinued,

and daily monitoring of ANC until it reaches 1,000/µl, then three times weekly until it is normal. Be aware that clozapine therapy should not be restarted unless the benefits outweigh future risks and if restarted, the patient should resume treatment as a new patient receiving drug for the first time.

- Monitor temperature. Expect to withhold clozapine if patient develops a fever of 38.5°C (101.3°F) or higher and obtain an ANC level immediately, as fever is often the first sign of neutropenic infection.
- Expect to check ANC weekly for at least 4 weeks after therapy ends or until ANC is 1,500/µl or more.
- Monitor patients, especially male patients and younger patients, for dystonia, particularly during the first few days of treatment. Be alert for complaints of neck spasms, which sometimes may progress to throat tightness, trouble swallowing or breathing, and tongue protrusion.
- Monitor patient for signs and symptoms of cardiomyopathy, mitral valve incompetence, or myocarditis such as chest pain, dyspnea, ECG changes, fever, flu-like symptoms, hypotension, palpitations, or tachycardia. If present, notify prescriber immediately and expect drug to be discontinued and a cardiac evaluation done promptly.
- Monitor patient's liver enzymes, as ordered. Report any signs of liver dysfunction such as anorexia, fatigue, jaundice, malaise, or nausea to prescriber. Expect clozapine to be discontinued if liver enzymes become elevated in combination with symptoms or patient develops hepatitis.
- Monitor patient for CNS and peripheral anticholinergic toxicity, especially at higher dosages or in overdose situation. Drug should be used cautiously in patients with a current or prior diagnosis of constipation, clinically significant prostatic hypertrophy, urinary retention, or other conditions in which anticholinergic effects can lead to significant adverse reactions.

PATIENT TEACHING

- Tell patient that he'll receive only a 1-week supply at a time.
- Instruct patient taking orally disintegrating tablets (Fazaclo) to leave tablet in blister pack until ready to take it. Tell him to peel foil

back to remove tablet (rather than pushing tablet through foil) and then to immediately place tablet in mouth and let it dissolve before swallowing. Explain that no water is needed.

- Instruct patient prescribed oral suspension form to shake container for 10 seconds before every administration. The oral dosing syringe provided with the product should be the only device used to measure dosage. Tell patient to firmly insert adapter into the neck of the bottle before the first use and keep it there. Instruct patient to first fill the syringe with air equivalent to the dose being withdrawn from the bottle. To withdraw the dose, he should insert the dosing syringe into the adapter and push air from syringe into the bottle. Then he should invert bottle and slowly pull back the plunger to the prescribed dose. After removing the syringe from the bottle adapter, the patient should be told to slowly squirt the suspension into his mouth. Then he should replace the cap over the adapter until next dose is due and rinse syringe well with warm water and dry.
- Inform patient that he'll need weekly blood tests. Review evidence of dyscrasias (fatigue, fever, sore throat, weakness); urge patient to report them to prescriber if they occur.
- Tell patient that drug-induced constipation may occur. Advise appropriate hydration, increased fiber intake, and physical activity. Patient should alert prescriber if constipation develops or other adverse effects such as abdominal distention or pain, nausea, or vomiting develop, because if left unchecked, severe complications could occur.
- Instruct patient to avoid hazardous activities until drug's CNS effects are known.
- Alert patient and family of increased risk for falls, especially if patient has other medical conditions or takes medication that may affect the nervous system.
- Tell patient to report any persistent, severe, or unusual adverse effects to prescriber immediately.
- Advise patient to rise slowly from lying or sitting position to minimize orthostatic hypotension.
- Warn patient that if he stops drug for more than 2 days, he will need to contact prescriber for instructions; dosage will have to be changed.

- Tell patient to consult prescriber before using alcohol or taking OTC drugs.
- Advise female patients of childbearing age to notify prescriber if pregnancy occurs or is suspected.

coagulation factor VIIa (recombinant)-jncw
Sevenfact

Class and Category
Pharmacologic class: Recombinant form of coagulation factor VIIa
Therapeutic class: Factor VIIa inhibitor antidote

Indications and Dosages
❋ *To control and treat bleeding episodes in patients with hemophilia A or B with inhibitors*

I.V. INFUSION
Adults and adolescents 12 years of age and older. *For mild and moderate bleeding of joint, mucous membranes, soft tissue, and superficial muscle:* 75 mcg/kg every 3 hr until hemostasis is achieved. Alternatively, 225 mcg/kg as initial dose followed 9 hr later if hemostasis is not achieved with additional 75 mcg/kg doses every 3 hr, as needed to achieve hemostasis. *For severe gastrointestinal or intracranial bleeding, life- or limb-threatening hemorrhage, iliopsoas and deep muscle with neurovascular injury, or retroperitoneal bleeding:* 225 mcg/kg initially, followed 6 hr later with 75 mcg/kg every 2 hours, as needed to achieve hemostasis.

Drug Administration
I.V.
- To reconstitute, first determine the prescribed dose and then obtain number of drug kits needed (each contains one vial of drug powder and one prefilled diluent syringe with one vial adapter), an infusion set, and alcohol swab. After taking items from kit, check that vial has a matching colored syringe.
- Allow vial powder and diluent syringe to come to room temperature, if refrigerated. Be aware that the specified volume of diluent corresponds to the amount of drug

powder as follows: 1-mg vial requires 1.1 ml Water for Injection diluent in prefilled syringe and 5-mg vial requires 5.2 ml Water for Injection diluent in prefilled syringe.

- Remove plastic cap on vial and cleanse the rubber stopper with alcohol swab and let dry. Peel back the protective paper from the vial adapter. Do not remove the vial adapter from the package.
- Place the drug vial on a flat surface. While holding the vial adapter package, place the vial adapter over the drug vial and press down firmly on the package until the vial adapter spike breaks through the rubber stopper. Lightly squeeze the plastic cover and lift up to remove it from the vial adapter. Know that the 5-mg vial adapter may not sit flat against the vial, but it is fully functional.
- Remove the syringe cap from the prefilled syringe by holding the syringe body to unscrew the syringe cap by turning to the left. While holding the edges of the vial adapter, screw on the prefilled syringe by turning to the right a few turns until it starts to tighten. Insert the plunger rod into the syringe, then screw a few turns turning to the right so that the plunger rod is attached to the gray rubber stopper in the syringe.
- Push the plunger rod to slowly inject all the diluent into the vial. Keep the plunger rod pressed down and swirl the vial gently until powder is dissolved. The solution should be clear to slightly opaque with no particles floating in the solution.
- Without withdrawing any drug back into the syringe, unscrew the syringe from the vial adapter by turning left until it is completely detached. Prepare number of vials needed for prescribed dose. Withdraw the drug solution from the vial(s), using an infusion syringe provided by the pharmacy; the syringe should be large enough to hold the prescribed dose. Each vial contains approximately 1 mg/ml.
- Infuse within 4 hours after reconstitution, discarding any unused solution after 4 hours. Infuse over 2 minutes or less as a bolus intravenous infusion.
- Prior to reconstitution, drug kit can be stored at room temperature or refrigerated. After reconstitution, drug can be stored at room temperature for up to 4 hr. Do not freeze or store in syringes.

- *Incompatibilities:* Other infusion drugs or solutions

Route	Onset	Peak	Duration
I.V.	Immediate	5 min	8 hr

Half-life: 1.41–1.7 hr

Mechanism of Action

In the presence of both calcium and phospholipids, Factor VIIa in a complex with tissue factor (TF) activates Factor X to Factor Xa, directly bypassing the reactions that require Factor VIII or IX. Factor Xa initiates the pathway of the coagulation cascade to form clot formation at the site of the hemorrhage.

Contraindications

Hypersensitivity to coagulation factor VIIa (recombinant)-jncw or its components; hypersensitivity to rabbits or rabbit proteins

Interactions

DRUGS

activated prothrombin complex concentrates: Increased risk of serious thrombotic events

Adverse Reactions

CNS: Dizziness, fever, headache
OTHER: Anticoagulation VIIa (recombinant)-jncw antibodies; hypersensitivity reactions (**anaphylaxis, difficulty breathing,** dizziness, fainting, **hypotension,** pruritus, rash, **swelling around the mouth and throat,** tightness of the chest, wheezing, urticaria); infusion-site discomfort, hematoma, or other infusion-related reactions (chest tightness, flushing, mild hypotension, shakiness, transient tachycardia)

Childbearing Considerations

PREGNANCY

- It is not known if drug can cause fetal harm.
- Use with caution only if benefit to mother outweighs potential risk to fetus.

LACTATION

- It is not known if drug is present in breast milk.
- Patient should check with prescriber before breastfeeding.

Nursing Considerations

- Be aware coagulation factor VIIa (recombinant)-jncw is not used to treat congenital Factor VII deficiency.

- Know that the site and severity will determine the duration of drug use for mild to moderate bleeding and additionally the use of other procoagulant therapies for severe bleeding.

! WARNING Monitor patients for signs and symptoms of thromboembolic events. Patients at increased risk include patients with a history of acquired or congenital hemophilia receiving concomitant treatment with activated or nonactivated prothrombin complex or other hemostatic agents; or a history of atherosclerotic disease, cerebrovascular disease, coronary artery disease, crush injury, septicemia, or thromboembolism. Be aware that the dose of coagulation factor VIIa (recombinant)-jncw should be reduced or drug discontinued if there is laboratory confirmation of intravascular coagulation or the presence of clinical thrombosis.

! WARNING Monitor patients for hypersensitivity reactions, which could be life-threatening. Patients at increased risk include patients with known IgE-based hypersensitivity to casein. If hypersensitivity occurs, notify prescriber, expect drug to be discontinued, and institute supportive treatment as prescribed.

- Be aware that neutralizing antibodies may occur with the use of coagulation factor VIIa (recombinant)-jncw. If treatment with drug does not produce adequate hemostasis, expect testing for neutralizing antibodies to be performed.
- Know that laboratory coagulation parameters, such as PT/INR, aPTT, and FVII:C, do not correlate with clinical response to coagulation factor VIIa (recombinant)-jncw treatment.

PATIENT TEACHING

- Inform patient that coagulation factor VIIa (recombinant)-jncw is given by an intravenous infusion with repeated doses, as needed.

! WARNING Review signs and symptoms of hypersensitivity with patient. Instruct patient to alert staff or seek immediate medical help, if present.

! WARNING Inform patient about the signs of thrombosis (altered consciousness or speech, loss of motor or sensory abilities, new-onset chest pain, new-onset swelling or pain in the abdomen or limbs, shortness of breath). Urge patient to seek immediate medical help, if present.

coagulation factor Xa, inactivated-zhzo
Andexxa

Class and Category
Pharmacologic class: Human coagulation factor Xa, recombinant
Therapeutic class: Factor Xa inhibitor antidote

Indications and Dosages
* *To reverse life-threatening or uncontrolled bleeding induced by apixaban or rivaroxaban therapy*

I.V. INFUSION, I.V. INJECTION

Adults. *For low dose (used if last dose of apixaban was 5 mg or less, rivaroxaban was 10 mg or less, and last dose of either drug was taken less than 8 hr or unknown):* 400 mg as an I.V. bolus, followed by 4 mg/min for up to 120 min. *For high dose (used if last dose of apixaban was greater than 5 mg or unknown or rivaroxaban was greater than 10 mg or unknown and last dose of either drug was taken less than 8 hr or unknown):* 800 mg as an I.V. bolus, followed by 8 mg/min for up to 120 min. If either drug was taken 8 hr or more, regardless of dosage, low-dose regimen used.

Drug Administration
I.V.

- Store unopened vials in refrigerator. Do not freeze.
- Prepare I.V. bolus by reconstituting each 200-mg vial of drug by slowly injecting 20 ml of Sterile Water for Injection, using a 20-gauge needle or higher and directing the solution onto the inside wall of the vial to minimize foaming. Gently swirl each vial until powder is completely dissolved. Do not shake, to avoid foaming. This takes about 3 to 5 minutes. Use a 60-ml syringe or larger with a 20-gauge needle to withdraw

the reconstituted solution from each of the vials until the required dosing volume is achieved. Transfer the solution from the syringe into an empty polyolefin or polyvinyl chloride I.V. bag with a volume of 250 ml or less. Use a 0.2- or 0.22-micron in-line polyethersulfone or equivalent low-protein-binding filter and administer the bolus at a rate of 30 mg/min.

- Prepare continuous I.V. infusion following the same procedure for I.V. bolus preparation. Use a 0.2- or 0.22-micron inline polyethersulfone or equivalent low-protein-binding filter. Within 2 minutes following the bolus dose, begin I.V. infusion and infuse for up to 120 minutes, as prescribed.
- Know that vials that have been reconstituted are stable at room temperature for up to 8 hours, or may be stored for up to 24 hours if refrigerated. Reconstituted solution in I.V. bags is stable at room temperature for up to 8 hours.
- *Incompatibilities:* None listed by manufacturer

Route	Onset	Peak	Duration
I.V.	2–5 min (bolus)	4 hr	2 hr (following infusion)

Half-life: 5–7 hr

Mechanism of Action

Binds and sequesters the factor Xa inhibitors apixaban and rivaroxaban, thereby exerting its procoagulant effect.

Contraindications

Hypersensitivity to coagulation factor Xa, inactivated-zhzo or its components

Interactions

DRUGS

None reported by manufacturer

Adverse Reactions

CV: Thromboembolic events
EENT: Altered sense of taste
GU: UTI
RESP: Cough, dyspnea, pneumonia
SKIN: Flushing, urticaria
Other: Anticoagulation factor Xa, inactivated-zhzo antibodies; feeling hot

Childbearing Considerations

PREGNANCY

- It is not known if drug can cause fetal harm.

- Use with caution during pregnancy only if benefit to mother outweighs potential risk to fetus.

LACTATION

- It is not known if drug is present in breast milk.
- Patient should check with prescriber before breastfeeding.

Nursing Considerations

- Be aware that the dosing of coagulation factor Xa, inactivated-zhzo is based on the specific drug that had been administered (apixaban or rivaroxaban), dose of the drug taken, and the time since the patient's last dose of the drug.

! **WARNING** Monitor patient closely for thrombosis, because patients treated with coagulation factor Xa, inactivated-zhzo have underlying disease states that predispose them to thromboembolic events that can occur up to 30 days after drug has been administered. Expect patient to resume anticoagulant therapy as soon as possible following use of coagulation factor Xa, inactivated-zhzo to reduce the risk of thrombosis.

PATIENT TEACHING

- Inform patient that coagulation factor Xa, inactivated-zhzo is administered in two steps: first, as an intravenous bolus; then followed by a continuous intravenous infusion that may last up to 2 hours after the bolus has been given.

! **WARNING** Inform patient that reversing the effects of the prescribed apixaban or rivaroxaban increases the risk of thromboembolic events for up to 30 days following the administration of coagulation factor Xa, inactivated-zhzo. Review the signs and symptoms of a blood clot that may occur in various areas of the body. Urge patient to seek immediate medical attention if a blood clot is suspected.

codeine sulfate

Class, Category, and Schedule

Pharmacologic class: Opioid

Therapeutic class: Antitussive, opioid analgesic
Controlled substance schedule: II

Indications and Dosages

✳ *To treat mild to moderate pain that requires opioid treatment and for which alternative treatment options (e.g., nonopioid analgesics or opioid combination products) are inadequate or not tolerated*

TABLETS

Adults. 15 to 60 mg (usual, 30 mg) every 4 hr, as needed. *Maximum:* 360 mg in 24 hours.

Drug Administration

P.O.

- Administer drug with food.
- Drug should not be discontinued abruptly after chronic use.

Route	Onset	Peak	Duration
P.O.	30–45 min	1 hr	4–6 hr

Half-life: 3 hr

Mechanism of Action

May produce analgesia through partial metabolism to morphine. Drug binds with delta, kappa, and mu receptors in the spinal cord and with $kappa_3$ and mu_1 receptors higher in the CNS, decreasing intracellular cAMP, which inhibits adenylate cyclase activity and prevents release of pain neurotransmitters, such as dopamine and substance P, and altering perception of and emotional response to pain.

Contraindications

Acute or severe bronchial asthma in an unmonitored setting or absence of resuscitative equipment, children under the age of 12 for all uses and adolescents under the age of 18 for use with cold and cough medications; gastrointestinal obstruction, including paralytic ileus; hypersensitivity to codeine, other opioids, or their components; significant respiratory depression; use of MAO inhibitors or within past 14 days; use for postoperative pain management in adolescents under the age of 18 who have undergone adenoidectomy and/or tonsillectomy

Interactions

DRUGS

anticholinergics: Increased risk of severe constipation and urinary retention

antihypertensives, diuretics: Potentiated hypotensive effects

benzodiazepines, CNS depressants, muscle relaxants, other opioids, sedating antihistamines, tricyclic antidepressants: Increased risk of severe respiratory depression and significant sedation and somnolence

buprenorphine, butorphanol, nalbuphine, pentazocine: Possibly reduces analgesic effect of codeine and/or precipitate withdrawal symptoms

CYP2D6 inhibitors (such as bupropion, fluoxetine, paroxetine, quinidine): Possibly decreased effectiveness of codeine that may cause some patients to experience opioid withdrawal

CYP2D6 inhibitor that is being discontinued: Possibly increase or prolong adverse reactions and potentially fatal respiratory depression

CYP3A4 inducers (such as carbamazepine, phenytoin, rifampin) or discontinuation of a CYP3A4 inhibitor (such as azole antifungals, macrolide antibiotics, protease inhibitors): Decreased plasma codeine concentration with possible decreased effectiveness, causing some patients to experience opioid withdrawal

CYP3A4 inhibitors or discontinuation of a CYP3A4 inducer: Increased plasma codeine concentration leading to increased or prolonged adverse reactions and potentially fatal respiratory depression

diuretics: Reduced effectiveness of diuretics

MAO inhibitors such as linezolid, tranylcypromine: Increased risk of unpredictable, severe, and sometimes fatal reactions

muscle relaxants: Possibly enhanced neuromuscular blocking action of skeletal muscle relaxants; increased severity of respiratory depression

naloxone: Antagonized codeine effect

naltrexone: Precipitated withdrawal symptoms in codeine-dependent patients

serotonergic drugs such as 5-HTA3 receptor antagonists, cyclobenzaprine, I.V. methylene blue, linezolid, MAO inhibitors, metaxalone, mirtazapine, selective serotonin reuptake inhibitors (SSRIs), serotonin and norepinephrine reuptake inhibitors (SNRIs), tramadol, trazodone, tricyclic antidepressants, triptans: Increased risk of serotonin syndrome

ACTIVITIES

alcohol use: Additive CNS effects, including severe respiratory depression and significant sedation and somnolence

☰ Adverse Reactions

CNS: **Coma**, delirium, depression, disorientation, dizziness, drowsiness, euphoria, hallucinations, headache, lack of coordination, lethargy, light-headedness, mental and physical impairment, mood changes, restlessness, sedation, **seizures**, tremor

CV: **Bradycardia**, **heart block**, hypertension, orthostatic hypotension, palpitations, tachycardia

EENT: Altered taste, blurred vision, diplopia, dry mouth, **laryngeal edema**, **laryngospasm**, miosis

ENDO: **Adrenal insufficiency (rare)**

GI: Abdominal cramps and pain, anorexia, constipation, flatulence, gastroesophageal reflux, ileus, indigestion, nausea, vomiting

GU: Decreased libido, difficult ejaculation, dysuria, erectile dysfunction, impotence, infertility with prolonged use, lack of menstruation, oliguria, ureteral spasm, urinary incontinence, urine retention

MS: Muscle rigidity

RESP: **Apnea**, **bronchoconstriction**, **bronchospasm**, **depressed cough reflex**, **respiratory depression**, **sleep-related breathing disorders (sleep apnea, sleep-related hypoxemia)**

SKIN: Diaphoresis, flushing, pallor, pruritus, rash, urticaria

Other: **Anaphylaxis**, **angioedema**, physical and psychological dependence

☰ Childbearing Considerations

PREGNANCY

- It is not known if drug can cause fetal harm, but drug does cross the placental barrier. However, prolonged use of drug during pregnancy may cause physical dependence in the neonate resulting in neonatal opioid withdrawal syndrome shortly after birth.
- Drug should be used with caution during pregnancy only if benefit to mother outweighs potential risk to fetus.

LABOR & DELIVERY

- Infants exposed to codeine during labor should be assessed for excess sedation and respiratory depression.

- An opioid antagonist, such as naloxone, must be readily available to reverse neonatal adverse effects, if present.

LACTATION

- Drug is present in breast milk.
- Breastfeeding is not recommended during drug therapy.
- If breastfeeding occurs, mother should monitor breastfed infant for breathing difficulties and drowsiness as well as withdrawal symptoms when breastfeeding ceases.

REPRODUCTION

- Chronic use of opioids such as codeine sulfate may reduce fertility in both men and women. It is not known if this effect is reversible.

☰ Nursing Considerations

- Evaluate patient's risk for abuse and addiction prior to the start of codeine therapy as excessive use of the drug may lead to abuse, addiction, misuse, overdose, and possibly death. Be prepared to monitor patient's intake throughout therapy. Because of the potential risks associated with codeine therapy, be aware that the FDA now requires a Risk Evaluation and Mitigation Strategy (REMS) for codeine use to educate the patient.

! **WARNING** Know that the safety and effectiveness of codeine therapy in pediatric patients have not been established. Codeine should not be given to children under the age of 12 for any reason and for adolescents under the age of 18 when used in cold or cough preparations, as well as following adenoidectomy and/or tonsillectomy. Also know that codeine should not be given to children age 12 to 18 if they have other risk factors that may increase their sensitivity to the respiratory depressant effects of codeine. Risk factors include conditions associated with hypoventilation such as concomitant use of other medications that cause respiratory depression or the presence of neuromuscular disease, obesity, obstructive sleep apnea, or severe pulmonary disease. In addition, codeine should not be given to patients who are known ultrarapid metabolizers of codeine, including mothers who are breastfeeding, as breastfed infants have died when exposed to high levels of morphine (codeine converts to morphine) in breast milk.

! WARNING Monitor any patient receiving codeine closely, especially the patient who has never received a narcotic like codeine or morphine, for signs of overdose such as confusion, extreme sleepiness, or shallow breathing, because patient may not know he is an ultrarapid metabolizer. Some patients are ultrarapid metabolizers because of a CYP2D6 polymorphism. How prevalent this phenotype is varies widely. It is estimated that 0.5% to 1% Chinese, Hispanics, and Japanese; 1% to 10% Caucasians; 3% African Americans; and 16% to 28% of Arabs, Ethiopians, and North Africans may carry the CYP2D6 genotype.

- Evaluate patient for therapeutic response, including decreased cough, facial grimacing, and pain.

! WARNING Be aware that opioid therapy like codeine should only be used concomitantly with benzodiazepine therapy in patients for whom other treatment options are inadequate. If prescribed together, expect dosing and duration of the opioid to be limited. Monitor patient closely for signs and symptoms of decrease in consciousness, including coma, profound sedation, and significant respiratory depression. Notify prescriber immediately and provide emergency supportive care, as death may occur.

- Take safety precautions, if needed.
- Monitor respiratory depth, effort, and rate, because codeine can cause respiratory depression that could become life-threatening. Notify prescriber immediately if respiratory rate drops below 10 breaths/min.
- Assess urine output to detect retention.
- Repeated injection in same site may cause tissue irritation, pain, and induration.
- Rotate sites for subcutaneous delivery.

! WARNING Know that many drugs may interact with opioids like codeine to cause serotonin syndrome. Monitor patient closely for signs and symptoms such as agitation, diaphoresis, diarrhea, fever, hallucinations, labile blood pressure, muscle twitching or stiffness, nausea, shakiness, shivering, tachycardia, trouble with coordination, or vomiting. Notify prescriber at once because serotonin syndrome may be life-threatening. Be prepared to discontinue drug, if possible, and provide supportive care.

- Monitor patient for adrenal insufficiency. Although rare, it can be life-threatening. Monitor patient for anorexia, dizziness, fatigue, hypotension, nausea, vomiting, or weakness. Notify prescriber if adrenal insufficiency is suspected and expect diagnostic testing to be done to determine if present. If diagnosis is confirmed, expect to administer corticosteroids and wean patient off codeine, if possible.
- Know that chronic maternal use of codeine during pregnancy can result in neonatal opioid withdrawal syndrome (NOWS), which may be life-threatening, if not recognized and treated appropriately. NOWS occurs when a newborn was exposed to opioid drugs like codeine for a prolonged period while in utero.

PATIENT TEACHING

- Instruct patient to take codeine exactly as prescribed and not to adjust dose or frequency without consulting prescriber, because misuse increases risk of addiction.
- Suggest that patient take drug with food to minimize nausea.
- Advise patient to avoid hazardous activities until drug's CNS effects are known.
- Caution patient to get up slowly from a sitting or lying position.
- Urge patient to consume plenty of fluids and high-fiber foods, if not contraindicated, to prevent constipation.

! WARNING Warn patient not to consume alcohol or take a benzodiazepine during codeine therapy without prescriber knowledge, as severe respiratory depression can occur and may lead to death.

! WARNING Inform patient about potentially fatal additive effects of combining codeine with a benzodiazepine. Instruct patient to inform all prescribers of codeine use.

- Advise patient to report difficulty breathing or shortness of breath.
- Urge breastfeeding women to notify prescriber before taking codeine because

drug appears in breast milk and could lead to overdose in infant.

- Inform patient that long-term use of opioids like codeine may decrease sex hormone levels, causing decreased libido, erectile dysfunction, impotence, infertility, or lack of menstruation. Encourage patient to report any such symptoms.
- Caution pregnant patient not to increase dosage or take codeine for a prolonged period, because infant may experience withdrawal when born.
- Warn patient to keep codeine out of the reach of children to prevent accidental ingestion that could be life-threatening.
- Instruct patient to tell all prescribers of codeine use and not to take any over-the-counter medication, including herbal medicines, without prescriber knowledge.
- Know that naloxone should be readily available to patient at home in the event of an opioid overdose, especially if patient uses concomitant CNS depressants, has a history of opioid use disorder, prior opioid overdose, or there are household members or other close contacts at risk for accidental ingestion or overdose. Provide instruction on how to administer naloxone.

colchicine

Colcrys, Gloperba, Mitigare

▤ Class and Category

Pharmacologic class: Colchicum alkaloid derivative
Therapeutic class: Antigout

▤ Indications and Dosages

✱ *To prevent gouty arthritis attacks*

CAPSULES, ORAL SOLUTION, TABLETS

Adults and adolescents age 16 and over.
0.6 mg once or twice daily. *Maximum:* 1.2 mg daily.

✱ *To treat acute gouty arthritis*

TABLETS (COLCRYS)

Adults. *Initial:* 1.2 mg at first sign of flare; then 0.6 mg 1 hr later. *Maximum:* 1.8 mg over a 1-hr period.

✱ *To treat familial Mediterranean fever (FMF)*

TABLETS (COLCRYS)

Adults and adolescents ages 12 and over.
1.2 mg to 2.4 mg daily, given in one to two divided doses, with dosage increments made in 0.3 mg/day to maximum dose or dosage decrements made in 0.3 mg/day for intolerable adverse reactions. *Maximum:* 2.4 mg daily in one or two divided doses.

Children ages 6 to 12. 0.9 to 1.8 mg daily, given in one or two divided doses.
Children ages 4 to 6. 0.3 to 1.8 mg daily, given in one or two divided doses.

±**DOSAGE ADJUSTMENT (Colcrys)** If treatment of a gout flare occurs during prophylactic treatment, dosage shouldn't exceed 1.2 mg at the first sign of flare, followed by 0.6 mg 1 hr later, and then prophylactic dose resumed 12 hr later. For patients taking strong CYP3A4 inhibitors (atazanavir, clarithromycin, indinavir, itraconazole, ketoconazole, nefazodone, nelfinavir, ritonavir, saquinavir, telithromycin) within 14 days, moderate CYP3A4 inhibitors (amprenavir, aprepitant, diltiazem, erythromycin, fluconazole, fosamprenavir, grapefruit juice, verapamil) within 14 days, P-gp inhibitors (cyclosporine, ranolazine) within 14 days, or protease inhibitors, dosage may be reduced, dosage interval may be increased, and dose not repeated for 3 days. For patients with severe renal impairment including patients receiving dialysis, dosage adjustment may be required and interval between treatment courses may be increased. For patients with severe hepatic impairment receiving colchicine prophylactically, dosage is decreased. For patients with severe hepatic impairment receiving colchicine treatment for acute gout flare, dosage is not adjusted but treatment course shouldn't be repeated more than once every 2 weeks.

▤ Drug Administration

P.O.

- If a dose is missed for patient taking drug for treatment of a gout flare during prophylaxis, the missed dose should be given immediately, then wait 12 hours, and resume previous dosing schedule. For all other missed doses, drug should be given as soon as possible. Dose should never be doubled.
- Do not administer drug with grapefruit juice.

Route	Onset	Peak	Duration
P.O.	18–24 hr	42–72 hr	Unknown

Half-life: 27–31 hr

Contraindications

Both hepatic and renal impairment present; concurrent use with strong CYP3A4 inhibitors or P-glycoprotein inhibitors in patients with hepatic or renal impairment; hypersensitivity to colchicine or its components

Interactions

DRUGS

clarithromycin, cyclosporin, ranolazine: Significant increase in colchicine plasma levels with possible fatal colchicine toxicity
digoxin; HMG-CoA reductase inhibitors, such as atorvastatin, fluvastatin, lovastatin, pravastatin, simvastatin; other lipid-lowering drugs, such as fibrates, gemfibrozil: Increased risk of myopathy and rhabdomyolysis

diltiazem, verapamil: Significant increase in colchicine plasma concentration with increased risk of colchicine toxicity; neuromuscular toxicity
moderate CYP3A4 inhibitors, such as amprenavir, aprepitant, erythromycin, fluconazole, fosamprenavir: Increased risk of colchicine toxicity
strong CYP3A4 inhibitors, such as atazanavir, darunavir/ritonavir, indinavir, itraconazole, ketoconazole, lopinavir/ritonavir, nefazodone, nelfinavir, ritonavir, saquinavir, telithromycin, tipranavir/ritonavir: Significant increase in colchicine plasma levels with high risk of toxicity

ACTIVITIES

alcohol use: Increased risk of adverse GI effects

FOOD

grapefruit juice: Increased risk of colchicine toxicity

Adverse Reactions

CNS: Peripheral neuropathy
GI: Abdominal pain, anorexia, diarrhea, nausea, vomiting
HEME: Agranulocytosis, aplastic anemia, thrombocytopenia
MS: Myopathy
SKIN: Alopecia, rash

Childbearing Considerations

PREGNANCY

- It is not known if drug can cause fetal harm but it does cross the placental barrier.
- Drug should be used with caution during pregnancy only if benefit to mother outweighs potential risk to fetus.

LACTATION

- Drug is present in breast milk.
- Patient should check with prescriber before breastfeeding.

REPRODUCTION

- Drug may cause infertility in males, although rare and possibly reversible.

Nursing Considerations

- Know that debilitated or elderly patients and those with a history of cardiac disease or impaired hepatic or renal function are at increased risk for cumulative toxicity.
- Expect to monitor CBC and platelet and reticulocyte counts at baseline and every 3 months after therapy starts.

Mechanism of Action

In gouty arthritis, leukocytes phagocytose urate crystals occuring in affected joints, a process that releases chemotactic factors, degradation enzymes, and other inflammatory substances. Colchicine helps stop this process, probably by disrupting microtubules in leukocytes. Normally, microtubules contribute to cell structure and movement. When colchicine binds to tubulin (protein from which microtubules are made), the microtubule falls apart, as shown. This process disrupts cell function and prevents leukocytes from invading joints and causing inflammation.

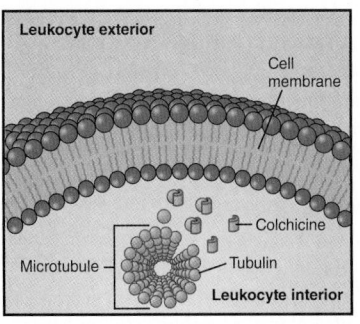

Leukocyte exterior

Cell membrane

Colchicine

Microtubule — Tubulin

Leukocyte interior

- Notify prescriber immediately and expect to stop colchicine if patient develops evidence of toxicity, such as abdominal pain, diarrhea, nausea, or vomiting.

PATIENT TEACHING

- Caution patient not to take drug with grapefruit juice. Review what to do if a dose is missed.
- Instruct patient to have blood tests every 3 months, as ordered, during therapy.
- Explain that gouty arthritis pain and swelling typically subside in 24 to 48 hours after therapy begins.
- Advise patient to notify prescriber immediately if abdominal pain, diarrhea, nausea, or vomiting occurs.
- Tell patient to inform all prescribers of colchicine therapy, especially if patient has kidney or liver dysfunction, because of potential drug interactions.

colesevelam hydrochloride
Welchol

Class and Category
Pharmacologic class: Bile acid sequestrant
Therapeutic class: Antilipemic, hypoglycemic

Indications and Dosages

✱ *As adjunct to diet and exercise to improve glycemic control in type 2 diabetes mellitus*

ORAL SUSPENSION, TABLETS
Adults. 3.75 g once daily.

✱ *As adjunct to diet and exercise to reduce elevated LDL cholesterol levels in patients with primary hypercholesterolemia and in boys and postmenarchal girls age 10 to 17 with heterozygous familial hypercholesterolemia who are unable to reach LDL-C target levels despite an adequate trial of dietary therapy and lifestyle modification*

ORAL SUSPENSION, TABLETS
Adults and children age 10 to 17. 3.75 g once daily.

Drug Administration

P.O.

- Administer 6 tablets once daily or 3 tablets twice daily with a meal and a beverage. Protect tablets from moisture.

- Administer oral suspension once daily with a meal. To prepare oral suspension, empty the entire contents of one packet into a glass, adding 8 ounces of diet soft drink, fruit juice, or water. Stir well and give patient to drink. Never administer the dry powder without mixing.
- Do not administer oral suspension to patients with PKU, as each 3.75-gram packet contains 27 mg of phenylalanine.
- Do not administer other drugs at the same time as colesevelam, because drug may interfere with absorption.

Route	Onset	Peak	Duration
P.O.	Unknown	2 wk	Unknown

Half-life: Not metabolized

Mechanism of Action
Binds with bile acids in intestine, preventing their absorption and forming an insoluble complex that's excreted in feces. This action decreases amount of bile acids returning through enterohepatic circulation to the liver. As a result, the liver must convert more cholesterol to bile acids, which increases liver's demand for cholesterol. This, in turn, causes increase in production and activity of the hepatic enzyme hydroxymethyl-glutaryl-coenzyme A (HMG-CoA) reductase, which is needed for cholesterol production. However, synthesis of cholesterol in the liver typically can't match the amount needed to synthesize bile acids. Because cholesterol levels can't be sustained, LDLs, lipoproteins composed mostly of cholesterol, are increasingly removed from the blood, thereby decreasing the LDL level in the blood.

How glycemic control is improved in patients with type 2 diabetes mellitus is unknown.

Contraindications
History of bowel obstruction or pancreatitis induced by hypertriglyceridemia, hypersensitivity to colesevelam or its components, serum triglyceride level greater than 500 mg/dl

Interactions

DRUGS

cyclosporine, drugs with narrow therapeutic index, fat-soluble vitamins, glimepiride, glipizide, glyburide, olmesartan, oral contraceptives containing ethinyl estradiol and

norethindrone, thyroid hormone replacement:
Possibly altered effectiveness of these drugs
metformin E.R.: Increased blood metformin
level, increasing risk of hypoglycemia
phenytoin: Decreased plasma phenytoin
levels, increasing risk of seizures
warfarin: Reduced INR, increasing risk of
clotting

Adverse Reactions

CNS: Asthenia, headache (children)
CV: Hypertension, hypertriglyceridemia
EENT: Oral blistering, pharyngitis, rhinitis
ENDO: Hypertriglyceridemia, hypoglycemia
GI: Abdominal distention or pain, bowel
or esophageal obstruction, constipation,
dyspepsia, dysphagia, elevated liver enzymes,
fecal impaction, indigestion, nausea,
pancreatitis, worsening of hemorrhoids,
vomiting (children)
MS: Myalgia
SKIN: Rash
Other: Elevated creatine phosphokinase
(children), fat-soluble vitamin deficiencies,
flu-like syndrome

Childbearing Considerations

PREGNANCY

- It is not known if drug can cause fetal harm.
  However, drug is not absorbed systemically
  and is not expected to result in fetal
  exposure.
- Drug should be used with caution during
  pregnancy only if benefit to mother
  outweighs potential risk to fetus.

LACTATION

- It is not known if drug is present in breast
  milk but is thought not to be since it is not
  absorbed systemically.
- Patient should check with prescriber before
  breastfeeding.

REPRODUCTION

- Females using oral contraceptives should
  take the contraceptive at least 4 hours
  before taking drug.

Nursing Considerations

- Know that colesevelam shouldn't be given
  to patients with gastroparesis or other GI
  motility disorders or to patients who had
  major GI tract surgery and are at risk for
  bowel obstruction from constipating effects.
- Use cautiously in patients with dysphagia
  or esophageal obstruction because size of

tablet can cause dysphagia or esophageal
obstruction.
- Use colesevelam cautiously in patients
  whose total triglycerides exceed 300 mg/dl;
  bile acid sequestrants can increase it.
- Evaluate patient's lipid levels before starting
  therapy for primary hyperlipidemia, again
  in 4 to 6 weeks, and then periodically,
  as ordered, during therapy. Expect drug
  to be discontinued if patient develops
  hypertriglyceridemia-induced pancreatitis
  or triglyceride level exceeds 500 mg/dl.
- Monitor diabetic patient's blood glucose
  level regularly, as ordered, to assess
  effectiveness of colesevelam therapy.
- Know that when giving colesevelam with a
  drug that has a narrow therapeutic index,
  expect to give that drug at least 4 hours
  before colesevelam to prevent reduced
  effectiveness.

! **WARNING** Monitor patients with preexisting
constipation, who are at increased risk for
developing fecal impaction.

- Monitor frequency of bowel movements
  and consistency of stools in patients with
  coronary artery disease or hemorrhoids
  because constipation may aggravate these
  conditions.

PATIENT TEACHING

- Instruct patient to take tablets with meals
  and drink plenty of liquids when taking it.
  Tell patient to protect tablets from moisture.

! **WARNING** Alert patient or caregiver
prescribed oral suspension form that it
contains phenylalanine and should not be
taken by anyone who has a PKU diagnosis.
If PKU is present, instruct patient not to take
oral suspension and notify prescriber to get a
different form of the drug.

- Instruct patient prescribed the oral
  suspension form to mix 1 packet with
  8 ounces of diet soft drinks, fruit juice, or
  water; stir well; and then drink immediately.
  Caution patient never to ingest the contents
  of the packet dry. Tell patient to take the
  drug, regardless of form, with a meal.
- Caution patient against changing prescribed
  dosage or stopping colesevelam abruptly
  because serum lipid level may increase
  significantly.

- Remind patient that drug therapy doesn't reduce the need for dietary changes.
- Urge patient to keep regularly scheduled appointments for follow-up blood tests.
- Instruct patient to take colesevelam separately from other drugs, as it may decrease or delay absorption of other drugs.
- Tell patient to promptly seek medical attention and stop taking colesevelam if severe abdominal pain with or without nausea and vomiting occurs or severe constipation.
- Advise patient to take oral contraceptives and vitamins at least 4 hours before taking colesevelam.

colestipol hydrochloride
Colestid

Class and Category
Pharmacologic class: Bile acid sequestrant
Therapeutic class: Antihyperlipidemic

Indications and Dosages
✳ *As adjunct to diet and exercise to reduce elevated serum total and LDL-C in patients with primary hypercholesterolemia*

GRANULES
Adults. *Initial:* 5 g once or twice daily. Then, increased, as needed, by 5 g per day at 1- to 2-month intervals. *Maximum:* 30 g daily.

TABLETS
Adults. *Initial:* 2 g once daily or in divided doses twice daily, increased every 1 to 2 months in 2-g increments once or twice daily. *Maximum:* 16 g daily.

Drug Administration
P.O.
- Give drug with meals.
- Mix granules in at least 3 ounces of water or a beverage such as a heavy or pulpy juice. Although carbonated beverages may be used, this mixture may cause GI upset. Stir mixture until drug is completely mixed. Know that granules will not be dissolved. After mixture is administered, rinse container with small amount of additional liquid and give to patient to drink.

- Granules may also be mixed with milk in hot or regular breakfast cereals, soups with a high fluid content, or pulpy fruits such as crushed pineapples, fruit cocktail, peaches, or pears.
- Never administer granules in dry form.
- Tablets must be taken one at a time and promptly swallowed whole. Give with plenty of water or other liquid.
- Tablets should not be chewed, crushed, or cut.
- Other drugs should be taken at least one hour before or 4 hours after drug.

Route	Onset	Peak	Duration
P.O.	24–48 hr	Unknown	Unknown

Half-life: Not metabolized

Mechanism of Action
Combines with bile acids in the intestine, preventing their absorption and forming an insoluble complex that's excreted in feces. Loss of bile acids increases hepatic production of cholesterol to form new bile acids and increases oxidation of cholesterol to bile acids. Depletion of cholesterol increases hepatic LDL receptor activity, which removes LDLs from the blood.

Contraindications
Complete biliary obstruction, hypersensitivity to colestipol or its components

Interactions
DRUGS
digoxin, hydrocortisone, oral phosphate supplements: Possible binding of these drugs decreasing their effectiveness
furosemide, gemfibrozil, penicillin G, propranolol, tetracycline, thiazide diuretics: Decreased absorption of these drugs
mycophenolic acid: Possibly reduced effectiveness of mycophenolic acid
oral drugs: Possibly decreased absorption of oral drugs
vancomycin (oral): Possibly marked decrease in vancomycin antibacterial action
vitamins (fat-soluble): Possibly interference with vitamin absorption

Adverse Reactions
CNS: Headache
GI: Abdominal distention and pain, constipation, diarrhea, eructation, esophageal reaction, fecal impaction, heartburn, nausea, vomiting

Childbearing Considerations
PREGNANCY
- It is not known if drug can cause fetal harm. However, drug is not absorbed systemically and is not expected to result in fetal exposure.
- Be aware that drug interferes with absorption of fat-soluble vitamins, which may make regular prenatal supplementation inadequate.
- Drug should be used with caution only if benefit to mother outweighs potential risk to fetus.

LACTATION
- It is not known if drug is present in breast milk.
- Patient should check with prescriber before breastfeeding.
- Be aware that the possibility of a lack of proper vitamin absorption may affect the breastfed infant.

Nursing Considerations
- Make sure patient has adequate fluid intake, and obtain an order for a stool softener or laxative to prevent constipation. To prevent impaction, expect to decrease dosage or discontinue drug if constipation occurs or worsens.
- Expect to discontinue drug if no response occurs after 3 months.
- Monitor patient's serum cholesterol level as appropriate, usually at baseline, 4 to 6 weeks after starting therapy, and then every 3 months. Expect to reduce monitoring frequency to every 4 months if response is adequate.
- Be aware that HDL and serum triglyceride levels may increase or remain unchanged during colestipol therapy.
- Keep in mind that adverse GI reactions are more common in patients over age 60.

PATIENT TEACHING
- Tell patient to mix granules in at least 3 ounces of water or a beverage such as a heavy or pulpy juice. Although carbonated beverages may be used, this mixture may cause GI upset. Mixture should be stirred until drug is completely mixed. Alert patient that granules will not be dissolved. After taking mixture, tell patient to add a small amount of additional liquid to the container and drink it.
- Advise patient that granules may also be mixed with milk in hot or regular breakfast cereals, soups with a high fluid content, or pulpy fruits such as crushed pineapples, fruit cocktail, peaches, or pears.
- Warn patient to never administer granules in dry form.
- Tell patient tablets must be taken one at a time and promptly swallowed whole. Tablets should not be chewed, crushed, or cut.
- Remind patient that colestipol doesn't reduce the importance of dietary changes.
- Caution patient not to decrease or increase prescribed dosage or to stop taking drug suddenly. Explain that stopping drug abruptly may significantly increase serum lipid levels.
- Instruct patient to keep appointments for follow-up blood tests.
- Teach patient how to prevent constipation, and advise him to contact prescriber if constipation occurs or worsens.

conivaptan hydrochloride
Vaprisol

Class and Category
Pharmacologic class: Arginine vasopressin antagonist
Therapeutic class: Aquaretic (sodium/water stabilizer)

Indications and Dosages
* *To treat euvolemic and hypervolemic hyponatremia in hospitalized patients*

I.V. INFUSION
Adults. *Loading dose:* 20 mg over 30 minutes followed by 20 mg as a continuous infusion over 24 hours. Additional 20 mg/24 hr, increased to 40 mg/24 hr, if needed, given by continuous infusion for 1 to 3 days. *Maximum:* 40 mg daily with total duration of therapy, after loading dose, not to exceed 4 days.
±**DOSAGE ADJUSTMENT** For patient with moderate hepatic impairment, loading dose decreased to 10 mg over 30 minutes followed by a decrease in daily dose to 10 mg/day as a continuous infusion for 2 to 4 days. If serum

sodium level does not rise, dosage may be titrated up to 20 mg/day.

Drug Administration

I.V.

- Store ampules in cardboard container, protected from light, until ready for use.
- Drug is supplied as ready-to-use with no further dilution necessary.
- Do not remove container from overwrap, which is a light and moisture barrier, until ready for use. When ready, tear overwrap down side at slit and remove solution container. Some opacity of the plastic may be present, but this is normal and will diminish gradually.
- Check for minute leaks by squeezing inner container firmly. Do not use if leaks are found or if solution is cloudy or a precipitate is present.
- Administer loading dose of 20 mg over 30 minutes through a large vein followed by a continuous infusion over 24 hours for 1 to 3 days.
- Drug is compatible with 5% Dextrose Injection and 0.9% Sodium Chloride Injection. When given with 0.9% Sodium Chloride Injection, drug is compatible for 48 hours when the two solutions are co-administered via a Y-site connection. Infusion rate for drug should be 4.2 ml/hr and the flow rate for 0.9% Sodium Chloride solution administered at either 2.1 ml/hr or 6.3 ml/hr, unless otherwise ordered.
- Do not use plastic containers in series connections.
- Change infusion site every 24 hours.
- Do not administer drug longer than 4 days.
- *Incompatibilities:* Furosemide injection and Lactated Ringer's Injection when mixed in same container; other drugs in same intravenous line or container

Route	Onset	Peak	Duration
I.V.	Unknown	Unknown	12 hr

Half-life: 5 hr

Mechanism of Action

Binds with arginine vasopressin V2 receptor sites in collecting ducts of kidneys. By doing so, drug blocks action of arginine vasopressin on V2 receptor, decreases water resorption in collecting ducts, increases excretion of free water (urine output), and increases serum sodium concentration, thus correcting water and sodium imbalance.

Incompatibilities

Don't mix with Lactated Ringer's Solution, normal saline solution, or other drugs.

Contraindications

Anuria; hypersensitivity to conivaptan or its components or to corn or corn products; patients with hypovolemic hyponatremia; use with potent CYP3A4 inhibitors such as clarithromycin, indinavir, itraconazole, ketoconazole, and ritonavir

Interactions

DRUGS

clarithromycin, indinavir, itraconazole, ketoconazole, ritonavir, and other strong CYP3A inhibitors: Increased blood conivaptan level
CYP3A substrates: Increased exposure of these drugs
digoxin: Possibly increased digoxin level and risk of digoxin toxicity
drugs metabolized by CYP3A, such as HMG-CoA reductase inhibitors; CYP3A substrates: Possibly increased risk of rhabdomyolysis

Adverse Reactions

CNS: Confusion, fever, headache, insomnia
CV: Atrial fibrillation, hypertension, hypotension, orthostatic hypotension, peripheral edema
EENT: Dry mouth, oral candidiasis, pharyngeal pain
ENDO: Hyperglycemia, hypoglycemia
GI: Constipation, diarrhea, nausea, thirst, vomiting
GU: Hematuria, pollakiuria, polyuria, UTI
HEME: Anemia
RESP: Pneumonia
SKIN: Erythema, pruritus
Other: Dehydration, hypokalemia, hypomagnesemia, hyponatremia, infusion-site reactions (erythema, pain, phlebitis, swelling)

Childbearing Considerations

PREGNANCY

- It is not known if drug can cause fetal harm.
- Drug should be used with caution during pregnancy only if benefit to mother outweighs potential risk to fetus.

LACTATION

- It is not known if drug is present in breast milk.
- Breastfeeding should not be undertaken during drug therapy because of the potential for serious adverse reactions such as electrolyte abnormalities, hypotension, and volume depletion in the breastfed infant.

☰ Nursing Considerations

- Know that conivaptan shouldn't be used to treat patients with heart failure, nor is it recommended in patients with severe renal impairment because of a high incidence of infusion-site phlebitis, which can reduce potential vascular access sites.
- Use cautiously in patients with hepatic or mild to moderate renal dysfunction because levels remain elevated longer in these patients.
- Be aware that drug may cause serious infusion-site reactions even when infused correctly. Inspect site regularly; change immediately if reactions occur.
- Monitor neurologic status and serum sodium level closely during therapy because rapid increase in serum sodium level (more than 12 mEq/L/24 hr) may result in serious neurologic impairment. If serum sodium level rises faster than expected, stop infusion temporarily and notify prescriber. If it keeps rising, expect conivaptan to be discontinued. If hyponatremia persists or recurs and patient has no neurologic abnormalities, drug may be resumed at a reduced rate.
- Monitor vital signs, and assess patient regularly for hypovolemia. If patient develops hypotension or hypovolemia while receiving conivaptan, stop infusion, notify prescriber, and provide supportive care, as prescribed. After hypotension and hypovolemia have been corrected, drug may be resumed at a reduced rate.

PATIENT TEACHING

- Instruct patient to report any infusion-site discomfort immediately.
- Tell patient that frequent laboratory tests will be performed to monitor his serum sodium level and volume status.

cortisone acetate

Cortisone Acetate (CAN), Cortone (CAN), Cortone Acetate

☰ Class and Category

Pharmacologic class: Glucocorticoid
Therapeutic class: Anti-inflammatory, corticosteroid replacement, immunosuppressant

☰ Indications and Dosages

✱ *To treat allergic and inflammatory disorders, collagen disorders, congenital adrenal hyperplasia, dermatologic disorders, edema (from nephrotic syndrome or systemic lupus erythematosus), endocrine disorders, GI disorders, hematologic disorders, multiple sclerosis (acute exacerbations), neoplastic diseases, ophthalmic disorders, primary or secondary adrenocortical insufficiency, respiratory disorders, rheumatic disorders, trichinosis with myocardial or neurologic involvement, and tuberculous meningitis*

TABLETS

Adults and adolescents. *Initial:* 25 to 300 mg once daily or equally divided and given twice daily. *Maintenance:* Dosage adjusted based on patient response.

☰ Drug Administration

P.O.

- Administer with food.

Route	Onset	Peak	Duration
P.O.	1–2 hr	2–4 hr	30–36 hr

Half-life: 30–60 min

☰ Mechanism of Action

Binds to intracellular glucocorticoid receptors and suppresses inflammatory and immune responses by:

- inhibiting neutrophil and monocyte accumulation at the inflammation site and suppressing their phagocytic and bactericidal activity
- stabilizing lysosomal membranes
- suppressing the antigen response of macrophages and helper T cells
- inhibiting synthesis of cellular mediators of inflammatory response, such as cytokines, interleukins, and prostaglandins

Contraindications

Hypersensitivity to cortisone or its components, idiopathic thrombocytopenic purpura (parenteral form), live-virus vaccine administration, systemic fungal infection

Interactions

DRUGS

ephedrine, phenobarbital, phenytoin, rifampin: Deceased blood levels of cortisone
oral anticoagulants: Possibly obstructed anticoagulant effects
potassium-wasting diuretics: Possibly hypokalemia

Adverse Reactions

CNS: Ataxia, behavior changes, depression, dizziness, euphoria, fatigue, headache, **increased intracranial pressure with papilledema,** insomnia, lassitude, malaise, mood swings, paresthesia, **seizures,** steroid psychosis, syncope, vertigo
CV: Arrhythmias, fat embolism, heart failure, hypertension, **hypotension,** thrombophlebitis
EENT: Exophthalmos, glaucoma, increased intraocular pressure, nystagmus, posterior subcapsular cataracts
ENDO: Adrenal insufficiency, Cushing's syndrome, diabetes mellitus, growth suppression in children, hyperglycemia, negative nitrogen balance from protein catabolism
GI: Abdominal distention, hiccups, increased appetite, nausea, **pancreatitis,** peptic ulcer, ulcerative esophagitis, vomiting
GU: Glycosuria, menstrual irregularities, perineal burning or tingling
HEME: Leukocytosis
MS: Arthralgia; aseptic necrosis of femoral and humeral heads; compression fractures; muscle atrophy, twitching, and weakness; myalgia; osteoporosis; spontaneous fractures; steroid myopathy; tendon rupture
SKIN: Acne; diaphoresis; ecchymosis; erythema; hirsutism; hyperpigmentation; hypopigmentation; necrotizing vasculitis; petechiae; purpura; rash; scarring; sterile abscesses; striae; subcutaneous fat atrophy; thin, fragile skin; urticaria
Other: Anaphylaxis, hypocalcemia, hypokalemia, hypokalemic alkalosis, impaired wound healing, masking of infection, **metabolic alkalosis,** suppressed skin test reaction, weight gain

Childbearing Considerations

PREGNANCY

- It is not known if drug can cause fetal harm.
- Drug should be used with caution during pregnancy only if benefit to mother outweighs potential risk to fetus.
- Monitor infant for hypoadrenalism if mother has received large doses of cortisone during pregnancy.

LACTATION

- Drug is present in breast milk.
- Breastfeeding should not be undertaken with drug therapy because of potential serious adverse reactions in breastfed infant.

Nursing Considerations

- Use cortisone cautiously in patients with ocular herpes simplex because corneal perforation may occur.
- Expect prescriber to order baseline ophthalmologic examination before therapy starts because prolonged use of cortisone may result in glaucoma, increased intraocular pressure, and damage to optic nerve.
- Assess patient for signs and symptoms of infection before giving cortisone, because drug may mask them. Be aware that new infections may develop during therapy because of risk of immunosuppression. If a new infection develops, expect to administer appropriate antibiotics.
- Obtain serum electrolyte levels before therapy, as ordered, and monitor results often during therapy to detect electrolyte imbalances. Increased calcium excretion, potassium depletion, and sodium and water retention may occur with large doses of cortisone. Anticipate the need for calcium and potassium supplementation and sodium restriction, if indicated.
- Keep in mind that prescriber will order lowest effective dose.
- Expect patient to receive concurrent antacid or antihistamine therapy to prevent peptic ulcer from cortisone.

! **WARNING** Be aware that live-virus vaccines shouldn't be given during cortisone therapy because patient may become immunosuppressed and develop the viral infection.

! WARNING Assess for adrenal suppression or insufficiency (fatigue, hypotension, lassitude, nausea, vomiting, and weakness) in patient exposed to stress or receiving prolonged cortisone therapy. Notify prescriber immediately if patient has evidence of this life-threatening adverse reaction.

- Watch for signs and symptoms of steroid psychosis (confusion, delirium, euphoria, insomnia, mood swings, personality changes, severe depression), which may develop 15 to 30 days after starting drug. Be prepared to stop drug if such signs occur. If stopping isn't possible, expect to administer a psychotropic drug.
- Watch for cushingoid signs, such as acne, buffalo hump, central obesity, ecchymosis, moon face, striae, and weight gain. Notify prescriber at once if they occur.
- Expect to taper oral cortisone dosage slowly to prevent withdrawal syndrome (abdominal or back pain, anorexia, dizziness, fever, headache, and syncope).

PATIENT TEACHING

- Instruct patient to take oral cortisone exactly as prescribed. Advise him to take it with food to prevent GI distress.
- Caution patient not to stop drug abruptly because doing so may lead to adrenal insufficiency, withdrawal symptoms, or both.
- Inform patient about adrenal insufficiency and need for possible dosage increases during stress. Advise him to notify prescriber immediately if signs or symptoms develop or if he's exposed to stress.
- Caution patient to avoid exposure to people with infections because cortisone can cause immunosuppression. Also, teach him to recognize and immediately report signs and symptoms of infection.
- Teach patient to recognize and report adverse reactions, including Cushing's syndrome.
- Urge patient receiving long-term cortisone therapy to carry medical identification.
- Recommend regular eye examinations.
- Urge patient to keep follow-up appointments with prescriber, which may include laboratory tests, to evaluate effects of therapy.

crizanlizumab-tmca
Adakveo

Class and Category
Pharmacologic class: Monoclonal antibody (P-selectin blocker)
Therapeutic class: Anti-vaso-occlusive

Indications and Dosages
* *To reduce the frequency of vaso-occlusive crises in patients with sickle cell disease*

I.V. INFUSION

Adults and adolescents age 16 and older.
5 mg/kg at wk 0, wk 2, and every 4 wk thereafter.

Drug Administration
I.V.

- Calculate the number of vials needed for administration. One vial is needed for every 100 mg (10 mL) of crizanlizumab-tmca. Bring vials to room temperature for a maximum of 4 hours prior to the start of preparation (piercing the first vial).
- Visually inspect vials. Solution should be clear to opalescent, colorless, or may have a slightly brownish yellow tint.
- Obtain a 100-ml 0.9% Sodium Chloride Injection or 5% Dextrose Injection infusion bag/container made of polyvinyl chloride (PVC), polyethylene (PE), or polypropylene (PP).
- Remove a volume of solution from the infusion bag/container that is equal to the required volume of the drug. Withdraw the necessary amount of drug solution and dilute by adding to the infusion bag/container. The volume added to the infusion bag/container should not exceed 96 ml.
- Gently invert infusion bag to mix diluted solution. Do not shake. Discard unused portion in drug vials.
- Administer diluted drug solution as soon as possible. If not administered immediately, store prepared solution at room temperature for no more than 4.5 hours from the start of preparation (piercing the first vial) to the completion of infusion, or refrigerate for no more than 24 hours from the start of preparation (piercing the first vial) to the completion of infusion. This includes storage of the diluted solution and time to warm up

C

to room temperature. Protect diluted solution from light during storage under refrigeration.

- Infuse diluted solution over a period of 30 minutes through an intravenous line, which must contain a sterile, nonpyrogenic 0.2-micron inline filter.
- After administration of drug, flush the line with at least 25 ml of 0.9% Sodium Chloride Injection or 5% Dextrose Injection.
- Adjust dosage schedule for missed doses. If a dose is missed, it should be administered as soon as possible. If drug is administered within 2 weeks after the missed dose, dosage schedule continues according to patient's original schedule. If dose is administered more than 2 weeks after it was missed, dosing is continued every 4 weeks thereafter.
- *Incompatibilities:* Other drugs through the same intravenous line

Route	Onset	Peak	Duration
I.V.	Unknown	Unknown	Unknown

Half-life: 10.6 days

Mechanism of Action

Binds to P-selectin to block interactions with its ligands, including P-selectin glycoprotein ligand 1. Binding P-selectin on the surface of the activated endothelium and platelets blocks interactions between endothelial cells, leukocytes, platelets, and red blood cells, which reduces vaso-occlusion.

Contraindications

Hypersensitivity to crizanlizumab-tmca or its components

Interactions

DRUGS

None reported by manufacturer

Adverse Reactions

CNS: Fever
EENT: Oropharyngeal pain
GI: Abdominal discomfort, pain, or tenderness; diarrhea; nausea; vomiting
GU: Vulvovaginal pruritus
MS: Arthralgia, back pain, musculoskeletal chest pain, myalgia
SKIN: Pruritus
Other: Crizanlizumab-tmca–induced antibodies, infusion-related reactions (chills, dizziness, fatigue, fever, nausea, pruritus, shortness of breath, sweating, urticaria,

vomiting, wheezing), infusion-site reactions (extravasation, pain, swelling)

Childbearing Considerations

PREGNANCY

- Drug has potential to cause fetal harm, based on animal studies.
- Use with caution only if benefit to mother outweighs potential risk to fetus.

LACTATION

- It is not known if drug is present in breast milk.
- Patient should check with prescriber before breastfeeding.

Nursing Considerations

- Know that crizanlizumab-tmca may be given with or without hydroxyurea.

! **WARNING** Monitor patient for infusion-related reactions. If severe, notify prescriber, discontinue infusion, and institute treatment protocol, as prescribed.

- Be aware that crizanlizumab-tmca interferes with automated platelet counts (platelet clumping), particularly when blood samples are collected in tubes containing EDTA, which may lead to unevaluable or falsely decreased platelet counts. Blood samples should be run within 4 hours of blood collection, or blood samples should be collected in tubes containing citrate. If needed, estimate platelet count via peripheral blood smear.

PATIENT TEACHING

- Inform patient that infusion-related reactions may occur. Review these reactions with patient. Advise patient to immediately report any signs or symptoms of an infusion-related reaction, including after leaving the healthcare facility.
- Instruct patient to inform healthcare provider that they are receiving crizanlizumab-tmca prior to any blood tests, due to the potential interference with laboratory tests used to measure platelet counts.

crofelemer
Mytesi

Class and Category

Pharmacologic class: Botanical
Therapeutic class: Antidiarrheal

☰ Indications and Dosages

❋ *To provide symptomatic relief of noninfectious diarrhea in patients with HIV/AIDS on antiretroviral therapy*

D.R. TABLETS

Adults. 125 mg twice daily.

☰ Drug Administration

P.O.

▪ D.R. tablets should be swallowed whole and not chewed, crushed, or split.

Route	Onset	Peak	Duration
P.O./E.R.	45–60 min	>2 hr	3–4 hr

Half-life: Not significantly absorbed

☰ Mechanism of Action

Inhibits both the cyclic adenosine monophosphate (cAMP)-stimulated cystic fibrosis transmembrane conductance regulator (CFTR) chloride ion channel, and the calcium-activated chloride channel (CaCC) at the luminal membrane of enterocytes. By blocking chloride secretion and accompanying high-volume water loss in diarrhea, the flow of chloride and water in the GI tract becomes normalized.

☰ Contraindications

Hypersensitivity to crofelemer or its components

☰ Interactions

None reported by manufacturer

☰ Adverse Reactions

CNS: Anxiety, depression, dizziness
EENT: Dry mouth, nasopharyngitis, sinusitis
GI: Abdominal distention or pain, constipation, dyspepsia, elevated bilirubin or liver enzymes, flatulence, gastroenteritis, giardiasis (intestinal parasitic infection), nausea
GU: Frequent daytime urination syndrome, nephrolithiasis, UTI
HEME: Leukopenia
MS: Arthralgia: back, extremity, or musculoskeletal pain
RESP: Bronchitis, cough, upper respiratory infection
SKIN: Acne, dermatitis
Other: Herpes zoster

☰ Childbearing Considerations

PREGNANCY

▪ It is not known if drug can cause fetal harm but because it is minimally absorbed systemically it is not expected to affect the fetus.

▪ Drug should be used with caution during pregnancy only if benefit to mother outweighs potential risk to fetus.

LACTATION

▪ It is not known if drug is present in breast milk.

▪ The Centers for Disease Control and Prevention recommends that HIV-1-infected mothers not breastfeed to avoid risking postnatal transmission of HIV-1 infection in HIV-negative infants or developing viral resistance in HIV-positive infants. They also do not recommend breastfeeding because of potential drug-induced adverse reactions in the infant.

☰ Nursing Considerations

▪ Be aware that crofelemer is used only to treat noninfectious diarrhea in patients with HIV/AIDS on antiretroviral therapy. Infectious etiologies should be ruled out before drug is started because crofelemer is not effective against infectious causes of diarrhea.

▪ Know that no dosage adjustment is needed related to the patient's CD4 cell count and HIV viral load.

PATIENT TEACHING

▪ Instruct patient to swallow tablet whole, avoiding chewing or crushing tablet.

▪ Inform patient that crofelemer may be taken with or without food.

▪ Advise patient to inform prescriber if no improvement in diarrhea is noted.

cyclobenzaprine hydrochloride

Amrix

☰ Class and Category

Pharmacologic class: Tricyclic antidepressant-like agent (TCA)
Therapeutic class: Skeletal muscle relaxant

☰ Indications and Dosages

❋ *As adjunct to rest and physical therapy for relief of muscle spasm associated with acute, painful musculoskeletal conditions*

TABLETS

Adults and adolescents age 15 and over.
5 mg three times daily, increased as needed

to 10 mg three times daily. *Maximum:* 30 mg daily for no more than 3 wk.

±**DOSAGE ADJUSTMENT** Dosage frequency reduced in elderly patients and those with hepatic impairment.

E.R. CAPSULES (AMRIX)

Adults. 15 mg once daily, increased to 30 mg once daily, as needed. *Maximum:* 30 mg once daily for no longer than 3 weeks.

Drug Administration

P.O.

- Tablets and E.R. capsules should be swallowed whole and not chewed or crushed. Tablets should not be split.
- If patient is unable to swallow E.R. capsule, contents of capsule may be mixed with applesauce. Have patient eat mixture immediately after mixing without chewing. Have patient rinse mouth and swallow afterwards.

Route	Onset	Peak	Duration
P.O.	1 hr	4 hr	12–24 hr
P.O./E.R.	1.5 hr	7–8 hr	Unknown
Half-life: 18–31 hr			

Mechanism of Action

Acts in the brain stem to reduce or abolish tonic muscle hyperactivity. Because cyclobenzaprine doesn't act at the neuromuscular junction or directly on skeletal muscle, it relieves muscle spasm without disrupting muscle function.

Contraindications

Acute recovery phase of MI; arrhythmias, including heart block and other conduction disturbances; heart failure; hypersensitivity to cyclobenzaprine or its components; hyperthyroidism; MAO inhibitor use within 14 days

Interactions

DRUGS

anticholinergics, antidyskinetics: Possibly potentiated anticholinergic effects of these drugs

bupropion, MAO inhibitors, meperidine, selective serotonin reuptake inhibitors (SSRIs), serotonin norepinephrine reuptake inhibitors (SNRIs), tramadol, tricyclic antidepressants,

verapamil: Possibly increased risk of serotonin syndrome

CNS depressants including barbiturates, tricyclic antidepressants: Possibly additive CNS depressant effects of these drugs, increased risk of adverse effects of antidepressants and cyclobenzaprine

guanadrel, guanethidine: Possibly decreased or blocked antihypertensive effects of these drugs

MAO inhibitors: Possibly hyperpyretic crisis, severe seizures, and death

tramadol: Increased risk of seizures

ACTIVITIES

alcohol use: Possibly additive CNS depression

Adverse Reactions

CNS: Aggression, agitation, anxiety, asthenia, ataxia, confusion, **CVA**, delusions, depression, disorientation, dizziness, drowsiness, EEG alterations, extrapyramidal symptoms, fatigue, fever, hallucinations, headache, hypertonia, insomnia, irritability, malaise, **neuroleptic malignant syndrome**, nervousness, paranoia, paresthesia, psychosis, **seizures**, **serotonin syndrome**, syncope, thirst, tremor, vertigo, weakness

CV: Arrhythmias, including tachycardia; **heart block**; hypertension; **hypotension**; MI; orthostatic hypotension; palpitations; peripheral neuropathy; vasodilation

EENT: Blurred vision, diplopia, dry mouth, parotid swelling, **tongue** discoloration or edema, stomatitis, tinnitus transient vision loss, unpleasant taste

ENDO: Breast enlargement, galactorrhea, gynecomastia, hyperglycemia, **hypoglycemia**, syndrome of inappropriate ADH syndrome (SIADH)

GI: Anorexia, cholestasis, constipation, diarrhea, elevated liver enzymes, flatulence, gastrointestinal pain, gastritis, **hepatitis**, hiccups, indigestion, jaundice, nausea, paralytic ileus, vomiting

GU: Libido changes, impotence, testicular swelling urinary frequency, urine retention

HEME: Bone marrow depression, eosinophilia, **leukopenia, thrombocytopenia**

MS: Dysarthria

RESP: Dyspnea

SKIN: Diaphoresis, facial flushing, pruritus, rash, urticaria

OTHER: Anaphylaxis, angioedema, weight changes

☰ Childbearing Considerations

PREGNANCY

- It is not known if drug can cause fetal harm.
- Drug should be used with caution during pregnancy only if benefit to mother outweighs potential risk to fetus.

LACTATION

- It is not known if drug is present in breast milk.
- Patient should check with prescriber before breastfeeding.

☰ Nursing Considerations

- Use cyclobenzaprine cautiously in patients with history of low seizure threshold.
- Be aware that drug is not recommended for use in the elderly because higher plasma levels of cyclobenzaprine occur in the elderly, increasing risk of serious adverse reactions.

! WARNING Monitor patient closely if cyclobenzaprine is being given with other serotonergic drug, especially when treatment is started and during dosage increases, because of the potential for life-threatening serotonin syndrome to develop. Assess patient for autonomic instability, mental status changes, and nervous system abnormalities. If present, stop both cyclobenzaprine and other serotonergic drugs immediately and notify prescriber. Provide supportive care, as ordered.

- Take safety precautions to prevent falls if patient is confused, dizzy, or weak.

PATIENT TEACHING

- Instruct patient that tablets and capsules should be swallowed whole and not chewed or crushed. Tablets should not be split. If patient cannot swallow capsules, they may be opened and contents sprinkled on a tablespoon of applesauce and swallowed immediately without chewing. Tell patient to follow drug with a drink of water.
- Urge patient to avoid alcohol and other CNS depressants during therapy.
- Inform patient about possible lack of alertness and dexterity.
- Advise patient to ask for assistance with walking, driving, or hazardous activities if he experiences dizziness or weakness.

cyclosporine
Sandimmune

cyclosporine (modified)
Gengraf, Neoral

☰ Class and Category

Pharmacologic class: Polypeptide
Therapeutic class: Antipsoriatic, antirheumatic, immunosuppressant

☰ Indications and Dosages

✳ *To prevent or treat organ rejection in heart, kidney, and liver allogenic transplantation*

CAPSULES, MODIFIED CAPSULES, MODIFIED ORAL SOLUTION, ORAL SOLUTION

Adults and children. *Initial:* 15 mg/kg as a single dose 4 to 12 hr before transplantation, followed by 15 mg/kg once daily postoperatively for 1 to 2 wk and then tapered by 5%/wk to maintenance dose. *Maintenance:* 5 to 10 mg/kg daily in divided doses every 12 hr.

I.V. INFUSION

Adults and children. 5 to 6 mg/kg daily starting 4 to 12 hr before surgery. Postoperatively 5 to 6 mg/kg once daily until patient can tolerate oral form of drug.

✳ *To treat severe rheumatoid arthritis in nonimmunocompromised patients who have failed to respond to at least one systemic therapy or in patients for whom other systemic therapies are contraindicated or cannot be tolerated*

MODIFIED CAPSULES, MODIFIED ORAL SOLUTION

Adults. 2.5 mg/kg daily in divided doses every 12 hr, increased by 0.5 to 0.75 mg/kg daily after 8 wk and again after 12 wk. *Maximum:* 4 mg/kg daily.

✳ *To treat severe plaque psoriasis in non-immunocompromised patients who have failed to respond to at least one systemic therapy or in patients for whom other systemic therapies are contraindicated, or cannot be tolerated*

MODIFIED CAPSULES, MODIFIED ORAL SOLUTION

Adults. *Initial:* 2.5 mg/kg daily in divided doses twice daily, increased by 0.5 mg/kg daily after 4 wk. Then dosage increased every 2 wk, if needed. *Maximum:* 4 mg/kg daily.

±**DOSAGE ADJUSTMENT** For patients with severe liver dysfunction, dosage reduced. For patients receiving cyclosporine to treat psoriasis or rheumatoid arthritis and experiencing serious adverse reactions, dosage reduced 25% to 50% in effort to bring adverse reactions under control.

☰ Drug Administration

- Intravenous and oral solutions contain alcohol and shouldn't be administered to patient who drinks heavily or has a history of alcohol dependence. In addition, these forms of cyclosporine should not be used with patients in whom alcohol intake should be avoided or minimized, such as breastfeeding or pregnant women, patients with epilepsy or liver disease, and children. Be aware that for an adult weighing 70 kg or 150 pounds, the maximum daily oral dose would deliver about 6% and a daily intravenous dose would deliver about 15% of the amount of alcohol contained in a standard drink.

P.O.

- Capsules and oral solution aren't interchangeable with modified capsules and modified oral solution. Modified forms have greater bioavailability.
- Neoral is not bioequivalent to Sandimmune and requires close monitoring of blood concentration to avoid the potential of underdosing if a conversion from Neoral to Sandimmune is ordered.
- Administer on a consistent schedule with regard to meals and time of day.
- Avoid giving with grapefruit juice.
- Capsules should not be chewed, crushed, or opened but swallowed whole.
- Administer oral solution doses in oral syringe. Clean outside of dosing syringe with a clean towel and replace protective cover after use. Do not rinse syringe with water or other cleaning agents. However, if syringe must be cleaned, it must be completely dry before reuse.
- To improve taste of Sandimmune oral solution, mix it with chocolate milk, milk, or orange juice. Gengraf or Neoral oral solution may be mixed with apple or orange juice that is at room temperature, but not milk. Don't add water to oral solution because it will alter drug's effectiveness.
- Use a glass container when mixing oral solution with other liquids and have patient drink the mixture at once. Do not let mixture stand before drinking. Rinse glass with more liquid and have patient drink again.

I.V.

- Protect drug from light.
- Prepare I.V. infusion immediately before administration by diluting each milliliter of concentrate in 20 to 100 ml of 0.9% Sodium Chloride Injection or 5% Dextrose Injection. Use glass containers because of possible leaching of diethylhexylphthalate from polyvinyl chloride bags into drug solution.
- Administer I.V. infusion slowly over 2 to 6 hr. Avoid rapid I.V. infusion which may cause acute nephrotoxicity.
- Discard diluted solution after 24 hours.
- *Incompatibilities:* Amphotericin B cholesteryl sulfate complex, magnesium sulfate

Route	Onset	Peak	Duration
P.O.	Unknown	1.5–2 hr	Unknown
I.V.	Unknown	Unknown	Unknown

Half-life: 8.5–27 hr

☰ Mechanism of Action

Causes immunosuppression by inhibiting the proliferation of T lymphocytes, the production and release of lymphokines, and the release of interleukin-2, responsible for organ rejection and in disease processes such as psoriasis and rheumatoid arthritis.

☰ Contraindications

Abnormal renal function, neoplastic diseases, and uncontrolled hypertension in patients with psoriasis or rheumatoid arthritis (modified capsules and oral solution); hypersensitivity to cyclosporine, its components, or polyoxyethylated castor oil (all indications; I.V. infusion for castor oil)

☰ Interactions

DRUGS

ACE inhibitors, angiotensin II receptor antagonists, potassium-sparing diuretics, potassium supplements: Increased risk of hyperkalemia

aliskiren, ambrisentan, bosentan, colchicine, CYP3A4 substrates, dabigatran, digoxin, daunorubicin, doxorubicin, etoposide, HMG-CoA reductase inhibitors (statins), methotrexate, mitoxantrone, NSAIDs, organic anion transporter protein substrates, P-glycoprotein substrates, prednisolone, repaglinide, sirolimus: Increased blood concentrations of these drugs and possible toxicity

allopurinol, amiodarone, azithromycin, bromocriptine, clarithromycin, colchicine, danazol, diltiazem, erythromycin, fluconazole, HIV protease inhibitors, imatinib, itraconazole, ketoconazole, methylprednisolone, metoclopramide, nefazodone, nicardipine, oral contraceptives, quinupristin and dalfopristin, verapamil, voriconazole: Increased cyclosporine level

amphotericin B, azapropazone, cimetidine, ciprofloxacin, colchicine, co-trimoxazole, diclofenac, fibric acid derivatives (bezafibrate, fenofibrate), gentamicin, ketoconazole, melphalan, naproxen, NSAIDs, sirolimus, sulindac, tacrolimus, tobramycin, vancomycin: Increased risk of nephrotoxicity

atorvastatin, fluvastatin, lovastatin, pravastatin, simvastatin: Risk of myotoxicity

bosentan, carbamazepine, nafcillin, octreotide, orlistat, oxcarbazepine, phenobarbital, phenytoin, rifampin, St. John's wort, sulfinpyrazone, terbinafine, ticlopidine: Decreased blood cyclosporine level and therapeutic response

methotrexate: Increased blood methotrexate level and risk of renal dysfunction

methylprednisolone (high dose): Increased risk of seizures

nifedipine: Increased risk of gingival hyperplasia

other immunosuppressants: Possibly excessive immunosuppression

repaglinide: Possibly increased repaglinide level and risk of hypoglycemia

vaccines (killed or live virus): Possibly suppressed immune response and increased adverse effects of vaccine

FOODS

grapefruit, grapefruit juice: Increased risk of nephrotoxicity; increased plasma concentration of cyclosporine

potassium-rich foods: Increased risk of hyperkalemia

Adverse Reactions

CNS: Altered level of consciousness, confusion, **encephalopathy**, headache, **intracranial hypertension**, lethargy, loss of motor function, migraine, **neurotoxicity**, paresthesia, **progressive multifocal leukoencephalopathy**, **posterior reversible encephalopathy syndrome** (PRES), psychiatric disturbances, **seizures**, tremor

CV: Chest pain, hypertension, **MI**

EENT: Gingival hyperplasia, optic disc edema, oral candidiasis, sinusitis, visual impairment including blindness

ENDO: Gynecomastia

GI: Cholestasis, diarrhea, **hepatitis**, **hepatotoxicity**, jaundice, **liver failure**, nausea, **pancreatitis**, vomiting

GU: Albuminuria, elevated serum creatinine and blood urea nitrogen levels, glomerular capillary thrombosis, hematuria, **nephropathy associated with BK virus**, **nephrotoxicity**, proteinuria, **renal failure**

HEME: Anemia, **leukopenia**, **thrombocytopenia**

MS: Lower extremity pain

SKIN: Acne, **cancer**, flushing, hirsutism, pruritus, rash

Other: **Anaphylaxis**; bacterial, fungal, protozoal, and viral infections including opportunistic infections such as polyomavirus; **hyperkalemia**; **hypomagnesemia**; **life-threatening infections**; **lymphoma and other malignancies**

Childbearing Considerations

PREGNANCY

- It is not known if drug can cause fetal harm.
- Drug should be used with caution during pregnancy only if benefit to mother outweighs potential risk to fetus.

LACTATION

- Drug is present in breast milk.
- A decision should be made to discontinue breastfeeding or the drug to avoid potential serious adverse reactions in the breastfed infant.

Nursing Considerations

- Don't draw blood to measure cyclosporine level through same I.V. tubing used to administer drug, even if line was flushed after administration. Blood level may be falsely elevated.

> **! WARNING** Monitor patient closely for hypersensitivity reactions, especially at the beginning of cyclosporine therapy and for at least the first 30 minutes following the start of an intravenous dose and then frequently thereafter. Know that while anaphylaxis may rarely occur, anaphylactic reactions have not occurred with the use of soft gelatin capsules or oral solution that did not contain Cremophor EL (polyoxyethylated castor oil). If anaphylaxis occurs, stop drug immediately and be prepared to administer epinephrine and oxygen, as ordered.

- Monitor blood pressure, especially in patients with a history of hypertension, because drug can worsen this condition. Expect to decrease dosage if hypertension develops.
- Monitor liver and renal function tests, as ordered, to detect decreased function. Be aware that it is not unusual for serum creatinine and BUN levels to be elevated during cyclosporine therapy. These elevations warrant investigation but do not always reflect kidney transplant rejection. If not related to rejection, a dosage reduction of cyclosporine often helps to decrease these levels.
- Be aware that there is an association between the development of interstitial fibrosis and higher cumulative doses or persistently high circulating through concentrations of cyclosporine, especially during first 6 months post-transplant, that may increase the risk of chronic nephrotoxicity.
- Be aware that although uncommon, cyclosporine may cause neurotoxicity, especially after liver transplantation. Watch for evidence of encephalopathy (impaired consciousness, loss of motor function, psychiatric disturbance, seizures, visual disturbance). Notify prescriber immediately if present, and expect cyclosporine dosage to be decreased or drug discontinued to increase possibility of a reversible or improvement of encephalopathy. Also monitor patients closely for seizures, especially if they are also receiving high-dose methylprednisolone therapy.

- Be aware that cyclosporine use may result in increased serum cholesterol levels.
- Be aware that St. John's wort may decrease blood cyclosporine level.
- Store capsules at 25°C (77°F) in prepackaged foil wrap to protect them from light.
- Expect about 50% of patients treated for psoriasis to relapse about 4 months after therapy stops. Know that patients with chronic plaque psoriasis may develop erythrodermic psoriasis or generalized pustular psoriasis when cyclosporine dose is reduced or drug is discontinued.

> **! WARNING** Watch for evidence of infection (such as cough, fever, malaise, pain) because patients receiving immunosuppressants such as cyclosporine are at increased risk for bacterial, fungal, parasitic, and viral infection. Watch for both generalized and localized infections, including worsening of preexisting infections, and be aware that these infections may become life-threatening. Activation of latent viral infections may also occur and include BK virus–associated nephropathy that can lead to decreased renal function and renal graft loss.

PATIENT TEACHING

- Instruct patient to take drug at same time each day and in same relation to type and timing of food intake to help increase compliance and maintain steady blood level.
- Tell patient capsules should not be chewed, crushed, or opened but swallowed whole.
- Tell patient to administer oral solution doses in oral syringe. Patient should clean outside of dosing syringe with a clean towel and replace protective cover after use. Tell patient not to rinse syringe with water or other cleaning agents. However, if syringe must be cleaned, it must be completely dry before reuse.
- Advise patient prescribed Sandimmune oral solution to mix with chocolate milk, milk, or orange juice; Gengraf or Neoral oral solution may be mixed with apple or orange juice that is at room temperature, but not milk. Warn patient not to mix any oral solution with grapefruit juice. Caution patient not to add water to oral solution because it will alter the drug's effectiveness.

- Tell patient to use a glass container when mixing oral solution with other liquids and to drink the mixture at once. Caution patient not to let mixture stand before drinking. After taking drug, tell patient to rinse glass with more liquid and drink again.
- Advise patient not to stop taking drug without consulting prescriber.

! WARNING Tell patient drug may cause an allergic reaction and to notify prescriber if present or to seek immediate emergency treatment, if reaction is severe.

- Instruct patient to avoid virus vaccines during therapy and people who have received such vaccines. Or, suggest wearing a protective mask when he's around them.
- Caution patient to avoid people who have infections during therapy because cyclosporine causes immunosuppression.
- Advise good dental hygiene because of risk of gingival hyperplasia.
- Advise patient to discard oral solution after it has been opened for 2 months.
- Inform patient with rheumatoid arthritis that drug effects may not appear for 4 to 6 weeks.
- Caution patient to avoid excessive exposure to ultraviolet light.

D

dabigatran etexilate mesylate
Pradaxa

☰ Class and Category
Pharmacologic class: Direct thrombin inhibitor
Therapeutic class: Anticoagulant

☰ Indications and Dosages
✳ *To reduce the risk of stroke and systemic embolism in patients with nonvalvular atrial fibrillation*

CAPSULES
Adults with creatinine clearance greater than 30 ml/min. 150 mg twice daily.
Adults with creatinine clearance between 15 and 30 ml/min. 75 mg twice daily.
±**DOSAGE ADJUSTMENT** For patient with a creatinine level between 30 and 50 ml/min and taking dronedarone or systemic ketoconazole concomitantly, dosage 75 mg twice daily.

✳ *To treat deep vein thrombosis and pulmonary emboli in patients who have been treated with a parenteral anticoagulant for 5 to 10 days; to reduce risk of recurrence of deep vein thrombosis and pulmonary emboli in patients who have been previously treated*

CAPSULES
Adults with creatinine clearance greater than 30 ml/min. 150 mg twice daily.

✳ *To prevent deep vein thrombosis and pulmonary embolism following a hip replacement*

CAPSULES
Adults with creatinine clearance greater than 30 ml/min. 110 mg 1 to 4 hr after surgery and after hemostasis has been achieved on first day, then 220 mg once daily for 28 to 35 days.

✳ *To treat venous thromboembolic events in children who have been treated with a parenteral anticoagulant for at least 5 days; to reduce risk of recurrence of venous thromboembolic events in children who have been previously treated*

CAPSULES
Children age 8 to less than 18 years who weigh 81 kg (178.2 lb) or greater. 260 mg twice daily.
Children age 8 to less than 18 years who weigh 61 kg (134.2 lb) to less than 81 kg (178.2 lb). 220 mg twice daily.
Children age 8 to less than 18 years who weigh 41 kg (90.2 lb) to less than 61 kg (134.2 lb). 185 mg twice daily.
Children age 8 to less than 18 years who weigh 26 kg (57.2 lb) to less than 41 kg (90.2 lb). 150 mg twice daily.
Children age 8 to less than 18 years who weigh 16 kg (35.2 lb) to less than 26 kg (57.2 lb). 110 mg twice daily.
Children age 8 to less than 18 years who weigh 11 kg (24.2 lb) to less than 16 kg (35.2 lb). 75 mg twice daily.

☰ Drug Administration
P.O.
▪ Capsule should be swallowed whole and not chewed, crushed, or opened.
▪ If a dose is missed, it should be given when discovered if on the same day of the missed dose, unless it is within 6 hours of the next dose.
▪ Keep bottle tightly closed when not in use and store in the original package to protect from moisture.
▪ Discard any remaining drug if not used within 4 months of initially opening the container.
▪ When patients convert to dabigatran from warfarin therapy, warfarin should be discontinued and dabigatran initiated when the INR is below 2.0.
▪ Expect patients converting from dabigatran to warfarin therapy to do so based on their creatinine clearance level. For adult patients who have a creatinine clearance level greater than 50 ml/min, expect warfarin to be started 3 days before dabigatran is discontinued. For adult patients who have a creatinine clearance level of 31 to 50 ml/min, expect warfarin to be started 2 days before dabigatran is discontinued. For adult patients who have a creatinine clearance level of 15 to 30 ml/min, expect warfarin to be started 1 day before dabigatran is discontinued. No recommendations are available for patients who have a creatinine clearance level of less than 15 ml/min or

children who have a creatinine clearance less than 50 ml/min.

- For patients who will begin dabigatran therapy currently receiving a parenteral anticoagulant, expect to start dabigatran therapy up to 2 hours before the time of the next dose of the parenteral drug or at the time of discontinuation of a continuously administered parenteral drug.
- For adult patients converting from dabigatran to a parenteral anticoagulant, expect to wait 12 hours for patient with a creatinine clearance of 30 ml/min or greater or wait 24 hours for patient with a creatinine clearance of less than 30 ml/min after the last dose of dabigatran before parenteral anticoagulant is initiated.
- For children converting from dabigatran to a parenteral anticoagulant, expect to wait 12 hours after the last dose before initiating the parenteral anticoagulant.

Route	Onset	Peak	Duration
P.O.	Rapid	1–2 hr	Unknown

Half-life: 12–17 hr

Mechanism of Action

Directly inhibits thrombin from converting fibrinogen into fibrin during the coagulation cascade. Inhibition of this activity prevents the development of a blood clot.

Contraindications

Active pathologic bleeding, hypersensitivity to dabigatran or its components, presence of mechanical prosthetic heart valve

Interactions
DRUGS

P-gp inducers such as rifampin: Decreased exposure to dabigatran
P-gp inhibitors such as dronedarone, ketoconazole: Increased exposure to dabigatran in patients with renal impairment; possibly increased exposure to dabigatran in children

Adverse Reactions

CNS: Intracranial or intraspinal hemorrhage
CV: Pericardial bleeding
EENT: Epistaxis, intraocular bleeding
GI: Diarrhea, dyspepsia, esophageal ulcer, gastritis-like symptoms, **gastrointestinal hemorrhage**, nausea, **retroperitoneal bleeding**, upper abdominal pain, vomiting
GU: Menorrhagia
HEME: **Agranulocytosis, bleeding (serious), neutropenia, thrombocytopenia**
MS: Intra-articular bleeding, intramuscular bleeding with compartment syndrome
SKIN: Alopecia, pruritus, rash, urticaria
Other: **Anaphylactic reaction or shock, angioedema**

Childbearing Considerations
PREGNANCY

- It is not known if drug causes fetal harm, although the use of anticoagulants such as dabigatran may increase risk of bleeding in the fetus.
- Drug should be used with caution during pregnancy only if benefit to mother outweighs potential risk to fetus.

LABOR & DELIVERY

- Drug may cause maternal bleeding and hemorrhage if given during labor and delivery.
- Know that drug should be temporarily withheld or a shorter acting anticoagulant substituted as delivery approaches or if neuraxial anesthesia is expected to be used during delivery.

LACTATION

- It is not known if drug is present in breast milk.
- Breastfeeding is not recommended during drug therapy.

REPRODUCTION

- Women of childbearing age should discuss pregnancy planning with prescriber because significant uterine bleeding, which may require surgical intervention, may occur with drug use.

Nursing Considerations

- Be aware that dabigatran should not be used in patients with triple-positive antiphospholipid syndrome because of increased risk for recurrent thrombosis.
- Assess renal function, as ordered, prior to beginning dabigatran therapy because dose is based on the patient's creatinine level. Continue to monitor the patient's serum creatinine level throughout therapy, as ordered, and expect frequency of serum creatinine tests to increase if patient

develops a condition that affects renal function, because a dosing adjustment may be required. Know that drug should be discontinued if the patient develops acute renal failure.

- Be aware that degree of anticoagulation does not have to be assessed by routine laboratory testing with dabigatran use. However, when necessary, expect the prescriber to use activated partial thromboplastin time (aPTT) or ecarin clotting time (ECT), and not INR, to assess for anticoagulant activity for the patient receiving dabigatran therapy.
- Know that dabigatran can elevate the patient's INR. Therefore, when patients are transitioned, dabigatran must be stopped for at least 2 days before the most accurate effects of warfarin can be known.
- Know that dabigatran therapy should be discontinued, if possible, 1 to 2 days before invasive or surgical procedures for patients with a creatinine clearance of 50 ml/min or more, and 3 to 5 days for patients whose creatinine clearance is less than 50 ml/min because of the increased risk for bleeding. Longer times may be required for patients undergoing major surgery, spinal puncture, or placement of a spinal or epidural catheter or port, in whom complete hemostasis is required. If surgery cannot be postponed, monitor patient closely for bleeding and assess bleeding risk with the ECT. If an ECT measurement is not possible, know that the aPTT can provide an approximation of dabigatran's anticoagulant activity.

activity of dabigatran. Instead, the prescriber may prescribe platelet concentrates if thrombocytopenia is present or the patient has been exposed to long-acting antiplatelet drugs. If bleeding is life-threatening or uncontrolled or emergency surgery or urgent procedures are necessary, expect to administer idarucizumab in adults to reverse the anticoagulant effect of dabigatran.

- Know that premature discontinuation of dabigatran increases the risk of thrombotic events. Be aware that patients receiving spinal/epidural anesthesia or a spinal puncture are at risk of developing an epidural or spinal hematoma, which can result in long-term or permanent paralysis. Monitor patient frequently for signs or symptoms of neurologic impairment. Notify prescriber immediately if patient complains of bladder or bowel dysfunction, midline back pain, or numbness, tingling, or weakness in the lower extremities.
- Assess patient closely for stroke if dabigatran therapy must be discontinued temporarily because of an active bleed, elective surgery, or an invasive procedure. Also, be aware that premature discontinuation of the drug increases risk of thrombotic events. Know that therapy should be restarted as soon as possible. If the drug must be discontinued for reasons other than pathological bleeding, expect patient to receive coverage with another anticoagulant to decrease the risk of thrombotic events, such as stroke.

! **WARNING** Monitor patient closely for bleeding because dabigatran increases risk for bleeding, which can become severe. Bleeding risk increases in patients taking concurrent antiplatelet drugs, fibrinolytic therapy, heparin, or with chronic use of NSAIDs. It also increases during labor and delivery. Monitor patient very closely. Promptly report any signs or symptoms of bleeding such as a drop in hemoglobin and/or hematocrit or the development of hypotension or overt bleeding. Expect to discontinue drug if active bleeding occurs and is persistent or serious. Know that protamine sulfate and vitamin K will not affect the anticoagulant

! **WARNING** Monitor patient closely for allergic reaction, such as pruritus, rash, and urticaria. If present, notify prescriber and if severe, provide supportive care, as prescribed.

! **WARNING** Be on the alert for an epidural or spinal hematoma formation in patients receiving dabigatran and neuraxial anesthesia or undergoing spinal puncture. This hematoma may result in long-term or permanent paralysis. Assess patient frequently for signs and symptoms of neurological impairment. If present, notify prescriber immediately, as urgent treatment is necessary.

PATIENT TEACHING

- Tell patient to take dabigatran exactly as prescribed.
- Instruct patient to swallow capsule whole without breaking, chewing, or emptying the contents of the capsule prior to ingestion.
- Tell patient that if she misses a dose, she should take it as soon as she remembers on the same day she missed the dose, unless it is within 6 hours of the next dose. She should never double a dose to make up for a missed dose.
- Instruct patient to keep bottle tightly closed when not in use and store in the original package to protect from moisture. Have patient date bottle when opened and tell her to discard any remaining drug if not used within 4 months of initially opening the bottle.
- Urge patient to take precautions against bleeding, such as using an electric shaver and a soft-bristled toothbrush.
- Caution patient to avoid activities that could cause traumatic injury and bleeding.
- Urge patient to notify prescriber immediately about unusual bleeding and any unexplained symptoms, such as abnormal vaginal bleeding, dizziness, easy bruising, gum bleeding, red or dark brown urine, stools that are black or tarry, vomiting blood or vomit that looks like coffee grounds, and weakness.

! **WARNING** Review signs and symptoms of an allergic reaction with patient. Tell patient to notify prescriber, if present. If signs and symptoms are severe, urge patient to seek immediate medical attention.

- Caution patient not to stop taking dabigatran abruptly.
- Urge patient to carry medical identification that reveals she is taking dabigatran.
- Tell patient to inform all healthcare providers that she is taking dabigatran and not to take any medication, including OTC drugs, without first consulting the prescriber.
- Warn mothers not to breastfeed while taking dabigatran because of increased risk of bleeding in the infant.

dalbavancin hydrochloride
Dalvance

Class and Category
Pharmacologic class: Lipoglycopeptide
Therapeutic class: Antibacterial antibiotic

Indications and Dosages
* *To treat acute bacterial skin and skin structure infections caused by* Enterococcus faecalis *(vancomycin-susceptible strains),* Staphylococcus aureus *(including methicillin-susceptible and methicillin-resistant strains),* Streptococcus agalactiae, S. anginosus group *(including* S. anginosus, S. constellatus, *and* S. intermedius*),* S. dysgalactiae, *and* S. pyogenes

I.V. INFUSION
Adults with a creatinine clearance of 30 ml/min or more. 1,500 mg infused as a single dose. Alternatively, 1,000 mg followed by 500 mg 1 wk later.
Children age 6 to less than 18 years with a creatinine clearance of 30 ml/min or more. 18 mg/kg (maximum 1,500 mg) as a single dose.
Neonates and children less than 6 years of age with a creatinine clearance of 30 ml/min or more. 22.5 mg/kg (maximum 1,500 mg) as a single dose.
±**DOSAGE ADJUSTMENT** For adult patients with renal impairment (creatinine clearance less than 30 ml/min) and who are not receiving hemodialysis, initial dosage reduced to 1,125 mg as a single dose or 750 mg, followed by 375 mg 1 wk later. There is insufficient information for dosage adjustment in neonates and children with renal impairment (creatinine clearance less than 30 ml/min).

Drug Administration
I.V.
- Reconstitute with 25 ml of either Sterile Water for Injection or 5% Dextrose Injection for each 500-mg vial.
- Avoid foaming by alternating between gently swirling and inverting the vial until contents are completely dissolved. Do not shake. Solution should appear clear and colorless to yellow.

- Once reconstituted, the vial may be refrigerated or stored at room temperature. Do not freeze.
- Further dilute reconstituted solution by transferring the required dose from the vial to an intravenous bag or bottle containing enough solution of 5% Dextrose Injection to provide a final concentration of 1 to 5 mg/ml. Discard any unused portion of the reconstituted solution.
- Once diluted, the intravenous bag or bottle may be refrigerated or stored at room temperature until administration as long as the total time from the vial being reconstituted until administration does not exceed 48 hours. Never freeze the diluted solution.
- Administer as an intravenous infusion over 30 minutes to minimize infusion reactions. If infusion reaction develops, stop or slow the infusion, as ordered, which may cause reaction to disappear.
- Flush intravenous line with 5% Dextrose Injection before and after administration if the line is used to administer other drugs.
- *Incompatibilities:* Other additives, drugs, or solutions including 0.9% Sodium Chloride Injection

Route	Onset	Peak	Duration
I.V.	Unknown	Unknown	Unknown

Half-life: 14.5 days

Mechanism of Action
Interferes with bacterial cell wall synthesis, which leads to impaired bacterial cell growth or cell death.

Contraindications
Hypersensitivity to dalbavancin or its components

Interactions
None reported by manufacturer

Adverse Reactions
CNS: Dizziness, fever (children), headache
EENT: Oral candidiasis
ENDO: Hypoglycemia
GI: Abdominal pain, *Clostridium difficile–associated colitis,* diarrhea, elevated liver enzymes, gastrointestinal hemorrhage, hepatotoxicity, melena, nausea, passage of bright red blood through anus
GU: Vulvovaginal mycotic infection

HEME: Anemia, elevated international normalized ratio (INR), eosinophilia, hemorrhagic anemia, leukopenia, neutropenia, spontaneous hematoma, thrombocytosis, thrombocytopenia
MS: Back pain
RESP: Bronchospasm
SKIN: Flushing of upper body, petechiae, pruritus, rash, urticaria
Other: Anaphylaxis, infusion reactions (back pain, flushing of upper body, pruritus, rash, urticaria), phlebitis, wound hemorrhage

Childbearing Considerations
PREGNANCY
- It is not known if drug causes fetal harm.
- Use with caution only if benefit to mother outweighs potential risk to fetus.

LACTATION
- It is not known if drug is present in breast milk.
- Patient should check with prescriber before breastfeeding.

Nursing Considerations
- Use cautiously in patients with a history of glycopeptides allergy because of a possibility of cross-sensitivity. Also, use cautiously in patients with hepatic impairment because it is not known if a dosage adjustment is needed.

! **WARNING** Monitor patient for hypersensitivity and skin reactions. If present, discontinue drug and notify prescriber. Provide supportive care, as needed and ordered.

- Use cautiously in patients with a history of hepatic impairment because dosing adjustments for dalbavancin in patients with moderate to severe hepatic impairment are not known. Dosage adjustment is not required for patients with mild hepatic impairment.
- Assess patient for signs of secondary infection, such as profuse, watery diarrhea. If such diarrhea develops, contact prescriber and expect to obtain a stool specimen to rule out pseudomembranous colitis caused by *C. difficile.* If diarrhea occurs, notify prescriber and expect to withhold dalbavancin and treat patient with an antibiotic effective against *C. difficile* along with electrolytes, fluids, and protein.

PATIENT TEACHING

- Emphasize importance of obtaining second dose of dalbavancin if patient was prescribed the two-dose regimen.

! WARNING Tell patient to immediately report any signs and symptoms of an allergic reaction. If reaction is serious, tell patient to seek immediate medical attention.

- Advise patient to report severe diarrhea to prescriber immediately.

dalteparin sodium

Fragmin

⦀ Class and Category

Pharmacologic class: Low-molecular-weight heparin
Therapeutic class: Anticoagulant

⦀ Indications and Dosages

✽ *To prevent ischemic complications in patients who receive aspirin as part of treatment for unstable angina and non-Q-wave MI*

SUBCUTANEOUS INJECTION

Adults. 120 international units/kg every 12 hr with aspirin (75 to 165 mg daily) until patient is stable, usually 5 to 8 days. *Maximum:* 10,000 international units/dose.

✽ *To prevent deep vein thrombosis in patients undergoing hip replacement surgery*

SUBCUTANEOUS INJECTION

Adults. *Initial:* 2,500 international units 4 to 8 hr after surgery (or later if hemostasis has not been achieved) and then 5,000 international units once daily for 5 to 10 days postoperatively or 2,500 international units 2 hr before surgery, repeated in 4 to 8 hr after surgery and then 5,000 international units once daily for 5 to 10 days postoperatively. Alternatively, 5,000 international units the evening before surgery followed by 5,000 international units 4 to 8 hr after surgery and then 5,000 international units once daily for 5 to 10 days postoperatively.

✽ *To prevent deep vein thrombosis in patients undergoing abdominal surgery who are at risk for thromboembolic complications*

SUBCUTANEOUS INJECTION

Adults. 2,500 international units daily, starting 1 to 2 hr before surgery and repeated once daily postoperatively for 5 to 10 days.

±**DOSAGE ADJUSTMENT** For patients at high risk (i.e., those with cancer), 5,000 international units the evening before surgery, repeated once daily postoperatively for 5 to 10 days; or alternatively for patients with cancer, 2,500 international units 1 to 2 hr before surgery followed by 2,500 international units 12 hr later and then 5,000 international units once daily postoperatively for 5 to 10 days.

✽ *To prevent deep vein thrombosis in patients with severe mobility restrictions during acute illness*

SUBCUTANEOUS INJECTION

Adults. 5,000 international units once daily for 12 to 14 days.

✽ *To provide extended treatment of symptomatic venous thromboembolism in patients with cancer*

SUBCUTANEOUS INJECTION

Adults. 200 international units/kg once daily for 30 days. Then 150 international units/kg once daily for 5 more months.
Maximum: 18,000 international units daily.

✽ *To treat symptomatic venous thromboembolism in pediatric patients*

SUBCUTANEOUS INJECTION

Children age 8 to less than 17 years. 100 international units/kg twice daily.
Children 2 years to less than 8 years. 125 international units/kg twice daily.
Infants 4 weeks to children less than 2 years. 150 international units/kg twice daily.

±**DOSAGE ADJUSTMENT** For adult patient with thrombocytopenia and cancer who experiences a platelet count between 50,000 and 100,000/mm^3, dosage reduced by 2,500 international units until platelet count recovers to or above 100,000 mm^3. For adult patient with thrombocytopenia and cancer who experiences a platelet count less than 50,000 mm^3, dalteparin withheld until platelet count is above 50,000 mm^3. For children 4 weeks and older, who experience a platelet count between 50,000 and 100,000 mm^3, dosage reduced by 50% until platelet count recovers to or above 100,000 mm^3. For children 4 weeks and older, who experience a platelet count less than 50,000 mm^3, dalteparin withheld until platelet count is above 50,000 mm^3. For adult patient needing extended treatment of acute symptomatic venous thrombosis and having severely impaired renal function (creatinine clearance below 30 ml/min), anti-Xa levels monitored to determine appropriate dose. Target anti-Xa range is 0.5 to 1.5 international units/ml.

Drug Administration

SUBCUTANEOUS

- Don't give drug by I.M. or I.V. injection.
- Needle shield on prefilled syringe may contain natural rubber latex and should not be handled by persons with a latex allergy.
- Administer drug deep into subcutaneous tissue in U-shaped area around navel, upper outer thigh, or upper outer quadrant of buttocks with patient seated or lying down. If using area around navel or on thigh, the skin fold must be lifted with thumb and forefinger while giving injection. Insert entire length of needle at a 45- to 90-degree angle.
- Rotate sites daily.
- After first penetration of rubber stopper, store multiple-dose vials at room temperature for up to 2 weeks.

Route	Onset	Peak	Duration
SubQ	1–2 hr	4 hr	12 hr

Half-life: 2–5 hr

Mechanism of Action

Binds to and accelerates the activity of antithrombin III, thus inhibiting thrombin and blocking the formation of fibrin clots.

Contraindications

Active major bleeding; history of heparin-induced thrombocytopenia or heparin-induced thrombocytopenia with thrombosis; hypersensitivity to dalteparin, heparin, or pork products; treatment for unstable angina and non-Q-wave MI or for prolonged venous thromboembolism prophylaxis while undergoing epidural/neuraxial anesthesia

Interactions

DRUGS

NSAIDs, oral anticoagulants, platelet aggregation inhibitors, thrombolytics: Possibly increased risk of hemorrhage and spinal or epidural hematoma

Adverse Reactions

EENT: Epistaxis
GI: Elevated liver enzymes
HEME: Hemorrhage, thrombocytopenia
MS: Osteoporosis
SKIN: Alopecia, bullous eruption, necrosis, pruritus, rash
Other: Anaphylaxis; injection-site bruising, hematoma, and pain

Childbearing Considerations

PREGNANCY

- It is not known if drug causes fetal harm although it has the potential for adverse effects on preterm infants when used in pregnancy if the 3.8-ml multiple-dose vial of the drug is used, because it contains 14 mg/ml of benzyl alcohol.
- Use with caution only if benefit to mother outweighs potential risk to fetus.

LACTATION

- Drug is present in breast milk.
- Patient should check with prescriber before breastfeeding.

Nursing Considerations

- Use dalteparin with extreme caution in patients with a history of heparin-induced thrombocytopenia; those at increased risk for hemorrhage (such as those who use a platelet inhibitor or have active ulcerative GI disorder, bacterial endocarditis, bleeding disorders, hemorrhagic stroke, or uncontrolled hypertension); and those with recent brain, eye, or spinal surgery.
- Use drug cautiously in patients with bleeding diathesis, diabetic retinopathy, platelet defects, recent GI bleeding, severe hepatic or renal insufficiency, or thrombocytopenia.
- Inform Jewish or Islamic patients that drug comes from porcine intestine before giving first dose.

! **WARNING** Question patient regarding use of aspirin and other NSAIDs, platelet inhibitors, or other anticoagulants prior to dalteparin therapy that may increase risk of bleeding.

- Be aware that risk factors for thromboembolic events include age over 40, cancer, history of deep vein thrombosis or pulmonary embolism, obesity, and planned use of anesthesia for more than 30 minutes.
- Know that routine coagulation tests and dosage adjustments usually aren't required. Instead, anti-Xa levels are measured, prior

to the fourth dose and as needed. Samples should be drawn 4 hours after drug administration. Dosages are then adjusted in increments of 25 international units/kg to achieve target anti-Xa level between 0.5 and 1 international units/ml. Thereafter anti-Xa levels are measured periodically for children and in adults with severe renal impairment or if abnormal coagulation parameters or bleeding occurs during drug therapy.

! **WARNING** Monitor patient receiving dalteparin and epidural or spinal anesthesia or spinal puncture because spinal hematomas can occur, causing long-term or permanent paralysis. Watch for evidence of neurologic impairment, such as changes in motor or sensory. If present, notify prescriber immediately; patient needs urgent care to minimize effect of hematoma. Use of indwelling epidural catheters; concurrent use of other drugs that affect hemostasis such as nonsteroidal anti-inflammatory drugs, platelet inhibitors, and other anticoagulants; a history of traumatic or repeated epidural or spinal punctures; or a history of spinal deformity or spinal surgery increase the risk of spinal or epidural hematoma in patients receiving dalteparin.

! **WARNING** Be aware that use of aspirin and other NSAIDs may enhance the risk of hemorrhage and should be discontinued prior to dalteparin therapy, if possible. If not, closely monitor patient's clinical and laboratory status throughout therapy.

PATIENT TEACHING

- Teach patient or caregiver administering drug at home how to select injection sites, give subcutaneous injections, and rotate sites daily. Tell patient to discard drug if it's discolored or contains particles. Review safe handling and disposal of syringes and needles. Inform patient with a latex allergy to notify prescriber if the prefilled syringe is ordered because the needle shield may contain natural rubber latex.
- Teach patient to store drug at room temperature, away from moisture and heat.
- Inform patient that bruising and/or bleeding occur more easily during dalteparin therapy.

- Urge patient to report adverse reactions, especially bleeding, and to seek help immediately if signs of blood clots develop, such as severe difficulty breathing or changes in mental status or motor or sensory abnormalities. Other adverse reactions to report include a rash of dark red spots under the skin.
- Instruct patient to inform all dentists and prescribers of dalteparin therapy. Tell patient who is receiving spinal anesthesia or a spinal puncture to alert medical staff immediately if he experiences muscular weakness, numbness (especially in his legs), or tingling following the procedure.
- Emphasize the importance of follow-up visits.

dapagliflozin propanediol
Farxiga

Class and Category
Pharmacologic class: Sodium glucose co-transporter 2 inhibitor
Therapeutic class: Antidiabetic

Indications and Dosages
* *Adjunct to diet and exercise to improve glycemic control in patients with type 2 diabetes mellitus*

TABLETS
Adults with an eGFR of 45 ml/min or greater. 5 mg once daily in morning, increased to 10 mg once daily in morning, as needed.

* *To reduce risk of hospitalization for heart failure in patients with type 2 diabetes mellitus and established cardiovascular disease or presence of multiple cardiovascular risk factors; to reduce risk of cardiovascular death and hospitalization for heart failure in patients with heart failure and reduced ejection fraction (NYHA class II–IV); to reduce the risk of sustained estimated glomerular filtration rate (eGFR) decline, end-stage kidney disease, cardiovascular death, and hospitalization for heart failure in adults with chronic kidney disease at risk of progression*

TABLETS
Adults with an eGFR of 25 ml/min or greater. 10 mg once daily.

Drug Administration

P.O.

- Administer in morning if being given for glucose control.

Route	Onset	Peak	Duration
P.O.	Unknown	2 hr	Unknown

Half-life: 12.9 hr

Mechanism of Action

Inhibits sodium glucose co-transporter 2 in the kidneys, which prevents glucose reabsorption. This decreases blood glucose levels.

Contraindications

Dialysis therapy, hypersensitivity to dapagliflozin or its components, severe renal impairment (glomerular filtration rate less than 30 ml/min) for treatment of glycemic control without established cardiovascular disease or multiple cardiovascular risk factors present

Interactions

DRUGS

insulin, insulin secretagogues: Increased risk of hypoglycemia

Adverse Reactions

CNS: Syncope
CV: Dyslipidemia, elevated low-density lipoprotein cholesterol, **hypotension**
EENT: Nasopharyngitis
ENDO: **Hypoglycemia (in patient with type 2 diabetes mellitus), ketoacidosis (in patient with type 2 diabetes mellitus)**
GI: Constipation, nausea
GU: **Acute kidney injury,** decreased eGFR, dysuria, elevated serum creatinine levels, genital mycotic infections, impaired renal function, increased urination, **necrotizing fasciitis of the perineum (Fournier's gangrene),** osmotic diuresis, **potential bladder cancer,** pyelonephritis, **urosepsis,** UTI
HEME: Elevated hematocrit level
MS: Back or extremity pain
SKIN: **severe cutaneous reactions,** urticaria
Other: **Anaphylaxis, angioedema,** flu-like symptoms, **hyperphosphatemia,** volume depletion

Childbearing Considerations

PREGNANCY

- It is not known if drug causes fetal harm.
- Drug is not recommended for use during the second and third trimesters of pregnancy because of potential fetal adverse renal effects as seen in animal studies.

LACTATION

- It is not known if drug is present in breast milk.
- Drug should not be used during breastfeeding because of the potential for adverse renal effects in the breastfed infant since renal maturation continues for up to 2 years after birth.

Nursing Considerations

- Know that dapagliflozin should not be given to patients with certain genetic forms of polycystic kidney disease, or who are taking or have recently received immunosuppressive therapy to treat kidney disease.
- Use drug cautiously in patients with chronic kidney insufficiency, congestive heart failure, decreased blood volume, and patients taking medications such as angiotensin-converting enzyme inhibitors, angiotensin receptor blockers, diuretics, and NSAIDs because these conditions and treatments may predispose the patient to acute kidney injury while receiving dapagliflozin. Ensure that kidney function has been assessed prior to starting dapagliflozin therapy and then periodically thereafter.
- Know that dapagliflozin should not be given to patients with active bladder cancer, as it is not known if the drug has an effect on preexisting bladder tumors. Use cautiously in patients with a history of bladder cancer. Monitor patient throughout therapy for hematuria, as this is a potential indicator for the presence of bladder tumor.
- Assess patient's kidney function and volume status and correct, if needed and as prescribed, prior to starting dapagliflozin therapy, because drug can cause intravascular volume contraction leading to acute kidney injury or symptomatic hypotension. Patients at highest risk include elderly patients, patients receiving loop diuretic therapy or drugs that interfere with the renin–angiotensin–aldosterone system, and patients who have low systolic blood

D

pressure or impaired renal function. Expect renal function to be evaluated periodically throughout drug therapy.

- Expect drug to be temporarily discontinued in patients who experience a reduced oral intake, such as with an acute illness or fasting, or who experience excessive fluid losses because of significant gastrointestinal illness or heat exposure, to reduce risk of acute kidney injury.
- Monitor patient's blood pressure and cholesterol level throughout dapagliflozin therapy. Be aware that patients with diabetes mellitus and renal dysfunction may be at increased risk to experience hypertension.

! **WARNING** Monitor patient for hypersensitivity reactions. Although rare, anaphylaxis, angioedema, and severe cutaneous adverse reactions have occurred. If present, stop drug immediately and notify prescriber. Provide care, as prescribed, according to the standard of care until signs and symptoms subside.

- Be aware that patients receiving insulin or insulin secretagogues may require a lower dose of these agents because dapagliflozin in combination increases risk of hypoglycemia. Monitor patient closely for hypoglycemia. If present, treat according to standard of care and notify prescriber.

! **WARNING** Monitor patient for a rare but serious and life-threatening necrotizing infection of the perineum called Fournier's gangrene. Notify prescriber immediately if patient develops erythema, pain, swelling, or tenderness in the genital or perineal area, along with fever or malaise. Expect treatment with broad-spectrum antibiotics and, if needed, surgical debridement of the area. Know that dapagliflozin will be discontinued if this occurs. Monitor patient's blood glucose levels closely and expect an alternative treatment for glycemic control.

- Monitor patients for genital mycotic infections, especially patients with a history of such infections. If present, notify prescriber and treat, as prescribed.

! **WARNING** Know that drug should not be used to treat type 1 diabetes mellitus.

Monitor patient closely for ketoacidosis that may occur despite the patient having type 2 diabetes and may be present even if a blood glucose level is less than 250 mg/dl. If signs and symptoms occur such as dehydration, fruity odor to breath, malaise, nausea, shortness of breath, and vomiting, notify prescriber and expect drug to be discontinued. Provide supportive care, as ordered.

PATIENT TEACHING

- Inform patient that dapagliflozin therapy is not a replacement for diet and exercise therapy.
- Tell patient to take drug in the morning if used to control blood glucose levels.
- Instruct patient if a dose is missed to take it as soon as it is remembered unless it is almost time for the next dose. Then patient should skip the missed dose and resume taking drug at the next regularly scheduled time. Warn patient never to double a dose to make up for a missed dose.
- Instruct patient on the signs and symptoms of hypoglycemia and how to treat it. Inform patient who is also receiving a sulfonylurea or insulin that the risk of hypoglycemia is greater. Tell patient to notify prescriber if hypoglycemia occurs frequently or is severe.
- Inform patient that dapagliflozin may have an adverse effect on the bladder, increasing the risk for bladder cancer. Tell patient to report blood in the urine immediately to the prescriber.
- Tell patient to monitor the blood glucose level using blood tests instead of urine tests because the drug increases urinary glucose excretion and will lead to positive urine glucose tests. Review signs and symptoms of ketoacidosis with patient and urge her to seek immediate medical attention, if present, even if blood glucose level is less than 250 mg/dl.

! **WARNING** Instruct patient to stop taking drug and seek immediate medical attention if an allergic reaction such as hives or facial or throat swelling occurs while taking dapagliflozin.

- Advise female patients to notify prescriber if pregnancy occurs or is suspected.

Also, inform female patients that drug may cause harm to infants who are breastfed.

- Advise patient to maintain adequate fluid intake throughout dapagliflozin therapy. However, tell patient to notify prescriber if he is unable to take a normal amount of daily fluids due to illness or fasting or experiences an excessive loss of fluids from excessive perspiration or gastrointestinal illnesses, as drug may have to be temporarily withheld.

! **WARNING** Warn patient to stop dapagliflozin and seek immediate medical attention if pain, redness, swelling, or tenderness occur in the genital or perineal area, along with fever or malaise because, although rare, this cluster of symptoms may become life-threatening.

- Advise patient to slowly rise from a sitting or lying position and to notify prescriber if symptoms of light-headedness or feeling faint occurs.

daptomycin
Cubicin, Cubicin RF

⬜ Class and Category
Pharmacologic class: Cyclic lipopeptide
Therapeutic class: Antibiotic

⬜ Indications and Dosages
⁕ *To treat complicated skin and skin structure infections caused by* Staphylococcus aureus *(including methicillin-resistant isolates),* Streptococcus agalactiae, S. dysgalactiae *subspecies* Enterococcus faecalis *(vancomycin-susceptible isolates only) and* equisimilis, S. pyogenes

I.V. INFUSION, I.V. INJECTION (CUBICIN, CUBICIN RF)
Adults. 4 mg/kg once daily for 7 to 14 days.
I.V. INFUSION (CUBICIN, CUBICIN RF)
Children ages 12 to 17. 5 mg/kg once every 24 hr for up to 14 days.
Children ages 7 to 11. 7 mg/kg once every 24 hr for up to 14 days.
Children ages 2 to 6. 9 mg/kg every 24 hr for up to 14 days.
Children ages 1 to less than 2 years. 10 mg/kg once every 24 hr for up to 14 days.

⁕ *To treat* Staphylococcus aureus *bloodstream infections (bacteremia), including right-sided infective endocarditis, caused by methicillin-susceptible and methicillin-resistant isolates*
I.V. INFUSION, I.V. INJECTION (CUBICIN, CUBICIN RF)
Adults. 6 mg/kg once daily for 2 to 6 wk.
⁕ *To treat pediatric patients with* S. aureus *bloodstream infections (bacteremia)*
I.V. INFUSION (CUBICIN)
Children ages 12 to 17. 7 mg/kg once daily for up to 42 days.
Children ages 7 to 11. 9 mg/kg once daily for up to 42 days.
Children ages 1 to 6. 12 mg/kg once daily for up to 42 days.
±**DOSAGE ADJUSTMENT** For adult patients with creatinine clearance less than 30 ml/min, dosage is 4 mg/kg every 48 hours for complicated skin or skin structure infections or 6 mg/kg for bacteremia once every 48 hr. No dosage adjustment has been established for children with renal impairment.

⬜ Drug Administration
I.V.
- The two formulations of the drug require different storage and methods of reconstitution.
- Reconstitute Cubicin by slowly transferring 10 ml of 0.9% Sodium Chloride Injection into vial and pointing needle (beveled sterile transfer 21-gauge needle or smaller or needleless device) toward wall of vial to minimize foaming. Then gently rotate vial until all powder is wet. Don't agitate or shake vial. Let vial stand undisturbed for 10 minutes, then gently rotate or swirl contents for a few minutes, as needed, to obtain a completely reconstituted solution. Remove reconstituted solution from vial slowly using same type of needle used to reconstitute drug.
- Reconstitute Cubicin RF with 10 ml of either Sterile Water for Injection or Bacteriostatic Water for Injection using a beveled sterile transfer needle that is 21 gauge or smaller in diameter. Saline-based diluents should not be used. Rotate or swirl vial contents for a few minutes, as needed, to obtain a completely reconstituted solution. Remove reconstituted solution from vial slowly using same type of needle used to reconstitute drug.

D

- For I.V. injection (only for adults), administer either formulation over a period of 2 minutes.
- For I.V. infusion, further dilute either formulation of reconstituted solution with 50 ml in an I.V. infusion bag containing 0.9% Sodium Chloride for Injection (25 ml for children age 1 to 6), and administer over 30 minutes for adults and children age 7 and older at a rate of 1.67 ml/min and 60 minutes for children 6 and under at a rate of 0.42 ml/min.
- Flush I.V. with a compatible intravenous solution before and after infusion of drug if the same I.V. line is being used for sequential infusion of other drugs.
- Do not infuse with the ReadyMED elastomeric infusion pumps, as drug is not as stable when stored in these pumps.
- Refer to manufacturer guidelines for storage information.
- *Incompatibilities:* Dextrose-containing solutions, other additives or drugs

Route	Onset	Peak	Duration
I.V.	Rapid	30–60 min	Unknown

Half-life: 8 hr

Mechanism of Action

Binds to bacterial membranes to cause rapid depolarization of membrane potential. This loss of membrane potential inhibits protein, DNA, and RNA synthesis, which results in bacterial cell death.

Contraindications

Hypersensitivity to daptomycin or its components

Interactions

DRUGS

HMG-CoA reductase inhibitors: Possibly increased CPK level and increased risk of myopathy

Adverse Reactions

CNS: Anxiety, asthenia, confusion, dizziness, dyskinesia, fatigue, fever, hallucination, headache, insomnia, mental status changes, paresthesia, peripheral neuropathy, rigors, weakness

CV: Atrial fibrillation or flutter, cardiac arrest or failure, chest pain, hypertension, hypotension, peripheral edema, supraventricular tachycardia

EENT: Blurred vision, dry mouth, eye irritation, gingival pain, hypoesthesia of mouth, oral candidiasis, pharyngolaryngeal pain, sore throat, stomatitis, taste disturbance, tinnitus, visual disturbances

ENDO: Hyperglycemia, hypoglycemia

GI: Abdominal distention or pain, anorexia, *Clostridium difficile*–associated diarrhea, constipation, diarrhea, dyspepsia, dysphagia, elevated liver enzymes or serum lactate dehydrogenase, GI hemorrhage, jaundice, nausea, vomiting

GU: Acute kidney injury, renal failure or insufficiency; proteinuria; tubulointerstitial nephritis; UTI; vaginal candidiasis

HEME: Anemia, decreased platelet count, eosinophilia, increased international normalized ratio (INR), leukocytosis, prolonged prothrombin time, thrombocythemia, thrombocytopenia, thrombocytosis

MS: Arthralgia, back or limb pain, elevated myoglobin level, muscle cramps or weakness, myalgia, myopathy, osteomyelitis, rhabdomyolysis

RESP: Cough, dyspnea, eosinophilic pneumonia, pleural effusion, pneumonia, pulmonary eosinophilia, shortness of breath

SKIN: Acute generalized exanthematous pustulosis, cellulitis, diaphoresis, eczema, erythema, flushing, pruritus, rash, Stevens–Johnson syndrome, toxic epidermal necrolysis (TEN), truncal erythema, urticaria, vesiculobullous rash

Other: Anaphylaxis, angioedema, bacteremia, drug reaction with eosinophilia and systemic symptoms (DRESS), electrolyte disturbance, elevated alkaline phosphatase or creatine phosphokinase levels, elevated serum sodium bicarbonate level, fungal infection, hyperkalemia, hypokalemia, hypomagnesemia, injection-site reactions, lymphadenopathy, sepsis

Childbearing Considerations

PREGNANCY

- It is not known if drug causes fetal harm.
- Use with caution only if benefit to mother outweighs potential risk to fetus.

LACTATION

- Drug is present in breast milk.
- Patient should check with prescriber before breastfeeding.

Nursing Considerations

- Use cautiously in adult patients with moderate to severe renal impairment and monitor drug effectiveness closely, as daptomycin may not be as effective in this patient population.
- Obtain blood samples for culture and sensitivity testing before starting daptomycin.
- Monitor results of the patient's bleeding studies, as ordered. Daptomycin may cause a significant false increase in PT and INR with some brands of laboratory assays. If this occurs during daptomycin therapy, draw blood sample just before next daptomycin dose and evaluate other causes of the increase.
- Monitor patient closely for diarrhea, which may herald pseudomembranous colitis caused by *C. difficile*. If diarrhea occurs, notify prescriber. If pseudomembranous colitis develops, expect to discontinue drug and give fluids, electrolytes, protein, and antibiotic effective against *C. difficile*.
- Monitor patient for evidence of superinfection, and inform prescriber if present. Expect to stop drug and provide care.
- Assess patient for muscle pain or weakness, especially of distal limbs. Expect to monitor creatine phosphokinase (CPK) level weekly or more often in patients recently or currently taking an HMG-CoA reductase inhibitor. Expect to stop daptomycin, as ordered, if patient has myopathy or marked rise in CPK level.
- Monitor patient's BUN and serum creatinine levels and patient's response to drug closely, especially if renal insufficiency is already present, because daptomycin may not be as effective in the presence of renal insufficiency as well as possibly causing tubulointerstitial nephritis.
- Expect to discontinue daptomycin therapy immediately if patient develops signs and symptoms of eosinophilic pneumonia, such as dyspnea with hypoxic respiratory insufficiency and diffuse pulmonary infiltrates or fever, and prepare to administer systemic steroids, as ordered.

! **WARNING** Monitor patient for serious hypersensitivity reactions such as anaphylaxis and angioedema as well as severe skin reactions such as DRESS exhibited by fever, skin rash, peripheral eosinophilia, and systemic organ impairment. If suspected, notify prescriber and expect drug to be discontinued and appropriate treatment given.

PATIENT TEACHING

- Inform patient that diarrhea may occur 2 months or more after daptomycin therapy stops. If severe or prolonged, advise patient to notify prescriber as soon as possible; additional treatment may be needed.
- Urge patient to report muscle pain, tenderness, or weakness, and other symptoms of myopathy immediately. Also tell patient to report breathlessness, cough, or a fever.

! **WARNING** Review signs and symptoms of an allergic reaction as well as serious skin reactions. Instruct patient to notify prescriber immediately if an allergic reaction or skin reactions occur, because drug may have to be discontinued.

darbepoetin alfa
Aranesp

Class and Category
Pharmacologic class: Recombinant human erythropoietin
Therapeutic class: Antianemic

Indications and Dosages
✽ *To treat anemia from chronic renal failure*

I.V. OR SUBCUTANEOUS INJECTION
Adults on dialysis other than hemodialysis. *Initial:* 0.45 mcg/kg as a single dose every wk. Alternatively, 0.75 mcg/kg once every 2 wk. *Maintenance:* Dosage individualized and increased monthly to maintain a hemoglobin level not to exceed 11 g/dl.
Adults not on dialysis. *Initial:* 0.45 mcg/kg as a single dose every 4 wk, as needed.
Children age 1 month and over on dialysis. 0.45 mcg/kg once every wk.
Children age 1 month and over not on dialysis. 0.75 mcg/kg once every 2 wk.

I.V. INJECTION
Adults on hemodialysis. *Initial:* 0.45 mcg/kg as a single dose every wk. Alternatively,

0.75 mcg/kg once every 2 wk. *Maintenance:* Dosage individualized and increased monthly to maintain a hemoglobin level not to exceed 11 g/dl.

± **DOSAGE ADJUSTMENT** Dosage reduced or therapy interrupted if hemoglobin level increases and approaches 12 g/dl for children, 11 g/dl for adults on dialysis, and 10 g/dl for adults not on dialysis. Dosage reduced by about 25% if hemoglobin level increases by more than 1 g/dl in a 2-wk period. Dosage increased by about 25% of previous dose if hemoglobin level increases less than 1 g/dl over 4 wk. Further increases made at 4-wk intervals until specified hemoglobin level is obtained.

± **DOSAGE ADJUSTMENT** For conversion from epoetin alfa to darbepoetin alfa, dosage administered every wk for patient who previously received epoetin alfa two to three times/wk and once every 2 wk for patient who previously received epoetin alfa once/wk. For conversion from epoetin alfa, 6.25 mcg/wk darbepoetin alfa given every wk for adult patients who received less than 1,500 units/wk of epoetin alfa; 6.25 mcg/week darbepoetin alfa given every wk for adult and pediatric patients who received 1,500 to 2,499 units/wk of epoetin alfa; 12.5 mcg/wk (10 mcg/wk for children) darbepoetin alfa every wk for patients who received 2,500 to 4,999 units/wk of epoetin alfa; 25 mcg/wk (20 mcg/wk for children) darbepoetin alfa every wk for adult and pediatric patients who received 5,000 to 10,999 units/wk of epoetin alfa; 40 mcg/wk darbepoetin alfa every wk for adult and pediatric patients who received 11,000 to 17,999 units/wk of epoetin alfa; 60 mcg/wk darbepoetin alfa every wk for adult and pediatric patients who received 18,000 to 33,999 units/wk of epoetin alfa; 100 mcg/wk darbepoetin alfa every wk for adult and pediatric patients who received 34,000 to 89,999 units/wk of epoetin alfa; 200 mcg/wk darbepoetin alfa every wk for adult and pediatric patients who received 90,000 or more units/wk of epoetin alfa.

* *To treat chemotherapy-induced anemia in patients with nonmyeloid malignancies and hemoglobin level less than 10 g/dl and if there is a minimum of 2 additional months of planned chemotherapy*

SUBCUTANEOUS INJECTION

Adults. *Initial:* 2.25 mcg/kg as a single dose every wk until completion of a chemotherapy course. Alternatively, 500 mcg every 3 wk until completion of a chemotherapy course. *Maintenance:* Dosage individualized to maintain a target hemoglobin level.

± **DOSAGE ADJUSTMENT** Dosage increased to 4.5 mcg/kg/wk (no dosage adjustment if patient is already receiving 500 mcg every 3 wk) if hemoglobin level increases less than 1.0 g/dl after 6 wk of therapy. If it increases more than 1.0 g/dl over 2 wk, dosage reduced by about 40%. If hemoglobin level exceeds a level needed to avoid RBC transfusion, dose withheld until hemoglobin approaches level when RBC transfusion may be required. Then, therapy is restarted at a dose about 40% less than last dose given.

Drug Administration

- Don't shake vial during preparation, to avoid denaturing drug and rendering it biologically inactive.
- Discard drug if discoloration or particulate matter is present.
- Don't dilute drug before giving it.
- Know that needle cover on prefilled syringe contains dry natural rubber and may cause allergic reaction in those with latex sensitivity.
- Discard unused portion of drug, because it contains no preservatives.
- Store drug at 2° to 8°C (36° to 46°F). Don't freeze, and do protect from light.

I.V.

- Manufacturer does not specify how long I.V. injection should be administered.
- *Incompatibilities:* Other drug solutions

SUBCUTANEOUS

- No special instructions given by manufacturer.

Route	Onset	Peak	Duration
I.V.	Unknown	Unknown	Unknown
SubQ	Slow	24–72 hr	Unknown

Half-life: 21 hr (I.V.); 49 hr (SubQ)

Mechanism of Action

Stimulates release of reticulocytes from the bone marrow into the bloodstream, where they develop into mature RBCs.

Contraindications

History of pure red cell aplasia that began after treatment with darbepoetin alfa or other erythropoietin protein drugs, hypersensitivity to darbepoetin alfa or its components, uncontrolled hypertension

Interactions

DRUGS

None reported by manufacturer

Adverse Reactions

CNS: Asthenia, CVA, dizziness, fatigue, fever, headache, seizures, transient ischemic attack

CV: Acute MI, angina, arrhythmias, cardiac arrest or death, chest pain, congestive heart failure, edema, hypertension, hypotension, peripheral edema, thromboembolic events, vascular access thrombosis

GI: Abdominal pain, constipation, diarrhea, nausea, vomiting

HEME: Low reticulocyte count, pure red cell aplasia, severe anemia

MS: Arthralgia, back pain, limb pain, muscle spasm, myalgia

RESP: Bronchitis, bronchospasm, cough, dyspnea, pneumonia, pulmonary embolism, upper respiratory tract infection

SKIN: Erythema multiforme, pruritus, rash, Stevens–Johnson syndrome, toxic epidermal necrolysis, urticaria

Other: Anaphylaxis, angioedema, dehydration, infection, flu-like symptoms, injection-site pain, sepsis

Childbearing Considerations

PREGNANCY

- It is not known if drug causes fetal harm.
- Use with caution only if benefit to mother outweighs potential risk to fetus.

LACTATION

- It is not known if drug is present in breast milk.
- Patient should check with prescriber before breastfeeding.

Nursing Considerations

- Ensure that patient has received the medication guide and patient instructions for darbepoetin alfa and that a written acknowledgment of a discussion of the risks involved with this type of therapy has been obtained before first dose is given.
- Know that before starting darbepoetin alfa therapy, expect to correct folic acid or vitamin B_{12} deficiencies because these conditions may interfere with drug's effectiveness.
- Be aware that darbepoetin alfa shouldn't be given to cancer patients when a cure is anticipated because drug may decrease survival rate and increase tumor progression in patients with certain types of cancers, such as breast, cervical, head and neck, lymphoid, and non-small-cell lung cancers. Be aware that all prescribers and hospitals must enroll in and comply with the ESA APPRISE oncology program to be able to prescribe and dispense the drug.
- Use extreme caution with darbepoetin alfa therapy in patients undergoing coronary artery bypass graft surgery because of increased risk of death, and in patients undergoing orthopedic procedures because of increased risk of deep venous thrombosis.
- Be aware that to ensure effective drug response, expect to obtain serum ferritin level and transferrin saturation before and during therapy, as ordered. If serum ferritin level is less than 100 mcg/L or serum transferrin saturation is less than 20%, expect to begin supplemental iron therapy.
- Monitor patient closely for hypertension during therapy. Expect to reduce dosage or withhold drug if blood pressure is poorly controlled with antihypertensive and dietary measures.
- Monitor hemoglobin level weekly, as ordered, until hemoglobin stabilizes and maintenance dosage has been achieved. Then monitor hemoglobin level regularly, as ordered. After each dosage adjustment, expect to check hemoglobin level weekly for 4 weeks until it stabilizes in response to dosage change.

! **WARNING** Know that if hemoglobin level increases more than about 1 g/dl during any 2-week period or it exceeds 12 g/dl for children, 11 g/dl for adult patient on dialysis, 10 g/dl for adult patient not on dialysis, or target range for cancer patient, the risk of acute MI, cardiac arrest, congestive heart failure, fluid overload with peripheral edema, seizures, shortened survival, stroke, tumor progression, vascular infarction, vascular ischemia, vascular thrombosis, and worsened hypertension increases. Expect to decrease dosage if this occurs.

- Expect to discontinue darbepoetin in cancer patients if hemoglobin level hasn't increased after 8 weeks or if patient continues to need transfusions despite therapy.
- Institute seizure precautions according to facility policy.
- Monitor patient for severe skin reactions that may include blistering and skin exfoliation. Notify prescriber immediately, if noted, and expect darbepoetin therapy to be discontinued. Prepare to provide supportive care, as ordered.
- Monitor renal function test results and fluid and electrolyte balance for signs of declining renal function in patients with renal impairment. If patient starts dialysis, monitor hemoglobin and blood pressure closely and expect dosage and route of administration to be adjusted, as needed, for type of dialysis.

PATIENT TEACHING

- Instruct patient how to administer a subcutaneous injection, rotate sites, and properly dispose of needles, syringes, or unused portions of single-dose vials.
- Ask patient about latex allergy because needle cover on prefilled syringe contains dry natural rubber and may cause allergic reaction in those with latex sensitivity.
- Advise patient that the risk of seizures is highest during the first 90 days of therapy. Discourage her from engaging in hazardous activities during this time.
- Emphasize the importance of complying with the dosage regimen and keeping follow-up medical and laboratory appointments.
- Advise patient to follow up with her prescriber for blood pressure monitoring.
- Encourage patient to eat adequate quantities of iron-rich foods.
- Review possible adverse reactions and urge patient to notify prescriber if she experiences serious adverse reactions such as chest pain, headache, rash, seizures, shortness of breath, or swelling of her face, lips, throat, or tongue.

darifenacin
Enablex

Class and Category

Pharmacologic class: Anticholinergic
Therapeutic class: Bladder antispasmodic

Indications and Dosages

✳ *To treat overactive bladder with symptoms of frequency, urge incontinence, or urgency*

E.R. TABLETS

Adults. *Initial:* 7.5 mg daily, increased to 15 mg daily after 2 wk as needed.

±**DOSAGE ADJUSTMENT** For patients with moderate hepatic impairment and those taking potent CYP3A4 inhibitors (such as clarithromycin, itraconazole, ketoconazole, nefazodone, nelfinavir, and ritonavir), daily dosage should not exceed 7.5 mg.

Drug Administration

P.O.

- E.R. tablets should be swallowed whole with water and not chewed, crushed, or split.

Route	Onset	Peak	Duration
P.O.	Unknown	7 hr	Unknown

Half-life: 13–19 hr

Mechanism of Action

Antagonizes effect of acetylcholine on muscarinic receptors in detrusor muscle, decreasing muscle spasms that cause inappropriate bladder emptying. This action increases bladder capacity and volume, which relieves sensations of frequency and urgency and enhances bladder control.

Contraindications

Gastric retention, hypersensitivity to darifenacin or its components, uncontrolled narrow-angle glaucoma, urinary retention, and patients at risk for these conditions

Interactions

DRUGS

CYP2D6 substrates such as flecainide, thioridazine, tricyclic antidepressants: Risk of toxicity with these drugs
potent CYP3A4 inhibitors (such as clarithromycin, itraconazole, ketoconazole,

nefazodone, nelfinavir, and ritonavir):
Decreased metabolism and increased effects of darifenacin, possibly increasing the risk of adverse reactions
other anticholinergics: Increased frequency and severity of anticholinergic adverse reactions

Adverse Reactions

CNS: Asthenia, confusion, dizziness, hallucinations, headache, somnolence
CV: Hypertension, palpitations, peripheral edema
EENT: Abnormal vision, dry eyes or mouth, pharyngitis, rhinitis, sinusitis
GI: Abdominal pain, constipation, diarrhea, indigestion, nausea, vomiting
GU: Urine retention, UTI, vaginitis
MS: Arthralgia, back pain
RESP: **Airway obstruction**, bronchitis
SKIN: Dry skin, **erythema multiforme**, interstitial granuloma annulare, pruritus, rash
Other: **Anaphylaxis**, **angioedema**, flu-like symptoms, **hypersensitivity reactions**, weight gain

Childbearing Considerations

PREGNANCY

- It is not known if drug causes fetal harm.
- Use with caution only if benefit to mother outweighs potential risk to fetus.

LACTATION

- It is not known if drug is present in breast milk.
- Patient should check with prescriber before breastfeeding.

Nursing Considerations

- Use darifenacin cautiously in patients with significant bladder outflow obstruction; they have increased risk of urine retention. Also use cautiously in patients with controlled narrow-angle glaucoma, as darifenacin therapy may worsen this condition.
- Use darifenacin cautiously in patients with myasthenia gravis, severe constipation, or ulcerative colitis, because it may decrease GI motility. Also use drug cautiously in obstructive GI disorders because it increases the risk of gastric retention.
- Monitor patient for signs of anticholinergic CNS effects such as confusion, hallucinations, headache, and somnolence, especially at beginning of therapy and with dosage increases.

! **WARNING** Monitor patient closely for serious adverse reactions that may become life-threatening, such as anaphylaxis and angioedema of the face, larynx, lips, and/or tongue that may occur even after just one dose. If present, withhold drug, notify prescriber immediately, and provide emergency supportive care, as indicated.

PATIENT TEACHING

- Tell patient to swallow tablets with liquid and not to break, crush, or split them.
- Advise patient to avoid exercising in hot weather because darifenacin decreases sweating, increasing the risk of heatstroke.
- Caution patient to avoid hazardous activities until drug's CNS effects are known.

! **WARNING** Warn patient to seek immediate medical attention if he experiences any signs of a serious drug reaction, including swelling of his face, lips, throat, and/or tongue.

deferoxamine mesylate
Desferal

Class and Category

Pharmacologic class: Iron chelator
Therapeutic class: Heavy metal chelator

Indications and Dosages

❋ *As adjunct to treat acute iron intoxication*

I.M. INJECTION

Adults and children age 3 and over who are not in shock. *Initial:* 1,000 mg, followed by 500 mg every 4 hr for 2 doses, if needed. Additional doses of 500 mg may be administered every 4 to 12 hr, as needed. *Maximum:* 6,000 mg in 24 hr.

I.V. INFUSION

Adults and children age 3 and over who are in shock. *Initial:* 1,000 mg followed by 500 mg every 4 hr for 2 doses, if needed. Additional doses of 500 mg may be administered every 4 to 12 hr, as needed. *Maximum:* 6,000 mg in 24 hr.

❋ *To treat chronic iron overload due to transfusion-dependent anemias*

I.M. INJECTION

Adults and children age 3 and over. 500 to 1,000 mg daily. *Maximum:* 1,000 mg daily.

I.V. INFUSION

Adults. 40 to 50 mg/kg/day for 5 to 7 days per week. *Maximum:* 60 mg/kg/day.
Children age 3 and over. 20 to 40 mg/kg/day. *Maximum:* 40 mg/kg/day.

SUBCUTANEOUS INFUSION

Adults and children age 3 and over. 20 to 40 mg/kg/day (1,000 to 2,000 mg/day) administered over 8 to 24 hr.

≣ Drug Administration

- Use within 3 hours after being reconstituted when stored at room temperature. Do not refrigerate. If product was reconstituted in a sterile laminar flow hood using aseptic technique, drug may be stored at room temperature for up to 24 hours before use.
- Color when reconstituted should be clear to slightly yellowish.
- Discard unused portion.
- *Incompatibilities:* Other solvents, turbid solutions

I.V.

- This route should be used only for patients in a state of cardiovascular collapse.
- Reconstitute by adding 5 ml of Sterile Water for Injection to a 500-mg vial or 20 ml of Sterile Water for Injection to a 2-g vial. Make sure drug is completely dissolved before the solution is withdrawn.
- Further dilute reconstituted solution with 0.45% or 0.9% Sodium Chloride Injection, Dextrose for Injection, or Ringer's Lactate solution.
- Administer only by slow infusion at a rate no greater than 15 mg/kg/hr and for the first 1,000 mg when treating acute iron intoxication. Subsequent doses, if needed, must be given at a slower rate, not to exceed 125 mg/hr.
- Never give as a rapid infusion.

I.M.

- Preferred route for all patients not in shock.
- Reconstitute by adding 2 ml of Sterile Water for Injection to a 500-mg vial or 8 ml of Sterile Water for Injection to a 2-g vial prior to administration.

SUBCUTANEOUS

- Reconstitute by adding 5 ml of Sterile Water for Injection to a 500-mg vial or 20 ml of

Sterile Water for Injection to a 2-g vial. Make sure drug is completely dissolved before the solution is withdrawn.

- Use a portable pump capable of providing continuous mini-infusion when administering drug by subcutaneous infusion.
- Administer over 8 to 24 hours, as rate must be individualized.

Route	Onset	Peak	Duration
I.V./I.M./SubQ	Unknown	Unknown	Unknown

Half-life: 1–6 hr

≣ Mechanism of Action

Binds iron by forming a stable complex with it. This prevents iron from entering into further chemical reactions. The chelate then passes through the kidneys and out of the body in urine, thereby decreasing the iron level in the body.

≣ Contraindications

Anuria, hypersensitivity to deferoxamine or its components, severe renal disease

≣ Interactions

DRUGS

prochlorperazine: Possibly impaired consciousness
vitamin C: Increased availability of iron for chelation by deferoxamine

≣ Adverse Reactions

CNS: Dizziness, **exacerbation or precipitation of aluminum-related dialysis encephalopathy**, fever, headache, paresthesias, peripheral neuropathy, **seizures**
CV: Hypotension, shock, tachycardia
EENT: Blurred vision, cataracts, decreased acuity, dyschromatopsia, high-frequency sensorineural hearing loss, loss of vision, night blindness, optic neuritis, retinopathy, scotoma, tinnitus, visual field defects
GI: Abdominal discomfort, diarrhea, **hepatic dysfunction**, increased liver enzymes, nausea, vomiting
GU: Acute renal failure, dysuria, increased serum creatinine, renal tubular disorder
HEME: Leukopenia, thrombocytopenia
MS: Arthralgia, growth retardation, metaphyseal dysplasia, myalgia
RESP: Acute respiratory distress syndrome, asthma

SKIN: Rash, urticaria

Other: Anaphylaxis; angioedema; infections with *Yersinia* or *Mucormycosis;* injection-site reactions such as localized irritation, pain, burning, swelling, induration, infiltration, pruritus, erythema, wheal formation, eschar, crust, vesicles, or local edema

Childbearing Considerations

PREGNANCY

- It is not known if drug causes fetal harm.
- Use with caution only if benefit to mother outweighs potential risk to fetus.

LACTATION

- It is not known if drug is present in breast milk.
- Patient should check with prescriber before breastfeeding.

Nursing Considerations

- Expect to administer other supportive measures, as ordered, when treating acute iron intoxication with deferoxamine because acute respiratory distress syndrome may occur. Supportive measures include control of shock with blood transfusions, intravenous fluids, oxygen, and vasopressors; correction of acidosis; gastric lavage; induction of emesis with syrup of ipecac; and suction and maintenance of a clear airway.
- Know that patients with thalassemia inadvertently given a high-dose or rapid intravenous infusion of deferoxamine may develop acute respiratory distress syndrome and other life-threatening disorders such as hypotension, CNS depression, and acute renal failure. Symptomatic treatment is required, as there is no specific antidote for deferoxamine, although the drug is readily dialyzable.
- Monitor patient closely for changes in hearing or vision, especially in patients receiving deferoxamine at high doses or over prolonged periods of time, or in patients who have low ferritin levels. If present, notify prescriber immediately and expect drug to be discontinued. Expect audiometry, fundoscopy, slit-lamp examinations, and visual acuity tests to be performed periodically in patients treated for prolonged periods of time. Early detection improves the possibility of reversal of these symptoms or test abnormalities.

- Monitor patient's serum creatinine level, and assess patient for symptoms of renal dysfunction, because deferoxamine has been associated with renal dysfunction.
- Assess children regularly for growth retardation, especially if high doses of the drug are being administered in the presence of low ferritin levels. Monitor the child's body weight and growth every 3 months. If abnormalities are detected, notify the prescriber because growth velocity may partially resume to pretreatment rates after a reduction of deferoxamine dosage occurs.

! WARNING Monitor patient, especially children, closely for signs and symptoms of respiratory distress, especially following treatment with excessively high intravenous doses of deferoxamine.

! WARNING Assess patient regularly for infections because either deferoxamine therapy or iron overload may enhance susceptibility to generalized infections. Some cases of mucormycosis have been fatal. If signs and symptoms occur, notify prescriber immediately and expect drug to be discontinued and appropriate treatment instituted.

- Expect to administer vitamin C with deferoxamine therapy because iron overload usually causes a vitamin C deficiency. However, be aware that high doses (more than 500 mg daily in adults, 100 mg in children age 10 and older, and 50 mg in children under age 10) may cause cardiac dysfunction. Therefore, make sure patient is not receiving vitamin C if he has cardiac failure, expect supplemental vitamin C therapy to begin only after an initial month of regular treatment with deferoxamine, and make sure the daily dose of vitamin C does not exceed 200 mg in adults, given in divided doses. Monitor all patients receiving deferoxamine and vitamin C therapy concomitantly for cardiac dysfunction and report any dysfunction immediately to prescriber.
- Be aware that patients with aluminum-related encephalopathy who are receiving dialysis may develop seizures as a result of deferoxamine therapy. Deferoxamine therapy may also precipitate the onset of dialysis

dementia in these patients, as well as cause a decrease in the patient's serum calcium levels and aggravate hyperparathyroidism, if present.

- Discontinue deferoxamine therapy, as ordered, 48 hours prior to scintigraphy because imaging results may be distorted as a result of the rapid urinary excretion of deferoxamine-bound gallium-67.

PATIENT TEACHING

- Inform patient that deferoxamine therapy is an adjunct to, and not a substitute for, standard measures used to treat acute iron intoxication.
- Advise patient not to exceed the recommended dose of daily vitamin C therapy prescribed.
- Caution patient not to perform hazardous activities such as driving until CNS, visual, and auditory adverse effects are known.
- Inform patient that his urine may have a reddish discoloration because of deferoxamine therapy.

delafloxacin meglumine
Baxdela

Class and Category

Pharmacologic class: Fluoroquinolone
Therapeutic class: Antibacterial

Indications and Dosages

✳ *To treat acute bacterial skin and skin structure infections (ABSSSI) caused by gram-negative organisms* (Enterobacter cloacae, Escherichia coli, Klebsiella pneumoniae, Pseudomonas aeruginosa) *and gram-positive organisms* (Enterococcus faecalis, Staphylococcus aureus, S. haemolyticus, S. lugdunensis, Streptococcus agalactiae, S. anginosus, S. pyogenes); *to treat community-acquired bacterial pneumonia (CABP) caused by* Chlamydia pneumoniae, E. coli, Haemophilus influenzae, H. parainfluenzae, K. pneumoniae, Legionella pneumophila, Mycoplasma pneumoniae, P. aeruginosa, S. aureus, *and* S. pneumoniae

TABLETS

Adults. 450 mg every 12 hr for 5 to 10 days (CABP) or 5 to 14 days (ABSSSI).

I.V. INFUSION, TABLETS

Adults. 300 mg I.V. every 12 hr for 5 to 10 days (CABP) and 5 to 14 days (ABSSSI). Alternatively, 300 mg I.V. every 12 hr switched to 450 mg P.O. every 12 hr at the discretion of the prescriber for a total of 5 to 10 days (CABP) and 5 to 14 days (ABSSSI).

±**DOSAGE ADJUSTMENT** For patients with an estimated glomerular filtration rate (eGFR) between 15 and 29 ml/min who are receiving the drug intravenously, dosage reduced to 200 mg every 12 hr or dosage reduced to 200 mg every 12 hr, then switched to 450 mg orally every 12 hr at the discretion of the prescriber.

Drug Administration

P.O.

- Administer tablets at least 2 hours before or 6 hours after antacids containing aluminum or magnesium, didanosine, iron preparations, multivitamins containing iron or zinc, or sucralfate.

I.V.

- Reconstitute drug powder by using 10.5 ml of 0.9% Sodium Chloride Injection or 5% Dextrose Injection for each 300-mg vial. Shake vial vigorously until contents are completely dissolved. Concentration will be 300 mg/12 ml. Solution should appear clear yellow to amber-colored.
- Further dilute to a total volume of 250 ml, using either 0.9% Sodium Chloride Injection or 5% Dextrose Injection to achieve a concentration of 1.2 mg/ml. To do so, withdraw 12 ml of reconstituted solution for a 300-mg dose and 8 ml of reconstituted solution for a 200-mg dose from vial and transfer to an intravenous bag.
- Discard any unused portion of the reconstituted solution.
- Reconstituted vials or diluted solution already added to an intravenous bag may be stored either in the refrigerator or at room temperature for up to 24 hours. The solution should not be frozen.
- Administer as an infusion over 60 minutes.
- If a common intravenous line is being used to administer other drugs in addition to delafloxacin, the line should be flushed before and after each delafloxacin infusion with 0.9% Sodium Chloride Injection or 5% Dextrose Injection.

- *Incompatibilities:* Other additives, drugs, or solutions except 0.9% Sodium Chloride Injection or 5% Dextrose Injection

Route	Onset	Peak	Duration
P.O.	Unknown	1 hr	Unknown
I.V.	Unknown	1 hr	Unknown

Half-life: 3.7 hr (I.V.); 4.2–8.5 hr (P.O.)

Mechanism of Action

Inhibits both bacterial topoisomerase IV and DNA gyrase enzymes, which are required for bacterial DNA recombination, repair, replication, and transcription.

Contraindications

Hypersensitivity to delafloxacin, other fluoroquinolones, or any of its components

Interactions

DRUGS

antacids containing aluminum or magnesium, didanosine, iron preparations, multivitamins containing iron or zinc, sucralfate: Significantly decreased absorption of oral delafloxacin

Adverse Reactions

CNS: Abnormal dreams, agitation, anxiety, confusion, delirium, depression, disorientation, disturbances in attention, dizziness, hallucinations, headache, hypoesthesia, **increased intracranial pressure,** insomnia, memory impairment, nervousness, nightmares, paresthesia, paranoia, peripheral neuropathy, **seizures, suicidal ideation,** syncope, tremors, toxic psychosis, vertigo
CV: **Aortic aneurysm and dissection, bradycardia,** hypertension, **hypotension,** palpitations, phlebitis, tachycardia, **ventricular extrasystoles**
EENT: Blurred vision, oral candidiasis, taste alteration, tinnitus
ENDO: Hyperglycemia, **hypoglycemia**
GI: Abdominal pain, *Clostridium difficile–associated diarrhea,* diarrhea, dyspepsia, elevated liver enzymes, nausea, vomiting
GU: Elevated blood creatinine levels, **renal failure,** renal impairment, vulvovaginal candidiasis
HEME: **Agranulocytosis,** anemia, **leukopenia, neutropenia, pancytopenia**
MS: Myalgia, tendinitis, tendon rupture
RESP: Dyspnea
SKIN: Dermatitis, flushing, pruritus, rash, urticaria
Other: **Anaphylaxis, angioedema,** elevated alkaline phosphatase and creatine phosphokinase levels, fungal infection, infusion-site reactions (bruising, discomfort, edema, erythema, irritation, pain, phlebitis, swelling, thrombosis)

Childbearing Considerations

PREGNANCY

- It is not known if drug causes fetal harm.
- Use with caution only if benefit to mother outweighs potential risk to fetus.

LACTATION

- It is not known if drug is present in breast milk.
- Patient should check with prescriber before breastfeeding.

Nursing Considerations

- Know that fluoroquinolones, including delafloxacin, may exacerbate muscle weakness in patients with myasthenia gravis and should not be given to patients with a history of myasthenia gravis.
- Be aware that studies have shown an increased risk for aortic aneurysm and dissection within 2 months following use of fluoroquinolones, especially in elderly patients. Drug should only be given to patients with an aortic aneurysm or who are at greater risk for an aortic aneurysm if there are no alternative antibacterial treatments.

! **WARNING** Know that fluoroquinolones like delafloxacin have been associated with disabling and potentially irreversible serious adverse reactions that have occurred together, including central nervous system effects, peripheral neuropathy, tendinitis, and tendon rupture. Fluoroquinolones also have been associated with an increased risk of increased intracranial pressure and seizures. At the first sign or symptom of any serious adverse reaction, withhold delafloxacin and notify prescriber. Expect delafloxacin to be discontinued.

- Monitor patients with severe renal impairment receiving intravenous delafloxacin by obtaining serum creatinine

D

levels and eGFR values, as ordered. Know that if serum creatinine level increases, prescriber should be notified; expect patient to be switched to oral form. Notify prescriber if patient's eGFR decreases to less than 15 ml/min and expect drug to be discontinued.

- Assess patient for evidence of peripheral neuropathy. Notify prescriber and expect to stop drug if patient complains of burning, numbness, pain, tingling, or weakness in extremities or if physical examination reveals deficits in light touch, motor strength, pain, position sense, temperature, or vibratory sensation.

- Monitor patients (especially patients over 60 years of age, patients receiving corticosteroids, and patients who have renal failure or who have had a heart, kidney, or lung transplant) for evidence of tendon rupture, such as inflammation, pain, and swelling at the site. Be aware that tendon rupture may occur within the first 48 hours of therapy, throughout therapy, or months after delafloxacin therapy. Notify prescriber about suspected tendon rupture, and have patient rest and refrain from exercise until tendon rupture has been ruled out. If present, expect to provide supportive care, as ordered.

- Monitor patient closely for changes in behavior or mood that may be caused by delafloxacin-induced depression or worsening psychotic reactions potentially resulting in self-injurious behavior, such as suicide. Be aware that these reactions may occur even after just one dose. Notify prescriber immediately and expect to discontinue delafloxacin therapy, if present, and institute precautions to keep patient safe until adverse effects have disappeared.

! **WARNING** Assess patient routinely for signs of rash or other hypersensitivity reactions, even after patient has received multiple doses. Stop drug at first sign of rash or other sign of hypersensitivity, and notify prescriber immediately. Be prepared to provide supportive emergency care.

- Monitor patient closely for diarrhea, which may reflect pseudomembranous colitis caused by *Clostridium difficile* infection.

If it occurs, notify prescriber and expect to withhold drug and treat diarrhea.

- Monitor patient's blood glucose levels, especially in diabetic patients, and for signs and symptoms of changes in blood glucose levels. Both symptomatic hyperglycemia and hypoglycemia may occur as a result of delafloxacin therapy. If present, alert prescriber and initiate appropriate treatment, as prescribed. Also be aware that severe hypoglycemia has occurred with other fluoroquinolones. If a hypoglycemic reaction occurs, discontinue administration immediately and initiate appropriate treatment for hypoglycemia.

PATIENT TEACHING

- Urge patient to complete the prescribed course of therapy, even if he feels better before it's finished.

- Tell patient that if he misses a dose, he should take it as soon as possible anytime up to 8 hours prior to the next dose. If less than 8 hours remain before the next dose, he should wait until the next scheduled dose.

- Instruct patient to take tablets at least 2 hours before or 6 hours after antacids containing aluminum or magnesium, didanosine, iron preparations, multivitamins containing iron or zinc, or sucralfate.

- Urge patient to avoid hazardous activities until CNS effects of drug are known.

- Advise patient to notify prescriber about changes in limb movement or sensation and about inflammation, pain, or swelling over a joint. Urge patient to rest the affected limb at the first sign of discomfort.

! **WARNING** Tell patient to stop taking drug and to notify prescriber at first sign of rash or other hypersensitivity reaction.

- Urge patient to report bloody, watery stools to prescriber immediately, even up to 2 months after drug therapy has ended.

- Urge caregivers to monitor patient closely for suicidal tendencies if patient develops depression or worsening of psychotic behavior during therapy and to notify prescriber.

- Instruct patient to report any persistent, severe, or unusual signs and symptoms to prescriber.

- Warn patients, especially diabetics, that delafloxacin may alter blood glucose levels. Review signs and symptoms of hyperglycemia and hypoglycemia. Tell patient to immediately report symptomatic changes in blood glucose levels to prescriber and review how to treat hypoglycemia.

denosumab
Prolia, Xgeva

≣ Class and Category
Pharmacologic class: Monoclonal antibody
Therapeutic class: Antiresorptive, antiosteoporotic

≣ Indications and Dosages
✳ *To treat men and postmenopausal women with osteoporosis at high risk for fracture; to treat bone loss in men receiving androgen deprivation therapy for nonmetastatic prostate cancer; to treat bone loss in women receiving adjuvant aromatase inhibitor therapy for breast cancer; to treat glucocorticoid-induced osteoporosis in men and women at high risk of fracture who are either initiating or continuing systemic glucocorticoids in a daily dosage equivalent to 7.5 mg or greater of prednisone and expected to remain on glucocorticoids for at least 6 months*

SUBCUTANEOUS INJECTION (PROLIA)
Adult. 60 mg once every 6 months.
✳ *To prevent skeletal-related events in patients with multiple myeloma and in patients with bone metastasis from solid tumors*

SUBCUTANEOUS INJECTION (XGEVA)
Adult. 120 mg every 4 wk.
✳ *To treat giant cell tumor of bone*

SUBCUTANEOUS INJECTION (XGEVA)
Adult and skeletally mature adolescents 12 to 16 years old. 120 mg every 4 wk with additional 120 mg doses on days 8 and 15 of the first month of therapy.
✳ *To treat hypercalcemia of malignancy refractory to bisphosphonate therapy*

SUBCUTANEOUS INJECTION (XGEVA)
Adults. 120 mg every 4 wk with additional 120 mg doses on days 8 and 15 for the first month of therapy.

≣ Drug Administration
SUBCUTANEOUS
▪ Drug solution may contain trace amounts of translucent to white proteinaceous particles. However, do not use if solution is discolored or cloudy, or if solution contains many particles or foreign particulate matter.
▪ Do not handle the gray needle cap on the prefilled syringe if allergic to latex.
▪ Remove drug from refrigerator and bring to room temperature, which generally takes 15 to 30 minutes. Do not warm drug any other way. Once removed from refrigerator, drug should not be exposed to temperatures above 25°C (77°F) or direct light.
▪ When using the single prefilled syringe, do not slide the green safety guard forward over the needle, as it will lock in place and prevent injection. Do so only after the injection to prevent an accidental needle stick.
▪ When using single-dose vials, withdraw solution using a 27G needle. Avoid vigorous shaking.
▪ Administer drug using a 27G needle and inject into the abdomen, thigh, or upper arm.
▪ Do not administer as an I.M. or I.V. injection.
▪ Discard if not used within 14 days after being taken from refrigerator.

Route	Onset	Peak	Duration
SubQ	Unknown	10 days	Unknown

Half-life: 25–28 days

≣ Mechanism of Action
Binds to RANKL, a transmembrane or soluble protein required for the formation, function, and survival of osteoclasts, the cells responsible for bone resorption. By preventing RANKL from activating its receptor, RANK, on the surface of osteoclasts, osteoclast formation, function, and survival are inhibited. This action decreases bone resorption and increases bone mass and strength in both cortical and trabecular bone.

≣ Contraindications
Hypersensitivity to denosumab and its components, hypocalcemia, pregnancy

≣ Interactions
DRUGS
other calcium-lowering drugs: Augmentation of calcium-lowering effect with possible severe hypocalcemia

≣ Adverse Reactions
CNS: Asthenia, headache, insomnia, sciatica, vertigo

CV: Angina pectoris, **atrial fibrillation, endocarditis,** hypercholesterolemia, peripheral edema, vasculitis
EENT: Ear infection, nasopharyngitis
ENDO: Increased serum parathyroid hormone levels (presence of severe renal impairment or dialysis)
GI: Abdominal pain, constipation, diarrhea, flatulence, gastroesophageal reflux disease, nausea, **pancreatitis,** upper abdominal pain
GU: Cystitis, UTI
HEME: Anemia, **thrombocytopenia**
MS: Arthralgia; atypical subtrochanteric and diaphyseal femoral fractures; back, bone, extremity including joint, or musculoskeletal pain; jaw osteonecrosis; myalgia; spinal osteoarthritis
RESP: Cough, dyspnea, pneumonia, upper respiratory infection
SKIN: Alopecia, cellulitis, dermatitis, eczema, erysipelas (infection of upper dermis and superficial lymphatics), erythema, lichenoid drug eruptions, pruritus, rash, urticaria
Other: **Anaphylaxis, angioedema,** antibodies to denosumab, **drug reaction with eosinophilia and systemic symptoms (DRESS),** herpes zoster, **hypercalcemia of malignancy, hypocalcemia, hypophosphatemia, malignancies (breast, gastrointestinal, reproductive),** serious infections

⊟ Childbearing Considerations

PREGNANCY

- Pregnancy status of females who are of childbearing potential should be verified before drug therapy is initiated.
- Drug may cause fetal harm.
- Drug is contraindicated during pregnancy.

LACTATION

- It is not known if drug is present in breast milk.
- Patient should check with prescriber before breastfeeding.

REPRODUCTION

- Females who are of childbearing potential should be advised to use effective contraception during therapy, and for at least 5 months after the last dose of the drug.

⊟ Nursing Considerations

- Know that preexisting hypocalcemia must be corrected prior to denosumab therapy.

- Ensure that a pregnancy test has been performed and is negative for all women of childbearing age before denosumab therapy is begun, because drug can be toxic to the fetus.

! WARNING Monitor patient closely for hypersensitivity reactions that may be severe such as dyspnea, hypotension, lip swelling, pruritus rash, upper airway edema, and urticaria. Also monitor patient for DRESS. If an allergic reaction or a rash is present, stop denosumab therapy immediately, notify prescriber, and provide supportive care, as needed and ordered.

! WARNING Monitor patient's calcium level, as ordered, especially in patients predisposed to hypocalcemia or disturbances of mineral metabolism, such as a history of excision of the small intestine, hypoparathyroidism, parathyroid or thyroid surgery, malabsorption syndromes, or severe renal impairment. Know that severe hypocalcemia has occurred with denosumab therapy resulting, in some cases, in death. Monitor patient closely for signs and symptoms of hypocalcemia such as neuromuscular irritability, and notify prescriber immediately if present. Expect drug to be discontinued, administer calcium replacement therapy, as ordered, and provide supportive care.

- Be aware that significant hypercalcemia has also occurred in patients with growing skeletons and patients with a giant cell tumor of the bone weeks to months after drug was discontinued. Monitor patient for signs of hypercalcemia (abdominal or bone pain, confusion, constipation, fatigue, frequent urination, muscle weakness, nausea, thirst, vomiting) and if present, notify prescriber and expect to treat, as prescribed.
- Know that fracture risk increases, including the risk of multiple vertebral fractures, when denosumab is discontinued. New vertebral fractures may occur as early as 7 months after the last dose. If denosumab therapy is discontinued, discuss possibility of patient transitioning to an alternative antiresorptive therapy with prescriber.
- Monitor patient for signs and symptoms of infection, because denosumab increases

risk, especially if patient is receiving immunosuppressant therapy or has an impaired immune system. Serious skin infections as well as infections of the abdomen, ear, and urinary tract have occurred. There has also been increased incidence of endocarditis in patients receiving denosumab. Notify prescriber if an infection is suspected.

PATIENT TEACHING

- Tell patient that if a dose of denosumab is missed, injection should be administered as soon as convenient. Thereafter, future injections should be scheduled from the date of the actual injection.
- Instruct patient to take a calcium supplement of 1,000 mg and at least 400 international units of vitamin D daily. Review signs and symptoms of hypocalcemia and instruct patient to seek medical care promptly, if present.

! **WARNING** Tell patient to stop taking denosumab and seek immediate emergency care if allergic reactions occur. If a rash develops, tell patient to notify prescriber immediately as drug may have to be discontinued.

- Advise patient to notify prescriber if signs and symptoms of infection occur, such as drainage, fever, pain, redness, or swelling.
- Inform patient to report bone, joint, and/or muscle pain, as drug may have to be discontinued depending on the severity.
- Tell patient to notify prescriber if severe adverse skin reactions occur, as drug may have to be discontinued.
- Instruct patient on proper oral hygiene and on the need to notify dentist of denosumab therapy before invasive dental procedures are performed.
- Instruct women of childbearing age to use effective contraception during treatment and for at least 5 months after the last dose of denosumab. Also tell patient to report suspected or confirmed pregnancy immediately, as drug may cause fetal harm and have to be discontinued. Also inform her that breastfeeding is not recommended while taking denosumab.
- Advise patient to report new or unusual groin, hip, or thigh pain or tingling or numbness in fingers and toes.

- Advise patient not to interrupt denosumab therapy without talking with prescriber, because of increased risk for multiple vertebral fractures.
- Advise patients with growing skeletons to report decreased alertness, headache, nausea, or vomiting following discontinuation of drug, as this could indicate a higher than normal calcium level requiring prompt treatment.

desipramine hydrochloride

Norpramin

D

Class and Category

Pharmacologic class: Tricyclic antidepressant
Therapeutic class: Antidepressant

Indications and Dosages

* *To treat depression*

TABLETS

Adults. *Initial:* 100 to 200 mg daily as single dose or divided doses. Increased gradually to 300 mg daily, if needed. *Maximum:* 300 mg daily.

Adolescents and elderly patients. *Initial:* 25 to 50 mg daily in divided doses. Increased gradually to 150 mg daily, if needed. *Maximum:* 150 mg daily.

Drug Administration

P.O.

- No special instructions given by manufacturer.

Route	Onset	Peak	Duration
P.O.	2–5 days	4–6 hr	Unknown

Half-life: 15–24 hr

Mechanism of Action

Blocks norepinephrine and serotonin reuptake by adrenergic nerves, which normally release these neurotransmitters from their storage sites when activated by a nerve impulse. By blocking reuptake, this tricyclic antidepressant increases norepinephrine and serotonin levels at nerve synapses, which may elevate mood and reduce depression.

⊞ Contraindications

Acute recovery phase of MI; hypersensitivity to desipramine, other tricyclic antidepressants (dibenzazepines), or their components; linezolid or I.V. methylene blue; MAO inhibitor therapy within 14 days

⊞ Interactions

DRUGS

barbiturates, CNS depressants: Increased CNS depression
clonidine: Increased risk of hypertensive crisis
MAO inhibitors: Increased risk of life-threatening adverse effects, such as hyperpyretic or hypertensive crisis and severe seizures
P450 2D6 inhibitors (cimetidine, quinidine), class 1C antiarrhythmics (flecainide, propafenone), many other antidepressants, phenothiazines, selective serotonin reuptake inhibitors: Increased blood level and adverse effects of desipramine; potential increased blood levels of and adverse reactions to these drugs
quinolones: Increased risk of arrhythmias, including torsades de pointes

ACTIVITIES

alcohol use: Possibly increased alcohol effects

⊞ Adverse Reactions

CNS: Agitation, akathisia, anxiety, ataxia, confusion, **CVA**, delusions, disorientation, dizziness, drowsiness, extrapyramidal reactions, fatigue, headache, hypomania, insomnia, lack of coordination, nervousness, nightmares, paresthesia, peripheral neuropathy, psychosis exacerbation, restlessness, **seizures**, **serotonin syndrome**, sleep disturbance, **suicidal ideation**, tremor, weakness
CV: Arrhythmias, including heart block; hypertension; **hypotension;** palpitations
EENT: Acute-angle glaucoma, black tongue, blurred vision, dry mouth, mydriasis, stomatitis, taste perversion, tinnitus
ENDO: Breast enlargement and galactorrhea (women), gynecomastia (men), hyperglycemia, **hypoglycemia**, syndrome of inappropriate ADH secretion
GI: Abdominal cramps, anorexia, constipation, diarrhea, elevated liver enzymes, elevated pancreatic enzyme levels, epigastric distress, **hepatitis**, ileus, increased appetite, nausea, vomiting

GU: Acute renal failure, impotence, libido changes, nocturia, painful ejaculation, testicular swelling, urinary frequency and hesitancy, urine retention
HEME: Agranulocytosis, eosinophilia, **thrombocytopenia**
SKIN: Acne, alopecia, dermatitis, diaphoresis, dry skin, flushing, petechiae, photosensitivity, pruritus, purpura, rash, urticaria
Other: Angioedema, drug fever, weight gain

⊞ Childbearing Considerations

PREGNANCY

- Pregnancy exposure registry: 1-844-405-6185 or https://womens mentalhealth.org/clinical-and -researchprograms/pregnancyregistry /antidepressants
- It is not known if drug causes fetal harm.
- Use with caution only if benefit to mother outweighs potential risk to fetus.

LACTATION

- Drug maybe present in breast milk.
- Patient should check with prescriber before breastfeeding.

⊞ Nursing Considerations

- Use desipramine with extreme caution in patients with cardiovascular disease, glaucoma, seizure disorder, thyroid disease, or urine retention or with a family history of sudden death, cardiac arrhythmias, or conduction disturbances.

! WARNING Be aware that desipramine increases risk of suicidal ideation in teens; monitor them closely for evidence.

! WARNING Expect drug to produce sedation and possibly to lower seizure threshold. Take safety and seizure precautions. Seizures may precede arrhythmias and death in some patients. Alert prescriber immediately if seizure activity occurs.

- Monitor blood glucose level often.
- Be prepared to obtain blood sample for leukocyte and differential counts if patient develops fever during therapy.
- Expect to discontinue drug as soon as possible before elective surgery because of its possible adverse cardiovascular effects.

! WARNING Monitor patient closely for evidence of serotonin syndrome, such as agitation, coma, diarrhea, hallucinations, hyperreflexia, hyperthermia, incoordination, labile blood pressure, nausea, tachycardia, or vomiting. Notify prescriber at once because serotonin syndrome maybe life-threatening. Be prepared to discontinue drug and provide supportive care.

PATIENT TEACHING

! **WARNING** Urge parents to watch teen closely and to report abnormal thinking or behavior, aggression, or hostility.

- Urge patient to use sunscreen outdoors and to avoid sunlamps and tanning beds.
- Instruct patient to notify prescriber immediately about fainting, a fast and pounding heartbeat, restlessness, severe agitation, and strange behavior or thoughts.
- Caution patient not to stop drug abruptly; doing so may cause dizziness, headache, hyperthermia, irritability, malaise, nausea, sleep disturbances, and vomiting.
- Advise against drinking alcohol because of increased risk of adverse CNS reactions.
- Advise patient to avoid hazardous activities until drug's CNS effects are known.
- Advise patient that drug may cause mild pupillary dilation, which may lead to an episode of acute-angle glaucoma. Encourage patient to have an eye exam before starting therapy to see if she is at risk.
- Urge diabetic patient to monitor blood glucose level often.

desmopressin acetate
DDAVP, Nocdurna, Stimate

≣ Class and Category
Pharmacologic class: Posterior pituitary hormone
Therapeutic class: Antidiuretic, hemostatic

≣ Indications and Dosages
✳ *To manage primary nocturnal enuresis*
TABLETS
Adults and children age 6 and over.
Initial: 0.2 mg, increased as needed.
Maximum: 0.6 mg daily.

✳ *To treat nocturia due to nocturnal polyuria in patients who awaken at least two times per night to void*
SUBLINGUAL TABLETS (NOCDURNA)
Women. 27.7 mcg once daily.
Men. 55.3 mcg once daily.
✳ *To control symptoms of central diabetes insipidus*
TABLETS
Adults. *Initial:* 0.05 mg twice daily, increased as needed. *Usual:* 0.1 to 1.2 mg in divided doses twice daily or three times daily. *Maximum:* 1.2 mg daily.
I.V. INFUSION, SUBCUTANEOUS INJECTION
Adults and adolescents. *Usual:* 2 to 4 mcg daily in divided doses twice daily. Dosage adjusted, as needed.
NASAL SPRAY (DDAVP)
Adults and adolescents. 10 mcg up to 40 mcg daily as a single dose in one nostril or in divided doses twice daily or three times daily. Dosage adjusted as needed. If daily dose is divided, each dose adjusted separately.
Children ages 4 to 12 years. 10 mcg up to 30 mcg daily as a single dose in one nostril or in divided doses twice daily. Dosage adjusted as needed. If daily dose is divided, each dose adjusted separately.
✳ *To prevent or manage bleeding episodes in hemophilia A or mild to moderate type I von Willebrand's disease*
I.V. INFUSION
Adults and children age 3 months and over. 0.3 mcg/kg. If used preoperatively, given 30 min before procedure.
NASAL SOLUTION (STIMATE)
Adults and children weighing 50 kg (110 lb) or more. 150 mcg in each nostril. If used preoperatively, given 2 hr before procedure.
Adults and children weighing less than 50 kg (110 lb). 150 mcg in one nostril. If used preoperatively, given 2 hr before procedure.

≣ Drug Administration
P.O.
- Sublingual tablet should be given 1 hour before bedtime and kept under the tongue until fully dissolved. Do not administer with water.
- Regular tablets should be given at bedtime when used to treat primary nocturnal enuresis.

D

I.V.

- Gently tap top of ampule to assist the flow of solution from the upper portion of ampule to the lower portion.
- Locate blue dot on upper portion of ampule. Below the dot is a small score on the neck of the ampule. Hold ampule with blue dot facing away.
- Cover ampule with an appropriate wipe. Apply pressure to the top and bottom portions of ampule to snap it open.
- For treatment of hemophilia A and von Willebrand's disease (Type 1), dilute drug in 0.9% Sodium Chloride. Use 50 ml in adults and children weighing more than 10 kg (22 lb) and 10 ml in children weighing 10 kg (22 lb) or less.
- Infuse over 15 to 30 minutes.
- *Incompatibilities:* None listed by manufacturer

SUBCUTANEOUS

- No special instructions given by manufacturer.

INTRANASAL

- Nasal passage should be clean and free of obstruction as well as intact before administration.
- Store in upright position.
- Prime Stimate spray bottle by pressing down on pump four times before first use. Store at room temperature. Discard after 25 sprays.
- Prime DDAVP spray bottle by pressing down four times before first use. Discard after 50 sprays.
- In children ages 4 to 12 being treated for central diabetes insipidus, who are receiving 30 mcg daily, dose divided into two doses; give larger dose (20 mcg) in the morning and smaller dose (10 mcg) at night.

Route	Onset	Peak	Duration
P.O.	1 hr	4–7 hr	6–14 hr
I.V.	30 min	1.5–2 hr	6–14 hr
Nasal	15–60 min	1–5 hr	6–14 hr

Half-life: 1.5–3.5 hr

⫶ Mechanism of Action

Exerts an antidiuretic effect similar to that of vasopressin by increasing cellular permeability of renal collecting ducts and distal tubules, thus enhancing water reabsorption, reducing urine flow, and increasing osmolality. As a hemostatic, drug increases blood level of clotting factor VIII (antihemophilic factor) and activity of von Willebrand factor (factor VII_{VWF}). It also may increase platelet aggregation and adhesion at injury sites by directly affecting blood vessel walls.

⫶ Contraindications

All forms: History or presence of hyponatremia, hypersensitivity to desmopressin or its components, moderate to severe renal impairment (creatinine clearance below 50 ml/min)
DDVAP, Minirin, and Noctiva only: Primary nocturnal enuresis
intranasal and sublingual forms: Concurrent therapy with inhaled or systemic glucocorticoids or loop diuretics, during illnesses that can cause fluid and electrolyte imbalance, polydipsia, syndrome of inappropriate antidiuretic hormone (SIADH) secretion
Nocdurna: Heart failure
Noctiva only: New York Heart Association Class II–IV congestive heart failure
Nocdurna and Noctiva: Uncontrolled hypertension

⫶ Interactions

DRUGS

carbamazepine, chlorpromazine, lamotrigine, NSAIDs, opioid analgesics, selective serotonin reuptake inhibitors, tricyclic antidepressants: Possibly increased risk of water intoxication with hyponatremia
vasopressor drugs: Possibly potentiated vasopressor effect of desmopressin

⫶ Adverse Reactions

CNS: Asthenia, chills, **CVA**, dizziness, headache
CV: Hypertension (with high doses), **MI**, **thrombosis**, transient hypotension
EENT: Conjunctivitis, epistaxis, lacrimation, nasal congestion (nasal form), ocular edema, pharyngitis, rhinitis, sore throat
GI: Abdominal cramps, nausea
GU: Vulvar pain (parenteral form)
RESP: Cough, upper respiratory infections
SKIN: Flushing
Other: Anaphylaxis, hyponatremia, injection-site pain and redness, water intoxication

Childbearing Considerations

PREGNANCY

- It is not known if drug causes fetal harm.
- Nocdurna is not recommended for use during pregnancy.
- Use with caution only if benefit to mother outweighs potential risk to fetus.

LACTATION

- Drug is present in breast milk but is poorly absorbed orally by the breastfed infant.
- Patient should check with prescriber before breastfeeding.

Nursing Considerations

- Use desmopressin cautiously in patients with conditions associated with fluid and electrolyte imbalance, such as cystic fibrosis, heart failure, and renal disorders; these patients are prone to hyponatremia.
- Also use cautiously in patients with habitual or psychogenic polydipsia; they may be more likely to drink excessive water, raising the risk of hyponatremia.
- Be aware that nasal cavity scarring, edema, and other abnormalities may cause erratic absorption and require a different administration route.
- Know that the recommended dose for women using the sublingual form of drug is lower than for men because women are more sensitive to the effects of the sublingual form and have a higher risk of hyponatremia with the 55.3-mcg dose.
- Check blood pressure often during therapy.

! **WARNING** Monitor patient closely for evidence of hyponatremia, such as changes in mental status, depressed reflexes, fatigue, headache, lethargy, nausea, restlessness, and vomiting. If left undetected, coma, respiratory arrest, and seizures may occur. Monitor patient's serum sodium level, and notify prescriber of abnormalities.

- Be aware that the nasal spray formulation is not used for the treatment of primary nocturnal enuresis due to a higher risk of hyponatremia and hyponatremic seizures.

PATIENT TEACHING

- Be aware that to prevent hyponatremia and water intoxication in a child or an elderly patient, family should be urged to restrict patient's fluids as prescribed.
- Tell patient to refrigerate nasal solution.
- Instruct patient who uses nasal spray to prime pump before first use by pressing down four times. Advise her to discard pump after 25 doses (Stimate) or 50 doses (DDAVP).
- Instruct patient taking sublingual tablets to keep tablet under the tongue until it is fully dissolved. Also instruct patient to empty the bladder immediately before bedtime and to limit fluids to a minimum from 1 hour before until 8 hours after taking drug.
- Teach patient or caregiver how to administer subcutaneous injection, if appropriate.
- Urge patient to report adverse reactions.

dexamethasone
Dexamethasone Intensol

dexamethasone acetate

dexamethasone sodium phosphate

Class and Category

Pharmacologic class: Glucocorticoid
Therapeutic class: Anti-inflammatory, diagnostic aid, immunosuppressant

Indications and Dosages

✴ *To treat inflammatory or neoplastic conditions*

ELIXIR, ORAL SOLUTION, TABLETS

Adults. Highly individualized dosage based on severity of disorder. *Usual:* 0.75 to 9 mg/day in divided doses.
Children. Highly individualized, based on severity of disorder. 0.02 to 0.3 mg/kg/day in three or four divided doses.

I.M. OR I.V. INJECTION

Adults. Highly individualized based on severity of disorder. *Usual:* 0.5 to 9 mg (one-third to one-half oral dose) in divided doses every 12 hr.
Children. Highly individualized based on severity of disorder: *Usual:* One-third to one-half of oral dosage in divided doses every 12 hr.

✴ *To manage adrenocortical insufficiency*

ELIXIR, ORAL SOLUTION, TABLETS

Adults. 0.5 to 9 mg daily as a single dose or in divided doses.

Children. 0.02 to 0.3 mg/kg/day in four divided doses.

✱ *To test for Cushing's syndrome*

ELIXIR, ORAL SOLUTION, TABLETS

Adults. 0.5 mg every 6 hr for 48 hr, followed by collection of 24-hr urine specimen to determine 17-hydroxycorticosteroid level. Or, 1 mg at 11 p.m., followed by plasma cortisol test performed at 8 a.m. the next day.

✱ *To distinguish Cushing's syndrome related to pituitary corticotropin excess from Cushing's syndrome from other causes*

ELIXIR, ORAL SOLUTION, TABLETS

Adults. 2 mg every 6 hr for 48 hr, followed by collection of 24-hr urine specimen to determine 17-hydroxycorticosteroid level.

✱ *To treat palliate management of inoperable or recurrent brain tumors*

ELIXIR, I.M. OR I.V. INJECTION, ORAL SOLUTION, TABLETS

Adults. 2 mg every 8 to 12 hr as maintenance after parenteral form has controlled initial symptoms.

✱ *To treat cerebral edema*

I.V. AND I.M. INJECTION

Adults. 10 mg I.V. followed by 4 mg I.M. every 6 hr. Decreased after 2 to 4 days, if needed, gradually tapering off over 5 to 7 days.

✱ *To treat unresponsive shock*

I.V. INFUSION AND INJECTION

Adults. 20 mg as a single dose, followed by 3 mg/kg over 24 hr as a continuous infusion. Alternatively, 40 mg as a single dose, followed by 40 mg every 2 to 6 hr, as needed; or 1 mg/kg to 6 mg/kg as a single dose. All regimens not used more than 3 days.

✱ *To treat acute exacerbation of multiple sclerosis*

ELIXIR, ORAL SOLUTION, TABLETS

Adults. 30 mg/day for 1 wk, followed by 4 to 12 mg every other day for 1 month.

✱ *To treat acute, self-limiting allergic disorder or exacerbation of chronic allergic disorder*

ELIXIR, I.M. INJECTION, ORAL SOLUTION, TABLETS

Adults. *Day 1:* 4 to 8 mg I.M. *Days 2 and 3:* 3 mg/day P.O. divided every 12 hr. *Day 4:* 1.5 mg/day P.O. divided every 12 hr. *Days 5 and 6:* 0.75 mg/day P.O. as a single dose.

✱ *To decrease localized inflammation*

INTRA-ARTICULAR INJECTION

Adults. 2 to 4 mg for large joint; 0.8 to 1 mg for small joint; 2 to 3 mg for bursae; 0.4 to 1 mg for tendon sheaths.

SOFT-TISSUE INJECTION

Adults. 2 to 6 mg; 1 to 2 mg for ganglia.

INTRALESIONAL INJECTION

Adults. 0.8 to 1.6 mg/injection site. Repeated, as needed, once every 3 to 5 days to once every 2 to 3 wk.

Drug Administration

- Taper drug rather than stopping it abruptly.

P.O.

- Give drug with food to decrease GI distress.
- Give once-daily dose in the morning.
- For concentrated oral solution, use calibrated dropper that is provided to measure doses. Mix dose well with liquid or semi-solid food such as applesauce or pudding. Administer immediately after mixing.
- Tablets may be crushed and mixed with semi-solid food. Administer immediately. Do not store mixture.

I.V.

- Use preservative-free dosage forms in neonates.
- For I.V. injection, inject undiluted directly into I.V. tubing of infusing compatible solution over at least 3 minutes (4 minutes for children).
- For I.V. infusion, dilute 1 to 50 mg with 50 ml of 0.9% Sodium Chloride Injection or Dextrose Injection and infuse over 30 minutes. Dilute 51 to 100 mg with 100 ml and infuse as directed.
- Use within 24 hours.
- *Incompatibilities:* Ciprofloxacin, daunorubicin, diphenhydramine with lorazepam and metoclopramide, fenoldopam mesylate, idarubicin, methotrexate, midazolam, topotecan

I.M.

- Shake I.M. solution before injecting deep into large muscle mass.
- Rotate sites.
- Avoid subcutaneous injection; it may cause atrophy and sterile abscess.

INTRA-ARTICULAR, INTRALESIONAL
- Avoid administering frequently, if possible, because damage to joint tissues may occur.

Route	Onset	Peak	Duration
P.O.	1–2 hr	1–2 hr	2.5 days
I.V.	Rapid	1 hr	Unknown
I.M.	1 hr	1–8 hr	6 days
Intra-articular	Unknown	Unknown	Unknown
Intralesional	Unknown	Unknown	Unknown

Half-life: 36–54 hr

Mechanism of Action

Binds to intracellular glucocorticoid receptors and suppresses inflammatory and immune responses by:
- inhibiting monocyte and neutrophil accumulation at inflammation site and suppressing bactericidal and phagocytic action
- stabilizing lysosomal membranes
- suppressing antigen response of helper T cells and macrophages
- inhibiting synthesis of inflammatory response mediators, such as cytokines, interleukins, and prostaglandins

Contraindications

Administration of live-virus vaccine to patient or family member, hypersensitivity to dexamethasone or its components (including sulfites), idiopathic thrombocytopenic purpura (I.M. administration), systemic fungal infections

Interactions

DRUGS

aminoglutethimide: Possibly diminished adrenal suppression by dexamethasone
amphotericin B (parenteral),
potassium-depleting drugs: Risk of hypokalemia
anticholinesterases: Decreased anticholinesterase effectiveness in myasthenia gravis producing severe weakness
aspirin, NSAIDs: Increased risk of adverse GI effects
cholestyramine: Increased dexamethasone clearance
cyclosporine: Increased activity of both drugs, possibly resulting in seizures
CYP3A4 inducers such as barbiturates, carbamazepine, phenytoin, rifampin: Possibly enhanced metabolism of dexamethasone requiring dosage increase
CYP3A4 inhibitors such as clarithromycin, cobicistat-containing drugs, itraconazole, ritonavir: Possibly increased plasma concentrations of dexamethasone with increased adverse reactions
CYP3A4 substrates such as erythromycin, indinavir: Possibly decreased plasma concentration of these drugs
digoxin: Increased risk of digitalis toxicity related to hypokalemia
ephedrine: Decreased half-life and increased clearance of dexamethasone
isoniazid: Decreased blood isoniazid level
macrolide antibiotics: Decreased dexamethasone clearance and increased dexamethasone effects
oral anticoagulants such as warfarin: Inhibition of response to oral anticoagulant
oral contraceptives including estrogens: Increased effect of oral contraceptives
phenytoin: Increased risk of seizures
thalidomide: Increased risk of toxic epidermal necrolysis
toxoids, vaccines: Decreased antibody response

ACTIVITIES

alcohol use: Increased risk of GI bleeding

Adverse Reactions

CNS: Depression, emotional lability, euphoria, fever, headache, **increased intracranial pressure (ICP) with papilledema**, insomnia, light-headedness, malaise, neuritis, neuropathy, paresthesia, psychosis, **seizures**, syncope, tiredness, vertigo, weakness
CV: Arrhythmias, bradycardia, edema, **fat embolism, heart failure,** hypercholesterolemia, hyperlipidemia, hypertension, **myocardial rupture,** tachycardia, **thromboembolism,** thrombophlebitis, vasculitis
EENT: Blurred vision, cataracts, epistaxis, glaucoma, loss of smell and taste, nasal burning and dryness, ocular infections, oral candidiasis, perforated nasal septum, pharyngitis, rebound nasal congestion, rhinorrhea
ENDO: Cushingoid symptoms, decreased iodine uptake, growth suppression in children, hyperglycemia, menstrual

irregularities, **secondary adrenocortical and pituitary unresponsiveness**
GI: Abdominal distention, bloody stools, elevated liver enzymes, heartburn, hepatomegaly, increased appetite, indigestion, **intestinal perforation, melena,** nausea, **pancreatitis,** peptic ulcer **with possible perforation,** ulcerative esophagitis, vomiting
GU: Glycosuria, increased or decreased number and motility of spermatozoa, perineal irritation, urinary frequency
HEME: Leukocytosis, **leukopenia**
MS: Aseptic necrosis of femoral and humeral heads; muscle atrophy, spasms, or weakness; myalgia; osteoporosis; pathologic fracture of long bones; tendon rupture (intra-articular injection); vertebral compression fracture
RESP: Bronchospasm
SKIN: Acne, allergic dermatitis, diaphoresis, ecchymosis, erythema, hirsutism, necrotizing vasculitis, petechiae, subcutaneous fat atrophy, striae, thin and fragile skin, urticaria
Other: Aggravated or masked signs of infection, **anaphylaxis, angioedema, hypernatremia, hypocalcemia, hypokalemia, hypokalemic alkalosis,** impaired wound healing, **metabolic acidosis,** suppressed skin test reaction, **tumor lysis syndrome,** weight gain

Childbearing Considerations

PREGNANCY

- It is not known if drug causes fetal harm. However, infants born of mothers who have received substantial doses of drug during pregnancy may develop hypoadrenalism.
- Use with caution only if benefit to mother outweighs potential risk to fetus.

LACTATION

- Drug is present in breast milk.
- A decision should be made to discontinue breastfeeding or the drug to avoid potential serious adverse reactions in the breastfed infant.

Nursing Considerations

- Use dexamethasone cautiously in patients with congestive heart failure, hypertension, or renal insufficiency because drug can cause sodium retention, which may lead to edema and hypokalemia.
- Also use cautiously in patients who have had intestinal surgery and in those with

diverticulitis, peptic ulcer, or ulcerative colitis because of the risk of perforation.
- Monitor fluid intake and output and daily weight, and watch for crackles, dyspnea, peripheral edema, and steady weight gain.
- Evaluate growth if patient is a child.
- Test stool for occult blood.
- Monitor results of hematology studies and blood glucose, cholesterol, lipids levels, and serum electrolyte. Dexamethasone may cause hyperglycemia, hypernatremia, hypocalcemia, hypokalemia, or leukopenia. It also may increase serum cholesterol and lipid levels, and it may decrease iodine uptake by the thyroid.
- Assess patient for evidence of Cushing's syndrome, osteoporosis, and other systemic effects during long-term use.
- Monitor neonate for signs of hypoadrenocorticism if mother received dexamethasone during pregnancy. Be aware that some preparations contain benzyl alcohol, which may cause a fatal toxic syndrome in neonates and immature infants.

! **WARNING** Watch for hypersensitivity reactions after giving acetate or sodium phosphate form; both may contain bisulfites or parabens, to which some people are allergic.

- Be aware that the use of corticosteroids such dexamethasone, especially for longer than 6 weeks, increases the risk of development of eye disorders, including cataracts and glaucoma, which can possibly damage the optic nerves, and ocular infections due to bacteria, fungi, or viruses. Know that patient should be referred to an ophthalmologist if patient develops ocular symptoms while taking dexamethasone.

PATIENT TEACHING

- Instruct patient not to store drug in damp or hot places and to protect liquid form from freezing.
- Instruct patient to take once-daily oral dose in the morning with food to help prevent GI distress.
- Caution against consuming alcohol during dexamethasone therapy because it increases the risk of GI bleeding.
- Advise patient to follow a low-sodium, high-potassium, high-protein diet, if prescribed, to help minimize weight gain,

which is common with dexamethasone therapy. Instruct her to inform prescriber if she's on a special diet.
- Instruct patient not to stop drug abruptly.
- Advise patient to notify prescriber if condition recurs or worsens after dosage is reduced or therapy stops.
- Urge patient to have regular eye examinations during long-term use and to report any eye abnormalities to prescriber.
- Advise patient on long-term therapy to carry medical identification and to notify all healthcare providers that she takes dexamethasone.
- Instruct patient (especially a child) to avoid close contact with anyone who has chickenpox or measles and to notify prescriber immediately if exposure occurs.
- Advise patient and family members to avoid live-virus vaccinations during therapy unless prescriber approves.
- Inform diabetic patient that drug may affect her blood glucose level.
- Instruct patient having drug injected into a joint to avoid putting excessive pressure on it and to notify prescriber if it becomes red or swollen.
- Tell patient to notify prescriber about anorexia, depression, light-headedness, malaise, muscle pain, nausea, vomiting, and early hyperadrenocorticism (abdominal distention, amenorrhea, easy bruising, extreme weakness, facial hair, increased appetite, moon face, weight gain). Tell patient and family about possible changes in appearance.
- Urge patient to notify prescriber about illness, surgery, or changes in stress level.

dexmethylphenidate hydrochloride
Focalin, Focalin XR

≣ Class, Category, and Schedule
Pharmacologic class: Methylphenidate derivative
Therapeutic class: CNS stimulant
Controlled substance schedule: II

≣ Indications and Dosages
* *To treat attention deficit hyperactivity disorder (ADHD)*

TABLETS (FOCALIN)
Adults and children age 6 and over who are new to methylphenidate or who are on stimulants other than methylphenidate. 2.5 mg twice daily at least 4 hr apart, increased weekly by 2.5 to 5 mg. *Maximum:* 10 mg twice daily.
Adults and children age 6 and over who take methylphenidate. Half of the current daily racemic methylphenidate dosage, increased weekly, as needed. *Maximum:* 10 mg twice daily at least 4 hr apart.

E.R. CAPSULES (FOCALIN XR)
Adults who are new to methylphenidate or who are on stimulants other than methylphenidate. 10 mg daily, increased weekly by 10 mg daily, as needed. *Maximum:* 40 mg daily.
Children age 6 and over who are new to methylphenidate or who are on stimulants other than methylphenidate. 5 mg daily, increased weekly as needed by 5-mg increments. *Maximum:* 30 mg daily.
Adults and children age 6 and over who take methylphenidate. Half of the current total daily racemic methylphenidate dosage increased weekly, as needed. *Maximum:* 40 mg daily (adults) and 30 mg daily (children).
±**DOSAGE ADJUSTMENT** Dosage decreased for paradoxical aggravation of symptoms or adverse reactions.

≣ Drug Administration
P.O.
- E.R. capsules may be swallowed whole or opened and contents sprinkled on a small amount of applesauce. Caution patient not to chew mixture. Do not store mixture but administer immediately.
- E.R. capsules should not be chewed, crushed, or contents divided.

Route	Onset	Peak	Duration
P.O.	Unknown	1–1.5 hr	Unknown
P.O./E.R.	Unknown	1–4 hr	Unknown

Half-life: 2–4.5 hr

≣ Mechanism of Action
May block reuptake of dopamine and norepinephrine into presynaptic neurons in cerebral cortex, which increases availability of dopamine and norepinephrine in extraneuronal space.

D

Contraindications

Hypersensitivity to dexmethylphenidate, methylphenidate, or their components; use within 14 days of MAO inhibitor

Interactions

DRUGS

antihypertensives: Decreased therapeutic effect of these drugs
halogenated anesthetics: Increased risk of sudden blood pressure and heart rate acceleration during surgery
MAO inhibitors: Increased adverse effects, risk of hypertensive crisis
risperidone: Increased risk of extrapyramidal symptoms when dosage changes for either drug
serotonergic drugs: Increased risk of serotonin syndrome

Adverse Reactions

CNS: Aggression, anxiety, **cerebral arteritis or occlusion, CVA,** depression, dizziness, drowsiness, dyskinesia, fever, headache, insomnia, motor or vocal tics, nervousness, psychosis, **seizures,** Tourette syndrome, toxic psychosis, tremor
CV: Angina, **arrhythmias,** decreased or increased pulse rate, hypertension, **hypotension, MI,** palpitations, peripheral vasculopathy including Raynaud's phenomenon, tachycardia, vasculitis
EENT: Accommodation abnormality, blurred vision, dry mouth, nasopharyngitis
ENDO: Suppression of growth (children)
GI: Abdominal pain, anorexia, dyspepsia, elevated liver enzymes, **hepatic dysfunction (may be severe),** nausea, vomiting
GU: Libido changes, priapism
HEME: Anemia, **leukopenia, thrombocytopenia, thrombocytopenic purpura**
MS: Arthralgia, muscle cramps, **rhabdomyolysis**
RESP: Cough
SKIN: Alopecia, **erythema multiforme,** excessive diaphoresis, **exfoliative dermatitis,** necrotizing vasculitis, pruritus, rash, urticaria
Other: **Anaphylaxis, angioedema,** physical and psychological dependence, weight loss (prolonged therapy in adults)

Childbearing Considerations

PREGNANCY

- Pregnancy exposure registry: 1-866-961-2388 or visit https://womensmentalhealth.org/adhd-medications/.
- It is not known if drug causes fetal harm but drug may cause vasoconstriction which may decrease placental perfusion.
- Use with caution only if benefit to mother outweighs potential risk to fetus.

LACTATION

- Drug is present in breast milk.
- Patient should check with prescriber before breastfeeding.
- If breastfeeding occurs, infant should be monitored for adverse reactions, such as agitation, anorexia, insomnia, and reduced weight gain.

Nursing Considerations

- Know that dexmethylphenidate should not be given to patients with cardiomyopathy, coronary artery disease, known serious structural cardiac abnormalities, serious heart rhythm abnormalities, and other serious heart problems because of risk of CVA, MI, or sudden death. Notify prescriber if patient develops arrhythmias, unexplained syncope, or exertional chest pain.

! **WARNING** Be aware that dexmethylphenidate may induce CNS stimulation, mania, and psychosis and may worsen behavior disturbances and thought disorders. Use drug cautiously in children with mania or psychosis. Be aware that withdrawal symptoms may occur with long-term use.

- Monitor blood pressure and pulse rate to detect hypertension and excessive stimulation. Notify prescriber if signs appear.

! **WARNING** Monitor patient for signs of physical or psychological dependence. Use drug cautiously in patients with a history of drug abuse, including alcoholism.

- Monitor CBC and differential and platelet counts, as ordered, during prolonged therapy.
- Expect to stop drug if seizures occur. Drug may lower seizure threshold, especially in patients with a history of seizures or EEG abnormalities.
- Assess patient for signs and symptoms of peripheral vasculopathy, including

Raynaud's phenomenon. Although mild and intermittent, know that digital ulceration and/or soft-tissue breakdown has occurred. Notify prescriber if present, as drug dosage may have to be reduced or drug discontinued.

! **WARNING** Question male patients, including male children, about painful and prolonged erections, especially after a dosage increase or during a period of drug withdrawal. Know that presence of priapism has sometimes required emergency surgical intervention, so report any findings to prescriber immediately.

- Monitor children on long-term dexmethylphenidate therapy for signs of growth suppression, which has been noted during long-term use of stimulants.

PATIENT TEACHING

- Tell patient that extended-release capsules should either be taken whole, without being chewed, crushed, or divided, or capsule contents should be sprinkled on a small amount of applesauce. Tablets should be swallowed whole.

! **WARNING** Stress importance of notifying prescriber if an irregular pulse, fainting, or chest pain on exertion develops.

- Urge patient to notify prescriber if she has excessive nervousness, fever, insomnia, nausea, palpitations, or rash while taking dexmethylphenidate.
- Caution patient with seizure disorder that drug may cause seizures.
- Teach patient (or parent) to watch for improvement in signs and symptoms of ADHD, such as decreased impulsiveness and increased attention. Stress the need for continued follow-up care, and suggest participation in an ADHD program.

! **WARNING** Inform male patients and parents or caregivers of male children that dexmethylphenidate may cause abnormally sustained or frequent and painful erections, especially when a dosage increase occurs or during a period of drug withdrawal. Advise immediate emergency care if this should occur.

- Instruct patient to inspect his fingers and toes daily for changes such as skin breakdown or ulcer formation. Although usually intermittent and mild, patient should contact prescriber if abnormalities occur, as drug may have to be discontinued or dosage reduced.

diazepam

Diastat, Diastat Acudial, Diazepam Intensol, Valium, Valtoco

≣ Class, Category, and Schedule

Pharmacologic class: Benzodiazepine
Therapeutic class: Anticonvulsant, anxiolytic, sedative-hypnotic, skeletal muscle relaxant
Controlled substance schedule: IV

≣ Indications and Dosages

✳ *To relieve anxiety*

ORAL SOLUTION, TABLETS

Adults. 2 to 10 mg twice daily to four times daily.

Children age 6 months and older. *Initial:* 1 to 2.5 mg three or four times daily, gradually increased as needed and tolerated.

I.V. OR I.M. INJECTION

Adults. *For moderate anxiety:* 2 to 5 mg every 3 to 4 hr, as needed. *For severe anxiety:* 5 to 10 mg, repeated in 3 to 4 hr, if needed.

✳ *To treat symptoms of acute alcohol withdrawal*

ORAL SOLUTION, TABLETS

Adults. 10 mg three times daily or four times daily during first 24 hr. Then 5 mg three times daily or four times daily, if needed.

I.V. OR I.M. INJECTION

Adults. 10 mg and then 5 to 10 mg in 3 to 4 hr, if needed.

✳ *As adjunct to treat muscle spasms*

ORAL SOLUTION, TABLETS

Adults. 2 to 10 mg three times daily or four times daily.

I.V. OR I.M. INJECTION

Adults. *Initial:* 5 to 10 mg, then repeated every 3 to 4 hr, as needed.

✳ *To treat seizures*

ORAL SOLUTION, TABLETS

Adults. 2 to 10 mg twice daily to four times daily.

Children age 6 months and over. *Initial:* 1 to 2.5 mg three times daily or four times daily. Increased gradually as needed and tolerated.

❋ *To treat acute, intermittent, stereotypic episodes of frequent seizure activity such as acute repetitive seizures or seizure clusters that are distinct from patient's usual seizure pattern in patients with epilepsy*

NASAL SPRAY (VALTOCO)

Adults and children age 12 years and older weighing 76 kg (167.2 lb) and up. 0.2 mg/kg given as a 20-mg single dose administered as one spray in each nostril using two 10-mg devices. Dosage repeated, if needed, after 4 hr.

Adults and children age 12 years and older weighing 51 kg (112.2 lb) to 75 kg (165 lb). 0.2 mg/kg given as a 15-mg single dose administered as one spray in each nostril using two 7.5-mg devices. Dosage repeated after 4 hr, if needed.

Adults and children age 12 and over weighing 28 kg (61.6 lb) to 50 kg (110 lb). 10 mg as a single dose administered as 1 spray in one nostril using one 10-mg device. Dosage repeated, after 4 hr, if needed,

Adults and children age 12 and over weighing 14 kg (30.8 lb) to 27 kg (59.4 lb). 5 mg as a single dose administered as one spray in one nostril using one 5-mg device. Dosage repeated after 4 hr, if needed.

Children age 6 to 11 years and weighing 56 kg (123.2 lb) to 74 kg (162.8 lb). 0.3 mg/kg given as 20-mg single dose administered as one spray in each nostril using two 10-mg devices. Dosage repeated after 4 hr, if needed.

Children age 6 to 11 years and weighing 38 kg (83.6 lb) to 55 kg (121 lb). 0.3 mg/kg given as a 15-mg dose single dose administered as one spray in each nostril using two 7.5-mg devices. Dosage repeated after 4 hr, if needed.

Children age 6 to 11 years and weighing 19 kg (19.8 lb) to 37 kg (81.4 lb). 0.3 mg/kg given as a 10-mg single dose administered as one spray in one nostril using one 10-mg device. Dosage repeated after 4 hr, if needed.

Children age 6 to 11 years and weighing 10 kg (22 lb) to 18 kg (39.6 lb). 0.3 mg/kg given as a 5-mg single dose administered as one spray in one nostril using one 5-mg device. Dosage repeated after 4 hr, if needed.

❋ *To treat status epilepticus and severe recurrent seizures*

I.V. INJECTION

Adults. 10 mg repeated every 10 to 15 min, as needed, up to a cumulative dose of 30 mg. Regimen repeated, if needed, in 2 to 4 hr. (Use I.M. route if I.V. access is unavailable.)

Children age 5 and over. 1 mg repeated every 2 to 5 min, as needed, up to a cumulative dose of 10 mg. Regimen repeated, if needed, in 2 to 4 hr.

Children ages 1 month to 5 years. 0.2 to 0.5 mg repeated every 2 to 5 min, as needed, up to a cumulative dose of 5 mg. Regimen repeated, if needed, in 2 to 4 hr.

❋ *As adjunct to manage bouts of increased seizure activity*

RECTAL GEL (DIASTAT ACUDIAL)

Adults and adolescents. 0.2 mg/kg rounded up to next available unit dose (or rounded down for debilitated or elderly patient). Repeated in 4 to 12 hr, if needed.

Children ages 6 to 12. 0.3 mg/kg rounded up to next available unit dose. Repeated in 4 to 12 hr, if needed.

Children ages 2 to 6. 0.5 mg/kg rounded up to next available unit dose. Repeated in 4 to 12 hr, if needed.

❋ *To provide preoperative sedation*

I.V. OR I.M. INJECTION

Adults. 10 mg 30 min before surgery with I.M. route preferred.

❋ *To reduce anxiety before cardioversion*

I.V. INJECTION

Adults. 5 to 15 mg 5 to 10 min before procedure.

❋ *To reduce anxiety before endoscopic procedures*

I.V. INJECTION

Adults. Up to 20 mg titrated to desired sedation and given immediately before procedure.

I.M. INJECTION

Adults. 5 to 10 mg 30 min before procedure if I.V. route cannot be used.

❋ *To treat tetanus*

I.V. OR I.M. INJECTION

Adults and children age 5 and over. *Initial:* 5 to 10 mg repeated every 3 to 4 hr, if needed. Sometimes larger doses are needed for adults.

Children ages 1 month to 5 years. 1 to 2 mg repeated every 3 to 4 hr, as needed.

±**DOSAGE ADJUSTMENT** For adult patients taking oral form and who are debilitated or elderly, dosage reduced to 2 to 2.5 mg one or two times daily. Then increased gradually as needed and tolerated. For adult patients who are debilitated and being treated for tetanus with an I.M. or I.V. injection, initial dose reduced to 2 to 5 mg and increased gradually as needed and tolerated.

Drug Administration

P.O.

- Use the calibrated dropper provided to measure dose of oral solution.
- Mix concentrated oral solution (Intensol) with a liquid such as juices, soda or soda-like beverages, water; or semi-solid foods such as applesauce or pudding. Stir the liquid or food gently for a few seconds after adding drug. Have patient consume immediately. Do not store once mixed.
- Protect oral solution from light. Discard open bottles after 90 days.

I.V.

- Have emergency resuscitation equipment and oxygen at bedside prior to administration.
- Solution should appear colorless to light yellow.
- Protect from light.
- Do not inject into small veins, such as those on the dorsum of the hand or wrist.
- Use extreme care to avoid intra-arterial administration or extravasation.
- Inject slowly, not exceeding 5 mg/min for adults and over 3 minutes in children not exceeding 0.25 mg/kg.
- If not feasible to administer as a direct I.V. injection, it may be injected slowly through the infusion tubing as close as possible to the vein insertion.
- I.V. therapy should be replaced with oral therapy as soon as possible.
- *Incompatibilities:* Other solutions or drugs in same infusion flask or syringe

I.M.

- Inject deeply into the muscle.

INTRANASAL

- Do not prime or attempt to use for more than one administration per device.

P.R.

- Lubricate rectal tip of syringe with lubricating jelly.

- Gently insert syringe tip into rectum. Rim should be snug against rectal opening.
- Slowly count to 3 while gently pushing plunger in until it stops.

Route	Onset	Peak	Duration
P.O.	30 min	0.25–2.5 hr	20–80 min
I.V.	1–5 min	1–5 min	15–60 min
I.M.	Unknown	1 hr	Unknown
Intranasal	Unknown	1.5 hr	Unknown
P.R.	2–10 min	90 min	Unknown

Half-life: 20–70 hr

Mechanism of Action

May potentiate effects of gamma-aminobutyric acid (GABA) and other inhibitory neurotransmitters by binding to specific benzodiazepine receptors in cortical and limbic areas of CNS. GABA inhibits excitatory stimulation, which helps control emotional behavior. Limbic system contains a dense area of benzodiazepine receptors, which may explain drug's antianxiety effects. Diazepam suppresses spread of seizure activity caused by seizure-producing foci in cortex, limbic, and thalamus structures.

Contraindications

For all forms: Acute angle-closure glaucoma, hypersensitivity to diazepam or its components, untreated open-angle glaucoma
For oral forms: Children under 6 months of age, myasthenia gravis, severe hepatic impairment, severe respiratory insufficiency, sleep apnea

Interactions

DRUGS

antacids: Altered rate of diazepam absorption
cimetidine, fluoxetine, fluvoxamine, ketoconazole, omeprazole Decreased diazepam metabolism, increased blood level and risk of adverse effects including prolonged sedation
CNS depressants including anesthetics, anticonvulsants, antipsychotics, anxiolytics, barbiturates, hypnotics, MAO inhibitors, narcotics, phenothiazines, sedatives including sedative antihistamines, and other antidepressants: Increased CNS depression and risk of falls and fractures

D

opioids: Increased risk of severe respiratory depression

phenytoin: Decreased metabolic elimination of phenytoin, increased risk of adverse reactions

ACTIVITIES

alcohol use: Increased CNS depression, including severe respiratory depression, significant sedation and somnolence, and increased risk of falls and fractures

Adverse Reactions

CNS: Anterograde amnesia, anxiety, ataxia, confusion, depression, dizziness, drowsiness, fatigue, headache, insomnia, lethargy, light-headedness, paradoxical reactions, psychiatric effects, sedation, sleepiness, slurred speech, **suicidal ideation**, tremor, vertigo

CV: Hypotension, palpitations, tachycardia

EENT: Blurred vision, diplopia, dry mouth, increased salivation

GI: Anorexia, constipation, diarrhea, elevated liver enzymes, jaundice, nausea, vomiting

GU: Libido changes, urinary incontinence, urine retention

HEME: Neutropenia

MS: Dysarthria, muscle weakness

RESP: Respiratory depression

SKIN: Dermatitis

Other: Physical and psychological dependence

Childbearing Considerations

PREGNANCY

- Pregnancy exposure registry: 1-888-233-2334 or http://aedpregnancyregistry.org.
- Drug may cause fetal harm. An increased risk of congenital malformations and other developmental abnormalities have occurred with benzodiazepines such as diazepam.
- Drug may also cause nonteratogenic issues after birth such as feeding difficulties, neonatal flaccidity, hypothermia, and respiratory problems.
- Know that if drug is given on a regular basis late in pregnancy, the neonate may experience withdrawal symptoms after birth.
- Drug should not be used during pregnancy, especially in the first and third trimester, unless there is no alternative and the benefit to the mother outweighs the risk to the fetus.

LABOR & DELIVERY

- Be aware that high single doses of the drug during labor and delivery may cause fetal heart rate irregularities and after birth hypotonia, hypothermia, poor sucking, and moderate respiratory depression.

LACTATION

- Drug is present in breast milk.
- Patient should not breastfed while taking drug.

Nursing Considerations

- Use diazepam with extreme caution in patients with a history of alcohol or drug abuse because it can cause physical and psychological dependence, and in patients with hepatic disorders such as hepatic fibrosis and hepatitis because of potentially significant increase in drug's half-life.
- Use diazepam cautiously in patients with hepatic or renal impairment.
- Expect to give a lower diazepam dose to patient with chronic respiratory insufficiency because of the risk of respiratory depression.
- Monitor patient for adverse reactions, especially if hypoalbuminemia is present, which increases the risk of sedation.

! WARNING Watch for signs of physical and psychological dependence (strong desire or need to continue taking diazepam, need to increase dose to maintain drug effects, and posttherapy withdrawal symptoms, such as abdominal cramps, insomnia, irritability, nervousness, and tremor).

- Monitor patient closely for increase in frequency or severity of grand mal seizures when diazepam is used with standard anticonvulsant therapy. Dosage of other anticonvulsants may have to be increased.
- Avoid abrupt withdrawal of diazepam, as ordered, when used as part of the patient's seizure control regimen because a transient increase in frequency or severity of seizures may occur.
- Monitor severely depressed patient or one with depression-related anxiety for suicidal tendencies, particularly when therapy starts and dosage changes; depression may worsen temporarily during these times.

- Watch for paradoxical and psychiatric reactions to diazepam, especially in children and the elderly. If reactions occur, notify prescriber and expect drug to be discontinued.
- Monitor patient for decreased drug effectiveness, especially with prolonged use.

! **WARNING** Be aware that benzodiazepine therapy like diazepam should only be used concomitantly with opioids in patients for whom other treatment options are inadequate. If prescribed together, expect dosing and duration of the opioid to be limited. Monitor patient closely for signs and symptoms of decrease in consciousness, including coma, profound sedation, and significant respiratory depression. Notify prescriber immediately and provide emergency supportive care, as death may occur.

- Check patient's blood counts and liver function periodically, as ordered, because prolonged diazepam therapy rarely causes jaundice and neutropenia.

PATIENT TEACHING
- Instruct patient not to take more drug, more often, or for a longer time than prescribed. Warn her that physical and psychological dependence can occur, and teach her to recognize the signs.
- Advise patient not to take drug to relieve everyday stress.
- Instruct patient to avoid hazardous activities until drug's CNS effects are known. Warn her that risk of falls and fractures increases when diazepam is taken with other sedatives or alcohol and to avoid this combination.
- Advise patient to avoid CNS depressants during therapy.

! **WARNING** Warn patient not to consume alcohol or take an opioid during diazepam therapy without prescriber knowledge, as severe respiratory depression can occur and may lead to death.

! **WARNING** Inform patient about potentially fatal additive effects of combining diazepam with an opioid. Instruct patient to inform all prescribers of diazepam use, especially if pain medication may be prescribed.

- Instruct patient not to stop taking drug abruptly without prescriber's supervision.

If patient has a history of seizures, warn that abrupt withdrawal may trigger them.
- Instruct patient to mix Diazepam Intensol with water, soda, or a similar beverage; applesauce; or pudding just before taking it. Caution her not to save the mixture for later. Tell her to use calibrated dropper that's provided to measure each dose.
- Teach patient how to self-administer a rectal form or intranasal form, if prescribed.

! **WARNING** Tell patients and caregivers not to administer a second dose of nasal spray if breathing difficulties arise or excessive sedation occurs. If severe, patient will require emergency rescue treatment.

- Instruct female patient of childbearing age to notify prescriber immediately if she is or could be pregnant because diazepam therapy will have to be discontinued.
- Urge family or caregiver to watch patient closely for suicidal tendencies, especially when therapy starts or dosage changes.

diazoxide
Proglycem

Class and Category
Pharmacologic class: Benzothiadiazine derivative
Therapeutic class: Antihypertensive, antihypoglycemic

Indications and Dosages
❋ *To manage hypoglycemia caused by hyperinsulinism*

CAPSULES, ORAL SUSPENSION (PROGLYCEM)
Adults and children. *Initial:* 1 mg/kg every 8 hr. *Maintenance:* 3 to 8 mg/kg daily in 2 or 3 equal doses given every 8 or 12 hr. *Maximum:* 15 mg/kg daily.
Infants and neonates. *Initial:* 3.3 mg/kg every 8 hr. *Maintenance:* 8 to 15 mg/kg daily in 2 or 3 equal doses given every 8 or 12 hr.
±**DOSAGE ADJUSTMENT** For patient with renal impairment, dosage reduced.

Drug Administration
P.O.
- Capsules should be swallowed whole and not chewed, crushed, or opened.

- Shake oral suspension container well before each use. Use dropper that comes with drug to measure dosage.
- Protect from light and store at room temperature.
- Do not interchange capsule and oral suspension mg for mg.

Route	Onset	Peak	Duration
P.O.	1 hr	Unknown	8 hr

Half-life: 24–36 hr

Mechanism of Action

Directly affects smooth-muscle cells of peripheral arteries and arterioles, causing them to dilate. This action decreases peripheral resistance, which helps reduce blood pressure. Diazoxide also inhibits insulin release from the pancreas, stimulates catecholamine release, and increases hepatic glucose release.

Contraindications

Acute aortic dissection; functional hypoglycemia (Polyglycem), hypersensitivity to diazoxide, thiazides, other sulfonamide derivatives, or their components; treatment of compensatory hypertension, as occurs with aortic coarctation or arteriovenous shunt (Hyperstat)

Interactions

DRUGS

antihypertensives, beta blockers, nitrates: Additive hypotensive effects
beta blockers: Increased hypotensive effects of diazoxide
diphenylhydantoin: Increased risk of loss of seizure control
diuretics, especially thiazides: Potentiated hyperglycemic, hyperuricemic, and antihypertensive effects of diazoxide
oral anticoagulants: Increased anticoagulation
peripheral vasodilators: Additive, possibly severe, hypotensive effects

Adverse Reactions

CNS: Anxiety, apprehension, **cerebral ischemia**, dizziness, euphoria, headache, insomnia, light-headedness, malaise, somnolence, weakness
CV: **Bradycardia**, chest pain, edema, **hypotension**, palpitations, tachycardia, transient hypertension

EENT: Blurred vision, dry mouth, increased salivation, taste perversion, tinnitus, transient hearing loss
ENDO: Transient hyperglycemia
GI: Abdominal pain, anorexia, constipation, diarrhea, ileus, nausea, vomiting
MS: Gout
RESP: **Pulmonary hypertension**
SKIN: Diaphoresis, flushing, pruritus, rash, sensation of warmth
Other: Extravasation with injection-site cellulitis and pain; **hypernatremia**

Childbearing Considerations
PREGNANCY

- Drug may cause fetal harm if given to mother just prior to delivery possibly causing altered carbohydrate metabolism, fetal or neonatal hyperbilirubinemia, thrombocytopenia, or other adverse effects.
- Use with caution only if benefit to mother outweighs potential risk to fetus.

LABOR & DELIVERY

- Be aware drug is not indicated for use during labor and delivery because it may cause cessation of uterine contractions.

LACTATION

- It is not known if drug is present in breast milk.
- A decision should be made to discontinue breastfeeding or the drug to avoid potential serious adverse reactions in the breastfed infant.

Nursing Considerations

- Use diazoxide cautiously in patients with uncompensated heart failure (can cause fluid retention and heart failure) and patients with impaired cardiac or cerebral circulation in whom abrupt blood pressure drop, mild tachycardia, and decreased blood perfusion may be harmful.
- Expect to adjust dosage if patient switches from oral suspension to capsules; suspension causes a higher blood diazoxide level.
- Monitor blood glucose level of all patients who receive diazoxide to see if drug has raised blood glucose level to normal.

! **WARNING** Monitor infants and neonates closely for pulmonary hypertension exhibited by respiratory distress. If present, notify prescriber immediately and expect drug to be discontinued because condition can be reversed when drug therapy is stopped.

PATIENT TEACHING

- Advise patient to protect oral suspension from light.
- Tell patient to take drug on a regular schedule and not to skip or double doses.
- Urge patient to monitor blood glucose level if she takes oral drug for hypoglycemia.
- Caution patient not to take antidiabetic drugs, unless prescribed.
- Advise patient to notify prescriber if she has signs of hyperglycemia, such as fatigue, or increased hunger, thirst, or urinary frequency.

diclofenac
Zorvolex

diclofenac epolamine
Flector Patch

diclofenac potassium
Cambia, Voltaren Rapide (CAN), Zipsor

diclofenac sodium
Apo-Diclo (CAN), Voltaren, Voltaren SR (CAN)

Class and Category
Pharmacologic class: NSAID
Therapeutic class: Analgesic, anti-inflammatory

Indications and Dosages
✽ *To manage signs and symptoms of rheumatoid arthritis*

TABLETS
Adults. 50 mg three or four times daily.

DELAYED-RELEASE TABLETS
Adults. *Initial:* 50 mg three times daily or four times daily or 75 mg twice daily. *Maximum:* 200 mg daily.

✽ *To manage signs and symptoms of osteoarthritis*

CAPSULES (ZORVOLEX)
Adults. 35 mg three times daily.

TABLETS
Adults. 50 mg two or three times daily.

DELAYED-RELEASE TABLETS
Adults. 50 mg twice daily or three times daily or 75 mg twice daily.

✽ *To relieve pain in patients with ankylosing spondylitis*

DELAYED-RELEASE TABLETS
Adults. 25 mg four times daily, with an extra 25 mg dose at bedtime, if needed.

✽ *To relieve pain and dysmenorrhea*

TABLETS
Adults. 50 mg three times daily, as needed; if needed, 100 mg for first dose only. *Maximum:* 200 mg for first day; 150 mg after first day.

✽ *To relieve mild to moderate acute pain*

CAPSULES (ZIPSOR)
Adults. 25 mg four times daily.

CAPSULES (ZORVOLEX)
Adults. 18 mg or 35 mg three times daily.

✽ *To treat acute migraine attacks*

ORAL SOLUTION (CAMBIA)
Adults. 50 mg (1 packet) per attack.

✽ *To relieve pain due to minor contusions, sprains, or strains*

TOPICAL PATCH 1.3%
Adults and children 6 years and over.
1 patch to the most painful area twice a day.

±**DOSAGE ADJUSTMENT** For patient prescribed Zorvolex with hepatic impairment, dosage no higher than 18 mg three times daily. For patient prescribed other drug forms with hepatic impairment, dosage may have to be reduced.

Drug Administration
P.O.

- Oral formulations are not interchangeable with other oral formulations even if the milligram strength is the same.
- Capsules and tablets should be swallowed whole and not be chewed, crushed, or opened.
- Empty packet (Cambia) into a cup containing 1 to 2 ounces of water, mix well, and have patient drink immediately. Do not use any other liquids to mix drug.
- Drug may be given with food except for Cambia or Zorvolex, which should be given on an empty stomach at least 1 hour before or 2 hours after a meal.

D

- Patient should not lie down for 15 to 30 minutes after administration of oral drug.

TOPICAL

- Do not apply patch to damaged or nonintact skin.
- If the patch begins to peel off, the edges may be taped down. If problems persist, overlay the patch with a mesh netting sleeve that allows air to pass through, where appropriate, such as ankles, elbows, or knees.
- Wash hands after applying, handling, or removing the patch and avoid eye contact with drug.

Route	Onset	Peak	Duration
P.O.	10 min	1 hr	8 hr
P.O./D.R.	30 min	2–3 hr	8 hr
P.O./E.R.	Unknown	5–6 hr	Unknown
Topical	Unknown	10–20 hr	Unknown

Half-life: 1–2 hr

Mechanism of Action

Blocks the activity of cyclooxygenase, the enzyme needed to synthesize prostaglandins, which mediate inflammatory response and cause local pain, swelling, and vasodilation. By blocking cyclooxygenase and inhibiting prostaglandins, diclofenac reduces inflammatory symptoms. This mechanism also relieves pain because prostaglandins promote pain transmission from periphery to spinal cord.

Contraindications

Active GI bleeding or ulcers; history of asthma attacks, rhinitis, or urticaria from aspirin or other NSAIDs; hypersensitivity to diclofenac, NSAIDs, or their components; pain management following coronary artery bypass graft (CABG) surgery; use on damaged or nonintact skin (topical system)

Interactions

DRUGS

angiotensin-converting enzyme (ACE) inhibitors, angiotensin receptor blockers (ARBs): Decreased antihypertensive effects of these drugs; decreased renal function in elderly patients or those with existing renal impairment or volume depletion
anticoagulants, antiplatelets, selective serotonin reuptake inhibitors (SSRIs),
serotonin norepinephrine reuptake inhibitors (SNRIs), thrombolytics: Prolonged PT, increased risk of bleeding
aspirin, other NSAIDs, salicylates: Increased GI irritability and bleeding, decreased diclofenac effectiveness with aspirin use
beta blockers: Impaired antihypertensive effect
cyclosporine, nephrotoxic drugs: Increased risk of nephrotoxicity
CYP2C9 inducers such as rifampin: Decreased effectiveness of diclofenac
CYP2C9 inhibitors such as voriconazole: Increased risk of diclofenac adverse reactions and toxicity
digoxin: Increased blood digoxin level
lithium: Increased risk of lithium toxicity
loop or thiazide diuretics: Decreased diuretic effects
methotrexate, pemetrexed: Increased risk of methotrexate or pemetrexed toxicity

FOODS

any food: Delayed absorption of delayed-release tablets

ACTIVITIES

alcohol use: Increased risk of GI irritability and bleeding

Adverse Reactions

CNS: Aseptic meningitis, cerebral hemorrhage, CVA, dizziness, drowsiness, headache
CV: Bradycardia and other arrhythmias, edema, heart failure, hypotension, MI, thrombotic events, vasculitis
EENT: Glaucoma, hearing loss, tinnitus
ENDO: Hypoglycemia
GI: Abdominal pain, constipation, diarrhea, dysphagia, elevated liver enzymes, esophageal ulceration, flatulence, GI bleeding or ulceration, hepatic failure, hepatitis, indigestion, jaundice, nausea, perforation of intestine or stomach
GU: Acute renal failure, interstitial nephritis
HEME: Agranulocytosis, anemia including aplastic anemia, bleeding events, eosinophilia, leukocytosis, leukopenia, pancytopenia, porphyria, thrombocytopenia
SKIN: Erythema multiforme, exfoliative dermatitis, pruritus, rash, Stevens–Johnson syndrome, toxic epidermal necrolysis
Other: Anaphylaxis, angioedema, hyperkalemia, hyperuricemia, hyponatremia, lymphadenopathy

Childbearing Considerations

PREGNANCY

- Drug may cause fetal harm if given during the third trimester of pregnancy by increasing the risk of premature closure of the fetal ductus arteriosus. Drug also can cause oligohydramnios and neonatal renal impairment if given at 20 weeks gestation or later.
- Drug should be avoided in pregnant women starting at 30 weeks of gestation. If absolutely needed between 20 and 30 weeks of gestation, drug should be given at lowest dose and for shortest time possible.

LACTATION

- Drug may be present in breast milk.
- Patient should check with prescriber before breastfeeding.

Nursing Considerations

- Be aware that NSAIDs like diclofenac should be avoided in patients with a recent MI because risk of reinfarction increases with NSAID therapy. If therapy is unavoidable, monitor patient closely for signs of cardiac ischemia.
- Be aware that the risk of heart failure increases with use of NSAIDs such as diclofenac. Diclofenac should not be given to patients with severe heart failure, but if unavoidable, monitor patient for worsening of heart failure.
- Use diclofenac with extreme caution and for shortest possible time in patients with a history of GI bleeding or ulcer disease because NSAIDs increase risk of GI bleeding and ulceration.
- Be aware that serious GI tract bleeding and ulceration, as well as perforation of intestine or stomach, can occur without warning or symptoms. Elderly patients are at greater risk. Monitor patient for signs of GI irritation and ulceration, especially if patient has a predisposing condition (such as a history of GI bleeding); takes an anticoagulant, NSAID (long-term), or oral corticosteroid; or has other factors such as being an alcoholic or smoker, has poor health, is over the age of 60; or tests positive for *Helicobacter pylori*. To minimize risk, give diclofenac with food. If patient develops GI distress, withhold drug and notify prescriber immediately.

- Use diclofenac cautiously in patients with hypertension, and monitor blood pressure closely; drug can cause or worsen hypertension.

! **WARNING** Know that use of NSAIDs like diclofenac increases risk of serious cardiovascular thrombotic events, including MI and stroke, which can be life-threatening. These events may occur early in treatment and risk increases with duration of use. Be aware that these events have occurred even in patients who do not have a history of or risk factors for cardiovascular disease. Monitor patient for warning signs such as chest pain, shortness of breath, slurring of speech, or weakness. If any signs and symptoms develop, withhold diclofenac, alert prescriber immediately, and provide supportive care as prescribed.

- Report signs of bleeding, such as bleeding gums, bloody or cloudy urine, ecchymoses, melena, and petechiae. Know that risk of bleeding is increased when patient is taking certain drugs like anticoagulants such as warfarin, antiplatelet agents such as aspirin, serotonin norepinephrine reuptake inhibitors, and serotonin reuptake inhibitors.
- Monitor BUN and serum creatinine levels in elderly patients, patients taking ACE inhibitors, ARDs, or diuretics, and patients with heart failure or impaired hepatic or renal function. These patients may have an increased risk of renal failure.
- Assess patient's skin routinely for rash or other signs of hypersensitivity reaction; drug may cause serious skin reactions without warning. At first sign of reaction, stop drug and notify prescriber.
- Know that because severe hepatic reactions may occur during diclofenac therapy, monitor liver enzymes and serum uric acid level as ordered. Liver enzyme elevations usually occur within 2 months of starting drug and should be reported promptly because dosage may have to be adjusted. Also monitor patient for evidence of hepatic dysfunction (diarrhea, fatigue, flu-like symptoms, jaundice, lethargy, nausea, pruritus, right upper quadrant tenderness).
- Report weight gain of more than 1 kg (2 lb) in 24 hours because it suggests fluid retention.

PATIENT TEACHING

- Advise patient not to chew, crush, or dissolve tablet, but to swallow it whole.
- Tell patient prescribed Cambia brand to mix packet in 1 to 2 ounces of water, mix well, and drink immediately. Caution patient not to use any other liquids to mix the drug. Remind patient taking this form of diclofenac that taking it with food may decrease its effectiveness.
- Instruct patient to take diclofenac with food to minimize GI distress unless he is prescribed Zorvolex, which should be taken on an empty stomach.
- Instruct patient not to lie down for 15 to 30 minutes after taking drug to decrease risk of esophageal ulceration.
- Teach patient prescribed a topical patch how to apply it. Tell patient if the patch begins to peel off, the edges may be taped down. If problems persist, patient may overlay the topical system with a mesh netting sleeve that allows air to pass through, where appropriate such as ankles, elbows, or knees. Stress importance of not applying patch to damaged or nonintact skin. Also, it should not be worn during bathing or showering. Warn patient not to use the patch at the same time as taking an oral NSAID unless instructed to do so. Tell patient to wash his hands after applying, handling, or removing the patch and to avoid eye contact.
- Warn patient to avoid hazardous activities until diclofenac's CNS effects are known.
- Urge patient to notify prescriber about dizziness, edema, impaired hearing, ringing or buzzing in ears, or unexplained weight gain.
- Advise patient to consult prescriber before taking aspirin or other OTC analgesics or drinking alcohol.
- Explain that diclofenac may increase risk of serious adverse cardiovascular reactions; urge patient to seek immediate medical attention for signs and symptoms such as chest pain, shortness of breath, slurred speech, and weakness.
- Inform patient that diclofenac therapy may increase risk of congestive heart failure. Instruct patient to promptly report to prescriber if edema, shortness of breath, or unexplained weight gain occurs.
- Tell patient that diclofenac also may increase risk of serious adverse GI reactions; stress need to seek immediate medical attention for such evidence as abdominal or epigastric pain, black or tarry stools, indigestion, and vomiting blood or material that looks like coffee grounds.
- Alert patient about possibly serious skin reactions and need to seek immediate medical attention for problems such as blisters, fever, itching, rash, and other signs of hypersensitivity such as difficulty breathing or swelling of face or throat.
- Urge patient to promptly report adverse liver effects (diarrhea, fatigue, flu-like symptoms, jaundice, lethargy, nausea, pruritus, right upper quadrant discomfort).
- Advise female patients to notify prescriber if pregnancy occurs or is suspected.
- Tell patient prescribed drug to treat migraine headaches not to overuse drug. Explain that this is because overuse, defined as using 10 or more days per month, may lead to exacerbation of headache. Inform patient that overuse headache may appear as migraine-like daily headaches or as a marked increase in frequency of migraine attacks. If this occurs, tell patient to notify prescriber, as a withdrawal period may be needed.

dicloxacillin sodium

Class and Category

Pharmacologic class: Penicillinase-resistant penicillin
Therapeutic class: Antibiotic

Indications and Dosages

✳ *To treat mild to moderate infections caused by penicillinase-producing staphylococci*

CAPSULES, ORAL SUSPENSION

Adults and children weighing 40 kg (88 lb) or more. 125 mg every 6 hr.
Children weighing less than 40 kg (less than 88 lb). 12.5 mg/kg daily divided into four equal doses and given every 6 hr.

✳ *To treat severe infections caused by penicillinase-producing staphylococci*

CAPSULES, ORAL SUSPENSION

Adults and children weighing 40 kg (88 lb) or more. 250 mg every 6 hr.

Children weighing less than 40 kg (less than 88 lb). 50 mg/kg daily divided into four equal doses and given every 6 hr.

Drug Administration

P.O.

- Drug should be administered on an empty stomach 1 hour before or 2 hours after meals. Do not administer drug at bedtime or when patient is supine.
- Administer with at least 4 ounces of water.
- Capsules should be taken whole and not chewed, crushed, or opened.
- Oral suspension should be shaken before each use.
- Use a calibrated device to measure oral suspension dose.
- Oral suspension may be kept at room temperature for 7 days or 14 days if kept refrigerated.
- Administer drug on an empty stomach at least 1 hour before or 2 hours after food. Have patient drink a glass of water when taking drug.

Route	Onset	Peak	Duration
P.O.	Unknown	0.5–2 hr	Unknown

Half-life: 0.6–0.8 hr

Mechanism of Action

Inhibits cell wall synthesis in susceptible bacteria, which assemble rigid, cross-linked cell walls in several steps. Dicloxacillin affects final cross-linking by inactivating penicillin-binding protein (the enzyme needed to link cell wall strands). This action inhibits cell wall synthesis and causes cell lysis and death.

Contraindications

Clostridium difficile infection; hypersensitivity to dicloxacillin, other penicillins, beta-lactamase inhibitors or their components

Interactions

DRUGS

aminoglycosides: Inactivation of aminoglycosides
oral contraceptives: Decreased contraceptive action
probenecid: Increased and prolonged blood dicloxacillin level
tetracyclines: Decreased dicloxacillin effectiveness
warfarin: Reduced anticoagulant effect

FOODS

all foods: Possibly delayed absorption

Adverse Reactions

CNS: Dizziness, fatigue, fever, insomnia
EENT: Black "hairy" tongue, dry mouth, glossitis, **laryngeal edema, laryngospasm,** stomatitis, taste perversion
GI: Abdominal pain, anorexia, diarrhea, flatulence, nausea, **pseudomembranous colitis,** transient hepatitis, vomiting
GU: Nephropathy, vaginitis
MS: Prolonged muscle relaxation
SKIN: Dermatitis, **erythema multiforme,** pruritus, rash, urticaria, vesicular eruptions
Other: **Anaphylaxis,** serum sickness-like reaction, superinfection

Childbearing Considerations

PREGNANCY

- It is not known if drug causes fetal harm.
- Use with caution only if benefit to mother outweighs potential risk to fetus.

LACTATION

- Drug is present in breast milk.
- Patient should check with prescriber before breastfeeding.

Nursing Considerations

- Expect to obtain body fluid and tissue samples for culture and sensitivity tests, as ordered, and review the results, if possible, before dicloxacillin therapy begins. Also check for history of sensitivity to cephalosporins, penicillins, and other substances.
- Notify prescriber if diarrhea develops; it could be the development of pseudomembranous colitis.

PATIENT TEACHING

- Instruct patient to take drug 1 hour before or 2 hours after meals.
- Instruct patient to take drug around the clock, not to miss a dose, and to complete the entire prescription unless directed otherwise by prescriber.
- Advise patient to take oral suspension with a full glass of water. Explain that suspension is effective for 7 days at room temperature and for 14 days if refrigerated.
- Caution patient not to open capsules and mix contents with food or liquids because an unpleasant taste and decreased drug absorption will result.

D

- Instruct patient to shake oral solution thoroughly and measure doses with a calibrated device for accuracy.
- Advise patient to notify prescriber if she experiences adverse GI reactions or signs of hypersensitivity or superinfection.
- Be aware that if patient takes an oral contraceptive, she should be advised to use an additional form of contraception during therapy.
- Instruct patient to store drug away from direct light, heat, and moisture and to refrigerate—but not freeze—oral solution.

dicyclomine hydrochloride
Bentyl, Protylol (CAN)

Class and Category
Pharmacologic class: Anticholinergic
Therapeutic class: Antispasmodic

Indications and Dosages
＊ *To treat functional or irritable bowel syndrome*

CAPSULES, SYRUP, TABLETS
Adults. *Initial:* 20 mg four times daily, increased as needed and tolerated after 1 wk to 40 mg four times daily. *Maximum:* 160 mg daily.

I.M. INJECTION
Adults. 10 to 20 mg four times daily. Dosage adjusted as needed and tolerated but not given longer than 1 or 2 days.

Drug Administration
P.O.
- Use calibrated device to measure dosage of syrup.
- Store in a tightly sealed container at room temperature, protected from moisture and direct light. Do not refrigerate syrup.

I.M.
- Aspirate the syringe before injecting drug to avoid intravascular injection, which could cause a thrombosis.
- Never administer I.V. or subcutaneously.

Route	Onset	Peak	Duration
P.O./I.M.	1–2 hr	1–1.5 hr	>4 hr

Half-life: 1.8 hr

Mechanism of Action
Inhibits acetylcholine's muscarinic actions at postganglionic parasympathetic receptors in CNS, secretory glands, and smooth muscles. These actions relax smooth muscles and diminish biliary, GI, and GU tract secretions.

Contraindications
Angle-closure glaucoma; breastfeeding; children less than 6 months old; GI obstruction; hemorrhagic shock; hypersensitivity to dicyclomine, other anticholinergic, or their components; ileus; myasthenia gravis; obstructive uropathy; reflux esophagitis; severe ulcerative colitis; toxic megacolon

Interactions
DRUGS
adsorbent antidiarrheals, antacids: Decreased dicyclomine absorption
amantadine, antihistamines, antipsychotics such as phenothiazines, benzodiazepines, Class 1 antiarrhythmics such as quinidine, MAO inhibitors, narcotic analgesics such as meperidine, nitrates and nitrites, other anticholinergics, sympathomimetic agents, tricyclic antidepressants: Increased dicyclomine effects
digoxin: Increased risk of digitalis toxicity
metoclopramide: Decreased effect of metoclopramide on GI motility
opioid analgesics: Increased risk of ileus, severe constipation, and urine retention

Adverse Reactions
CNS: Agitation, delirium, dizziness, drowsiness, dyskinesia, excitement, fever, insomnia, lethargy, light-headedness (I.M. use), nervousness, paresthesia, psychosis, syncope
CV: Palpitations, tachycardia
EENT: Blurred vision, cycloplegia, dry mouth, loss of taste, mydriasis, nasal congestion, photophobia
GI: Constipation, dysphagia, heartburn, ileus, vomiting
GU: Impotence, urine retention
SKIN: Decreased sweating, flushing, pruritus
Other: Heatstroke; injection-site pain, redness, and swelling

Childbearing Considerations
PREGNANCY
- It is not known if drug causes fetal harm.
- Use with caution only if benefit to mother outweighs potential risk to fetus.

LACTATION

- Drug is present in breast milk.
- A decision should be made to discontinue drug or breastfeeding.

☰ Nursing Considerations

- Assess patient for tachycardia before giving dicyclomine; heart rate may increase.
- Watch for symptoms of hypersensitivity, such as agitation and pruritus. They usually resolve within 48 hours of stopping drug.
- Assess patient during long-term use for chronic constipation and fecal impaction, and take corrective measures, as prescribed.
- Monitor patient, especially the elderly and/ or patients with mental illness, for delirium and psychosis. If present, notify prescriber and expect drug to be discontinued and symptoms to disappear within 12 to 24 hours.

PATIENT TEACHING

- Instruct patient to store dicyclomine in a tightly sealed container at room temperature, protected from moisture and direct light. Advise her not to refrigerate syrup.
- Inform patient that dicyclomine relieves symptoms but doesn't cure the disorder.
- Instruct patient to take drug 30 to 60 minutes before eating.
- Advise patient not to take an antacid or an antidiarrheal within 2 hours of dicyclomine.
- Inform patient that blurred vision, dizziness, or drowsiness may occur.
- Advise patient to eat high-fiber foods and drink at least eight glasses of water daily to prevent constipation.

! WARNING Urge patient to avoid getting overheated during exercise or in hot weather because heatstroke may result. Inform patient that hot baths or saunas may cause dizziness or fainting.

- Instruct patient to change position slowly to avoid light-headedness.
- Inform patient that stopping drug abruptly may cause dizziness and vomiting.
- Tell patient to take a missed dose as soon as she remembers, unless it's nearly time for the next dose. Caution against doubling the dose.
- Urge patient and family that if delirium or psychosis occurs, stop the drug and notify the prescriber. Inform them that these symptoms usually resolve within 12 to 24 hours after drug is discontinued.

didanosine
Videx, Videx EC

☰ Class and Category
Pharmacologic class: Nucleoside reverse transcriptase inhibitor (NRTI)
Therapeutic class: Antiretroviral

☰ Indications and Dosages
✱ *As adjunct to treat human immunodeficiency virus (HIV-1) infection*

ORAL SOLUTION
Adults weighing at least 60 kg (132 lb). 200 mg twice daily. Alternative (but less preferred) dosing, 400 mg once daily.
Adults weighing less than 60 kg (132 lb). 125 mg twice daily. Alternative (but less preferred) dosing, 250 mg once daily.
Children older than 8 months. 120 mg/m^2 twice daily.
Children 2 weeks to 8 months old. 100 mg/m^2 twice daily.

D.R. CAPSULES
Adults and children age 6 and older weighing at least 60 kg (132 lb). 400 mg once daily.
Adults and children age 6 and older weighing 25 kg (55 lb) to less than 60 kg (132 lb). 250 mg once daily.
Children age 6 and older weighing 20 kg (44 lb) to less than 25 kg (55 lb). 200 mg once daily.
±**DOSAGE ADJUSTMENT** *For oral solution:* For adult patient with a creatinine clearance between 30 and 59 ml/min and weighing at least 60 kg (132 lb), dosage decreased to 100 mg twice daily or 200 mg once daily; for adult patient weighing less than 60 kg (132 lb), dosage decreased to 75 mg twice daily or 150 mg once daily. For adult patient with a creatinine clearance between 10 and 29 ml/min and weighing at least 60 kg (132 lb), dosage decreased to 150 mg once daily; for adult patient weighing less than 60 kg (132 lb), dosage decreased to 100 mg once daily. For adult patient with a creatinine clearance less than 10 ml/min and weighing at least 60 kg (132 lb), dosage decreased to 100 mg once daily; for adult patient weighing less than 60 kg

(132 lb), dosage decreased to 75 mg once daily. For pediatric patients with renal insufficiency, dosage reduced, but specific dose adjustment is unknown due to insufficient data.

For D.R. capsules: For adult patient with a creatinine clearance between 59 and 30 ml/min and weighing at least 60 kg (132 lb), dosage decreased to 200 mg once daily; for adult patient weighing less than 60 kg (132 lb), dosage decreased to 125 mg once daily. For adult patient with a creatinine clearance between 10 and 29 ml/min regardless of weight, dosage decreased to 125 mg once daily. For adult patient with a creatinine clearance less than 10 ml/min and weighing at least 60 kg, dosage also reduced to 125 mg once daily. Drug discontinued for patient with a creatinine clearance less than 10 ml/min and weighing less than 60 kg (132 lb). For pediatric patients with renal insufficiency, dosage reduced, but specific dose adjustment is unknown due to insufficient data.

For adult patients taking tenofovir disoproxil fumarate concomitantly with either oral didanosine solution or D.R. didanosine capsules: For patient with a creatinine clearance of at least 60 ml/min and weighing at least 60 kg (132 lb), dosage reduced to 250 mg once daily; for patient weighing less than 60 kg (132 lb), dosage reduced to 200 mg once daily. The appropriate dosage reduction for patients taking tenofovir disoproxil with creatinine clearance levels less than 60 ml/min is not established.

Drug Administration

P.O.

- Administer on an empty stomach at least 30 minutes before or 2 hours after patient has eaten.
- Shake oral solution well before each dose.
- Use calibrated device to measure dose of oral solution.
- Store oral solution in refrigerator and discard after 30 days.
- Capsules must be swallowed whole and not chewed, crushed, or opened.

Route	Onset	Peak	Duration
P.O.	Unknown	15–90 min	Unknown
P.O./D.R.	Unknown	0.25–2 hr	Unknown

Half-life: 1.3–1.6 hr

Mechanism of Action

Inhibits the activity of HIV-1 reverse transcriptase in two ways. It competes with the natural substrate in the virus and it incorporates itself into the viral DNA causing termination of viral DNA chain elongation.

Contraindications

Concomitant therapy with allopurinol, ribavirin, and stavudine; hypersensitivity to didanosine or its components

Interactions

DRUGS

allopurinol, ganciclovir, ribavirin, tenofovir disoproxil fumarate: Increased plasma didanosine concentration increasing risk for serious didanosine adverse reactions such as pancreatitis, peripheral neuropathy, and symptomatic hyperlactatemia/lactic acidosis

antacids containing aluminum or magnesium: Potential for increased adverse reactions associated with antacids, such as constipation and diarrhea

azole antifungals (ketoconazole, itraconazole). quinolone antibiotics, tetracycline antibiotics: Potential for decreased concentration of these drugs

ciprofloxacin, delavirdine, indinavir: Decreased plasma levels of these drugs with potential for decreased effectiveness

drugs that may cause pancreatic toxicity: Potential for increased risk of pancreatitis

hydroxyurea: Potential for increased risk of fatal hepatotoxicity, pancreatitis, or severe peripheral neuropathy

methadone: Decreased plasma didanosine concentrations with potential for decreased effectiveness

neurotoxic drugs: Potential for increased risk of neuropathy

stavudine: Increased risk of fatal lactic acidosis in pregnant women

ACTIVITIES

alcohol use: Possibly increased risk of liver dysfunction

Adverse Reactions

CNS: Asthenia, chills, fever, headache, peripheral neuropathy

EENT: Dry eyes or mouth, inflamed salivary glands, optic neuritis, parotid gland enlargement, retinal changes

ENDO: Hyperglycemia, **hypoglycemia**
GI: Abdominal pain, anorexia, diarrhea, dyspepsia, elevated liver or pancreatic enzymes, flatulence, **hepatic toxicity, hepatitis, liver failure,** nausea, **non-cirrhotic portal hypertension, pancreatitis, severe hepatomegaly with steatosis,** vomiting
GU: **Acute renal failure**
HEME: Anemia, **leukopenia, thrombocytopenia**
MS: Arthralgia, myalgia, myopathy, **rhabdomyolysis**
SKIN: Alopecia, rash
Other: **Anaphylaxis,** generalized pain, **hyperlactatemia,** hyperuricemia, **lactic acidosis**

Childbearing Considerations

PREGNANCY

- Pregnancy exposure registry: 1-800-258-4263.
- Drug may cause fetal harm such as congenital malformations.
- Use with caution only if benefit to mother outweighs potential risk to fetus.
- Drug is contraindicated when used in conjunction with stavudine because of increased risk for fatal lactic acidosis in pregnant women.

LACTATION

- It is not known if drug is present in breast milk.
- The Centers for Disease Control and Prevention recommends that HIV-1 infected mothers not breastfeed to avoid risking postnatal transmission of HIV-1 infection to infants. They also do not recommend breastfeeding because of potential drug-induced adverse reactions in the infant.

Nursing Considerations

- Use didanosine with extreme caution in patients with risk factors for pancreatitis such as advanced HIV infection or renal impairment and in the elderly. Be aware that the use of didanosine with stavudine is contraindicated because the combination increases risk of pancreatitis. Know that the frequency of pancreatitis is dose related. Monitor patient for signs and symptoms of pancreatitis throughout therapy. Be aware that drug must be discontinued if pancreatitis is confirmed.

- Use didanosine cautiously in patients with known risk factors for liver disease. Be aware that the combined use of didanosine with hydroxyurea and stavudine is contraindicated because this combination has resulted in the highest number of fatal hepatic events. Monitor patient and liver enzymes for evidence of liver disease throughout therapy. If liver disease develops or becomes worse, expect drug to be discontinued and supportive care given.

! **WARNING** Know that lactic acidosis and severe hepatomegaly with steatosis have occurred with didanosine therapy, and death has occurred in some patients. Fatal lactic acidosis has been reported in pregnant women who received the combination of didanosine and stavudine with other antiretrovirals. Risk factors include presence of obesity, prolonged nucleoside exposure, and being female. However, know that lactic acidosis and severe hepatomegaly with steatosis have also occurred in patients with no known risk factors. Expect drug to be discontinued in any patient who develops clinical or laboratory findings suggestive of lactic acidosis or pronounced hepatotoxicity, even in the absence of marked transaminase elevations.

- Monitor patient for early signs of portal hypertension such as the presence of splenomegaly accompanied by thrombocytopenia, because didanosine has been linked to non-cirrhotic portal hypertension. Expect to monitor the patient with the following laboratory tests: complete blood count, international normalized ratio, liver enzymes, and serum albumin and bilirubin levels. Ultrasonography may be warranted as well. If confirmed, expect didanosine therapy to be discontinued.
- Assess patient for signs and symptoms of peripheral neuropathy such as complaints of numbness, pain, or tingling in the feet or hands. Risk factors for developing didanosine-related peripheral neuropathy include advanced HIV disease, history of neuropathy, or being treated with neurotoxic therapy. Report such complaints to prescriber, as drug may have to be discontinued.
- Ensure that patient has periodic retinal examinations while receiving didanosine,

because drug may cause optic neuritis and retinal changes.

- Be aware that immune reconstitution syndrome has occurred in patients treated with combination antiretroviral therapy, including didanosine. The inflammatory response predisposes susceptible patients to opportunistic infections such as cytomegalovirus, *Mycobacterium avium* infection, *Pneumocystis jiroveci* pneumonia, or tuberculosis. Autoimmune disorders such as Graves' disease, Guillain–Barré syndrome, or polymyositis have also occurred. Report sudden or unusual adverse reactions to prescriber.

PATIENT TEACHING

- Instruct patient to take didanosine exactly as prescribed. If a dose is missed, instruct patient to take it as soon as possible. Stress importance of taking drug on a regular schedule and not missing doses, if possible, to avoid the development of resistance to the drug.
- Tell patient to take drug on an empty stomach, at least 30 minutes before or 2 hours after eating.
- Warn patient to alert all prescribers of didanosine therapy, because drug may cause serious interactions with some other drugs. Also tell patient not to take any over-the-counter preparations, including herbal products, without consulting prescriber first.
- Stress importance of reporting persistent, severe, or unusual signs and symptoms to prescriber, because serious adverse reactions can occur with didanosine, especially affecting the liver and pancreas. Also stress the need to report any numbness, pain, or tingling in patient's feet or hands.
- Caution patient to be compliant with laboratory monitoring for early detection of adverse reactions associated with didanosine use.
- Inform patient to report any changes in vision, especially blurred vision, to prescriber. Stress importance of having regular eye examinations when taking didanosine.
- Tell patient to immediately report any symptoms of infections to prescriber.
- Inform patient that loss of body fat from his arms, face, or legs may occur while taking didanosine.

- Instruct patient to avoid alcohol while taking didanosine.
- Tell women of childbearing age to alert prescriber if pregnancy is suspected or known.
- Warn mothers with HIV infection not to breastfeed the infant, because the HIV-1 virus can be passed to the baby in breast milk.

difelikefalin
Korsuva

⬚ Class and Category
Pharmacologic class: Kappa opioid receptor agonist
Therapeutic class: Antipruritic

⬚ Indications and Dosages
∗ *To treat moderate to severe pruritus associated with chronic kidney disease in patients undergoing hemodialysis*

I.V. INJECTION
Adults. 0.5 mcg/kg at the end of each hemodialysis treatment.

⬚ Drug Administration
I.V.
- Do not mix or dilute difelikefalin prior to administration.
- Drug is supplied in a single-dose vial. Discard any unused product.
- Inspect solution, which should be clear, colorless, and free of particulate matter.
- Injection volume is based on patient's target dry body weight in kilograms. Use chart in manufacturer drug insert to determine injection volume. If patient's target dry body weight falls outside of the ranges given in the chart, use the formula: Total Injection Volume (ml) = Patient Target Dry Body Weight (kg) $\times$ 0.01, rounded to the nearest tenth (0.1 ml).
- Administer within 60 minutes of syringe preparation.
- Administer as an I.V. bolus into the venous line of the dialysis circuit at the end of the hemodialysis session. The dose may be administered either during or after the rinse back of the dialysis circuit. If the drug is given after rinse back, administer it into the venous line followed by at least 10 ml of

normal saline flush. If dose is given during rinse back, no additional normal saline is needed to flush the line.

- *Incompatibilities:* None listed by manufacturer

Route	Onset	Peak	Duration
I.V.	Unknown	Unknown	Unknown

Half-life: 23–31 hr

⊟ Mechanism of Action

The drug's ability to relieve pruritus is unknown.

⊟ Contraindications

Hypersensitivity to difelikefalin or its components

⊟ Interactions

None reported by the manufacturer

⊟ Adverse Reactions

CNS: Confusion, dizziness, gait disturbances, headache, mental status changes, somnolence
GI: Diarrhea, nausea
OTHER: Hyperkalemia

⊟ Childbearing Considerations

PREGNANCY

- It is not known if drug can cause fetal harm.
- Use with caution only if benefit to mother outweighs potential risk to fetus.

LACTATION

- It is not known if drug is present in breast milk.
- Patient should check with prescriber before breastfeeding.

⊟ Nursing Considerations

- Institute safety precautions because difelikefalin can cause adverse CNS reactions that could lead to patient falling, especially if patient is 65 years of age or older or is taking centrally acting depressants, opioid analgesics, or sedating antihistamines.
- Monitor patient's serum potassium level, as ordered, because difelikefalin may cause hyperkalemia.

PATIENT TEACHING

- Instruct patient on fall precautions, especially if somnolence occurs or patient is 65 years of age or older.
- Alert patient that other drugs such as those affecting the central nervous system, opioid analgesics, or sedating antihistamines taken concomitantly with difelikefalin can increase the risk of developing adverse central nervous system reactions. Patient should consult prescriber before taking these types of drugs.
- Caution patient to avoid potentially hazardous activities such as driving a car or operating heavy machinery until the effects of the drug are known.

digoxin

Lanoxin, Lanoxin Pediatric

⊟ Class and Category

Pharmacologic class: Cardiac glycoside
Therapeutic class: Antiarrhythmic, cardiotonic

⊟ Indications and Dosages

✳ *To treat mild to moderate heart failure with rapid digitalization*

I.V. INJECTION

Adults and children over age 10. *Loading:* 8 to 12 mcg/kg in 3 divided doses, with first dose equal to 50% of total dose and 25% of the total loading dose every 6 to 8 hr for two doses. *Maintenance:* 2.4 to 3.6 mcg/kg once daily.

Children ages 5 to 10. *Loading:* 15 to 30 mcg/kg in 3 divided doses, with first dose equal to 50% of total dose and 25% of the total loading dose given every 6 to 8 hr for two doses. *Maintenance:* 2.3 to 4.5 mcg/kg twice daily.

Children ages 2 to 5. *Loading:* 25 to 35 mcg/kg in 3 divided doses, with first dose equal to 50% of total dose and 25% of the total loading dose given every 6 to 8 hr for two doses. *Maintenance:* 3.8 to 5.3 mcg/kg twice daily.

Infants ages 1 to 24 months. *Loading:* 30 to 50 mcg/kg in 3 divided doses, with first dose equal to 50% of total dose and 25% of the total loading dose given every 6 to 8 hr for two doses. *Maintenance:* 4.5 to 7.5 mcg/kg twice daily.

Full-term neonates. *Loading:* 20 to 30 mcg/kg in 3 divided doses, with first dose equal to 50% of total dose and 25% of total loading dose given every 6 to 8 hr for two doses. *Maintenance:* 3 to 4.5 mcg/kg twice daily.

Premature neonates. *Loading:* 15 to 25 mcg/kg in 3 divided doses, with first dose equal to 50% of total dose and 25% of the total loading dose given every 6 to 8 hr for two doses. *Maintenance:* 1.9 to 3.1 mcg/kg twice daily.

ORAL SOLUTION, TABLETS

Adults and children over age 10. *Loading:* 10 to 15 mcg/kg total given in 3 divided doses every 6 to 8 hr, with first dose equal to 50% of total dose and subsequent two doses given each as 25% of the total loading dose. *Maintenance:* 3.4 to 5.1 mcg/kg (tablet) and 3 to 4.5 mcg/kg (oral solution) once daily.

Children ages 5 to 10. *Loading:* 20 to 45 mcg/kg (tablet) and 20 to 35 mcg/kg (oral solution) in 3 divided doses every 6 to 8 hr and subsequent two doses given each as 25% of the total loading dose. *Maintenance:* 3.2 to 6.4 mcg/kg (tablet) and 2.8 to 5.6 mcg/kg (oral solution) daily in 2 divided doses.

ORAL SOLUTION

Children ages 2 to 5. *Loading:* 30 to 45 mcg/kg in 3 divided doses every 6 to 8 hr, with first dose equal to 50% of total dose and each of remaining two doses equal to 25% of total dose. *Maintenance:* 4.7 to 6.6 mcg/kg daily in 2 divided doses.

Infants ages 1 to 24 months. *Loading:* 35 to 60 mcg/kg in 3 divided doses every 6 to 8 hr, with first dose equal to 50% of total dose and each of remaining two doses equal to 25% of total dose. *Maintenance:* 5.6 to 9.4 mcg/kg daily in 2 divided doses.

Full-term neonates. *Loading:* 25 to 35 mcg/kg in 3 divided doses every 6 to 8 hr, with first dose equal to 50% of total dose and each of remaining two doses equal to 25% of total dose. *Maintenance:* 3.8 to 5.6 mcg/kg daily in 2 divided doses.

Premature neonates. *Loading:* 20 to 30 mcg/kg in 3 divided doses every 6 to 8 hr, with first dose equal to 50% of total dose and each of remaining two doses equal to 25% of total dose. *Maintenance:* 2.3 to 3.9 mcg/kg daily in 2 divided doses.

✳ *To treat mild to moderate heart failure with gradual digitalization*

ORAL SOLUTION, TABLETS

Adults, children, infants, preterm infants. Eliminate loading dose and give only maintenance dosage as listed for rapid digitalization above.

✳ *To control ventricular response rate in chronic atrial fibrillation with rapid digitalization*

ORAL SOLUTION, TABLETS

Adults. *Loading:* 10 to 15 mcg/kg in 3 divided doses every 6 to 8 hr, with first dose equal to 50% of total loading dose and each of remaining two doses given as 25% of total loading dose. *Maintenance:* 3.4 to 5.1 mcg/kg once daily for tablets and 3.0 to 4.5 mcg/kg once daily for oral solution.

I.V. INJECTION

Adults. *Initial:* 8 to 12 mcg/kg every 6 to 8 hr, with first dose equal to 50% of total loading dose and each of remaining two doses given as 25% of total loading dose. *Maintenance:* 2.4 to 3.6 mcg/kg once daily.

✳ *To control ventricular response rate in chronic atrial fibrillation with gradual digitalization*

ORAL SOLUTION, TABLETS

Adults with normal renal function. 3.4 to 5.1 mcg/kg once daily for tablets and 3.0 to 4.5 mcg/kg once daily for oral solution and adjusted every 2 wk, as needed.

I.V. INJECTION

Adults with normal renal function. 2.4 to 3.6 mcg/kg once daily with dosage adjusted every 2 wk, as needed.

±**DOSAGE ADJUSTMENT** Dosage carefully adjusted for patients who are debilitated or elderly or have implanted pacemakers because toxicity may develop at doses tolerated by most patients.

⬚ Drug Administration

- Before administering a loading dose, obtain heart rate, heart rhythm, blood pressure, and electrolyte levels and question patient about the use of cardiac glycosides within the past 2 to 3 weeks.
- Take patient's apical pulse before giving each dose and notify prescriber if it's below 60 beats/minute (or other specified level).

P.O.

- Use the calibrated oral dosing syringe supplied by manufacturer to measure dosage of oral solution. However, if dosage is greater than 0.1 ml, use a separate measuring device.

I.V.

- I.V. route used only if oral administration is not feasible or a rapid therapeutic effect is necessary.
- Give undiluted, or dilute with a fourfold or greater volume of 0.9% Sodium Chloride for

Injection, 5% Dextrose in Water, or Sterile Water for Injection. Diluting with a smaller volume of diluent may cause precipitation of digoxin. Administer immediately, once diluted.

- Administer slowly over 5 minutes or longer. Rapid administration may cause coronary or systemic vasoconstriction to occur.
- Discard if solution is markedly discolored or contains precipitate.
- Do not administer as an I.M. injection because of severe local irritation and pain at site of injection.
- *Incompatibilities:* Other I.V. drugs

Route	Onset	Peak	Duration
P.O.	30–120 min	1–3 hr	3–4 days
I.V.	5–30 min	1–4 hr	3–4 days

Half-life: 36–48 hr

Mechanism of Action

Increases the force and velocity of myocardial contraction, resulting in positive inotropic effects. Digoxin produces antiarrhythmic effects by decreasing the conduction rate and increasing the effective refractory period of the AV node.

Contraindications

Hypersensitivity to digoxin or its components, presence of digitalis toxicity, ventricular fibrillation ventricular tachycardia unless heart failure occurs unrelated to digoxin therapy

Interactions

DRUGS

amiodarone, mirabegron, propafenone, quinine, verapamil: Increased digoxin concentration up to 50%, increasing risk of digitalis toxicity
beta blockers, calcium channel blockers: Increased additive effects of slowing heart rate, possibly producing bradycardia
calcium supplements given rapidly I.V.: Increased risk of serious arrhythmias
dofetilide: Increased risk for torsades de pointes
dronedarone: Increased risk of sudden death
ivabradine: Increased risk of bradycardia
nephrotoxic drugs: Increased risk of digitalis toxicity

neuromuscular blocking agents such as succinylcholine: Possibly sudden release of potassium from muscle cells increasing risk of arrhythmias
quinidine, ritonavir: Increased digoxin concentration by more than 50%, significantly increasing risk of digitalis toxicity
sotalol: Increased risk of proarrhythmias
sympathomimetics: Increased risk of arrhythmias
teriparatide: Transiently increases serum calcium which may cause digitalis toxicity
thyroid hormone: Decreased plasma digoxin level, requiring an increase in dosage

FOODS

high-fiber food: Decreased oral digoxin absorption

Adverse Reactions

CNS: Confusion, depression, drowsiness, extreme weakness, headache, syncope
CV: **Arrhythmias, heart block**
EENT: Blurred vision, colored halos around objects
GI: Abdominal discomfort or pain, anorexia, diarrhea, nausea, vomiting
Other: Electrolyte imbalances

Childbearing Considerations

PREGNANCY

- It is not known if drug causes fetal harm but drug does cross placenta.
- Use with caution only if benefit to mother outweighs potential risk to fetus.
- Dosage may have to be increased during pregnancy and decreased in the postpartum period.
- Upon birth, neonates should be monitored for signs and symptoms of digoxin toxicity.

LACTATION

- Drug is present in breast milk.
- Patient should check with prescriber before breastfeeding.

Nursing Considerations

- Be aware that digoxin therapy is not recommended in patients with acute cor pulmonale involving heart failure associated with amyloid heart disease, constrictive pericarditis, preserved left ventricular ejection fraction, or restrictive cardiomyopathy because of increased susceptibility to digoxin toxicity. The drug is also not recommended in patients with idiopathic hypertrophic subaortic stenosis because outflow obstruction may worsen because of the inotropic effects of digoxin.

- Expect to treat underlying thiamine deficiency in patients with beriberi heart disease because if left untreated, digoxin therapy may be ineffective.
- Monitor patient closely for signs of digitalis toxicity, such as altered mental status, arrhythmias, heart block, nausea, vision disturbances, and vomiting. If they appear, notify prescriber, check serum digoxin level as ordered, and expect to withhold drug until level is known. Monitor ECG tracing continuously.
- Be aware that because digoxin has a narrow therapeutic index and interacts with many different drugs, monitoring of serum digoxin levels is important when other drugs are prescribed or discontinued or dosages adjusted.
- Assess for drug effectiveness if patient has acute or unstable chronic atrial fibrillation. Ventricular rate may not normalize even when serum drug level falls within therapeutic range; raising the dosage probably won't produce a therapeutic effect and may lead to toxicity.
- Obtain frequent ECG tracings as ordered in elderly patients because of their smaller body mass and reduced renal clearance. Elderly patients, especially those with coronary insufficiency, are more susceptible to arrhythmias—particularly ventricular fibrillation—if digitalis toxicity occurs.
- Monitor patient's serum potassium level regularly because hypokalemia predisposes to digitalis toxicity and serious arrhythmias. Also monitor potassium level often when giving potassium salts because hyperkalemia in patients receiving digoxin can be fatal.
- Be aware that digoxin requirements may increase during pregnancy and decrease in the postpartum period. Expect digoxin levels to be monitored closely during pregnancy and the postpartum period. Also be aware that digoxin does cross the placenta. Monitor neonates of mothers taking digoxin during pregnancy for signs and symptoms of digoxin toxicity, including arrhythmias and vomiting.

PATIENT TEACHING

- Emphasize importance of taking digoxin exactly as prescribed. Warn about possible toxicity from taking too much and decreased effectiveness from taking too little.
- Instruct patient to take digoxin at same time each day to help increase compliance.
- Teach patient how to take her pulse, and instruct her to do so before each dose. Urge her to notify prescriber if pulse falls below 60 beats/minute or suddenly increases.
- Inform patient that small, white 0.25-mg tablets can easily be confused with other drugs. Caution against carrying digoxin in anything other than its original labeled container.
- Emphasize need to use special dropper supplied with elixir to ensure accurate dose measurement.
- Instruct patient to take a missed dose as soon as she remembers if within 12 hours of scheduled dose. If not, urge her to notify prescriber immediately.
- Urge patient to notify prescriber if she experiences adverse reactions, such as GI distress or pulse changes.
- Instruct patient to carry medical identification that indicates her need for digoxin.
- Advise patient to consult prescriber before using other drugs, including OTC products.

digoxin immune Fab (ovine)

Class and Category

Pharmacologic class: Antibody fragment
Therapeutic class: Cardiac glycoside antidote

Indications and Dosages

* *To treat acute ingestion of unknown amounts of digoxin and toxicity in the absence of a serum digitalis concentration or estimated ingestion amount*

I.V. INFUSION, I.V. INJECTION

Adults and children. *Initial:* 400 mg (10 vials) with a second dose of 400 mg (10 vials) given, if needed.

* *To treat acute ingestion of known amounts of digoxin*

I.V. INFUSION, I.V. INJECTION

Adults and children. Highly individualized based on the following formula: Amount of digoxin ingested (in mg) divided by 0.5 mg/vial equals dose (in vials).

✱ *To treat chronic digoxin toxicity in the absence of a serum digitalis concentration*

I.V. INFUSION, I.V. INJECTION

Adults and children weighing 20 kg (44 lb) or more. 240 mg (6 vials).

Infants and children weighing less than 20 kg (44 lb). 40 mg (1 vial).

✱ *To treat chronic digoxin toxicity with known serum digitalis concentration.*

I.V. INFUSION, I.V. INJECTION

Adults and children. Highly individualized based on the following formula: Serum digoxin ng/ml times weight in kg divided by 100.

±**DOSAGE ADJUSTMENT** Higher dose administered, as prescribed, if the dose based on ingested amount differs substantially from the dose based on serum digoxin or digitoxin level. Dose repeated after several hours, if needed.

⬒ Drug Administration

I.V.

- Expect each 40-mg vial of purified digoxin immune Fab to bind about 0.5 mg of digoxin.

Adults and children

- Reconstitute by dissolving powder in each vial with 4 ml of Sterile Water for Injection to yield 10 mg/ml. Mix gently.
- Use the reconstituted product immediately. If not used, it can be stored under refrigeration for up to 4 hours.
- Further dilute with 0.9% Sodium Chloride for Injection to proper volume for I.V. infusion.
- Give as an I.V. infusion through a 0.22-micron membrane filter slowly over at least 30 minutes. Keep in mind that drug may be given by rapid I.V. injection if cardiac arrest is imminent.

Infants

- Reconstitute digoxin immune Fab as ordered and administer undiluted with a tuberculin syringe. For very small doses, reconstituted vial can be diluted with an additional 36 ml of isotonic saline to achieve a concentration of 1 mg/ml.

- *Incompatibilities:* None listed by manufacturer

Route	Onset	Peak	Duration
I.V.	15–30 min	Unknown	Unknown

Half-life: 15–20 hr

⬒ Mechanism of Action

Binds with digoxin or digitoxin molecules. The resulting complex is excreted through the kidneys. As the free-serum digoxin level declines, tissue-bound digoxin enters the serum and also is bound and excreted.

⬒ Contraindications

Hypersensitivity to digoxin immune Fab or its components

DRUGS

None reported by manufacturer

⬒ Adverse Reactions

CV: Increased ventricular rate (in atrial fibrillation), worsening of heart failure or low cardiac output

Other: Allergic reaction, febrile reaction, hypokalemia

⬒ Childbearing Considerations

PREGNANCY

- It is not known if drug causes fetal harm.
- Use with caution only if benefit to mother outweighs potential risk to fetus.

LACTATION

- It is not known if drug is present in breast milk.
- Patient should check with prescriber before breastfeeding.

⬒ Nursing Considerations

! **WARNING** Monitor patient for an acute allergic reaction (angioedema, bronchospasm with cough or wheezing, erythema, hypotension, laryngeal edema, pruritus, stridor, tachycardia, or urticaria). If an anaphylactic reaction occurs during infusion, stop administration. Expect to treat all allergic reactions according to protocol. Be aware that patients with a history of hypersensitivity to papaya or papain are at high risk for an allergic reaction; digoxin immune Fab should be administered to this patient only if the benefits outweigh the risks. Also know that prior treatment with digoxin-specific Fab might increase the risk of diminished effects of the drug.

- Watch for fluid volume overload when administering drug to an infant or small child.
- Be aware that when giving a large dose, expect a faster onset but watch closely for febrile reaction.
- Monitor serum potassium level often, especially during first few hours of therapy. Potassium level may drop rapidly.

PATIENT TEACHING
- Inform patient of the purpose of digoxin immune Fab and how it will be given.
- Advise patient to immediately report any signs and symptoms associated with an allergic reaction.

dihydroergotamine mesylate

D.H.E. 45, Dihydroergotamine-Sandoz (CAN), Migranal, Trudhesa

Class and Category

Pharmacologic class: Ergot alkaloid
Therapeutic class: Antimigraine

Indications and Dosages

⁎ *To treat acute migraine with or without aura; to treat acute cluster headache episodes*

I.M. INJECTION, SUBCUTANEOUS INJECTION

Adults. 1 mg at first sign of headache, repeated after 30 to 60 minutes, if needed. *Maximum:* 3 mg/attack or /24 hr, 6 mg/wk.

I.V. INJECTION

Adults. 1 mg, repeated in 1 hr, if needed for migraine and 0.5 mg for cluster headaches. *Maximum:* 2 mg/24 hr, 6 mg/wk.

⁎ *To treat migraine headaches with or without aura*

NASAL SPRAY (MIGRANAL)

Adults. 1 spray (0.5 mg) in each nostril, repeated in 15 min for a total dose of 2 sprays in each nostril or 2 mg. *Maximum:* 3 mg/24 hr, 4 mg/wk.

NASAL SPRAY (TRUDHESA)

Adults. 1 spray (0.725 mg) in each nostril, repeated in 1 hr, if needed. *Maximum:* 2 doses/24 hr or 3 doses within 7 days.

Drug Administration

I.V.
- Give I.V. route as an injection slowly.

I.M. and Subcutaneous

- I.M. or subcutaneous injection administration does not require special administration instructions.
- Once drug ampul is opened, it must be administered within 1 hour or discarded.

NASAL SPRAY
Migranal
- Each vial contains one complete dose, which is 1 spray in each nostril followed 15 minutes later with 1 spray in each nostril.
- Assemble following manufacturer guidelines prior to use.
- Prime before initial use by pumping device four times and before each use. Do not pump more than four times.
- Spray once in each nostril. Do not have patient tilt their head back or sniff through their nose while spraying is taking place or immediately after. Wait 15 minutes and repeat dose.
- Once nasal spray applicator has been prepared, discard any remaining drug in opened vial after 8 hours.
- Store away from heat and light. Do not refrigerate or freeze.

Trudhesa
- Assemble following manufacturer guidelines prior to use. Use or discard within 8 hours once the vial has been opened or the product has been assembled.
- Always hold the device perfectly upright when priming and when administering.
- Prime the assembled device before each use by releasing four sprays. Administer immediately after priming. Tell patient sniffing is not necessary once drug has been administered.
- Discard used device after use. Open and prepare a new device if an additional dose is needed.

- Store drug in original packaging at room temperature.

Route	Onset	Peak	Duration
I.V.	5 min	15 min–2 hr	About 8 hr
I.M.,	15–30 min	Unknown	3–4 hr
SubQ	>30 min	30–60 min	8 hr
Nasal	30 min	30–60 min	8 hr

Half-life: 28 hr

Mechanism of Action

Produces intracranial and peripheral vasoconstriction by binding to all known 5-hydroxytryptamine$_1$ (5-HT$_1$) receptors, alpha$_1$- and alpha$_2$-adrenergic receptors, and dopaminergic receptors. Activation of 5-HT$_1$ receptors on intracranial blood vessels probably constricts large intracranial arteries and closes arteriovenous anastomoses to relieve cluster and migraine headaches. Activation of 5-HT$_1$ receptors on sensory nerves in the trigeminal system also may inhibit the release of proinflammatory neuropeptides. Peripherally, dihydroergotamine causes vasoconstriction by stimulating alpha-adrenergic receptors. At therapeutic doses, it inhibits norepinephrine reuptake, increasing vasoconstriction. Drug constricts veins more than arteries, increasing venous return while decreasing venous stasis and pooling.

Contraindications

Basilar or hemiplegic headaches; breastfeeding; concurrent use with central and peripheral vasoconstrictors; coronary artery disease, including vasospasm; hypersensitivity to dihydroergotamine, other ergot alkaloids, or their components; ischemic heart disease; peripheral arterial vascular disease or after vascular surgery; pregnancy; sepsis; severe hepatic or renal impairment; uncontrolled hypertension; use of macrolide antibiotics or protease inhibitors; use within 24 hours of 5-HT$_1$ agonist, ergotamine-containing or ergot-type drug, or methysergide

Interactions

DRUGS

beta blockers: Possibly peripheral vasoconstriction and peripheral ischemia, increased risk of gangrene

macrolides, protease inhibitors: Possibly increased risk of vasospasm, acute ergotism with peripheral ischemia

other ergot drugs, including ergoloid mesylates, ergonovine, methylergonovine, methysergide, and sumatriptan: Increased risk of serious adverse effects including coronary artery vasospasm

peripheral vasoconstrictors: Risk of severe hypertension

selective serotonin reuptake inhibitors such as fluoxetine, fluvoxamine, paroxetine, sertraline: Increased risk of hyperreflexia, incoordination, and weakness

ACTIVITIES

smoking: Possibly increased ischemic response to ergot therapy

Adverse Reactions

CNS: Anxiety, confusion, dizziness, fatigue, headache, paresthesia, somnolence, weakness
CV: Bradycardia, chest pain, peripheral vasospasm, tachycardia
EENT: Abnormal vision; dry mouth; epistaxis, nasal congestion or rhinitis, and sore nose (nasal spray); miosis; pharyngitis; sinusitis; taste perversion
GI: Diarrhea, nausea, vomiting
MS: Muscle stiffness
SKIN: Localized edema of face, feet, fingers, and lower legs; sensation of heat or warmth; sudden diaphoresis

Childbearing Considerations

PREGNANCY

- Drug may cause fetal harm.
- Drug is contraindicated during pregnancy.

LACTATION

- Drug may be present in breast milk and may cause diarrhea, unstable blood pressure, vomiting, or weak pulse in breastfed infants.
- Drug is contraindicated in women who are breastfeeding.

Nursing Considerations

! **WARNING** Monitor patient for signs of dihydroergotamine overdose, such as abdominal pain, confusion, delirium, dizziness, dyspnea, headache, nausea, pain in legs or arms, paresthesia, seizures, and vomiting.

- Assess patient's capillary refill, peripheral pulses, and skin sensation and warmth. After giving nasal dihydroergotamine, monitor patient for signs of widespread blood vessel constriction and adverse reactions caused by decreased circulation to many body areas.

PATIENT TEACHING

- Instruct patient to use nasal spray or give self a subcutaneous injection, if prescribed, when headache pain—not aura—begins.
- Teach her to prime spray pump by squeezing it four times.
- Advise patient to wait 15 minutes between each set of nasal sprays.
- Teach patient prescribed drug via subcutaneous route how to administer injection and how to properly dispose of needles.
- Encourage patient to lie down in a quiet, dark room after using drug.
- Instruct patient to use more dihydroergotamine if headache returns or worsens but not to exceed maximum prescribed amount or frequency.
- Remind patient to take drug only as needed, not on a daily basis.
- Instruct patient to discard residual nasal spray after 8 hours and an opened ampul after 1 hour.
- Caution her not to use dihydroergotamine and to notify prescriber if she experiences a different type of headache than drug prescribed to treat.
- Inform patient that nasal drug won't relieve pain other than throbbing headaches.
- Advise patient to avoid alcohol, which can cause or worsen headaches, and to avoid smoking, which may cause an ischemic response.

diltiazem hydrochloride

Cardizem, Cardizem CD, Cardizem LA, Cartia XT, Dilt-XR, Matzim LA, Taztia XT, Tiazac

≡ Class and Category

Pharmacologic class: Calcium channel blocker
Therapeutic class: Antianginal, antiarrhythmic, antihypertensive

≡ Indications and Dosages

✱ *To treat chronic stable angina and angina due to coronary artery spasm*

TABLETS (CARDIZEM)

Adults. *Initial:* 30 mg four times daily before meals and at bedtime, increased every 1 or 2 days as needed. *Maximum:* 360 mg daily in divided doses three times daily or four times daily.

E.R. CAPSULES OR TABLETS

Adults. *Initial:* 120 mg or 180 mg daily, increased every 7 to 14 days as needed. *Maximum:* 360 mg daily (Cardizem LA, Matzim LA), 480 mg (Cardizem CD, Cartia XT), and 540 mg (Taztia XT, Tiazac).

✱ *To improve exercise tolerance in patients with chronic stable angina*

E.R. TABLETS (CARDIZEM LA)

Adults. *Initial:* 180 mg once daily, increased in 7 to 14 days, as needed. *Maximum:* 360 mg daily.

✱ *To control hypertension*

E.R. CAPSULES

Adults and adolescents. *Initial:* 120 to 240 mg daily, increased in 7 to 14 days. *Maximum:* 480 mg daily (Cardizem CD, Cartia XT) or 540 mg daily (Taztia XT, Tiazac).

E.R. TABLETS (CARDIZEM LA)

Adults. *Initial:* 180 to 240 mg daily, increased after 14 days, as needed. *Maximum:* 540 mg daily.

✱ *To treat atrial fibrillation, atrial flutter, and paroxysmal supraventricular tachycardia*

I.V. INFUSION OR INJECTION

Adults. 0.25 mg/kg given by bolus. If response is inadequate after 15 min, 0.35 mg/kg given by bolus. Then 5 or 10 mg/hr after bolus, increased by 5 mg/hr, as needed. *Maximum:* 15 mg/hr for up to 24 hr.

≡ Drug Administration

P.O.

- E.R. capsules and tablets must be swallowed whole and not chewed, crushed, opened, or split.

I.V.

- For I.V. injection, administer undiluted and inject slowly over 2 min while monitoring blood pressure and ECG.
- For continuous I.V. infusion, dilute 100 ml of diluent for a final concentration of 1 mg/ml; 250 ml of diluent for a final concentration of

0.83 mg/ml; and 500 ml of diluent for a final concentration of 0.45 mg/ml.

- 0.9% Sodium Chloride Injection, 5% Dextrose Injection, or 5% Dextrose in Water, 0.45% Sodium Chloride Injection may be used as diluents.
- Mix thoroughly in a glass bottle or polyvinylchloride bag and use within 24 hours.
- Diluted solution may be stored in refrigerator or at room temperature for up to 24 hours before use.
- *Incompatibilities:* Acetazolamide, acyclovir, aminophylline, ampicillin, ampicillin sodium/sulbactam sodium, cefamandole, cefoperazone, diazepam, furosemide, hydrocortisone sodium succinate, insulin (regular 100 units/ml), methylprednisolone sodium succinate, mezlocillin, nafcillin, phenytoin, rifampin, and sodium bicarbonate

Route	Onset	Peak	Duration
P.O.	30–60 min	2–3 hr	6–8 hr
P.O./E.R. cap	2–3 hr	10–14 hr	12–24 hr
P.O./E.R. tab	3–4 hr	11–18 hr	Unknown
I.V.	>3 min	15 min	0.5–10 hr

Half-life: 3–4.5 hr

Contraindications

Acute MI; cardiogenic shock (I.V. administration); Lown–Ganong–Levine or Wolff–Parkinson–White syndrome (I.V. administration), second- or third-degree AV block, or sick sinus syndrome, unless artificial pacemaker is in place; pulmonary edema; systolic blood pressure below 90 mm Hg; ventricular tachycardia (wide complex) (I.V. administration); within a few hours of I.V. beta-blocker therapy (I.V. administration)

Interactions

DRUGS

anesthetic: Additive hypotension; possibly decreased cardiac contractility, conductivity, and automaticity
benzodiazepines: Increased risk of prolonged sedation
beta blockers: Possibly increased risk of adverse cardiovascular effects, especially AV block and bradycardia

buspirone: Increased effects and risk of buspirone toxicity
carbamazepine, quinidine: Decreased hepatic clearance and increased serum levels of these drugs, leading to toxicity
cimetidine: Decreased diltiazem metabolism, increased blood diltiazem level
clonidine: Increased risk of serious sinus bradycardia
cyclosporine: Possibly increased cyclosporine levels
digoxin: Increased blood digoxin level; increased risk of AV block or bradycardia
ivabradine: Increased ivabradine exposure which may exacerbate bradycardia and conduction disturbances
rifampin: Decreased blood diltiazem level to undetectable amounts
statins: Increased blood statin level with increased risk of myopathy and rhabdomyolysis

Adverse Reactions

CNS: Abnormal gait, amnesia, asthenia, depression, dizziness, dream disturbances, extrapyramidal reactions, fatigue, hallucinations, headache, insomnia, nervousness, paresthesia, personality change, somnolence, syncope, tremor, weakness
CV: Angina, **atrial flutter, AV block, bradycardia,** bundle-branch block, **ECG abnormalities, heart failure, hypotension,** palpitations, peripheral edema, **PVCs, sinus arrest,** sinus tachycardia, **ventricular fibrillation, ventricular tachycardia**
EENT: Amblyopia, dry mouth, epistaxis, eye irritation, gingival bleeding and hyperplasia, gingivitis, nasal congestion, retinopathy, taste perversion, tinnitus
ENDO: Hyperglycemia
GI: Anorexia, constipation, diarrhea, elevated liver enzymes, indigestion, nausea, thirst, vomiting
GU: **Acute renal failure,** impotence, nocturia, polyuria, sexual dysfunction
HEME: **Hemolytic anemia, leukopenia, prolonged bleeding time, thrombocytopenia**
MS: Arthralgia, muscle spasms, myalgia
RESP: Cough, dyspnea
SKIN: Acute generalized exanthematous pustulosis, alopecia, diaphoresis, **erythema multiforme, exfoliative dermatitis,** flushing, leukocytoclastic vasculitis, petechiae,

D

≣ Mechanism of Action

Diltiazem inhibits calcium movement into coronary and vascular smooth-muscle cells by blocking slow calcium channels in cell membranes, as shown. This action decreases intracellular calcium, which:

- inhibits smooth-muscle cell contractions
- decreases myocardial oxygen demand by relaxing coronary and vascular smooth muscle, reducing peripheral vascular resistance and systolic and diastolic blood pressures
- slows AV conduction time and prolongs AV nodal refractoriness
- interrupts the reentry circuit in AV nodal reentrant tachycardias.

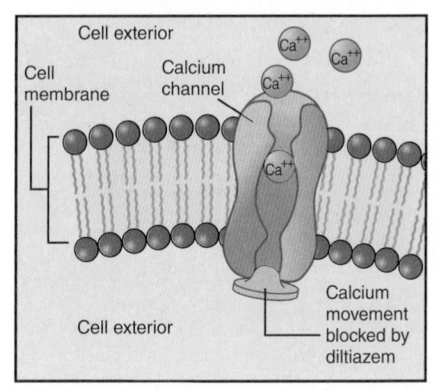

photosensitivity, pruritus, purpura, rash, **Stevens–Johnson syndrome, toxic epidermal necrolysis,** urticaria
Other: Angioedema, hyperuricemia, weight gain

≣ Childbearing Considerations

PREGNANCY

- It is not known if drug causes fetal harm.
- Use with caution only if benefit to mother outweighs potential risk to fetus.

LACTATION

- Drug is present in breast milk.
- A decision should be made to discontinue breastfeeding or the drug to avoid potential serious adverse reactions in the breastfed infant.

≣ Nursing Considerations

- Use diltiazem cautiously in patients with impaired hepatic or renal function, and monitor liver and renal function, as appropriate; drug is metabolized mainly in the liver and excreted by the kidneys.

! WARNING Monitor patient's blood pressure, heart rate and rhythm by continuous ECG, and pulse rate as appropriate during therapy. Keep emergency equipment and drugs available.

- Assess patient for signs and symptoms of heart failure.

- Watch for digitalis toxicity (nausea, vomiting, and visual color distortion) if patient takes digoxin and has an elevated serum digoxin level.
- Administer sublingual nitroglycerin, as prescribed, during diltiazem therapy.
- Expect to discontinue drug if adverse skin reactions, usually transient, persist although some may be severe.

PATIENT TEACHING

- Explain that capsules and E.R. tablets must be swallowed whole.

! WARNING Tell patient that stopping drug suddenly may have life-threatening effects.

- Advise patient to monitor blood pressure and pulse rate regularly and to report significant changes to prescriber.
- Urge patient to report chest pain, difficulty breathing, dizziness, fainting, irregular heartbeat, rash, or swollen ankles.
- Instruct patient to maintain good oral hygiene, perform gum massage, and see a dentist every 6 months to prevent gingival bleeding and hyperplasia and gingivitis.
- Inform all prescribers of diltiazem therapy. Tell patient to consult prescriber before taking any OTC medication.
- Tell patient to inform prescriber if pregnancy occurs or is suspected.

diphenhydramine hydrochloride

Allerdryl (CAN), Banophen, Benadryl, Sominex, Unisom

≣ Class and Category

Pharmacologic class: Antihistamine
Therapeutic class: Antianaphylactic adjunct, antidyskinetic, antiemetic, antihistamine, antitussive (syrup), antivertigo, sedative-hypnotic

≣ Indications and Dosages

✳ *To treat hypersensitivity reactions, such as perennial and seasonal allergic rhinitis, vasomotor rhinitis, allergic conjunctivitis due to food allergies, uncomplicated allergic skin eruptions, and transfusion reactions*

CAPSULES, CHEWABLE TABLETS, ELIXIR, ORAL SOLUTION, ORALLY DISINTEGRATING TABLETS, TABLETS

Adults and adolescents. 25 to 50 mg three or four times daily, as needed. *Maximum:* 300 mg daily.
Children ages 6 to 12 years. 12.5 to 25 mg three or four times daily, as needed. Alternatively, 5 mg/kg/24 hr. *Maximum:* 300 mg daily.

ELIXIR

Adults and adolescents. 25 to 50 mg every 4 to 6 hr, as needed. *Maximum:* 300 mg daily.
Children. 1.25 mg/kg every 4 to 6 hr. *Maximum:* 300 mg daily.

I.V. OR I.M. INJECTION

Adults and adolescents. 10 to 50 mg, up to 100 mg/dose, as needed. *Maximum:* 400 mg daily.
Children other than premature infants and neonates. 1.25 mg/kg (5 mg/kg/24 hr) divided into four doses.

✳ *To prevent or treat motion sickness*

CAPSULES, CHEWABLE TABLETS, ORAL SOLUTION, ORALLY DISINTEGRATING TABLETS, TABLETS

Adults and adolescents. 25 to 50 mg, with first dose given 30 min before exposure to motion and before meals and upon retiring for the duration of exposure.

✳ *To treat sleep disorders*

CAPSULES, CHEWABLE TABLETS, ORAL SOLUTION, ORALLY DISINTEGRATING TABLETS, TABLETS

Adults and adolescents. 50 mg 20 to 30 min before bedtime.

✳ *To provide antitussive effects*

ELIXIR

Adults and adolescents. 25 mg every 4 hr. *Maximum:* 150 mg/24 hr.

≣ Drug Administration

P.O.

- Give with food if drug upsets stomach.
- Use calibrated device to measure dosages of elixir and oral solution forms.
- Keep elixir container tightly closed.
- Chewable tablets should be chewed or allowed to dissolve on the tongue before swallowing.
- Oral solution should not be refrigerated.
- Protect all oral formulations from light and high humidity; film-coated tablets should also be kept from excessive heat.

I.V.

- Administer as an injection, not to exceed 25 mg/min.
- Protect from light.
- *Incompatibilities:* Allopurinol, amobarbital, amphotericin B, cefepime, dexamethasone, diatrizoate, foscarnet, furosemide, haloperidol, iodipamide, pentobarbital, phenobarbital, phenytoin, sodium phosphate with lorazepam and metoclopramide, thiopental

I.M.

- Administer as a deep I.M. injection.
- Do not exceed 25 mg per site.
- Protect from light.

Route	Onset	Peak	Duration
P.O.	15–60 min	2–4 hr	4–6 hr
I.V.	Immediate	1–3 hr	4–6 hr
I.M.	15–30 min	1–3 hr	4–6 hr

Half-life: 3.4–9.2 hr

≣ Mechanism of Action

Binds to central and peripheral H_1 receptors, competing with histamine for these sites and preventing it from reaching its site of action. By blocking histamine, diphenhydramine produces antihistamine effects, inhibiting GI, respiratory, and vascular smooth-muscle

D

contraction; decreasing capillary permeability, which reduces flares, itching, and wheals; and decreasing lacrimal and salivary gland secretions.

Diphenhydramine produces antidyskinetic effects, possibly by inhibiting acetylcholine in the CNS. It also produces antitussive effects by directly suppressing the cough center in the medulla oblongata in the brain. Diphenhydramine's antiemetic and antivertigo effects may be related to its ability to bind to CNS muscarinic receptors and depress vestibular stimulation and labyrinthine function. Its sedative effects are related to its CNS depressant action.

Contraindications

Breastfeeding; hypersensitivity to diphenhydramine, similar antihistamines, or their components; use in newborns or premature infants

Interactions

DRUGS

barbiturates, other CNS depressants: Possibly increased CNS depression
MAO inhibitors: Increased anticholinergic and CNS depressant effects of diphenhydramine

ACTIVITIES

alcohol use: Possibly increased CNS depression

Adverse Reactions

CNS: Confusion, dizziness, drowsiness
CV: Arrhythmias, palpitations, tachycardia
EENT: Blurred vision, diplopia
GI: Epigastric distress, nausea
HEME: Agranulocytosis, hemolytic anemia, thrombocytopenia
RESP: Thickened bronchial secretions
SKIN: Photosensitivity

Childbearing Considerations

PREGNANCY

- It is not known if drug causes fetal harm.
- Use with caution only if benefit to mother outweighs potential risk to fetus.

LACTATION

- Drug is present in breast milk.
- Drug as an antihistamine poses a higher risk of adverse reactions in breastfed infants.
- Drug is contraindicated in breastfeeding women.

Nursing Considerations

- Expect to give parenteral form of diphenhydramine only when oral ingestion isn't possible.
- Expect to discontinue drug at least 72 hours before skin tests for allergies because drug may inhibit cutaneous histamine response, thus producing false-negative results.

PATIENT TEACHING

- Instruct patient to take diphenhydramine at least 30 minutes before exposure to situations that may cause motion sickness.
- Advise her to take drug with food to minimize GI distress.
- Caution patient not to take higher than recommended dosage as euphoric highs, hallucinations, and other serious side effects could occur.
- Urge patient to avoid alcohol while taking diphenhydramine.
- Caution patient to avoid hazardous activities until drug's CNS effects are known.
- Instruct her to use sunscreen to prevent photosensitivity reactions.
- Advise patient to avoid taking other OTC drugs that contain diphenhydramine to prevent additive effects.

dipyridamole
Persantine

Class and Category

Pharmacologic class: Pyrimidine analogue
Therapeutic class: Antiplatelet

Indications and Dosages

* As adjunct to coumarin anticoagulants to prevent postoperative thromboembolic complications of cardiac valve replacement

TABLETS

Adults and adolescents. 75 to 100 mg four times daily with warfarin.

* To aid diagnosis during thallium perfusion imaging of myocardium

I.V. INFUSION

Adults. 0.57 mg/kg as a single dose.
Maximum: 60 mg.

⧉ Drug Administration

P.O.

- Administer at least 1 hour before or 2 hours after meals. However, if GI distress occurs, give with meals or milk.
- Administer drug at evenly spaced intervals.

I.V.

- Dilute in at least a 1:2 ratio with 0.45% or 0.9% Sodium Chloride Injection or 5% Dextrose Injection for a total volume of 20 to 50 ml.
- For use as a diagnostic drug, infuse over 4 minutes followed within 5 minutes by thallium-201 injection.
- Monitor blood pressure, pulse rate and rhythm, and breath sounds during I.V. infusion.
- Protect from direct light and do not freeze.
- *Incompatibilities:* Other drugs or solutions except for those used to dilute drug

Route	Onset	Peak	Duration
P.O.	Unknown	75 min	3 hr
I.V.	Unknown	Unknown	3 hr
Half-life: 10–12 hr			

⧉ Mechanism of Action

May increase the intraplatelet level of adenosine, which causes coronary vasodilation and inhibits platelet aggregation. Dipyridamole also may increase the intraplatelet level of cyclic adenosine monophosphate (cAMP) and may inhibit formation of the potent platelet activator stimulant thromboxane A_2, which decreases platelet activation. Vasodilation and increased blood flow occur preferentially in nondiseased coronary vessels, which results in redistribution of blood away from significantly diseased vessels. These changes in perfusion are observed during thallium imaging studies.

⧉ Contraindications

Hypersensitivity to dipyridamole or its components

⧉ Interactions

DRUGS

adenosinergic agents such as adenosine, regadenoson: Potentiated cardiovascular effects of adenosine

cholinesterase inhibitors: Decreased anticholinesterase effect, possibly aggravating myasthenia gravis
heparin, NSAIDs, thrombolytics: Possibly increased risk of bleeding
theophylline: Reversal of coronary vasodilation caused by dipyridamole, possibly false-negative thallium imaging result

⧉ Adverse Reactions

CNS: Dizziness, headache
CV: Angina, **arrhythmias, ECG changes (specifically ST-segment and T-wave changes)**
GI: Abdominal pain, diarrhea, nausea, vomiting
RESP: Dyspnea
SKIN: Flushing, pruritus, rash

⧉ Childbearing Considerations

PREGNANCY

- It is not known if drug causes fetal harm.
- Use with caution only if benefit to mother outweighs potential risk to fetus.

LACTATION

- Drug is present in breast milk.
- Patient should check with prescriber before breastfeeding.

⧉ Nursing Considerations

- Be aware that if patients taking oral dipyridamole are scheduled to undergo stress testing using intravenous dipyridamole or other adenosinergic agents, the oral dosage of dipyridamole should be withheld for 48 hours before the test because of increased risk for cardiovascular adverse reactions and possibly impaired sensitivity of the test.
- Expect adverse reactions to be minimal and transient at therapeutic doses. They typically resolve with long-term use.

PATIENT TEACHING

- Urge patient to take dipyridamole at least 1 hour before or 2 hours after meals for faster absorption. If she experiences GI distress, advise her to take drug with meals or milk.
- Advise patient to take drug at evenly spaced intervals.
- Inform patient that drug commonly is taken with warfarin. Tell patient that aspirin should not be administered concomitantly with warfarin.

D

- Urge her to keep appointments for coagulation tests.
- Instruct patient to seek immediate emergency treatment if chest pain occurs.
- Caution patient to consult prescriber before taking over-the-counter NSAIDs because of the possible increased risk of bleeding.
- Advise patient to notify all healthcare providers about dipyridamole use.

diroximel fumarate

Vumerity

Class and Category

Pharmacologic class: Nuclear factor-like 2 (Nrf2) activator
Therapeutic class: Immunomodulatory agent

Indications and Dosages

* *To treat relapsing forms of multiple sclerosis (MS), to include active secondary progressive disease, clinically isolated syndrome, and relapsing-remitting disease*

D.R. CAPSULES

Adults. *Initial:* 231 mg twice daily followed by dosage increase to 462 mg twice daily after 7 days. *Maintenance:* 462 mg twice daily.

± **DOSAGE ADJUSTMENT** For patient who cannot tolerate maintenance dosage, dosage reduced temporarily to 231 mg twice daily. Within 4 wk, dosage resumed at 462 mg twice daily.

Drug Administration

P.O.

- Administer nonenteric coated aspirin up to a dose of 325 mg 30 minutes before administering diroximel, as ordered, to reduce the incidence or severity of flushing. Administering with a light snack or meal may also help.
- Capsules should be swallowed whole and not chewed, crushed, or opened.
- A high-fat (more than 30 grams) or a high-calorie (more than 700 calories) meal or snack will interfere with the absorption of the drug.

Route	Onset	Peak	Duration
P.O./D.R.	Unknown	2.5–3 hr	Unknown
Half-life: 1 hr			

Mechanism of Action

Possibly activates the nuclear factor (erythroid-derived 2)-like 2 (Nrf2) pathway, which is involved in the cellular response to oxidative stress thought to be a factor in multiple sclerosis.

Contraindications

Concurrent use of dimethyl fumarate, hypersensitivity to diroximel fumarate, dimethyl fumarate, or any of their components

Interactions

DRUGS

dimethyl fumarate: Potentiated effect increasing risk of serious adverse reactions

ACTIVITIES

alcohol use: Possibly may reduce the plasma concentrations of monomethyl fumarate (MMF), the active metabolite of diroximel fumarate

Adverse Reactions

CNS: Progressive multifocal leukoencephalopathy
EENT: Rhinorrhea
GI: Abdominal pain, diarrhea, dyspepsia, elevated liver enzymes, nausea, vomiting
GU: Albumin present in urine
HEME: Lymphopenia
SKIN: Erythema, flushing, pruritus, rash
Other: Anaphylaxis, angioedema, herpes zoster infections

Childbearing Considerations

PREGNANCY

- It is not known if drug causes fetal harm.
- Use with caution only if benefit to mother outweighs potential risk to fetus.

LACTATION

- It is not known if drug is present in breast milk.
- Patient should check with prescriber before breastfeeding.

Nursing Considerations

- Expect to obtain laboratory test results for alkaline phosphatase; complete blood cell count (CBC), including lymphocyte count; serum aminotransferase; and total bilirubin levels prior to starting diroximel.
- Obtain an MRI at baseline and as clinically indicated to assess for signs of PML.

- Be aware that diroximel is not recommended for patients with moderate or severe renal impairment.

! **WARNING** Monitor patient closely for hypersensitivity reactions such as anaphylaxis and angioedema, which have occurred as early as after the first dose and throughout the duration of drug therapy.

- Obtain a CBC, including lymphocyte count, 6 months after drug therapy has begun and then every 6 to 12 months thereafter, as indicated and ordered. Also expect to obtain laboratory results for alkaline phosphatase, serum aminotransferase, and total bilirubin levels during drug therapy, as indicated and ordered.

! **WARNING** Monitor patient for signs and symptoms of progressive multifocal leukoencephalopathy (PML) such as changes in memory, orientation, or thinking leading to confusion and personality changes, as well as clumsiness of limbs, progressive weakness on one side of the body, and visual disturbances. Although no reports of PML have occurred with cladribine for treating relapsing forms of MS, it is a possibility. At first sign of PML, notify prescriber, expect cladribine to be withheld, and ensure that appropriate diagnostic evaluation is done. Know that MRI findings may reveal PML before clinical signs or symptoms are apparent.

- Monitor patient for signs and symptoms of infections, which could become serious because drug decreases the lymphocyte count. Know that drug therapy may have to be interrupted if lymphocyte counts less than 0.5×10^9/L persist for more than 6 months or if serious infections such as herpes zoster occur (until infections are resolved).
- Know that although liver injury has not been reported with diroximel therapy, it is a high possibility because drug contains the same active metabolite as dimethyl fumarate, which has caused liver injury. Expect to monitor patient's alkaline phosphatase, serum aminotransferase, and total bilirubin throughout drug therapy. If significant liver injury is suspected, drug will have to be discontinued.

PATIENT TEACHING

- Instruct patient to take a nonenteric coated aspirin, up to a dose of 325 mg, 30 minutes before administering diroximel, if ordered to reduce the incidence or severity of flushing caused by the drug. Taking drug with food may also help reduce the incidence of flushing.
- Tell patient to swallow capsule whole and not to chew, crush, or sprinkle capsule contents on food.
- Remind patient to avoid taking drug with a high-fat, high-calorie meal/snack; meal or snack should contain no more than 700 calories and no more than 30 grams of fat.
- Advise patient to avoid coadministration of drug with alcohol.

! **WARNING** Advise patient to stop taking drug and seek emergency medical care if signs and symptoms of an allergic reaction occur.

- Instruct patient to report any unexplained or unusual signs and symptoms to prescriber. Also instruct patient to report persistent and/or severe GI reactions or flushing or signs and symptoms of an infection.
- Stress importance of being compliant with scheduled laboratory tests.

disulfiram
Antabuse

⩶ Class and Category
Pharmacologic class: Aldehyde dehydrogenase inhibitor
Therapeutic class: Alcohol deterrent

⩶ Indications and Dosages
⁎ *As adjunct to maintain sobriety in treatment of chronic alcoholism*
TABLETS
Adults. *Initial:* 250 to 500 mg daily for 1 to 2 wk. *Maintenance:* 125 to 500 mg daily. *Maximum:* 500 mg daily.

⩶ Drug Administration
P.O.
- Check alcohol content of patient's other drugs before starting therapy.

- Don't give drug within 14 days of patient's ingestion of an alcohol-containing substance.
- Crush tablet and mix with fluids before administration, if needed.
- Administer daily dose in morning, or if sedation occurs, administer at bedtime.

Route	Onset	Peak	Duration
P.O.	2–12 hr	Unknown	>14 days

Half-life: 60–120 hr

Mechanism of Action

Interferes with the enzyme responsible for hepatic oxidation of acetaldehyde to acetate, which occurs during alcohol catabolism. Ingestion of even a small amount of alcohol after taking disulfiram raises the blood acetaldehyde level to 5 to 10 times normal. Disulfiram doesn't alter the rate of alcohol elimination. Its major metabolite, diethyldithiocarbamate, inhibits norepinephrine synthesis and may be responsible for the drug's hypotensive effect.

Contraindications

Alcohol intoxication; coronary artery occlusion; hypersensitivity to disulfiram, other thiuram derivatives used in pesticides and rubber vulcanization, or their components; psychosis; recent use of alcohol, alcohol-containing preparations, metronidazole, or paraldehyde; severe myocardial disease

Interactions

DRUGS

alcohol-containing preparations, amitriptyline: Increased sensitivity to alcohol in product, resulting in disulfiram–alcohol reaction
barbiturates: Increased blood barbiturate concentration possibly resulting in barbiturate toxicity
isoniazid: Increased risk of behavioral changes, incoordination, marked changes in mental status, psychotic reactions, or unsteady gait
metronidazole: Risk of CNS toxicity, resulting in confusion and psychosis
oral anticoagulants: Possibly increased anticoagulant effects
phenytoin: Possibly increased blood phenytoin level and risk of phenytoin toxicity

ACTIVITIES

alcohol use: Increased sensitivity to alcohol, resulting in disulfiram–alcohol reaction

FOOD

caffeine (ingested in large amounts): Possibly exaggerated or prolonged caffeine effects

Adverse Reactions

CNS: Drowsiness, headache, peripheral neuropathy, psychotic reaction, tiredness
EENT: Blurred vision, garlic or metallic taste, optic atrophy, optic neuritis
GU: Impotence
SKIN: Rash

Childbearing Considerations

PREGNANCY

- It is not known if drug causes fetal harm.
- Use with caution only if benefit to mother outweighs potential risk to fetus.

LACTATION

- Drug maybe present in breast milk.
- A decision should be made to discontinue breastfeeding or the drug to avoid potential serious adverse reactions in the breastfed infant.

Nursing Considerations

- Keep in mind that disulfiram is given only to patients who are highly motivated to stop drinking and who are receiving psychotherapy or substance abuse counseling.
- Know that the alcohol content of patient's other drugs should be checked before starting therapy.

! **WARNING** Never give drug to patient without her knowledge or if she is intoxicated.

- Expect alcohol ingestion during disulfiram therapy to produce a severe reaction that lasts from 30 minutes to several hours. Symptoms may include angina, anxiety, blurred vision, confusion, diaphoresis, dyspnea, heart failure, hypotension, nausea, palpitations, sinus tachycardia, syncope, thirst, throbbing headache, throbbing in neck, vertigo, vomiting, and weakness. A deep sleep usually follows.

! **WARNING** Be aware that the ingestion of three or more alcoholic beverages with a disulfiram dose greater than 500 mg daily may cause respiratory depression, arrhythmias, and cardiac arrest.

- Know that if patient takes phenytoin, monitor blood phenytoin level before and during disulfiram therapy, and adjust dosage of either drug as prescribed. Interactions may not occur if disulfiram therapy starts before phenytoin therapy. A subtherapeutic phenytoin level may result if disulfiram therapy stops.
- Be aware that if patient takes an oral anticoagulant, monitor PT before and during disulfiram therapy, and adjust anticoagulant dosage as prescribed. Drug interactions may not occur if disulfiram therapy starts before warfarin therapy. If disulfiram therapy stops, be prepared to adjust warfarin dosage to avoid loss of hypoprothrombinemic effects.
- Expect some adverse reactions, such as drowsiness, headache, and impotence, to subside over time or with a brief dosage reduction.
- Know that because one-fifth of a disulfiram dose may stay in the body for 1 week or longer, alcohol ingestion may continue to produce unpleasant symptoms for up to 2 weeks after therapy stops.
- Expect therapy to last months to years, depending on patient's ability to abstain from alcohol.

PATIENT TEACHING

- Teach patient's household and family members about precautions needed and risks associated with disulfiram therapy.
- Explain that drug doesn't cure alcoholism but does help deter alcohol consumption.
- Advise her to take drug at bedtime if she reports daytime drowsiness.
- Warn patient to avoid alcohol-containing substances, such as cough syrup, sauces, and vinegar during therapy because a disulfiram–alcohol reaction may occur after ingesting as little as 15 ml of 100-proof alcohol. Urge her to avoid alcohol-containing liniments and lotions as well.
- Teach patient what to expect if disulfiram–alcohol reaction occurs. Inform her that a deep sleep usually follows the reaction.
- Advise patient that a reaction can occur up to 14 days after therapy stops and that

a severe reaction may cause arrhythmias, cardiac arrest, and respiratory depression.

- Instruct patient to carry medical identification that indicates drug, describes possible reactions, and lists someone to notify in case of emergency.

dobutamine hydrochloride

D

≡ Class and Category

Pharmacologic class: Sympathomimetic
Therapeutic class: Inotropic

≡ Indications and Dosages

❋ *To provide inotropic support short-term in patients with cardiac decompensation due to depressed contractility resulting either from organic heart disease or from cardiac surgical procedures*

I.V. INFUSION

Adults. *Initial:* 0.5 to 1 mcg/kg/min adjusted every couple of minutes according to hemodynamic response. *Usual maintenance:* 2 to 20 mcg/kg/min. *Maximum:* 40 mcg/kg/min.

≡ Drug Administration

I.V.

- Expect to administer a digitalis preparation prior to start of therapy if patient has atrial fibrillation with a rapid ventricular response or a suitable volume expander if hypovolemia is present.
- Dilute concentrate with at least 50 ml of a compatible I.V. solution such as 0.9% Sodium Chloride Injection or 5% Dextrose Injection (see manufacturer information for other suitable diluents). Solution should be clear.
- Discard diluted solution after 24 hours.
- Give as a continuous infusion through a central venous line or large peripheral vein using an infusion pump.
- Monitor blood pressure continuously during therapy, preferably by continuous intra-arterial monitoring; systolic increase of 10 to 20 mm Hg may indicate dobutamine-induced increase in cardiac output.
- Expect to reduce dosage or discontinue drug if hypotension develops.

- *Incompatibilities:* 5% Sodium Bicarbonate Injection or other strongly alkaline solutions, other agents or diluents containing both ethanol and sodium bisulfite, other drugs mixed in same solution

Route	Onset	Peak	Duration
I.V.	1–2 min	10 min	>5 min
Half-life: 2 min			

Mechanism of Action

Mainly stimulates beta$_1$-adrenergic receptors, and mildly stimulates beta$_2$- and alpha$_1$-adrenergic receptors. Beta$_1$-receptor stimulation produces a positive inotropic effect on the myocardium, increasing cardiac output by boosting myocardial contractility and stroke volume. Increased myocardial contractility raises coronary blood flow and myocardial oxygen consumption. Systolic blood pressure typically rises as a result of increased stroke volume. Other hemodynamic effects include decreased systemic vascular resistance, which reduces afterload, and decreased ventricular filling pressure, which reduces preload.

Contraindications

Hypersensitivity to dobutamine or its components, idiopathic hypertrophic subaortic stenosis

Interactions

DRUGS

catechol-O-methyltransferase (COMT) inhibitors such as entacapone: Possibly increased incidence of arrhythmias, changes in blood pressure, and heart rate
nitroprusside: Increased cardiac output and lowered pulmonary wedge pressure

Adverse Reactions

CNS: Fever, headache, nervousness, restlessness
CV: Angina, **bradycardia**, hypertension, **hypotension**, nonspecific chest pain, palpitations, **PVCs, stress cardiomyopathy** (with cardiac stress testing), tachycardia
GI: Nausea, vomiting
RESP: Dyspnea, shortness of breath
SKIN: Extravasation with tissue necrosis and sloughing, rash
Other: Hypokalemia

Childbearing Considerations

PREGNANCY

- It is not known if drug causes fetal harm.
- Use with caution only if benefit to mother outweighs potential risk to fetus.

LACTATION

- It is not known if drug is present in breast milk.
- Due to critical nature of situation, breastfeeding would not be done during drug therapy. Patient should check with prescriber before breastfeeding after receiving the drug.

Nursing Considerations

- Avoid giving dobutamine to patients with acute MI because it can intensify or extend myocardial ischemia.
- Use drug cautiously in patients allergic to sulfites because drug may cause anaphylactic-like signs and symptoms; commercially available dobutamine injections contain sodium bisulfite. Also use drug cautiously in patients with atrial fibrillation because drug increases AV conduction. Keep in mind that patient should be adequately digitalized before administration.
- Monitor heart rate and rhythm via ECG recordings continuously for PVCs, which may result from drug's stimulatory effect on heart's conduction system, and sinus tachycardia, which results from positive chronotropic effect of beta stimulation and may increase heart rate by 5 to 15 beats/minute.
- Monitor hemodynamic parameters, such as cardiac output, central venous pressure, and pulmonary artery wedge pressure, as indicated, to assess drug's effectiveness.

! **WARNING** Monitor serum potassium level to check for hypokalemia, a rare result of beta$_2$ stimulation that causes electrolyte imbalance.

- Monitor urine output hourly, as appropriate, to check for improved renal blood flow.
- Know that dobutamine isn't indicated for long-term treatment of heart failure because it may not be effective and may increase the risk of hospitalization and death.

PATIENT TEACHING

- Explain the need for frequent hemodynamic monitoring.

dofetilide
Tikosyn

Class and Category
Pharmacologic class: Class III antiarrhythmic
Therapeutic class: Antiarrhythmic

Indications and Dosages
⁎ *To convert symptomatic atrial fibrillation or flutter to normal sinus rhythm or to maintain normal sinus rhythm in patients converted from symptomatic atrial fibrillation or flutter*

CAPSULES
Adults. Highly individualized based on creatinine clearance and QTc (QT interval used if heart rate is below 60 beats per min). *Usual:* 500 mcg twice daily for patients with creatinine clearance above 60 ml/min. *Maximum:* 500 mcg twice daily.

±**DOSAGE ADJUSTMENT** For patient with renal impairment, initial dose reduced to 250 mcg twice daily if creatinine clearance is 40 to 60 ml/min and to 125 mcg twice daily if clearance is 20 to 39 ml/min, as prescribed. If, 2 to 3 hr after initial dose, QTc interval has increased by at least 15% or is more than 500 milliseconds (msec) (550 msec in patients with ventricular conduction abnormalities), dosage decreased by 50%, as prescribed. However, for patients receiving lowest initial dose of 125 mcg twice daily, dosage reduced to 125 mcg daily, as prescribed. If at any time after second dose, QTc interval increases to more than 500 msec (550 msec in patients with ventricular conduction abnormalities), expect to discontinue drug, as prescribed.

Drug Administration
P.O.
- Capsules should be swallowed whole with water. Capsules should not be chewed, crushed, or opened.
- Do not administer with grapefruit juice.

Route	Onset	Peak	Duration
P.O.	2 hr	2–3 hr	4 hr
Half-life: 10 hr			

Mechanism of Action
Selectively blocks potassium channels in myocardial cell membranes involved in cardiac repolarization. By blocking potassium channels, dofetilide prolongs action potential duration, effective refractory period, and ventricular refractoriness (widens QT interval). These actions terminate or prevent reentrant tachyarrhythmias, such as atrial fibrillation, atrial flutter, and ventricular tachycardia.

Contraindications
Acquired or congenital QT prolongation syndrome; concurrent therapy with cimetidine, dolutegravir, hydrochlorothiazide, ketoconazole, megestrol, prochlorperazine, trimethoprim, or verapamil; hypersensitivity to dofetilide or its components; severe renal impairment (creatinine clearance less than 20 ml/min)

Interactions
DRUGS
amiloride, cimetidine, cotrimoxazole, ketoconazole, megestrol, metformin, sulfamethoxazole-trimethoprim, triamterene, trimethoprim: Possibly increased blood dofetilide level

azole antifungals, cannabinoids, diltiazem, nefazodone, norfloxacin, protease inhibitors, quinine, selective serotonin reuptake inhibitors, zafirlukast: Possibly increased blood dofetilide level and risk of dofetilide toxicity

bepridil, cisapride, macrolide antibiotics, phenothiazines, selected fluoroquinolones, tricyclic antidepressants: Possibly prolonged QT interval

class I and III antiarrhythmics, especially amiodarone: Possibly prolonged QT interval and increased risk of dofetilide-induced proarrhythmias

diuretics (potassium-depleting): Increased risk of torsades de pointes in patients with hypokalemia or hypomagnesemia

hydrochlorothiazide, verapamil: Possibly increased blood dofetilide level and increased risk of torsades de pointes

FOODS
grapefruit juice: Increased dofetilide level

Adverse Reactions
CNS: Cerebral ischemia, CVA, dizziness, facial or flaccid paralysis, headache, insomnia, paresthesia, slurred speech, syncope
CV: AV block, bradycardia, cardiac arrest, chest pain, edema, MI, tachycardia,

ventricular arrhythmias (including torsades de pointes and ventricular tachycardia)
GI: Abdominal pain, diarrhea, **hepatic dysfunction**, jaundice, nausea
MS: Back pain, muscle weakness
RESP: Cough, dyspnea, respiratory tract infection
SKIN: Rash
Other: Angioedema, flu-like symptoms, weight gain

≣ Childbearing Considerations

PREGNANCY
- It is not known if drug causes fetal harm.
- Use with caution only if benefit to mother outweighs potential risk to fetus.

LACTATION
- It is not known if drug is present in breast milk.
- A decision should be made to discontinue breastfeeding during drug therapy.

≣ Nursing Considerations

! WARNING Be aware that dofetilide shouldn't be started if patient has previously received amiodarone until blood amiodarone level is less than 0.3 mcg/ml or until amiodarone has been withdrawn for at least 3 months.

- Evaluate and document QTc interval before and during dofetilide therapy.
- Place patient on continuous ECG monitoring for at least 3 days, as ordered, during dofetilide therapy.

! WARNING Know that if patient does not convert to normal sinus rhythm within 24 hours of starting dofetilide, expect possible synchronized electrical cardioversion.

- Be prepared to reevaluate renal function and QTc interval every 3 months, as ordered, during dofetilide therapy.
- Monitor continuous ECG for at least 30 hours, as ordered when switching to dofetilide from class I or class III antiarrhythmics, or after withdrawing antiarrhythmic treatment.
- Be aware that if patient requires a drug that may interact with dofetilide, expect to discontinue dofetilide, as prescribed, for 2 or more days before starting the other drug.

! WARNING Monitor laboratory test results for hypokalemia or hypomagnesemia, especially in patients taking diuretics, because of the increased risk of dofetilide-induced torsades de pointes.

- Monitor women often for adverse reactions, including prolonged QTc interval and torsades de pointes; they have 12% to 18% lower renal clearance of drug than men and therefore a greater risk of adverse reactions.

PATIENT TEACHING
- Advise patient to swallow capsules whole with water and not to chew, crush, or open capsules.
- Instruct patient to avoid drinking grapefruit juice while taking this drug.
- Inform patient that she may be hospitalized for at least 3 days if dofetilide dosage is increased.
- Teach patient to measure blood pressure and pulse rate during dofetilide therapy.
- Urge patient to report chest discomfort, fluttering, or palpitations immediately.
- Tell patient to notify prescriber immediately if she experiences loss of appetite, severe diarrhea, unusual sweating, or vomiting, or if she develops excessive thirst that may occur as a result of certain drug interactions that cause an electrolyte imbalance.
- Advise patient to consult prescriber before using any OTC drugs, nutritional supplements, or herbal products.
- Instruct patient to keep follow-up appointments to monitor heart rhythm.

donepezil hydrochloride
Aricept, Aricept ODT

≣ Class and Category
Pharmacologic class: Acetylcholinesterase inhibitor
Therapeutic class: Antidementia

≣ Indications and Dosages
* *To treat mild to moderate Alzheimer's disease*

ORAL SOLUTION, ORALLY DISINTEGRATING TABLETS, TABLETS

Adults. *Initial:* 5 mg once daily. After 4 to 6 wk, dosage increased to 10 mg once daily, as indicated. *Maximum:* 10 mg daily.

✱ *To treat moderate to severe Alzheimer's disease*

ORAL SOLUTION, ORALLY DISINTEGRATING TABLETS, TABLETS

Adults. *Initial:* 5 mg once daily. After 4 to 6 wk, dosage increased to 10 mg once daily, as indicated. Dosage may be further increased, as needed, after 3 months to 23 mg daily if not using oral solution or orally disintegrating tablet form. *Maximum:* 10 mg daily for oral solution and orally disintegrating tablets, 23 mg daily for tablets.

Drug Administration

P.O.

- Administer the once-daily dose at bedtime.
- Immediate-release tablet should not be chewed, crushed, or split.
- When administering oral disintegrating tablets, tell patient not to swallow the tablet whole but to allow it to dissolve on the tongue and follow with a drink of water.
- Use a calibrated device when measuring oral solution dosage. Each 5 ml equals a 5-mg dose.

Route	Onset	Peak	Duration
P.O.	Unknown	3–4 hr	Unknown

Half-life: 70 hr

Mechanism of Action

Reversibly inhibits acetylcholinesterase and improves acetylcholine's concentration at cholinergic synapses. Raising acetylcholine level in the cerebral cortex may improve cognition. Donepezil becomes less effective as Alzheimer's disease progresses and number of intact cholinergic neurons declines.

Contraindications

Hypersensitivity to donepezil, piperidine derivatives, or their components

Interactions

DRUGS

anticholinergics: Possibly interference with activity of these drugs

cholinergic agonists, succinylcholine and similar neuromuscular blockers: Possibly synergistic effects of these drugs

Adverse Reactions

CNS: Abnormal gait, agitation, aggression, anxiety, asthenia, confusion, depression, dizziness, dream disturbances, fatigue, fever, hallucinations, headache, hostility, insomnia, nervousness, **neuroleptic malignant syndrome, seizures,** somnolence, syncope, tremor

CV: **Abnormal ECG, AV block, bradycardia,** chest pain, edema, **heart failure,** hypertension, **hypotension, prolonged QT interval, torsades de pointes**

EENT: Pharyngitis

ENDO: Hyperglycemia

GI: Abdominal pain, anorexia, cholecystitis, constipation, diarrhea, dyspepsia, fecal incontinence, gastroenteritis, **hepatitis,** nausea, **pancreatitis,** vomiting

GU: Cystitis, glycosuria, hematuria, urinary frequency or incontinence, UTI

HEME: Anemia, **hemolytic hemorrhage**

MS: Arthralgia, back pain, elevated creatine kinase level, muscle cramps or spasms, **rhabdomyolysis**

RESP: Bronchitis, increased cough, pneumonia

SKIN: Ecchymosis, eczema, pruritus, rash, ulceration

Other: Angioedema, dehydration, elevated alkaline phosphatase or lactate dehydrogenase level, flu-like syndrome, hyponatremia, weight loss

Childbearing Considerations

PREGNANCY

- It is not known if drug causes fetal harm.
- Use with caution only if benefit to mother outweighs potential risk to fetus.

LACTATION

- It is not known if drug is present in breast milk.
- Patient should check with prescriber before breastfeeding.

Nursing Considerations

- Use donepezil cautiously in patients with bladder obstruction because drug's weak peripheral cholinergic effect could obstruct outflow.
- Use drug cautiously in patients with asthma, COPD, or other pulmonary

disorders because it has weak affinity for peripheral cholinesterase, which may increase bronchoconstriction and bronchial secretions.

- Know that if patient has cardiac disease, monitor heart rate and rhythm for bradycardia, which may result from increased vagal tone caused by drug's inhibition of peripheral cholinesterase. Reduced heart rate may be especially significant if patient has bradycardia, sick sinus syndrome, or other supraventricular arrhythmia.
- Take safety precautions if patient is dizzy or has other adverse CNS reactions.

PATIENT TEACHING

- Advise patient to take donepezil only once per day just before going to bed.
- Inform her that drug may be taken with or without food.
- Tell patient prescribed oral disintegrating tablets not to swallow the tablet whole but to allow it to dissolve on the tongue and follow with a drink of water.
- Instruct patient to avoid hazardous activities, such as driving, until drug's CNS effects are known. Urge her to take safety precautions to prevent falling if she has adverse reactions, such as dizziness.
- Tell patient who has a history of gastric irritation or peptic ulcer disease that drug may aggravate these conditions by increasing gastric acid secretion.
- Alert patient that drug may cause decreased appetite, diarrhea, fatigue, insomnia, muscle cramps or spasms, nausea, or vomiting as some of the adverse reactions associated with drug use. Tell patient to notify prescriber if signs or symptoms are bothersome, persistent, or severe.

dopamine hydrochloride

Class and Category

Pharmacologic class: Adrenergic
Therapeutic class: Vasopressor

Indications and Dosages

∗ *To correct hypotension due to inadequate cardiac output; to correct hemodynamic imbalances present in shock syndrome due to chronic cardiac decompensation, endotoxic septicemia, MI, open-heart surgery, renal failure, or trauma*

I.V. INFUSION

Adults. *Initial:* 2 to 5 mcg/kg/min, increased gradually in increments of 5 to 10 mcg/kg/min, as needed. *Usual:* Less than 20 mcg/kg/min.

Adults who are more seriously ill. *Initial:* 5 mcg/kg/min, increased gradually by 5 to 10 mcg/kg/min up to a rate of 20 to 50 mcg/kg/min, as needed. *Maximum:* 50 mcg/kg/min

±**DOSAGE ADJUSTMENT** Initial dosage reduced to 10% of usual amount if patient has taken MAO inhibitor in previous 2 to 3 wk.

Drug Administration

I.V.

- Ensure adequate fluid resuscitation before giving drug.
- When using the single-dose plastic containers, the solution does not have to be diluted further. Be aware that the overwrap is a moisture and oxygen barrier. Do not remove unit from overwrap until ready for use. Be aware that a sulfur dioxide odor may occur upon removal of drug from the overwrap Viaflex container. This does not pose a risk to the patient.
- Visually inspect the container. If the administration port protector is damaged, detached, or not present, discard container, because solution's sterility may be impaired. Solution should be slightly yellow in color. If darker or discolored, discard container.
- Dilute concentrate with a compatible I.V. solution before administering, such as 0.9% Sodium Chloride Injection or 5% Dextrose Injection (see manufacturer guidelines for other suitable solutions). Using a 250-ml diluting solution, add 5 ml of drug (40 mg/ml) to obtain a concentration of 800 mcg/ml or 10 ml of drug to obtain a concentration of 1,600 mcg/ml; using a 500-ml solution, add 5 ml of drug (40 mg/ml) to obtain a concentration of 400 mcg/ml or 10 ml of drug to obtain a concentration of 800 mcg/ml; and using a 1,000-ml solution, add 5 ml of drug (40 mg/ml) to obtain a concentration of

200 mcg/ml or 10 ml of drug to obtain a concentration of 400 mcg/ml.

- Give drug by I.V. infusion using a precision volume control infusion set and an infusion pump. When infusion rate exceeds 20 mcg/kg/min, monitor patient for excessive vasoconstriction and loss of renal vasodilating effects.
- Administer infusion through a central catheter to avoid extravasation and tissue necrosis. If drug must be given via peripheral line, administer through a large vein and inspect site often for signs of extravasation and necrosis. If such signs are detected, start a new I.V. line for infusion, discontinue previous I.V. line, and notify prescriber immediately.
- Titrate dopamine gradually to minimize hypotension, especially after a high infusion rate.
- Never administer as an I.V. bolus.
- Discard diluted solution after 24 hours.
- *Incompatibilities:* Alkaline solutions such as sodium bicarbonate, blood products, iron salts, other drugs mixed in same solution

Route	Onset	Peak	Duration
I.V.	>5 min	Unknown	Up to 10 min

Half-life: 2 min

Mechanism of Action

Stimulates dopamine$_1$ (D$_1$) and dopamine$_2$ (D$_2$) postsynaptic receptors. D$_1$ receptors causing vasodilation in cerebral, coronary, mesenteric, and renal blood vessels. D$_2$ receptors inhibit norepinephrine release. In higher doses, dopamine also stimulates alpha$_1$ and alpha$_2$ receptors, causing vascular smooth-muscle contraction.

It also causes increased renal blood flow, improved GFR, and increased urine output. At doses of 2 to 10 mcg/kg/min, dopamine stimulates beta$_1$-adrenergic receptors, increasing cardiac output while maintaining dopaminergic-induced vasodilation. At doses of 10 mcg/kg/min or more, alpha-adrenergic agonism takes over, causing increased peripheral vascular resistance and renal vasoconstriction.

Contraindications

Hypersensitivity to dopamine or its components, pheochromocytoma,

uncorrected ventricular fibrillation, ventricular tachycardia, and other tachyarrhythmias

Interactions

DRUGS

alpha blockers: Antagonized peripheral vasoconstriction with high doses of dopamine

beta blockers: Antagonized beta receptor–mediated inotropic effects of dopamine

cyclopropane, halogenated hydrocarbon anesthetics: Increased cardiac autonomic irritability with possible increased risk of hypertension and ventricular arrhythmias

diuretics: Possibly increased diuretic effects of dopamine or diuretic

haloperidol: Suppression of dopaminergic mesenteric vasodilation occurs with low rates of dopamine infusion

MAO inhibitors: Prolonged and intensified cardiac stimulation and vasopressor effect

oxytocic drugs, other vasopressors, vasoconstricting agents: Possibly severe persistent hypertension

phenytoin: Possibly sudden bradycardia and hypotension

tricyclic antidepressants: Possibly potentiated pressor response to dopamine

Adverse Reactions

CNS: Anxiety, headache

CV: Angina, **atrial fibrillation, bradycardia, cardiac conduction abnormalities, ectopic beats,** hypertension, **hypotension,** palpitations, peripheral vasoconstriction, sinus tachycardia, **ventricular arrhythmias, widened QRS complex**

GI: Nausea, vomiting

GU: Azotemia

RESP: Dyspnea

SKIN: Extravasation with tissue necrosis, piloerection

Childbearing Considerations

PREGNANCY

- It is not known if drug causes fetal harm.
- Use with caution only if benefit to mother outweighs potential risk to fetus.

LABOR & DELIVERY

- Be aware that if a vasopressor drug such as dopamine is given during labor and delivery, an interaction with some oxytocic drugs may result in severe hypertension.

LACTATION
- It is not known if drug is present in breast milk.
- Due to critical nature of situation, breastfeeding would not be done during drug therapy. Patient should check with prescriber about breastfeeding once condition is stable.

Nursing Considerations
- Avoid, if possible, giving dopamine to patients with occlusive vascular disease, such as atherosclerosis, Buerger's disease, diabetic endarteritis, or Raynaud's disease, because of risk of decreased peripheral circulation. Also, be aware that high doses of dopamine given for a prolonged period of time increase the risk of decreased peripheral circulation and could lead to gangrene in the patient's extremities.
- Use drug cautiously in patients with cardiac disease, particularly coronary artery disease, because dopamine increases myocardial oxygen demand. Also use drug cautiously in patients allergic to sulfites, which are contained in some forms of dopamine.
- Monitor blood pressure continuously with an intra-arterial line, as indicated.
- Place patient on continuous ECG monitoring, and assess heart rate and rhythm for arrhythmias.
- Monitor patient's hemodynamic parameters, such as cardiac output, central venous pressure, and pulmonary artery wedge pressure, as indicated, to assess effectiveness of dopamine therapy.
- Monitor urine output hourly as appropriate to assess patient for improved renal blood flow.

PATIENT TEACHING
- Explain the need for frequent hemodynamic monitoring.

doravirine
Pifeltro

Class and Category
Pharmacologic class: Non-nucleoside reverse transcriptase inhibitor (NRTI)
Therapeutic class: Antiretroviral

Indications and Dosages
* *As adjunct to treat human immunodeficiency virus (HIV-1) infection in patients with no prior antiretroviral treatment history; to replace the current antiretroviral regimen in patients who are virologically suppressed (HIV-1 RNA less than 50 copies/ml) on a stable antiretroviral regimen with no history of treatment failure and no known substitutions associated with resistance to doravirine*

TABLETS
Adults and children weighing at least 35 kg (77 lb). 100 mg once daily.
±**DOSAGE ADJUSTMENT** For patient taking rifabutin concomitantly, dosage increased to 100 mg twice daily and given about 12 hours apart.

Drug Administration
P.O.
- Keep bottle tightly closed and do not remove the desiccant.
- Administer at about the same time every day.

Route	Onset	Peak	Duration
P.O.	Unknown	2 hr	Unknown

Half-life: 15 hr

Mechanism of Action
Inhibits HIV-1 replication by noncompetitive inhibition of HIV-1 reverse transcriptase.

Contraindications
Coadministration with carbamazepine, enzalutamide, mitotane, oxcarbazepine, phenobarbital, phenytoin, rifampin, rifapentine, or St. John's wort; hypersensitivity to doravirine or its components

Interactions
DRUGS
CYP3A inducers such as carbamazepine, efavirenz, etravirine, enzalutamide, mitotane, nevirapine, oxcarbazepine, phenobarbital, phenytoin, rifabutin, rifampin, rifapentine, St. John's wort: Decreased concentration of doravirine with decreased effectiveness
CYP3A inhibitors: Possibly increased concentration of doravirine, increasing risk of adverse reactions

Adverse Reactions
CNS: Abnormal dreams, depression, dizziness, fatigue, headache, insomnia, somnolence, **suicidal ideation**

CV: Elevated lipid levels
GI: Abdominal pain, diarrhea, elevated lipase and liver enzymes, nausea
GU: Elevated bilirubin and creatinine levels
MS: Elevated creatine kinase level
SKIN: Rash
Other: Elevated alkaline phosphatase, immune reconstitution syndrome

Childbearing Considerations
PREGNANCY
- Pregnancy exposure registry: 1-800-258- 4263.
- It is not known if drug causes fetal harm.
- Use with caution only if benefit to mother outweighs potential risk to fetus.

LACTATION
- It is not known if drug is present in breast milk.
- The Centers for Disease Control and Prevention recommends that HIV-1 infected mothers not breastfeed to avoid risking postnatal transmission of HIV-1 infection to infants. They also do not recommend breastfeeding because of potential drug-induced adverse reactions in the infant.

Nursing Considerations
- Obtain cholesterol and triglyceride levels before doravirine therapy is begun and periodically throughout therapy, because drug may cause an increase in lipid levels.
- Monitor patient's mood and emotional status, as doravirine may cause significant depression, mood changes, and suicidal ideation. Report any changes to prescriber.
- Be aware that immune reconstitution syndrome has occurred in patients treated with combination antiretroviral therapy, including doravirine. The inflammatory response predisposes susceptible patients to opportunistic infections such as cytomegalovirus, *Mycobacterium avium* infection, *Pneumocystis jiroveci* pneumonia, or tuberculosis. Autoimmune disorders such as Graves' disease, Guillain–Barré syndrome, or polymyositis have also occurred. Report sudden or unusual adverse reactions to prescriber.

PATIENT TEACHING
- Advise patient to avoid missing doses of doravirine. If she misses a dose, she should take it as soon as she remembers, but should not double the next dose or take more than prescribed.
- Instruct patient to alert prescriber of all medications taken, including over-the-counter products and any newly prescribed medication from other prescribers.
- Encourage women of childbearing age to report known or suspected pregnancy.
- Alert mothers that breastfeeding is not recommended during doravirine therapy.
- Instruct patient to report any persistent, severe, or unusual signs and symptoms.
- Tell patient or caregiver to report any signs of depression, mood changes, sleep disorders, or suicidal thoughts to prescriber.

doxazosin mesylate
Cardura, Cardura XL

Class and Category
Pharmacologic class: Alpha blocker
Therapeutic class: Antihypertensive, benign prostatic hyperplasia therapeutic agent

Indications and Dosages
✳ *To manage hypertension*
TABLETS
Adults. *Initial:* 1 mg once daily titrated upward by doubling dose each time to maximum dosage to achieve desired blood pressure, as needed. *Maximum:* 16 mg daily.

✳ *To treat benign prostatic hyperplasia (BPH)*
TABLETS
Adults. *Initial:* 1 mg once daily. Doubled every 1 to 2 wk, if needed, based on signs and symptoms. *Maximum:* 8 mg daily

E.R. TABLETS
Adults. *Initial:* 4 mg once daily, increased to 8 mg after 3 to 4 wk, as needed.

Drug Administration
P.O.
- Tablets should be swallowed whole and not chewed, crushed, or split.
- Immediate-release tablets to treat BPH can be given in the morning or evening; extended-release tablets should be given with breakfast.

D

- If therapy is interrupted for either indication for more than several days, dosage should be restarted at 4 mg once daily.

Route	Onset	Peak	Duration
P.O.	1–2 hr	2–3 hr	24 hr

Half-life: 15–22 hr

Mechanism of Action

Competitively inhibits alpha$_1$-adrenergic receptors in the sympathetic nervous system, causing peripheral vasodilation and reduced peripheral vascular resistance. This action decreases blood pressure, especially when the patient stands. Doxazosin also relaxes smooth muscle of the bladder neck, prostate, and prostate capsule, which reduces urethral resistance and pressure and urinary outflow resistance.

Contraindications

Hypersensitivity to doxazosin, other quinazolines such as prazosin or terazosin, or their components

Interactions

DRUGS

diuretics, phosphodiesterase-5 inhibitors, other antihypertensives, strong CYP3A4 inhibitors: Enhanced hypotensive effects

Adverse Reactions

CNS: Dizziness, drowsiness, headache, nervousness, restlessness, vertigo
CV: Arrhythmias, first-dose orthostatic hypotension, palpitations, peripheral edema, sinus tachycardia
EENT: Intraoperative floppy iris syndrome, rhinitis
GI: GI obstruction, nausea
GU: Priapism
RESP: Dyspnea

Childbearing Considerations

PREGNANCY

- It is not known if drug causes fetal harm.
- Use with caution for treatment of hypertension only if benefit to mother outweighs potential risk to fetus.

LACTATION

- Drug may be present in breast milk.
- Patient should check with prescriber before breastfeeding if prescribed for hypertension.

Drug used to treat benign prostatic hypertrophy is not used for women.

Nursing Considerations

- Know that drug should not be given to hypotensive patients.
- Be aware that Cardura XL is not for use in female patients and is not to be used to treat hypertension.
- Use doxazosin cautiously in patients with hepatic disease (because normal dosage may cause exaggerated effects) and in elderly patients (because hypotensive response may be more pronounced).

! WARNING Monitor patient for orthostatic hypotension (which may cause syncope) early in therapy, especially after exercise and in patients with hypovolemia.

- Monitor blood pressure for 2 to 6 hours after first dose and with each increase because orthostatic hypotension commonly occurs at this time. Adjust dose as prescribed, based on standing blood pressure.
- Carefully monitor patients with renal disease for exaggerated effects, such as first-dose orthostatic hypotension.
- Monitor urination, checking for difficulty urinating and urine retention, to assess drug's effects on BPH.

PATIENT TEACHING

- Inform patient prescribed drug to treat BPH that he may take immediate-release tablets in the morning or evening but extended-release tablets should be taken with breakfast. Tablets should be swallowed whole and not chewed, crushed, or split.
- Instruct patient to change position slowly to minimize orthostatic hypotension.
- Advise patient to avoid exercising, going outside in hot weather, standing for long periods, and using alcohol; these activities may worsen orthostatic hypotension.
- Advise patient to avoid hazardous activities until drug's CNS effects are known.
- Tell patient to inform surgeon that he is taking doxazosin therapy if cataract surgery is required because drug may cause intraoperative floppy iris syndrome with this procedure.
- Inform the patient taking drug for benign prostatic hyperplasia that he may become dizzy or faint if he takes an oral erectile

dysfunction medicine during doxazosin therapy. Therefore, he should not use an oral erectile dysfunction medicine until he has discussed its use with the prescriber. Also alert him to the rare possibility of developing a painful penile erection caused by doxazosin therapy that could last for hours and require immediate medical attention, if it occurs.

doxepin hydrochloride
Silenor

Class and Category
Pharmacologic class: Tricyclic antidepressant
Therapeutic class: Antidepressant

Indications and Dosages
* To treat very mild depression or anxiety accompanying organic disease

CAPSULES, ORAL SOLUTION
Adults. 25 to 50 mg once daily (may be given at bedtime) or in divided doses. *Maximum:* 150 mg daily.
* To treat mild to moderate depression or anxiety

CAPSULES, ORAL SOLUTION
Adults. 75 to 150 mg once daily or in divided doses. *Maximum:* 150 mg daily.
* To treat severe depression or anxiety

CAPSULES, ORAL SOLUTION
Adults. 50 mg three times daily, gradually increased to 300 mg daily, as needed. *Maximum:* 300 mg daily.
* To treat insomnia characterized by difficulty with sleep maintenance

TABLET (SILENOR)
Adults. 3 to 6 mg. *Maximum:* 6 mg daily.
±**DOSAGE ADJUSTMENT** For elderly patients age 65 and over taking Silenor, dosage reduced to 3 mg within 30 min of bedtime but may be increased to 6 mg daily, as needed.

Drug Administration
P.O.
- When used to treat insomnia, administer within 30 minutes of bedtime.
- When used to treat anxiety or depression, once-daily dose is administered at bedtime

because drug may cause dizziness and drowsiness.
- Mix oral solution in 120 ml of juice such as grapefruit, orange, pineapple, or tomato; milk; or water, if desired.

Route	Onset	Peak	Duration
P.O.	2–3 hr	3.5 hr	Unknown

Half-life: 15 hr

Mechanism of Action
May block norepinephrine and serotonin reuptake by adrenergic nerves. In this way, the tricyclic antidepressant raises norepinephrine and serotonin levels at nerve synapses, which may elevate mood and reduce depression. It is unknown how doxepin maintains sleep, but is thought to be due to its antagonism of the H1 receptor.

Contraindications
Hypersensitivity to doxepin, other tricyclic antidepressants, or their components; severe urinary retention; untreated narrow-angle glaucoma; use of MAO inhibitor within 14 days

Interactions
DRUGS
cimetidine, flecainide, other tricyclic antidepressants, phenothiazines, propafenone, quinidine, selective serotonin reuptake inhibitors: Increased blood doxepin level from inhibited systemic clearance, resulting in increased risk of toxicity
CNS depressants, sedating antihistamines: Possibly potentiated CNS depression, hypotension, and respiratory depression
MAO inhibitors: Possibly hyperpyrexia, hypertension, seizures, and death
tolazamide: Possibly severe hypoglycemia

ACTIVITIES
alcohol use: Possibly enhanced CNS depression, hypotension, and respiratory depression

Adverse Reactions
CNS: Confusion, delirium, dream disturbances, drowsiness, fatigue, hallucinations, headache, nervousness, Parkinsonism, restlessness, sedation, **seizures, suicidal ideation (especially teens),** tremor
CV: **ECG changes,** orthostatic hypotension, palpitations

EENT: Blurred vision, dry mouth, taste perversion
ENDO: Hyperglycemia, **hypoglycemia**
GI: Constipation, diarrhea, heartburn, ileus, increased appetite, jaundice, nausea, vomiting,
GU: Decreased libido, ejaculation disorders
SKIN: Diaphoresis
Other: Weight gain

Childbearing Considerations

PREGNANCY
- It is not known if drug causes fetal harm.
- Use with caution only if benefit to mother outweighs potential risk to fetus.

LACTATION
- Drug is present in breast milk.
- Drug use is not recommended during breastfeeding as it may cause apnea, drowsiness, and hypotonia in the breastfed infant.

REPRODUCTION
- Drug may reduce fertility and it is not known if this effect is reversible.

Nursing Considerations
- Expect to observe adverse reactions within a few hours after giving drug.
- Evaluate patient for therapeutic response, such as decreased anxiety, apprehension, depression, fear, guilt, somatic symptoms, and worry; increased energy; and more restful sleep.

! **WARNING** Monitor patients, especially young adults, closely for evidence of suicidal thinking and behavior because doxepin increases the risk in this group of suicidal thinking.

- Keep in mind that abrupt withdrawal of doxepin after prolonged therapy can cause cholinergic rebound effects, including diarrhea, nausea, and vomiting.
- Plan to discontinue drug, as prescribed, several days before elective surgery to avoid hypertension.
- Monitor elderly patients for Parkinsonism, especially with high-dose therapy.
- Be alert for seizures. Patients with seizure disorder may need increased anticonvulsant dosage to maintain seizure control.
- Know that for patients with asthma or sulfite sensitivity, doxepin tablets may aggravate asthma or cause allergic reactions because they contain sulfites.
- Follow diabetic patient's serum glucose level closely; drug may alter glucose metabolism.

PATIENT TEACHING
- Instruct patient taking drug to treat mild to moderate anxiety or depression that he may divide the daily dose or take it once daily, which could be at bedtime.
- Tell patient taking drug for insomnia to take it within 30 minutes of bedtime.
- Tell patient to mix oral solution in 120 ml of juice such as grapefruit, orange, pineapple, or tomato; milk; or water, if desired.

! **WARNING** Alert parents of young adults to watch them closely for abnormal thinking or behavior and increased aggression or hostility. Emphasize importance of notifying prescriber about unusual changes.

- Instruct patient to avoid alcohol during doxepin therapy because mental alertness may decrease.
- Advise diabetic patient to measure serum glucose level more often than usual.

doxycycline
Oracea

doxycycline calcium
Vibramycin

doxycycline hyclate
Acticlate, Acticlate CAP, Alti-Doxycycline (CAN), Atridox, Doryx, Doryx MPC, Doxycin (CAN), Morgidox, Vibramycin

doxycycline monohydrate
Monodox, Vibramycin

Class and Category
Pharmacologic class: Tetracycline
Therapeutic class: Antibiotic
✳ *To treat inhalation anthrax post exposure*

CAPSULES, DELAYED-RELEASE TABLETS, ORAL SUSPENSION, SYRUP, TABLETS
Adults and children age 8 and over weighing 45 kg (99 lb) or more. 100 mg (120 mg Doryx MPC) twice daily for 60 days. **Children age 8 and over weighing less than 45 kg (99 lb).** 2.2 mg/kg (2.6 mg/kg Doryx MPC) twice daily for 60 days.
* *To treat inflammatory lesions (papules and pustules) of rosacea*
E.R. CAPSULES (ORACEA)
Adults. 40 mg once daily in the morning on an empty stomach.
* *To treat endocervical, rectal, and urethral infections caused by* Chlamydia trachomatis
CAPSULES, DELAYED-RELEASE TABLETS, ORAL SUSPENSION, SYRUP, TABLETS
Adults. 100 mg (120 mg Doryx MPC) twice daily for 7 days.
* *To treat uncomplicated gonococcal infections except anorectal infections in men*
CAPSULES, DELAYED-RELEASE TABLETS, ORAL SUSPENSION, SYRUP, TABLETS
Adults. 100 mg (120 mg Doryx MPC) twice a day for 7 days. Alternatively, 300 mg (360 mg Doryx MPC) followed in 1 hr by a second 300 mg (360 mg Doryx MPC) dose.
* *To treat epididymo orchitis caused by* C. trachomatis *or* Neisseria gonorrhoeae
CAPSULES, DELAYED-RELEASE TABLETS, ORAL SUSPENSION, SYRUP, TABLETS
Adults. 100 mg (120 mg Doryx MPC) twice daily for at least 10 days.
* *To prevent malaria*
CAPSULES, DELAYED-RELEASE TABLETS, ORAL SUSPENSION, SYRUP, TABLETS
Adults. 100 mg (120 mg Doryx MPC) daily starting 1 to 2 days before travel, continued daily during travel, and then daily for 4 wk after travel ends. **Children over age 8.** 2 mg/kg (2.4 mg/kg Doryx MPC) daily starting 1 to 2 days before travel, continued daily during travel, and daily for 4 wk after travel ends.
* *To treat early syphilis in penicillin-allergic patients*
CAPSULES, DELAYED-RELEASE TABLETS, ORAL SUSPENSION, SYRUP, TABLETS
Adults. 100 mg (120 mg Doryx MPC) twice daily for 2 wk.
* *To treat syphilis of more than 1 year duration in penicillin-allergic patients*

CAPSULES, DELAYED-RELEASE TABLETS, ORAL SUSPENSION, SYRUP, TABLETS
Adults. 100 mg (120 mg Doryx MPC) twice daily for 4 wk.
* *To treat all other infections caused by susceptible organisms*
CAPSULES, DELAYED-RELEASE TABLETS, ORAL SUSPENSION, SYRUP, TABLETS
Adults and children over age 8 weighing 45 kg (99 lb) or more. 100 mg (120 mg Doryx MPC) every 12 hr on day 1 and then 100 mg (120 mg Doryx MPC) once daily or 50 mg twice daily. For severe infections, 100 mg continued every 12 hr.
Children over age 8 weighing less than 45 kg (99 lb). 2.2 mg/kg (2.6 mg/kg Doryx MPC) twice daily on day 1 and then 2.2 mg/kg (2.6 mg/kg Doryx MPC) once daily or 1.1 to 2.2 mg/kg (1.3 mg/kg Doryx MPC) twice daily.
I.V. INFUSION
Adults and children over age 8 weighing more than 45 kg. 200 mg once daily or 100 mg every 12 hr on day 1 and then 100 to 200 mg once daily or 50 to 100 mg every 12 hr.
Children over age 8 weighing 45 kg (99 lb) or less. *For severe or life-threatening infections:* 2.2 mg/kg every 12 hr. *For less severe infections:* 4.4 mg/kg divided into two doses on day 1 and then 2.2 to 4.4 mg/kg once daily or 1.1 to 2.2 mg/kg every 12 hr.

Drug Administration
P.O.
- Doryx and Doryx MPC are not interchangeable. Doryx 100 mg equals 120 mg of Doryx MPC. Also Doryx MPC cannot be interchanged with other oral doxycyclines on a milligram-per-milligram basis.
- Shake oral liquid container before measuring dose. Use a calibrated device when measuring dosage of oral suspension or syrup.
- Give Oracea 1 hour before or 2 hours after morning meal with a full glass of water. Other products can be taken with food or milk if GI upset occurs.
- Do not administer drug within 1 hour of bedtime because of possible esophageal irritation or ulceration.
- D.R. capsules can be opened and D.R. tablets broken (not crushed) and sprinkled

over cold, soft applesauce followed by a cool glass of water. Do not store mixture. Mixture should not be chewed but swallowed.

- Immediate-release capsules and tablets should be swallowed whole followed by a glass of water. However, for emergency administration of doxycycline hyclate for patients unable to swallow pills, do the following. Take one tablet and put in 4 ounces of water. Soak at least 10 minutes. Crush tablet with back of spoon. Stir. Then measure dose with a calibrated device and squirt it in another container. Mix with 3 teaspoons of milk, formula, chocolate milk, or apple juice that has had 2 to 4 teaspoons of sugar added to it (or add to chocolate pudding). Mix well and administer immediately.

I.V.

- Never administer drug I.M. or subcutaneously.
- Reconstitute with Sterile Water for Injection (see manufacturer guidelines for other suitable solutions) using 10 ml for a 100-mg vial or 20 ml for a 200-mg vial.
- Further dilute (see manufacturer guidelines for suitable diluents) as follows: Dilute 100 mg of drug with 100 to 1,000 ml of solution; 200 mg of drug with 200 to 2,000 ml of solution. This will result in a concentration of 0.1 to 1.0 mg/ml. Concentrations lower than 0.1 mg/ml or higher than 1.0 mg/ml should not be used.
- Don't expose diluted solution to light. Protect it from direct sunlight during infusion.
- Infusion time varies with dose prescribed, but most range from 1 to 4 hours. Do not infuse rapidly. Storage times also vary depending on solution used for dilution.
- *Incompatibilities:* Allopurinol, drugs that are unstable in an acidic solution, erythromycin lactobionate, heparin, meropenem, nafcillin, penicillin G potassium, piperacillin-tazobactam, riboflavin, sulfonamides

Route	Onset	Peak	Duration
P.O.	Unknown	1.5–4 hr	Unknown
P.O./D.R.	Unknown	2–4 hr	Unknown
I.V.	Immediate	Unknown	Unknown

Half-life: 18–22 hr

Mechanism of Action

Exerts a bacteriostatic effect against a wide variety of gram-positive and gram-negative organisms. Doxycycline is more lipophilic than other tetracyclines, which allows it to pass more easily through the bacterial lipid bilayer, where it binds reversibly to 30S ribosomal subunits. Bound doxycycline blocks the binding of aminoacyl transfer RNA to messenger RNA, thus inhibiting bacterial protein synthesis.

Contraindications

Hypersensitivity to doxycycline, other tetracyclines, or their components

Interactions

DRUGS

antacids that contain aluminum, calcium, magnesium, or zinc; calcium supplements; choline and magnesium salicylates; iron-containing preparations, laxatives that contain magnesium: Decreased doxycycline absorption and effects

barbiturates, carbamazepine, phenytoin: Increased clearance and decreased effects of doxycycline

methoxyflurane: Increased risk of severe or fatal renal toxicity

oral anticoagulants: Possibly increased hypoprothrombinemic effects of these drugs

oral contraceptives: Decreased effectiveness of estrogen-containing oral contraceptives, increased risk of breakthrough bleeding

penicillin: Possibly interference with bactericidal action of penicillin

Adverse Reactions

CNS: Headache, **intracranial hypertension,** paresthesia

CV: Pericarditis, phlebitis

EENT: Black "hairy" tongue, glossitis, hoarseness, oral candidiasis, pharyngitis, stomatitis, tooth discoloration, visual disturbances

GI: Anorexia; bulky, loose stools; *Clostridium difficile*–associated diarrhea; diarrhea; dysphagia; enterocolitis; epigastric distress; esophageal ulceration; esophagitis; **hepatotoxicity,** inflammatory lesions in anogenital region; nausea; **pancreatitis; pseudomembranous colitis;** rectal candidiasis; vomiting

GU: Anogenital lesions, dark yellow or brown urine, elevated BUN level, vaginal candidiasis

HEME: Eosinophilia, **hemolytic anemia, neutropenia, thrombocytopenia, thrombocytopenic purpura**
MS: Inhibition of bone growth in infants and children
SKIN: Dermatitis, **erythema multiforme,** erythematous and maculopapular rashes, **exfoliative dermatitis,** photosensitivity, rash, skin hyperpigmentation, **Stevens–Johnson syndrome, toxic epidermal necrolysis,** urticaria
Other: Anaphylaxis, angioedema, drug reaction with eosinophilia and systemic symptoms (DRESS), exacerbation of systemic lupus erythematosus, injection-site phlebitis, Jarisch–Herxheimer (systemic inflammatory response) reaction in presence of spirochete infections, serum sickness

Childbearing Considerations

PREGNANCY

- Drug causes fetal harm, especially retardation of skeleton and permanent discoloration of deciduous teeth if given during second and third trimesters of pregnancy.
- Drug is not recommended for use during pregnancy unless absolutely necessary and there is no alternative drug therapy available.

LACTATION

- Drug is present in breast milk.
- A decision should be made to discontinue breastfeeding or the drug to avoid potential serious adverse reactions in the breastfed infant.

Nursing Considerations

- Avoid giving doxycycline to breastfeeding women because of the risk of enamel hypoplasia, inhibited linear skeletal growth, oral and vaginal candidiasis, photosensitivity reactions, and tooth discoloration in breastfeeding infant.
- Avoid giving drug to children age 8 and under, if possible; it may cause discoloration and enamel hypoplasia of developing teeth that may be permanent.
- Observe patient often for injection-site phlebitis, a common adverse reaction to I.V. administration.
- Monitor liver function test results as appropriate to detect hepatotoxicity.
- Expect doxycycline to increase risk of oral, rectal, or vaginal candidiasis—especially in debilitated or elderly patients and those

on prolonged therapy—by changing the normal balance of microbial flora.

! **WARNING** Monitor patient for signs and symptoms of intracranial hypertension, such as blurred vision, diplopia, headache, and vision loss; papilledema may be seen on fundoscopy. Patients at greater risk include women of childbearing age who are overweight or have a history of intracranial hypertension. If patient complains of visual changes, notify prescriber to obtain an immediate ophthalmologic evaluation because permanent visual loss can occur. Be aware that intracranial pressure may remain elevated for weeks after doxycycline therapy has been discontinued and warrants close follow-up.

- Monitor patient closely for diarrhea, which may indicate pseudomembranous colitis. If diarrhea occurs, notify prescriber and expect to withhold doxycycline. Expect to treat pseudomembranous colitis with electrolytes, fluids, protein, and an antibiotic effective against *Clostridium difficile.*

! **WARNING** Monitor patient for allergic reactions and adverse skin reactions, because doxycycline has caused allergic reactions and severe skin reactions that could be life-threatening. Notify prescriber as soon as possible; if allergic or skin adverse reactions occur, provide supportive care, as ordered, and expect drug to be discontinued.

PATIENT TEACHING

- Instruct patient not to take doxycycline just before bed because it may not dissolve properly when she's recumbent and may cause esophageal burning and ulceration.
- Instruct patient taking doxycycline for rosacea to take the capsule in the morning on an empty stomach with a full glass of water.
- Advise patient to avoid antacids containing aluminum, calcium, or magnesium.
- Instruct patient to drink plenty of fluids while taking doxycycline to reduce the risk of esophageal burning and ulceration.
- Inform patient that her urine may become dark yellow or brown during therapy.
- Urge patient to avoid sun exposure and ultraviolet light as much as possible during therapy and to use sunscreen or sunblock as needed. If patient develops phototoxicity,

such as skin eruption, tell her to stop drug and notify prescriber.

! **WARNING** Tell patient to notify prescriber if allergic or skin adverse reactions occur, because reactions may become severe and drug may have to be discontinued.

- Advise patients who take an oral contraceptive to use an additional contraceptive method during therapy. Also advise all women of childbearing age to notify prescriber immediately if pregnancy occurs or is suspected, as drug may cause retardation of skeletal development in the fetus.
- Know that if patient is being treated for a sexually transmitted disease, her partner may need treatment as well.
- Tell patient to notify prescriber immediately about anorexia, epigastric distress, nausea, or vomiting as well as any visual changes during therapy.
- Urge patient to report bloody, watery stools to prescriber immediately, even up to 2 months after drug therapy has ended.
- Alert female patients that doxycycline may increase risk of vaginal candidiasis. Tell her to notify prescriber if she develops vaginal discharge or itching.
- Inform mothers wishing to breastfeed their infant during doxycycline therapy that it is not recommended because effects are unknown.
- Advise patient prescribed Lymepak to notify prescriber if fever, intensification of skin rash, and shaking chills occurs, a systemic reaction known as Jarisch–Herxheimer reaction. Reassure patient that symptoms usually resolve within several hours with fluid intake and antipyretic treatment.

dronabinol
(delta-9-tetrahydro-cannabinol, THC)
Marinol, Syndros

Class, Category, and Schedule
Pharmacologic class: Cannabinoid
Therapeutic class: Antiemetic, appetite stimulant
Controlled substance schedule: II (Syndros), III (Marinol)

Indications and Dosages

✱ *To prevent nausea and vomiting caused by chemotherapy and unresponsive to other antiemetics*

CAPSULES (MARINOL)
Adults and children. 5 mg/m^2 1 to 3 hr before chemotherapy and then every 2 to 4 hr after chemotherapy for a total of 4 to 6 doses daily, increased by 2.5 mg/m^2 increments, as needed. *Maximum:* 15 mg/m^2/dose for a total of 4 to 6 doses daily.

ORAL SOLUTION (SYNDROS)
Adults. 4.2 mg/m^2 1 to 3 hr before chemotherapy and then every 2 to 4 hr after chemotherapy for a total of 4 to 6 doses daily, increased, as needed, in increments of 2.1 mg/m^2. *Maximum:* 12.6 mg/m^2 per dose for 4 to 6 doses daily.

±**DOSAGE ADJUSTMENT** For elderly patients prescribed Marinol, initial dosage may be reduced to 2.5 mg/m^2 1 to 3 hr before chemotherapy to reduce CNS adverse reactions. For elderly patients prescribed Syndros and all patients who experience persistent or severe adverse reactions, dosage reduced to 2.1 mg/m^2 1 to 3 hr before chemotherapy.

✱ *To stimulate appetite in AIDS patients*

CAPSULES (MARINOL)
Adults. *Initial:* 2.5 mg twice daily 1 hr before lunch and dinner, increased as needed. *Maximum:* 10 mg twice daily.

ORAL SOLUTION (SYNDROS)
Adults. 2.1 mg twice daily 1 hr before lunch and dinner. Increased to 2.1 mg 1 hr before lunch and 4.2 mg 1 hr before dinner, if needed. Then further increased to 4.2 mg 1 hr before lunch and 4.2 mg 1 hr before dinner, if needed. *Maximum:* 8.4 mg twice daily.

±**DOSAGE ADJUSTMENT** Dosage for capsule form (Marinol) reduced to 2.5 mg before dinner or at bedtime for the elderly and patients who can't tolerate 5 mg daily. Dosage maintained for oral solution form (Syndros) at 2.1 mg, but dosage frequency reduced to once daily 1 hr before dinner or bedtime in the elderly and patients who can't tolerate a twice-daily dosage.

Drug Administration
P.O.
- Administer 1 to 3 hours before chemotherapy for the first dose. Although

first dose should be given on an empty stomach at least 30 minutes before patient eats, the remainder of doses can be given without regard to meals. The timing of dosing in relation to meal times should be kept consistent for each chemotherapy cycle.

- Administer 1 hour before lunch and dinner if given to treat anorexia and weight loss in patients with AIDS. Administering drug later in the day may reduce the frequency of CNS adverse reactions.
- Give drug with at least 6 to 8 ounces of water.
- Always use the calibrated oral dosing syringe that comes with drug to measure oral solution doses. If dose is greater than 5 mg, divide the total dose into 2 or more portions using the oral syringe.
- Oral solution may be administered by a feeding tube that is silicone only and equal to or greater than a 14 French. Tubes consisting of polyurethane should not be used. Draw up the prescribed dose of drug using the calibrated dosing syringe packaged with drug. After administering drug via feeding tube, flush feeding tube with 30 ml of water using a catheter-tip syringe.
- Discard after 42 days from opening container or if unused oral solution remains.

Route	Onset	Peak	Duration
P.O.	30–60 min	2–4 hr	6–24 hr

Half-life: 25–36 hr

Mechanism of Action

May exert antiemetic effect by inhibiting the vomiting control mechanism in the medulla oblongata. As the main psychoactive substance in marijuana (*Cannabis sativa* L.), dronabinol's effects may be mediated by cannabinoid receptors in neural tissues.

Contraindications

For Marinol: Hypersensitivity to dronabinol, its components, other cannabinoids, or sesame oil; *For Syndros:* Hypersensitivity reaction to dronabinol, its components, or alcohol; use of disulfiram- or metronidazole-containing products within past 14 days

Interactions

DRUGS

amphotericin B, cyclosporine, warfarin, other drugs highly bound to plasma proteins with a narrow therapeutic index: Possibly increased risk of adverse reactions associated with these drugs
CNS depressants (such as benzodiazepines), sedatives, tricyclic antidepressants: Additive CNS effects
CYP2C9 inhibitors such as amiodarone, CYP2C9 and CYP3A4 inducers: Possibly decreased dronabinol exposure and effectiveness of fluconazole
CYP3A4 inhibitors such as clarithromycin, erythromycin, itraconazole, ketoconazole, ritonavir: Possibly increased dronabinol-related adverse reactions from increased exposure
disulfiram, metronidazole (Syndros only): Possible disulfiram-like reaction

ACTIVITIES

alcohol use: Additive CNS depressant effects

Adverse Reactions

CNS: Altered mental state, amnesia, asthenia, anxiety, ataxia, chills, cognitive impairment, confusion, delirium, delusions, depersonalization, depression, disorientation, dizziness, drowsiness, euphoria, exacerbation of mania or schizophrenia, fatigue, hallucinations, headache, insomnia, irritability, loss of consciousness, malaise, mood changes, movement disorder, nervousness, nightmares, panic attack, paranoid reaction, **seizures**, sleep disturbance, speech difficulties, somnolence, syncope
CV: Orthostatic hypotension, palpitations, sinus tachycardia, vasodilation
EENT: Lip swelling, oral lesions, rhinitis, sinusitis, throat tightness, tinnitus, vision difficulties
GI: Abdominal pain, anorexia, diarrhea, elevated liver enzymes, fecal incontinence, nausea, vomiting
MS: Myalgias
RESP: Cough
SKIN: Diaphoresis, disseminated rash, facial flushing, skin burning, urticaria
Other: Physical and psychological dependence

Childbearing Considerations

PREGNANCY

- Drug may cause fetal harm such as fetal growth restriction, low birth weight, preterm birth, small for gestational age, and stillbirth.

- Drug use should be avoided in pregnant women.

LACTATION

- Drug may be present in breast milk.
- The Centers for Disease Control and Prevention recommends that HIV-1 infected mothers not breastfeed to avoid risking postnatal transmission of HIV-1 infection to infants. They also do not recommend breastfeeding because of potential drug-induced adverse reactions in the infant.
- Mothers receiving drug for treatment of nausea and vomiting related to cancer chemotherapy should not breastfeed during treatment and for 9 days after the last dose.

≣ Nursing Considerations

! **WARNING** Know that dronabinol shouldn't be discontinued abruptly; if it is, withdrawal syndrome may occur.

- Be aware that patients should be screened for depression, mania, and schizophrenia prior to treatment, because dronabinol can exacerbate these conditions. Use with extreme caution, if usage cannot be avoided, in these patients. Monitor patient for new or worsening psychiatric symptoms during therapy. Also know that concomitant use with other drugs associated with similar psychiatric effects should be avoided.
- Be aware that oral solution contains alcohol, which can produce disulfiram-like reactions when co-administered with disulfiram or other drugs that produce this reaction. Know that these products should be discontinued at least 14 days before starting oral solution form of dronabinol and not administered for at least 7 days after therapy with dronabinol has ceased.
- Use cautiously in patients with history of seizures because drug may lower seizure threshold. Notify prescriber of seizures immediately, and expect to stop drug.
- Be aware that patients with a history of substance abuse or dependence are at higher risk for abusing dronabinol. Assess patient's risk for abuse or misuse prior to dronabinol therapy and monitor patient throughout for evidence of abuse or misuse.

- Be aware that patients under age 45 may tolerate drug better than those over age 45.
- Anticipate higher risk of cardiovascular reactions, such as blood pressure changes (especially orthostatic hypotension) and increased heart rate, at higher doses and in patients with cardiac conditions. Monitor patient's vital signs closely, especially when drug is initiated or when dosage is increased.

! **WARNING** Expect tolerance to drug to develop over time, especially if patient has smoked marijuana.

- Be aware that short-term, low-dose therapy doesn't typically lead to physical and psychological dependence, which may occur with long-term, high-dose therapy.
- Alert prescriber if patient experiences changes in mental state or cognitive impairment, because dosage will have to be reduced or drug discontinued. Know that elderly patients may be more sensitive to the neurological and psychoactive effects of dronabinol.
- Expect drug to alter REM sleep pattern, even after therapy stops.
- Be aware that paradoxical abdominal pain, nausea, and vomiting can occur with chronic, long-term use of dronabinol.

PATIENT TEACHING

- Caution patient not to stop drug abruptly because withdrawal symptoms may occur.
- Instruct patient to take dronabinol with a full glass of water (6 to 8 ounces).
- Instruct patient taking oral solution to use only the calibrated syringe that comes with drug to measure dose.
- Tell patient taking drug to prevent nausea and vomiting to take drug 1 to 3 hours before chemotherapy and that first dose should be taken on an empty stomach at least 30 minutes before eating. The same time frame should be followed for each chemotherapy cycle.
- Tell AIDS patient to take drug 1 hour before lunch and dinner.
- Urge patient not to use alcohol while taking dronabinol because it may enhance CNS depression.
- Instruct patient to rise slowly to sitting or standing position to minimize effects of orthostatic hypotension.

- Advise patient to avoid hazardous activities until drug's CNS effects are known.
- Inform patient that sleep pattern may be adversely affected during therapy and for some time afterward.
- Inform women of childbearing age to notify prescriber if pregnancy is known or suspected, because dronabinol may cause fetal harm. Also advise mothers not to breastfeed.
- Monitor elderly patients closely, especially if dementia is present, because they may be more sensitive to the neuropsychiatric and postural hypotensive effects of the drug and be at increased risk of falls.

dronedarone
Multaq

Class and Category
Pharmacologic class: Benzofuran derivative
Therapeutic class: Antiarrhythmic

Indications and Dosages
* *To reduce risk of hospitalization for atrial fibrillation in patients in sinus rhythm with a history of paroxysmal or persistent atrial fibrillation*

TABLETS
Adults. 400 mg twice daily.

Drug Administration
P.O.
- Administer drug with breakfast and dinner.
- Do not administer drug with grapefruit juice.

Route	Onset	Peak	Duration
P.O.	Unknown	3–6 hr	Unknown

Half-life: 13–19 hr

Mechanism of Action
Although specific effect on heart rhythm is unknown, dronedarone possesses properties of all four Vaughn–Williams antiarrhythmic classes.

Contraindications
Bradycardia less than 50 beats/minute; breastfeeding; concurrent use of drugs or herbal products that prolong QT interval, such as class I and III antiarrhythmics, phenothiazine antipsychotics, oral macrolide antibiotics (selected), and tricyclic antidepressants or strong CYP3A inhibitors, such as clarithromycin, cyclosporine, ketoconazole, itraconazole, nefazodone, ritonavir, telithromycin, and voriconazole; hypersensitivity to dronedarone or its components; liver or lung toxicity related to previous use of amiodarone; pregnancy; PR interval greater than 280 msec or QTc Bazett interval of 500 msec or more; permanent atrial fibrillation; second- or third-degree atrioventricular block or sick sinus syndrome (except when used with a functioning pacemaker); severe hepatic impairment (Child–Pugh class C); symptomatic heart failure with recent decompensation requiring hospitalization or NYHA Class IV symptoms

Interactions
DRUGS
beta blockers: Increased risk of bradycardia
calcium channel blockers: Possibly increased dronedarone effects on conduction
calcium channel blockers, such as diltiazem, nifedipine, and verapamil; CYP3A substrates with narrow therapeutic range such as sirolimus and tacrolimus; CYP2D6 substrates, such as beta blockers, selective serotonin reuptake agents, and tricyclic antidepressant; statins, such as simvastatin: Increased effects of these drugs with possibly increased risk of adverse reactions
class I and III antiarrhythmics, macrolide antibiotics, phenothiazines, tricyclic antidepressants: Possibly increased QT interval
CYP3A inducers, such as carbamazepine, phenobarbital, phenytoin, rifampin, St. John's wort: Decreased dronedarone effects
CYP3A inhibitors, such as clarithromycin, cyclosporine, ketoconazole, itraconazole, nefazodone, ritonavir, telithromycin, and voriconazole: Increased dronedarone effects
digoxin and other P-gp substrates such as dabigatran: Increased effect of these drugs with risk of toxicity
warfarin: Possible increased risk of bleeding and INR

FOODS
grapefruit juice: Increased dronedarone effects

Adverse Reactions

CNS: Asthenia
CV: Bradycardia, heart failure, prolonged QT interval, vasculitis
GI: Abdominal pain, diarrhea, dyspepsia, liver injury, nausea, vomiting
GU: Increased serum creatinine levels
RESP: Dyspnea, interstitial lung disease such as pneumonitis and pulmonary fibrosis, nonproductive cough, pulmonary toxicity
SKIN: Allergic dermatitis, dermatitis, eczema, photosensitivity, pruritus, rash
Other: Anaphylaxis, angioedema, hypokalemia, hypomagnesemia

Childbearing Considerations

PREGNANCY

- Drug may cause fetal harm.
- Drug is contraindicated in women who are or who may become pregnant during drug therapy.

LACTATION

- It is not known if drug is present in breast milk.
- A decision should be made to discontinue breastfeeding or the drug to avoid potential serious adverse reactions in the breastfed infant.

REPRODUCTION

- Women of childbearing age should use an effective contraceptive during drug therapy.

Nursing Considerations

- Check that patient has stopped taking any drug contraindicated with dronedarone, as prescribed, before giving first dose. Also check that patient is receiving appropriate antithrombotic therapy prior to giving first dose because patients are at increased risk for stroke, especially in the first 2 weeks of therapy. In addition, check patient's serum potassium and magnesium levels prior to initiating therapy and throughout therapy because of increased risk of deficiency and arrhythmias, especially if patient is also taking a potassium-depleting diuretic.
- Assess patient for evidence of heart failure, such as dependent edema, increasing shortness of breath, or weight gain. If present, notify prescriber; dronedarone may have to be discontinued.

- Review patient's electrocardiogram at least once every 3 months, as ordered to determine patient's rhythm. If atrial fibrillation is found, prepare patient for cardioversion, as ordered or expect dronedarone therapy to be discontinued. Monitor patient's PR and QT interval, as ordered, to see if conduction is delayed. If so, notify prescriber immediately. Dronedarone will have to be stopped.
- Monitor patient's serum creatinine levels, as ordered. Elevation may occur rapidly, plateau after 7 days, and usually is reversible after therapy stops.
- Monitor patient's liver function, as ordered, because severe liver injury may occur with dronedarone therapy. If liver enzymes become elevated or the patient develops symptoms of liver dysfunction such as anorexia, dark urine, fatigue, fever, itching, jaundice, malaise, nausea, right upper quadrant pain, or vomiting, notify prescriber and expect drug to be discontinued immediately.
- Monitor patient for dyspnea or nonproductive cough as possible development of pulmonary toxicity. If confirmed, expect drug to be discontinued.

PATIENT TEACHING

- Inform patient that dronedarone must be taken with breakfast and dinner.
- Warn patient that dronedarone should not be taken with grapefruit juice, nor should grapefruit juice be part of patient's diet during drug therapy.
- Urge patient to contact prescriber if he develops evidence of heart failure, such as dependent edema, increasing shortness of breath or weight gain, because dronedarone may have to be discontinued.
- Inform women of childbearing age of need for contraception if sexually active because drug is contraindicated during pregnancy and breastfeeding. If pregnancy occurs, she should notify prescriber immediately.
- Tell patient to inform all prescribers that she is taking dronedarone and to check with prescriber before taking any herbal product with dronedarone, newly prescribed drug, or OTC product.
- Review symptoms of liver dysfunction with patient and urge her to seek immediate medical attention, if present, and to stop taking dronedarone.

droxidopa
Northera

Class and Category
Pharmacologic class: Norepinephrine prodrug
Therapeutic class: Vasoconstrictor

Indications and Dosages
＊ *To treat symptomatic neurogenic orthostatic hypotension caused by dopamine beta-hydroxylase deficiency, nondiabetic autonomic neuropathy, and primary autonomic failure seen in multiple-system atrophy, Parkinson's disease, and pure autonomic failure*

CAPSULES
Adults. *Initial:* 100 mg three times daily. Dosage then titrated to symptomatic response in increments of 100 mg three times daily every 24 to 48 hr to maximum dosage. *Maximum:* 600 mg three times daily.

Drug Administration
P.O.
- Monitor supine blood pressure before initiating therapy and after dosage increases.
- Administer drug when patient awakes in the morning, at midday, and in late afternoon at least 3 hours before bedtime. Elevate head of bed when giving last dose of the day to reduce potential for supine hypertension during the night.
- Capsule should be swallowed whole and not chewed, crushed, or opened.

Route	Onset	Peak	Duration
P.O.	Unknown	1–4 hr	Unknown

Half-life: 2.5 hr

Mechanism of Action
Produces peripheral arterial and venous vasoconstriction, which increases blood pressure.

Contraindications
Hypersensitivity to droxidopa or its components

Interactions
DRUGS
dopa-decarboxylase inhibitors: Possibly altered plasma droxidopa levels

ephedrine, midodrine, norepinephrine, triptans and other drugs that increase blood pressure: Increased risk of supine hypertension
nonselective MAO inhibitors such as rasagiline, selegiline; linezolid: Possibly increased blood pressure

Adverse Reactions
CNS: Agitation, confusion, **CVA**, delirium, dizziness, fatigue, fever, hallucination, headache, memory disorder, **neuroleptic malignant syndrome-like complex,** psychosis, syncope
CV: Chest pain, **exacerbation of arrhythmias, congestive heart failure, ischemic heart disease,** hypertension, supine hypertension
EENT: Blurred vision
GI: Abdominal pain, diarrhea, nausea, **pancreatitis,** vomiting
GU: UTI
RESP: Bronchospasm
SKIN: Rash, urticaria
Other: Anaphylaxis, **angioedema,** falls

Childbearing Considerations
PREGNANCY
- It is not known if drug causes fetal harm.
- Use with caution only if benefit to mother outweighs potential risk to fetus.

LACTATION
- It is not known if drug is present in breast milk.
- A decision should be made to discontinue breastfeeding or drug therapy.

Nursing Considerations

! WARNING Notify prescriber if supine hypertension occurs and expect dosage to be reduced or drug discontinued, because it can increase the risk of cardiovascular events, especially stroke.

- Know that, although rare, droxidopa may cause a symptom complex resembling neuroleptic malignant syndrome (NMS). Observe patients carefully when dosage is changed or when concomitant levodopa is reduced abruptly or discontinued, especially if patient is receiving neuroleptics. Monitor patient for signs and symptoms such as altered consciousness, fever, hyperthermia, involuntary movements,

D

mental status changes, and muscle rigidity. Notify prescriber immediately; an early diagnosis is important because NMS can be life-threatening.

! WARNING Monitor patient for hypersensitivity reactions that may include anaphylaxis, angioedema, bronchospasm, rash, and urticaria. If present, withhold droxidopa, notify prescriber, provide emergency supportive care as ordered, and expect drug to be discontinued.

- Be aware that droxidopa contains FD&C Yellow No. 5 (tartrazine), which may cause an allergic-type reaction such as bronchial asthma. Risk is higher in patients who also have an aspirin hypersensitivity.

PATIENT TEACHING

- Tell patient to take droxidopa three times a day: upon arising in the morning, at midday, and in the late afternoon at least 3 hours prior to bedtime to reduce the potential for supine hypotension during sleep.
- Instruct patient to swallow capsules whole and not to chew, crush, or open capsule. Advise her that if a dose is missed to wait and take the next scheduled dose. Tell her doses should never be doubled to make up for a missed dose.
- Advise patient to elevate the head of her bed when resting or sleeping to minimize effects of supine hypertension.
- Tell patient to inform prescriber of all new medications, including over-the-counter preparations, prior to taking them.

! WARNING Instruct patient to stop taking droxidopa and seek emergency medical attention if signs and symptoms of an allergic reaction occur, such as difficulty breathing, hives, rash, or swelling.

---

dulaglutide
Trulicity

Class and Category
Pharmacologic class: Glucagon-like peptide-1 receptor agonist
Therapeutic class: Antidiabetic

Indications and Dosages

* *Adjunct to diet and exercise to improve glycemic control in patients with type 2 diabetes mellitus*

SUBCUTANEOUS INJECTION
Adults. 0.75 mg once weekly, increased to 1.5 mg once weekly, as needed. Then, increased to 3 mg once weekly after 4 wk on the 1.5-mg dose, as needed, and then increased to 4.5 mg once weekly after 4 wk on the 3-mg dose, as needed. *Maximum:* 4.5 mg once weekly.

* *To reduce the risk of major cardiovascular events (cardiovascular death, non-fatal MI or CVA) in adults with type 2 diabetes mellitus who have established cardiovascular disease or multiple cardiovascular risk factors*

SUBCUTANEOUS INJECTION
Adults. 0.75 mg once weekly.

Drug Administration
SUBCUTANEOUS

- Solution should appear clear and colorless in the single-dose pen.
- Administer any time of day with or without food.
- Inject into patient's abdomen, thigh, or upper arm following manufacturer guidelines. It is important when injecting drug to press and hold the green injection button, which should produce a loud click. Continue holding against patient's skin until a second click is heard in about 5 to 10 seconds. The pen can then be removed.
- Rotate injection sites with each dose.
- Never administer as an I.M. or I.V. injection.
- When administering drug with insulin, separate injections and never mix. However, both can be injected into the same body region, but the injections should not be adjacent to each other.
- If a dose is missed and there are at least 3 days (72 hours) until next scheduled dose, drug can be administered. If less than 3 days (72 hours) remains, skip missed dose and administer next dose as scheduled. In either case, a once-weekly dosing schedule can be resumed.
- The day of weekly administration can be changed as long as the last dose was administered 3 or more days before.

- Store drug in refrigerator. If needed, each single-dose pen can be kept at room temperature for up to 2 weeks.
- Never freeze drug, and protect from light by storing in original carton until time of administration.

Route	Onset	Peak	Duration
SubQ	Unknown	24–72 hr	Unknown

Half-life: 5 days

Mechanism of Action

Activates the GLP-1 receptor to increase intracellular cyclic AMP (cAMP) in beta cells, causing a glucose-dependent insulin release. Insulin then lowers blood glucose levels. Dulaglutide also decreases glucagon secretion and slows gastric emptying to further decrease blood glucose levels.

Contraindications

Hypersensitivity to dulaglutide or its components, personal or family history of medullary thyroid carcinoma or multiple endocrine neoplasia syndrome type 2, preexisting severe gastrointestinal disease

Interactions

DRUGS

insulin, insulin secretagogues: Increased risk of hypoglycemia
orally administered drugs: Possibly decreased absorption of the orally administered drugs

Adverse Reactions

CNS: Asthenia, fatigue, malaise
CV: First-degree AV block, sinus tachycardia
ENDO: Hypoglycemia
EENT: Diabetic retinopathy occurrence or progression
GI: Abdominal distention or pain, anorexia, cholecystitis, cholelithiasis, constipation, diarrhea, dyspepsia, elevated pancreatic enzymes, flatulence, gastroesophageal reflux disease, nausea, **pancreatitis**, vomiting
GU: **Acute renal failure**, elevated creatinine level, **worsening chronic renal failure**
SKIN: Pruritus, rash, urticaria
Other: Angioedema, anti-drug antibody formation, **hypersensitivity reactions**, injection-site reactions such as erythema and rash

Childbearing Considerations

PREGNANCY

- It is not known if drug causes fetal harm.
- Use with caution only if benefit to mother outweighs potential risk to fetus.

LACTATION

- It is not known if drug is present in breast milk.
- Patient should check with prescriber before breastfeeding.

Nursing Considerations

- Know that dulaglutide should not be used as first-line therapy for patients who have inadequately controlled their blood glucose levels on diet and exercise alone.
- Use caution when beginning dulaglutide therapy or titrating dose in patients with renal impairment. Monitor renal function in these patients if they experience severe adverse gastrointestinal reactions. Also use cautiously in patients with hepatic impairment, because the effect of dulaglutide therapy on the liver is unknown, and in patients with gastroparesis, because drug slows gastric emptying.
- Be aware that dulaglutide may potentially be linked to the development of thyroid C-cell tumors. While elevated serum calcitonin is a biological marker, its value in routine monitoring is unclear. If an elevated serum calcitonin level is found at any time during therapy, expect patient to be referred to an endocrinologist for further evaluation.
- Monitor patient for signs and symptoms of pancreatitis, such as persistent severe abdominal pain, sometimes radiating to the back, which may or may not be accompanied by vomiting. If confirmed, expect dulaglutide to be discontinued.
- Monitor patient also receiving insulin or insulin secretagogue therapy concomitantly for hypoglycemia. The dosage of insulin or insulin secretagogue may have to be lowered to reduce the risk of hypoglycemia. If hypoglycemia occurs, treat it according to policy and notify prescriber.

! **WARNING** Monitor patient for signs of hypersensitivity such as pruritus, rash, or urticaria. If present, withhold drug, notify prescriber. and expect drug to be discontinued.

- Monitor patient for signs of diarrhea, dehydration, nausea or vomiting, which may suggest renal impairment. If present, notify prescriber because the frequency of these gastrointestinal symptoms may increase as renal function declines.
- Monitor patient for change in vision, as diabetic retinopathy may occur or worsen during drug therapy. Most patients experience diabetic retinopathy complications if condition was present before drug was started. If visual changes occur, notify prescriber. However, know that a temporary worsening of diabetic retinopathy may occur with rapid improvement in glucose control.
- Keep patient hydrated, especially if adverse gastrointestinal reactions occur, because dehydration increases risk of renal dysfunction.

PATIENT TEACHING

- Inform patient that drug may be administered at any time of day without regard to meals but that it should be administered on the same day each week. However, if the day of the week needs to be changed, that change may be made, as long as the last dose was administered 4 or more days earlier.
- Instruct patient that if a dose is missed it should be administered when remembered if there are at least 3 days (72 hours) until the next schedule dose. If it is within 1 to 2 days of his next regularly scheduled dose, he should administer at the regularly scheduled time.
- Teach patient to administer the injection into the abdomen, thigh, or upper arm region. Instruct patient that if the same body region is being used each week, the sites of injection should be rotated within that region. Tell patient how to safely dispose of the used pen and needle.

! WARNING Instruct patient to stop taking dulaglutide and seek immediate emergency care if any of the following allergic reactions occurs: difficulty breathing or swallowing; dizziness, fainting; feeling itching; rapid heartbeat; severe rash; or swelling of face, lips, tongue, or throat.

- Ensure that patient has been informed of the potential risk for developing thyroid tumors before starting dulaglutide therapy. Tell patient to report any symptoms of thyroid tumors such as a mass in the neck, difficulty swallowing or breathing, or persistent hoarseness.
- Instruct patient on the signs and symptoms of hypoglycemia and how to treat it. Inform patient who is also receiving an insulin secretagogue or insulin that the risk of hypoglycemia is greater. Tell patient to notify prescriber if hypoglycemia occurs frequently or is severe.
- Tell patient to notify prescriber if any orally administered drugs appear to be losing their effectiveness, as dulaglutide causes a delay of gastric emptying and has the potential to affect the absorption of drugs taken by mouth. Also tell prescriber about any new prescribed medication or over-the-counter preparation before using.
- Stress importance of reporting visual changes to prescriber.

duloxetine hydrochloride
Cymbalta, Drizalma Sprinkle

☰ Class and Category
Pharmacologic class: Selective serotonin and norepinephrine reuptake inhibitor
Therapeutic: Antidepressant, neuropathic and musculoskeletal pain reliever

☰ Indications and Dosages
✳ *To treat major depressive disorder*
DELAYED-RELEASE CAPSULES
Adults. *Initial:* 20 mg twice daily to 60 mg (given either once daily or as 30 mg twice daily), and then increased as needed. Alternatively, 30 mg once daily for 1 wk before increasing, as needed. *Maintenance:* 60 mg/day. *Maximum:* 120 mg/day.
✳ *To relieve neuropathic pain associated with diabetic peripheral neuropathy*
DELAYED-RELEASE CAPSULES
Adults. 60 mg once daily.
✳ *To treat generalized anxiety disorder*
DELAYED-RELEASE CAPSULES
Adults less than 65 years of age. *Initial:* 60 mg once daily, increased in 30-mg increments weekly, as needed. Alternatively,

30 mg once daily for 1 wk, then increased to 60 mg once daily with further increases in 30-mg increments, as needed. *Maximum:* 120 mg once daily.

Adults 65 years of age and older. *Initial:* 30 mg once daily for 2 weeks, before dosage increased to 60 mg once daily. Further increases in dosage made in 30-mg increments weekly, as needed. *Maximum:* 120 mg once daily.

Children age 7 to 17 years of age. *Initial:* 30 mg once daily for 2 wk, then increased in 30-mg increments weekly, as needed. *Maximum:* 120 mg daily.

✱ *To treat fibromyalgia; to treat chronic musculoskeletal pain*

DELAYED-RELEASE CAPSULES

Adults. *Initial:* 30 mg once daily for 1 wk; then increased to 60 mg once daily.

Adolescents age 13 to 17. *Initial:* 30 mg once daily, increased to 60 mg once daily, as needed.

Drug Administration

P.O.

- Cymbalta capsules should be swallowed whole and not chewed, crushed, or opened.
- Drizalma Sprinkle capsules may be swallowed whole without chewing or crushing capsule or opened and sprinkled on applesauce. Have patient swallow mixture immediately and do not store mixture.
- To administer Drizalma Sprinkle capsules via a nasogastric tube, open capsule and add contents to an all-plastic catheter-tip syringe and add 50 ml of water. Gently shake syringe for about 10 seconds. Promptly deliver through a 12 French or larger nasogastric tube. Check that no pellets are left in the syringe. Rinse with about 15 ml of water, if needed.

Route	Onset	Peak	Duration
P.O.	Unknown	6 hr	Unknown

Half-life: 12 hr

Mechanism of Action

Inhibits dopamine, neuronal serotonin, and norepinephrine reuptake to potentiate noradrenergic and serotonergic activity in the CNS. These activities may elevate mood and inhibit pain signals stemming from peripheral nerves adversely affected by chronically elevated serum glucose level.

Contraindications

Chronic liver disease including cirrhosis, hypersensitivity to duloxetine or its components severe renal impairment (glomerular filtration rate less than 30 ml/min), use of linezolid or intravenous methylene blue, use of MAO inhibitors within 5 days of stopping duloxetine or within 14 days of stopping MAO inhibitors

Interactions

DRUGS

amphetamines, buspirone, fentanyl, intravenous methylene blue, lithium, linezolid, MAO inhibitors, selective serotonin reuptake inhibitors, serotonin norepinephrine reuptake inhibitors, St. John's Wort, tramadol, tricyclic antidepressants, triptans, tryptophan: Increased risk of serotonin syndrome

aspirin, NSAIDs, warfarin: Possibly increased risk of bleeding

cimetidine, fluoxetine, fluvoxamine, paroxetine, quinidine, quinolones: Increased blood duloxetine level

CNS drugs: Increased effect of duloxetine

CYP1A2, CYP2D6 inhibitors: Altered duloxetine metabolism

drugs that raise gastrointestinal pH: Possibly early release of duloxetine

phenothiazines, tricyclic antidepressants (such as amitriptyline, imipramine, nortriptyline), type 1C antiarrhythmics (such as flecainide, propafenone): Increased plasma levels of these drugs with possible increase in adverse reactions

thioridazine: Increased plasma thioridazine levels increasing risk of serious ventricular arrhythmias and sudden death

ACTIVITIES

alcohol use: Increased risk of hepatotoxicity

Adverse Reactions

CNS: Abnormal dreams, aggression, agitation, anger, anxiety, asthenia, chills, dizziness, extrapyramidal disorder, fatigue, fever, hallucinations, headache, insomnia, migraine, nervousness, **neuroleptic malignant syndrome**, paresthesia, peripheral neuropathy, restless legs syndrome, **seizures, serotonin syndrome**, somnolence, **suicidal ideation**, syncope, tremor, vertigo

CV: Hypertension, **hypertensive crisis,** **MI,** orthostatic hypotension, palpitations, paresthesia, peripheral edema or coldness, **supraventricular arrhythmia,** tachycardia, **Takotsubo cardiomyopathy**

EENT: Acute-angle glaucoma, blurred vision, dry mouth, glaucoma, nasopharyngitis, oropharyngeal pain, pharyngitis, taste alteration, tinnitus

ENDO: Galactorrhea, hot flashes, hyperglycemia, hyperprolactinemia

GI: **Acute pancreatitis,** abdominal pain, anorexia, cholestatic jaundice, colitis, constipation, diarrhea, dyspepsia, elevated liver enzymes, flatulence, **hepatitis,** **hepatotoxicity,** indigestion, jaundice, nausea, upper abdominal pain, vomiting

GU: Abnormal orgasm; decreased libido; erectile or ejaculatory dysfunction; **gynecological bleeding;** urinary frequency, hesitancy, or retention; UTI

HEME: **Bleeding episodes** (may range from mild to **life-threatening**), **leukopenia,** **thrombocytopenia**

MS: Arthralgia, back or neck pain, extremity pain, muscle cramp or spasm, myalgia

RESP: Cough, upper respiratory tract infection

SKIN: Cutaneous vasculitis, diaphoresis, **erythema multiforme,** flushing, hyperhidrosis, pruritus, rash, **Stevens–Johnson syndrome,** urticaria

Other: **Anaphylaxis, angioedema,** discontinuation syndrome, flu-like symptoms, **hyponatremia,** weight gain or loss

Childbearing Considerations

PREGNANCY

- Pregnancy exposure registry: *For Cymbalta:* 1-866-814-6975 or www .cymbaltapregnancyregistry.com. *For Drizalma Sprinkle:* 1-844-405-6185 or https://womensmentalealth.org/clinical -and-research-programs/pregnancy registry/antidepressants/.
- It is not known if drug causes fetal harm. However, be aware that neonates exposed to the drug during pregnancy may develop serious and life-threatening adverse reactions, which can arise immediately following birth. These adverse reactions may require prolonged hospitalization, respiratory support, and tube feeding.

- Use with caution only if benefit to mother outweighs potential risk to fetus.
- Use of drug in the month before delivery may increase risk of postpartum hemorrhage.

LACTATION

- Drug is present in breast milk.
- Patient should check with prescriber before breastfeeding.
- If breastfeeding occurs, infant should be monitored for drowsiness, poor feeding, and poor weight gain.

Nursing Considerations

- Know that duloxetine should not be given to patients with severe renal impairment or end-stage renal disease that requires hemodialysis because blood drug levels increase significantly in these patients. Also know that duloxetine should be avoided in patients with hepatic insufficiency or who use alcohol excessively because drug is metabolized by the liver.
- Screen patients for a personal or family history of bipolar disorder, mania, or hypomania, which drug may activate.
- Use duloxetine cautiously in patients with delayed gastric emptying because drug's enteric coating resists dissolution until it reaches an area where pH exceeds 5.5.
- Give cautiously to patients with a seizure disorder because drug effects aren't known in these patients.
- Obtain patient's baseline blood pressure before duloxetine therapy starts, and assess it periodically thereafter for changes. If orthostatic hypotension occurs during therapy, notify prescriber and anticipate that drug may have to be discontinued.

! WARNING Monitor patient for bleeding events because drug increases risk. Bleeding events can range from ecchymoses, epistaxis, hematomas, and petechiae to life-threatening hemorrhages. Know that concomitant use of aspirin, NSAIDs, or other drugs that affect coagulation increases risk.

- Inspect patient's skin and mucous membranes often because drug can cause serious skin reactions that could become life-threatening. Notify prescriber immediately if patient develops skin blisters or peeling as well as hives, rash, sores in the mouth, or any other allergic reaction.

- Monitor patient's serum sodium level, as ordered, especially if patient is elderly, is taking a diuretic, or has volume depletion, because drug may lower serum sodium level.
- Monitor patient's hepatic function, as ordered, because drug may increase the risk of hepatotoxicity. Expect to discontinue duloxetine, as ordered, if patient develops jaundice or other serious liver dysfunction manifestation.
- Watch closely for evidence of suicidal thinking or behavior, especially when therapy starts or dosage changes.
- Avoid stopping duloxetine therapy abruptly, if possible, because withdrawal symptoms such as anxiety, diarrhea, dizziness, fatigue, headache, hyperhidrosis, insomnia, irritability, nausea, nightmares, paresthesia, vertigo, and vomiting, may occur. Taper dosage gradually, as ordered.

! WARNING Monitor patient for serotonin syndrome, characterized by agitation, chills, confusion, diaphoresis, diarrhea, fever, hyperactive reflexes, poor coordination, restlessness, shaking, talking or acting with uncontrolled excitement, tremor, and twitching. In its most severe form, serotonin syndrome can resemble neuroleptic malignant syndrome, which includes autonomic instability with possible fluctuations in vital signs, high fever, mental status changes, and muscle rigidity.

! WARNING Know that treatment with linezolid or I.V. methylene blue is not recommended while patient is taking duloxetine because of increased risk of serotonin syndrome. However, if prescriber feels benefits outweigh the risks, expect duloxetine to be discontinued promptly if serotonin syndrome occurs. Monitor patient closely for serotonin syndrome for 5 days or until 24 hours after the last dose of linezolid or I.V. methylene blue, whichever comes first. Know that therapy with duloxetine may be resumed 24 hours after the last dose of linezolid or I.V. methylene blue.

PATIENT TEACHING

- Tell patient to take Cymbalta capsule whole and not to chew it, crush it, or sprinkle contents on food or liquids, because doing so alters enteric coating and may affect drug absorption.
- Tell patient prescribed Drizalma Sprinkle capsules that they may be swallowed whole without chewing or crushing or it can be opened and sprinkled on applesauce. Tell patient to swallow mixture immediately and do not store mixture.
- Inform patient that full effect of duloxetine may take weeks to occur; emphasize the importance of continuing to take the drug as directed.
- Caution patient against excessive alcohol consumption while taking duloxetine because it may increase risk of hepatic dysfunction. Also tell him to report a yellowing of skin immediately, as drug may have to be discontinued.
- Advise patient not to stop duloxetine abruptly because adverse reactions may occur. Explain that drug will be stopped gradually.
- Instruct patient to notify prescriber if any serious or troublesome adverse effects develop, especially if they are persistent, severe, or unusual.

! WARNING Stress importance of notifying prescriber if skin blisters or peeling occurs, as well as hives, rash, sores in the mouth, or any other allergic reactions.

- Advise patient that drug may increase risk of bleeding. Tell patient to notify prescriber if mild bleeding occurs or seek immediate medical attention if severe. Tell patient to consult prescriber before taking aspirin or NSAIDs.
- Advise patient to avoid hazardous activities until drug's CNS effects are known.
- Advise patient that drug may cause mild pupillary dilation, which may lead to an episode of acute-angle glaucoma. Encourage him to have an eye exam before starting therapy to see if he is at risk.
- Instruct patient to rise from a lying or sitting position slowly to minimize drug's effect on lowering blood pressure, which may possibly lead to falls or cause patient to faint.
- Urge caregivers to watch closely for evidence of suicidal tendencies, especially when therapy starts or dosage changes.
- Instruct female patients of childbearing age to notify prescriber if they are, could be, or

wish to become pregnant. Alert pregnant women that there is a risk of relapse if an antidepressant is discontinued.

> ! WARNING Tell patient to stop taking duloxetine and notify prescriber immediately at the first sign of blisters, mucosal erosions, peeling rash, or any other sign of hypersensitivity, as drug will have to be discontinued.

- Instruct patient with diabetes to monitor his blood glucose levels more closely, as duloxetine therapy can alter control.
- Tell patient to notify prescriber of any new medication, including over-the-counter preparations, before using duloxetine.
- Advise patient to discuss any sexual dysfunction concerns with prescriber.

dutasteride
Avodart

Class and Category
Pharmacologic class: 5-alpha-reductase enzyme inhibitor
Therapeutic class: Benign prostatic hyperplasia agent

Indications and Dosages
✱ *To treat symptomatic benign prostatic hyperplasia (BPH); as adjunct with tamsulosin therapy to treat symptomatic BPH*

CAPSULES
Adult men. 0.5 mg daily.

Drug Administration
P.O.
- Handle drug carefully, as it is a known teratogen. Female medical personnel who are pregnant or suspect pregnancy should not touch capsules. Follow institutional policies for handling and disposal procedure.
- Capsules should be swallowed whole and not chewed, crushed, or opened.

Route	Onset	Peak	Duration
P.O.	Unknown	2–3 hr	Unknown

Half-life: 5 wk

Contraindications
Children; hypersensitivity to dutasteride other 5-alpha reductase inhibitors or their components; pregnancy; women of childbearing age

Interactions
DRUGS
CYP3A4 inhibitors such as cimetidine, ciprofloxacin, diltiazem, ketoconazole, ritonavir, verapamil: Increased dutasteride exposure and enhanced effects including increased risk of adverse reactions

Adverse Reactions
CNS: Depression, dizziness
ENDO: Gynecomastia, increased serum testosterone and thyroid-stimulating hormone levels, **male breast cancer**
GU: Decreased ejaculatory volume, decreased libido, **high-grade prostate cancer**, impotence, testicular pain and swelling
SKIN: Localized edema, pruritus, rash, serious skin reactions, urticaria
Other: Angioedema, hypersensitivity reactions, male breast cancer

Childbearing Considerations
PREGNANCY
- Drug may cause fetal harm such as abnormalities in the genitalia of male fetuses if pregnant women come in contact with drug.
- Drug is not given to women.

REPRODUCTION
- Be aware that drug's effect on fertility of male patients is unknown. However, there is some evidence to suggest drug may decrease sperm count.
- Patient or female partner should use an effective contraceptive during drug therapy as drug appears in semen.

Nursing Considerations

> ! WARNING Be aware that dutasteride is absorbed through the skin, so female healthcare workers should not handle dutasteride capsules if of childbearing age or pregnant.

- Know that patient should be evaluated for other urologic conditions, including

☰ Mechanism of Action

Dutasteride reduces prostate gland enlargement by inhibiting conversion of testosterone to its active metabolite, 5-alpha dihydrotestosterone (DHT). DHT is the main hormone that stimulates prostate cells to grow. As men age, they may become more sensitive to DHT, resulting in excessive growth of prostatic cells and enlargement of the prostate. This condition, benign prostatic hyperplasia, may cause nocturia, urinary hesitancy, and urinary urgency.

Two forms of the intracellular enzyme 5-alpha-reductase (5α-R types 1 and 2) in liver, prostate, and skin, convert testosterone to DHT, as shown below left. Dutasteride, a dual 5α-R inhibitor, deactivates both forms. When 5α-R is inhibited by dutasteride, production of DHT is suppressed, as shown below right. With less circulating DHT, the prostate gland shrinks and symptoms improve.

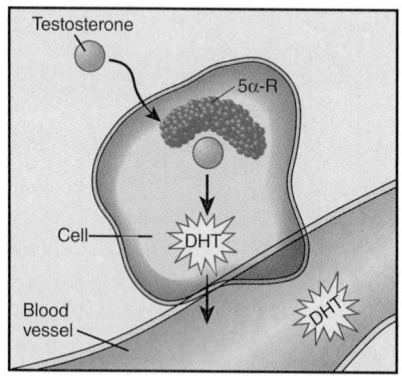

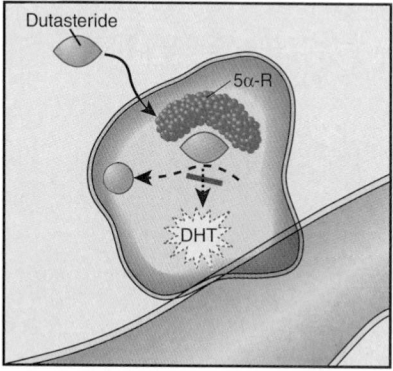

prostate cancer, before dutasteride therapy starts because dutasteride therapy increases risk of patient developing high-grade prostate cancer.

- Expect patient to undergo a digital rectal examination of the prostate before and periodically during dutasteride therapy.
- Anticipate need to obtain a new baseline prostate-specific antigen (PSA) value after 3 to 6 months of dutasteride treatment because drug can decrease PSA concentration by 40% to 50%. Dutasteride also can decrease serum PSA level in the presence of prostate cancer. Any PSA reading in a patient receiving dutasteride should be doubled for comparison with normal values in untreated men. If value still falls within the normal range for men not taking a 5-alpha-reductase inhibitor, further evaluation should still be done to rule out prostate cancer.

PATIENT TEACHING

! WARNING Urge patient and female partners to use reliable contraceptive method during

dutasteride therapy because semen of men who take drug can harm male fetuses. Caution women and children against handling capsules.

- Advise patient to inform prescriber if he has liver disease.
- Explain how to take drug properly, and advise patient to follow instructions that accompany drug. Instruct him to swallow capsule whole and to notify pharmacist if capsules are cracked or leaking.
- Inform patient that drug may decrease ejaculatory volume and libido and may cause impotence.
- Instruct patient to postpone blood donations for 6 months after final dose to avoid transmitting dutasteride to a pregnant woman during a blood transfusion.
- Urge patient to have periodic follow-up appointments.

E F

edoxaban tosylate
Savaysa

Class and Category
Pharmacologic class: Factor Xa inhibitor
Therapeutic class: Anticoagulant

Indications and Dosages
* *To reduce risk of stroke and systemic embolism in nonvalvular atrial fibrillation*

TABLETS
Adults. 60 mg once daily.

±**DOSAGE ADJUSTMENT** For patients with impaired renal failure (creatinine clearance between 15 and 50 ml/min), dosage reduced to 30 mg once daily.

* *To treat deep vein thrombosis and pulmonary embolism*

TABLETS
Adults weighing more than 60 kg (132 lb). 60 mg once daily following 5 to 10 days of initial therapy with a parenteral anticoagulant.

±**DOSAGE ADJUSTMENT** For patients with impaired renal failure (creatinine clearance between 15 and 50 ml/min), patients who weigh less than or equal to 60 kg (132 lb), or patients who are taking selected concomitant P-gp inhibitors, dosage reduced to 30 mg once daily.

Drug Administration
P.O.
- Do not administer to a patient who has a creatinine clearance greater than 95 ml/min because of an increased risk of ischemic stroke.
- For a patient unable to swallow tablets, crush tablet and mix with 60 to 90 ml of water and immediately administer by mouth or gastric tube. Crushed tablet may also be mixed with applesauce and immediately given by mouth. Do not store mixture.

Route	Onset	Peak	Duration
P.O.	Unknown	1–2 hr	Unknown

Half-life: 10–14 hr

Mechanism of Action
Inhibits free FXa and prothrombinase activity and inhibits thrombin-induced platelet aggregation. By inhibiting FXa in the coagulation cascade, thrombin generation and formation is reduced.

Contraindications
Active pathological bleeding, hypersensitivity to edoxaban or its components

Interactions
DRUGS
anticoagulants, antiplatelets, aspirin or aspirin-containing products, NSAIDs (long-term use), selective serotonin reuptake inhibitors, serotonin norepinephrine reuptake inhibitors, thrombolytics: Increased risk of bleeding
rifampin: Decreased effectiveness of edoxaban
quinidine, verapamil, or short-term concomitant administration of azithromycin, clarithromycin, erythromycin, oral itraconazole or oral ketoconazole: Increased blood level with increased risk of bleeding in patients being treated for deep venous thrombosis or pulmonary embolism

Adverse Reactions
CNS: Dizziness, headache, **intracranial bleeding**
EENT: Epistaxis, intraocular bleeding
GI: Abdominal pain, elevated liver enzymes, **GI bleeding**
GU: Hematuria, uterine or vaginal bleeding
HEME: Anemia, **bleeding, thrombocytopenia**
RESP: Interstitial lung disease
SKIN: Rash, urticaria
Other: Angioedema, hypersensitivity reactions

Childbearing Considerations
PREGNANCY
- Drug may cause fetal harm because use of drug may increase risk of bleeding in the fetus and neonate.
- Use with caution only if benefit to mother outweighs potential risk to fetus.

LABOR & DELIVERY
- Drug withheld, if possible, and replaced with a shorter-acting anticoagulant as delivery approaches because of increased risk of bleeding.

E
F

LACTATION

- It is not known if drug is present in breast milk.
- Breastfeeding is not recommended during drug therapy.

REPRODUCTION

- Women of childbearing age should discuss pregnancy plans with prescriber because drug may cause significant uterine bleeding that may require surgical intervention.

☰ Nursing Considerations

- Keep in mind that edoxaban is not recommended for use in patients with a mechanical heart valve or who have moderate to severe mitral stenosis, because the effects of edoxaban in these patients are unknown. Drug is also not recommended for use in patients with triple positive antiphospholipid syndrome because of an increased risk for thrombosis.
- Be aware that edoxaban should be withheld for at least 24 hours before invasive or surgical procedures are performed to reduce the risk of bleeding. If it is not possible to delay the procedure, monitor patient closely for bleeding. If edoxaban was withheld, know that it may be restarted after the invasive or surgical procedure as soon as the patient has achieved adequate hemostasis. Be prepared to administer a parenteral anticoagulant if oral medication cannot be initially taken and then when oral medication can be taken, the patient may be switched to edoxaban.
- Know that when a patient is being transitioned to edoxaban from warfarin or other vitamin K antagonist, warfarin should be discontinued and edoxaban started when the INR is 2.5 or less; transitioned from oral anticoagulants other than warfarin or other vitamin K antagonists, the current oral anticoagulant should be discontinued and edoxaban started at the time of the next scheduled dose of the other oral anticoagulant; transitioned from low-molecular-weight heparin, the low-molecular-weight heparin should be discontinued and edoxaban started at the time of the next scheduled administration of the low-molecular-weight heparin; or transitioned from unfractionated heparin, the unfractionated heparin infusion should

be discontinued and edoxaban started 4 hours later.
- Be aware that when a patient is being transitioned from edoxaban (60-mg dose) to warfarin, the dose of edoxaban should be reduced to 30 mg and warfarin begun concomitantly. When a patient is being transitioned from edoxaban (30-mg dose) to warfarin, the dose of edoxaban should be reduced to 15 mg and warfarin begun concomitantly. When a stable INR of 2 or greater is achieved in either situation, edoxaban should be discontinued. Know that a second method of transitioning a patient from edoxaban to warfarin may be used. In this method, edoxaban should be discontinued and a parenteral anticoagulant and warfarin administered, as ordered, at the same time of the next scheduled edoxaban dose. Once a stable INR of 2 or greater is achieved, the parenteral anticoagulant should be discontinued and warfarin therapy continued. Be aware that when a patient is being transitioned from edoxaban to a non-vitamin K dependent oral anticoagulant, edoxaban should be discontinued and the other oral anticoagulant started at the time of the next dose of edoxaban. Know that when a patient is being transitioned from edoxaban to a parenteral anticoagulant, edoxaban should be discontinued and the parenteral anticoagulant should be started at the time of the next dose of edoxaban.

! WARNING Monitor patient receiving edoxaban and epidural or spinal anesthesia or spinal puncture because spinal hematomas can occur, causing long-term or permanent paralysis. Watch for evidence of neurologic impairment, such as changes in motor or sensory function. If present, notify prescriber immediately; patient needs urgent care to minimize effect of hematoma. Use of indwelling epidural catheters; concurrent use of other drugs that affect hemostasis such as nonsteroidal anti-inflammatory drugs, platelet inhibitors, and other anticoagulants; a history of traumatic or repeated epidural or spinal punctures; or a history of spinal deformity or spinal surgery increases the risk of epidural or spinal hematoma in patients receiving edoxaban.

- Expect to receive another anticoagulant, as ordered, if edoxaban must be discontinued for reasons other than the presence of active bleeding or therapy is no longer needed. This is because premature discontinuation of edoxaban increases the risk of ischemic events.
- Monitor patient closely for bleeding. If present, notify prescriber immediately because there is no antidote to reverse the anticoagulation effects of edoxaban, which may last for up to 24 hours after the last dose. Know that patients who take other drugs that affect hemostasis, such as aspirin and other antiplatelet agents, chronic use of nonsteroidal anti-inflammatory drugs, fibrinolytic therapy, or other antithrombotic drugs, are at increased risk for bleeding.
- Know that the use of anticoagulants, including edoxaban, may increase the risk of bleeding in the fetus and neonate. Monitor neonate for bleeding if mother was taking edoxaban prior to birth.

PATIENT TEACHING

- Tell patient that if she misses a dose of edoxaban, she should take the dose as soon as possible on the same day and resume the dosing for the next day at the normal time. However, if she forgets the dose until the next day, she should not double the dose to make up for the missed dose.
- Inform patient unable to swallow tablets that edoxaban may be crushed and mixed with 2 to 3 ounces of water or mixed in applesauce and immediately taken by mouth.
- Instruct patient on bleeding precautions. If bleeding occurs, tell her to report any unusual bleeding immediately to the prescriber.
- Caution patient not to stop taking edoxaban without talking to her prescriber first.
- Tell patient to alert all healthcare providers and dentists that she is taking edoxaban and to consult the prescriber before taking any new drugs, including OTC drugs.
- Stress importance for females of childbearing age to notify prescriber if pregnancy occurs or is suspected. This is because anticoagulants, including edoxaban, may increase the risk of bleeding in the fetus and neonate. Tell mother who took edoxaban during late pregnancy to watch neonate for bleeding.

- Advise mothers that breastfeeding is not recommended during edoxaban therapy because of the potential risk of serious adverse reactions.

! **WARNING** Alert patient who is having neuraxial anesthesia or spinal puncture to immediately report signs and symptoms suggestive of epidural or spinal hematomas such as back pain, muscle weakness, numbness (especially in the lower limbs), stool or urine incontinence, and tingling.

efavirenz

Sustiva

Class and Category

Pharmacologic class: Non-nucleoside reverse transcriptase inhibitor
Therapeutic class: Antiretroviral

Indications and Dosages

* *As adjunct to treat human immunodeficiency virus type 1 (HIV-1) in combination with other antiretroviral agents*

CAPSULES, TABLETS

Adults and children age 3 months and older and weighing 40 kg (88 lb) or more. 600 mg once daily.
Children age 3 months and older and weighing 32.5 kg (71.5 lb) to less than 40 kg (88 lb). 400 mg once daily.
Children age 3 months and older and weighing 25 kg (55 lb) to less than 32.5 kg (71.5 lb). 350 mg once daily.
Children age 3 months and older and weighing 20 kg (44 lb) to less than 25 kg (55 lb). 300 mg once daily.
Children age 3 months and older and weighing 15 kg (33 lb) to less than 20 kg (44 lb). 250 mg once daily.
Children age 3 months and older and weighing 7.5 kg (16.5 lb) to less than 15 kg (33 lb). 200 mg once daily.
Children age 3 months and older and weighing 5 kg (11 lb) to less than 7.5 kg (16.5 lb). 150 mg once daily.
Children age 3 months and older and weighing 3.5 kg (7.7 lb) to less than 5 kg (11 lb). 100 mg once daily.

±DOSAGE ADJUSTMENT For adult patients weighing 50 kg (110 lb) and also receiving rifampin, dosage increased to 800 mg once daily. For adult patients receiving voriconazole concurrently, dosage decreased to 300 mg once daily.

Drug Administration

P.O.

- Administer on an empty stomach at bedtime.
- Tablets and capsules should be swallowed whole and not chewed or crushed.
- For patients who cannot swallow capsules or tablets, have prescriber order capsule form because capsule can be opened and sprinkled on 1 to 2 teaspoons of soft food (applesauce, grape jelly, or yogurt) and mixed gently. Administer within 30 minutes.
- For infants, mix contents of capsule with 10 ml of reconstituted infant formula that is at room temperature. Draw up mixture in a 10-ml oral dosing syringe and administer. Add 10 ml of formula to cup used to make mixture and stir. Draw up in a 10-ml oral dosing syringe and administer. Use mixture within 30 minutes.
- Do not give patient any food or formula for 2 hours after administration.

Route	Onset	Peak	Duration
P.O.	Unknown	3–5 hr	Unknown
Half-life: 40–76 hr			

Mechanism of Action

Inhibits HIV integrase by binding to the integrase active site and blocking the strand transfer step of retroviral DNA integration, which is needed for the HIV replication cycle.

Contraindications

Concurrent therapy with elbasvir and grazoprevir, hypersensitivity to efavirenz or its components

Interactions

DRUGS

artemether, atazanavir, atorvastatin, atovaquone, boceprevir, bupropion, clarithromycin, cyclosporine, dihydroartemisinin, diltiazem, ethinyl estradiol/norgestimate, etonogestrel implant, felodipine, fosamprenavir, hydroxyitraconazole, immunosuppressants, indinavir, ketoconazole, itraconazole, lopinavir, lumefantrine, maraviroc, methadone, nicardipine, nifedipine, posaconazole, pravastatin, proguanil, rifabutin, saquinavir, sertraline, simeprevir, simvastatin, sirolimus, tacrolimus, velpatasvir/sofosbuvir, velpatasvir/sofosbuvir/voxilaprevir, verapamil: Decreased effectiveness of these drugs

carbamazepine, phenobarbital, phenytoin: Decreased plasma levels of both drugs

CYP3A inducers: Decreased plasma levels of efavirenz with decreased effectiveness

elbasvir/grazoprevir, pibrentasvir/glecaprevir: Possibly loss of virologic response and reduced therapeutic effect

other non-nucleoside reverse transcriptase inhibitors: Decreased or increased plasma levels of both drugs without added efficacy

psychoactive drugs: Possibly additive central nervous system effects

QT prolongation drugs such as artemether/lumefantrine, clarithromycin: Increased risk of torsades de pointes

rifabutin: Decreased plasma levels of both drugs decreasing effectiveness

rifampin: Decreased plasma efavirenz levels with possible decrease in effectiveness

ritonavir: Increased plasma levels of both efavirenz and ritonavir, possibly leading to elevated liver enzymes and other adverse reactions

voriconazole: Decreased voriconazole level and increased plasma efavirenz

warfarin: Decreased or increased warfarin levels, requiring close monitoring of INR and adjustment of warfarin dosage as needed

ACTIVITIES

alcohol use: Possibly increased additive central nervous system effects

Adverse Reactions

CNS: Abnormal dreams, aggression, agitation, amnesia, anxiety, asthenia, ataxia, catatonia, cerebellar balance and coordination disturbances, confusion, delusions, depersonalization, depression (severe), dizziness, emotional lability, **encephalopathy**, euphoria, fatigue, fever, hallucinations, headache, hypoesthesia, impaired concentration, insomnia, paranoid behavior, manic reactions, nervousness, neuropathy, neurosis, paranoia, paresthesia, psychosis-like behavior, **seizures**, somnolence, stupor, **suicidal ideation**, tremor, vertigo

CV: Elevated cholesterol and triglyceride levels, palpitations, **QT prolongation**

EENT: Abnormal vision, tinnitus

ENDO: Cushingoid appearance, fat redistribution, gynecomastia, hyperglycemia

GI: Abdominal pain, anorexia, constipation, diarrhea, dyspepsia, elevated amylase or liver enzymes, **hepatic failure**, **hepatitis**, **hepatotoxicity**, malabsorption, nausea, **pancreatitis**, vomiting

HEME: Neutropenia

MS: Arthralgia, myalgia, myopathy

RESP: Dyspnea

SKIN: Blisters, **erythema multiforme**, flushing, moist desquamation, photoallergic dermatitis, pruritus, rash, **Stevens–Johnson syndrome**, ulcerations

Other: Allergic reactions, nonspecific pain, immune reconstitution syndrome

Childbearing Considerations

PREGNANCY

- Pregnancy exposure registry: 1-800-258-4263.
- Be aware pregnancy testing should be done in women of childbearing age prior to initiation of drug therapy.
- It is not known if drug causes fetal harm. However, there are retrospective reports of neural tube defects in infants whose mothers were exposed to an efavirenz-containing regimen in the first trimester of pregnancy.
- Drug should not be given during the first trimester of pregnancy.

LACTATION

- It is not known if drug is present in breast milk.
- The Centers for Disease Control and Prevention recommends that HIV-1 infected mothers not breastfeed to avoid risking postnatal transmission of HIV-1 infection to infants. They also do not recommend breastfeeding because of potential drug-induced adverse reactions in the infant.

REPRODUCTION

- Effective contraceptive measures should be in place prior to beginning drug therapy as well as throughout therapy and for 12 weeks after drug is discontinued.
- Barrier contraception should always be used in combination with other methods of contraception.
- Know that hormonal methods of contraception that contain progesterone may not be as effective.

Nursing Considerations

- Be aware that efavirenz should not be used as a single agent in treating HIV infection, because resistant virus emerges quickly when drug is used alone.
- Know that efavirenz therapy is not recommended with the combination drug Atripla, which contains efavirenz, unless needed for dose adjustment when coadministered with rifampin.
- Know that drug should not be used in patients taking other medications with a known risk of torsades de pointes or in patients at higher risk of torsades de pointes, because efavirenz may cause QT prolongation.
- Obtain liver enzymes before therapy begins, as ordered, in patients with marked transaminase elevations, patients treated with other medications associated with liver toxicity, and patients with underlying hepatic disease, including hepatitis B or C infections. Also monitor liver enzymes throughout therapy, as ordered, on all patients, because efavirenz may cause hepatotoxicity. Know that persistent elevations of serum transaminase levels greater than five times the upper limit of the normal range may require efavirenz therapy to be discontinued.
- Obtain cholesterol and triglyceride levels before efavirenz is begun and periodically throughout therapy, because drug may cause an increase in total cholesterol and triglycerides.
- Use efavirenz cautiously in patients with a history of seizures, as drug may increase risk of seizures. Know that if patient is also taking anticonvulsant medications metabolized by the liver, such as phenobarbital or phenytoin, periodic monitoring of plasma levels of these drugs may be required.

! WARNING Monitor patient for rash. While usually mild to moderate, occurring within the first 2 weeks of therapy, and resolving within a month, a rash rarely may evolve into more serious skin conditions that could become life-threatening and should be reported. Know that it is recommended that children be given antihistamines and/or corticosteroids before initiating therapy, as a prophylactic measure.

- Monitor patient for serious psychiatric adverse reactions such as aggressive behavior, manic reactions, paranoia, severe depression, or suicidal ideation. Patients at increased risk include patients with drug addiction (injected) or psychiatric history including use of psychiatric drugs.
- Monitor patient for nervous system symptoms that commonly occur with efavirenz use. Be especially watchful for abnormal dreams, dizziness, hallucinations, impaired concentration, insomnia, and somnolence. Be aware that these symptoms usually occur within a day or two of starting therapy and usually resolve in the first 2 to 4 weeks. However, know that late-onset neurotoxicity, including ataxia and encephalopathy, may occur months to years after beginning efavirenz therapy.
- Be aware that immune reconstitution syndrome has occurred in patients treated with combination antiretroviral therapy, including efavirenz. The inflammatory response predisposes susceptible patients to opportunistic infections such as cytomegalovirus, *Mycobacterium avium* infection, *Pneumocystis jiroveci* pneumonia, or tuberculosis. Autoimmune disorders such as Graves' disease, Guillain–Barré syndrome, or polymyositis have also occurred. Report sudden or unusual adverse reactions to prescriber.

PATIENT TEACHING

- Inform patient that efavirenz is administered with other antiretroviral agents and to follow administration instructions as ordered, noting that drug should be taken on an empty stomach at bedtime.
- Instruct patient or parent that if patient is unable to swallow capsule form, it may be opened and sprinkled on 1 to 2 teaspoonfuls of food such as applesauce, grape jelly, or yogurt. The capsule should be opened carefully so as not to spill any of the contents or disperse drug into the air. To accomplish this, tell patient to hold capsule horizontally over a small container and carefully twist open. If infant is unable to consume food, the entire capsule contents may be gently mixed into 2 teaspoons of reconstituted room temperature infant formula, stirred gently with a small spoon, and then drawn up into a 10-ml oral dosing syringe for administration. After administration, an additional 2 teaspoons of formula should be added to the empty mixing container, stirred, and administered. Caution that the food or formula mixture should be administered within 30 minutes of mixing and no additional food should be consumed for 2 hours after the drug is given.
- Inform patient that efavirenz therapy may cause changes in his body appearance because of fat redistribution. Prepare him for the possibility of developing breast enlargement, central obesity, dorsocervical fat enlargement (buffalo hump), facial wasting, and peripheral wasting.
- Instruct patient to report a rash. Also alert patient that drug may cause nervous system symptoms or psychiatric symptoms. Review these symptoms with patient and urge patient to report to prescriber if present. Advise him also to report any persistent, severe, or unusual signs and symptoms.
- Warn family or caregiver to watch patient closely for evidence of suicidal behavior or thinking.
- Inform patient that neurological adverse reactions such as abnormal dreams, drowsiness, dizziness, impaired concentration, and insomnia may occur in the first weeks of efavirenz therapy but taking drug at bedtime will help and symptoms should diminish with continued therapy. Alert patient to the possibility of late-onset neurotoxicity that may occur months to years after beginning efavirenz therapy. Encourage patient to report any abnormal neurological signs and symptoms regardless of how long efavirenz therapy has been taken.
- Advise patient to contact prescriber before taking any new drugs, including over-the-counter preparations and herbals.
- Caution patient to avoid hazardous activities such as driving until nervous system effects are known and abated.

- Warn women of childbearing age that efavirenz may cause fetal harm when administered during the first trimester of pregnancy. Stress importance of using reliable birth control and tell patient to alert prescriber immediately if pregnancy occurs or is suspected.
- Inform mothers that breastfeeding should not be done while taking efavirenz.

eletriptan hydrobromide
Relpax

Class and Category
Pharmacologic class: Triptan
Therapeutic class: Antimigraine agent

Indications and Dosages
✳ *To relieve acute migraine attacks with or without aura*

TABLETS
Adults. *Initial:* 20 or 40 mg as a single dose. Repeated in 2 hr, as needed.
Maximum: 40 mg as single dose, 80 mg daily; and no more than three treated migraines in 30-day period.

Drug Administration
P.O.
- Tablets should be swallowed whole and not chewed, crushed, or divided.
- Following administration, have patient drink a full glass of water.

Route	Onset	Peak	Duration
P.O.	0.5 hr	1.5–2 hr	Unknown

Half-life: 4 hr

Mechanism of Action
May stimulate 5-HT$_1$ receptors, causing selective vasoconstriction of dilated and inflamed cranial blood vessels in carotid circulation, which decreases carotid arterial blood flow and relieves acute migraines.

Contraindications
Bibasilar or hemiplegic migraine, cardiovascular disease (significant), cerebrovascular syndromes (stroke, transient ischemic attack), hepatic impairment (severe), hypersensitivity to eletriptan or components, ischemic bowel disease, ischemic or vasospastic coronary artery disease (CAD), peripheral vascular disease, uncontrolled hypertension, use within 24 hours of another serotonin 5-HT$_1$ receptor agonist or ergot-type drug, use within 72 hours of a potent CYP3A4 inhibitor (clarithromycin, itraconazole, ketoconazole, nefazodone, nelfinavir, ritonavir, troleandomycin), Wolff–Parkinson–White syndrome or arrhythmias associated with other cardiac accessory conduction pathway disorders

Interactions
DRUGS
clarithromycin, ketoconazole, itraconazole, nefazodone, nelfinavir, ritonavir, troleandomycin, and other potent CYP3A4 inhibitors: Increase blood eletriptan level significantly
ergot-containing drugs, 5-HT$_1$ receptor agonists: Possibly additive or prolonged vasoconstrictive effects
MAO inhibitors, selective serotonin norepinephrine reuptake inhibitors, selective serotonin reuptake inhibitors, tricyclic antidepressants: Increased risk of serotonin syndrome

Adverse Reactions
CNS: Asthenia, chills, dizziness, headache, hypertonia, hypesthesia, paresthesia, **seizures**, somnolence, tiredness, weakness, vertigo
CV: Chest tightness, pain, or pressure; **coronary artery vasospasm**; hypertension, **MI**, or myocardial ischemia (transient); palpitations; **shock**; **ventricular fibrillation or tachycardia**
EENT: Dry mouth, pharyngitis, **throat tightness**
GI: Abdominal pain, cramps, discomfort, or pressure; dysphagia; indigestion; nausea, vomiting
MS: Back pain
SKIN: Diaphoresis, flushing
Other: **Allergic reaction**; **angioedema**; feeling of warmth, pain, or pressure

Childbearing Considerations
PREGNANCY
- It is not known if drug causes fetal harm.
- Use with caution only if benefit to mother outweighs potential risk to fetus.

E
F

- Women with migraine may be at increased risk of gestational hypertension and preeclampsia during pregnancy.

LACTATION

- Drug is present in breast milk.
- Patient should check with prescriber before breastfeeding.
- Infant exposure can be minimized by avoiding breastfeeding for 24 hours after treatment.

Nursing Considerations

- Ensure that patients who are at risk for CAD undergo a satisfactory CV evaluation before administering the first dose of eletriptan and that they have a periodic reevaluation of their cardiac status during intermittent long-term therapy.
- Obtain an ECG immediately after first dose of drug in patients who have CV risk factors but who have had a satisfactory CV evaluation because of the drug's potential to cause coronary vasospasm.
- Evaluate patient for CV signs and symptoms after administration of eletriptan and notify prescriber if they occur. Expect drug to be withheld, as ordered, while patient undergoes an extensive CV workup, and discontinued if abnormalities are detected.
- Monitor patient's blood pressure during therapy because of drug's potential to increase blood pressure.

PATIENT TEACHING

- Advise patient to take eletriptan as soon as possible after onset of migraine symptoms.
- Urge patient to contact prescriber and avoid taking drug if headache symptoms aren't typical.
- Advise against exceeding prescribed dose.

! **WARNING** Instruct patient to seek emergency care for chest, jaw, or neck tightness after taking drug because these may indicate adverse CV reactions; subsequent doses may require ECG monitoring.

- Urge patient to report palpitations.
- Advise patient to avoid hazardous activities until drug's CNS effects are known.
- Advise yearly ophthalmic examinations during prolonged eletriptan therapy.
- Instruct patient to inform prescriber of all drugs he's taking, including OTC products and herbal remedies.

eltrombopag olamine
Promacta

Class and Category

Pharmacologic class: Thrombopoietin receptor agonist
Therapeutic class: Thrombopoietin agonist

Indications and Dosages

∗ *To treat thrombocytopenia in patients with persistent or chronic immune (idiopathic) thrombocytopenic purpura and who have had an insufficient response to corticosteroids, immunoglobulins, or splenectomy*

ORAL SUSPENSION, TABLETS

Adults and children ages 6 yr and older.
Initial: 50 mg daily, increased as needed to maintain a platelet count of 50×10^9/L or greater. *Maximum:* 75 mg daily.
Children ages 1 to 5. *Initial:* 25 mg once daily, increased as needed to maintain a platelet count of 50×10^9/L or greater.
±**DOSAGE ADJUSTMENT** For adult and pediatric patients 6 years and older of Asian ancestry or patients with hepatic impairment, starting dose of 25 mg daily. For patients of Asian ancestry who also have hepatic impairment, starting dose of 12.5 mg daily. For patients with a platelet count less than 50×10^9/L following at least 2 weeks of therapy, dosage increased by 25 mg daily to maximum of 75 mg/day unless patient started therapy at 12.5 mg daily, then dosage increased to 25 mg daily before increasing the dose amount by 25 mg, as needed. For patients with a platelet count equal to or greater than 200×10^9/L but equal to or less than 400×10^9/L, dosage decreased by 25 mg daily or 12.5 mg if patient was taking 25 mg daily for at least 2 weeks before further dosage adjustment made. For patient with a platelet count greater than 400×10^9/L, drug should be withheld until platelet count is less than 150×10^9/L and then restarted at a daily dose reduced by 25 mg, unless patient had been taking 25 mg daily, then dosage restarted at 12.5 mg daily.

∗ *To treat thrombocytopenia in patients with chronic hepatitis C infection to allow the initiation and maintenance of interferon-based therapy*

TABLETS

Adults. *Initial:* 25 mg daily, increased in increments of 25 mg daily every 2 wk, as needed, to achieve the target platelet count required to initiate antiviral therapy. *Maximum:* 100 mg daily.

±**DOSAGE ADJUSTMENT** For patients with a platelet count less than 50×10^9/L following at least 2 weeks of therapy, daily dose increased by 25 mg daily to maximum of 100 mg/day. For patients with a platelet count equal to or greater than 200×10^9/L but equal to or less than 400×10^9/L, dosage decreased by 25 mg for at least 2 weeks before further dosage adjustment made. For patient with a platelet count greater than 400×10^9/L, drug should be withheld until platelet count is less than 150×10^9/L and then restarted at a daily dose reduced by 25 mg, unless patient had been taking 25 mg daily, then dosage restarted at 12.5 mg daily. For patient receiving antiviral therapy, dosage adjusted, as needed, to avoid dose reductions of peginterferon.

* *As adjunct with immunosuppressive therapy for first-line treatment of severe aplastic anemia*

ORAL SUSPENSION, TABLETS

Adults and children 12 years and over. 150 mg once daily for 6 months.
Children age 6 to 11 years. 75 mg once daily for 6 months.
Children age 2 to 5 years. 2.5 mg/kg once daily for 6 months.

±**DOSAGE ADJUSTMENT** For patients of Asian ancestry or patients with hepatic impairment, initial dosage decreased by 50%. For patients with a platelet count greater than 400×10^9/L, drug withheld for 1 week. Once platelet count is less than 200×10^9/L, drug restarted at a daily dosage reduced by 25 mg for adults and 12.5 mg for children under age 12. For patients with a platelet count greater than 200×10^9 but equal to or less than 400×10^9, daily adult dose decreased by 25 mg every 2 weeks to lowest dose that maintains platelet count equal to or greater than 50×10^9/L, and for children under the age of 12, dosage decreased by 12.5 mg.

* *To treat refractory severe aplastic anemia in patients who have had an insufficient response to immunosuppressive therapy*

ORAL SUSPENSION, TABLETS

Adults. *Initial:* 50 mg once daily, increased as needed in 50-mg increments every 2 wk. *Maximum:* 150 mg daily.

±**DOSAGE ADJUSTMENT** For patients of Asian ancestry or patients with any degree of hepatic impairment, initial dosage decreased to 25 mg daily. For patients with a platelet count less than 50×10^9/L following at least 2 weeks of therapy, dosage increased by 50 mg daily to maximum of 150 mg daily. For patients taking 25 mg once daily, dosage increased to 50 mg once daily before dosage increased by 50 mg. For patients with a platelet count equal to or greater than 200×10^9/L but equal to or less than 400×10^9/L, dosage decreased by 50 mg daily for at least 2 weeks before further dosage adjustment made. For patient with a platelet count greater than 400×10^9/L, drug should be withheld for 1 week and until platelet count is less than 150×10^9/L and then drug restarted at a daily dose reduced by 50 mg.

▤ Drug Administration

P.O.

- Administer without a meal or a meal low in calcium (containing 50 mg or less).
- Administer at least 2 hours before or 4 hours after other medications such as antacids; calcium-rich foods (more than 50 mg of calcium) such as dairy products, calcium-fortified juices, and certain fruits and vegetables; or supplements containing polyvalent cations such as aluminum, calcium, iron, magnesium, selenium, and zinc.
- Administer tablet whole and not chewed, crushed, or split nor mixed with food or liquids.
- For oral suspension, prepare only with water following instructions that come with drug. Do not use hot water. Use a new single-use syringe to prepare each dose. Do not reuse the syringe. Discard any suspension not administered within 30 minutes after preparation.

Route	Onset	Peak	Duration
P.O.	1–2 wk	2–6 hr	1–2 wk
Half-life: 21–32 hr			

Mechanism of Action

Interacts with the transmembrane domain of the thrombopoietin receptor to signal cascades that induce differentiation and proliferation of megakaryocytes from bone marrow progenitor cells. This action increases platelet production, which is abnormally low in patients with aplastic anemia, chronic hepatitis C, and thrombocytopenic purpura.

Contraindications

Hypersensitivity to eltrombopag or its components

Interactions

DRUGS

antacids and mineral supplements containing aluminum, calcium, iron, magnesium, selenium, or zinc: Decreased eltrombopag absorption
BCRP substrates (imatinib, irinotecan, lapatinib, methotrexate, mitoxantrone, rosuvastatin, sulfasalazine, topotecan), OATP1B1 substrates (atorvastatin, bosentan, ezetimibe, fluvastatin, glyburide, olmesartan, pitavastatin, pravastatin, rosuvastatin, repaglinide, rifampin, simvastatin acid, valsartan): Possibly increased risk of adverse reactions related to excessive exposure to these drugs

FOODS

all foods, especially dairy: Decreased absorption of eltrombopag

Adverse Reactions

CNS: Asthenia, chills, dizziness, fatigue, fever, headache, insomnia, paresthesia
CV: **Arterial and venous thromboembolism,** peripheral edema, **primary portal venous system thromboses** (in presence of chronic liver disease)
EENT: Cataracts, conjunctival hemorrhage, nasopharyngitis, oropharyngeal pain, pharyngitis, rhinitis, rhinorrhea, toothache
GI: Abdominal pain, anorexia, diarrhea, dyspepsia, elevated bilirubin or liver enzymes, **hepatotoxicity,** nausea, vomiting
GU: **Acute renal failure with thrombotic microangiopathy,** menorrhagia, UTI
HEME: Anemia, **aplastic anemia, febrile neutropenia, hemorrhage, thrombocytopenia**
MS: Arthralgia, back or extremity pain, muscle spasm, myalgia
RESP: Cough, dyspnea, upper respiratory tract infection
SKIN: Alopecia, ecchymosis, pruritus, rash, skin discoloration including hyperpigmentation and skin yellowing
Other: Flu-like symptoms

Childbearing Considerations

PREGNANCY

- Drug can cause fetal harm based on animal studies.
- Drug is not recommended for use during pregnancy.

LACTATION

- It is not known if drug is present in breast milk.
- Breastfeeding is not recommended during drug therapy.

REPRODUCTION

- Sexually active females of childbearing age should use effective contraception that results in less than 1% pregnancy rates during drug therapy and for at least 7 days after drug is discontinued.

Nursing Considerations

- Know that eltrombopag should not be used to treat any other kind of thrombocytopenia because of the risk of hematologic malignancies or portal venous system thromboses in patients with chronic liver disease. Also, know the drug should not be used to treat myelodysplastic syndromes because of an increased risk of progression to acute myeloid leukemia which could be fatal.
- Be aware that eltrombopag can be used only through a restricted distribution program called *Promacta Cares*. Patient, pharmacy, and prescriber must all be enrolled before therapy begins.
- Use cautiously in patients with hepatic impairment because drug may cause hepatotoxicity and arterial and venous thrombosis, although most are portal venous system thromboses. This is especially important if patient with hepatic impairment also has risk factors present for thromboembolism.
- Monitor bilirubin level and liver enzymes, as ordered, before starting eltrombopag, every 2 weeks during dosage adjustment, and monthly once dose is stable except for treatment for first-line treatment of severe

aplastic anemia. For this indication, monitor bilirubin level and liver enzymes, as ordered, before starting eltrombopag, every other day while hospitalized for horse antithymocyte globulin (h-ATG) therapy, and then every 2 weeks during treatment. If abnormalities occur, repeat testing within 3 to 5 days and then weekly until liver enzymes return to baseline. Expect to discontinue drug if alanine aminotransferase level (ALT) increases to 3 or more times the upper normal limit, progresses or persists for 4 or more weeks, or is accompanied by an increase in direct bilirubin or clinical symptoms of liver injury.

- Know that there is an increased risk of hepatic decomposition when eltrombopag is used in combination with interferon and ribavirin in patients with chronic hepatitis C. Monitor these patients closely for evidence of hepatic dysfunction.
- Expect to monitor platelet counts every week prior to starting antiviral therapy, as ordered, for patient with hepatitis C. Once antiviral therapy has started, expect to monitor CBCs with differentials including platelet counts weekly during antiviral therapy until a stable platelet count is achieved. Thereafter, monitor platelet counts monthly, as ordered.
- Know that patient should have a baseline eye examination, as ordered, before starting eltrombopag and periodically throughout therapy, because drug may cause cataracts.
- Be aware that dosage adjustments are based on platelet count response and are not used to normalize platelet counts in order to prevent or minimize thrombotic complications.
- Expect to discontinue drug for patient with persistent or chronic thrombocytopenia if improvement doesn't occur within 4 weeks at maximum dose of 75 mg daily or if the platelet count remains greater than 400×10^9/L after 2 weeks of therapy at the lowest dose of eltrombopag. Expect to discontinue drug for patient with hepatitis C if the platelet count remains greater than 400×10^9/L after 2 weeks of therapy at the lowest dose of eltrombopag or when antiviral therapy is discontinued. Expect to discontinue drug for patient with severe aplastic anemia if improvement doesn't occur after 16 weeks of therapy.

- Monitor patient for hematologic malignancies because eltrombopag stimulates thrombopoietin receptor on the surface of hematopoietic cells, which increases risk of malignancies.
- Monitor patient for increased bleeding after stopping eltrombopag because thrombocytopenia may worsen, increasing bleeding risk, especially if patient is on anticoagulants or antiplatelet therapy. If bleeding occurs, obtain weekly CBC, including platelet count, for at least 4 weeks after therapy stops, and provide supportive care, as indicated and ordered.

PATIENT TEACHING

- Inform patient that before eltrombopag therapy can begin, he must be enrolled in the *Promacta Cares* program, which provides comprehensive education about the drug.
- Urge patient to tell prescriber about all health conditions and all prescribed drugs, OTC drugs, herbs, and supplements taken.
- Tell patient to prepare the prescribed oral suspension using water only, but not hot water, and to ingest immediately after preparation. Any suspension not used should be discarded within 30 minutes. Remind patient that a new oral dosing syringe should be used to prepare every dose of oral suspension.
- Instruct patient to take eltrombopag on an empty stomach with a full glass of water or take drug with a meal low in calcium and at least 2 hours before or 4 hours after eating calcium-rich foods such as calcium-fortified juices, certain fruits and vegetables, and dairy products.
- Tell patient to separate use of other drugs by administering 2 hours before or 4 hours after other medications (such as antacids and iron and vitamin supplements) which may interfere with eltrombopag absorption.
- Instruct patient to take drug at the same time every day because no more than one dose should be taken within any 24-hour period because too much of the drug may cause blood clots.
- Encourage patient to have regular eye exams because drug may increase the development of cataracts.
- Urge patient to report any adverse reactions, especially signs and symptoms of liver problems such as confusion, right upper

E
F

stomach area pain or swelling, tiredness or unusual darkening of the urine, or yellowing of the skin or the whites of the eyes, to prescriber. In addition, tell patient to keep all appointments for blood work and follow-up.

- Review bleeding precautions with patient. Tell him that he may be at increased risk for bleeding and should follow bleeding precautions even after drug is discontinued, especially if he is also taking a drug that affects the ability to clot. He should seek medical attention if serious bleeding occurs.
- Inform women of childbearing age to use effective contraception throughout eltrombopag therapy and for at least 7 days after drug is discontinued, because drug may cause fetal harm. If pregnancy is suspected or occurs, prescriber should be notified immediately.
- Tell mothers wishing to breastfeed that breastfeeding is not recommended during eltrombopag therapy.

eluxadoline
Viberzi

Class, Category, and Schedule
Pharmacologic class: Mu-opioid receptor agonist
Therapeutic class: Antidiarrheal
Controlled substance sche*du*le: IV

Indications and Dosages
∗ *To treat irritable bowel syndrome with diarrhea (IBS-D)*

TABLETS
Adults. 100 mg twice daily.

±**DOSAGE ADJUSTMENT** For patients who are unable to tolerate the 100-mg dose, who are receiving concomitant OATP1B1 inhibitors, have moderate to severe renal impairment including end-stage renal disease, or who have mild to moderate hepatic impairment, dosage reduced to 75 mg twice daily.

Drug Administration
P.O.
- Administer drug with food.

Route	Onset	Peak	Duration
P.O.	Unknown	1.5–2 hr	Unknown

Half-life: 3.7–6 hr

Mechanism of Action
Interacts with opioid receptors in the intestines to relieve diarrhea.

Contraindications
Absence of a gallbladder, alcoholism, or patients who drink more than three alcoholic beverages daily, biliary duct obstruction, history of pancreatitis or structural disease of the pancreas, history of chronic or severe constipation, hypersensitivity to eluxadoline or its components, known or suspected mechanical gastrointestinal obstruction, severe hepatic impairment, sphincter of Oddi disease, or dysfunction

Interactions
DRUGS
alosetron, anticholinergics, opioids, or other drugs that cause constipation: Increased risk of constipation and constipation-related adverse reactions
OATP1B1 inhibitors such as antivirals, cyclosporine, eltrombopag, gemfibrozil, rifampin: Increased exposure to eluxadoline increasing risk of adverse reactions
rosuvastatin: Increased exposure to rosuvastatin with increased risk for myopathy and rhabdomyolysis

ACTIVITIES
alcohol use: Increased risk for acute pancreatitis

Adverse Reactions
CNS: Dizziness, euphoria, fatigue, sedation, sensation of feeling drunk, somnolence
CV: Chest pain or tightness
EENT: Nasopharyngitis, **throat tightness**
GI: Abdominal distention or pain, constipation (which may become severe), elevated liver enzymes, flatulence, gastroesophageal reflux disease, nausea, **pancreatitis**, sphincter of Oddi spasm, vomiting
RESP: Asthma, bronchitis, **bronchospasm**, dyspnea, **respiratory failure**, upper respiratory infection, wheezing
SKIN: Pruritus, rash, urticaria
Other: Anaphylaxis, angioedema

Childbearing Considerations
PREGNANCY
- It is not known if drug causes fetal harm.
- Use with caution only if benefit to mother outweighs potential risk to fetus.

E
F

LACTATION

- It is not known if drug is present in breast milk.
- Patient should check with prescriber before breastfeeding.

☰ Nursing Considerations

- Assess patient's alcohol intake prior to starting eluxadoline therapy. Also, question patient about gallbladder removal surgery, as drug is contraindicated in patients without a gallbladder.

! WARNING Monitor patient closely for hypersensitivity reactions that could include anaphylaxis, angioedema, difficulty breathing or swallowing, and skin reactions such as itching, rash, or urticaria. If present, notify prescriber immediately, stop administering drug, and provide emergency supportive care, as ordered.

- Monitor patient closely for acute abdominal pain, especially during the first few weeks of therapy, because mu-opioid receptor agonism increases risk for sphincter of Oddi spasm, which could result in elevated liver enzymes or pancreatitis. If present, notify prescriber and expect eluxadoline to be discontinued.
- Monitor patient's liver enzymes, as ordered and report any elevations to prescriber.
- Notify prescriber if patient develops severe constipation and expect drug to be discontinued. Severe cases of fecal impaction or intestinal obstruction or perforation have occurred with severe constipation, requiring emergency intervention.

PATIENT TEACHING

- Instruct patient to take drug with food.
- Tell patient that if she misses a dose to take the next dose at the regular time and not to double up the dose to make up for a missed dose.
- Warn patient against acute excessive or chronic alcohol intake while taking eluxadoline.

! WARNING Instruct patient to stop taking eluxadoline and immediately seek medical attention if she experiences acute epigastric or right, upper quadrant abdominal pain that may radiate to the back or shoulder and may be accompanied by nausea and vomiting.

Also tell patient to seek immediate medical attention if a serious allergic reaction occurs.

- Tell patient to notify prescriber immediately if she develops severe constipation and not to use other drugs that may cause constipation during eluxadoline therapy.
- Advise patient to inform all prescribers of eluxadoline therapy.
- Tell patient not to take other drugs to treat diarrheal symptoms unless prescribed and the prescriber is aware of eluxadoline use.

empagliflozin
Jardiance

☰ Class and Category

Pharmacologic class: Sodium glucose cotransporter 2 inhibitor
Therapeutic class: Antidiabetic

☰ Indications and Dosages

✳ *Adjunct to diet and exercise to improve glycemic control in patients with type 2 diabetes mellitus*

TABLETS

Adults with an estimated glomerular filtration rate of 30 ml/min or greater.
10 mg once daily, increased to 25 mg once daily as needed

✳ *To reduce risk of cardiovascular death in patients with type 2 diabetes mellitus who have established cardiovascular disease*

TABLETS

Adults with an estimated glomerular filtration rate of 30 ml/min or greater.
10 mg once daily.

✳ *To reduce the risk of cardiovascular death plus hospitalization for heart failure in adults with heart failure and reduced ejection fraction*

TABLETS

Adults with an estimated glomerular filtration rate of 20 ml/min or greater.
10 mg once daily.

☰ Drug Administration

P.O.

- Administer drug in the morning.
- Ensure that patient is well hydrated when administering drug; otherwise drug may have to be temporarily withheld.

Route	Onset	Peak	Duration
P.O.	Unknown	1.5 hr	3 days

Half-life: 12.4 hr

Mechanism of Action

Inhibits sodium glucose cotransporter 2 in the kidneys, which prevents glucose reabsorption. This decreases blood glucose levels.

Contraindications

Dialysis therapy, end-stage renal disease, hypersensitivity to empagliflozin or its components, severe renal impairment

Interactions

DRUGS

diuretics: Increased risk of acute kidney injury and renal impairment in presence of dehydration

insulin, insulin secretagogues: Increased risk of hypoglycemia

Adverse Reactions

CNS: Syncope
CV: Dyslipidemia, elevated low-density lipoprotein cholesterol, **hypotension**
ENDO: **Ketoacidosis**
GI: Nausea
GU: **Acute kidney injury**, decreased estimated glomerular filtration rate, dysuria, elevated serum creatinine levels, genital mycotic infections, impaired renal function, increased urination, **necrotizing fasciitis of the perineum (Fournier's gangrene)**, osmotic diuresis, **pyelonephritis**, **urosepsis**, UTI
MS: Arthralgia, increased risk of bone fracture
RESP: Upper respiratory tract infection
SKIN: Rash, urticaria
Other: **Angioedema**, dehydration

Childbearing Considerations

PREGNANCY

- Drug may cause adverse renal effects to the developing fetus.
- Drug is not recommended for use during the second and third trimester of pregnancy.

LACTATION

- It is not known if drug is present in breast milk.
- Women should not breastfeed their infant while taking drug because kidney maturation continues through the first 2 years of life.

Nursing Considerations

- Assess patient's volume status and correct, if needed and as prescribed, prior to starting empagliflozin therapy because drug can cause intravascular volume contraction leading to symptomatic hypotension and acute kidney injury. Continue to monitor patient throughout therapy for dehydration and renal dysfunction. Patients at highest risk include the elderly and patients with chronic renal insufficiency, congestive heart failure, and hypovolemia or patients who take diuretics. Notify prescriber immediately if patient has fluid losses or reduced oral intake, as acute kidney injury may occur. Expect that drug may be temporarily withheld until fluid balance can be restored.
- Obtain serum creatinine level, as ordered, prior to starting empagliflozin therapy because empagliflozin can cause adverse renal effects. Be aware that the elderly and patients with existing impaired renal function are at higher risk for these adverse effects. Monitor renal function throughout therapy.

! **WARNING** Monitor patient for hypersensitivity reactions that could be serious, such as the development of angioedema. If present, withhold drug, notify prescriber immediately, and be prepared to provide emergency supportive care, as ordered.

- Monitor patient's blood pressure and cholesterol level throughout empagliflozin therapy.
- Be aware that patients receiving insulin or insulin secretagogues may require a lower dose of these agents because empagliflozin in combination increases risk of hypoglycemia. Monitor patient closely for hypoglycemia. If present, treat according to standard of care and notify prescriber.

! **WARNING** Monitor patient closely for ketoacidosis that has occurred in patients with type 2 diabetes being treated with empagliflozin. Be aware that ketoacidosis can become life-threatening quickly even when blood glucose levels are less than 250 mg/dl. Notify prescriber immediately if ketoacidosis is suspected and expect drug to be discontinued. Be prepared to treat patient's ketoacidosis, as ordered. Be aware that patients at higher risk include patients with a history of alcohol abuse or who have a pancreatic insulin deficiency from any cause or have reduced caloric intake. Expect drug to be temporarily discontinued if patient must undergo prolonged fasting due to acute illness or surgery.

- Monitor patients for genital mycotic infections or urinary tract infections, especially those with a history of such. If present, notify prescriber and treat, as prescribed.

! **WARNING** Monitor patient for a rare but serious and life-threatening necrotizing infection of the perineum called Fournier's gangrene. Notify prescriber immediately if patient develops erythema, pain, swelling, or tenderness in the genital or perineal area, along with fever or malaise. Expect treatment with broad-spectrum antibiotics and, if needed, surgical debridement of the area. Know that empagliflozin will be discontinued if this occurs. Monitor patient's blood glucose levels closely and expect an alternative treatment for glycemic control.

PATIENT TEACHING
- Inform patient that empagliflozin therapy is not a replacement for diet and exercise therapy.
- Instruct patient to take drug in the morning.

! **WARNING** Tell patient that drug may cause an allergic reaction such as swelling of the eyes, face, throat, and tongue. It may also cause skin reactions such as a rash or hives. If present, stress importance of stopping drug and seeking immediate emergency medical treatment.

- Instruct patient on the signs and symptoms of hypoglycemia and how to treat it. Inform patient who is also receiving insulin or a sulfonylurea that the risk of hypoglycemia is greater. Tell patient to notify prescriber if hypoglycemia occurs frequently or is severe.
- Tell patient to monitor the blood glucose level using blood tests instead of urine tests because

drug increases urinary glucose excretion and will lead to positive urine glucose tests.
- Review signs and symptoms of ketoacidosis with patient and urge her to seek immediate medical attention, if present, even if blood glucose level is less than 250 mg/dl.
- Advise female patients to notify prescriber if pregnancy occurs or is suspected. Also advise women that breastfeeding is not recommended while taking empagliflozin.
- Advise patient to maintain adequate fluid intake throughout empagliflozin therapy. However, tell patient to notify prescriber if she is unable to take a normal amount of daily fluids due to fasting or illness or experiences an excessive loss of fluids from excessive perspiration or gastrointestinal illnesses. Drug may have to be temporarily withheld.
- Stress importance of notifying prescriber if patient develops dehydration, has onset of hunger or thirst, or notices a sudden change in mental status. Tell patient not to belittle these symptoms and seek medical attention quickly.

! **WARNING** Warn patient to stop empagliflozin and seek immediate medical attention if pain, redness, swelling, or tenderness occurs in the genital or perineal area, along with fever or malaise because, although rare, this cluster of symptoms may become life-threatening.

- Teach patient to take fall precautions and other safety measures because drug may increase risk of bone fracture as early as 12 weeks after empagliflozin therapy is begun.
- Warn patient that drug may increase risk for urinary tract and yeast infections for both men and women. Review signs and symptoms and advise patient to notify prescriber if present.

emtricitabine
Emtriva

≡ Class and Category
Pharmacologic class: Nucleoside analogue
Therapeutic class: Antiretroviral

≡ Indications and Dosages
* As adjunct to treat human immunodeficiency virus type 1 (HIV-1) infection

CAPSULES, ORAL SOLUTION

Adults. 200 mg (capsule) or 240 mg (oral solution) once daily.

CAPSULES

Children ages 3 months to 18 years who weigh more than 33 kg (72.6 lb) and can swallow an intact capsule. 200 mg once daily.

ORAL SOLUTION

Children ages 3 months to 18 years. 6 mg/kg up to maximum of 240 mg once daily.
Newborns and infants up to 3 months. 3 mg/kg once daily.

± **DOSAGE ADJUSTMENT** For adult patients with a creatinine clearance of 30 to 49 ml/min, dosage interval increased to every 48 hr if using capsules or dosage reduced to 120 mg once daily if using oral solution. For adult patients with a creatinine clearance of 15 to 29 ml/min, dosage interval increased to every 72 hr if using capsules or dosage reduced to 80 mg once daily if using oral solution. For adult patients with a creatinine clearance of less than 15 ml/min or who are on hemodialysis, dosage interval increased to every 96 hr if using capsules or dosage reduced to 60 mg once daily if using oral solution. For pediatric patients with renal impairment, there is insufficient data to recommend a specific dose adjustment, but a reduction in dose and/or an increase in dosing interval similar to adults may be considered.

Drug Administration

P.O.

- Keep in original container tightly closed.
- Capsules should be swallowed whole and not opened.
- Use calibrated device to measure oral solution dosage. Solution should be clear but orange to dark orange in color.
- Oral solution should be refrigerated. However, if stored at room temperature, discard after 3 months.

Route	Onset	Peak	Duration
P.O.	Unknown	1–2 hr	Unknown

Half-life: 10 hr

Mechanism of Action

Phosphorylated by cellular enzymes, emtricitabine then inhibits the activity of the HIV-1 reverse transcriptase by competing with the natural substrate and by being incorporated into the nascent viral DNA, which leads to chain termination of the HIV virus.

Contraindications

Hypersensitivity to emtricitabine or its components

Interactions

DRUGS

None reported by manufacturer

Adverse Reactions

CNS: Abnormal dreams, asthenia, depression, dizziness, fatigue, fever, headache, insomnia, neuropathy, paresthesia, peripheral neuritis
CV: Elevated cholesterol and triglycerides
EENT: Nasopharyngitis, otitis media, rhinitis, sinusitis
ENDO: Cushingoid appearance, fat redistribution, hyperglycemia
GI: Abdominal pain; diarrhea; dyspepsia; elevated amylase, bilirubin, lipase, and liver enzymes; gastroenteritis; nausea; **severe acute exacerbations of hepatitis B; severe hepatomegaly with steatosis;** vomiting
GU: Glycosuria, hematuria, new onset or worsening of renal impairment
HEME: Anemia, decreased hemoglobin, **neutropenia**
MS: Arthralgia, elevated creatine kinase, myalgia
RESP: Increased cough, pneumonia, upper respiratory infections
SKIN: Hyperpigmentation on palms and/or soles, pruritus, rash, urticaria
Other: Elevated alkaline phosphatase, immune reconstitution syndrome, infection, **lactic acidosis**

Childbearing Considerations

PREGNANCY

- Pregnancy exposure registry: 1-800-258-4263.
- It is not known if drug causes fetal harm.
- Use with caution only if benefit to mother outweighs potential risk to fetus.

LACTATION

- Drug may be present in breast milk.
- The Centers for Disease Control and Prevention recommends that HIV-1 infected mothers not breastfeed to avoid

risking postnatal transmission of HIV-1 infection to infants. They also do not recommend breastfeeding because of potential drug-induced adverse reactions in the infant.

≣ Nursing Considerations

- Expect to test patient for hepatitis B virus (HBV) prior to starting emtricitabine, as ordered. This is because acute exacerbations of hepatitis B have occurred after patient has discontinued the drug. Know that in some cases the exacerbation resulted in liver failure.
- Monitor patient's liver enzymes throughout therapy and for several months after drug is discontinued, because lactic acidosis and severe hepatomegaly with steatosis have occurred with emtricitabine therapy, as have acute exacerbations of hepatitis B with patients coinfected. Know that most cases of lactic acidosis and severe hepatomegaly with steatosis have occurred in women with prolonged nucleoside exposure and obesity. Report abnormal liver function signs and symptoms to prescriber, such as abdominal discomfort, jaundice, nausea, vomiting, or weakness.
- Perform a complete drug history on patient, because combination drugs containing emtricitabine (Atripla, Complera, Truvada) should not be given concurrently with emtricitabine therapy. Also, expect not to coadminister drugs containing lamivudine (Combivir, Epivir, Epivir-HBV, Epzicom, Trizivir) because of the similarities between emtricitabine and lamivudine.
- Monitor patient's renal function, because drug is primarily eliminated by the kidney and dosage alterations are necessary for those with impaired kidney function.
- Be aware that immune reconstitution syndrome has occurred in patients treated with combination antiretroviral therapy, including emtricitabine. The inflammatory response predisposes susceptible patients to opportunistic infections such as cytomegalovirus, *Mycobacterium avium* infection, *Pneumocystis jiroveci* pneumonia, or tuberculosis. Autoimmune disorders such as Graves' disease, Guillain–Barré syndrome, or polymyositis have also occurred. Report sudden or unusual adverse reactions to prescriber.

PATIENT TEACHING

- Instruct patient or caregiver that a calibrated device should be used to measure dose of oral solution, not a household spoon. Also tell patient to store oral solution in refrigerator; if stored at room temperature, it should be discarded after 3 months.
- Tell patient or caregiver to swallow capsule whole and not to chew, crush, or open it.
- Inform patient that emtricitabine will be prescribed along with other antiviral drugs.
- Review signs and symptoms of liver dysfunction (belly discomfort, nausea, vomiting, weakness, yellowing of skin or whites of eyes) and stress importance of reporting any occurrence to prescriber.
- Instruct patient to remind all prescribers of emtricitabine therapy.
- Inform patient that emtricitabine therapy may cause changes in his body appearance because of fat redistribution. Prepare him for the possibility of developing breast enlargement, central obesity, dorsocervical fat enlargement (buffalo hump), facial wasting, and peripheral wasting.
- Instruct patient to report any persistent, severe, or unusual signs and symptoms.
- Alert mothers that breastfeeding is not recommended during emtricitabine therapy.

enalapril maleate
Epaned, Vasotec

enalaprilat

≣ Class and Category
Pharmacologic class: Angiotensin-converting enzyme (ACE) inhibitor
Therapeutic class: Antihypertensive, vasodilator

≣ Indications and Dosages
⁜ *To control hypertension*

ORAL SOLUTION, TABLETS
Adults. *Initial:* 5 mg daily, increased after 1 to 2 wk, as needed. *Maintenance:* 10 to 40 mg once daily or in divided doses twice daily. *Maximum:* 40 mg daily.
Children older than 1 month. 0.08 mg/kg daily, titrated according to blood pressure

response up to 5 mg daily. *Maximum:*
0.58 mg/kg/dose (40 mg).

I.V. INFUSION, I.V. INJECTION

Adults. 1.25 mg every 6 hr.

±**DOSAGE ADJUSTMENT** Initial dose reduced
to 2.5 mg P.O. or 0.625 mg I.V. for patients
who have sodium and water depletion from
diuretic therapy, are receiving diuretics, or
adults who have a creatinine clearance below
30 ml/min (not used in children who have a
glomerular filtration rate below 30 ml/min).
For patient who is receiving a diuretic, if
response to I.V. dose is inadequate after 1 hr,
I.V. dose of 0.625 mg repeated and therapy
continued at 1.25 mg every 6 hr.

✱ *To convert from I.V. to oral dosage form*
Adults. *Initial:* 5 mg once daily, then
increased as needed.

±**DOSAGE ADJUSTMENT** For patient with a
creatinine clearance of 30 ml/min or less,
dosage reduced to 2.5 mg once daily.

✱ *To convert from oral to I.V. dosage form*
Adults. *Initial:* 1.25 mg every 6 hr.

✱ *To treat symptomatic heart failure*

ORAL SOLUTION, TABLETS

Adults. *Initial:* 2.5 mg twice daily, increased
after 1 to 2 wk, as needed. *Maintenance:* 5 to
40 mg daily in 2 divided doses. *Maximum:*
40 mg daily in 2 divided doses.

±**DOSAGE ADJUSTMENT** For patients with
hyponatremia (serum sodium less than
130 mEq/L) or serum creatinine greater than
1.6 mg/dl, initial dosage reduced to 2.5 mg
once daily.

✱ *To treat asymptomatic left ventricular*
dysfunction, to decrease the rate of
development of overt heart failure and reduce
hospitalization for heart failure

ORAL SOLUTION, TABLETS

Adults. *Initial:* 2.5 mg twice daily, increased
to 20 mg daily in 2 divided doses, as tolerated.

☰ Drug Administration

P.O.

- Tablets are to be swallowed whole and not
chewed, crushed, or split.
- Ask for oral solution reconstituted by
pharmacist for patient who cannot swallow
tablets.
- Use a calibrated device to measure oral
solution dosage. No shaking needed prior to
measuring each dose.

- Store oral solution at room temperature.
Discard oral solution after 60 days.

I.V.

- May be administered undiluted or diluted
with up to 50 ml of a compatible diluent
such as 0.9% Sodium Chloride Injection, 5%
Dextrose Injection, 0.9% Sodium Chloride
Injection with 5% Dextrose, or 5% Dextrose
in Lactated Ringer's Injection, or Isolyte*E.
- Solution should be clear and colorless.
- Administer, if undiluted, as an I.V. injection
slowly over at least 5 minutes or if diluted,
administer as an I.V. infusion slowly over
5 minutes or longer. Administer up to
one hour for patients at risk of excessive
hypotension, as ordered.
- I.V. administration usually not
recommended for more than 7 days.
- *Incompatibilities:* Y-site administration of
amphotericin B, cefepime, phenytoin

Route	Onset	Peak	Duration
P.O.	1 hr	4–6 hr	24 hr
I.V.	15 min	1–4 hr	6 hr

Half-life: 11 hr

☰ Mechanism of Action

May reduce blood pressure and development
of heart failure by affecting the renin–
angiotensin–aldosterone system. By
inhibiting angiotensin-converting enzyme
(ACE), enalapril:

- prevents conversion of angiotensin I to
angiotensin II, a potent vasoconstrictor that
also stimulates the adrenal cortex to secrete
aldosterone
- may inhibit renal and vascular production
of angiotensin II
- decreases the serum angiotensin II level
and increases serum renin activity, which
decreases aldosterone secretion and slightly
increases serum potassium level and fluid loss
- decreases vascular tone and blood pressure
- inhibits aldosterone release, which reduces
sodium and water reabsorption and
increases their excretion, further reducing
blood pressure and development of heart
failure.

☰ Contraindications

Concurrent aliskiren therapy in patients
with diabetes; concurrent therapy with a

neprilysin inhibitor such as sacubitril, history of hereditary or idiopathic angioedema; hypersensitivity to enalapril, enalaprilat, other ACE inhibitors, or their components; use within 36 hours of sacubitril/valsartan therapy

Interactions

DRUGS

aliskiren, angiotensin receptor blockers, other ACE inhibitors: Increased risk of hyperkalemia, hypotension, and renal dysfunction
diuretics, other antihypertensives: Additive hypotensive effects
lithium: Increased blood lithium level and lithium toxicity
mTOR inhibitors (everolimus, sirolimus, temsirolimus); neprilysin inhibitor (sacubitril): Increased risk of angioedema
NSAIDs including selective cyclooxygenase-2 inhibitors: Possibly reduced antihypertensive effects of enalapril and enalaprilat; possibly increased risk of renal dysfunction, especially in the elderly or who are volume-depleted or already have compromised renal function
potassium-sparing diuretics, potassium supplements: Increased risk of hyperkalemia
sodium aurothiomalate: Increased risk of nitritoid reactions, such as facial flushing, nausea, vomiting, and hypotension
thiazide diuretics: Increased loss of potassium

FOODS

potassium-containing salt substitutes: Increased risk of hyperkalemia

Adverse Reactions

CNS: Ataxia, confusion, **CVA**, depression, dizziness, dream disturbances, fatigue, headache, insomnia, nervousness, peripheral neuropathy, somnolence, syncope, vertigo, weakness
CV: Angina, **arrhythmias**, **cardiac arrest**, **hypotension**, **MI**, orthostatic hypotension, palpitations, Raynaud's phenomenon
EENT: Blurred vision, conjunctivitis, dry eyes and mouth, glossitis, hoarseness, lacrimation, loss of smell, pharyngitis, rhinorrhea, stomatitis, taste perversion, tinnitus
ENDO: Gynecomastia
GI: Abdominal pain, anorexia, constipation, diarrhea, **hepatic failure**, **hepatitis**, ileus, indigestion, **melena**, nausea, **pancreatitis**, vomiting
GU: Flank pain, impotence, oliguria, **renal failure**, UTI
MS: Muscle spasms
RESP: Asthma, bronchitis, **bronchospasm**, cough, dyspnea, pneumonia, **pulmonary edema**, **pulmonary embolism and infarction**, **pulmonary infiltrates**, upper respiratory tract infection
SKIN: Alopecia, diaphoresis, **erythema multiforme**, **exfoliative dermatitis**, flushing, pemphigus, photosensitivity, pruritus, rash, **Stevens–Johnson syndrome**, **toxic epidermal necrolysis**, urticaria
Other: **Anaphylaxis**, **angioedema**, herpes zoster, **hyperkalemia**

Childbearing Considerations

PREGNANCY

- Drug may cause adverse renal effects to the developing fetus, especially in the second and third trimester.
- Drug should be discontinued when pregnancy is known.

LACTATION

- Drug is present in breast milk.
- Women should not breastfeed their infant while taking drug because kidney maturation continues through the first 2 years of life.

Nursing Considerations

- Use enalapril and enalaprilat cautiously in patients with impaired renal function.
- Measure patient's blood pressure immediately after first dose and frequently for at least 2 hours thereafter. If hypotension develops, place patient in a supine position and expect to give I.V. 0.9% Sodium Chloride Injection or other volume expander, as prescribed. If hypotension requires a dosage reduction, monitor blood pressure frequently for 2 hours after reduced dosage is administered and for another hour after blood pressure has stabilized.
- Monitor patient's heart rate and rhythm. Expect to obtain repeated 12-lead ECG tracings.
- Monitor laboratory test results to check hepatic and renal function, leukocyte count, and serum potassium level.

E
F

! WARNING Monitor patient closely for angioedema of the face, glottis, larynx, limbs, lips, and tongue. Notify prescriber and stop drug administration immediately. Expect to give an antihistamine, as prescribed. If glottis, larynx, or tongue is involved, assess patient for airway obstruction and prepare to give epinephrine 1:1,000 (0.3 to 0.5 ml) subcutaneously and maintain a patent airway.

PATIENT TEACHING

- Advise patient to take drug at the same time each day.
- Instruct patient not to chew, crush, or split tablets.
- Tell patient oral solution may be stored at room temperature, with any remaining solution discarded after 6 months. Advise patient to use a calibrated device when measuring dose.
- Inform patient that fainting and light-headedness may occur, especially during first few days of therapy. Advise him to change position slowly and avoid hazardous activities until drug's CNS effects are known.
- Inform patient that diarrhea, excessive sweating, vomiting, and other conditions may cause dehydration, which can lead to dizziness, fainting, and very low blood pressure during therapy. Urge sufficient fluid intake to prevent dehydration and related adverse reactions. If diarrhea or vomiting is severe or prolonged, instruct patient to notify prescriber.

! WARNING Urge patient to stop taking drug and immediately seek emergency care if swelling of extremities, face, lips, throat, or tongue occurs. Also tell patient to notify prescriber if other adverse reactions, including persistent dry cough, occur.

- Advise patient to consult prescriber before using potassium supplements, salt substitutes, or other drugs (including OTC drugs) while taking drug.

! WARNING Caution women of childbearing age that they should use a reliable form of contraception and should notify prescriber immediately if pregnancy is suspected.

enfuvirtide
Fuzeon

Class and Category
Pharmacologic class: Fusion inhibitor
Therapeutic class: Antiretroviral

Indications and Dosages
* As adjunct to treat human immunodeficiency virus type 1 (HIV-1) infection in treatment-experienced patients with HIV-1 replication despite ongoing antiretroviral therapy

SUBCUTANEOUS INJECTION
Adults. 90 mg twice daily.
Children weighing at least 11 kg (24.2 lb). 2 mg/kg twice daily. *Maximum:* 90 mg twice daily.

Drug Administration
SUBCUTANEOUS

- Reconstitute with 1 ml of Sterile Water for Injection provided in the convenience kit. Then gently tap vial for 10 seconds, followed by gently rolling vial between hands to avoid foaming and to ensure that all particles of drug are in contact with the liquid. Let vial stand until powder is completely dissolved, which may take up to 45 minutes. If the solution is foamy or jelled, allow more time for it to dissolve.
- Once reconstituted, use immediately or keep refrigerated in the original vial for up to 24 hours. If refrigerated, allow reconstituted solution to come to room temperature before administration and recheck that drug is still fully dissolved and appears clear, colorless, and without bubbles or particulate matter.
- Administer into patient's abdomen, anterior thigh, or upper arm using the Biojector 2000 needle-free device or a needle and syringe.
- Rotate site of injections, avoiding injecting into any anatomical areas where large nerves course close to the skin; directly over a blood vessel; or into skin abnormalities such as bruises, burn sites, moles, near the navel, scar tissue, surgical scars, or tattoos.

Route	Onset	Peak	Duration
SubQ	Unknown	4–8 hr	Unknown

Half-life: 3.8 hr

Mechanism of Action

Interferes with the entry of HIV-1 into cells to inhibit fusion of cellular membranes with the virus. It does this by binding to the viral envelope glycoprotein and preventing the conformational changes required for the fusion.

Contraindications

Hypersensitivity to enfuvirtide or its components

Interactions

DRUGS

None reported by manufacturer

Adverse Reactions

CNS: Anxiety, asthenia, chills, depression, fatigue, fever, **Guillain–Barré syndrome**, insomnia, peripheral neuropathy, rigors, sixth nerve palsy, **suicidal ideation**
CV: Elevated triglycerides, **hypotension, unstable angina pectoris**
EENT: Conjunctivitis, dry mouth, sinusitis, taste disturbance
ENDO: Hyperglycemia
GI: Anorexia; constipation; diarrhea; elevated amylase, lipase, and liver enzymes; hepatic steatosis; nausea; **pancreatitis; toxic hepatitis**; upper abdominal pain; vomiting
GU: Glomerulonephritis, renal failure or insufficiency, tubular necrosis
HEME: Eosinophilia, **neutropenia, thrombocytopenia**
MS: Elevated creatine phosphokinase, extremity pain, myalgia
RESP: Cough, pneumonia (bacterial), respiratory distress
SKIN: Cutaneous amyloidosis at injection site, folliculitis, pruritus, rash
Other: Formation of anti-enfuvirtide antibodies, flu-like symptoms, herpes simplex infection, immune reconstitution syndrome, local injection-site reactions (bruising, cyst formation, discomfort, ecchymosis, erythema, hematomas, **hypersensitivity reaction**, induration, infection, neuralgia, nodule formation, pain, paresthesia, pruritus), lymphadenopathy, post-injection bleeding, **sepsis**, weight loss

Childbearing Considerations

PREGNANCY

- Pregnancy exposure registry: 1-800-258-4263.
- It is not known if drug causes fetal harm.

- Use with caution only if benefit to mother outweighs potential risk to fetus.

LACTATION

- It is not known if drug is present in breast milk.
- The Centers for Disease Control and Prevention recommends that HIV-1 infected mothers not breastfeed to avoid risking postnatal transmission of HIV-1 infection to infants. They also do not recommend breastfeeding because of potential drug-induced adverse reactions in the infant.

Nursing Considerations

- Assess patient's injection site for local adverse reactions, because most patients experience at least one local injection-site reaction. Be especially alert for infection such as cellulitis or a local infection. Provide supportive care, as ordered, to manage injection-site reactions.
- Monitor patient's respiratory status closely, as bacterial pneumonia may occur and be serious enough to warrant hospitalization. Be especially alert for pneumonia in patients with a high initial viral load, history of intravenous drug use, low initial CD4 lymphocyte count, prior history of lung disease, or who are smokers.

! **WARNING** Monitor patient for hypersensitivity reactions, which may be come life-threatening. Be alert for systemic hypersensitivity reactions associated with enfuvirtide therapy, which may include chills, fever, hypotension, nausea, rash, rigors, and vomiting. Elevated liver enzymes may also occur. If present, notify prescriber, expect drug to be discontinued and provide emergency care, as prescribed.

- Know that enfuvirtide may cause formation of anti-enfuvirtide antibodies, which may result in a false positive HIV test with an ELISA assay.
- Be aware that immune reconstitution syndrome has occurred in patients treated with combination antiretroviral therapy, including enfuvirtide. The inflammatory response predisposes susceptible patients to opportunistic infections such as cytomegalovirus, *Mycobacterium avium* infection, *Pneumocystis jiroveci* pneumonia,

E
F

or tuberculosis. Autoimmune disorders such as Graves' disease, Guillain–Barré syndrome, or polymyositis have also occurred. Report sudden or unusual adverse reactions to prescriber.

- Watch patient closely for suicidal ideation.

PATIENT TEACHING

- Inform patient that enfuvirtide therapy will be used in conjunction with other antiretroviral agents.
- Review how to reconstitute enfuvirtide and how to properly store it if not used immediately. Remind patient that drug does not contain a preservative and therefore must be refrigerated and used within 24 hours after being reconstituted. If refrigerated, tell patient that drug must be brought naturally to room temperature before administering.
- Instruct patient on how to properly use the Biojector 2000 device used to administer enfuvirtide subcutaneously, if needed. Otherwise, instruct her on how to use a needle and syringe and how to give a subcutaneous injection.
- Tell patient that drug should only be injected into her abdomen, front of her thigh, or in her upper arms. Sites must be rotated and drug should not be injected into any abnormal skin area, including tattoos, not near the navel, and not over blood vessels or large nerves close to the skin such as the back or side of thigh or near the elbow, groin, or knee. Advise patient how to safely discard used equipment such as needles and syringes.
- Advise patient to alert prescriber to persistent or severe local injection-site adverse reactions, including any signs or symptoms of infection. Inform her that almost all patients experience at least one injection-site reaction.

! **WARNING** Review signs and symptoms of an allergic reaction with patient and stress importance of seeking immediate medical attention.

- Alert patient that enfuvirtide may produce antibodies that could give a false positive for HIV testing. Remind her to alert all healthcare professionals of enfuvirtide therapy.
- Instruct patient to report any persistent, severe, or unusual signs and symptoms.

- Encourage women of childbearing age to report known or suspected pregnancy.
- Alert mothers that breastfeeding is not recommended during enfuvirtide therapy.
- Tell patient to seek medical attention if she develops signs or symptoms suggestive of pneumonia, such as cough with fever, rapid breathing, or shortness of breath.
- Caution patient and family that drug may cause suicidal thoughts. If present, prescriber should be notified.

enoxaparin sodium
Lovenox

⬚ Class and Category
Pharmacologic class: Low-molecular-weight heparin
Therapeutic class: Anticoagulant

⬚ Indications and Dosages
✱ *To prevent deep vein thrombosis (DVT) after hip or knee replacement and for continued prophylaxis after hospitalization for hip replacement*

SUBCUTANEOUS INJECTION
Adults. 30 mg every 12 hr, starting 12 to 24 hr after surgery for 7 to 10 days. Or, 40 mg daily, starting 9 to 15 hr before hip replacement surgery and then daily for up to 3 wk.

±**DOSAGE ADJUSTMENT** For patients with severe renal impairment (creatinine clearance less than 30 ml/min), dosage interval increased to once daily if 30 mg is taken twice daily or dosage reduced from 40 mg to 30 mg and dosage interval increased to once daily.

✱ *To prevent deep vein thrombosis (DVT) after abdominal surgery for patients with thrombo-embolic risk factors*

SUBCUTANEOUS INJECTION
Adults. *Initial:* 40 mg once daily, starting 2 hr before surgery and continued 24 hr after initial dose for 7 to 10 days.

±**DOSAGE ADJUSTMENT** For patients with severe renal impairment (creatinine clearance less than 30 ml/min), dosage reduced to 30 mg once daily.

✱ *To prevent DVT in medical patients who are at risk for thromboembolic complications due to severely restricted mobility during acute illness*

SUBCUTANEOUS INJECTION

Adults. 40 mg once daily for 6 to 11 days.

±**DOSAGE ADJUSTMENT** For patients with severe renal impairment (creatinine clearance less than 30 ml/min), dosage reduced to 30 mg once daily.

✳ *To treat acute DVT for inpatients with or without pulmonary embolism*

SUBCUTANEOUS INJECTION

Adults. 1 mg/kg every 12 hr or 1.5 mg/kg once daily for a minimum of 5 days after warfarin therapy has been initiated and a therapeutic oral anticoagulant effect has been achieved. *Usual duration:* 7 days.

±**DOSAGE ADJUSTMENT** For patient with severe renal impairment (creatinine clearance less than 30 ml/min) and taking warfarin concomitantly, dosage reduced or kept at 1 mg/kg and dosage interval increased to once daily.

✳ *To treat acute DVT as outpatient without pulmonary embolism*

SUBCUTANEOUS INJECTION

Adults. 1 mg/kg every 12 hr for a minimum of 5 days after warfarin therapy has been initiated and a therapeutic oral anticoagulant effect has been achieved. *Usual duration:* 7 days.

±**DOSAGE ADJUSTMENT** For patients with severe renal impairment (creatinine clearance less than 30 ml/min) and taking warfarin concomitantly, dosage interval increased to once daily.

✳ *To prevent ischemic complications of unstable angina and non-Q-wave MI*

SUBCUTANEOUS INJECTION

Adults. 1 mg/kg every 12 hr with 100 to 325 mg of aspirin P.O. daily for 2 to 8 days or until condition is stable.

±**DOSAGE ADJUSTMENT** For patients with severe renal impairment (serum creatinine less than 30 ml/min) when administered in conjunction with aspirin, dosage interval increased to once daily.

✳ *To treat acute ST-segment–elevation MI (STEMI)*

I.V. INJECTION, THEN SUBCUTANEOUS INJECTION

Adults. 30 mg I.V. as a single dose plus 1 mg/kg subcutaneously. Then, 1 mg/kg subcutaneously every 12 hr (maximum 100 mg for first 2 doses) with aspirin 75 to 325 mg P.O. once daily.

±**DOSAGE ADJUSTMENT** For patient with STEMI who is also receiving a thrombolytic, enoxaparin should be given between 15 min before and 30 min after fibrinolytic therapy starts. If STEMI patient has percutaneous coronary intervention, expect to give 0.3-mg/kg I.V. bolus if last enoxaparin dose was given more than 8 hr before balloon inflation. For patients less than 75 years of age with STEMI and severe renal impairment (less than 30 ml/min) when administered in conjunction with aspirin, 30 mg as a single I.V. bolus plus a 1 mg subcutaneous dose followed by 1 mg/kg subcutaneously once daily. For elderly patients with STEMI who are 75 years of age and older, initial I.V. bolus eliminated and initial subcutaneous injection dosage reduced to 0.75 mg/kg every 12 hr (maximum 75 mg for the first 2 doses only, followed by 0.75 mg/kg for remaining doses). For elderly patients 75 years and older who also have severe renal impairment (creatinine clearance less than 30 ml/min) and concurrent aspirin therapy is taken, dosage interval increased to once daily.

☰ Drug Administration

- Use of multidose vials should be avoided, if at all possible, in pregnant women because benzyl alcohol may cross the placenta and cause fetal harm.
- Use a tuberculin syringe or equivalent when using multiple-dose vials to ensure correct dose is withdrawn.

I.V.

- Solution should appear clear, colorless to pale yellow.
- Always flush I.V. access with 0.9% Sodium Chloride Injection or 5% Dextrose Injection before and after administration.
- Administer bolus as an I.V. injection.
- Don't give drug by I.M. injection.
- *Incompatibilities:* Other drugs and solutions (except for 0.9% Sodium Chloride Injection or 5% Dextrose Injection)

SUBCUTANEOUS

- Administer by first putting patient in a supine position.
- Do not expel the air bubble from prefilled syringes before the injection, to avoid the loss of drug.
- Administer as a deep subcutaneous injection by introducing the whole length

of needle into a skin fold held between the thumb and forefinger; hold the skin fold throughout the injection.

- Do not rub the injection site after injection, to minimize bruising.
- The prefilled syringe safety system will only be activated once the syringe is empty and removed from patient. Activation may cause a minimal splatter of fluid, so activate the system while holding syringe downward and away from people.
- Rotate sites.
- Monitor for site bleeding.

Route	Onset	Peak	Duration
SubQ	Unknown	3–5 hr	24 hr
I.V.	Unknown	Unknown	Unknown

Half-life: 4.5–7 hr

Mechanism of Action

Potentiates the action of antithrombin III, a coagulation inhibitor. By binding with antithrombin III, enoxaparin rapidly binds with and inactivates clotting factors (primarily factor Xa and thrombin). Without thrombin, fibrinogen can't convert to fibrin and thrombus can't form.

Contraindications

Active major bleeding; history of immune-mediated heparin-induced thrombocytopenia (HIT) within past 100 days or in the presence of circulating antibodies, which may persist for several years; hypersensitivity to benzyl alcohol (if only the multidose vial is available), enoxaparin, heparin (including low-molecular-weight heparins), pork products or their components

Interactions

DRUGS

NSAIDs; oral anticoagulants; platelet aggregation inhibitors, such as aspirin, dipyridamole, salicylates, sulfinpyrazone, and ticlopidine; thrombolytics, such as alteplase, anistreplase, streptokinase, and urokinase: Possibly increased risk of bleeding

Adverse Reactions

CNS: Confusion, **CVA**, epidural or spinal hematoma, fever, headache, paralysis
CV: Atrial fibrillation, congestive heart failure, hyperlipidemia, peripheral edema, **thrombosis**

EENT: Epistaxis
GI: Bloody stools, **cholestatic and hepatocellular liver injury**, diarrhea, elevated liver enzymes, **hematemesis**, **melena**, nausea, vomiting
GU: Hematuria, menstrual irregularities
HEME: Anemia, eosinophilia, **hemorrhage, heparin-induced thrombocytopenia or immune-mediated thrombocytopenia, purpura, thrombocytopenia purpura, thrombocytopenia**, thrombocytosis
MS: Osteoporosis (with long-term therapy)
RESP: Dyspnea, pneumonia, **pulmonary edema or embolism**
SKIN: Alopecia, cutaneous vasculitis, ecchymosis, persistent bleeding or oozing from mucous membranes or surgical wounds, pruritus, skin necrosis at injection site or distant from injection site, urticaria, vesiculobullous rash
Other: Anaphylaxis including shock; hyperkalemia; injection-site erythema, hematoma, inflammation, irritation, nodules, oozing, and pain

Childbearing Considerations

PREGNANCY

- It is not known if drug causes fetal harm.
- Use with caution only if benefit to mother outweighs potential risk to fetus.
- Be aware that all patients receiving anticoagulants, including pregnant women, are at risk for bleeding.
- Know that the multiple-dose vial of the drug contains 15 mg benzyl alcohol per 1 ml as a preservative. Cases of gasping syndrome have occurred in premature infants when large amounts of benzyl alcohol have been administered (99 to 405 mg/kg/day) to the mother.

LABOR & DELIVERY

- Be aware that drug therapy may be changed to a shorter-acting anticoagulant as delivery approaches to decrease bleeding risk for both mother and fetus.

LACTATION

- It is not known if drug is present in breast milk.
- Patient should check with prescriber before breastfeeding.

Nursing Considerations

- Use enoxaparin with extreme caution in patients with a history of heparin-induced thrombocytopenia (HIT). Know that enoxaparin should only be used in these patients if more than 100 days have elapsed since the prior HIT episode and no circulating antibodies are present.

- Use also extreme caution in patients with an increased risk of hemorrhage, as from active ulcerative or angiodysplastic GI disease; bacterial endocarditis; congenital or acquired bleeding disorder; concurrent treatment with a platelet inhibitor; hemorrhagic stroke; or recent brain, ophthalmologic, or spinal surgery.
- Use cautiously in those with bleeding diathesis, diabetic retinopathy, hepatic or renal impairment, recent GI hemorrhage or ulceration, or uncontrolled hypertension. Expect delayed elimination in elderly patients and those with renal insufficiency.
- Be aware that drug isn't recommended for patients with prosthetic heart valves, especially pregnant women, because of risk of prosthetic valve thrombosis. If enoxaparin is needed, monitor peak and trough antifactor Xa levels often and adjust dosage as needed.

! WARNING Know that if patient is receiving enoxaparin with epidural or spinal anesthesia or spinal puncture, watch closely for development of spinal hematoma, which may cause long-term or permanent paralysis. If evidence of neurologic impairment, such as changes in sensory or motor function, occurs, notify prescriber immediately because urgent care is needed to minimize hematoma's effect. Risk of epidural or spinal hematoma during enoxaparin therapy is increased by indwelling epidural catheters, concurrent use of other drugs that affect hemostasis, a history of traumatic or repeated epidural or spinal punctures, or a history of spinal deformity or spinal surgery. Know that placement or removal of a catheter should be delayed for at least 12 hours after administration of lower doses of enoxaparin (30 mg once or twice daily or 40 mg once daily) and at least 24 hours after the administration of higher doses. (0.75 mg/kg twice daily, 1 mg/kg twice daily, or 1.5 mg/kg once daily). However, for patients with creatinine clearance of less than 30 ml/min, timing of removal should be doubled because enoxaparin elimination is more prolonged in renal dysfunction.

- Expect to give drug with aspirin to patient with unstable angina, STEMI, and non-Q-wave MI. To minimize risk of bleeding after vascular procedures, give enoxaparin at recommended intervals.
- Know that after a percutaneous revascularization procedure, it is important to achieve hemostasis at the puncture site. A closure device may be removed right away; however, if a manual compression method is used, the sheath should be removed 6 hours after last enoxaparin dose. If enoxaparin therapy will continue, give next scheduled dose no sooner than 6 to 8 hours after sheath removal.
- Watch closely for bleeding. Notify prescriber immediately if platelet count falls below 100,000/mm^3. Expect to stop drug and start treatment if patient has a thromboembolic event, such as a stroke.
- Test stool for occult blood, as ordered.
- Keep protamine sulfate nearby in case of accidental overdose.
- Check serum potassium level for elevation, especially in patients with renal impairment or who are currently using potassium-sparing diuretics.

PATIENT TEACHING

- Advise patient to notify prescriber about adverse reactions, especially bleeding. Inform patient that taking aspirin or other NSAIDs may increase risk for bleeding and to use only if prescribed.
- Instruct patient to seek immediate help for evidence of thromboembolism, such as neurologic changes and severe shortness of breath. Also tell patient to report any unusual bleeding, bruising, or rash of dark red spots under the skin to prescriber.
- Emphasize the importance of complying with follow-up visits with prescriber.
- Teach patient or family member how to give enoxaparin at home, if needed. Show how to give drug by deep subcutaneous injection while lying down. Instruct him not to expel air bubble from a prefilled syringe to avoid losing some of the drug. Tell him to insert the entire needle into a skin fold held between the thumb and forefinger and then push plunger to bottom of syringe. Remind

him to alternate injection sites between the left and right anterolateral abdominal wall.

- Caution patient not to rub the site after giving the injection, to minimize bruising.
- Review safe handling and disposal of syringes and needles.
- Instruct patient to alert all healthcare providers, but especially those administering anesthesia, about enoxaparin therapy. If neuraxial anesthesia or spinal puncture is necessary, and especially if taking other drugs that could affect bleeding, tell patient to watch for signs and symptoms of epidural or spinal bleeding such as muscle weakness or numbness or tingling in lower extremities.
- Inform patient that he may bruise and/ or bleed more easily and that it may take longer than usual to stop bleeding while taking enoxaparin. Review bleeding precautions with patient.

entecavir

Baraclude

≡ Class and Category

Pharmacologic class: Nucleoside analogue
Therapeutic class: Antiviral

≡ Indications and Dosages

❋ *To treat chronic hepatitis B virus infection in patients with evidence of active viral replication and either evidence of persistent elevations in serum aminotransferases (ALT or AST) or histologically active disease*

ORAL SOLUTION, TABLETS

Adults and adolescents ages 16 and over who are nucleoside-inhibitor-treatment-naïve with compensated liver disease. 0.5 mg once daily.

Adults and adolescents ages 16 and over who have a history of hepatitis B viremia while receiving lamivudine or have experienced known lamivudine or telbivudine resistance substitutions; adults with compensated liver disease. 1 mg once daily.

Adults with decompensated liver disease. 1 mg once daily.

Children ages 2 and over weighing more than 30 kg (66 lb). 0.5 mg (10 ml oral solution) once daily if treatment-naïve or 1 mg (20-ml oral solution) once daily if lamivudine-experienced.

ORAL SOLUTION

Children ages 2 and over weighing more than 26 kg (57.2 lb) but less than 30 kg (66 lb). 9 ml once daily if treatment-naïve or 18 ml once daily if lamivudine-experienced.

Children ages 2 and over weighing more than 23 kg (50.6 lb) but less than 26 kg (57.2 lb). 8 ml once daily if treatment-naïve or 16 ml once daily if lamivudine-experienced.

Children ages 2 and over weighing more than 20 kg (44 lb) but less than 23 kg (50.6 lb). 7 ml once daily if treatment-naïve or 14 ml once daily if lamivudine-experienced.

Children ages 2 and over weighing more than 17 kg (37.4 lb) but less than 20 kg (44 lb). 6 ml once daily if treatment-naïve or 12 ml once daily if lamivudine-experienced.

Children ages 2 and over weighing more than 14 kg (30.8 lb) but less than 17 kg (37.4 lb). 5 ml once daily if treatment-naïve or 10 ml once daily if lamivudine-experienced.

Children ages 2 and over weighing more than 11 kg (24.2 lb) but less than 14 kg (30.8 lb). 4 ml once daily if treatment-naïve or 8 ml once daily if lamivudine-experienced.

Children ages 2 and over weighing at least 10 kg (22 lb) but less than 11 kg (24.2 lb). 3 ml once daily if treatment-naïve or 6 ml once daily if lamivudine-experienced.

±**DOSAGE ADJUSTMENT** For adult patient with a creatinine clearance between 30 and less than 50 ml/min, dosage reduced to 0.25 mg once daily or 0.5 mg every 48 hr, and dosage reduced to 0.5 mg once daily or 1 mg every 48 hr if lamivudine-refractory or decompensated liver disease is present. For adult patient with a creatinine clearance between 10 and less than 30 ml/min, dosage reduced to 0.15 mg once daily or 0.5 mg every 72 hr, and dosage reduced to 0.3 mg once daily or 1 mg every 72 hr if lamivudine-refractory or decompensated liver disease is present. For adult patient with a creatinine clearance less than 10 ml/min or who is on dialysis, dosage reduced to 0.05 mg once daily or 0.5 mg every 7 days (given after hemodialysis), and dosage reduced to 0.1 mg once daily or 1 mg every 7 days (given after hemodialysis) if lamivudine-refractory or decompensated liver disease is present. For pediatric patients with renal impairment, there is insufficient data to recommend a specific dose adjustment but a reduction in dose and/or an increase in dosing interval similar to adults may be considered.

Drug Administration

P.O.

- Administer on an empty stomach 2 hours before or after a meal.
- Tablets should be swallowed whole and not chewed, crushed, or split.
- To measure oral solution dosage, hold the dosing spoon in a vertical position and fill it gradually to the mark corresponding to the prescribed dose.
- Administer oral solution for doses less than 0.5 mg.
- Rinse dosing spoon after each use with water.

Route	Onset	Peak	Duration
P.O.	Unknown	0.5–1.5 hr	Unknown

Half-life: 5–6 hr

Mechanism of Action

Inhibits all three activities of the hepatitis B virus (HBV) reverse transcriptase which are base priming, reverse transcription of the negative strand from the pregenomic messenger RNA, and synthesis of the positive strand of HBV DNA. This lowers the ability of HBV to multiply and infect new liver cells.

Contraindications

Hypersensitivity to entecavir or its components

Interactions

DRUGS

drugs that reduce renal function or compete for active tubular secretion: Possibly increased serum concentrations of either entecavir or the coadministered drug, increasing risk of adverse reactions

Adverse Reactions

CNS: Dizziness, fatigue, fever, headache, **hepatic encephalopathy**, insomnia, somnolence
CV: Peripheral edema
EENT: Taste abnormality
ENDO: Hyperglycemia

GI: Abdominal pain, ascites, diarrhea, dyspepsia, elevated liver and pancreatic enzymes, **exacerbation of hepatitis** (after discontinuation of therapy), **gastrointestinal hemorrhage, hepatic failure, hepatorenal syndrome,** hyperalbuminemia, hyperbilirubinemia, nausea, **severe hepatomegaly with steatosis,** vomiting
GU: Elevated creatinine level, glycosuria, hematuria, **renal failure**
HEME: Decreased platelet count
RESP: Upper respiratory infection
SKIN: Alopecia, rash
Other: Anaphylaxis, decreased serum bicarbonate level, lactic acidosis

Childbearing Considerations

PREGNANCY

- Pregnancy exposure registry: 1-800-258-4263.
- It is not known if drug causes fetal harm.
- Use with caution only if benefit to mother outweighs potential risk to fetus.

LACTATION

- It is not known if drug is present in breast milk.
- Patient should check with prescriber before breastfeeding.

Nursing Considerations

- Ensure that patient has been tested for HIV infection before entecavir therapy begins, because resistance to HIV therapy may develop when entecavir is administered to treat chronic hepatitis B virus infection in patients who also have an HIV infection that is not being treated. Know that entecavir therapy is not recommended for coinfected patients who are not receiving treatment.

! **WARNING** Know that lactic acidosis and severe hepatomegaly with steatosis have occurred with entecavir therapy and death has occurred in some patients. Risk factors include the presence of obesity, prolonged nucleoside exposure, and being a woman. However, know that lactic acidosis and severe hepatomegaly with steatosis have also occurred in patients with no known risk factors. Monitor patient's liver enzymes as ordered. Expect entecavir to be discontinued in any patient who develops clinical or laboratory findings suggestive of lactic acidosis or pronounced hepatotoxicity, even in the absence of marked transaminase elevations.

- Expect patient to be closely monitored for at least several months after entecavir has been discontinued, because severe acute exacerbation of hepatitis may occur.

PATIENT TEACHING

- Instruct patient with hepatitis B on the importance of testing for HIV before therapy begins and then periodically throughout therapy to avoid development of resistance to HIV treatment.
- Instruct patient to take entecavir once daily on an empty stomach either 2 hours before or after a meal.
- Tell patient tablets should be swallowed whole and not chewed, crushed, or split.
- Teach patient or caregiver how to measure oral solution using the provided dosing spoon.
- Instruct patient using the oral solution to hold the dosing spoon in a vertical position and fill it gradually to the mark corresponding to the prescribed dose. The dosing spoon should be rinsed after each daily dose.
- Remind patient if he misses a dose to take it as soon as he remembers but not to double the next dose or take more than the prescribed dose.
- Tell patient that entecavir therapy does not reduce the transmission of HBV to others through blood contamination or sexual contact.
- Warn patient with hepatitis B that acute severe exacerbations of hepatitis B may occur following discontinuation of entecavir. He should not discontinue drug without prescriber knowledge. Tell patient to report any reappearance of signs and symptoms of hepatitis B.
- Instruct mothers not to breastfeed while receiving entecavir therapy.
- Advise female patient to notify prescriber if pregnancy occurs or is suspected.

! WARNING Alert patient that severe conditions may develop while taking entecavir. Encourage him to stop taking drug and seek medical attention immediately if he experiences any persistent, severe, or unusual symptoms.

epinephrine
(adrenaline)
Adrenalin, Auvi-Q, EpiPen, EpiPen Jr., Symjepi

Class and Category
Pharmacologic class: Sympathomimetic
Therapeutic class: Antianaphylactic, bronchodilator, cardiac stimulant, vasopressor

Indications and Dosages
❋ *To treat anaphylaxis*

I.M. OR SUBCUTANEOUS INJECTION
Adults and children weighing 30 kg (66 lb) or more. 0.3 to 0.5 mg, repeated every 5 to 10 min, as needed.
Children weighing less than 30 kg (66 lb). 0.01 mg/kg up to maximum of 0.3 mg per injection, repeated every 5 to 10 min, as needed.

❋ *To provide emergency treatment of allergic reactions (Type I), including anaphylaxis to allergen immunotherapy, biting and stinging insects, diagnostic testing substances, drugs, foods, and other allergens, as well as exercise-induced or idiopathic anaphylaxis*

I.M. INJECTION, SUBCUTANEOUS INJECTION
Adults and children weighing 30 kg (66 lb) or more who are at increased risk for anaphylaxis. 0.3 mg immediately upon exposure.
Adults and children weighing 15 to 30 kg (33 to 66 lb) who are at increased risk of anaphylaxis. 0.15 mg immediately upon exposure.

I.M. INJECTION, SUBCUTANEOUS INJECTION (AUVI-Q)
Children weighing 7.5 to 15 kg (16.5 to 33 lb) who are at increased risk of anaphylaxis. 0.1 mg immediately upon exposure.

❋ *To treat hypotension associated with septic shock*

I.V. INFUSION
Adults. 0.05 mcg/kg/min to 2 mcg/kg/min, titrated to achieve desired mean arterial pressure by adjusting dose every 10 to 15 min, in increments of 0.05 to 0.2 mcg/kg/min.

✴ To induce and maintain mydriasis during intraocular surgery

INTRAOCULAR (ADRENALIN)

Adults. 10 mcg/ml to 1 mcg/ml used as an irrigating solution during eye surgery.

⬚ Drug Administration

- Some preparations contain sulfites, which may cause allergic-type reactions. However, the presence of sulfites in epinephrine should not deter its use in a patient with anaphylaxis, even if patient is sensitive to sulfites.
- Protect solution from light.

INTRAOCULAR

- If the Adrenalin brand of epinephrine is used during intraocular surgery to induce and maintain mydriasis, the 30-ml multiple-dose vial of the drug should not be used because it contains chlorobutanol, which may be harmful to the corneal endothelium.
- The Adrenalin 1-ml single-use vial must be diluted before intraocular use. Dilute in 100 ml to 1000 ml of an ophthalmic irrigation fluid to obtain a concentration of 1:100,000 to 1:1,000,000 (10 mcg/ml to 1 mcg/ml).

I.M. AND SUBCUTANEOUS

- When given by these routes, the drug is intended for use as emergency supportive therapy only and is not a substitute for immediate medical care.
- Inspect epinephrine solution before use. If it's pink or brown, air has entered a multidose vial. If it's discolored or contains particles, discard it. Also discard unused portions.
- Do not administer by intra-arterial injection because marked vasoconstriction may cause gangrene. Also, accidental injection of drug into patient's feet, fingers, or hands may result in loss of blood flow to the affected area.
- NEVER inject drug into the buttocks or use the deltoid muscle for injection.
- Inject drug only into the anterolateral aspect of the thigh, through clothing, if necessary.
- When administering drug to a child, hold the leg firmly in place and limit movement prior to and during an injection to minimize the risk of injury related to the injection or inadvertently injecting drug into the buttocks.

- Remember to rotate sites because repeated injections in the same site may cause vasoconstriction and localized necrosis.
- Assess injection site periodically after administration of drug for signs of infection such as persistent redness, swelling, tenderness, or warmth because, although rare, serious skin and soft-tissue infections, including myonecrosis and necrotizing fasciitis caused by *Clostridia* (gas gangrene), have been reported at the injection site, especially if drug was inadvertently injected into buttocks. Cleaning the site with alcohol before injecting drug does not kill bacterial spores and therefore does not reduce the risk.

I.V.

- Prepare I.V. infusion by diluting 1 mg of epinephrine to 1,000 ml of a 5% Dextrose or 5% Dextrose and 0.9% Sodium Chloride Injection solution to produce a 1 mcg/ml dilution. Administration in 0.9% Sodium Chloride Injection alone is not recommended.
- Administer as a continuous infusion only to treat hypotension associated with septic shock. Do not use autoinjectors I.V.
- When possible, administer I.V. infusion through a central line or, if not possible, a large vein. Avoid using a catheter tie-in technique, because the obstruction to blood flow around the tubing may cause stasis and increased local concentration of drug.
- Avoid injecting into the veins of the leg in elderly patients or in those suffering from occlusive vascular diseases.
- Avoid extravasation of epinephrine into the tissues to prevent local necrosis. Assess infusion site frequently for free flow and look for blanching along the course of the infused vein which may indicate some leakage from the vein wall. If blanching occurs, change infusion site. To prevent sloughing and necrosis in areas in which extravasation has taken place, obtain an order to infiltrate the area with 10 to 15 ml of saline solution containing 5 to 10 mg phentolamine. Using a syringe with a fine hypodermic needle, infiltrate the area liberally, which is easily identified by its cold, hard, and pallid appearance.

E
F

- The diluted solution may be stored up to 4 hours at room temperature and 24 hours if refrigerated.
- *Incompatibilities:* Alkaline solutions, aminophylline, hyaluronidase, sodium bicarbonate, mephentermine, thiopental

Route	Onset	Peak	Duration
I.V.	Immediate	5 min	Short
I.M.	Rapid	Unknown	Short
SubQ	5–15 min	30 min	Short

Half-life: < 2 min

Mechanism of Action

Acts on alpha and beta receptors. This nonselective adrenergic agonist stimulates:

- alpha$_1$ receptors, which constricts arteries and may decrease bronchial secretions
- presynaptic alpha$_2$ receptors, which inhibits norepinephrine release by way of negative feedback
- postsynaptic alpha$_2$ receptors, which constricts arteries
- beta$_1$ receptors, which induces positive chronotropic and inotropic responses
- beta$_2$ receptors, which dilates arteries, relaxes bronchial smooth muscles, increases glycogenolysis, and prevents mast cells from secreting histamine and other substances, thus reversing bronchoconstriction and edema.

Contraindications

Cerebral arteriosclerosis, coronary insufficiency, dilated cardiomyopathy, general anesthesia with halogenated hydrocarbons or cyclopropane, hypersensitivity to epinephrine or its components, labor, angle-closure glaucoma, organic brain damage, shock (nonanaphylactic)

Interactions

DRUGS

alpha blockers such as phentolamine: Antagonized pressor effects of epinephrine
antiarrhythmics, cardiac glycosides, diuretics: Increased risk of cardiac arrhythmias
antihistamines (chlorpheniramine, diphenhydramine, tripelennamine), levothyroxine, MAO inhibitors, tricyclic antidepressants: Increased risk of potentiated effect of epinephrine
beta-adrenergic blockers such as propranolol: Antagonized bronchodilating and cardiostimulating effects of epinephrine

ergot alkaloids: Possibly reverse pressor effects of epinephrine

Adverse Reactions

CNS: Anxiety, apprehensiveness, chills, **CVA**, disorientation, dizziness, drowsiness, excitability, fever, hallucinations, headache, impaired memory, insomnia, light-headedness, nervousness, panic, psychomotor agitation, restlessness, **seizures**, sleepiness, temporary worsening of Parkinson's disease, tingling, tremor, weakness
CV: Angina (in presence of coronary artery disease); **arrhythmias, including ventricular fibrillation**; chest discomfort or pain; fast, irregular, or slow heartbeat; increased cardiac output; **myocardial ischemia**; palpitations; peripheral vasoconstriction; **severe hypertension**; **stress cardiomyopathy**; tachycardia; vasoconstriction; **ventricular ectopy**
EENT: Blurred vision, dry mouth or throat, miosis
ENDO: Hyperglycemia in diabetics
GI: Anorexia, heartburn, nausea, vomiting
GU: Dysuria, oliguria, renal impairment
MS: Muscle twitching, severe muscle spasms
RESP: Dyspnea, **pulmonary edema**
SKIN: Cold skin, diaphoresis, ecchymosis, flushed or red face or skin, pallor, tissue necrosis
Other: **Hyperkalemia**; **hypokalemia**; injection-site coldness, hypoesthesia, infections (*Clostridia*), pain, pallor, and stinging

Childbearing Considerations

PREGNANCY

- It is not known if drug causes fetal harm.
- Use with caution only if benefit to mother outweighs potential risk to fetus.

LABOR & DELIVERY

- May delay second stage of labor because drug usually inhibits spontaneous or oxytocin-induced contractions. It may also cause a prolonged period of uterine atony with hemorrhage.
- Drug should be avoided during second stage of labor and in patients with a blood pressure that exceeds 130/80 mm/Hg.
- While drug may improve maternal hypotension associated with anaphylaxis and septic shock, it may cause decreased

uterine blood flow, fetal anoxia, and uterine vasoconstriction.

LACTATION
- It is not known if drug is present in breast milk.
- Patient should check with prescriber before breastfeeding after receiving epinephrine.

▤ Nursing Considerations

- Use epinephrine with extreme caution in patients with angina, arrhythmias, asthma, degenerative heart disease, or emphysema. Epinephrine's inotropic effect equals that of dopamine and dobutamine; its chronotropic effect exceeds that of both.
- Use drug cautiously in elderly patients and those with cardiovascular disease (other than listed above), diabetes mellitus, hypertension, hyperthyroidism, prostatic hypertrophy, and psychoneurologic disorders.
- Monitor patient's blood pressure frequently and titrate I.V. dosages to avoid excessive increases in blood pressure.
- Monitor patient for cardiac arrhythmias and myocardial ischemia, especially patients suffering from cardiomyopathy or coronary artery disease.
- Monitor patient for potassium imbalances. Initially, hyperkalemia occurs when hepatocytes release potassium. Hypokalemia may quickly follow as skeletal muscles take up potassium.

PATIENT TEACHING
- Teach patient and family how to administer epinephrine subcutaneously in an emergency. Tell them to inject drug only into anterolateral aspect of the thigh, through the clothing if necessary. If injecting drug into a child, stress importance of holding the leg firmly in place and limiting movement prior to and during the injection, to prevent injury.

! **WARNING** Instruct patient and family never to give epinephrine in the buttocks, as absorption may be hindered. Also, a serious infection (gas gangrene) may occur if injected in the buttocks. In addition, tell patient and family to inspect the thigh for signs of infection at the injection site and report if persistent redness, swelling, tenderness, and warmth develop.

- Remind patient or family that drug used in an emergency situation to treat anaphylaxis is intended for emergency supportive therapy only. Stress importance of seeking immediate care after drug is administered.
- Explain that solution is light sensitive and should be stored in the carrying case and at room temperature. Tell them not to refrigerate drug or keep it in overheated areas such as a closed car and to replace solution if it discolors.
- Caution patient to avoid accidentally injecting drug into his fingers, hands, toes, or feet because epinephrine is a strong vasoconstrictor and could cause loss of blood flow to the area, resulting in gangrene.
- Instruct patient using an EpiPen to never put fingers, hand, or thumb over the orange tip and not to press or push the orange tip with fingers, hand, or thumb because the needle comes out of the orange tip. If accidental injection occurs in any of these areas, instruct patient to go immediately to nearest emergency room.

! **WARNING** Tell patient using an EpiPen or EpiPen Jr to always check to make sure the blue safety release is not raised, which means it has been activated and is useless. Tell him he should never flip the blue safety release off using a thumb or by pulling it sideways, or bending and twisting the blue safety release. This may cause the device to activate by accident: a "click" is heard, the orange tip is extended, and the window is blocked. Once activated, the device cannot be used in an emergency. A new pen should be obtained in either case.

- Remind patient or caregiver using the EpiPen or EpiPen Jr that the pen delivers a fixed dose of epinephrine and the autoinjectors cannot be reused. Offer reassurance that it is normal for some of the drug to remain in the autoinjector after the dose has been injected. The dose has been injected if the orange tip is extended and the window is blocked.
- Instruct patient never to throw away expired, unwanted, or unused epinephrine injections into household trash. Instead, drug should be disposed of in an FDA-cleared sharps disposal container or

E
F

a container made of heavy-duty plastic, leak-resistant, able to stand upright during use, close with a tight-fitting, puncture-resistant lid, without sharps being able to protrude out and properly labeled to warn of hazardous waste inside the container. Dispose of container when almost full according to state regulations. If not sure, tell patient to go to the FDA's website at: http://fda.gov/safesharpsdisposal.

- Remind patient or caregiver to keep drug away from young children.
- Advise patient to notify prescriber immediately if he has blurred vision, chest pain, fast or irregular heartbeat, increased sweating, or trouble breathing.
- Inform patient with diabetes that epinephrine may cause hyperglycemia. Inform patient with Parkinson's disease that symptoms may temporarily worsen but this should not deter use of drug.

eplerenone
Inspra

▤ Class and Category
Pharmacologic class: Aldosterone receptor blocker
Therapeutic class: Antihypertensive

▤ Indications and Dosages
✳ *To improve survival of stable patients with symptomatic heart failure with reduced ejection fraction (equal to or less than 40%) after an acute myocardial infarction*

TABLETS
Adults. *Initial:* 25 mg daily, increased to 50 mg daily within 4 wk, as needed. Then dosage adjusted based on the serum potassium level.
±**DOSAGE ADJUSTMENT** Dosage adjusted based on the serum potassium level. If potassium level is less than 5.0 mEq/L and patient is taking 25 mg every other day, dosage interval increased to daily; if patient is taking 25 mg once daily, dosage increased to 50 mg once daily. If potassium level is 5.0 to 5.4 mEq/L, no adjustment needed. If potassium level is between 5.5 and 5.9 mEq/L and patient is taking 50 mg once daily, dosage reduced to 25 mg once daily, or if patient is taking 25 mg once daily, dosage interval increased to 25 mg every other day;

if already taking 25 mg every other day or potassium level is 6.0 mEq/L or higher, drug withheld until potassium level returns to acceptable level. Dosage then restarted at 25 mg every other day. For patients taking moderate CYP450 3A4 inhibitors, such as erythromycin, fluconazole, saquinavir, and verapamil, dosage not to exceed 25 mg once daily.

✳ *To treat hypertension alone or with other antihypertensive drugs*

TABLETS
Adults. *Initial:* 50 mg daily, increased to 50 mg twice daily after 4 wk, if needed.
±**DOSAGE ADJUSTMENT** For patients taking moderate CYP450 3A4 inhibitors, such as erythromycin, fluconazole, saquinavir, and verapamil, initial dosage for hypertension reduced to 25 mg daily. If patient's blood pressure is not controlled with this dose, dosing increased to maximum of 25 mg twice daily.

▤ Drug Administration
P.O.
- Drug may be given without regard to meals.

Route	Onset	Peak	Duration
P.O.	Unknown	1.5–2 hr	Unknown
Half-life: 4–6 hr			

▤ Mechanism of Action
Blocks the binding of aldosterone at its mineralocorticoid receptor sites located in the blood vessels, brain, heart, and kidneys. This action decreases blood pressure by preventing aldosterone from inducing sodium reabsorption and possibly other mechanisms that contribute to raising blood pressure.

▤ Contraindications
For all patients: Concurrent therapy with strong CYP3A inhibitors, creatinine clearance 30 ml/min or less, hyperkalemia (greater than 5.5 mEq) at initiation, hypersensitivity to eplerenone or its components
For patients with hypertension: Concurrent therapy with potassium supplements or potassium-sparing diuretics, creatinine level greater than 2 mg/dl in males and greater than 1.8 mg/dl in females, creatinine

clearance less than 50 ml/min, type 2 diabetes mellitus with microalbuminuria

Interactions

DRUGS

ACE inhibitors, angiotensin II receptor antagonists: Increased risk of hyperkalemia
CYP3A inhibitors: Increased blood level and effect of eplerenone
lithium: Possibly lithium toxicity
NSAIDs: Possibly reduced antihypertensive effect of eplerenone; severe hyperkalemia in patients with impaired renal function

Adverse Reactions

CNS: Dizziness, fatigue, headache
CV: Angina pectoris, hypercholesterolemia, hypertriglyceridemia, MI
ENDO: Gynecomastia, mastodynia
GI: Abdominal pain, diarrhea, increased liver enzymes
GU: Albuminuria, elevated BUN and serum creatinine levels, vaginal bleeding
RESP: Cough
Other: Flu-like symptoms, hyperkalemia, hyponatremia, increased uric acid level

Childbearing Considerations

PREGNANCY

- It is not known if drug causes fetal harm.
- Use with caution only if benefit to mother outweighs potential risk to fetus.

LACTATION

- It is not known if drug is present in breast milk.
- Patient should check with prescriber before breastfeeding.

REPRODUCTION

- Male fertility may become compromised with drug therapy based on animal studies.

Nursing Considerations

- Monitor patient's blood pressure regularly to evaluate eplerenone effectiveness.
- Be aware that patients with diabetes, impaired renal function, or proteinuria or who take an ACE inhibitor or an angiotensin II receptor antagonist during eplerenone therapy have an increased risk of hyperkalemia.
- Monitor patient's serum potassium level before start of therapy, within the first week of therapy, at one month, and periodically thereafter, as ordered. Notify prescriber

of abnormalities, as dosage will have to be adjusted.
- Monitor patients over 65 closely, because the risk of hyperkalemia may be increased because of age-related decreases in creatine clearance.

PATIENT TEACHING

- Caution patient not to use potassium salt substitutes or potassium-containing supplements because increased potassium levels can lead to serious adverse reactions to eplerenone.
- Urge patient to tell all prescribers about eplerenone use because of possible interactions.

epoetin alfa
(EPO, erythropoietin alfa, recombinant erythropoietin, r-HuEPO)
Epogen, Eprex (CAN), Procrit

epoetin alfa-epbx
Retacrit

Class and Category

Pharmacologic class: Erythropoietin
Therapeutic class: Antianemic

Indications and Dosages

✳ *To treat anemia due to chronic kidney disease for patients on dialysis and who have a hemoglobin less than 10 g/dl; to treat anemia due to chronic kidney disease for patients not on dialysis but have a hemoglobin less than 10 g/dl, the rate of decline of hemoglobin level indicates patient will need an RBC transfusion, and the treatment goal is to reduce the risk of alloimmunization and other RBC transfusion-related risks*

I.V. OR SUBCUTANEOUS INJECTION

Adults. *Initial:* 50 to 100 units/kg 3 times/wk, increased as needed by 25% at 4-wk intervals or longer. *Maintenance:* Dosage highly individualized to lowest dose that keeps hemoglobin below 11 g/dl.
Neonates age 1 month and older and children. 50 units/kg 3 times/wk; increased as needed by 25% at 4-wk intervals or longer.

Maintenance: Dosage highly individualized to lowest dose that keeps hemoglobin below 12 g/dl.

± **DOSAGE ADJUSTMENT** For patients with anemia from renal failure on dialysis, dosage temporarily reduced or drug discontinued if hemoglobin approaches or exceeds 11 g/dl (12 g/dl for children). For patients with anemia from renal failure not on dialysis, dosage temporarily reduced or drug discontinued if hemoglobin exceeds 10 g/dl (12 g/dl for children). For patients with anemia from renal failure with or without dialysis, dosage reduced 25% or more if hemoglobin rises rapidly (more than 1 g/dl in any 2-week period).

* *To treat anemia in HIV-infected patients due to zidovudine administered at 4,200 mg or more each week and patient's endogenous serum erythropoietin level is 500 mU/ml or less.*

I.V. OR SUBCUTANEOUS INJECTION

Adults. *Initial:* 100 units/kg 3 times/wk, increased by 50 to 100 units/kg every 4 to 8 wk after 8 wk of therapy. *Maintenance:* Dosage gradually titrated to maintain desired response, based on such factors as variations in zidovudine dosage and occurrence of infection or inflammation. *Maximum:* 300 units/kg 3 times/wk or hemoglobin has reached a level needed to avoid RBC transfusions.

± **DOSAGE ADJUSTMENT** For patients with a hemoglobin that exceeds 12 g/dl, drug withheld and resumed at a dose 25% below the previous dose when hemoglobin has declined to less than 11 g/dl.

* *To treat anemia from chemotherapy*

SUBCUTANEOUS INJECTION

Adults with a hemoglobin less than 10 g/dl, and there is a minimum of two additional months of planned chemotherapy. *Initial:* 150 units/kg 3 times/wk or 40,000 units weekly until completion of a chemotherapy course. Dosage increased to 300 units/kg 3 times/wk or 60,000 units weekly after 4 wk if response is inadequate.
Maximum: 300 units/kg 3 times/wk; or 60,000 units weekly.

I.V. INJECTION

Children ages 5 to 18 with a hemoglobin less than 10 g/dl, and if there is a minimum of two additional months of planned chemotherapy. 600 units/kg until completion of a chemotherapy course. Dosage increased to 900 units/kg weekly after initial 4 wk of therapy if hemoglobin increases by less than 1 g/dl and remains below 10 g/dl. *Maximum:* 900 units/kg (60,000 units) weekly.

± **DOSAGE ADJUSTMENT** For adults and children, dosage decreased by 25% if hemoglobin level approaches a level needed to avoid RBC transfusion or increases more than 1 g/dl in any 2-wk period. Dose withheld if hemoglobin exceeds a level needed to avoid RBC transfusion and resumed at 25% less than previous dose when hemoglobin approaches a level where RBC transfusions may be required.

* *To reduce need for allogeneic red blood cell transfusions in patients undergoing elective, noncardiac, nonvascular surgery*

SUBCUTANEOUS INJECTION

Adults. 300 units/kg daily for 10 days before surgery, on day of surgery, and 4 days after surgery; or 600 units/kg/wk on 21, 14, and 7 days before surgery and on the day of surgery. Dose of 300 units/kg repeated on day of surgery.

▤ Drug Administration

- Don't shake vial while preparing, to avoid inactivating drug.
- Discard unused portion of single-dose vial because it contains no preservatives. Store multidose vial in refrigerator and discard unused portion after 21 days.
- Do not use multidose vials, which contain benzyl alcohol for pregnant or breastfeeding patients, neonates, or infants.
- Protect drug vials from light.
- Do not use if drug vial has been frozen or shaken. Also, do not use if the green area of the freeze strip indicator on Retacrit vials appears cloudy or white.

I.V.

- Administer as an injection undiluted. Manufacturer does not specify rate of administration. However, preservative-free drug from a single-dose vial may be mixed in a syringe with bacteriostatic 0.9% Sodium Chloride Injection with benzyl alcohol 0.9% (bacteriostatic saline) in a 1:1 ratio at the time of administration. Do not use this mixture in pregnant or breastfeeding women, neonates, or infants.

- I.V. is the preferred route for patients on hemodialysis. Inject into the venous port of the hemodialysis tubing.
- *Incompatibilities:* Other I.V. drugs

SUBCUTANEOUS

- Injection sites that can be used include abdomen (except for 2-inch area around the navel), front of thighs, outer area of upper arms, and upper outer area of buttocks.
- Administer as an injection undiluted while pinching a fold of skin. Do not inject into an area that is bruised, hard, red, tender or has scars or stretch marks.
- Rotate sites.

Route	Onset	Peak	Duration
I.V.	Immediate	15 min	2 wk
SubQ	Unknown	5–24 hr	2 wk

Half-life: 4–13 hr

⬚ Mechanism of Action

Stimulates the release of reticulocytes from the bone marrow into the bloodstream, where they develop into mature RBCs.

⬚ Contraindications

Hypersensitivity to epoetin alfa, epoetin alfa-epbx, or its components; pure red cell aplasia that began after treatment with epoetin alfa, epoetin alfa-epbx, or other erythropoietin protein drugs; uncontrolled hypertension; use of multidose vials in infants, neonates, or women who are breastfeeding or pregnant

⬚ Interactions

DRUGS

None reported by manufacturer

⬚ Adverse Reactions

CNS: Anxiety, asthenia, **CVA**, dizziness, fatigue, fever, headache, insomnia, paresthesia, **seizures**
CV: Chest pain, **congestive heart failure, deep vein thrombosis**, edema, hypertension, **MI**, tachycardia, **thromboembolic events**
GI: Constipation, diarrhea, indigestion, nausea, vomiting
GU: UTI
HEME: Polycythemia
MS: Arthralgia, bone pain, muscle weakness
RESP: Cough, dyspnea, **pulmonary congestion**, upper respiratory tract infection

SKIN: Erythema multiforme, rash, pruritus, **Stevens–Johnson syndrome, toxic epidermal necrolysis**, urticaria
Other: Flu-like symptoms, **hyperkalemia**, injection-site reaction, trunk pain

⬚ Childbearing Considerations

PREGNANCY

- It is not known if drug causes fetal harm.
- Use with caution only if benefit to mother outweighs potential risk to fetus.
- Know that use of the multiple-dose vials of the drug are contraindicated for use in pregnant women because it contains benzyl alcohol. A benzyl alcohol-free formulation should be used instead, such as the single-dose vial.
- Do not mix drug with bacteriostatic saline containing benzyl alcohol when administering to pregnant women.

LACTATION

- It is not known if drug is present in breast milk.
- Advise patient to check with prescriber before breastfeeding if drug will be administered from a single-dose vial.
- Use of the multiple-dose vial of the drug is contraindicated in women who are breastfeeding.
- Do not mix drug with bacteriostatic saline containing benzyl alcohol being administering to a woman who is breastfeeding.
- Inform breastfeeding women that if drug is administered using a multiple-dose vial, breastfeeding should be withheld for at least 2 weeks after the last dose.

⬚ Nursing Considerations

- Be aware that epoetin alfa shouldn't be given to cancer patients when a cure is anticipated because drug may decrease survival rate and increase tumor progression in patients with certain types of cancers, such as breast, non-small-cell lung, head and neck, lymphoid, and cervical cancers. All prescribers and hospitals must enroll and comply with the ESA APPRISE Oncology program to be able to prescribe and dispense the drug.
- Ensure that patient has received the medication guide and patient instructions for epoetin alfa and that a written acknowledgment of a discussion of the risks

E
F

involved with this type of therapy has been obtained before first dose is given.

- Evaluate the patient's serum iron level before and during treatment, as ordered. Expect to give an iron supplement (I.V. iron dextran, if needed) because iron requirements rise when erythropoiesis consumes existing iron stores.

- Use epoetin alfa cautiously in patients who have conditions that could decrease or delay response to drug, such as aluminum intoxication, folic acid deficiency, hemolysis, infection, inflammation, iron deficiency, malignant neoplasm, osteitis (fibrosa cystica), or vitamin B_{12} deficiency.

- Also use drug cautiously in patients with cardiovascular disorders caused by hypertension, a history of porphyria or seizures, vascular disease, or a hematologic disorder, such as hypercoagulation, myelodysplastic syndrome, or sickle cell disease.

- Know that lowest possible dose should be used in cancer patients because drug has shortened survival rate and increased tumor progression in patients with certain types of cancers, such as breast, non-small-cell lung, head and neck, and lymphoid cancers. Drug should only be used to treat anemia caused by myelosuppressive chemotherapy in cancer patients.

- Be aware that baseline hemoglobin level should be above 10 but below 13 g/dl if drug is given to patient scheduled for surgery. Watch closely throughout surgical period for deep vein thrombosis, especially in patients not receiving prophylactic anticoagulation, because risk increases.

- Evaluate the patient's serum iron level before and during treatment, as ordered. Expect to give an iron supplement (I.V. iron formulation, if needed) because iron requirements rise when erythropoiesis consumes existing iron stores.

- Check hemoglobin levels, as ordered, with twice-weekly measurements recommended for chronic renal failure patients, until stable and then monthly thereafter and weekly measurements recommended for zidovudine-treated HIV-infected and cancer patients.

! WARNING Know that hemoglobin shouldn't exceed 11 g/dl when treating anemia in patients with chronic renal failure on dialysis and 10 g/dl for patients not on dialysis. Exceeding these parameters increases risk of life-threatening adverse cardiovascular effects.

- Expect to increase heparin dose if patient receives hemodialysis because epoetin alfa can increase the RBC volume, which could cause clots to form in the dialyzer, hemodialysis vascular access, or both.

- Monitor patient for hypertensive or thrombotic complications, especially if hemoglobin is approaching target goal.

- Monitor patient throughout therapy for skin reactions which may include blistering and skin exfoliation that could be severe. If present, notify prescriber at once and expect drug to be discontinued.

PATIENT TEACHING

- Ensure that patient has been instructed on the serious adverse effects related to epoetin alfa therapy before therapy begins.

- Teach patient how to administer drug and how to dispose of needles properly. Caution him against reusing needles.

- Emphasize the importance of complying with the dosage regimen and keeping follow-up medical appointments and appointments for laboratory tests.

- Encourage patient to eat iron-rich foods.

- Review possible adverse reactions, and urge patient to notify prescriber if he experiences chest pain, headache, hives, rapid heartbeat, rash, seizures, shortness of breath, or swelling. Also inform patient of the possibility of severe skin reactions such as blistering and exfoliation. Stress importance of stopping drug and alerting prescriber immediately if present.

- Advise women of childbearing age to use effective contraception during therapy if pregnancy isn't desired because menses may resume during epoetin alfa therapy.

eptifibatide
Integrilin

Class and Category
Pharmacologic class: Glycoprotein IIb/IIIa inhibitor
Therapeutic class: Antiplatelet

Indications and Dosages

* *To treat acute coronary syndrome (unstable angina and non-ST-elevation MI)*

I.V. INFUSION, I.V. INJECTION

Adults. *Initial:* 180 mcg/kg as soon as possible after diagnosis, followed by 2 mcg/kg/min immediately after initial dose and continuing until discharge or coronary artery bypass grafting (CABG), up to 72 hr. If patient is to undergo PCI, infusion continued until hospital discharge or up to 18 to 24 hr after the procedure, whichever comes first, allowing for up to 96 hr of therapy.

±**DOSAGE ADJUSTMENT** For patient with serum creatinine level less than 50 ml/min, initial bolus remains unchanged at 180 mcg/kg but continuous infusion decreased to 1.0 mcg/kg/min.

* *To treat patients undergoing percutaneous transluminal coronary angioplasty (PTCA), including intracoronary stenting*

I.V. INFUSION, I.V. INJECTION

Adults. *Initial:* 180 mcg/kg immediately before procedure, immediately followed by 2 mcg/kg/min, and a second 180 mcg/kg bolus administered 10 minutes after the first bolus. The continuous infusion continued until hospital discharge, or for up to 18 to 24 hr, whichever comes first. A minimum of 12 hr of infusion recommended. For patient undergoing CABG surgery, infusion discontinued prior to surgery.

±**DOSAGE ADJUSTMENT** For patient with serum creatinine level less than 50 ml/min, initial and subsequent bolus remains unchanged at 180 mcg/kg but continuous infusion decreased to 1.0 mcg/kg/min.

Drug Administration

I.V.

- Protect drug from light before administration.
- May administer in the same I.V. line as alteplase, atropine, dobutamine, heparin, lidocaine, meperidine, metoprolol, midazolam, morphine, nitroglycerin, or verapamil.
- May also administer drug in same I.V. line with 0.9% Sodium Chloride Injection or 0.9% Sodium Chloride Injection and 5% Dextrose Injection solution. Infusion may also contain up to 60 mEq/L of potassium chloride.
- Withdraw bolus dose from a 10-ml (2 mg/ml) vial into a syringe.
- Administer I.V. injection as a bolus over 1 to 2 minutes. Immediately follow with a continuous infusion.
- Using vented I.V. infusion set, give continuous infusion directly from the 100-ml (0.75 mg/ml) vial undiluted, using an infusion pump. Be sure to center the spike in the circle on top of vial stopper. Administer infusion rate according to the patient's weight.
- Drug should be given concomitantly with heparin.
- If patient requires thrombolytic therapy, drug should be discontinued.
- Vials should be stored in refrigerator. Vials may be stored at room temperature but must be discarded if not used within 2 months.
- *Incompatibilities:* None listed by manufacturer

Route	Onset	Peak	Duration
I.V.	Immediate	5 min	4 hr

Half-life: 2.5–2.8 hr

Mechanism of Action

Reversibly inhibits platelet aggregation by preventing fibrinogen, von Willebrand factor, and other adhesive ligands from binding to glycoprotein IIb/IIIa receptors on activated platelets. As a result, eptifibatide disrupts final cross-linking stage of platelet aggregation—and thrombus formation.

Contraindications

Active bleeding, bleeding diathesis, or stroke during prior 30 days, current or planned administration of another parenteral GP IIb/IIIa inhibitor, dependency on dialysis, history of hemorrhagic stroke, hypersensitivity to eptifibatide or its components, major surgery during previous 6 weeks, severe uncontrolled hypertension (systolic pressure above 200 mm Hg, diastolic pressure above 110 mm Hg)

Interactions

DRUGS

anticoagulants, other antiplatelet agents, other platelet aggregation inhibitors (especially inhibitors of platelet receptor glycoprotein IIb/IIIa, such as abciximab) thrombolytics:

Increased risk of additive pharmacologic effects, increased risk of bleeding

Adverse Reactions
CNS: Intracranial hemorrhage
CV: Hypotension
GI: GI hemorrhage, hematemesis
GU: Hematuria
HEME: Bleeding that may be severe, decreased hemoglobin level, immune-mediated thrombocytopenia, thrombocytopenia
RESP: Pulmonary hemorrhage
Other: Anaphylaxis

Childbearing Considerations
PREGNANCY
- It is not known if drug causes fetal harm.
- Use with caution only if benefit to mother outweighs potential risk to fetus.

LACTATION
- It is not known if drug is present in breast milk.
- Patient should check with prescriber before breastfeeding.

Nursing Considerations
- Expect to obtain APTT and PT as a baseline and hematocrit and hemoglobin, platelet count, and serum creatinine during therapy.
- Expect to keep APTT between 50 and 70 seconds or per facility protocol during therapy unless patient has PTCA.
- Be aware that if patient has PTCA, expect to maintain activated clotting time between 200 and 250 seconds during the procedure.
- Avoid arterial and venous punctures, I.M. injections, urinary catheters, nasotracheal or nasogastric intubation, and use of noncompressible I.V. sites, such as subclavian and jugular veins during therapy.
- Expect to discontinue eptifibatide and heparin and monitor patient closely if platelet count falls below 100,000/mm^3.
- Plan to stop drug, as prescribed, if patient undergoes coronary artery bypass surgery.

PATIENT TEACHING
- Instruct patient to immediately report bleeding during eptifibatide therapy.
- Reassure patient that he'll be monitored closely throughout therapy.
- Advise patient to avoid activities that may lead to bruising and bleeding.

eptinezumab-jjmr
Vyepti

Class and Category
Pharmacologic class: Monoclonal antibody (calcitonin gene-related peptide antagonist)
Therapeutic class: Antimigraine

Indications and Dosages
✳ *To prevent migraine*
I.V. INFUSION
Adults. 100 mg every 3 months; dosage increased to 300 mg every 3 months, if needed.

Drug Administration
I.V.
- Must be diluted before administration. Dilute dose with 100 ml of 0.9% Sodium Chloride Injection. The infusion bag of 0.9% Sodium Chloride Injection must be made of polyvinyl chloride (PVC), polyethylene (PE), or polyolefin (PO).
- Discard any unused portion remaining in drug vial because it contains no preservative.
- Gently invert the drug solution to mix completely. Do not shake.
- Must be infused within 8 hours after being mixed.
- Infuse over approximately 30 minutes using an intravenous infusion set with a 0.2-micron or 0.22-micron inline or add-on sterile filter.
- After infusion is complete, flush the line with 20 ml of 0.9% Sodium Chloride Injection.
- Never administer as a bolus injection or intravenous push.
- May be stored at room temperature. Do not freeze.
- *Incompatibilities:* Other drugs or solutions other than 0.9% Sodium Chloride Injection

Route	Onset	Peak	Duration
I.V.	Unknown	30 min	Unknown

Half-life: 27 days

Mechanism of Action
Binds to calcitonin gene-related peptide ligand and blocks its binding to the receptor, which interferes with pain mechanism in migraine headaches.

Contraindications
Hypersensitivity to eptinezumab-jjmr or its components

Interactions
DRUGS
None reported by manufacturer

Adverse Reactions
EENT: Nasopharyngitis
ENDO: Hot flashes
SKIN: Facial flushing, pruritus, rash, urticaria
OTHER: Anaphylaxis, angioedema, hypersensitivity reactions

Childbearing Considerations
PREGNANCY
- It is not known if drug can cause fetal harm.
- Use with caution only if benefit to mother outweighs potential risk to fetus.
- Be aware that women with migraine may be at increased risk of gestational hypertension and preeclampsia during pregnancy.

LACTATION
- It is not known if drug is present in breast milk.
- Patient should check with prescriber before breastfeeding.

Nursing Considerations
! **WARNING** Monitor patient for hypersensitivity reactions that may become serious. Reactions such as angioedema, facial flushing, rash, and urticaria may occur. Hypersensitivity reactions usually occur during the infusion of eptinezumab-jjmr rather than after drug administration. If a reaction occurs, notify prescriber, expect drug to be discontinued, and institute appropriate therapy, as ordered and needed.

- Be aware that, as with all therapeutic proteins, there is a potential for the development of anti-eptinezumab-jjmr antibodies.

PATIENT TEACHING
! **WARNING** Review signs and symptoms of hypersensitivity reactions. Advise patient to seek emergency medical treatment, if present.

- Instruct female patients of childbearing age to notify prescriber if pregnancy occurs

or is being planned or if breastfeeding is planned because effects of drug on the fetus or neonate are unknown.

eravacycline
Xerava

Class and Category
Pharmacologic class: Tetracycline
Therapeutic class: Antibiotic

Indications and Dosages
* *To treat complicated intra-abdominal infections caused by* Bacteroides *species,* Citrobacter freundii, Clostridium perfringens, Enterobacter cloacae, Enterococcus faecalis, Enterococcus faecium, Escherichia coli, Klebsiella pneumoniae, Klebsiella oxytoca, Parabacteroides distasonis, Staphylococcus aureus, Streptococcus anginosus *group*

I.V. INFUSION
Adults. 1 mg/kg every 12 hr for 4 to 14 days, depending on location and severity of infection and clinical response.
±**DOSAGE ADJUSTMENT** For patients with severe hepatic impairment, dosage remains at 1 mg/kg every 12 hr for day 1, followed by 1 mg/kg every 24 hr starting on day 2 and continued for duration of therapy. For patients using a strong CYP3A inducer, dosage increased to 1.5 mg/kg every 12 hr for duration of therapy.

Drug Administration
I.V.
- To reconstitute, use the appropriate number of vials for dosage prescribed and reconstitute each vial with 5 ml of Sterile Water for Injection or 0.9% Sodium Chloride Injection, which will deliver 10 mg/ml for 50-mg vial and 20 mg/ml for 100-mg vial.
- Swirl vial gently until powder is dissolved. Avoid shaking or rapid movement, as it may cause foaming. Solution should be a clear, pale yellow to orange solution. Dilute further within 1 hour of reconstitution.
- Further dilute reconstituted solution from each vial for dosage prescribed. Then add reconstituted solution to a 0.9% Sodium Chloride Injection infusion bag to

generate an infusion solution with a target concentration of 0.3 mg/ml (within range of 0.2 to 0.6 mg/ml). Do not shake bag.

- Expect to use diluted solutions within 24 hours if stored at room temperature or within 10 days if refrigerated.
- Administer over 60 minutes through a dedicated line or through a Y-site. If same line is used for other drugs, flush line before and after infusion of eravacycline with 0.9% Sodium Chloride Injection, USP.
- *Incompatibilities:* Other drugs or I.V. infusion solutions except for 0.9% Sodium Chloride Injection

Route	Onset	Peak	Duration
I.V.	Unknown	Unknown	Unknown

Half-life: 20 hr

≣ Mechanism of Action

Disrupts bacterial protein synthesis by binding to the 30S ribosomal subunit, which prevents the incorporation of amino acid residues into elongating peptide chains needed for bacterial action.

≣ Contraindications

Hypersensitivity to eravacycline, tetracycline-class antibacterial drugs, or their components

≣ Interactions

DRUGS

anticoagulants: Depressed plasma prothrombin activity
CYP3A inducers (strong): Decreases exposure of eravacycline, which may reduce effectiveness

≣ Adverse Reactions

CNS: Anxiety, depression, dizziness, insomnia
CV: Chest pain, **hypotension**, palpitations
EENT: Taste distortion, tooth discoloration
GI: **Acute pancreatitis or necrosis,** *Clostridium difficile*–**associated diarrhea,** diarrhea, elevated liver and pancreatic enzymes, nausea, vomiting
GU: Elevated creatinine levels
HEME: **Leukopenia, neutropenia, prolonged activated partial thromboplastin time**
MS: Bone growth inhibition
RESP: Dyspnea, pleural effusion
SKIN: Excessive diaphoresis, rash

OTHER: Hypersensitivity reactions, hypocalcemia, infusion-site reactions, wound dehiscence

≣ Childbearing Considerations

PREGNANCY

- Drug can cause fetal harm such as adverse effects on skeletal and tooth development.
- Use of drug during the second or third trimesters of pregnancy may cause permanent discoloration of the child's teeth.
- Drug should not be used during pregnancy unless there is no alternative available.

LACTATION

- It is not known if drug is present in breast milk, although other tetracyclines are.
- Breastfeeding should not occur during drug therapy and for 4 days after the last dose.

REPRODUCTION

- Drug may possibly lead to impaired spermiation and sperm maturation, resulting in abnormal sperm morphology and poor motility.

≣ Nursing Considerations

- Know that eravacycline should not be used to treat complicated urinary tract infections.
- Be aware that drug may cause permanent tooth discoloration if given during tooth development and therefore should be avoided in pregnant women during the last half of the pregnancy and in children younger than 8 years.

> **! WARNING** Monitor patient for hypersensitivity reactions that may be life-threatening. If an allergic reaction occurs, stop drug therapy, notify prescriber, and provide supportive measures, as prescribed.

- Monitor patient for signs and symptoms of *Clostridium difficile*–associated diarrhea. If suspected or confirmed, notify prescriber, expect that eravacycline may be discontinued, and provide supportive care, as ordered and needed (antibacterial drug treatment of *C. difficile*, fluid and electrolyte therapy, protein supplementation, and possibly surgical evaluation, as needed).

> **! WARNING** Monitor patient for tetracycline-class adverse reactions because eravacycline as a tetracycline may cause similar reactions. Know that adverse reactions such as

anti-anabolic action, photosensitivity, and pseudotumor cerebri, have occurred with tetracycline use. Anti-anabolic action may lead to abnormal liver enzymes, acidosis, azotemia, hyperphosphatemia, and pancreatitis. If any of these serious adverse reactions occur, notify prescriber, and expect drug to be discontinued.

- Monitor patient for overgrowth of nonsusceptible organisms, including fungi, because eravacycline therapy may result in overgrowth. If such infections occur, notify prescriber; expect drug to be discontinued and appropriate therapy instituted.

PATIENT TEACHING

! **WARNING** Tell patient to notify staff or seek immediate medical attention if serious allergic reactions occur.

- Advise women not to breastfeed during eravacycline therapy and for 4 days after the last dose.
- Inform women of childbearing age to notify prescriber if pregnant.
- Tell patient that diarrhea is a common problem with antibiotic therapy including eravacycline and usually ends when drug is discontinued. However, sometimes watery and bloody stools can occur, which signals something more serious. This can occur even as late as 2 or more months after therapy was discontinued. Prescriber should be contacted as soon as possible if this occurs.
- Instruct patient on tetracycline-class adverse reactions and tell patient to notify prescriber promptly if present.
- Warn patient that eravacycline may cause an overgrowth of other micro-organisms. If another infection develops, instruct patient to notify prescriber.

erenumab-aooe
Aimovig

Class and Category
Pharmacologic class: Human monoclonal antibody
Therapeutic class: Antimigraine

Indications and Dosages
✴ *To prevent migraine headaches*
SUBCUTANEOUS INJECTION
Adults. 70 mg to 140 mg (given as two 70-mg consecutive injections) monthly.

Drug Administration
SUBCUTANEOUS
- Needle shield within the white cap of the prefilled autoinjector and the gray needle cap of the prefilled syringe contain dry natural rubber, a derivative of latex. Handling the caps may cause allergic reactions in individuals sensitive to latex.
- Store in refrigerator in original container until ready to use, protecting from light.
- Allow erenumab-aooe to sit at room temperature for at least 30 minutes protected from direct sunlight prior to administration. Drug should not be warmed by using a heat source such as hot water or a microwave.
- Do not shake solution.
- Inspect solution and do not use if solution is cloudy or discolored or contains flakes or particles.
- Both prefilled autoinjector and prefilled syringe are single dose; give entire contents. If patient is prescribed a 140-mg dose, give as two 70-mg consecutive injections.
- Administer in the abdomen, thigh, or upper arm. Do not inject into areas where the skin is bruised, hard, red, or tender.
- Once removed from refrigerator, keep in original container at room temperature for up to 7 days. Discard, if not used, after 7 days.
- If a dose is missed, give as soon as possible and then reschedule monthly dose from that dose.

Route	Onset	Peak	Duration
SQ	Unknown	4–6 days	Unknown

Half-life: 28 days

Mechanism of Action
Binds to the calcitonin gene-related peptide (CGRP) receptor. The CGRP receptor is thought to be responsible for transmitting signals that can cause incapacitating pain. By binding to the CGRP receptor, the drug antagonizes its function, preventing pain signals from being transmitted.

Contraindications

Hypersensitivity to erenumab-aooe or its components

Interactions

DRUGS

None reported by manufacturer

Adverse Reactions

CV: Hypertension
EENT: Mucosal ulceration
GI: Constipation (may become severe)
MS: Muscle cramps or spasms
SKIN: Alopecia, rash
Other: Anaphylaxis, angioedema, erenumab-aooe antibody formation, injection-site reactions (erythema, pain, pruritus)

Childbearing Considerations

PREGNANCY

- It is not known if drug causes fetal harm.
- Use with caution only if benefit to mother outweighs potential risk to fetus.
- Know that women with migraine may be at increased risk of preeclampsia during pregnancy.

LACTATION

- It is not known if drug is present in breast milk.
- Patient should check with prescriber before breastfeeding.

Nursing Considerations

- Monitor effectiveness of drug to relieve migraine headaches.

! WARNING Monitor patient for hypersensitivity reactions, which usually are not serious and occurs within hours of administration. However, some have occurred more than one week after administration and some have been serious or severe. Be prepared to initiate appropriate treatment if serious or severe and expect drug to be discontinued.

- Monitor patient for constipation, which could become severe with serious complications requiring hospitalization. Patients who are taking drugs that decrease gastrointestinal motility are at increased risk.
- Monitor patient's blood pressure because hypertension may develop or worsen if preexisting. Hypertension may occur at any time, but most commonly occurs

within 7 days of dose administration. Notify prescriber, as drug may have to be discontinued.

PATIENT TEACHING

- Instruct patient how to prepare and administer erenumab-aooe as a subcutaneous injection using the single-dose prefilled autoinjector or single-dose prefilled syringe.
- Warn patient that the needle shield within the white cap of the prefilled autoinjector and the gray needle cap of the prefilled syringe contain dry natural rubber, a derivative of latex. Handling the caps may cause allergic reactions in individuals sensitive to latex.
- Tell patient to allow drug to sit at room temperature for at least 30 minutes protected from direct sunlight. Caution patient not to warm drug by using a heat source such as hot water or a microwave. Also caution patient not to shake the syringe. Instruct patient to inspect solution for discoloration or particulate matter prior to administration. Tell him not to use solution if it is cloudy or discolored or contains flakes or particles. Remind him that both the prefilled autoinjector and prefilled syringe are single dose and to deliver the entire contents with each injection.
- Inform patient prescribed the 140-mg dose to administer the drug once a month as two separate but consecutive subcutaneous injections of 70 mg each.
- Instruct patient to administer the injection in the abdomen, thigh, or upper arm subcutaneously. Advise patient not to inject into areas where the skin is bruised, hard, red, or tender.
- Inform patient that drug may cause injection-site reactions such as itching, pain, or redness. Also tell patient that muscle cramps or spasms may occur, as well as constipation.
- Instruct patient that if a dose is missed, he should administer drug as soon as possible. Thereafter, drug can be given monthly from the date of that dose.

! WARNING Alert patient that hypersensitivity reactions may occur even as late as one week after administration. Although most are not serious, stress importance of seeking immediate medical attention if difficulty breathing or swallowing occurs.

- Inform patient that constipation is one of the most common adverse reactions related to drug use. However, tell patient to report constipation that is prolonged or severe because a bowel obstruction could occur if left untreated.
- Tell patient that blood pressure may become elevated during therapy, but most commonly within 7 days of dosage administration. Have patient monitor blood pressure, if possible, and notify prescriber if blood pressure becomes elevated.

ertapenem sodium
Invanz

☰ Class and Category
Pharmacologic class: Carbapenem
Therapeutic class: Antibiotic

☰ Indications and Dosages
❋ *To treat moderate to severe infections, such as acute pelvic infections (including postpartum endomyometritis, postsurgical gynecologic infections, or septic abortion) due to* Bacteroides fragilis, Escherichia coli, Peptostreptococcus *species,* Prevotella bivia, Porphyromonas asaccharolytica, *or* Streptococcus agalactiae; *community-acquired pneumonia due to* Haemophilus influenzae *(beta-lactamase-negative strains only),* Moraxella catarrhalis, *or* Streptococcus pneumoniae *(penicillin-susceptible strains only, including cases with concurrent bacteremia); complicated intra-abdominal infections due to* B. distasonis, B. fragilis, B. ovatus, B. thetaiotaomicron, B. uniformis, Clostridium clostridioforme, E. coli, Eubacterium lentum, *or* Peptostreptococcus *species; complicated skin and skin structure infections, including diabetic foot infections without osteomyelitis, due to* B. fragilis, E. coli, Klebsiella pneumoniae, Peptostreptococcus *species,* Porphyromonas asaccharolytica, P. bivia, Proteus mirabilis, Staphylococcus aureus, S. agalactiae, *or* S. pyogenes; *and complicated UTI (including pyelonephritis) due to* E. coli *(including cases with concurrent bacteremia) or* K. pneumoniae

I.V. INFUSION
Adults and adolescents. 1 g daily, 3 to 10 days for acute pelvic infections, 10 to 14 days for community-acquired pneumonia, 5 to 14 days for complicated intra-abdominal infections, 7 to 14 days for complicated skin and skin structure infections including diabetic foot infections, and 10 to 14 days for complicated urinary tract infections.
Children ages 3 months to 12 years. 15 mg/kg twice daily, for 3 to 10 days for acute pelvic infections, 10 to 14 days for community-acquired pneumonia, 5 to 14 days for complicated intra-abdominal infections, 7 to 14 days for complicated skin and skin structure infections including diabetic foot infections, and 10 to 14 days for complicated urinary tract infections. *Maximum:* 1 g daily.

I.M. INJECTION
Adults and adolescents. 1 g daily for up to 7 days.
Children ages 3 months to 13 years. 15 mg/kg twice daily for up to 7 days. *Maximum:* 1 g daily.
❋ *To provide prophylaxis of surgical site infection following elective colorectal surgery*

I.V. INFUSION
Adults. 1 g given 1 hr prior to surgical incision.
±**DOSAGE ADJUSTMENT** Dosage decreased to 500 mg daily for patients with advanced renal insufficiency (creatinine clearance less than or equal to 30 ml/min) or end-stage renal insufficiency (creatinine clearance less than or equal to 10 ml/min). For patients on hemodialysis who have received 500 mg of ertapenem within 6 hr of hemodialysis, supplemental dose of 150 mg given after hemodialysis.

☰ Drug Administration
I.V.
- Reconstitute 1 g with 10 ml 0.9% Sodium Chloride Injection, Bacteriostatic Water for Injection, or Sterile Water for Injection. Don't use solutions that contain dextrose.
- Shake well to dissolve.
- For adults, immediately transfer reconstituted drug to 50 ml of 0.9% Sodium Chloride Injection solution. For children 3 months to 12 years, immediately withdraw a volume equal to 15 mg/kg (not to exceed 1 g/day), then dilute in 0.9% Sodium Chloride Injection to a final concentration of 20 mg/ml.

E
F

- Infuse over 30 minutes.
- Store reconstituted and diluted solution at room temperature and use within 6 hours or store in refrigerator and use within 4 hours after removal from refrigerator. Do not freeze.
- *Incompatibilities:* Dextrose solutions, other drugs

I.M.

- Reconstitute 1 g of drug with 3.2 ml of 1% Lidocaine Hydrochloride Injection (without epinephrine). Shake thoroughly.
- Use within 1 hour after preparation.
- For adults, withdraw contents of vial and inject deep into a large muscle mass such as the gluteal muscle or lateral part of thigh. For children 3 months to 13 years, withdraw a volume equal to 15 mg/kg (not to exceed 1 g/day) and inject deep into a large muscle mass such as the gluteal muscles or lateral part of the thigh.
- Don't give reconstituted I.M. solution by I.V. route because of possible adverse reaction to lidocaine hydrochloride injection used to reconstitute drug.

Route	Onset	Peak	Duration
I.V.	Immediate	30 min	24 hr
I.M.	Unknown	2 hr	24 hr

Half-life: 4 hr

Mechanism of Action

Inhibits bacterial cell wall synthesis by binding to specific penicillin-binding proteins inside the cell wall. Penicillin-binding proteins are responsible for various steps in bacterial cell wall synthesis. By binding to these proteins, ertapenem leads to bacterial cell wall lysis.

Contraindications

Hypersensitivity to ertapenem, beta-lactams, other drugs in the same class, or their components; hypersensitivity to local anesthetics of the amide type (I.M. injection)

Interactions

DRUGS

probenecid: Increased ertapenem half-life, increased and prolonged blood ertapenem level

valproic acid: Possibly decreased serum valproic acid level and increased risk of breakthrough seizures

Adverse Reactions

CNS: Abnormal coordination, aggression, agitation, anxiety, asthenia, confusion, delirium, depressed level of consciousness, disorientation, dizziness, dyskinesia, fatigue, fever, gait disturbance, hallucinations, headache, hypothermia, insomnia, mental changes, myoclonus, **seizures**, somnolence, stupor, tremor

CV: Chest pain, edema, hypersensitivity vasculitis, hypertension, **hypotension**, tachycardia, thrombophlebitis

EENT: Nasopharyngitis, oral candidiasis, rhinitis, rhinorrhea, teeth staining, viral pharyngitis

ENDO: Hyperglycemia

GI: Abdominal pain, acid regurgitation, anorexia, **Clostridium difficile–associated diarrhea**, constipation, diarrhea, elevated liver enzymes, indigestion, nausea, **small intestine obstruction**, vomiting

GU: Dysuria, elevated serum creatinine level, genital rash, proteinuria, RBCs and WBCs in urine, UTI, vaginitis

HEME: Anemia, decreased hematocrit, eosinophilia, leukocytosis, **leukopenia**, **neutropenia**, **prolonged PT**, **thrombocytopenia**, thrombocytosis

MS: Arthralgia, leg pain, muscle weakness

RESP: **Atelectasis**, cough, crackles, dyspnea, pleural effusion, pneumonia, **respiratory distress**, upper respiratory tract infection, wheezing

SKIN: Acute generalized exanthematous pustulosis, cellulitis, dermatitis, erythema, extravasation, pruritus, rash

Other: **Anaphylaxis; death; drug reaction with eosinophilia and systemic symptoms (DRESS); hyperkalemia;** hypokalemia; infusion-site induration, pain, phlebitis, pruritus, redness, swelling, or warmth

Childbearing Considerations

PREGNANCY

- It is not known if drug causes fetal harm.
- Use with caution only if benefit to mother outweighs potential risk to fetus.

LACTATION

- Drug is present in breast milk.
- Patient should check with prescriber before breastfeeding.

≣ Nursing Considerations

- Obtain sputum, urine, or other specimens for culture and sensitivity testing, as ordered, before giving ertapenem. Expect to start therapy before results are available.

! WARNING Monitor patient closely for a life-threatening anaphylactic reaction. Patients with a history of hypersensitivity to cephalosporins, penicillin, other allergens or other beta-lactams are at increased risk. Know that if drug triggers an anaphylactic reaction, stop drug, notify prescriber immediately, and provide appropriate therapy. Anaphylaxis requires immediate treatment with epinephrine as well as airway management and administration of I.V. corticosteroids and oxygen, as needed.

- Be aware that patients with a history of seizures, other CNS disorders that predispose them to seizures (such as brain lesions), or compromised renal function may be at increased risk for seizures. Administer anticonvulsant, as ordered.
- Monitor patient for diarrhea during and for at least 2 months after drug therapy; diarrhea may signal pseudomembranous colitis caused by *C. difficile*. If diarrhea occurs, notify prescriber and expect to withhold ertapenem and treat with an antibiotic effective against *C. difficile,* electrolytes, fluids, and protein.

PATIENT TEACHING

! WARNING Instruct patient receiving ertapenem to immediately report signs of anaphylaxis, such as itching, rash, or shortness of breath; or signs of superinfection, such as severe diarrhea or white patches on tongue or in mouth.

- Urge patient to tell prescriber about diarrhea that's severe or lasts longer than 3 days. Remind patient that watery or bloody stools can occur 2 or more months after antibiotic therapy and can be serious, requiring prompt treatment.
- Alert patient taking divalproex or valproic acid for seizure control to notify prescriber of this type of concurrent therapy because ertapenem may interfere with these drugs' effectiveness to control seizures.

ertugliflozin
Steglatro

≣ Class and Category
Pharmacologic class: Sodium glucose-dependent cotransporter inhibitor
Therapeutic class: Antidiabetic

≣ Indications and Dosages
∗ *As adjunct to improve glycemic control in patients with type 2 diabetes mellitus*
TABLETS
Adults. *Initial:* 5 mg once daily, increased as needed. *Maximum:* 15 mg once daily.

≣ Drug Administration
P.O.
- Administer in the morning.
- Drug may have to be temporarily discontinued if dehydration occurs.

Route	Onset	Peak	Duration
P.O.	Unknown	1 hr	Unknown

Half-life: 16.6 hr

≣ Mechanism of Action
Inhibits sodium glucose link transporter-2 to reduce renal reabsorption of filtered glucose and lower the renal threshold for glucose. These actions increase urinary glucose excretion and lower blood glucose levels.

≣ Contraindications
Dialysis, end-stage renal disease, hypersensitivity to ertugliflozin or its components, severe renal impairment

≣ Interactions
DRUGS
insulin, insulin secretagogues: Increased risk of hypoglycemia

≣ Adverse Reactions
CNS: Headache, thirst
CV: Elevated low-density lipoprotein cholesterol, **hypotension**
EENT: Nasopharyngitis
ENDO: **Ketoacidosis**
GU: **Acute kidney injury and impairment, acute prerenal failure,** decreased estimated glomerular filtration rate, elevated serum creatinine levels, genital mycotic infections,

E
F

increased urination, **necrotizing fasciitis of the perineum (Fournier's gangrene)**, **pyelonephritis, urosepsis,** UTI, vaginal pruritus
HEME: Increased hemoglobin level
MS: Back pain
Other: Angioedema, dehydration, **hyperphosphatemia,** weight loss

Childbearing Considerations

PREGNANCY

- Drug may cause fetal harm, especially on the renal system.
- Drug is not recommended during the second and third trimesters of pregnancy.

LACTATION

- It is not known if drug is present in breast milk.
- Breastfeeding is not recommended because kidney maturation continues through the first 2 years of life.

Nursing Considerations

- Know that volume depletion should be corrected before ertugliflozin therapy is begun.
- Assess patient for factors that may predispose patient to acute kidney injury before ertugliflozin therapy is begun. Risk factors may include presence of chronic renal insufficiency, congestive heart failure, and hypovolemia and use of drugs such as ACE inhibitors, ARBs, diuretics, and NSAIDs. Be aware that ertugliflozin should not be initiated in patients who have an estimated glomerular filtration rate (eGFR) below 45 ml/min. Assess renal function before ertugliflozin is initiated and periodically throughout drug therapy, as ordered.
- Review patient's history for any risk factors that may predispose patient to need a lower-limb amputation, such as presence of diabetic foot ulcers, neuropathy, peripheral vascular disease, or a prior amputation, before ertugliflozin therapy is begun. This is because an increased risk for lower-limb amputation has been found with another drug in the same class as ertugliflozin.
- Monitor patient's blood pressure closely because ertugliflozin causes intravascular volume contraction. Those at greater risk include the elderly and patients with impaired renal function or low systolic blood pressure or with concomitant use of diuretics.

! WARNING Monitor patient for signs and symptoms of metabolic acidosis. If present, also assess patient for ketoacidosis. Know that patient may have ketoacidosis even if her blood glucose level is less than 250 mg/dl. If ketoacidosis is suspected, notify prescriber. If confirmed, expect ertugliflozin to be discontinued and treatment with carbohydrate, fluid, and insulin replacement to be given.

- Expect ertugliflozin to be withheld when oral intake is reduced, such as in acute illness or fasting, or when fluid losses occur, such as excessive heat exposure or gastrointestinal illness. This is because dehydration increases risk of kidney impairment that could be quite serious.
- Monitor patient for signs and symptoms of infection, new pain or tenderness, sores, or ulcers involving the lower limbs. If present, notify prescriber and expect drug to be discontinued.
- Monitor patients also receiving insulin or an insulin secretagogue such as a sulfonylurea for hypoglycemia. Dosage of these drugs may have to be reduced to minimize the risk of hypoglycemia.
- Assess both men and women for genital mycotic infections, which may occur with ertugliflozin therapy. Patients at higher risk include those with a history of genital mycotic infections or men who are uncircumcised.

! WARNING Monitor patient for a rare but serious and life-threatening necrotizing infection of the perineum called Fournier's gangrene. Notify prescriber immediately if patient develops erythema, pain, swelling, or tenderness in the genital or perineal area, along with fever or malaise. Expect treatment with broad-spectrum antibiotics and, if needed, surgical debridement of the area. Know that ertugliflozin will be discontinued if this occurs. Monitor patient's blood glucose levels closely and expect an alternative treatment for glycemic control.

PATIENT TEACHING

- Advise patient to take ertugliflozin exactly as prescribed and to take drug in the morning. Tell her if a dose is missed to take it as soon as it's remembered unless it is close to the next dose. Warn patient never to double the dose.

- Inform patients also prescribed insulin or antidiabetic agents known to cause hypoglycemia to monitor blood glucose level closely, as hypoglycemia may occur. Also review the signs and symptoms of hypoglycemia and how to treat.
- Instruct patient to maintain adequate fluid intake, as dehydration increases the risk of the blood pressure dropping. Advise patient to notify prescriber if he experiences dizziness or light-headedness and weakness.

! WARNING Teach patient how to check urine for ketones and review signs and symptoms of ketoacidosis with patient. Remind patient that ketoacidosis may occur even when her blood glucose is not elevated. Tell patient to seek immediate medical attention if she experiences abdominal pain, labored breathing, nausea, tiredness, and vomiting and ketones are present in urine.

- Instruct patient to report any persistent, severe, or unusual signs and symptoms to prescriber, especially if changes in kidney function occur.
- Inform patient of the potential for an increased risk of amputations. Review preventative foot care with patient. Tell patient to report any infection, new pain or tenderness, sore, or ulcer involving the foot or leg to prescriber and seek immediate medical attention.
- Tell patient to seek medical care if a urinary tract infection occurs, because it can become serious if left untreated.
- Review signs and symptoms of genital mycotic infection such as itching, rash, or redness in the area. Tell patient to notify prescriber if present.

! WARNING Warn patient to stop ertugliflozin and seek immediate medical attention if pain, redness, swelling, or tenderness occurs in the genital or perineal area along with fever or malaise because, although rare, this cluster of symptoms may become life-threatening.

- Remind patient to monitor her diabetes by testing blood glucose, as she will test positive for glucose in the urine while taking ertugliflozin.

- Advise women of childbearing age to notify prescriber if pregnancy occurs, because ertugliflozin therapy is not recommended during the second and third trimesters of pregnancy.
- Tell women considering breastfeeding that it is not recommended during ertugliflozin therapy.

erythromycin base
E-Mycin, Erybid (CAN), ERY-C, Ery-Tab

erythromycin ethylsuccinate
E.E.S., EryPed

erythromycin lactobionate
Erythrocin

erythromycin stearate
Erythro-S (CAN), Erythrocin Stearate

Class and Category
Pharmacologic class: Macrolide
Therapeutic class: Antibiotic

Indications and Dosages
* *To treat mild to moderate respiratory tract infections caused by* Haemophilus influenzae, Streptococcus pneumoniae, *or* Streptococcus pyogenes *(group A beta-hemolytic streptococcus)*

CAPSULES, CHEWABLE TABLETS, DELAYED-RELEASE CAPSULES, DELAYED-RELEASE TABLETS, ORAL SUSPENSION, TABLETS

Adults. 250 (base) or 400 mg to 800 mg (ethylsuccinate) every 6 hr for 10 days. Alternatively, 500 mg (base) every 12 hr or one-half of total daily dose (ethylsuccinate) every 12 hr or one-third total daily dose (ethylsuccinate) every 8 hr.
Children. 30 to 50 mg (base)/kg daily in divided doses every 6 hr for 10 days.

For more severe infection, dosage may be doubled. For *H. influenzae* infections, erythromycin ethylsuccinate is administered with 150 mg/kg daily of sulfisoxazole.

✳ *To treat severe respiratory tract infections caused by* H. influenzae, S. pneumoniae, *or* S. pyogenes *(group A beta-hemolytic streptococcus)*

I.V. INFUSION (ERYTHROMYCIN LACTOBIONATE)

Adults. 1 to 4 g daily continuously or in divided doses every 6 hr for 10 days.
Children. 15 to 20 mg/kg daily in divided doses every 4 to 6 hr for 10 days.

✳ *To treat respiratory tract infections caused by* Mycoplasma pneumoniae

CAPSULES, CHEWABLE TABLETS, DELAYED-RELEASE CAPSULES, DELAYED-RELEASE TABLETS, ORAL SUSPENSION, TABLETS

Adults with mild to moderate infection. 250 to 500 mg (base) or 400 to 800 mg (ethylsuccinate) every 6 hr for up to 3 wk.

I.V. INFUSION (ERYTHROMYCIN LACTOBIONATE)

Adults with severe infection. 1 to 4 g daily continuously or in divided doses every 6 hours.

✳ *To treat skin and soft-tissue infections caused by* S. pyogenes *or* Staphylococcus aureus

CAPSULES, CHEWABLE TABLETS, DELAYED-RELEASE CAPSULES, DELAYED-RELEASE TABLETS, ORAL SUSPENSION, TABLETS

Adults with mild to moderate infection. 250 mg to 500 mg or 400 mg to 800 mg (ethylsuccinate) every 6 hr.

I.V. INFUSION (ERYTHROMYCIN LACTOBIONATE)

Adults with severe infection. 1 to 4 g (lactobionate) daily continuously or in divided doses every 6 hr for up to 3 wk.

✳ *To treat pertussis (whooping cough) caused by* Bordetella pertussis

CAPSULES, CHEWABLE TABLETS, DELAYED-RELEASE CAPSULES, DELAYED-RELEASE TABLETS, ORAL SUSPENSION, TABLETS

Adults and children. 40 to 50 mg (base)/kg daily in divided doses every 6 hr for 5 to 14 days.

✳ *To treat intestinal amebiasis caused by* Entamoeba histolytica

CAPSULES, CHEWABLE TABLETS, DELAYED-RELEASE CAPSULES, DELAYED-RELEASE TABLETS, ORAL SUSPENSION, TABLETS

Adults. 250 mg (base or stearate) or 400 mg (ethylsuccinate) every 6 hr or 500 mg (base, stearate) every 12 hr for 10 to 14 days.
Children. 30 to 50 mg (base or ethylsuccinate)/kg daily in divided doses for 10 to 14 days.

✳ *To treat pelvic inflammatory disease caused by* Neisseria gonorrhoeae

CAPSULES, CHEWABLE TABLETS, DELAYED-RELEASE CAPSULES, DELAYED-RELEASE TABLETS, ORAL SUSPENSION, TABLETS, I.V. INFUSION

Adults. 500 mg I.V. (lactobionate) every 6 hr for 3 days and then 250 mg to 500 mg (base) P.O. every 6 hr for 7 days.

✳ *To treat conjunctivitis in newborns*

ORAL SUSPENSION

Neonates. 50 mg (base)/kg daily in 4 divided doses for 14 days.

✳ *To treat pneumonia in neonates caused by* Chlamydia trachomatis

I.V. INFUSION (ERYTHROMYCIN LACTOBIONATE)

Neonates. 15 to 20 mg/kg daily continuously or in divided doses every 6 hr.

ORAL SUSPENSION

Neonates. 50 mg/kg (base, stearate) daily in 4 divided doses for at least 3 wk.

✳ *To treat urogenital infections caused by* C. trachomatis *during pregnancy*

CAPSULES, CHEWABLE TABLETS, DELAYED-RELEASE CAPSULES, DELAYED-RELEASE TABLETS, ORAL SUSPENSION, TABLETS

Adults. 500 mg (base, stearate) every 6 hr for 7 days; or 250 mg (base, stearate) every 6 hr for at least 14 days.

✳ *To treat nongonococcal urethritis or uncomplicated urethral, endocervical, or rectal infections caused by* C. trachomatis

CAPSULES, CHEWABLE TABLETS, DELAYED-RELEASE CAPSULES, DELAYED-RELEASE TABLETS, ORAL SUSPENSION, TABLETS

Adults. 500 mg (base, stearate) every 6 hr for 7 days. If patient can't tolerate high doses, 250 mg (base stearate) every 6 hr for 14 days.

Alternatively, 400 to 800 mg (ethylsuccinate) every 6 hr for 7 to 14 days.

✳ *To treat Legionnaire's disease*

CAPSULES, CHEWABLE TABLETS, DELAYED-RELEASE CAPSULES, DELAYED-RELEASE TABLETS, ORAL SUSPENSION, TABLETS, I.V. INFUSION

Adults. 1 to 4 g (base, stearate) daily in divided doses every 6 hr for 10 to 14 days. I.V. (lactobionate) dosage infused continuously or, dosage divided and given every 6 hr.

✳ *To prevent rheumatic fever*

CAPSULES, CHEWABLE TABLETS, DELAYED-RELEASE CAPSULES, DELAYED-RELEASE TABLETS, ORAL SUSPENSION, TABLETS

Adults. 250 mg (base, stearate) or 400 mg (ethylsuccinate) every 12 hr.

Children. 250 mg (base, stearate) twice daily.

▤ Drug Administration

P.O.

- Chewable tablets should be thoroughly chewed before swallowing. They are not to be swallowed whole.
- Capsules or tablets should be swallowed whole and not chewed, crushed, or split/opened.
- For oral suspension, use the calibrated measuring device provided to ensure accurate doses. Shake the suspension before measuring a dose.
- Administer with a full glass of water.
- Nonenteric forms should be administered 2 hours before or after a meal. Enteric-coated forms and oral suspension (ethylsuccinate) can be given with food, if GI upset occurs.

I.V.

- Don't use diluent with benzyl alcohol if drug is being given to a neonate.
- Reconstitute by adding 10 ml of preservative-free Sterile Water for Injection to each 500-mg vial. Do not use other diluents. Each ml contains 50 mg. Reconstituted solution is stable for 24 hours if stored at room temperature or 2 weeks if refrigerated.
- Dilute the reconstituted solution to a concentration of 1 to 5 mg/ml for intermittent infusion and 1 mg/ml for

continuous infusion using 0.9% Sodium Chloride Solution, Lactated Ringer's solution, or other solutions recommended by manufacturer. Diluted solution must be administered within 8 hours.

- Dextrose solutions should only be used if they are first buffered with 4% Sodium Bicarbonate.
- Infuse intermittent infusions over 20 to 60 minutes.
- Don't store infusions prepared in the ADD-Vantage system.
- Do not use flexible containers in series connections.

Route	Onset	Peak	Duration
P.O.	Unknown	2.5–4 hr	Unknown
I.V.	Unknown	Immediate	Unknown

Half-life: 1.5–2 hr

▤ Mechanism of Action

Binds with the 50S ribosomal subunit of the 70S ribosome in many types of aerobic, anaerobic, gram-negative, and gram-positive organisms. This action inhibits RNA-dependent protein synthesis in bacterial cells, causing them to die.

▤ Contraindications

Astemizole, cisapride, dihydroergotamine, ergotamine, lovastatin, pimozide, simvastatin, or terfenadine therapy; hypersensitivity to erythromycin, other macrolide antibiotics, or their components

▤ Interactions

DRUGS

alfentanil: Decreased alfentanil clearance, prolonged alfentanil action

amiodarone, dofetilide, procainamide, quinidine, sotalol: Increased risk of prolonged QT interval

astemizole, cisapride, pimozide, terfenadine: Increased risk of cardiotoxicity, prolonged QT interval, torsades de pointes, ventricular tachycardia, and death

calcium channel blockers such as amlodipine, diltiazem, verapamil: Increased risk of hypotension

carbamazepine, valproic acid: Possibly inhibited metabolism of these drugs, increasing their blood levels and risk of toxicity *clindamycin:* Antagonized effects of these drugs

colchicine: Possible life-threatening colchicine toxicity

cyclosporine: Increased risk of nephrotoxicity

digoxin: Increased serum digoxin level and risk of digitalis toxicity

dihydroergotamine, ergotamine: Decreased ergotamine metabolism, increased risk of ergot toxicity with ischemia and vasospasm

HMG-CoA reductase inhibitors such as atorvastatin, lovastatin, simvastatin: Possibly increased risk of rhabdomyolysis

midazolam, triazolam, and other related benzodiazepines: Increased pharmacologic effects of these drugs

oral anticoagulants: Increased anticoagulant effects, especially in the elderly

oral contraceptives: Decrease or loss of effectiveness of oral contraceptive

sildenafil: Increased effects of sildenafil

verapamil: Increased risk of bradyarrhythmias, hypotension, and lactic acidosis

xanthines (except dyphylline): Increased serum theophylline level with high doses and risk of theophylline toxicity

ACTIVITIES

alcohol use: Increased alcohol level (by 40%) with I.V. erythromycin

Adverse Reactions

CNS: Fatigue, fever, malaise, weakness
CV: Prolonged QT interval, torsades de pointes, ventricular arrhythmias
EENT: Hearing loss, oral candidiasis
GI: Abdominal cramps and pain, *Clostridium difficile*–associated diarrhea, diarrhea, hepatotoxicity, infantile hypertrophic pyloric stenosis, jaundice, nausea, vomiting
GU: Interstitial nephritis, vaginal candidiasis
MS: New or aggravated myasthenia gravis syndrome
SKIN: Erythema, pruritus, rash
Other: Fluid overload (from I.V. infusion), injection-site inflammation and phlebitis

Childbearing Considerations

PREGNANCY

- It is not known if drug causes fetal harm.
- Use with caution only if benefit to mother outweighs potential risk to fetus.

LACTATION

- Drug is present in breast milk.
- Patient should check with prescriber before breastfeeding.

Nursing Considerations

- Be aware that erythromycin should not be used in patients with history of QT interval prolongation or in patients with ongoing proarrhythmic conditions such as uncorrected hypokalemia or hypomagnesemia, serious bradycardia, and in patients receiving Class IA or Class III antiarrhythmic agents. Monitor the elderly closely as well because they are more susceptible to drug effects on the QT interval.
- Use erythromycin cautiously in patients with impaired hepatic function because drug is metabolized by the liver.
- Use erythromycin cautiously in elderly patients, especially those with renal or hepatic dysfunction, because these patients are at increased risk of hearing loss and torsades de pointes. They're also at increased risk of bleeding if taking an oral anticoagulant.
- Expect to obtain body fluid or tissue sample for culture and sensitivity testing before giving first erythromycin dose.
- Monitor liver enzymes periodically to detect hepatotoxicity, which is most common with erythromycin estolate. Signs typically appear within 2 weeks after continuous therapy starts and resolve when it stops.
- Assess hearing regularly, especially in elderly patients and those who receive 4 g or more daily or have hepatic or renal disease. Hearing impairment begins 36 hours to 8 days after treatment starts and usually begins to improve 1 to 14 days after it stops.
- Watch for evidence of fluid overload, such as acute dyspnea and crackles, during I.V. therapy.
- Monitor infants for vomiting or irritability with feeding because infantile hypertrophic pyloric stenosis has been reported.
- Assess myasthenia gravis patients for weakness because drug may aggravate it. Keep in mind that myasthenic syndrome may arise in patients previously undiagnosed with myasthenia gravis.
- Watch closely for signs and symptoms of superinfection. If they occur, notify prescriber and expect to stop drug and provide appropriate therapy.

- Monitor patient for diarrhea during and for at least 2 months after erythromycin therapy; diarrhea may signal pseudomembranous colitis caused by *Clostridium difficile.* If diarrhea occurs, notify prescriber and expect to withhold drug and treat with fluids, electrolytes, protein, and an antibiotic effective against *C. difficile.*
- Know that if patient receives an order for urine catecholamine analysis, notify prescriber because erythromycin interferes with fluorometric measurement of urine catecholamines.

PATIENT TEACHING
- Urge patient to complete prescribed therapy, even if he feels better before it's finished.
- Tell patient to notify prescriber if symptoms worsen or don't improve after a few days.
- Teach patient how to administer prescribed form of erythromycin. Instruct him to swallow capsules or tablets whole. Caution patient to chew the chewable tablets and not swallow chewable tablets whole. For an oral suspension, teach him to use the calibrated measuring device provided to ensure accurate doses. Remind him to shake the suspension before measuring a dose.
- Advise patient to take oral form of erythromycin with a full glass of water on an empty stomach.
- Instruct patient to take enteric-coated oral form with food if GI distress occurs.

! **WARNING** Instruct patient to promptly notify prescriber if he develops allergic reactions, hearing changes, or signs of hepatic dysfunction.

- Urge patient to tell prescriber about diarrhea that's severe or lasts longer than 3 days. Remind patient that watery or bloody stools can occur 2 or more months after antibiotic therapy and can be serious, requiring prompt treatment.

escitalopram oxalate
Lexapro

Class and Category
Pharmacologic class: Selective serotonin reuptake inhibitor (SSRI)
Therapeutic class: Antidepressant

Indications and Dosages
* *To treat acute generalized anxiety disorder*
ORAL SOLUTION, TABLETS
Adults. *Initial:* 10 mg once daily increased to 20 mg once daily after 1 or more wk, as needed.
* *To provide treatment and maintenance for major depression*
ORAL SOLUTION, TABLETS
Adults. *Initial:* 10 mg once daily, increased to 20 mg once daily after 1 wk, as needed.
Adolescents ages 12 to 17. *Initial:* 10 mg once daily, increased to 20 mg once daily after 3 wk, as needed.
±**DOSAGE ADJUSTMENT** Dosage shouldn't exceed 10 mg daily for elderly patients and those with hepatic impairment.

Drug Administration
P.O.
- Administer drug in the morning or evening.

Route	Onset	Peak	Duration
P.O.	Unknown	5 hr	Unknown
Half-life: 27–32 hr			

Mechanism of Action
Inhibits reuptake of the neurotransmitter serotonin by CNS neurons, thereby increasing the amount of serotonin available in nerve synapses. An elevated serotonin level may result in elevated mood and reduced anxiety or depression.

Contraindications
Concomitant therapy with pimozide; hypersensitivity to escitalopram, citalopram or its components; use within 14 days of MAO inhibitor therapy including intravenous methylene blue or linezolid

Interactions
DRUGS
amphetamines, buspirone, fentanyl, lithium, St. John's wort, tramadol, tricyclic antidepressants, triptans, tryptophan: increased risk of serotonin syndrome
aspirin, NSAIDs, warfarin: Possibly increased risk of bleeding
carbamazepine: Possibly increased clearance of escitalopram
cimetidine: Possibly increased plasma escitalopram level
CNS drugs: Additive CNS effects

lithium: Possible enhancement of the serotonergic effects of escitalopram

MAO inhibitors: Possibly hyperpyretic episodes, hypertensive crisis, serotonin syndrome, and severe seizures

metoprolol: Increased plasma metoprolol levels with decreased cardioselectivity of metoprolol

pimozide: Increased risk of QT prolongation

sumatriptan: Increased risk of hyperreflexia, incoordination, and weakness

triptans: Increased risk of serotonin syndrome

ACTIVITIES

alcohol use: Possibly increased cognitive and motor effects of alcohol

Adverse Reactions

CNS: Abnormal gait, acute psychosis, aggression, akathisia, delirium, dizziness, dyskinesia, dystonia, extrapyramidal effects, fatigue, headache, hypomania, insomnia, lethargy, mania, myoclonus, **neuroleptic malignant syndrome**, paresthesia, **seizures, serotonin syndrome**, somnolence, **suicidal ideation**

CV: Atrial fibrillation, cardiac failure, deep vein thrombosis, hypotension, MI, prolonged QT interval, torsades de pointes, ventricular arrhythmias

EENT: Acute-angle glaucoma, diplopia, dry mouth, nystagmus, rhinitis, sinusitis, toothache, visual hallucinations

ENDO: Diabetes mellitus, hyperprolactinemia, syndrome of inappropriate ADH secretion

GI: Abdominal pain, constipation, decreased appetite, diarrhea, flatulence, **GI bleeding or hemorrhage, hepatic necrosis, hepatitis**, indigestion, nausea, **pancreatitis, rectal hemorrhage**, vomiting

GU: Acute renal failure, anorgasmia, decreased libido, ejaculation disorders, impotence, priapism

HEME: Bleeding, decreased prothrombin time, hemolytic anemia, leukopenia, thrombocytopenia

MS: Neck or shoulder pain, **rhabdomyolysis**

RESP: Pulmonary embolism

SKIN: Ecchymosis, **erythema multiforme**, increased sweating, photosensitivity, **Stevens–Johnson syndrome, toxic epidermal necrolysis**, urticaria

Other: Anaphylaxis, angioedema, flu-like symptoms, **hyponatremia**

Childbearing Considerations

PREGNANCY

- Pregnancy exposure registry: 1-844-405 -6185 or https://womensmentalhealth .org/clinical-and-research-programs /pregnancyregistry/antidepressants/
- It is not known if drug causes fetal harm. However, be aware that neonates exposed to the drug late in the third trimester of pregnancy may develop serious and life-threatening adverse reactions, which can arise immediately following birth. These adverse reactions may require prolonged hospitalization, respiratory support, and tube feeding.
- Use with caution only if benefit to mother outweighs potential risk to fetus.

LACTATION

- Drug is present in breast milk.
- Patient should check with prescriber before breastfeeding.
- If breastfeeding occurs, infant should be monitored for agitation, excessive drowsiness, poor feeding, restlessness, and weight loss.

Nursing Considerations

- Use escitalopram cautiously in patients with history of mania or seizures, patients with severe renal impairment, and those with diseases or conditions that produce altered metabolism or hemodynamic responses.
- Be aware that patients should be assessed for bipolar disorder before escitalopram therapy begins, because its use in treating depression may precipitate a mixed/manic episode.

! **WARNING** Know that when escitalopram dosage increases, monitor patient for possible serotonin syndrome, which may include agitation, chills, confusion, diaphoresis, diarrhea, fever, hyperactive reflexes, poor coordination, restlessness, shaking, talking or acting with uncontrolled excitement, tremor, and twitching. In its most severe form, serotonin syndrome can resemble neuroleptic malignant syndrome, which includes autonomic instability with possible changes in vital signs, a high fever, muscle rigidity, and mental status changes.

- Be aware that escitalopram should not be given to patients with bradycardia, congenital long QT syndrome, hypokalemia or hypomagnesemia, recent acute myocardial infarction, or uncompensated heart failure because of increased risk of prolonged QT interval and torsades de pointes. It should also not be given to patients who are taking other drugs that prolong the QT interval. Expect hypokalemia and hypomagnesemia to be corrected before escitalopram therapy is begun.

- Monitor patient—especially elderly patient—for hypo-osmolarity of serum and urine and for hyponatremia (headache, impaired memory, trouble concentrating, unsteadiness, weakness) because they may indicate escitalopram-induced syndrome of inappropriate ADH secretion.
- Watch for signs of abuse or misuse; drug's potential for physical and psychological dependence is unknown.
- Monitor patient for bleeding, especially if patient is also taking an anticoagulant, aspirin, or an NSAID. Bleeding can range from ecchymoses, epistaxis, hematomas, and petechiae to life-threatening hemorrhages.
- Expect prescriber to reassess patient periodically to determine the continued need for therapy and evaluate dosage.
- Know that if patient (particularly an adolescent) takes escitalopram for depression, she must be watched closely for suicidal tendencies, especially when therapy starts or dosage changes, because depression may worsen temporarily.
- Expect to taper dosage to avoid serious adverse reactions when therapy is no longer needed.

PATIENT TEACHING

- Instruct patient to take drug either in the morning or evening.
- Inform patient that alcohol use isn't recommended during escitalopram therapy because it may decrease his ability to think clearly and perform motor skills.
- Advise patient to avoid hazardous activities until drug's CNS effects are known.
- Instruct patient that drug shouldn't be taken with citalopram hydrobromide because of potentially additive effects.
- Tell patient that improvement may not be noticed for 1 to 4 weeks after therapy

begins. Emphasize the importance of continuing therapy as prescribed.

- Urge caregivers to watch closely for suicidal tendencies, especially in adolescents and young adults and when therapy starts or dosage changes.
- Warn patient not to stop taking drug abruptly. Explain that gradual tapering helps to avoid withdrawal symptoms.
- Urge patient to inform prescriber of any OTC drugs he takes because of potential for interactions.
- Review signs and symptoms of hyponatremia, and instruct patient to report them to prescriber.
- Advise patient that drug may cause mild pupillary dilation, which may lead to an episode of acute-angle glaucoma. Encourage patient to have an eye exam before starting therapy to see if he is at risk.
- Warn patient that escitalopram increases bleeding risk if taken with an anticoagulant, aspirin, or an NSAID and that bleeding events could range from mild to severe. Tell patient to seek emergency care for serious or prolonged bleeding.
- Instruct patient to notify prescriber promptly of any persistent, severe, or unusual signs and symptoms.
- Stress importance of notifying prescriber if pregnancy occurs.

esketamine
Spravato

≡ Class and Category

Pharmacologic class: Ionotropic glutamate receptor
Therapeutic class: Antidepressant
Controlled substance schedule: III

≡ Indications and Dosages

* *As adjunct with an oral antidepressive for treatment-resistant depression*

NASAL SPRAY

Adults. *Induction phase (wks 1–4):* 56 mg on day 1; 56 or 84 mg twice a wk through wk 4. *Maintenance phase (wks 5–8):* 56 mg or 84 mg once a wk. *Maintenance phase (wk 9 and thereafter):* 56 mg or 84 mg every 2 wk unless weekly dosing is needed.

* As adjunct to treat depressive symptoms in patients with major depressive disorder with acute suicidal ideation or behavior

NASAL SPRAY

Adults. 84 mg twice a wk for 4 wk.

± **DOSAGE ADJUSTMENT** For patient unable to tolerate 84-mg dosage, dosage reduced to 56 mg twice a week for 4 wk.

Drug Administration

NASAL SPRAY

- Administration of esketamine should be at least 2 hours after patient ate and at least 30 minutes after patient had something to drink, because drug may cause nausea and vomiting after administration.
- Assess patient's blood pressure prior to administration. If baseline blood pressure is elevated (greater than 140 mmHg systolic, greater than 90 mmHg diastolic), drug should not be administered if the increase in blood pressure poses a serious risk.
- Do not prime nasal spray before use. Expect to use 2 devices for a 56-mg dose or 3 devices for an 84-mg dose, with a 5-minute rest period between use of each device. (Each device delivers two sprays containing a total of 28 mg of esketamine.)
- Administer drug by first having patient blow their nose. Peel blister and remove device. Check that indicator shows 2 green dots. If not, dispose of device and get a new one. Hand device to patient. Instruct patient to hold device with thumb gently supporting the plunger. Patient should not press the plunger yet. Instruct patient to recline head at about 45 degrees during administration to keep drug inside nose. Then have patient insert the device tip straight into the first nostril. The device nose rest should touch the skin between the nostrils. Instruct patient to close opposite nostril and breathe through nose while pushing plunger all the way up until it stops.
- Encourage patient to sniff gently after spraying to keep drug inside nose. Then instruct patient to switch hands to insert tip into the second nostril and repeat the same procedure.
- After administration, take device from patient and check that indicator shows no green dots. If a green dot is visible, have

patient spray again into the second nostril. Check again to confirm that device is empty.
- Have patient rest in a comfortable position (preferably semi-reclined) for 5 minutes before using next device. If liquid drips out, have patient dab nose with a tissue.
- Warn patient not to blow nose.
- Discard used devices per facility procedure for a schedule III drug.
- Reassess blood pressure about 40 minutes after administration and subsequently as clinically warranted. If blood pressure is decreasing and patient appears stable for at least 2 hours, patient may be discharged at the end of the post-dose monitoring period; if not, continue to monitor.

Route	Onset	Peak	Duration
Intranasal	2–24 hr	20–40 min*	Unknown

Half-life: 7–12 hr

*After last nasal spray dose

Mechanism of Action

The mechanism by which esketamine exerts its antidepressant effect is unknown.

Contraindications

Aneurysmal vascular disease (including abdominal and thoracic aorta, intracranial, and peripheral arterial vessels) or arteriovenous malformation; history of intracerebral hemorrhage; hypersensitivity to esketamine, ketamine, or any of their components

Interactions

DRUGS

CNS depressants (benzodiazepines, opioids): Increased sedation
MAOIs, psychostimulants (amphetamines, armodafinil, methylphenidate, modafinil): Possibly increased blood pressure

ACTIVITIES

alcohol use: Increased sedation

Adverse Reactions

CNS: Anxiety, cognitive impairment, depersonalization, depression, derealization, dissociation, dizziness, euphoria, feeling intoxicated, headache, hypoesthesia, insomnia, lethargy, mental impairment, panic attacks, sedation, **suicidal ideation**, tremor, vertigo

CV: Hypertension, tachycardia

EENT: Dry mouth, nasal discomfort, oropharyngeal pain, taste alteration, throat irritation
GI: Constipation, diarrhea, nausea, vomiting
GU: Interstitial or ulcerative cystitis, pollakiuria
MS: Dysarthria, muscular weakness
SKIN: Diaphoresis

Childbearing Considerations

PREGNANCY

- Pregnancy exposure registry: 1-844-405 -6185 or https://womensmentalhealth .org/clinical -and-research-programs /pregnancyregistry/antidepressants.
- Drug may cause fetal harm, based on animal studies.
- Drug therapy is not recommended during pregnancy.

LACTATION

- Drug is present in breast milk.
- Breastfeeding is not recommended during drug therapy because of the potential for neurotoxicity in infant.

REPRODUCTION

- Women of childbearing age should use effective contraception throughout drug therapy.

Nursing Considerations

- Know that esketamine is available only through a restricted program called the Spravato REMS. To receive drug, patient must be enrolled in the Spravato REMS program prior to administration.
- Be aware that esketamine must be administered with an oral antidepressant.
- Assess patient for psychosis before drug administration because of the potential for dissociation and perceptual changes to occur after administration. Also, assess patient for a history of drug abuse or dependency, because drug is a schedule III controlled substance. Monitor patient for signs of abuse or dependence after esketamine therapy is started.

! **WARNING** Know that concomitant use with psychostimulants or MAOIs increases risk of blood pressure elevation. Promptly seek emergency assistance if patient displays symptoms of a hypertensive crisis or hypertensive encephalopathy. Also be aware that up to 19% of patients in clinical studies experienced an increase of greater than or equal to 40 mmHg in systolic blood pressure and/or 25 mmHg in diastolic blood pressure in the first 1.5 hours after administration at least once during the first four weeks of therapy.

- Be aware that if patient misses treatment sessions and there is worsening of depression, prescriber may consider returning to patient's previous dosing schedule, such as from every 2 weeks to weekly or weekly to twice weekly.
- Administer a prescribed nasal corticosteroid or nasal decongestant to treat other conditions on an esketamine dosing day at least 1 hour before administering esketamine.
- Monitor patient for suicidal tendencies, particularly when therapy starts and when dosage changes are made.
- Monitor patient for signs and symptoms of cystitis, because esketamine use may increase risk of lower urinary tract symptoms.

PATIENT TEACHING

- Inform patient that esketamine is available only through a restricted program called the Spravato REMS. Review the program requirements with patient.
- Tell patient that drug will be prepared for administration by a healthcare professional. Drug cannot be self-administered at home.
- Caution patient to avoid performing activities that are considered hazardous (such as driving or operating machinery) until the next day after a restful sleep, as more than half of all patients experience sedation following administration of esketamine.
- Instruct patient that dissociation or perceptual changes (including illusions or distortion of time or space) are the most common psychological effects, which is why patient must be monitored for 2 hours after drug administration.
- Inform patient that drug use may increase risk of physical or psychological dependency. Instruct patient to discuss concerns with prescriber.
- Urge family or caregiver to watch patient closely for suicidal tendencies, especially when therapy starts or dosage changes.

E
F

- Alert women of childbearing age to use effective contraception during drug therapy, as esketamine may cause fetal harm.
- Inform women that breastfeeding is not recommended during drug therapy.

eslicarbazepine acetate

Aptiom

Class and Category
Pharmacologic class: Carboxamide derivative
Therapeutic class: Anticonvulsant

Indications and Dosages
* *Adjunct or monotherapy to treat partial-onset seizures*

TABLETS
Adults. *Initial:* 400 or 800 mg once daily, increased weekly in increments of 400 to 600 mg, as needed. *Maintenance:* 800 mg once daily when used as monotherapy and patient unable to tolerate a 1,200 mg daily dose; 1,600 mg once daily when used as adjunctive therapy and patient did not achieve a satisfactory response with a 1,200 mg daily dose. *Maximum:* 1,600 mg once daily.
Children age 4 to 17 weighing more than 38 kg (83.6 lb). *Initial:* 400 mg once daily, increased as needed by no more than 400 mg weekly. *Maintenance:* 800 to 1,200 mg daily. *Maximum:* 1,200 mg daily.
Children age 4 to 17 weighing 32 kg (70.4 lb) to 38 kg (83.6 lb). *Initial:* 300 mg once daily, increased as needed by no more than 300 mg weekly. *Maintenance:* 600 to 900 mg daily. *Maximum:* 900 mg daily.
Children age 4 to 17 weighing 22 kg (48.4 lb) to 31 kg (68.2 lb). *Initial:* 300 mg once daily, increased as needed by no more than 300 mg weekly. *Maintenance:* 500 to 800 mg daily. *Maximum:* 800 mg daily.
Children age 4 to 17 weighing 11 kg (24.2 lb) to 21 kg (46.2 lb). *Initial:* 200 mg once daily, increased as needed by no more than 200 mg weekly. *Maintenance:* 400 to 600 mg daily. *Maximum:* 600 mg daily.
±**DOSAGE ADJUSTMENT** For patients with moderate and severe renal impairment (creatinine clearance less than 50 ml/min), dosage decreased by half beginning with initial dosage and including titration and maintenance dosages. For patients receiving carbamazepine, phenobarbital, phenytoin, or primidone concomitantly, dosage may have to be increased.

Drug Administration
P.O.
- Tablets can be swallowed whole or as crushed tablets.

Route	Onset	Peak	Duration
P.O.	Rapid	1–4 hr	Unknown

Half-life: 13–30 hr

Mechanism of Action
Possibly inhibits voltage-gated sodium channels to exert anticonvulsant effect.

Contraindications
Hypersensitivity to eslicarbazepine acetate or oxcarbazepine and their components

Interactions
DRUGS
carbamazepine, phenobarbital, phenytoin, primidone: Decreased plasma concentration of eslicarbazepine
clobazam, omeprazole, phenytoin: Increased plasma levels of these drugs
lovastatin, simvastatin: Decreased plasma concentration of these drugs
oral contraceptives: Decreased effectiveness of oral contraceptives

Adverse Reactions
CNS: Amnesia, aphasia, asthenia, ataxia, attention deficits, confusion, coordination abnormality, depression, disorientation, dizziness, fatigue, gait disturbance, headache, insomnia, lethargy, malaise, memory impairment, psychomotor disturbances, somnolence, **suicidal ideation**, tremor, vertigo
CV: Hypertension, peripheral edema
EENT: Blurred vision, diplopia, impaired vision, nystagmus
ENDO: Decreased serum T3 and T4 levels, syndrome of inappropriate antidiuretic hormone secretion
GI: Abdominal pain, constipation, diarrhea, elevated liver enzymes, gastritis, **liver dysfunction**, nausea, vomiting
GU: UTI

HEME: Agranulocytosis, leukopenia, megaloblastic anemia, pancytopenia, thrombocytopenia
MS: Dysarthria
RESP: Cough
SKIN: Rash, Stevens–Johnson syndrome, toxic epidermal necrolysis
Other: Anaphylaxis, angioedema, drug reaction with eosinophilia and systemic symptoms (DRESS), hypochloremia, hyponatremia

☰ Childbearing Considerations

PREGNANCY
- Pregnancy exposure registry: 1-888-233-2334 or http://www.aedpregnancyregistry.org.
- Drug may cause fetal harm based on animal studies.
- Use with caution only if benefit to mother outweighs potential risk to fetus.

LACTATION
- Drug is present in breast milk.
- Patient should check with prescriber before breastfeeding.

REPRODUCTION
- Women using hormonal contraceptives will need to use additional or alternative nonhormonal contraceptives.
- Drug may affect impairment of female fertility based on animal studies.

☰ Nursing Considerations
- Be aware that eslicarbazepine should not be given as adjunctive therapy with oxcarbazepine.

! **WARNING** Monitor patient closely for adverse reactions because many of them are serious and some can become life-threatening, such as DRESS multi-organ hypersensitivity. Notify prescriber immediately, expect drug to be discontinued, and provide emergency supportive care, as ordered.

- Monitor patient closely for evidence of suicidal thinking or behavior, especially when therapy starts or dosage changes.
- Monitor patient's electrolytes, especially sodium level, as ordered. Hyponatremia may occur as an adverse reaction to eslicarbazepine therapy, especially in the elderly and patients treated with diuretics. Assess patient regularly for signs and symptoms of hyponatremia such as confusion, difficulty concentrating, headache, memory impairment, unsteadiness, and weakness. If present, notify prescriber and expect drug to be discontinued.
- Withdraw eslicarbazepine slowly when discontinued and as ordered to minimize risk of seizures and status epilepticus.

PATIENT TEACHING
- Instruct patient to take eslicarbazepine exactly as prescribed and not to abruptly stop taking drug without consulting prescriber.
- Advise patient that tablets can be swallowed whole or crushed.
- Warn patient about possible dizziness and unsteadiness that may develop while taking eslicarbazepine. Discourage performing hazardous activities such as driving until the neurologic effects of the drug are known.

! **WARNING** Tell patient to discontinue drug immediately and seek emergency medical care if patient develops difficulty breathing, fever, or a rash or experiences facial or throat swelling. Also instruct patient to promptly report other skin reactions such as blistering or exfoliation or other persistent, severe, or unusual signs and symptoms.

- Instruct caregivers to watch patient closely for evidence of suicidal tendencies, especially when therapy starts or dosage changes, and to report such tendencies to prescriber immediately.
- Tell female patients taking oral contraceptives to use additional or alternative nonhormonal birth control.
- Advise patient to report symptoms of low sodium such as confusion, irritability, muscle weakness or spasms, tiredness, or more frequent or severe seizure activity.

esmolol hydrochloride
Brevibloc

☰ Class and Category
Pharmacologic class: Beta blocker
Therapeutic class: Antiarrhythmic, antihypertensive

≡ Indications and Dosages

∗ *To treat supraventricular tachycardia including atrial fibrillation and atrial flutter; to control heart rate in noncompensatory sinus tachycardia*

I.V. INFUSION

Adults. The dosage is titrated in a step-wise fashion as follows: *Step 1:* Optional loading dose of 500 mcg/kg given over 1 min, followed by a maintenance infusion of 50 mcg/kg/min given over 4 min. If response is not adequate, step 2 initiated. *Step 2:* Optional loading dose of 500 mcg/kg given over 1 min followed by a maintenance infusion of 100 mcg/kg/min given over 4 min. If response is not adequate, step 3 initiated. *Step 3:* Optional loading dose of 500 mcg/kg given over 1 min followed by a maintenance dose of 150 mcg/kg/min given over 4 min. If response is not adequate, step 4 initiated. *Step 4:* Maintenance dose increased to a continuous infusion of 200 mcg/kg/min and continued for up to 48 hr, as needed.

∗ *To treat intraoperative and postoperative hypertension and tachycardia*

I.V. INFUSION

Adults. *For immediate control:* 1 mg/kg given over 30 seconds, followed by an infusion of 150 mcg/kg/min, if needed and adjusted to maintain desired blood pressure and heart rate. *For gradual control:* 500 mcg/kg given over 1 min, then a maintenance infusion of 50 mcg/kg/min given over 4 min. If response is inadequate, another 500 mcg/kg may be given over 1 min followed by a maintenance infusion of 100 mcg/kg/min given over 4 min. If response is inadequate, another 500 mcg/kg given over 1 min followed by a maintenance infusion of 150 mcg/kg/min given over 4 min. If response is inadequate, maintenance dose increased to a continuous infusion of 200 mcg/kg/min and continued until maximum dose reached, if needed. *Maximum:* 200 mcg/kg/min for tachycardia; 300 mcg/kg/min for hypertension.

±**DOSAGE ADJUSTMENT** When transitioning from esmolol infusion to alternative drugs, esmolol infusion rate reduced by 50% 30 minutes following the first dose of the alternative drug. After administration of the second dose of the alternative drug, if patient's response is satisfactory and maintained for the first hour, esmolol infusion discontinued.

≡ Drug Administration

I.V.

- Drug is available in a premixed bag and ready-to-use vial; don't dilute either one.
- Do not remove premixed bag from overwrap until ready to use. Tear overwrap at notch and remove premixed bag. Some opacity of the plastic due to moisture absorption during the sterilization process may be observed and will diminish gradually. This is normal and does not affect the solution quality or safety.
- Check for minute leaks by squeezing the inner bag firmly. If a leak is present, discard. Solution should be colorless to light yellow and the seal intact.
- When using the premixed bag, use the medication port solely for withdrawing an initial bolus from the bag. Do not add any additional drugs to the bag.
- The ready-to-use vial may be used to administer a loading dose by hand-held syringe while the maintenance infusion is being prepared.
- Once drug has been withdrawn from the ready-to-use bag, the bag should be used within 24 hours, with any unused portion discarded.
- Do not use plastic containers in series connections when administering drug.
- Don't give more than 10 mg/ml into a small vein or using a butterfly catheter.
- Administer loading or bolus doses of 1 mg/kg dose over 30 seconds and 500 mcg/kg over 1 minute using an infusion-control device.
- Inspect site often for thrombophlebitis (pain, redness, swelling at site). Infusion of 20 mg/ml is more likely to cause serious vein irritation than 10 mg/ml. Extravasation of 20 mg/ml may cause a serious local reaction and skin necrosis and so should be administered through a central line.
- *Incompatibilities:* Furosemide, 5% Sodium Bicarbonate Injection

Route	Onset	Peak	Duration
I.V.	Immediate	2–6 min	10–20 min

Half-life: 9 min

Mechanism of Action

Inhibits stimulation of beta$_1$ receptors mainly in the heart, which decreases cardiac excitability, cardiac output, and myocardial oxygen demand. Esmolol also decreases renin release from kidneys, which helps reduce blood pressure.

Contraindications

Cardiogenic shock; decompensated heart failure; hypersensitivity to esmolol, other beta-blockers and their components; I.V. administration of cardiodepressant calcium channel antagonists (i.e., verapamil) and esmolol close together while cardiac effects from other drug are still present; pulmonary hypertension; second- or third-degree heart block; severe sinus bradycardia; sick sinus syndrome

Interactions

DRUGS

anticholinesterases such as mivacurium, succinylcholine: Prolonged clinical duration and recovery of mivacurium and prolonged duration of succinylcholine-induced neuromuscular blockage
calcium channel antagonists: Increased risk of fatal cardiac arrest in patients with depressed myocardial function
clonidine, guanfacine, moxonidine: Increased risk of withdrawal rebound hypertension
digitalis glycosides: Increased risk of bradycardia
positive inotropic and vasoconstrictive agents such as dopamine, epinephrine, or norepinephrine: Increased risk of reducing cardiac contractility in presence of high systemic resistance
sympathomimetics that have beta-adrenergic agonist activity: May counter effects of esmolol

Adverse Reactions

CNS: Anxiety, confusion, depression, dizziness, fatigue, fever, headache, syncope
CV: **Bradycardia**, chest pain, decreased peripheral circulation, **heart block**, **hypotension**
GI: Nausea, vomiting
RESP: Dyspnea, wheezing
SKIN: Diaphoresis, flushing, pallor
Other: Infusion-site pain, redness, and swelling

Childbearing Considerations

PREGNANCY

- Drug may cause fetal bradycardia if given during the last trimester of pregnancy.
- Use with caution only if benefit to mother outweighs potential risk to fetus.

LABOR & DELIVERY

- Drug may cause fetal bradycardia if given during labor and delivery, which may continue after drug is discontinued.
- Use with caution only if benefit to mother outweighs potential risk to fetus.

LACTATION

- It is not known if drug is present in breast milk.
- A decision should be made to discontinue breastfeeding or the drug to avoid potential serious adverse reactions in the breastfed infant.

Nursing Considerations

- Use esmolol cautiously if patient has supraventricular arrhythmias with decreased cardiac output, hypotension, or other hemodynamic compromise or is taking drugs that decrease contractility, impulse generation, myocardial filling, or peripheral resistance.
- Also use drug cautiously in patients with impaired renal function because drug is excreted by the kidneys. Patients with end-stage renal disease have an increased risk of adverse reactions.
- Be aware that esmolol should not be given for intraoperative or postoperative hypertension caused by hypothermia-induced vasoconstriction.
- Expect to give lowest possible dose to patients with allergies, asthma, bronchitis, or emphysema. If patient develops bronchospasm, expect to discontinue infusion immediately and give a beta$_2$-stimulating drug, as ordered.
- Monitor blood pressure and heart rate often during therapy. Hypotension can occur at any dose but usually is dose related. It typically reverses within 30 minutes after dose is decreased or infusion stopped.

PATIENT TEACHING

- Urge patient to report adverse reactions immediately.
- Reassure patient that his blood pressure, heart rate, and response to therapy will be monitored throughout esmolol therapy.

E
F

esomeprazole magnesium

Nexium, Nexium 24 HR

esomeprazole sodium

Nexium I.V.

esomeprazole strontium

Class and Category

Pharmacologic class: Proton pump inhibitor
Therapeutic class: Antiulcerative

Indications and Dosages

* *To treat symptomatic gastroesophageal reflux disease (GERD)*

DELAYED-RELEASE CAPSULES, DELAYED-RELEASE SUSPENSION (NEXIUM)

Adults. 20 mg daily for 4 wk, with cycle repeated once more, if needed.
Adolescents ages 12 to 17. 20 mg once daily for 4 wk.
Children ages 1 to 11. 10 mg once daily for up to 8 wk.

DELAYED-RELEASE CAPSULES (ESOMEPRAZOLE STRONTIUM)

Adults. 24.65 mg once daily for 4 wk.

* *To promote healing of erosive esophagitis in patient with GERD*

DELAYED-RELEASE CAPSULES, DELAYED-RELEASE SUSPENSION (NEXIUM)

Adults. 20 or 40 mg once daily for 4 to 8 wk, with cycle repeated once more if healing has not taken place after first 8 wk. *Maintenance:* 20 mg once daily for up to 6 months.
Adolescents ages 12 to 17. 20 or 40 mg once daily for 4 to 8 wk.
Children ages 1 to 11 weighing 20 kg(44 lb) or more. 10 or 20 mg once daily for 8 wk.
Children ages 1 to 11 weighing less than 20 kg (44 lb). 10 mg once daily for 8 wk.

DELAYED-RELEASE CAPSULES (ESOMEPRAZOLE STRONTIUM)

Adults. 24.65 or 49.3 mg once daily for 4 to 8 wk, with cycle repeated once more if healing has not taken place after first 8 wk. *Maintenance:* 24.65 mg once daily for up to 6 months.

* *To treat erosive esophagitis due to acid-mediated GERD*

ORAL SUSPENSION

Infants age 1 month to less than 1 year weighing 7.5 kg (16.5 lb) to 12 kg (26.4 lb). 10 mg once daily for up to 6 wk.
Infants age 1 month to less than 1 year weighing 5 kg (11 lb) to 7.5 kg (16.5 lb). 5 mg once daily for up to 6 wk.
Infants age 1 month to less than 1 year weighing 3 kg (6.6 lb) to 5 kg (11 lb). 2.5 mg once daily for up to 6 wk.

* *To treat GERD in a patient with erosive esophagitis who can't take drug by mouth*

I.V. INJECTION

Adults. 20 or 40 mg once daily up to 10 days with switch to oral therapy as soon as possible.

I.V. INFUSION

Adults. 20 or 40 mg once daily up to 10 days with switch to oral therapy as soon as possible.
Children ages 1 to 17 weighing 55 kg (121 lb) or more. 20 mg daily up to 10 days with switch to oral therapy as soon as possible.
Children ages 1 to 17 weighing less than 55 kg (121 lb). 10 mg daily up to 10 days with switch to oral therapy as soon as possible.
Children ages 1 month to less than 1 year. 0.5 mg/kg daily up to 10 with switch to oral therapy as soon as possible.
± **DOSAGE ADJUSTMENT** For adult patient with severe liver impairment, dosage should not exceed 20 mg once daily.

* *As adjunct to treat duodenal ulcer associated with* Helicobacter pylori

DELAYED-RELEASE CAPSULES (NEXIUM), DELAYED-RELEASE SUSPENSION (NEXIUM)

Adults. 40 mg daily with amoxicillin 1,000 mg twice a day and clarithromycin 500 mg twice a day for 10 days.

DELAYED-RELEASE CAPSULES (ESOMEPRAZOLE STRONTIUM)

Adults. 49.3 mg once daily with amoxicillin 1,000 mg twice daily and clarithromycin 500 mg twice daily for 10 days.

✱ *To reduce the risk of gastric ulcer formation in patients who are receiving continuous NSAID therapy and who either are 60 and older or have a history of gastric ulcer*

DELAYED-RELEASE CAPSULES (NEXIUM), DELAYED-RELEASE SUSPENSION (NEXIUM)

Adults. 20 or 40 mg daily for up to 6 months.

DELAYED-RELEASE CAPSULES (ESOMEPRAZOLE STRONTIUM)

Adults. 24.65 or 49.3 mg once daily for up to 6 months.

✱ *To treat pathological hypersecretory conditions, including Zollinger–Ellison syndrome*

DELAYED-RELEASE CAPSULES, DELAYED-RELEASE SUSPENSION

Adults. 40 mg twice daily.

±**DOSAGE ADJUSTMENT** For patients with severe hepatic insufficiency, maximum 20 mg daily.

DELAYED-RELEASE CAPSULES (ESOMEPRAZOLE STRONTIUM)

Adults. 49.3 mg twice daily.

✱ *To reduce risk of rebleeding of duodenal or gastric ulcers following therapeutic endoscopy for acute-bleeding duodenal or gastric ulcers*

I.V. INFUSION

Adults. *Initial:* 80 mg followed by 8 mg per hour for 71.5 hr after initial dose is completed.

±**DOSAGE ADJUSTMENT** For patients with mild to moderate liver impairment, maximum continuous infusion should not exceed 6 mg/hr; for patients with severe liver impairment, maximum continuous infusion should not exceed 4 mg/hr.

≡ Drug Administration

P.O.

- Give oral drug at least 1 hour before meals because food decreases bioavailability.
- Use delayed-release capsules or oral suspension specific for nasogastric tube administration and delayed-release oral suspension specific for nasogastric or gastric tube administration when administering to a patient with a nasogastric or gastric tube.
- Delayed-release capsules or tablets should be swallowed whole and not chewed, crushed, or split/opened. However, if patient has difficulty swallowing capsules, tell patient to open the delayed-release capsules and sprinkle contents onto 1 tablespoon of cool applesauce and mix. Caution him not to use any other food and not to chew or crush the granules.
- Mix oral suspension by adding 5 ml of water to the contents of a 2.5- or 5-mg packet or 15 ml of water to 10-, 20-, or 40-mg packet. Let mixture sit for 2 to 3 minutes to thicken. Stir and give to patient to drink within 30 minutes. Use calibrated device when measuring oral suspension dosage.

I.V.

- Always flush I.V. line with 0.9% Sodium Chloride Injection, 5% Dextrose Injection, or Lactated Ringer's Injection before and after giving drug.
- For I.V. injection, reconstitute each vial with 5 ml of 0.9% Sodium Chloride Injection. Administer I.V. injection over at least 3 minutes.
- For intermittent I.V. infusion, reconstitute each vial with 5 ml of 0.9% Sodium Chloride Injection, then further dilute reconstituted solution with 45 ml of 0.9% Sodium Chloride Injection. Administer over 10 to 30 minutes. Prepare the continuous infusion in the same manner but administer over 71.5 hours at a rate of 8 mg/hr or decrease rate to 6 mg/hr for mild to moderate liver impairment and to 4 mg/hr for severe liver impairment, as ordered.
- Reconstituted drug may be stored at room temperature up to 6 hours if mixed with 5% Dextrose Injection or up to 12 hours if mixed with 0.9% Sodium Chloride Injection or Lactated Ringer's Injection.
- I.V. therapy should be switched to oral form as soon as possible.
- *Incompatibilities:* Other I.V. drugs

Route	Onset	Peak	Duration
P.O.	Immediate	1.5 hr	13–17 hr
I.V.	Unknown	Unknown	Unknown
Half-life: 1–1.5 hr			

Mechanism of Action

Interferes with gastric acid secretion by inhibiting the hydrogen–potassium–adenosine triphosphatase (H^+–K^+–ATPase) enzyme system, or proton pump, in gastric parietal cells. Normally, the proton pump uses energy from hydrolysis of ATPase to drive H^+ and chloride (Cl^-) out of parietal cells and into the stomach lumen in exchange for potassium (K^+), which leaves the stomach lumen and enters parietal cells. After this exchange, H^+ and Cl^- combine in the stomach to form hydrochloric acid (HCl). Esomeprazole irreversibly inhibits the final step in gastric acid production by blocking exchange of intracellular H^+ and extracellular K^+, thus preventing H^+ from entering the stomach and additional HCl from forming.

Contraindications

Concurrent therapy with rilpivirine-containing products, hypersensitivity to esomeprazole, substituted benzimidazoles, or their components

Interactions

DRUGS

atazanavir, dasatinib, erlotinib, ketoconazole, iron salts, itraconazole, mycophenolate mofetil, nelfinavir nilotinib, rilpivirine: Decreased blood levels of these drugs
cilostazol: Possibly increased blood cilostazol levels
citalopram: Increased exposure of citalopram leading to an increased risk of QT prolongation
clopidogrel: Reduced effectiveness of clopidogrel
digoxin: Possibly increased risk of digoxin toxicity
methotrexate: Increased risk of methotrexate toxicities
rifampin, St. John's wort: Decreased blood esomeprazole level
saquinavir: Increased plasma saquinavir level with increased toxicity
tacrolimus: Increased serum tacrolimus level
voriconazole: Increased esomeprazole exposure and risk of adverse effects
warfarin: Possibly increased INR and PT, leading to abnormal bleeding

FOODS

all foods: Decreased bioavailability of esomeprazole

Adverse Reactions

CNS: Agitation, aggression, depression, dizziness, fever, headache, hallucinations, encephalopathy (hepatic), vertigo
EENT: Blurred vision, dry mouth, mucosal discoloration, sinusitis, stomatitis, taste disturbance
ENDO: Gynecomastia
GI: Abdominal pain; Barrett's esophagus; benign polyps or nodules; candidiasis; *Clostridium difficile*–associated diarrhea; constipation; diarrhea; duodenitis; dyspepsia; esophagitis; esophageal stricture, ulceration, or varices; flatulence; fundic gland polyps; gastric ulcer; gastritis; hepatic failure; hepatitis; jaundice; microscopic colitis; nausea; pancreatitis
GU: Acute tubulointerstitial nephritis
HEME: Agranulocytosis, pancytopenia
MS: Bone fracture, muscle weakness, myalgia
RESP: Bronchospasm, cough, respiratory tract infection
SKIN: Alopecia, cutaneous lupus erythematosus, diaphoresis, erythema multiforme, photosensitivity, pruritus, Stevens–Johnson syndrome, toxic epidermal necrolysis
Other: Anaphylaxis, cyanocobalamin deficiency (prolonged use), hypocalcemia, hypokalemia, hypomagnesemia, infusion-site reactions (erythema, inflammation, phlebitis, pruritus, swelling), systemic lupus erythematosus, vitamin B_{12} deficiency

Childbearing Considerations

PREGNANCY

- It is not known if drug causes fetal harm.
- Use with caution only if benefit to mother outweighs potential risk to fetus.

LACTATION

- Drug may be present in breast milk.
- Patient should check with prescriber before breastfeeding.

Nursing Considerations

! **WARNING** Be aware that if patient takes drug with amoxicillin or clarithromycin for *H. pylori*-related ulcer, severe diarrhea may indicate pseudomembranous colitis. Obtain stool cultures, as ordered.

- Monitor patients for bone fractures, especially in patients who are receiving multiple daily doses for a year or longer, as proton pump inhibitors such as esomeprazole have been associated with an increased risk for osteoporosis-related fractures of the hip, spine, or wrist.

- Monitor patient's magnesium level, as ordered, because hypomagnesemia may occur with esomeprazole therapy that has lasted longer than 3 months, although most cases have occurred after therapy had been given for more than a year. Notify prescriber if magnesium level drops below normal as hypomagnesemia may cause tetany, arrhythmias, and seizures. Expect patient to receive magnesium replacement and esomeprazole to be discontinued.
- Be aware that esomeprazole therapy may have to be temporarily halted for at least 14 days if patient is undergoing testing for neuroendocrine tumors, because drug may cause false positive results in diagnostic testing.
- Monitor patient for diarrhea, because esomeprazole therapy may increase the risk of *Clostridium difficile*–associated diarrhea. Know that the lowest dose possible for the shortest amount of time should be used to decrease this risk. If diarrhea occurs, expect to obtain a stool specimen to determine if diarrhea is *C. difficile* so that it may be treated appropriately.
- Monitor patient for signs and symptoms of cutaneous and systemic lupus erythematosus or exacerbation of these conditions if already present. Notify prescriber if present and expect serological testing to be done. If results are positive, expect drug to be discontinued. Symptoms are usually relieved in most patients within 4 to 12 weeks.
- Be aware that patients who take esomeprazole long term, especially after 1 year, are at increased risk for developing fundic gland polyps.

PATIENT TEACHING

- Inform patient that drug should be taken at the lowest dose possible and for the shortest time to decrease risk of adverse effects. Tell him he should never increase dosage or take it long term without consulting prescriber.
- Instruct patient to take drug 1 hour before eating.

- Tell patient to swallow capsules and tablets whole and not chew or crush. If he has trouble swallowing esomeprazole capsules, tell him to open capsule and sprinkle pellets with a tablespoon of cool applesauce and mix. Tell him not to chew or crush the pellets when taking drug in this manner.
- Instruct patient or caregiver how to mix oral suspension and to use a calibrated device to measure oral suspension dosage.
- Remind patient that esomeprazole, including the over-the-counter preparation, is not intended for immediate relief of heartburn; the drug may take up to 4 days before the full effect is experienced.

! **WARNING** Instruct patient to seek immediate medical attention if he experiences an allergic reaction to esomeprazole.

- Urge patient to tell prescriber if he takes antacids or any other OTC or prescription drug.
- Advise patient to contact prescriber if he develops abdominal pain, diarrhea, and fever that does not improve, especially if he has recently taken or is taking an antibiotic. Also advise patient to report any other persistent or serious signs and symptoms that occur while taking esomeprazole. Instruct patient to stop taking drug if he develops joint pain or rash and to see his doctor for an evaluation of these symptoms.
- Advise patient that drug may increase risk for osteoporosis-related fractures of the hip, spine, or wrist. Instruct him to take fall precautions and have bone health evaluated regularly.
- Review the signs and symptoms of hypomagnesemia if taking drug longer than 3 months or vitamin B-12 deficiency if taking drug longer than 3 years.

estazolam

Class, Category, and Schedule

Pharmacologic class: Benzodiazepine
Therapeutic class: Sedative-hypnotic
Controlled substance schedule: IV

Indications and Dosages

＊ *To treat insomnia short-term*

TABLETS

Adults. 1 to 2 mg once daily.
Elderly adults. 1 mg once daily.
± **DOSAGE ADJUSTMENT** Starting dose 0.5 mg for small or debilitated elderly patients.

☰ Drug Administration

P.O.

- Administer drug at bedtime.

Route	Onset	Peak	Duration
P.O.	Unknown	2 hr	Variable

Half-life: 10–24 hr

☰ Mechanism of Action

May potentiate effects of gamma-amino-butyric acid (GABA) and other inhibitory neurotransmitters by binding to specific benzodiazepine receptors in cortical and limbic areas of CNS. By binding to these receptors, estazolam increases GABA's inhibitory effects and blocks cortical and limbic arousal.

☰ Contraindications

Concurrent therapy with itraconazole or ketoconazole; hypersensitivity to estazolam, other benzodiazepines, or their components; pregnancy

☰ Interactions

DRUGS

anticonvulsants, antihistamines, barbiturates, CNS depressants, MAO inhibitors, narcotics, phenothiazines, psychotropics: Possibly potentiated action of estazolam
barbiturates, carbamazepine, phenytoin, rifampin: Possibly decreased estazolam level
cimetidine, diltiazem, fluvoxamine, isoniazid, itraconazole, ketoconazole, nefazodone, selected macrolide antibiotics: Possibly increased blood level and impaired hepatic metabolism of estazolam
opioids: Possibly significant respiratory depression and sedation

ACTIVITIES

alcohol use: Possibly potentiated CNS depression, including respiratory depression and sedation
smoking: Increased clearance of estazolam

☰ Adverse Reactions

CNS: Amnesia, anxiety, ataxia, confusion, delusions, depression, dizziness, drowsiness, euphoria, headache, hypokinesia, irritability, malaise, nervousness, slurred speech, tremor
CV: Chest pain, palpitations, tachycardia
EENT: Blurred vision, dry mouth, increased salivation, photophobia
GI: Abdominal pain, constipation, diarrhea, nausea, thirst, vomiting
GU: Libido changes
RESP: Respiratory depression
SKIN: Diaphoresis
Other: Physical or psychological dependence

☰ Childbearing Considerations

PREGNANCY

- Drug may cause fetal harm.
- Drug is contraindicated in pregnant women.
- Be aware that if mother takes drug prior to delivery, neonate may experience withdrawal symptoms during the postnatal period.

LACTATION

- It is not known if drug is present in breast milk.
- Breastfeeding should not be undertaken during drug therapy.

☰ Nursing Considerations

- Use estazolam with extreme caution in patients with a history of alcohol or drug abuse because of risk of addiction. Expect to give drug for no more than 12 weeks.
- Use cautiously in debilitated or elderly patients and those with depression or impaired hepatic, renal, or respiratory function.
- Expect to stop drug gradually to prevent withdrawal symptoms. Avoid stopping abruptly if patient has history of seizures.
- Monitor respiratory status, especially in patients with respiratory compromise, who are at increased risk for respiratory depression.
- Be aware that if patient takes estazolam for depression, watch for suicidal tendencies, especially when therapy starts or dosage changes.

PATIENT TEACHING

- Instruct patient to take drug at bedtime.
- Warn patient not to exceed prescribed time because of risk of addiction.
- Advise patient to avoid hazardous activities until CNS effects of the drug are known.

- Advise patient not to drink alcohol or take other CNS depressants during therapy because of the risk of additive effects.
- Warn debilitated or elderly patients and those with impaired hepatic or renal function about risk of excessive sedation or mental impairment and need to report them.
- Tell patient that if he takes 2-mg dosage for a long time, he should not stop drug abruptly.

estradiol
Divigel 1%, Elestrin, Estrace, Estring, Estrogel, Evamist, Imvexxy, Vagifem, Yuvafem

estradiol acetate
Femring

estradiol cypionate
Depo-Estradiol

estradiol transdermal system
Alora, Climara, Dotti, Menostar, Minivelle, Vivelle, Vivelle-Dot

estradiol valerate
Delestrogen, Femogex (CAN)

Class and Category
Pharmacologic class: Estrogen
Therapeutic class: Hormone

Indications and Dosages
✷ *To treat menopausal symptoms*

TABLETS (ESTRADIOL)
Adult menopausal and postmenopausal women. *Initial:* 0.5 to 2 mg once daily and then adjusted to control symptoms.

VAGINAL RING (ESTRADIOL ACETATE [FEMRING])
Adult women. One ring (0.05 or 0.1 mg of estradiol/24 hr) inserted into upper third of vaginal vault and replaced every 3 months.

I.M. INJECTION (ESTRADIOL CYPIONATE IN OIL)
Adult women. 1 to 5 mg as a single dose every 3 to 4 wk as needed.

I.M. INJECTION (ESTRADIOL VALERATE IN OIL)
Adult women. 10 to 20 mg every 4 wk as needed.

TRANSDERMAL (ALORA)
Adult menopausal and postmenopausal women. *Initial:* 0.05 mg continuously with one patch replaced twice/wk if uterus is not present or in cycles of 3 wk on (patch replaced twice/wk), 1 wk off (no patch applied) if uterus is intact. Dosage adjusted to control symptoms, as prescribed.

TRANSDERMAL (VIVELLE, VIVELLE-DOT)
Adult menopausal and postmenopausal women. *Initial:* 0.0375 mg/day with one patch applied to trunk or buttocks and replaced twice/wk (every 3 to 4 days). Dosage adjusted to control symptoms, as prescribed.

TRANSDERMAL (CLIMARA)
Adult women. *Initial:* 0.025 mg daily. One patch applied to trunk or buttocks, replaced every wk. Dosage titrated to control symptoms, as prescribed.

TRANSDERMAL (ESTROGEL)
Adult women. 1.25 g daily applied in thin layer from wrist to shoulder on inside and outside of one arm.

✷ *To treat postmenopausal moderate to severe symptoms of vulvar and vaginal atrophy*

TABLETS (ESTRADIOL)
Adult women. 1 to 2 mg once daily. Dosage adjusted to control symptoms, as needed.

VAGINAL CREAM (ESTRACE)
Adult women. *Initial:* 2 to 4 g daily for 1 to 2 wk. Then, dosage gradually reduced to half of initial dose, as prescribed, for 1 to 2 wk. *Maintenance:* 1 g daily 1 to 3 times/wk.

VAGINAL RING (ESTRING)
Adult women. One ring (7.5 mcg of estradiol/24 hr) inserted into upper third of vaginal vault and replaced every 3 months.

VAGINAL RING (FEMRING)
Adult women. One ring (0.05 or 0.1 mg of estradiol/24 hr) inserted into upper third of vaginal vault and replaced every 3 months.

✷ *To treat atrophic vaginitis due to menopause*

VAGINAL INSERT (VAGIFEM)

Adult women. *Initial:* 10-mcg insert daily for 2 wk, followed by 1 insert twice/wk.

∗ *To treat moderate to severe dyspareunia*

VAGINAL INSERT (IMVEXXY)

Adult women. *Initial:* 4 mcg (1 insert) daily for 2 wk, followed by 4 mcg (1 insert) twice weekly. Dosage increased to 10 mcg (1 insert), as needed.

∗ *To treat moderate to severe vasomotor symptoms due to menopause*

TRANSDERMAL (MINIVELLE)

Adult women. 0.0375 mg daily with patch replaced twice/wk. Dosage adjusted as needed.

GEL (DIVIGEL 0.1%)

Adult women. *Initial:* 0.25 mg once daily to skin of left or right upper thigh and then dosage increased, as needed.

GEL (ELESTRIN 0.06%)

Adult women. 1 pump of gel (0.52 mg) once per day applied to the upper arm. Dosage increased to 2 pumps of gel (1.04 mg) once per day applied to the upper arm, if needed.

TRANSDERMAL SPRAY (EVAMIST)

Adult women. *Initial:* 1.53 mg (1 spray) daily to the inner surface of the forearm, starting near the elbow, increased to 2 sprays (3.06 mg), as needed and further increased to 3 sprays (4.59 mg), as needed.

∗ *To prevent osteoporosis secondary to estrogen deficiency due to either natural or surgical menopause*

TRANSDERMAL (ALORA)

Adult women. Initial: 0.025 mg daily with one patch applied to lower abdomen or buttocks and replaced twice/wk if uterus is not present or in cycles of 3 wk on (patch replaced twice/wk), 1 wk off (no patch applied) if uterus is intact. Dosage adjusted to control symptoms, as prescribed.

TRANSDERMAL (MINIVELLE, VIVELLE-DOT)

Adult women. 0.025 mg daily.

TRANSDERMAL (CLIMARA)

Adult women. *Initial:* 0.025 mg daily. One patch applied to trunk or buttocks and replaced every wk. Dosage adjusted to control symptoms.

TRANSDERMAL (MENOSTAR)

Adult women. *Initial:* 0.014 mg daily. One patch applied to lower abdomen and replaced every wk.

∗ *To treat estrogen deficiency due to oophorectomy, primary ovarian failure, or female hypogonadism*

TABLETS (ESTRADIOL)

Adult women. 1 to 2 mg daily.

I.M. INJECTION (ESTRADIOL CYPIONATE IN OIL)

Adult women. 1.5 to 2 mg every month (for female hypogonadism only).

I.M. INJECTION (ESTRADIOL VALERATE IN OIL)

Adult women. 10 to 20 mg every month as needed.

TRANSDERMAL (ALORA, ESTRADERM)

Adult women. *Initial:* 0.05 mg daily with one patch applied to trunk or buttocks and replaced twice/wk. Dosage titrated to control symptoms, as prescribed. A cyclic schedule is followed unless patient has had a hysterectomy.

TRANSDERMAL (VIVELLE)

Adult women. 0.0375 mg daily with one patch applied to trunk or buttocks and replaced twice/wk. Dosage titrated to control symptoms, as prescribed. A cyclic schedule is followed unless patient has had a hysterectomy.

TRANSDERMAL (CLIMARA)

Adult women. *Initial:* 0.025 mg daily. One patch applied to trunk or buttocks and replaced every wk. Dosage adjusted to control symptoms, as prescribed.

∗ *To provide palliative treatment for inoperable, progressive breast cancer in selected men and postmenopausal women*

TABLETS (ESTRADIOL)

Adults. 10 mg 3 times daily for at least 3 months.

∗ *To treat advancing, inoperable prostate cancer*

TABLETS (ESTRADIOL)

Adult men. 1 to 2 mg or 3 times daily, adjusted or continued, as prescribed, according to patient response.

I.M. INJECTION (ESTRADIOL VALERATE)

Adult men. 30 mg every 1 to 2 wk, adjusted or continued, as prescribed, according to patient response.

☰ Drug Administration

P.O.

- Administer oral preparations with or immediately after food to decrease nausea.
- Avoid administering with grapefruit juice.

I.M.

- Roll vial and syringe between palms of hands to evenly disperse drug. Use at least a 21 G needle (estradiol cypionate) or a 20 G needle (estradiol valerate).
- Inject deep into upper outer quadrant of gluteal muscle.
- Rotate sites.
- Never administer I.V.

TRANSDERMAL

- If patient is converting from oral estrogen to transdermal system, oral estrogen should be stopped 1 week before skin patches are applied.
- Apply patch to the area designated by product being used. Apply patch to clear, dry, intact skin that is hairless on abdomen or buttock. Hold in place for at least 10 seconds.
- Do not apply patch to breasts, waistline, or other areas where it may not adhere properly.
- Rotate application sites at least weekly and remove old patch before applying new one.
- If patch falls off, reapply it to another area or apply a new patch and continue the original treatment schedule. Patient may bathe while wearing the patch. Discard used patch according to institutional protocol.
- Prime spray pump by holding pump upright and vertical and spraying 3 sprays with cover on before initial use. Apply spray in the morning to adjacent, nonoverlapping areas on the inner surfacer of the forearm, starting near the elbow. Do not apply anywhere else. Allow area to dry for at least 2 minutes before covering area with clothing. Do not wash site for at least an hour after application.

TOPICAL

- Apply to clean, dry skin in area designated by product being used. Wash hands with soap and water afterward.
- Never apply gel to breasts.
- Rotate Divigel gel to the opposite site on alternating days. Application surface area should be about 5 to 7 inches (about the size of two palm prints). The entire contents of a unit-dose packet should be applied each day. Gel should never be applied to the breasts, face, irritated skin, or in or around vagina. After application, let gel dry before patient gets dressed. Do not wash the site

for 1 hour after application. Wash hands after application.

VAGINAL

- Patient should remain recumbent for at least 30 minutes after applying estradiol vaginal cream. She may use a sanitary napkin (but not a tampon) to protect clothing after application.
- Imvexxy vaginal inserts are inserted with the smaller end first for a depth of about two inches into the vaginal canal. Each insert should be inserted at about the same time every day.
- When a vaginal ring is to be inserted, have patient squeeze sides of ring together and insert into upper third of her vagina where it will stay for 90 days, and then removed and a new ring inserted. If it is removed during the 90-day dosage period, patient should rinse it with lukewarm (not hot or boiling) water, and reinsert it as needed for personal hygiene. Patient shouldn't be able to feel the ring when it's in place. If she does, she should use a finger to push the ring farther into her vagina. If vaginal wall ulceration or erosion occurs, suggest that patient leave ring out, as ordered, and not replace it until healing is complete, to keep ring from adhering to healing tissue.

Route	Onset	Peak	Duration
All routes	Unknown	Unknown	Unknown

Half-life: Unknown

☰ Mechanism of Action

Increases the rate of DNA and RNA synthesis in cells of female reproductive organs, pituitary gland, hypothalamus, and other target organs. In the hypothalamus, estrogens reduce release of gonadotropin-releasing hormone, which decreases pituitary release of follicle-stimulating hormone and luteinizing hormone. In women, these hormones are required for normal genitourinary and other essential body functions.

At the cellular level, estrogens increase cervical secretions, cause endometrial cell proliferation, and improve uterine tone. Estrogen replacement helps maintain genitourinary function and reduces vasomotor symptoms when estrogen production declines as a result of menopause, surgical removal of ovaries, or other estrogen deficiency states. Estrogen replacement also helps prevent osteoporosis by inhibiting bone resorption.

In men, estrogens inhibit pituitary secretion of luteinizing hormone and decrease testicular secretion of testosterone. These actions may decrease prostate tumor growth and lower the level of prostate-specific antigen (PSA).

Contraindications

Active deep vein thrombosis, pulmonary embolism, or history of these conditions; active or recent (within past year) arterial thromboembolic disease, such as MI or stroke; hepatic dysfunction or disease; history of anaphylactic reaction or angioedema to estradiol; history of jaundice with previous oral contraceptive use; hypersensitivity to estradiol, ethinyl estradiol, or their components; hypersensitivity to tartrazine dye (contained in 0.02-mg estradiol and ethinyl estradiol tablets); known or suspected breast cancer or history of breast cancer except in appropriately selected patients being treated for metastatic disease; known or suspected estrogen-dependent cancer; known protein C, protein S, or antithrombin deficiency, or other known thrombophilic disorders; uncontrolled diabetes mellitus with hypertension or vascular involvement; pregnancy; liver tumors; uncontrolled diabetes mellitus with hypertension or vascular involvement; undiagnosed abnormal genital bleeding

Interactions

DRUGS

aromatase inhibitors: Possible interference with aromatase inhibitor's effectiveness
corticosteroids: Increased therapeutic and toxic effects of corticosteroids
cyclosporine: Increased risk of hepatotoxicity and nephrotoxicity
CYP3A4 inducers such as carbamazepine, phenobarbital, rifampin, St. John's wort: Possibly reduced plasma concentration of estradiol affecting therapeutic effects
CYP3A4 inhibitors such as clarithromycin, erythromycin, itraconazole, ketoconazole, ritonavir: Possibly increased plasma concentration of estradiol increasing risk of adverse effects
hepatotoxic drugs, such as isoniazid: Increased risk of hepatitis and hepatotoxicity

insulin, oral antidiabetic drugs: Decreased therapeutic effects of these drugs
tamoxifen: Possibly decreased therapeutic effects of tamoxifen
thyroid hormone replacement: Decreased effectiveness
warfarin: Decreased anticoagulant effect

FOODS

grapefruit juice: Decreased estradiol metabolism and possibly increased adverse effects

ACTIVITIES

smoking: Increased risk of pulmonary embolism, stroke, thrombophlebitis, and transient ischemic attack

Adverse Reactions

CNS: Affect liability, chorea, CVA, dementia, depression, dizziness, emotional lability, fatigue, headache, insomnia, irritability, malaise, migraine headache, mood swings, nervousness, paresthesia
CV: Deep venous thrombosis, hypertension, MI, palpitations, peripheral edema, thromboembolism, thrombophlebitis, thromboembolism, unstable angina
EENT: Intolerance of contact lenses, oral paresthesia, pharyngeal edema, retinal vascular thrombosis, swollen lip or tongue, vision changes
ENDO: Breast enlargement, pain, tenderness, or tumors; breast cancer, elevated estrogen levels, exacerbation of hypothyroidism, fibrocystic breast changes; gynecomastia; hyperglycemia; nipple discharge or nipple and areola discoloration
GI: Abdominal cramps or pain, anorexia, bloating, bowel obstruction (vaginal ring), cholelithiasis, constipation, diarrhea, elevated liver enzymes, enlargement of abdomen or hepatic hemangiomas, gallbladder disease, gallbladder obstruction, GI hemorrhage, hepatitis, increased appetite, jaundice, nausea, pancreatitis, portal vein thrombosis, vomiting
GU: Amenorrhea, breakthrough bleeding, cervical or vaginal erosion, clear vaginal discharge, decreased libido, dysmenorrhea, endometrial hyperplasia or cancer, genital edema or itching, impotence, increased libido (females), ovarian cancer, pelvic pain, prolonged or heavy menstrual bleeding, ring adherence to vaginal wall, testicular atrophy, urinary frequency, uterine leiomyomata,

vaginismus, vaginitis, vaginal abrasion or ulceration (ring), vaginal candidiasis or discharge, vulvovaginal discomfort (burning sensation, pain, rash, swelling), worsening of endometriosis
MS: Arthralgia, leg cramps, muscle spasms
RESP: Dyspnea, **pulmonary embolism**
SKIN: Acne, alopecia, diaphoresis, discoloration or dry skin, **erythema multiforme**, erythema nodosum, facial pigmentation, hirsutism, melasma, oily skin, pruritus, purpura, rash, seborrhea, urticaria
Other: **Angioedema**, application-site reactions (transdermal), folic acid deficiency, **hypercalcemia** (in metastatic bone disease), **hypersensitivity reactions, hypocalcemia (in presence of hypoparathyroidism), toxic shock syndrome** (vaginal ring), weight gain or loss

Childbearing Considerations

PREGNANCY

- Drug is not known to cause fetal harm if inadvertently taken during early pregnancy.
- Drug has no therapeutic use during pregnancy and is contraindicated in pregnancy.

LACTATION

- Drug is present in breast milk and decreases the quality and quantity of breast milk but is less likely to do so once breastfeeding is well established.
- Patient should check with prescriber before breastfeeding.

Nursing Considerations

- Use estradiol cautiously in patients with asthma, chorea, diabetes mellitus, epilepsy, migraine headaches, porphyria, systemic lupus erythematosus, or hepatic hemangiomas because estradiol may worsen these disorders.
- Expect to begin prophylaxis treatment against osteoporosis at the start of menopause.
- Be aware that estrogen therapy should be given cyclically or combined with a progestin for 10 to 14 days per month in women with an intact uterus to minimize the risk of endometrial hyperplasia.

! **WARNING** Be aware that severe hypercalcemia may occur in patients with bone metastasis due to breast cancer because estrogens influence the metabolism of calcium and phosphorus. Monitor for toxic effects of increased calcium absorption in patients who are predisposed to hypercalcemia or nephrolithiasis. Also monitor patient with hypoparathyroidism for hypocalcemia.

! **WARNING** Assess patient for possible contact lens intolerance or changes in vision or visual acuity because estrogens can cause keratoconus, leading to increased curvature of the cornea. Be prepared to discontinue drug immediately, as prescribed, if patient experiences sudden partial or complete loss of vision or sudden onset of diplopia, migraine, or proptosis.

- Monitor PT test results of patients receiving warfarin for loss of anticoagulant effect because estrogens increase production of clotting factors VII, VIII, IX, and X and promote platelet aggregation.
- Watch for elevated liver enzymes because estrogens may worsen such conditions as acute intermittent or variegate hepatic porphyria.
- Closely monitor patient's blood pressure. A few patients may experience a substantial increase in blood pressure as an idiosyncratic reaction to estrogen. Monitor patients who already have hypertension for increases in blood pressure because estrogens may cause fluid retention. Also monitor patients with asthma, heart disease, migraines, renal disease, or seizure disorder for exacerbation of these conditions.
- Watch for peripheral edema or mild weight gain because estrogens can cause sodium and fluid retention.
- Monitor serum glucose level frequently in patients who have diabetes mellitus because estrogens may decrease insulin sensitivity and alter glucose tolerance.

! **WARNING** Expect to stop estrogen therapy in any woman who develops signs or symptoms of cancer; cardiovascular disease, such as MI, pulmonary embolism, stroke; dementia; or venous thrombosis.

- Be aware that women at risk for arterial vascular disease include those with diabetes mellitus, hypercholesterolemia, hypertension, obesity, tobacco use, or venous thromboembolism. Know that these factors, if present, should be addressed and brought under control.

- Be aware that exogenous estradiol and progestins may worsen mood disorders, including depression. Monitor patient for anxiety, depression, dizziness, fatigue, insomnia, or mood changes.
- Assess skin for melasma (tan or brown patches), which may develop on forehead, cheeks, temples, and upper lip. These patches may persist after drug is stopped.
- Check patient's triglyceride level routinely because, in patients with hypertriglyceridemia, estrogen therapy may increase serum triglyceride level enough to cause pancreatitis and other complications.
- Monitor serum PSA level in patients with inoperable prostate cancer to determine if patient is responding to hormone therapy. If patient responds (usually within 3 months), expect therapy to continue until disease is significantly advanced.
- Expect to stop estrogen therapy several weeks before patient undergoes major surgery, as prescribed, because certain procedures are associated with prolonged immobilization and therefore pose a risk of thromboembolism.
- Be aware that if patient takes thyroid hormone replacement therapy, monitor her for increased signs and symptoms of hypothyroidism because estradiol may increase thyroid-binding globulin levels, which may make the patient's current dose of thyroid hormone insufficient.
- Be aware that women with residual endometriosis posthysterectomy are at increased risk for malignant transformation of residual endometrial implants. Expect progesterone therapy to be given along with estradiol. Also, estradiol may exacerbate symptoms of many other conditions including angioedema, asthma, diabetes mellitus, epilepsy, migraine, porphyria, systemic lupus erythematosus, and hepatic hemangiomas. Monitor these patients closely.

! WARNING Monitor patient closely for signs of anaphylaxis, which may occur any time during therapy and may require emergency medical treatment. Monitor patient with history of hereditary angioedema closely because estradiol may exacerbate symptoms of angioedema.

PATIENT TEACHING

- Inform patient of risks involved in estrogen therapy before therapy starts. These risks may include increased risk of breast, endometrial, or ovarian cancer; cardiovascular disease; dementia (if age 65 or over); gallbladder disease; and vision abnormalities.
- Advise patient to remain recumbent for at least 30 minutes after applying estradiol vaginal cream. Inform her that she may use a sanitary napkin (but not a tampon) to protect clothing after application.
- Teach patient proper application and use of transdermal patch. Instruct her not to apply patch to breasts, waistline, or other areas where it may not adhere properly. Advise her to rotate application sites at least weekly and to remove old patch before applying new one. If patch falls off, instruct her to reapply it to another area or to apply a new patch and continue the original treatment schedule. Caution her not to expose patch to sun for long periods. Explain that she may bathe while wearing the patch. Instruct patient to discard used patch in household trash in a way that prevents accidental application or ingestion by children, pets, or others.
- Teach patient to apply Estrogel to clean, dry skin of one arm, using applicator. Emphasize importance of transferring all of the gel from applicator to arm. Tell patient to spread gel as thinly as possible over entire inside and outside of arm from wrist to shoulder. Advise her to wash her hands with soap and water afterward and to avoid fire and smoking until gel has dried because it's flammable. Tell patient never to apply gel to breasts. Warn that gel is alcohol-based and that patient should avoid fire, flame, or smoking until gel has dried.
- Instruct patient to apply Divigel to either the left or right upper thigh once daily, but to rotate to the opposite site on alternating days. Explain that the application surface area should be about 5 to 7 inches (about

the size of two palm prints). The entire contents of a unit-dose packet should be applied each day. Remind patient that gel should never be applied to her breasts, face, irritated skin, or in or around her vagina. After application, tell patient to let gel dry before dressing and not to wash the site for 1 hour after application. Instruct patient to wash her hands after applying gel.

- Tell patient using Imvexxy vaginal inserts to insert the smaller end up for a depth of about two inches into the vaginal canal. Each insert should be inserted at about the same time every day.

- Teach patient proper use of estradiol vaginal ring. Instruct her to insert ring in upper third of vagina, to keep it there for 90 days, and then to remove it and insert a new ring. Or she may remove it during the 90-day dosage period, rinse it with lukewarm (not hot or boiling) water, and reinsert it as needed for personal hygiene. Remind patient that she shouldn't be able to feel the ring when it's in place. If she does, she should use a finger to push the ring farther into her vagina. If vaginal wall ulceration or erosion occurs, suggest that patient leave ring out and not replace it until healing is complete, to keep ring from adhering to healing tissue.

- Instruct patient using estradiol vaginal ring to remove ring immediately and contact prescriber if she develops fever, nausea, vomiting, diarrhea, muscle pain, dizziness, faintness, or a sunburn rash on face or body that may suggest a rare but serious bacterial infection called toxic shock syndrome. Also urge patient to seek prompt medical care if ring becomes attached to vaginal wall (rare), making removal difficult.

- Inform patient receiving estradiol treatment that she should have an annual pelvic examination to screen for cervical dysplasia and be followed closely for other types of cancers and disorders associated with estradiol use.

- Tell patient who has an intact uterus and is prescribed transdermal Menostar that she will need to receive progestin for 14 days every 6 to 12 months and have an endometrial biopsy yearly.

- Advise patient that less serious but common side effects of estradiol therapy include abdominal or stomach cramps, bloating, breast pain or tenderness, fluid retention, hair loss, irregular vaginal bleeding or spotting, nausea and vomiting, and vaginal yeast infection.

- Tell patient using Elestrin not to apply sunscreen to the application site for at least 25 minutes.

- Urge patient to report any vaginal bleeding to prescriber.

estrogens
(conjugated)
Premarin

⁞ Class and Category
Pharmacologic class: Estrogen
Therapeutic class: Hormone

⁞ Indications and Dosages
✳ *To treat moderate to severe vasomotor menopausal symptoms; to treat vaginal and vulvar atrophy*

TABLETS
Adult women. 0.3 mg daily or cyclically 25 days on, 5 days off. Dosage increased as needed to control symptoms.

✳ *To treat atrophic vaginitis and kraurosis*

VAGINAL CREAM
Adult women. 0.5 to 2 g once daily in cycles of 3 wk on, 1 wk off.

✳ *To treat moderate to severe dyspareunia, a symptom of vulvar and vaginal atrophy in menopause*

VAGINAL CREAM
Adult women. 0.5 g twice/wk. Or, 0.5 g daily for 21 days followed by 7 days off, with cycle repeated every 28 days.

✳ *To prevent postmenopausal osteoporosis*

TABLETS
Adult women. 0.3 mg daily continuously or in cycles of 25 days on, 5 days off. Dosage increased as needed to control symptoms.

✳ *To provide palliative treatment for advanced androgen-dependent prostate cancer*

TABLETS
Adult men. 1.25 to 2 mg 3 times daily.

✳ *To provide palliative treatment for metastatic breast cancer*

TABLETS

Adult women. 10 mg 3 times daily for 3 months or longer.

* *To treat dysfunctional uterine bleeding*

I.V. INJECTION, I.M. INJECTION

Adult women. 25 mg, repeated in 6 to 12 hr as needed.

* *To treat estrogen deficiency from oophorectomy or primary ovarian failure*

TABLETS

Adult women. 1.25 mg daily in cycles of 3 wk on, 1 wk off. Dosage adjusted as needed.

* *To treat female hypogonadism*

TABLETS

Adult women. 0.3 to 0.625 mg daily in cycles of 3 wk on, 1 wk off. Dosage adjusted as needed.

Drug Administration

P.O.

- Administer drug at the same time every day.

I.V.

- I.V. is preferred route over I.M. route.
- Keep drug refrigerated before reconstituting.
- Reconstitute by adding 5 ml of Sterile Water for Injection to drug vial by directing stream slowly against the side of the vial and agitate gently. Do not shake.
- Administer immediately after reconstitution as an I.V. injection, injected slowly to prevent a flushing reaction.
- Compatible with 0.9% Sodium Chloride Injection, 5% Dextrose Injection, and invert sugar solutions.
- *Incompatibilities:* Ascorbic acid, protein hydrolysate, or any solution with an acid pH

I.M.

- Follow manufacturer guidelines for preparing drug for I.M. injection.
- Inject deeply into a large muscle such as in the buttocks or thigh.
- Rotate sites.

VAGINAL

- Place patient in a supine position.
- Clean vaginal area with soap and water.
- Insert applicator into the vagina about two-thirds the length of the applicator.
- Push plunger to release drug.
- Have patient remain supine for 30 minutes after administration.
- Store at room temperature.

Route	Onset	Peak	Duration
P.O.	Unknown	7 hr	Unknown
I.V./I.M.	Unknown	Unknown	Unknown
Vaginal	Unknown	7 hr	Unknown

Half-life: 17 hr

Mechanism of Action

Increases the rate of DNA and RNA synthesis in the cells of female reproductive organs, hypothalamus, pituitary glands, and other target organs. In the hypothalamus, estrogens reduce the release of gonadotropin-releasing hormone, which decreases pituitary release of follicle-stimulating hormone and luteinizing hormone. In women, these hormones are required for normal genitourinary and other essential body functions. At the cellular level, estrogens increase cervical secretions, cause endometrial cell proliferation, and increase uterine tone. Estrogen replacement helps maintain genitourinary function and reduce vasomotor symptoms when estrogen production declines from menopause, surgical removal of ovaries, or other estrogen deficiency. Estrogen also helps prevent osteoporosis by keeping bone resorption from exceeding bone formation. In men, estrogens inhibit pituitary secretion of luteinizing hormone and decrease testicular secretion of testosterone. These actions may decrease prostate tumor growth and lower the level of prostate-specific antigen.

Contraindications

Active deep vein thrombosis, pulmonary embolism, or history of these conditions; active or recent (within past year) arterial thromboembolic disease such as MI or stroke; history of anaphylactic reaction or angioedema to estradiol; hypersensitivity to estrogens or their components; known or suspected breast cancer or history of breast cancer; known or suspected estrogen-dependent cancer; known protein C, protein S, or antithrombin deficiency or other known thrombophilic disorders; pregnancy; liver impairment or disease; undiagnosed abnormal genital bleeding

Interactions

DRUGS

aromatase inhibitors: Possibly interference with aromatase inhibitor's effectiveness
barbiturates, carbamazepine, hydantoins, rifabutin, rifampin: Possibly reduced activity of estrogen and medroxyprogesterone
corticosteroids: Increased therapeutic and toxic effects of corticosteroids
cyclosporine: Increased risk of hepatotoxicity and nephrotoxicity
hepatotoxic drugs (such as isoniazid): Increased risk of hepatitis and hepatotoxicity
insulin, oral antidiabetic drugs: Decreased therapeutic effects of these drugs
tamoxifen: Possibly interference with tamoxifen's therapeutic effects
thyroid hormone replacement: Decreased effectiveness
warfarin: Decreased anticoagulant effect

ACTIVITIES

smoking: Increased risk of pulmonary embolism, stroke, thrombophlebitis, and transient ischemic attack

Adverse Reactions

CNS: Asthenia, CVA, dementia, depression, dizziness, growth benign meningioma, headache, insomnia, migraine headache, mood disturbance, nervousness, paresthesia
CV: Deep vein thrombosis, hypertension, MI, peripheral edema, thromboembolism, thrombophlebitis, vasodilation
EENT: Intolerance of contact lenses, pharyngitis, retinal vascular thrombosis, rhinitis, sinusitis
ENDO: Breast enlargement, pain, tenderness, or tumors; gynecomastia (men); hot flashes; hyperglycemia
GI: Abdominal cramps or pain, abdominal distention, anorexia, cholestatic jaundice, constipation, diarrhea, flatulence, gallbladder disease, gallbladder obstruction, hepatic hemangioma enlargement, hepatitis, increased appetite, ischemic colitis, nausea, pancreatitis, vomiting
GU: Amenorrhea, breakthrough bleeding, cervical erosion, clear vaginal discharge, decreased libido (men), dysmenorrhea, endometrial cancer or hyperplasia, impotence, increased libido (women), leukorrhea, ovarian cancer, prolonged or heavy menstrual bleeding, testicular atrophy, uterine leiomyomata enlargement, vaginal candidiasis, vaginitis, vaginal-site reactions (vaginal administration only such as burning, irritation, and genital pruritus)
MS: Arthralgias, back pain, muscle spasms
RESP: Bronchitis, increased cough, pulmonary embolism
SKIN: Acne, alopecia, chloasma, erythema multiforme, erythema nodosum, hemorrhagic eruption, hirsutism, melasma, oily skin, pruritus, purpura, rash, seborrhea, urticaria
Other: Anaphylaxis, angioedema, flu-like syndrome, folic acid deficiency, hypercalcemia (in metastatic bone disease), weight gain

Childbearing Considerations

PREGNANCY

- Drug is not known to cause fetal harm if inadvertently taken during early pregnancy.
- Drug is contraindicated in pregnancy.

LACTATION

- Drug decreases the quality and quantity of breast milk.
- Breastfeeding should not be undertaken during drug therapy.

Nursing Considerations

- Use conjugated estrogens cautiously in patients with severe hypocalcemia because a sudden increase in serum calcium level may cause adverse reactions.

! **WARNING** Monitor serum calcium level to detect severe hypercalcemia in patients with bone metastasis from breast cancer.

! **WARNING** Monitor patient closely, especially within minutes to hours of taking first dose, as anaphylaxis may occur, requiring emergency intervention. Be aware that estrogen therapy may exacerbate symptoms of angioedema in women with hereditary angioedema. Monitor for signs of swelling of the face, lips, throat, or tongue, and provide emergency care, as needed.

- Watch for elevated liver enzymes because estrogen and progestins may worsen such conditions as acute intermittent or variegate hepatic porphyria.
- Assess hypertensive patients for increases in blood pressure because estrogens may cause fluid retention.

- Monitor patients with asthma, diabetes mellitus, endometriosis, heart disease, lupus erythematosus, migraine headaches, renal disease, or seizure disorder for worsening of these conditions.
- Assess PT for loss of anticoagulant effects if patient takes warfarin, because estrogens increase production of clotting factors and promote platelet aggregation.
- Expect to stop drug during periods of immobilization, 4 weeks before elective surgery, and if jaundice develops.

! **WARNING** Expect to stop estrogen therapy in any woman who develops signs or symptoms of cancer; cardiovascular disease, such as MI, pulmonary embolism, stroke, venous thrombosis; or dementia.

- Check triglyceride level routinely because, in hypertriglyceridemia, estrogen therapy may increase triglycerides enough to cause pancreatitis and other complications.
- Know that if patient takes thyroid hormone replacement therapy, monitor her for increased signs and symptoms of hypothyroidism because estrogen may increase thyroid-binding globulin level, which may make the patient's current dose of thyroid hormone insufficient.
- Be aware that estrogen may worsen mood disorders, including depression. Monitor patient for depression, fatigue, insomnia, or mood changes.

PATIENT TEACHING

- Explain the risks of estrogen therapy, including increased risk of breast, endometrial, or ovarian cancer; cardiovascular disease; dementia; and gallbladder disease.
- Instruct patient taking oral form to take drug at the same time every day.
- Instruct patient how to administer vaginal cream, if ordered. Tell patient to wash vaginal area with soap and water and then lie down. Then tell patient to insert the applicator into the vagina about two-thirds the length of the applicator and then push the plunger to release the cream. Stress importance of lying down for 30 minutes after administration. Inform patient to store drug at room temperature.

! **WARNING** Review signs and symptoms of an allergic reaction that could become severe. Urge patient to stop drug, notify prescriber, or seek immediate medical help if serious.

- Urge patient to immediately report breakthrough bleeding to prescriber.
- Instruct patient to perform monthly breast self-examination and to comply with all prescribed follow-up examinations.
- Warn female patient that long-term use may increase risk of breast or endometrial cancer, dementia, gallbladder disease, heart disease, and stroke.
- Inform patient that estrogen vaginal cream may alter effectiveness of cervical caps, condoms, or diaphragms made of latex or rubber.
- Instruct patient to notify prescriber if she sees something that resembles a tablet in her stool.

eszopiclone
Lunesta

☰ Class, Category, and Schedule
Pharmacologic class: Pyrrolopyrazine derivative
Therapeutic class: Sedative-hypnotic
Controlled substance schedule: IV

☰ Indications and Dosages
✳ *To treat insomnia when at least 7 or 8 hours are remaining before the planned time of awakening*

TABLETS
Adults. *Initial:* 1 mg. May be increased to 2 or 3 mg as needed. *Maximum:* 3 mg.
±**DOSAGE ADJUSTMENT** For patients with severe hepatic impairment, patients who take potent CYP3A4 inhibitors, or patients who are debilitated or elderly, dosage should not exceed 2 mg. Dosage adjustment may be needed if other CNS depressants are also being taken.

☰ Drug Administration
P.O.
- Administer immediately before bedtime.
- Avoid administering after a heavy, high-fat meal.

Route	Onset	Peak	Duration
P.O.	Unknown	1 hr	Unknown

Half-life: 6–9 hr

Mechanism of Action

May potentiate effects of the inhibitory neurotransmitter gamma-aminobutyric acid (GABA) by binding close to or with benzodiazepine receptors in cortical and limbic areas of the CNS. By binding to these receptor sites and areas, eszopiclone increases GABA's inhibitory effects and blocks cortical and limbic arousal, thereby inducing and maintaining sleep.

Contraindications

Complex sleep behaviors with eszopiclone past administration, hypersensitivity to eszopiclone or its components

Interactions

DRUGS

CYP3A inducers such as rifampin: Decreased eszopiclone level
CYP3A inhibitors such as clarithromycin, itraconazole, ketoconazole, nefazodone, nelfinavir, ritonavir, troleandomycin: Increased eszopiclone level
other CNS depressants: Possibly additive effects

ACTIVITIES

alcohol use: Additive effect on psychomotor performance

FOOD

Heavy, high-fat meal: Possibly reduced effectiveness of eszopiclone

Adverse Reactions

CNS: Aggressiveness that seems out of character, agitation, anxiety, bizarre behavior such as sleep driving or walking, confusion decreased level of consciousness, depersonalization, depression with possible suicidal ideation, dizziness, drowsiness, hallucinations, headache (including migraine), nervousness, neuralgia, next day psychomotor impairment, somnolence, unusual dreams
CV: Chest pain, peripheral edema
EENT: Dry mouth; smell distortion; swelling of glottis, larynx, or tongue; taste perversion
ENDO: Gynecomastia
GI: Diarrhea, hepatitis, indigestion, nausea, vomiting

GU: Decreased libido, dysmenorrhea, UTI
RESP: Asthma, respiratory tract infection
SKIN: Pruritus, rash
Other: Angioedema, generalized pain, heatstroke, viral infection

Childbearing Considerations

PREGNANCY

- It is not known if drug causes fetal harm.
- Use with caution only if benefit to mother outweighs potential risk to fetus.

LACTATION

- It is not known if drug is present in breast milk.
- Patient should check with prescriber before breastfeeding.

Nursing Considerations

- Use eszopiclone cautiously in patients with severe mental depression or reduced respiratory function; drug may intensify mental depression and lead to respiratory depression.
- Institute safety and prevention of fall measures because of the adverse CNS effects of the drug.

PATIENT TEACHING

- Instruct patient not to exceed prescribed eszopiclone dosage and not to stop drug abruptly, because withdrawal symptoms may occur.
- Advise patient to take drug immediately before bedtime and to avoid taking drug after a heavy, high-fat meal.
- Warn patient, especially if debilitated or elderly, that drug may impair motor and/or cognitive performance increasing risk of falls. Advise patient to avoid potentially hazardous activities until drug's CNS effects are known.
- Urge patient to avoid alcohol and CNS depressants because of additive effects.
- Explain that sleep may be disturbed for the first few nights after therapy stops.
- Warn patient and caregiver that some patients have performed bizarre activities after taking drug, such as driving the car, preparing and eating food, making phone calls, or having sex while not fully awake and often with no memory of the event. These episodes usually occur in patients who have taken the drug with alcohol or other CNS depressant, who have taken the drug with less than a full night of sleep remaining (7 to 8 hours), or who have

E
F

exceeded the recommended dose. If such an episode occurs, the prescriber should be notified and eszopiclone therapy discontinued immediately.

etanercept
Enbrel

etanercept-szzs
Erelzi

etanercept-ykro
Eticovo

Class and Category
Pharmacologic class: Tumor necrosis factor (TNF) blocker
Therapeutic class: Immunosuppressant

Indications and Dosages
✲ *To treat rheumatoid arthritis alone or in combination with methotrexate; to treat psoriatic arthritis alone or in combination with methotrexate; to treat active ankylosing spondylitis*

SUBCUTANEOUS INJECTION
Adults. 50 mg once/wk on same day each wk. *Maximum:* 50 mg/wk.

✲ *To treat chronic moderate to severe plaque psoriasis in candidates for systemic therapy or phototherapy*

SUBCUTANEOUS INJECTION
Adults. *Initial:* 50 mg twice/wk 3 to 4 days apart for 3 months; then reduced to 50 mg/wk. Alternatively but less common, 25 mg or 50 mg/wk.
Children ages 4 and older weighing 63 kg (138 lb) or more. 50 mg once/wk on same day each wk.

SUBCUTANEOUS INJECTION (ENBREL)
Children ages 4 and older weighing less than 63 kg (138 lb). 0.8 mg/kg/wk.

✲ *To reduce signs and symptoms of moderately to severely active polyarticular juvenile idiopathic arthritis*

SUBCUTANEOUS INJECTION
Children ages 2 to 17 weighing 63 kg (138 lb) or more. 50 mg once/wk on same day each wk.

SUBCUTANEOUS INJECTION (ENBREL)
Children ages 2 to 17 weighing less than 63 kg (138 lb). 0.8 mg/kg/wk. *Maximum:* 50 mg/wk.

Drug Administration
SUBCUTANEOUS
- Store in refrigerator in original carton and protect from light. However, for short-term use, drug may be stored at room temperature for a maximum of 14 days (Enbrel) or 28 days (Erelzi) protected from sources of heat and light. Once drug has been stored at room temperature, do not place back into refrigerator.
- It is normal for small white particles of protein to be present in the solution but the solution should not be discolored, cloudy, or contain foreign particulate matter.
- When taking drug from refrigerator for administration, leave at room temperature for 15 to 30 minutes for Enbrel single-dose prefilled syringe or 30 minutes for Enbrel single-dose vial, SureClick autoinjector, or AutoTouch reusable autoinjector single-dose prefilled cartridge, or Eticovo prefilled syringe, before administering. Do not remove the needle cover or purple cap while drug is reaching room temperature.
- Rotate injection sites among abdomen, middle front of thigh, and upper back of arms and avoid areas that are bruised, hard, red, or tender. Keep each site at least 1 inch away from a previous site.
- Injection site should not be rubbed after drug is administered.

Enbrel
- Avoid handling needle cover of the prefilled syringe, within the white cap of the SureClick autoinjector, or inside the purple cap of the Mini cartridge if latex allergy is present. These components contain dry natural rubber.
- When using the Enbrel single-dose prefilled syringe, check to see if the amount of liquid falls between the two purple fill level indicator lines on the syringe. If not, discard and obtain a new syringe.
- If using a single-dose vial, use a 1-ml Luer-Lock syringe, a withdrawal needle with a Luer-Lock connection that is a 22G 1½-inch needle to withdraw solution and then change to a 27G, 1/2-inch needle for

≣ Mechanism of Action

Etanercept reduces inflammation by binding with tumor necrosis factor (TNF), a cytokine, or protein that plays an important role in normal inflammatory and immune responses.

The immune and inflammatory process triggers release of TNF, mainly from macrophages. TNF then binds to TNF receptors on cell membranes, as shown below left. This action renders TNF biologically active and triggers a cascade of inflammatory events that results in increased inflammation, release of destructive lysosomal enzymes, and joint destruction.

Etanercept binds to TNF and prevents it from binding with TNF receptors on the cell membranes, as shown below right. This action renders bound TNF biologically inactive, prevents TNF-mediated cellular responses, and significantly reduces inflammatory activity.

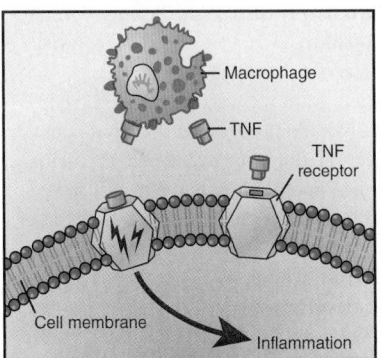

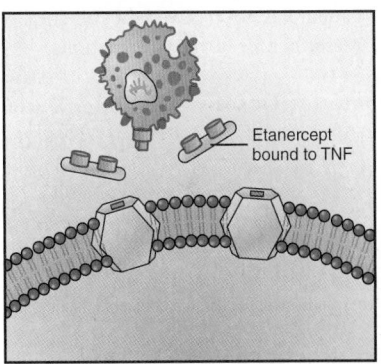

administration. Two vials may be required to administer the total dose. If so, use a new syringe for each vial. Discard unused portions in vial.

- If preparing dose from a multidose vial, reconstitute with 1 ml of supplied Bacteriostatic Water for Injection. Inject the solution slowly into vial. Use a 25G needle rather than the supplied vial adapter if the vial will be used for multiple doses. (If using the vial adapter, twist the vial adapter onto the diluent syringe. Then, place the vial adapter over the drug vial and insert the vial adapter into the vial stopper. Push down on the plunger to inject the diluent into the drug vial.) Gently swirl during dissolution rather than shaking vial. It may take up to 10 minutes for the powder to be dissolved. Resulting solution contains 25 mg/1 ml. Use a 27G needle for injection. Use drug as soon as possible after dissolving powder. Dissolved powder must be kept in refrigerator for up to 14 days. Discard if not used within that time frame. Do not mix one vial of drug solution with another vial of drug solution. Also do not add any other drugs to the solutions or use other diluents. Do not filter reconstituted solution during preparation.

- When using the SureClick autoinjector, the window turns yellow when the injection is complete. If after removing the autoinjector, the window has not turned yellow or it appears drug is still injecting, patient has not received the full dose. Notify prescriber for further instructions.

- To use AutoTouch reusable autoinjector, open the door by pushing the door button and inserting the mini single-dose prefilled cartridge into AutoTouch. It should slide freely and completely into the door. Close the door and inject drug.

- The AutoTouch makes sounds to help guide the injection. To turn sound off, slide the sound switch up (red bar visible). However, even when the sound is turned off, it still will produce the noise of the motor during the injection and will provide error alerts. Follow manufacturer guidelines on what to do if an error alert occurs and how to reset the AutoTouch.

Eticovo

- Solution in prefilled syringe should be clear or almost clear, colorless to pale yellow and may contain small white or almost clear particles, which is normal.
- When removing needle cover there may be a drop of liquid at the end of the needle, which is normal.

Erelzi

- When using the Sensoready Pen, the window will turn green when injection is complete. If window has not turned green, or if it looks like drug is still injecting, patient has not received the full dose. Notify prescriber for further instructions.

Route	Onset	Peak	Duration
SubQ	1–2 wk	72 hr	Unknown

Half-life: 4–5 days

Contraindications

Hypersensitivity to etanercept or its components, sepsis or risk of it

Interactions

DRUGS

abatacept: Increased risk of adverse reactions, especially infections
cyclophosphamide: Possibly increased risk of malignancy
live vaccines: Possibly increased risk of secondary transmission of infection from live vaccine
sulfasalazine: Possibly decreased neutrophil count

Adverse Reactions

CNS: Asthenia, chills, demyelination including both central and peripheral nervous systems, dizziness, fever, headache, multiple sclerosis, paresthesias, seizures
CV: Chest pain, congestive heart failure, hypertension, hypotension, peripheral edema, systemic vasculitis
EENT: Optic neuritis, pharyngitis, rhinitis, scleritis, sinusitis, uveitis
GI: Abdominal abscess or pain, autoimmune hepatitis, cholecystitis, diarrhea, elevated liver enzymes, gastroenteritis, indigestion, inflammatory bowel disease, nausea, noninfectious hepatitis, reactivation of hepatitis B, vomiting
GU: Pyelonephritis

HEME: Anemia, aplastic anemia, leukemia, leukopenia, neutropenia, pancytopenia, thrombocytopenia
MS: Osteomyelitis, septic arthritis, transverse myelitis
RESP: Bronchitis, cough, interstitial lung disease, pneumonia, upper respiratory tract infection
SKIN: Cellulitis, cutaneous lupus erythematosus or vasculitis, erythema multiforme, foot abscess, leg ulceration, melanoma and nonmelanoma skin cancers, Merkel cell carcinoma, new or worsening psoriasis, pruritus, rash, Stevens–Johnson syndrome, toxic epidermal necrolysis, urticaria
Other: Angioedema; bacterial, fungal, mycobacterial, parasitic, and viral infections; injection-site bruising, edema, erythema, itching, and pain; etanercept-induced antibodies; lymphadenopathy; lupus-like syndrome; macrophage activation syndrome; malignancy, such as lymphoma; sarcoidosis; sepsis

Childbearing Considerations

PREGNANCY

- It is not known if drug causes fetal harm.
- Use with caution only if benefit to mother outweighs potential risk to fetus.
- Safety of administering live or live attenuated vaccines in infants exposed to drug in utero is unknown.

LACTATION

- Drug is present in breast milk in low levels.
- Patient should check with prescriber before breastfeeding.

Nursing Considerations

- Be aware that etanercept should not be given to patients with granulomatosis with polyangiitis because of a higher incidence of noncutaneous solid malignancies with no improved outcome.
- Screen patient for latent tuberculosis with a tuberculin skin test before starting etanercept therapy. If test is positive, expect to give treatment, as ordered, before starting etanercept. Also screen patient for hepatitis B. If present, expect etanercept therapy to be withdrawn because antirheumatic therapies like etanercept may reactivate hepatitis B.

- Be aware that patients treated with tumor necrosis factor-alpha blockers such as etanercept are at increased risk for developing serious infections due to bacterial (including *Legionella* and *Listeria*), fungal, mycobacterial, parasitic, and viral pathogens. These infections can become life-threatening and involve multiple organ systems. Monitor patient closely throughout therapy.
- Know that tumor necrosis factor antagonists shouldn't be given with etanercept because doing so increases the risk of serious infection.
- Use cautiously in patients with a history of recurrent infection, underlying conditions that may predispose them to infections, or an existing chronic, latent, or localized infection because etanercept increases their risk of infection.
- Use cautiously in patients with COPD, and monitor respiratory status closely because etanercept therapy may increase patient's risk of adverse respiratory reactions.
- Use cautiously in patients with preexisting or recent onset CNS demyelinating disorders because drug may worsen these conditions. Also use cautiously in patients with heart failure or who have a history of serious hematologic abnormalities because drug may worsen these conditions.

! **WARNING** Expect to stop etanercept if patient develops sepsis. Also monitor patient for hypersensitivity reactions, which could become severe.

- Avoid giving live-virus vaccines to patients who are taking etanercept because drug decreases immune response and increases risk of secondary transmission of vaccine virus. Ensure that children are up to date on immunizations prior to etanercept being initiated.
- Monitor immunosuppressed patients for evidence of acute or chronic infection, including chills, fever, and tachycardia, because etanercept decreases defenses against infection. It also increases the risk of developing malignant tumors.
- Continue giving corticosteroids, NSAIDs, and other analgesics, as prescribed, during etanercept therapy.
- Be aware that malignancies, especially leukemias and lymphomas, have been reported rarely in patients taking tumor necrosis factor blockers such as etanercept. Children, adolescents, and patients with rheumatoid arthritis, especially those with very active disease, are at greatest risk. Monitor closely.

PATIENT TEACHING

- Reassure patient or caregiver that other medications such as analgesics, NSAIDs, and steroid therapy may be continued while patient is receiving etanercept.
- Inform patient that etanercept is given by a small injection into the skin, and teach him proper injection technique if needed.
- Alert patient using Enbrel brand of drug and SureClick autoinjector that the window turns yellow or if using Erelzi the window turns green, when the injection is complete. If after removing the autoinjector the window has not turned yellow or green, respectively, or it appears drug is still injecting, stress that patient has not received the full dose. If this happens, tell patient to notify prescriber.
- Alert patient using the AutoTouch reusable autoinjector with Enbrel Mini single-dose prefilled cartridge that the AutoTouch makes sounds to help guide the injection. If patient wants to turn the sounds off, she should slide the sound switch up (red bar visible). However, remind patient that even when the sound is turned off, she will still hear the noise of the motor during the injection and also error alerts. Instruct her what to do if an error alert occurs and how to reset the AutoTouch.
- Instruct patient to rotate injection sites among abdomen, thigh, and upper arms and to avoid areas that are bruised, hard, red, or tender. Advise him to keep each site at least 1 inch away from a previous site. Tell patient injection site should not be rubbed after drug is administered.
- Urge patient to use needles and syringes only once and discard in puncture-proof container.

! **WARNING** Stress importance of seeking immediate medical care if a severe allergic reaction occurs.

- Alert patients who are latex sensitive that the needle cover of the prefilled syringe, the needle cover within the white cap of the SureClick autoinjector, and inside the purple cap of the Enbrel Mini cartridge all contain dry natural rubber, which is a derivative of latex.

- Caution patient that the risk of malignancies such as leukemia and lymphoma may be higher in those who take etanercept, especially children and adolescents. Tell him to seek medical attention promptly for any suspicious signs and symptoms.
- Urge patient to consult prescriber immediately if he develops an infection because drug may decrease the body's infection-fighting ability.
- Caution patient who hasn't had chickenpox to contact prescriber right away if he's exposed because he may develop a more serious infection.
- Urge patient to seek immediate emergency care if he develops a bleeding, bruising, persistent fever or pallor while taking drug.
- Instruct patient to seek medical attention promptly for any unusual or persistent adverse signs or symptoms.
- Advise mother to alert pediatrician if she had received drug while pregnant.

ethacrynic acid
Edecrin

ethacrynate sodium
Edecrin

Class and Category
Pharmacologic class: Loop diuretic
Therapeutic class: Diuretic

Indications and Dosages
⁎ *To promote diuresis in heart failure, hepatic cirrhosis; renal disease; ascites of short duration caused by cancer, idiopathic edema, or lymphedema; and edema in hospitalized children other than infants, with congenital heart disease or nephrotic syndrome*

TABLETS
Adults. *Initial:* 50 to 100 mg daily as a single dose or in divided doses. Dosage increased by 25 to 50 mg daily, as needed. *Maintenance:* 50 to 200 mg daily and given continuously or on an intermittent schedule after effective diuresis is obtained.

Children (except infants). *Initial:* 25 mg daily. Dosage increased in 25-mg increments daily, as needed.

± **DOSAGE ADJUSTMENT** For patients who are sensitive to diuretic therapy, the following schedule may be used: Day 1, 50 mg once daily; day 2, 50 mg twice daily, if needed; and day 3, 100 mg in morning and 50 to 100 mg following the afternoon or evening meal, depending on the response of the morning dose.

⁎ *To provide rapid onset of diuresis, when needed, in acute pulmonary edema or when gastrointestinal absorption is impaired or oral medication is not practicable.*

I.V. INJECTION
Adults. *Initial:* 50 mg or 0.5 to 1 mg/kg. Dose repeated in 2 to 4 hr, if needed. *Maximum:* 100 mg as single dose.

Drug Administration

P.O.
- Administer once-daily dosing in the morning or last dose of the day several hours before bedtime.
- Administer after meals.

I.V.
- Reconstitute with 50 ml of 0.9% Sodium Chloride Injection or 5% Dextrose Injection. Be aware that some 5% Dextrose solutions may have a low pH resulting in a hazy or opalescent appearance. If this occurs, do not use.
- Administer slowly through the tubing of a running infusion or by direct intravenous injection over several minutes at 10 mg/min.
- Discard unused reconstituted solution after 24 hours.
- If second injection is needed, choose a new injection site to avoid possible thrombophlebitis. Do not give drug subcutaneously or intramuscularly.
- Discard unused portion after 24 hours.
- *Incompatibilities:* Hydralazine, procainamide, ranitidine, tolazoline, triflupromazine, whole blood, or its derivatives

Route	Onset	Peak	Duration
P.O.	30 min	2 hr	6–8 hr
I.V.	5 min	15–30 min	2 hr

Half-life: 1–4 hr

Mechanism of Action

Probably inhibits the sulfhydryl-catalyzed enzyme systems that cause sodium and chloride resorption in the proximal and distal tubules and the ascending limb of the loop of Henle. These inhibitory effects increase urinary excretion of sodium, chloride, and water, causing profound diuresis. Drug also increases the ammonium, bicarbonate, calcium, excretion of potassium, hydrogen, magnesium, and phosphate.

Contraindications

Anuria; hypersensitivity to ethacrynic acid, ethacrynate sodium, or their components; infancy; severe diarrhea

Interactions

DRUGS

aminoglycosides, some cephalosporins: Increased risk of ototoxicity
digoxin: Increased risk of digitalis toxicity
lithium: Increased risk of lithium toxicity
NSAIDs: Possibly decreased effects of ethacrynic acid
warfarin: Increased risk of bleeding

Adverse Reactions

CNS: Confusion, fatigue, headache, malaise, nervousness
CV: Orthostatic hypotension
EENT: Blurred vision, hearing loss, ototoxicity (ringing or buzzing in ears), sensation of fullness in ears, yellow vision
ENDO: Hyperglycemia, **hypoglycemia**
GI: Abdominal pain, anorexia, diarrhea, dysphagia, **GI bleeding (I.V.)**, nausea, vomiting
GU: Hematuria (I.V. form), interstitial nephritis, polyuria
HEME: Agranulocytosis, severe neutropenia, thrombocytopenia
SKIN: Rash
Other: Hyperuricemia, **hypochloremic alkalosis, hypokalemia, hypomagnesemia, hyponatremia,** hypovolemia, infusion-site irritation and pain

Childbearing Considerations

PREGNANCY

- It is not known if drug causes fetal harm.
- Use with caution only if benefit to mother outweighs potential risk to fetus.

LACTATION

- It is not known if drug is present in breast milk.

- A decision should be made to discontinue breastfeeding or the drug to avoid potential serious adverse reactions in the breastfed infant.

Nursing Considerations

! **WARNING** Give ethacrynic acid and ethacrynate sodium cautiously in patients with advanced hepatic cirrhosis, especially those with a history of electrolyte imbalance or hepatic encephalopathy because drug may lead to lethal hepatic coma.

- Weigh patient daily, and assess him for signs and symptoms of dehydration and electrolyte imbalances.
- Monitor blood pressure and fluid intake and output, and check laboratory test results.
- Report significant changes. Prescriber may reduce dosage or temporarily stop drug.
- Know that if hypokalemia develops, administer replacement potassium, as ordered.
- Monitor serum glucose level frequently, especially if patient has diabetes mellitus; both forms of drug may cause hyperglycemia or hypoglycemia.
- Notify prescriber if patient experiences hearing loss; buzzing, sense of fullness, or ringing in his ears; or vertigo. Drug may have to be discontinued.

PATIENT TEACHING

- Instruct patient to take the last dose of ethacrynic acid several hours before bedtime to avoid sleep interruption from diuresis. If patient receives once-daily dosing, advise him to take the dose in the morning to avoid sleep disturbance caused by nocturia.
- Suggest that patient take ethacrynic acid after a meal to reduce the likelihood of GI distress.
- Advise patient to change position slowly to minimize effects of orthostatic hypotension, especially if he also takes an antihypertensive.
- Urge patient to eat more high-potassium foods unless contraindicated and to take a potassium supplement, if prescribed, to prevent hypokalemia.
- Caution patient not to drink alcohol, stand for prolonged periods, or exercise during hot weather because these activities may exacerbate orthostatic hypotension.

E
F

- Instruct patient to notify prescriber if he has buzzing, fullness, or ringing in his ears; diarrhea; hearing loss; severe nausea; vertigo; or vomiting. Drug may have to be discontinued.
- Remind diabetic patients to check their serum glucose levels often for changes.

ethambutol hydrochloride
Etibi (CAN), Myambutol

Class and Category
Pharmacologic class: Synthetic antituberculotic
Therapeutic class: Antituberculotic

Indications and Dosages
✱ *As adjunct to treat pulmonary tuberculosis caused by* Mycobacterium tuberculosis

TABLETS
Adults and adolescents who haven't received previous antituberculotic therapy. 15 mg/kg daily.
Adults and adolescents who have received antituberculotic therapy. 25 mg/kg daily; after 60 days, decreased to 15 mg/kg daily.

Drug Administration
P.O.
- Administer with food if GI distress occurs.

Route	Onset	Peak	Duration
P.O.	Unknown	2–4 hr	Unknown

Half-life: 2.5–3.5 hr

Mechanism of Action
May suppress bacterial multiplication by interfering with RNA synthesis in susceptible bacteria that are actively dividing.

Contraindications
Hypersensitivity to ethambutol or its components, inability to report changes in vision, optic neuritis

Interactions
DRUGS
antacids that contain aluminum hydroxide: Decreased absorption of ethambutol

Adverse Reactions
CNS: Burning sensation or weakness in arms and legs, confusion, disorientation, dizziness, fever, headache, malaise, paresthesia, peripheral neuritis
EENT: Blurred vision, decreased visual acuity, eye pain, optic neuritis, red-green color blindness
GI: Abdominal pain, anorexia, **hepatic dysfunction**, nausea, vomiting
HEME: **Leukopenia, neutropenia, thrombocytopenia**
MS: Arthralgia, gouty arthritis, joint pain
RESP: **Pulmonary infiltrates**
SKIN: Dermatitis, **erythema multiforme, exfoliative dermatitis**, pruritus, rash
Other: **Anaphylaxis, hypersensitivity syndrome**, lymphadenopathy

Childbearing Considerations
PREGNANCY
- It is not known if drug causes fetal harm. However, there are reports of neonatal ophthalmic abnormalities born to women who took drug during pregnancy.
- Use with caution only if benefit to mother outweighs potential risk to fetus.

LACTATION
- Drug is present in breast milk.
- Patient should check with prescriber before breastfeeding.

Nursing Considerations
- Expect prescriber to refer patient for an ophthalmologic examination that includes tests for acuity, red-green color blindness, and visual fields before taking ethambutol and monthly thereafter. This is especially likely if therapy is prolonged or dosage exceeds 15 mg/kg daily.

! **WARNING** Notify prescriber immediately if patient develops vision changes, and expect ethambutol to be stopped if they occur.

- Expect to give patient at least one other antituberculotic with ethambutol, as prescribed, because bacteria may become resistant quickly to a single drug.
- Monitor laboratory test results for changes in liver function or for increased serum uric acid level if patient has gouty arthritis or impaired renal function. Notify prescriber of any abnormalities.
- Obtain a monthly sputum specimen, as ordered, to check bacteriologic response in sputum-positive patient.

- Know that successful ethambutol therapy typically takes 6 to 12 months but may take years.

PATIENT TEACHING

- Teach patient to recognize possible adverse reactions to ethambutol.
- Advise patient to take drug with food if he experiences adverse GI reactions.
- Instruct patient to take a missed dose as soon as he remembers, unless it's nearly time for the next dose, but not to double dose.
- Explain that ethambutol therapy may last months or years and that compliance is essential.
- Advise patient to notify prescriber if no improvement occurs within 3 weeks of starting ethambutol therapy; if bothersome or severe adverse reactions occur; if his vision changes; or if a fever, joint pain, or rash (possible hypersensitivity) develops.

ethosuximide
Zarontin

Class and Category
Pharmacologic class: Succinimide
Therapeutic class: Anticonvulsant

Indications and Dosages
✳ *To manage absence (petit mal) seizures*

CAPSULES, ORAL SOLUTION

Adults and children age 6 and over. *Initial:* 500 mg daily. *Maintenance:* Increased by 250 mg every 4 to 7 days until control is achieved with minimal adverse reactions. *Optimal:* 20 mg/kg/day.

Children ages 3 to 6. *Initial:* 250 mg daily. *Maintenance:* Increased by 250 mg every 4 to 7 days until control is achieved with minimal adverse reactions. *Optimal:* 20 mg/kg/day.

Drug Administration
P.O.

- Capsule should be swallowed whole and not chewed, crushed, or opened.
- Use a measuring device to measure dose when administering oral solution. Store oral solution at room temperature protected from light.

Route	Onset	Peak	Duration
P.O.	Unknown	4 hr	Unknown

Half-life: 60 hr

Mechanism of Action
Elevates the seizure threshold and reduces the frequency of attacks by depressing the motor cortex and elevating the threshold of CNS response to convulsive stimuli.

Contraindications
Hypersensitivity to ethosuximide, other succinimides, or their components

Interactions
DRUGS

phenytoin: Possibly increased blood phenytoin level
valproic acid: Increased or decreased blood ethosuximide level

Adverse Reactions
CNS: Aggressiveness, ataxia, decreased concentration, depression, dizziness, drowsiness, euphoria, fatigue, headache, hyperactivity, irritability, lethargy, light-headedness, nightmares, paranoid psychosis, psychosis, sleep disturbance, **suicidal ideation**, unsteadiness when walking
EENT: Gingival hypertrophy, myopia, **tongue swelling**
GI: Abdominal and epigastric pain, abdominal cramps, anorexia, diarrhea, hiccups, indigestion, nausea, vomiting
GU: Increased libido, microscopic hematuria, vaginal bleeding
HEME: **Agranulocytosis**, aplastic anemia, eosinophilia, **leukopenia, pancytopenia, thrombocytopenia including drug-induced immune thrombocytopenia**
SKIN: Erythematous and pruritic rashes, hirsutism, **Stevens–Johnson syndrome,** urticaria
Other: **Drug reaction with eosinophilia and systemic symptoms (DRESS), hypersensitivity reaction,** systemic lupus erythematosus, weight loss

Childbearing Considerations
PREGNANCY

- Pregnancy exposure registry: 1-888-233-2334 or http://www.aedpregnancyregistry.org/.
- Drug may cause fetal harm as reports indicate a potential increase risk of birth defects.
- Use with caution only if benefit to mother outweighs potential risk to fetus.

LACTATION

- Drug is present in breast milk.
- Patient should check with prescriber before breastfeeding.

REPRODUCTION

- Women of childbearing age should use an effective contraceptive throughout drug therapy.

☰ Nursing Considerations

- Use ethosuximide with extreme caution in patients with hepatic or renal disease.
- Give other anticonvulsants concurrently, as prescribed, to control generalized tonic–clonic seizures.
- Monitor CBC and platelet count and assess for signs of infection, such as cough, fever, and pharyngitis, as drug can cause blood dyscrasias and drug-induced immune thrombocytopenia, which could become life-threatening. Report abnormal signs and symptoms to prescriber. Also routinely evaluate liver and renal function test results.
- Take safety precautions because drug may cause adverse CNS reactions, such as dizziness and drowsiness.
- Monitor patient closely for evidence of suicidal thinking or behavior, especially when therapy starts or dosage changes.
- Assess patient regularly for signs of skin adverse effects. Stop ethosuximide immediately at first sign of rash and notify prescriber.

PATIENT TEACHING

- Emphasize the importance of complying with ethosuximide regimen.
- Tell patient to swallow capsule whole and not to chew, crush, or open it. If using oral solution, advise patient to use a calibrated device to measure dose and to store drug at room temperature protected from light.
- Advise patient to take a missed dose as soon as he remembers, unless it's nearly time for the next dose. Warn him not to double the dose.
- Instruct patient not to engage in potentially hazardous activities until drug's CNS effects are known.
- Caution patient not to stop taking drug abruptly; doing so increases the risk of absence seizures.
- Inform patient that the most common side effects of ethosuximide therapy include diarrhea, dizziness or light-headedness, fatigue, headache, hiccups, indigestion, loss of concentration or appetite, nausea, stomach pain, unsteadiness when walking, vomiting, and weight loss.
- Urge caregivers to watch patient closely for evidence of suicidal tendencies, especially when therapy starts or dosage changes, and to report any concerns immediately to prescriber.
- Advise patient or caregiver that prescriber should be notified immediately if a skin rash develops. Also tell patient to notify prescriber if persistent or serious adverse effects develop while taking ethosuximide.
- Caution female patient of childbearing age to use effective contraception methods while taking ethosuximide and to alert prescriber if pregnancy is suspected or known, as drug may cause fetal harm.

etravirine
Intelence

☰ Class and Category

Pharmacologic class: Non-nucleoside reverse transcriptase inhibitor (NNRTI)
Therapeutic class: Antiretroviral

☰ Indications and Dosages

⁎ *As adjunct to treat HIV-1 infection in patients who are antiretroviral treatment-experienced*

TABLETS

Adults, pregnant women, and children ages 2 to 18 weighing 30 kg (66 lb) or more. 200 mg twice daily.
Children ages 2 to 18 yr weighing 25 kg (55 lb) to less than 30 kg (66 lb). 150 mg twice daily.
Children ages 2 to 18 yr weighing 20 kg (44 lb) to less than 25 kg (55 lb). 125 mg twice daily.
Children ages 2 to 18 yr weighing 10 kg (22 lb) to less than 20 kg (44 lb). 100 mg twice daily.

☰ Drug Administration

P.O.

- Administer drug after meals.
- Tablet should be swallowed whole with a liquid and not chewed, crushed, or split.
- For patient unable to swallow tablets, dissolve tablet in 5 ml of water and stir

well until the water looks milky. Then add 15 ml of milk, orange juice, or water (not carbonated beverages, grapefruit juice, or warm liquids). Have patient drink mixture immediately and then add more milk, orange juice, or water to glass and have patient drink it. Do this several times to ensure that patient has received the entire dose.

Route	Onset	Peak	Duration
P.O.	Unknown	2.5–4 hr	Unknown

Half-life: 21–61 hr

Mechanism of Action

Binds directly to reverse transcriptase and blocks the RNA-dependent and DNA-dependent DNA polymerase activities by causing a disruption of the enzyme's catalytic site.

Contraindications

Hypersensitivity to etravirine or its components

Interactions

DRUGS

amiodarone, artemether, atazanavir, atazanavir/ritonavir, atorvastatin, bepridil, buprenorphine, clopidogrel, cyclosporine, dihydroartemisinin, disopyramide, dolutegravir, dolutegravir/darunavir/ritonavir, dolutegravir/ lopinavir/ritonavir, flecainide, indinavir, lidocaine (systemic), lovastatin, lumefantrine, maraviroc, mexiletine, propafenone, quinidine, rilpivirine, sildenafil, simvastatin, sirolimus, tacrolimus, telaprevir, warfarin: Decreased plasma concentrations of these drugs with possible decreased effectiveness

boceprevir: Decreased plasma concentration of etravirine with possible decreased effectiveness; increased plasma concentration of boceprevir with possible increased risk of adverse reactions

carbamazepine, darunavir/ritonavir, dexamethasone (systemic), efavirenz, lopinavir/ritonavir, nevirapine, phenobarbital, phenytoin, rifampin, rifapentine, ritonavir, St. John's wort, saquinavir/ritonavir, tipranavir/ ritonavir: Decreased plasma concentration of etravirine and its effectiveness

clarithromycin, itraconazole, ketoconazole: Decreased plasma concentrations of these drugs with possible decreased effectiveness; increased plasma concentration of etravirine

delavirdine: Increased plasma concentration of etravirine with possible increased risk of serious adverse reactions

diazepam, digoxin, fluvastatin, fosamprenavir, fosamprenavir/ritonavir, maraviroc/ darunavir/ritonavir, nelfinavir, pitavastatin: Increased plasma concentration of these drugs with possible increased risk of serious adverse reactions

rifabutin: Decreased plasma concentration of both etravirine and rifabutin with possible decreased effectiveness of both drugs

voriconazole: Increased plasma concentrations of both etravirine and voriconazole with possible increased risk of serious adverse reactions

Adverse Reactions

CNS: Abnormal dreams, amnesia, anxiety, confusion, **CVA**, difficulty concentrating, disorientation, fatigue, fever, general malaise, hypoesthesia, nervousness, nightmares, paresthesia, peripheral neuropathy, **seizures**, sleep disorders, sluggishness, somnolence, syncope, tremor, vertigo

CV: Angina pectoris, **atrial fibrillation**, dyslipidemia, elevated cholesterol and triglyceride levels, **MI**

EENT: Blurred vision, conjunctivitis, dry mouth, oral lesions, stomatitis

ENDO: Cushingoid appearance, diabetes mellitus, fat redistribution, gynecomastia, hyperglycemia

GI: Abdominal distention, anorexia, constipation, elevated liver or pancreatic enzymes, flatulence, gastroesophageal reflux disease, gastritis, hematemesis, **hepatic failure**, hepatic steatosis, **hepatitis**, hepatomegaly, **pancreatitis**, vomiting

GU: **Acute renal failure**, elevated creatinine level

HEME: Decreased hemoglobin eosinophilia, **hemolytic anemia, leukopenia, neutropenia, thrombocytopenia**

MS: Joint or muscle aches, **rhabdomyolysis**

RESP: **Bronchospasm**, exertional dyspnea

SKIN: Blisters, diaphoresis, dry skin, **erythema multiforme**, lipohypertrophy, night sweats, **Stevens–Johnson syndrome, toxic epidermal necrolysis**

Other: Angioedema, **drug reaction with eosinophilia and systemic symptoms (DRESS)**, immune reconstitution syndrome, lipodystrophy

E
F

☰ Childbearing Considerations

PREGNANCY

- Pregnancy exposure registry: 1-800-258-4263.
- It is not known if drug causes fetal harm.
- Use with caution only if benefit to mother outweighs potential risk to fetus.

LACTATION

- Drug is present in breast milk.
- The Centers for Disease Control and Prevention recommends that HIV-1 infected mothers not breastfeed to avoid risking postnatal transmission of HIV-1 infection to infants. They also do not recommend breastfeeding because of potential drug-induced adverse reactions in the infant.

☰ Nursing Considerations

! **WARNING** Assess patient for skin alterations, especially a rash that may occur anytime but most commonly within the first 6 weeks of treatment because, although uncommon, etravirine has caused severe skin and hypersensitivity reactions. Notify prescriber immediately if rash and other symptoms that may accompany the rash (such as angioedema, blisters, fatigue, jaundice, joint or muscle aches, or oral lesions) occur. Expect to check patient's liver enzymes and drug to be discontinued if rash is serious. Know that symptoms can evolve into a life-threatening reaction if drug is not promptly discontinued.

- Be aware that immune reconstitution syndrome has occurred in patients treated with combination antiretroviral therapy, including etravirine. The inflammatory response predisposes susceptible patients to opportunistic infections such as cytomegalovirus, *Mycobacterium avium* infection, *Pneumocystis jiroveci* pneumonia, or tuberculosis. Autoimmune disorders such as Graves' disease, Guillain–Barré syndrome, or polymyositis have also occurred. Report sudden or unusual adverse reactions to prescriber.
- Observe patient for redistribution of body fat, including breast enlargement, central obesity, development of buffalo hump, facial wasting, and peripheral wasting, which may produce a cushingoid-type appearance.

PATIENT TEACHING

- Tell patient to take etravirine twice daily following a meal. Tell her not to chew the tablets but to swallow them whole and take with a liquid.
- Instruct patient unable to swallow tablet to do the following: place tablet in a glass containing 1 teaspoon of water; stir well until water is milky looking; add more water or alternatively milk or orange juice, if needed (milk or orange juice should only be used after water has been used first); drink immediately; add milk, orange juice, or water to glass and drink. Repeat this procedure several times to ensure that entire dose has been taken. Caution patient not to use carbonated beverages, grapefruit juice, or warm liquids to dissolve drug.
- Advise patient that if a dose is missed and it is less than 6 hours from the time it is usually taken, she should take the drug following the intake of a meal. However, if it is longer than 6 hours, tell her to skip the dose and resume her normal dosing schedule with the next dose.
- Tell mothers not to breastfeed their infants while receiving etravirine.
- Alert patient to the possibility of fat distribution with the appearance of a buffalo hump, thin extremities and face, and breast enlargement.
- Instruct patient to inform all prescribers of etravirine therapy and not to take any drugs, including over-the-counter drugs and herbal medicines, without prescriber consent, because etravirine interacts with many drugs.

! **WARNING** Tell patient to notify prescriber immediately of any alteration in skin but especially a rash that may be associated with other symptoms. Drug will have to be discontinued if serious.

everolimus

Afinitor, Afinitor Disperz, Zortress

☰ Class and Category

Pharmacologic class: mTOR kinase inhibitor
Therapeutic class: Immunosuppressant

≡ Indications and Dosages

* As adjunct to prevent organ rejection in renal transplantation

TABLETS (ZORTRESS)

Adults. *Initial:* 0.75 mg twice daily in combination with reduced-dose cyclosporine, administered as soon as possible after transplantation.

* As adjunct to prevent organ rejection in liver transplantation

TABLETS (ZORTRESS)

Adults. *Initial:* 1 mg twice daily in combination with reduced-dose tacrolimus begun 30 days post-transplant.

±**DOSAGE ADJUSTMENT** For patient taking Zortress, dosage adjusted at 4- to 5-day intervals, as needed, according to everolimus blood concentrations, tolerability, change in concomitant medications, the clinical situation, and individual response. For patients with mild hepatic impairment, initial daily dose reduced by one-third, and for patients with moderate or severe hepatic impairment, initial daily dose is reduced by 50% with further adjustments made according to everolimus blood concentration levels.

* To treat advanced hormone receptor-positive, HER2-negative breast cancer in postmenopausal women in combination with exemestane after failure of treatment with anastrozole or letrozole; to treat progressive neuroendocrine tumors of pancreatic origin or are progressive, well-differentiated, nonfunctional tumors of gastrointestinal or lung origin that are locally advanced, metastatic, or unresectable; to treat renal cell carcinoma after failure of treatment with sorafenib or sunitinib; to treat renal angiomyolipoma and tuberous sclerosis complex that does not require immediate surgery

TABLETS (AFINITOR)

Adults. 10 mg once daily. Treatment continued until disease progression or unacceptable toxicity occurs.

* To treat tuberous sclerosis complex-associated subependymal giant cell astrocytoma (SEGA)

ORAL SUSPENSION (AFINITOR DISPERZ), TABLETS (AFINITOR)

Adults and children age 1 year and over. 4.5 mg/m^2 once daily until disease progresses or unacceptable toxicity occurs.

* As adjunct to treat tuberous sclerosis complex-associated partial-onset seizures

ORAL SUSPENSION (AFINITOR DISPERZ)

Adults and children age 2 years and over. 5 mg/m^2 once daily until disease progresses or unacceptable toxicity occurs.

±**DOSAGE ADJUSTMENT** For patients taking Afinitor or Afinitor Disperz, dosage adjusted according to degree of adverse reactions present. Also, for patients with breast cancer, neuroendocrine tumors, renal cell carcinoma, or tuberous sclerosis complex-associated renal angiomyolipoma and mild hepatic impairment, dosage reduced to 7.5 mg once daily or 5 mg once daily if higher dose is not tolerated; for moderate hepatic impairment, dosage reduced to 5 mg once daily or 2.5 mg once daily if higher dose is not tolerated; and for patients with severe hepatic impairment, dosage reduced to 2.5 mg once daily. For patients with tuberous sclerosis complex-associated subependymal giant cell astrocytoma or tuberous sclerosis complex-associated partial-onset seizures and severe hepatic impairment, dosage reduced to 2.5 mg/m^2 once daily. For patient taking a P-gp and moderate CYP3A inhibitors and who has breast cancer, neuroendocrine tumor, renal cell carcinoma, or tuberous sclerosis complex-associated renal angiomyolipoma, dosage reduced to 2.5 mg once daily, with dosage then increased to 5 mg once daily, if tolerated. For patients taking P-gp and moderate CYP3A inhibitors and who have tuberous sclerosis complex-associated subependymal giant cell astrocytoma or tuberous sclerosis complex-associated partial-onset seizures, daily dosage reduced by 50%. For patients taking a P-gp and strong CYP3A4 inducers and who have any indication treated by everolimus, dosage doubled using increments of 5 mg or less.

≡ Drug Administration

P.O.

- Zortress brand of everolimus isn't recommended in transplants other than kidney or liver transplantation. Everolimus therapy should not begin until 30 days after liver transplant because of patient's increased risk of developing hepatic artery thrombosis, which may lead to graft loss or death.

- Another form of everolimus under the trade names of Afinitor and Afinitor Disperz are used only to treat certain cancers. The three brands are not interchangeable. To avoid a medication error, make sure the right brand is being used for indication being treated.
- Tablets should be swallowed whole and given with a glass of water and not chewed or crushed before ingesting.
- Wear gloves when preparing and administering oral suspension. Prepare suspension with only water following manufacturer guidelines.
- Use a calibrated device to measure oral suspension dose. Administer immediately after preparation. Discard within 60 minutes if not administered.
- Twice-daily dosages should be consistently taken approximately 12 hours apart and at the same time as the prescribed cyclosporine or tacrolimus dose, if prescribed.

Route	Onset	Peak	Duration
P.O.	Unknown	1–2 hr	Unknown

Half-life: 30 hr

Mechanism of Action

Causes immunosuppression by inhibiting antigenic and interleukin (IL-2 and IL-15) stimulated activation and proliferation of B and T lymphocytes.

Contraindications

Hypersensitivity to everolimus, other rapamycin derivatives, or their components

Interactions

DRUGS

ACE inhibitors: Possibly increased risk of angioedema
amprenavir, aprepitant, atazanavir, clarithromycin, cyclosporine, digoxin, diltiazem, erythromycin, fluconazole, fosamprenavir, indinavir, itraconazole, ketoconazole, macrolide antibiotics, nefazodone, nelfinavir, nicardipine, ritonavir, saquinavir, telithromycin, verapamil, voriconazole: Possible increased blood everolimus level
anticonvulsants, carbamazepine, efavirenz, nevirapine, phenobarbital, phenytoin, rifabutin, rifampin, rifapentine, St. John's wort: Possibly decreased blood everolimus level

lovastatin, simvastatin: Possible development of rhabdomyolysis and other adverse reactions
octreotide (depot): Increased octreotide levels
live vaccines: Possibly increased risk of contracting disease from live virus; decreased therapeutic effect of vaccine

FOODS

grapefruit, grapefruit juice: Possibly decreased metabolism of everolimus increasing everolimus level

Adverse Reactions

CNS: Aggression, agitation, anxiety, asthenia, chills, dizziness, fatigue, fever, headache, insomnia, **progressive multiple leukoencephalopathy (PML)**, multiple, paresthesia, reflex sympathetic dystrophy
CV: **Arterial thrombotic events**, chest pain, **congestive heart failure, deep vein thrombosis**, hyperlipidemia, hypertension, **pericardial effusion**, peripheral edema, tachycardia, **thrombotic microangiopathy**
EENT: Conjunctivitis, dry mouth, epistaxis, eyelid pain, oropharyngeal pain, rhinorrhea, stomatitis
ENDO: Hot flashes, hyperglycemia, new-onset diabetes mellitus
GI: Abdominal pain, anorexia, ascites, cholecystitis, cholelithiasis, constipation, diarrhea, elevated bilirubin or liver enzymes, gastroenteritis, **hepatic artery thrombosis** (liver transplant), nausea, **pancreatitis**
GU: **Acute renal failure**, amenorrhea, azoospermia, **BK virus-associated nephropathy**, elevated creatinine level, **kidney graft thrombosis, nephrotoxicity**, oligospermia, proteinuria, UTI
HEME: Anemia, **bleeding, elevated partial thromboplastin time, elevated prothrombin time, leukopenia, lymphopenia, neutropenia, thrombocytopenia**
MS: Arthralgia; back, extremity, or jaw pain; muscle spasm; myalgia
RESP: Cough, dyspnea, **interstitial lung disease**, noninfectious pneumonitis, pleural effusion, **pulmonary embolism**, upper respiratory infection
SKIN: Acne, alopecia, dermatitis, erythema, nail disorders, pruritus, rash, **skin cancer**
Other: Angioedema; **decreased bicarbonate level**; delayed wound healing; elevated alkaline phosphatase; **hyperkalemia; hypersensitivity**

reactions; hypocalcemia; hypokalemia; hyponatremia; hypophosphatemia; infections such as bacterial, fungal, protozoal, and viral; lymphedema; **lymphomas and other malignancies**; opportunistic infections including polyoma virus; radiation sensitization and radiation recall (cancer treatment); **sepsis**; **septic shock**; weight loss

Childbearing Considerations

PREGNANCY

- A negative pregnancy test result is required before starting drug therapy.
- Drug may cause fetal harm based on animal studies.
- Use with caution only if benefit to mother outweighs potential risk to fetus.

LACTATION

- It is not known if drug is present in breast milk.
- Breastfeeding should not occur during drug therapy.

REPRODUCTION

- Advise women of childbearing potential to use highly effective contraception methods while receiving drug and up to 8 weeks after drug is discontinued.
- Advise male patients with female partners of childbearing potential to use effective contraception during treatment and for 4 weeks after the last dose.
- Drug therapy may cause both female and male infertility.

Nursing Considerations

- Know that patients with galactose intolerance, glucose–galactose malabsorption, or Lapp lactase deficiency should not receive everolimus therapy because this may result in diarrhea and malabsorption.
- Expect female patient of childbearing age to undergo a pregnancy test prior to initiating everolimus therapy, because drug can cause fetal harm.
- Assess patient's renal function before therapy with Afinitor or Afinitor Disperz brand of everolimus is begun, and annually thereafter unless patient has underlying risk factors for renal failure. Renal evaluation in these patients should be done every 6 months.

! WARNING Monitor patient closely for hypersensitivity reactions that could be severe. These may include anaphylaxis, angioedema, chest pain, dyspnea, or flushing. At the first sign of a reaction, notify prescriber, expect to administer emergency treatment according to institutional protocol, and expect drug to be discontinued.

- Measure whole blood trough concentrations of both cyclosporine and everolimus in patient with kidney transplant or tacrolimus and everolimus in liver transplant because of increased risk of nephrotoxicity when either combination of drugs are used or when drug is used to treat malignancies or tuberous sclerosis complex-associated partial-onset seizures. Everolimus levels, ideally drawn 4 to 5 days after a previous dosing change, will also reveal if the therapeutic range has been achieved (3 to 8 ng/ml).
- Know that dosage adjustments of everolimus can be made, as needed. In addition, everolimus levels should be obtained during concomitant administration of CYP3A4 inducers or inhibitors, when switching cyclosporine formulations, and/or when cyclosporine dosing is reduced as well as in patients with hepatic impairment. Know that there is little to no pharmacokinetic interaction of tacrolimus on everolimus. Therefore, there is no need to alter everolimus dosing if tacrolimus dosing is altered.
- Monitor patient's incision, as everolimus delays wound healing and increases the occurrence of wound-related complications such as wound dehiscence, wound infection, incisional hernia, lymphocele, and seroma.

! WARNING Watch for evidence of infection (such as cough, fever, pain, malaise) because patients receiving immunosuppressants such as everolimus are at increased risk for bacterial, fungal, parasitic, or viral infection. Watch for both generalized and localized infections, including worsening of preexisting infections, and be aware that these infections may become life-threatening. Activation of latent viral infections may also occur and include BK-virus-associated nephropathy that can lead to decreased renal function and renal graft loss.

- Be aware that interstitial lung disease may occur in patients with symptoms consistent with infectious pneumonia but usually only becomes apparent when patient does not respond to antibiotic therapy and other causes have been ruled out. If this occurs, expect everolimus therapy to be interrupted until the noninfectious pneumonitis has been resolved. Know that glucocorticoid therapy may also be prescribed to help resolve it.
- Monitor cancer patient receiving radiation during or sequentially with everolimus therapy as radiation sensitization and recall involving cutaneous and visceral organs may occur, resulting in worsening adverse effects of radiation therapy. Adverse effects may become severe.
- Monitor patient, especially within the first 30 days post transplantation, for evidence of kidney arterial and venous thrombosis (kidney transplant) or hepatic artery thrombosis (liver transplant) resulting in graft loss.
- Monitor patient's lipid levels routinely because hyperlipidemia may occur as a result of everolimus therapy. If hyperlipidemia drug therapy is required, be aware that lovastatin or simvastatin should not be used to treat it for patient with a kidney transplant because of a potential interaction with cyclosporine.
- Monitor patient's CBC and platelet count, as ordered, routinely because of increased risk of hemolytic uremic syndrome, thrombotic microangiopathy, or thrombotic thrombocytopenic purpura that may occur with combined everolimus and cyclosporine therapy used with kidney transplantation. Also know that drug causes myelosuppression, which may lead to hematologic disorders such as anemia, lymphopenia, neutropenia, and thrombocytopenia.
- Report abnormalities promptly to prescriber.
- Monitor patient's blood glucose levels regularly because everolimus therapy may increase the risk of new-onset diabetes mellitus after transplant.

PATIENT TEACHING

- Instruct patient to swallow tablets whole with a glass of water and not chew or crush before ingesting. Tell patient taking oral suspension how to mix the suspension and to use a calibrated device to measure dosage. Stress importance of taking drug immediately after mixing.
- Tell patient that ideally twice-daily dosages should be consistently taken approximately 12 hours apart and at the same time as his cyclosporine or tacrolimus dose, if prescribed.

! WARNING Advise patient to report an allergic reaction or signs and symptoms of an infection to prescriber, but if serious tell patient to seek immediate medical attention.

- Instruct patient to report any, persistent, severe, or unusual symptoms to prescriber.
- Caution patient to avoid excessive exposure to ultraviolet light, to wear protective clothing when outdoors, and use a sunscreen with a high protection factor.
- Inform patient that stomatitis most often occurs within the first 8 weeks of treatment. Instruct patient that he will be prescribed a dexamethasone alcohol-free oral solution and to use it as a swish-and-spit mouthwash. Caution him to avoid alcohol-, hydrogen peroxide-, iodine-, or thyme-containing products.
- Advise patient to avoid immunizations that use live vaccines such as BCG, intranasal influenza, measles, mumps, rubella, oral polio, TY21a typhoid, varicella, and yellow fever.
- Emphasize importance of avoiding grapefruit and grapefruit juice while receiving concomitant therapy with everolimus and cyclosporine.
- Urge women of childbearing age to use a highly effective birth control method throughout everolimus therapy and for 8 weeks after the drug has been discontinued.
- Alert both men and women that drug may affect fertility.
- Inform mothers that they should not breastfeed while taking everolimus.

evinacumab-dgnb
Evkeeza

⬚ Class and Category
Pharmacologic class: Recombinant human monoclonal antibody (angiopoietin-like 3 inhibitor)
Therapeutic class: Antilipemic

⬚ Indications and Dosages
⁎ *As adjunct to treat homozygous familial hypercholesterolemia*

I.V. INFUSION
Adults and children age 12 and older.
15 mg/kg every 4 wk.

⬚ Drug Administration
I.V.
- Calculate the dose in mg, total drug volume in ml required, and the number of vials needed based on patient's current body weight.
- Solution should be clear to slightly opalescent, colorless to pale yellow. Discard if it is discolored, looks cloudy, or has particulate matter in it.
- Be aware that the drug vials are single-dose vials and do not contain a preservative.
- Do not shake the vial. Withdraw the required volume from the drug vial(s) and transfer into an I.V. infusion bag containing a maximum volume of 250 ml of 0.9% Sodium Chloride Injection or 5% Dextrose Injection. Mix the diluted solution by gentle inversion; do not shake. The final concentration of the diluted solution should be between 0.5 mg/ml and 20 mg/ml, depending on the patient's weight.
- Administer the drug immediately after preparation and discard any unused solution left in drug vial.
- If drug cannot be administered immediately, store the diluted solution in refrigerator for no more than 24 hours from the time of preparation or at room temperature for no more than 6 hours from the time of preparation. Never freeze the diluted solution.
- Allow refrigerated solution to come to room temperature before administration.
- Do not mix other medications or administer other medications concomitantly in the same infusion line.
- Administer as an I.V. infusion over 60 minutes using an I.V. line containing a sterile, inline or add-on 0.2-micron to 5-micron filter.

Route	Onset	Peak	Duration
I.V.	Unknown	Unknown	Unknown

Half-life: Not constant

⬚ Mechanism of Action
Binds and inhibits ANGPTL3, which is expressed primarily in the liver and helps to regulate lipid metabolism by inhibiting lipoprotein lipase and endothelial lipase. Inhibition of ANGPTL3 causes a reduction in LDL-C, HDL-C, and triglycerides.

⬚ Contraindications
Hypersensitivity to evinacumab-dgnb or its components

⬚ Interactions
None reported by manufacturer

⬚ Adverse Reactions
CNS: Asthenia, dizziness
CV: Increased heart rate, mild increased diastolic pressure
EENT: Nasal congestion, nasopharyngitis, rhinorrhea
GI: Abdominal pain, constipation, nausea
MS: Extremity pain
RESP: Predisposition to upper respiratory tract infection
OTHER: Anaphylaxis, anti-evinacumab-dgnb antibody formation, flu-like illness, infusion reactions (muscle weakness, pruritus, pyrexia)

⬚ Childbearing Considerations
PREGNANCY
- Pregnancy exposure registry: 1-833-385-3392.
- Drug may cause fetal harm based on animal studies.
- Use with caution only if benefit to mother outweighs potential risk to fetus.

LACTATION
- It is not known if drug is present in breast milk.
- Patient should check with prescriber before breastfeeding.

REPRODUCTION
- Women of childbearing age should use effective contraception during treatment

E
F

with drug and for at least 5 months following the last dose of drug.

NURSING CONSIDERATIONS

- Ensure that all women of childbearing age have a negative pregnancy test result prior to initiating treatment with evinacumab-dgnb.

! **WARNING** Monitor patient for serious hypersensitivity reactions. If present, notify prescriber and expect to provide supportive care as needed and ordered. Monitor patient until the signs and symptoms of the hypersensitivity reaction are resolved.

PATIENT TEACHING

! **WARNING** Advise patients to seek immediate emergency care if a serious allergic reaction occurs.

- Women of childbearing age should use effective contraception during treatment with drug and for at least 5 months following the last dose of drug.

exenatide

Bydureon, Bydureon BCise, Byetta

☰ Class and Category

Pharmacologic class: Glucagon-like peptide-1 (GLP-1) receptor agonist
Therapeutic class: Antidiabetic

☰ Indications and Dosages

⁎ *Adjunct treatment to diet and exercise to improve blood glucose levels in patients with type 2 diabetes mellitus*

SUBCUTANEOUS INJECTION (BYETTA)

Adults. *Initial:* 5 mcg twice daily. After 1 month, increased, as needed, to 10 mcg twice daily.

SUBCUTANEOUS INJECTION (BYDUREON, BYDUREON BCISE)

Adults and children age 10 and older. 2 mg once every 7 days.

☰ Drug Administration

SUBCUTANEOUS

- Administer drug into patient's abdomen, thigh, or upper arm. Rotate sites.
- Prior to first use, store in refrigerator, protected from light.

Byetta
- Administer within 60 minutes before morning and evening meals or before two main meals that are about 6 hours or more apart.
- Drug should not be administered after a meal.
- Once pen is used, it can be kept at room temperature protected from light.
- Discard pen after 30 days from first use, even if some drug remains in the pen.

Bydureon Vial
- Drug can be administered at any time during the day and without regard to meals.
- Expect to discontinue any other exenatide product before Bydureon is begun.
- Bydureon comes in a single-dose tray or a single-dose pen.
- To use single-dose tray, remove from refrigerator, peel back the corner to open, and remove all the items.
- Pick up needle and twist off the blue cap. Tap drug vial several times against a hard surface to loosen the powder, then remove the green cap on the vial.
- Pick up vial connector package and peel off the paper cover. Do not touch the orange connector inside. Holding the vial connector package in one hand, pick up vial in the other hand. Press the top of the vial firmly into the orange connector. Then lift the vial with the orange connector now attached out of the package. Put it aside.
- Pick up the syringe and firmly grasp the 2 gray squares on the white cap and break off the cap. Do not push in the plunger. Then twist the orange connector onto the syringe until snug. Do not overtighten.
- With thumb, push down the plunger until it stops. Holding the plunger down, shake the syringe hard. Keep shaking until the liquid and powder are mixed well. When mixed well, it should appear cloudy. If clumps are seen, keep shaking with plunger pushed down until well mixed.
- After mixing, hold vial upside down so the syringe is pointing up. Continue to hold the plunger in place. Gently tap vial with other hand. Pull the plunger down beyond the black dashed dose line. Bubbles are normal. While holding plunger in, twist the orange connector to remove it from the syringe.
- Twist needle onto syringe until snug. Slowly push in the plunger so the top of the

⬚ Mechanism of Action

Normally, when serum glucose level rises, insulin is secreted within 10 minutes. This first-phase insulin response is absent in patients with type 2 diabetes. Exenatide, an incretin mimetic, restores the first-phase insulin response and improves the second-phase response that immediately follows. It does so by promoting incretins that spur insulin synthesis and release from beta cells by binding and activating human GLP-1 receptors to reduce fasting and postprandial serum glucose levels.

The drug also suppresses inappropriately elevated glucagon secretion. Lower serum glucagon level leads to decreased hepatic glucose output and decreased insulin demand. It also slows gastric emptying and thus the rise of serum glucose level.

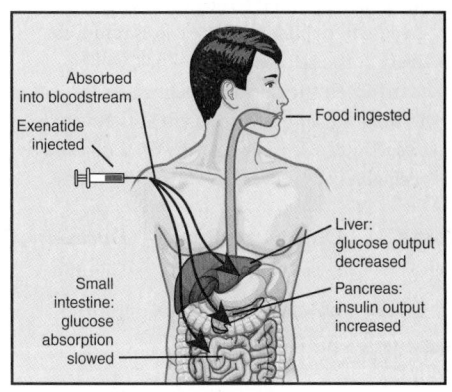

Labels in figure:
- Absorbed into bloodstream
- Exenatide injected
- Food ingested
- Liver: glucose output decreased
- Pancreas: insulin output increased
- Small intestine: glucose absorption slowed

plunger lines up with the black dashed dose line, then take thumb off the plunger.
- Remove needle cover (do not twist).
- Inject into site selected.

Bydureon Pen
- Drug may be given at any time during the day and without regard to meals.
- Pen may be kept at room temperature for up to 4 weeks, if needed.
- Allow pen to come to room temperature, if stored in refrigerator, for at least 15 minutes.
- Pull up on the corner of the tray and remove the pen and needle.
- Check pen solution; it should be clear and free of particles. Some bubbles in the liquid are normal.
- Attach needle to pen by pushing and twisting clockwise until it is tight. Keep needle cover on.
- While holding pen straight up, slowly turn knob and stop when a click is heard and the green label disappears.
- Holding pen by the end with the orange label, tap pen firmly against the palm of a hand. Do not twist the white knob. Rotate pen every 10 taps. Taps of 80 times or more may be needed. Check solution by holding pen up to the light and looking through both sides of the mixing window. There should be no clumps and solution should appear uniformly cloudy. Do not administer until solution is mixed well.

- When solution is mixed well, hold pen with the needle pointing straight up and turn the white knob until the orange label disappears and the injection button is released. Do not push the injection button yet.
- Remove the needle cover by pulling it straight off, not twisting it.
- Insert the needle into the injection site and press the injection button with thumb until a click is heard. Keep holding the button down and slowly count to 10 to inject the full dose.

Bydureon BCise
- Expect to discontinue any other exenatide product before Bydureon BCise is begun.
- Store flat in original package in refrigerator protected from light. Or it can be kept at room temperature for no more than 4 weeks total.
- Remove from refrigerator, if stored there, and let autoinjector come to room temperature for 15 minutes.
- Mix drug by shaking the autoinjector hard until drug is mixed evenly and no white powder is seen. It will appear cloudy. Shake at least 15 seconds, but shake longer if it was not stored flat.
- Hold the autoinjector straight up with the orange cap toward the ceiling. Unlock the autoinjector by turning knob from the lock to unlock position until a click is heard.

- While holding the autoinjector straight up, firmly unscrew the orange cap. The cap may have to be turned a few times before it loosens. If a clicking sound is heard, it is being turned in the wrong direction. A green shield will pop up after the cap is removed.
- Inject at the selected site. A click will be heard when the injection begins. Keep holding the autoinjector against the skin for 15 seconds to ensure that the total dose has been given.

Route	Onset	Peak	Duration
SubQ	Immediate	2.1 hr	Unknown
SubQ/E.R.	Unknown	6–7 wk	10 wk

Half-life: 2.5 hr; E.R. unknown

Contraindications

History of drug-induced immune-mediated thrombocytopenia, hypersensitivity to exenatide or its components, personal or family history of medullary thyroid carcinoma or multiple endocrine neoplasia syndrome type 2 (Bydureon, Bydureon BCise)

Interactions

DRUGS

oral antidiabetics such as meglitinides or sulfonylureas, insulin: Increased risk of hypoglycemia
oral drugs: May decrease rate and extent of absorption of these drugs
warfarin: Possibly increased INR with increased risk of bleeding

Adverse Reactions

CNS: Asthenia, dizziness, fatigue, headache, jitteriness, somnolence
CV: Chest pain
EENT: Decreased taste
ENDO: Hypoglycemia
GI: Abdominal distention or pain, anorexia, cholecystitis, cholelithiasis, constipation, diarrhea, dyspepsia, flatulence, gastroesophageal reflux, indigestion, nausea, pancreatitis (including life-threatening hemorrhagic or necrotizing), vomiting
GU: Acute renal failure, decreased renal function, elevated serum creatinine level, kidney transplant dysfunction, worsening chronic renal failure
HEME: Drug-induced thrombocytopenia
RESP: Chronic hypersensitivity pneumonitis

SKIN: Alopecia, diaphoresis, macular or papular rash, pruritus, rash, urticaria
Other: Anaphylaxis, angioedema, dehydration, elevated antiexenatide antibody level, hematoma, injection-site reactions (abscess, cellulitis, hematoma, necrosis, pruritus, redness, subcutaneous nodules), weight loss

Childbearing Considerations

PREGNANCY

- It is not known if drug causes fetal harm. However, animal studies suggest drug may increase risk for fetal harm.
- Use with caution only if benefit to mother outweighs potential risk to fetus.

LACTATION

- It is not known if drug is present in breast milk.
- Patient should check with prescriber before breastfeeding.

Nursing Considerations

- Know that exenatide isn't recommended for patients with severe GI disease, patients with creatinine clearance less than 30 ml/min, or patients having dialysis because of adverse GI or renal effects.
- Use exenatide cautiously in a renal transplant patient or patient with moderate renal disease when dosage of Byetta is increased from 5 to 10 mcg or the extended-release formulations (Bydureon or Bydureon BCise) are used. Monitor renal function throughout therapy, especially in the elderly, and notify prescriber of abnormalities because drug can cause acute kidney injury, especially if patient becomes hypovolemic from drug-induced nausea and vomiting. Know that drug is not recommended for use in patients with an estimated glomerular filtration rate below 45 ml/min.
- Be aware that exenatide may induce acute gallbladder disease. If cholelithiasis is suspected, expect gallbladder studies to be ordered and appropriate follow-up to occur.
- Be aware that if patient also takes a sulfonylurea or insulin, patient may be at higher risk for hypoglycemia, which could become severe and may require the insulin or sulfonylurea dosage to be decreased to reduce the risk of hypoglycemia. Usually, no dosage adjustment is needed for a patient taking metformin.

- Monitor patient's blood glucose level. If control decreases despite the patient's best efforts, drug may have to be discontinued because of the possibility that anti-exenatide antibodies have formed. Be aware that if patient is already taking the rapid-release form of exenatide (Byetta) and is switching to the extended-release form of exenatide (Bydureon or Bydureon BCise), Byetta must be discontinued first. Also know that he may experience a transient elevation in his blood glucose levels for about 2 weeks as his body adjusts to the extended-release form.
- Monitor patient for evidence of acute pancreatitis, such as persistent, severe abdominal pain accompanied by vomiting, especially when drug is started or dosage increased. Notify prescriber, and expect to stop exenatide and give supportive care.
- Know that the immediate-release form of exenatide (Byetta) may be used concomitantly with insulin glargine (Lantus), which is a long-acting insulin to help improve the patient's blood glucose control. Byetta should not be used with any other type of insulin. If the patient is susceptible to hypoglycemia, expect the insulin glargine dosage to be decreased when used with Byetta.
- Be aware that Bydureon extended-release for injectable suspension can be used as an add-on to basal insulin in adults with type 2 diabetes who have inadequate glycemic control.

! **WARNING** Monitor patient for bleeding because drug can induce immune-mediated thrombocytopenia, which can be fatal. If suspected, notify prescriber immediately and expect drug to be discontinued. Also monitor patient for hypersensitivity reactions, which could become severe.

PATIENT TEACHING

- Instruct patient on how to prepare the type of exenatide product prescribed. Also teach patient how to give a subcutaneous injection.
- Inform patient that exenatide may be administered in the abdomen, thigh, or upper arm. Stress the need to rotate injection sites.
- Tell patient to inspect injection site daily and to report any adverse effects at site that are persistent or appear serious.

- Emphasize the need to use immediate-release form of drug (Byetta) within 60 minutes before morning and evening meals or the two main meals of the day, about 6 hours or more apart, never after a meal.
- Know that if patient misses a dose of Byetta, tell him to resume treatment with the next scheduled dose. If patient is prescribed Bydureon or Bydureon BCise and misses a dose, tell him to administer the drug as soon as he remembers as long as his regularly scheduled dose is at least 3 days later. If the time frame is less than this, tell patient to wait until his next regularly scheduled dose. Make patient aware that he may change the day of weekly administration of Bydureon as long as the last dose was administered 3 or more days before.
- Caution patient not to share his pen or needles with anyone else.
- Alert patient that pen doesn't come with needles and that he'll need to buy them.
- Warn patient that nausea may occur at the beginning of therapy but usually subsides over time.
- Inform patient taking a sulfonylurea or insulin glargine to be alert for hypoglycemic reactions because risk increases with both drugs. Review ways to treat such reactions, and tell patient to alert prescriber if they occur often or are severe.

! **WARNING** Stress importance of notifying prescriber if bleeding occurs and stop taking drug. If bleeding is serious, tell patient to seek immediate emergency care.

- Tell patient to seek emergency care for persistent, severe abdominal pain and vomiting.
- Caution patient that exenatide doesn't replace diet and exercise measures.

! **WARNING** Urge patient to stop taking drug and seek immediate emergency care if signs and symptoms of an allergic reaction occur, such as difficulty breathing or swallowing, hoarseness, or a lump in neck.

- Tell patient that kidney function may become impaired, especially if dehydration occurs, and to let prescriber know if patient becomes dehydrated.

E
F

ezetimibe
Zetia

Class and Category
Pharmacologic class: Cholesterol absorption inhibitor
Therapeutic class: Antilipemic

Indications and Dosages
* *To reduce elevated total-C, LDL-C, Apo B, and non-HDL-C in patients with primary hyperlipidemia, alone or in combination with an HMG-CoA reductase inhibitor (statin); to reduce elevated total-C, LDL-C, Apo B, and non-HDL-C in patients with mixed hyperlipidemia in combination with fenofibrate; to reduce elevated total-C and LDL-C in patients with homozygous familial hypercholesterolemia (HoFH), in combination with atorvastatin or simvastatin; to reduce elevated sitosterol and campesterol in patients with homozygous sitosterolemia*

TABLETS
Adults and children age 10 and older.
10 mg daily.

Drug Administration

P.O.
- Administer 2 hours before or 4 hours after giving bile acid sequestrant or cholestyramine.
- Can be administered at the same time as fenofibrate or an HMG-CoA reductase inhibitor.

Route	Onset	Peak	Duration
P.O.	<1 wk	4–12 hr	Unknown

Half-life: 22 hr

Contraindications
Active liver disease or unexplained persistent elevations in hepatic transaminase levels (with concurrent statin use), breastfeeding (with concurrent statin use), hypersensitivity to ezetimibe or its components, pregnancy (with concurrent statin use)

Interactions

DRUGS
cholestyramine: Reduced effects of ezetimibe
cyclosporine: Increased blood cyclosporine and ezetimibe levels

Mechanism of Action
Reduces blood cholesterol by inhibiting its absorption through the small intestine.

Normally, in the intestinal lumen, lipids break down to cholesterol and other substances that create smaller droplets called micelles, as shown below left. The micelles enter intestinal epithelial cells called enterocytes, where they combine with cholesterol, triglycerides, and other substances to form chylomicrons. Chylomicrons then pass through to the lymphatic system to be carried to the blood.

Ezetimibe blocks cholesterol absorption into enterocytes and keeps cholesterol from moving through the intestinal wall, as shown below right. Reduced cholesterol absorption from the intestine decreases chylomicron and LDL cholesterol content.

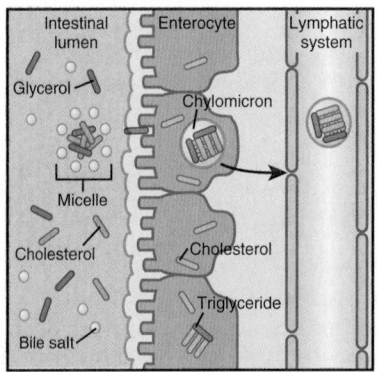

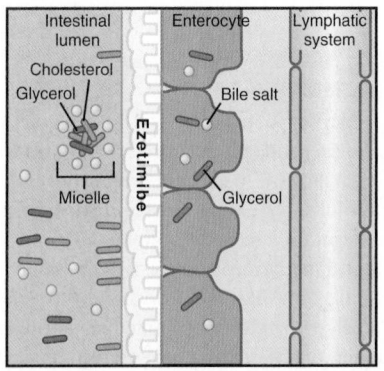

fibrates: Increased cholesterol excretion into the bile, leading possibly to cholelithiasis
warfarin: Possibly altered international normalized ratio (INR)

Adverse Reactions

CNS: Depression, dizziness, fatigue, headache, paresthesia
CV: Chest pain
EENT: Pharyngitis, sinusitis
GI: Abdominal pain, cholelithiasis, cholecystitis, diarrhea, elevated enzymes, **hepatitis**, nausea, **pancreatitis**
HEME: **Thrombocytopenia**
MS: Arthralgia, back or limb pain, elevated creatinine kinase level, myalgia, myopathy, **rhabdomyolysis**
RESP: Cough, upper respiratory tract infection
SKIN: **Erythema multiforme**, rash, urticaria
Other: **Anaphylaxis**, **angioedema**, flu-like symptoms, viral infection

Childbearing Considerations

PREGNANCY

- It is not known if drug causes fetal harm.
- Use with caution only if benefit to mother outweighs potential risk to fetus.
- Know that all statins are contraindicated in pregnancy. If a statin is combined with ezetimibe, the resulting combination is a contraindication for use during pregnancy.

LACTATION

- It is not known if drug is present in breast milk.
- Use with caution only if benefit to mother outweighs potential risk to her breastfed infant.
- Breastfeeding is contraindicated if a statin is given concurrently.

Nursing Considerations

- Monitor liver enzymes before and during ezetimibe therapy, as ordered.

PATIENT TEACHING

- Direct patient to follow a low-cholesterol diet as an adjunct to ezetimibe therapy. Recommend weight loss and exercise programs, as appropriate.
- Tell him to take ezetimibe either 2 hours before or at least 4 hours after taking a bile acid sequestrant, to prevent drug interactions.
- Advise patient to report unexplained muscle pain, tenderness, or weakness.

famciclovir

Class and Category

Pharmacologic class: Nucleoside analogue
Therapeutic class: Antiviral

Indications and Dosages

✳ *To treat recurrent episodes of herpes labialis*

TABLETS

Immunocompetent adults. 1,500 mg as a single dose at first sign of burning, itching, lesion formation, pain, or tingling.

✳ *To treat recurrent episodes of genital herpes*

TABLETS

Immunocompetent adult. 1,000 mg twice a day for 1 day beginning at the first sign of a recurrent episode (burning, itching, lesion formation, pain, or tingling).

✳ *To suppress chronic recurrent episodes of genital herpes*

TABLETS

Immunocompetent adults. 250 mg twice daily.

✳ *To treat herpes zoster*

TABLETS

Immunocompetent adults. 500 mg every 8 hr for 7 days.

✳ *To treat recurrent episodes of genital or orolabial herpes in HIV-infected patients*

TABLETS

Adults. 500 mg twice daily for 7 days beginning at the first sign of a recurrent episode (burning, itching, lesion formation, pain, tingling).

±**DOSAGE ADJUSTMENT** For patient with renal impairment, dosage decreased and/or dosage interval increased depending on what patient's creatinine clearance level is at the time of treatment and the herpes condition being treated.

Drug Administration

P.O.

- Administer drug without regard to meals.

Route	Onset	Peak	Duration
P.O.	Unknown	1 hr	Unknown

Half-life: 2.4 hr as penciclovir

Mechanism of Action

Selectively inhibits herpes viral DNA synthesis and replication.

E
F

Contraindications

Hypersensitivity to famciclovir or its components, use of penciclovir cream

Interactions

DRUGS

drugs eliminated by active renal tubular secretion such as probenecid: Possibly increased plasma concentration of famciclovir, with increased risk of adverse reactions

Adverse Reactions

CNS: Confusion, dizziness, fatigue, hallucinations, headache, migraine, paresthesia, **seizures**, somnolence
CV: Hypersensitivity vasculitis, palpitations
GI: Abdominal pain, cholestatic jaundice, diarrhea, elevated bilirubin levels, elevated liver or pancreatic enzymes, flatulence, nausea, vomiting
GU: Acute renal failure, dysmenorrhea, elevated serum creatinine
HEME: Anemia, **leukopenia, neutropenia, thrombocytopenia**
SKIN: Erythema multiforme, pruritus, rash, **Stevens–Johnson syndrome, toxic epidermal necrolysis**, urticaria
Other: Anaphylaxis, angioedema

Childbearing Considerations

PREGNANCY

- Pregnancy exposure registry: 1-888-669-6682.
- It is not known if drug causes fetal harm.
- Use with caution only if benefit to mother outweighs potential risk to fetus.

LACTATION

- It is not known if drug is present in breast milk.
- Patient should check with prescriber before breastfeeding.
- Women with HIV infection should not breastfeed.

Nursing Considerations

- Use cautiously in patients with renal impairment because of the risk of acute renal failure and hepatic impairment, because conversion of famciclovir to its active metabolite may be impaired, resulting in a lower plasma concentration and possibly decreased effectiveness of the drug.

! **WARNING** Be aware that dosage adjustment must be made in patients with renal impairment. Acute renal failure has occurred in patients with underlying renal disease who have received inappropriately high doses of famciclovir for their level of renal function.

- Monitor patient's liver and renal function closely, and laboratory test values as ordered.

! **WARNING** Monitor patient for hypersensitivity reactions that could become serious. If present, notify prescriber, expect drug to be discontinued, and provide supportive care, as needed and ordered.

PATIENT TEACHING

- Remind patient that famciclovir should be initiated as soon as possible after a recurrent onset of a herpes-related condition exhibited by sensations of burning, itching, pain, or tingling or when a lesion has appeared.

! **WARNING** Tell patient with renal impairment to remind prescriber of this condition when famciclovir is prescribed and when dosage adjustments are made.

! **WARNING** Advise patient to get immediate emergency medical treatment if she develops any signs of an allergic reaction, such as difficulty breathing, hives, or swelling of face, lips, tongue, or throat.

- Inform patient that famciclovir is not a cure for herpes. Because genital herpes is a sexually transmitted disease, instruct patient to avoid contact with lesions or intercourse when lesions and/or symptoms are present, to avoid infecting partners. Remind patient, however, that genital herpes is frequently transmitted in the absence of symptoms and therefore patient should always engage in safe sex practices.
- Instruct patient to notify prescriber at once if she experience serious adverse reactions such as confusion, feeling short of breath, increased thirst, pounding heartbeats, swelling, urinating less than usual or not at all, weakness, or weight gain.
- Alert patient that famciclovir does contain lactose and famciclovir usage should be discussed with patients who experience lactose intolerance or who have galactose intolerance or glucose–galactose malabsorption.

famotidine
Pepcid, Pepcid AC

⬛ Class and Category
Pharmacologic class: Histamine-2 blocker
Therapeutic class: Antiulcer agent

⬛ Indications and Dosages
✳ *To provide short-term treatment of active duodenal ulcer*

ORAL SUSPENSION
Adults. 40 mg once daily or 20 mg twice daily up to 8 wk.

CHEWABLE TABLETS, TABLETS
Adults and children weighing 40 kg (88 lb) or greater. 40 mg once daily or 20 mg twice daily up to 8 wk.

✳ *To prevent recurrence of duodenal ulcer*

CHEWABLE TABLETS, ORAL SUSPENSION, TABLETS
Adults. 20 mg once daily up to 1 yr.

✳ *To provide short-term treatment for active, benign gastric ulcer*

ORAL SUSPENSION
Adults. 40 mg once daily up to 8 wk.

CHEWABLE TABLETS, TABLETS
Adults and children weighing 40 kg (88 lb) or more. 40 mg once daily up to 8 wk.

✳ *To treat gastroesophageal reflux disease (GERD)*

ORAL SUSPENSION
Adults. 20 mg twice daily for up to 6 wk.
Children ages 1 to 17. 1 mg/kg daily in divided doses twice daily for 6 to 12 wk. *Maximum:* 40 mg twice daily.
Infants age 3 months to 1 year. *Initial:* 0.5 mg/kg twice daily for up to 8 wk, increased to 1 mg/kg twice daily, if needed. *Maximum:* 40 mg/day.
Infants age less than 3 months. 0.5 mg/kg once daily for up to 8 wk, increased to 1 mg/kg once daily, if needed.

✳ *To treat symptomatic nonerosive GERD*

CHEWABLE TABLETS, TABLETS
Adults and children weighing 40 kg (88 lb) or more. 20 mg twice daily for up to 6 wk.

✳ *To treat erosive esophagitis caused by gastroesophageal reflux*

ORAL SUSPENSION
Adults. 20 to 40 mg twice daily for up to 12 wk

✳ *To treat erosive esophagitis due to GERD diagnosed by endoscopy.*

ORAL SUSPENSION
Adults. 20 or 40 mg twice daily for up to 12 wk.

CHEWABLE TABLETS, TABLETS
Adults and children weighing 40 kg (88 lb) or more. 20 or 40 mg twice daily for up to 12 wk.

✳ *To treat pediatric peptic ulcer disease*

CHEWABLE TABLETS, ORAL SUSPENSION, TABLETS
Children age 1 to 17 years. *Initial:* 0.5 mg/kg once daily or 0.25 mg/kg twice daily for 8 wk, increased to 1 mg/kg once daily or 0.5 mg/kg twice daily, as needed. *Maximum:* 40 mg/day.

✳ *To treat gastric hypersecretory conditions, such as Zollinger–Ellison syndrome*

CHEWABLE TABLETS, ORAL SUSPENSION, TABLETS
Adults. *Initial:* 20 mg every 6 hr. Dosage adjusted, if needed, based on patient response. *Maximum:* 160 mg every 6 hr.

✳ *To treat hospitalized patients with intractable ulcers or pathological hypersecretory conditions; to treat patients who are unable to take oral medication*

I.V. INFUSION OR INJECTION
Adults. 20 mg every 12 hr.
Children ages 1 to 16. *Initial:* 0.25 mg/kg every 12 hr. *Maximum:* 40 mg daily.

✳ *To prevent heartburn and indigestion*

CHEWABLE TABLETS, TABLETS
Adults. 10 mg 1 hr before eating. *Maximum:* 20 mg every 24 hr for up to 2 wk.

✳ *To treat heartburn and indigestion*

CHEWABLE TABLETS, TABLETS
Adults. 10 mg at onset of symptoms. *Maximum:* 20 mg every 24 hr for up to 2 wk unless prescribed otherwise.

±**DOSAGE ADJUSTMENT** Oral or parenteral dosage reduced or dosing interval increased (to 48 hr), if needed, in patients with renal insufficiency and creatinine clearance less than 60 ml/min.

⬛ Drug Administration
P.O.
- Drug should be taken once daily at bedtime or twice daily in the morning and before bedtime.
- Reconstitute oral suspension by slowly adding 46 ml of Purified Water.

E
F

Shake vigorously for 5 to 10 seconds immediately after adding the water and immediately before use. Store at room temperature. Discard after 30 days.

- Chewable tablets should be chewed thoroughly before swallowing.
- Tablets should be swallowed whole and not chewed, crushed, or split.

I.V.

- Store drug in refrigerator until ready to administer.
- For I.V. injection, dilute with 2 ml of 0.9 Sodium Chloride for Injection, 5% or 10% Dextrose Injection, 5% Sodium Bicarbonate Injection, or Lactated Ringer's Injection to a total volume of either 5 or 10 ml. Inject over no less than 2 minutes.
- For I.V. infusion, dilute in 100 ml of 5% Dextrose Injection or other compatible intravenous solution mentioned earlier. Infuse over 15 to 30 minutes. Diluted solution may be stored for 7 days at room temperature.
- Drug also comes as a premixed solution ready for infusion administration. Check container for minute leaks prior to use by squeezing the bag firmly. Solution must be clear and seal intact to use. Do not administer with plastic containers in series connections.
- *Incompatibilities:* Amphotericin B, azithromycin, cefepime, furosemide (at 2 mg/ml), piperacillin-tazobactam

Route	Onset	Peak	Duration
P.O.	<1 hr	1–4 hr	10–12 hr
I.V.	<30 min	20 min	10–12 hr

Half-life: 2.5–3.5 hr

☰ Contraindications

Hypersensitivity to famotidine, other H_2-receptor antagonists, or their components

☰ Interactions

DRUGS

drugs dependent on gastric pH for absorption: Reduced absorption of these drugs
tizanidine: Possibly substantial increase in blood tizanidine levels with increased risk of adverse reactions

☰ Adverse Reactions

CNS: Agitation (infants), anxiety, asthenia, confusion, delirium, depression, dizziness, fatigue, fever, hallucinations, headache, insomnia, lethargy, mental or mood changes, paresthesia, **seizures**, somnolence

☰ Mechanism of Action

In normal digestion, parietal cells in the gastric epithelium secrete hydrogen (H^+) ions, which combine with chloride ions (Cl^-) to form hydrochloric acid (HCl), as shown below left. However, HCl can inflame, ulcerate, and perforate gastric and intestinal mucosa normally protected by mucus. Famotidine, an H_2-receptor antagonist, reduces HCl formation by preventing histamine from binding with H_2 receptors on the surface of parietal cells, as shown below right. By doing so, the drug helps prevent peptic ulcers from forming and helps heal existing ones.

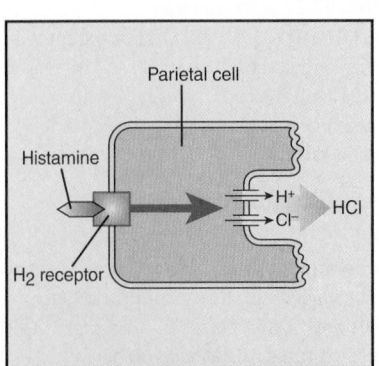

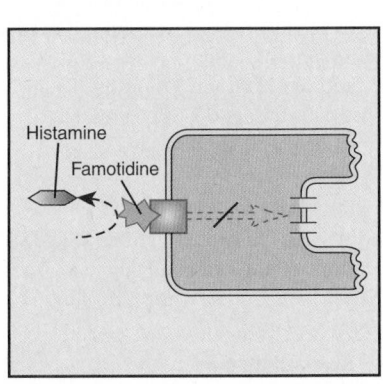

CV: **Arrhythmias, AV block**, palpitations, **prolonged QT interval**
EENT: Dry mouth, **laryngeal edema**, taste alteration, tinnitus
GI: Abdominal pain, anorexia, cholestatic jaundice, constipation, diarrhea, elevated liver enzymes, **hepatitis**, jaundice, nausea, vomiting
GU: Decreased libido, impotence
HEME: **Agranulocytosis, aplastic anemia, leukopenia, neutropenia, pancytopenia, thrombocytopenia**
MS: Arthralgia, muscle cramps, musculoskeletal pain, **rhabdomyolysis**
RESP: **Bronchospasm**, dyspnea, **interstitial pneumonia**, wheezing
SKIN: Acne, alopecia, dry skin, **erythema multiforme, exfoliative dermatitis**, flushing, pruritus, rash, **Stevens–Johnson syndrome, toxic epidermal necrolysis**, urticaria
Other: **Anaphylaxis, angioedema**, hyperuricemia

Childbearing Considerations

PREGNANCY
- It is not known if drug causes fetal harm.
- Use with caution only if benefit to mother outweighs potential risk to fetus.

LACTATION
- Drug is present in breast milk.
- Patient should check with prescriber before breastfeeding.

Nursing Considerations

! **WARNING** Be aware that Pepcid AC chewable tablets contain aspartame, which can be dangerous for patients who have phenylketonuria.

- Know that adult patients who have a suboptimal response or an early symptomatic relapse after completing famotidine therapy, should be evaluated for gastric malignancy.

PATIENT TEACHING
- Instruct patient to store famotidine oral suspension at room temperature (below 86° F [30° C]) and to protect it from freezing. Tell her to shake the bottle vigorously, right before use, for 5 to 10 seconds.
- Instruct patient to carefully chew chewable tablets thoroughly before swallowing. Tablets should be swallowed whole and not chewed, crushed, or split.

- Caution patient to avoid alcohol and smoking during famotidine therapy because they irritate the stomach and can delay ulcer healing.
- Advise patient to notify prescriber if she develops pain, has trouble swallowing, or if she has bloody vomit or black stools.
- Caution patient not to take famotidine with other acid-reducing products.
- Caution patient, especially the elderly and patients with renal impairment, to avoid hazardous activities until drug's CNS effects are known.

febuxostat
Uloric

Class and Category
Pharmacologic class: Xanthine oxidase inhibitor
Therapeutic class: Antigout

Indications and Dosages
✽ *To treat chronic hyperuricemia in patients with gout, in patients who have an inadequate response to a maximally titrated dose of allopurinol, who are intolerant to allopurinol, or for whom treatment with allopurinol is not advisable*

TABLETS
Adults. *Initial:* 40 mg once daily, increased after 2 wk to 80 mg once daily, if needed.
±**DOSAGE ADJUSTMENT** For patient with severe renal impairment, dosage limited to 40 mg once daily.

Drug Administration
P.O.
- Tablets can be taken without regard to food or antacid use.

Route	Onset	Peak	Duration
P.O.	Unknown	1–1.5 hr	Unknown

Half-life: 5–8 hr

Mechanism of Action
Inhibits the action of xanthine oxidase, the key enzyme responsible for purine breakdown. Xanthine oxidase catalyzes conversion of xanthine to uric acid, thereby increasing uric acid levels. High uric acid levels cause gout attacks. Inhibiting xanthine oxidase causes uric acid levels to drop, decreasing the risk of gout attack.

Contraindications

Concurrent use of azathioprine or mercaptopurine, hypersensitivity to febuxostat or its components

Interactions

DRUGS

azathioprine, mercaptopurine, theophylline: Possibly increased serum levels of these drugs, leading to toxicity

Adverse Reactions

CNS: Aggression, CVA, dizziness, hemiparesis, lacunar infarction, psychotic behavior, transient ischemic attack
CV: Angina, chest pain or discomfort, ECG abnormalities, MI
EENT: Blurred vision, deafness, epistaxis, nasal dryness, paranasal sinus hypersecretion, pharyngeal edema, sneezing, taste disturbance, throat irritation, tinnitus
ENDO: Breast pain, gynecomastia, hot flashes, hypoglycemia
GI: Diarrhea, dyspepsia, elevated liver enzymes, GI discomfort, hepatic failure, hepatomegaly, jaundice, nausea, vomiting
GU: Decreased libido, erectile dysfunction, hematuria, nephrolithiasis, pollakiuria, proteinuria, renal failure or insufficiency, tubulointerstitial nephritis, urgency
HEME: Agranulocytosis, anemia, eosinophilia, idiopathic thrombocytopenic purpura, leukocytosis, leukopenia, neutropenia, pancytopenia, splenomegaly, thrombocytopenia
MS: Arthralgia, joint stiffness or swelling, rhabdomyolysis
RESP: Upper respiratory tract infection
SKIN: Dermatitis, eczema, erythema multiforme, flushing, hair color or growth changes, hyperhidrosis, peeling skin, petechiae, photosensitivity, pruritis, rash, Stevens–Johnson syndrome, toxic epidermal necrolysis, urticaria
Other: Anaphylaxis, drug reaction with eosinophilia and systemic symptoms (DRESS), gout flares, hypersensitivity reactions

Childbearing Considerations

PREGNANCY

- It is not known if drug causes fetal harm.
- Use with caution only if benefit to mother outweighs potential risk to fetus.

LACTATION

- It is not known if drug is present in breast milk.
- Patient should check with prescriber before breastfeeding.

Nursing Considerations

- Know that febuxostat therapy isn't recommended for patients in whom rate of urate formation is greatly increased, as in malignancy and its treatment or Lesch–Nyhan syndrome.
- Obtain a liver test panel, as ordered, prior to initiating febuxostat therapy and then periodically thereafter. Monitor patient for signs and symptoms of liver dysfunction such as anorexia, dark urine, fatigue, jaundice, or right upper abdominal discomfort throughout therapy. If signs and symptoms occur or if abnormal liver tests occur, especially an elevated serum alanine aminotransferase level greater than 3 times the upper normal limit, notify prescriber and expect drug to be withheld until underlying cause is determined. If no other cause can be found other than febuxostat therapy, expect drug to be discontinued permanently.
- Monitor patient's serum uric acid level, as prescribed, to determine drug effectiveness. Expect it to take about 2 weeks for uric acid level to be therapeutically altered. Dose may be increased from 40 to 80 mg daily if target serum uric acid level fails to fall below 6 mg/dl.
- Monitor patient for gout flares, which may occur after therapy is started because of changing serum uric acid levels that result in mobilization of urate from tissue deposits. Expect prescriber to order colchicine or an NSAID when febuxostat therapy starts. If patient has a gout flare-up during treatment, notify prescriber, and expect symptoms to be managed. Know that febuxostat therapy usually isn't discontinued during this time.

! WARNING Monitor patient with established cardiovascular disease because use of febuxostat increases the risk of death from cardiovascular conditions. Also monitor patient for evidence of cardiovascular thrombosis, such as acute MI or stroke, because drug may increase patient's risk of developing these disorders, which may result in death.

- Assess patient's skin for abnormalities. At first sign of rash or other skin abnormality, notify prescriber and expect drug to be discontinued if serious skin reactions are suspected or occur, because febuxostat may cause severe skin reactions. Also know that patients who have experienced hypersensitivity reactions to allopurinol may be at increased risk of developing serious skin reactions to febuxostat.

PATIENT TEACHING

- Inform patient that a gout attack may occur when febuxostat therapy starts and that colchicine or an NSAID may be prescribed, usually along with febuxostat, to treat it.
- Instruct patient to seek immediate emergency care for signs or symptoms of a heart attack or stroke.
- Tell patient that periodic blood tests will be needed to determine drug's effectiveness and to detect adverse effects.
- Advise patient to notify prescriber at first sign of a rash or other skin abnormality.

felodipine
Plendil

Class and Category
Pharmacologic class: Calcium channel blocker
Therapeutic class: Antihypertensive

Indications and Dosages
* *To manage mild to moderate essential hypertension alone or with other antihypertensives*

E.R. TABLETS
Adults. *Initial:* 5 mg daily. Dosage adjusted every 2 wk. *Maintenance:* 2.5 to 10 mg daily based on patient response.
±**DOSAGE ADJUSTMENT** For patients who are over age 65, initial dosage reduced to 2.5 mg daily. For patients with impaired liver function, dosage may have to be reduced based on blood pressure.

Drug Administration
P.O.
- Administer on an empty stomach or with a light meal.
- Do not administer with grapefruit juice.
- Tablets should be swallowed whole and not chewed, crushed, or split.

- Store drug at room temperature and protect it from light.

Route	Onset	Peak	Duration
P.O.	2–5 hr	2.5–5 hr	24 hr

Half-life: 11–16 hr

Mechanism of Action
May slow the movement of extracellular calcium into myocardial and vascular smooth-muscle cells by deforming calcium channels in cell membranes, inhibiting ion-controlled gating mechanisms, and interfering with calcium release from the sarcoplasmic reticulum. The effect of these actions is a decrease in intracellular calcium ions, which inhibits contraction of smooth-muscle cells and dilates coronary and systemic arteries. As with other calcium channel blockers, felodipine's actions result in increased oxygen to the myocardium and reduced afterload, blood pressure, and peripheral resistance.

Contraindications
Hypersensitivity to felodipine, other dihydropyridine calcium channel blockers, or their components

Interactions
DRUGS
antihypertensives: Increased risk of hypotension
cimetidine, erythromycin itraconazole, ketoconazole: Increased felodipine level and effects
clarithromycin: Increased risk of acute kidney injury in elderly patients
CYP3A4 inducers (long-term) such as carbamazepine, phenobarbital, phenytoin: Decreased felodipine levels
CYP3A4 substrates such as benzodiazepines, flecainide, imipramine, propafenone, terfenadine, theophylline: Increased felodipine plasma concentrations
metoprolol: Possible altered pharmacokinetics of metoprolol
tacrolimus: Possibly increased blood tacrolimus level and risk of adverse effects

ACTIVITIES
alcohol use: Induced vasodilation enhancing the effects of felodipine and increasing risk of hypotension

E
F

FOODS
grapefruit juice: Significant increase in felodipine levels, increasing risk of hypotension
high carbohydrate or fat diet: Significantly increased felodipine bioavailability with increased risk of hypotension

⊟ Adverse Reactions
CNS: Asthenia, dizziness, drowsiness, fatigue, headache, paresthesia, syncope, weakness
CV: Chest pain, **hypotension**, palpitations, peripheral edema, tachycardia
EENT: Gingival hyperplasia, pharyngitis, rhinitis
GI: Abdominal cramps, constipation, diarrhea, indigestion, nausea
HEME: Agranulocytosis
MS: Back pain
RESP: Cough
SKIN: Flushing, rash

⊟ Childbearing Considerations
PREGNANCY
- It is not known if drug causes fetal harm. However, animal studies have shown the possibility of digital anomalies.
- While manufacturer makes no recommendations regarding use during pregnancy, some authorities recommend not to use the drug during pregnancy.

LACTATION
- It is not known if drug is present in breast milk.
- Drug should be discontinued or breastfeeding should be discontinued.

REPRODUCTION
- Women of childbearing age should use effective contraception throughout drug therapy.

⊟ Nursing Considerations
- Use felodipine cautiously in patients with heart failure or reduced ventricular function.
- Monitor blood pressure during dosage titration and throughout felodipine therapy, especially in elderly patients.

! **WARNING** Be aware that felodipine may cause severe hypotension with syncope, which may lead to reflex tachycardia. This can precipitate angina in patients with coronary artery disease or a history of angina.

- Watch for signs of overdose, such as excessive peripheral vasodilation, marked hypotension, and, possibly, bradycardia. If they appear, place patient in supine position with legs elevated and give I.V. fluids, as ordered. Expect to give I.V. atropine for bradycardia.

PATIENT TEACHING
- Instruct patient to swallow tablets whole and not to crush or chew them. Also tell patient to take drug on an empty stomach and with a light meal.
- Caution patient not to drink grapefruit juice during therapy.
- Advise patient to store felodipine at room temperature and to protect it from light.
- Instruct patient to monitor her pulse rate and blood pressure.
- Teach patient how to minimize gingival hyperplasia.
- Advise patient to notify prescriber immediately if she has palpitations, pronounced dizziness, or swelling of hands or feet.
- Instruct women of childbearing age to notify prescriber if pregnancy occurs or is suspected and not to breastfeed.

fenofibrate
Antara, Fenoglide, Lipofen, Tricor, Triglide

fenofibrate choline
Trilipix

fenofibric acid
Fibricor

⊟ Class and Category
Pharmacologic class: Fibrate
Therapeutic class: Antilipemic

⊟ Indications and Dosages
✳ *To treat primary hypercholesterolemia or mixed hyperlipidemia*
CAPSULES (LIPOFEN)
Adults. 150 mg daily.
CAPSULES (ANTARA)
Adults. 90 mg daily.

DELAYED-RELEASE CAPSULES (TRILIPIX)
Adults. 135 mg daily.
TABLETS (TRICOR)
Adults. 145 mg daily.
TABLETS (FIBRICOR)
Adults. 105 mg daily.
TABLETS (TRIGLIDE)
Adults. 160 mg daily.
TABLETS (FENOGLIDE)
Adults. 120 mg daily.
✱ *As adjunct to diet to treat severe
hypertriglyceridemia*
CAPSULES (ANTARA)
Adults. *Initial:* 30 to 90 mg daily, increased
as needed at 4- to 8-wk intervals. *Maximum:*
90 mg daily.
CAPSULES (LIPOFEN)
Adults. *Initial:* 50 to 150 mg daily, increased
as needed at 4- to 8-wk intervals. *Maximum:*
150 mg daily.
DELAYED-RELEASE CAPSULES (TRILIPIX)
Adults. *Initial:* 45 to 135 mg once daily,
increased as needed at 4- to 8-wk intervals.
Maximum: 135 mg daily.
TABLETS (FIBRICOR)
Adults. *Initial:* 35 to 105 mg daily, increased
as needed at 4- to 8-wk intervals. *Maximum:*
105 mg daily.
TABLETS (TRICOR)
Adults. *Initial:* 48 to 145 mg daily, increased
as needed at 4- to 8-wk intervals. *Maximum:*
160 mg daily.
TABLETS (TRIGLIDE)
Adults. 160 mg daily, *Maximum:* 160 mg
daily.
TABLETS (FENOGLIDE)
Adults. 40 to 120 mg daily, increased as
needed at 4- to 8-wk intervals. Maximum:
120 mg daily.
±**DOSAGE ADJUSTMENT** For patients with
mild to moderate renal impairment or elderly
patients, dosage limited for all indications
to lowest dosage prescribed for treatment of
severe hypertriglyceridemia with increase
only after drug's therapeutic and renal effects
are known.

Drug Administration
P.O.
- Administer drug consistently with or
  without food except for Fenoglide and

Lipofen, which have to be given with food
to enhance absorption.
- Administer drug 1 hour before or 4 hours
  after bile acid sequestrants.
- Capsules and tablets must be swallowed
  whole and not chewed, crushed, or
  split/opened. Do not administer broken or
  chipped tablets.
- Protect from moisture. Fibricor, Lipofen, and
  Triglide should also be protected from light.

Route	Onset	Peak	Duration
P.O.	2 wk	6–8 wk	Unknown

Half-life: 20 hr

Mechanism of Action
May increase the lipolysis of triglyceride-rich
lipoproteins and decrease the synthesis of
fatty acids and triglycerides by enhancing
the activation of lipoprotein lipase and
acyl-coenzyme A synthetase. Fenofibrate
also may:
- increase hepatic elimination of cholesterol
  as bile salts
- promote the catabolism of larger, less
  dense LDLs with a high-binding affinity for
  cellular LDL receptors.

Contraindications
Active liver disease; breastfeeding; Active
liver disease; breastfeeding; gallbladder
disease; hypersensitivity to fenofibrate,
fenofibric acid, or their components; severe
renal impairment

Interactions
DRUGS
bile acid sequestrants: Decreased fenofibrate
absorption
colchicine: Increased risk of myopathy and
rhabdomyolysis
coumarin anticoagulants: Increased risk of
bleeding
*immunosuppressants such as cyclosporine and
tacrolimus:* Increased risk of nephrotoxicity
FOODS
all foods: Increased fenofibrate bioavailability
when given in capsule form

Adverse Reactions
CNS: Asthenia, fatigue, headache
CV: **Deep vein thrombosis**, severely
depressed HDL cholesterol levels
EENT: Rhinitis

GI: Abdominal pain, cholelithiasis, **cirrhosis,** constipation, diarrhea, elevated bilirubin or liver enzymes, **hepatitis, hepatotoxicity,** nausea, **pancreatitis**

GU: Acute renal failure, increased serum creatinine level

HEME: Agranulocytosis, anemia, **leukopenia, thrombocytopenia**

MS: Arthralgia, back pain, elevated creatinine phosphokinase, muscle spasms, myalgia, myopathy, myositis, **rhabdomyolysis**

RESP: Interstitial lung disease, pulmonary embolus

SKIN: Photosensitivity, rash, **Stevens–Johnson syndrome, toxic epidermal necrolysis,** urticaria

Other: Anaphylaxis, angioedema, delayed hypersensitivity reactions, drug reaction with eosinophilia and systemic symptoms (DRESS), flu-like symptoms

Childbearing Considerations

PREGNANCY

- It is not known if drug causes fetal harm.
- Use with caution only if benefit to mother outweighs potential risk to fetus.

LACTATION

- It is not known if drug is present in breast milk.
- Drug is contraindicated in breastfeeding women. Women should not breastfeed during drug therapy; some manufacturers recommend to also avoid breastfeeding for 5 days after final dose.

Nursing Considerations

- Be aware that all drugs that increase serum triglycerides, such as beta-blockers, estrogens, and thiazides, should be stopped, and baseline lipid levels obtained before starting fenofibrate.
- Monitor results of liver function tests. If liver enzyme levels rise to more than 3 times the upper limit of normal and persist, or if the patient develops gallstones, expect to stop drug.
- Monitor patient's renal function, as elevations in serum creatinine levels have occurred with fenofibrate therapy.
- Monitor serum cholesterol and triglyceride levels at 4- to 8-week intervals, as ordered. If levels don't decrease after 2 months at maximum dosage, expect therapy to be discontinued.

! **WARNING** Monitor patient closely for acute hypersensitivity reactions, including severe rash, and notify prescriber if they occur. Patient may need inpatient corticosteroids. Also monitor patient for delayed cutaneous hypersensitivity reactions that may be severe and can occur days to weeks after fenofibrate therapy is initiated.

- Assess blood counts periodically, as ordered, during first 12 months of therapy to detect adverse hematologic effects.
- Watch closely for evidence of deep vein thrombosis (pain, redness in extremity, or swelling) or pulmonary embolus (sudden onset of anxiety, restlessness, or shortness of breath) because risk is higher in patients taking fenofibrate. Notify prescriber immediately, and start emergency treatment, as prescribed.

PATIENT TEACHING

- Emphasize that drug will be effective only if patient carefully follows prescriber's instructions about diet and exercise.
- Instruct patient to take Fenoglide and Lipofen with food and other brands consistently with or without food.
- Instruct patient to swallow capsules and tablets whole and not to break, chew, or crush them. Also tell patient prescribed tablet form to store the tablets in their original, desiccant-containing bottle and to avoid taking any chipped or broken tablets.
- Inform patient that it is important to protect drug from moisture and Fibricor, Lipofen, and Triglide should also be protected from light.
- Advise patient to have laboratory tests, as directed, to determine drug's effectiveness. They typically include liver function tests after 3 to 6 months, hematocrit and hemoglobin levels, and WBC counts periodically during first year.
- Urge patient to notify prescriber immediately about chills, fever, or sore throat, as well as skin changes such as appearance of blisters or a rash. Also urge her to tell prescriber about unexplained muscle pain, tenderness, or weakness, especially if accompanied by fatigue or fever and signs and symptoms of liver injury such as abdominal pain, abnormal stool, dark urine, itching, malaise, or yellowing of skin or white portion of eyes.

- Tell patient to seek emergency treatment if he develops pain, swelling, and redness in his limb or sudden shortness of breath, anxiety, and restlessness.
- Instruct patient to use sunscreen and protective clothing while in sun and to limit time spent in sun because photosensitivity may occur weeks to months after drug is initiated.

fentanyl citrate
Abstral, Actiq, Fentora, Lazanda, Onsolis, Sublimaze, SUBSYS

fentanyl transdermal system
Duragesic

≡ Class, Category, and Schedule
Pharmacologic class: Opioid
Therapeutic class: Opioid analgesic
Controlled substance schedule: II

≡ Indications and Dosages
❋ *To provide surgical premedication*
I.M. INJECTION (SUBLIMAZE)
Adults. 0.05 to 0.1 mg 30 to 60 min before surgery.
❋ *As adjunct to regional anesthesia*
I.V. OR I.M. INJECTION (SUBLIMAZE)
Adults. 0.05 to 0.1 mg.
❋ *To induce and maintain anesthesia*
I.V. OR I.M. INJECTION (SUBLIMAZE)
Children age 2 to 12. 2 to 3 mcg/kg.
❋ *To manage postoperative emergence delirium, pain, or tachypnea in postanesthesia care unit*
I.M. INJECTION (SUBLIMAZE)
Adults. 0.05 to 0.1 mg. Repeated in 1 to 2 hr, if needed.
❋ *As adjunct to general anesthesia*
I.V. INJECTION (SUBLIMAZE)
Adults. *For low-dose therapy:* 0.002 mg/kg followed by 0.002 mg/kg, as needed. *For moderate-dose therapy:* 0.002 to 0.02 mg/kg, followed by 0.025 to 0.1 mg, as needed. *For high-dose therapy:* 0.02 to 0.05 mg/kg followed by 0.025 mg to one-half initial loading dose, as needed.

❋ *To treat breakthrough pain in cancer patients who are receiving around-the-clock opioid therapy and have developed tolerance to it*

TRANSMUCOSAL LOZENGE (ACTIQ)
Adults and adolescents 16 years and older. *Initial:* 200 mcg and allowed to dissolve, followed by second dose 15 min after first dose is dissolved, as needed. Dosage increased according to patient's needs. *Maximum:* 2 doses of same strength per episode with at least 4 hr between episodes treated; once successful dosage has occurred, no more than 4 lozenges/day.

SUBLINGUAL TABLETS (ABSTRAL)
Adults. *Initial:* 100 mcg followed by second dose 30 min after first dose, if needed. Dosage increased in 100-mcg increments, as needed, until 400-mcg dosage reached, then increased in increments of 200 mcg, as needed, until maximum dosage of 800 mcg per dose is reached. No more than two doses of same strength may be used to treat an episode of breakthrough pain and 2 hr has elapsed between each episode. *Maximum:* 800 mcg given twice 30 min apart per episode of breakthrough pain; dosage interval between episodes of breakthrough pain must be at least 2 hr; only four episodes of breakthrough pain treated per day.

BUCCAL FILM (ONSOLIS)
Adults. *Initial:* One 200-mcg film. Increased in increments of 200 mcg with each subsequent episode. Only 1 film of the appropriate dose used for each episode and doses separated by at least 2 hr, as needed. If patient's pain is still not controlled at a dose of 800 mcg and patient is tolerating the 800-mcg dose, one 1,200-mcg film may be used with next episode. *Maximum:* 1,200-mcg film/episode given at least 2 hr apart.

BUCCAL TABLETS (FENTORA)
Adults. *Initial:* 100 mcg, followed by second dose 30 min after first dose, as needed. Dosage increased to 200 mcg, as needed. Further increased to 400 mcg, as needed. Further titration done in multiples of 200 mcg, if needed, until maximum dose of 800 mcg per dose is reached. *Maximum:* 800 mcg given twice 30 min apart 4 times daily with at least 4 hr between each episode treated.

E
F

NASAL SPRAY (LAZANDA)

Adults. *Initial:* 100 mcg. Increased, as needed, to 200 mcg, then 300 mcg, then 400 mcg, then 600 mcg, and finally to 800 mcg with doses spaced at least 2 hr apart. *Maximum:* 800 mcg 4 times daily with a dosing interval of at least 2 hr between each episode.

SUBLINGUAL SPRAY (SUBSYS)

Adults. *Initial:* 100 mcg (200 or 400 mcg or more if patient is converting from Actiq) followed by 100 mcg 30 minutes later, if needed. Increased, as needed, to 200 mcg (titration increased using multiples of strength used initially if converting from Actiq), then 400 mcg, then 600 mcg, then 800 mcg, then 1,200 mcg, then 1,600 mcg with doses spaced at least 4 hr apart. A second dose of same strength may be taken 30 minutes after the first dose, as needed and counted as 1 breakthrough episode. *Maximum:* 1,600 mcg given twice 30 minutes apart 4 times daily with doses spaced at least 4 hr apart.

✳ *To relieve severe chronic pain in opioid-tolerant patient who doesn't respond to less potent drugs and requires around-the-clock opioid administration for an extended time*

TRANSDERMAL SYSTEM (DURAGESIC)

Adults and children age 2 and over. *Initial:* Highly individualized and based on current opioid therapy. Each patch may be worn for 48 to 72 hr. Dosage increased after first 72 hr and then every 6 days, as needed. For more than 100 mcg/hr, more than one patch required.

±**DOSAGE ADJUSTMENT** For cachectic, debilitated, or elderly patients, initial dosage should not exceed 25 mcg/hr, unless patient is already receiving more of an equivalent dose of another opioid. For patients receiving long-term opioid therapy, dosage adjusted based on previous day's drug requirement. For patients with mild to moderate hepatic or renal failure, initial dosage decreased by 50%.

▤ Drug Administration

- Do not substitute buccal, intranasal, sublingual, or transmucosal forms for any other fentanyl product, and do not substitute for each other. Do not convert dosage to or from other products on a microgram-per-microgram basis because doing so may result in a fatal overdose.

P.O.

- For Actiq transmucosal form, open package just before use and save plastic cap for discarding the unused part of the lozenge. Have patient place lozenge between the cheek and gum and suck, not chew, on it for 15 minutes. Show her how to move lozenge from one side of her mouth to the other using the handle provided separately.

- For Onsolis buccal film, have patient wet the inside of cheek or rinse mouth with water to wet the area for placement of the film. Place the entire film near the tip of a gloved, dry finger with the printed side facing up and hold in place. Then, place the printed side of film against the inside of patient's cheek. Press and hold for 5 seconds. Patient may drink liquids after 5 minutes. Film should not be chewed and swallowed nor should it be cut or torn prior to use. Film will dissolve within 30 minutes. Warn patient not to manipulate the film with tongue or finger. Eating food should be avoided until the film is dissolved. If using 200-mcg film strength, do not administer more than 4 films at one time and do not place multiple films on top of each other.

- For Fentora buccal tablets, have patient place tablet between the upper cheek and gum or under the tongue and allow to dissolve, which may take from 14 to 25 minutes. Tablet should not be chewed, crushed, sucked on, or swallowed. Do not have patient eat or drink anything until tablet is completely dissolved. However, if after 30 minutes, some remnants of the tablet(s) remain, the patient may swallow some water. If two tablets are needed, place one tablet on each side of mouth in buccal cavity. If four tablets are needed, place two tablets on each side of mouth in buccal cavity.

- For Abstral sublingual tablets, place tablet on the floor of the mouth directly under the tongue immediately after removing tablet from the blister unit. Tablet should not be chewed, sucked, or swallowed but allowed to dissolve completely in the mouth. Do not have patient eat or drink anything until the tablet is completely dissolved.

- For Subsys sublingual spray, open the blister package with scissors immediately prior to drug use. Never use a blister package that has been opened. Have patient swallow any saliva in mouth. Hold the spray unit upright and point the nozzle into patient's mouth under the tongue. Spray contents of the unit into mouth carefully. Have patient hold the medicine under tongue for 30 to 60 seconds. Tell patient not to spit or rinse mouth immediately after administration.

I.V.

- Administered only by persons specifically trained in the use of intravenous anesthetics.
- Have emergency resuscitative equipment and naloxone close at hand.
- As an I.V. injection, administer slowly over 1 to 2 minutes directly into a vein or into the tubing of a freely flowing I.V. solution. If injected too rapidly, apnea may occur.
- *Incompatibilities:* None listed by manufacturer

I.M.

- Administered only by persons specifically trained in the use of anesthetics.
- Inject into a large muscle.

TRANSDERMAL

- Choose a site with intact (not irritated or irradiated) skin on a flat surface, such as the chest, back, flank, or upper arm.
- If needed, clip, not shave, hair from the site and clean site with water (no soaps, lotions, oils, or alcohol). Dry area completely before applying patch.
- Do not apply transdermal patch if seal has been broken or the patch has been cut, damaged, or changed in any way, because drug may be released too rapidly.
- Apply by pressing patch firmly in place with palm of hand for 30 seconds, making sure edges are sealed. If applying more than one patch, the edges shouldn't touch or overlap.
- Wash hands immediately after application with soap and water.
- If patch loosens, tape edges down but do not cover the entire patch.
- When removing patch after 72 hours, fold it in half with adhesive sides together, and discard.
- Do not reuse a site for at least 3 days.

INTRANASAL

- For nasal spray (Lazanda), prime the device before use by spraying into the pouch

4 sprays in total. If device has not been used for 5 days, reprime by spraying once. To use, have patient insert the nozzle of the Lazanda bottle a short distance (about 1/2 inch) into the nose and point toward the bridge of the nose, tilting the bottle slightly. Have patient press down firmly on the finger grips until a "click" is heard and the number in the counting window advances by 1. The fine mist spray is not always felt on the nasal mucosal membrane, but advancement of the dose counter confirms that a spray has been administered.

Route	Onset	Peak	Duration
P.O.	1–3 min	Unknown	15–45 min
I.V.	1–2 min	3–5 min	30–60 min
I.M.	7–15 min	20–30 min	1–2 hr
Intranasal	10 min	15–21 min	30–60 min
Transdermal	12–24 hr	24–72 hr	1–4 days
Transmucosal	3–5 min	20–30 min	2–3 hr

Half-life: 7–18 hr

☰ Mechanism of Action

Binds to opioid receptor sites in the CNS, altering perception of and emotional response to pain by inhibiting ascending pain pathways. Fentanyl may alter neurotransmitter release from afferent nerves responsive to painful stimuli, and it causes respiratory depression by acting directly on respiratory centers in the brain stem.

☰ Contraindications

All forms: Hypersensitivity to fentanyl, alfentanil, sufentanil, or their components; intermittent pain; opioid nontolerance; significant respiratory depression; treatment of mild to moderate pain responsive to nonopioid drugs; upper airway obstruction
Transdermal form: Hypersensitivity to adhesives; management of postoperative pain or pain that may be acute, intermittent, or mild, or pain in patients requiring opioid therapy for a short period of time; patients who are not opioid-tolerant
Transmucosal form: Acute or chronic pain, including postoperative pain

☰ Interactions

anticholinergics: Increased risk of severe constipation and urinary retention

antimigraine agents; cyclobenzaprine; dextromethorphan; dolasetron; granisetron; linezolid; MAO inhibitors; metaxalone; methylene blue (I.V.); ondansetron; palonosetron; selected psychiatric drugs such as amoxapine, buspirone, lithium, mirtazapine, nefazodone, trazodone, vilazodone; selective serotonin reuptake inhibitors; serotonin norepinephrine reuptake inhibitors; St. John's wort; tramadol; tricyclic antidepressants; triptans; tryptophan: Increased risk of serotonin syndrome

benzodiazepines, CNS depressants, muscle relaxants, other opioids, sedating antihistamines, tricyclic antidepressants: Increased risk of sedation and somnolence and severe respiratory depression

buprenorphine, butorphanol, nalbuphine, pentazocine: Decreased analgesic effect of fentanyl and possibly precipitation of withdrawal symptoms

CYP3A4 inducers such as barbiturates, carbamazepine, efavirenz, glucocorticoids, modafinil, nevirapine, oxcarbazepine, phenytoin, pioglitazone, rifabutin, rifampin, St. John's wort, troglitazone: Possibly induced metabolism and increased clearance of fentanyl with decreased effectiveness and potential development of withdrawal syndrome in dependent patients

CYP3A4 inhibitors such as amiodarone, amprenavir, aprepitant, cimetidine, clarithromycin, diltiazem, erythromycin, fluconazole, fosamprenavir, indinavir, itraconazole, ketoconazole, nefazodone, nelfinavir, ritonavir, saquinavir, telithromycin, troleandomycin, verapamil: Possibly increased opioid effect, leading to increased or prolonged adverse effects, including severe respiratory depression

diuretics: Possibly decreased efficacy of diuretics

MAO inhibitors: Possibly unpredictable or fatal effects if taken within 14 days

FOODS
grapefruit juice: Increased blood fentanyl level

ACTIVITIES
alcohol use: Increased serum fentanyl level, possibly resulting in fatal overdose from CNS and respiratory depression and hypotension

Adverse Reactions
CNS: Agitation, amnesia, anxiety, asthenia, ataxia, confusion, delusions, depression, dizziness, drowsiness, euphoria, fever, hallucinations, headache, lack of coordination, light-headedness, nervousness, paranoia, sedation, seizures, sleep disturbance, slurred speech, syncope, tremor, weakness, yawning

CV: Asystole, bradycardia, chest pain, edema, hypotension, orthostatic hypotension, tachycardia

EENT: Blurred vision, dental caries, dry mouth, gum-line erosion, laryngospasm, rhinitis, sneezing, tooth loss

ENDO: Adrenal insufficiency (rare)

GI: Anorexia, constipation, elevated serum amylase levels, ileus, indigestion, nausea, spasm of the sphincter of Oddi, vomiting

GU: Anorgasmia, decreased libido, ejaculatory difficulty, impotence, infertility, lack of menstruation, urinary hesitancy, urine retention

RESP: Apnea, depressed cough reflex, dyspnea, hypoventilation, respiratory depression

SKIN: Diaphoresis, exfoliative dermatitis, localized skin redness and swelling (with transdermal form), pruritus, rash

Other: Anaphylaxis, drug tolerance, physical or psychological dependence with long-term use, weight loss

Childbearing Considerations
PREGNANCY
- It is not known if drug causes fetal harm. However, prolonged use during pregnancy may cause neonatal opioid withdrawal syndrome.
- Use with caution only if benefit to mother outweighs potential risk to fetus.

LABOR & DELIVERY
- Drug may prolong labor.
- Drug crosses the placental barrier and may produce excessive sedation and respiratory depression in the neonate.
- Drug should not be used during labor and delivery.

LACTATION
- Drug is present in breast milk.
- Breastfeeding is not recommended during drug therapy.

Nursing Considerations
- Be aware that fentanyl is now only available through a restricted program called Risk Evaluation and Mitigation Strategy (REMS)

because of the risk of accidental exposure, abuse, addiction, misuse, and overdose. In addition, under the Transmucosal Immediate-Release Fentanyl (TIRF) REMS program, healthcare professionals, outpatient departments, and pharmacies must enroll in the program to prescribe the drug to outpatients. Inpatient pharmacies must have policies and procedures in place to verify opioid tolerance for inpatients who require a transmucosal immediate-release type of fentanyl while hospitalized.

! **WARNING** Know that fentanyl transdermal system should be used only in patients already receiving opioid therapy and with demonstrated opioid tolerance (taking for a week or longer at least 60 mg of morphine daily, 30 mg of oral oxycodone daily, 8 mg of oral hydromorphone daily, or an equianalgesic dose of another opioid), and require at least a fentanyl dosage of 25 mcg/hour to manage their pain.

- Be aware that opioids like fentanyl should not be given to women during pregnancy and labor and while breastfeeding as the newborn or infant may experience neonatal opioid withdrawal syndrome (NOWS) which may be life-threatening and is exhibited as poor feeding, rapid breathing, trembling, and excessive or high-pitched crying.
- Use with extreme caution in patients with significant chronic obstructive pulmonary disease or cor pulmonale, and in patients having a substantially decreased respiratory reserve, hypoxia, hypercapnia, or preexisting respiratory depression, because even therapeutic doses of fentanyl may decrease respiratory drive in these patients to the point of apnea.
- Use with extreme caution in patients who may be susceptible to the intracranial effects of carbon dioxide retention such as those with brain tumors, head injury, increased intracranial pressure, or impaired consciousness. Monitor these patients closely for signs of sedation and respiratory depression.
- Use caution when titrating fentanyl dosage in elderly, cachectic, and debilitated patients, especially when using I.V. route, because these patients are more sensitive to the drug's effects.

- Use cautiously in patients at risk for opioid abuse, such as those with mental illness or personal or family history of substance abuse. Monitor patient throughout therapy for fentanyl abuse or addiction. Be aware that excessive use of fentanyl may lead to abuse, addiction, misuse, overdose, and possibly death. Monitor patient's intake of drug closely.
- Expect the blood fentanyl level to be prolonged if patient chews or swallows the transmucosal form because drug is absorbed slowly from GI tract.
- Be aware that 100 mcg of fentanyl is equivalent in potency to 10 mg of morphine.
- Know that to achieve optimum pain control with the lowest possible fentanyl dose, also plan to give a nonopioid analgesic, such as acetaminophen, as prescribed.
- Be aware that fentanyl should only be used concomitantly with benzodiazepines or other CNS depressants in patients for whom other treatment options are inadequate. If prescribed together, expect dosing and duration of opioid to be limited. Monitor patient closely for signs and symptoms of a decrease in consciousness, including coma, profound sedation, and significant respiratory depression. Notify prescriber immediately and provide emergency supportive care, as death may occur.

! **WARNING** Monitor patient's respiratory status closely, especially during the first 24 to 72 hours after therapy starts or with dosage increases, because severe hypoventilation may occur without warning at any time during therapy. Patients at increased risk include the elderly, cachectic, or debilitated patients. Respiratory depression can occur in patients even if the drug is not misused or abused. Be aware that significant amounts of fentanyl can be absorbed from the skin for 24 hours or more after a transdermal patch is removed. Monitor patient for at least 72 hours after patch has been removed for respiratory depression. Have emergency equipment available including an opioid antagonist.

- Monitor cancer patients receiving sublingual spray form of fentanyl closely for oral mucositis because exposure to the drug

E
F

in this form has been found to be greater than in patients without mucositis. If Grade 1 mucositis is present, the risk of respiratory or CNS depression increases, especially when therapy is initiated. Expect to avoid use of sublingual spray in cancer patients with Grade 2 mucositis or higher.

- Monitor patient closely who is receiving concurrent CYP3A4 inhibitor therapy along with fentanyl because these drugs may result in an increase in plasma fentanyl concentrations, which could increase or prolong adverse drug effects and may cause sedation and potentially fatal respiratory depression. Notify prescriber immediately, if present. Be aware that discontinuation of CYP3A4 inducers can result in a fatal overdose of fentanyl. Monitor these patients closely as well.

! **WARNING** Know that many drugs may interact with opioids like fentanyl to cause serotonin syndrome. Monitor patient closely for signs and symptoms such as agitation, diaphoresis, diarrhea, fever, hallucinations, labile blood pressure, muscle twitching or stiffness, nausea, shakiness, shivering, tachycardia, trouble with coordination, or vomiting. Notify prescriber at once because serotonin syndrome may be life-threatening. Be prepared to discontinue drug, if possible and ordered, and provide supportive care.

- Monitor patient for adrenal insufficiency. Although rare, it can be life-threatening. Monitor patient for anorexia, dizziness, fatigue, hypotension, nausea, vomiting, or weakness. Notify prescriber if adrenal insufficiency is suspected and expect diagnostic testing to be done. If diagnosis is confirmed, expect to administer corticosteroids and wean patient off fentanyl, if possible.
- Know that to prevent withdrawal symptoms after long-term use, expect to taper drug dosage gradually, as prescribed. Assess patient for withdrawal symptoms after dosage reduction or conversion to another opioid analgesic.
- Monitor patient who is receiving the drug via a transdermal system and who develops a fever for opioid adverse effects because a fever may increase fentanyl release from the system and increase skin permeability.

If symptoms occur, notify prescriber and anticipate dosage may be decreased.
- Be aware that for a patient with bradycardia, implement cardiac monitoring, as ordered, and assess heart rate and rhythm frequently during fentanyl therapy because drug may further slow heart rate.

! **WARNING** Expect respiratory depressant effects to last longer than analgesic effects. Also be prepared for residual drug to potentiate effects of subsequent doses. Residual drug can be detected for at least 6 hours after I.V. dose and 17 hours after other forms. Monitor patient closely for at least 24 hours after therapy ends.

! **WARNING** Assess patient for evidence of overdose, such as cardiopulmonary arrest, hypoventilation, pupil constriction, respiratory and CNS depression, seizures, and shock. Give naloxone (possibly in repeated doses), as prescribed. Be prepared to assist with endotracheal intubation and mechanical ventilation and to provide fluids.

- Monitor blood glucose level of diabetic patient receiving transdermal fentanyl because each unit contains about 2 g of sugar.

PATIENT TEACHING

- Warn patient not to take more drug than prescribed and not to take it longer than absolutely needed because excessive or prolonged use can lead to abuse, addiction, misuse, overdose, and possibly death.
- Instruct patient or caregiver on the proper use of fentanyl product prescribed and safe guidelines to follow with administration.
- Advise patient not to stop taking drug unless directed by prescriber because withdrawal symptoms may occur. Warn against increasing dose or frequency without consulting prescriber because drug can cause dependency.
- Tell patient not to stop drug abruptly, as dosage must be tapered to prevent return of pain or withdrawal symptoms.
- Instruct patient to dispose of expired, unwanted, or unused drug by flushing down the toilet if a drug take-back option is not readily available.
- Instruct patient to avoid alcohol and other CNS depressants including benzodiazepines during fentanyl therapy unless prescribed.

- Remind patient to keep used and unused dosage units out of reach of children and to dispose of drug properly. For buccal tablets, patient should flush leftover drug down the toilet when no longer needed. For sublingual spray, remind patient to dispose of any used or unneeded units immediately in the disposal bottle provided with every dispensed carton. For transdermal patch, patient should fold in half and flush down toilet.
- Caution patient that accidentally exposing others to transdermal fentanyl could cause serious adverse reactions that may become life-threatening, especially in children, even with one dose. If accidental exposure occurs, the person should remove the patch, wash the area well with water, and seek medical attention.
- Inform patient that long-term use of opioids like fentanyl may decrease sex hormone levels, causing decreased libido, erectile dysfunction, impotence, infertility, or lack of menstruation. Encourage patient to report any such symptoms to prescriber.
- Caution patient to avoid hazardous activities until drug's CNS effects are known.
- Inform patient about potentially fatal additive effects of combining fentanyl with a benzodiazepine. Tell patient to inform all prescribers of fentanyl use.
- Tell patient to increase fiber and fluid intake, unless contraindicated, because drug may cause severe constipation. If it persists or becomes severe, urge patient to notify prescriber.

ferric carboxymaltose
Injectafer

Class and Category
Pharmacologic class: Hematinic
Therapeutic class: Antianemic

Indications and Dosages
∗ *To treat iron-deficiency anemia in patients who are intolerant to oral iron or have had unsatisfactory response to oral iron; to treat iron-deficiency anemia in patients who have nondialysis-dependent chronic kidney disease*

I.V. INFUSION, I.V. INJECTION
Adults weighing 50 kg (110 lb) or more. 750 mg followed by a second dose of 750 mg given no sooner than 7 days later. Alternatively, 15 mg/kg up to 1,000 mg given as a single-dose treatment course.
Children age 1 year and older weighing 50 kg (110 lb) or more. 750 mg followed by a second dose of 750 mg given no sooner than 7 days later.
Adults and children age 1 year and older weighing less than 50 kg (110 lb). 15 mg/kg followed by a second dose of 15 mg/kg given no sooner than 7 days later.

∗ *To treat iron-deficiency anemia in patients who have nondialysis-dependent chronic kidney disease*

I.V. INFUSION, I.V. INJECTION
Adults weighing 50 kg (110 lb) or more. 750 mg followed by a second dose of 750 mg given no sooner than 7 days later. Alternatively, 15 mg/kg up to 1,000 mg given as a single-dose treatment course.
Adults weighing less than 50 kg (110 lb). 15 mg/kg followed by a second dose of 15 mg/kg given no sooner than 7 days later.

Drug Administration
I.V.
- For I.V. injection, administer undiluted by slow intravenous push given at a rate of 100 mg (2 ml) per minute.
- For I.V. infusion, dilute up to 1,000 mg of iron in no more than 250 ml of 0.9% Sodium Chloride Injection, so that the concentration of the infusion is not less than 2 mg of iron per ml. Infuse over at least 15 minutes.
- Infusion solution at concentrations ranging from 2 mg to 4 mg of iron per ml can be stored at room temperature for 72 hours.
- *Incompatibilities:* None listed by manufacturer

Route	Onset	Peak	Duration
I.V.	Unknown	15 min–1.21 hr	Unknown

Half-life: 7–12 hr

Mechanism of Action
Releases iron as a colloidal iron (III) hydroxide in complex with carboxymaltose, a carbohydrate polymer to increase hemoglobin formation.

Contraindications

Hypersensitivity to ferric carboxymaltose or its components

Interactions

DRUGS

None reported by manufacturer

Adverse Reactions

CNS: Chills, dizziness, fever, headache, paresthesia, syncope
CV: Chest pain, hypertension, **hypotension,** tachycardia
EENT: Nasopharyngitis, sneezing, taste distortion
GI: Abdominal pain, constipation, diarrhea, elevated liver enzymes, nausea, vomiting
HEME: Decreased platelet and white blood cell counts
MS: Arthralgia, back pain
RESP: Dyspnea
SKIN: Erythema, flushing, hot flash, pruritus, rash, urticaria
OTHER: Anaphylaxis including shock, angioedema, hypersensitivity reactions, hypophosphatemia, injection-site discoloration or irritation

Childbearing Considerations

PREGNANCY

- It is not known if drug can cause fetal harm but maternal hypersensitivity reactions to the drug may cause fetal bradycardia, especially in the second and third trimesters.
- Use with caution only if benefit to mother outweighs potential risk to fetus.

LACTATION

- Drug is present in breast milk.
- Patient should check with prescriber before breastfeeding.
- If breastfeeding occurs, infant should be monitored for constipation or diarrhea.

Nursing Considerations

! **WARNING** Monitor patient for hypersensitivity reactions that may become life-threatening, such as anaphylaxis, collapse, shock, and significant hypotension, during and for at least 30 minutes after completion of infusion or until clinically stable. If present, stop infusion or injection if still being administered, notify prescriber, and provide supportive care, as prescribed and needed.

- Monitor serum phosphate levels, as ordered in patients at risk for low serum phosphate who require a repeat course of treatment. Possible risk factors for hypophosphatemia include concurrent or prior use of medications that affect proximal renal tubular function or a history of gastrointestinal disorders associated with malabsorption of fat-soluble vitamins or phosphate, hyperparathyroidism, or vitamin D deficiency and malnutrition.
- Monitor patient for transient hypertension following each administration of ferric carboxymaltose. Assess patient's blood pressure and monitor patient for accompanying signs and symptoms of dizziness, facial flushing, or nausea that usually occur immediately after dosing and resolve within 30 minutes.
- Be aware that in the 24 hours after administration of drug, laboratory assays may overestimate serum iron and transferring bound iron.

PATIENT TEACHING

- Urge patient to inform prescriber if patient had experienced a prior history of allergies to parenteral iron products.

! **WARNING** Stress importance of reporting any signs and symptoms of an allergic reaction such as breathing problems, dizziness, itching, light-headedness, rash, or swelling.

- Alert patient that a long-lasting brown discoloration may occur at the site of injection. Tell patient to alert staff immediately if pain or swelling occurs at the injection site.

ferric citrate
Auryxia

Class and Category

Pharmacologic class: Ferric iron-based phosphate binder
Therapeutic class: Phosphate binder

Indications and Dosages

✳ *To control serum phosphorus levels in patients with chronic kidney disease on dialysis*

TABLETS

Adults. *Initial*: 2 tablets (420 mg ferric iron, equivalent to 2 g ferric citrate) 3 times a day, increased or decreased by 1 to 2 tablets per day at 1-wk or longer intervals, as needed. *Maximum*: 12 tablets (12 g ferric citrate) daily.

✱ *To treat iron-deficiency anemia in patients with chronic kidney disease not on dialysis*

TABLETS

Adults. 1 tablet (210 ferric iron, equivalent to 1 g ferric citrate) 3 times a day, titrated to achieve and maintain hemoglobin at target levels. *Maximum*: 12 tablets (12 g ferric citrate) daily.

☰ Drug Administration

P.O.

- Administer with meals.
- Tablets should be swallowed whole, and not chewed, crushed, or split.
- Protect from moisture during storage.

Route	Onset	Peak	Duration
P.O.	Unknown	Unknown	Unknown

Half-life: Unknown

☰ Mechanism of Action

Binds dietary phosphate in the gastrointestinal (GI) tract and precipitates as ferric phosphate, which is then excreted in the stool. By binding phosphate in the GI tract and decreasing absorption, serum phosphate levels are reduced. Also, replaces iron stores in body.

☰ Contraindications

Hypersensitivity to ferric citrate or its components, iron overload syndromes

☰ Interactions

DRUGS

ciprofloxacin, doxycycline: Decreased effectiveness of these drugs

☰ Adverse Reactions

GI: Abdominal pain, constipation, diarrhea, discolored stools, nausea, vomiting
HEME: Increased serum ferritin and transferrin saturation levels
RESP: Cough
Other: Hyperkalemia

☰ Childbearing Considerations

PREGNANCY

- It is not known if drug causes fetal harm. However, an overdose of iron in pregnant women may carry a risk for fetal malformation or spontaneous abortion.
- Use with caution only if benefit to mother outweighs potential risk to fetus.

LACTATION

- Drug is present in breast milk.
- Patient should check with prescriber before breastfeeding.

☰ Nursing Considerations

- Be aware that ferric citrate produces dark stools because of its iron content, but this effect does not affect laboratory tests for occult bleeding.
- Know that iron absorption from ferric citrate therapy may cause an excessive elevation in iron stores. Assess patients' serum ferritin and transferrin saturation levels before initiating ferric citrate therapy, as ordered, and monitor throughout therapy.
- Expect that patients receiving iron intravenously may need a reduction in dose or discontinuation of I.V. iron therapy.

☰ Patient Teaching

- Instruct patient to take ferric citrate exactly as ordered with meals and to swallow tablets whole because chewed or crushed tablets may discolor mouth and teeth.

! **WARNING** Remind patient that accidental overdose of iron-containing products is a leading cause of death in children under age 6. Stress the importance of keeping ferric citrate tablets out of the reach of children. If accidental overdose occurs, the poison control center should be called and immediate emergency treatment sought for the child.

---

ferric derisomaltose
Monoferric

☰ Class and Category

Pharmacologic class: Hematinic
Therapeutic class: Antianemic

☰ Indications and Dosages

✱ *To treat iron-deficiency anemia in patients who are intolerant to oral iron or have had unsatisfactory response to oral iron; to treat iron-deficiency anemia in patients who have nonhemodialysis-dependent chronic kidney disease*

I.V. INFUSION

Adults weighing 50 kg (110 lb) or more. 1,000 mg infused as a single dose. Dose repeated if iron-deficiency anemia reoccurs. **Adults weighing less than 50 kg (110 lb).** 20 mg/kg infused as a single dose. Dose repeated if iron-deficiency anemia reoccurs.

Drug Administration

I.V.

- To dilute, withdraw the appropriate volume of drug and inject into 100 ml to 500 ml of 0.9% Sodium Chloride Injection. Final diluted concentration should be more than 1 mg iron/ml.
- Infuse over at least 20 minutes.
- Following dilution, drug solution may be stored at room temperature for up to 8 hours.
- *Incompatibilities:* Other drugs

Route	Onset	Peak	Duration
I.V.	Unknown	7 days	Unknown

Half-life: 1–4 days

Mechanism of Action

Releases iron, which then binds to transferrin for transport to erythroid precursor cells to be incorporated into hemoglobin.

Contraindications

Hypersensitivity to ferric derisomaltose or its components

Interactions

DRUGS

None reported by manufacturer

Adverse Reactions

CNS: Anxiety, chills, dizziness, fatigue, fever, headache, loss of consciousness, paresthesia, **seizures**, syncope
CV: Chest pain, hypertension, **hypotension**, tachycardia
EENT: Taste distortion
GI: Abnormal pain, constipation, diarrhea, elevated liver enzymes, nausea, vomiting
HEME: Iron overload
MS: Arthralgia, back pain, muscle spasms, myalgia
RESP: Cough, dyspnea

SKIN: Diaphoresis, discoloration of skin, erythema, flushing, pruritus, rash, urticaria
OTHER: **Anaphylactic reaction including shock**, extravasation (long-lasting brown discoloration, irritation), Fishbane reaction (chest tightness, facial flushing, truncal myalgia and/or joint pains), flu-like symptoms, **hypersensitivity reactions (may be severe)**, **hypophosphatemia**, injection-site reactions such as phlebitis

Childbearing Considerations

PREGNANCY

- It is not known if drug can cause fetal harm. However, maternal hypersensitivity reaction may cause fetal bradycardia, especially in the second and third trimesters.
- Use with caution only if benefit to mother outweighs potential risk to fetus.

LACTATION

- Drug is present in breast milk.
- Patient should check with prescriber before breastfeeding.
- If breastfeeding occurs, infant should be monitored for constipation or diarrhea.

Nursing Considerations

- Know that the dosage of ferric derisomaltose is expressed in mg of elemental iron. Each ml of drug contains 100 mg of elemental iron.
- Expect to monitor the hematologic response to ferric derisomaltose, such as hemoglobin and hematocrit and iron parameters (serum ferritin, transferring saturation). Excessive therapy with parenteral iron can lead to excess iron storage and possibly iatrogenic hemosiderosis or hemochromatosis.

! WARNING Monitor patient for hypersensitivity reactions that may become life-threatening, such as anaphylaxis, collapse, shock, and significant hypotension, during and for at least 30 minutes after infusion or until clinically stable. If present, stop infusion if still being administered, notify prescriber, and provide supportive care, as prescribed and needed.

! WARNING Know that ferric derisomaltose should not be given to patients with iron overload.

PATIENT TEACHING

- Urge patient to inform prescriber if patient had experienced a prior history of allergies to parenteral iron products.

! **WARNING** Stress importance of reporting any signs and symptoms of an allergic reaction, such as breathing problems, dizziness, itching, light-headedness, rash, or swelling.

- Alert patient that a long-lasting brown discoloration may occur at the site of injection. Tell patient to alert staff immediately if pain or swelling occurs at the injection site.

ferric maltol
Accrufer

▤ Class and Category
Pharmacologic class: Iron agent
Therapeutic class: Hematinic

▤ Indications and Dosages
✳ *To treat iron deficiency*

CAPSULES
Adults. 30 mg twice daily until iron stores are replenished.

▤ Drug Administration
P.O.
- Administer on an empty stomach at least 1 hour before or 2 hours after meals.
- Capsules should be swallowed whole and not chewed, crushed, or opened.

Route	Onset	Peak	Duration
P.O.	Unknown	1.5–3 hr	Unknown

Half-life: 0.7 hr

▤ Mechanism of Action
Delivers iron for uptake across the intestinal wall and transfer to transferrin and ferritin.

▤ Contraindications
Hemochromatosis and other iron overload syndromes, hypersensitivity to ferric maltol or its components, repeated blood transfusions

▤ Interactions
DRUGS
dimercaprol: Possibly increased risk of nephrotoxicity

oral drugs: Possibly decreased absorption of these drugs

▤ Adverse Reactions
GI: Abdominal discomfort, distension, pain; constipation; diarrhea; discolored feces; flatulence; increased risk of inflammation in gastrointestinal tract; nausea, vomiting
HEME: Iron overload

▤ Childbearing Considerations
PREGNANCY
- Drug is not absorbed systemically and maternal use is not expected to result in fetal exposure.
- Overdose of iron in pregnant women may carry a risk for fetal malformation, gestational diabetes, or spontaneous abortion.

LACTATION
- It is not known if drug is present in breast milk, but presence is not expected because drug is not absorbed systemically.
- Patient should check with prescriber before breastfeeding.

▤ Nursing Considerations
- Know that ferric maltol should be avoided in patients with an active inflammatory bowel disease flare, because drug has the potential to increase inflammation in the gastrointestinal tract.
- Be aware that ferric maltol should not be given to patients with evidence of iron overload or patients receiving intravenous iron to avoid excess storage of iron.
- Expect to monitor iron parameters, as ordered, during therapy.

▤ Patient Teaching
- Instruct patient to take drug on an empty stomach 1 hour before or 2 hours after meals and not break, chew, or open the capsules.
- Inform patient that treatment duration will depend on the severity of iron deficiency but that generally at least 12 weeks of therapy are required. However, treatment will continue as long as necessary until ferritin levels are within normal range.
- Urge patient to keep ferric maltol out of reach of children, as accidental overdose of iron-containing products is a leading cause of fatal poisoning in children under age 6.

ferrous salts
ferrous fumarate
Ferretts, Ferrocite, Fumerin, Hemocyte, Iron Fumarate, Neo-Fer (CAN), Novofumar (CAN), Palafer (CAN)

ferrous gluconate
Ferate, Fergon, Ferralet, Ferralet Slow Release, Fertinic (CAN), Novo-Ferrogluc (CAN), Simron

ferrous sulfate

iron, carbonyl
Feosol Natural Release, Ferra-Cap, Icar

☰ Class and Category
Pharmacologic class: Hematinic
Therapeutic class: Antianemic, nutritional supplement

☰ Indications and Dosages
✳ *To prevent iron deficiency based on recommended daily allowances*

CAPLETS, CAPSULES, CHEWABLE TABLETS, DRIED CAPSULES, DRIED E.R. CAPSULES, DRIED E.R. TABLETS, DRIED TABLETS, ELIXIR, ENTERIC-COATED TABLETS, E.R. CAPSULES, E.R. TABLETS, ORAL SOLUTION, ORAL SUSPENSION, SYRUP, TABLETS

Adults age 51 and over. 8 mg daily.
Adult females age 19 to 50. 18 mg daily.
Adult men age 19 to 50. 8 mg daily.
Pregnant women. 27 mg daily.
Breastfeeding women. 9 to 10 mg daily.
Boys age 14 to 18. 11 mg daily.
Girls age 14 to 18. 15 mg daily.
Children age 9 to 13. 8 mg daily.
Children age 4 to 8. 10 mg daily.
Children age 1 to 3. 7 mg daily.
Infants age 7 to 12 months. 11 mg daily.
Newborns to age 6 months. 0.27 mg daily.
✳ *To replace iron in deficiency states*

CAPLETS, CAPSULES, CHEWABLE TABLETS, DRIED CAPSULES, DRIED E.R. CAPSULES, DRIED E.R. TABLETS, DRIED TABLETS, ELIXIR, ENTERIC-COATED TABLETS, E.R. CAPSULES, E.R. TABLETS, ORAL SOLUTION, ORAL SUSPENSION, SYRUP, TABLETS

Adults and adolescents. 300 to 325 mg daily. Alternatively, 100 to 200 mg of elemental iron daily and divided into three equal doses and given every other day. *Maintenance:* 325 mg daily or 60 mg up to 3 times daily or every other day for several wk or mo.
Infants and children. *For mild to moderate iron-deficiency anemia:* 3 mg elemental iron/ kg/day in 1 to 2 divided doses. *For severe iron-deficiency anemia:* 4 to 6 mg elemental iron/kg/day in 3 divided doses.
Premature neonates. 2 to 4 mg elemental iron/kg/day divided every 12 to 24 hr. *Maximum:* 15 mg daily.
✳ *To provide iron supplementation during pregnancy*

CAPLETS, CAPSULES, CHEWABLE TABLETS, DRIED CAPSULES, DRIED E.R. CAPSULES, DRIED E.R. TABLETS, DRIED TABLETS, ELIXIR, ENTERIC-COATED TABLETS, E.R. CAPSULES, E.R. TABLETS, ORAL SOLUTION, ORAL SUSPENSION, SYRUP, TABLETS

Pregnant women. 30 mg elemental iron daily.
± **DOSAGE ADJUSTMENT** Dosage increased if needed for elderly patients, who may not absorb iron as easily as younger adults do.

☰ Drug Administration
P.O.
- Administer iron salts 1 hour before or 2 hours after meals. If GI irritation occurs, give with or just after meals.
- Don't give antacids, coffee, dairy products, eggs, tea, or whole-grain breads or cereals within 1 hour before or 2 hours after iron.
- Tablets and capsules should be given with a full glass of juice or water. Don't crush enteric-coated tablets or open capsules.
- Chewable tablets should be chewed thoroughly before swallowing.
- Dilute and administer drops with a straw or place drops in back of patient's throat, because iron solutions may stain teeth.

- Mix elixir form in water.
- Use a measuring device to measure dosage of liquid forms.
- Protect liquid form from freezing.

Route	Onset	Peak	Duration
P.O.	4–7 days	5–8 days	Unknown

Half-life: Variable

Mechanism of Action

Acts to normalize RBC production by binding with hemoglobin or by being oxidized and stored as hemosiderin or aggregated ferritin in reticuloendothelial cells of the bone marrow, liver, and spleen. Iron is an essential component of hemoglobin, myoglobin, and several enzymes, including catalase, cytochromes, and peroxidase. Iron is needed for catecholamine metabolism and normal neutrophil function.

Contraindications

Hemochromatosis, hemolytic anemias, hemosiderosis, hypersensitivity to iron salts or their components, other anemic conditions unless accompanied by iron deficiency

Interactions

DRUGS

antacids: Possibly decreased absorption of iron salts
bisphosphonates, dolutegravir, integrase inhibitors: Decreased absorption of these drugs
dimercaprol: Increased risk of nephrotoxic effect of iron salts
levodopa: Possibly chelation with iron, decreasing levodopa absorption and blood level
levothyroxine: Decreased levothyroxine effectiveness and, possibly, hypothyroidism
methyldopa: Decreased methyldopa absorption and efficacy
quinolones, tetracyclines: Decreased effectiveness of these antibiotics

FOODS

coffee; eggs; foods that contain bicarbonates, carbonates, oxalates, or phosphates; milk and milk products; tea that contains tannic acid; whole-grain breads and cereals and other high-fiber foods: Decreased iron absorption and effectiveness

ACTIVITIES

alcohol abuse (acute or chronic): Increased serum iron level

Adverse Reactions

CNS: Chills, dizziness, fever, headache, paresthesia, syncope
CV: Chest pain, hypertension, **hypotension**, tachycardia
EENT: Metallic taste, tooth discoloration
GI: Abdominal cramps, constipation, epigastric pain, nausea, stool discoloration, vomiting
HEME: Hemochromatosis, **hemolysis**, hemosiderosis
MS: Arthralgia, back pain, hypophosphatemic osteomalacia (rare)
RESP: Dyspnea, wheezing
SKIN: Diaphoresis, erythema, flushing, pruritus, rash, urticaria
Other: Angioedema

Childbearing Considerations

PREGNANCY

- It is not known if drug causes fetal harm.
- Use with caution only if benefit to mother outweighs potential risk to fetus.

LACTATION

- Drug is present in breast milk.
- Patient should check with prescriber before breastfeeding.

Nursing Considerations

- Be aware that at usual dosages, serum hemoglobin level usually normalizes in about 2 months unless blood loss continues. Treatment may last for 3 to 6 months to help replenish iron stores.

! **WARNING** Monitor patient for signs of iron overdose, which may include abdominal pain, diarrhea (possibly bloody), nausea, severe vomiting, and sharp abdominal cramps. In case of iron toxicity or accidental iron overdose (a leading cause of fatal poisoning in children under age 6), give deferoxamine, as prescribed. As few as 3 adult iron tablets can cause serious poisoning in young children.

- Remember that unabsorbed iron turns stool black or green and can mask blood in stool. Check stool for occult blood, as ordered.

PATIENT TEACHING

- Instruct patient to take iron on an empty stomach unless adverse GI reactions occur, which may require taking iron with a small amount of food. Tell patient not to chew any solid form of iron except for chewable tablets and to take iron with a full glass of water or juice.
- Instruct patient to use a calibrated device to measure liquid forms.
- Tell patient to minimize tooth stains from liquid iron, by mixing dose with, fruit juice, tomato juice, or water and to drink it with a straw. If patient must take liquid iron by dropper, direct her to place drops well back on the tongue and to follow with water or juice. Tell her that iron stains can be removed by brushing with baking soda (sodium bicarbonate).
- Urge patient to eat chicken, fish, lean red meat, and turkey, as well as foods rich in vitamin C (such as citrus fruits and fresh vegetables) to improve iron absorption.
- Urge patient to avoid foods that impair iron absorption, including dairy products, eggs, spinach, and high-fiber foods, such as whole-grain breads and cereals and bran. Also advise her to avoid drinking coffee or tea within 1 hour of iron intake.
- Caution patient not to take antacids or calcium supplements within 1 hour before and 2 hours after taking iron supplement.
- Inform patient that stool should become dark green or black during therapy. Advise her to notify prescriber if it doesn't.
- Advise patient to consult prescriber before taking large amounts of iron for longer than 6 months.
- Warn patient about high risk of accidental poisoning, and urge her to keep iron preparations out of the reach of children.

fesoterodine fumarate

Toviaz

≣ Class and Category

Pharmacologic class: Muscarinic receptor antagonist
Therapeutic class: Antispasmodic

≣ Indications and Dosages

⁎ *To treat overactive bladder with symptoms of urinary frequency, incontinence, and urgency*

E.R. TABLETS

Adults. *Initial:* 4 mg daily, increased to 8 mg, as needed. *Maximum:* 8 mg daily.

⁎ *To treat neurogenic detrusor overactivity in pediatric patients*
E.R. Tablets
Children age 6 and older weighing more than 35 kg (77 lb). *Initial:* 4 mg once daily then increased to 8 mg once daily after 1 wk.
Children age 6 and older weighing more than 25 kg (55 lb) but up to 35 kg (77 lb). *Initial:* 4 mg once daily then increased to 8 mg once daily, if needed.

±**DOSAGE ADJUSTMENT** For adult patients with severe renal insufficiency (creatinine clearance less than 30 ml/min) or who are taking potent CYP3A4 inhibitors (such as clarithromycin, itraconazole, and ketoconazole), dosage shouldn't exceed 4 mg once daily. For pediatric patients weighing more than 35 kg (77 lb) who have a creatinine clearance between 15 and 29 ml/min or are taking potent CYP3A4 inhibitors, dosage shouldn't exceed 4 mg once daily; for a creatinine clearance less than 15 ml/min or if dialysis is required, use is not recommended. For pediatric patients who weigh more than 25 kg (55 lb) to 35 kg (77 lb) with severe renal insufficiency (creatinine clearance less than 30 ml/min), require dialysis, or who are taking strong CYP3A4 inhibitors, use is not recommended.

≣ Drug Administration

P.O.

- E.R. tablets should be swallowed whole and not chewed, crushed, or split.
- Administer drug with a full glass of water.

Route	Onset	Peak	Duration
P.O.	<1 hr	5 hr	24 hr

Half-life: 7–8 hr

≣ Mechanism of Action

Exerts antimuscarinic (atropine-like) and potent direct antispasmodic (papaverine-like) actions on smooth muscle in the bladder. The result is increased bladder capacity and a decreased urge to void. Fesoterodine has an active metabolite that inhibits bladder contraction and decreases detrusor pressure.

Contraindications

Gastric retention; hypersensitivity to fesoterodine, tolterodine tartrate extended-release capsules or immediate-release tablets, or their components; uncontrolled narrow-angle glaucoma; urine retention

Interactions

DRUGS

other antimuscarinic agents: Possibly increased anticholinergic effects; possibly altered absorption of oral drugs taken concurrently
potent CYP3A4 inhibitors, such as clarithromycin, itraconazole, ketoconazole: Possibly increased serum fesoterodine level and increased risk of adverse effects

FOODS

caffeine: May aggravate bladder symptoms

ACTIVITIES

alcohol use: Increased drowsiness

Adverse Reactions

CNS: Dizziness, drowsiness, headache, insomnia, somnolence
CV: Angina, chest pain, palpitations, peripheral edema, **QT interval prolongation**
EENT: Accommodation disorder, blurred vision; dry eyes, mouth, or throat; myopia
GI: Constipation, decreased gastrointestinal motility, diarrhea, diverticulitis, dyspepsia, elevated liver enzymes, gastroenteritis, irritable bowel syndrome, nausea, upper abdominal pain
GU: Dysuria, urine retention, UTI
MS: Back pain
RESP: Cough, upper respiratory tract infection
SKIN: Decreased sweating, pruritus, rash, urticaria
Other: **Hypersensitivity reactions including angioedema with airway obstruction,** weight gain

Childbearing Considerations

PREGNANCY

- It is not known if drug causes fetal harm.
- Use with caution only if benefit to mother outweighs potential risk to fetus.

LACTATION

- It is not known if drug is present in breast milk.
- Patient should check with prescriber before breastfeeding.

Nursing Considerations

- Be aware drug is not recommended in patients with significant bladder outlet obstruction because fesoterodine can cause urine retention. It is also not recommended for patients with decreased gastrointestinal motility.
- Use cautiously in patients with controlled narrow-angle glaucoma or myasthenia gravis, because drug can make these conditions worse.
- Use cautiously in patients taking other drugs with anticholinergic effects, such as antihistamines.

! **WARNING** Monitor patient closely for angioedema, which may occur after the first dose. If present, discontinue fesoterodine therapy immediately, as ordered, and provide emergency supportive care, including maintaining a patent airway, as needed.

- Monitor patient for CNS anticholinergic effects, especially after beginning fesoterodine therapy or increasing the dose. If present, notify prescriber, as dosage may have to be reduced or drug discontinued. Know that patients who are 75 years and older have a higher rate of antimuscarinic adverse reactions.

PATIENT TEACHING

- Instruct patient to take drug exactly as prescribed.
- Tell patient to take drug with a full glass of water and not to cut, crush, or chew tablets.
- Explain that drug can cause adverse effects such as constipation and urine retention. If they occur and are severe or prolonged, patient should notify prescriber.

! **WARNING** Tell patient to seek immediate emergency medical attention if he experiences difficulty breathing or any swelling of his face, lips, throat, or tongue.

E
F

- Advise patient to avoid alcohol consumption during fesoterodine therapy.
- Tell patient to avoid hazardous activities until drug's CNS effects are known.
- Caution patient to avoid strenuous exercise and excessive sun exposure because of increased risk of heatstroke.
- Advise patient to limit caffeine consumption during drug therapy.
- Explain that full benefits of fesoterodine therapy may take 2 to 3 months.
- Inform patient that chewing sugarless gum or sucking hard candy (especially lemon drops) may help ease dry mouth.

fidaxomicin
Dificid

Class and Category
Pharmacologic class: Macrolide
Therapeutic class: Antibiotic

Indications and Dosages
⚹ *To treat* Clostridium difficile–*associated diarrhea (CDAD)*

TABLET
Adults and children weighing at least 12.5 kg (27.5 lb) and able to swallow tablets. 200 mg twice daily for 10 days.

ORAL SUSPENSION
Children age 6 months and older weighing 9 kg (19.8 lb) to less than 12.5 kg (27.5 lb). 160 mg (4 ml) twice daily for 10 days.
Children age 6 months and older weighing 7 kg (15.4 lb) to less than 9 kg (19.8 lb). 120 mg (3 ml) twice daily for 10 days.
Children age 6 months and older weighing 4 kg (8.8 lb) to less than 7 kg (15.4 lb). 80 mg (2 ml) twice daily for 10 days.

Drug Administration
P.O.
- Tablets should be swallowed whole and not chewed, crushed, or split.
- To reconstitute oral suspension, shake bottle to loosen powder. Measure 130 ml of Purified Water, add to the glass bottle, and cap tightly. Hold bottle in a horizontal position and shake vigorously for at least 2 minutes. Verify that a homogeneous

suspension is obtained. If not, repeat shaking. Once homogeneous suspension is visually confirmed, shake an additional 30 seconds. Let bottle stand for 1 minute. Verify that suspension is still homogeneous. If not, shake for at least 2 minutes, then 30 seconds and let bottle stand again for 1 minute. Once reconstituted, oral suspension appears white to yellowish white in color.
- Remove oral suspension from refrigerator 15 minutes before administration. Shake vigorously until suspension has an even consistency. Use an oral dosing syringe to measure dose.
- Store in refrigerator and discard after 12 days.

Route	Onset	Peak	Duration
P.O.	<1 hr	1–5 hr	Unknown

Half-life: 12 hr

Mechanism of Action
Inhibits RNA synthesis in *Clostridium difficile* bacterial cells by RNA polymerases, causing the cells to die.

Contraindications
Hypersensitivity to fidaxomicin or its components

Interactions
DRUGS
cyclosporine: Possible increased blood fidaxomicin level

Adverse Reactions
CNS: Fever
ENDO: Hyperglycemia
GI: Abdominal distention or pain, constipation, diarrhea, dyspepsia, dysphagia, elevated liver enzymes, flatulence, **GI hemorrhage, intestinal obstruction, megacolon,** nausea, vomiting
HEME: Anemia, **neutropenia, thrombocytopenia**
RESP: Dyspnea
SKIN: Drug eruption, pruritus, rash, urticaria
Other: **Acute hypersensitivity reactions, angioedema, decreased blood bicarbonate,** elevated blood alkaline phosphatase, **metabolic acidosis**

Childbearing Considerations

PREGNANCY

- It is not known if drug causes fetal harm.
- Use with caution only if benefit to mother outweighs potential risk to fetus.

LACTATION

- It is not known if drug is present in breast milk.
- Patient should check with prescriber before breastfeeding.

Nursing Considerations

- Be aware that fidaxomicin should only be used to treat infections that are caused or strongly suspected to be caused by *Clostridium difficile.*
- Know that fidaxomicin and other drugs for *C. difficile*–associated diarrhea are most effective when patients are not taking other antibiotics. If other antibiotics can be stopped safely, expect them to be withheld during the 10 days of fidaxomicin therapy.

! **WARNING** Monitor patient for hypersensitivity reactions that may include angioedema, dyspnea, pruritus, or rash. Patients with a history of allergy to other macrolides are at increased risk. If a severe reaction occurs, discontinue fidaxomicin immediately and notify prescriber. Provide supportive care, as needed and ordered.

- Monitor patient for adverse effects and notify prescriber, if present.

PATIENT TEACHING

- Instruct patient to take fidaxomicin exactly as prescribed and for the full 10 days, regardless of how he is feeling.
- Tell patient or caregiver to take suspension out of the refrigerator 15 minutes before measuring dose, shake the bottle well, and use an oral syringe to measure dose. Bottle should be stored in refrigerator between doses and discarded after 12 days.

! **WARNING** Tell patient to seek immediate emergency care if an allergic reaction occurs during fidaxomicin therapy.

- Tell patient to notify prescriber if symptoms worsen at any time or don't improve after a few days.

filgrastim
(granulocyte colony-stimulating factor, G-CSF)
Grastofil (CAN), Neupogen

filgrastim-aafi
Nivestym

filgrastim-sndz
(granulocyte colony-stimulating factor, G-CSF)
Zarxio

tbo-filgrastim
Granix

Class and Category

Pharmacologic class: Colony-stimulating factor
Therapeutic class: Hematopoietic

Indications and Dosages

* *To reduce infection in patients with nonmyelid malignancies after myelosuppressive chemotherapy associated with a significant incidence of severe neutropenia with fever; to reduce neutrophil recovery time and duration of fever following induction or consolidation chemotherapy in patients with acute myeloid leukemia*

I.V. INFUSION (GRASTOFIL, NEUPOGEN, NIVESTYM, ZARXIO)

Adults and children. *Initial:* 5 mcg/kg daily for up to 2 wk or until absolute neutrophil count (ANC) has reached 10,000/mm^3 following the expected chemotherapy-induced neutrophil nadir beginning 24 hr or more after cytotoxic chemotherapy. Increased, as needed, by 5 mcg/kg with each chemotherapy cycle.

SUBCUTANEOUS INJECTION (GRASTOFIL, NEUPOGEN, NIVESTYM, ZARXIO)

Adults and children. *Initial:* 5 mcg/kg daily for up to 2 wk or until ANC has reached

10,000/mm^3 following the expected chemotherapy-induced neutrophil nadir beginning 24 hr or more after cytotoxic chemotherapy. Increased, as needed, by 5 mcg/kg with each chemotherapy cycle.

* *To reduce the duration of severe neutropenia in patients with nonmyeloid malignancies after receiving myelosuppressive chemotherapy associated with a significant incidence of febrile neutropenia*

SUBCUTANEOUS INJECTION (GRANIX)

Adults and children age 1 month and older. 5 mcg/kg daily starting no earlier than 24 hr after myelosuppressive chemotherapy and continued until the neutrophil count has recovered to normal.

* *To reduce duration of neutropenia in patients with nonmyeloid malignancies undergoing myeloablative chemotherapy followed by bone marrow transplantation*

I.V. INFUSION (GRASTOFIL, NEUPOGEN, NIVESTYM, ZARXIO)

Adults. *Initial:* 10 mcg/kg daily as a continuous infusion for no longer than 24 hr beginning at least 24 hr after bone marrow infusion and cytotoxic chemotherapy. Dosage adjusted according to ANC response.

* *To mobilize autologous hematopoietic progenitor cells into the peripheral blood for collection by leukapheresis*

SUBCUTANEOUS INJECTION (GRASTOFIL, NEUPOGEN, NIVESTYM, ZARXIO)

Adults. 10 mcg/kg daily starting at least 4 days before first leukapheresis and continuing until last day of leukapheresis.

* *To reduce occurrence and duration of severe neutropenia in congenital neutropenia*

SUBCUTANEOUS INJECTION (GRASTOFIL, NEUPOGEN, NIVESTYM, ZARXIO)

Adults and children. *Initial:* 6 mcg/kg twice daily. Dosage adjusted, as needed.

* *To reduce the occurrence and duration of severe neutropenia in idiopathic or cyclic neutropenia*

SUBCUTANEOUS INJECTION (GRASTOFIL, NEUPOGEN, ZARXIO)

Adults and children. *Initial:* 5 mcg/kg daily. Dosage adjusted as needed.

* *To treat patients acutely exposed to myelosuppressive doses of radiation*

SUBCUTANEOUS INJECTION (NEUPOGEN)

Adults. 10 mcg/kg daily beginning as soon as possible after exposure to radiation doses

greater than 2 gray and continued until ANC remains greater than 1,000/mm^3 for 3 consecutive CBCs or exceeds 10,000/mm^3 after a radiation-induced nadir.

* *To prevent and treat neutropenia in patients with HIV infection*

SUBCUTANEOUS INJECTION (GRASTOFIL)

Adults. *Initial:* 1 mcg/kg/day or 300 mcg three times weekly and continued with dosage adjustment, as needed, until a normal neutrophil count is reached and ANC is maintained at or greater than 2 3 10^9/L.

±**DOSAGE ADJUSTMENT** Dosage adjusted according to CBC with differential and platelet count response.

☰ Drug Administration

- Remove drug from refrigeration and allow drug to come to room temperature (minimum 30 minutes, maximum 24 hours) before administering. Discard drug if stored longer than 24 hours at room temperature. Solution should be clear and colorless.
- Withdraw only one dose from a vial; don't repuncture the vial.
- Don't shake the solution.
- Be aware that needle cover on single-use prefilled syringe contains dry natural rubber (except for the brands Granix and Nivestym) and may cause sensitivity reaction. It shouldn't be handled by people allergic to latex.
- Don't give within 24 hours before or after cytotoxic chemotherapy.

I.V.

- Dilute with 5% Dextrose Injection to a concentration between 5 and 15 mcg/ml. Never dilute with 0.9% Sodium Chloride Injection and do not dilute to less than 5 mcg/ml.
- Administer by continuous infusion over 24 hours or by intermittent infusion over 15 to 30 minutes daily.
- Protect absorption in plastic materials by the addition of albumin (human) at a concentration of 2 mg/ml making solution compatible with PVC or polyolefin intravenous bags. If albumin is not added to solution, a glass bottle must be used.
- Diluted solution can be stored at room temperature for up to 24 hours, which includes infusion and storage time.
- *Incompatibilities:* Saline solutions

SUBCUTANEOUS
- For subcutaneous dose larger than 1 ml, divide and give in more than one site.
- For direct administration of doses less than 0.3 ml, the single-dose vial should be used to ensure accuracy.
- Inject in abdomen, outer upper arms or outer areas of buttock, or thighs.
- Inject only in normal-appearing skin.
- Rotate injection sites.
- Nivestym prefilled syringe with BD UltraSafe Plus Passive Needle Guard cannot be used for doses less than 0.3 ml (180 mcg), because the spring mechanism of the needle guard apparatus affixed to the prefilled syringe interferes with the visibility of the graduation markings on the syringe barrel corresponding to 0.1 ml and 0.2 ml.
- Be aware that the brand Granix's prefilled syringe has a safety needle guard device for use by healthcare professionals only. To safely use the device, hold the syringe assembly by the open sides of the device and remove the needle shield. Expel any extra volume depending on dose needed. Inject Granix into site and push plunger as far as it will go to inject all of the drug. Injection of the entire prefilled syringe contents is needed to activate the needle guard. With the plunger still pressed all the way down, remove the needle from the skin. Slowly let go of the plunger and allow the empty syringe to move up inside the device until the entire needle is guarded. Discard the syringe assembly in an approved container.

Route	Onset	Peak	Duration
I.V.	1–2 days	Unknown	4 days
SubQ	1–2 days	2–8 hr	4 days
SubQ	3–5 days	4–6 hr	21 days

(tbo-filgrastim)

Half-life: 3–3.5 hr

Mechanism of Action

Is pharmacologically identical to human granulocyte colony-stimulating factor, an endogenous hormone synthesized by endothelial cells, fibroblasts and monocytes. Filgrastim induces formation of neutrophil progenitor cells by binding directly to receptors on the surface of granulocytes, which then divide and differentiate. It also potentiates the effects of mature neutrophils, which reduces fever and the risk of infection raised by severe neutropenia.

Contraindications

Hypersensitivity to filgrastim, other human granulocyte colony-stimulating factors such as pegfilgrastim, or their components

Interactions

DRUGS

None reported by manufacturer

Adverse Reactions

CNS: Fever, headache
CV: Aortitis, **capillary leak syndrome**, transient **supraventricular tachycardia**
GI: **Splenic rupture**, splenomegaly
GU: **Glomerulonephritis**
HEME: Acute myeloid leukemia, leukocytosis, **myelodysplastic syndrome** (patients with congenital neutropenia), **thrombocytopenia**
MS: Arthralgia; decreased bone density (children with chronic treatment); myalgia; pain in arms, legs, lower back, or pelvis: osteoporosis (children with chronic therapy)
RESP: **Acute respiratory distress syndrome (ARDS)**, **alveolar hemorrhage**, dyspnea, **hemoptysis**, wheezing
SKIN: Cutaneous vasculitis, pruritus, rash, Sweet's syndrome (acute febrile neutrophilic dermatosis)
Other: **Anaphylaxis**, **angioedema**, injection-site pain and redness, sickle cell crisis

Childbearing Considerations

PREGNANCY

- Pregnancy exposure registry: Enroll women prescribed Neupogen in Amgen's Pregnancy Surveillance Program by calling 1-800-77-AMGEN.
- It is not known if drug causes fetal harm.
- Use with caution only if benefit to mother outweighs potential risk to fetus.

LACTATION

- Drug is present in breast milk.
- Patient should check with prescriber before breastfeeding.

Nursing Considerations

- Expect to monitor CBC, hematocrit, and platelet count 2 or 3 times weekly.
- Inform prescriber and expect to stop drug if leukocytosis develops or absolute

neutrophil count consistently exceeds 10,000/mm^3.

- Anticipate decreased response to drug if patient has received extensive radiation therapy or long-term chemotherapy.

! **WARNING** Monitor patient for hypersensitivity reactions that could be severe. If present, stop drug therapy, notify prescriber, and provide supportive care as needed and prescribed.

- Know that aortitis has occurred in patients receiving filgrastim, occurring as early as the first week after start of therapy. Monitor patient for generalized signs and symptoms such as abdominal pain, back pain, fever, and malaise. Increased inflammatory markers (e.g., C-reactive protein and white blood cell count) help to confirm the diagnosis. Expect drug to be discontinued if aortitis is suspected.
- Monitor patient's renal function, as ordered, because drug may cause glomerulonephritis. If abnormalities occur, expect dosage to be reduced or drug discontinued.
- Monitor patients with congenital neutropenia for signs and symptoms of myelodysplastic syndrome (MDS) and acute myeloid leukemia (AML). Also know that patients with breast or lung cancer who are receiving chemotherapy and/or radiotherapy are at higher risk for developing MDS and AML.

! **WARNING** Monitor patients with sickle cell anemia receiving filgrastim, as sickle cell crisis can occur that can be life-threatening. Notify prescriber immediately if sickle cell crisis occurs. Expect drug to be discontinued.

PATIENT TEACHING

- Review possible serious side effects (allergic reactions, capillary leak syndrome, hematological abnormalities, inflammation of blood vessels, kidney injury, respiratory distress syndrome, and sickle cell crises) with patient before drug is given and determine patient's understanding. Tell her the most common side effect is aching in the bones and muscles.
- Teach patient how to prepare, administer, and store drug. Caution her not to reuse needle, syringe, or vial.

- Advise patient prescribed single-use prefilled syringe to notify prescriber if she has an allergy to latex, unless she is using the brands Granix or Nivestym, because needle cover may cause sensitivity reaction.
- Instruct patient who is self-injecting drug to notify prescriber if a dose is missed, to obtain instructions on when to take the next dose.

! **WARNING** Advise patient to promptly report pain in left upper quadrant of abdomen or shoulder-tip pain. Also tell patient to report any persistent, severe, or unusual signs and symptoms to prescriber and seek emergency medical attention, if needed. For example, tell her that difficulty breathing, facial swelling, rash, or wheezing require immediate attention.

- Emphasize the importance of returning for follow-up laboratory tests.
- Instruct patient to inform all prescribers of filgrastim, filgrastim-aafi, filgrastim-sndz, or tbo-filgrastim use. Patient should not take any over-the-counter preparations until after speaking to prescriber.

finasteride
Propecia, Proscar

≡ Class and Category
Pharmacologic class: 5-alpha reductase inhibitor
Therapeutic class: Benign prostatic hyperplasia agent, hair growth stimulant

≡ Indications and Dosages
✳ *To treat symptomatic benign prostatic hyperplasia; to reduce the risk of symptomatic progression of benign prostatic hyperplasia when given with doxazocin*

TABLETS (PROSCAR)
Adults. 5 mg daily.

✳ *To treat male-pattern baldness*

TABLETS (PROPECIA)
Adults. 1 mg daily.

≡ Drug Administration
P.O.

- Drug is a potential teratogen. Handle and dispose of according to institutional protocol.

- Do not handle broken or crushed tablets if pregnant or suspect pregnancy, because of adverse effects on male fetus.

Route	Onset	Peak	Duration
P.O.*	Unknown	2–6 hr	Unknown
P.O.†	3 mo	Unknown	12 mo

Half-life: 6 hr

* For benign prostatic hyperplasia

† For male-pattern baldness

≡ Mechanism of Action

Inhibits 5-alpha reductase, an intracellular enzyme that converts testosterone to its metabolite (5-alpha dihydrotestosterone) in liver, prostate, and skin. The metabolite is a potent androgen partially responsible for benign prostatic hyperplasia and hair loss.

≡ Contraindications

Females, hypersensitivity to finasteride or its components

≡ Interactions

DRUGS

None reported by manufacturer

≡ Adverse Reactions

CNS: Asthenia, depression, dizziness, headache, **progressive multifocal leukoencephalopathy** (extremely rare)
CV: **Hypotension**, peripheral edema
EENT: Lip swelling, rhinitis
ENDO: Gynecomastia, **male breast cancer**
GI: Abdominal pain, diarrhea
GU: Altered prostate-specific antigen level, blood in semen, decreased ejaculatory volume, decreased libido, erectile dysfunction, **high-grade prostate cancer**, impotence, male infertility, testicular pain
MS: Back pain
RESP: Dyspnea
SKIN: Pruritus, rash, urticaria
Other: Angioedema

≡ Childbearing Considerations

PREGNANCY

- Drug is known to cause fetal harm in the male fetus by preventing normal development of male genitalia.
- Drug is not indicated for use in women and is contraindicated in pregnant women and women of childbearing age.

- Women of childbearing age or who are pregnant should not handle crushed or broken tablets because of the possibility of absorption and subsequent potential risk to a male fetus.

LACTATION

- It is not known if drug is present in breast milk.
- Drug is not indicated for use in women.

REPRODUCTION

- Patient and female partner of childbearing age should use an effective contraceptive during drug therapy.

≡ Nursing Considerations

- Be aware that patient should have a urologic evaluation prior to starting finasteride therapy and periodically throughout therapy because drug can increase the risk of prostate cancer, especially high-grade prostate cancer.
- Expect patient to have a digital rectal examination of the prostate before and periodically during finasteride therapy.
- Be aware that finasteride therapy affects PSA levels. For example, drug may decrease levels even in the presence of prostate cancer. Any increases, no matter how slight or even if increase is still within normal limits, warrant further evaluation because of finasteride's risk of high-grade prostate cancer.
- Be aware that pregnant female healthcare workers should not handle broken finasteride tablets because of potential adverse effect on male fetus.

PATIENT TEACHING

! **WARNING** Urge patient and female partners to use reliable contraception during therapy because semen of men who take drug can harm male fetuses. Caution women and children not to handle broken tablets.

- Explain how to take drug, and urge patient to follow instructions that accompany it.
- Inform patient that drug may cause a variety of sexual dysfunction problems including decreased libido, erectile dysfunction, and male infertility, which may continue after drug is discontinued.
- Urge patient to have periodic follow-up to determine drug effectiveness.
- Caution patient that noncompliance with therapy may affect PSA test results.

E
F

finerenone
Kerendia

Class and Category
Pharmacologic class: Nonsteroidal mineralocorticoid receptor (MR) antagonist
Therapeutic class: Selected steroid blocker

Indications and Dosages
* *To reduce the risk of cardiovascular death, end-stage kidney disease, hospitalization for heart failure, nonfatal myocardial infarction, and sustained estimated glomerular filtration rate (eGFR) decline in patients with chronic kidney disease associated with type 2 diabetes*

TABLETS
Adults with an eGFR greater than 60 ml/min. *Initial:* 20 mg once daily. *Maintenance:* 20 mg once daily.

Adults with an eGFR greater than 25 but less than 60 ml/min. *Initial:* 10 mg once daily. Target dose: 20 mg once daily.

±**DOSAGE ADJUSTMENT** For patients with a serum potassium level greater than 5.5 mEq/L, drug withheld until serum potassium drops to 5.0 mEq/L or less, then drug restarted at 10 mg once daily. For patients with a serum potassium level 4.8 mEq/L or less and patient is taking 10 mg once daily, dosage increased to 20 mg once daily.

Drug Administration
P.O.
- Administer drug once daily at about the same time each day.
- For patient unable to swallow tablets, crush tablet and mix with water or soft foods such as applesauce immediately before administration.

Route	Onset	Peak	Duration
P.O.	Unknown	0.5 to 1.25 hr	Unknown

Half-life: 2–3 hr

Mechanism of Action
MR overactivation is believed to help cause fibrosis and inflammation. Blocks MR-mediated sodium reabsorption and MR overactivation in both epithelial tissues such as the kidney and nonepithelial tissues such as the heart and blood vessels.

Contraindications
Adrenal insufficiency, concomitant therapy with strong CYP3A4 inhibitors, hypersensitivity to finerenone or its components

Interactions
DRUGS
CYP3A4 inducers: Decreased finerenone exposure, decreasing effectiveness of drug
CYP3A4 inhibitors: Increased finerenone exposure, increasing risk of adverse reactions
drugs and supplements affecting serum potassium: Possibly increased serum potassium level

FOODS
grapefruit, grapefruit juice: Increased finerenone exposure, increasing risk of adverse reactions

Adverse Reactions
CV: Hypotension
GU: Mild decrease in estimated glomerular filtration rate
OTHER: Hyperkalemia, hyponatremia

Childbearing Considerations
PREGNANCY
- It is not known if drug can cause fetal harm. However, animal studies suggest a fetal risk.
- Use with caution only if benefit to mother outweighs potential risk to fetus.

LACTATION
- It is not known if drug is present in breast milk.
- Mother should avoid breastfeeding during drug therapy and for 1 day after drug is discontinued.

Nursing Considerations

! **WARNING** Check serum potassium level before finerenone therapy is started and periodically during drug therapy because drug may cause hyperkalemia. Know that drug should not be initiated if serum potassium is greater than 5.0 mEq/L until level decreases below 5.0 mEq/L. Also know that during drug therapy, notify prescriber if serum potassium level becomes greater than 5.5 mEq/L, as drug will have to be withheld and dosage restarted at 10 mg once daily when serum potassium is 5.0 mEq/L or less. Patients at risk for hyperkalemia are those with decreasing kidney function. Risk is greater in patients who have higher baseline serum potassium levels or other risk factors for hyperkalemia such as patients on concomitant drugs that impair potassium excretion or increase serum potassium levels. These patients may require increased monitoring.

- Be aware that patients with moderate hepatic impairment may require increased serum potassium monitoring. Know that drug should not be given to patients with severe hepatic impairment.

PATIENT TEACHING

- Stress importance of patient being compliant for required periodic blood work to measure her serum potassium level.
- Advise patient to avoid using potassium supplements or salt substitutes containing potassium without consulting prescriber first.
- Instruct patient not to eat grapefruit or drink grapefruit juice during finerenone therapy.
- Inform mothers that breastfeeding is not recommended during finerenone therapy and for 1 day after drug is discontinued.

! **WARNING** Review signs and symptoms of hyperkalemia with patient. If present, urge patient to contact prescriber, as the patient's serum potassium level must be checked and possible medical intervention may be required.

---

fingolimod hydrochloride
Gilenya

Class and Category
Pharmacologic class: Sphingosine 1-phosphate receptor modulator
Therapeutic class: Antimultiple sclerotic

Indications and Dosages
∗ *To treat relapsing forms of multiple sclerosis (MS), including active secondary progressive disease, clinically isolated syndrome, and relapsing-remitting disease*

CAPSULES

Adults and children age 10 and over weighing more than 40 kg (88 lb). 0.5 mg once daily.
Children age 10 and over weighing 40 kg (88 lb) or less. 0.25 mg once daily.

Drug Administration
P.O.

- Capsules should be swallowed whole and not chewed, crushed, or opened.
- After first dose, monitor patient for 6 hours for symptomatic bradycardia. Obtain hourly blood pressure and pulse checks and, if warranted, ECG monitoring. If an abnormality occurs, monitor for an additional 6 hours. Patient may need to stay overnight for additional monitoring. If abnormalities occurred with first dose, monitoring repeated for second dose.
- When restarting drug after treatment interrupted, perform first-dose monitoring again, because of potential effects on heart rate and AV conduction.

Route	Onset	Peak	Duration
P.O.	Unknown	12–16 hr	Unknown

Half-life: 6–9 days

Mechanism of Action
Possibly involves reduction of lymphocyte migration into the central nervous system to produce improved physical mobility.

Contraindications
Baseline QTc interval equal to or greater than 500 msec; experience within past 6 months of class III or IV heart failure, decompensated heart failure requiring hospitalization, MI, stroke, TIA, or unstable angina; history or presence of Mobitz Type II second-degree or third-degree atrioventricular block or sick sinus syndrome unless patient has functioning pacemaker in place; hypersensitivity to fingolimod or its components; presence of arrhythmias requiring the use of Class IA or Class III antiarrhythmic drugs

Interactions
DRUGS

antineoplastics, immunosuppressives, immunomodulators: Increased immunosuppression

beta-blockers, calcium channel blockers such as diltiazem or verapamil, digoxin: Possibly increased severity of bradycardia or slowing of atrioventricular conduction
chlorpromazine, citalopram, erythromycin, haloperidol, methadone: Possibly increased risk for prolonged QT interval which may lead to torsades de pointes
ketoconazole: Increased fingolimod levels
live attenuated vaccines: Increased risk of contracting disease from live virus
vaccines: Decreased effectiveness of vaccines during and up to 2 months after fingolimod therapy

Adverse Reactions

CNS: Asthenia, depression, dizziness, headache, migraine, paresthesia, **posterior reversible encephalopathy syndrome, progressive multifocal leukoencephalopathy, seizures, status epilepticus**, syncope, tumefactive demyelinating lesions
CV: Atrioventricular blocks, bradycardia, elevated blood triglycerides, hypertension, **transient asystole**
EENT: Blurred vision, eye pain, macular edema, sinusitis
GI: Diarrhea, elevated liver enzymes, gastroenteritis, **liver injury**
HEME: Hemolytic anemia, leukopenia, lymphopenia, thrombocytopenia
MS: Arthralgia, back pain, myalgia, severe increase in disability with discontinuation of therapy
RESP: Bronchitis, cough, dyspnea, pulmonary dysfunction
SKIN: Alopecia, **basal cell carcinoma,** eczema, **melanoma, Merkel cell carcinoma,** pruritus, rash, **squamous cell carcinoma**, tinea infections, urticaria
Other: Angioedema; flu-like symptoms; increased severity of herpes viral infections, including human papilloma viral infections; infections such as bacterial, fungi, and viral; **lymphomas**; weight loss

Childbearing Considerations

PREGNANCY

- Pregnancy exposure registry: 1-877-598-7237; email: gpr@quintiles.com, or website: www.gilenyapregnancyregistry.com.
- Pregnancy status of women of childbearing age should be determined before drug therapy is started.

- Drug may cause fetal harm. Animal studies suggest an increased risk of developmental toxicity.
- Use with caution only if benefit to mother outweighs potential risk to fetus.

LACTATION

- It is not known if drug is present in breast milk.
- Patient should check with prescriber before breastfeeding.

REPRODUCTION

- Women of childbearing age should use effective contraception during drug therapy and for 2 months after drug is discontinued.
- Women who plan to become pregnant need to have drug discontinued 2 months before planned conception.

Nursing Considerations

- Be aware that fingolimod therapy should not begin in a patient with an active acute or chronic infection until the infection is resolved, because drug causes a dose-dependent reduction in peripheral lymphocyte count up to 30% of baseline values.
- Immunize patient against the varicella zoster virus if he is antibody negative, as ordered. Be aware that fingolimod therapy will have to be postponed for 1 month to allow the full effect of vaccination to occur.
- Expect patient to be vaccinated against human papilloma virus (HPV) prior to fingolimod therapy taking into account vaccination recommendations because infections caused by HPV have occurred during drug therapy. Cancer screening, including Papanicolaou test, should be done routinely.
- Obtain an electrocardiogram on patients receiving antiarrhythmic therapy including beta-blockers and calcium channel blockers, those with cardiac risk factors, and those who have an irregular or slow heartbeat prior to beginning fingolimod therapy because drug may cause bradycardia and increased risk for atrioventricular block, especially in the first 24 hours of therapy.
- Obtain a recent complete blood count (within past 6 months) prior to starting therapy, as ordered, because drug increases risk of infection, especially bacterial, fungi,

and viral, that may become serious and life-threatening. Monitor patient throughout drug therapy for signs and symptoms of infection. If present, notify prescriber, and expect drug to be discontinued if serious and infection treated according to standard of care.

- Expect patient to have an ophthalmologic evaluation prior to beginning drug therapy and then again 3 to 4 months after therapy has begun to assess for macular edema. Patients with diabetes mellitus or a history of uveitis should have ongoing evaluations because they are at increased risk for macular edema. Report any visual disturbances to prescriber during drug therapy and expect additional ophthalmologic evaluation to be performed, if present, and drug discontinued. Visual acuity loss may persist even after resolution of macular edema in some patients.

- Obtain a recent liver enzyme evaluation (within past 6 months) prior to initiating fingolimod therapy, as ordered, because drug may cause elevation of liver enzymes. Monitor periodically throughout therapy and expect drug to be discontinued if liver enzymes exceed 5 times the upper limit of normal. Also evaluate in patient who develops symptoms suggestive of hepatic dysfunction, such as unexplained abdominal pain, anorexia, dark urine, fatigue, jaundice, nausea, and vomiting. Know that patients with preexisting liver disease may be at increased risk for developing elevated liver enzymes during fingolimod therapy.

! **WARNING** Monitor patient for hypersensitivity reactions such as angioedema, rash, or urticaria following administration. Prepare to provide supportive care if present and expect drug to be discontinued.

- Observe patient for 24 hours after the first dose of fingolimod for signs and symptoms of bradycardia. Heart rate usually begins to decrease within an hour of the first dose. The maximal decline in heart rate usually occurs within 6 hours and recovers but not to baseline level within 10 hours after the first dose. A second decline may occur after the first within the first 24 hours after the first dose. Monitor patient closely because the second decline may be more pronounced than the first. If patient develops chest pain, dizziness, fatigue, hypotension, or palpitations, notify prescriber, initiate appropriate management, as ordered, and continue observation until the symptoms have resolved. Know that with continued drug use, the heart rate returns to baseline within one month. Also observe patient closely for cardiac effects after drug is reinitiated if treatment is discontinued or interrupted for certain periods, as well as after dosage increases.

- Monitor patient for dyspnea throughout fingolimod therapy because drug may reduce diffusion lung capacity for carbon monoxide (DLCO) and forced expiratory volume over 1 second. Expect to perform spirometric evaluations of respiratory function and evaluation of DLCO during therapy, if clinically indicated.

- Monitor patient's blood pressure regularly to detect development of hypertension.

- Assess patient's skin for abnormalities, as drug may increase risk of basal cell carcinoma, melanoma, and Merkel cell carcinoma. Promptly report any suspicious looking lesions.

- Be aware that tumefactive demyelinating lesions may occur within the first 9 months after fingolimod has begun and may also occur within 4 months after drug is discontinued. Expect prompt imaging evaluation and initiation of appropriate treatment in patients who develop a severe multiple sclerosis relapse during fingolimod therapy.

- Be aware that it takes about 2 months for drug effects to be gone after therapy is discontinued requiring patient to be monitored for adverse effects during this time. Also be aware that severe increase in disability may occur after discontinuation of drug, which may occur up to 24 weeks after drug is stopped. Assess patient's level of function during this time and expect appropriate treatment to be given, as needed.

PATIENT TEACHING

- Inform patient that he will need to be observed for at least 6 hours after the first dose. He will need to repeat this observation period again for 6 hours if treatment is interrupted for more than 1 day within the first 2 weeks of therapy, if treatment is interrupted for more than 7 days during week 3 and 4 of therapy, or if treatment is discontinued for more than 14 days and then treatment is reinitiated, as well as any time dosage is increased.

- Instruct patient to swallow capsules whole and not to chew, crush, or open them.
- Tell patient to report any adverse signs and symptoms of infection or any other persistent or serious abnormalities to prescriber promptly, even up to 2 months after drug has been discontinued.
- Advise patient to examine his skin regularly for skin abnormalities, because drug may increase risk of skin cancer, including melanoma. Tell patient to report any suspicious skin lesion to prescriber for evaluation. Remind patient to limit exposure to sunlight and ultraviolet light and to wear protective clothing and use a sunscreen with a high protection factor when going outdoors.
- Instruct female patients to use effective contraception to avoid pregnancy during and for 2 months after fingolimod therapy is discontinued because of potential fetal harm. Stress importance of notifying prescriber immediately if pregnancy is suspected or occurs.
- Instruct patient how to check his pulse and tell him to notify prescriber if his pulse rate drops below 60 beats per minute or becomes irregular.

! **WARNING** Advise patient to notify prescriber immediately if difficulty breathing or other signs of an allergic reaction occur and if visual changes occur.

- Tell patient to notify prescriber if he notices symptoms suggestive of liver dysfunction, such as unexplained abdominal pain, anorexia, dark urine, fatigue, jaundice, nausea, or vomiting.
- Alert patient of the need to have periodic blood work done during fingolimod therapy and urge him to be compliant with these evaluations.

flavoxate hydrochloride

Class and Category
Pharmacologic class: Flavone derivative
Therapeutic class: Urinary tract antispasmodic

Indications and Dosages
✷ *To relieve dysuria; nocturia; suprapubic pain; urinary frequency, incontinence, and urgency caused by cystitis, prostatitis, urethritis, urethrocystitis, or urethrotrigonitis*

TABLETS
Adults and adolescents. 100 to 200 mg 3 times daily or 4 times daily. Dosage reduced with improvement.

Drug Administration
P.O.
- Protect drug from light by keeping it in a tight, light-resistant container.

Route	Onset	Peak	Duration
P.O.	55 min	112 min	Unknown

Half-life: 2–3.5 hr

Mechanism of Action
Relaxes muscles by cholinergic blockade and counteracts smooth-muscle spasms in the urinary tract.

Contraindications
Achalasia; duodenal or pyloric obstruction; GI hemorrhage; hypersensitivity to flavoxate or its components; obstructive intestinal lesions or ileus; obstructive uropathies of the lower urinary tract

Interactions
DRUGS
bethanechol, metoclopramide: Possibly antagonized GI motility effects of these drugs

Adverse Reactions
CNS: Confusion, decreased concentration, dizziness, drowsiness, fever, headache, nervousness, vertigo
CV: Palpitations, tachycardia
EENT: Accommodation disturbances, blurred vision, dry mouth, eye pain, photophobia, worsening of glaucoma

GI: Constipation, nausea, vomiting
GU: Dysuria
HEME: Eosinophilia, **leukopenia**
SKIN: Decreased sweating, dermatoses, urticaria

Childbearing Considerations

PREGNANCY

- It is not known if drug causes fetal harm.
- Use with caution only if benefit to mother outweighs potential risk to fetus.

LACTATION

- It is not known if drug is present in breast milk.
- Patient should check with prescriber before breastfeeding.

Nursing Considerations

- Monitor for eye pain if patient has glaucoma because flavoxate's anticholinergic effects may worsen glaucoma.

PATIENT TEACHING

- Caution patient about possible dry mouth and photophobia. Advise her to wear sunglasses outdoors, and suggest sugarless candy or gum, ice chips, saliva substitute, or sips of water for dry mouth.
- Advise patient to avoid hazardous activities until CNS effects of flavoxate are known.
- Caution patient not to become overheated or to take hot baths or saunas during therapy because drug reduces sweating, which can lead to dizziness, fainting, or heatstroke.
- Instruct patient to notify prescriber immediately if she experiences confusion, drowsiness, dysuria, headache, high fever, hives, nausea, nervousness, palpitations, rash, tachycardia, vertigo, vision problems, vomiting, or worsening dry mouth.

flecainide acetate

Tambocor

Class and Category

Pharmacologic class: Benzamide derivative
Therapeutic class: Class IC antiarrhythmic

Indications and Dosages

✱ *To prevent and suppress recurrent life-threatening ventricular tachycardia*

TABLETS

Adults. *Initial:* 100 mg every 12 hr. Increased by 50 mg twice daily every 4 days, as needed, until response occurs. *Maintenance:* Up to 150 mg every 12 hr. *Maximum:* 400 mg daily.

✱ *To prevent paroxysmal atrial fibrillation or flutter or paroxysmal supraventricular tachycardia associated with disabling symptoms*

TABLETS

Adults. *Initial:* 50 mg every 12 hr. Increased by 50 mg twice daily every 4 days, as needed, until response occurs. *Maintenance:* Up to 150 mg every 12 hr. *Maximum:* 300 mg daily.

±**DOSAGE ADJUSTMENT** Initial dose reduced to 100 mg daily or 50 mg every 12 hr for patients with creatinine clearance less than 35 ml/min.

Drug Administration

P.O.

- Take patient's pulse before each dose.
- Heart rate may have to be monitored with an ECG during the first few doses.

Route	Onset	Peak	Duration
P.O.	Unknown	1–6 hr	Unknown

Half-life: 12–27 hr

Mechanism of Action

Achieves antiarrhythmic effect by inhibiting fast sodium channels of myocardial cell membranes, which increase myocardial recovery after repolarization, and by depressing the upstroke of the action potential. Flecainide also produces its antiarrhythmic effect by:

- slowing intracardiac conduction, which slightly increases the duration of the action potential in atrial and ventricular muscle, thus prolonging the PR interval, QRS complex, and QT interval
- shortening the action potential of Purkinje fibers without affecting surrounding myocardial tissue
- inhibiting extracellular calcium influx (at high doses)
- stopping paroxysmal reentrant supraventricular tachycardias by acting on antegrade pathways of dysfunctional AV conduction
- decreasing conduction in accessory pathways in those with Wolff–Parkinson–White syndrome.

E
F

Contraindications

Cardiogenic shock, hypersensitivity to flecainide or its components, recent MI, right bundle-branch block associated with left hemiblock or second- or third-degree AV block unless pacemaker is present

Interactions

DRUGS

amiodarone: Increased blood flecainide level
antiretrovirals: Possibly increased flecainide levels
beta-blockers such as propranolol: Possibly myocardial depression and increased blood levels of both drugs
digoxin: Possibly increased blood digoxin level
quinidine: Possibly increased plasma flecainide concentrations in patients on chronic flecainide therapy, especially if these patients are extensive metabolizers

FOODS

acidic juices, foods that decrease urine pH below 5.0: Increased flecainide elimination and decreased therapeutic effects
foods that increase urine pH above 7.0, strict vegetarian diet: Decreased flecainide elimination and increased therapeutic effects

ACTIVITIES

smoking: Increased flecainide clearance

Adverse Reactions

CNS: Anxiety, depression, dizziness, drowsiness, fatigue, headache, light-headedness, tremor, weakness
CV: Arrhythmias, chest pain, **heart failure, hypotension**
EENT: Blurred vision
GI: Abdominal pain, anorexia, constipation, **hepatic dysfunction**, nausea, vomiting
RESP: Dyspnea
SKIN: Rash

Childbearing Considerations

PREGNANCY

- It is not known if drug causes fetal harm.
- Use with caution only if benefit to mother outweighs potential risk to fetus.

LACTATION

- Drug is present in breast milk.
- A decision may be made to discontinue breastfeeding or the drug to avoid potential serious adverse reactions in the breastfed infant.

Nursing Considerations

- Monitor urine pH beginning at the start of flecainide therapy.
- Check blood pressure, fluid intake and output, and weight regularly during therapy.
- Monitor trough flecainide level, as needed; therapeutic level is 0.2 to 1 mcg/ml.
- Expect drug to cause mild to moderate negative inotropic effects, minimal cardiovascular effects, and no effect on blood pressure, heart rate, and left ventricular function.

! WARNING Know that because hypokalemia or hyperkalemia may interfere with flecainide's therapeutic effects, serum potassium level must be monitored before and during therapy as ordered, and notify prescriber immediately if potassium imbalance develops. Also monitor for and notify prescriber about prolonged PR interval, QRS complex, or QT interval; chest pain; hypotension; and signs of heart failure. Keep in mind that drug can cause fatal proarrhythmias, which is why it isn't considered a first-line antiarrhythmic.

- Expect prolonged flecainide therapy to raise blood alkaline phosphatase level.

PATIENT TEACHING

- Instruct patient to take flecainide at regular intervals to keep a constant blood level.
- Advise patient to take a missed dose as soon as she remembers if it's within 6 hours of the scheduled time.
- Teach patient how to take her pulse, and instruct her to record it daily, along with her weight. Advise her to bring record to follow-up visits.
- Encourage family members to obtain instruction in basic cardiac life support.
- Advise patient to notify prescriber immediately about chest pain, difficulty breathing, and dizziness.
- Caution patient not to stop taking flecainide suddenly but to taper dosage gradually according to prescriber's instructions.

fluconazole
Diflucan

Class and Category
Pharmacologic class: Azole antifungal
Therapeutic class: Antifungal

Indications and Dosages
✴ *To treat oropharyngeal candidiasis*

ORAL SUSPENSION, TABLETS, I.V. INFUSION

Adults and adolescents. *Initial:* 200 mg on day 1 followed by 100 mg daily for at least 2 wk.

Children. *Initial:* 6 mg/kg on day 1, followed by 3 mg/kg daily for at least 2 wk.

✴ *To treat esophageal candidiasis*

ORAL SUSPENSION, TABLETS, I.V. INFUSION

Adults and adolescents. *Initial:* 200 mg on day 1 followed by 100 mg daily and given for at least 3 wk and for at least 2 wk following resolution of symptoms. Dosage increased, as needed. *Maximum:* 400 mg/day.

Children. *Initial:* 6 mg/kg on day 1, followed by 3 mg/kg daily and increased, as needed, and given for at least 3 wk and for at least 2 wk after esophageal symptoms resolve. *Maximum:* 12 mg/day.

✴ *To treat cryptococcal meningitis*

ORAL SUSPENSION, TABLETS, I.V. INFUSION

Adults and adolescents. *Initial:* 400 mg on day 1, followed by 200 to 400 mg daily based on patient's response, and continued for 10 to 12 wk after CSF culture is negative. *Maintenance:* 200 mg daily to suppress relapse.

Children. *Initial:* 12 mg/kg on day 1, followed by 6 to 12 mg/kg daily and continued for 10 to 12 wk after CSF culture is negative. *Maintenance:* 6 mg/kg daily to suppress relapse.

✴ *To prevent candidiasis after bone marrow transplantation in patients who receive cytotoxic chemotherapy and/or radiation*

ORAL SUSPENSION, TABLETS, I.V. INFUSION

Adults. 400 mg daily starting several days before procedure if severe neutropenia is expected and continued for 7 days after absolute neutrophil count exceeds 1,000/mm^3.

✴ *To treat vaginal candidiasis*

ORAL SUSPENSION, TABLETS

Adults. 150 mg as a single dose.

± **DOSAGE ADJUSTMENT** After initial loading dose, dosage reduced for all indications except to treat vaginal candidiasis by 50% for patients with creatinine clearance of 50 ml/min or less. For patient on hemodialysis, usual dosage given after each hemodialysis; on nondialysis days, dosage reduced according to the patient's creatinine clearance.

Drug Administration
P.O.
- Tablets should be swallowed whole.
- Prepare oral suspension by first tapping bottle until all the powder flows freely. Reconstitute by adding 24 ml of Distilled Water or Purified Water to bottle and shake vigorously.
- Shake suspension well before administering. Use a measuring device for determining dosage.
- Store suspension at room temperature and discard after 2 weeks.
- Protect drug from freezing.

I.V.
- Discard I.V. solution that's cloudy or contains precipitate.
- Do not remove unit from overwrap until ready for use. Tear overwrap down side at slit and remove solution container. Some opacity of the plastic may occur but does not affect solution quality or safety. The opacity will diminish gradually.
- Check for minute leaks by squeezing inner bag firmly. If leaks are found, discard.
- Do not use plastic containers in series connections.
- Don't infuse more than 200 mg/hr.
- Use an infusion pump for administration.
- *Incompatibilities:* Other I.V. drugs

Route	Onset	Peak	Duration
P.O./I.V.	Unknown	1–2 hr	Unknown

Half-life: 20–50 hr

Mechanism of Action
Damages fungal cells by interfering with a cytochrome P-450 enzyme needed

to convert lanosterol to ergosterol, an essential part of the fungal cell membrane. Decreased ergosterol synthesis causes increased cell permeability, which allows cell contents to leak. Fluconazole also may inhibit endogenous respiration, interact with membrane phospholipids, inhibit transformation of yeasts to mycelial forms, inhibit purine uptake, and impair biosynthesis of triglycerides and phospholipids.

Contraindications

Coadministration of drugs known to prolong QT interval and which are metabolized via the enzyme CYP3A4 (erythromycin, pimozide, or quinidine), hypersensitivity to fluconazole or its components

Interactions

DRUGS

alfentanil, amitriptyline, astemizole, celecoxib, cyclosporine, halofantrine, methadone, nortriptyline, olaparib, phenytoin, rifabutin, saquinavir, sirolimus, theophylline, tofacitinib, triazolam, zidovudine: Increased blood levels of these drugs with possible increase in adverse reactions

amiodarone, astemizole, cisapride, erythromycin, pimozide, quinidine: Increased risk of QT interval prolongation possibly leading to torsades de pointes

benzodiazepines (short-acting): Possibly increased benzodiazepine level and psychomotor effects

calcium channel blockers: Possibly increased systemic exposure of calcium channel blockers causing adverse effects

carbamazepine: Possibly increased risk of carbamazepine toxicity

cyclophosphamide: Increased serum bilirubin and creatinine levels

fentanyl: Possibly elevated fentanyl concentration that may lead to respiratory depression

glipizide, glyburide, tolbutamide and other sulfonylurea oral hypoglycemic agents: Increased risk of hypoglycemia

HMG-CoA reductase inhibitors: Increased risk of myopathy and rhabdomyolysis

hydrochlorothiazide: Increased fluconazole level from decreased excretion

ibrutinib: Possibly increased plasma ibrutinib concentrations and increased risk of adverse reactions from ibrutinib administration

lemborexant: Increased plasma concentration of lemborexant increasing risk of adverse reactions

losartan: Possibly decreased hypotensive effect of losartan

NSAIDs: Increased systemic exposure of NSAIDs

oral anticoagulants: Increased anticoagulant effects

prednisone: Possibly increased risk of acute adrenal cortex insufficiency

rifampin: Decreased serum fluconazole level

tacrolimus: Increased tacrolimus levels, possibly leading to nephrotoxicity

terfenadine: Increased risk of serious cardiac arrhythmias; increased terfenadine levels when dosage of terfenadine is 400 mg/day or greater

tolvaptan: Increased plasma exposure to tolvaptan with possible significant increase in risk of tolvaptan-induced adverse reactions

vinca alkaloids: Possibly increased plasma vinca alkaloids, which may lead to neurotoxicity

vitamin A: Possible adverse CNS effects

voriconazole: Increased risk of toxicity

Adverse Reactions

CNS: Chills, dizziness, drowsiness, fever, headache, **seizures**

CV: Prolonged QT interval, torsades de pointes

ENDO: Adrenal insufficiency

GI: Abdominal pain, anorexia, constipation, diarrhea, **hepatic failure,** nausea, vomiting

HEME: Agranulocytosis, leukopenia, thrombocytopenia

SKIN: Acute generalized exanthematous pustulosis, alopecia, diaphoresis, drug eruption, **exfoliative dermatitis,** photosensitivity, pruritus, rash, **Stevens–Johnson syndrome, toxic epidermal necrolysis**

Other: Anaphylaxis, angioedema, drug reaction with eosinophilia and systemic symptoms (DRESS)

Childbearing Considerations

PREGNANCY

- Drug can cause fetal harm such as distinct congenital anomalies in infants exposed in utero to high doses of the drug (400 to 800 mg per day) during most or all of the first trimester. Spontaneous abortions and congenital abnormalities may be potential risks even with 150 mg of the drug given as a single or repeated dose during the first trimester.

- Drug should be avoided in pregnancy except in patients with severe or potentially life-threatening fungal infections in whom the beneficial use of the drug outweighs the potential risk to the fetus.

LACTATION

- Drug is present in breast milk.
- Patient should check with prescriber before breastfeeding.

REPRODUCTION

- Advise women of childbearing age to use effective contraceptive measures during drug therapy and for about 1 week after the final dose when prescribed 400 to 800 mg of the drug daily.

≡ Nursing Considerations

- Use fluconazole cautiously in patients with potentially proarrhythmic conditions because drug may prolong the QT interval, which can lead to life-threatening torsades de pointes.
- Expect to obtain BUN and serum creatinine levels, as well as culture, sensitivity, and liver enzymes, as ordered, before therapy starts.
- Monitor hepatic and renal function periodically during therapy, and notify prescriber if you detect signs of dysfunction.
- Assess for rash every 8 hours during therapy, and notify prescriber if rash occurs.
- Monitor coagulation test results and assess patient for bleeding if patient is receiving an oral anticoagulant.
- Monitor patient for symptoms of overdose, such as hallucinations and paranoia. If they occur, provide supportive treatment, gastric lavage, and, possibly, hemodialysis, which can reduce blood fluconazole level by half after about 3 hours.

PATIENT TEACHING

- Inform patient that tablets should be swallowed whole. If patient is using oral suspension, instruct patient to shake bottle well before each use and to use a calibrated device to measure dosage, not a household spoon. Also tell patient to store oral suspension at room temperature and to discard after 2 weeks.

- Advise patient to complete entire course of therapy, even if she feels better.
- Tell patient to inform all prescribers of fluconazole use and not to take any over-the-counter preparations, including herbal preparations, without consulting prescriber first, as drug can interact with many other drugs and substances.
- Urge patient to monitor blood glucose level often if she takes an oral antidiabetic drug, because of increased risk of hypoglycemia.
- Alert patient that fluconazole may change the taste of food.
- Encourage patient to notify prescriber immediately about diarrhea, headache, nausea, rash, right-upper-quadrant abdominal pain, yellow skin or whites of eyes, or vomiting. Also tell patient to notify prescriber of fever, skin rash, swollen glands, or other persistent, severe, or unusual adverse reactions such as chronic fatigue, loss of appetite, muscle weakness, or weight loss.
- Urge women of childbearing age to notify prescriber immediately if pregnancy is suspected or known, as drug may have to be discontinued.

flumazenil

≡ Class and Category

Pharmacologic class: Imidazobenzodiazepine derivative
Therapeutic class: Benzodiazepine antidote

≡ Indications and Dosages

* *To reverse conscious sedation or general anesthesia from benzodiazepine therapy*

I.V. INJECTION

Adults. *Initial:* 0.2 mg given over 15 sec, repeated after 45 sec if response is inadequate and then repeated every 1 min, if needed, up to maximum dose. If sedation recurs, regimen is repeated every 20 min or more. *Maximum:* 1 mg given in 0.2 mg increments over 15 sec every 1 min over 5-min cycle. For reoccurrence of sedation, no more than 1 mg (0.2 mg/min) administered at any one time every 20 min 3 times for a total of 3 mg over 1 hr.

* *To reverse conscious sedation in children*

I.V. INJECTION

Children age 1 and older. *Initial:* 0.01 mg/kg (up to 0.2 mg) given over 15 sec, repeated after 45 sec if response is inadequate and then repeated every 1 min, if needed, up to 4 additional doses. *Maximum:* 5 doses total, not exceeding accumulative dosage of 0.05 mg/kg or 1 mg, whichever is lower.

* *To reverse benzodiazepine toxicity or suspected overdose*

I.V. INJECTION

Adults. *Initial:* 0.2 mg given over 30 sec followed by 0.3 mg given over 30 sec after waiting 30 sec if response is inadequate and then 0.5 mg given over 30 sec at 1-min intervals, if needed, to maximum dose. If sedation recurs, regimen is repeated every 20 min. *Maximum:* Cycle repeated every 20 min 3 times for a total of 3 mg in 1-hr period.

Drug Administration

I.V.

- Do not remove drug from drug vial until ready for administration.
- Give undiluted or diluted in a syringe with 0.9% Sodium Chloride Injection, 5% Dextrose Injection, or Lactated Ringer's solution.
- Avoid aerosol generation when preparing syringes for injection, If drug splatters onto skin, wash area with cool water.
- Administer over 15 seconds to reverse conscious sedation or general anesthesia and over 30 seconds to reverse benzodiazepine toxicity or suspected overdose. Inject directly into tubing of a free-flowing compatible I.V. solution.
- Use a large vein, if possible, to minimize pain at site. Avoid extravasation because drug may irritate tissue.
- If drug is stored in a syringe diluted or undiluted, discard after 24 hours.
- *Incompatibilities:* None listed by manufacturer

Route	Onset	Peak	Duration
I.V.	1–2 min	6–10 min	Variable
Half-life: 40–80 min			

Mechanism of Action

Antagonizes CNS effects of benzodiazepines by competing for their binding sites.

Contraindications

Evidence of tricyclic antidepressant overdose; hypersensitivity to flumazenil, benzodiazepines, or their components; use of benzodiazepine to control intracranial pressure, status epilepticus, or a potentially life-threatening condition

Interactions

DRUGS

benzodiazepines: Benzodiazepine withdrawal symptoms, including seizures
nonbenzodiazepine agonists: Loss of effectiveness of these drugs
tetracyclic or tricyclic antidepressant overdose: High risk of seizures

Adverse Reactions

CNS: Agitation, anxiety, ataxia, confusion, dizziness, drowsiness, emotional lability, fatigue, headache, hypoesthesia, insomnia, paresthesia, resedation, **seizures**, tremor, vertigo
CV: Hypertension, palpitations
EENT: Blurred vision, diplopia, dry mouth
GI: Nausea, vomiting
RESP: Dyspnea, hyperventilation, **hypoventilation**
SKIN: Diaphoresis, flushing, rash
Other: Injection-site pain and thrombophlebitis

Childbearing Considerations

PREGNANCY

- It is not known if drug causes fetal harm.
- Use with caution only if benefit to mother outweighs potential risk to fetus.

LABOR & DELIVERY

- Not recommended for use during labor and delivery.

LACTATION

- It is not known if drug is present in breast milk.
- Patient should check with prescriber before breastfeeding.

Nursing Considerations

- Use flumazenil cautiously in patients with cardiac disease. Assess for increased anxiety or stress from benzodiazepine withdrawal because patient's blood pressure may rise.
- Be aware that drug may cause signs of benzodiazepine withdrawal in drug-dependent patient. Also, abrupt awakening

from benzodiazepine overdose can cause agitation, dysphoria, and increased adverse reactions.

- Be aware that benzodiazepine reversal may cause an anxiety or a panic attack for patient with a history of these episodes. Expect to adjust dosage carefully.
- Monitor patient for signs of hypoventilation or resedation for at least 2 hours after giving flumazenil because drug has a short half-life. Be aware that patient shouldn't be discharged until the risk of resedation has resolved.

PATIENT TEACHING

- Caution patient to avoid alcohol and OTC drugs for 10 to 24 hours after receiving drug.
- Advise patient to avoid hazardous activities for 18 to 24 hours after discharge.
- Inform patient and family that agitation, emotional lability, fear, and panic attack (if patient has a history of them) may occur. Tell them to seek medical care if patient has depression, flushing, hyperventilation, insomnia, palpitations, tremor, or trouble breathing.
- Provide written instructions or instructions to caregiver even if patient is alert, because drug doesn't always reverse postprocedure amnesia.

fluoxetine hydrochloride
Prozac, Sarafem

⬚ Class and Category

Pharmacologic class: Selective serotonin reuptake inhibitor (SSRI)
Therapeutic class: Antidepressant

⬚ Indications and Dosages

✳ *To treat acute depression; to provide maintenance therapy for depression*

CAPSULES, ORAL SOLUTION, TABLETS (PROZAC)

Adults. *Initial:* 20 mg once daily in the morning. Dosage increased every couple of weeks, as needed. Doses above 20 mg daily given once daily in the morning or divided and given in morning and at noon. *Maximum:* 80 mg daily.

Children ages 8 and older. *Initial:* 10 mg once daily. Increased after 1 wk or longer to 20 mg daily, if needed.

✳ *To treat acute obsessive–compulsive disorder (OCD); to provide maintenance therapy for OCD*

CAPSULES, ORAL SOLUTION, TABLETS (PROZAC)

Adults. *Initial:* 20 mg daily. Dosage increased every couple of wk, as needed. Doses above 20 mg daily given once daily in the morning or divided and given in morning and at noon. *Maximum:* 80 mg daily.

Children ages 7 and older. *Initial:* 10 mg daily. Dosage increased after 2 wk to 20 mg daily. Subsequent dosage increased, as needed, at intervals of at least several wk. *Maintenance:* 20 to 60 mg daily.

✳ *To treat moderate to severe bulimia nervosa; to provide maintenance therapy for bulimia nervosa*

CAPSULES, ORAL SOLUTION, TABLETS (PROZAC)

Adults. 60 mg once daily in the morning. Alternatively, dosage titrated up to 60 mg once daily over several days.

✳ *To treat acute panic disorder with or without agoraphobia*

CAPSULES, ORAL SOLUTION, TABLETS (PROZAC)

Adults. *Initial:* 10 mg daily. Dosage increased in 1 wk to 20 mg daily, as needed. Dosage further increased after several wk, as needed. *Maximum:* **60 mg daily.**

✳ *As adjunct to treat acute depressive episodes associated with bipolar I disorder*

CAPSULES, ORAL SOLUTION, TABLETS (PROZAC)

Adults. *Initial:* 20 mg given with 5 mg olanzapine once daily in the evening. Dosage adjusted, as needed. *Usual:* 20 to 50 mg with 5 to 12.5 mg olanzapine.

Children age 10 and older. *Initial:* 20 mg given with 2.5 mg olanzapine once daily in the evening. Dosage adjusted, as needed. *Maximum:* 50 mg given with 12 mg of olanzapine once daily in the evening.

✳ *As adjunct to treat resistant depression*

CAPSULES, ORAL SOLUTION, TABLETS (PROZAC)

Adults. *Initial:* 20 mg with 5 mg olanzapine once daily in the evening. Dosage adjusted, as needed, *Usual:* 20 to 50 mg with 5 to 20 mg olanzapine once daily in the evening.

±**DOSAGE ADJUSTMENT** For all indications with Prozac, dose or frequency reduced for adult patients with concurrent illness or hepatic impairment, those who take multiple medications, and for elderly patients. For lower-weight children taking drug for OCD, dosage increased above 10 mg daily only if clinical improvement remains insufficient after several weeks. Maintenance dosage for such children should not exceed 30 mg daily. For lower-weight children taking drug for depression, dosage increased to 20 mg daily only if improvement insufficient after several weeks.

＊ *To treat premenstrual dysmorphic disorder*

TABLETS (SARAFEM)

Adults. 20 mg once daily given continuously or intermittently in relation to menstrual cycle. Dosage increased as needed. *Maximum:* 80 mg daily.

±**DOSAGE ADJUSTMENT** Dose or frequency reduced for patients with concurrent illness or hepatic impairment, or those who take multiple medications.

Drug Administration

P.O.

- Give Prozac prescribed once daily in morning and twice-daily doses in morning and at noon, except for acute depressive episodes associated with bipolar I disorder. In this indication, Prozac once-daily dose should be given in the evening.
- Use calibrated device when measuring dose using Prozac oral solution. Store oral solution at room temperature.
- Give Sarafem continuously (every day of the menstrual cycle) or intermittently (starting daily dose 14 days prior to the anticipated onset of menstruation through the first full day of menses and repeated with each new cycle).

Route	Onset	Peak	Duration
P.O.	2–4 wk	6–8 hr	Unknown

Half-life: 1–6 days

Mechanism of Action

Selectively inhibits reuptake of the neurotransmitter serotonin by CNS neurons and increases the amount of serotonin available in nerve synapses. An elevated serotonin level may result in elevated mood and, consequently, reduce depression, lessen obsessive–compulsive behavior, and diminish panic symptoms, as well as relieve premenstrual dysmorphic discomfort.

Contraindications

Concurrent therapy with pimozide or thioridazine; hypersensitivity to fluoxetine, other selective serotonin reuptake inhibitors or their components; use within 14 days of MAO inhibitor therapy, including linezolid or intravenous methylene blue.

Interactions

DRUGS

alprazolam, diazepam: Possibly prolonged half-life of these drugs
anticonvulsants: Increased anticonvulsant levels with potential for toxicity
aspirin, NSAIDs, warfarin: Increased anticoagulant activity and risk of bleeding
benzodiazepines, CNS depressants: Increased CNS effect and development of adverse effects
CYP2D6-metabolized drugs, such as antiarrhythmics (especially flecainide, propafenone), antidepressants (tricyclics), antipsychotics (phenothiazines and most atypicals), thioridazine, and vinblastine: Increased plasma levels of these drugs and increased risk of serious adverse reactions
buspirone, fentanyl, intravenous methylene blue, linezolid, serotonergics (such as amphetamines and other psychostimulants, antidepressants, and dopamine agonists), St. John's wort, tramadol, tricyclic antidepressants, triptans, tryptophan: Increased risk of serotonin syndrome
highly protein-bound drugs: Possibly increased risk of elevated plasma levels of drugs increasing risk of adverse effects
lithium: Decreased or increased lithium levels; potential for serotonergic effects
MAO inhibitors: Possibly severe and life-threatening adverse effects; increased risk of serotonin syndrome
olanzapine: Increased blood olanzapine levels with decreased clearance resulting in possible increased risk for adverse reactions
phenytoin: Increased blood phenytoin level and risk of toxicity
pimozide, thioridazine, or other drugs that may prolong QT interval: Increased blood

levels of these drugs; possibly increased risk of prolonged QT interval

Adverse Reactions

CNS: Akathisia, anxiety, ataxia, balance disorder, chills, depersonalization, dream disturbances, drowsiness, emotional lability, euphoria, fatigue, fever, headache, hypertonia, hypomania, insomnia, mania, myoclonus, nervousness, **neuroleptic malignant syndrome**, paranoid reaction, restlessness, **seizures**, **serotonin syndrome**, somnolence, **suicidal ideation**, tremor, vertigo, weakness, yawning
CV: Arrhythmias, hypotension, palpitations, **prolonged QT interval, torsades de pointes, ventricular arrhythmias**
EENT: Abnormal vision, angle-closure glaucoma, dry mouth, mydriasis, pharyngitis, sinusitis, taste perversion, teeth grinding
ENDO: Galactorrhea, gynecomastia, **hypoglycemia**, syndrome of inappropriate antidiuretic hormone secretion (SIADH)
GI: Anorexia, diarrhea, dysphagia, gastritis, gastroenteritis, indigestion, **melena**, nausea, stomach ulcer
GU: Decreased or increased libido, delayed or absent orgasm (females), dysuria, ejaculation disorders, erectile dysfunction, gynecological bleeding, impotence, micturition disorder
HEME: Altered platelet function, unusual bleeding
MS: Arthralgia, myalgia
RESP: Dyspnea
SKIN: Alopecia, diaphoresis, ecchymosis, pruritus, rash, urticaria
Other: Flu-like symptoms, **hyponatremia**, weight loss

Childbearing Considerations

PREGNANCY

- Pregnancy exposure registry: 1-844-405-6185 or https://womenshealth.org/clinical-and -research-programs/pregnancyregistry /antidepressants/.
- Drug may cause fetal harm if administered late in the third trimester.
- Neonates exposed to drug late in the third trimester may develop serious complications after birth requiring prolonged hospitalization, respiratory support, and tube feeding.
- Use with caution only if benefit to mother outweighs potential risk to fetus.

LACTATION

- Drug is present in breast milk.
- Patient should check with prescriber before breastfeeding.
- If breastfeeding occurs, infant should be monitored for agitation, irritability, poor feeding, and poor weight gain.

Nursing Considerations

- Use fluoxetine cautiously in patients with a history of seizures and in children, because of potential for adverse effects.
- Use fluoxetine cautiously in patients with congenital long QT syndrome, previous history of QT prolongation, or family history of long QT syndrome or sudden cardiac death. In addition, use caution in presence of other conditions that increase risk of QT prolongation and ventricular arrhythmia, such as concurrent drug therapy with drugs known to prolong the QT interval, hypokalemia, hypomagnesemia, recent MI, significant arrhythmias, uncompensated heart failure and conditions that predispose patient to increased fluoxetine exposure, such as hepatic impairment or concurrent use of drugs known to increase blood fluoxetine levels such as CYP2D6 inhibitors, CYP2D6 poor metabolizer status, or use of other highly protein-bound drugs. Obtain an ECG recording, as ordered, before fluoxetine begins in these patients and periodically throughout therapy. Expect fluoxetine to be discontinued if the QT interval becomes prolonged or patient develops a ventricular arrhythmia.

⚠ **WARNING** Avoid giving fluoxetine within 14 days of an MAO inhibitor or starting MAO inhibitor therapy within 5 weeks of discontinuing fluoxetine.

- Know that patients with depression should be screened for bipolar disorder before fluoxetine therapy is started, because treating depression alone in these patients may precipitate a manic or mixed episode.
- Monitor patient for depression (especially children, adolescents, and young adults) and watch closely for suicidal tendencies, particularly when therapy starts and dosage changes, because depression may worsen temporarily during those times.

E
F

- Monitor patient closely for evidence of GI bleeding, especially if patient takes another drug known to increase the risk, such as aspirin, an NSAID, or warfarin.
- Monitor patient—especially an elderly patient—for hypoosmolarity of serum and urine and for hyponatremia (difficulty concentrating, headache, memory impairment, unsteadiness, weakness), which may indicate fluoxetine-induced SIADH.
- Expect to taper drug when being discontinued, as ordered, to minimize adverse reactions.

! **WARNING** Monitor patient for possible serotonin syndrome, characterized by agitation, chills, confusion, diaphoresis, diarrhea, fever, hyperactive reflexes, poor coordination, restlessness, shaking, talking or acting with uncontrolled excitement, tremor, and twitching, especially if patient is receiving another drug that raises serotonin level (such as amphetamine, dopamine agonist, MAO inhibitor, tryptophan, or other antidepressant or psychostimulant). In its most severe form, serotonin syndrome can resemble neuroleptic malignant syndrome, which includes autonomic instability, high fever, muscle rigidity, and possible fluctuations in vital signs and mental status.

- Monitor patient with diabetes mellitus for altered blood glucose level because drug may cause hypoglycemia during therapy and hyperglycemia when it stops. Expect to adjust dosage of antidiabetic drug, as prescribed.
- Expect patient to be reevaluated periodically to determine continued need for therapy.

PATIENT TEACHING

- Instruct patient when to take daily dose(s). Tell patient prescribed oral solution to use a calibrated device to measure dosage, not a household spoon, and to store solution at room temperature.
- Inform patient that drug may take several weeks to achieve full effects.

! **WARNING** Tell patient that drug increases risk of serotonin syndrome, a rare but serious complication, especially when taken with certain other drugs. Teach patient to recognize its signs and symptoms, and advise her to notify prescriber immediately if they occur.

- Urge family or caregiver to watch patient closely for suicidal tendencies, especially when therapy starts or dosage changes, and particularly if patient is a child, teenager, or young adult.
- Caution patient to avoid hazardous activities until CNS effects of drug are known.
- Caution against stopping fluoxetine abruptly because serious adverse effects may result.
- Instruct patient to notify prescriber of any persistent, severe, or unusual signs or symptoms while taking fluoxetine.
- Inform patient that drug may cause mild pupillary dilation, which may lead to an episode of acute-angle glaucoma. Encourage patient to have an eye exam prior to starting fluoxetine therapy to see if she is at risk.
- Advise patient to consult prescriber before taking OTC or prescription drugs, if hives or a rash develop.
- Urge women of childbearing age to notify prescriber if pregnancy is suspected or occurs, because fluoxetine therapy may increase risk of serious adverse effects in the newborn. Also tell mothers breastfeeding to monitor infant for agitation, irritability, poor feeding, and poor weight gain.
- Alert patient that drug may cause sexual dysfunction. Advise patient to discuss sexual dysfunction with prescriber.

fluphenazine decanoate

fluphenazine hydrochloride

Class and Category

Pharmacologic class: Phenothiazine
Therapeutic class: Antipsychotic

Indications and Dosages

＊ *To control psychotic disorders*

ELIXIR, ORAL SOLUTION, TABLETS (FLUPHENAZINE HYDROCHLORIDE)

Adults and adolescents. *Initial:* 2.5 to 10 mg/day in divided doses every 6 to 8 hr. *Maintenance:* 1 to 5 mg daily in divided doses every 6 to 8 hr or as a single daily dose. *Maximum:* 40 mg/day.

±**DOSAGE ADJUSTMENT** For elderly or debilitated patients, initial oral dosage reduced to 1 to 2.5 mg daily in divided doses every 6 to 8 hr.

I.M. INJECTION (FLUPHENAZINE HYDROCHLORIDE)

Adults. 1/3 to 1/2 oral daily dosage divided and given every 6 to 8 hr. *Maximum:* 10 mg daily.

I.M. OR SUBCUTANEOUS INJECTION (FLUPHENAZINE DECANOATE)

Adults. *Initial:* 12.5 to 25 mg given every 3 to 4 weeks or longer depending on patient's needs. *Maximum:* 100 mg/dose.

≡ Drug Administration

P.O.

- Mix liquid concentrate with 60 ml of uncaffeinated drinks, milk, or tomato or fruit juice. Don't mix with beverages that contain caffeine, such as coffee and cola; pectins, such as apple juice; or tannins, such as tea. They're physically incompatible.
- Protect drug from light.
- Measure dosage of elixir or oral solution with a calibrated device and not with household teaspoon.

I.M.

- For hydrochloride parenteral formulation, inject only as an I.M. injection. Solution should be clear to light amber; do not administer if darker or discolored.
- For decanoate formulation, use at least a 21G needle for administration. Needle and syringe should be dry; a wet needle or syringe may cause solution to become cloudy. Do not administer a cloudy solution. Administer as a deep I.M. injection, using Z-track technique, into the gluteal muscle, although the deltoid muscle has been used.

SUBCUTANEOUS

- Administer only decanoate formulation via this route.
- Use with dry syringe and needle that is 21G or greater to administer.
- Do not administer if solution is cloudy.

Route	Onset	Peak	Duration
P.O.	<1 hr	2 hr	6–8 hr
I.M.*	<1 hr	90–120 min	6–8 hr
I.M.†	24–72 hr	8–10 hr	4 wk
SubQ†	Unknown	Unknown	Unknown

Half-life: 15 hours (hydrochloride); 14 days (decanoate)

* For hydrochloride.

† For decanoate.

≡ Mechanism of Action

May block postsynaptic dopamine receptor sites in the CNS. This action may depress areas of the brain that control activity and aggression, including the cerebral cortex, hypothalamus, and limbic system.

≡ Contraindications

Blood dyscrasias; coma; concomitant use of large amounts of another CNS depressant; hepatic dysfunction; hypersensitivity to fluphenazine, other phenothiazines, or their components; narrow-angle glaucoma; poorly controlled seizure disorder, severe cardiovascular disease, CNS depression or hypertension; subcortical brain damage

≡ Interactions

DRUGS

adsorbent antidiarrheals, aluminum- or magnesium-containing antacids: Possibly inhibited absorption of fluphenazine
anticholinergics: Possibly intensified adverse effects of both drugs
antihypertensives: Possibly severe hypotension
barbiturates, CNS depressants, opioids: Possibly prolonged and intensified CNS depression and respiratory depression
lithium: Possibly neurotoxicity (disorientation, extrapyramidal reactions, unconsciousness)

ACTIVITIES

alcohol use: Possibly increased CNS and respiratory depression that may become severe

≡ Adverse Reactions

CNS: Ataxia, cerebral edema, dizziness, drowsiness, headache, insomnia,

E
F

light-headedness, nervousness, **seizures,** slurred speech, syncope, worsening psychotic symptoms

CV: AV conduction disorders, bradycardia, cardiac arrest, hypercholesterolemia, hypertension, orthostatic hypotension, **QT interval prolongation, shock, ST-segment depression,** tachycardia

EENT: Blurred vision, dry mouth, glaucoma, increased salivation, **laryngeal edema, laryngospasm,** miosis, mydriasis, nasal congestion, papillary hypertrophy of the tongue, parotid gland enlargement, photophobia, pigmentary retinopathy, ptosis

ENDO: Breast engorgement (females), galactorrhea, hyperglycemia, **hypoglycemia,** mastalgia, syndrome of inappropriate ADH secretion

GI: Anorexia, constipation, diarrhea, fecal impaction, ileus, increased appetite, jaundice, nausea, vomiting

GU: Amenorrhea, bladder paralysis, decreased libido, enuresis, menstrual irregularities, polyuria, urinary frequency, urinary incontinence, urine retention

HEME: Anemia, **aplastic anemia,** eosinophilia, **leukopenia, nonthrombocytopenic or thrombocytopenic purpura, thrombocytopenia**

RESP: Bronchospasm, dyspnea, increased respiratory depth

SKIN: Contact dermatitis, dry skin, eczema, erythema, photosensitivity, pruritus, seborrhea

Other: Heatstroke, hyponatremia, lupus-like symptoms, weight gain

≣ Childbearing Considerations

PREGNANCY

- It is not known if drug causes fetal harm but may have an adverse effect on the fetus if administered during the third trimester of pregnancy.
- Use with caution only if benefit to mother outweighs potential risk to fetus.

LABOR & DELIVERY

- Neonates exposed to antipsychotics during the third trimester of pregnancy may develop extrapyramidal and withdrawal signs and symptoms after delivery.

LACTATION

- Drug maybe present in breast milk.
- Patient should check with prescriber before breastfeeding.

≣ Nursing Considerations

- Be aware that fluphenazine shouldn't be used to treat dementia-related psychosis in elderly patients, because of an increased mortality risk.
- Use fluphenazine cautiously in patients with a history of glaucoma or renal impairment.
- Monitor temperature; a significant, unexplained rise can indicate intolerance and a need to discontinue drug. Notify prescriber immediately if this occurs.
- Watch for signs of hepatic failure, such as jaundice.
- Notify prescriber about worsening psychotic symptoms: agitation, catatonic state, confusion, depression, hallucinations, lethargy, paranoid reactions.

PATIENT TEACHING

- Instruct patient prescribed elixir form of fluphenazine to keep it in an amber or opaque bottle because drug is sensitive to light. Tell patient to use a calibrated device when measuring dosage, not a household spoon.
- Instruct patient to mix concentrated solution with 2 ounces of uncaffeinated beverages, milk, or tomato or fruit juice. Advise patient not to mix oral solution with beverages that contain caffeine (coffee, cola), pectins (apple juice), or tannins (tea). Tell patient to use a calibrated device when measuring dosage, not a household spoon.
- Caution patient about possible dizziness or light-headedness.
- Teach patient how to prevent heatstroke, orthostatic hypotension, and photosensitivity reactions.
- Warn against stopping drug abruptly.

flurazepam hydrochloride

≣ Class, Category, and Schedule

Pharmacologic class: Benzodiazepine
Therapeutic class: Sedative-hypnotic
Controlled substance schedule: IV

≣ Indications and Dosages

✳ *To treat insomnia characterized by difficulty falling asleep, frequent nocturnal awakenings, or early-morning awakening*

CAPSULES

Adult women. *Initial:* 15 mg, increased to 30 mg, as needed.

Adult men. *Initial:* 15 or 30 mg. Dosage may be increased to 30 mg, as needed, if initial dose was 15 mg.

±**DOSAGE ADJUSTMENT** Initial dose not to exceed 15 mg for elderly or debilitated men until individual response is known.

Drug Administration

P.O.

- Administer drug at bedtime.

Route	Onset	Peak	Duration
P.O.	15–45 min	30–60 min	7–8 hr

Half-life: 2.3 hr

Mechanism of Action

May potentiate the effects of gamma-aminobutyric acid (GABA) and other inhibitory neurotransmitters by binding to specific benzodiazepine receptor sites in the cortical and limbic areas of the CNS. As a result, flurazepam increases GABA's inhibitory effects and blocks cortical and limbic arousal.

Contraindications

Hypersensitivity to flurazepam, other benzodiazepines, or their components

Interactions

DRUGS

CNS depressants: Possibly potentiated CNS depression
opioids: Increased risk of profound CNS and respiratory depression and sedation

ACTIVITIES

alcohol use: Possibly potentiated CNS and respiratory depression

Adverse Reactions

CNS: Amnesia, anxiety, ataxia, bizarre behavior (such as sleep driving), confusion, delusions, depression, dizziness, drowsiness, euphoria, headache, hypokinesia, irritability, malaise, nervousness, slurred speech, tremor
CV: Chest pain, palpitations, tachycardia
EENT: Blurred vision, dry mouth, increased salivation, photophobia
GI: Abdominal pain, constipation, diarrhea, nausea, thirst, vomiting
GU: Libido changes
SKIN: Diaphoresis

Other: Anaphylaxis, angioedema, physical or psychological dependence

Childbearing Considerations

PREGNANCY

- Pregnancy exposure registry: 1-888-233-2334 or http://www.aedpregnancyregistry.org/.
- Infants born to mothers who have taken the drug during the later stages of pregnancy can develop dependence, and subsequently withdrawal, during the postnatal period.
- Use with extreme caution only if benefit to mother outweighs potential risk to fetus. If possible, drug should not be used during pregnancy.

LABOR & DELIVERY

- Administration of drug immediately prior to or during childbirth can result in a syndrome of hypothermia, hypotonia, respiratory depression, and difficulty feeding for the infant.

LACTATION

- It is not known if drug is present in breast milk.
- Patient should check with prescriber before breastfeeding.

Nursing Considerations

- Use flurazepam cautiously in patients with severe mental depression or reduced respiratory function; drug may intensify mental depression and lead to respiratory depression.
- Expect to use lowest effective dose in debilitated or elderly patients to minimize the risk of ataxia, confusion, dizziness, and oversedation.
- Monitor liver function test results, as appropriate.

PATIENT TEACHING

- Tell patient to take drug at bedtime. Instruct patient not to exceed prescribed dosage and not to stop drug abruptly.

! **WARNING** Warn patient that, although rare, drug may cause swelling of the oral cavity or throat, which could cause airway obstruction. If swelling occurs, patient should seek emergency care immediately and never take flurazepam again.

- Caution patient about possible morning dizziness or drowsiness.

- Advise patient to avoid hazardous activities until drug's CNS effects are known.
- Caution patient to avoid alcohol and CNS depressants during therapy.
- Advise patient to notify prescriber if she becomes or intends to become pregnant during therapy.
- Inform patient that sleep may be disturbed for the first few nights after stopping drug.
- Warn patient and caregiver that some patients have performed bizarre activities after taking drug, such as driving a car, eating food, having sex, or making phone calls while not fully awake and often with no memory of the event. These episodes usually occur in patients who have taken the drug with alcohol or other CNS depressant or who have exceeded the recommended dose. If such an episode occurs, the prescriber should be notified and flurazepam therapy discontinued immediately.

fluticasone propionate

Armonair Respiclick, Flonase, Flonase Allergy Relief, Flovent Diskus, Flovent HFA, Xhance

fluticasone furoate

Arnuity Ellipta, Flonase Sensimist

☰ Class and Category

Pharmacologic class: Corticosteroid
Therapeutic class: Antiasthmatic, anti-inflammatory

☰ Indications and Dosages

✳ *To prevent asthma attacks, alone or with oral corticosteroids as maintenance therapy*

INHALATION AEROSOL (FLOVENT HFA)

Adults and children age 12 and over not on an inhaled corticosteroid. *Initial:* 88 mcg twice daily. After 2 wk, dosage may be increased, as needed. *Maximum:* 880 mcg twice daily.

Adults and children age 12 and over previously taking other corticosteroids. Initial dosage highly individualized and based on previous asthma therapy and severity. After 2 wks, dosage may be increased, as needed. *Maximum:* 880 mcg twice daily.

Children ages 4 to 11 regardless of previous therapy. 88 mcg inhaled twice daily. *Maximum:* 88 mcg twice daily.

INHALATION AEROSOL (FLOVENT DISKUS)

Adults and children age 12 and over not on an inhaled corticosteroid. *Initial:* 100 mcg twice daily, about 12 hr apart. After 2 wk, dosage may be increased, as needed. *Maximum:* 1,000 mcg twice daily.

Adults and children age 12 and over previously taking other corticosteroids. Initial dosage highly individualized and based on previous asthma therapy and severity. After 2 wks, dosage may be increased, as needed. *Maximum:* 1,000 mcg twice daily.

Children ages 4 to 11 not taking an inhaled corticosteroid. *Initial:* 50 mcg inhaled twice daily, increased as needed to 100 mcg twice daily. *Maximum:* 100 mcg inhaled twice daily.

Children ages 4 to 11 taking other corticosteroids. Initial dosage highly individualized based on previous asthma therapy and severity. After 2 wks, dosage may be increased to 100 mcg twice daily. *Maximum:* 100 mcg twice daily.

INHALATION AEROSOL (ARMONAIR RESPICLICK)

Adults and children age 12 and older not on inhaled corticosteroids. 55 mcg inhaled twice daily.

Adults and children age 12 and older switching from another inhaled corticosteroid. Individualized based upon strength of previous inhaled corticosteroid and disease severity. Dosage may be low at 55 mcg inhaled twice daily, medium at 113 mcg inhaled twice daily, or high at 232 mcg inhaled twice daily, with dosage increase from lower dosages after 2 wk, if needed. *Maximum:* 232 mg inhaled twice daily.

Children age 4 to 11 years not taking inhaled corticosteroids. 30 mcg twice daily.

Children age 4 to 11 years switching from another inhaled corticosteroid. 30 mcg or 55 mcg twice daily based on the strength of the previous inhaled corticosteroid. *Maximum:* 55 mcg twice daily.

INHALATION AEROSOL (ARNUITY ELLIPTA)

Adults and children age 12 and older not on inhaled corticosteroid therapy. 100 mcg inhaled once daily, increased after 2 wk to 200 mcg once daily, as needed. *Maximum: 200 mcg once daily.*

Adults and children age 12 and older receiving other drug treatments for asthma. Highly individualized based on patient's previous asthma drug therapy and disease severity.

Children age 5 to 11. 50 mcg inhaled once daily.

✳ *To manage nasal symptoms of perennial nonallergic rhinitis*

NASAL SUSPENSION (FLONASE, FLONASE ALLERGY RELIEF)

Adults. *Initial:* 100 mcg (2 sprays) in each nostril once daily or 50 mcg (1 spray) in each nostril twice daily. *Maximum:* 100 mcg (2 sprays) in each nostril daily.

Children ages 4 and over. 50 mcg (1 spray) in each nostril, daily, increased, as needed, to 100 mcg (2 sprays) in each nostril, daily. *Maximum:* 100 mcg (2 sprays) in each nostril daily.

✳ *To treat perennial and seasonal allergic rhinitis*

NASAL SUSPENSION (FLONASE SENSIMIST)

Adults and children ages 12 and over. *Initial:* 55 mcg (2 sprays) in each nostril once daily for 1 wk. Beginning wk 2 through 6 mo, 27.5 or 55 mcg (1 to 2 sprays) in each nostril once daily.

Children ages 2 to 11. 27.5 mcg (1 spray) in each nostril.

✳ *To treat nasal polyps*

NASAL SPRAY (XHANCE)

Adults. 1 spray (93 mcg) in each nostril twice daily, increased to 2 sprays (186 mcg) in each nostril twice daily, if needed. *Maximum:* 2 sprays (186 mcg) in each nostril twice daily for total daily dose of 744 mcg.

▤ Drug Administration

- If two doses are prescribed daily, space doses about 12 hours apart and administer at the same time every day.
- Avoid exposing inhalers and nasal sprays to extreme cold, heat, and humidity.

INHALATION

- Follow manufacturer guidelines for administering product prescribed. Check to see if product has to be primed before first use and if not used for a period of time.
- Do not use spacer or volume holding chamber with Armonair Respiclick.
- If patient is prescribed 2 inhalations, wait at least 1 minute between them.
- If patient is prescribed more than 1 inhaler, use fluticasone last, at least 5 minutes after previous inhaler.
- Have patient gargle and rinse mouth after each dose of an oral inhaler to help prevent dry mouth and throat, oropharyngeal yeast infection, and throat irritation.
- Clean inhaler according to manufacturer guidelines at least once a week after evening dose. However, when using Armonair Respiclick brand, never wash or put any part of inhaler in water, as routine maintenance is not required. If the mouthpiece should be cleaned, gently wipe mouthpiece with a dry cloth or tissue.
- When counter reaches 000 or 0, discard the inhaler. Flovent Diskus should be discarded after 6 weeks for 50-mcg strength or 2 months for 100- and 250-mcg strengths after opening the foil pouch or when counter reads 0, whichever comes first.

INTRANASAL

- Shake container well before each use.
- Prime the container before using for the first time by pressing the bottle six times (Flonase) or seven times (Xhance) or until a fine mist appears. If the container is not used for 7 days or more, container will have to be reprimed with six sprays for Flonase and two sprays for Xhance.
- To administer Flonase, have patient blow nose. Then have patient close one nostril while tilting head slightly forward and keeping bottle upright. Then have patient carefully insert the nasal applicator into the other nostril. Tell patient to press firmly and quickly down 1 time on the applicator while breathing in through the nose. Repeat steps if two sprays are needed with other nostril.
- Wipe nasal applicator with a clean tissue and replace cover.
- To administer Xhance, have patient insert the tip of the nosepiece deep into one nostril and form a tight seal between the nosepiece and nostril. Next, have patient place the mouthpiece into mouth, bending it, if needed, to maintain a tight seal. Have

E
F

patient blow hard into the mouthpiece, and while continuing to blow, have patient push the bottle up to actuate the spray pump. Repeat the process in the other nostril.

- Although Xhance container does not have to be cleaned, it can be wiped after each use with a clean, dry, lint-free cloth.
- Protect Xhance from light and discard after using 120 sprays after initial priming.

Route	Onset	Peak	Duration
Inhalation	24 hr	Unknown	Unknown
Nasal	< 12 hr	Unknown	24 hr

Half-life: 11–12 hr

Mechanism of Action

Inhibits cells involved in the inflammatory response of asthma, such as basophils, eosinophils, lymphocytes, macrophages, mast cells, and neutrophils. Fluticasone also inhibits production or secretion of chemical mediators, such as cytokines eicosanoids, histamine, and leukotrienes. These actions also relieve nasal symptoms of rhinitis.

Contraindications

Hypersensitivity to fluticasone or its components, or to milk proteins; primary treatment of status asthmaticus or other acute asthma episodes that require intensive measures (inhalation form); untreated nasal mucosal infection (nasal suspension)

Interactions

DRUGS

strong CYP3A4 inhibitors such as atazanavir, clarithromycin, indinavir, itraconazole, ketoconazole, nefazodone, nelfinavir, ritonavir, saquinavir, telithromycin: Possibly increased fluticasone level with increased risk of corticosteroid adverse effects

Adverse Reactions

CNS: Aggressiveness, agitation, anxiety, depression, difficulty speaking, dizziness, fatigue, fever, headache, insomnia, irritability, malaise, restlessness

EENT: Allergic rhinitis, blurred vision, cataracts, central serous chorioretinopathy, conjunctivitis, dental caries, difficulty speaking, dry mouth and throat, ear infection, epistaxis, esophageal candidiasis, eye irritation, facial and **oropharyngeal edema**, glaucoma, hoarseness, impaired nasal wound healing, laryngitis, loss of voice, nasal *Candida* infection, nasal congestion or discharge, nasal discomfort (burning, dryness, irritation, soreness), nasal sinus pain, nasal septal perforation or ulceration, nasopharyngitis, oropharyngeal candidiasis, otitis media, pharyngitis, rhinitis, sinusitis, throat irritation, tonsillitis, tooth discoloration

ENDO: Adrenal insufficiency, cushingoid symptoms, hyperglycemia, slower growth in children

GI: Abdominal pain, diarrhea, indigestion, nausea, vomiting

GU: Dysmenorrhea

HEME: Churg–Strauss syndrome, easy bruising, eosinophilia

MS: Arthralgia, back pain, bone mineral density reduction (long-term use), myalgia, osteoporosis

RESP: Asthma exacerbation, bronchitis, **bronchospasm,** chest congestion and tightness, cough, dyspnea, pneumonia, upper respiratory tract infection, wheezing

SKIN: Dermatitis, ecchymosis, pruritus, rash, urticaria

Other: Anaphylaxis, angioedema, flu-like symptoms, immunosuppression, infections, weight gain

Childbearing Considerations

PREGNANCY

- It is not known if drug causes fetal harm.
- Use with caution only if benefit to mother outweighs potential risk to fetus.

LACTATION

- It is not known if drug is present in breast milk.
- Patient should check with prescriber before breastfeeding.

Nursing Considerations

- Use fluticasone cautiously in patients with ocular herpes simplex, pulmonary tuberculosis, or untreated systemic bacterial, fungal, parasitic, or viral infection. Monitor patient throughout therapy for signs and symptoms of infection, as drug causes immunosuppression and increased risk of infections. Also, use cautiously in patients with moderate or severe hepatic impairment.

! **WARNING** Monitor patient closely at start of therapy for a hypersensitivity reaction, especially if patient has severe allergy to milk. If hypersensitivity reaction occurs, notify prescriber, expect drug to be discontinued, and provide supportive care, as prescribed.

- Know that if patient takes a systemic corticosteroid, expect to taper dosage by no more than 2.5 mg daily at weekly intervals, starting 1 week after fluticasone therapy begins.

! **WARNING** Be aware that if patient is switched from systemic corticosteroid to fluticasone, assess for adrenal insufficiency (fatigue, hypotension, lassitude, nausea, vomiting, weakness) early in therapy and when patient has infection, stress, surgery, trauma, or other electrolyte-depleting conditions or procedures. Notify prescriber immediately if signs or symptoms develop. Also, be aware that the patient should be weaned slowly from systemic corticosteroid use. For example, expect to reduce daily prednisone dose by 2.5 mg on a weekly basis with fluticasone therapy.

- Administer a fast-acting inhaled bronchodilator, as ordered, if bronchospasm occurs immediately after fluticasone use. Expect to stop fluticasone and start another drug therapy.
- Expect to titrate fluticasone to lowest effective dosage after asthma has stabilized.
- Notify prescriber if patient develops ocular adverse reactions because fluticasone therapy may cause many (cataracts, increased intraocular pressure, and glaucoma) that should be checked by an ophthalmologist.

PATIENT TEACHING
- Urge patient to use fluticasone regularly, as prescribed, and stress that drug is not for acute bronchospasm. Instruct her to have a rescue inhaler accessible if acute bronchospasm occurs.
- Teach patient how to administer drug according to the form prescribed (nasal spray or oral inhaler) and product being used.
- Tell patient prescribed 2 inhalations to wait at least 1 minute between them.
- Instruct patient to gargle and rinse her mouth after each dose of an oral inhaler

to help prevent dry mouth and throat and oropharyngeal yeast infection and relieve throat irritation.

- Instruct patient prescribed more than 1 inhaler to use fluticasone last, at least 5 minutes after previous inhaler.
- Instruct patient to clean inhaler according to manufacturer guidelines at least once a week after her evening dose. Alert patient prescribed Armonair Respiclick brand never to wash or put any part of the inhaler in water, as routine maintenance is not required. Tell patient that if the mouthpiece needs cleaning, gently wipe the mouthpiece with a dry cloth or tissue.
- Inform patient that, when counter reads 000 or 0, she should discard the inhaler.
- Explain that symptoms may improve within 2 days but that full improvement may not occur for 1 to 2 weeks or longer.
- Caution patient not to increase dosage but to contact prescriber after 1 week if symptoms continue or worsen.

! **WARNING** Urge patient to tell prescriber immediately if asthma attacks don't respond to bronchodilators during fluticasone therapy or if an allergic reaction occurs.

- Know that if patient is switching from an oral corticosteroid to fluticasone, urge her to carry medical identification indicating the need for supplemental systemic corticosteroids during stress or severe asthma attack.
- Caution patient to avoid people who have infections because fluticasone suppresses the immune system, increasing the risk of infection. Instruct patient to notify prescriber about exposure to chickenpox, measles, or other infections because additional treatment may be needed.
- Instruct patient to report ocular adverse reactions to prescriber.

fluvastatin sodium
Lescol XL

⦀ Class and Category
Pharmacologic class: HMG-CoA reductase inhibitor
Therapeutic class: Antilipemic

E
F

Indications and Dosages

＊ *As adjunct to lower cholesterol level in primary hypercholesterolemia (heterozygous familial and nonfamilial) and mixed dyslipidemia (Fredrickson Type IIa and II b) in patients whose response to dietary restriction and other nonpharmacologic measures has been inadequate; to decrease progression of coronary atherosclerosis; to reduce risk in patients with coronary artery disease undergoing coronary revascularization*

CAPSULES

Adults. 20 to 40 mg daily, increased up to 40 mg twice daily, as needed. *Maximum:* 40 mg twice daily.

E.R. TABLETS

Adults. 80 mg once daily. *Maximum:* 80 mg daily.

＊ *As adjunct to lower cholesterol level in children with heterozygous familial hypercholesterolemia whose LDL-C remains 190 ml/dl or greater or whose LDL-C remains 160 mg/dl or greater combined with a positive family history of premature cardiovascular disease or two or more other cardiovascular disease risk factors are present*

CAPSULES, E.R. TABLETS

Boys and girls (who are at least 1 year past menarche) ages 10 to 16. *Initial:* 20 mg once daily (immediate-release capsule), increased every 6 wk, as needed. *Maximum:* 40 mg twice daily (immediate-release capsule) or 80 mg once daily (E.R. tablet).

±**DOSAGE ADJUSTMENT** For patients taking cyclosporine or fluconazole, dosage not to exceed 20 mg twice daily.

Drug Administration

P.O.

- Capsules and tablets should be swallowed whole and not chewed, crushed, or split/opened.
- Administer immediate-release capsules in the evening. Do not administer two 40-mg capsules at the same time.
- Administer E.R. tablets at any time of day, but be consistent.

Route	Onset	Peak	Duration
P.O.	Unknown	1 hr	Unknown
P.O. (E.R.)	Unknown	3 hr	Unknown

Half-life: 3–9 hr

Mechanism of Action

Interferes with the hepatic enzyme hydroxymethylglutaryl-coenzyme A reductase, reducing formation of mevalonic acid (a cholesterol precursor) and interrupting the pathway by which cholesterol is synthesized. When cholesterol level declines in hepatic cells, LDLs are consumed, which reduces circulating total cholesterol and serum triglycerides.

Contraindications

Acute hepatic disease, hypersensitivity to fluvastatin or its components, pregnancy or in women who may become pregnant, unexplained persistently elevated liver enzyme levels

Interactions

DRUGS

colchicine, cyclosporine, erythromycin, gemfibrozil, niacin, other fibrates: Increased risk of severe myopathy and rhabdomyolysis
cyclosporine, fluconazole, glyburide, phenytoin: Increased drug levels of these drugs
protease inhibitors: Possible increased blood fluvastatin level; possible increased risk of myopathy and rhabdomyolysis
rifampin: Significantly decreased blood fluvastatin level, increased plasma clearance
warfarin: Possibly increased bleeding and/or increased prothrombin times

ACTIVITIES

alcohol use: Increased risk of liver dysfunction

Adverse Reactions

CNS: Dizziness, fatigue, headache, hypoesthesia, insomnia, memory loss, weakness
EENT: Pharyngitis, rhinitis, sinusitis
ENDO: Adrenal insufficiency, decreased gonadal steroid hormone production, elevated hemoglobin A1c levels, hyperglycemia
GI: Abdominal cramps and pain, anorexia, cirrhosis, constipation, diarrhea, elevated liver enzymes, flatulence, fulminant hepatic necrosis, hepatic failure, hepatitis, hepatoma, hyperbilirubinemia, indigestion, jaundice, nausea, pancreatitis, vomiting
GU: UTI
MS: Arthritis, back pain, immune-mediated necrotizing myopathy, muscle pain, myalgia, myopathy, myositis, rhabdomyolysis

RESP: Bronchitis, cough, **interstitial lung disease**, upper respiratory tract infection
SKIN: Pruritus, rash

Childbearing Considerations

PREGNANCY

- Drug may cause fetal harm because cholesterol and cholesterol derivatives are needed for normal fetal development.
- Drug is contraindicated in pregnant women or women who may become pregnant.

LACTATION

- Drug is present in breast milk.
- Breastfeeding is not recommended during drug therapy.

Nursing Considerations

! **WARNING** Expect to stop drug if CK level rises sharply or myopathy is suspected.

- Expect liver enzymes to be checked before fluvastatin therapy starts and then thereafter as clinically necessary.
- Assess patient for signs and symptoms of hepatic dysfunction such as dark urine or jaundice, fatigue, and/or elevation in liver enzymes to more than 3 times the upper limit of normal. Also look for hyperbilirubinemia. If present, notify prescriber and expect fluvastatin to be discontinued until cause of liver dysfunction has been identified. If no cause can be found, expect the drug to be discontinued permanently.
- Monitor patient for hyperglycemia, especially diabetic patients, and for other endocrine signs and symptoms. Notify prescriber, if present.

PATIENT TEACHING

- Instruct patient to take once-daily immediate-release capsule in the evening and E.R. capsule any time of day, but to be consistent. Also tell patient taking two 40-mg capsules daily to separate the doses by several hours.
- Urge patient to comply with monthly laboratory tests early in treatment.
- Tell patient to follow prescribed low-fat diet.
- Encourage patient to notify prescriber promptly about muscle pain or unexplained weakness.
- Instruct patient with diabetes to monitor his blood glucose level more closely.

fluvoxamine maleate

Class and Category

Pharmacologic class: Selective serotonin reuptake inhibitor (SSRI)
Therapeutic class: Antidepressant

Indications and Dosages

✱ *To treat obsessive–compulsive disorder*

TABLETS

Adults. *Initial:* 50 mg daily at bedtime, increased by 50 mg every 4 to 7 days, as needed. *Maximum:* 300 mg daily, with doses greater than 100 mg daily given as 2 divided doses.
Children ages 8 to 17. *Initial:* 25 mg daily at bedtime, increased by 25 mg every 4 to 7 days, as needed. *Maximum:* 200 mg daily (children ages 8 to 11) and 300 mg daily (children ages 11 to 17), with doses greater than 50 mg daily divided into 2 doses.

E.R. CAPSULES

Adults. *Initial:* 100 mg daily at bedtime, increased by 50 mg weekly, if needed. *Maximum:* 300 mg daily.

±**DOSAGE ADJUSTMENT** For elderly patients or those with hepatic impairment, initial dosage decreased for immediate-release form and dosage increases made more slowly for both immediate-release and extended-release forms.

Drug Administration

P.O.

- Administer once-daily dosage at bedtime; twice-daily dosage, once in the morning and once at bedtime.
- Capsules and tablets should be swallowed whole and not chewed, crushed, or opened.

Route	Onset	Peak	Duration
P.O.	Unknown	3–8 hr	Unknown
P.O./E.R.	Unknown	Unknown	Unknown

Half-life: 9–28 hr

Mechanism of Action

May potentiate serotonin's action by blocking its reuptake at neuronal membranes. An elevated serotonin level may elevate mood and decrease depression and anxiety, which often accompany obsessive–compulsive disorder.

Contraindications

Alosetron, pimozide, thioridazine, or tizanidine therapy; hypersensitivity to fluvoxamine maleate or its components; use within 14 days of MAO inhibitor, including intravenous methylene blue and linezolid

Interactions

DRUGS

alosetron, antipsychotics, benzodiazepines, tacrine, ramelteon, tricyclic antidepressants: Elevated plasma levels of these drugs with increased risk of adverse reactions
amphetamines, buspirone, fentanyl, linezolid, lithium, methylene blue (intravenous), other serotonergic drugs, St. John's wort, tramadol, tricyclic antidepressants, triptans, tryptophan: Increased risk of serotonin syndrome
aspirin, NSAIDs, warfarin: Risk of bleeding
astemizole, cisapride, pimozide, terfenadine, thioridazine: Possibly fatal QT prolongation
carbamazepine: Increased risk of carbamazepine toxicity
clozapine: Increased blood clozapine level increasing risk of orthostatic hypotension and seizures
diltiazem: Increased risk of bradycardia
lithium: Possibly increased serotonin reuptake action of fluvoxamine and increased risk of seizures
MAO inhibitors: Possibly serious or fatal reactions (such as agitation, autonomic instability, coma, delirium, fluctuating vital signs, hyperthermia, myoclonus, and rigidity); increased risk of serotonin syndrome
methadone: Possibly significantly increased blood methadone level, increased risk of methadone toxicity
metoprolol, propranolol, and other beta-blockers: Increased blood levels of these drugs, possibly reduced diastolic blood pressure and heart rate induced by these drugs
mexiletine: Possibly decreased clearance of mexiletine
pimozide, thioridazine: Increased plasma levels of these drugs with increased risk of QT interval associated with serious ventricular arrhythmias
sumatriptan: Increased risk of hyperreflexia, incoordination, and weakness

theophylline: Decreased theophylline clearance, increased risk of theophylline toxicity
tizanidine: Increased risk of serious adverse effects, such as hypotension and profound sedation
tryptophan: Enhanced effect of tryptophan and possibly induced severe vomiting
warfarin: Significant increased plasma level of warfarin with prolonged prothrombin time

ACTIVITIES

alcohol: Possibly increased CNS effects
smoking: Increased fluvoxamine metabolism

Adverse Reactions

CNS: Agitation, anxiety, apathy, chills, confusion, depression, dizziness, drowsiness, fatigue, headache, hypomania, insomnia, malaise, mania, nervousness, **neuroleptic malignant syndrome**, sedation, **serotonin syndrome**, **suicidal ideation**, tremor, vertigo, yawning
CV: Palpitations, tachycardia, vasculitis, **ventricular tachycardia**
EENT: Acute-angle glaucoma, altered taste, blurred vision, dry mouth
GI: Anorexia, constipation, diarrhea, flatulence, **hepatitis**, ileus, indigestion, nausea, **pancreatitis**, **upper GI bleeding**, vomiting
GU: **Acute renal failure**, amenorrhea, decreased libido, delayed or absent orgasm (females), erectile dysfunction, ejaculation disorders, impotence, urinary frequency, urine retention
HEME: **Agranulocytosis, aplastic anemia, bleeding events**
MS: Muscle twitching
RESP: Dyspnea, upper respiratory tract infection
SKIN: Bullous eruption, diaphoresis, Henoch-Schoenlein purpura, rash, **Stevens–Johnson syndrome, toxic epidermal necrolysis**
Other: Anaphylaxis, **angioedema**, flu-like symptoms, weight gain

Childbearing Considerations

PREGNANCY

- Pregnancy exposure registry: 1-844-405-6185 or https://womensmentalhealth.org/clinical-and-research-programs/pregnancyregistry/antidepressants/.
- It is not known if drug causes fetal harm but may have adverse effects if given late in third trimester.

- Use with caution only if benefit to mother outweighs potential risk to fetus.

LABOR & DELIVERY

- Fetal exposure to drug late in third trimester may cause neonatal complications as soon as birth.
- Complications such as persistent pulmonary hypertension of the newborn may require prolonged hospitalization, respiratory support, and tube feeding.

LACTATION

- Drug is present in breast milk.
- Patient should check with prescriber before breastfeeding.
- If breastfeeding occurs, infant should be monitored for agitation, decreased sleep, diarrhea, and vomiting.

REPRODUCTION

- Fertility may be impaired while taking drug according to animal studies.

Nursing Considerations

- Use fluvoxamine cautiously in patients with cardiovascular disease, impaired hepatic or renal function, mania, seizures, or suicidal tendencies.

! **WARNING** Be aware that fluvoxamine shouldn't be given within 14 days of an MAO inhibitor.

! **WARNING** Monitor patient for possible serotonin syndrome, characterized by agitation, chills, confusion, diaphoresis, diarrhea, fever, hyperactive reflexes, poor coordination, restlessness, shaking, talking or acting with uncontrolled excitement, tremor, and twitching, especially if patient is receiving another drug that raises serotonin level (such as amphetamine, dopamine agonist, MAO inhibitor, tryptophan, or other antidepressant or psychostimulant). In its most severe form, serotonin syndrome can resemble neuroleptic malignant syndrome, which includes autonomic instability, a high fever, muscle rigidity, and possible fluctuations in vital signs and mental status.

- Watch patient closely (especially children, adolescents, and young adults), for suicidal tendencies, particularly when therapy starts and dosage changes, because depression may worsen temporarily during these times and lead to suicidal ideation.

- Monitor patient for bleeding, especially if patient also takes aspirin, an anticoagulant, or NSAID. Bleeding can range from ecchymoses, epistaxis, hematomas, and petechiae to life-threatening hemorrhage.
- Discontinue fluvoxamine therapy gradually, as ordered, to prevent unpleasant adverse reactions.

PATIENT TEACHING

- Instruct patient to take once-a-day dose at bedtime.
- Tell patient capsules and tablets must be swallowed whole and not chewed, crushed, or split/opened.
- Caution patient not to drink alcohol during fluvoxamine therapy.
- Urge patient to avoid potentially hazardous activities until drug's CNS effects are known.

! **WARNING** Inform patient that fluvoxamine increases the risk of a rare but serious problem: serotonin syndrome. Encourage her to notify prescriber immediately if symptoms develop.

- Caution patient not to stop taking drug abruptly. Explain that gradual tapering helps avoid withdrawal symptoms.
- Urge family or caregiver to watch patient closely for suicidal tendencies, especially when therapy starts or dosage changes and particularly if patient is a child, teenager, or young adult.
- Warn patient that fluvoxamine increases bleeding risk if taken with an anticoagulant, aspirin, or an NSAID and that bleeding events could range from mild to severe. Tell patient to seek emergency care for serious or prolonged bleeding.
- Advise patient that drug may cause mild pupillary dilation, which may lead to an episode of acute-angle glaucoma. Encourage patient to have an eye exam before starting therapy to see if she is at risk.
- Alert patient that drug may cause sexual dysfunction and to discuss concerns with prescriber.

! **WARNING** Advise pregnant patient to consult with prescriber before her third trimester about ongoing fluvoxamine therapy because of an increased risk to her unborn child.

fondaparinux sodium
Arixtra

Class and Category
Pharmacologic class: Activated factor X inhibitor
Therapeutic class: Anticoagulant

Indications and Dosages
* *To provide prophylaxis against deep vein thrombosis, which may lead to pulmonary embolism in patients undergoing abdominal surgery, hip fracture surgery, hip replacement surgery, or knee replacement surgery in patients at risk for thromboembolic complications*

SUBCUTANEOUS INJECTION
Adults. *Initial:* After hemostasis has been established, 2.5 mg 6 to 8 hr after surgery, followed by 2.5 mg daily for 5 to 9 days, except for hip fracture surgery which may be given up to 24 additional days for a total of 32 days.

* *To treat acute deep vein thrombosis (with warfarin); to treat acute pulmonary embolism (with warfarin) in a hospital setting*

SUBCUTANEOUS INJECTION
Adults weighing more than 100 kg (220 lb). 10 mg once daily for at least 5 days and until INR is between 2.0 and 3.0 (usually in 5 to 9 days).
Adults weighing 50 kg (110 lb) to 100 kg (220 lb). 7.5 mg once daily for at least 5 days and until INR is between 2.0 and 3.0 (usually in 5 to 9 days).
Adults weighing less than 50 kg (110 lb). 5 mg once daily for at least 5 days and until INR is between 2.0 and 3.0 (usually in 5 to 9 days).

Drug Administration
SUBCUTANEOUS
* Do not handle needle guard on prefilled syringe if latex sensitive, because it contains dry natural latex rubber.
* Never administer as an I.M. injection.
* Don't give initial dose less than 6 hours after surgery.
* Don't expel air bubble from prefilled syringe before injection, to prevent expelling drug from syringe.
* Alternate injection sites using left and right anterolateral or left and right posterolateral abdominal wall.

* After injecting drug, the plunger should be released. The plunger will then rise automatically while the needle is withdrawn from the skin and retracted into the security sleeve. To be certain the syringe safety feature has worked, listen or feel for a soft click when the plunger rod is released fully. When the needle is pulled back into the security sleeve, the white safety indicator will appear above the upper body.
* Store drug at a controlled room temperature.

Route	Onset	Peak	Duration
SubQ	Unknown	2–3 hr	Unknown

Half-life: 17–21 hr

Mechanism of Action
Selectively binds to antithrombin III, which enhances the inactivation of clotting factor Xa by antithrombin III. Inactivation of factor Xa interrupts the blood coagulation pathway, which then inhibits thrombin formation. Without thrombin, fibrinogen can't convert to fibrin and clots can't form.

Contraindications
Active major bleeding; bacterial endocarditis; body weight less than 50 kg (110 lb) for venous thromboembolism prophylaxis; fondaparinux-induced thrombocytopenia associated with a positive in vitro test for antiplatelet antibodies; hypersensitivity to fondaparinux or its components; severe renal impairment (creatinine clearance less than 30 ml/min)

Interactions
DRUGS
drugs that increase risk of bleeding: Increased risk of hemorrhage and epidural or spinal hematoma

Adverse Reactions
CNS: Confusion, dizziness, fever, headache, insomnia
CV: Edema, **hypotension**
GI: Constipation, diarrhea, elevated liver enzymes, indigestion, nausea, vomiting
GU: Urine retention, UTI
HEME: Anemia, **bleeding, elevated activated partial thromboplastin time,** hematoma, **hemorrhage, thrombocytopenia, thrombocytopenia with thrombosis**

SKIN: Bullous eruption, increased wound drainage, purpura, rash
Other: Anaphylaxis; **angioedema**; generalized pain; **hypokalemia**; injection-site bleeding, pruritus, and rash

Childbearing Considerations

PREGNANCY

- It is not known if drug causes fetal harm but drug does cross the placental barrier, which may increase risk of bleeding in the fetus and neonate.
- Use with caution only if benefit to mother outweighs potential risk to fetus.

LABOR & DELIVERY

- Increased risk of bleeding during labor and delivery and epidural or spinal hematoma formation if neuraxial anesthesia is used.
- A shorter-acting anticoagulant may be substituted as delivery approaches.

LACTATION

- It is not known if drug is present in breast milk.
- Patient should check with prescriber before breastfeeding.

Nursing Considerations

- Use fondaparinux cautiously in elderly patients, especially those weighing less than 50 kg (110 lb) and are receiving the drug for pulmonary embolism or deep vein thrombosis, because the risk of drug-induced bleeding increases with age.

! **WARNING** Know that if patient is receiving fondaparinux with epidural or spinal anesthesia or spinal puncture, patient must be watched closely for development of spinal hematoma, which may cause long-term or permanent paralysis. If evidence of neurologic impairment, such as changes in motor or sensory function occurs, notify prescriber immediately because urgent care is needed to minimize hematoma's effect. Risk of spinal or epidural hematoma during fondaparinux therapy is increased by concurrent use of other drugs that affect hemostasis, a history of traumatic or repeated epidural or spinal punctures, or a history of spinal deformity or spinal surgery as well as indwelling epidural catheters. Be aware that optimal timing between the administration of fondaparinux and neuraxial procedures is unknown.

- Closely monitor patient for bleeding (such as ecchymosis, epistaxis, hematemesis, hematuria, and melena), especially those at risk for decreased drug elimination (such as elderly patients and patients with mild to moderate renal impairment) and those at increased risk for bleeding (such as patients with acquired or congenital bleeding disorders; active ulcerative and angiodysplastic GI disease; diabetic retinopathy; hemorrhagic stroke; uncontrolled arterial hypertension; recent brain, spinal, or ophthalmologic surgery; history of heparin-induced thrombocytopenia; and those being treated concomitantly with platelet inhibitors). Also monitor neonates born to mothers taking fondaparinux for bleeding, because drug does cross the placenta.
- Perform periodic CBC, including platelet count, as ordered. Expect prescriber to discontinue drug if platelet count falls below 100,000/mm^3. Be aware that routine coagulation tests, such as INR and PT, are not used to monitor fondaparinux therapy; an anti-Xa assay may be used instead. Also, test stools for occult blood, as ordered.
- Monitor patient with thrombocytopenia for evidence of thrombosis that may appear similar to heparin-induced thrombocytopenia even when no exposure to heparin has taken place. If patient's platelet count falls below 100,000/mm^3, fondaparinux should be discontinued.
- Monitor renal function test results, as ordered. Expect to discontinue drug if labile renal function or severe renal impairment occurs during fondaparinux therapy because the risk of hemorrhage increases as renal function decreases.

PATIENT TEACHING

- Inform patient that fondaparinux can't be taken orally.
- Teach patient or family member how to administer fondaparinux by subcutaneous injection, if needed. Instruct her not to expel air bubble from a prefilled syringe to avoid expelling some of the drug. Tell her to insert the entire needle into a skinfold held between thumb and forefinger, and remind her to alternate administration sites.
- Review safe handling and disposal of syringes and needles.

! WARNING Instruct patient to seek immediate help if she experiences signs of thromboembolism, such as neurologic changes and severe shortness of breath.

- Inform patient about the increased risk of bleeding. Instruct her or family member to watch for and report abdominal or lower back pain, black stools, bleeding gums, bloody urine, or severe headaches.
- Review safe handling and disposal of syringes and needles.
- Advise patient to have follow-up appointments and prescribed laboratory tests.
- Tell patient that fondaparinux may cause serious side effects and to report any persistent, severe, or unusual signs and symptoms to prescriber.

! WARNING Know that if patient is receiving fondaparinux with epidural or spinal anesthesia or spinal puncture, patient must be watched closely for development of spinal hematoma, which may cause long-term or permanent paralysis. If evidence of neurologic impairment, such as changes in sensory or motor function, occurs, notify prescriber immediately, because urgent care is needed to minimize hematoma's effect. Risk of epidural or spinal hematoma during fondaparinux therapy is increased by concurrent use of other drugs that affect hemostasis, a history of traumatic or repeated epidural or spinal punctures, or a history of spinal deformity or spinal surgery. The risk is also increased with indwelling epidural catheters.

- Advise patient to alert prescriber about any new drugs being taken, including over-the-counter drugs and especially drugs that affect clotting such as aspirin or NSAIDs.

formoterol fumarate
Oxeze Turbuhaler (CAN), Perforomist

☰ Class and Category
Pharmacologic class: Selective beta₂-adrenergic agonist
Therapeutic class: Bronchodilator

☰ Indications and Dosages
✳ *To prevent exercise-induced bronchospasm*

POWDER FOR ORAL INHALATION (OXEZE TURBUHALER)
Adults and children age 6 and over. 6 or 12 mcg at least 15 min before exercise every 12 hr as needed. *Maximum:* 24 mcg daily (children) and 48 mcg daily (adults).
✳ *To provide long-term treatment of bronchospasm in patients with chronic obstructive pulmonary disease (COPD), including chronic bronchitis and emphysema*

POWDER FOR ORAL INHALATION (OXEZE TURBUHALER)
Adults. 6 or 12 mcg every 12 hr through inhaler device, dosage increased, as needed. *Maximum:* 48 mcg daily.

SOLUTION FOR ORAL INHALATION (PERFOROMIST)
Adults. 20 mcg twice daily by nebulization. *Maximum:* 40 mcg daily.

☰ Drug Administration
INHALATION
Perforomist
- Administer solution only by oral inhalation.
- Store drug in its original packaging, and open immediately before use.
- Give inhalation solution only by standard jet nebulizer and air compressor.

Oxeze turbuhaler
- If using for the first time, prime inhaler. Hold the inhaler upright and turn the greenish-blue grip as far as it will go in one direction, then turn in the opposite direction. Repeat turning process one more time. At some point in the process a click will be heard; this is part of the process. After initial priming, inhaler need not be reprimed even if the inhaler is not used regularly.
- To load a dose, hold container in an upright position. Turn the greenish-blue grip as far as it will go in one direction and then turn in the opposite direction. A dose has now been loaded. At some point a clicking sound will be heard; this is part of the process. Do not interrupt the turning process. If inhaler is dropped or shaken or if patient breathes out into the turbuhaler, the dose will be lost and the loading steps will have to be repeated.
- To administer, hand loaded inhaler to patient and have patient breathe out away from mouthpiece, then close the

mouthpiece gently between the teeth, and close lips over the mouthpiece. The mouthpiece should not be bitten or chewed. Tell patient to inhale as deeply and strongly as possible. Remove mouthpiece before exhalation. Repeat loading and administration steps if more than one dose has been prescribed.
- Mouthpiece should be cleaned once a week with a dry tissue. Never use water or any other fluid.
- For the last 10 doses, the dose indicator will become a dash instead of a number. When the 0 appears, discard.

Route	Onset	Peak	Duration
Oral inhalation	<15 min	1–3 hr	12 hr

Half-life: 7–10 hr

Mechanism of Action

Selectively attaches to beta$_2$ receptors on bronchial membranes, stimulating the intracellular enzyme adenyl cyclase to convert adenosine triphosphate to cAMP. The resulting increase in the intracellular cAMP level inhibits histamine release, relaxes bronchial smooth-muscle cells, and stabilizes mast cells.

Contraindications

Hypersensitivity to formoterol fumarate or its components, patients who also have asthma and are not taking an inhaled corticosteroid, treatment of asthma as monotherapy

Interactions
DRUGS

adrenergics: Possibly increased sympathetic effects of formoterol
beta-blockers: Decreased effects of both beta-blockers and formoterol
corticosteroids, diuretics, xanthine derivatives: Possibly increased hypokalemic effect of formoterol
disopyramide, macrolides, MAO inhibitors, phenothiazines, procainamide, quinidine, tricyclic antidepressants: Possibly prolonged QT interval, increasing risk of ventricular arrhythmias

Adverse Reactions

CNS: Anxiety, dizziness, fatigue, fever, headache, insomnia, malaise, tremor
CV: Angina, **arrhythmias**, chest pain, hypertension, **hypotension**, palpitations, **prolonged QT interval**, tachycardia

EENT: Dry mouth, laryngeal irritation, **laryngeal spasm or swelling**, hoarseness, pharyngitis, rhinitis and tonsillitis (in children), sinusitis
ENDO: Hyperglycemia
GI: Abdominal pain, gastroenteritis, indigestion (in children); nausea
MS: Back pain, leg cramps, muscle spasms
RESP: **Asthma exacerbation**, bronchitis, **bronchospasm**, cough, dyspnea, increased sputum production, **paradoxical bronchospasm**, upper respiratory tract infection
SKIN: Dermatitis, pruritus, rash, urticaria
Other: **Anaphylaxis, angioedema, hypokalemia, metabolic acidosis**

Childbearing Considerations
PREGNANCY
- It is not known if drug causes fetal harm.
- Use with caution only if benefit to mother outweighs potential risk to fetus.

LABOR & DELIVERY
- It is not known if drug affects a pregnant woman or fetus during labor and delivery. However, other beta-agonists may interfere with uterine contractility.
- Use of drug should be restricted to patients during labor and delivery only if benefits outweighs the risks.

LACTATION
- It is not known if drug is present in breast milk.
- Patient should check with prescriber before breastfeeding.

Nursing Considerations
- Know that formoterol therapy should not be used in patients as monotherapy to treat asthma. If asthma is present, patient must be on an inhaled corticosteroid before receiving formoterol because of an increased risk of hospitalization and death. There does not appear to be an increased risk of death with use of formoterol in patients with COPD.

! **WARNING** Be aware that formoterol therapy should not be initiated in patients with acutely deteriorating COPD, which may be a life-threatening condition, nor should it be administered for the relief of acute symptoms.

- Use caution when administering formoterol to patients with cardiovascular disorders such as aneurysm, arrhythmias, coronary insufficiency, hypertension, or pheochromocytoma; in patients with seizure disorders or thyrotoxicosis; and in patients who are unusually responsive to sympathomimetic amines.
- Expect inhaled, short-acting beta$_2$-agonists taken by the patient on a regular basis to be discontinued and used only for symptomatic relief of acute respiratory symptoms when formoterol therapy is begun. If an inhaled, short-acting beta$_2$-agonist has not been prescribed for symptomatic relief of acute respiratory symptoms, expect one to be prescribed.

! **WARNING** Watch closely for paradoxical bronchospasm; if this occurs, discontinue formoterol immediately and notify prescriber. Also monitor patient for hypersensitivity reactions.

- Notify prescriber of any significant increases in pulse rate or blood pressure or worsening of chronic conditions because formoterol may produce cardiovascular reactions, including angina, arrhythmias, hypertension or hypotension, palpitations, and tachycardia. Drug may have to be discontinued if such reactions occur.

PATIENT TEACHING

- Advise patient, especially if she has a significant cardiac history, to inform prescriber of any other drugs she takes before beginning formoterol therapy to prevent harmful drug interactions.
- Instruct patient to use manufacturer's device for inhaling powder form of formoterol and not to use a spacer.
- Teach patient proper use of powdered formoterol delivery system. Emphasize that she should only inhale, not exhale, through device.
- For solution form, teach patient how to use, clean, and store nebulizer equipment. Tell her to leave the vial in its original foil pack until just before use.
- Instruct patient who currently uses inhaled or oral corticosteroids to continue using them, as prescribed, even if she feels better after starting formoterol.

- Caution patient not to increase formoterol dosage or frequency without consulting prescriber because she may need a rapid-acting bronchodilator and excessive use may result in an overdose.
- Urge patient to notify prescriber if her symptoms worsen, if formoterol becomes less effective, or if she needs more inhalations of short-acting beta$_2$-agonist than usual. This may indicate that her asthma is worsening.

! **WARNING** Instruct patient to notify prescriber immediately if she experiences chest pain, nervousness, palpitations, rapid heart rate, or tremor while taking formoterol because dosage may have to be adjusted. Also, alert patient to stop drug and seek immediate emergency care if allergic reaction occurs, such as the presence of difficulty breathing or swallowing, hives, itching, rash, or swelling.

- Ensure that patient has been informed that long-acting beta-agonists, such as formoterol, increase the risk of asthma-related death and should not be used without a long-term asthma control drug prior to starting formoterol therapy.

foscarnet sodium
Foscavir

☰ Class and Category
Pharmacologic class: Pyrophosphate analogue
Therapeutic class: Antiviral

☰ Indications and Dosages
❋ *To treat cytomegalovirus (CMV) retinitis in patients with acquired immunodeficiency syndrome (AIDS)*

I.V. INFUSION
Adults. *Initial:* 90 mg/kg every 12 hr or 60 mg/kg every 8 hr for 2 to 3 wks, depending on clinical response. *Maintenance:* 90 mg/kg/day to 120 mg/kg/day.

❋ *To treat acyclovir-resistant mucocutaneous herpes simplex virus (HSV) infections in immunocompromised patients*

I.V. INFUSION
Adults. 40 mg/kg given either every 8 or 12 hr for 2 to 3 wk or until healing has taken place.

± **DOSAGE ADJUSTMENT** For patients with renal impairment, dosage calculated individually when creatinine clearance becomes 1.4 ml/min/kg or less.

Drug Administration

I.V.

- Calculate each dose, even in the presence of a normal serum creatinine, to reduce risk of nephrotoxicity.
- Maintain adequate hydration of patient to reduce the risk of nephrotoxicity. Expect to administer 750 to 1,000 ml of 0.9% Sodium Chloride Injection or 5% Dextrose Injection prior to the first infusion to establish diuresis. With subsequent infusions, expect to infuse 750 to 1,000 ml of hydration fluid with a dose of 90 to 120 mg/kg of foscarnet and 500 ml of hydration fluid with a dose of 40 to 60 mg/kg. Oral hydration may be used instead if patient is able to drink the required amount of fluid.
- Do not administer drug by bolus or rapid intravenous injection.
- The standard 24-mg/ml solution may be used with or without dilution when using a central venous catheter for infusion. If a peripheral vein catheter is used, the standard 24-mg/ml solution must be diluted to a 12-mg/ml concentration with 0.9% Sodium Chloride Injection or 5% Dextrose Injection prior to administration to avoid local irritation of peripheral veins.
- Use an infusion pump to control the rate of infusion.
- Administer at a rate not exceeding 1 mg/kg/min and over a minimum of at least 1 hour (doses of 90 mg/kg and higher given over at least 1.5 to 2 hr).
- Discard diluted solution within 24 hours.
- Flush eyes or skin with water if accidental contact with drug occurs, because a burning sensation and local irritation may occur.
- *Incompatibilities:* 30% dextrose, acyclovir sodium, amphotericin, diazepam, digoxin, divalent cations, ganciclovir, leucovorin, midazolam, pentamidine isethionate, phenytoin, prochlorperazine, solutions containing calcium such as Ringer's lactate and total parenteral nutrition, trimethoprim/sulfamethoxazole, trimetrexate glucuronate, vancomycin

Route	Onset	Peak	Duration
I.V.	Unknown	Unknown	Unknown

Half-life: 2–4 hr

Mechanism of Action

Selectively inhibits the pyrophosphate binding site on virus-specific DNA polymerases, which inhibits herpes virus replication.

Contraindications

Hypersensitivity to foscarnet sodium or its components

Interactions

DRUGS

acyclovir, aminoglycosides, amphotericin B, cyclosporine, loop diuretics, methotrexate, pentamidine (intravenous), ritonavir, ritonavir and saquinavir, tacrolimus: Increased risk of renal dysfunction

class IA antiarrhythmics (procainamide, quinidine), class III antiarrhythmics (amiodarone, dofetilide, sotalol), phenothiazines, selected fluoroquinolones and macrolides, tricyclic antidepressants: Increased risk of QT prolongation and possible torsades de pointes

pentamidine (intravenous) and other drugs known to influence serum calcium levels: Possibly hypocalcemia

Adverse Reactions

CNS: Abnormal coordination, aggressive reaction, agitation, amnesia, anxiety, aphasia, asthenia, ataxia, **coma**, confusion, dementia, depression, dizziness, EEG abnormalities, fatigue, fever, hallucination, headache, hypoesthesia, insomnia, malaise, **meningitis**, nervousness, neuropathy, paresthesia, rigors, **seizures including grand mal**, sensory disturbances, somnolence, **status epilepticus**, stupor, thirst, tremors

CV: **Cardiac arrest**, chest pain, nonacute ECG abnormalities (first-degree AV block, nonspecific ST-T segment changes, sinus tachycardia), edema, elevated gamma GT level, hypertension, **hypotension**, palpitations, **prolonged QT interval**, **torsades de pointes, thrombosis, ventricular arrhythmia**

EENT: Conjunctivitis, dry mouth, eye abnormalities or pain, pharyngitis, rhinitis, sinusitis, **stridor**, taste perversions, vision abnormalities, ulcerative stomatitis

ENDO: Diabetes insipidus (usually nephrogenic), syndrome of inappropriate antidiuretic hormone secretion

GI: Abdominal pain, abnormal albumin-to-globulin ratio, anorexia, cachexia,

E
F

constipation, diarrhea, dyspepsia, dysphagia, elevated liver or pancreatic enzymes, esophageal ulceration, flatulence, **GI hemorrhage, hepatic dysfunction, melena,** nausea, **pancreatitis, rectal hemorrhage,** vomiting

GU: Acute renal failure, acquired Fanconi syndrome, albuminuria, crystal-induced nephropathy, decreased creatinine clearance, dysuria, elevated BUN or serum creatinine level, **glomerulonephritis,** hematuria, **nephrotic syndrome, nephrotoxicity,** nocturia, polyuria, renal calculus or impairment, **renal tubular acidosis or necrosis,** urethral disorder, urinary retention, UTI

HEME: Anemia, **granulocytopenia, leukopenia, neutropenia, pancytopenia, thrombocytopenia**

MS: Arthralgia, back pain, generalized spasms, involuntary muscle contractions, leg cramps, muscle weakness, myalgia, myositis, **rhabdomyolysis**

RESP: Bronchospasm, coughing, dyspnea, **hemoptysis,** pneumonia, **pneumothorax, pulmonary infiltration, respiratory insufficiency**

SKIN: Diaphoresis, **erythema multiforme,** erythematous or maculopapular rash, flushing, pruritus, rash, seborrhea, skin discoloration or ulceration, **Stevens–Johnson syndrome, toxic epidermal necrolysis,** urticaria

Other: Acidosis, **anaphylaxis, angioedema,** dehydration, elevated alkaline phosphatase or LDH, flu-like symptoms, generalized pain, **hypercalcemia, hypernatremia,** hyperphosphatemia, **hypocalcemia, hypokalemia, hypomagnesemia, hypophosphatemia,** hypoproteinemia, infections (bacterial, fungal, moniliasis), injection-site inflammation or pain, localized edema, lymphadenopathy, **lymphoma-like disorder, sarcoma, sepsis,** weight loss

Childbearing Considerations

PREGNANCY

- It is not known if drug causes fetal harm.
- Use with caution only if benefit to mother outweighs potential risk to fetus.

LACTATION

- It is not known if drug is present in breast milk

- The Centers for Disease Control and Prevention recommends that HIV-1 infected mothers not breastfeed to avoid risking postnatal transmission of HIV-1 infection to infants. They also do not recommend breastfeeding because of potential drug-induced adverse reactions in the infant.
- For women with HSV, breastfeeding or the drug should be discontinued.

Nursing Considerations

- Know that foscarnet therapy should not be used in patients on a controlled sodium diet, because of the sodium content of the drug.
- Use cautiously in patients with history of prolonged QT interval, in patients taking drugs known to prolong the QT interval, in patients with electrolyte disturbances, or in patients who have other risk factors for QT prolongation, as QT prolongation and torsades de pointes have occurred with foscarnet therapy. Expect prescriber to order routine electrocardiograms and measure patient's electrolytes before foscarnet therapy is begun and periodically throughout therapy.
- Use foscarnet cautiously in patients with neurologic abnormalities (especially seizure disorders), and patients with decreased total calcium or other electrolyte abnormalities before treatment, as well as in patients receiving other drugs known to influence serum calcium levels.
- Assess patient's estimated or measured creatinine clearance before foscarnet therapy is begun, 2 to 3 times a week during initial therapy, and once weekly during maintenance therapy, as ordered, because most patients will experience some decrease in renal function as a result of foscarnet therapy. Know also that a 24-hour creatinine clearance should be determined before therapy is begun and periodically thereafter to ensure correct dosing. Expect foscarnet to be discontinued if creatinine clearance drops below 0.4 ml/min/kg.
- Determine patient's serum calcium, magnesium, phosphorus, and potassium levels before foscarnet therapy is begun, 2 to 3 times a week during initial therapy, and once weekly during maintenance therapy, as ordered, because foscarnet can chelate

divalent metal ions and alter levels of serum electrolytes.

- Know that combination therapy with foscarnet and ganciclovir is indicated for patients who have relapsed after monotherapy with either drug used to treat CMV retinitis.
- Monitor patient for symptoms of electrolyte abnormalities (mild: perioral numbness or paresthesias; severe: seizures) regularly. If present, notify prescriber and expect serum electrolyte and mineral levels to be assessed as soon as possible and treatment initiated if abnormalities are revealed.

! **WARNING** Assess patient closely for hypersensitivity reactions to foscarnet. Serious acute hypersensitivity reactions have occurred in patients exposed to foscarnet. If present, notify prescriber immediately, expect foscarnet to be discontinued, and provide supportive care, as indicated and ordered.

PATIENT TEACHING

- Advise patient that foscarnet is not a cure for either CMV retinitis or mucocutaneous acyclovir-resistant HSV infection.
- Tell patient that it is important to maintain hydration during foscarnet therapy.
- Inform patient that the major adverse reactions related to foscarnet therapy are electrolyte abnormalities, kidney dysfunction, and seizures. Stress importance of reporting any abnormal, persistent, severe, or unusual signs and symptoms to prescriber, as dosage may have to be adjusted or drug discontinued.

! **WARNING** Advise patient to get immediate emergency medical treatment if she develops any signs of an allergic reaction, such as difficulty breathing, hives, or swelling of her face, lips, tongue, or throat.

- Instruct patient to notify prescriber at once if she experiences serious adverse reactions such as confusion, feeling short of breath, increased thirst, pounding heartbeats, swelling, urinating less than usual or not at all, weakness, or weight gain.
- Caution patient to avoid performing hazardous activities such as driving until the effects of the drug on her nervous system are known and have been resolved.

- Inform mothers that breastfeeding is not recommended during foscarnet therapy, to prevent potentially serious adverse events in the nursing infant.
- Encourage patient being treated for CMV retinitis to have regular ophthalmologic examinations.

fosinopril sodium

☰ Class and Category

Pharmacologic class: Angiotensin-converting enzyme (ACE) inhibitor
Therapeutic class: Antihypertensive, vaso-dilator

☰ Indications and Dosages

✱ *To manage blood pressure, alone or with other antihypertensives*

TABLETS

Adults. *Initial:* 10 mg daily. *Maintenance:* 20 to 40 mg daily or in divided doses. *Maximum:* 80 mg daily.

Children age 6 to 16 years of age and weighing more than 50 kg (110 lb). 5 to 10 mg daily as monotherapy.

✱ *As adjunct to treat heart failure*

TABLETS

Adults. 10 mg daily with dosage increased over several weeks, if needed. *Maintenance:* 20 to 40 mg daily. *Maximum:* 40 mg daily.

±**DOSAGE ADJUSTMENT** Initial dosage reduced to 5 mg daily, if needed, for patients with heart failure who have moderate to severe renal failure or recent aggressive diuresis.

☰ Drug Administration

P.O.

- Observe patient being treated for heart failure for at least 2 hours after giving drug, to detect hypotension or orthostatic hypotension. If either develops, notify prescriber and monitor patient until blood pressure stabilizes. Keep in mind that orthostatic hypotension is unlikely to develop in patient with a systolic blood pressure over 100 mm Hg who has received a 10-mg dose.
- Separate administration times between antacids and fosinopril by at least 2 hours.

Route	Onset	Peak	Duration
P.O.	1 hr	2–6 hr	24 hr

Half-life: 12 hr

Mechanism of Action

May reduce blood pressure by affecting renin–angiotensin–aldosterone system. By inhibiting angiotensin-converting enzyme, fosinopril:

- prevents conversion of angiotensin I to angiotensin II, a potent vasoconstrictor that also stimulates the adrenal cortex to secrete aldosterone
- may inhibit renal and vascular production of angiotensin II
- decreases serum angiotensin II level and increases serum renin activity, which decreases aldosterone secretion, slightly increasing the serum potassium level and fluid loss
- decreases vascular tone and blood pressure
- inhibits aldosterone release, which reduces sodium and water reabsorption and increases their excretion, further reducing blood pressure and symptoms of heart failure.

Contraindications

Hypersensitivity to fosinopril, other ACE inhibitors, or their components

Interactions

DRUGS

antacids: Impaired fosinopril absorption
diuretics, other antihypertensives: Possibly additive hypotension
lithium: Increased blood lithium level and risk of lithium toxicity
potassium-sparing diuretics, potassium supplements: Increased risk of hyperkalemia
sodium aurothiomalate: Nitritoid reactions, including facial flushing, hypotension, nausea, and vomiting

FOODS

salt substitutes: Increased risk of hyperkalemia

Adverse Reactions

CNS: Confusion, depression, dizziness, drowsiness, fatigue, fever, headache, insomnia, mood changes, sleep disturbance, syncope, tremor, vertigo, weakness
CV: Angina, **arrhythmias (including AV conduction disorders, bradycardia**, and tachycardia), claudication, **hypotension, MI**, orthostatic hypotension, palpitations
EENT: Dry mouth, epistaxis, eye irritation, hoarseness, rhinitis, sinus problems, taste perversion, tinnitus, vision changes

GI: Abdominal distention and pain, anorexia, constipation, diarrhea, flatulence, **hepatic failure, hepatitis**, hepatomegaly, jaundice, nausea, **pancreatitis**, vomiting
GU: Decreased libido, flank pain, **renal insufficiency**, sexual dysfunction, urinary frequency
MS: Arthralgia, gout, myalgia
RESP: Asthma; bronchitis; **bronchospasm**; dry, persistent, tickling cough; dyspnea; tracheobronchitis; upper respiratory tract infection
SKIN: Diaphoresis, photosensitivity, pruritus, rash, urticaria
Other: Anaphylaxis, angioedema, hyperkalemia, weight gain

Childbearing Considerations

PREGNANCY

- Drug may cause fetal harm during second and third trimester. Anuria, hypotension, neonatal skull hypoplasia, oligohydramnios, and reversible and irreversible renal failure have occurred along with fetal demise.
- Drug should be discontinued as soon as pregnancy is known.

LACTATION

- Drug is present in breast milk.
- A decision should be made to discontinue breastfeeding or the drug to avoid potential serious adverse reactions in the breastfed infant.

Nursing Considerations

- Monitor serum potassium level before and during fosinopril therapy, as appropriate.
- Know that if patient also receives a diuretic or another antihypertensive, you should expect to reduce its dosage over 2 to 3 days before starting fosinopril. If blood pressure isn't controlled with fosinopril alone, other antihypertensive therapy may resume, as prescribed. If so, observe for excessive hypotension.

! WARNING Know that if angioedema affects the face, glottis, larynx, limbs, lips, mucous membranes, or tongue, prescriber must be notified immediately. Expect to discontinue fosinopril and start appropriate therapy at once. If airway obstruction threatens, promptly give 0.3 to 0.5 ml of epinephrine solution 1:1,000 subcutaneously, as prescribed.

PATIENT TEACHING

- Instruct patient to take fosinopril at same time each day to improve compliance and maintain drug's therapeutic effect.
- Emphasize the importance of taking fosinopril as prescribed, even if patient feels well. Caution her not to stop taking drug without consulting prescriber.
- Explain that drug helps control—but doesn't cure—hypertension and that patient may need lifelong therapy.

! **WARNING** Urge patient to seek immediate medical attention for difficulty breathing or swallowing, hoarseness, or swelling of the face, lips, throat, or tongue.

- Instruct patient to notify prescriber about persistent, severe diarrhea, nausea, and vomiting; resulting dehydration may lead to hypotension.
- Advise patient not to take other drugs or use salt substitutes without consulting prescriber.
- Encourage patient to keep scheduled appointments with prescriber to monitor blood pressure, blood test results, and effects of therapy.
- Caution patient about possible dizziness.
- Advise patient to rise slowly from a lying or sitting position and to dangle legs over bed for several minutes before standing to minimize effects of orthostatic hypotension.
- Reinforce prescriber's recommendations for lifestyle changes, such as alcohol avoidance, dietary improvements, smoking cessation, regular exercise, and stress reduction.
- Urge women of childbearing age to use contraception during therapy because drug may harm fetus.
- Advise patient to use caution during exercise and hot weather because of the increased risk of dehydration from excessive sweating.

fosphenytoin sodium
Cerebyx

☰ Class and Category
Pharmacologic class: Hydantoin derivative
Therapeutic class: Anticonvulsant

☰ Indications and Dosages
✻ *To treat generalized tonic–clonic status epilepticus*

I.V. INFUSION, I.M. INJECTION
Adults. *Emergent loading dose:* 15 to 20 mg of phenytoin equivalent (PE)/kg I.V. infused at a rate of 100 to 150 PE/min. *Maintenance:* 4 to 6 mg PE/kg daily in divided doses I.V. infused at a rate no greater than 150 mg PE/min or given I.M.

I.V. INFUSION
Neonates, infants, children, and adolescents to age 17 years. *Emergent loading dose:* 15 to 20 mg PE/kg infused at a rate of 2 mg PE/kg/min or 150 mg PE/min, whichever is slower.

✻ *To prevent or treat seizures during neurosurgery*

I.V. INFUSION, I.M. INJECTION
Adults. *Nonemergent loading dose:* 10 to 20 mg PE/kg, not to exceed 150 mg PE/min for I.V. administration. *Maintenance:* 4 to 6 mg PE/kg in divided doses at an I.V. rate no greater than 150 mg/PE/min or given I.M.

I.V. INFUSION
Neonates, infants, children, and adolescents to age 17 years. *Nonemergent loading dose:* 10 to 15 mg PE/kg at a rate of 1 to 2 mg PE/kg/min or 150 mg PE/min, whichever is slower. *Maintenance:* 2 to 4 mg PE/kg given 12 hr after initial dose and then continued every 12 hr at a rate of 1 to 2 mg PE/kg/min or 100 mg PE/min, whichever is slower.

✻ *To substitute for oral phenytoin therapy when administration of oral phenytoin is not possible.*

I.V. INFUSION, I.M. INJECTION
Adults. Same total daily phenytoin sodium equivalents (PE) dose. I.V. infusion rate should not exceed 150 mg PE/min.

I.V. INFUSION
Neonates, infants, children, and adolescents to age 17. Same total daily phenytoin sodium equivalents (PE) dose. I.V. infusion rate should not exceed 2 mg PE/kg/min or 150 mg PE/min, whichever is slower.

±**DOSAGE ADJUSTMENT** For patients who are intermediate or poor metabolizers of CYP2C9 substrates, initial dosage started at lower dosage range.

☰ Drug Administration
- Usually stored in refrigerator. If stored at room temperature, discard after 48 hours.
- Injection vials are single dose only.

E
F

▪ The dosage, concentration, and infusion rate of drug are expressed in phenytoin sodium equivalents (PE) units. Do not confuse the concentration of drug with the total amount of drug in the vial. Misreading an order or a label could result in massive overdose.

I.V.

▪ Dilute drug in 0.9% Sodium Chloride Injection or 5% Dextrose in Water to a concentration of 1.5 to 25 mg PE/ml.
▪ Don't administer solution faster than 150 mg PE/min in adults. Pediatric infusion rate is 2 mg PE/kg/min or 150 mg PE/min, whichever is slower for emergent dosing and 1–2 mg PE/kg/min or 150 mg PE/min, whichever is slower for nonemergent dosing. Do not exceed these rates because of the risk of cardiac arrhythmias and severe hypotension.
▪ Expect to give an I.V. benzodiazepine (such as diazepam or lorazepam), as prescribed, with fosphenytoin; otherwise, drug's full antiepileptic effect won't be immediate.
▪ Monitor patient throughout the infusion for adverse signs and symptoms of cardiovascular toxicity. If present, notify prescriber and expect infusion rate to be slowed or drug discontinued.
▪ Monitor blood pressure, ECG, and respiratory function for 10 to 20 minutes after infusion ends.
▪ Patient should be switched to oral phenytoin as soon as possible because of the risks of cardiac and local toxicity associated with I.V. administration.
▪ Monitor patient for signs of sensory disturbances during the infusion, such as severe burning, itching, and/or paresthesia, especially in the groin. Know that the intensity of discomfort can be lessened by slowing or temporarily stopping the infusion.
▪ Expect to obtain blood fosphenytoin (phenytoin) level 2 hours after I.V. infusion. Therapeutic level generally ranges from 10 to 20 mcg/ml; steady state may take several days to several weeks to reach.
▪ *Incompatibilities:* Other I.V. drugs

I.M.

▪ Be aware that loading doses shouldn't be given I.M. because I.V. route allows faster onset and peak. Use only if I.V. access is impossible.

▪ Do not administer I.M. injection in children unless I.V. access is impossible.
▪ Expect to obtain blood fosphenytoin (phenytoin) level 4 hours after I.M. injection.

Route	Onset	Peak	Duration
I.V.	Unknown	End of infusion	Unknown
I.M.	Unknown	30 min	Unknown

Half-life: 15 min to convert to phenytoin

Mechanism of Action

Is converted from fosphenytoin (a prodrug) to phenytoin, which limits the spread of seizure activity and the start of new seizures. Phenytoin does so by regulating voltage-dependent sodium and calcium channels in neurons, inhibiting calcium movement across neuronal membranes, and enhancing the sodium–potassium–adenosine triphosphatase activity in glial cells and neurons. These actions may stem from phenytoin's ability to slow the recovery rate of inactivated sodium channels.

Contraindications

Adams-Stokes syndrome, concurrent delavirdine use; history of prior acute hepatotoxicity caused by fosphenytoin or phenytoin: hypersensitivity to fosphenytoin, phenytoin, other hydantoins, or their components; second- or third-degree A-V block; sino-atrial block; sinus bradycardia

Interactions

DRUGS

acyclovir: Decreased blood phenytoin level, loss of seizure control
alfentanil: Increased clearance and decreased effectiveness of alfentanil
albendazole, antiepileptics (carbamazepine, felbamate, lamotrigine, topiramate, oxcarbazepine), antilipidemics (atorvastatin, fluvastatin, simvastatin), antivirals (efavirenz, lopinavir/ritonavir, indinavir, nelfinavir, ritonavir, saquinavir), calcium channel blockers (nifedipine, nimodipine, verapamil), chlorpropamide, clozapine, cyclosporine, digoxin, disopyramide, folic acid, methadone, mexiletine, praziquantel, quetiapine: Decreased blood levels of these drugs

amiodarone, calcium channel blockers, capecitabine, chloramphenicol, chlordiazepoxide, cimetidine, disulfiram, estrogen, ethosuximide, felbamate, fluconazole, fluorouracil, fluoxetine, fluvastatin, fluvoxamine, isoniazid, itraconazole, ketoconazole, methylphenidate, miconazole, omeprazole, oxcarbazepine, phenothiazines, salicylates, sertraline, sulfadiazine, sulfamethizole, sulfamethoxazole-trimethoprim, sulfaphenazole, ticlopidine, tolbutamide, topiramate, trimethoprim, voriconazole, warfarin: Possibly increased blood phenytoin level and risk of toxicity
antineoplastics, carbamazepine, diazepam, diazoxide, folic acid, fosamprenavir, nelfinavir, reserpine, rifampin, ritonavir, St. John's wort, theophylline, vigabatrin: Increased phenytoin metabolism and decreased phenytoin level
antineoplastic agents (irinotecan, paclitaxel, teniposide), azoles (fluconazole, ketoconazole, itraconazole, posaconazole, voriconazole), corticosteroids, delavirdine, doxycycline, estrogens, furosemide, neuromuscular blocking agents (cisatracurium, pancuronium, rocuronium, vecuronium), oral contraceptives, paroxetine, quinidine, rifampin, sertraline, theophylline, vitamin D, warfarin: Decreased effectiveness of these drugs
lithium: Increased risk of lithium toxicity
methadone: Possibly increased methadone
phenobarbital, valproate sodium, valproic acid: Possible decrease or increase in phenytoin serum levels
tricyclic antidepressants: Possibly lowered seizure threshold and decreased therapeutic effects of phenytoin; possibly decreased blood antidepressant level
valproic acid: Increased blood valproic acid level

ACTIVITIES

alcohol use: Possibly decreased or increased phenytoin effectiveness

▤ Adverse Reactions

CNS: Agitation, amnesia, asthenia, ataxia, **cerebral edema**, chills, **coma**, confusion, **CVA**, decreased or increased reflexes, delusions, depression, dizziness, dyskinesia, emotional lability, **encephalitis**, **encephalopathy**, extrapyramidal reactions, fever, headache, hemiplegia, hostility, hypoesthesia, lack of coordination, malaise, **meningitis**, nervousness, neurosis, paralysis, paresthesia, personality disorder, positive Babinski's sign, **seizures**, somnolence, speech disorders, stupor, **subdural hematoma**, syncope, transient paresthesia, tremor, vertigo

CV: **Atrial flutter**, **bradycardia**, bundle-branch block, **cardiac arrest**, **cardiomegaly**, edema, **heart failure**, hypertension, **hypotension**, orthostatic hypotension, palpitations, **PVCs**, **serious arrhythmias**, **shock**, tachycardia, thrombophlebitis, vasodilation

EENT: Amblyopia, conjunctivitis, diplopia, dry mouth, earache, epistaxis, eye pain, gingival hyperplasia, hearing loss, hyperacusis, increased salivation, loss of taste, mydriasis, nystagmus, pharyngitis, photophobia, rhinitis, sinusitis, taste perversion, tinnitus, **tongue swelling**, visual field defects

ENDO: Decreased dexamethasone, metyrapone, or T4 levels; diabetes insipidus; hyperglycemia; **ketosis**

GI: Anorexia, constipation, diarrhea, dysphagia, elevated liver enzymes, flatulence, gastritis, **GI bleeding**, **hepatic necrosis**, **hepatitis**, ileus, indigestion, nausea, vomiting

GU: Albuminuria, dysuria, incontinence, oliguria, polyuria, **renal failure**, urine retention, vaginal candidiasis

HEME: **Agranulocytosis**, anemia, easy bruising, **granulocytopenia**, **leukopenia**, lymphadenopathy, **pancytopenia**, **thrombocytopenia**

MS: Arthralgia, back or pelvic pain, dysarthria, leg cramps, muscle twitching, myalgia, myasthenia, myoclonus, myopathy

RESP: **Apnea**, **asthma**, **atelectasis**, bronchitis, dyspnea, **hemoptysis**, hyperventilation, **hypoxia**, increased cough, increased sputum production, pneumonia, **pneumothorax**

SKIN: Acute generalized exanthematous pustulosis (AGEP), contact dermatitis, diaphoresis, maculopapular or pustular rash, photosensitivity, pruritus, skin discoloration, skin nodule, **Stevens–Johnson syndrome**, **toxic epidermal necrolysis**, urticaria

Other: Anaphylaxis; angioedema; cachexia; **cryptococcosis**; dehydration; **drug reaction with eosinophilia and systemic symptoms (DRESS)**; elevated alkaline phosphatase;

flu-like symptoms; **hyperkalemia**; **hypokalemia**; **hypophosphatemia**; infection; injection-site reaction such as edema, discoloration, and pain distal to the site of injection; lymphadenopathy; porphyria; **sepsis**

Childbearing Considerations

PREGNANCY

- Pregnancy exposure registry: 1-888-233-2334 or http://www.aedpregnancyregistry.org/.
- Drug may cause fetal harm increasing risk for congenital malformations and other adverse developmental outcomes, including hydantoin syndrome. In addition, malignancies, including neuroblastoma have been reported in children whose mothers received drug during pregnancy.
- A potentially life-threatening bleeding disorder may occur in neonates exposed to drug in utero.
- Drug is not recommended in pregnancy unless absolutely necessary and no other alternative is available.

LACTATION

- It is not known if drug is present in breast milk, but the active metabolite of the drug is present in human milk.
- Patient should check with prescriber before breastfeeding.

REPRODUCTION

- Women of childbearing age should use effective contraception throughout drug therapy.

Nursing Considerations

- Know that antiepileptic drugs such as fosphenytoin should not be discontinued abruptly, because of the possibility of increased seizure frequency, including status epilepticus.
- Remember that when switching between phenytoin and fosphenytoin, small differences in phenytoin bioavailability can lead to significant changes in blood phenytoin level and an increased risk of toxicity.
- Monitor CBC for leukopenia or thrombocytopenia—signs of hematologic toxicity. Also monitor serum albumin level and results of liver and renal function tests.
- Anticipate increased frequency and severity of adverse reactions after I.V. administration in patients with hepatic or renal impairment or hypoalbuminemia. Know that the phosphate load contained in fosphenytoin should be kept in mind when patients

with severe renal impairment who require phosphate restriction are treated.

! WARNING Discontinue drug, as ordered, if signs of hypersensitivity develop: acute hepatotoxicity (hepatic necrosis and hepatitis), fever, lymphadenopathy, and skin reactions during first 2 months of therapy. Expect to rapidly substitute drug with alternative therapy not belonging to the hydantoin chemical class because abrupt withdrawal of fosphenytoin may increase risk of seizures, including status epilepticus.

- Monitor phenytoin level to detect early signs of toxicity, such as diplopia, nausea, severe confusion, slurred speech, and vomiting. Expect to reduce or stop drug.

! WARNING Monitor patient for seizures; at toxic levels, phenytoin is excitatory.

! WARNING Know that if patient has bradycardia or heart block rhythm, you must notify prescriber and expect to withhold drug; severe cardiovascular reactions and death have occurred.

- Expect to provide vitamin D supplement if patient has inadequate dietary intake and is receiving long-term anticonvulsant treatment.
- Document onset, characteristics, and type of seizures and response to treatment.
- Monitor patient for injection-site reactions such as local toxicity known as Purple Glove syndrome, exhibited by discoloration, edema, and pain distal to the site of injection. Know that this may occur without extravasation being present and up to several days after injection. If present, notify prescriber and expect drug to be discontinued.

! WARNING Know that patients of Asian ancestry who have the genetic allelic variant HLA-B 1502 or CYP2C9*3 variant develop serious and sometimes fatal dermatologic reactions 10 times more often than people without this variant when given carbamazepine, another antiepileptic drug. Because early data suggest a similar effect with fosphenytoin, this drug shouldn't be used as a substitute for carbamazepine in these patients.

- Monitor all patients' skin for skin reactions, because serious and sometimes fatal dermatologic reactions may occur, usually within the first 28 days of treatment. Notify prescriber at the first sign of a rash or other skin abnormalities.

PATIENT TEACHING

- Inform patient that fosphenytoin typically is used for short-term treatment.

! **WARNING** Urge patient to seek immediate medical care if allergic reactions occur, especially swelling of face, lips, or upper airway making breathing difficult.

- Inform patient that some sensory discomfort may be felt during fosphenytoin administration. Advise patient to alert the nurse, as slowing the infusion can decrease the discomfort.
- Instruct patient to notify prescriber immediately about bothersome symptoms, especially rash and swollen glands or local reaction at injection site, including discoloration, edema, and pain distal to the site, and swelling. Also notify prescriber immediately if persistent, severe, or unusual signs and symptoms occur as well as a skin rash.
- Tell patient to inform prescriber of all drugs being used, including over-the-counter preparations and alcohol products, before using.
- Emphasize need for good oral hygiene and gum massage because gingival hyperplasia may develop during long-term therapy when oral phenytoin therapy is not feasible.
- Urge patient to consume adequate amounts of vitamin D.
- Advise female patient to use effective contraceptive and to notify prescriber immediately if pregnancy is suspected or occurs.

fostemsavir
Rukobia

Class and Category
Pharmacologic class: Glycoprotein (gp) 120 attachment inhibitor
Therapeutic class: HIV-1 antiretroviral

Indications and Dosages

✱ *As adjunct to treat HIV-1 infection in heavily treatment-experienced patients with multidrug-resistant HIV-1 infection who are failing their current antiretroviral regimen due to resistance, intolerance, or safety considerations*

E.R. TABLETS
Adults. 600 mg twice daily.

Drug Administration
P.O.
- Tablets should be swallowed whole and not chewed, crushed, or split.
- Tablets may have a slight vinegar smell to them.

Route	Onset	Peak	Duration
P.O.	Unknown	2 hr	Unknown

Half-life: 11 hr

Mechanism of Action
By attaching to the gp120 protein on the outer surface of the human immunodeficiency virus type 1, the virus is blocked from getting into and infecting the immune cells.

Contraindications
Concurrent therapy with strong CYP3A inducers such as androgen receptor inhibitor (enzalutamide), anticonvulsants (carbamazepine, phenytoin), antimycobacterial (rifampin), antineoplastic (mitotane), or herbal product (St. John's wort); hypersensitivity to fostemsavir or its components

Interactions
DRUGS
CYP3A strong inducers (carbamazepine, enzalutamide, mitotane, phenytoin, rifampin, St. John's wort): Significantly decreases temsavir (active ingredient of fostemsavir) concentrations, which may lead to loss of virologic response
drugs with known risk of torsades de pointes: Increased risk of torsades de pointes
ethinyl estradiol: Increased concentration of ethinyl estradiol, possibly leading to increased adverse reactions
grazoprevir, voxilaprevir: Possibly increased plasma concentrations of these drugs, possibly leading to increased adverse reactions

E
F

statins (atorvastatin, fluvastatin, pitavastatin, rosuvastatin, simvastatin): Increased concentrations of statins, possibly leading to increased adverse reactions

Adverse Reactions

CNS: Abnormal dreams, asthenia, dizziness, fatigue, headache, insomnia, peripheral neuropathy, sleep disturbance, somnolence
CV: Elevated cholesterol and triglyceride levels, **QT prolongation**
EENT: Taste disturbance
ENDO: Hyperglycemia
GI: Abdominal discomfort or pain; diarrhea; dyspepsia; elevated bilirubin, liver, and pancreatic enzymes; nausea; vomiting
GU: Elevated creatinine level
HEME: Decreased hemoglobin, **neutropenia**
MS: Myalgia
SKIN: Allergic dermatitis, pruritus, rash
OTHER: Elevated creatine kinase or urate levels, immune reconstitution inflammatory syndrome

Childbearing Considerations

PREGNANCY

- Pregnancy exposure registry: 1-800-258-4263.
- It is not known if drug causes fetal harm.
- Use with caution only if benefit to mother outweighs potential risk to fetus.

LACTATION

- It is not known if drug is present in breast milk.
- The Centers for Disease Control and Prevention recommends that HIV-1 infected mothers not breastfeed, to avoid risking postnatal transmission of HIV-1 infection to infant. They also do not recommend breastfeeding because of potential drug-induced adverse reactions in the infant.

Nursing Considerations

- Use fostemsavir cautiously in patients with a history of QT interval prolongation, when coadministered with a drug with a known risk of torsades de pointes, or in patients with relevant preexisting cardiac disease, because of risk of QT prolongation. Know that elderly patients may be more susceptible to drug-induced QT interval prolongation.
- Expect to monitor liver enzymes in patients with hepatitis B or C viral co-infection

because elevations may signal hepatitis B reactivation, particularly in patients when antihepatitis therapy has been withdrawn. Be aware that caution should be used when patient begins or is maintaining effective hepatitis B therapy and starting fostemsavir therapy.

- Become familiar with patient's current medications because significant drug interactions may occur, which may cause a loss of therapeutic effect of fostemsavir. In addition, drug may cause possible development of resistance due to reduced exposure to the active ingredient (temsavir) or possible prolongation of QT interval from increased exposure to temsavir.

! WARNING Be aware that immune reconstitution syndrome has occurred in patients treated with combination antiretroviral therapy, including fostemsavir. The inflammatory response predisposes susceptible patients to opportunistic infections such as cytomegalovirus, *Mycobacterium avium* infection, *Pneumocystis jiroveci* pneumonia, or tuberculosis. Autoimmune disorders, such as Graves' disease, Guillain–Barré syndrome, or polymyositis, have also occurred. Report sudden or unusual adverse reactions to prescriber.

PATIENT TEACHING

- Stress to patient that missed doses could cause resistance. Tell patient to take dose as soon as remembered but not to double dose or take more than prescribed.

! WARNING Tell patient to notify prescriber if an abnormal rhythm, dizziness. Lightheadedness or loss of consciousness occurs.

! WARNING Advise patient to inform prescriber immediately of any signs and symptoms of infection, as inflammation from previous infection may occur soon after combination antiretroviral therapy is started.

- Inform patients coinfected with hepatitis B or C that routine laboratory tests will be performed and stress importance of taking drugs prescribed for hepatitis B or C while taking fostemsavir.
- Advise patient to report to prescriber the use of any other prescription or

nonprescription drugs, including herbal products such as St. John's wort.

- Tell female patients that mothers with HIV-1 should not breastfeed.

fremanezumab-vfrm
Ajovy

Class and Category
Pharmacologic class: Calcitonin gene-related peptide antagonist
Therapeutic class: Antimigraine

Indications and Dosages
✱ *To prevent migraine headaches*

SUBCUTANEOUS INJECTION
Adults. 225 mg monthly. Alternatively, 675 mg every 3 months given as 3 consecutive injections of 225 mg each.

Drug Administration
SUBCUTANEOUS
- Remove drug from refrigerator and allow it to sit at room temperature for 30 minutes protected from direct sunlight prior to administration. Do not warm drug using a heat source such as hot water or a microwave. Discard if drug (kept in original carton) has been left at room temperature for 7 days or longer.
- Do not use if solution appears to be cloudy, discolored, or contains particles.
- Inject drug into the abdomen, thigh, or upper arm in an area that is not bruised, indurated, red, or tender. If giving 3 consecutive injections, the same body site may be used, but not the exact location.
- Do not coadminister drug with other injectable drugs at the same injection site.

Route	Onset	Peak	Duration
SQ	Unknown	5 to 7 days	Unknown

Half-life: 31 days

Mechanism of Action
Binds to the calcitonin gene-related peptide (CGRP) receptor. The CGRP receptor is thought to be responsible for transmitting signals that can cause incapacitating pain. By binding to the CGRP receptor, drug antagonizes its function, preventing pain signals from being transmitted.

Contraindications
Hypersensitivity to fremanezumab-vfrm or its components

Interactions
DRUGS
None reported by manufacturer

Adverse Reactions
SKIN: Pruritus, rash, urticaria
Other: Anaphylaxis, angioedema, fremanezumab-vfrm antibody formation, injection-site reactions (induration, pain, redness)

Childbearing Considerations
PREGNANCY
- Pregnancy exposure registry: 1-833-927-2605 or www.tevamigraine pregnancyregistry.com
- It is not known if drug causes fetal harm.
- Use with caution only if benefit to mother outweighs potential risk to fetus.
- Know that women with migraine may be at increased risk of gestational hypertension and preeclampsia during pregnancy.

LACTATION
- It is not known if drug may be present in breast milk.
- Patient should check with prescriber before breastfeeding.

Nursing Considerations

! **WARNING** Monitor patient for an allergic reaction such as hives, itching, or a rash, although anaphylaxis and angioedema may also occur. Be aware that most allergic reactions occur within hours to 1 month after administration. Know that if an allergic reaction occurs, the drug may have to be discontinued and signs and symptoms treated.

- Know that when switching dosage options, the first dose of the new regimen should be administered on the next scheduled date of administration.

PATIENT TEACHING
- Teach patient how to prepare and administer drug subcutaneously using syringe or autoinjector, if self-injecting.
- Instruct patient to remove fremanezumab-vfrm from refrigerator and allow it to sit at room temperature for 30 minutes protected

E
F

from direct sunlight prior to administration. Warn patient not to warm drug using a heat source such as hot water or a microwave. Tell patient to discard drug if it has been left at room temperature for 24 hours or longer.

- Tell patient to inspect solution for discoloration or particles and not to use if solution appears to be cloudy, discolored, or contains particles.
- Instruct patient to administer fremanezumab-vfrm subcutaneously into the abdomen, thigh, or upper arm in an area that is not bruised, indurated, red, or tender. If giving 3 consecutive injections, tell patient that the same body site may be used, but not the exact location of the previous injection. Warn patient not to coadminister drug with other injectable drugs at the same injection site.
- Tell patient that if a dose is missed, she should administer it as soon as she remembers. Thereafter, the next dose can be scheduled from the date of that dose.
- Inform patient that when switching dosage options, first dose of the new regimen should be administered on the next scheduled date of administration.
- Stress importance of keeping prefilled autoinjector or prefilled syringe out of the reach of small children.

! **WARNING** Advise patient that drug may cause an allergic reaction within hours to up to 1 month following administration. If hives, itching, or a rash occurs, tell patient to notify prescriber immediately, because more serious reactions may develop requiring drug to be discontinued. The allergic reaction may require additional treatment.

frovatriptan succinate
Frova

Class and Category
Pharmacologic class: Serotonin 5-HT1 receptor agonist
Therapeutic class: Antimigraine

Indications and Dosages
❋ *To treat acute migraine headache*

TABLETS

Adults. 2.5 mg, as needed. If migraine returns, 2.5-mg dose repeated providing there is at least a 2-hr interval between the 2 doses. *Maximum:* 7.5 mg (three 2.5-mg doses) per 24 hr; treatment of more than four migraines over 30 days.

Drug Administration
P.O.
- Do not exceed maximum dosage.

Route	Onset	Peak	Duration
P.O.	Unknown	2–4 hr	Unknown
Half-life: 26 hr			

Mechanism of Action
Binds to 5-HT1 receptors on intracranial blood vessels and sensory nerves of the trigeminal system to produce cranial vessel constriction and inhibition of proinflammatory neuropeptide release, which causes pain relief.

Contraindications
Arrhythmias associated with cardiac accessory conduction pathway disorders such as Wolff–Parkinson–White syndrome; history of basilar or hemiplegic migraine, stroke, or transient ischemic attack; hypersensitivity to frovatriptan or its components; ischemic coronary artery disease or coronary artery vasospasm; ischemic bowel disease; peripheral vascular disease; uncontrolled hypertension; use within 24 hours of another 5-HT$_1$ agonist or an ergotamine-containing or ergot-type drug such as dihydroergotamine or methysergide

Interactions
DRUGS
ergot-containing or ergot-type drugs such as dihydroergotamine, methysergide: Increased risk of prolonged vasospastic reaction
MAO inhibitors, selective serotonin reuptake inhibitors, serotonin norepinephrine reuptake inhibitors, tricyclic antidepressants: Possible development of serotonin syndrome
other 5-HT1 agonists: Potential additive effects increasing risk of serious adverse reactions

Adverse Reactions
CNS: Anxiety; **cerebral hemorrhage, CVA, and other cerebrovascular events;** dizziness;

dysesthesia; exacerbation of headache; fatigue; hypoesthesia; insomnia; palpitations; paresthesia; **seizure; serotonin syndrome; subarachnoid hemorrhage**

CV: Arrhythmias, including ventricular fibrillation or tachycardia; chest, jaw, neck, or throat pain, pressure, or tightness; **MI; myocardial ischemia;** peripheral vascular ischemia; Prinzmetal's angina; Raynaud's syndrome

EENT: Abnormal vision, blindness (transient or permanent), dry mouth, partial vision loss, rhinitis, sinusitis, tinnitus

GI: Abdominal pain, bloody diarrhea, diarrhea, dyspepsia, **gastrointestinal vascular infarction or ischemia,** splenic infarction, vomiting

RESP: Bone pain

SKIN: Diaphoresis, flushing

Other: Anaphylaxis, angioedema, generalized pain, sensation of being cold or hot

Childbearing Considerations

PREGNANCY

- It is not known if drug causes fetal harm.
- Use with caution only if benefit to mother outweighs potential risk to fetus.
- Know that women with migraine may be at increased risk of preeclampsia during pregnancy.

LACTATION

- It is not known if drug is present in breast milk.
- Patient should check with prescriber before breastfeeding.

Nursing Considerations

- Expect triptan-naïve patient with multiple cardiovascular risk factors such as diabetes, increased age, hypertension, obesity, smoking, or strong family history of coronary artery disease to have a cardiovascular evaluation prior to frovatriptan being prescribed, because drug can cause serious cardiovascular disorders such as myocardial infarction or ischemia and Prinzmetal's angina. In patients who have a negative cardiovascular evaluation, know that the first dose of frovatriptan may be administered in a medically supervised setting with an EKG performed immediately following administration to detect adverse effects. Expect periodic cardiovascular evaluations to be performed throughout frovatriptan therapy. Also expect drug to be immediately discontinued if patient develops arrhythmias, because of potential life-threatening consequences.

- Know that if patient complains of chest, jaw, neck, or throat pain, pressure, or tightness, an immediate cardiovascular evaluation should be performed even though these symptoms are usually noncardiac in nature.

- Monitor patient for signs and symptoms of cerebrovascular events, because drug use increases risk of CVAs and cerebrovascular hemorrhage.

- Monitor patient for noncardiovascular vasospasm events such as gastrointestinal vascular infarction and ischemia (abdominal pain, bloody diarrhea), peripheral vascular ischemia, Raynaud's syndrome, or splenic infarction. If suspected, notify prescriber immediately, stop frovatriptan therapy, and be prepared to provide emergency supportive care according to institutional protocol.

! WARNING Monitor patient for evidence of serotonin syndrome, such as agitation, chills, confusion, diaphoresis, diarrhea, fever, hyperactive reflexes, poor coordination, restlessness, shaking, talking or acting with uncontrolled excitement, tremor, and twitching. Be aware that risk is greater during coadministration with monoamine oxidase inhibitors, selective serotonin reuptake inhibitors, serotonin norepinephrine reuptake inhibitors, and tricyclic antidepressants. Onset of symptoms usually occurs within minutes to hours of receiving a new or a greater dose of a serotonergic medication. If serotonin syndrome is suspected, notify prescriber immediately, expect drug to be discontinued, and provide symptomatic supportive care, as prescribed.

- Monitor patient's blood pressure, because significant elevation in blood pressure, including hypertensive crisis, has been reported in patients treated with other 5-HT1 agonists.

! WARNING Monitor patient for hypersensitivity reactions to frovatriptan. These reactions may be life-threatening and include anaphylaxis and angioedema. Stop drug therapy immediately and notify prescriber if a hypersensitivity reaction occurs. Provide supportive care, as prescribed.

PATIENT TEACHING

- Tell patient to take drug exactly as prescribed and not to overuse drug by using it 10 days or more in a month, because medication-overuse headache may develop. If patient begins to experience daily migraine-like headaches or a marked increase in frequency of headaches, tell him to notify prescriber. Inform him that a period of detoxification may be necessary.

! **WARNING** Alert patient that frovatriptan therapy may cause allergic reactions that may become severe. Tell patient to notify prescriber at the first sign of an allergic reaction and to seek immediate medical attention if difficulty breathing, or swelling, especially of eyes, face, or throat, occurs.

- Advise patient to notify all prescribers of frovatriptan therapy, because serious drug interactions can occur with certain medications when taken concomitantly with frovatriptan.

! **WARNING** Inform patient that drug has the potential to cause a heart attack or stroke or other forms of vasospastic disorders. Instruct patient to seek immediate emergency treatment if he experiences chest pain, shortness of breath, slurring of speech, or weakness, or if he develops persistent, severe, or unusual signs and symptoms.

furosemide

Lasix, Lasix Special (CAN)

Class and Category

Pharmacologic class: Loop diuretic
Therapeutic class: Antihypertensive, diuretic

Indications and Dosages

＊ *To reduce edema caused by cirrhosis, heart failure, and renal disease, including nephrotic syndrome*

ORAL SOLUTION, TABLETS

Adults. 20 to 80 mg as a single dose, increased by 20 to 40 mg every 6 to 8 hr until desired response occurs. *Maintenance:* Effective dose given once or divided and given twice daily (8 am and 2 pm). *Maximum:* 600 mg daily.

Children. 2 mg/kg as a single dose, increased by 1 to 2 mg/kg every 6 to 8 hr until desired response occurs. *Maximum:* 6 mg/kg/dose.

I.V. INFUSION, I.V. OR I.M. INJECTION

Adults. 20 to 40 mg as a single dose, increased by 20 mg every 2 hr until desired response occurs.

I.V. OR I.M. INJECTION

Children. 1 mg/kg as a single dose, increased by 1 mg/kg every 2 hr until desired response occurs. *Maximum:* 6 mg/kg/dose, (children), 1 mg/kg/day (premature infants).

＊ *To treat acute pulmonary edema*

I.V. INJECTION

Adults. 40 mg with dosage repeated but increased to 80 mg after 1 hr, as needed.

＊ *To manage hypertension*

ORAL SOLUTION, TABLETS

Adults. *Initial:* 40 mg twice daily, adjusted until desired response occurs.

± **DOSAGE ADJUSTMENT** Dosage for elderly patients started at the low end of dosing range.

Drug Administration

P.O.

- Administer once-daily doses in morning and twice-daily doses in morning and early afternoon 6 hours apart (e.g., 8 am and 2 pm).
- Protect from light, which may cause a slight discoloration. Do not administer discolored tablets.
- Use a calibrated measuring device to obtain accurate dosing of oral solution.

I.V.

- Use only when patient is unable to take oral medication or in emergency situations. Replace with oral therapy as soon as possible.
- Do not use solution if discolored.
- For I.V. injection, inject undiluted directly or into tubing of actively running I.V. slowly over 1 to 2 minutes to prevent ototoxicity.
- For I.V. infusion, prepare drug for infusion with 0.9% Sodium Chloride Injection, 5%

Dextrose Injection, or Lactated Ringer's solution after pH has been adjusted to above 5.5. Administer with an infusion pump at a rate not to exceed 4 mg/min in adults as an intermittent infusion. Use prepared solution within 24 hours.

- *Incompatibilities:* Other I.V. drugs except for cimetidine, epinephrine, heparin, nitroglycerin, potassium chloride, verapamil; for Y-site: other I.V. drugs except for epinephrine, fentanyl, heparin, norepinephrine, nitroglycerin, potassium chloride, vitamins B and C

I.M.

- Used only if oral or I.V. administration is not feasible.
- Do not administer drug I.M. for treatment of pulmonary edema or if solution is discolored.

Route	Onset	Peak	Duration
P.O.	20–60 min	1–2 hr	6–8 hr
I.V.	5 min	30 min	2 hr
I.M.	30 min	Unknown	Unknown

Half-life: 0.5–2 hr

☰ Mechanism of Action

Inhibits sodium and water reabsorption in the loop of Henle and increases urine formation. As the body's plasma volume decreases, aldosterone production increases, which promotes sodium reabsorption and the loss of potassium and hydrogen ions. Furosemide also increases the excretion of ammonium, bicarbonate, calcium, magnesium, and phosphate. By reducing intracellular and extracellular fluid volume, the drug reduces blood pressure and decreases cardiac output. Over time, cardiac output returns to normal.

☰ Contraindications

Anuria, hypersensitivity to furosemide or its components

☰ Interactions

DRUGS

ACE inhibitors, angiotensin II receptor blockers: Possibly first-dose hypotension, severe hypotension, deterioration in renal function
aminoglycosides, cisplatin, ethacrynic acid: Increased risk of ototoxicity

cephalosporins: Increased risk of cephalosporin-induced nephrotoxicity
chloral hydrate: Possibly diaphoresis, hot flashes, and hypertension
cyclosporine: Increased risk of gouty arthritis
ganglionic or peripheral adrenergic blocking agents: Increased furosemide effects
indomethacin: Possibly reduced natriuretic and antihypertensive effects of furosemide
lithium: Increased risk of lithium toxicity
methotrexate and other drugs that undergo significant renal tubular secretion: Possibly decreased therapeutic effects of furosemide
norepinephrine: Possibly decreased arterial response to norepinephrine
NSAIDs: Possibly increased BUN, serum creatinine and serum potassium levels; weight gain
phenytoin: Possibly decreased therapeutic effects of furosemide
succinylcholine: Increased action of succinylcholine
sucralfate: Possibly reduced natriuretic and antihypertensive effects of furosemide
thiazide diuretics: Possibly profound diuresis and electrolyte imbalances
thyroid hormones: Possibly overall decrease in total thyroid hormone levels with high doses (greater than 80 mg) of furosemide
tubocurarine: Antagonized skeletal muscle relaxing effect of tubocurarine

☰ Adverse Reactions

CNS: Dizziness, drowsiness, fever, headache, lethargy, paresthesia, restlessness, vertigo, weakness
CV: Arrhythmias, elevated cholesterol and triglyceride levels, orthostatic hypotension, shock, tachycardia, **thromboembolism**, thrombophlebitis, vertigo
EENT: Blurred vision, deafness, dry mouth, oral irritation, ototoxicity, stomatitis, tinnitus, hearing loss (rapid I.V. injection), yellow vision
ENDO: Hyperglycemia
GI: Abdominal cramps, anorexia, constipation, diarrhea, elevated liver enzymes, gastric irritation, **hepatocellular insufficiency**, indigestion, jaundice, nausea, **pancreatitis**, vomiting
GU: Azotemia, bladder spasms, glycosuria, oliguria

E
F

HEME: Agranulocytosis (rare), anemia, aplastic anemia (rare), eosinophilia, hemolytic anemia, leukopenia, thrombocytopenia
MS: Muscle pain or spasms
SKIN: Acute generalized exanthematous pustulosis, bullous pemphigoid, erythema multiforme, exfoliative dermatitis, photosensitivity, pruritus, purpura, rash, Stevens–Johnson syndrome, toxic epidermal necrolysis, urticaria
Other: Allergic reaction, anaphylaxis, dehydration, drug reaction with eosinophilia and systemic symptoms (DRESS), hyperuricemia, hypocalcemia, hypochloremia, hypokalemia, hypomagnesemia, hyponatremia, hypovolemia, thirst

Childbearing Considerations

PREGNANCY

- It is not known if drug causes fetal harm.
- Use with caution only if benefit to mother outweighs potential risk to fetus.
- If drug is used during pregnancy, fetal growth should be monitored.

LACTATION

- Drug is present in breast milk and as a diuretic partially inhibits lactation.
- Patient should check with prescriber before breastfeeding.

Nursing Considerations

! **WARNING** Use furosemide cautiously in patients with advanced hepatic cirrhosis, especially those who also have a history of electrolyte imbalance or hepatic encephalopathy; drug may lead to lethal hepatic coma.

- Be aware that patients who are allergic to sulfonamides may also be allergic to furosemide. Monitor patient closely.
- Know that furosemide may precipitate nephrocalcinosis/nephrolithiasis in premature infants. Know that in patients with nephrotic syndrome who are hypoproteinemic, furosemide therapy may be less effective and its ototoxicity potentiated. Drug may also increase the risk of persistence of patent ductus arteriosus in premature infants.
- Obtain patient's weight before and periodically during furosemide therapy to monitor fluid loss.

- Be aware that concomitant therapy with aminoglycoside antibiotics, ethacrynic acid, or other ototoxic drugs increases risk of ototoxicity.
- Expect patient to have periodic hearing tests during prolonged or high-dose I.V. therapy.
- Monitor blood pressure and hepatic and renal function as well as BUN, blood glucose, and serum creatinine, electrolyte, and uric acid levels, as appropriate.
- Be aware that elderly patients are more susceptible to hypotensive and electrolyte-altering effects and thus are at greater risk for shock and thromboembolism.
- Monitor patient for hypokalemia which may occur with brisk diuresis, inadequate oral electrolyte intake, or when cirrhosis is present. It may also occur during concomitant use of ACTH or corticosteroid therapy, intake of large amounts of licorice, or prolonged use of laxatives. Digoxin may exaggerate the metabolic effects of hypokalemia, especially cardiac effects. If patient is at high risk for hypokalemia, give potassium supplements along with furosemide, as prescribed.
- Expect to discontinue furosemide at maximum dosage if oliguria persists for more than 24 hours.
- Be aware that furosemide may worsen left ventricular hypertrophy, systemic lupus erythematosus, or renal retention and adversely affect glucose tolerance and lipid metabolism as well as increase risk of decreased renal function in patients at high risk for radiocontrast nephropathy after a procedure.
- Be aware that patients with hypoproteinemia, such as occurs with nephrotic syndrome, may weaken effect of furosemide and increase its ototoxicity potential.
- Notify prescriber if patient experiences hearing loss, vertigo, or ringing, buzzing, or sense of fullness in her ears. Drug may have to be discontinued.

PATIENT TEACHING

- Instruct patient to take furosemide at the same time each day to maintain therapeutic effects. Urge her to take it as prescribed, even if she feels well.
- Instruct patient to take the last dose of furosemide several hours before bedtime

to avoid sleep interruption from diuresis. If patient receives once-daily dosing, advise her to take the dose in the morning.

- Advise patient to change position slowly to minimize effects of orthostatic hypotension.
- Caution patient about drinking alcoholic beverages, standing for prolonged periods, and exercising in hot weather because these actions increase the hypotensive effect of furosemide.
- Emphasize the importance of weight and diet control, especially limiting sodium intake.
- Unless contraindicated, urge patient to eat more high-potassium foods and to take a potassium supplement, if prescribed, to prevent hypokalemia.
- Instruct patient to keep follow-up appointments with prescriber to monitor progress. Urge her to notify prescriber about persistent, severe nausea, vomiting, and diarrhea, because they may cause dehydration.
- Inform diabetic patient that furosemide may increase blood glucose level, and advise her to check her blood glucose level frequently.

G H I

gabapentin
Gralise, Neurontin

gabapentin enacarbil
Horizant

≡ Class and Category
Pharmacologic class: 1-amino-methyl cyclohexaneacetic acid
Therapeutic class: Anticonvulsant

≡ Indications and Dosages
✱ *To manage postherpetic neuralgia*

CAPSULES, ORAL SOLUTION, TABLETS (NEURONTIN)

Adults. *Initial:* 300 mg on day 1, increased to 300 mg twice daily on day 2, increased to 300 mg three times daily on day 3, and increased gradually thereafter according to pain response, up to 600 mg three times daily. *Maximum:* 1,800 mg daily.

TABLETS (GRALISE)

Adults. *Initial:* 300 mg once daily on day 1, 600 mg once daily on day 2, 900 mg once daily on days 3 through 6, 1,200 mg once daily on days 7 through 10, 1,500 mg once daily on days 11 through 14, and 1,800 mg once daily on day 15 and thereafter.

E.R. TABLETS (HORIZANT)

Adults. *Initial:* 600 mg once daily for 3 days, followed by 600 mg twice daily. *Maximum:* 600 mg twice daily.

±**DOSAGE ADJUSTMENT** For patients taking Gralise who have a reduced creatinine clearance of 30 to 60 ml/min, dosage must be individualized and may have to be reduced. Patients with a creatinine clearance of less than 30 ml/min or who are receiving hemodialysis should not receive Gralise. For patients taking Neurontin who have a reduced creatinine clearance, including patients on hemodialysis, dosage reduced but reduction is highly individualized. For patients taking Horizant with a creatinine clearance between 30 and 59 ml/min, dosage reduced to 300 mg once daily for 3 days, followed by 300 mg twice daily with further increase to 600 mg twice daily, as needed. For patients taking Horizant with a creatinine clearance between 15 and 29 ml/min, dosage reduced to 300 mg once daily on days 1 and 3, followed by 300 mg once daily with further increase to 300 mg twice daily, if needed. For patient with a creatinine clearance less than 15 ml/min and not on dialysis, dosage reduced to 300 mg once daily every other day, followed by 300 mg once daily, if needed. For patient with a creatinine clearance less than 15 ml/min and on hemodialysis, 300 mg following every dialysis with further increase to 600 mg following every dialysis, if needed.

✱ *As adjunct to treat partial seizures*

CAPSULES, ORAL SOLUTION, TABLETS (NEURONTIN)

Adults and children 12 years and older. *Initial:* 300 mg three times daily, increased gradually according to clinical response. *Maintenance:* 300 to 600 mg three times daily. *Maximum:* 3,600 mg daily with maximum time between doses not to exceed 12 hr. **Children ages 3 to 11:** *Initial:* **10 to 15 mg/kg/day divided into 3 doses, increased, as needed, over a period of 3 days.** *Maintenance for ages 3 to 4:* 40 mg/kg/day, given in 3 divided doses. *Maintenance for ages 5 to 11:* 25 to 35 mg/kg/day, given in 3 divided doses. *Maximum:* 50 mg/kg/day, given in 3 divided doses with maximum time between doses not to exceed 12 hr.

±**DOSAGE ADJUSTMENT** For patients taking Neurontin who have a reduced creatinine clearance, including patients on hemodialysis, dosage reduced but reduction is highly individualized.

✱ *To treat moderate to severe primary restless legs syndrome*

E.R. TABLETS (HORIZANT)

Adults. 600 mg once daily at about 5 pm.

±**DOSAGE ADJUSTMENT** For patients with a creatinine clearance between 30 and 59 ml/min, dosage reduced to 300 mg daily and then increased to 600 mg, as needed. For patients with a creatinine clearance between 15 and 29 ml/min, dosage reduced to 300 mg daily and not increased. For patients with a creatinine clearance of less than 15 ml/min and not on hemodialysis, dosage reduced to 300 mg every other day. Patients with a creatinine clearance of less than 15 ml/min and receiving hemodialysis should not receive Horizant.

Drug Administration
P.O.
- Brands of gabapentin aren't interchangeable.
- Capsules and E.R. tablets should be swallowed whole with water and not chewed, crushed, or split/opened.
- Immediate-release tablets should be swallowed whole with water and not chewed or crushed. However, the 600- and 800-mg Neurontin immediate-release tablets are scored and may be divided. Administer the unused half-tablet as the next dose. Half-tablets not used within 28 days of dividing should be discarded.
- Oral solution should be refrigerated. Use a calibrated measuring device for dosing to ensure an accurate dose.
- Administer Gralise brand with evening meal.
- Administer Horizant with food in the morning except for treatment of restless leg syndrome, which requires administration at about 5:00 p.m. with food.
- Give drug at least 2 hours after an antacid.
- Don't exceed 12 hours between doses on a three-times-a-day schedule.

Route	Onset	Peak	Duration
P.O.	Unknown	2–4 hr	Unknown
P.O./E.R.	Unknown	8 hr	Unknown

Half-life: 5–7 hr

Mechanism of Action
Gabapentin is structurally like gamma-aminobutyric acid (GABA), the main inhibitory neurotransmitter in the brain. Although gabapentin's exact mechanism of action is unknown, GABA inhibits the rapid firing of neurons associated with seizures. It also may prevent exaggerated responses to painful stimuli and pain-related responses to a normally innocuous stimulus to account for its effectiveness in relieving postherpetic neuralgia and restless legs syndrome symptoms.

Contraindications
Hypersensitivity to gabapentin or its components

Interactions
DRUGS
aluminum- and magnesium-containing antacids: Decreased gabapentin bioavailability
CNS depressants: Increased CNS depression
hydrocodone: Decreased hydrocodone exposure
morphine: Increased CNS depression
opioids such as buprenorphine, hydrocodone, morphine, oxycodone: Increased risk of decreased awareness, respiratory depression, and severe sleepiness

ACTIVITIES
alcohol: Increased risk of CNS and respiratory depression, which may become severe

Adverse Reactions
CNS: Agitation, altered proprioception, amnesia, anxiety, apathy, aphasia, asthenia, ataxia, cerebellar dysfunction, chills, **CNS tumors**, delusions, depersonalization, depression, disappearance of aura, dizziness, dream disturbances, dysesthesia, dystonia, emotional lability, euphoria, facial paralysis, fatigue, fever, hallucinations, headache, hemiplegia, hostility, hyperkinesia, hyperreflexia, hypoesthesia, hypotonia, **intracranial hemorrhage**, lack of coordination, malaise, migraine headache, movement disorder, nervousness, occipital neuralgia, paranoia, paresis, paresthesia, positive Babinski's sign, psychosis, reflexes (absent or decreased), sedation, **seizures**, somnolence, **status epilepticus**, stupor, **subdural hematoma**, **suicidal ideation**, syncope, tremor, vertigo, **withdrawal precipitated seizure**
CV: Angina, hypertension, **hypotension**, murmur, palpitations, peripheral edema, peripheral vascular insufficiency, tachycardia, vasodilation
EENT: Abnormal vision, amblyopia, blepharospasm, cataracts, conjunctivitis, diplopia, dry eyes and mouth, earache, epistaxis, eye hemorrhage, eye pain, gingival bleeding, gingivitis, glossitis, hearing loss, hoarseness, increased salivation, inner ear infection, loss of taste, nystagmus, pharyngitis, photophobia, ptosis (bilateral or unilateral), rhinitis, sensation of fullness in ears, stomatitis, taste perversion, tinnitus, tooth discoloration, visual field defects

ENDO: Breast hypertrophy, hyperglycemia, **hypoglycemia**

GI: Abdominal pain, anorexia, constipation, diarrhea, elevated liver enzymes, fecal incontinence, flatulence, gastroenteritis, hemorrhoids, **hepatitis**, hepatomegaly, increased appetite, indigestion, jaundice, **melena**, nausea, thirst, vomiting

GU: **Acute renal failure**, anorgasmia, decreased libido, ejaculation disorders, impotence

HEME: Anemia, **coagulation defect**, **leukopenia**, **thrombocytopenia**

MS: Arthralgia, arthritis, back pain, bone fractures, dysarthria, elevated creatine kinase level, joint stiffness or swelling, muscle twitching, myalgia, positive Romberg test, **rhabdomyolysis**, tendinitis

RESP: **Apnea**, cough, dyspnea, pneumonia, pseudocroup, **respiratory depression**

SKIN: Acne, alopecia, bullous pemphigoid, cyst, diaphoresis, dry skin, eczema, **erythema multiforme**, hirsutism, pruritus, purpura, rash, seborrhea, **Stevens–Johnson syndrome**, urticaria

Other: Anaphylaxis, **angioedema**, dehydration, **drug reaction with eosinophilia and systemic symptoms (DRESS)**, **hyponatremia**, increased risk of viral infection, lymphadenopathy, weight gain or loss

⁞ Childbearing Considerations

PREGNANCY
- Pregnancy exposure registry: 1-888-233-2334 or http://www.aedpregnancyregistry.org/.
- It is not known if drug causes fetal harm.
- Use with caution only if benefit to mother outweighs potential risk to fetus.

LACTATION
- Drug is present in breast milk except for Horizant, which is unknown.
- Patient should check with prescriber before breastfeeding.

⁞ Nursing Considerations
- Be aware that routine monitoring of blood gabapentin level isn't needed.

! **WARNING** Know that to discontinue drug used to treat seizures or switch to a different anticonvulsant, expect to change gradually over at least 1 week, as prescribed, to avoid loss of seizure control. When gabapentin is discontinued after treating other indications, expect to reduce dosage, as ordered, over 1 week.

- Monitor renal function test results, as ordered, and expect to adjust dosage, if needed.
- Monitor patient closely for evidence of suicidal thinking or behavior, especially when therapy starts or dosage changes.

! **WARNING** Monitor patient for hypersensitivity, such as fever or lymphadenopathy suggestive of DRESS. Although rare, DRESS may be life-threatening. If suspected, notify prescriber immediately and expect gabapentin to be discontinued.

! **WARNING** Monitor patient who is receiving concomitant opioid therapy for respiratory depression and sedation, which may be life-threatening or even fatal. Patients at higher risk are those who have an underlying respiratory impairment. Know that Neurontin brand should be started at a lower dose.

PATIENT TEACHING
- Tell patient taking gabapentin capsules and immediate-release and extended-release tablets to swallow the capsule/tablet whole and not to chew, crush, or split/open. However, tell patient the exception is if he is taking 600- or 800-mg Neurontin immediate-release tablets because these tablets are scored and can be divided with the unused half-tablet taken as the next dose. Tell patient half-tablets not used within 28 days of dividing should be discarded.
- Tell patient taking oral solution to store drug in refrigerator and to use a calibrated measuring device, not a household spoon, to measure dosage.
- Instruct patient taking Gralise brand to take it with an evening meal. Tell patient taking Horizant brand to take it in the morning with food unless used to treat restless leg syndrome; then he should take it with food at about 5:00 p.m.
- Instruct patient not to take drug within 2 hours after taking an antacid.

G
H
I

- Urge patient to take a missed dose as soon as he remembers. If the next dose is in less than 2 hours, tell him to resume his regular schedule. Caution against doubling the dose.
- Caution patient not to stop drug abruptly.

! **WARNING** Inform patient that an allergic reaction may occur after the first dose but it may also occur at any time. If he experiences difficulty breathing or swelling of his lips, throat, or tongue, he should seek immediate emergency treatment and notify prescriber, as drug will have to be discontinued.

! **WARNING** Urge patient to seek immediate medical care if breathing problems, decreased awareness, and severe sleepiness occur. Tell him to inform all prescribers of over-the-counter and prescribed drugs being taken, especially drugs that affect the central nervous systems (CNS depressants or opioids).

- Inform patient about possible ataxia, dizziness, drowsiness, and nystagmus. Advise him to avoid hazardous activities until drug's CNS effects are known.
- Instruct patient how to prevent complications from adverse oral reactions (such as gingivitis) by encouraging patient to use good oral hygiene and to seek routine dental care.
- Explain that adverse effects usually are mild to moderate and decline with time.
- Urge patient to keep follow-up appointments with prescriber to check progress.
- Urge caregivers to watch closely for evidence of suicidal tendencies, especially when therapy starts or dosage changes, and to report concerns immediately.

galantamine hydrobromide

Razadyne, Razadyne ER

☰ Class and Category

Pharmacologic class: Cholinesterase inhibitor
Therapeutic class: Antidementia agent

☰ Indications and Dosages

＊ *To treat mild to moderate Alzheimer's-type dementia*

ORAL SOLUTION, TABLETS

Adults. *Initial:* 4 mg twice daily. Dosage increased to 8 mg twice daily after 4 wk, if tolerated and further increased to 12 mg twice a day after an additional 4 wk, if tolerated. *Maximum:* 12 mg twice daily.

E.R. CAPSULES

Adults. *Initial:* 8 mg daily. Dosage increased to 16 mg daily in 4 wk if tolerated, with further increase to 24 mg daily after another 4 wk, if tolerated. *Maximum:* 24 mg daily.

±**DOSAGE ADJUSTMENT** For patients who are taking E.R. capsules and have moderately impaired hepatic function or a creatinine clearance between 9 and 59 ml/min, maximum dosage shouldn't exceed 16 mg daily.

☰ Drug Administration

P.O.

- Give tablets and oral solution twice daily with morning and evening meals, and ensure adequate fluid intake to prevent GI symptoms. Tablets should be swallowed whole and not chewed, crushed, or split.
- Oral solution dosage should be measured using the pipette which comes with drug. Insert the pipette into the bottle and invert. Hold it tightly with one hand by the lower ring and with the other hand pull the upper ring of the pipette until the correct quantity of the drug is visible on the barrel. Turn bottle upright and draw the pipette carefully from the bottle, holding it tightly by the lower ring. Administer into a glass containing 3 to 4 ounces of a nonalcoholic liquid and then stir mixture. Have patient drink immediately.
- Give E.R. capsules once daily with food in the morning. Capsules should be swallowed whole and not chewed, crushed, or opened.
- Know that if therapy is interrupted for several days, expect to restart drug at lowest dose because benefits are lost when dosage is interrupted.

Route	Onset	Peak	Duration
P.O.	Unknown	1 hr	Unknown

Half-life: 7 hr

☰ Mechanism of Action

Reduces acetylcholine metabolism by competitively and reversibly inhibiting the brain enzyme acetylcholinesterase.

Acetylcholine-producing neurons degenerate in the brains of patients with Alzheimer's disease. Inhibition of acetylcholinesterase increases the amount of acetylcholine, which is needed for nerve impulse transmission.

Contraindications

Hypersensitivity to galantamine hydrobromide or its components

Interactions

DRUGS

anticholinergics: Possibly interference with cholinesterase activity

cholinergic agonists such as bethanechol, cholinesterase inhibitors, neuromuscular blockers: Possibly exaggerated effects of these drugs and galantamine

Adverse Reactions

CNS: Aggression, asthenia, **CVA**, depression, dizziness, dysgeusia, extrapyramidal disorder, fatigue, fever, hallucinations, headache, hypersomnia, insomnia, lethargy, malaise, **seizures**, somnolence, **suicidal ideation**, syncope, tremor

CV: AV block (including complete), **bradycardia**, chest pain, hypertension, **MI**, myocardial ischemia

EENT: Blurred vision, rhinitis, tinnitus

GI: Abdominal pain, anorexia, diarrhea, elevated liver enzymes, flatulence, **GI bleeding**, **hepatitis**, indigestion, nausea, vomiting

GU: Hematuria, incontinence, **renal failure or insufficiency**, UTI

HEME: Anemia

SKIN: Acute generalized exanthematous pustulosis, **erythema multiforme, Stevens–Johnson syndrome**

Other: Dehydration, **hypersensitivity reactions, hypokalemia**, weight loss

Childbearing Considerations

PREGNANCY

- It is not known if drug causes fetal harm.
- Use with caution only if benefit to mother outweighs potential risk to fetus.

LACTATION

- Drug is not present in breast milk.
- Patient should check with prescriber before breastfeeding.

Nursing Considerations

- Monitor patient's cardiovascular status closely because cholinesterase inhibitors like galantamine may have a depressive effect AV and sinoatrial nodes and may lead to AV block and bradycardia.
- Monitor patient for progressive deterioration of mental status because drug is less effective as Alzheimer's disease progresses and intact cholinergic neurons decrease.

PATIENT TEACHING

- Instruct patient to take or caregiver to give regular-strength drug with morning and evening meals. Extended-release capsules should be given once in the morning, preferably with food. Instruct patient taking oral solution how to remove drug from bottle. Tell patient to mix in 3 to 4 ounces of a nonalcoholic drink. Tell patient to drink mixture immediately after stirring.
- Tell patient or caregiver to stop drug immediately at the first sign of a skin rash and to notify the prescriber.
- Tell patient or caregiver to notify prescriber immediately if therapy stops for several days. Prescriber may restart at lowest dose.
- Instruct patient to maintain adequate fluid intake throughout galantamine therapy.
- Advise patient not to drive or perform activities requiring alertness, especially during first weeks of treatment, because drug may cause dizziness and drowsiness.
- Inform patient and family members that drug isn't a cure for Alzheimer's disease.

galcanezumab-gnlm

Emgality

Class and Category

Pharmacologic class: Calcitonin gene-related peptide (CGRP) humanized monoclonal antibody

Therapeutic class: Antimigraine

Indications and Dosages

✱ *To prevent migraine headaches*

SUBCUTANEOUS INJECTION

Adults. *Loading:* 240 mg given as 2 consecutive injections of 120 mg each, followed by 120 mg monthly.

✱ *To treat episodic cluster headache*

SUBCUTANEOUS INJECTION

Adults. 300 mg (administered as three consecutive injections of 100 mg each) at the onset of the cluster period, and then monthly until the end of the cluster period.

Drug Administration

SUBCUTANEOUS

- Use the single-dose prefilled pen or single-dose prefilled syringe.
- Protect drug from direct sunlight.
- Prior to injection, remove from refrigerator and allow drug to sit at room temperature for 30 minutes. Do not warm drug by using a heat source such as hot water or a microwave. Also, do not shake the pen or syringe.
- Do not use if solution looks cloudy or has visible particles.
- Inject drug into patient's abdomen, back of the upper arm, buttocks, or thigh.
- Do not inject into areas where the skin is bruised, hard, red, or tender.
- For patient receiving a 240-mg dose, two consecutive injections of 120 mg each given; for a 300-mg dose, three consecutive injections of 100 mg each given.
- Store pen or syringe in refrigerator.

Route	Onset	Peak	Duration
SQ	Unknown	5 days	Unknown

Half-life: 27 days

Mechanism of Action

Binds to calcitonin gene-related peptide ligand to block its binding to the receptor as a means of pain relief.

Contraindications

Hypersensitivity to galcanezumab-gnlm or its components

Interactions

DRUGS

None reported by manufacturer

Adverse Reactions

RESP: Dyspnea
SKIN: Rash, urticaria
Other: Anaphylaxis, angioedema, antibody formation to galcanezumab-gnlm, injection-site reactions (erythema, pain, pruritus)

Childbearing Considerations

PREGNANCY

- Pregnancy exposure registry: 1-833-464-4724 or www .migrainepregnancyregistry.com.

- It is not known if drug causes fetal harm.
- Use with caution only if benefit to mother outweighs potential risk to fetus.
- Know that women with migraines may be at increased risk of preeclampsia during pregnancy.

LACTATION

- It is not known if drug is present in breast milk.
- Patient should check with prescriber before breastfeeding.

Nursing Considerations

! WARNING Monitor patient for hypersensitivity reactions such as dyspnea, rash, or urticaria. If a serious or severe reaction occurs such as anaphylaxis or angioedema, notify prescriber, expect drug to be discontinued, and initiate supportive therapy, as prescribed. Know that a hypersensitivity reaction may occur days after administration and that reaction may be prolonged.

PATIENT TEACHING

- Instruct patient on how to administer a subcutaneous injection using the single-dose prefilled pen or single-dose prefilled syringe. Tell patient to protect drug from direct sunlight. Have patient allow drug to sit at room temperature for 30 minutes before injection. Caution patient not to warm drug by using a heat source such as hot water or a microwave. Also caution patient not to shake the pen or syringe. Tell patient to look for discoloration and particulate matter in the solution before injecting drug. Tell patient not to use if solution looks cloudy or has visible particles.
- Tell patient to administer drug into her abdomen or thigh subcutaneously. Reinforce that she should not inject into areas where the skin is bruised, hard, red, or tender. Tell patient to dispose of pen or syringe and needle in an appropriate container.
- Instruct patient receiving drug to prevent migraines that a loading dose requiring two consecutive injections will be given followed by a monthly dose. Instruct patient receiving drug to treat episodic cluster headache that an initial dose requiring

three consecutive injections will be given at the onset of the cluster period and then monthly until the end of the cluster period.

- Advise patient that if a dose is missed, to administer drug as soon as it is remembered and then schedule the next monthly dose from the date delayed dose was given.

! **WARNING** Instruct patient to seek medical attention if difficulty breathing, hives, rash, or swelling of face, lips, or throat occurs. Inform patient that an allergic reaction can occur days after administration and not to delay seeking treatment, as reaction may become prolonged and life-threatening.

ganciclovir sodium
Cytovene-I.V.

Class and Category

Pharmacologic class: Nucleoside analogue
Therapeutic class: Antiviral

Indications and Dosages

* *To treat cytomegalovirus (CMV) retinitis in immunocompromised patients, including patients with acquired immunodeficiency syndrome (AIDS)*

I.V. INFUSION

Adults. *Induction:* 5 mg/kg every 12 hr for 14 to 21 days. *Maintenance:* 5 mg/kg once daily for 7 days per wk. Alternatively, 6 mg/kg once daily for 5 days every wk.

* *To prevent CMV disease in transplant recipients at risk for CMV disease*

I.V. INFUSION

Adults. *Induction:* 5 mg/kg infused every 12 hr for 7 to 14 days. *Maintenance:* 5 mg/kg once daily for 7 days per wk for 100 to 120 days post-transplantation. Alternatively, 6 mg/kg once daily for 5 days every wk for 100 to 120 days post-transplantation.

±**DOSAGE ADJUSTMENT** For patient with a creatinine clearance between 50 and 69 ml/min, dosage for induction and maintenance reduced by 50%. For patient with a creatinine clearance between 25 and 49 ml/min, dosage for induction reduced by half and dosage interval increased to every 24 hr while maintenance dosage reduced to 1.25 mg/kg every 24 hr. For patient with a

creatinine clearance between 10 and 24 ml/min, induction dosage reduced to 1.25 mg/kg and dosage interval increased to every 24 hr while maintenance dosage reduced to 0.625 mg/kg every 24 hr. For patient with a creatinine clearance of less than 10 ml/min, induction dosage reduced to 1.25 mg/kg with dosage interval increased to only 3 times per wk following hemodialysis while maintenance dosage decreased to 0.625 mg/kg with dosage interval increased to only 3 times per wk following hemodialysis.

Drug Administration

I.V.

- Wear disposable gloves during reconstitution and when wiping the outer surface of vial and table after reconstitution. Avoid direct contact of the skin or mucous membranes with drug. If contact occurs, wash thoroughly with soap and water; rinse eyes thoroughly with plain water. Guidelines issued for antineoplastic drugs should be considered in the handling and disposal of drug because it shares some of the properties of antitumor agents.
- To reconstitute, inject 10 ml of Sterile Water for Injection (never use Bacteriostatic Water) into 500-mg vial to provide a concentration of 50 mg/ml. Gently swirl vial until a clear solution is obtained. Look for particulate matter and discoloration prior to proceeding with infusion. Discard vial, if present.
- Do not refrigerate or freeze reconstituted solution. It may be kept at room temperature for 12 hours.
- Remove the appropriate volume of reconstituted solution and add to 100 ml of 0.9% Sodium Chloride Injection, 5% Dextrose Injection, Lactated Ringer's Injection, or Ringer's Injection.
- Infusion concentrations greater than 10 mg/ml are not recommended.
- Diluted infusion solution should be refrigerated if not used immediately. Use within 24 hours.
- Administer, using an infusion pump, as an intravenous infusion over 1 hour, preferably with a plastic cannula, into a vein with adequate blood flow.
- Do not administer drug by rapid or bolus injection, which may increase toxicity; do not administer drug intramuscularly or

subcutaneously because it may cause severe tissue irritation.

- Do not exceed the recommended dosage and infusion rate.
- *Incompatibilities:* Bacteriostatic Water

Route	Onset	Peak	Duration
I.V.	Unknown	Unknown	Unknown

Half-life: 3.5 hr

Mechanism of Action

Initially, drug is phosphorylated and then slowly metabolized intracellularly into virus-infected cells. There it inhibits the viral DNA polymerase pUL54 to prevent replication of human CMV.

Contraindications

Hypersensitivity to ganciclovir, valganciclovir, or their components

Interactions

DRUGS

amphotericin B, cyclosporine: Increased risk of renal dysfunction

dapsone, doxorubicin, flucytosine, hydroxyurea, pentamidine, tacrolimus, trimethoprim/sulfamethoxazole, vinblastine, vincristine, zidovudine: Increased risk of myelosuppression or nephrotoxicity

didanosine: Increased risk of didanosine toxicity

imipenem-cilastatin: Increased risk of generalized seizures

mycophenolate mofetil: Increased risk for hematologic and renal toxicity

probenecid: Increased serum ganciclovir concentration with increased risk of ganciclovir toxicity

Adverse Reactions

CNS: Agitation, amnesia, anxiety, aphasia, asthenia, chills, confusion, **CVA**, depression, dizziness, dream abnormality, dysesthesia, **encephalopathy**, extrapyramidal disorder, facial paralysis, fatigue, fever, hallucinations, headache, hypoesthesia, insomnia, **intracranial hypertension**, irritability, malaise, paresthesia, peripheral neuropathy, psychotic disorder, **seizures**, somnolence, thinking abnormality, third cranial nerve paralysis, tremor

CV: **Arrhythmias, cardiac arrest**, chest pain, **conduction disorder**, edema, elevated triglycerides, hypertension, **hypotension**, peripheral ischemia, phlebitis, **torsades de pointes**, vasculitis, vasodilatation, **ventricular tachycardia**

EENT: Cataracts, conjunctivitis, deafness, dry eyes or mouth, ear pain, loss of smell, macular edema, mouth ulceration, retinal detachment, taste disturbance, tinnitus, visual impairment, vitreous disorders

ENDO: Inappropriate antidiuretic hormone secretion

GI: Abdominal distention or pain, anorexia, cholelithiasis, cholestasis, constipation, diarrhea, dyspepsia, dysphagia, elevated liver enzymes, eructation, flatulence, **gastrointestinal perforation, hepatic dysfunction or failure, hepatitis**, intestinal ulcer, nausea, **pancreatitis**, vomiting

GU: Abnormal kidney function, decreased creatinine clearance, elevated serum creatinine, hematuria, **hemolytic uremic syndrome**, infertility, **kidney failure**, renal tubular disorder, testicular hypotrophy, urinary frequency

HEME: Agranulocytosis, anemia including hemolytic, **bone marrow failure, decreased platelet count, granulocytopenia, leukopenia, pancytopenia, thrombocytopenia**

MS: Arthralgia, arthritis, back pain, leg cramps, muscle spasms, myalgia, myasthenia, myelopathy, **rhabdomyolysis**

RESP: Bronchospasm, cough, dyspnea, **pulmonary fibrosis**

SKIN: Alopecia, dermatitis, diaphoresis, dry skin, **exfoliative dermatitis**, pruritus, rash, **Stevens–Johnson syndrome**, urticaria

Other: Acidosis, **anaphylaxis**, elevated blood alkaline phosphatase, generalized pain, **hypercalcemia, hyponatremia**, infection including *Candida*, injection-site inflammation, **multiple organ failure, sepsis**, weight loss

Childbearing Considerations

PREGNANCY

- Drug may cause fetal harm such as mutagenic and teratogenic effects based on animal studies.
- A negative pregnancy test in women of childbearing age should be obtained before starting drug therapy.
- Use with extreme caution only if benefit to mother outweighs potential risk to fetus.

LACTATION

- It is not known if drug is present in breast milk.
- Breastfeeding should not be undertaken.

REPRODUCTION

- Women of childbearing age should use effective contraception during drug therapy and for at least 30 days following the last dose of the drug.
- Men should use condoms during drug therapy and for at least 90 days after the last dose of the drug when engaging in sexual activity.
- Drug may cause permanent or temporary female and male infertility.

Nursing Considerations

- Be aware that ganciclovir is not recommended if the absolute neutrophil count is less than 500 cells/µL, hemoglobin is less than 8 g/dl, or the platelet count is less than 25,000 cells/µL.
- Use cautiously in patients with preexisting cytopenias and in patients receiving myelosuppressive drugs or irradiation, because ganciclovir can cause hematologic toxicities. Also use cautiously in patients with impaired renal function, because ganciclovir levels will increase in these patients, requiring dosage adjustments.
- Expect female patients of childbearing age to have a pregnancy test done prior to receiving ganciclovir.
- Obtain a serum creatinine or creatinine clearance prior to starting ganciclovir therapy, as ordered, to establish a baseline for renal function, and then frequently throughout therapy to determine need for and degree of dosage adjustment.
- Ensure that patient has adequate hydration while receiving ganciclovir to reduce adverse effects on renal function. Monitor patient's serum creatinine levels during therapy and assess patient for signs and symptoms of renal dysfunction, especially elderly and those patients receiving concurrent therapy with nephrotoxic drugs such as amphotericin B or cyclosporine.
- Monitor patient's complete blood counts with differential and platelet counts frequently throughout therapy, especially in patients in whom ganciclovir therapy or other nucleoside analogues have previously caused cytopenias, or in whom absolute neutrophil counts are less than 1,000 cells/µL at the beginning of treatment. Granulocytopenia usually occurs during the first or second week of treatment, but may occur at any time during treatment. Notify prescriber of hematologic abnormalities and expect possibility that drug will be discontinued. Cell counts usually begin to recover within 3 to 7 days after drug is discontinued. Colony-stimulating factors may be helpful in increasing neutrophil and white blood cell counts.
- Expect patient to have frequent ophthalmologic examinations during treatment to monitor ganciclovir effectiveness.

! **WARNING** Be aware that ganciclovir has the potential to cause cancer.

PATIENT TEACHING

- Inform patient that frequent blood tests will have to be done throughout ganciclovir therapy because drug may cause blood toxicities. Stress importance of not missing any appointments. In addition, review signs and symptoms of anemia and infections and instruct patient to notify prescriber if present.
- Instruct patient to notify prescriber of persistent, severe, or unusual adverse effects, because drug can cause many adverse reactions, some of which could be serious.
- Stress importance of maintaining adequate hydration throughout ganciclovir therapy, because of potential adverse effect of drug on the kidneys.
- Inform patient that drug may cause temporary or permanent infertility and to discuss this with prescriber if concerned.
- Instruct women of childbearing age to use effective contraception during treatment and for at least 30 days following treatment, because drug may cause fetal toxicity. Instruct men to practice barrier contraception during and for at least 90 days following treatment.
- Tell patient to inform all prescribers of ganciclovir therapy, because drug can interact with other drugs.
- Advise patient not to perform any hazardous activities, such as driving, if cognitive impairment is present.

- Remind patient that ganciclovir is not a cure for CMV retinitis and that it is important to comply with ophthalmologic follow-up examinations.
- Advise mothers not to breastfeed infant while taking ganciclovir.

gemfibrozil
Lopid

Class and Category
Pharmacologic class: Fibric acid derivative
Therapeutic class: Antilipemic

Indications and Dosages
❋ *As adjunct (with diet) to treat hyperlipidemia types IV and V; to reduce risk of coronary artery disease (CAD) in patients with type IIb hyperlipidemia who do not have a history of or symptoms of existing CAD, who have had an inadequate response to lifestyle changes or other pharmacologic agents, and have the following triad of lipid abnormalities: low HDL-cholesterol levels, elevated LDL-cholesterol levels, and elevated triglycerides*

TABLETS
Adults. 600 mg twice daily.

Drug Administration
P.O.
- Administer 30 minutes before morning and evening meals.
- Protect from light and humidity.

Route	Onset	Peak	Duration
P.O.	2–5 days	1–2 hr	Unknown

Half-life: 5–9 hr

Mechanism of Action
May decrease hepatic triglyceride production by decreasing hepatic extraction of free fatty acids, inhibiting peripheral lipolysis, and reducing VLDL synthesis. Gemfibrozil also may inhibit synthesis and increase clearance of apolipoprotein B, a carrier molecule for VLDL. In addition, it may accelerate turnover and removal of total cholesterol from the liver while increasing cholesterol excretion in the feces. As a result, total cholesterol, triglyceride, and VLDL levels decrease; the HDL level increases; and the LDL level is unaffected.

Contraindications
Concurrent therapy with dasabuvir, repaglinide, selexipag, or simvastatin; gallbladder disease; hepatic or severe renal dysfunction, including primary biliary cirrhosis; hypersensitivity to gemfibrozil or its components

Interactions
DRUGS
colchicine: Increased toxicity of either drug; risk of myopathy, including rhabdomyolysis
CYP2C8 substrates such as dabrafenib, loperamide, montelukast, paclitaxel, pioglitazone, rosiglitazone, selexipag: Increased plasma concentration of these drugs
dasabuvir: Increased dasabuvir plasma concentration increasing risk of QT prolongation
enzalutamide: Increased enzalutamide plasma concentration increasing risk of seizures
HMG-CoA reductase inhibitors: Increased risk of acute renal failure and rhabdomyolysis
OATP1B1 substrates such as atrasentan, atorvastatin, bosentan, ezetimibe, fluvastatin, glyburide, olmesartan, pitavastatin, pravastatin, rifampin, rosuvastatin, SN-38 (active metabolite of irinotecan), simvastatin, valsartan: Increased plasma concentrations of these drugs
oral anticoagulants such as warfarin: Increased anticoagulation
repaglinide: Increased serum repaglinide level and risk of severe hypoglycemia
resin-granule drugs such as colestipol: Decreased blood gemfibrozil levels

Adverse Reactions
CNS: Chills, fatigue, headache, hypoesthesia, paresthesia, **seizures**, somnolence, syncope, vertigo
CV: Vasculitis
EENT: Blurred vision, cataracts, hoarseness, retinal edema, taste perversion
GI: Abdominal or epigastric pain, cholelithiasis, colitis, diarrhea, flatulence, heartburn, **hepatoma**, jaundice, nausea, **pancreatitis**, vomiting
GU: Decreased male fertility, dysuria, impotence
HEME: Anemia, **bone marrow hypoplasia**, eosinophilia, **leukopenia, thrombocytopenia**

MS: Arthralgia, back pain, myalgia, myasthenia, myopathy, myositis, **rhabdomyolysis,** synovitis
RESP: Cough
SKIN: Eczema, pruritus, rash
Other: Anaphylaxis, angioedema, increased risk of bacterial and viral infections, lupus-like symptoms, weight loss

Childbearing Considerations

PREGNANCY

- It is not known if drug causes fetal harm.
- Use with caution only if benefit to mother outweighs potential risk to fetus.

LACTATION

- It is not known if drug is present in breast milk.
- A decision should be made to discontinue breastfeeding or the drug to avoid potential serious adverse reactions in the breastfed infant.

Nursing Considerations

- Monitor serum triglyceride and cholesterol levels, as appropriate.
- Periodically review CBC and liver enzymes, during therapy, as ordered.
- Know that if serum cholesterol and triglyceride levels don't improve within 3 months, expect to switch to a different drug, as prescribed.
- Monitor patient's prothrombin time, as ordered, if patient is also receiving warfarin therapy because gemfibrozil therapy may cause a drug interaction with warfarin. Warfarin dosage may have to be decreased to maintain prothrombin time at a level needed to prevent adverse bleeding effects.

PATIENT TEACHING

- Instruct patient to take gemfibrozil 30 minutes before breakfast and 30 minutes before dinner.
- Advise patient to take a missed dose as soon as he remembers, unless it's nearly time for the next dose. Caution against doubling the dose.
- Emphasize importance of alcohol avoidance, a low-fat diet, regular exercise, and smoking cessation, as appropriate.
- Caution patient to avoid hazardous activities until drug's CNS effects are known.
- Instruct patient to notify prescriber if he experiences chills; cough; fever; hoarseness; lower back, side, or muscle pain; painful or

difficult urination; severe abdominal pain with nausea and vomiting; tiredness; or weakness.
- If patient also takes an oral anticoagulant, urge him to report unusual bleeding or bruising; anticoagulant dosage may have to be reduced.
- Advise patient to keep scheduled appointments with prescriber to check progress.

gemifloxacin mesylate
Factive

Class and Category
Pharmacologic class: Fluoroquinolone
Therapeutic class: Antibiotic

Indications and Dosages
* *To treat acute bacterial exacerbation of chronic bronchitis caused by* Haemophilus influenzae, H. parainfluenzae, Moraxella catarrhalis, *or* Streptococcus pneumoniae

TABLETS
Adults. 320 mg daily for 5 days.
* *To treat mild to moderate community-acquired pneumonia caused by* Chlamydia pneumoniae, H. influenzae, Klebsiella pneumoniae, M. catarrhalis, Mycoplasma pneumoniae, *or* S. pneumoniae *including multidrug-resistant strains*

TABLETS
Adults. 320 mg daily for 5 days (when due to *C. pneumoniae, H. influenzae, M. pneumoniae,* or *S. pneumoniae*) or 7 days (when due to *K. pneumoniae, M. catarrhalis,* or multidrug-resistant *S. pneumoniae*).
±**DOSAGE ADJUSTMENT** Dosage should be decreased to 160 mg daily in patients with creatinine clearance of 40 ml/min or less.

Drug Administration
P.O.
- Tablets should be swallowed whole and not chewed, crushed, or split. Administer with a full glass of water.
- Administer drug 2 hours before or 3 hours after administering an antacid, multivitamin, or other products that contain aluminum, iron, magnesium, or zinc; didanosine; or sucralfate.

G
H
I

Route	Onset	Peak	Duration
P.O.	Unknown	0.5–2 hr	Unknown

Half-life: 5–9 hr

Mechanism of Action

Inhibits actions of the enzymes DNA gyrase and topoisomerase IV, which are required for bacterial growth, thereby causing bacterial cells to die.

Contraindications

Hypersensitivity to gemifloxacin, other fluoroquinolones, or their components; myasthenia gravis

Interactions

DRUGS

aluminum and magnesium antacids, didanosine as buffered or chewable tablets or pediatric powder for oral solution, ferrous sulfate, sucralfate, zinc or other metal cations: Reduced blood gemifloxacin level
antipsychotics; class IA antiarrhythmics, such as procainamide and quinidine; class III antiarrhythmics, such as amiodarone and sotalol; erythromycin; tricyclic antidepressants: Possibly prolonged QT interval
probenecid: Increased blood gemifloxacin level
warfarin: Possibly enhanced warfarin anticoagulant effects

Adverse Reactions

CNS: Agitation, anxiety, confusion, delirium, depression, disorientation, disturbance in attention, dizziness, fever, hallucinations, headache, **increased intracranial pressure**, insomnia, light-headedness, memory impairment, nervousness, paranoia, peripheral neuropathy, restlessness, **seizures, suicidal ideation**, syncope, toxic psychosis, transient ischemic attack, tremors
CV: **Aortic aneurysm and dissection**, peripheral edema, **prolonged QT interval**, **supraventricular tachycardia**, vasculitis
EENT: Taste perversion
ENDO: Hyperglycemia, **hypoglycemia**
GI: Abdominal pain, **acute hepatic necrosis or failure**, diarrhea, elevated liver enzymes, **hepatitis**, jaundice, nausea, **pseudomembranous colitis**, vomiting
GU: **Acute renal insufficiency or failure**, interstitial nephritis

HEME: **Agranulocytosis, aplastic or hemolytic anemia, elevated international normalized ratio (INR), hemorrhage, leukopenia, pancytopenia, thrombocytopenia**, thrombocytosis
MS: Arthralgia, muscle weakness, myalgia, tendinitis, tendon rupture
RESP: **Hypersensitivity pneumonitis**
SKIN: **Erythema multiforme**, exfoliation, photosensitivity, rash, **Stevens–Johnson syndrome, toxic epidermal necrolysis**, urticaria
Other: **Anaphylaxis, angioedema**, serum sickness

Childbearing Considerations

PREGNANCY

- Drug may cause fetal harm based on animal studies.
- Use with caution only if benefit to mother outweighs potential risk to fetus.

LACTATION

- It is not known if drug is present in breast milk.
- Patient should check with prescriber before breastfeeding.

Nursing Considerations

- Review patient's medical history before giving gemifloxacin, which shouldn't be used in patient with a history of prolonged QT interval, patient with uncorrected electrolyte disorders, or patient receiving class IA or III antiarrhythmics because of increased risk of prolonged QT interval. Monitor elderly patients closely because they may be more susceptible to prolonged QT interval.
- Be aware that an increased rate of aortic aneurysm and dissection may occur within 2 months of gemifloxacin therapy, especially in the elderly. Patients with known aortic aneurysm or patients who are at greater risk for aortic aneurysms should not receive gemifloxacin unless there are no alternative antibacterial treatments available.
- Use cautiously in patients with CNS disorders, such as epilepsy, or in those prone to seizures because gemifloxacin has caused increased intracranial pressure, seizures, and toxic psychosis. Monitor patient closely; if CNS alterations occur, notify prescriber immediately and expect drug to be discontinued.

! **WARNING** Monitor patient closely for hypersensitivity reaction, which may occur as soon as first dose. If patient has such evidence as angioedema, bronchospasm, dyspnea, itching, rash, shortness of breath, and urticaria, notify prescriber immediately and expect drug to be discontinued.

- Monitor patients prone to tendinitis, such as athletes, the elderly, and those taking corticosteroids, for reports of tendon inflammation, pain, or rupture. If present, notify prescriber. Expect gemifloxacin to be discontinued, patient placed on bed rest with no exercise of affected limb, and diagnostic tests ordered to confirm rupture.
- Notify prescriber about severe or prolonged diarrhea; it may indicate pseudomembranous colitis caused by *Clostridium difficile.* If diarrhea occurs, notify prescriber and expect to withhold gemifloxacin and treat with electrolytes, fluids, protein, and an antibiotic effective against *C. difficile.*
- Monitor patients, especially women under age 40 and postmenopausal women receiving hormone replacement therapy, for rash. It may appear days after therapy starts and resolve in 7 days. Notify prescriber immediately if rash occurs because it can be severe in about 10% of patients.
- Assess patient for evidence of peripheral neuropathy. Notify prescriber and expect to stop drug if patient complains of burning, numbness, pain, tingling, or weakness in extremities or if physical examination reveals deficits in light touch, motor strength, pain, position sense, temperature, or vibratory sensation.
- Monitor coagulation status, as ordered, for patient who takes warfarin because adding gemifloxacin may increase risk of bleeding.
- Know that fluoroquinolones like gemifloxacin have caused disabling and potentially irreversible serious adverse reactions from different body systems that can occur together in the same patient. These reactions can occur within hours to weeks after starting the drug and usually cause central nervous system effects, peripheral neuropathy, tendinitis, and tendon rupture. All ages of patients and patients without any preexisting risk factors have experienced these reactions.

Notify prescriber and expect to discontinue gemifloxacin immediately at the first sign or symptom of any serious adverse reactions.

- Monitor patient's blood glucose levels, especially in diabetic patients, and for signs and symptoms of changes in blood glucose levels. Both symptomatic hyperglycemia and hypoglycemia may occur as a result of gemifloxacin therapy. If present, alert prescriber and initiate appropriate treatment, as prescribed. Also be aware that severe hypoglycemia has occurred with other fluoroquinolones. If a hypoglycemic reaction occurs, discontinue gemifloxacin administration immediately and initiate appropriate treatment for hypoglycemia.
- Monitor patient closely for changes in behavior or mood that may be caused by gemifloxacin-induced depression or worsening psychotic reactions potentially resulting in self-injurious behavior, such as suicide. Be aware that these reactions may occur even after just one dose. If present, notify prescriber immediately and expect to discontinue gemifloxacin therapy and institute precautions to keep patient safe until adverse effects have resolved.

PATIENT TEACHING

- Tell patient to swallow tablet whole and take with a full glass of liquid.
- Inform patient that drug should be taken 2 hours before or 3 hours after taking aluminum and/or magnesium antacids; didanosine (Videx) buffered or chewable tables and pediatric powder for oral solution (if prescribed); multivitamins containing zinc or other metal cations; and products containing iron.
- Warn patient not to increase dose because doing so may cause life-threatening cardiac arrhythmias.
- Instruct patient to complete entire course of therapy, even if symptoms decrease before prescription is finished.
- Caution patient to avoid sun exposure as much as possible while taking gemifloxacin. Patient who can't avoid sun exposure should apply sunscreen and wear a hat, sunglasses, and long sleeves to cover as much skin as possible.
- Urge caregivers to monitor patient closely for suicidal tendencies; if patient develops depression or worsening of psychotic

G
H
I

behavior during therapy, instruct them to notify prescriber.

- Instruct patient to maintain adequate hydration throughout therapy to keep urine from becoming too concentrated. Tell patient to increase fluid intake if urine darkens or amount voided decreases.
- Caution patient to avoid hazardous activities until CNS effects of drug are known.

> ! **WARNING** Instruct patient to seek medical attention and notify prescriber immediately if he has tendon pain, tenderness, or rupture; evidence of hypersensitivity reaction, such as difficulty breathing, facial swelling, rash, or urticaria; or fainting spells or palpitations. Also advise patient to stop taking gemifloxacin immediately and notify prescriber if any other persistent, serious, or worsening adverse effects occur.

- Urge patient to tell prescriber about diarrhea that's severe or lasts longer than 3 days. Explain that bloody or watery stools can occur 2 or more months after therapy and can be serious, requiring prompt treatment.
- Tell patient to consult prescriber before starting any new medications, including OTC products, because gemifloxacin may interact adversely.
- Inform patient that drug should be taken 2 hours before or 3 hours after taking aluminum and/or magnesium antacids; didanosine (Videx) buffered or chewable tables and pediatric powder for oral solution (if prescribed); multivitamins containing zinc or other metal cations; and products containing iron.
- Warn patient, especially diabetics, that gemifloxacin may alter blood glucose levels. Review signs and symptoms of hyperglycemia and hypoglycemia. Tell patient to immediately report symptomatic changes in blood glucose levels to prescriber and review how to treat hypoglycemia.

gentamicin sulfate
Cidomycin (CAN)

☰ Class and Category
Pharmacologic class: Aminoglycoside
Therapeutic class: Antibiotic

☰ Indications and Dosages
✴ *To treat serious bacterial infections caused by* Citrobacter *species,* Escherichia coli, Klebsiella-Enterobacter-Serratia species, Proteus *species (indole negative and indole positive),* Pseudomonas aeruginosa, Staphylococcus *species*

I.V. INFUSION, I.M. INJECTION
Adults and adolescents. 3 mg/kg/day divided into 3 equal doses every 8 hr for 7 to 10 days. For life-threatening infections: Up to 5 mg/kg/day divided into 3 or 4 equal doses for 7 to 10 days or longer with dosage reduced as soon as possible to 3 mg/kg/day.
Children. 2 to 2.5 mg/kg every 8 hr for 7 to 10 days.
Infants and neonates over age 1 week. 2.5 mg/kg every 8 hr for 7 to 10 days.
Premature or full-term neonates up to age 1 week. 2.5 mg/kg every 12 hr for 7 to 10 days.

±**DOSAGE ADJUSTMENT** For adults with impaired renal function, highly individualized and dependent on degree of renal function and drug level. For adult patients receiving dialysis, 1 to 1.7 mg/kg at the end of each dialysis period has been suggested. For children receiving dialysis, a dose of 2 mg/kg at the end of each dialysis period has been suggested.

☰ Drug Administration
I.V.
- May be the preferred route for patients with bacterial septicemia or those in shock. It may also be the preferred route for patients with congestive heart failure, hematologic disorders, severe burns, or those with reduced muscle mass.
- Dilute each dose with 50 to 200 ml of 0.9% Sodium Chloride Injection or 5% Dextrose in Water. In children, infants, and neonates, the volume of diluent should be less.
- Administer as an intermittent infusion slowly over 30 minutes to 2 hours.
- Flush I.V. line before and after I.V. infusion with either 0.9% Sodium Chloride Injection or 5% Dextrose in Water.
- Expect to adjust dosage based on peak and trough blood drug levels.
- *Incompatibilities:* Other drugs

I.M.
- Inject deeply into a large muscle.
- Rotate sites.

Route	Onset	Peak	Duration
I.V.	Immediate	30–60 min	Unknown
I.M.	Unknown	30–90 min	Unknown

Half-life: 2–3 hr

Mechanism of Action

Binds to negatively charged sites on the outer cell membrane of bacteria, thereby disrupting the membrane's integrity. Gentamicin also binds to bacterial ribosomal subunits and inhibits protein synthesis. Both actions lead to cell death.

Contraindications

Hypersensitivity to gentamicin, other aminoglycosides, or their components

Interactions

DRUGS

loop diuretics (ethacrynic acid, furosemide), other aminoglycosides (kanamycin, neomycin, streptomycin): Increased risk of nephrotoxicity and ototoxicity
neuromuscular blockers: Prolonged respiratory depression, increased neuromuscular blockade
other nephrotoxic drugs: Increased risk of nephrotoxicity
penicillins: Inactivation of gentamicin by certain penicillins, increased risk of nephrotoxicity

Adverse Reactions

CNS: Acute organic mental syndrome, confusion, depression, fever, headache, increased protein in cerebrospinal fluid, lethargy, myasthenia gravis-like syndrome, **neurotoxicity**, peripheral neuropathy or **encephalopathy**, **pseudotumor cerebri**, **seizures**
CV: Hypertension, **hypotension**, palpitations
EENT: Blurred vision, increased salivation, **laryngeal edema**, ototoxicity, stomatitis, vision changes
GI: Anorexia, nausea, splenomegaly, transient hepatomegaly, vomiting
GU: **Nephrotoxicity**
HEME: Anemia, eosinophilia, **granulocytopenia**, increased or decreased reticulocyte count, **leukopenia**, **thrombocytopenia**
MS: Arthralgia, leg cramps

RESP: **Pulmonary fibrosis, respiratory depression**
SKIN: Alopecia, generalized burning sensation, pruritus, purpura, rash, urticaria
Other: **Anaphylaxis**, injection-site pain, superinfection, weight loss

Childbearing Considerations

PREGNANCY

- Aminoglycosides, such as gentamicin, may cause fetal harm as they cross the placental barrier and may cause irreversible deafness and severe muscle weakness in the neonate.
- Drug is usually not recommended during pregnancy except in life-threatening situations.

LACTATION

- Drug is present in breast milk.
- A decision should be made to discontinue breastfeeding or the drug to avoid potential serious adverse reactions in the breastfed infant.

Nursing Considerations

- Expect to obtain a body fluid or tissue specimen for culture and sensitivity testing, as ordered, before gentamicin therapy begins, or check test results, if available.
- Know that drug should not be given to a pregnant patient because it can cause hearing loss in fetus.
- Know that any report of dizziness, hearing loss, or ringing in the ears should be taken very seriously. Hold drug with any report of these problems.

! **WARNING** Be alert for allergic reactions—including anaphylaxis and possibly life-threatening asthmatic episodes. Notify prescriber and expect to discontinue drug and provide supportive care, as ordered.

- Assess patient for evidence of other infections, because gentamicin may cause overgrowth of nonsusceptible organisms.
- Be aware that premature infants, neonates, and elderly patients have an increased risk of nephrotoxicity.

PATIENT TEACHING

- Emphasize importance of completing full course of gentamicin therapy.

G
H
I

! **WARNING** Review signs and symptoms of an allergic reaction and emphasize importance of reporting an allergic reaction to the prescriber and seeking immediate emergency care, if severe.

- Instruct patient to immediately report adverse reactions, such as hearing loss, to avoid permanent effects.

glimepiride
Amaryl

Class and Category
Pharmacologic class: Sulfonylurea
Therapeutic class: Antidiabetic

Indications and Dosages
* *As adjunct to control blood glucose level in type 2 diabetes mellitus*

TABLETS
Adults. *Initial:* 1 to 2 mg once daily. Dosage increased by 1 to 2 mg every 1 to 2 wk as needed for blood glucose control. *Maximum:* 8 mg once daily.

±**DOSAGE ADJUSTMENT** Initial dosage reduced to 1 mg daily and dosage titrated more slowly for the elderly and patients with renal impairment.

Drug Administration
P.O.
- Administer with first meal of the day.

Route	Onset	Peak	Duration
P.O.	1 hr	2–3 hr	>24 hr

Half-life: 5–9 hr

Mechanism of Action
Stimulates insulin release from beta cells in pancreas. Glimepiride also increases peripheral tissue sensitivity to insulin, either by enhancing insulin binding to cellular receptors or by increasing the number of insulin receptors.

Contraindications
Hypersensitivity to glimepiride, sulfonamide derivatives, or their components

Interactions
DRUGS
ACE inhibitors, anabolic steroids, androgens, azole antifungals, bromocriptine, chloramphenicol, clarithromycin, clonidine, cyclophosphamide, disopyramide, fibric acid derivatives, fluconazole, fluoxetine, guanethidine, H₂-receptor antagonists, insulin, magnesium salts, MAO inhibitors, methyldopa, NSAIDs, octreotide, oral anticoagulants, other oral hypoglycemic agents, oxyphenbutazone, pentoxifylline, phenylbutazone, phenyramidol, pramlintide, probenecid, propoxyphene, quinidine, quinolones, reserpine, salicylates, somatostatin analogs, sulfonamides, tetracyclines, theophylline, tricyclic antidepressants, urinary acidifiers: Increased risk of hypoglycemia
asparaginase, barbiturates, calcium channel blockers, cholestyramine, clonidine, clozapine, colesevelam, corticosteroids, danazol, diazoxide, estrogens, glucagon, hydantoins, isoniazid, laxatives, lithium, morphine, nicotinic acid, olanzapine, oral contraceptives, phenothiazines, phenytoin, protease inhibitors, reserpine, rifabutin, rifampin, somatropin, sympathomimetics, thiazide and other diuretics, thyroid hormones, urinary alkalinizers: Increased risk of hyperglycemia
beta-blockers, clonidine, reserpine: Possibly hyperglycemia or masking of hypoglycemia signs
miconazole (oral): Increased risk of severe hypoglycemia
sympatholytic drugs such as beta-blockers, clonidine, guanethidine, reserpine: Reduced or absent hypoglycemic signs and symptoms

ACTIVITIES
alcohol use: Altered blood glucose control (usually hypoglycemia)

Adverse Reactions
CNS: Abnormal gait, anxiety, asthenia, chills, depression, dizziness, fatigue, headache, hypertonia, hypoesthesia, insomnia, malaise, migraine headache, nervousness, paresthesia, somnolence, syncope, tremor, vertigo
CV: **Arrhythmias**, edema, hypertension, vasculitis
EENT: Blurred vision, conjunctivitis, eye pain, pharyngitis, retinal hemorrhage, rhinitis, taste perversion, tinnitus
ENDO: **Hypoglycemia**, increased release of antidiuretic hormone secretion (SIADH)
GI: Anorexia, cholestasis, constipation, diarrhea, elevated liver enzymes, epigastric discomfort or fullness, flatulence, heartburn, hepatic porphyria, **hepatotoxicity**, hunger,

jaundice, **liver failure,** nausea, proctocolitis, trace blood in stool, vomiting

GU: Darkened urine, decreased libido, dysuria, polyuria

HEME: Agranulocytosis, aplastic anemia, eosinophilia, **hemolytic anemia, leukopenia, pancytopenia, thrombocytopenia, thrombocytopenic purpura**

MS: Arthralgia, leg cramps, myalgia

RESP: Dyspnea

SKIN: Allergic skin reactions, alopecia, diaphoresis, eczema, **erythema multiforme, exfoliative dermatitis,** flushing, lichenoid reactions, maculopapular or morbilliform rash, photosensitivity, pruritus, **Stevens–Johnson syndrome,** urticaria

Other: Anaphylaxis, angioedema, disulfiram-like reaction, **hyponatremia**

☰ Childbearing Considerations

PREGNANCY

- It is not known if drug can cause fetal harm. However, it may cause neonatal hypoglycemia.
- Drug is not recommended during pregnancy because abnormal blood glucose levels during pregnancy are associated with a higher incidence of congenital abnormalities, making insulin the preferred drug of choice during pregnancy.

LABOR & DELIVERY

- At birth, neonate may experience birth injury, respiratory distress, and prolonged severe hypoglycemia, lasting 4 to 10 days, if mother receives drug at time of delivery.
- If drug is used during pregnancy, expect it to be discontinued at least 2 weeks before expected delivery.

LACTATION

- It is not known if drug is present in breast milk.
- Patient should check with prescriber before breastfeeding.
- If breastfeeding occurs, infant should be monitored for signs and symptoms of hypoglycemia.

☰ Nursing Considerations

- Use cautiously in patients with glucose 6-phosphate dehydrogenase (G6PD) deficiency because glimepiride is a sulfonylurea, and sulfonylureas can cause hemolytic anemia in these patients.

- Monitor fasting blood glucose level to determine response to glimepiride. Expect to check glycosylated hemoglobin level every 3 to 6 months to evaluate long-term blood glucose control, or as ordered.
- Expect to switch patient to insulin therapy, as prescribed, during physical stress, such as infection, surgery, and trauma.

! **WARNING** Expect a higher risk of hypoglycemia when giving glimepiride to a debilitated or malnourished patient or one with adrenal, hepatic, pituitary, or renal insufficiency. Also be aware that hypoglycemia may be more difficult to recognize in patients with autonomic neuropathy, the elderly, and patients taking beta-blockers or other sympatholytic agents. Monitor blood glucose level closely.

- Be aware that patients taking the sulfonylurea, tolbutamide, may have an increased risk of dying from cardiovascular disease. Glimepiride has not been studied for cardiovascular mortality, but because it is also a sulfonylurea, monitor patients closely.

! **WARNING** Monitor patient closely for allergic reactions that could become life-threatening. If allergic reaction occurs, stop drug immediately and notify prescriber. Provide supportive care, as ordered. Give glimepiride at least 4 hours before administering colesevelam, if prescribed, to patient because colesevelam decreases exposure to glimepiride.

PATIENT TEACHING

- Instruct patient to take glimepiride just before first meal of the day. Caution him not to skip the meal after taking drug.
- Urge patient not to skip doses or increase dosage without consulting prescriber.
- Alert patient prescribed both glimepiride and colesevelam of the need to take glimepiride 4 hours before colesevelam.

! **WARNING** Urge patient to seek immediate emergency care and stop taking glimepiride if an allergic reaction occurs.

- Urge patient to report signs of hypoglycemia, such as anxiety, confusion, dizziness, excessive sweating, headache, and nausea.

G
H
I

- Encourage patient to carry hard candy or other simple sugars to treat mild hypoglycemia.
- Advise patient to consult prescriber before taking any OTC drug.
- Urge patient to carry identification indicating that he has diabetes.
- Teach patient how to monitor his blood glucose level.
- Teach patient about diet, exercise, foot care, hygiene, signs of hyperglycemia and hypoglycemia, and ways to avoid infection.
- Instruct patient to notify prescriber about darkened urine, difficulty controlling his blood glucose level, easy bruising, fever, rash, sore throat, or unusual bleeding.
- Instruct patient to avoid direct sunlight and to wear sunscreen.
- Tell women of childbearing age to notify prescriber if pregnancy is suspected or occurs.
- Have mothers who are breastfeeding while taking glimepiride monitor their infant for signs of low blood sugar. If present, ensure mother knows how to treat it, including reporting infant hypoglycemia to prescriber. Breastfeeding or drug may have to be discontinued.

glipizide
Glucotrol, Glucotrol XL

Class and Category
Pharmacologic class: Sulfonylurea
Therapeutic class: Antidiabetic

Indications and Dosages
✱ *As adjunct to control blood glucose level in type 2 diabetes mellitus*

E.R. TABLETS
Adults. *Initial:* 5 mg once daily. Dosage increased, as needed, based on patient's glucose response. *Maximum:* 20 mg daily.

TABLETS
Adults. *Initial:* 5 mg once daily. Dosage adjusted by 2.5 to 5 mg every 2 to 3 days and given as a single dose, if dosage is 15 mg or less or given in 2 divided doses, if dosage exceeds 15 mg daily. *Maximum:* 40 mg daily in divided doses.

✱ *To replace insulin therapy in type 2 diabetes mellitus*

TABLETS
Adults who receive 20 units of insulin or less. Insulin discontinued and 5 mg given once daily. Dosage adjusted, by 2.5 to 5 mg as needed, every 3 to 4 days.

Adults who receive more than 20 units insulin daily. *Initial:* 5 mg once daily given while insulin dosage decreased by one-half. Dosage adjusted by 2.5 to 5 mg, as needed, every 3 to 4 days. Further insulin reductions are made based on clinical response.

±**DOSAGE ADJUSTMENT** Initial dosage reduced to 2.5 mg daily if needed for patients over age 65, patients who are debilitated or malnourished, and those with impaired hepatic or renal function.

Drug Administration
P.O.
- Give as a single dose if dosage is 15 mg or less or divided; give twice daily if dosage exceeds 15 mg daily.
- Administer immediate-acting tablets 30 minutes before the first meal of the day if given once daily and 30 minutes before meals if given in divided doses.
- Administer X.L. tablets with the first main meal of the day. X.L. tablets should be swallowed whole and not chewed, crushed, or split.

Route	Onset	Peak	Duration
P.O.	30 min	1–3 hr	12–24 hr
P.O./X.L.	2–3 hr	6–12 hr	24 hr
Half-life: 2–5 hr			

Mechanism of Action
Stimulates insulin release from beta cells in pancreas. Glipizide also increases peripheral tissue sensitivity to insulin, either by increasing insulin binding to cellular receptors or by increasing number of insulin receptors.

Contraindications
Hypersensitivity to glipizide, sulfonylureas, or their components; ketoacidosis; sole therapy for type 1 diabetes mellitus

Interactions
DRUGS
ACE inhibitors, anabolic steroids, androgens, angiotensin II receptor blocking agents, azole antifungals (selected), beta-blockers,

bromocriptine, chloramphenicol, coumarins, disopyramide, fibric acid derivatives, fluconazole, fluoxetine, guanethidine, H₂-receptor antagonists, insulin and other antidiabetic drugs, magnesium salts, MAO inhibitors, methyldopa, NSAIDs, octreotide, oral anticoagulants, oxyphenbutazone, pentoxifylline, phenylbutazone, pramlintide, probenecid, propoxyphene, quinidine, quinolones, salicylates, sulfonamide antibiotics, tetracycline, theophylline, tricyclic antidepressants, urinary acidifiers, voriconazole: Increased risk of hypoglycemia
asparaginase, atypical antipsychotics, calcium channel blockers, cholestyramine, clonidine, colesevelam, corticosteroids, danazol, diazoxide, estrogen, glucagon, hydantoins, isoniazid, lithium, morphine, niacin, nicotinic acid, oral contraceptives, phenothiazines, phenytoin, protease inhibitors, rifabutin, rifampin, somatropin, sympathomimetics, thiazides and other diuretics, thyroid drugs, urinary alkalinizers: Increased risk of hyperglycemia
beta-blockers, clonidine, reserpine: Possibly hyperglycemia or hypoglycemia
miconazole (oral): Possibly severe hypoglycemia
sympatholytic drugs such as beta-blockers, clonidine, guanethidine, reserpine: Possible masking of hypoglycemia signs

FOODS
all foods: Possibly delayed absorption of immediate-release tablets if taken within 30 minutes of meal

ACTIVITIES
alcohol use: Altered blood glucose control (usually hypoglycemia)

Adverse Reactions
CNS: Abnormal gait, anxiety, asthenia, chills, depression, dizziness, fatigue, headache, hypertonia, hypoesthesia, insomnia, malaise, migraine headache, nervousness, paresthesia, somnolence, syncope, tremor, vertigo
CV: **Arrhythmias**, edema, hypertension, vasculitis
EENT: Blurred vision, conjunctivitis, eye pain, pharyngitis, retinal hemorrhage, rhinitis, taste perversion, tinnitus
ENDO: **Hypoglycemia**
GI: Abdominal pain, anorexia, cholestatic jaundice, constipation, diarrhea, elevated liver, enzymes, epigastric discomfort or

fullness, flatulence, heartburn, hepatic porphyria, **hepatitis**, hunger, jaundice, nausea, proctocolitis, trace blood in stool, vomiting
GU: Darkened urine, decreased libido, dysuria, polyuria
HEME: **Agranulocytosis**, **aplastic anemia**, eosinophilia, **hemolytic anemia**, **leukopenia**, **pancytopenia**
MS: Arthralgia, leg cramps, myalgia
RESP: Dyspnea
SKIN: Allergic skin reactions, diaphoresis, eczema, **erythema multiforme**, **exfoliative dermatitis**, flushing, lichenoid reactions, maculopapular or morbilliform rash, photosensitivity, urticaria
Other: Disulfiram-like reaction

Childbearing Considerations
PREGNANCY
- It is not known if drug can cause fetal harm. However, it may cause neonatal hypoglycemia.
- Drug is not recommended during pregnancy because abnormal blood glucose levels during pregnancy are associated with a higher incidence of congenital abnormalities, making insulin the preferred drug of choice during pregnancy.

LABOR & DELIVERY
- At birth, neonate may experience birth injury, respiratory distress, and prolonged severe hypoglycemia, lasting 4 to 10 days if mother receives drug at time of delivery.
- If drug is used during pregnancy, expect it to be discontinued at least 4 weeks before expected delivery.

LACTATION
- It is not known if drug is present in breast milk.
- Drug or breastfeeding should be discontinued because of risk for infant hypoglycemia.

Nursing Considerations
- Use cautiously in patients with glucose 6-phosphate dehydrogenase deficiency because hemolytic anemia may develop. Monitor patient's CBC closely.
- Check blood glucose level at least three times daily for a patient switching from insulin to glipizide. Patients who take more than 40 units of insulin daily may need hospitalization during transition.

G
H
I

- Monitor fasting blood glucose level to determine response to drug. Expect to check glycosylated hemoglobin every 3 to 6 months or as ordered to evaluate long-term blood glucose control.
- Expect to switch patient to insulin therapy, as prescribed, during physical stress, such as infection, surgery, or trauma.

! WARNING Be aware that the risk of hypoglycemia is higher when giving glipizide to a debilitated or malnourished patient or one with adrenal, hepatic, pituitary, or renal insufficiency.

PATIENT TEACHING

- Tell patient to take immediate-release form of glipizide 30 minutes before the first meal of the day or, if taking twice daily, to take 30 minutes before meals. Tell patient prescribed the extended-release form of glipizide to take it with breakfast, swallowing tablet whole. Caution him not to skip the meal after taking drug.
- Advise patient not to skip doses or increase the dosage without consulting prescriber.

! WARNING Urge patient to report evidence of hypoglycemia, such as anxiety, confusion, dizziness, excessive sweating, headache, and nausea.

- Encourage patient to carry hard candy or other simple sugars to treat mild hypoglycemia.
- Caution patient to consult prescriber before taking any OTC drugs.
- Urge patient to carry identification indicating that he has diabetes.
- Teach patient how to monitor his blood glucose level.
- Teach patient about diet, exercise, foot care, hygiene, signs of hyperglycemia and hypoglycemia, and ways to avoid infection.
- Instruct patient to notify prescriber if he experiences darkened urine, easy bruising, fever, hypoglycemia or hyperglycemia, rash, sore throat, and unusual bleeding.
- Instruct patient to avoid direct sunlight and to wear sunscreen.
- Alert patient prescribed both extended-release form of glipizide and colesevelam of the need to take glipizide extended-release 4 hours before colesevelam.
- Advise pregnant women that glipizide will have to be temporarily withheld for about 4 weeks before expected delivery to prevent infant hypoglycemia, which could be severe.
- Tell mothers breastfeeding or the drug will have to be discontinued because of the risk for infant hypoglycemia.

glucagon
Baqsimi, Gvoke HypoPen, Gvoke PFS

glucagon hydrochloride
GlucaGen, Glucagon Diagnostic Kit, Glucagon Emergency Kit

Class and Category
Pharmacologic class: Pancreatic hormone
Therapeutic class: Antihypoglycemic, diagnostic aid adjunct

Indications and Dosages
* *To provide emergency treatment of severe hypoglycemia*

I.V., I.M., OR SUBCUTANEOUS INJECTION (GLUCAGEN, GLUCAGON)

Adults and children weighing more than 20 kg (44 lb) or, with GlucaGen, more than 25 kg (55 lb) and for children 6 years and older of unknown weight. 1 mg, repeated in 15 min as needed.

Children weighing 20 kg (44 lb) or less or, with GlucaGen, 25 kg (55 lb) or less or for children who are less than 6 years of unknown weight. 0.5 mg repeated in 15 min, as needed.

SUBCUTANEOUS INJECTION (GVOKE)

Adults and children 12 years and older. 1 mg, repeated in 15 min, if needed.

Children age 2 to less than 12 years weighing 45 kg (99 lb) or more. 1 mg, repeated in 15 min, if needed.

Children age 2 to less than 12 years weighing less than 45 kg (99 lb). 0.5 mg, repeated in 15 min, if needed.

NASAL SPRAY (BAQSIMI)

Adults and children age 4 and over. 3 mg (1 spray) into one nostril. If no response after 15 minutes, dosage repeated.

✳ *To provide diagnostic assistance by inhibiting bowel peristalsis in radiologic examination of GI tract*

I.M. INJECTION (GLUCAGEN, GLUCAGON)

Adults. *For relaxing duodenum, small bowel, or stomach:* 1 mg before procedure. *For relaxing colon:* 1 to 2 mg before procedure.

I.V. INJECTION (GLUCAGEN, GLUCAGON)

Adults. *For relaxing duodenum, small bowel, or stomach:* 0.25 to 0.5 mg before procedure. *For relaxing colon:* 0.5 to 0.75 mg before procedure.

≡ Drug Administration

- Don't mix parenteral preparations of glucagon with 0.9% Sodium Chloride Injection or solutions that have a pH of 3.0 to 9.5; use with dextrose solutions instead.
- Store drug at room temperature.

I.V. (GLUCAGEN, GLUCAGON)

- Reconstitute 1-mg vial with 1 ml of diluent, either supplied or Sterile Water for Injection. Shake vial gently until powder is completely dissolved. Reconstituted fluid should be clear and colorless. Concentration should be 1 mg/ml.
- Use drug immediately after reconstitution.
- Place unconscious patient on his side before injecting drug, to prevent aspiration of vomitus when he regains consciousness.
- Administer by slow I.V. injection over 1 minute to decrease risk of adverse reactions, such as tachycardia and vomiting.
- Give I.V. dextrose, as ordered, if patient doesn't respond to drug or oral carbohydrates once responsive.
- *Incompatibilities:* Electrolyte-containing solutions such as Sodium Chloride or Potassium Chloride

I.M. (GLUCAGEN, GLUCAGON)

- Reconstitute 1-mg vial of drug with 1 ml of supplied diluent or Sterile Water for Injection. Shake vial gently until powder is completely dissolved. Solution should be clear and colorless. Concentration should be 1 mg/ml. Use immediately.
- Place unconscious patient on his side before injecting drug, to prevent aspiration of vomitus when he regains consciousness.
- Inject into buttocks, outer thigh, or outer upper arm.
- Give I.V. dextrose, as ordered, if patient doesn't respond to glucagon or oral carbohydrates once responsive.

SUBCUTANEOUS (GLUCAGEN, GLUCAGON, GVOKE)

Glucagen or Glucagon
- Same instructions as for I.M. injection.

GVOKE

- Gvoke comes as either an autoinjector or prefilled syringe. Do not open foil pouch until ready to administer. Follow instructions printed on foil pouch label, carton, or the Instructions for Use. Solution should be clear and colorless to pale yellow.
- Place unconscious patient on his side before injecting drug to prevent aspiration of vomitus when he regains consciousness.
- Inject into the lower abdomen, outer thigh, or outer upper arm.
- Each autoinjector or prefilled syringe contains one dose of glucagon and cannot be reused. If a repeat dose is needed, a new device must be used.
- Give I.V. dextrose, as ordered, if patient doesn't respond to drug or oral carbohydrates once responsive.

INTRANASAL (BAQSIMI)

- The plunger should not be pushed or tested prior to use.
- Administer dose by inserting the device tip into one nostril and pressing the device plunger all the way in until the green line is no longer showing. The dose does not have to be inhaled.
- Each device contains one dose of glucagon and cannot be reused. If a repeat dose is needed, a new device must be used.

Route	Onset	Peak	Duration
I.V.	Immediate	5–20 min	1–2 hr
I.M.	8–10 min	30 min	1–2 hr
SubQ	<10 min	30 min	1–2 hr
Intranasal	Unknown	15 min	Unknown

Half-life: <35 min

≡ Mechanism of Action

Increases production of adenylate cyclase, which catalyzes conversion of adenosine triphosphate to cAMP, a process that in turn activates phosphorylase. Phosphorylase promotes breakdown of glycogen to glucose (glycogenolysis) in the liver. As a result, blood glucose level increases and GI smooth muscles relax.

Contraindications

Glucagonoma (when used as a diagnostic aid), hypersensitivity to glucagon or its components, insulinoma, pheochromocytoma

Interactions

DRUGS

anticholinergic drugs: Increased gastrointestinal adverse reactions
beta-blockers: Transient increase in blood pressure and pulse
indomethacin: Possibly loss of effectiveness to raise blood glucose; possibly even produce hypoglycemia
insulin: Antagonistic toward glucagon
oral anticoagulants: Possibly increased anticoagulant effects

Adverse Reactions

CNS: Asthenia, dizziness, headache, somnolence
CV: Hypertension, **hypotension**, tachycardia
EENT: *Nasal form:* Altered taste, eye itchiness or redness, itchy ears or throat, nasal congestion or itching, running nose, sneezing, watery eyes
ENDO: **Hyperglycemia** (presence of diabetes mellitus during diagnostic testing), **hypoglycemia** (presence of glucagonoma or insulinoma)
GI: Abdominal pain, diarrhea, nausea, vomiting
RESP: **Bronchospasm, respiratory distress,** upper respiratory irritation (nasal form)
SKIN: **Necrolytic migratory erythema,** pallor, pruritus (nasal form), urticaria
Other: Hypersensitivity reactions (**anaphylactic shock, breathing difficulties,** generalized rash, **hypotension**), injection-site reactions (discomfort, redness, swelling)

Childbearing Considerations

PREGNANCY

- It is not known if drug causes fetal harm.
- Use with caution only if benefit to mother outweighs potential risk to fetus.

LACTATION

- It is not known if drug is present in breast milk.

- Patient should check with prescriber before breastfeeding.

Nursing Considerations

- Rouse patient as quickly as possible because prolonged hypoglycemia can cause cerebral damage.
- Monitor patients with diabetes mellitus receiving glucagon for diagnostic purposes for hyperglycemia and treat according to institutional protocol.

! WARNING Prepare patient for cardiac monitoring when glucagon is used as a diagnostic aid because glucagon may increase blood pressure, myocardial oxygen demand, and pulse rate, which may become life-threatening in patients with cardiac disease.

- Keep in mind that glucagon isn't effective in patients with depleted hepatic glycogen stores caused by such conditions as adrenal insufficiency, chronic hypoglycemia, and starvation.

! WARNING Be aware hypersensitivity reactions have occurred with glucagon use. Although a generalized rash has occurred, anaphylactic shock with breathing difficulties and hypotension have also occurred. Monitor patient closely.

- Expect to administer 5 to 10 mg of phentolamine mesylate intravenously, as ordered, if glucagon is administered to a patient with undiagnosed pheochromocytoma and substantial increase in blood pressure occurs.
- Monitor patient for necrolytic migratory erythema, a skin rash common with glucagonomas that may present with bullae, erosions, and scaly, pruritic erythematous plaques following continuous glucagon infusion. These lesions may appear on patient's face, groin, legs, or perineum or may become more widespread. Notify prescriber and expect glucagon infusion to be discontinued, if possible. Know that treatment with corticosteroids is not effective in treating necrolytic migratory erythema.

PATIENT TEACHING

- Instruct patient to monitor blood glucose level, especially with signs of hypoglycemia.

- Teach patient and family members how to recognize signs of hypoglycemia and when to notify prescriber.
- Advise patient to carry hard candy or other simple sugars to treat early hypoglycemia.
- Make sure unstable diabetic patients and family members know how to give glucagon subcutaneously, if prescribed, in case of hypoglycemia. Instruct family members to keep patient on his side and give him both a fast-acting and long-acting carbohydrate when he awakens. Advise against giving fluids by mouth until patient is fully conscious.
- Teach family/caregivers how to administer nasal spray form of glucagon, if ordered. Tell them to administer dose by inserting the device tip into one nostril and pressing the device plunger all the way in until the green line is no longer showing. The dose does not have to be inhaled. Each device contains one dose of glucagon and cannot be reused. If a repeat dose is needed, tell them to use a new device. The plunger should not be pushed or tested prior to use.
- Teach family how to use the Gvoke autoinjector/prefilled syringes, if prescribed.
- Instruct patient and family members to call for emergency medical assistance after glucagon treatment, especially if patient can't ingest oral glucose or if he's taking the sulfonylurea, chlorpropamide, in case secondary hypoglycemia occurs.

! **WARNING** Urge patient to seek immediate emergency care if allergic reactions occur such as difficulty breathing, feeling light-headed, or a rash develops.

---

glyburide
(glibenclamide)
DiaBeta, Euglucon (CAN), Glynase

⬛ Class and Category
Pharmacologic class: Sulfonylurea
Therapeutic class: Antidiabetic

⬛ Indications and Dosages
✽ *As adjunct to control blood glucose level in type 2 diabetes mellitus*

TABLETS (GLYNASE)
Adults. *Initial:* 1.5 to 3 mg daily, increased by up to 1.5 mg at weekly intervals, if needed. *Maintenance:* 0.75 to 12 mg as a single dose or in divided doses. *Maximum:* 12 mg daily.

TABLETS (DIABETA)
Adults. *Initial:* 2.5 to 5 mg daily, increased by up to 2.5 mg at weekly intervals, if needed. *Maintenance:* 1.25 to 20 mg daily as a single dose or in divided doses. *Maximum:* 20 mg daily.

±**DOSAGE ADJUSTMENT** For conversion from insulin to glyburide for adults who use more than 40 units of insulin daily, glyburide started at 5 mg (Diabeta) or 3 mg (Glynase) as a single dose with 50% of usual insulin dose; glyburide dosage increased gradually, as needed. For adults who use less than 40 units but more than 20 units of insulin, glyburide started at 5 mg (Diabeta) or 3 mg (Glynase) daily as a single dose and insulin stopped. If patient is taking less than 20 units of insulin daily, usual glyburide dosage is used and insulin discontinued.

For elderly patients or patients more sensitive to hypoglycemic drugs, initial glyburide dosage possibly reduced to 1.25 mg (Diabeta) daily, gradually increased by 2.5 mg/wk, as needed; or reduced to 0.75 mg (Glynase) daily, gradually increased by 1.5 mg/wk, as needed.

⬛ Drug Administration
P.O.
- Give as a single dose before first meal of the day. If patient takes more than 10 mg of glyburide (Diabeta) or more than 6 mg of glyburide (Glynase) or develops severe GI distress, give in 2 divided doses before meals.
- Ensure patient eats after drug has been administered.
- Diabeta tablets aren't equal to Glynase tablets; they contain smaller particles, which affects drug bioavailability.
- Do not administer Diabeta with a high-fat meal because it may reduce glyburide bioavailability.

Route	Onset	Peak	Duration
P.O.*	1 hr	2–3 hr	24 hr
P.O.†	2 hr	3–4	24 hr

Half-life: 4–10 hr

* Glynase
† Diabeta

G
H
I

Mechanism of Action

Stimulates insulin release from beta cells in the pancreas. Glyburide also increases peripheral tissue sensitity to insulin either by enhancing insulin binding to cellular receptors or by increasing the number of insulin receptors.

Contraindications

Concurrent therapy with bosentan; diabetic ketoacidosis; hypersensitivity to glyburide, sulfonylureas, or their components; type 1 diabetes mellitus

Interactions

DRUGS

ACE inhibitors, anabolic steroids, azole antifungals, chloramphenicol, clarithromycin, disopyramide, drugs highly protein bound, fluoxetine, guanethidine, MAO inhibitors, NSAIDs, oxyphenbutazone, phenylbutazone, probenecid, quinolones, salicylates, sulfonamides: Increased risk of hypoglycemia
calcium channel blockers, colesevelam, corticosteroids, estrogens, isoniazid, nicotinic acid, oral contraceptives, phenothiazines, phenytoin, sympathomimetics, thiazide diuretics and other diuretics, thyroid drugs: Increased risk of hyperglycemia
beta-blockers: Possibly hyperglycemia or masking of hypoglycemia signs
bosentan: Increased risk of elevated liver enzymes
cyclosporine: Increased cyclosporine plasma level and toxicity
CYP2C9 and CYP3A4 inducers or inhibitors: Possibly altered blood glucose levels
miconazole (oral): Possibly severe hypo-glycemia
oral anticoagulants: Possibly potentiated or weakened anticoagulant effects; increased risk of hypoglycemia
rifampin: Decreased glyburide effectiveness

FOODS

high-fat foods: Reduced bioavailability of nonmicronized glyburide

ACTIVITIES

alcohol use: Altered blood glucose control (usually hypoglycemia)

Adverse Reactions

CNS: Abnormal gait, anxiety, asthenia, chills, depression, dizziness, fatigue, headache, hypertonia, hypoesthesia, insomnia, malaise, migraine headache, nervousness, paresthesia, somnolence, syncope, tremor, vertigo
CV: Arrhythmias, edema, hypertension, vasculitis
EENT: Blurred vision, changes in accommodation, conjunctivitis, eye pain, pharyngitis, retinal hemorrhage, rhinitis, taste perversion, tinnitus
ENDO: Hypoglycemia
GI: Anorexia, constipation, cholestatic jaundice, diarrhea, elevated liver enzymes, epigastric discomfort or fullness, flatulence, heartburn, **hepatic failure** or porphyria, **hepatitis,** hunger, jaundice, nausea, proctocolitis, trace blood in stool, vomiting
GU: Decreased libido, dysuria, polyuria
HEME: Agranulocytosis, aplastic anemia, eosinophilia, **hemolytic anemia, leukopenia, pancytopenia,** purpura, **thrombocytopenia**
MS: Arthralgia, leg cramps, myalgia
RESP: Dyspnea
SKIN: Allergic skin reactions, bullous reactions, diaphoresis, eczema, erythema, **erythema multiforme, exfoliative dermatitis,** flushing, lichenoid reactions, maculopapular or morbilliform rash, photosensitivity, porphyria cutanea tarda, pruritus, urticaria
Other: Angioedema, disulfiram-like reaction, **hyponatremia,** weight gain

Childbearing Considerations

PREGNANCY

- It is not known if drug can cause fetal harm. However, it may cause neonatal hypoglycemia.
- Drug is not recommended during pregnancy because abnormal blood glucose levels during pregnancy are associated with a higher incidence of congenital abnormalities, making insulin the preferred drug of choice during pregnancy.

LABOR & DELIVERY

- At birth, neonate may experience birth injury, respiratory distress, and prolonged severe hypoglycemia, lasting 4 to 10 days if mother receives drug at time of delivery.
- If drug is used during pregnancy, expect it to be discontinued at least 2 weeks before expected delivery.

LACTATION

- It is not known if drug is present in breast milk.

- Drug or breastfeeding should be discontinued.

Nursing Considerations

- Use cautiously in patients with glucose 6-phosphate dehydrogenase deficiency because hemolytic anemia may develop. Monitor patient's CBC closely.
- Monitor fasting blood glucose level to determine patient's response to glyburide. Expect to check glycosylated hemoglobin every 3 to 6 months or as ordered to evaluate long-term blood glucose control.
- Know that when patient switches from insulin to glyburide, check blood glucose level three times daily before meals.

! WARNING Expect a higher risk of hypoglycemia when giving drug to a debilitated or malnourished patient or one with adrenal, hepatic, pituitary, or renal insufficiency. Also be aware that hypoglycemia may be more difficult to recognize in patients with autonomic neuropathy, the elderly, and patients who are taking beta-blockers or other sympatholytic agents. Monitor blood glucose level closely.

! WARNING Monitor patient with history of allergies to other sulfonamide derivatives closely because of increased risk of allergy to glyburide. If allergic reactions persist or worsen, expect drug to be discontinued.

- Administer insulin as needed and prescribed during periods of increased stress, such as infection, surgery, and trauma.
- Arrange for diabetic teaching and consultation between patient and dietitian, if appropriate.

PATIENT TEACHING

- Instruct patient to take glyburide with first meal of the day or, if taking drug twice daily, to take with meals. Caution him not to skip the meal after taking drug.
- Advise patient not to take Diabeta with a high-fat meal because it may reduce glyburide bioavailability.
- Caution patient to avoid skipping doses, discontinuing glyburide, or taking OTC drugs without first consulting prescriber.
- Teach patient how to monitor his blood glucose level and when to notify prescriber about changes.

- Urge patient to report signs of hypoglycemia: anxiety, confusion, dizziness, excessive sweating, headache, and nausea.
- Suggest that patient carry candy or other simple sugars to treat mild hypoglycemia.
- Urge patient to avoid alcohol because it increases the risk of hypoglycemia.
- Advise patient to carry identification indicating that he has diabetes.
- Teach patient about diet, exercise, foot care, hygiene, signs of hyperglycemia and hypoglycemia, and ways to avoid infection.
- Instruct patient to notify prescriber if he experiences easy bruising, fever, hypoglycemia or hyperglycemia, rash, sore throat, and unusual bleeding.
- If photosensitivity is a problem, instruct patient to avoid direct sunlight and to wear sunscreen.

glycopyrrolate
Cuvposa, Dartisla ODT, GLYRX-PF, Lonhala Magnair, Seebri

Class and Category
Pharmacologic class: Anticholinergic
Therapeutic class: Antiarrhythmic, anticholinergic, bronchodilator, cholinergic adjunct

Indications and Dosages
* *As adjunct to treat peptic ulcer disease*

ODT TABLETS (DARTISLA ODT)
Adults. 1.7 mg two or three times daily. Maximum: 6.8 mg daily.

TABLETS (GLYRX-PF)
Adults and adolescents using 1-mg tablet. *Initial:* 1 mg three times daily with some adults requiring a 2-mg dose in evening at bedtime. *Maintenance:* 1 mg twice a day.
Adults and adolescents using the 2-mg tablet. 2 mg twice daily or three times daily.

I.M. OR I.V. INJECTION (GLYRX-PF)
Adults and adolescents. 0.1 to 0.2 mg every 4 hr, as needed. *Maximum:* 3 to 4 doses daily.
* *To reduce gastric acid and respiratory secretions before anesthesia*

I.M. INJECTION (GLYRX-PF)
Adults and children over age 2. 0.004 mg/kg 30 to 60 min before anesthesia or when preanesthesia sedative or opioid is given.

Infants age 1 month to 2 years. Up to 0.009 mg/kg 30 to 60 min before anesthesia or when preanesthesia sedative or opioid is given.

* *To counteract intraoperative and anesthesia-induced arrhythmias*

I.V. INJECTION (GLYRX-PF)

Adults and adolescents. 0.1 mg, repeated every 2 to 3 min, if needed.

Children over age 2. 0.004 mg/kg. Dose repeated every 2 to 3 min, if needed. *Maximum:* 0.1 mg as a single dose.

* *To reverse neuromuscular blockade due to nondepolarizing muscle relaxants*

I.V. INJECTION (GLYRX-PF)

Adults and children over age 2. 0.2 mg glycopyrrolate for each 1 mg neostigmine or 5 mg pyridostigmine.

* *To reduce chronic severe drooling in patients with neurologic conditions associated with problem drooling, such as cerebral palsy*

ORAL SOLUTION (CUVPOSA)

Children ages 3 to 16. *Initial:* 0.02 mg/kg three times daily increased in increments of 0.02 mg/kg every 5 to 7 days, as needed and based on response and adverse reactions. *Maximum:* 0.1 mg/kg three times daily not to exceed 1.5 to 3 mg per dose based on weight of child.

* *To provide long-term, maintenance treatment of airflow obstruction in patients with chronic obstructive pulmonary disease, including chronic bronchitis and/or emphysema*

ORAL INHALATION (LONHALA MAGNAIR)

Adults. 25 mcg (1 vial) inhaled using the Magnair device twice daily.

ORAL INHALATION (SEEBRI)

Adults. 15.6 mcg using the Neohaler device twice daily.

Drug Administration

P.O.

- Give 1-mg dose used to treat peptic ulcers 3 times daily in morning, afternoon, and evening. A 2-mg oral dose may be needed at bedtime to ensure overnight control of symptoms, as prescribed.
- Give drug used to treat drooling 1 hour before or 2 hours after meals.
- Administer oral solution 1 hour before meals or 2 hours after meals. Use a calibrated device to measure dosage.

- Place an ODT tablet with a gloved, dry hand on the patient's tongue, let it dissolve, and then have patient swallow without water.

I.V.

- Do not administer to neonates, as drug solution contains benzyl alcohol.
- Administer by direct injection with or without diluting. Inject into tubing of flowing I.V. solution.
- *Incompatibilities:* Solution containing an alkaline drug or sodium bicarbonate, Lactated Ringer's Solution; glycopyrrolate mixed in same syringe as chloramphenicol, diazepam, methohexital sodium, pentobarbital sodium, secobarbital sodium, sodium bicarbonate, or thiopental sodium.

I.M.

- Do not administer to neonates, as drug solution contains benzyl alcohol.
- Administer undiluted into a deep muscle.
- Rotate sites.

INHALATION

Lonhala Magnair

- Administer once in the morning and once in the evening using the Magnair device. The device should not be used to administer any other medication.
- Store vials in the sealed foil pouch and open pouch only to remove a vial immediately before use. Unopened vials should be returned to the opened foil pouch and used for the next treatment.
- Discard if not used within 7 days, as the drug may be ineffective.
- Do not administer 2 vials at one time and do not administer more than 2 vials in a day.

Seebri

- Administer once in the morning and once in the evening using the Neohaler device. The device should not be used to administer any other medication.
- Follow manufacturer guidelines on how to load the capsule into the inhaler and how to use the Neohaler device. Remove the capsule from the blister immediately before use and do not pierce the capsule more than once.
- The Neohaler need not be cleaned and it should be kept dry. The Neohaler should not be taken apart.

Route	Onset	Peak	Duration
P.O.	60 min	3 hr	8–12 hr
Inhaled	Immediate	5–20 min	Unknown
I.V.	1 min	Unknown	2–4 hr
I.M.	15–30 min	30–45 min	2–3 hr

Half-life: Variable from 2.8 hr to 33–53 hr

Mechanism of Action

Inhibits acetylcholine's action on postganglionic muscarinic receptors throughout the body. Depending on the receptors' location, glycopyrrolate produces various effects, such as:

- reducing the volume and acidity of gastric secretions
- controlling excessive bronchial, pharyngeal, and tracheal secretions and dilating the bronchi
- inhibiting vagal stimulation of the heart
- relaxing smooth muscle in the GI, GU, and respiratory tracts.

Contraindications

For all forms: Hypersensitivity to glycopyrrolate or its components; *For Cuvposa:* Angle-closure glaucoma; concomitant use of solid oral dosage forms of potassium chloride; hemorrhage with unstable cardiovascular status; ileus; intestinal atony; myasthenia gravis; severe ulcerative colitis; toxic megacolon; *For generic glycopyrrolate in treatment of peptic ulcer:* glaucoma, intestinal atony in the debilitated or elderly patient, myasthenia gravis, obstructive GI or uropathy disorders, paralytic ileus, severe ulcerative colitis, toxic megacolon complicating ulcerative colitis, unstable cardiovascular status in acute hemorrhage

Interactions

DRUGS

amantadine, other anticholinergics: Increased anticholinergic effects of glycopyrrolate
anticholinergics, antiparkinsonian drugs, phenothiazines, tricyclic antidepressants: Possibly increased anticholinergic effects
atenolol, metformin: Increased effects of these drugs; possibly potentiated atenolol effects
digoxin (slow dissolution oral tablets): Possibly potentiated digoxin effects
potassium chloride (Cuvposa): Possibly arrested or decreased passage of potassium chloride through the GI tract

potassium chloride in a wax matrix (generic glycopyrrolate): Possibly increased severity of potassium chloride-induced GI lesions

Adverse Reactions

CNS: Confusion, difficulty speaking, dizziness, drowsiness, headache, insomnia, nervousness, weakness
CV: **Bradycardia** (low doses), **heart block**, palpitations, **prolonged QT interval**, tachycardia (high doses)
EENT: Blurred vision, cycloplegia, dilated pupils, dry mouth, increased intraocular pressure, loss of taste, mydriasis, nasal congestion, nasopharyngitis, oropharyngeal pain, photophobia, sinusitis, taste perversion
GI: Abdominal distention, constipation, dysphagia, nausea, vomiting
GU: Impotence, urinary hesitancy, urine retention, UTI
RESP: Dyspnea, **paradoxical bronchospasm**
SKIN: Decreased sweating (**heat exhaustion**), dry skin, flushing, pruritus, rash, urticaria
Other: Anaphylaxis, angioedema

Childbearing Considerations

PREGNANCY

- It is not known if drug causes fetal harm.
- Use with caution only if benefit to mother outweighs potential risk to fetus.

LACTATION

- It is not known if drug is present in breast milk. However, it may suppress lactation.
- Patient should check with prescriber before breastfeeding.

Nursing Considerations

- Know that inhalation form of glycopyrrolate should not be used in patients during acutely deteriorating or potentially life-threatening episodes of COPD, nor should it be used for relief of acute symptoms.
- Use glycopyrrolate cautiously in patients with autonomic neuropathy, hepatic disease, hiatal hernia, mild to moderate ulcerative colitis, narrow-angle glaucoma, or prostatic hypertrophy because drug's anticholinergic effect can worsen these conditions; gastric ulcer because drug may delay gastric emptying; and renal disease because drug excretion may be altered.

G
H
I

! WARNING Monitor patient closely after administration for an immediate hypersensitivity reaction such as patient experiencing difficulty breathing or swallowing; rash; swelling of the patient's face, lips, or throat; or urticaria. Notify prescriber at once, expect drug to be discontinued, and be prepared to provide emergency supportive care, as ordered.

- Notify prescriber if patient using inhalation form of glycopyrrolate is experiencing lack of control of respiratory symptoms exhibited by increased bronchoconstriction or patient's prescribed short-acting beta$_2$-agonist becomes less effective or patient needs to use it more, as these are markers of deterioration of the patient's respiratory status indicating that glycopyrrolate may no longer be effective.
- Use continuous cardiac monitoring, as ordered, to assess patient for arrhythmias during drug administration.

! WARNING Check all doses carefully because even a slight overdose can lead to toxicity.

- Adjust the room temperature and make sure patient is well hydrated to prevent overheating caused by decreased sweating.

PATIENT TEACHING
- Advise patient to take glycopyrrolate exactly as prescribed.
- Instruct patient how to administer inhalation form of drug using the correct device.
- Inform patient that the prescribed inhalation form of drug is not to be used to treat acute respiratory symptoms. If patient needs to use his rescue inhaler more often or his symptoms worsen, he should notify prescriber. If acute bronchospasms occur, he should stop taking drug immediately, seek emergency medical treatment, and notify prescriber, as drug must be discontinued.

! WARNING Alert patient that an allergic reaction may occur. Advise patient to notify prescriber and to seek immediate emergency care, if serious.

- Instruct patient to consult prescriber before taking any over-the-counter drugs.

- Caution patient about possible dizziness and drowsiness and need to avoid hazardous activities until drug's effects are known.
- Suggest that patient use sugarless hard candy, ice, or saliva substitute to relieve dry mouth.
- Instruct patient to avoid exertion and hot environments because he's prone to heat exhaustion while taking glycopyrrolate.
- Urge patient to drink at least eight glasses of water daily, unless contraindicated.
- Tell patient to notify prescriber about abdominal distention, eye pain, irregular heartbeat, sensitivity to light, severe constipation, or trouble breathing or urinating.
- Advise patient to wear sunglasses in bright light.
- Advise patient to void before taking each dose, if urinary hesitancy occurs and to notify prescriber.

golimumab
Simponi, Simponi Aria

≡ Class and Category
Pharmacologic class: Tumor necrosis factor (TNF) blocker
Therapeutic class: Biologic disease-modifying antirheumatic drug (DMARD)

≡ Indications and Dosages
∗ *To treat active psoriatic arthritis; to treat ankylosing spondylitis with or without methotrexate or other nonbiologic disease-modifying antirheumatic drugs (DMARDs); to treat moderate to severe rheumatoid arthritis with methotrexate*

SUBCUTANEOUS INJECTION (SIMPONI)
Adults. 50 mg monthly.

I.V. INFUSION (SIMPONI ARIA)
Adults. 2 mg/kg at weeks 0 and 4, then every 8 wk thereafter.

∗ *To treat polyarticular juvenile idiopathic arthritis and psoriatic arthritis*

I.V. INFUSION (SIMPONI ARIA)
Children age 2 and older. 80 mg/m^2 at wks 0 and 4, and every 8 wks thereafter.

∗ *To treat moderate to severe active ulcerative colitis in patients who have demonstrated corticosteroid dependence or who have had an inadequate response to or failed to tolerate 6-mercaptopurine, azathioprine, oral aminosalicylates, or oral corticosteroid*

SUBCUTANEOUS INJECTION (SIMPONI)

Adults. *Initial:* 200 mg at week 0, followed by 100 mg at week 2. *Maintenance:* 100 mg every 4 wk.

⬚ Drug Administration

I.V.

- Each 4-ml vial contains 50 mg of golimumab. Solution should appear colorless to light yellow. Dilute the total volume of the drug solution with 0.45% or 0.9% Sodium Chloride Injection to a final volume of 100 ml. Gently mix.
- Discard any unused solution remaining in the vials.
- Use within 4 hours, keeping diluted solution at room temperature.
- Inspect diluted solution prior to infusion for particulate matter or discoloration. Do not use if present.
- Use only an infusion set with an in-line, low-protein-binding, nonpyrogenic, sterile filter (pore size 0.22 micrometer or less).
- Infuse the diluted solution over 30 minutes.
- Do not infuse concomitantly in the same intravenous line with other drugs.
- *Incompatibilities:* Other drugs

SUBCUTANEOUS

- Needle cover of syringe contains dry rubber and should not be handled by anyone with a latex allergy.
- Take prefilled syringe or autoinjector out of the refrigerator 30 minutes before giving injection to allow time for drug to warm up to room temperature. Never warm drug in any other way.
- Solution should be clear to slightly opalescent to light yellow.
- Do not inject drug into areas that are bruised, hard, red, or tender.
- When using autoinjector, do not pull the device away from the skin until a first "click" and then a second "click" is heard, indicating the injection is finished. It may take up to 15 seconds before second click is heard. If device is pulled away from the skin before the second click, a full dose may not have been given.
- Rotate injection sites. If more than one subcutaneous injection is required, administer the injections at different sites on the body.

- Discard any leftover product remaining in the prefilled syringe or autoinjector.

Route	Onset	Peak	Duration
I.V.	Unknown	Unknown	Unknown
SubQ	Unknown	2–6 days	Unknown

Half-life: 12–14 days

⬚ Mechanism of Action

Binds to a cytokine protein, tumor necrosis factor-alpha (TNF-alpha), to block interaction with its receptors, which prevents biological activity of TNF-alpha. Elevated TNF-alpha levels in the blood, joints, and synovium may play an important role in pathophysiology of such inflammatory diseases as ankylosing spondylitis, psoriatic arthritis, rheumatoid arthritis, and ulcerative colitis. Reduced TNF-alpha activity in these disorders improves signs and symptoms.

⬚ Contraindications

Hypersensitivity to golimumab or its components

⬚ Interactions

DRUGS

abatacept, anakinra, rituximab: Possibly increased risk of serious infection
cytochrome P-450 substrates such as cyclosporine, theophylline, warfarin: Effects or blood levels of these drugs may change when golimumab therapy starts or stops
live vaccines, therapeutic infectious agents such as BCG bladder instillation for treatment of cancer: Increased risk of adverse vaccine effects
methotrexate: Decreased clearance of golimumab

⬚ Adverse Reactions

CNS: Demyelinating disorders both central and peripheral, dizziness, fever, paresthesia
CV: Congestive heart failure, hypertension
EENT: Nasopharyngitis, oral herpes, pharyngitis, rhinitis, sinusitis
GI: Elevated liver enzymes, nausea
HEME: Agranulocytosis, aplastic anemia, leukemia, leukopenia, neutropenia, thrombocytopenia
RESP: Bronchitis, dyspnea, **interstitial lung disease**, pneumonia, tuberculosis, upper respiratory tract infection
SKIN: Bullous skin reactions, cellulitis, lichenoid reactions, **melanoma, Merkel cell**

G
H
I

carcinoma, new or worsening psoriasis, pruritus, rash, skin exfoliation, urticaria
Other: Abscess; **anaphylaxis**; antibody formation to golimumab; bacterial (including *Legionella* and *Listeria*), fungal (including invasive), mycobacterial, parasitic, or viral infections (including **reactivation of hepatitis B infection** in chronic carriers); injection-site erythema; lupus-like syndrome; **malignancies such as lymphomas**; sarcoidosis; **sepsis**

Childbearing Considerations
PREGNANCY
- It is not known if drug causes fetal harm. However, it does cross the placenta during the third trimester of pregnancy and may affect immune response of the infant after birth.
- If drug is given during pregnancy, know that infant is at increased risk for infection. Administration of live vaccines to infants exposed to drug in utero is not recommended for 6 months following the mother's last dose during pregnancy.

LACTATION
- It is not known if drug is present in breast milk.
- Patient should check with prescriber before breastfeeding.

Nursing Considerations
- Make sure patient has a tuberculin skin test before therapy starts. If skin test is positive, treatment of latent tuberculosis must start before golimumab therapy starts, as prescribed. Also, antituberculosis therapy may be started if patient has a history of active or latent tuberculosis, if adequate therapy can't be confirmed, or if patient has a negative test for latent tuberculosis but also has risk factors for tuberculosis.

! **WARNING** Know that if patient has evidence of an active infection when drug is prescribed, golimumab therapy shouldn't start until infection has been treated. Monitor all patients for bacterial (including *Legionella* and *Listeria*), fungal, mycobacterial, parasitic, or viral infections during therapy, especially those receiving immunosuppressants. Know that the infection could become life-threatening and affect multiple organs. If a serious infection, an opportunistic

infection, or sepsis develops, expect prescriber to stop drug and start appropriate antimicrobial therapy. Monitor patient closely for tuberculosis throughout golimumab therapy because active tuberculosis has occurred in patients during and after treatment of latent tuberculosis.

- Know that patients with a history of cancer, except those successfully treated for nonmelanoma skin cancer, should be thoroughly evaluated before golimumab therapy starts because treatment may pose more risks than benefits. Patients with rheumatoid arthritis may have a higher risk than the general population for developing leukemia while taking a TNF blocker such as golimumab.
- Use golimumab cautiously in patients with congestive heart failure, demyelinating disorders such as multiple sclerosis, and hematologic cytopenias because these disorders may develop or become worse with golimumab therapy.
- Use golimumab cautiously in patients with recurrent infection or increased risk of infection, patients who live in regions where histoplasmosis and tuberculosis are endemic, and patients with a history of hepatitis B infection, because drug increases risk of infection.
- Ensure that patient is current on immunizations before therapy is begun.
- Monitor patient, especially young adult males, for signs and symptoms of malignancies. Although lymphomas account for about half of all malignancies associated with golimumab therapy, leukemia and rare malignancies, including melanomas and Merkel cell carcinoma, have also occurred. Report any persistent or unusual signs and symptoms to prescriber.

PATIENT TEACHING
- Explain that first injection of golimumab given subcutaneously must be administered with a health care professional present.
- Teach patient or caregiver how to give golimumab as a subcutaneous injection at home, if applicable. Tell him to let prefilled syringe or autoinjector sit at room temperature outside carton for 30 minutes before injecting. Tell him not to warm drug in any other way and not to remove needle cover or cap while letting golimumab warm up.

- Teach patient using autoinjector not to pull the device away from his skin until he hears a first "click" and then a second "click" indicating the injection is finished. Remind patient it may take up to 15 seconds before second click is heard and, if device is pulled away from the skin before the second click, a full dose may not have been given.
- Emphasize need to inject full amount in prefilled syringe to obtain correct dose. Instruct patient to discard any drug left in prefilled syringe or autoinjector.
- Tell patient requiring multiple injections to administer the injections at different sites on the body.
- Alert patient that needle cover contains natural dry rubber and should not be handled by anyone with a latex allergy.
- Instruct patient or caregiver to use a puncture-resistant container to dispose of needles and syringes at home.
- Inform patient that drug must be refrigerated (not frozen) for storage.
- Urge patient to check expiration dates and not to use outdated drug.
- Teach patient to rotate injection sites and never to give injection into an area where skin is bruised, hard, red, or tender.
- Explain that tuberculosis may occur during golimumab therapy. Instruct him to report low-grade fever, persistent cough, and wasting or weight loss, to prescriber.
- Teach patient how to recognize evidence of bleeding disorders and infection and to tell prescriber if they occur; drug may have to be stopped. Advise patient to avoid people with infections and to have all prescribed laboratory tests performed.
- Inform patient that golimumab therapy increases the risk of certain kinds of cancer, especially leukemias and lymphomas. Emphasize the importance of having follow-up visits and reporting unusual or sudden onset of signs or symptoms. Also, encourage patient to have regular skin examinations, as melanomas and Merkel cell carcinoma have occurred with golimumab therapy.
- Instruct patient to check with prescriber before receiving any vaccines. Live vaccines should be avoided.
- Tell patient to report lupus-like signs and symptoms that, although rare, may occur during therapy, such as chest pain that doesn't go away, joint pain, a rash on arms or cheeks that's sensitive to the sun or shortness of breath. Explain that drug may have to be discontinued if these occur.
- Advise patient to tell all health care providers about golimumab therapy and to tell prescriber about any OTC drugs, herbal remedies, and mineral and vitamin supplements being taken.
- Inform mothers who received golimumab therapy during pregnancy to monitor their infant for infections and not to have their infant receive live vaccines for 6 months following the mother's last golimumab dose during the pregnancy.

granisetron
Sancuso, Sustol

granisetron hydrochloride

☰ Class and Category
Pharmacologic class: Serotonin blocker (5-HT$_3$ receptor antagonist)
Therapeutic class: Antiemetic

☰ Indications and Dosages
❋ *To prevent nausea and vomiting caused by emetogenic chemotherapy, including high-dose cisplatin*

TABLETS
Adults. 1 mg up to 1 hr before chemotherapy, repeated 12 hr later. Or, 2 mg up to 1 hr before chemotherapy.

I.V. INFUSION, I.V. INJECTION
Adults and children ages 2 and over. 10 mcg/kg starting 30 min before chemotherapy.

❋ *To prevent nausea and vomiting associated with moderately and/or highly emetogenic chemotherapy regimens of up to 5 consecutive days duration*

TRANSDERMAL (SANCUSO)
Adults. 3.1 mg/24 hr patch 24 to 48 hr before chemotherapy and worn up to 7 days. Patch removed no sooner than 24 hr after chemotherapy is completed.

❋ *As adjunct with other antiemetics to prevent acute and delayed nausea and vomiting*

G
H
I

associated with initial and repeat course of moderately emetogenic chemotherapy or anthracycline and cyclophosphamide combination chemotherapy regimens

E. R. SUBCUTANEOUS INJECTION (SUSTOL)

Adults. 10 mg in combination with dexamethasone at least 30 min before chemotherapy on day 1. *Maximum:* 10 mg once every 7 days.

± **DOSAGE ADJUSTMENT** For patients with a creatinine clearance of between 30 to 59 ml/min, Sustol brand dosage interval increased to once every 14 days.

＊ *To prevent nausea and vomiting caused by radiation therapy, including fractionated abdominal radiation and total body irradiation*

TABLETS

Adults. 2 mg daily given 1 hr before radiation therapy.

☰ Drug Administration

P.O.

- May give drug on an empty stomach, if preferred.
- Give tablets up to 1 hour before chemotherapy or 1 hour before radiation.

I.V.

- For I.V. injection, administer undiluted over 30 seconds, 30 minutes before chemotherapy.
- For I.V. infusion, dilute with 0.9% Sodium Chloride or 5% Dextrose Injection to total volume of 20 to 50 ml. Infuse over 5 minutes, 30 minutes before chemotherapy. Mixture may be stored up to 24 hours. Use only on days when chemotherapy is given.
- *Incompatibilities:* Other drugs

SUBCUTANEOUS

- Know that the Sustol brand is the only granisetron that can be administered subcutaneously and comes as a refrigerated kit. Do not substitute nonkit components for any of the components from the kit.
- Remove kit at least 60 minutes prior to administration. Unpack kit to allow the syringe containing drug as well as all other contents to warm to room temperature. Activate one of the syringe warming pouches, and wrap the warming pouch

around the syringe containing the drug for 5 to 6 minutes.

- Inspect the syringe containing drug prior to administration for particulate matter and discoloration. Know that the syringe is amber-colored glass. Do not use if particulate matter or discoloration is seen, the tip cap is missing or has been tampered with, or if the Luer fitting is missing or dislodged.
- A topical anesthetic may be applied to the injection site prior to administration.
- Administer at least 30 minutes before chemotherapy on day 1.
- To administer, inject into abdomen at least one inch away from the umbilicus or into the back of the upper arm. Avoid injecting drug into areas that are burned, hardened, inflamed, swollen, or otherwise compromised.
- Inject as a slow, sustained injection that may take up to 30 seconds. Pressing the plunger harder will not expel the drug faster.
- Once drug has been removed from refrigerator, it can remain at room temperature for up to 7 days. Otherwise, store in refrigerator and protect from light. Do not freeze.

TRANSDERMAL

- Apply immediately after opening pouch containing the patch.
- Do not cut the patch.
- Apply transdermal patch to patient's upper outer arm 24 to 48 hours before chemotherapy, and don't remove it until at least 24 hours after chemotherapy is completed.

Route	Onset	Peak	Duration
P.O.	Unknown	Unknown	24 hr
I.V.	< 30 min	Unknown	< 24 hr
SubQ	Unknown	24 hr	7 days
Transdermal	Unknown	48 hr	Unknown

Half-life: 5–24 hr

☰ Mechanism of Action

Has a high affinity for serotonin receptors along vagal nerve endings in intestines. Because of this affinity, granisetron prevents nausea and vomiting that usually result when serotonin is released by damaged enterochromaffin cells.

≡ Contraindications

Hypersensitivity to granisetron, its components, or any other 5-HT$_3$ receptor antagonists

≡ Interactions

DRUGS

drugs that prolong the QT interval: Increased risk of QT interval prolongation
serotonin and nonadrenaline reuptake inhibitors (SNRIs), selective serotonin reuptake inhibitors (SSRIs): Increased risk of serotonin syndrome

≡ Adverse Reactions

CNS: Asthenia, chills, CNS stimulation, drowsiness, fever, headache, insomnia, **serotonin syndrome**, somnolence
CV: Bradycardia, chest pain, hypertension, palpitations, **prolonged QT interval, sick sinus syndrome**
EENT: Taste perversion
GI: Abdominal pain, anorexia, constipation, diarrhea, elevated liver enzymes, gastric distention, nausea, progressive ileus, vomiting
HEME: Anemia, **leukopenia, thrombocytopenia**
SKIN: Alopecia, reactions at patch application site (burns, discoloration, irritation, pruritus, rash, redness, vesicles, urticaria)
Other: Anaphylaxis; subcutaneous injection-site reactions such as bleeding, bruising, hematomas, infections, nodules, pain, or tenderness

≡ Childbearing Considerations

PREGNANCY

- It is not known if drug causes fetal harm.
- Use with caution only if benefit to mother outweighs potential risk to fetus.

LACTATION

- It is not known if drug is present in breast milk.
- Patient should check with prescriber before breastfeeding.

≡ Nursing Considerations

- Use cautiously in patients with arrhythmias or cardiac conduction disorders because granisetron may prolong QT interval. Patients especially at risk include those with cardiac disease or electrolyte abnormalities and those receiving cardiotoxic chemotherapy or therapy with another drug that prolongs QT interval.
- Be aware that if Sustol brand is used with an NK$_1$ receptor antagonist, the dosage for dexamethasone may be different. Check the prescribing information for the NK$_1$ receptor antagonist for recommended dexamethasone dosage.
- Assess patient receiving subcutaneous granisetron for injection-site reactions following administration. Know that some of the reactions, such as bruising, hematoma, and infection, may develop up to 2 weeks or more after the injection. Monitor patients receiving anticoagulants or antiplatelet agents closely, as bruising or hematoma formation may be more severe.

! **WARNING** Monitor patient for serotonin syndrome, characterized by agitation, chills, confusion, diaphoresis, diarrhea, fever, hyperactive reflexes, poor coordination, restlessness, shaking, talking tremor, twitching or uncontrolled excitement behavior.

! **WARNING** Monitor patient for hypersensitivity reactions. Know that because the Sustol brand has extended-release properties, a reaction may not occur until 7 days or longer following administration and may take longer to resolve.

- Monitor patient for persistent or severe gastrointestinal effects such as constipation, gastric distention, or progressive ileus that may become severe and require hospitalization. Monitor patient closely, especially if patient is also receiving opioid medications. Consult with prescriber about using a bowel regimen, if needed. Know that the drug may mask gastric distention and/or a progressive ileus, especially in patients with recent abdominal surgery. Assess patient for decreased bowel sounds regularly.

PATIENT TEACHING

- Inform patient that granisetron is given I.V., orally, subcutaneously, or by patch before chemotherapy or orally before radiation to help prevent nausea.
- Instruct patient to take granisetron tablet without food, if preferred.
- Teach patient to apply patch to clean, dry, nearly hairless, intact, healthy skin on the upper arm. Advise patient wearing granisetron patch to cover it with clothing

if there's a risk of exposure to sunlight or artificial light such as sunlamps. Tell patient to continue covering application site with clothing for 10 days after removal of patch. Also, tell patient not to put a heating pad over or in vicinity of the patch.

- Teach patient to fold the used transdermal system in half, when removed, with the sticky side together. Discard in a manner that prevents accidental contact or ingestion by children, pets, or others.
- Advise patient to report constipation, fever, severe diarrhea, or severe headache. Also caution about possible drowsiness and need to take safety measures until effects of drug are known.

! **WARNING** Review signs and symptoms of an allergic reaction. Tell patient to seek immediate emergency care if present. Inform patient receiving drug subcutaneously to watch for allergic reactions for 7 days or longer because drug may be present in his body for up to 7 days following administration.

- Inform patient receiving drug subcutaneously about possible injection-site reactions that can occur and that these reactions may occur up to 2 weeks or more after the injection. Instruct patient to seek immediate medical care if bleeding occurs and is severe or lasts for longer than one day or the site looks infected. Tell him to notify prescriber if he experiences bruising, hematoma, persistent nodule at the injection site, or pain or tenderness severe enough to interfere with activities of daily living or for him to take pain medication.

! **WARNING** Instruct patient to seek immediate medical attention if the following symptoms occur: autonomic instability, changes in mental status, or neuromuscular symptoms, with or without gastrointestinal symptoms.

---

guselkumab
Tremfya

Class and Category
Pharmacologic class: Monoclonal antibody
Therapeutic class: Antipsoriatic

Indications and Dosages
∗ *To treat moderate to severe plaque psoriasis in patients who are candidates for systemic therapy or phototherapy; to treat active psoriatic arthritis*

SUBCUTANEOUS INJECTION

Adults. 100 mg at wk 0, wk 4, and every 8 wks thereafter.

Drug Administration
SUBCUTANEOUS

- Remove prefilled syringe or single-dose One-Press injector from refrigerator and allow to warm to room temperature, keeping needle cap in place until ready to use.
- Inspect solution. It should be clear and colorless to light yellow and may contain small translucent particles. Do not use if the liquid contains large particles, is discolored, or is cloudy.
- Inject the full amount of solution in the prefilled syringe or injector.
- Do not inject into an area where the skin is bruised, hard, scaly, tender, thick, or affected by psoriasis.
- Discard any unused product remaining in the prefilled syringe or injector, because it does not contain preservatives.

Route	Onset	Peak	Duration
SubQ	Unknown	5.5 days	Unknown

Half-life: 15–18 days

Mechanism of Action
Selectively binds to the p19 subunit of interleukin 23 (IL-23) and inhibits its interaction with the IL-23 receptor, which prevents the release of proinflammatory chemokines and cytokines.

Contraindications
Hypersensitivity to guselkumab or its components

Interactions
DRUGS

CYP450 substrates: Possibly decreased effectiveness of these drugs
live vaccines: Possible decreased response to vaccine

Adverse Reactions
CNS: Headache, migraine

EENT: Nasopharyngitis, oral herpes, pharyngitis
GI: Diarrhea, elevated liver enzymes, gastroenteritis
GU: Genital herpes
MS: Arthralgia
RESP: Upper respiratory infections
SKIN: Rash, tinea infections, urticaria
Other: Antibody formation to guselkumab; candidal infections; herpes simplex infections; **hypersensitivity reactions** (**angioedema**, chest or **throat tightness**, **difficulty breathing**, hives, rash), injection-site reactions of bruising, discoloration, edema, erythema, hematoma, hemorrhage, induration, inflammation, pain, pruritus, swelling, urticaria

Childbearing Considerations
PREGNANCY
- Pregnancy exposure registry: 1-877-311-8972.
- It is not known if drug causes fetal harm. However, human IgG antibodies are known to cross the placental barrier and therefore may be transmitted to the fetus.
- Use with caution only if benefit to mother outweighs potential risk to fetus.

LACTATION
- It is not known if drug is present in breast milk.
- Patient should check with prescriber before breastfeeding.

Nursing Considerations
- Assess patient for tuberculosis before guselkumab therapy is begun. Expect treatment for latent tuberculosis to be given prior to starting guselkumab therapy.
- Know that all age-appropriate immunizations should be done before guselkumab therapy begins.

! **WARNING** Monitor patient closely for hypersensitivity reactions after administration, such as angioedema, chest or throat tightness, difficulty breathing, hives, or rash. If present, notify prescriber and provide supportive emergency care, as prescribed.

- Monitor patient for infections, as guselkumab increases risk. Institute infection precautions. Be aware that if infection occurs and is severe or

does not respond to appropriate treatment, guselkumab will probably be discontinued.

PATIENT TEACHING
- Instruct patient on how to administer a subcutaneous injection. Tell patient to remove prefilled syringe or single-dose One-Press patient-controlled injector from refrigerator and allow to warm to room temperature, keeping needle cap in place until ready to administer the injection. Tell him to inject the full amount of solution in the prefilled syringe or injector. Warn patient not to inject into an area where the skin is bruised, hard, scaly, tender, thick, or affected by psoriasis.
- Review how to properly dispose of used needles and syringes.
- Tell patient to take a missed dose as soon as he remembers and then take the next dose at the scheduled time.

! **WARNING** Urge patient that if an allergic reaction occurs to stop taking drug and seek immediate emergency care, as reactions can become serious enough to warrant hospitalization.

- Review infection prevention practices with patient. Emphasize importance of notifying prescriber if an infection should occur.

haloperidol

haloperidol decanoate
Haldol Decanoate, Haldol LA (CAN)

haloperidol lactate
Haldol Concentrate

Class and Category
Pharmacologic class: Butyrophenone derivative
Therapeutic class: Antipsychotic

Indications and Dosages
∗ *To treat psychosis and schizophrenia*

G
H
I

ORAL SOLUTION, TABLETS

Adults and adolescents. *Initial:* 0.5 to 2 mg every 8 to 12 hr, increased to 3 to 5 mg every 8 to 12 hr, as needed.

Children ages 3 to 12 weighing 15 kg (33 lb) to 40 kg (88 lb). *Initial:* 0.5 mg daily in divided doses twice daily or three times daily. Increased by 0.5 mg every 5 to 7 days, as needed. *Maintenance:* 0.05 to 0.15 mg/kg/day given in 2 to 3 divided doses.

±**DOSAGE ADJUSTMENT** For debilitated or elderly patients, initial dosage reduced to 0.5 to 2 mg twice daily or three times daily, as needed.

✳ *To treat nonpsychotic behavior disorders*

ORAL SOLUTION, TABLETS

Children ages 3 to 12 weighing 15 kg (33 lb) to 40 kg (88 lb). *Initial:* 0.5 mg daily in divided doses twice daily or three times daily. Increased by 0.5 mg every 5 to 7 days, if needed and then reduced to lowest effective maintenance dose. *Maintenance:* 0.05 to 0.075 mg/kg daily divided into two or three doses.

✳ *To treat Tourette's syndrome*

ORAL SOLUTION, TABLETS

Adults and adolescents weighing more than 40 kg (88 lb). *Initial:* 0.5 to 2 mg every 8 to 12 hr. Increased to 3 to 5 mg every 8 to 12 hr, if needed. *Maximum:* 100 mg daily in divided doses.

Children ages 3 to 12 weighing 15 kg (33 lb) to 40 kg (88 lb). *Initial:* 0.5 mg daily, increased by 0.5 mg every 5 to 7 days, as needed. *Maintenance:* 0.05 to 0.075 mg/kg daily divided into 2 or 3 doses.

✳ *To treat acutely agitated schizophrenic patient*

PROMPT-ACTING I.M. INJECTION

Adults and adolescents. *Initial:* 2 to 5 mg, with subsequent doses every 60 min, as needed. Or, if symptoms are controlled, dose may be repeated every 4 to 8 hr. First oral dose may be given 12 to 24 hr after last parenteral dose. *Maximum:* 20 mg daily.

✳ *To provide long-term antipsychotic therapy for patients with schizophrenia who require conversion from oral therapy to parenteral therapy*

LONG-ACTING I.M. (DECANOATE) INJECTION

Adults. *Initial:* 10 to 20 times the previous daily oral dose up to 100 mg. Repeated every 4 wk. *Usual maintenance:* 10 to 15 times the previous daily dose. *Maximum:* Initial dose should not exceed 100 mg. If conversion requires more than 100 mg as an initial dose, dose should be administered in 2 injections, the first at the maximum of 100 mg, followed by the balance in 3 to 7 days.

±**DOSAGE ADJUSTMENT** For patients who are debilitated or elderly or who are stable on low doses of oral haloperidol (up to 10 mg/day), a range of 10 to 15 times the previous daily dose in oral equivalents may be used for initial conversion.

≡ Drug Administration

P.O.

- Tablets may be administered with or without food.
- Protect concentrate from light. Slight yellowing is common and doesn't affect potency. Discard very discolored solution.
- Measure oral solution dosage with the dropper that comes with the bottle. Do not use other droppers, as dosage may not be accurate.
- Dilute oral solution with a beverage, such as apple, orange, or tomato juice; cola; or water. Administer immediately.

I.M.

- Be sure right parenteral formulation is being used; there is a prompt-acting one and a long-acting one.
- Know that a slight yellow discoloration of injection solution doesn't affect potency.
- Do not administer parenteral form intravenously.
- Administer by deep I.M. injection into gluteal muscle using Z-track technique and 21G needle.
- Don't give more than 3 ml per site.

Route	Onset	Peak	Duration
P.O.	Unknown	2–6 hr	Unknown
I.M. (lactate)	30–60 min	10–20 min	Unknown
I.M. (decanoate)	Unknown	6 days	2–4 wk

Half-life: 18 hr; 3 wk (decanoate)

≡ Mechanism of Action

May block postsynaptic dopamine receptors in the limbic system and increase brain turnover of dopamine, producing an antipsychotic effect.

Contraindications

Dementia with Lewy bodies, hypersensitivity to haloperidol or its components, Parkinson's disease, severe toxic CNS comatose states or depression

Interactions

DRUGS

anticholinergics: Increased anticholinergic effect

buspirone, CYP2D6 inhibitors (chlorpromazine, promethazine, quinidine, paroxetine, sertraline, venlafaxine), CYP3A4 inhibitors (alprazolam, itraconazole, ketoconazole, nefazodone, ritonavir), combined CYP2D6 and CYP3A4 inhibitors (fluoxetine, fluvoxamine, ritonavir): Increased haloperidol plasma concentrations and increased risk of adverse events, including prolonged QT interval

carbamazepine, phenobarbital, phenytoin, rifampin, St. John's wort: Decreased plasma haloperidol levels

citalopram, class IA and 3 antiarrhythmics, corticosteroids, diuretics, erythromycin, ketoconazole, levofloxacin, methadone, paroxetine, ziprasidone: Possibly increased risk of QT prolongation

CNS depressants such as anesthetics and opiates: Increased CNS depression and risk of respiratory depression and hypotension

levodopa and other dopamine agonists: Possibly decreased therapeutic effects of these drugs

tricyclic antidepressants such as desipramine, imipramine: Increased plasma concentrations of these drugs with increased risk of adverse reactions

ACTIVITIES

alcohol use: Increased CNS depression and risk of hypotension and respiratory depression

Adverse Reactions

CNS: Agitation, akinesia, anxiety, cogwheel rigidity, confusion, depression, dizziness, drowsiness, dystonia, euphoria, extrapyramidal reactions that may be irreversible, **hypothermia**, insomnia, masked facies, **neuroleptic malignant syndrome**, opisthotonus, Parkinsonism, restlessness, **seizures**, slurred speech, somnolence, tremor, vertigo

CV: **Cardiac arrest**, edema, **extrasystoles**, hypertension, hypersensitivity vasculitis, orthostatic hypotension, **QT interval prolongation**, **ventricular arrhythmias**, tachycardia, **torsades de pointes**

EENT: Blurred vision, dry mouth, increased salivation (all drug forms), **laryngeal edema**, **laryngospasm**, nystagmus, oculogyric crisis, stomatitis (oral solution)

ENDO: Breast discomfort and engorgement, galactorrhea, gynecomastia, hyperprolactinemia, inappropriate antidiuretic hormone secretion

GI: **Acute hepatic failure**, cholestasis, constipation, elevated liver enzymes, **hepatitis**, jaundice, nausea, vomiting

GU: Decreased or loss of libido, difficult ejaculation, impotence, menstrual irregularities, priapism, urinary retention

HEME: **Agranulocytosis**, anemia, leukocytosis, **leukopenia**, **neutropenia**, **pancytopenia**, **thrombocytopenia**

MS: Muscle rigidity or twitching, **rhabdomyolysis**, torticollis, trismus

RESP: **Bronchospasm**, dyspnea

SKIN: Acneiform skin reactions, diaphoresis, **exfoliative dermatitis**, photosensitivity, pruritis, rash, urticaria

Other: **Anaphylaxis**, **angioedema**, **heatstroke**, **hypersensitivity reactions**, weight gain or loss

Childbearing Considerations

PREGNANCY

- Drug may cause fetal harm with a potential increase risk for limb malformations when given during the first trimester of pregnancy.
- Neonates exposed to antipsychotic drugs such as haloperidol during the third trimester of pregnancy are at risk for extrapyramidal and/or withdrawal symptoms at birth.
- Use with caution only if benefit to mother outweighs potential risk to fetus.

LACTATION

- Drug is present in breast milk.
- Breastfeeding should not be undertaken during drug therapy.

Nursing Considerations

- Be aware that haloperidol shouldn't be used to treat dementia-related psychosis in the elderly because of an increased mortality risk.

G
H
I

- Use haloperidol cautiously in patients with a history of prolonged QT interval, patients with uncorrected electrolyte disturbances, and patients receiving class IA or III antiarrhythmics because of an increased risk of prolonged QT interval. Monitor elderly patients closely because they may have an increased risk of prolonged QT interval.
- Be aware that haloperidol concentrations may increase in hepatically impaired patients. Monitor closely for adverse reactions.
- Assess patient for fall risks, such those who are elderly and those with conditions or diseases, or taking drugs that exacerbate central nervous system adverse effects such as motor instability, orthostatic hypotension, and somnolence. Use fall precautions in patients at risk.
- Watch for tardive dyskinesia (potentially irreversible involuntary movements) in patients receiving long-term therapy, especially elderly women who take large doses.
- Monitor CBC, especially if patient has a low WBC count or history of drug-induced leukopenia or neutropenia, often during the first few months of therapy, as ordered. If WBC count drops, especially if neutrophil count drops below 1,000/mm³, expect haloperidol to be discontinued. If neutropenia is significant, also monitor patient for fever or other symptoms of infection and provide appropriate treatment, as prescribed.
- Know that if extrapyramidal reactions occur during the first few days of treatment, dosage should be reduced as prescribed. If symptoms persist, drug may be discontinued. Dystonia also may occur during first few days of treatment, especially in patients receiving higher doses and in males and younger age-groups. Notify prescriber.
- Avoid stopping haloperidol abruptly unless severe adverse reactions occur, because withdrawal emergent dyskinesia may occur.
- Monitor for signs of neuroleptic malignant syndrome, a rare but possibly fatal disorder linked to antipsychotic drugs. Signs include altered mental status, arrhythmias, fever, and muscle rigidity.

! **WARNING** Know that QT interval prolongation, sudden death, and torsades de pointes, although uncommon, may occur in patients receiving haloperidol despite the lack of such predisposing factors.

! **WARNING** Be aware that if patient develops hypotension while receiving haloperidol therapy, and a vasopressor is required, epinephrine must not be used, because haloperidol may block its vasopressor activity and paradoxically cause hypotension to worsen.

PATIENT TEACHING

- Advise patient to take haloperidol exactly as prescribed and not to stop abruptly, because withdrawal symptoms may occur.
- Instruct patient to dilute liquid form with cola, juice, or water before taking it, to prevent oral mucosal irritation. Tell patient when measuring oral solution dosage to only use the dropper that comes with it.
- Caution patient to avoid skin contact with oral solution because it may cause a rash.
- Advise patient to take tablets with food or a full glass of milk if GI distress occurs.
- Instruct patient to consume adequate fluids and to take precautions against heatstroke.
- Urge patient not to drink alcohol during therapy.
- Caution patient to avoid driving and other hazardous activities if sedation occurs. Also warn patient to take measures to avoid falls because of adverse effects.
- Instruct patient to report repetitive movements, tremor, and vision changes.

heparin sodium
Heparin Lock Flush, Heparin Sodium Injection

Class and Category
Pharmacologic class: Anticoagulant
Therapeutic class: Anticoagulant

Indications and Dosages
* *To prevent and treat pulmonary embolism and venous thrombosis; to prevent postoperative deep venous thrombosis and pulmonary embolism in patients undergoing*

major abdominothoracic surgery or who, for other reasons, are at risk of developing thromboembolic disease; to treat atrial fibrillation with embolization; to treat acute and chronic consumptive coagulopathies (disseminated intravascular coagulation)

FULL-DOSE I.V. INJECTION, FULL-DOSE I.V. INFUSION

Adults receiving continuous intravenous therapy. *Initial:* 5,000 units by I.V. injection followed by 20,000 to 40,000 units infused per 24 hr.

Children age 1 year and older. *Initial:* 75 to 100 units/kg by I.V. injection over 10 min followed by infusion of 18 to 20 units/kg/hr.

Infants ages 2 months to one year. *Initial:* 75 to 100 units/kg by I.V. injection given over 10 min followed by infusion of 25 to 30 units/kg/hr.

Infants less than 2 months. *Initial:* 75 to 100 mg/kg by I.V. injection given over 10 min followed by individualized infusion with average of 28 units/kg/hr.

Adults receiving intermittent intravenous therapy. *Initial:* 10,000 units followed by 5,000 to 10,000 units every 4 to 6 hr.

FULL-DOSE SUBCUTANEOUS INJECTION

Adults. *Initial:* 5,000 units by I.V. injection and 10,000 to 20,000 units subcutaneously with a concentrated solution; then 8,000 to 10,000 units subcutaneously every 8 hr or 15,000 to 20,000 units subcutaneously every 12 hr.

✳ *To prevent postoperative thromboembolism*

LOW-DOSE SUBCUTANEOUS INJECTION

Adults. 5,000 units 2 hr before surgery and then 5,000 units every 8 to 12 hr for 7 days or until patient is fully ambulatory, whichever is longer.

✳ *To prevent clots in patients undergoing cardiovascular surgery*

I.V. INFUSION OR INJECTION

Adults. *Initial:* Not less than 150 units/kg. *Usual:* 300 units/kg for procedures that last less than 60 min; 400 units/kg for procedures that last longer than 60 min.

✳ *To provide anticoagulation with blood transfusions*

I.V. INFUSION

Adults. 400 to 600 units/100 ml of whole blood.

✳ *To provide anticoagulation with extracorporeal dialysis*

I.V. INFUSION, I.V. INJECTION

Adults. *Loading:* 25 to 30 units/kg by I.V. injection followed by infusion of 1,500 to 2,000 units/hr.

✳ *To maintain heparin lock patency*

I.V. INJECTION

Adults. 10 to 100 units/ml heparin flush solution (enough to fill device) after each use of device.

±**DOSAGE ADJUSTMENT** Dosage possibly decreased in patients over 60 years of age, especially women, because of an increased risk of bleeding.

☰ Drug Administration

- Revision has been made to state the strength of the entire container of heparin, followed by how much heparin is in 1 ml. To lessen risk of a drug error, look for the red cautionary label that extends above the main label. Read and confirm that the correct medication and strength have been selected. Remove red cautionary label prior to removing the flip-off cap.
- Never administer heparin by I.M. route.
- Don't use heparin sodium injection as a catheter-lock flush, because fatal errors have occurred in children when 1-ml heparin sodium injection vials were confused with 1-ml catheter-lock flush vials. Always examine vial labels closely to ensure that correct product is being used.
- Some heparin products contain benzyl alcohol and should not be used in pregnant women, neonates or infants, or mothers who are breastfeeding; instead use preservative-free Heparin Sodium Injection.

I.V.

Heparin Sodium Injection

- Concentrated heparin solutions contain more than 100 units/ml, which can irritate blood vessels.
- For continuous infusion, invert container at least 6 times to ensure adequate mixing and to prevent drug from pooling. Solution should appear clear and the seal intact.
- Use an infusion pump.
- During continuous I.V. therapy, expect to obtain APTT before therapy begins to obtain a baseline and then every 4 hours, or

G
H
I

as appropriate after therapy begins. Use the arm opposite the infusion site.

- For I.V. injection, expect to adjust dose based on coagulation test results performed 30 minutes before each injection during initiation and then at appropriate intervals. Therapeutic range is typically 1.5 to 2.5 times the control.
- Expect to adjust the heparin dose based on frequent blood coagulation tests, as ordered, when patient is receiving a full-dose heparin regimen. If coagulation test is unduly prolonged or hemorrhage occurs, heparin should be discontinued immediately.
- Do not piggyback other drugs while heparin infusion is being administered and do not mix other drugs with heparin in the same syringe when giving heparin as an I.V. injection.

Heparin Lock Flush
- Make sure product being used is heparin lock flush and not heparin sodium injection.
- Use enough flush to fill entire device.
- If a drug is known to be incompatible with heparin, the entire device should be flushed with 0.9% Sodium Chloride Injection before and after the medication is given; followed by a second saline flush. Then a heparin lock flush should be reinstilled into the device.
- Clear heparin solution from device before withdrawing blood sample if heparin may interfere with test results.
- *Incompatibilities:* Alteplase, amikacin sulfate, atracurium besylate, ciprofloxacin, cytarabine, daunorubicin, droperidol, erythromycin lactobionate, gentamicin sulfate, idarubicin, kanamycin sulfate, mitoxantrone HCl, polymyxin B sulfate, promethazine HCl, streptomycin sulfate, tobramycin sulfate

SUBCUTANEOUS
- Inject into anterior abdominal wall, above the iliac crest, and 5 cm (2 inches) or more away from the umbilicus.
- To minimize subcutaneous tissue trauma, lift adipose tissue away from deep tissues; don't aspirate for blood before injecting drug; don't move needle while injecting drug; and don't massage injection site before or after injection. Apply gentle pressure to the site after withdrawing needle.

- Alternate injection sites, and watch for signs of bleeding and hematomas.
- Expect blood samples to be drawn 4 to 6 hours after each injection to determine adequacy of dosage.

Route	Onset	Peak	Duration
I.V.	Immediate	Immediate	2–6 hr
SubQ	20–60 min	2–4 hr	8–12 hr

Half-life: 60–90 min

⅀ Mechanism of Action
Binds with antithrombin III, enhancing antithrombin III's inactivation of the coagulation enzymes thrombin (factor IIa) and factors Xa and XIa. At low doses, heparin inhibits factor Xa and prevents conversion of prothrombin to thrombin. Thrombin is needed for conversion of fibrinogen to fibrin; without fibrin, clots can't form. At high doses, heparin inactivates thrombin, preventing fibrin formation and existing clot extension.

⅀ Contraindications
Breastfeeding, infants, neonates, or pregnant woman (heparin sodium injection, USP, preserved with benzyl alcohol); history of heparin-induced thrombocytopenia or heparin-induced thrombocytopenia and thrombosis, or thrombocytopenia with pentosan polysulfate; hypersensitivity to heparin, pork, or its components; inability to monitor coagulation parameters when full-dose heparin is used; uncontrolled active bleeding, except in disseminated intravascular coagulation (DIC)

⅀ Interactions
DRUGS
antihistamines, digoxin, nicotine, tetracyclines: Decreased anticoagulant effect of heparin
antithrombin III (human): Increased risk of bleeding
aspirin, dextran, dipyridamole, glycoprotein IIb/IIIa antagonists, hydroxychloroquine, NSAIDs, phenylbutazone, platelet aggregation inhibitors, thienopyridines: Increased platelet inhibition and risk of bleeding
dicumarol, warfarin: Possibly invalid prothrombin time if blood drawn sooner than 5 hours after last intravenous dose or 24 hours after last subcutaneous dose of heparin
ethacrynic acid, glucocorticoids, salicylates: Increased risk of bleeding

ACTIVITIES
smoking: Decreased anticoagulant effect

Adverse Reactions

CNS: Chills, dizziness, fever, headache, peripheral neuropathy
CV: Chest pain, rebound hyperlipemia, **thrombosis**
EENT: Epistaxis, gingival bleeding, rhinitis
ENDO: Adrenal hemorrhage causing acute adrenal insufficiency
GI: Abdominal distention and pain, elevated liver enzymes, **hematemesis, melena,** nausea, **retroperitoneal hemorrhage,** vomiting
GU: Hematuria, hypermenorrhea, **ovarian hemorrhage,** priapism
HEME: Delayed onset of heparin-induced thrombocytopenia, easy bruising, **excessive bleeding from wounds, hemorrhage, heparin-induced thrombocytopenia, heparin-induced thrombocytopenia and thrombosis, thrombocytopenia**
MS: Back pain, myalgia, osteoporosis (long-term use of high doses)
RESP: Asthma, dyspnea, wheezing
SKIN: Alopecia, cutaneous necrosis following subcutaneous injection, cyanosis, petechiae, pruritus, urticaria
Other: Anaphylaxis; heparin resistance; histamine-like reactions at injection site, including necrosis of the skin; **hypersensitivity reactions;** subcutaneous deep injection-site hematoma, irritation, pain, redness, and ulceration

Childbearing Considerations

PREGNANCY
- It is not known if drug causes fetal harm.
- Use with caution only if benefit to mother outweighs potential risk to fetus.
- Use preservative-free Heparin Sodium Injection during pregnancy.

LACTATION
- It is not known if drug is present in breast milk.
- Patient should check with prescriber before breastfeeding.
- If mother is breastfeeding, use preservative-free Heparin Sodium Injection.

Nursing Considerations

- Use heparin cautiously in alcoholics; menstruating women; patients over age 60, especially women; and patients with conditions that increase risk of hemorrhage, such as certain cardiovascular conditions (severe hypertension, subacute bacterial endocarditis), gastrointestinal conditions (continuous tube drainage of small intestine or stomach, ulcerative lesions), hematologic conditions that increase risk of bleeding (hemophilia, thrombocytopenia, some vascular purpuras), liver disease with impaired hemostasis, presence of hereditary antithrombin III deficiency in patients receiving concurrent antithrombin III therapy, or presence of indwelling catheters, severe renal disease, and during or immediately following major surgery (especially involving the brain, eye, or spinal cord) or following spinal anesthesia or spinal tap. Also use cautiously in patients with a history of allergies or asthma.
- Avoid injecting any drugs by I.M. route during heparin therapy, to decrease risk of bleeding and hematoma.

> **! WARNING** Know that bleeding is a major adverse effect of heparin therapy. Take safety precautions to prevent bleeding, such as having patient use a soft-bristled toothbrush and an electric razor. Bleeding may occur at any site and also may indicate an underlying problem, such as GI or urinary tract bleeding. Other sites of bleeding that could be fatal and require immediate attention include adrenal, ovarian, and retroperitoneal hemorrhage.

- Expect to periodically monitor patient's hematocrit, platelet counts, and occult blood in stool during the entire course of heparin therapy, regardless of the route of administration.
- Be aware that heparin-induced thrombocytopenia (HIT) can occur in patients exposed to heparin, including delayed onset, and is due to the development of antibodies to a platelet factor 4-heparin complex. It may progress to the development of arterial and venous thromboses. Monitor blood test results, and observe for signs of bleeding, such as ecchymosis, epistaxis, hematemesis, hematuria, melena, and petechiae. Thrombocytopenia of any degree can occur 2 to 20 days following the onset of heparin therapy, so patient should be monitored closely. If platelet count drops below 100,000/mm^3 or recurrent thrombosis

G
H
I

develops, notify prescriber and expect heparin to be discontinued.

- Be aware that heparin resistance may occur, especially in patients with antithrombin III deficiency, cancer, fever, infections with thrombosing tendencies, MI, thrombophlebitis, or thrombosis and postsurgery. Monitor coagulation tests closely in these patients and expect an adjustment in the heparin dose, as needed.
- Make sure all health care providers know that patient is receiving heparin.
- Keep protamine sulfate on hand to use as an antidote for heparin. Be aware that each milligram of protamine sulfate neutralizes 100 units of heparin.
- Be aware that prescriber may order oral anticoagulants before discontinuing heparin to avoid increased coagulation caused by heparin withdrawal. Heparin may be discontinued when full therapeutic effect of oral anticoagulant is achieved.
- Know that women over age 60 have highest risk of hemorrhage during therapy.
- Watch closely if patient is receiving heparin therapy and nitroglycerin I.V. because PTT may decrease and then rebound after nitroglycerin is discontinued. Monitor PTT closely, and be prepared to adjust heparin dose, as prescribed.

! WARNING Know that delayed-onset, heparin-induced thrombocytopenia may occur several weeks after heparin is discontinued and may progress to heparin-induced thrombocytopenia thrombosis, causing arterial and venous thromboses, including thrombus formation on a prosthetic cardiac valve.

PATIENT TEACHING
- Explain that heparin can't be taken orally.
- Inform patient about increased risk of bleeding; urge her to avoid injuries and to use a soft-bristled toothbrush and an electric razor.
- Urge patient to report any abnormal sign or symptom to prescriber, even weeks after heparin has been discontinued, because of the potential for delayed adverse reactions.
- Advise patient to avoid drugs that interact with heparin, such as aspirin and ibuprofen.
- Instruct patient and family to watch for and report abdominal or lower back pain, black stools, bleeding gums, bloody urine, excessive menstrual bleeding, nosebleeds, and severe headaches. Also tell patient to report any persistent, severe, or unusual signs and symptoms to prescriber immediately. Alert patient receiving heparin subcutaneously that necrosis of the skin has been reported following subcutaneous administration of heparin and to alert prescriber if any abnormalities occur at injection sites.
- Explain that temporary hair loss may occur.
- Advise patient to wear or carry appropriate medical identification.

hydralazine hydrochloride
Apresoline (CAN)

☰ Class and Category
Pharmacologic class: Vasodilator
Therapeutic class: Antihypertensive

☰ Indications and Dosages
* *To manage essential hypertension, alone or with other antihypertensives*

TABLETS
Adults. *Initial:* 10 mg four times daily for first 2 to 4 days and then increased to 25 mg four times daily for remainder of first wk. Further increased to 50 mg four times daily beginning wk 2 and thereafter. *Maintenance:* 50 to 200 mg daily in divided doses. *Maximum:* 300 mg daily.

Children. *Initial:* 0.75 mg/kg daily in divided doses four times daily. Increased gradually over 3 to 4 wk. *Maximum:* 7.5 mg/kg daily, not to exceed 200 mg/day.

* *To manage severe essential hypertension when drug can't be taken orally or when need to reduce blood pressure is urgent*

I.V. OR I.M. INJECTION
Adults. 20 to 40 mg, repeated as needed.
Children. *Initial:* 1.7 to 3.5 mg/kg/day in 4 to 6 divided doses.

± **DOSAGE ADJUSTMENT** For adults with marked renal impairment, dosage may have to be reduced. For slow acetylators, dosage may have to be reduced or dosage frequency changed.

☰ Drug Administration

P.O.

- Do not use if blister is torn or broken.
- Do not administer with food, as higher plasma levels may occur.

I.V.

- I.V. route used only if oral administration is not feasible.
- Solution may become discolored if in contact with metal. If solution is discolored, discard.
- Administer immediately after vial is opened. Inject undiluted rapidly.
- *Incompatibilities:* Infusion solutions; manufacturer does not list any other drug incompatibilities

I.M.

- Administer undiluted.
- Rotate sites.

Route	Onset	Peak	Duration
P.O.	20–30 min	1–2 hr	3–8 hr
I.V.	5–20 min	10–80 min	1–4 hr
I.M.	10–30 min	1 hr	2–6 hr

Half-life: 3–7 hr

☰ Mechanism of Action

May act in a manner that resembles organic nitrates and sodium nitroprusside, except that hydralazine is selective for arteries. It:

- exerts a direct vasodilating effect on vascular smooth muscle
- interferes with calcium movement in vascular smooth muscle by altering cellular calcium metabolism
- dilates arteries, not veins, which minimizes orthostatic hypotension and increases cardiac output and cerebral blood flow
- causes reflex autonomic response that increases, cardiac output, heart rate, and left ventricular ejection fraction
- has a positive inotropic effect on the heart.

☰ Contraindications

Coronary artery disease, hypersensitivity to hydralazine or its components, mitral valvular rheumatic heart disease

☰ Interactions

DRUGS

diazoxide, MAO inhibitors, other antihypertensives: Risk of severe hypotension
NSAIDs: Decreased hydralazine effects

FOODS

all foods: Possibly increased bioavailability of hydralazine

☰ Adverse Reactions

CNS: Chills, fever, headache, peripheral neuritis
CV: Angina, edema, orthostatic hypotension, palpitations, tachycardia
EENT: Lacrimation, nasal congestion
GI: Anorexia, constipation, diarrhea, nausea, vomiting
RESP: Dyspnea
SKIN: Blisters, flushing, pruritus, rash, urticaria
Other: Lupus-like symptoms, especially with high doses; lymphadenopathy

☰ Childbearing Considerations

PREGNANCY

- It is not known if drug causes fetal harm.
- Use with caution only if benefit to mother outweighs potential risk to fetus.

LACTATION

- Drug is present in breast milk.
- Patient should check with prescriber before breastfeeding.

☰ Nursing Considerations

- Monitor ANA titer, CBC, and lupus erythematosus cell preparation before therapy and periodically as ordered during long-term treatment.
- Monitor blood pressure and pulse rate regularly and weigh patient daily during therapy.
- Check blood pressure with patient in lying, sitting, and standing positions, and watch for signs of orthostatic hypotension. Expect orthostatic hypotension to be most common in the morning, during hot weather, and with exercise.

! **WARNING** Expect to discontinue drug immediately if patient has lupus-like symptoms, such as arthralgia, fever, myalgia, pharyngitis, and splenomegaly.

- Expect prescriber to withdraw hydralazine gradually to avoid a rapid increase in blood pressure.
- Expect to treat peripheral neuritis with pyridoxine.

PATIENT TEACHING

- Instruct patient to not take hydralazine tablets with food, as it may increase incidence of adverse reactions.

G
H
I

- Advise patient to change position slowly, especially in the morning. Caution that hot showers may increase hypotension.
- Instruct patient to immediately notify prescriber about fever, joint and muscle aches, and sore throat.
- Urge patient to report numbness and tingling in limbs, which may require treatment with another drug.
- Caution patient against stopping drug abruptly because doing so may cause severe hypertension.

hydrochlorothiazide
Microzide, Urozide (CAN)

☰ Class and Category
Pharmacologic class: Thiazide diuretic
Therapeutic class: Diuretic

☰ Indications and Dosages
✴ *To manage hypertension as monotherapy or adjunct with other antihypertensive drugs in more severe forms of hypertension*

CAPSULES
Adults. *Initial:* 12.5 to 25 mg daily increased, as needed, to 50 mg daily given as a single dose or 2 divided doses. *Maximum:* 50 mg daily.

TABLETS
Adults. *Initial:* 25 mg daily, increased to 50 mg daily, as needed, and given as a single dose or in divided doses twice daily.
Children age 2 to 12 years. 1 to 2 mg/kg daily as a single dose or divided into 2 doses. *Maximum:* 100 mg daily.
Children age 6 months to 2 years. 1 to 2 mg/kg daily as a single dose or divided into 2 doses. *Maximum:* 37.5 mg daily.
Infants less than 6 months of age. Up to 3 mg/kg daily divided into two doses.
✴ *As adjunct to treat edema caused by cirrhosis, corticosteroids, estrogen, heart failure, or renal disorders*

TABLETS
Adults. 25 to 100 mg daily given as a single dose or divided and given twice daily.
Children age 2 to 12 years. 1 to 2 mg/kg daily as a single dose or divided into 2 doses. *Maximum:* 100 mg daily.

Children age 6 months to 2 years. 1 to 2 mg/kg daily as a single dose or divided into 2 doses. *Maximum:* 37.5 mg daily.
Infants less than 6 months of age. Up to 3 mg/kg daily divided into two doses.

☰ Drug Administration
P.O.
- Capsules and tablets should be swallowed whole and not chewed, crushed, or opened.
- Administer once-daily dose in morning; twice-daily dose in morning and late afternoon.
- Administer with food or milk if GI upset occurs.

Route	Onset	Peak	Duration
P.O.	2 hr	4 hr	6–12 hr

Half-life: 6–15 hr

☰ Contraindications
Anuria; hypersensitivity to hydrochlorothiazide, other thiazides, sulfonamide derivatives, or their components

☰ Interactions
DRUGS
ACTH, corticosteroids: Increased electrolyte depletion, especially potassium
antihypertensives: Increased antihypertensive effects
barbiturates, opioids: Possibly orthostatic hypotension
cholestyramine, colestipol: Reduced GI absorption of hydrochlorothiazide
insulin, oral antidiabetic drugs: Possibly increased blood glucose level
lithium: Decreased lithium clearance, increased risk of lithium toxicity
nondepolarizing skeletal muscle relaxants: Possibly increased response to muscle relaxants
NSAIDs: Decreased diuretic effect of hydrochlorothiazide, increased risk of renal failure

ACTIVITIES
alcohol use: Possibly orthostatic hypotension

☰ Adverse Reactions
CNS: Asthenia, dizziness, fever, headache, insomnia, paresthesia, restlessness, vertigo, weakness
CV: Elevated cholesterol and triglycerides levels, **hypotension**, orthostatic hypotension, vasculitis

EENT: Acute myopia, acute angle-closure glaucoma, blurred vision, dry mouth
ENDO: Hyperglycemia
GI: Abdominal cramps, anorexia, constipation, diarrhea, indigestion, jaundice, nausea, **pancreatitis**, vomiting
GU: Decreased libido, impotence, interstitial nephritis, nocturia, polyuria, **renal failure**
HEME: Agranulocytosis, aplastic anemia, bone marrow failure, hemolytic anemia, leukopenia, neutropenia, thrombocytopenia
MS: Muscle spasms and weakness
RESP: Pneumonitis, pulmonary edema
SKIN: Alopecia, cutaneous vasculitis, **erythema multiforme, exfoliative dermatitis, nonmelanoma skin cancer,** photosensitivity, purpura, rash, **Stevens–Johnson syndrome, toxic epidermal necrolysis,** urticaria
Other: Anaphylaxis, dehydration, **hypercalcemia,** hyperuricemia, hypochloremia, **hypokalemia, hypomagnesemia, hyponatremia, hypovolemia, metabolic alkalosis,** weight loss

Childbearing Considerations

PREGNANCY
- It is not known if drug causes fetal harm but because it crosses the placental barrier, there is a risk of fetal or neonatal jaundice, thrombocytopenia, and possibly other adverse reactions.
- Use with caution only if benefit to mother outweighs potential risk to fetus.

LACTATION
- Drug is present in breast milk.
- A decision should be made to discontinue breastfeeding or the drug to avoid potential serious adverse reactions in the breastfed infant.

Nursing Considerations
- Monitor blood pressure, daily weight, fluid intake and output, and serum levels of electrolytes, especially potassium.
- Assess for evidence of hypokalemia, such as muscle spasms and weakness.
- Check blood glucose level often, as ordered, in diabetic patients, and expect to increase antidiabetic dosage, as needed and prescribed.
- Know that if patient has gouty arthritis, expect increased risk of gout attacks during therapy.
- Monitor BUN and serum creatinine levels, as ordered, especially in patients with chronic kidney disease, renal artery stenosis, severe congestive heart failure, or volume depletion, because of increased risk of acute renal failure with hydrochlorothiazide therapy. Notify prescriber if serum creatinine levels become elevated, as drug may have to be withheld or discontinued.
- Monitor patient for decreased visual acuity or ocular pain, especially within hours to weeks of beginning drug therapy and in patients with a history of penicillin or sulfonamide allergy, as acute myopia and acute angle-closure glaucoma may develop.

Mechanism of Action

A thiazide diuretic, hydrochlorothiazide promotes movement of sodium (Na^+), chloride (Cl^-), and water (H_2O) from blood in peritubular capillaries into nephron's distal convoluted tubule, as shown. Initially, it may decrease cardiac output, extracellular fluid volume, or plasma volume, which helps explain blood pressure reduction. It also may reduce blood pressure by direct arterial dilation. After several weeks, cardiac output, extracellular fluid volume, and plasma volume return to normal, and peripheral vascular resistance remains decreased.

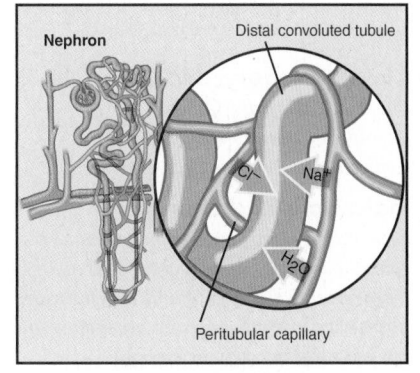

Nephron

Distal convoluted tubule

Cl^- Na^+

H_2O

Peritubular capillary

If left untreated, permanent blindness may occur. If present, notify prescriber immediately, expect to discontinue hydrochlorothiazide, and assist with prompt medical or surgical intervention, as indicated.

> ! **WARNING** Be aware that even minor alterations in fluid and electrolyte balance may precipitate hepatic coma in patients with impaired hepatic function.

PATIENT TEACHING

- Advise patient to take hydrochlorothiazide in morning and early evening to avoid awakening during the night to urinate.
- Instruct patient to take drug with food or milk if adverse GI reactions occur.
- Tell patient to weigh herself at the same time each day wearing the same amount of clothing and to notify prescriber if she gains more than 0.9 kg (2 lb) per day or 2.3 kg (5 lb) per week.
- Instruct patient to eat a diet high in potassium-rich food, including bananas, citrus fruits, dates, and tomatoes.
- Advise patient to change position slowly to minimize effects of orthostatic hypotension.
- Urge patient to report decreased urination, muscle cramps and weakness, and unusual bleeding or bruising.
- Advise patient to protect skin from the sun and undergo regular skin cancer screening.

hydrocodone bitartrate

Hysingla ER, Zohydro ER

≣ Class, Category, and Schedule

Pharmacologic class: Opioid
Therapeutic class: Opioid analgesic
Controlled substance schedule: II

≣ Indications and Dosages

∗ To *manage severe pain in patients requiring continuous, around-the-clock opioid analgesia for an extended period of time and for which alternative treatment options are inadequate*

E.R. CAPSULES (ZOHYDRO ER)

Adults who are opioid naïve or opioid nontolerant. *Initial:* 10 mg every 12 hr, increased, as needed, in increments of 10 mg every 12 hr every 3 to 7 days to effective and tolerable dose. *Maximum:* 40 mg/dose or 80 mg total daily dose.

Adults who are opioid tolerant and converting from another opioid. Highly individualized.

±**DOSAGE ADJUSTMENT** For patients with severe hepatic impairment, a single dose of 10 mg given, followed by close monitoring for respiratory depression and sedation. If single dose tolerated, 10 mg every 12 hr as needed and titrated carefully.

E.R. TABLETS (HYSINGLA ER)

Adults who are opioid naïve or opioid nontolerant. *Initial:* 20 mg every 24 hr, increased, as needed, in increments of 10 to 20 mg daily every 3 to 5 days to effective and tolerable dose. *Maximum:* 80 mg every 24 hr.

Adults who are opioid tolerant and converting from another opioid. Highly individualized.

±**DOSAGE ADJUSTMENT** For patient with moderate or severe renal impairment, including end-stage renal disease or severe hepatic impairment, initial dosage decreased by half.

≣ Drug Administration

P.O.

- Tablets and capsules should be swallowed whole and not chewed, crushed, dissolved, or split/opened.
- Administer with enough water to ensure complete swallowing immediately after patient places drug in mouth.
- Have patient take tablets one at a time.
- Naloxone should always be readily available with hydrocodone administration.

Route	Onset	Peak	Duration
P.O./E.R. tab	Unknown	6–30 hr	Unknown
P.O./E.R. cap	Unknown	5 hr	Unknown

Half-life: 7–12 hr

≣ Mechanism of Action

Binds to and activates opioid receptors at sites in the periaqueductal and periventricular gray matter, the ventromedial medulla, and the spinal cord to produce pain relief.

Contraindications

Acute or severe bronchial asthma (in an unmonitored setting or in the absence of resuscitative equipment); hypersensitivity to hydrocodone bitartrate or any of its components; known or suspected gastrointestinal obstruction, including paralytic ileus; significant respiratory depression

Interactions

DRUGS

5-HT3 receptor antagonists, drugs that affect the serotonin neurotransmitter system (mirtazapine, trazodone, tramadol), linezolid, methylene blue (I.V.), selective serotonin reuptake inhibitors, serotonin and norepinephrine reuptake inhibitors, tricyclic antidepressants triptans, tryptophan: Increased risk of serotonin syndrome
anticholinergics: Increased risk of urinary retention or severe constipation, which may lead to paralytic ileus
antipsychotics, anxiolytics, benzodiazepines and other CNS depressants, general anesthetics, muscle relaxants, other opioids and sedatives/hypnotics, sedating antihistamines, tranquilizers, tricyclic antidepressants: Increased risk of coma, hypotension, profound sedation, and severe respiratory depression
CYP3A4 inducers: Increased clearance of hydrocodone with decreased effectiveness
CYP2D6 inhibitors, CYP3A4 inhibitors: Decreased clearance of hydrocodone resulting in increased or prolonged opioid effects
diuretics: Possible reduction of the effectiveness of diuretics
mixed agonist/antagonist analgesics such as buprenorphine, butorphanol, nalbuphine, pentazocine: Possible reduced hydrocodone effectiveness or precipitation of withdrawal symptoms
MAO inhibitors: Increased risk of serotonin syndrome or opioid toxicity
muscle relaxants: Enhanced neuromuscular blocking action of skeletal muscle relaxants producing increased degree of respiratory depression

ACTIVITIES

alcohol use: Possibly increased hydrocodone plasma levels with potentially fatal overdose

Adverse Reactions

CNS: Anxiety, CNS depression, coma, depression, dizziness, fatigue, fever, headache, insomnia, lethargy, migraine, paresthesia, seizures, somnolence, syncope, tremor
CV: Hypercholesterolemia, hypotension, peripheral edema
EENT: Dry mouth
ENDO: Adrenal insufficiency (rare), hot flashes
GI: Abdominal discomfort or pain, constipation (may be severe), elevated liver enzymes, gastroesophageal reflux disease, nausea, spasm of the Sphincter of Oddi, vomiting
GU: Decreased libido, erectile dysfunction, impotence, infertility, lack of menstruation, UTI
MS: Arthralgia; back, extremity, musculoskeletal, or neck pain; muscle spasms
RESP: Cough, dyspnea, respiratory depression
SKIN: Pruritis, rash, sweating including night sweats
Other: Dehydration, hypokalemia, noncardiac chest pain, physical and psychological dependence

Childbearing Considerations

PREGNANCY

- Drug may cause fetal harm.
- Prolonged use of drug during pregnancy can result in neonatal opioid withdrawal syndrome (NOWS) after birth, which may be life-threatening if not recognized and treated.
- Prolonged use during pregnancy should be avoided. Use with caution only if benefit to mother outweighs potential risk to fetus.

LABOR & DELIVERY

- Drug is not recommended for use in pregnant women immediately before or during labor. Opioids may alter length of time of labor.
- Opioids cross the placental barrier and may produce respiratory depression and psycho-physiologic effects in the newborn. Monitor newborn closely for signs of excess sedation and respiratory depression.
- An opioid antagonist, such as naloxone, must be available at the time of delivery in the event it is needed to reverse

G
H
I

opioid-induced respiratory depression in the neonate.

LACTATION

- Drug is present in breast milk.
- Breastfeeding should not be undertaken during drug therapy.

REPRODUCTION

- Chronic use of opioids may reduce fertility in females and males.

Nursing Considerations

- Be aware that hydrocodone increases the risk of abuse, addiction, and misuse. Know that to ensure that the benefits of hydrocodone therapy outweigh the risks, a Risk Evaluation and Mitigation Strategy (REMS) is required.
- Know that hydrocodone should not be given to a patient with impaired consciousness, nor should the drug be administered on an as-needed basis.
- Be aware that opioids like hydrocodone should not be given to women during pregnancy, while in labor, or when breastfeeding, as the newborn or infant may experience neonatal opioid withdrawal syndrome (NOWS), which could be life-threatening. This syndrome may exhibit as excessive or high-pitched crying, poor feeding, rapid breathing, or trembling. If not recognized and treated appropriately, it can become life-threatening.
- Know that hydrocodone is contraindicated in children under the age of 18 when used in cold or cough preparations.
- Use extreme caution when administering hydrocodone to patients with significant chronic obstructive pulmonary disease or cor pulmonale, and in patients having a substantially decreased respiratory reserve, hypoxia, hypercapnia, or preexisting respiratory depression, especially when initiating or titrating therapy. These patients may develop respiratory depression, even with usual therapeutic doses, because hydrocodone may decrease the patient's respiratory drive to the point of apnea.
- Use hydrocodone cautiously in cachectic, debilitated or elderly patients, especially when initiating and titrating therapy, as

they are at increased risk for adverse effects, especially respiratory depression.

- Be aware that opioid therapy like hydrocodone should only be used concomitantly with benzodiazepines and other CNS depressants in patients for whom other treatment options are inadequate. If prescribed together, expect dosing and duration of hydrocodone to be limited. Monitor patient closely for signs and symptoms of decrease in consciousness, including coma, profound sedation, and significant respiratory depression. Notify prescriber immediately and provide emergency supportive care, as death may occur.
- Be aware that patients who are considered opioid tolerant are those who have received for 1 week or longer, at least 8 mg of oral hydromorphone per day, 60 mg of oral morphine daily, 30 mg of oral oxycodone per day, 25 mg of oral oxymorphone per day, 25 micrograms transdermal fentanyl per hour, or an equianalgesic dose of another opioid.
- Do not administer hydrocodone to a patient wearing a transdermal fentanyl patch until the patch has been removed for 18 hours. Also know that close monitoring is especially important for a patient converting from methadone because methadone has a long half-life and tends to accumulate in the blood.

! **WARNING** Be aware that hydrocodone available as an extended-release formulation increases risk of overdose and death because of larger amount of drug present in this form. Also know that crushing, chewing, snorting, or injecting the contents of the Hysingla E.R. tablet dissolved in a liquid base will result in the uncontrolled delivery of hydrocodone and can result in overdose and death. Be aware that Zohydro E.R. capsules are made with a formulation that deters abuse because it forms an immediate inactive viscous gel when crushed or dissolved in liquids or solvents.

! **WARNING** Monitor patient for respiratory depression, especially when initiating therapy or when increasing dosage, even when the drug has been used as prescribed and not abused or misused. Be aware that overestimating hydrocodone dose when converting patients from another opioid medication can result in fatal overdose with the first dose. To avoid this, know that it is recommended to underestimate a patient's 24-hour oral hydrocodone requirement and provide rescue medication, as needed, until the right dose is determined. Keep resuscitation equipment nearby.

- Be aware that drug can cause sleep-related breathing disorders, including central sleep apnea and sleep-related hypoxemia, that may require a dosage decrease, if present.
- Monitor patients closely who may be susceptible to the intracranial effects of carbon dioxide retention from respiratory depression caused by hydrocodone therapy, such as patients with head injuries or those who have a preexisting elevation in intracranial pressure.
- Monitor patients with a seizure history or disorder because hydrocodone may cause or worsen seizures.
- Monitor effectiveness of hydrocodone in relieving pain; consult prescriber as needed.
- Assess patient for constipation and provide a high-fiber diet and adequate fluid intake, if not contraindicated, because constipation can become severe.
- Monitor patient for evidence of physical dependence or abuse. Know that addiction can occur not only in those who obtain the drug illicitly but also in patients who are appropriately prescribed the drug at recommended doses. Be aware that excessive use of hydrocodone may lead to abuse, addiction, misuse, overdose, and possibly death. Monitor patient's intake of drug closely.
- Notify prescriber if serious adverse reactions occur with hydrocodone therapy and expect dosage to be reduced.
- Expect to taper hydrocodone dosage gradually every 2 to 4 days when patient no longer requires therapy, to prevent withdrawal symptoms in the physically dependent patient. Know that hydrocodone should not be discontinued abruptly.

- Monitor patient's vital signs closely, especially after initiating or titrating dose of hydrocodone. Know that in addition to respiratory depression, hydrocodone may cause severe hypotension, especially in patients whose blood pressure is already compromised by a depleted blood volume or after concurrent administration of drugs that decrease blood pressure.
- Be aware that concomitant use with CYP3A4 inhibitors or discontinuation of CYP3A inducers can result in a fatal overdose of hydrocodone.

! **WARNING** Know that many drugs may interact with opioids like hydrocodone to cause serotonin syndrome. Monitor patient closely for signs and symptoms such as agitation, diaphoresis, diarrhea, fever, hallucinations, labile blood pressure, muscle twitching or stiffness, nausea, shakiness, shivering, tachycardia, trouble with coordination, or vomiting. Notify prescriber at once because serotonin syndrome may be life-threatening. Be prepared to discontinue drug, if possible and ordered, and provide supportive care.

- Monitor patient for adrenal insufficiency. Although rare, it can be life-threatening. Monitor patient for anorexia, dizziness, fatigue, hypotension, nausea, vomiting, or weakness. Notify prescriber if adrenal insufficiency is suspected and expect diagnostic testing to be done. If diagnosis is confirmed, expect to administer corticosteroids and wean patient off of hydrocodone, if possible.
- Monitor patient for decreased bowel motility in postoperative patients receiving hydrocodone, as drug may obscure the development of acute abdominal conditions.

PATIENT TEACHING

- Warn parents that children under age 18 should not receive hydrocodone when mixed with cold or cough preparations.
- Instruct patient to take drug exactly as ordered and not to adjust dosage without speaking to prescriber first. Warn patient of possibility of addiction even when taken as prescribed. Inform him that

excessive or prolonged use can also lead to addiction, misuse, overdose, and possibly death.

- Inform patient that capsules and tablets should be taken whole and never chewed, crushed, dissolved, or snorted. In addition, enough water should be taken with the capsule or tablet to ensure complete swallowing immediately after placing drug in mouth.
- Instruct family/caregiver on how to use naloxone and to have it readily available while patient is taking hydrocodone.
- Warn patient to keep hydrocodone away from the reach of children, as accidental consumption of even one capsule or tablet can cause significant respiratory depression and death.
- Caution patient to avoid ingesting alcohol, including medications containing alcohol, as the combination increases the risk of overdose, respiratory depression, and death, as does taking other types of depressants, including benzodiazepines, together with hydrocodone therapy. Patient should notify all prescribers of hydrocodone use.
- Advise women of childbearing age to notify prescriber if pregnancy occurs or is suspected. Also advise women not to breastfeed while taking oxycodone.
- Caution patient to avoid hazardous activities until drug's CNS effects are known.
- Instruct patient to rise slowly from a lying or sitting position and to lie or sit down if he experiences light-headedness. If effect is frequent or severe, tell him to notify prescriber.
- Urge patient to consume plenty of fluids and high-fiber foods, if not contraindicated, to prevent constipation.
- Inform patient that long-term use of opioids like hydrocodone may decrease sex hormone levels, causing decreased libido, erectile dysfunction, impotence, infertility, or lack of menstruation. Encourage patient to report any such symptoms.
- Instruct patient to notify all prescribers of hydrocodone use.
- Advise patients to take unused drug to a proper disposal place when drug is no longer needed.

hydrocortisone
(cortisol)
Alkindi Sprinkle, Cortef, Cortenema

hydrocortisone acetate
Cortifoam

hydrocortisone sodium succinate
Solu-Cortef

☰ Class and Category
Pharmacologic class: Glucocorticoid
Therapeutic class: Adrenocorticoid replacement, anti-inflammatory

☰ Indications and Dosages
* *To treat severe inflammation related to collagen and dermatologic diseases, endocrine dysfunction, hematologic disorders, hypersensitivity states, nervous system disorders, palliative care of certain cancers, respiratory conditions, and rheumatoid disorders*

TABLETS (CORTEF)
Adults. 20 to 240 mg daily as a single dose or in divided doses.

±**DOSAGE ADJUSTMENT** Dosage increased to more than 240 mg daily if needed to treat acute disease.

I.V. INFUSION; I.V. OR I.M. INJECTION (SOLU-CORTEF)
Adults. 100 to 500 mg every 2, 4, or 6 hr.
Children. 0.56 to 8 mg/kg daily divided into 3 or 4 doses.

* *To treat acute exacerbations of multiple sclerosis*

TABLETS (CORTEF)
Adults. 200 mg daily for 1 wk followed by 80 mg every other day for 1 month.

I.V. INFUSION, I.V. OR I.M. INJECTION (SOLU-CORTEF)
Adults. 800 mg for 1 wk followed by 320 mg every other day for 1 month.

* *To treat pediatric adrenocortical insufficiency*

ORAL GRANULES (ALKINDI SPRINKLE)

Children. *Initial:* 8 to 10 mg/m^2 daily and divided into 3 equal doses for younger children and divided into 2 or 3 equal doses for older children. Round dose to nearest 0.5 or 1 mg. Individualized for dosage increases.

✱ *As adjunct to treat ulcerative proctitis of the distal portion of the rectum in patients who can't retain hydrocortisone or other corticosteroid enemas*

RECTAL AEROSOL (CORTIFOAM)

Adult men. *Initial:* 1 applicatorful once or twice daily for 2 to 3 wk; then every other day thereafter. *Maintenance:* Highly individualized.

✱ *As adjunct to treat nonspecific inflammatory diseases involving the rectum, sigmoid, and left colon such as idiopathic ulcerative colitis, ulcerative proctitis, regional enteritis with left side involvement, proctitis, proctocolitis, and radiation proctitis*

ENEMA (CORTENEMA)

Adults. 100 mg every night for 14 to 21 days and then every other evening until condition improves.

Drug Administration

P.O.

- Administer drug in the morning.
- Give drug with food or milk to prevent GI upset.
- To administer oral granules, hold the capsule so that the printed strength is at the top and tap to ensure that all the granules are in the lower half of the capsule. Squeeze the bottom of the capsule gently and twist off the top of the capsule. Pour directly onto child's tongue, or pour onto a spoon and place in child's mouth, or sprinkle onto a spoonful of cold or room temperature soft food (such as fruit puree or yogurt). Administer granules and have child swallow them within 5 minutes after capsule is opened to avoid a bitter taste. Do not wet the capsule on the tongue or soft food prior to administration but immediately follow administration with a beverage to ensure all the granules have been swallowed. Capsules should not be chewed or crushed, nor should the contents be administered in a gastric or nasogastric tube.

I.V.

- Reconstitute with no more than 2 ml of Bacteriostatic Water or Bacteriostatic Saline solution for each drug vial to be given by I.V. injection; use only Bacteriostatic Water for Injection if giving as an infusion.
- The ACT-O-VIAL system does not contain any preservative. To use the ACT-O-VIAL system, press down on plastic activator to force diluent into the lower compartment. Gently agitate. Remove plastic tab covering center of stopper. Sterilize top of stopper and insert needle squarely through center of stopper until tip is just visible. Invert vial and withdraw dose.
- For I.V. injection after reconstitution, rate of administration is dependent on dosage. For example, administer over 30 seconds for doses up to 100 mg and 10 minutes for doses of 500 mg or more.
- For intermittent I.V. infusion after reconstitution, dilute with 0.9% Sodium Chloride Injection, 5% Dextrose Injection, or 5% Dextrose/0.9% Sodium Chloride Injection. The 100-mg reconstituted solution may be added to 100 to 1,000 ml of diluent, 250-mg solution may be added to 250 to 1,000 ml; 500-mg solution may be added to 500 to 1,000 ml; and 1,000-mg solution may be added to 1,000 ml of diluent. If patient requires fluid restriction, 100 to 3,000 mg of drug may be added to 50 ml of the above diluents. Diluted solution is stable for at least 4 hours. Rate of administration is dependent on dosage.
- *Incompatibilities:* Solutions other than 0.9% Sodium Chloride Injection, 5% Dextrose in Water, 5% Dextrose in Water/0.9% Sodium Chloride Injection; other drugs

I.M.

- Reconstitute with no more than 2 ml of Bacteriostatic Water or Bacteriostatic Saline solution for each vial, or use the ACT-O-VIAL system as described above.
- Inject I.M. deep into gluteal muscle.
- Rotate injection sites to prevent muscle atrophy.

P.R.

- Shake foam container vigorously for 5 to 10 seconds before each use. Do not remove container cap during use of product. Gently place tip of the applicator onto the nose

G
H
I

of the container cap while container is upright on a level surface. Pull plunger past the fill line on the applicator barrel. Press firmly down on cap flanges, hold for 1–2 seconds and release. Pause 5 to 10 seconds to allow foam to expand in applicator barrel. Repeat until foam reaches fill line. Remove applicator from cap. Allow some foam to remain on the applicator tip. Hold applicator firmly by barrel, making sure thumb and middle finger are positioned securely underneath and resting against barrel wings. Place index finger over the plunger. Gently insert tip into anus. Once in place, push plunger to expel foam, then withdraw applicator. Never insert any part of the aerosol container directly into the anus. After each use, wash applicator, container cap, and underlying tip with warm water.

- For enema administration, have patient lie on the left side for administration and for 30 minutes afterward. Administer enema using normal procedure. Encourage patient to retain enema for at least an hour, and preferably all night.

Route	Onset	Peak	Duration
P.O.	Unknown	1–2 hr	Unknown
I.V.	1 hr	1–2 hr	Unknown
I.M./P.R.	Variable	Variable	Variable

Half-life: 1–3 hr

Mechanism of Action

Binds to intracellular glucocorticoid receptors and suppresses inflammatory and immune responses by:

- inhibiting monocyte and neutrophil accumulation at inflammation site and suppressing their bactericidal and phagocytic activity
- stabilizing lysosomal membranes
- suppressing antigen response of helper T cells and macrophages
- inhibiting synthesis of cellular mediators of inflammatory response, such as cytokines, interleukins, and prostaglandins.

Contraindications

Hypersensitivity to hydrocortisone or its components, idiopathic thrombocytopenic purpura (I.M.), intestinal conditions prohibiting intrarectal steroids (P.R.), systemic fungal infection

Interactions

DRUGS

aspirin, NSAIDs: Increased risk of GI distress and bleeding; increased risk of salicylate toxicity with chronic high doses of aspirin
phenobarbital, phenytoin, rifampin: Decreased blood hydrocortisone level
insulin, oral antidiabetic drugs: Possibly increased blood glucose level
ketoconazole, troleandomycin: Decreased clearance of hydrocortisone with increased plasma levels and higher risk of adverse reactions
oral anticoagulants: May decrease or increase anticoagulant effect
vaccines (live attenuated): Decreased antibody response and increased risk of neurologic complications

ACTIVITIES

alcohol use: Increased risk of GI distress and bleeding

Adverse Reactions

CNS: Ataxia, behavioral changes, depression, dizziness, epidural lipomatosis, euphoria, fatigue, headache, **increased intracranial pressure with papilledema**, insomnia, malaise, mood changes, paresthesia, **seizures**, steroid psychosis, syncope, vertigo
CV: Arrhythmias, fat embolism, heart failure, hypertension, **hypertrophic cardiomyopathy, hypotension, thromboembolism**, thrombophlebitis
EENT: Central serous chorioretinopathy, exophthalmos, glaucoma, increased intraocular pressure, nystagmus, posterior subcapsular cataracts
ENDO: Adrenal insufficiency during stress, cushingoid symptoms (buffalo hump, central obesity, moon face, supraclavicular fat pad enlargement), diabetes mellitus, growth suppression in children, hyperglycemia, negative nitrogen balance from protein catabolism
GI: Abdominal distention; hiccups; increased appetite; nausea; **pancreatitis**; peptic ulcer; rectal abnormalities, such as **bleeding**, blistering, burning, itching, or pain (rectal form); ulcerative esophagitis; vomiting
GU: Amenorrhea, glycosuria, menstrual irregularities, perineal burning or tingling
HEME: Easy bruising, leukocytosis
MS: Arthralgia; aseptic necrosis of femoral and humeral heads; compression fractures;

muscle atrophy, twitching, or weakness; myalgia; osteoporosis; spontaneous fractures; steroid myopathy; tendon rupture

SKIN: Acne; altered skin pigmentation; diaphoresis; erythema; hirsutism; necrotizing vasculitis; petechiae; purpura; rash; scarring; sterile abscess; striae; subcutaneous fat atrophy; thin, fragile skin; urticaria

Other: **Anaphylaxis**, **hypocalcemia**, **hypokalemia**, **hypokalemic alkalosis**, impaired wound healing, masking of signs of infection, **metabolic alkalosis**, **pheochromocytoma crisis** (in presence of pheochromocytoma), suppressed skin test reaction, weight gain

⋮ Childbearing Considerations

PREGNANCY

- Drug has the potential to cause fetal harm, as it does cross the placental barrier.
- Infants born of mothers who have received substantial doses of corticosteroids during pregnancy must be observed for signs of adrenal insufficiency. Cataracts have also been observed in mothers undergoing long-term treatment with corticosteroids during pregnancy.
- Use with caution only if benefit to mother outweighs potential risk to fetus.

LACTATION

- Drug is present in breast milk and could suppress infant growth.
- Patient should check with prescriber before breastfeeding.

REPRODUCTION

- Drug may alter male fertility.

⋮ Nursing Considerations

- Know that systemic hydrocortisone shouldn't be given to immunocompromised patients, such as those with fungal and other infections, including amebiasis, hepatitis B, tuberculosis, vaccinia, and varicella.
- Be aware that high-dose therapy shouldn't be given for longer than 48 hours. Be alert for depression and psychotic episodes.
- Monitor blood pressure, electrolyte levels, and weight regularly during therapy.
- Expect hydrocortisone to worsen infections or mask signs and symptoms.
- Monitor blood glucose level in diabetic patients, and increase insulin or oral antidiabetic drug dosage, as prescribed.

- Know that elderly patients are at high risk for osteoporosis during long-term therapy.
- Anticipate the possibility of acute adrenal insufficiency with stress, such as emotional upset, fever, surgery, or trauma. Increase hydrocortisone dosage, as prescribed.

! **WARNING** Avoid withdrawing drug suddenly after long-term therapy, because adrenal crisis can result. Expect to reduce dosage gradually and monitor response.

PATIENT TEACHING

- Advise patient to take daily dose of hydrocortisone in morning.
- Instruct patient to take tablets with food or milk.
- Instruct patient or caregiver how to use Alkindi sprinkles, if prescribed.
- Teach patient how to use enema or foam, if prescribed.
- Caution patient not to stop drug abruptly without first consulting prescriber.
- Instruct patient to report early evidence of adrenal insufficiency: anorexia, difficulty breathing, dizziness, fainting, fatigue, joint pain, muscle weakness, and nausea.
- Inform patient that he may bruise easily.
- Advise patient on long-term therapy to have periodic eye examinations.
- If patient receives long-term therapy, urge him to carry or wear medical identification.
- Caution patient to avoid people with infections because drug can suppress immune system, increasing risk of infection. If patient comes into contact with chickenpox or measles, instruct him to call prescriber because he may need prophylactic care.

hydromorphone hydrochloride
(dihydromorphinone)
Dilaudid

⋮ Class, Category, and Schedule

Pharmacologic class: Opioid
Therapeutic class: Opioid analgesic
Controlled substance schedule: II

≣ Indications and Dosages

✳ *To relieve pain severe enough to require opioid treatment and for which alternative treatment options such as nonopioid analgesics or opioid combination products are inadequate or not tolerated*

ORAL SOLUTION (DILAUDID)

Adults. 2.5 to 10 mg every 3 to 6 hr, as needed.

TABLETS (DILAUDID)

Adults. 2 to 4 mg every 4 to 6 hr, as needed.

I.V. INJECTION (DILAUDID)

Adults. 0.2 to 1 mg every 2 to 3 hr, as needed.

I.M. OR SUBCUTANEOUS INJECTION (DILAUDID)

Adults. 1 or 2 mg every 2 to 3 hr, as needed.

SUPPOSITORIES (DILAUDID)

Adults. 3 mg every 6 to 8 hr, as needed.

± **DOSAGE ADJUSTMENT** For patients with hepatic or renal impairment, initial dosage is given at 25 to 50% of normal dosage. For debilitated or elderly patients, I.V. dosage kept at 0.2 mg.

✳ *To treat moderate to severe pain for opioid-tolerant patients who require higher doses of opioids*

I.M., I.V., OR SUBCUTANEOUS INJECTION (DILAUDID-HP)

Adults who are not opioid naïve. Highly individualized and dependent on patient's previous total daily 24-hour opioid use. *Usual for I.M. or subcutaneous injection:* 1 to 2 mg every 2 to 3 hr, as needed, with dosage adjusted according to clinical response. *Usual for I.V. injection:* 0.2 to 1 mg every 2 to 3 hr, depending on dose.

± **DOSAGE ADJUSTMENT** For debilitated or elderly patient, I.V. injection initial dosage may be kept at 0.2 mg.

✳ *To manage moderate to severe pain in opioid-tolerant patients requiring continuous, around-the-clock opioid analgesia for an extended period of time and for which alternative treatment options are inadequate*

E.R. TABLETS

Adults. Highly individualized and dependent on patient's previous total 24-hour opioid use and risk factors for abuse, addiction, and misuse. Once dosage is determined, drug is given once daily. Dosage may be increased by 4 to 8 mg every 3 to 4 days, as needed.

± **DOSAGE ADJUSTMENT** For patients with hepatic or renal impairment, dosage started at 25% of normal dosage for moderate hepatic impairment or for severe renal impairment if extended-release tablets are used. Dosage started at 50% of normal dosage for moderate renal impairment.

≣ Drug Administration

- Administer before pain becomes intense.
- Have naloxone readily available.

P.O.

- Use a calibrated device when measuring oral solution dosage.
- Tablets should be swallowed whole and not chewed, crushed, or split.
- Administer with food if GI upset occurs.

I.V.

- Inspect solution. A slight yellowish discoloration may develop in ampuls but potency is not affected.
- The prefilled syringe does not have to be diluted before administration.
- Administer as an injection slowly over at least 2 to 3 minutes.
- *Incompatibilities:* None listed by manufacturer

I.M.

- Do not dilute drug in a prefilled syringe before administration.
- Rotate sites.

SUBCUTANEOUS

- Do not dilute drug in a prefilled syringe before administration.
- Rotate sites.

P.R.

- Keep suppositories in refrigerator until ready to administer.

Route	Onset	Peak	Duration
P.O.	15–30 min	30–60 min	3–4 hr
P.O./E.R.	6 hr	12–16 hr	13 hr
I.V.	5 min	10–20 min	3–4 hr
I.M.	15 min	30–60 min	4–5 hr
SubQ	15 min	30–90 min	4 hr

Half-life: 2–3 hr; 11 hr E.R.

≣ Mechanism of Action

May bind with opioid receptors in the spinal cord and higher levels in the CNS. In this way, hydromorphone is believed to stimulate kappa and mu receptors, thus altering the perception of and emotional response to pain.

Contraindications

Acute asthma (in an unmonitored setting or in the absence of resuscitative equipment); history of narrowing of the GI tract or presence of blind loops in the GI tract, or GI obstruction, including paralytic ileus; hypersensitivity to hydromorphone, hydromorphone salts, sulfite-containing drugs, or their components; opioid nontolerant patients (Dilaudid-HP, Exalgo); paralytic ileus; severe respiratory depression

Interactions

DRUGS

5-HT3 receptor antagonists, drugs that affect the serotonin neurotransmitter system (mirtazapine, trazodone, tramadol), linezolid, methylene blue (I.V.), selective serotonin reuptake inhibitors, serotonin and norepinephrine reuptake inhibitors, tricyclic antidepressants, triptans, tryptophan: Increased risk of serotonin syndrome
anticholinergics: Increased risk of ileus, severe constipation, or urine retention
anxiolytics, antipsychotics, benzodiazepines and other CNS depressants, general anesthetics, muscle relaxants, other opioids and sedative/hypnotics, sedating antihistamines, tranquilizers, tricyclic antidepressants: Increased risk of coma, hypotension, profound sedation, and severe respiratory depression
diuretics: Reduced effects of diuretics
mixed agonist/antagonist, partial agonist opioid analgesics such as buprenorphine, butorphanol, nalbuphine, pentazocine: Possibly reduced analgesic effect of hydromorphone; may precipitate withdrawal symptoms
MAO inhibitors: Increased risk of serotonin toxicity; increased risk of opioid toxicity
muscle relaxants: Possibly enhanced neuromuscular blocking action of skeletal muscle relaxants producing increased degree of respiratory depression

ACTIVITIES

alcohol use: Increased CNS and respiratory depression, which may become severe

Adverse Reactions

CNS: Anxiety, **CNS depression,** confusion, dizziness, drowsiness, euphoria, hallucinations, headache, nervousness, restlessness, sedation, somnolence, tremor, weakness
CV: Hypertension, orthostatic hypotension, palpitations, tachycardia
EENT: Blurred vision, diplopia, dry mouth, **laryngeal edema, laryngeal spasms,** nystagmus, tinnitus
ENDO: Adrenal insufficiency
GI: Abdominal cramps, anorexia, biliary tract spasm, constipation, **hepatotoxicity,** nausea, vomiting
GU: Decreased libido, dysuria, erectile dysfunction, impotence, infertility, lack of menstruation, urine retention
RESP: Dyspnea, **respiratory depression,** wheezing
SKIN: Diaphoresis, flushing
Other: Injection-site pain, redness, and swelling; physical and psychological dependence

Childbearing Considerations

PREGNANCY

- Drug may cause fetal harm.
- Prolonged use of drug during pregnancy can result in neonatal opioid withdrawal syndrome (NOWS), which may be life-threatening if not recognized and treated.
- Avoid prolonged use during pregnancy. Use with caution only if benefit to mother outweighs potential risk to fetus.

LABOR & DELIVERY

- Drug is not recommended for use in pregnant women immediately before or during labor. Opioids may alter length of time of labor.
- Opioids cross the placental barrier and may produce respiratory depression and psycho-physiologic effects in the newborn. Monitor newborn closely for signs of excess sedation and respiratory depression.
- An opioid antagonist, such as naloxone, must be available at the time of delivery in the event it is needed to reverse opioid-induced respiratory depression in the neonate.

LACTATION

- Drug is present in breast milk.
- Patient should check with prescriber before breastfeeding.
- If breastfeeding occurs, infant should be monitored for excess drowsiness and respiratory depression.

REPRODUCTION

- Chronic use of opioids may reduce fertility.

Nursing Considerations

- Be aware that hydromorphone therapy increases risk of abuse, addiction, and misuse. A Risk Evaluation and Mitigation Strategy (REMS) is required. Monitor patient closely throughout therapy for abuse, addiction, or misuse.
- Know that chronic maternal use of hydromorphone during pregnancy can result in neonatal opioid withdrawal syndrome (NOWS), which may be life-threatening, if not recognized and treated appropriately. NOWS occurs when a newborn has been exposed to opioid drugs for a prolonged period while in utero.
- Use extreme caution when administering hydromorphone to patients with cor pulmonale or significant chronic obstructive pulmonary disease, and in patients having a substantially decreased respiratory reserve, hypercapnia, hypoxia, or preexisting respiratory depression, especially when initiating and titrating therapy. These patients may develop respiratory depression, even with usual therapeutic doses, because hydromorphone may decrease the patient's respiratory drive to the point of apnea.
- Use hydromorphone cautiously in cachectic, debilitated, or elderly patients, especially when initiating and titrating therapy, as they are at increased risk for adverse effects, especially respiratory depression.
- Use hydromorphone cautiously in patients whose ability to maintain a normal blood pressure is already compromised by a reduced blood volume or concurrent administration of certain CNS depressant drugs; the drug may cause severe hypotension in these patients, especially when initiating or titrating the dose of hydromorphone.
- Be aware that hydromorphone should only be used concomitantly with benzodiazepines and other CNS depressants in patients for whom other treatment options are inadequate. If prescribed together, expect dosing and duration of hydromorphone to be limited. Monitor patient closely for signs and symptoms of decrease in consciousness, including coma, profound sedation, and significant respiratory depression. Notify prescriber immediately, expect drug to be discontinued, and provide emergency supportive care, as death may occur.

! **WARNING** Monitor patient for respiratory depression, especially within the first 72 hours of initiating therapy or when increasing dosage, even when the drug has been used as prescribed and not abused or misused. Patients who are especially vulnerable include the elderly and those who are cachectic or debilitated. Be aware that overestimating hydromorphone dose when converting patients from another opioid medication can result in fatal overdose with the first dose. To avoid this, know that it is recommended to underestimate a patient's 24-hour oral hydromorphone requirement and provide rescue medication, as needed, until the right dose is determined. Keep resuscitation equipment and naloxone nearby.

- Be aware that drug can cause sleep-related breathing disorders including central sleep apnea and sleep-related hypoxemia that may require a dosage decrease, if present.
- Monitor patient for coma, hypotension, profound sedation, or respiratory depression when administering hydromorphone around-the-clock; these reactions can occur if alcohol or illicit drugs are being used without the prescriber's knowledge.

! **WARNING** Know that many drugs may interact with opioids like hydromorphone to cause serotonin syndrome. Monitor patient closely for signs and symptoms such as agitation, diaphoresis, diarrhea, fever, hallucinations, labile blood pressure, muscle twitching or stiffness, nausea, shakiness, shivering, tachycardia, trouble with coordination, or vomiting. Notify prescriber at once because serotonin syndrome may be life-threatening. Be prepared to discontinue drug, if possible and ordered, and provide supportive care.

- Monitor patient for adrenal insufficiency. Although rare, it can be life-threatening. Monitor patient for anorexia, dizziness, fatigue, hypotension, nausea, vomiting, or weakness. Notify prescriber if adrenal insufficiency is suspected and expect to do diagnostic testing. If diagnosis is confirmed, expect to administer corticosteroids and wean patient off hydromorphone, if possible.

- Monitor patients with seizure disorders because hydromorphone therapy may aggravate or induce convulsions.
- Monitor effectiveness of hydromorphone in relieving pain; consult prescriber as needed.
- Assess patient for constipation.
- Monitor patient for evidence of physical abuse or dependence. Be aware that excessive use of opioids such as hydromorphone may lead to abuse, addiction, misuse, overdose, and possibly death. Monitor patient's intake of drug closely.
- Anticipate that drug may mask or worsen gallbladder pain.
- Be aware that all other around-the-clock opioid analgesics should be stopped when E.R. tablets are prescribed. Expect to give immediate-release nonopioid analgesics for exacerbation of pain and for preventing pain during certain activities.
- Know that E.R. tablets may be visible on abdominal X-rays under certain circumstances, especially when digital enhancing techniques are utilized, because the tablet is nondeformable and does not change much in shape in the GI tract.
- Expect to taper dosages of hydromorphone that have been administered for an extended period of time to the opioid-tolerant patient gradually by 25 to 50% every 2 to 3 days, down to a dose of 8 mg before the drug is discontinued. This will help prevent signs and symptoms of withdrawal.

PATIENT TEACHING

- Instruct patient to take drug exactly as prescribed and before pain is severe. Also, tell her not to take more drug than prescribed and not to take it longer than absolutely needed, because excessive or prolonged use can lead to abuse, addiction, misuse, overdose, and possibly death.
- Alert patient that drug is a controlled substance. She should take steps to protect drug from theft.
- Advise patient to take drug with food to avoid GI distress.
- Tell patient not to break, chew, crush, or dissolve tablets, but to swallow them whole.

- Instruct family/caregiver on use of naloxone and importance of having drug available in case of an overdose.
- Inform patient about potentially fatal additive effects of combining hydromorphone with a benzodiazepine. In addition, other serious drug reactions can occur. Instruct patient to inform all prescribers of hydromorphone use.
- Caution patient to avoid alcohol and OTC drugs during therapy, unless prescriber approves.
- Instruct patient to report constipation, difficulty breathing, severe nausea, or vomiting.
- Inform patient that drug may cause drowsiness and sedation. Advise her to avoid hazardous activities until drug's CNS effects are known.
- Tell patient to change position slowly to minimize orthostatic hypotension.
- Instruct physically dependent patient not to stop taking hydromorphone abruptly, to avoid withdrawal.
- Warn patient to keep drug out of reach of children, as accidental ingestion may cause death.
- Advise women of childbearing age to notify prescriber immediately if they suspect they are pregnant or become pregnant.
- Advise patients when hydromorphone tablets or solution are no longer needed to remit to authorities at a certified drug take-back program.
- Inform patient that long-term use of opioids like hydromorphone may decrease sex hormone levels, causing decreased libido, erectile dysfunction, impotence, infertility, or lack of menstruation. Encourage patient to report any such symptoms.

hydroxychloroquine sulfate

Plaquenil

Class and Category

Pharmacologic class: Aminoquinoline
Therapeutic class: Antimalarial, antirheumatic, lupus erythematosus suppressant

Indications and Dosages

* *To prevent malaria*

TABLETS

Adults. 400 mg the same day of each week starting 2 wk before entering endemic area and continued for 4 wk after departure from endemic area.

Children weighing 31 kg (68.2 lb) or more. 6.5 mg/kg weekly on the same day of each week, starting 2 wk before entering endemic area and continued for 4 wk after departure from endemic area. *Maximum:* 400 mg once weekly.

* *To treat uncomplicated malaria caused by* Plasmodium falciparum, P. malariae, P. ovale, *or P. vivax*

TABLETS

Adults. *Initial:* 800 mg, followed by 400 mg in 6 hr, 24 hr, and 48 hr after initial dose.

Children weighing 31 kg (68.2 lb) or more. *Initial:* 13 mg/kg (up to 800 mg), then 6.5 mg/kg (up to 400 mg) at 6 hr, 24 hr, and 48 hr after initial dose.

* *To treat chronic discoid and systemic lupus erythematosus*

TABLETS

Adults. 200 mg once daily or 400 mg once daily or in 2 divided doses. *Maximum:* 400 mg daily.

* *To treat acute or chronic rheumatoid arthritis*

TABLETS

Adults. *Initial:* 400 to 600 mg daily as a single dose or in 2 divided doses. Following a good response, dosage reduced by 50%. *Maintenance:* 200 mg once daily or 400 mg daily as a single dose or in 2 divided doses.

±**DOSAGE ADJUSTMENT** For patients with hepatic or renal disease or for patients who are taking medications known to affect these organs, dosage may have to be reduced.

Drug Administration

P.O.

- Administer with a meal or a glass of milk.
- Tablets should not be chewed, crushed, or split.

Route	Onset	Peak	Duration
P.O.	Unknown	3–4 hr	Unknown

Half-life: 40–50 days

Mechanism of Action

May mildly suppress the immune system, inhibiting production of rheumatoid factor and acute phase reactants. Hydroxychloroquine accumulates in WBCs, stabilizing lysosomal membranes and inhibiting enzymes such as collagenase and proteases that cause cartilage breakdown. These actions may decrease symptoms of rheumatoid arthritis and lupus erythematosus. Hydroxychloroquine also binds to and alters DNA of malaria parasite to prevent it from reproducing. It also may increase the pH of acid vesicles, which interferes with vesicle function and may inhibit parasitic phospholipid metabolism in erythrocytes, thereby halting plasmodial activity.

Contraindications

Hypersensitivity to hydroxychloroquine, other 4-aminoquinoline compounds, or their components

Interactions

DRUGS

ampicillin: Possibly significant decrease in bioavailability of ampicillin, decreasing its effectiveness

antacids, kaolin: Possibly reduced absorption of hydroxychloroquine

antidiabetic drugs, insulin: Possibly increased risk of hypoglycemia

antiepileptics, mefloquine, other drugs that lower seizure threshold: Increased risk of seizures

cimetidine: Possibly increased plasma hydroxychloroquine levels

cyclosporin: Increased plasma cyclosporin levels

digoxin: Increased digoxin concentrations

drugs that prolong QT interval, including other arrhythmogenic drugs: Increased risk of arrhythmias

hepatotoxic or nephrotoxic drugs: Possibly increased risk of kidney or liver toxicity

methotrexate: Possibly increased risk of adverse reactions

praziquantel: Possibly reduced bioavailability of praziquantel affecting its effectiveness

Adverse Reactions

CNS: Abnormal nerve conduction, ataxia, dizziness, emotional lability, fatigue, extrapyramidal disorders, headache, irritability, lassitude, nervousness, neuromuscular sensory abnormalities, nightmares, psychosis, **seizures, suicidal ideation,** vertigo

CV: Atrioventricular blocks, bundle branch block, **cardiac failure, cardiomyopathy** (prolonged high doses), **prolonged QT interval, sick sinus syndrome, torsades de pointes, ventricular arrhythmias**

EENT: Abnormal pigmentation (bullseye appearance) or colored vision, blurred vision, central scotoma with decreased visual acuity, corneal deposits or edema, decreased corneal sensitivity, decreased dark adaptation, diplopia, irreversible retinal damage, halo vision, lassitude, macular atrophy or edema, macular degeneration, nerve-related hearing loss, nystagmus, paracentral or pericentral scotoma, photophobia, retinal fundus changes, retinopathy, sensorineural hearing loss, tinnitus, visual abnormalities including visual fields

ENDO: Hypoglycemia

GI: Abdominal cramps or pain, **acute or fulminant hepatic failure,** anorexia, diarrhea, elevated liver enzymes, nausea, vomiting

HEME: Agranulocytosis, anemia, **aplastic anemia, bone marrow depression, hemolysis** (in patients with glucose-6 phosphate dehydrogenase [G6PD] deficiency), **leukopenia,** porphyria, **thrombocytopenia**

MS: Atrophy of proximal skeletal muscle groups, depressed tendon reflexes, muscle weakness, myopathy

RESP: Bronchospasm, pulmonary hypertension

SKIN: Acute generalized exanthematous pustulosis, alopecia, altered mucosal and skin pigmentation, bleaching of hair, dermatitis (including bullous and **exfoliative dermatitis**), **erythema multiforme,** hyperpigmentation, non-light-sensitive psoriasis, photosensitivity, pruritus, psoriasis exacerbation, rash, **Stevens–Johnson syndrome, toxic epidermal necrolysis,** urticaria

Other: Angioedema, drug reaction with eosinophilia and systemic symptoms (DRESS), porphyria including worsening, weight loss

Childbearing Considerations
PREGNANCY
- Pregnancy exposure registry: 1-877-311-8972.
- It is not known if drug may cause fetal harm.
- Use with caution only if benefit to mother outweighs potential risk to fetus.

LACTATION
- Drug is present in breast milk.
- Patient should check with prescriber before breastfeeding.

Nursing Considerations
- Use hydroxychloroquine cautiously in patients with G6PD deficiency, patients with alcoholism or hepatic or renal disease, and patients taking hepatotoxic drugs. Also use cautiously in patients with blood, gastrointestinal, or neurological disorders and in patients who are sensitive to quinine.
- Monitor children closely for adverse reactions because they're especially sensitive to 4-aminoquinoline compounds.
- Observe patients with psoriasis closely because hydroxychloroquine may lead to severe psoriasis attack. Also monitor patients with porphyria closely because hydroxychloroquine may worsen it. Expect to use hydroxychloroquine in patients with porphyria or psoriasis only after risks and benefits have been considered.
- Obtain periodic blood cell counts, as ordered, during prolonged therapy to detect adverse hematologic effects. Expect to stop drug if severe adverse effects occur.
- Monitor patient's vision when giving hydroxychloroquine, because irreversible retinal damage may occur in some patients during high-dose or long-term therapy. Ask regularly about vision abnormalities, such as light flashes or streaks that may indicate retinopathy. Expect patient to have an initial ophthalmologic examination, followed by examinations every 3 months. Be aware that in patients of Asian descent, retinal toxicity may first be noticed outside the macula. Report changes to prescriber immediately, and expect drug to be stopped. Retinal changes may progress even after therapy stops.
- Monitor patient on long-term therapy for muscle weakness and abnormal ankle and knee reflexes. If present, notify prescriber and expect drug to be stopped.
- Expect drug to be stopped if patient with rheumatoid arthritis shows no

improvement, such as reduced joint swelling or increased mobility, in 6 months.
- Notify prescriber immediately if serious adverse reactions occur. Expect drug to be stopped. Also expect to give ammonium chloride (8 g daily in divided doses for adults) 3 or 4 days weekly for several months because acidification of urine increases renal excretion of drug.

! **WARNING** Be aware that drug has not been approved for use by the FDA to treat the COVID-19 virus.

PATIENT TEACHING
- Instruct patient to take drug with meals or milk to minimize stomach upset.
- Tell patient to take hydroxychloroquine exactly as prescribed because taking too much may cause serious adverse reactions and taking too little or skipping doses decreases effectiveness.
- Caution patient to notify prescriber about troublesome adverse reactions. Hydroxychloroquine dosage may have to be adjusted or drug stopped.
- Caution patient about possible visual reactions and the need for periodic eye examinations. Tell patient to notify prescriber about abnormal visual changes, including blurred vision, halos around lights, and light flashes or streaks; explain that drug will have to be stopped.
- Tell patient receiving prolonged therapy about the need for periodic blood tests to detect adverse effects.
- Advise patient to notify prescriber if muscle weakness develops.
- Review early signs and symptoms of toxicity. Tell patient to notify prescriber immediately, if present.
- Inform mothers wishing to breastfeed to discuss breastfeeding with prescriber before doing so.
- Warn patient to keep drug out of reach of children, as fatalities have occurred when drug has been accidentally ingested, even in small amounts.

! **WARNING** Inform patients that drug has not been approved by the FDA for treatment of COVID-19 virus.

---

hydroxyzine hydrochloride
Atarax (CAN)

hydroxyzine pamoate
Vistaril

Class and Category
Pharmacologic class: Piperazine derivative
Therapeutic class: Anxiolytic, antiemetic, antihistamine, sedative-hypnotic

Indications and Dosages
✴ *To relieve anxiety and tension associated with psychoneurosis; adjunct in organic disease states in which anxiety is manifested*

CAPSULES, ORAL SUSPENSION, SYRUP, TABLETS
Adults. 50 to 100 mg four times daily.
Children age 6 and over. 50 to 100 mg daily in divided doses.
Children under 6 years of age. 50 mg daily in divided doses.

I.M. INJECTION
Adults. 50 to 100 mg every 4 to 6 hr, as needed.

✴ *To treat pruritus due to allergic conditions*

CAPSULES, ORAL SUSPENSION, SYRUP, TABLETS
Adults. 25 mg three times daily or four times daily, as needed.
Children age 6 and over. 50 to 100 mg daily in divided doses.
Children under 6 years of age. 50 mg daily in divided doses.

✴ *To treat nausea and vomiting excluding nausea and vomiting of pregnancy*

I.M. INJECTION
Adults. 25 to 100 mg.
Children. 0.5 mg/kg dose.

✴ *As a sedative when used as premedication and following general anesthesia*

CAPSULES, ORAL SUSPENSION, SYRUP, TABLETS
Adults. 50 to 100 mg.
Children. 0.6 mg/kg.

I.M. INJECTION
Adults. 25 to 100 mg.
Children. 0.5 mg/kg dose.
±**DOSAGE ADJUSTMENT** For elderly patients, treatment is started at lowest possible dosage.

⬚ Drug Administration
P.O.
- Capsules and tablets should be swallowed whole and not chewed, crushed, or split/opened.
- Use a calibrated device when measuring oral suspension or syrup, to ensure an accurate dose.
- Shake suspension well before measuring dose.

I.M.
- Do not dilute before administration.
- Never administer intra-arterially, I.V., or subcutaneously.
- Aspirate carefully before pushing plunger to avoid an inadvertent I.V. injection.
- Inject deeply into a large muscle (preferred sites are the gluteus maximus or mid-lateral thigh for adults; mid-lateral thigh for children) using the Z-track method.

Route	Onset	Peak	Duration
P.O.	15–60 min	2 hr	4–6 hr
I.M.	Rapid	Unknown	4–6 hr

Half-life: 20 hr

⬚ Mechanism of Action
Competes with histamine for histamine$_1$ receptor sites on surfaces of effector cells. This suppresses results of histaminic activity, including edema, flare, and pruritus. Sedative actions occur at subcortical level of CNS and are dose related.

⬚ Contraindications
Early pregnancy; hypersensitivity to cetirizine, hydroxyzine, levocetirizine or their components; prolonged QT interval

⬚ Interactions
DRUGS
antibiotics such as azithromycin, erythromycin, clarithromycin, gatifloxacin, or moxifloxacin; antidepressants such as citalopram or fluoxetine; antipsychotics such as chlorpromazine, clozapine, iloperidone, quetiapine, or ziprasidone; class IA antiarrhythmics such as procainamide or quinidine; class III antiarrhythmics such as amiodarone or sotalol; droperidol; methadone; ondansetron; pentamidine: Increased risk of QT prolongation
CNS depressants: Increased CNS depression

ACTIVITIES
alcohol use: Increased CNS depression

⬚ Adverse Reactions
CNS: Drowsiness, hallucinations, headache, involuntary motor activity, **seizures**, tremor
CV: Prolonged QT interval, torsades de pointes
EENT: Dry mouth
SKIN: Fixed drug eruptions, pruritus, rash, urticaria
Other: Hypersensitivity reactions, injection-site pain

⬚ Childbearing Considerations
PREGNANCY
- Drug may cause fetal harm.
- Drug is contraindicated in early pregnancy.

LACTATION
- It is not known if drug is present in breast milk.
- Breastfeeding should not be undertaken during drug therapy.

⬚ Nursing Considerations
- Use hydroxyzine cautiously in patients with risk factors for QT prolongation such as concomitant arrhythmogenic drug use, electrolyte imbalance, or preexisting heart disease. Also use cautiously in patients with bradyarrhythmias, congenital or family history of long QT syndrome, other conditions that predispose patient to QT prolongation and ventricular arrhythmia, recent MI, or uncompensated heart failure.
- Observe for oversedation if patient takes another CNS depressant.

PATIENT TEACHING
- Tell patient capsules and tablets should be swallowed whole and not chewed, crushed, or split/opened.
- Tell patient to shake suspension well before measuring dose.
- Instruct patient to use a calibrated device, not a household spoon, when measuring oral suspension or syrup, to ensure an accurate dose.
- Urge patient to avoid alcohol.

- Caution patient about drowsiness; tell her to avoid hazardous activities until drug's CNS effects are known.
- Instruct woman to tell prescriber if she is or could be pregnant because drug is contraindicated in early pregnancy. Breastfeeding is not recommended during therapy.

ibalizumab-uiyk
Trogarzo

Class and Category
Pharmacologic class: CD4-directed post-attachment HIV-1 inhibitor
Therapeutic class: Antiretroviral

Indications and Dosages
* *As adjunct to treat human immunodeficiency virus (HIV) type 1 infection in heavily treatment-experienced patients with multidrug-resistant HIV-1 infection who are failing their current antiretroviral regimen*

I.V. INFUSION
Adults. *Loading:* 2,000 mg followed by 800 mg 2 wk later. *Maintenance:* 800 mg every 2 wk.

Drug Administration
I.V.
- Use 10 vials to prepare the loading dose of 2,000 mg and 4 vials to prepare each maintenance dose of 800 mg.
- To prepare, insert sterile syringe needle into each vial through center of stopper, withdraw 1.33 ml of drug, and transfer into a 250-ml intravenous bag of 0.9% Sodium Chloride Injection. Do not use any other diluent solutions.
- Once diluted, administer immediately or store at room temperature for up to 4 hours or refrigerated for up to 24 hours. If refrigerated, allow diluted drug solution to stand at room temperature for at least 30 minutes but no more than 4 hours prior to administration.
- Administer infusion in the cephalic vein of patient's left or right arm. If this vein is not accessible, know that an appropriate vein located elsewhere can be used.
- Never administer drug as an I.V. bolus or I.V. push.
- Infuse loading dose over at least 30 minutes or more. Observe patient for 1 hour after loading-dose infusion is complete. If no infusion-associated adverse reactions occur, time of observation can be decreased to 15 minutes for subsequent maintenance infusions.
- After infusion is complete, flush intravenous line with 30 ml of 0.9% Sodium Chloride Injection.
- If a maintenance dose is missed by 3 days or longer beyond the scheduled dosing day, a loading dose of 2,000 mg should be administered as early as possible and the maintenance dosing of 800 mg resumed 2 weeks later.

Route	Onset	Peak	Duration
I.V.	Unknown	Unknown	Unknown

Half-life: 2.7–64 hr (dose dependent)

Mechanism of Action
Blocks HIV-1 from infecting CD4 T cells by binding to domain 2 of CD4 and interfering with post-attachment steps required for entry of HIV-1 virus particles into host cells. Also prevents the viral transmission that occurs via cell–cell infusion.

Contraindications
Hypersensitivity to ibalizumab-uiyk or its components

Interactions
DRUGS
None reported by manufacturer

Adverse Reactions
CNS: Dizziness
ENDO: Hyperglycemia
GI: Diarrhea, elevated bilirubin and lipase levels, nausea
GU: Elevated creatinine level
HEME: Anemia, decreased platelet count, leukopenia, neutropenia
SKIN: Pruritus, rash
Other: Antibody formation to ibalizumab-uiyk, elevated uric acid level, hypersensitivity reactions (anaphylaxis, angioedema, chest pain or tightness, cough, dyspnea, hot flush, nausea, vomiting), immune reconstitution inflammatory syndrome, infusion reactions

⊟ Childbearing Considerations
PREGNANCY

- Pregnancy exposure registry: 1-800-258-4263.
- Drug may cause fetal harm based on animal studies because drug does cross placental barrier increasingly as pregnancy progresses and may cause reversible immunosuppression in infants exposed to drug in utero.
- Use with caution only if benefit to mother outweighs potential risk to fetus.

LACTATION

- It is not known if drug is present in breast milk.
- The Centers for Disease Control and Prevention recommends that HIV-1 infected mothers not breastfeed to avoid risking postnatal transmission of HIV-1 infection to infants. They also do not recommend breastfeeding because of potential drug-induced adverse reactions in the infant.

⊟ Nursing Considerations

! WARNING Monitor patient for hypersensitivity reactions such as anaphylaxis, angioedema, chest pain or tightness, cough, dyspnea, hot flush, nausea, vomiting). If present, notify prescriber, as drug must be discontinued, and initiate appropriate emergency treatment.

- Monitor patient for signs and symptoms of infection, which could be caused by immune reconstitution inflammatory syndrome. Although rare, this syndrome may occur in combination with other antiretroviral therapy in patients whose immune systems respond during the initial phase causing an inflammatory reaction to indolent or residual opportunistic infections. If present, further evaluation and treatment will be needed.
- Know that the safety of administering live or live-attenuated vaccines in infants exposed to drug in utero is unknown.

PATIENT TEACHING

- Stress importance of compliance with dosage schedule of every 2 weeks. Remind patient that if dose is missed for 3 days or longer, a loading dosage will have to be repeated before maintenance dosing can be reestablished.

! WARNING Alert patient to possibility of an allergic reaction that could be severe. If an allergic reaction occurs, tell patient to seek immediate emergency treatment.

- Instruct patient to immediately report any signs and symptoms of an infection to prescriber.
- Advise mothers not to breastfeed their infant while receiving ibalizumab-uiyk and to alert pediatrician if she received drug during her pregnancy.

ibandronate sodium
Boniva

⊟ Class and Category
Pharmacologic class: Bisphosphonate
Therapeutic class: Antiosteoporotic

⊟ Indications and Dosages
✴ *To prevent osteoporosis in postmenopausal women*

TABLETS
Adult women. 150 mg once monthly.

✴ *To treat osteoporosis in postmenopausal women*

TABLETS
Adult women. 150 mg once monthly.

I.V. INJECTION
Adults. 3 mg every 3 mo.

⊟ Drug Administration
P.O.

- Tablet should be swallowed whole and not chewed, crushed, split, or sucked on.
- Administer with 6 to 8 ounces of plain water, at least 60 minutes before the first food, beverage, or medication of the day.
- Ensure that patient does not lie down for at least 60 minutes after drug is administered.
- Do not administer with any other medication and ensure that patient does not drink anything except water for 60 minutes after drug is administered.
- Administer tablets same day of each month.

I.V.

- Administer undiluted over 15 to 30 seconds as an I.V. injection using the prefilled syringe and needle supplied by manufacturer.

G
H
I

- Take care not to administer drug intra-arterially or paravenously, as this can lead to tissue damage.
- Do not administer by I.M. or subcutaneously.
- Administer a missed dose as soon as possible when realized and schedule future doses from that date, not the original date.
- *Incompatibilities:* Calcium-containing solutions or other I.V. drugs

Route	Onset	Peak	Duration
P.O.	Unknown	0.5–2 hr	Unknown
I.V.	Rapid	Unknown	Unknown

Half-life: 4.5–25.5 hr

Mechanism of Action

Based on its affinity for hydroxyapatite, which is part of the mineral matrix of bone, osteoclast activity is inhibited and bone resorption and turnover are reduced. In postmenopausal women, the elevated rate of bone turnover is reduced leading to, on average, a net gain in bone mass.

Contraindications

Esophageal abnormalities that delay esophageal emptying, such as achalasia or stricture (oral form); hypersensitivity to ibandronate or its components; inability to stand or sit upright for at least 60 minutes (oral form); uncorrected hypocalcemia

Interactions

DRUGS

aspirin, NSAIDs: Increased risk of GI irritation
products containing calcium and other multivalent cations such as aluminum, magnesium, iron: Impaired absorption of ibandronate

FOODS

all foods: Decreased ibandronate bioavailability

Adverse Reactions

CNS: Asthenia, depression, dizziness, fatigue, headache, insomnia, nerve root lesion, vertigo
CV: Hypercholesterolemia, hypertension
EENT: Nasopharyngitis, pharyngitis, tooth disorder
GI: Abdominal pain, constipation, diarrhea, dyspepsia, gastritis, gastroenteritis, nausea, vomiting

GU: Cystitis, UTI
MS: Arthralgia; arthritis; atypical subtrochanteric and diaphyseal femoral fractures; back, bone, extremity, joint, or muscle pain; joint disorder; localized osteoarthritis; myalgia; osteonecrosis of jaw and other orofacial sites
RESP: Asthma exacerbations, bronchitis, bronchospasm, pneumonia, upper respiratory infection
SKIN: Dermatitis bullous, erythema multiforme, rash, Stevens–Johnson syndrome
Other: Anaphylaxis, angioedema, flu-like symptoms, hypersensitivity reactions, hypocalcemia, infection, injection-site reactions such as redness or swelling

Childbearing Considerations

PREGNANCY

- It is not known if drug causes fetal harm.
- Drug is not indicated for use in women of reproductive potential.

LACTATION

- It is not known if drug is present in breast milk.
- Drug is not indicated for use in women of reproductive potential.

Nursing Considerations

- Be aware that hypocalcemia, hypovitaminosis D, and other disturbances of bone and mineral metabolism must be effectively treated before starting ibandronate therapy.
- Know that ibandronate should not be administered to patients with severe renal impairment or to women who are not postmenopausal.
- Use cautiously in patients with active upper gastrointestinal problems (such as known Barrett's esophagus, dysphagia, other esophageal diseases, duodenitis, gastritis, ulcers), because drug may cause local irritation of the upper gastrointestinal mucosa.
- Make sure patient has had a dental checkup before having invasive dental procedures during ibandronate therapy, especially if patient has cancer; is receiving chemotherapy, head or neck radiation, or a corticosteroid; or has poor oral hygiene, because the risk of jaw osteonecrosis has increased in these patients taking other

bisphosphonates, a class of drugs of which ibandronate is a member.

- Obtain serum creatinine level in patients receiving injection form of ibandronate prior to administering each dose because other bisphosphonates have been associated with serious renal toxicity. If renal deterioration occurs, expect drug to be withheld.

PATIENT TEACHING

- Instruct patient prescribed oral ibandronate to take the tablet at least 1 hour before first food or drink of day (except water) while in an upright position and with 6 to 8 oz of water. Caution against lying down for at least 60 minutes after taking drug to keep it from lodging in esophagus and causing irritation. Also instruct patient not to chew or suck on tablet because doing so may irritate mouth or throat.
- Inform patient of need and importance of taking supplemental calcium and vitamin D on daily basis.
- Instruct patient to take calcium supplements at least 2 hours before or after oral ibandronate.
- Advise patient to stop taking drug and to notify prescriber if GI symptoms appear or become worse.
- Alert patient that drugs in the same class as ibandronate have caused severe bone, joint, or muscle pain. If such symptoms appear while taking ibandronate, advise patient to contact prescriber. Also, tell him to report new or worsening groin or thigh pain.
- Tell patient to stop taking drug and notify prescriber if he develops dysphagia, pain while swallowing, retrosternal pain, or new or worsening heartburn.
- Instruct patient on proper oral hygiene and on the need to notify prescriber about invasive dental procedures because risk of developing osteonecrosis of the jaw decreases in the absence of bisphosphonate therapy.

ibrexafungerp
Brexafemme

≡ Class and Category

Pharmacologic class: Triterpenoid antifungal
Therapeutic class: Azole antifungal

≡ Indications and Dosages

✳ *To treat vulvovaginal candidiasis*

TABLETS

Adult females and postmenarchal pediatric females. 300 mg (two 150 mg tablets) given twice in one 24-hr period. *Maximum:* 600 mg in one 24-hr period.

±**DOSAGE ADJUSTMENT** For patients taking a strong CYP3A inhibitor, dosage decreased to 150 mg and given twice in one 24-hr period.

≡ Drug Administration

P.O.

- Verify pregnancy status prior to administering drug.
- Administer the two doses of drug about 12 hrs apart, preferably in the morning and evening. However, if first dose is administered in the afternoon or evening, the second dose should be taken the following morning.

Route	Onset	Peak	Duration
P.O.	Unknown	4–6 hr	Unknown

Half-life: 20 hr

≡ Mechanism of Action

Inhibits glucan synthase, an essential component for the development of the fungal cell wall, causing fungicidal activity against *Candida* species.

≡ Contraindications

Hypersensitivity to ibrexafungerp or its components, pregnancy

≡ Interactions

DRUGS

CYP3A strong and moderate inducers such as bosentan, carbamazepine, efavirenz, etravirine, long-acting barbiturates, phenytoin, rifampin, St. John's wort: Possibly significant reduction in plasma concentration of ibrexafungerp, thereby reducing effectiveness

CYP3A strong inhibitors such as itraconazole, ketoconazole: Significantly increases plasma concentration of ibrexafungerp, which increases risk of adverse reactions

≡ Adverse Reactions

CNS: Dizziness

GI: Abdominal pain, diarrhea, elevated liver enzymes, flatulence, nausea, vomiting

G
H
I

GU: Dysmenorrhea, vaginal bleeding
MS: Back pain
SKIN: Rash
OTHER: Hypersensitivity reaction

Childbearing Considerations

PREGNANCY

- Pregnancy exposure registry: 888-982-7299.
- Drug may cause fetal harm based on animal studies.
- Drug is contraindicated in pregnancy.

LACTATION

- It is not known if drug is present in breast milk.
- Patient should check with prescriber before breastfeeding.

REPRODUCTION

- Pregnancy status must be determined and only if a negative result is found should drug be given.
- Women of childbearing age should use effective contraception during drug treatment and for 4 days after last dose.

NURSING CONSIDERATIONS

- Be aware that ibrexafungerp should not be given to premenarchal pediatric females.

! **WARNING** Monitor patient for hypersensitivity reaction. If present, notify prescriber and provide supportive care as needed and ordered.

PATIENT TEACHING

- Review with patient how tablets are to be taken. Tell patient a total treatment course is two doses (2 tablets each dose) to be taken about 12 hours apart either in the morning and evening or in the afternoon or evening with the second dose taken the following morning.
- Instruct patient that a pregnancy test will be required before drug can be given because drug may cause fetal harm.
- Advise patient to use effective contraception while taking drug and for 4 days after the last dose.
- Tell patient to inform prescriber if she is taking any other drugs, including over-the-counter drugs such as St. John's wort, before taking ibrexafungerp.

! **WARNING!** Instruct patient to notify prescriber if an allergic reaction occurs such as a rash.

ibuprofen
Actiprofen Caplets (CAN), Advil, Advil Migraine, Caldolor, Children's Advil, Children's Motrin, Excedrin, Motrin

ibuprofen lysine
NeoProfen

Class and Category
Pharmacologic class: NSAID
Therapeutic class: Analgesic, anti-inflammatory, antipyretic

Indications and Dosages

✳ *To relieve pain in rheumatoid arthritis and osteoarthritis*

CAPSULES, CHEWABLE TABLETS, ORAL SUSPENSION, TABLETS

Adults. 300 mg four times daily; or 400, 600, or 800 mg three times daily or four times daily. *Usual:* 1.2 to 3.2 g daily. *Maximum:* 3.2 g daily.

✳ *To relieve pain in juvenile arthritis*

CAPSULES, CHEWABLE TABLETS, ORAL SUSPENSION, TABLETS

Children ages 6 months and over. 20 to 40 mg/kg daily in 3 or 4 divided doses. *Maximum:* **50 mg/kg daily.**

✳ *To relieve mild to moderate pain*

CAPSULES, CHEWABLE TABLETS, ORAL SUSPENSION, TABLETS

Adults. 200 to 400 mg every 4 to 6 hr, as needed.
Children age 12 and older. 200 to 400 mg every 4 to 6 hr, as needed. *Maximum:* 1.2 g.

CHEWABLE TABLETS, ORAL SUSPENSION

Children age 11 weighing 33 kg (72 lb) to 43 kg (95 lb). 300 mg every 6 to 8 hr, as needed.
Children ages 9 and 10 weighing 27 kg (59 lb) to 32 kg (70 lb). 250 mg every 6 to 8 hr, as needed.
Children ages 6 to 8 weighing 22 kg (48 lb) to 27 kg (59 lb). 200 mg every 6 to 8 hr, as needed.
Children ages 4 and 5 weighing 16 kg (35 lb) to 21 kg (46 lb). 150 mg every 6 to 8 hrs, as needed.
Children ages 2 and 3 weighing 11 kg (24 lb) to 16 kg (35 lb). 100 mg every 6 to 8 hrs, as needed.

ORAL DROPS

Children ages 12 to 23 months weighing 8.18 kg (18 lb) to 10.45 kg (23 lb). 75 mg every 6 to 8 hrs, as needed.

Children ages 6 to 11 months weighing 5.45 kg (12 lb) to 7.73 kg (17 lb). 50 mg every 6 to 8 hrs, as needed.

I.V. INFUSION (CALDOLOR)

Adults. 400 to 800 mg every 6 hr, as needed. *Maximum:* 3,200 mg daily.

Adolescents. 400 mg every 4 to 6 hr, as needed. *Maximum:* 2,400 mg daily.

Children ages 6 months to 12 years. 10 mg/kg up to 400 mg maximum every 4 to 6 hr, as needed. *Maximum:* 40 mg/kg or 2,400 mg daily, whichever is less.

✴ *To relieve moderate to severe pain as an adjunct to opioid analgesics*

I.V. INFUSION (CALDOLOR)

Adults. 400 to 800 mg every 6 hr, as needed.

Adolescents. 400 mg every 4 to 6 hr, as needed. *Maximum:* 2,400 mg daily.

Children ages 6 months to 12 years. 10 mg/kg up to 400 mg maximum for single dose every 4 to 6 hr, as needed. *Maximum:* 40 mg/kg or 2,400 mg daily, whichever is less.

✴ *To reduce fever*

CAPSULES, CHEWABLE TABLETS, ORAL SUSPENSION, TABLETS

Adults and adolescents. 200 to 400 mg every 4 to 6 hr, as needed.

CHEWABLE TABLETS, ORAL SUSPENSION

Children age 11 weighing 33 kg (72 lb) to 43 kg (95 lb). 300 mg every 6 to 8 hr, as needed.

Children ages 9 and 10 weighing 27 kg (59 lb) to 32 kg (70 lb). 250 mg every 6 to 8 hr, as needed.

Children ages 6 to 8 weighing 22 kg (48 lb) to 27 kg (59 lb). 200 mg every 6 to 8 hr, as needed.

Children ages 4 and 5 weighing 16 kg (35 lb) to 21 kg (46 lb). 150 mg every 6 to 8 hr, as needed.

Children ages 2 and 3 weighing 11 kg (24 lb) to 16 kg (35 lb). 100 mg every 6 to 8 hr, as needed.

ORAL DROPS

Children ages 12 to 23 months weighing 8.18 kg (18 lb) to 10.45 kg (23 lb). 75 mg every 6 to 8 hrs, as needed.

Children ages 6 to 11 months weighing 5.45 kg (12 lb) to 7.73 kg (17 lb). 50 mg every 6 to 8 hrs, as needed.

I.V. INFUSION (CALDOLOR)

Adults. 400 mg, followed by 400 mg every 4 to 6 hr. Or, 100 to 200 mg every 4 hr, as needed. *Maximum:* 3,200 mg daily.

Adolescents. 400 mg every 4 to 6 hr, as needed. *Maximum:* 2,400 mg daily.

Children ages 6 months to 12 years. 10 mg/kg up to 400 mg maximum for single dose every 4 to 6 hr, as needed. *Maximum:* 40 mg/kg or 2,400 mg daily, whichever is less.

✴ *To treat patent ductus arteriosus*

I.V. INFUSION (NEOPROFEN)

Gestational age 32 weeks or less and weighing between 500 and 1,500 g. *Initial:* 10 mg/kg (based on birth weight) followed by 5 mg/kg 24 hr later and 5 mg/kg 24 hr after second dose.

✴ *To relieve migraine pain and related symptoms, like nausea and sensitivity to light and sound.*

CAPSULES (ADVIL MIGRAINE)

Adults. 400 mg as a single dose. *Maximum:* 400 mg/24 hr.

☰ Drug Administration

P.O.

- Administer with food or after meals to reduce GI distress.
- Give drug with a full glass of water.
- Ensure that patient does not lie down for 15 to 30 minutes, to prevent esophageal irritation.
- Shake oral suspension and drops well before measuring dosage. Use a calibrated measuring device to measure dosage.

I.V.

Caldolor

- Dilute to final concentration of 4 mg/ml or less using 0.9% Sodium Chloride Injection, 5% Dextrose Injection, or Lactated Ringer's solution. For an 800-mg dose, dilute 8 ml in at least 200 ml diluent; for a 400-mg dose, dilute 4 ml in at least 100 ml of diluent; for a 200-mg dose, dilute 2 ml in at least 100 ml of diluent; and for a 100-mg dose, dilute 1 ml in at least 100 ml of diluent.
- Diluted solutions may be kept at room temperature up to 24 hours.
- Infuse at least over 30 minutes for adults and 10 minutes for children.

G
H
I

Neoprofen
- Withdraw drug from vial and discard any remaining drug in vial because it does not contain a preservative. Dilute to an appropriate volume with 0.9% Sodium Chloride Injection or 5% Dextrose Injection.
- Administer within 30 minutes of preparation.
- Administer via the I.V. port that is nearest the insertion site. Infuse over 15 minutes.
- *Incompatibilities:* Total Parenteral Nutrition in the same I.V. line

Route	Onset	Peak	Duration
P.O.	30–60 min	1–2 hr	4–6 hr
I.V.	Unknown	Unknown	Unknown

Half-life: 2–4 hr

Mechanism of Action

Blocks activity of cyclooxygenase, the enzyme needed to synthesize prostaglandins, which mediate inflammatory response and cause local pain, swelling, and vasodilation. By inhibiting prostaglandins, this NSAID reduces inflammatory symptoms and relieves pain. Ibuprofen's antipyretic action probably stems from its effect on the hypothalamus, which increases peripheral blood flow, causing vasodilation and encouraging heat dissipation.

Contraindications

For all forms except ibuprofen lysine: Angioedema, asthma, bronchospasm, nasal polyps, rhinitis, or urticaria caused by hypersensitivity to aspirin or other NSAIDs; hypersensitivity to ibuprofen or its components; pain with coronary artery bypass graft (CABG) surgery
For ibuprofen lysine: Bleeding (especially active intracranial hemorrhage or gastrointestinal bleeding), coagulation defects, congenital heart disease where patency of the patent ductus arteriosus is necessary for satisfactory pulmonary or systemic blood flow (pulmonary atresia, severe coarctation of the aorta, severe tetralogy of Fallot), hypersensitivity to ibuprofen or its components, known or suspected infection or necrotizing enterocolitis, significant renal impairment, thrombocytopenia

Interactions

DRUGS

angiotensin-converting enzyme (ACE) inhibitors, angiotensin receptor blockers (ARBs), beta-blockers (including propranolol): Possibly diminished antihypertensive effect of these drugs
aspirin: Possibly decreased cardioprotective and stroke-preventive effects of aspirin; increased risk of bleeding and adverse GI effects
cyclosporine: Increased risk of nephrotoxicity
digoxin: Increased blood digoxin level and risk of digitalis toxicity
diuretics (loop, potassium-sparing, and thiazide): Decreased diuretic and antihypertensive effects
heparin, oral anticoagulants, selective serotonin reuptake inhibitors, serotonin norepinephrine reuptake inhibitors, thrombolytics: Increased anticoagulant effects, increased risk of hemorrhage
lithium: Increased blood lithium level
methotrexate: Decreased methotrexate clearance and increased risk of toxicity
other NSAIDs, salicylates: Increased risk of GI toxicity
pemetrexed: Increased risk of GI and renal toxicity; myelosuppression

ACTIVITIES

alcohol use: Increased risk of adverse GI effects

Adverse Reactions

CNS: **Aseptic meningitis**, **CVA**, dizziness, headache, nervousness, **seizures**
CV: Fluid retention, **heart failure**, hypertension, **MI**, peripheral edema, tachycardia
EENT: Amblyopia, epistaxis, stomatitis, tinnitus
GI: Abdominal cramps, distention, or pain; anorexia; constipation; diarrhea; diverticulitis; dyspepsia; dysphagia; elevated liver enzymes; epigastric discomfort; esophagitis; flatulence; gastritis; gastroenteritis; gastroesophageal reflux disease; **GI bleeding, hemorrhage, perforation**, or ulceration; heartburn; hemorrhoids; **hepatic failure; hepatitis**; hiatal hernia; indigestion; **melena**; nausea; **necrotizing enterocolitis**; vomiting
GU: Cystitis, hematuria, **renal failure (acute)**

HEME: Agranulocytosis, anemia, **aplastic anemia,** eosinophilia, **hemolytic anemia, leukopenia, neutropenia, pancytopenia, prolonged bleeding time,** thrombocytopenia

RESP: Bronchospasm, dyspnea, **pulmonary hypertension (neonates),** wheezing

SKIN: Blisters, **erythema multiforme,** photosensitivity, pruritus, rash, **Stevens–Johnson syndrome, toxic epidermal necrolysis,** urticaria

Other: **Anaphylaxis, angioedema, drug reaction with eosinophilia and systemic symptoms (DRESS),** flu-like symptoms, hypokalemia, weight gain

Childbearing Considerations

PREGNANCY
- Drug increases risk of premature closure of the fetal ductus arteriosus if given at 30 weeks or later during pregnancy.
- Neonatal renal impairment and oligohydramnios may occur if drug is given at 20 weeks gestation or later. Drug should only be administered between 20 and 30 weeks gestation if absolutely necessary with the lowest dose and shortest duration possible.

LACTATION
- Drug is present in breast milk.
- Breastfeeding is not recommended because maturation of renal system in infant may take up to 2 years.

REPRODUCTION
- Drug may delay or prevent rupture of ovarian follicles, which may cause reversible infertility in some women.

Nursing Considerations
- Be aware that NSAIDs like ibuprofen should be avoided in patients with a recent MI because risk of reinfarction increases with NSAID therapy. If therapy is unavoidable, monitor patient closely for signs of cardiac ischemia.
- Know that the risk of heart failure increases with use of NSAIDs such as ibuprofen. Ibuprofen should not be used in patients with severe heart failure but, if unavoidable, monitor patient for worsening of heart failure.
- Use ibuprofen with extreme caution in patients with a history of GI bleeding or ulcer disease because NSAIDs, such as ibuprofen, increase risk of GI bleeding and ulceration. Expect to use ibuprofen for shortest time possible in these patients.

! WARNING Be aware that the risk of serious cardiovascular thrombotic events such as MI or stroke increases the longer ibuprofen is used. Expect to give drug for shortest time possible. These events may occur early in treatment and happen even in patients who do not have a history of or risk factors for cardiovascular disease. Monitor patient for warning signs such as chest pain, slurring of speech, shortness of breath, or weakness. If any signs and symptoms develop, withhold ibuprofen, alert prescriber immediately, and provide supportive care as prescribed.

- Keep in mind that serious GI tract bleeding, perforation, and ulceration may occur without warning symptoms. Elderly patients are at greater risk. To minimize risk, give oral drug with food. If GI distress occurs, withhold drug and notify prescriber immediately.
- Use ibuprofen cautiously in patients with hypertension, and monitor blood pressure closely throughout therapy. Drug may cause hypertension or worsen it.

! WARNING Monitor patient closely for thrombotic events, including MI and stroke, because NSAIDs increase the risk.

- Monitor patient—especially if he's elderly or receiving long-term oral ibuprofen therapy—for less common but serious adverse GI reactions, including anorexia, constipation, diverticulitis, dysphagia, esophagitis, gastritis, gastroenteritis, gastroesophageal reflux disease, hemorrhoids, hiatal hernia, melena, stomatitis, and vomiting.
- Monitor liver enzymes, as ordered, because, in rare cases, elevations may progress to severe hepatic reactions, including fatal hepatitis, hepatic failure, or liver necrosis.
- Monitor BUN and serum creatinine levels in elderly patients, patients taking ACE inhibitors or diuretics, and patients with heart failure, hepatic dysfunction, or impaired renal function; drug may cause renal failure.
- Monitor CBC for decreased hemoglobin and hematocrit. Drug may worsen anemia.

G
H
I

! **WARNING** Be aware that if patient has bone marrow suppression or is receiving an antineoplastic drug, monitor laboratory results (including WBC count), and watch for evidence of infection. Ibuprofen's anti-inflammatory and antipyretic actions may mask signs and symptoms, such as fever and pain.

! **WARNING** Assess patient's skin regularly for signs of rash or other hypersensitivity reaction because ibuprofen is an NSAID and may cause serious skin reactions without warning, even in patients with no history of NSAID sensitivity. At first sign of reaction, stop drug and notify prescriber.

- Expect higher doses for rheumatoid arthritis than for osteoarthritis.
- Be aware that ibuprofen oral suspension may contain sucrose, which may affect blood glucose level in diabetic patients.

PATIENT TEACHING

- Advise parents to consult prescriber before giving OTC ibuprofen to a child if the child has any of the following: asthma; bleeding problems; heart or kidney disease; high blood pressure; need for diuretic therapy; persistent stomach problems, such as heartburn, stomach pain, or upset stomach; serious adverse effects from previous use of fever reducers or pain relievers; or ulcers.
- Instruct patient to take tablets with a full glass of water, and caution him not to lie down for 15 to 30 minutes, to prevent esophageal irritation.
- Tell patient prescribed liquid form of drug to shake container before measuring dose and to use a calibrated device, not a spoon, to measure dosage.
- Advise patient to take drug with food or after meals to reduce GI distress.
- Urge patient not to take higher doses of drug or for a longer time than prescribed because stomach bleeding may occur and risk of MI or stroke may increase.
- Instruct patient to consult prescriber if he needs to take drug for more than 3 days for fever or 10 days for pain; if stomach problems (heartburn, pain, or upset) occur; if liver problems occur (diarrhea, fatigue, "flu-like" symptoms, itchiness, lethargy, nausea, right upper abdominal

tenderness, and yellowing of skin and whites of his eyes); if he has a history of bleeding problems, heart or renal disease, hypertension, or ulcers; if he takes a diuretic; or if he's over age 65.
- Inform patient with phenylketonuria that Motrin chewable tablets contain aspartame.
- Inform patient that full therapeutic effect for arthritis may take 2 weeks or longer.
- Urge patient to avoid taking two different NSAIDs at the same time, unless directed, and to alert prescriber before taking ibuprofen if he has ever had an allergic reaction to any other analgesic or fever-reducing drug or has a history of asthma.
- Urge patient to avoid alcohol, aspirin, and corticosteroids while taking ibuprofen, unless prescribed. If patient takes aspirin as prevention of MI or stroke, explain that ibuprofen may interfere with this effect.
- Suggest that patient wear sunscreen and protective clothing when outdoors.
- Advise patient to report flu-like symptoms, rash, signs of GI bleeding, swelling, vision changes, and weight gain.

! **WARNING** Urge parents to seek medical care and to tell prescriber promptly if child receiving drug develops headache, high fever, nausea, persistent diarrhea, severe persistent sore throat, or vomiting or hasn't been drinking fluids.

! **WARNING** All ibuprofen products should be kept out of reach of children. If an overdose occurs, instruct parents/caregivers to get immediate medical help or contact a Poison Control Center immediately.

- Caution pregnant patient not to take oral ibuprofen at 20 weeks of gestation or more because of adverse effects on fetal renal system and potential for premature closure of the ductus arteriosus to occur after 30 weeks gestation.

! **WARNING** Explain that ibuprofen may increase risk of serious adverse cardiovascular reactions; urge patient to seek immediate medical attention if signs or symptoms arise, such as chest pain, edema, shortness of breath, slurring of speech, swelling in legs, unexplained weight gain, or weakness.

! **WARNING** Alert patient to rare but serious skin reactions. Urge him to seek immediate medical attention for blisters, fever, itching, rash, or other indications of hypersensitivity.

ibutilide fumarate
Corvert

Class and Category
Pharmacologic class: Methane sulfonanilide derivative
Therapeutic class: Class III antiarrhythmic

Indications and Dosages
⁕ *To rapidly convert recent-onset atrial flutter or fibrillation to sinus rhythm*

I.V. INFUSION

Adults weighing 60 kg (132 lb) or more.
1 mg. Dose repeated 10 min after first dose is finished if arrhythmia persists.
Adults weighing less than 60 kg (132 lb).
0.01 mg/kg. Dose repeated 10 min after first dose is completed if arrhythmia persists.
±**DOSAGE ADJUSTMENT** Infusion stopped if arrhythmia is terminated or if nonsustained or sustained ventricular tachycardia or prolonged QT or QTc interval develops.

Drug Administration
I.V.
- Give drug undiluted or diluted in 50 ml of 0.9% Sodium Chloride Injection or 5% Dextrose Injection by adding contents of one 10-ml vial (0.1 mg/ml) to form a concentration of about 0.017 mg/ml.
- Use polyvinyl chloride plastic bags or polyolefin bags for admixtures.
- Give drug within 24 hours if stored at room temperature or 48 hours if refrigerated.
- Infuse over 10 minutes.
- Immediately stop infusion if conversion occurs or patient develops marked prolongation of QT interval or ventricular tachycardia.
- *Incompatibilities:* None listed by manufacturer

Route	Onset	Peak	Duration
I.V.	<90 min	Unknown	24 hr

Half-life: 6 hr

Mechanism of Action
May promote sodium movement through slow inward sodium channels in myocardial cell membranes. Ibutilide also may inhibit potassium channels in myocardial cell membranes involved in cardiac repolarization. These actions prolong cardiac action potential by delaying repolarization and increasing atrial and ventricular refractoriness. As a result, sinus rate slows and AV conduction is delayed.

Contraindications
Hypersensitivity to ibutilide or components

Interactions
DRUGS
antihistamine drugs (selective) such as H1 receptor antagonists, class Ia antiarrhythmics (disopyramide, procainamide, quinidine), class III antiarrhythmics (amiodarone, sotalol), phenothiazines, tetracyclic or tricyclic antidepressants: Possibly increased risk of prolonged QT interval, leading to increased risk of proarrhythmias
digoxin: Possibly masking cardiotoxicity associated with excessive digoxin levels

Adverse Reactions
CNS: Headache, syncope
CV: AV block, bradycardia, bundle branch block, heart failure, hypertension, hypotension, idioventricular rhythm, orthostatic hypotension, palpitations, prolonged QT interval, sinus tachycardia, supraventricular arrhythmias, ventricular arrhythmias
GI: Nausea
GU: Renal failure

Childbearing Considerations
PREGNANCY
- Drug may cause fetal harm, according to animal studies.
- Use with caution only if benefit to mother outweighs potential risk to fetus.

LACTATION
- It is not known if drug is present in breast milk.
- Breastfeeding should not be undertaken during drug therapy.

Nursing Considerations
- Know that before giving ibutilide, check serum electrolyte levels and expect to correct abnormalities, as prescribed.

G
H
I

Be especially alert for hypokalemia and hypomagnesemia, which can lead to arrhythmias.

- As ordered, monitor patient's cardiac rhythm continuously during infusion and for at least 4 hours afterward—longer if arrhythmias appear or if patient has abnormal hepatic function. Observe patient for ventricular ectopy.
- Make sure defibrillator and drugs to treat sustained ventricular tachycardia are available during therapy and when monitoring patient after therapy.

PATIENT TEACHING

- Inform patient that ibutilide will be given by I.V. infusion and that his heart rhythm will be monitored continuously.
- Ask patient to report chest pain, faintness, numbness, palpitations, shortness of breath, and tingling.
- Advise patient to keep follow-up appointments to monitor heart rhythm.

icosapent ethyl
Vascepa

Class and Category
Pharmacologic class: Lipid-regulating agent
Therapeutic class: Antilipemic

Indications and Dosages
∗ *Adjunct to diet to reduce triglyceride levels in patients with severe (equal to or greater than 500 mg/dl) hypertriglyceridemia; adjunct to maximally tolerated statin therapy to reduce the risk of coronary revascularization, myocardial infarction, stroke, and unstable angina requiring hospitalization in patients with elevated triglyceride levels of 150 mg/dl or greater and diabetes mellitus and two or more additional risk factors for cardiovascular disease or patients with established cardiovascular disease*

CAPSULES
Adults. 2 g twice daily.

Drug Administration
P.O.
- Capsules should be swallowed whole and not chewed, crushed, dissolved, or opened.
- Administer with food.

Route	Onset	Peak	Duration
P.O.	Unknown	5 hr	Unknown

Half-life: 89 hr

Mechanism of Action
Reduces very low-density lipoprotein triglycerides (VLDL-TG) synthesis and/or secretion in the liver and enhances triglyceride clearance from circulating VLDL particles. Mechanisms used to accomplish this may include decreased lipogenesis in the liver, increased beta oxidation, increased lipoprotein lipase activity, and inhibition of acyl-CoA:1,2-diacylglycerol acyltransferase. These mechanisms work together to lower triglyceride levels.

Contraindications
Hypersensitivity to icosapent ethyl or its components

Interactions
DRUGS
anticoagulants, antiplatelet drugs: Possibly increased bleeding time

Adverse Reactions
CV: **Atrial fibrillation** or **flutter**, elevated blood triglycerides, peripheral edema
EENT: Oropharyngeal pain
GI: Abdominal discomfort, constipation, diarrhea
HEME: **Increased risk of bleeding**
MS: Arthralgia, extremity or musculoskeletal pain
Other: Gout

Childbearing Considerations
PREGNANCY
- It is not known if drug causes fetal harm.
- Use with caution only if benefit to mother outweighs potential risk to fetus.

LACTATION
- Drug is present in breast milk.
- Patient should check with prescriber before breastfeeding.

Nursing Considerations

! **WARNING** Use icosapent ethyl cautiously in patients with a known hypersensitivity to fish and/or shellfish because the drug contains ethyl esters of the omega-3 fatty acid obtained from the oil of fish.

- Be aware that patient should have been placed on a lipid-lowering diet and exercise regimen before starting icosapent ethyl therapy.
- Know that efforts should be made to control conditions that may increase lipid abnormalities, such as alcohol intake, diabetes mellitus, and hypothyroidism.
- Expect medications known to exacerbate hypertriglyceridemia, such as beta-blockers, estrogen therapy, and immunosuppressants, to be changed or discontinued prior to icosapent ethyl therapy.
- Obtain lipid levels prior to initiating icosapent ethyl therapy, as ordered, to determine a baseline. Monitor lipid levels periodically throughout icosapent ethyl therapy to determine effectiveness.
- Monitor alanine aminotransferase and aspartate aminotransferase levels periodically, as ordered, in patients with hepatic impairment.
- Monitor patient for an irregular or fast heart rate because icosapent ethyl therapy increases the risk of atrial fibrillation or flutter that may be severe enough to require hospitalization. Incidence is greater in patients with a previous history of these arrhythmias.
- Institute bleeding precautions because icosapent ethyl increases risk of bleeding, especially if patient is taking antithrombotic drugs, such as aspirin, clopidogrel, or warfarin.

PATIENT TEACHING

- Tell patient that icosapent ethyl therapy is not a substitute for diet and exercise but that these lifestyle changes should continue during icosapent ethyl therapy.
- Instruct patient to take capsules whole and not to break, chew, crush, or open the capsules.

! **WARNING** Advise patient with known hypersensitivity to fish and/or shellfish about the potential for allergic reactions to icosapent ethyl. Tell patient to discontinue drug and seek medical attention if any reactions occur.

- Inform patient that periodic blood tests will be needed to monitor effectiveness of icosapent ethyl therapy.

- Teach patient how to take a pulse and to report an irregular or fast pulse immediately to prescriber.
- Review bleeding precautions with patient.

idarucizumab
Praxbind

≣ Class and Category
Pharmacologic class: Humanized monoclonal antibody fragment
Therapeutic class: Antidote

≣ Indications and Dosages
∗ *To reverse anticoagulant effects of dabigatran needed in emergency surgery, life-threatening bleeding, urgent procedures, or uncontrolled bleeding*

I.V. INFUSION, I.V. INJECTION
Adults. 5 g given in two 2.5-g doses consecutively, and repeated one time, as needed.

≣ Drug Administration
I.V.
- Administer drug solution immediately after it is removed from vial. Solution should be clear and colorless to slightly yellow.
- Use two 2.5-g/50 ml vials and administer drug as 2.5-g doses back to back either as an intravenous infusion or injection.
- Flush intravenous line with 0.9% Sodium Chloride Injection prior to administering drug.
- Drug vial solution may be stored at room temperature but must be used within 6 hours.
- *Incompatibilities:* Other drugs in the same intravenous line

Route	Onset	Peak	Duration
I.V.	Rapid	Unknown	24 hr

Half-life: 10.3 hr

≣ Mechanism of Action
Binds to dabigatran and its acyl-glucuronide metabolites with higher affinity than the binding of dabigatran to thrombin, thereby neutralizing their anticoagulant effect and reversing the effects of dabigatran.

G
H
I

Contraindications

Hypersensitivity to idarucizumab or its components

Interactions

DRUGS

None reported by manufacturer

Adverse Reactions

CNS: Delirium, fever
CV: Thrombotic events
GI: Constipation
RESP: Bronchospasm, hyperventilation, pneumonia
SKIN: Pruritus, rash
Other: Anaphylaxis, formation of idarucizumab antibodies, hypokalemia

Childbearing Considerations

PREGNANCY

- It is not known if drug causes fetal harm.
- Use with caution only if benefit to mother outweighs potential risk to fetus.

LACTATION

- Drug is present in breast milk.
- Patient should check with prescriber before breastfeeding.

Nursing Considerations

- Use extreme caution when administering idarucizumab to a patient with hereditary fructose intolerance because idarucizumab contains 4 g of sorbitol. The amount of sorbitol that may cause serious or even fatal adverse reactions is not known.
- Provide standard supportive measures to control dabigatran-induced bleeding, as needed, in conjunction with idarucizumab treatment.
- Monitor patient's coagulation parameters such as activated partial thromboplastin time (aPTT) or ecarin clotting time (ECT), as ordered.

! **WARNING** Monitor patient closely for thrombotic events because reversing dabigatran with idarucizumab increases the risk of such events. Know that resumption of anticoagulant therapy should be done as soon as possible. For example, dabigatran may be resumed 24 hours after the administration of idarucizumab.

! **WARNING** Monitor patient for an allergic reaction to idarucizumab. If present,

stop administration immediately, notify prescriber, and provide emergency supportive care, as indicated.

PATIENT TEACHING

! **WARNING** Instruct patient to alert medical personnel immediately if she experiences difficulty breathing or develops skin reactions such as itchiness or a rash during or after idarucizumab has been administered.

- Alert patient that she will continue to need anticoagulant therapy once the bleeding episode has been resolved to prevent future blood clots. She may be able to resume dabigatran therapy 24 hours after idarucizumab therapy is given, if ordered.
- Tell her she will need blood tests to monitor effectiveness of idarucizumab therapy and that a second dose of idarucizumab may be required if bleeding reoccurs or an emergency procedure or surgery is required.

iloperidone
Fanapt

Class and Category

Pharmacologic class: Atypical antipsychotic
Therapeutic class: Second-generation antipsychotic

Indications and Dosages

✳ *To treat schizophrenia*

TABLETS

Adults. *Initial:* 1 mg twice daily, adjusted to target dosage range as follows: 2 mg twice daily on day 2, 4 mg twice daily on day 3, and 6 mg twice daily on day 4. Dosage may be further increased, as needed, as follows: 8 mg twice daily on day 5, 10 mg twice daily on day 6, and 12 mg twice daily on day 7. *Maximum:* 12 mg twice daily.

±**DOSAGE ADJUSTMENT** For patients taking strong CYP2D6 inhibitors, such as fluoxetine and paroxetine, CYP3A4 inhibitors, such as clarithromycin and ketoconazole, or are poor metabolizers of CYP2D6, dosage reduced by half. For patients with moderate hepatic impairment, dose reduced, if needed.

Drug Administration
P.O.
- Expect to restart dosage adjustment schedule in patients who have been off drug for more than 3 days.
- Protect from light and moisture when stored.

Route	Onset	Peak	Duration
P.O.	Unknown	2–4 hr	Unknown

Half-life: 18–33 hr

Mechanism of Action
Selectively blocks dopamine type 2 (D_2) and serotonin type 2 (5-HT_2) receptors in CNS, thereby suppressing psychotic symptoms.

Contraindications
Hypersensitivity to iloperidone or its components

Interactions
DRUGS
antibiotics such as fluoroquinolones or macrolides, class IA antiarrhythmics such as procainamide or quinidine, class III antiarrhythmics such as amiodarone or sotalol, other antipsychotic drugs such as chlorpromazine or thioridazine, or any other drug that affects the QT interval, such as methadone or pentamidine: Possibly prolonged QT interval
antihypertensive drugs: Increased antihypertensive effects
CNS depressants: Possibly additive CNS effects
CYP2D6 inhibitors such as fluoxetine or paroxetine, CYP3A4 inhibitors such as ketoconazole: Increased plasma iloperidone level
dextromethorphan: Increased blood dextromethorphan level

ACTIVITIES
alcohol: Possibly increased CNS effects

Adverse Reactions
CNS: Aggression, delusion, dizziness, extrapyramidal effects, fatigue, lethargy, **neuroleptic malignant syndrome**, restlessness, **seizures**, somnolence, **suicidal ideation**, tremor
CV: Congestive heart failure, dyslipidemia, orthostatic hypotension, palpitations, **QT interval prolongation**, tachycardia
EENT: Blurred vision, conjunctivitis, dry mouth, nasal congestion, nasopharyngitis, **oropharyngeal swelling**, **throat tightness**, upper respiratory tract infection
ENDO: Diabetic ketoacidosis, elevated prolactin levels, hyperglycemia, **hyperosmolar coma**
GI: Abdominal discomfort, diarrhea, nausea
GU: Ejaculation failure, erectile dysfunction, priapism, urinary incontinence
HEME: Leukopenia
MS: Arthralgia, musculoskeletal stiffness, spasms, myalgia
RESP: Dyspnea
SKIN: Pruritus, rash, urticaria
Other: Anaphylaxis, angioedema, weight gain

Childbearing Considerations
PREGNANCY
- Pregnancy exposure registry: 1-866-961-2388 or http://womensmentalhealth.org/clinical -and-research-programs/pregnancyregistry/.
- Drug may cause fetal harm.
- Exposure during third trimester increases risk of fetus developing extrapyramidal and/or withdrawal symptoms following delivery.
- Use with caution only if benefit to mother outweighs potential risk to fetus.

LACTATION
- It is not known if drug is present in breast milk.
- Breastfeeding is not recommended during drug therapy.

Nursing Considerations
- Know that iloperidone shouldn't be used in patients with a history of cardiovascular disease such as cardiac arrhythmias, QT interval prolongation, recent MI, or uncompensated heart failure. It also shouldn't be used in patients taking other drugs known to prolong the QT interval and in patients with hepatic impairment.

! **WARNING** Be aware that iloperidone shouldn't be used to treat patients with dementia-related psychosis, especially elderly patients, because of an increased risk of death.

- Use cautiously in patients who have a history of seizures or who have conditions that lower the seizure threshold, such as

G
H
I

Alzheimer's dementia. Also use cautiously in patients who are at risk for aspiration pneumonia or who have moderate hepatic impairment (not recommended for use in patients with severe hepatic impairment).

- Obtain baseline serum magnesium and potassium levels in patients at risk for electrolyte imbalances, and then monitor periodically throughout therapy, as ordered, because electrolyte imbalances increase risk of prolonged QT interval or arrhythmia. If patient reports dizziness, palpitations, or syncope, notify prescriber and expect further evaluation to be done.

! **WARNING** Know that neuroleptic malignant syndrome has occurred in patients taking other antipsychotic drugs. Monitor patient for altered mental status, autonomic instability, hyperpyrexia, and muscle rigidity. If present, notify prescriber immediately, expect drug to be discontinued, and start intensive treatment, as prescribed. Watch for recurrence if patient resumes antipsychotic therapy.

- Monitor patient for tardive dyskinesia, which has occurred with other antipsychotic drugs. If patient develops involuntary, dyskinetic movements, notify prescriber and expect to discontinue drug.
- Monitor blood glucose level, especially in patients with diabetes mellitus, because iloperidone may alter blood glucose enough to induce life-threatening hyperosmolar coma or ketoacidosis.
- Monitor patient's CBC periodically, as ordered, especially during first few months of therapy, because iloperidone may cause neutropenia. Also, be aware that other antipsychotic drugs have caused sometimes fatal agranulocytosis and leukopenia. If patient's WBC count decreases, expect drug to be discontinued.
- Monitor patient closely for abnormal tendencies that may suggest suicidal thinking, especially when iloperidone therapy starts or dosage is changed.

PATIENT TEACHING

- Inform patient that when iloperidone therapy starts, dosage must be adjusted for up to a week to reach target level. Also explain that adjustment process will have to be repeated if she skips drug for more than 3 days.
- Advise patient or caregiver to notify prescriber about persistent, severe, or unusual adverse reactions because drug may have to be discontinued.
- Urge patient or caregiver to report evidence of abnormal thinking, especially when therapy starts or dosage changes.
- Tell diabetic patient to monitor blood glucose levels closely and to report persistent elevations immediately to prescriber.
- Caution patient to avoid hazardous activities until CNS effects of drug are known. Patient should also avoid alcohol.
- Instruct patient to avoid activities that might raise body temperature, such as being exposed to extreme heat, being subjected to dehydration, doing strenuous exercise, or taking other drugs with anticholinergic activity.
- Emphasize the need to comply with follow-up appointments and laboratory tests.
- Tell patient to rise slowly from lying to sitting position and from sitting position to standing to avoid dizziness or light-headedness during therapy.
- Advise female patient of childbearing age to notify prescriber if she intends to become or suspects that she is pregnant during therapy and that breastfeeding is not recommended during drug therapy.

imipramine hydrochloride
Tofranil

imipramine pamoate

⬚ Class and Category
Pharmacologic class: Tricyclic antidepressant (TCA)
Therapeutic class: Antidepressant

⬚ Indications and Dosages
✻ *To treat depression*
CAPSULES
Hospitalized adults. *Initial:* 100 to 150 mg once daily, gradually increased as needed and

tolerated, to 200 mg once daily or in divided doses, as needed. Further increased to 250 to 300 mg once daily or in divided doses after 2 wk, if needed. *Maximum:* 300 mg once daily or in divided doses.

Outpatient adults. *Initial:* 75 mg once daily, increased to 150 mg once daily or in divided doses and further increased to 200 mg once daily or in divided doses, if needed. *Maintenance:* 75 to 150 mg once daily. Doses above 75 mg may be given in divided doses. *Maximum:* 200 mg daily.

CAPSULES, TABLETS

Adolescents and elderly. *Initial:* 25 to 50 mg once daily as tablets and then increased, as needed. Once 75-mg dosage reached, capsules may be used. *Maximum:* 100 mg daily.

TABLETS

Hospitalized adults. *Initial:* 100 mg daily in divided doses, gradually increased as needed and tolerated, to 200 mg daily in divided doses as needed. Further increased to 250 to 300 mg daily in divided doses after 2 wk, if needed. *Maximum:* 300 mg daily in divided doses.

Outpatient adults. *Initial:* 75 mg daily, increased to 150 mg daily and further increased to 200 mg daily, if needed. *Maintenance:* 50–150 mg daily. *Maximum:* 200 mg daily.

Adolescents and elderly. *Initial:* 30 to 40 mg daily as a single dose or in divided doses, adjusted as needed and tolerated. *Maximum:* 100 mg daily.

✷ *As adjunct to treat childhood enuresis*

TABLETS

Children age 6 and over. *Initial:* 25 mg once daily. Increased to 50 mg once daily if no response occurs within 1 wk and child is under age 12; increased to 75 mg once daily if child is age 12 or over. *Maximum:* 2.5 mg/kg daily.

▤ Drug Administration

P.O.

- For depression, administer once-daily dose at bedtime.
- For childhood enuresis, administer 1 hour before bedtime. For early night bedwetters, administer drug earlier and in divided amounts, such as 25 mg in afternoon and repeated at bedtime.
- Capsules and tablets should be swallowed whole and not chewed, crushed, or opened.

Route	Onset	Peak	Duration
P.O.	1–2 wk	1–2 hr	Unknown

Half-life: 8–19 hr

▤ Mechanism of Action

May interfere with reuptake of serotonin (and possibly other neurotransmitters) at presynaptic neurons, thus enhancing serotonin's effects at postsynaptic receptors. Mood elevation may result from restoration of normal levels of neurotransmitters at nerve synapses. This tricyclic antidepressant also blocks acetylcholine receptors, which may explain how it relieves enuresis.

▤ Contraindications

Acute recovery period after MI; hypersensitivity to imipramine, other tricyclic antidepressants, or their components; use within 14 days of MAO inhibitor therapy, including intravenous methylene blue and linezolid

▤ Interactions

DRUGS

anticholinergics, antiparkinsonian drugs: Risk of increased anticholinergic effects, including confusion, hallucinations, and nightmares
barbiturates, phenytoin: Possibly decreased imipramine level and effects
CNS depressants: Increased CNS depression, hypotension, and respiratory depression
P450 2D6 inhibitors such as cimetidine, class IC antiarrhythmics (flecainide, propafenone), other antidepressants, phenothiazines, quinidine, selective serotonin reuptake inhibitors (fluoxetine, paroxetine, sertraline): Increased concentrations of both drugs
MAO inhibitors: Increased risk of hypertensive crisis, severe seizures, and death
oral anticoagulants: Possibly increased anticoagulant activity
sympathomimetics containing epinephrine or norepinephrine such as decongestants, local anesthetics: Potentiated effects of catecholamines

ACTIVITIES

alcohol use: Increased CNS depression

▤ Adverse Reactions

CNS: Anxiety, ataxia, chills, confusion, CVA, delirium, dizziness, drowsiness, excitation, extrapyramidal reactions, fever, hallucinations, headache, insomnia, nervousness, nightmares,

Parkinsonism, **seizures, serotonin syndrome, suicidal ideation**, tremor
CV: Arrhythmias, orthostatic hypotension, palpitations
EENT: Blurred vision, dry mouth, increased intraocular pressure, pharyngitis, taste perversion, tinnitus, tongue swelling
ENDO: Gynecomastia, syndrome of inappropriate ADH secretion
GI: Constipation, diarrhea, heartburn, ileus, increased appetite, jaundice, nausea, vomiting
GU: Impotence, libido changes, testicular swelling, urine retention
HEME: Agranulocytosis, bone marrow depression
RESP: Wheezing
SKIN: Alopecia, diaphoresis, photosensitivity, pruritus, rash, urticaria
Other: Angioedema, hypersensitivity reactions, weight gain

Childbearing Considerations
PREGNANCY
- Drug may cause fetal harm, possibly increasing risk of congenital malformations.
- Use with caution only if benefit to mother outweighs potential risk to fetus.

LACTATION
- Drug may be present in breast milk.
- Breastfeeding is not recommended during drug therapy.

Nursing Considerations
- Use imipramine cautiously in patients with a history of angle-closure glaucoma or urine retention because drug's anticholinergic effects may cause increased intraocular pressure and urine retention.

! **WARNING** Know that MAO inhibitors should not be given within 2 weeks of imipramine, including intravenous methylene blue and linezolid. Patient may experience hypertensive crisis, seizures, and death.

! **WARNING** Monitor patient for possible serotonin syndrome, characterized by agitation, chills, confusion, diaphoresis, diarrhea, fever, hyperactive reflexes, poor coordination, restlessness, shaking, talking or acting with uncontrolled excitement, tremor, and twitching. Notify prescriber immediately if serotonin syndrome is suspected because

it can become life-threatening. Expect to discontinue imipramine therapy if serotonin syndrome is confirmed.

- Assess patient frequently for adverse reactions during first 2 hours of therapy.
- Check standing and supine blood pressure for orthostatic hypotension before and during imipramine therapy and before dosage increases.
- Anticipate increased risk of arrhythmias in patients with a history of cardiac disease.
- Know that when drug is used for depression, expect mood elevation to take 2 to 3 weeks. Watch patient closely for suicidal tendencies, especially children and adolescents and especially when therapy starts or dosage changes, because depression may worsen temporarily at these times.
- Avoid abrupt withdrawal of drug in patients on long-term therapy. Such withdrawal may cause headache, malaise, nausea, sleep disturbance, and vomiting.
- Taper drug gradually, as ordered, a few days before surgery to avoid risk of hypertension during surgery.
- Obtain CBC, as ordered, if patient experiences signs and symptoms of infection, such as fever or pharyngitis.
- Limit amount of drug given to potentially suicidal patient.

PATIENT TEACHING
- Instruct patient being treated for depression to take drug at bedtime if taking once daily. Tell parents of a child being treated for bedwetting to administer drug 1 hour before bedtime unless child is an early night bedwetter. In that case, dosage divided in two with first dose given in the afternoon and the second dose given at bedtime.
- Advise patient to take imipramine exactly as prescribed. Warn that stopping drug abruptly may cause headache, malaise, nausea, trouble sleeping, and vomiting.
- Caution parents to monitor child or adolescent closely for suicidal tendencies, especially when therapy starts or dosage changes.
- Urge patient to report chills, dizziness, excess sedation, fever, palpitations, signs of allergic reaction, sore throat, and trouble urinating.

- Caution patient to avoid hazardous activities until drug's CNS effects are known.
- Urge patient to avoid alcohol during imipramine therapy because it increases alcohol effects and CNS depression.
- Suggest that patient eat frequent, small meals to help relieve nausea.
- Instruct patient to avoid prolonged exposure to sunlight because of the risk of photosensitivity.
- Inform male patient about possible impotence and decreased or increased libido.
- If patient reports dry mouth, suggest sugarless candy or gum to relieve it. Tell him to check with prescriber if dry mouth persists after 2 weeks.

immune globulin intramuscular (human)
(gamma globulin, IG)
GamaSTAN S/D 5%

immune globulin intravenous (human)
(IGIV)
Asceniv 10%, Bivigam Liquid 10%, Flebogamma DIF 5% and 10%, Gammagard Liquid 10%, Gammagard S/D 5%, Gammaplex 5% and 10%, Gamunex-C 10%, Octagam 5%, Panzyga 10%, Privigen 10%

immune globulin subcutaneous (human)
Cutaquig 16.5%, Cuvitru 20%, Gammagard Liquid 10%, Gamunex-C 10%, Hizentra 20%, HyQvia 10%, Xembify 20%

☰ Class and Category
Pharmacologic class: Immune serum
Therapeutic class: Antibody production stimulator

☰ Indications and Dosages
✳ *To treat primary immunodeficiency*

I.V. INFUSION (GAMMAGARD S/D 5%)
Adults. 300 to 600 mg/kg every 3 to 4 wk. If response is inadequate, dose or frequency may be adjusted. Initially infused at 0.5 ml/kg/hr, then gradually increased as tolerated to maximum rate of 4 ml/kg/hr.

SUBCUTANEOUS INFUSION (HYQVIA 10%)
Adults. Highly individualized. Consult manufacturer guidelines for initial ramp-up schedule given for first 7 wk. *For patients previously on another IgG treatment*: First dose administered about 1 wk after last infusion of previous treatment. *For adults naïve to IgG therapy or switching from another IgG subcutaneous therapy*: After initial ramp-up schedule given over 7 wk, 300 to 600 mg/kg every 3 to 4 wk. *For adults switching from IGIV therapy*: After initial ramp-up schedule given over 7 wk, same dose and frequency given as the previous IGIV therapy every 3 to 4 wk. Consult manufacturer guidelines for subsequent dose adjustments.

✳ *To treat primary immunodeficiency disorders associated with defects in humoral immunity*

I.V. INFUSION (FLEBOGAMMA DIF 5%, GAMMAGARD LIQUID 10%)
Adults and children ages 2 and over. 300 to 600 mg/kg every 3 to 4 wk. Initially infused at 0.5 mg/kg/min and gradually increased to 5 mg/kg/min for maintenance rate for Flebogamma DIF 5% and initially infused at 0.8 mg/kg/min for 30 min, then increased every 30 min up to 8 mg/kg/min for maintenance rate for Gammagard Liquid 10%.

I.V. INFUSION (FLEBOGAMMA DIF 10%)
Adults. 300 to 600 mg/kg every 3 to 4 wk. Initially infused at 1 mg/kg/min and gradually increased to 8 mg/kg/min.

I.V. INFUSION (GAMUNEX-C 10%)
Adults and children ages 2 and over. 300 to 600 mg/kg every 3 or 4 wk. Initially infused at 1 mg/kg/min and increased as tolerated to maintenance infusion rate of 8 mg/kg/min.

I.V. INFUSION (OCTAGAM 5%)
Adults. *Initial:* 300 to 600 mg/kg every 3 to 4 wk and adjusted as needed. Initially infused at 0.5 mg/kg/min for first 30 min; increased, if tolerated, to 1 mg/kg/min for second

30 min and, if tolerated, to 2 mg/kg/min for another 30 min. Maintenance infused up to 3.33 mg/kg/min.

±**DOSAGE ADJUSTMENT** For patient with risk of developing renal dysfunction, infusion rate should not exceed 3.33 mg/kg/min.

I.V. INFUSION (PANZYGA 10%)

Adults and children age 2 and over. 300 to 600 mg/kg every 3 to 4 wk. Initially infused for first 30 min at 1 mg/kg/min and then adjusted. Infusion rate should not exceed 14 mg/kg/min.

I.V. INFUSION (PRIVIGEN 10%)

Adults. 200 to 800 mg/kg every 3 to 4 wk. Initially infused at 0.5 mg/kg/min and gradually increased, as tolerated, to 8 mg/kg/min for maintenance infusion rate.

I.V. INFUSION (BIVIGAM LIQUID 10%)

Adults. 300 to 800 mg/kg every 3 to 4 wk. Infuse 0.5 mg/kg/min for the first 10 min, then increase infusion rate every 20 min, if tolerated, by 0.8 mg/kg/min up to 6 mg/kg/min.

I.V. INFUSION (ASCENIV 10%)

Adults and adolescents. 300 to 800 mg/kg every 3 to 4 wk. Infused at 0.5 mg/kg/min for the first 15 min, then increased gradually every 15 min up to 8 mg/kg/min, if tolerated.

I.V. INFUSION (GAMMAPLEX 5% AND 10%)

Adults and children age 2 and older. 300 to 800 mg/kg once every 3 to 4 wk. *For 5% solution*: Initially infused at 0.5 mg/kg/min for 15 min and then gradually increased every 15 min, if tolerated, to final infusion rate of 4 mg/kg/min. *For 10% solution*: Initially infused at 0.5 mg/kg/min for 15 min followed by gradual rate increase every 15 min, if tolerated, to maintenance infusion rate of 8 mg/kg/min.

SUBCUTANEOUS INFUSION (HIZENTRA 20%)

Adults and children age 2 and over. Highly individualized and administered at regular intervals from daily up to every 2 wk. *For patients switching from IGIV*: Initial weekly dosage started 1 wk after patient's last IGIV infusion. Initial weekly dosage obtained by dividing the previous IGIV dose in grams by the number of weeks between doses during the patient's previous IGIV treatment, followed by multiplying the result by 1.37.

To calculate dose in grams to milliliters, multiply the calculated dose by 5.

SUBCUTANEOUS INFUSION (XEMBIFY 20%)

Adults and children age 2 and over. Highly individualized. *For patients switching from IGIV*: Initial weekly dosage started 1 wk after patient's last IGIV infusion. Initial weekly dosage obtained by dividing the previous IGIV dose in grams by the number of weeks between doses during the patient's previous IGIV treatment. Then multiply the result by 1.37. To convert dose in grams to milliliters, multiply the calculated dose by 5.

SUBCUTANEOUS INFUSION (GAMMAGARD LIQUID 10%, GAMUNEX-C 10%)

Adults and children age 2 and over. Highly individualized. *For patients switching from IGIV*: Initial weekly dosage started 1 wk after patient's IGIV infusion. Initial weekly dosage obtained by dividing the previous IGIV dose in grams by the number of weeks between doses during the patient's previous IGIV treatment, followed by multiplying the number by 1.37. To convert dose in grams to milliliters, multiply by 10.

SUBCUTANEOUS INFUSION (CUTAQUIG 16.5%)

Adults and children age 2 and over. Highly individualized and started 1 wk after patient's last IGIV infusion, with initial weekly dosage obtained by dividing the previous IGIV dose in grams by the number of weeks between intravenous doses. Then multiply this number by 1.30. Multiply the calculated dose by 6 to convert the dose calculated in grams to milliliters.

±**DOSAGE ADJUSTMENT** See manufacturer guidelines if drug is to be administered more or less frequently and to determine rate of infusion, which is based on patient's age.

SUBCUTANEOUS INJECTION (CUVITRU 20%)

Adults and children ages 2 and over. Highly individualized and administered at regular intervals from daily up to every 2 wk. *For patient switching from IGIV or adult patients switching from Hyqvia*: First dosage administered 1 wk after patient's last IGIV infusion or adult's last dose of Hyqvia. Initial weekly dosage obtained by dividing the previous IGIV or Hyqvia dose in grams by the number of weeks between intravenous doses. Then multiply this number by 1.30. Multiply the calculated dose by 5 to convert the dose calculated in grams to milliliters.

＊ *To treat thrombocytopenic purpura (ITP)*

I.V. INFUSION (GAMMAPLEX 5% AND 10%)

Adults. 1 g/kg for 2 consecutive days. *For 5% solution*: Initially infused at 0.5 mg/kg/min for 15 min and then gradually increased every 15 min, if tolerated, to final infusion rate of 4 mg/kg/min. *For 10% solution*: Initially infused at 0.5 mg/kg/min for 15 min followed by gradual rate increase every 15 min, if tolerated, to maintenance infusion rate of 8 mg/kg/min.

I.V. INFUSION (PRIVIGEN 10%)

Adults and adolescents age 15 and over. 1 g/kg daily for 2 consecutive days. Initially infused at 0.5 mg/kg/min and then gradually increased to 4 mg/kg/min for maintenance infusion rate.

I.V. INFUSION (FLEBOGAMMA DIF 10%)

Adults and children ages 2 and over. 1 g/kg daily for 2 consecutive days. Initially infused at a rate of 1 mg/kg/min with rate adjusted, as tolerated, to 8 mg/kg/min.

I.V. INFUSION (OCTAGAM 10%)

Adults. 1 g/kg (10 ml/kg) daily for 2 consecutive days. Initially infuse at 1 mg/kg/min for 30 min. If tolerated, increase infusion rate to 2 mg/kg/min for next 30 min. If tolerated, further increase infusion rate to 4 mg/kg/min for 30 min. If tolerated, further increase infusion rate to 8 mg/kg/min for 30 min. If tolerated, infusion rate may be increased up to 12 mg/kg/min for remainder of infusion.

I.V. INFUSION (GAMUNEX-C 10%)

Adults. 2 g/kg divided into 2 doses of 1 g/kg and given on 2 consecutive days or divided into 5 doses of 0.4 g/kg each and given on 5 consecutive days. Initially infused at 1 mg/kg/min and increased gradually, as tolerated, to maintenance infusion rate of 8 mg/kg/min.

I.V. INFUSION (GAMMAGARD S/D 5%)

Adults. 1 g/kg as a single dose. If response is inadequate, up to 3 separate doses may be administered on alternate days. Initially infused

at 0.5 ml/kg/hr and then gradually increased, as tolerated, up to a maximum of 4 ml/kg/hr.

I.V. INFUSION (PANZYGA 10%)

Adults. 2 g/kg divided into 2 doses of 1 g/kg and given on 2 consecutive days. Initially infused at 1 mg/kg/min over first 30 min and then rate adjusted. Maximum infusion rate should not exceed 8 mg/kg/min.

I.V. INFUSION (GAMMAPLEX LIQUID 5%)

Adults. 1 g/kg on 2 consecutive days, initially infused at 0.5 mg/kg/min and then gradually rate increased every 15 min, if tolerated, to final infusion rate of 4 mg/kg/min.

±**DOSAGE ADJUSTMENT** In acute ITP of childhood, I.V. Carimune NF therapy may be discontinued after second day of 5-day course if initial platelet count response is adequate (30,000 to 50,000/mm^3). In chronic ITP, an additional I.V. infusion of 400 mg/kg (Carimune NF or Gamimune) may be prescribed if platelet count falls below 30,000/mm^3 or if patient develops significant bleeding. If response remains inadequate, an additional I.V. infusion of 800 to 1,000 mg/kg may be given. In chronic ITP, dosage of Gammaplex 5% liquid may have to be reduced in patients at risk for thrombosis, hemolysis, acute kidney injury, or volume overload.

＊ *To prevent coronary artery aneurysms associated with Kawasaki syndrome*

I.V. INFUSION (GAMMAGARD S/D 5%)

Children. 1 g/kg as a single dose or 400 mg/kg daily for 4 consecutive days and started within 7 days of onset of fever. Administered with aspirin 80 to 100 mg/kg/day in 4 divided doses. Initially infused at a rate of 0.5 ml/kg/hr and then gradually increased to maximum of 4 ml/kg/hr, as tolerated.

＊ *To treat chronic inflammatory demyelinating polyneuropathy (CIDP)*

I.V. INFUSION (GAMUNEX-C 10%)

Adults. *Loading dose:* 2 g/kg given in divided doses over 3 to 4 consecutive days with infusion rate of 2 mg/kg/min. *Maintenance dose:* 1 g/kg every 3 wk infused over 1 day or divided into 2 doses of 0.5 g/kg and given on 2 consecutive days with infusion rate gradually increased to 8 mg/kg/min, as tolerated.

G
H
I

INTRAVENOUS INFUSION (PRIVIGEN 10%)

Adults. *Loading dose:* 2 g/kg given in divided doses over 2 to 5 consecutive days. Initially infused at 0.5 mg/kg/min and, if tolerated, rate gradually increased up to a maximum of 8 mg/kg/min. *Maintenance:* 1 g/kg as a single infusion or divided into 2 doses given on 2 consecutive days, every 3 wk for up to 6 months. Minimum infusion rate is 0.5 mg/kg/min and maximum infusion rate is 8 mg/kg/min.

I.V. INFUSION (PANZYGA 10%)

Adults. *Loading dose:* 1 g/kg twice daily on 2 consecutive days. Initially infused at 1 mg/kg/min over first 30 min and then adjusted. Infusion rate should not exceed 12 mg/kg/min. *Maintenance:* 0.5 to 1 g/kg twice daily on 2 consecutive days every 3 wk.

SUBCUTANEOUS INFUSION (HIZENTRA 20%)

Adults. 0.2 g/kg/wk administered in 1 or 2 sessions over 1 or 2 consecutive days, increased to 0.4 g/kg/wk administered in 2 sessions over 1 or 2 consecutive days. Dosage increased to 0.4 g/kg/wk given in 2 sessions per wk over 1 or 2 consecutive days.

✱ *To prevent bacterial infections in hypogammaglobulinemia and/or recurrent bacterial infections associated with B-cell chronic lymphocytic leukemia*

I.V. INFUSION (GAMMAGARD S/D 5%)

Adults. 400 mg/kg every 3 to 4 wk. Initially infused at 0.5 ml/kg/hr and then gradually increased to maximum of 4 ml/kg/hr, as tolerated.

✱ *To improve muscle strength and disability as maintenance therapy in patients with multifocal motor neuropathy*

I.V. INFUSION (GAMMAGARD LIQUID 10%)

Adults. 0.5 to 2.4 g/kg/mo, based on clinical response. Initially infused at 0.8 mg/kg/min with rate increased, as needed, up to 9 mg/kg/min.

✱ *To treat dermatomyositis (OCTAGAM 10%)*

Adults. 2 g/kg divided in equal doses given over 2 to 5 consecutive days every 4 wk. Initially infused at 1 mg/kg/min and then increased as tolerated to maintenance infusion rate up to 4 mg/kg/min.

✱ *To treat hepatitis A exposure*

I.M. INJECTION (GAMASTAN S/D 5%)

Adults and children. 0.02 ml/kg as a single dose for household and institutional hepatitis A contact, as soon as possible after exposure.

✱ *To prevent hepatitis A when traveling in areas where hepatitis A is common*

I.M. INJECTION (GAMASTAN S/D 5%)

Adults and children staying in area less than 3 months. 0.02 ml/kg as a single dose. **Adults and children staying in area 3 months or longer.** 0.06 ml/kg as a single dose and repeated every 4 to 6 months while in the area.

✱ *To prevent or modify measles in a susceptible person exposed fewer than 6 days previously*

I.M. INJECTION (GAMASTAN S/D 5%)

Adults and children. 0.25 ml/kg as a single dose as soon as possible after exposure. **Immunocompromised children.** 0.5 ml/kg (maximum dose 15 ml) as a single dose.

✱ *To modify varicella infection when Varicella-Zoster Immune Globulin is unavailable*

I.M. INJECTION (GAMASTAN S/D 5%)

Adults and children. 0.6 to 1.2 ml/kg as a single dose given as soon as possible after exposure.

✱ *To lessen effects of rubella exposure*

I.M. INJECTION (GAMASTAN S/D 5%)

Women in first trimester of pregnancy. 0.55 ml/kg as a single dose as soon as possible after exposure.

▤ Drug Administration

- When preparing immune globulin, verify that appropriate form is being used— either immune globulin intramuscular for I.M. injection, immune globulin intravenous for I.V. infusion, or immune globulin subcutaneous for subcutaneous infusion.

- To reconstitute drug, if required, follow manufacturer's guidelines and use only diluent recommended by manufacturer. Don't shake solution; excessive shaking causes foaming. If drug or diluent is cold, drug may take up to 20 minutes to dissolve.

- Know that if drug is reconstituted outside of sterile laminar airflow conditions, administer it immediately and discard unused portions.

I.V.

- An in-line filter may be required for intravenous infusion of drug. Check manufacturer's guidelines for specific product being used.
- Consult manufacturer's guidelines to determine appropriate flow rate for infusion.
- *Incompatibilities:* Check manufacturer guidelines for specific product being used

I.M.

- Inject only into deltoid muscle of upper arm or anterolateral aspect of upper thigh.
- If giving a dose larger than 5 ml, divide it and administer at separate sites.

SUBCUTANEOUS

- Use an infusion pump to administer drug.
- Infusion sites should be at least 2 inches apart and sites changed each week.
- Consult manufacturer guidelines to determine number of sites that can be used simultaneously and infusion flow rate.

Route	Onset	Peak	Duration
I.V.	Immediate	< 30 min	Unknown
I.M.	Unknown	2 days	Unknown
SubQ	Unknown	Unknown	Unknown

Half-life: 16–31 days

Mechanism of Action

Releases antibody-specific globulins to produce an antibody–antigen reaction that results in bacterial lysis and facilitates bacterial phagocytosis. In treatment of ITP, immune globulin blocks iron receptors on macrophages to increase immunoglobulin action. Immune globulin also increases cytokine production and improves B-cell immune function by regulating macrophage and T-cell activity. Newly formed antigen–antibody complexes produce split complement components that cause bacterial lysis.

In Kawasaki disease and bacterial infections with B-cell chronic lymphocytic leukemia, immune globulin neutralizes bacterial and viral toxins that harm immune and inflammatory responses.

Contraindications

Hypersensitivity to immune globulin (human) or its components; IgA deficiency in patients with known antibody to IgA

Interactions

DRUGS

live-virus vaccines: Possibly decreased response to vaccine

Adverse Reactions

CNS: **Aseptic meningitis** (rare), headache, malaise
CV: Chest discomfort, hypertension, tachycardia, **thrombotic events**, **volume overload**
EENT: Blurred vision, oropharyngeal pain
GI: Nausea, vomiting
GU: **Acute renal dysfunction or failure,** osmotic nephrosis
HEME: **Acute hemolysis, delayed hemolytic anemia, disseminated intravascular coagulation (DIC),** positive Coombs' test
MS: Arthralgia, back or extremity pain, muscle spasms or weakness, myalgia
RESP: Dyspnea, **pulmonary edema or embolism**
Other: Hyperproteinemia, **hyponatremia,** increased serum viscosity

Childbearing Considerations

PREGNANCY

- It is not known if drug causes fetal harm although immune globulins increasingly cross the placental barrier after 30 weeks' gestation.
- Use with caution only if benefit to mother outweighs potential risk to fetus.

LACTATION

- Drug may be present in breast milk.
- Patient should check with prescriber before breastfeeding.

Nursing Considerations

- Know that before giving immune globulin, monitor patient's fluid volume and BUN and serum creatinine levels, as ordered, to determine risk for acute renal failure. Those at increased risk include patients with diabetes mellitus, paraproteinemia, renal insufficiency, sepsis, or volume depletion; those taking nephrotoxic drugs; and those over age 65. Expect drug to be discontinued if renal function deteriorates.
- Use caution when administering immune globulin, regardless of the route of administration, because of risk for thrombosis. Monitor closely patients with increased risk of thrombosis such as advanced age, coagulation disorders,

a history of atherosclerosis, impaired cardiac output, multiple cardiovascular risk factors, or prolonged periods of immobilization, and/or hyperviscosity. In such patients, obtain a baseline assessment of blood viscosity, as ordered. Ensure patient is adequately hydrated prior to administration. When administering drug intravenously, expect to infuse at the lowest rate possible. Report any signs and symptoms suggestive of a thrombotic event immediately to prescriber and be prepared to administer treatment, as ordered.

! **WARNING** Watch for an acute inflammatory reaction in patients who have never received immune globulin therapy before, in those whose last treatment was more than 8 weeks before, and in those whose initial infusion rate exceeded 1 ml/min. Within 30 minutes to 1 hour after beginning infusion, assess for chills, diaphoresis, dizziness, facial flushing, feeling of tightness in chest, fever, hypotension, nausea, and vomiting. Notify prescriber immediately if such symptoms occur, and be prepared to stop infusion until symptoms have subsided.

- Monitor patient closely for signs and symptoms of hemolysis, especially patients with risk factors. For patients at increased risk, expect to obtain a baseline measurement of hematocrit or hemoglobin prior to infusion and within 36 to 96 hours post infusion. Notify prescriber of any abnormalities.

! **WARNING** Be aware that after immune globulin administration, monitor patient closely for aseptic meningitis. Notify prescriber if patient develops drowsiness, fever, nausea, nuchal rigidity, painful eye movements, photophobia, severe headache, or vomiting.

- Be aware that immune globulin intravenous is made from human plasma and therefore may contain infectious agents, such as viruses. Risk of transmitting a virus by infusion has been reduced by inactivating or removing certain viruses from the product, screening blood donors, or testing donated blood.

PATIENT TEACHING

- Review with patient how immune globulin will be administered.
- Instruct patient to report immediately any symptoms he experiences after receiving immune globulin.
- Inform patient to postpone live-virus vaccinations for up to 11 months after receiving immune globulin, because drug may delay or inhibit response to vaccine.

inclisiran

Leqvio

≣ Class and Category
Pharmacologic class: Small interfering ribonucleic acid (siRNA)
Therapeutic class: Antipipemic

≣ Indications and Dosages
٭ *As adjunct to diet and maximally tolerated statin therapy in patients with heterozygous familial hypercholesterolemia*

SUBCUTANEOUS INJECTION
Adults. *Initial:* 284 mg as a single dose, repeated in 3 months and then again after 6 months of last dose. *Maintenance:* 284 mg every 6 months.

≣ Drug Administration
SUBCUTANEOUS INJECTION

- Inspect solution before injecting. Solution should be clear, colorless to pale yellow with no particulate matter.
- Inject into abdomen, thigh, or upper arm. Do not inject into areas of skin disease or injury.
- If a planned dose is missed in less than 3 months, maintain dosing schedule.
- If a planned dose is missed longer than 3 months, restart dosing schedule with an initial dose followed by a dose in 3 months and then every 6 months thereafter.

Route	Onset	Peak	Duration
SQ	Unknown	4 hr	Unknown

Half-life: 9 hr

Mechanism of Action

After entering hepatocytes, breakdown of mRNA for PCSK9 occurs resulting in an increase in LDL-C uptake. This lowers LDL-C levels in circulation.

Contraindications

Hypersensitivity to inclisiran or its components

Interactions

DRUGS

None reported by manufacturer

Adverse Reactions

GI: Diarrhea
GU: UTI
MS: Arthralgia, extremity pain
RESP: Bronchitis, dyspnea
OTHER: Anti-inclisiran antibody formation, injection-site reaction (redness, pain, and rash)

Childbearing Considerations

PREGNANCY

- Drug may cause fetal harm.
- Drug should not be given during pregnancy.

LACTATION

- It is not known if drug is present in breast milk.
- Patient should check with prescriber before breastfeeding.

Nursing Considerations

- Be aware that inclisiran should only be given by a health care professional.
- Monitor patient for decreased effectiveness that may indicate anti-inclisiran antibody formation is occurring.
- Monitor patient's lipid levels to assess effectiveness of the drug.
- Assess injection site for redness or rash and determine if pain is present at the injection site.

PATIENT TEACHING

- Inform patient that the subcutaneous injection must be administered by a health care professional.
- Instruct patient to inform prescriber if pain, rash, or redness occurs at the injection site.
- Tell women of childbearing age to notify prescriber immediately if pregnancy is suspected or known, as drug will have to be discontinued during pregnancy.

indacaterol maleate

Onbrez Breezhaler (CAN)

Class and Category

Pharmacologic class: Long-acting beta$_2$-adrenergic agonist
Therapeutic class: Bronchodilator

Indications and Dosages

＊ *To alleviate airflow obstruction in patients with chronic obstructive pulmonary disease (COPD), including chronic bronchitis and/or emphysema*

ORAL INHALATION

Adults. 75 mcg once daily.

Drug Administration

INHALATION

- Drug capsules are only for use in the Onbrez Breezhaler and should never be swallowed.
- To use device, place capsule in well of inhaler device and then press and release buttons on side of device only once to pierce capsule. A click-type sound will occur. Then have him place the inhaler into his mouth and inhale rapidly and deeply through mouthpiece; drug is dispersed into airways as patient inhales. During inhalation, expect to hear a whirring sound. Alert patient that he may taste the drug as he inhales. After inhalation, open the inhaler to see if any powder is left in the capsule. If powder is present, repeat the steps again. Then remove the empty capsule and discard.
- Never wash inhaler with water or take it apart. To clean inhaler, wipe the mouthpiece inside and outside with a clean, dry, lint-free cloth.
- Store capsules in their original packaging and open immediately before use.

Route	Onset	Peak	Duration
Inhalation	Within 5 min	2–4 hr	24 hr

Half-life: 40–56 hr

Mechanism of Action

Selectively attaches to beta$_2$ receptors on bronchial membranes, stimulating the intracellular enzyme adenyl cyclase to

G
H
I

convert adenosine triphosphate to cAMP. The resulting increase in the intracellular cAMP level relaxes bronchial smooth muscle cells, which allows greater airflow through the airways.

Contraindications

Hypersensitivity to indacaterol or its components; presence of asthma without use of an inhaled corticosteroid

Interactions

DRUGS

adrenergic drugs: Potentiated sympathetic effects
beta-blockers: Possible interference with the effect of beta-blockers and indacaterol
diuretics, steroids, xanthine derivatives: Possible increased risk of hypokalemic effect
MAO inhibitors, tricyclic antidepressants: Potentiated adrenergic action on the cardiovascular system
non–potassium-sparing diuretics: Increased risk of ECG changes or hypokalemia
QT prolonging drugs: Increased risk of ventricular arrhythmias

Adverse Reactions

CNS: Dizziness, headache, nervousness, tremor
CV: Angina, **atrial fibrillation**, peripheral edema, palpitations, tachycardia
EENT: Nasopharyngitis, oropharyngeal pain, sinusitis
ENDO: Hyperglycemia
GI: Nausea
MS: Muscle spasm, musculoskeletal pain
RESP: COPD exacerbation, cough, dyspnea, **paradoxical bronchospasm**, pneumonia, upper respiratory tract infection
SKIN: Pruritus, rash, urticaria
Other: **Angioedema, hypokalemia, immediate hypersensitivity reactions**

Childbearing Considerations

PREGNANCY

- It is not known if drug causes fetal harm.
- Use with caution only if benefit to mother outweighs potential risk to fetus.

LABOR & DELIVERY

- There is the potential that drug may interfere with uterine contractions because it is a beta-agonist.
- Use of drug during labor and delivery should be restricted to those patients in whom the benefits clearly outweigh the risks.

LACTATION

- It is not known if drug is present in breast milk.
- Patient should check with prescriber before breastfeeding.

Nursing Considerations

- Be aware that indacaterol should not be given to patients with acutely deteriorating COPD, nor should it be used for relief of acute symptoms. Instead, acute symptoms should be treated with an inhaled short-acting beta$_2$-agonist.

! **WARNING** Know that indacaterol is not used to treat asthma but may be used in patients with asthma who also have COPD as long as the patient is also receiving inhaled corticosteroid therapy. This is because the use of long-acting beta$_2$-adrenergic agonists such as indacaterol without inhaled corticosteroid therapy in patients with asthma increases the risk of serious asthma-related events requiring hospitalization and intubation and possibly ending in death.

- Use cautiously in patients with cardiovascular disorders, especially cardiac arrhythmias, coronary insufficiency, and hypertension, because drug can increase blood pressure, pulse rate, and cause ECG changes, such as flattening of the T wave, prolongation of the QT interval, and ST segment depression.
- Use cautiously in patients with convulsive disorders or thyrotoxicosis, or in patients who are unusually responsive to sympathomimetic amines, as drug may aggravate these conditions.
- Monitor the patient's vital signs for an increase in blood pressure or pulse rate. If such effects occur, notify prescriber, as indacaterol may have to be discontinued.

! **WARNING** Monitor patient for immediate hypersensitivity reactions after administering indacaterol that may include difficulties in breathing or swallowing; rash; swelling of face, lips, and tongue; or urticaria. If present, discontinue drug immediately, notify prescriber, and provide supportive care, as indicated.

- Instruct patient who has been taking inhaled, short-acting beta$_2$-agonists on a regular basis to discontinue the regular use of these drugs, as directed by prescriber, and use them only for symptomatic relief of acute respiratory symptoms, as ordered.
- Tell patient indacaterol capsules are only for use in inhaler device and should never be swallowed.
- Instruct patient to store capsules in their original packaging and to open immediately before use.
- Teach patient how to use delivery system. Tell him to place capsule in well of inhaler device and then to press and release buttons on side of device only once to pierce capsule. A click-type sound will occur. Have patient place the inhaler into his mouth. Then have him inhale rapidly and deeply through the mouthpiece; drug is dispersed into airways as patient inhales. A whirring noise should be heard when inhaling. If not, the capsule may be stuck in the capsule cavity. If this occurs, have patient open the inhaler and carefully loosen the capsule by tapping the base of the device. Tell him not to press the piercing buttons to loosen the capsule. Have him repeat these steps, if needed.
- Remind patient that indacaterol is not to be used to relieve acute symptoms. Instead, he should use his short-acting beta$_2$-agonist.

! **WARNING** Tell patient to seek immediate medical care if an allergic reaction occurs right after drug is administered and reaction is serious, such as difficulty breathing or swelling of face, lips, or tongue.

- Inform patient to notify prescriber if any of the following situations occur: if indacaterol no longer seems to control his symptoms, if he needs to use his short-acting beta$_2$-agonist more often than usual, or if the short-acting beta$_2$-agonist becomes less effective.

indinavir sulfate
Crixivan

Class and Category
Pharmacologic class: Protease inhibitor
Therapeutic class: Antiretroviral

Indications and Dosages
* *As adjunct to treat human immunodeficiency virus (HIV) infection*

CAPSULES
Adults. 800 mg every 8 hr.
± **DOSAGE ADJUSTMENT** For patient who has mild to moderate hepatic insufficiency due to cirrhosis and for patients who are taking delavirdine at a dosage of 400 mg three times daily, itraconazole at a dosage of 200 mg twice daily, or ketoconazole, dosage reduced to 600 mg every 8 hr. For patients taking rifabutin concomitantly, dosage increased to 1,000 mg every 8 hr with rifabutin dosage reduced by half.

Drug Administration
P.O.
- Administer drug 1 hour before or 2 hours after a meal with water. Alternatively, drug can be administered with other liquids such as coffee, juice, skim milk, or tea or with a light meal (such as dry toast with jelly or cereal with skim milk and sugar). A meal high in calories, fat, and protein reduces the absorption of indinavir.
- Store drug in original container and keep desiccant in the bottle because the capsules are sensitive to moisture.

Route	Onset	Peak	Duration
P.O.	Rapid	< 1 hr	Unknown

Half-life: 1.5–2 hr

Mechanism of Action
Binds to the protease active site to inhibit the activity of the HIV-1 protease enzyme. This inhibition prevents cleavage of the viral polyproteins, resulting in the formation of immature noninfectious viral particles.

Contraindications
Concurrent therapy with alfuzosin, alprazolam, amiodarone, cisapride, dihydroergotamine, ergonovine, ergotamine, lovastatin, methylergonovine, midazolam (oral), pimozide, sildenafil (when used to treat pulmonary arterial hypertension), simvastatin, or triazolam; hypersensitivity to indinavir or its components

Interactions
DRUGS
alfuzosin: Possibly increased alfuzosin concentrations leading to hypotension

G
H
I

alprazolam, midazolam (oral), triazolam: Possible risk of increased or prolonged respiratory depression or sedation

amiodarone, cisapride: Increased risk for serious or life-threatening adverse reactions such as cardiac arrhythmias

atazanavir: Increased risk of unconjugated hyperbilirubinemia

atorvastatin, bepridil, bosentan, calcium channel blockers, colchicine, fluticasone, lidocaine (systemic), midazolam (parenteral), quetiapine, quinidine, rosuvastatin, trazodone: Increased concentration of these drugs

carbamazepine, efavirenz, nevirapine, phenobarbital, phenytoin, venlafaxine: Decreased indinavir concentration, lowering effectiveness

clarithromycin: Increased concentrations of both clarithromycin and indinavir

cyclosporine, sirolimus, tacrolimus: Increased immunosuppressant effects

delavirdine, itraconazole, ketoconazole, nelfinavir, ritonavir, saquinavir: Increased indinavir concentration, increasing risk of adverse reactions

didanosine: Possibly interference with absorption of indinavir

dihydroergotamine, ergonovine, ergotamine, methylergonovine: Possible acute ergot toxicity

lovastatin, simvastatin: Increased risk of myopathy and rhabdomyolysis

lurasidone, pimozide: Possibly increased risk of serious or life-threatening adverse reactions

rifabutin: Decreased indinavir concentration and effectiveness; increased rifabutin concentration and possibly adverse reactions

rifampin, St. John's wort: Possible loss of virologic response and resistance to indinavir

salmeterol: Possibly increased risk of cardiovascular adverse effects such as palpitations, prolonged QT, and sinus tachycardia

sildenafil (used to treat of pulmonary arterial hypertension), tadalafil, vardenafil: Possible increased risk of PDE5-inhibitor-induced adverse reactions such as hypotension, prolonged erection, syncope, and visual disturbances

Adverse Reactions

CNS: Asthenia, **cerebrovascular disorders**, depression, dizziness, fatigue, fever, headache, malaise, somnolence

CV: Angina pectoris, elevated cholesterol and triglyceride levels, **MI**, vasculitis

EENT: Oral paresthesia, pharyngitis, taste perversion

ENDO: Cushingoid appearance, exacerbation of preexisting diabetes mellitus, fat redistribution, hyperglycemia, new-onset diabetes mellitus

GI: Abdominal distention or pain, acid regurgitation, anorexia, diarrhea, dyspepsia, elevated amylase or liver enzymes, **hepatic dysfunction or failure, hepatitis**, hyperbilirubinemia, increased appetite, jaundice, nausea, **pancreatitis**, vomiting

GU: **Acute renal failure**, dysuria, elevated creatinine level, flank pain, hematuria, interstitial nephritis, leukocyturia, nephrolithiasis, pyelonephritis, **renal insufficiency**, urolithiasis

HEME: **Acute hemolytic anemia**, anemia, decreased hemoglobin, **neutropenia**, **spontaneous bleeding in patients with hemophilia, thrombocytopenia**

MS: Arthralgia, back pain, periarthritis

RESP: Cough, dyspnea, shortness of breath, upper respiratory infection

SKIN: Alopecia, dry skin, **erythema multiforme**, hyperpigmentation, paronychia, pruritus, rash, **Stevens–Johnson syndrome**, urticaria

Other: Anaphylaxis

Childbearing Considerations

PREGNANCY

- Pregnancy exposure registry: 1-800-258-4263.
- It is not known if drug causes fetal harm.
- Use with caution only if benefit to mother outweighs potential risk to fetus.

LACTATION

- It is not known if drug is present in breast milk.
- The Centers for Disease Control and Prevention recommends that HIV-1 infected mothers not breastfeed to avoid risking postnatal transmission of HIV-1 infection infants. They also do not recommend breastfeeding because of potential drug-induced adverse reactions in the infant.

Nursing Considerations

- Review patient's drug history before starting indinavir therapy, because drug interacts with many other drugs, some of which are contraindicated during indinavir use.

- Monitor patient for signs and symptoms of nephrolithiasis or urolithiasis, such as flank pain with or without hematuria. Notify prescriber if patient complains of flank pain or exhibits hematuria. Expect drug to be temporarily stopped for up to 3 days or discontinued. Ensure that patient receives adequate hydration throughout therapy.
- Monitor patient's complete blood count, because acute hemolytic anemia has occurred with indinavir therapy, ending in death for some patients. Report any change in complete blood count and signs and symptoms of anemia to prescriber. Be prepared to provide supportive care as ordered. Expect indinavir to be discontinued.
- Monitor patient's liver enzymes and assess patient for signs and symptoms of liver dysfunction, because hepatitis including hepatic failure has occurred with indinavir therapy.
- Check patient's blood glucose levels routinely, because indinavir therapy may cause hyperglycemia and exacerbate glucose control in patients with diabetes or even induce diabetes mellitus in patients not diagnosed with diabetes mellitus before therapy was begun.
- Be aware that immune reconstitution syndrome has occurred in patients treated with combination antiretroviral therapy, including indinavir. The inflammatory response predisposes susceptible patients to opportunistic infections such as cytomegalovirus, *Mycobacterium avium* infection, *Pneumocystis jiroveci* pneumonia, or tuberculosis. Autoimmune disorders such as Graves' disease, Guillain–Barré syndrome, or polymyositis have also occurred. Report sudden or unusual adverse reactions to prescriber.
- Perform a urinalysis periodically, as ordered. Notify prescriber if leukocyturia occurs, as further evaluation and possible discontinuation of indinavir may be needed.

PATIENT TEACHING

- Instruct patient to take indinavir 1 hour before or 2 hours after a meal with water. Tell patient that alternatively, she may take the drug with other liquids such as coffee, juice, skim milk, or tea, or with a light meal such as dry toast with jelly or cereal with skim milk and sugar.
- Tell patient to store drug in original container and that the desiccant should remain in the bottle because the capsules are sensitive to moisture.
- Inform patient that she must maintain adequate hydration throughout therapy. She should drink at least 48 ounces of liquids daily.
- Instruct patient who is also taking didanosine to take the two drugs 1 hour apart on an empty stomach.
- Advise patient to notify all prescribers of indinavir therapy, because of potential drug interactions, and advise patient not to take over-the-counter preparations (including herbal drugs and preparations) without consulting prescriber first.
- Warn male patient of the danger of taking drugs used to treat erectile dysfunction, because very serious adverse reactions can occur if taken with indinavir.
- Inform patient that indinavir therapy may cause changes in her body appearance because of fat redistribution. Prepare her for the possibility of developing breast enlargement, central obesity, dorsocervical fat enlargement (buffalo hump), facial wasting, and peripheral wasting.
- Instruct patient to report any persistent, severe, or unusual signs and symptoms.
- Alert mothers that breastfeeding is not recommended during indinavir therapy.
- Inform patients with hemophilia that indinavir may cause spontaneous bleeding and to seek immediate medical attention if bleeding occurs.

indomethacin
Indocin, Tivorbex

indomethacin sodium trihydrate
Indocin I.V.

⦀ Class and Category

Pharmacologic class: NSAID
Therapeutic class: Analgesic

▤ Indications and Dosages

＊ *To relieve moderate to severe symptoms of ankylosing spondylitis, osteoarthritis, and rheumatoid arthritis*

CAPSULES, ORAL SUSPENSION

Adults and adolescents over age 14.
25 mg twice daily or three times daily, increased by 25 or 50 mg daily every wk, as needed. *Maximum:* 200 mg daily. After adequate response, dosage reduced as low as possible.

E.R. CAPSULES

Adults and adolescents over age 14. 75 mg daily, increased to 75 mg twice daily, if needed.

SUPPOSITORIES

Adults and adolescents over age 14. 50 mg up to three times daily.

＊ *To relieve symptoms of acute gouty arthritis*

CAPSULES, ORAL SUSPENSION, SUPPOSITORIES (INDOCIN)

Adults. 50 mg three times daily until gout attack relieved, and then drug rapidly reduced to complete cessation.

＊ *To treat inflammation and relieve acute shoulder pain from bursitis or tendinitis*

CAPSULES, ORAL SUSPENSION

Adults and adolescents over age 14. 75 to 150 mg daily in divided doses three times daily or four times daily for 7 to 14 days.

E.R. CAPSULES

Adults and adolescents over age 14. 75 mg once or twice daily for 7 to 14 days.

SUPPOSITORIES

Adults and adolescents over age 14. 50 mg up to four times daily for 7 to 14 days. *Maximum:* 200 mg daily. ·

＊ *To treat mild to moderate acute pain*

CAPSULES (TIVORBEX)

Adults. 20 mg three times daily or 40 mg two or three times daily.

±**DOSAGE ADJUSTMENT** Dosage reduced for elderly patients.

＊ *To treat hemodynamically significant patent ductus arteriosus in premature infants weighing 500 to 1,750 g (1 to 3.9 lb)*

I.V. INFUSION (INDOCIN I.V.)

Infants over age 7 days. *Initial:* 200 mcg/kg (0.2 mg/kg) over 20 to 30 min; 2 additional doses of 250 mcg/kg (0.25 mg/kg) given at 12- to 24-hr intervals. A second course may be repeated if ductus arteriosus reopens.

Neonates ages 2 to 7 days. *Initial:* 200 mcg/kg (0.2 mg/kg) over 20 to 30 min; 2 additional doses of 200 mcg/kg (0.2 mg/kg) given at 12- to 24-hr intervals. A second course may be repeated if ductus arteriosus reopens.

Neonates under age 48 hours. *Initial:* 200 mcg/kg (0.2 mg/kg) over 20 to 30 min; 2 additional doses of 100 mcg/kg (0.1 mg/kg) given at 12- to 24-hr intervals. A second course may be repeated if ductus arteriosus reopens.

▤ Drug Administration

P.O.

- Administer drug immediately after meals or with food.
- Capsules should be swallowed whole without chewing, crushing, or opening. Administer capsules with a full glass of water.
- Shake suspension well before giving it. Use a calibrated device to measure dosage.
- Ensure that patient does not lie down for at least 15 minutes after drug has been administered.

I.V.

- To reconstitute, add 1 to 2 ml of preservative-free 0.9% Sodium Chloride Injection or preservative-free Sterile Water to drug vial. Solution made with 1 ml diluent contains 100 mcg (0.1 mg) indomethacin/0.1 ml. Solution made with 2 ml diluent contains 50 mcg (0.05 mg) indomethacin/0.1 ml. Solution should be clear, slightly yellow, and essentially free from visible particles. Do not dilute further.
- Use solution immediately because it contains no preservatives. Discard unused portion.
- Infuse over 20 to 30 minutes.
- Scheduled I.V. doses may be withheld if neonate has anuria or a significant decrease in urine output (less than 0.6 ml/kg/hr).
- Avoid extravasation to protect surrounding tissue.
- Anticipate a second course (3 more doses) if patent ductus arteriosus reopens. After 2 courses, surgery may be performed.

- *Incompatibilities:* Other I.V. infusion solutions except for preservative-free 0.9% Sodium Chloride Injection or preservative-free Sterile Water for Injection

P.R.

- If suppository is too soft, put in refrigerator for 15 minutes or run it under cold water while still wrapped.
- Make sure suppository stays in rectum at least 1 hour to improve absorption.
- Be aware that suppositories can be substituted for capsule administration in the treatment of ankylosing spondylitis, osteoarthritis, and rheumatoid arthritis but only if necessary, because there is a significant difference in blood levels between the two dosage forms.

Route	Onset	Peak	Duration
P.O.	30 min	2 hr	4–6 hr
P.O./E.R.	30 min	2 hr	Unknown
I.V.	Unknown	Unknown	Unknown
P.R.	Unknown	Unknown	4–6 hr

Half-life: 2.6–11.2 hr

Mechanism of Action

Blocks activity of cyclooxygenase, the enzyme needed to synthesize prostaglandins, which mediate inflammatory response and cause local pain, swelling, and vasodilation. By blocking cyclooxygenase and inhibiting prostaglandins, this NSAID reduces inflammatory symptoms and helps relieve pain.

Contraindications

History of asthma, urticaria, or other allergic-type reactions after taking aspirin or other NSAIDs; hypersensitivity to indomethacin, other NSAIDs, or their components; history of proctitis or recent rectal bleeding (suppositories); postoperative pain with coronary artery bypass graft (CABG) surgery

Interactions

DRUGS

Note: All effects listed are for oral forms and suppositories unless indicated.

angiotensin-converting enzyme (ACE) inhibitors, angiotensin receptor blockers (ARBs), or beta-blockers (including propranolol): Decreased antihypertensive effects of these drugs; in the elderly or patients with renal impairment or who are volume-depleted, increased risk of acute renal failure

anticoagulants such as warfarin, antiplatelets such as aspirin, selective serotonin reuptake inhibitors, serotonin norepinephrine reuptake inhibitors: Increased risk of serious bleeding

aspirin, other NSAIDs, other salicylates: Increased risk of adverse GI effects and non-GI bleeding

cyclosporine: Increased risk of nephrotoxicity

digoxin: Increased blood digoxin level and risk of digitalis toxicity (all forms)

diuretics (loop, potassium-sparing, and thiazide): Decreased antihypertensive and diuretic effects; increased risk of hyperkalemia with potassium-sparing diuretics

lithium: Increased blood lithium level and risk of toxicity

methotrexate: Increased risk of methotrexate toxicity

pemetrexed: Increased risk of myelosuppression; increased risk of GI and renal toxicity

probenecid: Increased blood level and effectiveness of indomethacin, increased risk of indomethacin toxicity

ACTIVITIES

alcohol use: Increased risk of adverse GI effects

Adverse Reactions

Note: All reactions are for oral forms and suppositories unless indicated.

CNS: Confusion, **CVA**, depression, dizziness, drowsiness, fatigue, hallucinations, headache, **intraventricular hemorrhage (I.V.)**, peripheral neuropathy, **seizures**, syncope, vertigo

CV: Arrhythmias, chest pain, edema, fluid retention (all forms), **heart failure**, hypertension, **MI**, **pulmonary hypertension (I.V.)**, tachycardia

EENT: Blurred vision, corneal and retinal damage, epistaxis, hearing loss, stomatitis, tinnitus

ENDO: Hypoglycemia (I.V.)

GI: Abdominal cramps or pain, abdominal distention (I.V.), anorexia, constipation, diarrhea, diverticulitis, dyspepsia,

dysphagia, elevated liver enzymes, epigastric discomfort, esophagitis, gastritis, gastroenteritis, gastroesophageal reflux disease, **GI bleeding** and ulceration (all forms), hemorrhoids, **hepatic dysfunction (I.V.), hepatic failure,** hiatal hernia, ileus (I.V.), indigestion, **melena,** nausea, **necrotizing enterocolitis (I.V.), pancreatitis,** peptic ulcer, **perforation of intestine or stomach,** vomiting (all forms)
GU: Acute renal failure, hematuria, interstitial nephritis, **nephrotic syndrome,** oliguria (I.V.), proteinuria, renal dysfunction (I.V.), vaginal bleeding
HEME: Agranulocytosis, anemia, **aplastic anemia, bone marrow depression, decreased platelet aggregation (I.V.), disseminated intravascular coagulation (DIC),** hemolytic anemia, iron deficiency anemia, **leukopenia, neutropenia, pancytopenia, thrombocytopenia, unusual bleeding** or bruising (all forms)
RESP: Asthma, respiratory depression
SKIN: Ecchymosis, **erythema multiforme,** erythema nodosum, photosensitivity, pruritus, rash, **Stevens–Johnson syndrome, toxic epidermal necrolysis,** urticaria
Other: Anaphylaxis, angioedema, drug reaction with eosinophilia and systemic symptoms (DRESS), hyperkalemia (I.V.), hyponatremia (I.V.), injection-site irritation

☰ Childbearing Considerations

PREGNANCY

- Drug increases risk of premature closure of the fetal ductus arteriosus if given during the third trimester of pregnancy and may cause fetal renal dysfunction, leading to oligohydramnios and neonatal renal impairment if given at 20 weeks or thereafter.
- Drug should be avoided in pregnant women starting at 30 weeks of gestation and onward and the lowest dose for the shortest period of time only should be used between 20 and 30 weeks gestation if absolutely necessary.

LACTATION

- Drug may be present in breast milk.
- Patient should check with prescriber before breastfeeding because many manufacturers do not recommend drug use during breastfeeding.

REPRODUCTION

- Drug may delay or prevent rupture of ovarian follicles, which has been associated with reversible infertility in some women.

☰ Nursing Considerations

- Be aware that NSAIDs like indomethacin should be avoided in patients with a recent MI because risk of reinfarction increases with NSAID therapy. If therapy is unavoidable, monitor patient closely for signs of cardiac ischemia.
- Know that the risk of heart failure increases with indomethacin use because it is an NSAID. This class of drugs should not be used in patients with severe heart failure but, if unavoidable, monitor patient for worsening of heart failure.
- Use indomethacin with extreme caution in patients with history of GI bleeding or ulcer disease because NSAIDs, such as indomethacin, increase risk of GI bleeding and ulceration. Expect to use drug for shortest time possible in these patients.
- Be aware that serious GI tract, bleeding, perforation, and ulceration may occur without warning symptoms. Elderly patients are at greater risk. To minimize risk, give oral indomethacin with an antacid, food, or a full glass of water (not suspension), to reduce GI distress.
- Know that if GI distress occurs, withhold drug and notify prescriber immediately.
- Use indomethacin cautiously in patients with hypertension, and monitor blood pressure closely throughout therapy. Drug may cause hypertension or worsen it.

! WARNING Monitor patient closely for thrombotic events, including MI and stroke, because NSAIDs increase the risk. These events may occur early in treatment and risk increases with duration of use. Be aware that these events have occurred even in patients who do not have a history or risk factors for cardiovascular disease. Monitor patient for warning signs such as chest pain, slurring of speech, shortness of breath, or weakness. If any signs and symptoms develop, withhold indomethacin, alert prescriber immediately, and provide supportive care as prescribed.

- Monitor patient—especially if he's elderly or receiving long-term indomethacin therapy—for less common but serious adverse GI reactions, including anorexia, constipation, diverticulitis, dysphagia, esophagitis, gastritis, gastroenteritis, gastroesophageal reflux disease, hemorrhoids, hiatal hernia, melena, stomatitis, and vomiting.

- Monitor liver enzymes because, rarely, elevations may progress to severe hepatic reactions, including fatal hepatitis, hepatic failure, and liver necrosis.
- Monitor BUN and serum creatinine levels in elderly patients, those taking ACE inhibitors or diuretics, and those with heart failure, hepatic dysfunction, or impaired renal function; drug may cause renal failure.
- Monitor CBC for decreased hemoglobin and hematocrit. Drug may worsen anemia.

! WARNING Know that if patient has bone marrow suppression or is receiving an antineoplastic drug, monitor laboratory results (including WBC count), and watch for evidence of infection because anti-inflammatory and antipyretic actions of indomethacin may mask signs and symptoms, such as fever and pain.

! WARNING Assess patient's skin regularly for signs of rash or other hypersensitivity reaction because indomethacin is an NSAID and may cause serious skin reactions (including DRESS) without warning, even in patients with no history of NSAID sensitivity. At first sign of reaction, stop drug and notify prescriber.

- Monitor weight and blood pressure, especially if patient has hypertension, because indomethacin causes sodium retention.
- Keep in mind that when drug is used to treat gouty arthritis, significant swelling will gradually disappear over 3 to 5 days.
- Assess for improved joint mobility and reduced pain and inflammation to evaluate drug effectiveness.
- Expect patient to have intermittent checkups during long-term therapy and an ophthalmologic examination if vision changes.

PATIENT TEACHING

- Urge patient to take indomethacin capsules with a full glass of water and to avoid lying down for 15 to 30 minutes afterward. This helps prevent drug from lodging in esophagus and causing irritation. Caution patient not to chew, crush, or open capsules. Tell patient to shake suspension well before taking it and to use a calibrated device to measure dosage, not a household spoon.
- Instruct patient to take drug immediately after meals or with food to reduce GI distress.
- Instruct patient to make sure suppository stays in rectum at least 1 hour.
- Urge patient to avoid alcohol during indomethacin therapy.
- Remind patient that improvement may not occur for 2 to 4 weeks after starting indomethacin to treat arthritis or ankylosing spondylitis and that he should continue taking drug, as prescribed.
- Caution against prolonged sun exposure during therapy.
- Urge patient to notify prescriber immediately about changes in hearing or vision, fever, itching, rash, sore throat, or swelling in arms or legs.
- Emphasize importance of having ordered laboratory tests and eye examinations during long-term therapy.
- Caution pregnant patient not to take NSAIDs such as indomethacin during last trimester because they may cause premature closure of the ductus arteriosus.

! WARNING Explain that indomethacin may increase risk of serious adverse cardiovascular reactions; urge patient to seek immediate medical attention if signs or symptoms arise, such as chest pain, edema, shortness of breath, slurring of speech, unexplained weight gain, or weakness.

- Explain that indomethacin may increase risk of serious adverse GI reactions; emphasize need to seek immediate medical attention for such signs and symptoms as abdominal or epigastric pain, black or tarry stools, indigestion, or vomiting blood or material that looks like coffee grounds.

! WARNING Alert patient to rare but serious skin reactions as well as allergic reactions. Urge him to seek immediate medical attention for blisters, fever, itching, rash, or other indications of hypersensitivity.

infliximab
Remicade

infliximab abda
Renflexis

infliximab axxq
Avsola

infliximab dyyb
Inflectra

infliximab-qbtx
Ixifi

☰ Class and Category
Pharmacologic class: Monoclonal antibody (tumor necrosis factor [TNF] blocker)
Therapeutic class: Anti-inflammatory

☰ Indications and Dosages
* *To control moderate to severe Crohn's disease long-term; to reduce number of draining enterocutaneous and rectovaginal fistulas; to maintain fistula closure in patients with fistulizing Crohn's disease; to treat active ankylosing spondylitis; to treat psoriatic arthritis with or without methotrexate; to treat moderate to severe active ulcerative colitis in patients who have had an inadequate response to conventional therapy; to treat chronic severe plaque psoriasis in patients who are candidates for systemic therapy and when other systemic therapies are medically less appropriate*

I.V. INFUSION
Adults. *Initial:* 5 mg/kg, repeated 2 and 6 wk after first infusion. *Maintenance:* 5 mg/kg every 6 wk (active ankylosing spondylitis) or 8 wk (other indications).

±**DOSAGE ADJUSTMENT** For adults who respond to treatment for Crohn's disease and then lose response, dosage may be increased to 10 mg/kg.

* *To treat moderate to severe pediatric Crohn's disease; to treat moderate to severe pediatric active ulcerative colitis*

I.V. INFUSION
Children ages 6 and over. 5 mg/kg, repeated 2 and 6 wk after first infusion. *Maintenance:* 5 mg/kg every 8 wk.

* *As adjunct to treat moderate to severe active rheumatoid arthritis along with methotrexate*

I.V. INFUSION
Adults. *Initial:* 3 mg/kg, repeated 2 and 6 wk after first infusion. *Maintenance:* 3 mg/kg every 8 wk.

±**DOSAGE ADJUSTMENT** For adults who have an incomplete response for treatment of rheumatoid arthritis, dosage increased up to 10 mg/kg per infusion or treatment frequency increased to every 4 wk.

☰ Drug Administration
I.V.
- Store unopened drug vials in a refrigerator. If needed, unopened drug vials may be stored at room temperature for a single period of up to 6 months but not exceeding expiration date. Once removed from refrigerator, do not return to refrigerator.
- Expect to premedicate patient, as prescribed, with acetaminophen, antihistamines, and/or corticosteroids to decrease an infusion reaction.
- Calculate dose, total volume of reconstituted drug solution required, and the number of vials needed. More than one vial may be needed for a full dose.
- Reconstitute drug by using a 21G (or smaller) needle to add 10 ml Sterile Water for Injection to each 100-mg drug vial. Concentration will be 10 mg/ml.
- Swirl to mix; don't shake. Let reconstituted solution stand for 5 minutes. Solution may foam and should be clear or light yellow.
- Do not store reconstituted solution.
- Withdraw volume equal to amount of reconstituted drug from a 250-ml bottle or bag of 0.9% Sodium Chloride Injection. Then slowly add reconstituted drug to bottle to dilute to 250 ml. Gently invert bag to mix. Infusion concentration should range between 0.4 mg/ml (minimum concentration) and 4 mg/ml (maximum concentration). For volumes greater than 250 ml, either use a larger infusion bag (e.g., 500 ml) or multiple 250-ml infusion bags to ensure that the concentration of the infusion solution does not exceed 4 mg/ml.

- Use within 3 hours.
- Infuse over at least 2 hours using infusion set and in-line, sterile, nonpyrogenic, low–protein-binding filter with pores 1.2 microns or less.
- If a mild to moderate infusion reaction occurs, notify prescriber and expect to slow or suspend infusion. If infusion was suspended, know that once the reaction has been resolved, the infusion may be restarted at a lower infusion rate and patient premedicated if not done before.
- If a severe infusion reaction occurs, know that infusion should be stopped and drug permanently discontinued. Be prepared to provide supportive emergency care according to protocol.
- *Incompatibilities:* Diluents except for 0.9% Sodium Chloride Injection; other I.V. drugs infused in the same I.V. line

Route	Onset	Peak	Duration
I.V.	Unknown	Unknown	Unknown

Half-life: 7.7–9.5 days

Mechanism of Action

Binds with cytokine tumor necrosis factor-alpha (TNF-alpha), preventing it from binding with its receptors. As a result, TNF-alpha can't produce proinflammatory cytokines and endothelial permeability. Infiltration of inflammatory cells declines.

Contraindications

Doses greater than 5 mg/kg in patients with moderate to severe heart failure; hypersensitivity to infliximab, murine proteins, or their components

Interactions

DRUGS

abatacept, anakinra, etanercept, tocilizumab: Increased risk of neutropenia and serious infections

CYP450 substrates such as cyclosporine, theophylline, warfarin: May normalize formation of CYP450 enzymes which could affect dosage requirements of these drugs

immunosuppressants: Fewer infusion reactions in patients treated for Crohn's disease

live vaccines, therapeutic infectious agents such as BCG in bladder instillation: Increased risk of adverse vaccine effects

methotrexate: Decreased incidence of anti-infliximab antibody production and increased infliximab product concentrations

Adverse Reactions

CNS: Chills, **CVA**, central nervous system demyelinating disorders, dizziness, fatigue, fever, headache, **meningitis**, neuritis, neuropathies, numbness, paresthesia, peripheral demyelinating disorders, **seizures**, syncope, tingling

CV: **Arrhythmias**, **bradycardia**, chest pain, edema, **heart failure**, hypertension, **hypotension**, **MI**, myocardial ischemia, myelitis, neuropathies, **pericardial effusion**, systemic vasculitis, thrombophlebitis

EENT: **Laryngeal/pharyngeal edema**, oral candidiasis, pharyngitis, rhinitis, sinusitis, transient vision loss, visual changes

GI: Abdominal hernia; abdominal pain; **acute hepatic failure**; cholecystitis; cholestasis; constipation; diarrhea; dyspepsia; elevated liver enzymes; **GI hemorrhage**; **hepatitis**, **hepatotoxicity**; ileus; **intestinal obstruction**, **perforation**, or **stenosis**; jaundice; **melena**; nausea; **pancreatitis**; splenic infarction; splenomegaly; vomiting

GU: **Cervical cancer**, kidney infection, **renal failure**, ureteral obstruction, UTI, vaginal candidiasis, vaginitis

HEME: **Agranulocytosis**, anemia, **aplastic anemia**, **hemolytic anemia**, **leukemia**, **leukopenia**, **neutropenia**, **pancytopenia**, **thrombocytopenia**, **thrombocytopenic purpura**, **thrombotic thrombocytopenic purpura**

MS: Ankylosing spondylitis, arthralgia, back pain, limb weakness, myalgia, psoriatic arthritis, transverse myelitis

RESP: **Adult respiratory distress syndrome**, bronchitis, **bronchospasms (severe)**, cough, dyspnea, **interstitial lung disease**, pleurisy, pneumonia, **pulmonary edema**, tuberculosis, respiratory tract infection, **severe bronchospasm**, wheezing

SKIN: Acute generalized exanthematous pustulosis, cellulitis, cutaneous vasculitis, diaphoresis, **erythema multiforme**, facial flushing, lichenoid reactions, linear IgA bullous dermatosis, **melanoma, Merkel cell cancer**, pruritus, psoriasis (new or worsening), rash, **Stevens–Johnson syndrome, toxic epidermal necrolysis,** urticaria

G
H
I

Other: Anaphylaxis; antibody formation to infliximab; bacterial (including *Legionella* and *Listeria*), fungal, mycobacterial, parasitic, or viral infections; dehydration; infusion reaction; lupus-like symptoms; lymphadenopathy; **malignancies, such as lymphomas, including hepatosplenic T-cell lymphoma**; sarcoidosis; **sepsis**; serum sickness; vaccine breakthrough infection

Childbearing Considerations

PREGNANCY

- It is not known if drug causes fetal harm but it does cross the placental barrier and cases of agranulocytosis in infants exposed to drug in utero have been reported as well as an increased risk of infection that can become fatal.
- Use with caution only if benefit to mother outweighs potential risk to fetus.
- Know that a six-month waiting period following birth is recommended before live vaccines should be administered to the infant.

LACTATION

- Drug may be present in breast milk at low levels.
- Patient should check with prescriber before breastfeeding.

Nursing Considerations

- Update patient's vaccinations with current vaccination guidelines prior to initiating infliximab.
- Know that infliximab therapy shouldn't be started in a patient with an active infection, including serious localized infection.
- Know that because drug increases risk of developing tuberculosis or reactivating latent tuberculosis, expect prescriber to evaluate patient's risk and start tuberculosis treatment, as needed, before starting infliximab.
- Use with extreme caution if patient has a history of chronic or recurrent infection, known exposure to tuberculosis, an underlying condition that predisposes to infection, or residence or travel to areas of endemic tuberculosis or mycoses, such as blastomycosis, coccidioidomycosis, or histoplasmosis.
- Use with extreme caution in patients with heart failure because drug can worsen heart failure and increase mortality in these patients. Also know that new heart failure can develop in patients without known preexisting cardiovascular disease. Closely monitor patient throughout infliximab therapy for signs and symptoms of heart failure. If new or worsening symptoms of heart failure occur, expect drug to be discontinued.

- Use cautiously in elderly patients because they have a higher risk of infection than younger patients taking infliximab.
- Use cautiously in patients with previous or ongoing hematologic abnormalities because infliximab may cause serious or even life-threatening adverse hematologic effects. Monitor patient's CBC regularly, as ordered. If adverse effects occur, expect drug to be discontinued.
- Use cautiously in patients with CNS demyelinating disorders such as multiple sclerosis and optic neuritis; use cautiously in patients with peripheral demyelinating disorders such as Guillain–Barré syndrome. If these disorders develop or worsen, expect drug to be discontinued.
- Be aware that use of TNF-blocking therapy, including infliximab, may reactivate hepatitis B virus in patients who are chronic carriers of this virus. Ensure that patient has been tested for hepatitis B infection before infliximab therapy is begun. For patients who develop reactivation of hepatitis B, know that therapy should be stopped and antiviral therapy with appropriate supportive treatment begun.

! **WARNING** Be aware that infliximab increases risk of serious or fatal opportunistic infections, including invasive fungal infections, as well as bacterial (including *Legionella* and *Listeria*), mycobacterial, parasitic, and viral infections. The most common ones include aspergillosis, blastomycosis, candidiasis, coccidioidomycosis, cryptococcosis, histoplasmosis, legionellosis, listeriosis, pneumocystis, salmonellosis, and tuberculosis.

! **WARNING** Watch for other infections, especially if patient receives immunosuppressant therapy or has a chronic infection. Upper respiratory tract infections and UTIs are most common, but sepsis and fatal infections have occurred. If infection is suspected, notify prescriber, and if a serious infection is confirmed, expect drug to be discontinued.

! **WARNING** Monitor patient for a hypersensitivity or infusion reaction, which usually occurs during or within 2 hours of infliximab infusion. However, a reaction may occur 2 hours to 12 days after infusion. If present, notify prescriber and expect drug to be discontinued for severe hypersensitivity reactions. Provide supportive care, as prescribed.

- Monitor patient closely for the first 24 hours after the initial drug infusion because serious cardiovascular and cerebrovascular reactions, such as CVA, MI, seizures, or severe bronchospasms, may occur during and after infusion. Also, monitor patient for transient visual loss during or within 2 hours of infusion.
- Monitor liver function because severe hepatic reactions may occur. Expect to stop drug if jaundice develops or liver enzymes are five times or more the upper limit of normal.
- Be aware that infliximab is a tumor necrosis factor (TNF) blocker. Malignancies, especially leukemia and such rare lymphomas as hepatosplenic T-cell lymphoma, have been reported in patients, particularly children and adolescents, receiving TNF blockers. Patients at increased risk of leukemia are those with rheumatoid arthritis. Patients at increased risk of lymphomas are those with ankylosing spondylitis, Crohn's disease, plaque psoriasis, psoriatic arthritis, and rheumatoid arthritis, especially those with long-term or very active disease. Other malignancies, such as cervical cancer and skin cancer, have also occurred. Monitor them closely.

PATIENT TEACHING

- Urge patient to report evidence of infection, such as cough, painful urination, and sore throat. Infusion reaction (chest pain, chills, dyspnea, facial flushing, fever, itching, headache, rash) may occur for up to 12 days.
- Explain that infliximab increases the risk of lymphoma and other malignancies; urge prompt medical attention for suspicious

signs or symptoms. Also, advise patient to have regular skin examinations because drug increases risk of skin cancer and for female patients to have periodic screening for cervical cancer.

- Review signs and symptoms of heart failure, hepatotoxicity, and hematologic reactions as well as neurologic abnormalities that may occur, and instruct patient to notify prescriber if any develops. Stress importance of seeking immediate medical attention if patient experiences heart or stroke signs and symptoms within 24 hours of drug administration.

! **WARNING** Tell patient to seek immediate medical attention if an allergic reaction occurs.

- Advise patient not to receive vaccinations using live vaccines or infectious agents. Also advise parents not to have their infant exposed to live vaccines for up to 6 months after birth if the mother was taking infliximab during the pregnancy.

insulin, inhaled
(rapid-acting)
Afrezza

Class and Category
Pharmacologic class: Human insulin
Therapeutic class: Antidiabetic

Indications and Dosages
* *To improve glycemic control in patients with diabetes mellitus*

ORAL INHALATION
Adults who are not currently taking insulin. *Initial:* 4 units at each meal with dosage increased, as needed.
Adults converting from subcutaneous mealtime (prandial) insulin. Dosage dependent upon subcutaneous insulin dosage as follows: 4 units with each meal, if up to 4 units of subcutaneous mealtime insulin was being used; 8 units with each meal, if 5 to 8 units of subcutaneous mealtime insulin were used; 12 units with each meal, if 9 to 12 units of subcutaneous mealtime insulin were used; 16 units with each meal, if 13 to 16 units of subcutaneous mealtime insulin were used;

20 units with each meal, if 17 to 20 units of subcutaneous mealtime insulin were used; and 24 units with each meal, if 21 to 24 units of subcutaneous mealtime insulin were used. *Maintenance*: Dosage based on blood glucose monitoring results, glycemic control goal, and metabolic needs.

Adults converting from subcutaneous premixed insulin. Both basal and mealtime dosages required for conversion. *Mealtime dosage*: Beginning-of-mealtime injected dose estimated by dividing half of the total daily injected premixed insulin dose equally among the three meals of the day. Then each estimated injected mealtime dose converted as follows: 4 units if up to 4 units of subcutaneous premixed insulin were used; 8 units if 5 to 8 units of subcutaneous premixed insulin were used; 12 units if 9 to 12 units of subcutaneous premixed insulin were used; 16 units if 13 to 16 units of subcutaneous premixed insulin were used; 20 units if 17 to 20 units of subcutaneous premixed insulin were used; and 24 units if 21 to 24 units of subcutaneous premixed insulin were used. *Basal dosage*: The remaining half of the total daily injected premixed dose injected as a basal insulin dose. *Maintenance*: Mealtime and basal dosages based on blood glucose monitoring results, glycemic control goal, and metabolic needs.

±**DOSAGE ADJUSTMENT** Dosage may have to be decreased if patient is taking any of the following drugs concurrently: angiotensin-converting enzyme (ACE) inhibitors, angiotensin II receptor blocking agents, disopyramide, fibrates, fluoxetine, monoamine oxidase inhibitors, other antidiabetic agents, pentoxifylline, pramlintide, propoxyphene, salicylates, somatostatin analogues, or sulfonamide antibiotics. Dosage may have to be increased if patient is taking any of the following drugs concurrently: atypical antipsychotics, corticosteroids, danazol, diuretics, estrogens, glucagon, isoniazid, niacin, oral contraceptives, phenothiazines, progestogens, protease inhibitors, somatropin, sympathomimetic agents, or thyroid hormones. Dosage may have to be increased or decreased if patient is taking any of the following concurrently: alcohol, beta-blockers, clonidine, lithium, or pentamidine.

Drug Administration
INHALATION
- Administer inhaled insulin using only the Afrezza inhaler. Each cartridge provides a single inhalation. Cartridges left over in an opened strip must be used within 3 days.
- Doses that exceed 12 units per mealtime will require more than one cartridge.
- Administer at the beginning of meals. Cartridges and inhaler should be at room temperature for 10 minutes before use.
- To load a cartridge into the inhaler, keep the inhaler level in one hand with the white mouthpiece on top and the purple base on the bottom. Open inhaler by lifting the white mouthpiece to a vertical position. Hold the cartridge with the cup facing down. Line up the cartridge with the opening in the inhaler. The pointed end of the cartridge should line up with the pointed end in the inhaler. Place the cartridge into the inhaler, making sure the cartridge lies flat in the inhaler. Lower the mouthpiece to close the inhaler. A snap should be felt when the inhaler is closed.
- Loss of drug effect can occur if the inhaler is turned upside down, held with the mouthpiece pointing down, or shaken (or dropped) after the cartridge has been inserted but before the dose has been administered. If any of these events occurs, replace the cartridge before use.
- Have the patient hold the inhaler away from mouth and fully exhale. Then have patient, while keeping head level, place the mouthpiece in his mouth and tilt the inhaler down toward his chin. He should close his lips to form a seal. With his mouth closed around the mouthpiece, have patient inhale deeply through the inhaler. Have him hold his breath as long as comfortable while removing the inhaler from his mouth. After holding his breath, the patient can then exhale and continue to breathe normally.
- Replace the purple mouthpiece cover onto the inhaler. Open the inhaler by lifting up the white mouthpiece and remove cartridge from purple base. Discard used cartridge.
- If more than one cartridge is needed for dose, repeat the steps again for each cartridge used.
- Discard Afrezza inhaler after 15 days.

Route	Onset	Peak	Duration
Inhalation	1–2 min	15–20 min	2.5–3 hr
Half-life: 28–29 min			

Mechanism of Action

Lowers blood glucose levels by stimulating peripheral glucose uptake by fat and skeletal muscle, and by inhibiting hepatic glucose production. Also enhances protein synthesis, inhibits lipolysis in adipocytes, and inhibits proteolysis.

Contraindications

Chronic lung disease (asthma, chronic obstructive pulmonary disease), during episodes of hypoglycemia, hypersensitivity to regular human insulin or any of its components

Interactions

DRUGS

angiotensin-converting enzyme (ACE) inhibitors, angiotensin II receptor blocking agents, disopyramide, fibrates, fluoxetine, monoamine oxidase inhibitors, other antidiabetic agents, pentoxifylline, pramlintide, propoxyphene, salicylates, somatostatin analogues, sulfonamide antibiotics: Increased risk of hypoglycemia
atypical antipsychotics, corticosteroids, danazol, diuretics, estrogens, glucagon, isoniazid, niacin, oral contraceptives, phenothiazines, progestogens, protease inhibitors, somatropin, sympathomimetic agents, thyroid hormones: Decreased effectiveness of inhaled insulin
beta-blockers, clonidine, lithium, or pentamidine: Possibly decreased or increased blood glucose levels
beta-blockers, clonidine, guanethidine, reserpine: Blunted hypoglycemic signs and symptoms
thiazolidinediones: Increased risk of fluid retention and heart failure

ACTIVITIES

alcohol use: Possibly decreased or increased blood glucose levels

Adverse Reactions

CNS: Confusion, dizziness, drowsiness, fatigue, headache
CV: Tachycardia
EENT: Throat irritation or pain
ENDO: **Diabetic ketoacidosis,** hypoglycemia

GI: Diarrhea, nausea
GU: UTI
RESP: **Acute bronchospasm,** bronchitis, cough, decline in pulmonary function, dyspnea, **lung cancer** (rare), shortness of breath
SKIN: Diaphoresis, rash
Other: **Anaphylaxis, angioedema,** anti-insulin antibodies, **hypokalemia,** weight gain

Childbearing Considerations

PREGNANCY

- It is not known if drug causes fetal harm.
- Use with caution only if benefit to mother outweighs potential risk to fetus.

LACTATION

- It is not known if drug is present in breast milk.
- Patient should check with prescriber before breastfeeding.

Nursing Considerations

- Be aware that inhaled insulin is not a substitute for long-acting insulin and must be used in combination with long-acting insulin in patients with type 1 diabetes mellitus.
- Know that inhaled insulin should not be used to treat diabetic ketoacidosis, nor should it be used in patients who smoke or who have recently stopped smoking. Also know that drug is not recommended in patients with active lung cancer or who have a prior history of lung cancer or risk factors for lung cancer because, although rare, lung cancer has occurred in nonsmokers prescribed inhaled insulin.
- Ensure that patient has had a complete medical history, physical examination, and spirometry before inhaled insulin therapy is begun, to identify potential lung disease, as the drug is contraindicated in patients with chronic lung disease. Spirometry should be repeated after the first 6 months of therapy and annually thereafter. Expect drug to be discontinued if patient experiences a 20% or more decline in pulmonary function.

! **WARNING** Monitor patient closely for signs and symptoms of hypoglycemia, which could become severe, causing seizures or even death. If present, withhold inhaled insulin, treat according to standard of care, and notify prescriber.

G
H
I

- Monitor patient's blood glucose level closely to detect need for dosage adjustment, as ordered. Expect dosage adjustments with changes in patient's hepatic or renal function, meal patterns, and physical activity, or during acute illness.

! **WARNING** Monitor patient for hypersensitivity reactions. If present, withhold drug, treat according to standard of care, and monitor patient closely until signs and symptoms resolve. Notify prescriber and expect drug to be discontinued and replaced with subcutaneous forms of insulin therapy.

- Monitor patient's serum potassium levels throughout inhaled insulin therapy in patients at risk for hypokalemia, such as those using drugs sensitive to serum potassium concentrations, intravenously administered insulin, or potassium-lowering drugs.

PATIENT TEACHING
- Teach patient how to use the inhaler device.
- Tell patient that doses that exceed 12 units per mealtime will require more than one cartridge.
- Instruct patient to keep the inhaler level, the white mouthpiece on the top, and the purple base on the bottom after a cartridge has been inserted into the inhaler. Remind patient that loss of drug effect can occur if the inhaler is turned upside down, held with the mouthpiece pointing down, or shaken (or dropped) after the cartridge has been inserted but before the dose has been administered. If any of these events occurs, tell patient to replace the cartridge before use.

! **WARNING** Review signs and symptoms of hypoglycemia and how to treat them. If frequent or severe, tell patient to notify prescriber, as dosage may have to be adjusted. Stress importance of monitoring blood glucose levels.

- Stress importance of not ingesting alcoholic beverages or smoking while using inhaled insulin.

! **WARNING** Advise patient to notify prescriber if an allergic reaction occurs and to seek immediate medical care if reaction is severe,

such as having difficulty breathing or swelling occurs in face, throat, or tongue.

- Tell patient to avoid performing hazardous activities such as driving until the effects of inhaled insulin on her nervous system is known.

ipratropium bromide
Atrovent HFA, Ipravent (CAN)

☰ Class and Category
Pharmacologic class: Anticholinergic
Therapeutic class: Bronchodilator

☰ Indications and Dosages
✳ *To provide maintenance treatment for bronchospasm associated with chronic obstructive pulmonary disease (COPD), including chronic bronchitis and emphysema*

INHALATION AEROSOL (ATROVENT HFA)
Adults. *Initial:* 2 inhalations four times daily, increased, as needed. *Maximum:* Up to 12 inhalations/24 hr.

INHALATION SOLUTION FOR NEBULIZER (IPRAVENT)
Adults and adolescents. 500 mcg dissolved in preservative-free sterile normal saline solution every 6 to 8 hr.

✳ *To treat perennial and allergic rhinitis*

NASAL SPRAY
Adults and children age 6 and over. 2 sprays of 0.03% (21 mcg/spray) per nostril twice daily or three times daily. *Maximum:* 12 sprays (252 mcg)/24 hr.

✳ *To treat rhinorrhea caused by seasonal allergic rhinitis*

NASAL SPRAY
Adults and children age 5 and over. 2 sprays of 0.06% (42 mcg/spray) per nostril four times daily. *Maximum:* 16 sprays (672 mcg)/24 hr.

✳ *To treat rhinorrhea associated with the common cold*

NASAL SPRAY
Adults and adolescents. 2 sprays of 0.06% (42 mcg/spray) per nostril three or four times daily for up to 4 days.
Children ages 5 to 11. 2 sprays of 0.06% (42 mcg/spray) per nostril three times daily for up to 4 days.

⬛ Mechanism of Action

After acetylcholine is released from cholinergic fibers, ipratropium prevents it from attaching to muscarinic receptors on membranes of smooth muscle cells, as shown here. By blocking acetylcholine's effects in bronchi and bronchioles, ipratropium relaxes smooth muscles and causes bronchodilation.

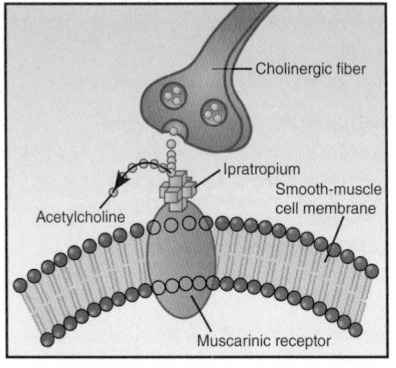

leaking out around mask and causing blurred vision or eye pain.

- Protect vials from light and keep unused vials in foil pouch until ready to use.

Inhaler

- Inhaler should be initially primed with 2 test sprays; if not used for more than 3 days, repeat priming. There is no need to shake inhaler before administration. Wait 15 seconds between inhalations. Attach spacer device to inhaler to improve delivery, if needed. Have patient rinse mouth after inhaling drug. Wash mouthpiece once a week for 30 seconds in warm water and let air-dry. Discard inhaler after the labeled number of actuations has been used, which is usually 200 actuations. The canister may not be completely empty but should be discarded.

Route	Onset	Peak	Duration
Inhalation	15 min	1–2 hr	2–8 hr
Nasal	15 min	Unknown	Unknown

Half-life: 1.6–2 hr

⬛ Drug Administration

INTRANASAL

- Before using for first time, prime nasal spray by pumping bottle 7 times or until a fine spray comes out.
- Have patient blow his nose.
- Have patient insert tip into one nostril while holding opposite nostril closed and leaning head slightly forward.
- Have patient then spray and sniff deeply, then breathe out through his mouth. After administration, have patient lean his head backward for a few seconds. Then repeat in the other nostril.
- If spray pump gets clogged, hold tip of bottle under warm running water for about 1 minute. Dry the pump and prime again.
- If spray bottle is not used for more than 24 hours, prime it again by releasing 2 sprays. If bottle is not used for more than 7 days, prime bottle again by releasing 7 sprays.

INHALATION

Nebulizer

- Inhalation solution is for use with an oral nebulizer. See manufacturer guidelines for administration. When using the nebulizer, apply a mouthpiece to prevent drug from

⬛ Contraindications

Hypersensitivity to atropine, ipratropium bromide, or their components

⬛ Interactions

DRUGS

anticholinergics: Increased anticholinergic effects

⬛ Adverse Reactions

CNS: Dizziness, insomnia
CV: **Atrial fibrillation** (oral inhalation), **bradycardia** (nasal spray), edema, hypertension, palpitations, **supraventricular tachycardia** (oral inhalation), tachycardia
EENT: Acute eye pain, dry mouth or pharyngeal area, increased intraocular pressure, **laryngospasm**, taste perversion, **oropharyngeal edema** (all drug forms); blurred vision, conjunctival and corneal congestion, eye irritation and pain, mydriasis, visual halos (if nasal spray comes in contact with eyes); epistaxis, mydriasis, nasal dryness and irritation, pharyngitis, rhinitis, sinusitis, tinnitus (with nasal spray)
GI: **Bowel obstruction**, constipation, diarrhea, ileus, nausea, vomiting
GU: Prostatitis, urine retention
MS: Arthritis

G
H
I

RESP: Bronchitis, **bronchospasm,** cough, dyspnea, increased sputum production, wheezing
SKIN: Dermatitis, pruritus, rash, urticaria
Other: Anaphylaxis, angioedema, flu-like symptoms

☰ Childbearing Considerations
PREGNANCY
- It is not known if drug causes fetal harm.
- Use with caution only if benefit to mother outweighs potential risk to fetus.

LACTATION
- It is not known if drug is present in breast milk.
- Patient should check with prescriber before breastfeeding.

☰ Nursing Considerations
- Use ipratropium cautiously in patients with angle-closure glaucoma, benign prostatic hyperplasia, or bladder neck obstruction and in patients with hepatic or renal dysfunction.

! **WARNING** Monitor patient for hypersensitivity reactions that could be life-threatening. If present, stop drug use immediately, notify prescriber, and provide supportive care, as needed.

PATIENT TEACHING
- Caution patient not to use ipratropium inhaler to treat acute bronchospasm.
- Teach patient to use inhaler, nasal spray, or nebulizer.
- Advise patient to keep spray out of his eyes because it may irritate them or blur his vision. If spray comes in contact with eyes, instruct patient to flush them with cool tap water for several minutes and to contact prescriber.
- Instruct patient to rinse mouth after each nebulizer or inhaler treatment to help minimize throat dryness and irritation.
- Teach patient to track canister contents in inhaler by counting and recording number of doses.

! **WARNING** Warn patient that an allergic reaction, which could become severe, may occur after using drug. If present, tell patient to immediately discontinue use of drug and notify prescriber if not severe, or seek immediate emergency attention if difficulty breathing or swelling occurs.

- Advise patient to report decreased response to ipratropium as well as difficulty voiding, eye pain, nasal dryness, nose bleeds, palpitations, and vision changes.

irbesartan
Avapro

☰ Class and Category
Pharmacologic class: Angiotensin II receptor antagonist
Therapeutic class: Antihypertensive

☰ Indications and Dosages
∗ *To manage hypertension, alone or with other antihypertensives*

TABLETS
Adults and adolescents. *Initial:* 150 mg once daily, and increased, as needed. *Maximum:* 300 mg daily.

∗ *To treat nephropathy in type 2 diabetes mellitus in patients with hypertension, an elevated serum creatinine, and proteinuria*

TABLETS
Adults. 300 mg once daily.
±**DOSAGE ADJUSTMENT** Initial dosage reduced to 75 mg daily for patients with hyponatremia or hypovolemia from such causes as hemodialysis or vigorous diuretic therapy.

☰ Drug Administration
P.O.
- Administer drug at the same time each day to maintain its therapeutic effect.

Route	Onset	Peak	Duration
P.O.	Unknown	1.5–2 hr	24 hr

Half-life: 11–15 hr

☰ Mechanism of Action
Selectively blocks binding of the potent vasoconstrictor angiotensin (AT) II to AT_1 receptor sites in many tissues, including adrenal glands and vascular smooth muscle. This inhibits the aldosterone-secreting and vasoconstrictive effects of AT II, which reduces blood pressure.

☰ Contraindications
Concurrent aliskiren use in patients with diabetes, hypersensitivity to irbesartan or its components

Interactions

DRUGS

aliskiren (patients with diabetes or renal impairment), angiotensin-converting enzyme (ACE) inhibitors, other angiotensin receptor blockers: Increased risk of hyperkalemia, hypotension, and renal dysfunction

lithium: Possibly increased serum lithium level

NSAIDs: Possible decreased renal function in patients who are elderly, volume-depleted, or have a compromised renal function

potassium-sparing diuretics, potassium supplements, or salt substitutes containing potassium: Possible hyperkalemia

Adverse Reactions

CNS: Anxiety, dizziness, fatigue, headache, nervousness

CV: Chest pain, **hypotension**, peripheral edema, tachycardia

EENT: Pharyngitis, rhinitis, tinnitus

ENDO: **Hypoglycemia** (in diabetic patients)

GI: Abdominal pain, diarrhea, elevated liver enzymes, heartburn, **hepatitis**, indigestion, jaundice, nausea, vomiting

GU: Impaired renal function, **renal failure**, UTI

HEME: Anemia**, thrombocytopenia**

MS: Increased CPK level, musculoskeletal pain, **rhabdomyolysis**

RESP: Upper respiratory tract infection

SKIN: Rash, urticaria

Other: **Anaphylaxis including shock, angioedema, hyperkalemia**

Childbearing Considerations

PREGNANCY

- Drug can cause fetal harm, especially if exposure occurs during the second or third trimester.
- Drug reduces fetal renal function leading to anuria and renal failure and increases fetal and neonatal morbidity and death. It can also cause fetal lung hypoplasia, hypotension, and skeletal deformations such as skull hypoplasia.
- Drug is contraindicated in pregnant women and should be discontinued as soon as possible when pregnancy is known.

LACTATION

- It is not known if drug is present in breast milk.
- A decision should be made to discontinue breastfeeding or the drug to avoid potential serious adverse reactions including hyperkalemia, hypotension, and renal impairment in the breastfed infant.

Nursing Considerations

- Know that if patient has known or suspected hypovolemia, provide treatment, such as I.V. 0.9% Sodium Chloride Injection, as prescribed, to correct this condition before beginning irbesartan therapy. Or expect to begin therapy with a lower dosage.
- Check blood pressure often to evaluate drug's effectiveness.
- Be aware that if blood pressure isn't controlled with irbesartan alone, expect to also give a diuretic, such as hydrochlorothiazide, as prescribed.

! **WARNING** Be alert for hypotension in a patient who receives a diuretic or another antihypertensive during irbesartan therapy. Frequently monitor blood pressure. If patient experiences symptomatic hypotension, expect to stop drug temporarily. Immediately place him in supine position and prepare to give I.V. normal saline solution, as prescribed. Expect to resume drug therapy after blood pressure stabilizes.

- Be aware that if patient receives a diuretic, provide adequate hydration, as appropriate, to help prevent hypovolemia. Also monitor patient for signs and symptoms of hypovolemia, such as dizziness, fainting, and hypotension.
- Monitor patients with diabetes mellitus for hypoglycemia.

! **WARNING** Monitor patient for increased BUN and serum creatinine levels if he has heart failure or impaired renal function because drug may cause acute renal failure. If increases are significant or persistent, notify prescriber immediately.

PATIENT TEACHING

- Advise patient to take drug at the same time each day to maintain its therapeutic effect.
- Explain importance of regular exercise, proper diet, and other lifestyle changes in controlling hypertension.
- Caution patient to avoid hazardous activities until drug's CNS effects are known.

G
H
I

- Instruct patient to consult prescriber before taking any new drug.
- To reduce risk of dehydration and hypotension, advise patient to drink adequate fluids during hot weather and exercise.
- Advise patients with diabetes mellitus to be alert for signs and symptoms of hypoglycemia and to treat immediately. If hypoglycemia occurs frequently or is severe, tell patient to notify prescriber.
- Instruct patient to contact prescriber if diarrhea, severe nausea, or vomiting occurs and continues, because of the risk of dehydration and hypotension.

! **WARNING** Advise female patient to notify prescriber immediately about known or suspected pregnancy. Explain that if she becomes pregnant, prescriber may replace irbesartan with another antihypertensive that's safe to use during pregnancy.

- Urge patient to keep follow-up appointments with prescriber to monitor progress.

iron dextran
(contains 50 mg of elemental iron per milliliter)
Dexiron (CAN), InFeD

Class and Category
Pharmacologic class: Iron mineral
Therapeutic class: Hematinic

Indications and Dosages
✳ *To treat iron deficiency anemia when oral administration is impossible or unsatisfactory*

I.M. OR I.V. INJECTION
Adults and children weighing more than 15 kg (33 lb). Calculated using following formula: Dose (ml) = 0.0442 (desired hemoglobin − observed hemoglobin) × lean body weight (LBW) in kg (Males = 50 kg + 2.3 kg for each inch of patient's height over 5 feet. Females = 45.5 kg + 2.3 kg for each inch of patient's height over 5 feet.) + (0.26 × LBW). Or, consult dosage table in package insert. *Test dose on day 1:* 0.5 ml followed in 1 hr or more with remainder of dose, if no reaction occurs. Total dosage repeated once daily thereafter. *Maximum:* 100 mg daily.

Children over age 4 months weighing 5 to 15 kg (11 to 33 lb). Calculated using following formula: Dose (ml) = 0.0442 (desired hemoglobin − observed hemoglobin) × weight in kg + (0.26 × weight in kg). Or, consult dosage table in package insert. *Test dose on day 1:* 0.5 ml followed in 1 hr or more with remainder of dose, if no reaction occurs. Total dosage repeated once daily thereafter. *Maximum daily dosage:* 2 ml (100 mg for heavier children and adults); 1 ml (50 mg for children weighing less than 10 kg); 0.5 ml (25 mg for infants weighing less than 5 kg)

✳ *To replace iron lost in blood loss*

I.V. INJECTION
Adults. Replacement iron (mg) = Blood loss (ml) × hematocrit divided by 50 mg/ml.

Drug Administration
I.V.
- Infuse undiluted slowly, at no more than 1 ml/minute (50 mg/minute).
- Flush with 10 ml of 0.9% Sodium Chloride Injection after administration.
- *Incompatibilities:* Other drugs, or parenteral nutrition solutions for I.V. infusion

I.M.
- Change needle after drawing up iron dextran into syringe.
- Administer using Z-track method using a 2- to 3-inch, 19G or 20G needle.
- Inject deep into the upper outer quadrant of patient's buttock. Do not inject drug into any other site.

Route	Onset	Peak	Duration
I.V./I.M.	1–2 days	7–9 days	Unknown

Half-life: 6 hr

Mechanism of Action
Restores hemoglobin and replenishes iron stores. Iron, an essential component of hemoglobin, myoglobin, and several enzymes (including catalase, cytochromes, and peroxidase), is needed for catecholamine metabolism and normal neutrophil function. In iron dextran therapy, iron binds to available protein parts after the drug has been split into dextran and iron by cells of the reticuloendothelial system. The bound iron forms hemosiderin or ferritin, physiologic forms of iron, and transferrin, which

replenish hemoglobin and deplete iron stores. Dextran is metabolized or excreted.

Contraindications

Anemia other than iron deficiency, hypersensitivity to iron dextran or its components

Interactions

DRUGS

angiotensin-converting enzyme inhibitors: Possibly increased risk for anaphylactic-type reaction

Adverse Reactions

CNS: Chills, disorientation, dizziness, fever, headache, malaise, paresthesia, **seizures**, syncope, unconsciousness, weakness
CV: Arrhythmias, bradycardia, chest pain, hypertension, **hypotension, shock**, tachycardia
EENT: Altered taste
GI: Abdominal pain, diarrhea, nausea, vomiting
GU: Hematuria
HEME: Leukocytosis
MS: Arthralgia, arthritis, backache, myalgia, **rhabdomyolysis**
RESP: Bronchospasm, cyanosis, dyspnea, **respiratory arrest**, wheezing
SKIN: Diaphoresis, rash, pruritus, purpura, urticaria
Other: Anaphylaxis, infusion-site phlebitis

Childbearing Considerations

PREGNANCY

- It is not known if drug causes fetal harm. However, fetal bradycardia may occur, especially in the second and third trimester, if mother develops a severe hypersensitivity reaction to the drug.
- Use with caution only if benefit to mother outweighs potential risk to fetus.

LACTATION

- Drug is present in breast milk in trace amounts.
- Patient should check with prescriber before breastfeeding.

Nursing Considerations

- Be aware that iron dextran is given only when oral therapy isn't feasible.
- Expect to monitor hematocrit, hemoglobin level, serum ferritin level, and transferrin saturation, as ordered, before, during, and after iron dextran therapy.

! WARNING Expect with first dose to administer a test dose as prescribed, and monitor patient closely for anaphylactic reaction. Expect to wait 1 or more hours before giving remainder of dose if no reaction occurs.

! WARNING Monitor patient closely for signs and symptoms of anaphylaxis (such as collapse, dyspnea, loss of consciousness, seizures, and severe hypotension) during and after drug administration. Patients with a history of allergies or asthma or who take angiotensin-converting enzyme inhibitors are at increased risk for anaphylaxis, possibly death. Institute emergency resuscitation measures as needed, including epinephrine administration, as prescribed.

! WARNING Assess blood pressure often after iron dextran administration, especially if given intravenously, because hypotension is a common adverse effect that may be related to infusion rate; avoid rapid infusion.

- Be aware that patient may have adverse reactions, including arthralgia, backache, chills, and vomiting, 1 to 2 days after drug therapy. Symptoms should resolve within 3 to 4 days.
- Assess patients with a history of rheumatoid arthritis for exacerbation of joint pain and swelling.
- Know that if patient has cardiovascular disease, watch for worsening from drug's adverse effects.
- Assess patient for iron overload, characterized by bleeding in GI tract and lungs, decreased activity, pale eyes, and sedation.
- Be aware iron dextran may give a brown color to serum from a blood sample drawn 4 hours after administration and may cause falsely elevated serum bilirubin and falsely decreased values of serum calcium. Serum iron determinations may not be accurate for 23 weeks following iron dextran administration, especially if done by colorimetric assays.

PATIENT TEACHING

- Instruct patient to report immediately signs of adverse reaction, such as rash, shortness of breath, or wheezing, during iron dextran therapy.

G
H
I

- Advise patient not to take any oral iron without first consulting prescriber.
- Urge patient to plan periods of activity and rest to avoid excessive fatigue.
- Emphasize need to follow dosage regimen and keep follow-up medical and laboratory appointments.

iron sucrose

(contains 100 mg of elemental iron per 5 ml)
Venofer

Class and Category
Pharmacologic class: Iron mineral
Therapeutic class: Hematinic

Indications and Dosages

✳ *To treat iron deficiency anemia in patients with hemodialysis dependent-chronic kidney disease*

I.V. INJECTION, I.V. INFUSION

Adults. *Initial:* 100 mg elemental iron injected undiluted over 2 to 5 min early during dialysis. Alternatively, 100 mg elemental iron infused diluted and infused over at least 15 min early during dialysis. *Usual:* 100 mg elemental iron every wk to 3 times/wk to total dose of 1,000 mg. Dosage repeated as needed to maintain target levels of hemoglobin and hematocrit and acceptable blood iron level. *Maximum:* 100 mg/dose.

✳ *To treat iron deficiency anemia patients with peritoneal dialysis–dependent chronic kidney disease*

I.V. INFUSION

Adults. *Initial:* 300 mg elemental iron infused diluted over 1.5 hr on days 1 and 14, followed by 400 mg elemental iron infused over 2.5 hr on day 28. Dosage repeated as needed to maintain target levels of hemoglobin and hematocrit and acceptable blood iron level. *Maximum:* 1,000 mg/28 days.

✳ *To maintain iron therapy in children with chronic kidney disease who are nondialysis-dependent receiving erythropoietin or who are peritoneal dialysis–dependent receiving erythropoietin; to maintain iron therapy in children with hemodialysis dependent-chronic kidney disease (HDD-CKD)*

I.V. INJECTION, I.V. INFUSION

Children age 2 years and over. 0.5 mg/kg, not to exceed 100 mg/dose, every 2 wk (HDD-CKD) or 4 wk (other indications) for 12 wk given undiluted over 5 min as an I.V. injection or diluted and infused over 5 to 60 min as an I.V. infusion. Treatment repeated, as needed.

✳ *To treat iron deficiency anemia in nondialysis patients with chronic renal disease (NDD-CKD).*

I.V. INJECTION, I.V. INFUSION

Adults. *Initial:* 200 mg elemental iron injected undiluted over 2 to 5 min and repeated 4 more times over a 14-day period for a total dose of 1,000 mg. Alternatively, 200 mg elemental iron infused diluted over at least 15 min or 500 mg elemental iron infused diluted over 3.5 to 4 hr on day 1 and day 14. Dosage repeated as needed to maintain target levels of hemoglobin and hematocrit and acceptable blood iron level. *Maximum:* 1,000 mg/14 days.

Drug Administration

I.V.

- Follow guidelines given under each indication for administration times for both injection and infusion, as there are differences based on indication.
- If given during hemodialysis, administer early during the dialysis session (usually within the first hour).
- For I.V. injection, administer undiluted.
- For I.V. infusion in adults, dilute 100 mg or 200 mg elemental iron in maximum of 100 ml 0.9% Sodium Chloride Injection; 300 or 400 mg in maximum of 250 ml of 0.9% Sodium Chloride Injection. Dilute immediately before infusion.
- For I.V. infusion in children, dilute with 0.9% Sodium Chloride Injection to a concentration of 1 to 2 mg/ml. Do not dilute to concentrations below 1 mg/ml. Dilute immediately before infusion.
- Discard any unused diluted solution.
- Store in original carton at controlled room temperature.
- Drug diluted or undiluted can be stored in a plastic syringe or mixed in I.V. infusion bags (PVC or non-PVC) containing 0.9% Sodium Chloride Injection for 7 days at controlled room temperature. Drug in plastic syringe can also be stored in refrigerator.

▪ *Incompatibilities:* Other I.V. drugs, parenteral nutrition solutions

Route	Onset	Peak	Duration
I.V.	Unknown	Unknown	Unknown

Half-life: 6 hr

Mechanism of Action

Acts to replenish iron stores lost during dialysis because of increased erythropoiesis and insufficient absorption of iron from GI tract. Iron is an essential component of hemoglobin, myoglobin, and several enzymes, including catalase, cytochromes, and peroxidase, and is needed for catecholamine metabolism and normal neutrophil function. Iron sucrose also normalizes RBC production by binding with hemoglobin or being stored as ferritin in reticuloendothelial cells of the bone marrow, liver, or spleen.

Contraindications

Anemia other than iron deficiency, hypersensitivity to iron components, iron overload

Interactions

DRUGS

oral iron preparations: Possibly reduced absorption of oral iron supplements

Adverse Reactions

CNS: Asthenia, **collapse**, confusion, dizziness, fatigue, fever, headache, hypoesthesia, light-headedness, loss of consciousness, malaise, **seizures**
CV: Bradycardia, chest pain, edema, **heart failure**, hypertension, **hypotension**, peripheral edema, **shock**
EENT: Conjunctivitis, ear pain, nasal congestion, nasopharyngitis, rhinitis, sinusitis, taste perversion
ENDO: Hyperglycemia, **hypoglycemia**
GI: Abdominal pain, constipation, diarrhea, elevated liver enzymes, nausea, occult-positive feces, peritoneal infection, vomiting
GU: Chromaturia, UTI
MS: Arthralgia, arthritis, back pain, joint swelling, leg cramps, muscle pain or weakness, myalgia
RESP: Bronchospasm, cough, dyspnea, pneumonia, upper respiratory tract infection

SKIN: Hyperhidrosis, pruritus, rash
Other: Anaphylaxis; angioedema; iron overload; gout; infusion or injection-site burning, pain, redness, or skin discoloration (with extravasation); **sepsis**

Childbearing Considerations

PREGNANCY

▪ It is not known if drug causes fetal harm. However, fetal bradycardia may occur, especially in the second and third trimester, if mother develops a severe hypersensitivity reaction to drug.
▪ Use with caution only if benefit to mother outweighs potential risk to fetus.

LACTATION

▪ Drug is present in breast milk.
▪ Patient should check with prescriber before breastfeeding.
▪ If breastfeeding occurs, infant should be monitored for gastrointestinal toxicity (constipation, diarrhea).

Nursing Considerations

! **WARNING** Monitor patient closely for evidence of anaphylaxis, such as collapse, dyspnea, loss of consciousness, seizures, or severe hypotension during and for at least 30 minutes after therapy. Institute emergency resuscitation measures as needed.

! **WARNING** Assess blood pressure often after drug administration because hypotension is a common adverse reaction that may be related to infusion rate (avoid rapid infusion) or total cumulative dose.

▪ Expect to monitor hematocrit, hemoglobin, serum ferritin, and transferrin saturation, as ordered, before, during, and after iron sucrose therapy. Test serum iron level 48 hours after last dose, as ordered. Notify prescriber and expect to stop therapy if blood iron levels are normal or elevated, to prevent iron toxicity.
▪ Watch for evidence of iron overload, such as bleeding in GI tract and lungs, decreased activity, pale eyes, and sedation.

PATIENT TEACHING

▪ Tell patient to inform prescriber if she has a prior history of reactions to parenteral iron products before drug is given.
▪ Inform patient that symptoms of iron deficiency may include decreased stamina,

fatigue, learning problems, and shortness of breath.

! **WARNING** Instruct patient to report any of the following signs and symptoms of an allergic reaction that may develop during and following the infusion of iron sucrose: breathing problems, dizziness, itching, light-headedness, rash, and swelling.

- Tell mothers who are breastfeeding while receiving iron sucrose to monitor their infant for constipation or diarrhea. If present, pediatrician should be notified, as this may indicate gastrointestinal toxicity.

isoniazid
(isonicotinic acid hydrazide, INH)
Isotamine (CAN), PDP-Isoniazid (CAN)

⊟ Class and Category
Pharmacologic class: Isonicotinic acid derivatives
Therapeutic class: Antitubercular agent

⊟ Indications and Dosages
⁎ *To prevent tuberculosis*

ORAL SOLUTION, TABLETS
Adults over 30 kg (66 lb). 300 mg daily for 6 to 12 mo.
Infants and children. 10 mg/kg once daily (up to 300 mg) for up to 1 yr. Alternatively when daily compliance is uncertain, 20 to 30 mg/kg (not to exceed 900 mg) twice weekly under direct observation of a health care worker.

⁎ *As adjunct to treat active tuberculosis*

ORAL SOLUTION, TABLETS, I.M. INJECTION
Adults. 5 mg/kg up to 300 mg once daily or 15 mg/kg (up to 900 mg) 2 or 3 times/wk.
Infants and children. 10 to 15 mg/kg (up to 300 mg) once daily or 20 to 40 mg/kg (up to 900 mg) 2 or 3 times/wk.

⊟ Drug Administration
- Expect to administer drug with other antitubercular drugs to prevent development of resistant organisms.

P.O.
- Give oral drug 1 hour before or 2 hours after meals to promote absorption.

- If patient has trouble swallowing tablets, obtain oral solution.
- Use a calibrated device, such as a dropper or syringe, to measure dosage of oral solution.
- If patient should vomit within 30 minutes of drug administration, repeat dose; if more than 30 minutes after administration, do not repeat dose.

I.M.
- Use reserved for when patient cannot take oral form of drug.
- Solution may crystallize at low temperatures. If this occurs, warm vial to room temperature before administering to redissolve the crystals.
- Inject deeply into a large muscle mass.

Route	Onset	Peak	Duration
P.O./I.M.	Unknown	1–2 hr	Unknown

Half-life: 0.5–5 hr

⊟ Mechanism of Action
Interferes with lipid and nucleic acid synthesis in actively growing tubercule bacilli cells. Isoniazid also disrupts bacterial cell wall synthesis and may interfere with mycolic acid synthesis in mycobacterial cells.

⊟ Contraindications
History of severe adverse reactions (acute liver disease of any etiology, including drug-induced hepatitis; arthritis; chills; drug fever); hypersensitivity to isoniazid or its components

⊟ Interactions
DRUGS
acetaminophen: Increased risk of hepatotoxicity
carbamazepine: Increased blood carbamazepine level and toxicity
hepatotoxic drugs, rifampin: Increased risk of hepatotoxicity
ketoconazole: Possibly decreased blood ketoconazole level and resistance to antifungal treatment
phenytoin: Increased blood phenytoin level, increased risk of phenytoin toxicity
theophylline, valproate: Increased levels of these drugs

FOODS
all food: Decreased absorption of isoniazid
histamine-containing foods, such as tuna, skipjack, and other tropical fish: Inhibited

action of the enzyme diamine oxidase in foods, possibly resulting in flushing, headache, hypotension, palpitations, and sweating.

tyramine-containing foods, such as cheese and fish: Increased response to tyramine in foods, possibly resulting in chills; diaphoresis; headache; light-headedness; and red, itchy, clammy skin

ACTIVITIES

alcohol use: Increased risk of hepatotoxicity

Adverse Reactions

CNS: Clumsiness, confusion, dizziness, **encephalopathy**, fatigue, fever, hallucinations, **neurotoxicity**, paresthesia, peripheral neuritis, psychosis, **seizures**, weakness
CV: Vasculitis
EENT: Optic neuritis
ENDO: Gynecomastia, hyperglycemia
GI: Abdominal pain, anorexia, elevated liver enzymes, epigastric distress, **hepatitis**, jaundice, nausea, **pancreatitis**, vomiting
GU: Glycosuria
HEME: **Agranulocytosis**, **aplastic anemia**, eosinophilia, **hemolytic anemia**, sideroblastic anemia, **thrombocytopenia**
MS: Arthralgia, joint stiffness
SKIN: **Pruritus**, rash, **Stevens–Johnson syndrome**, **toxic epidermal necrolysis**
Other: Anaphylaxis, **drug reaction with eosinophilia and systemic symptoms (DRESS)**, **hypocalcemia**, **hypophosphatemia**, injection-site irritation, lupus-like symptoms, lymphadenopathy

Childbearing Considerations

PREGNANCY

- Drug may be used to treat active tuberculosis in pregnant women.
- Drug should be deferred to treat latent tuberculosis until after delivery to avoid risk to fetus.
- Be aware that risk of fatal maternal isoniazid-associated hepatitis may be increased, especially during the postpartum period.

LACTATION

- Drug is present in breast milk.
- Breastfeeding may take place during drug therapy.

Nursing Considerations

- Administer isoniazid cautiously to alcoholic, diabetic, or malnourished patients and those at risk for peripheral neuritis.
- Monitor liver enzyme studies, which may be ordered monthly, because isoniazid can cause severe (possibly fatal) hepatitis.
- Know that about 50% of patients metabolize isoniazid slowly, which may lead to increased toxic effects. Watch for adverse reactions, such as peripheral neuritis; if they occur, expect to decrease dosage.
- Be aware that patients with advanced HIV infection may experience more severe adverse reactions in greater numbers.
- Follow patient compliance with the Potts-Cozart test, which is a simple colorimetric method of checking drug in the urine. Additionally, isoniazid test strips are also available to check compliance.

PATIENT TEACHING

- Instruct patient to take isoniazid exactly as prescribed and not to stop without first consulting prescriber. Explain that treatment may take months or years.
- Direct patient to take drug on an empty stomach 1 hour before or 2 hours after meals.
- Tell patient unable to swallow tablets to switch to oral solution. Advise patient to use a calibrated device, such as a dropper or syringe, to measure dosage of oral solution.
- Instruct patient that if he should vomit within 30 minutes of drug administration, repeat dose; if more than 30 minutes after administration, do not repeat dose.
- Advise patient to report signs of hepatic dysfunction, including dark urine, decreased appetite, fatigue, and jaundice.
- Caution patient not to drink alcohol while taking isoniazid because alcohol increases the risk of hepatotoxicity.
- Give patient a list of tyramine-containing foods to avoid when taking isoniazid, such as cheese, fish, red wine, salami, and yeast extracts. Explain that consuming these foods during isoniazid therapy may cause unpleasant adverse reactions, such as chills, pounding heartbeat, and sweating.
- Tell patient to avoid histamine-containing foods such as tuna, skipjack, and other tropical fish during therapy to avoid such

G
H
I

adverse reactions as flushing, headache, low blood pressure, rapid heartbeat, and sweating. Tell patient to also avoid foods containing tyramine such as aged cheese or red wine.

- Tell patient that he'll need periodic laboratory tests and physical examinations.
- Urge patient to report fever, nausea, numbness and tingling in arms and legs, rash, vision changes, vomiting, and yellowing skin.

isosorbide dinitrate
Dilatrate-SR, ISDM (CAN), Isordil Titradose

isosorbide mononitrate
Apo-ISMN (CAN), Monoket

Class and Category
Pharmacologic class: Nitrate
Therapeutic class: Antianginal

Indications and Dosages
* *To prevent angina*

E.R. TABLETS
Adults. *Initial:* 30 to 60 mg (mononitrate) once daily, increased after several days to 120 once daily and then after several more days to 240 mg once daily, as needed.

TABLETS
Adults. *Initial:* 5 to 20 mg (dinitrate) two or three times daily. *Maintenance:* 10 to 40 mg two or three times daily.

* *To prevent or treat nonacute angina pectoris due to coronary artery disease*

TABLETS
Adults. *Initial:* 5 to 20 mg (mononitrate) twice daily given 7 hr apart.

Drug Administration
P.O.
- Give immediate-acting drug 30 minutes before or 2 hours after meals.
- E.R. tablets should be swallowed whole and not chewed, crushed, or split and administered once daily in the morning.
- For dinitrate immediate-release dosages given more than once daily, calculate

administration time to allow for a daily nitrate-free interval of at least 14 hours, although the optimal interval will vary with patient, dosage, and drug regimen. Immediate-release mononitrate tablets administered twice daily and given 7 hr apart.

- Protect drug from heat and light.

Route	Onset	Peak	Duration
P.O.	7.5–45 min	30–60 min	2–6 hr
P.O. (E.R.)	60–90 min	3–4.5 hr	10–14 hr
P.O. (S.L.)	5–20 min	Unknown	45–120 min

Half-life: 5 hr

Mechanism of Action
Isosorbide may interact with nitrate receptors in vascular smooth muscle cell membranes. By interacting with receptors' sulfhydryl groups, drug is reduced to nitric oxide. Nitric oxide activates the enzyme guanylate cyclase, increasing intracellular formation of cyclic guanosine monophosphate (cGMP). An increased cGMP level may relax vascular smooth muscle by forcing calcium out of muscle cells, causing vasodilation. This improves cardiac output by reducing mainly preload but also afterload.

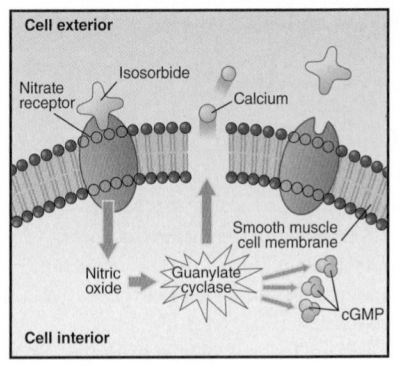

Contraindications
Concurrent use of phosphodiesterase inhibitors (sildenafil, tadalafil, vardenafil) or riociguat; hypersensitivity to isosorbide, other nitrates, or their components

Interactions

DRUGS
phosphodiesterase inhibitors such as sildenafil, tadalafil, vardenafil: Increased risk of hypotension, myocardial ischemia, syncope, and possibly death
riociguat: Increased risk of hypotension
vasodilators: Additive effects

ACTIVITIES
alcohol use: Increased risk of orthostatic hypotension

Adverse Reactions
CNS: Agitation, confusion, dizziness, headache, insomnia, restlessness, syncope, vertigo, weakness
CV: Arrhythmias, orthostatic hypotension, palpitations, peripheral edema, tachycardia
EENT: Blurred vision, diplopia (all forms); sublingual burning (S.L. form)
GI: Abdominal pain, diarrhea, indigestion, nausea, vomiting
GU: Dysuria, impotence, urinary frequency
HEME: Hemolytic anemia
MS: Arthralgia, muscle twitching
RESP: Bronchitis, pneumonia, upper respiratory tract infection
SKIN: Diaphoresis, flushing, rash

Childbearing Considerations

PREGNANCY
- It is not known if drug causes fetal harm.
- Use with caution only if benefit to mother outweighs potential risk to fetus.

LACTATION
- It is not known if drug is present in breast milk.
- Patient should check with prescriber before breastfeeding.

Nursing Considerations
- Use isosorbide cautiously in patients with hypovolemia or mild hypotension. Monitor patient for increased hypotension and reduced cardiac output.
- Know that patient may experience daily headaches from isosorbide's vasodilating effects. Give acetaminophen, as prescribed, to relieve pain.

! **WARNING** Be aware that stopping drug abruptly may cause angina and increase the risk of MI.

- Monitor blood pressure often during isosorbide therapy, especially in elderly patients; drug may cause severe hypotension.

PATIENT TEACHING
- Teach patient and family to recognize signs and symptoms of angina, including chest pain, fullness, or pressure, which commonly is accompanied by nausea and sweating. Pain may radiate down the left arm or into the neck or jaw. Inform female patients and those with diabetes mellitus or hypertension that they may experience only fatigue and shortness of breath.
- Caution patient not to crush or chew isosorbide E.R. tablets.
- Advise patient on length of time to follow if drug is to be taken more than once daily.
- Caution patient that abrupt drug discontinuation may cause angina and increase the risk of MI.
- Instruct patient to notify prescriber about blurred vision, fainting, increased angina attacks, rash, and severe or persistent headaches.
- Teach patient to reduce the effects of orthostatic hypotension by changing position slowly. Advise him to lie down if he becomes dizzy.
- Inform patient that drug commonly causes headache, which typically resolves after a few days of continuous therapy. Suggest that patient take acetaminophen as needed and as prescribed.
- Advise patient to avoid potentially hazardous activities until drug's CNS effects are known.
- Urge patient to avoid alcohol consumption.
- Instruct patient to store drug in a tightly closed container and protect from heat and light.
- Advise male patient with erectile dysfunction to alert prescriber that he is taking isosorbide because sildenafil, tadalafil, and vardenafil can cause fatal reactions when taken with isosorbide.

isotretinoin
Absorica, Absorica LD, Amnesteem, Claravis, Myorisan, Zenatane

Class and Category
Pharmacologic class: Retinoid
Therapeutic class: Acne inhibitor

Indications and Dosages

* *To treat severe recalcitrant nodular acne unresponsive to conventional therapy*

CAPSULES (AMNESTEEM, CLARAVIS, MYORISAN, ZENATANE)

Adults. *Initial:* 0.5 mg to 1 mg/kg daily in 2 divided doses, increased as needed up to 2 mg/kg daily given in 2 divided doses. *Maximum:* 2 mg/kg daily. Course of therapy given for 15 to 20 wk with second course given, as needed, after a period of 2 mo or more off therapy.

Adolescents age 12 and over. 0.5 mg to 1 mg daily in 2 divided doses for 15 to 20 wk.

CAPSULES (ABSORICA)

Adults and adolescents age 12 and over. 0.5 to 1 mg/kg daily in 2 divided doses for 15 to 20 wk. Second course of therapy given, as needed, after a period of 2 months or more off therapy.

Adults with severe scarring or primarily manifested on the trunk. Up to 2 mg/kg/day in two divided doses for 15 to 20 wk. Second course of therapy given, as needed, after a period of 2 months or more off therapy.

CAPSULES (ABSORICA LD)

Adults and adolescents age 12 and over. 0.4 to 0.8 mg/kg daily in 2 divided doses for 15 to 20 wk. Second course of therapy may be given, as needed, after a period of 2 months or more off therapy.

Adults with severe scarring or primarily manifested on the trunk. Up to 1.6 mg/kg/day in two divided doses for 15 to 20 wk. Second course of therapy given, as needed, after a period of 2 months or more off therapy.

Drug Administration

P.O.

- Administer drug with food or milk except for Absorica or Absorica LD brands, which may be taken with or without food.
- Capsules should be swallowed whole and not chewed, crushed, or opened.
- The brands Absorica and Absorica LD are not interchangeable.

Route	Onset	Peak	Duration
P.O.	Unknown	3–5 hr	Unknown

Half-life: 22 hr

Mechanism of Action

Inhibits sebaceous gland function and keratinization, which results in diminished nodular formation associated with recalcitrant nodular acne.

Contraindications

Hypersensitivity to isotretinoin parabens, vitamin A, or any of their components, pregnancy

Interactions

DRUGS

corticosteroids (systemic): Possibly increased risk of osteoporosis
hormonal contraceptives including levonorgestrel implants, medroxyprogesterone injection, microdosed progesterone preparations: Possibly decreased effectiveness of contraceptive
phenytoin: Possibly increased risk of osteomalacia
tetracyclines: Increased risk of benign intracranial hypertension
vitamin A supplements: Increased risk of additive toxic effects

Adverse Reactions

CNS: Aggressive or **violent** behavior, anger, anxiety, **CVA**, depression, dizziness, drowsiness, emotional instability, euphoria, fatigue, hallucinations, headache, insomnia, irritability, lethargy, malaise, nervousness, panic attack, paresthesias, **pseudotumor cerebri**, psychosis, **seizures**, **suicidal ideation**, syncope, weakness
CV: Chest pain, decreased high-density lipoprotein level, edema, hypercholesteremia, hypertriglyceridemia, palpitation, tachycardia, **vascular thrombotic disease**, vasculitis
ENDO: Abnormal menses, hyperglycemia, **hypoglycemia**
EENT: Bleeding and inflammation of gums, blurred vision, cataracts, color vision disorder, conjunctivitis, corneal opacities, decreased night vision, dry eyes, dry mouth or nose, epistaxis, eye irritation or pruritus, eye strain, eyelid inflammation, hearing impairment, keratitis, nasal dryness, nasopharyngitis, optic neuritis, photophobia, reduced visual acuity, stye, tinnitus, visual disturbances, voice alteration
GI: Colitis, **hepatitis**, ileitis, inflammatory bowel disease, elevated liver enzymes, nausea, **pancreatitis**

GU: Abnormal menses, decreased libido, erectile dysfunction, **glomerulonephritis**, hematuria, proteinuria, sexual dysfunction, WBCs in urine

HEME: Anemia, **agranulocytosis**, **elevated platelet count**, **leukopenia**, **neutropenia**, sedimentation rate elevation, **thrombocytopenia**, thrombocytosis

MS: Arthralgia, arthritis, back or musculoskeletal pain, bone abnormalities, calcification of ligaments and tendons, musculoskeletal stiffness, myalgia, premature epiphyseal closure, **rhabdomyolysis**, skeletal hyperostosis, tendinitis

RESP: Bronchospasms, respiratory infection

SKIN: Alopecia, bruising, contact dermatitis, diaphoresis, disseminated herpes simplex, dry lips or skin, eczema, eruptive xanthomas, **erythema multiforme**, facial erythema, flushing, fulminant acne, hair abnormalities, hirsutism, hyperpigmentation, hypopigmentation, increased sunburn susceptibility, infections, nail dystrophy, paronychia, peeling of palms and soles, photoallergic or photosensitizing reactions, pruritus, pyogenic granuloma, rash, seborrhea, skin fragility, **Stevens–Johnson syndrome, toxic epidermal necrolysis**, urticaria

Other: Abnormal wound healing, alkaline phosphatase increase, **disseminated herpes simplex**, elevated creatine phosphokinase levels, **hypersensitivity reactions (may become severe)**, hyperuricemia, lymphadenopathy, weight loss

☰ Childbearing Considerations
PREGNANCY
- Pregnancy exposure registry: 1-866-495-0654 or www.ipledgeprogam. com; or MedWatch at 1-800-FDA-1088.
- Drug causes fetal harm, especially severe congenital defects, spontaneous abortions, and premature births. Drug must be discontinued immediately if pregnancy occurs. Pregnancy registry should also be notified.
- It is contraindicated in pregnant women and women of childbearing age who are not using reliable contraception during drug therapy and for at least 1 month following drug discontinuation.

- Women of childbearing age must meet all of the following conditions before drug can be prescribed:
- Patient agrees to participate in the "iPLEDGE" program.
- Patient understands that no more than a 30-day supply of the drug will be given at any one time.
- Patient agrees to talk about effective birth control methods with health care provider and agrees to use two separate methods of effective birth control at the same time 1 month before, while taking the drug, and for 1 month after drug is discontinued.
- Patient has a negative monthly pregnancy test before prescription is refilled.
- Patient agrees to have a pregnancy test done 30 days after drug is discontinued.
- Patient understands drug may interfere with the contraceptive effect of microdosed progestin preparations and knows that microdosed "minipill" is not recommended for use with the drug.
- Patient expresses an understanding that it is not known if there is an interaction between the drug and combined oral contraceptives.
- Patient agrees not to use St. John's wort during drug therapy because it may make hormonal birth control pills be less effective.
- Patient agrees not to donate blood during and for at least 1 month following the completion of therapy because women of childbearing potential must not receive blood from patients being treated with drug.

LACTATION
- It is not known if drug is present in breast milk.
- A decision should be made to discontinue breastfeeding or the drug to avoid potential serious adverse reactions in infant.

☰ Nursing Considerations
- Ensure that women of childbearing age have met the iPLEDGE restricted program requirements before drug therapy begins.

! WARNING Notify prescriber if elevated serum triglyceride levels can't be controlled or if symptoms of pancreatitis occur (abdominal pain, nausea, vomiting). Drug may have to be discontinued because fatal hemorrhagic pancreatitis has occurred with drug use.

- Obtain serum lipid level before therapy and periodically thereafter, as ordered, to detect elevated lipid levels that result from isotretinoin therapy.
- Monitor liver enzyme levels periodically, as ordered, because drug can cause hepatitis.
- Assess patient frequently for adverse reactions and report to prescriber any that occur; drug may have serious adverse effects that require discontinuation.

PATIENT TEACHING

- Inform patient that drug is available only through a restricted program. Review criteria and question patient regarding understanding and willingness to comply.

! WARNING Alert patient that Absorica brand of isotretinoin contains the color additive FD&C Yellow No. 5 (tartrazine), which may cause allergic reactions, especially in patients with an allergy to aspirin or who have asthma. Tell patient that if an allergic reaction occurs, regardless of brand taken, to seek immediate medical attention, if severe, and to stop taking isotretinoin.

- Instruct patient to take isotretinoin with food or milk except for Absorica or Absorica LD brands, which may be taken with or without food.
- Advise women of childbearing age that two forms of contraceptives must be used simultaneously (unless absolute abstinence is the chosen method) 1 month before therapy and for 1 month after therapy has stopped because of potential for fetal harm. Inform women who use oral contraceptives that drug may lessen effectiveness of oral contraceptives. Urge patient to notify prescriber immediately if pregnancy occurs.
- Urge patient to report headache, nausea, vomiting and visual disturbances immediately to prescriber, because drug will have to be discontinued immediately and patient referred to a neurologist.
- Caution patient and family that isotretinoin may cause aggressive or violent behavior, depression, psychosis, and suicidal ideation. Instruct patient to notify prescriber immediately if changes in mood occur.
- Tell patient to report hearing changes or tinnitus; painful or trouble swallowing; rectal bleeding; severe abdominal, bowel, or chest pain; severe diarrhea or skin reactions to prescriber because drug may have to be discontinued.
- Advise patient to avoid hazardous activities until drug's CNS effects are known. Caution that changes in night vision may occur suddenly.
- Caution patient not to donate blood during therapy and for 1 month after therapy has stopped, because blood might be given to a pregnant woman.
- Warn patient that transient exacerbation of acne may occur, especially during initial therapy and to notify prescriber if this occurs.
- Instruct patient to avoid wax epilation and skin resurfacing procedures during therapy and for at least 6 months thereafter because of scarring potential.
- Caution patient to avoid exposure to direct sunlight or UV light and to wear sunscreen when outdoors.
- Inform patient that contact lens tolerance may decrease during and after isotretinoin therapy and night vision may decrease as well.
- Alert patient to the potential for mild musculoskeletal adverse reactions, which usually clear rapidly after drug is discontinued. Urge patient to notify prescriber if symptoms become bothersome or serious because drug may have to be discontinued. Inform adolescents and their families that participation in sports with repetitive impact may increase their risk of hip growth plate injuries or spondylolisthesis.
- Advise patient not to take vitamin A supplements while on isotretinoin therapy because of potentially additive toxic effects. Also advise female patients of childbearing age not to self-treat depression with the herbal, St. John's wort, because it may interfere with hormonal contraceptives being used.
- Instruct patient to notify all prescribers of isotretinoin use because of the risk of interactions.
- Inform patient of need for frequent laboratory tests and importance of complying with scheduled appointments.

isradipine

Class and Category
Pharmacologic class: Calcium channel blocker
Therapeutic class: Antihypertensive

Indications and Dosages
✻ *To manage essential hypertension as monotherapy or adjunct with a thiazide diuretic*

CAPSULES
Adults. *Initial:* 2.5 mg twice daily, increased by 5 mg every 2 to 4 wk, as needed. *Maximum:* 20 mg daily.

Drug Administration
P.O.
- Capsules should be swallowed whole and not chewed, crushed, or opened.

Route	Onset	Peak	Duration
P.O.	30–60 min	2–3 hr	12 hr

Half-life: 8–9 hr

Mechanism of Action
Inhibits calcium movement into coronary vascular smooth muscle cells by blocking the slow calcium channels in their membranes. By decreasing intracellular calcium level, isradipine inhibits smooth muscle cell contractions. The result is decreased peripheral vascular resistance, reduced diastolic and systolic blood pressure, and relaxation of coronary and vascular smooth muscle, all of which decrease myocardial oxygen demand.

Contraindications
Hypersensitivity to isradipine or its components

Interactions
DRUGS
cimetidine: Increased blood level and bioavailability of isradipine
fentanyl anesthesia: Increased risk of severe hypotension
rifampicin: Decreased isradipine concentration and effectiveness

Adverse Reactions
CNS: Asthenia, CVA, dizziness, fatigue, headache, paresthesia, somnolence, syncope, transient ischemic attack, weakness

CV: Angina, **atrial fibrillation**, **heart failure**, **hypotension**, **MI**, orthostatic hypotension, palpitations, peripheral edema, tachycardia, **ventricular fibrillation**
EENT: Gingival hyperplasia, pharyngitis, rhinitis
GI: Abdominal cramps, constipation, diarrhea, elevated liver enzymes, indigestion, nausea, vomiting
HEME: **Leukopenia**
MS: Back pain
RESP: Cough
SKIN: Flushing, photosensitivity, rash, urticaria
Other: **Angioedema**

Childbearing Considerations
PREGNANCY
- It is not known if drug causes fetal harm.
- Use with caution only if benefit to mother outweighs potential risk to fetus.

LACTATION
- It is not known if drug is present in breast milk.
- A decision should be made to discontinue breastfeeding or the drug to avoid potential serious adverse reactions in the breastfed infant.

Nursing Considerations
- Monitor blood pressure and heart rate often during isradipine therapy.
- Monitor patient with impaired hepatic or renal function for an increased blood isradipine level.
- Observe for mild peripheral edema caused by vasodilation of small blood vessels. Know that this type of edema doesn't result from fluid retention or heart failure.

PATIENT TEACHING
- Inform patient that isradipine therapy will be long-term and will require laboratory tests and follow-up visits to monitor drug effects.
- Instruct patient to take drug exactly as prescribed and to swallow capsules whole, not chewing or crushing them.
- Instruct patient to take a missed dose as soon as he remembers it unless it's nearly time for the next dose. In that case, advise him to wait and take next scheduled dose, but not to double the dose. If more than one dose is missed, tell him to contact prescriber.

G
H
I

! **WARNING** Urge patient not to stop taking drug suddenly. Doing so may lead to life-threatening problems.

- Inform patient that fragments of capsules may be visible in stool.
- Urge patient to avoid potentially hazardous activities until isradipine's CNS effects are known.
- Caution patient to change position slowly to minimize orthostatic hypotension.
- Urge patient to contact prescriber if he experiences chest pain, fainting, irregular heartbeat, rash, or swollen ankles while taking isradipine.
- Instruct patient to maintain good oral hygiene, perform gum massage, and see a dentist every 6 months to prevent gum bleeding and gum disorders.
- Caution patient to avoid direct sunlight and to wear protective clothing and apply sunscreen when outdoors.
- Instruct patient to store drug at room temperature in a dry place.

istradefylline
Nourianz

Class and Category
Pharmacologic class: Adenosine A_{2A} receptor antagonist
Therapeutic class: Anti-Parkinson agent, central nervous system agent

Indications and Dosages
* *As adjunct to treat patients with Parkinson's disease on levodopa/carbidopa experiencing "off" episodes*

TABLETS
Adults. 20 mg once daily, increased to 40 mg if needed. *Maximum:* 40 mg once daily.
±**DOSAGE ADJUSTMENT** For patients taking strong CYP3A4 inhibitors or patients with moderate hepatic impairment, maximum dosage should not exceed 20 mg once daily. For patients who smoke 20 or more cigarettes per day (or use the equivalent of another tobacco product), dosage is initiated and maintained at 40 mg once daily.

Drug Administration
P.O.
- Store drug at room temperature.

Route	Onset	Peak	Duration
P.O.	Unknown	4 hr	Unknown

Half-life: 83 hr

Mechanism of Action
The precise mechanism in which a therapeutic effect is exerted in Parkinson's disease is unknown, although it is thought to be related to its adenosine A_{2A} receptor antagonist action.

Contraindications
Hypersensitivity to istradefylline or its components

Interactions
DRUGS
drugs to treat Parkinson's disease: May cause impulse control issues
strong CYP3A4 inducers such as carbamazepine, phenytoin, rifampin, St. John's wort: Decreased istradefylline levels and effectiveness
strong CYP3A4 inhibitors such as clarithromycin, itraconazole, ketoconazole: Increased istradefylline levels with increased risk of adverse reactions
CYP3A4 substrates such as atorvastatin, P-gp substrates such as digoxin: Increased CYP3A4 substrate level with increased risk of adverse reactions

ACTIVITIES
smoking 20 cigarettes a day or more (or equivalent use of another tobacco product): Decreased effectiveness of istradefylline

Adverse Reactions
CNS: Dizziness, dyskinesia, hallucination, insomnia
ENDO: Hyperglycemia
GI: Constipation, decreased appetite, diarrhea, nausea
GU: Elevated blood urea, increased libido
RESP: Upper respiratory tract inflammation
SKIN: Rash

Childbearing Considerations
PREGNANCY
- It is not known if drug causes fetal harm. However, animal studies suggest it might cause fetal harm.
- Use is not recommended during pregnancy.

LACTATION
- It is not known if drug may be present in breast milk.

- Patient should check with prescriber before breastfeeding.

REPRODUCTION
- Women of childbearing potential should use contraception during treatment.

▤ Nursing Considerations
- Know that patient with a major psychotic disorder should not be administered istradefylline, because of the potential risk of exacerbating psychosis.
- Monitor patient for adverse reactions, especially central nervous system adverse effects. The most common effect leading to discontinuation of drug is dyskinesia.
- Monitor patient for hallucinations or psychotic behavior. If present, expect dosage to be decreased or drug discontinued.
- Be aware that patients taking istradefylline and one or more medications for the treatment of Parkinson's disease (including levodopa) may develop intense urges to binge-eat, gamble, have sex, or spend money excessively. If patient develops an impulse control disorder, notify prescriber. Dosage may have to be reduced or discontinued.
- Expect to monitor liver function tests. Dosage may require adjustment.
- Confirm smoking status in patients. Educate patients who smoke to inform prescribers.

PATIENT TEACHING
- Advise patient that when istradefylline is taken with one or more drugs to treat Parkinson's disease (including levodopa), impulse control problems or compulsive behaviors may develop, such as intense urges to binge-eat, gamble, have sex, or spend money excessively. Tell patient to notify prescriber if an impulse control disorder occurs. Also educate caregivers and family that this may occur and have them contact prescriber if present and patient is unaware of a lack of control.
- Tell a woman of childbearing potential that she should use contraception while taking istradefylline.
- Inform patient that drug may cause dyskinesia or exacerbate preexisting dyskinesia and to notify prescriber if present.
- Warn patient that istradefylline may cause hallucinations or psychotic behavior. If present, advise patient or family/caregiver to notify prescriber.
- Tell patient to inform prescribers of all medications taken, including over-the-counter drugs and herbal products such as St. John's wort.

itraconazole
Sporanox, Tolsura

▤ Class and Category
Pharmacologic class: Triazole derivative
Therapeutic class: Antifungal

▤ Indications and Dosages
✱ *To treat blastomycosis caused by* Blastomyces dermatitidis *and histoplasmosis caused by* Histoplasma capsulatum

CAPSULES (SPORANOX)
Adults. *Initial:* 200 mg daily, increased, in 100-mg increments, as needed. *Maximum:* 400 mg daily, with dosage greater than 200 mg given in divided doses twice daily.

CAPSULES (TOLSURA)
Adults. *Initial:* 130 mg once daily, increased in increments of 65 mg to maximum of 130 mg twice daily. *Maximum:* 260 mg daily in two divided doses.

✱ *To treat aspergillosis unresponsive to amphotericin B*

CAPSULES (SPORANOX)
Adults. 200 to 400 mg daily, with dosage greater than 200 mg daily given in divided doses twice daily.

CAPSULES (TOLSURA)
Adults. *Initial:* 130 mg once daily. Maximum: 260 mg daily in two divided doses.

✱ *To treat life-threatening aspergillosis, blastomycosis, or histoplasmosis infections*

CAPSULES (SPORANOX)
Adults. *Loading dose:* 200 mg given three times a day for 3 days followed by usual dosage for specific fungal infection and continued for a minimum of 3 months and until clinical parameters and laboratory tests indicate the active fungal infection has subsided.

CAPSULES (TOLSURA)
Adults. *Loading dose:* 130 mg three times daily for first 3 days, followed by usual dosage for specific fungal infection and

G
H
I

continued for a minimum of 3 months and until clinical parameters and laboratory tests indicate the active fungal infection has subsided.

✴ *To treat oropharyngeal candidiasis*

ORAL SOLUTION (SPORANOX)
Adults and adolescents. 200 mg once a day for 7 to 14 days.

✴ *To treat fluconazole-resistant oropharyngeal candidiasis*

ORAL SOLUTION (SPORANOX)
Adults and adolescents. 100 mg twice daily for 2 to 4 wk.

✴ *To treat esophageal candidiasis*

ORAL SOLUTION (SPORANOX)
Adults. 100 mg daily increased to 200 mg daily, if needed, for a minimum of 3 wk, with treatment continued for 2 wk following resolution of symptoms.

✴ *To treat onychomycosis of toenails only or of toenails and fingernails in non-immunocompromised patients*

CAPSULES (SPORANOX)
Adults. 200 mg daily for 12 wk.

✴ *To treat onychomycosis of fingernails only in non-immunocompromised patients*

CAPSULES (SPORANOX)
Adults. 200 mg twice daily for 7 days; then repeated after 3 wk.

✴ *To treat onychomycosis of toenails only in non-immunocompromised patients*

CAPSULES (SPORANOX)
Adults. 200 mg once daily for 12 wk.

±**DOSAGE ADJUSTMENT** For some immunocompromised patients taking capsule form of drug, dosage may have to be increased because oral bioavailability of capsule form may be decreased.

≣ Drug Administration

P.O.
- Capsules should be swallowed whole with a full meal and not chewed, crushed, or split/opened.
- Capsules are not interchangeable with oral solution.
- Tablets are not interchangeable with oral solution.
- Use a calibrated device when measuring dosage of oral solution.
- Oral solution concentration is 10 mg/ml. Have patient vigorously swish 10 ml at a

time of oral solution for several seconds in the mouth and then swallow.

Route	Onset	Peak	Duration
P.O.	Unknown	3–7 hr	Unknown

Half-life: 20–30 hr

≣ Mechanism of Action
Inhibits the synthesis of ergosterol, an essential component of fungal cell membranes, by binding with a cytochrome P-450 enzyme needed to convert lanosterol to ergosterol. Lack of ergosterol results in increased cellular permeability and leakage of cell contents. Itraconazole also may lead to fungal cell death by inhibiting fungal respiration under aerobic conditions.

≣ Contraindications
Concurrent therapy with avanafil, cisapride, disopyramide, dofetilide, dronedarone, eplerenone, ergot alkaloids, felodipine, HMG-CoA inhibitors (lovastatin and simvastatin), irinotecan, isavuconazole, ivabradine, levomethadyl, lomitapide, lovastatin, lurasidone, methadone, naloxegol, oral midazolam, pimozide, quinidine, ranolazine, simvastatin, ticagrelor, or triazolam; concurrent therapy with colchicine, fesoterodine, or solifenacin in patients with hepatic or renal impairment; concurrent therapy with eliglustat in patients who are poor or intermediate metabolizers of CYP2D6 or are taking moderate or strong CYP2D6 inhibitors; evidence of ventricular dysfunction, as in congestive heart failure (CHF) or a history of it (onychomycosis treatment); hypersensitivity to itraconazole or its components; pregnancy or contemplating pregnancy during onychomycosis treatment

≣ Interactions
DRUGS
alfentanil, budesonide, buspirone, busulfan, carbamazepine, cyclosporine, dexamethasone, digoxin, docetaxel, felodipine, fluticasone, indinavir, methylprednisolone, phenytoin, pimozide, rifabutin, ritonavir, saquinavir, sirolimus, tacrolimus, trimetrexate, vinca alkaloids: Possibly increased blood levels of these drugs and serious adverse effects

alprazolam, diazepam, oral midazolam, triazolam: Elevated blood levels and possibly prolonged sedative effects of these drugs
atorvastatin, lovastatin, simvastatin: Increased blood levels of these drugs; possibly rhabdomyolysis
avanafil, cisapride, colchicine, dofetilide, dronedarone, eplerenone, ergot alkaloids, felodipine, fesoterodine, halofantrine, irinotecan, isavuconazole, ivabradine, levomethadyl, lovastatin, lurasidone, methadone, midazolam (oral), naloxegol, pimozide, quinidine, ranolazine, simvastatin, solifenacin, ticagrelor, triazolam: Possibly increased plasma levels of these drugs leading to potentially life-threatening cardiovascular complications such as cardiac arrest, prolonged QT interval, torsades de pointes, ventricular tachycardia, and sudden death
calcium channel blockers: Possibly edema and increased risk of CHF; increased blood levels of these drugs
carbamazepine, isoniazid, nevirapine, phenobarbital, phenytoin, rifabutin, rifampin: Possibly decreased blood itraconazole level
cilostazol; eletriptan; glucocorticosteroids such as budesonide, dexamethasone, fluticasone, and methylprednisolone; trimetrexate: Possibly inhibited metabolism increasing concentrations of these drugs
clarithromycin, erythromycin, indinavir, ritonavir: Possibly increased blood itraconazole level
ergot alkaloids: Possibly increased plasma ergot alkaloid elevation, leading to cerebral ischemia and ischemia of the extremities
fentanyl: Possibly increased plasma fentanyl level, causing potentially fatal respiratory depression
oral antidiabetic drugs such as repaglinide, saxagliptin: Possibly increased blood levels of these drugs and risk of hypoglycemia
systemic contraceptive hormones: Increased concentrations of these contraceptives
warfarin: Increased anticoagulant effect of warfarin

Adverse Reactions

CNS: Chills, confusion, dizziness, drowsiness, fatigue, fever, headache, hypoesthesia, paresthesia, peripheral neuropathy, tremor, vertigo
CV: **Cardiac failure,** chest pain, **congestive heart failure,** hypertension, hypertriglyceridemia, **hypotension, left ventricular failure,** peripheral edema, tachycardia
EENT: Altered sense of taste, blurred vision, diplopia, dysphonia, transient or permanent hearing loss, tinnitus
ENDO: Hyperglycemia
GI: Abdominal pain, anorexia, constipation, diarrhea, elevated liver enzymes, flatulence, **hepatic failure, hepatitis, hepatotoxicity,** hyperbilirubinemia, indigestion, jaundice, nausea, **pancreatitis,** vomiting
GU: Erectile dysfunction, menstrual irregularities, pollakiuria, renal impairment, urinary incontinence
HEME: **Leukopenia, neutropenia, thrombocytopenia**
MS: Arthralgia, myalgia
RESP: Cough, dyspnea, **pulmonary edema**
SKIN: Acute generalized exanthematous pustulosis, alopecia, diaphoresis, **erythema multiforme, exfoliative dermatitis,** leukocytoclastic vasculitis, photosensitivity, pruritus, rash, **Stevens–Johnson syndrome, toxic epidermal necrolysis,** urticaria
Other: **Anaphylaxis, angioedema, hyperkalemia, hypokalemia, hypomagnesemia,** serum sickness

Childbearing Considerations
PREGNANCY

- Drug may cause fetal harm such as congenital abnormalities.
- Drug should be used to treat systemic fungal infections in pregnancy only if the benefit outweighs the potential risk.
- Drug should not be used to treat onychomycosis in pregnant patients or in women contemplating pregnancy.

LACTATION

- Drug is present in breast milk.
- Mother who is HIV negative should check with prescriber before breastfeeding.
- The Centers for Disease Control and Prevention recommends that HIV-1 infected mothers not breastfeed to avoid risking postnatal transmission of HIV-1 infection to infants. They also do not recommend breastfeeding because of potential drug-induced adverse reactions in the infant.

REPRODUCTION

- Drug should not be used in women of childbearing age for treatment of onychomycosis unless they are using effective measures to prevent pregnancy and they begin therapy on the second or third day following the onset of menses.

- Highly effective contraception should be continued throughout drug therapy and for 2 months following drug discontinuation.

▤ Nursing Considerations

- Know that itraconazole should not be used for the treatment of onychomycosis in patients with evidence of ventricular dysfunction such as congestive heart failure (CHF) or a history of CHF. If signs and symptoms of CHF develops during therapy, notify prescriber immediately and expect drug to be discontinued.
- Use itraconazole with extreme caution in patients with risk factors for CHF, such as ischemic or valvular heart disease, renal failure and other edematous disorders, or significant pulmonary disease such as chronic obstructive pulmonary disease because of increased risk of developing CHF during itraconazole treatment.
- Use itraconazole cautiously in patients with hypersensitivity to other azole antifungals (because cross-hypersensitivity is unknown) and in patients with hepatic or renal impairment.
- Know that because itraconazole has been linked to serious adverse cardiac and hepatic effects, expect to send appropriate nail specimens for laboratory testing to confirm onychomycosis before beginning therapy.

! **WARNING** Keep in mind that itraconazole is a potent inhibitor of the cytochrome P-450 3A4 (CYP3A4) isoenzyme system, which may increase blood levels of drugs metabolized by this system. Patients taking such drugs as cisapride with itraconazole or other CYP3A4 inhibitors have experienced life-threatening cardiovascular complications, such as prolonged QT interval, torsades de pointes, and ventricular tachycardia, as well as sudden death.

- Keep in mind that a patient with AIDS may have hypochlorhydria, which reduces drug absorption. For such a patient, expect to administer higher doses of itraconazole.

- Monitor liver enzymes in patients with impaired hepatic function and those who have experienced hepatotoxicity with other drugs.
- Be aware that if patient develops signs and symptoms of peripheral neuropathy or CHF, such as dyspnea, fatigue, and peripheral edema, expect to discontinue drug.
- Assess patient for rash every 8 hours during therapy; notify prescriber if rash occurs.
- Know that if patient also receives warfarin, monitor PT and assess patient for signs and symptoms of bleeding.
- Keep in mind that if patient also receives digoxin, monitor blood digoxin level as appropriate to detect toxic level, and assess patient for signs and symptoms of digitalis toxicity, such as nausea and yellow vision.
- Know that if a patient with cystic fibrosis does not respond to itraconazole therapy, alternative therapy should be considered.

PATIENT TEACHING

- Instruct patient to take itraconazole capsules with a full meal and to swallow them whole and not chew, crush, or split/open them. Oral solution should be vigorously swished in mouth for several seconds and then swallowed 10 ml at a time.
- Tell patient with diabetes who takes an oral antidiabetic drug to check his blood glucose level often because of the increased risk of hypoglycemia.
- Advise patient to avoid taking antacids with oral itraconazole.
- Advise patient to notify prescriber immediately of changes in other drugs, such as new drugs and dosage changes.
- Advise patient to notify prescriber immediately about abdominal pain, diarrhea, headache, hearing loss, nausea, peripheral neuropathy, or vomiting.

! **WARNING** Instruct patient to stop itraconazole and notify prescriber immediately if he experiences an allergic reaction.

- Tell him to stop itraconazole and notify prescriber immediately if he notices fluid retention.
- Instruct patient to notify prescriber if he experiences signs of liver problems, such as abdominal pain, dark urine, fatigue, loss

of appetite, pale stools, weakness, or yellow eyes or skin.

- Caution patient to avoid performing hazardous activities such as driving until CNS effects such as dizziness or change in vision are not present.
- Tell women of childbearing age to begin therapy on the second or third day following the onset of menses. Also, advise patient to use effective contraception to prevent pregnancy during itraconazole therapy and for 2 months following the end of treatment. Tell patient to notify prescriber immediately if pregnancy is suspected or occurs. Inform women of childbearing age that itraconazole should not be given to pregnant women or women contemplating pregnancy for the treatment of onychomycosis.

ivabradine
Corlanor

Class and Category
Pharmacologic class: Nucleotide-gated channel blocker
Therapeutic class: Cardiac pacemaker regulator

Indications and Dosages
✳ *To reduce risk of hospitalization for worsening heart failure in patients with stable, symptomatic chronic heart failure who have a left ventricular ejection fraction of 35% or less, who are in sinus rhythm with a resting heart rate of 70 beats/minute or more and either are on maximally tolerated doses of beta-blockers or have a contraindication to beta-blocker use*

ORAL SOLUTION, TABLETS
Adults. *Initial:* 5 mg twice daily followed by a dosage adjustment in 2 weeks to achieve a resting heart rate between 50 and 60 beats/minute. *Maximum:* 7.5 mg twice daily.
±**DOSAGE ADJUSTMENT** For a patient with a resting heart rate greater than 60 beats/minute, dosage increased by 2.5 mg given twice daily up to a maximum dose of 7.5 mg twice daily, as needed. For a patient with a heart rate between 50 and 60 beats/min, dose maintained. For a patient with a resting heart rate below 50 beats/minute

or who experience signs and symptoms of bradycardia, dosage decreased by 2.5 mg given twice daily; if current dose is already 2.5 mg twice daily, drug discontinued.
✳ *To treat stable symptomatic heart failure due to dilated cardiomyopathy in children who are in sinus rhythm with an elevated heart rate*

ORAL SOLUTION, TABLETS
Children weighing 40 kg (88 lb) or greater. *Initial:* 2.5 mg twice daily. Dose adjusted at 2-wk intervals by 2.5 mg to target a heart rate reduction of at least 20%, if tolerated. *Maximum:* 7.5 mg twice daily.

ORAL SOLUTION
Children age 6 months and older weighing less than 40 kg (88 lb). *Initial:* 0.05 mg/kg twice daily. Dose adjusted at 2-wk intervals by 0.05 mg/kg to target a heart rate reduction of at least 20%, if tolerated. *Maximum:* 0.2 mg/kg twice daily (patients 6 months to less than 1 yr); 0.3 mg/kg twice daily (patients 1 yr and older) up to 7.5 mg twice daily.
±**DOSAGE ADJUSTMENT** For children who develop bradycardia, dosage reduced to previous titration step. If child is at the recommended initial dosage, dosage reduced to 0.02 mg/kg twice daily.

Drug Administration
P.O.
- Instruct patient to take drug with meals.
- Give oral solution to younger children and patients who have difficulty swallowing tablets.
- Use a calibrated oral syringe to draw up drug dosage from a medicine cup to avoid dosing errors.
- Drug dose should not be doubled up if child spits out the drug.
- Medicine cup should be thrown away after drug is drawn up in the syringe.

Route	Onset	Peak	Duration
P.O.	Unknown	1–2 hr	Unknown

Half-life: 6 hr

Mechanism of Action
Blocks the hyperpolarization-activated cyclic nucleotide-gated (HCN) channel responsible for the cardiac pacemaker, which regulates heart rate. This results in a reduction in heart rate.

Contraindications

Acute decompensated heart failure; clinically significant bradycardia or hypotension; concomitant use of strong cytochrome P-450 3A4 (CYP3A4) inhibitors; hypersensitivity to ivabradine or its components; pacemaker dependence; severe hepatic impairment; sick sinus syndrome, sinoatrial block, or third degree AV block, unless a functioning demand pacemaker is present

Interactions
DRUGS

CYP3A4 inducers such as barbiturates, phenytoin, rifampicin, St. John's wort: Decreased ivabradine plasma concentrations decreasing effectiveness

moderate and strong CYP3A4 inhibitors such as azole antifungals, diltiazem, HIV protease inhibitors, macrolide antibiotics, nefazodone, verapamil: Increased ivabradine plasma concentrations, which may exacerbate bradycardia and conduction disturbances

negative chronotropes such as amiodarone, beta-blockers, digoxin: Increased risk of bradycardia

FOODS

grapefruit juice: Increased ivabradine plasma concentrations, which may exacerbate bradycardia and conduction disturbances

Adverse Reactions

CNS: Syncope, vertigo
CV: **Atrial fibrillation, bradycardia,** conduction disturbances, hypertension, **hypotension, sinus arrest, torsades de pointes, ventricular fibrillation and tachycardia**
EENT: Colored bright lights, diplopia, halos, image decomposition such as kaleidoscopic or stroboscopic effects, multiple images, transiently enhanced brightness in a limited area of the visual field, visual impairment
SKIN: Erythema, pruritus, rash, urticaria
Other: Angioedema

Childbearing Considerations
PREGNANCY

- Drug may cause fetal harm based on animal studies.
- Use with caution only if benefit to mother outweighs potential risk to fetus.
- Be aware that pregnant women with congestive heart failure, who are started on drug, especially during the first trimester, should be followed closely for destabilization that could result from a decreased heart rate.
- Monitor pregnant women with chronic heart failure in third trimester for preterm birth.

LACTATION

- It is not known if drug is present in breast milk.
- Breastfeeding is not recommended during drug therapy.

REPRODUCTION

- Advise women of childbearing age to use effective contraception during drug therapy.

Nursing Considerations

- Be aware that ivabradine should not be given to patients with demand pacemakers set to a rate of 60 beats/minute or greater because these patients will not be able to achieve a target heart rate of less than 60 beats/minute.
- Know that although drug is not contraindicated, it is not recommended for use in patients with a second-degree heart block unless a functioning demand pacemaker is in place.
- Monitor patient's cardiac rhythm regularly because ivabradine increases the risk of atrial fibrillation and conduction disturbances. Also monitor patient's heart rate, because drug may cause bradycardia. Risk factors for bradycardia include conduction defects, sinus node dysfunction, ventricular dysfunction, and use of other negative chronotropic drugs such as amiodarone, digoxin, diltiazem, or verapamil. Be aware that bradycardia may increase risk of prolonged QT interval, which may lead to life-threatening ventricular arrhythmias. Notify prescriber if arrhythmias such as atrial fibrillation or conduction disturbances occurs or the patient's heart rate drops below 50 beats/minute. Expect drug to be discontinued in these situations.

PATIENT TEACHING

- Instruct patient to take ivabradine with meals.
- Inform patients having difficulty swallowing tablets that an oral solution is available. If oral solution is used,

teach patient how to administer oral solution (children should not be self-administering). Remind patient and parents/caregivers to use a calibrated oral syringe and a medicine cup to avoid dosing errors. Drug dose should not be doubled up if child spits out the drug or drug is forgotten to be taken at the prescribed time. Medicine cup should be thrown away after drug is drawn up in the syringe.

> **! WARNING** Advise female patients of childbearing age that ivabradine may cause fetal toxicity and an effective contraceptive must be used during therapy. Tell patient to notify prescriber immediately if pregnancy is suspected or occurs.

- Instruct patient to notify all prescribers of ivabradine therapy.
- Tell patient to notify prescriber if pulse becomes irregular or less than 50 beats/minute or visual disturbances occur.

ixekizumab
Taltz

≣ Class and Category
Pharmacologic class: Interleukin-17 A antagonist
Therapeutic class: Immunomodulator

≣ Indications and Dosages
✳ *To treat moderate to severe plaque psoriasis in patients who are candidates for phototherapy or systemic therapy*

SUBCUTANEOUS INJECTION
Adults. *Initial:* 160 mg (two 80-mg injections) at wk 0, followed by 80 mg at wks 2, 4, 6, 8, 10, and 12; then 80 mg every 4 wk.
Children age 6 and older weighing more than 50 kg (110 lb). 160 mg (two 80-mg injections) and then 80 mg every 4 wk.
Children age 6 and older weighing 25 kg (55 lb) up to and including 50 kg (110 lb). 80 mg and then 40 mg every 4 wk.
Children age 6 and older weighing less than 25 kg (55 lb). 40 mg and then 20 mg every 4 wk.
✳ *To treat active psoriatic arthritis; to treat active ankylosing spondylitis*

SUBCUTANEOUS INJECTION
Adults. *Initial:* 160 mg (two 80-mg injections), followed by 80 mg every 4 wk.
± DOSAGE ADJUSTMENT For patient with psoriatic arthritis with coexistent moderate to severe plaque psoriasis, the dosing regimen for plaque psoriasis should be used.
✳ *To treat active non-radiographic axial spondyloarthritis with objective signs of inflammation*

SUBCUTANEOUS INJECTION
Adults. 80 mg every 4 wk.

≣ Drug Administration
SUBCUTANEOUS
- Remove autoinjector or prefilled syringe from refrigerator and allow about 30 minutes for drug to reach room temperature. Don't remove the needle cap during this time.
- Inspect solution for particulate matter or discoloration. Solution should appear clear and colorless to slightly yellow.
- Administer drug to adults and children who weigh more than 50 kg using either the autoinjector or prefilled syringe. Don't shake. Inject the full amount (1 ml), which provides 80 mg, into any quadrant of the abdomen or any area of the thighs, or upper arms.
- Administer drug to children who weigh 50 kg or less by expelling the entire contents of the prefilled syringe into the sterile vial. Do not shake or swirl the vial. No other medications should be added. Using a 0.5-ml or 1-ml disposable syringe and sterile needle, withdraw the prescribed dose from the vial (0.25 ml for a 20-mg dose; 0.5 ml for a 40-mg dose). Remove the needle from the syringe and replace it with a 27G needle prior to administering. Prepared solution may be stored at room temperature for up to 4 hours from first puncturing the sterile vial.
- Discard any unused solution, because the solution does not contain a preservative.
- Rotate injection sites and do not inject into areas where the skin is affected by psoriasis or is bruised, erythematous, or indurated.

Route	Onset	Peak	Duration
SubQ	Unknown	4 days	Unknown

Half-life: 13 days

G
H
I

Mechanism of Action

Selectively binds with the interleukin 17A cytokine and inhibits its interaction with the IL-17 receptor. This inhibits the release of proinflammatory cytokines and chemokines involved in normal inflammatory and immune responses. Binding of IL-17 receptors prevents inflammation-related signals from being relayed, which reduces the inflammatory response and relieves signs and symptoms of inflammatory disorders.

Contraindications

Hypersensitivity to ixekizumab or its components

Interactions

DRUGS

CYP450 substrates with a narrow therapeutic index such as cyclosporine, warfarin: Possibly decreased plasma levels of these drugs with decreased effectiveness
live vaccines: Increased risk of adverse vaccine effects

Adverse Reactions

EENT: Conjunctivitis, oral candidiasis, rhinitis
GI: Crohn's disease (new onset or exacerbation), nausea, ulcerative colitis (new onset or exacerbation)
HEME: Neutropenia, thrombocytopenia
RESP: Upper respiratory infections
SKIN: Tinea infections, urticaria
Other: Anaphylaxis, angioedema, anti-ixekizumab antibodies, flu-like symptoms, infections including fungal infections and activation of latent infections such as tuberculosis, injection-site reactions such as erythema and pain

Childbearing Considerations

PREGNANCY

- It is not known if drug causes fetal harm.
- Use with caution only if benefit to mother outweighs potential risk to fetus.

LACTATION

- It is not known if drug is present in breast milk.
- Patient should check with prescriber before breastfeeding.

Nursing Considerations

- Check patient's immunization history and make sure all age-appropriate immunizations according to current guidelines have been administered prior to initiating ixekizumab therapy. Live vaccines should be avoided during ixekizumab therapy.
- Make sure patient has a tuberculin skin test before therapy starts. If skin test is positive, tuberculosis treatment will have to be started before ixekizumab therapy can begin. Even patients who have tested negative for tuberculosis may develop tuberculosis during therapy. Monitor patient for low-grade fever, persistent cough, and wasting or weight loss; report such findings to prescriber.
- Know that if patient has evidence of an active infection when drug is prescribed, therapy shouldn't start until infection has been treated. Monitor patients for the development of infections such as conjunctivitis, oral candidiasis, tinea infections, and upper respiratory tract infections during therapy; report such findings to prescriber. Know that if a patient develops a serious infection or does not respond to treatment prescribed for the infection, ixekizumab may have to be temporarily withheld until the infection is resolved.

! WARNING Monitor patient closely for hypersensitivity. If a serious reaction occurs, such as angioedema or urticaria, discontinue drug immediately, notify prescriber, and provide supportive care, as prescribed.

- Monitor patient closely for evidence of inflammatory bowel disease. Know that Crohn's disease and ulcerative colitis may occur. During treatment, monitor patient for onset or exacerbation of inflammatory bowel disease.

PATIENT TEACHING

- Instruct patient or caregiver on how to administer drug subcutaneously, if self-administration is prescribed. Children who weigh less than 50 kg will need to have drug administered by a healthcare provider. Provide instructions on how to use the autoinjector or prefilled syringe correctly. Tell patient how to dispose of syringe or autoinjector properly and to keep out of reach of children and pets, including those already used.

- Tell patient to keep drug refrigerated in between doses but to allow the drug to warm to room temperature for about 30 minutes before administering. Tell adult patient to inject the full amount of the drug into any quadrant of the abdomen, thighs, or upper arms. Stress importance of avoiding areas where the skin is affected by psoriasis or is bruised, indurated, or red and to rotate sites. Alert him to the possibility of experiencing redness or pain at injection site, but advise him that these are not usually severe.

! **WARNING** Review the signs and symptoms of an allergic reaction (difficulty breathing, hives, swollen face) and tell patient to seek emergency care immediately if these occur.

- Inform patient that infections, including activation of latent infections such as tuberculosis, may occur during ixekizumab therapy. Instruct him to report persistent, severe, or unusual signs and symptoms to prescriber. Advise patient to avoid people with infections.
- Alert patient that irritable bowel syndrome may occur or be aggravated by ixekizumab therapy. Tell him to notify prescriber of adverse reactions such as abdominal distention or pain or diarrhea that is persistent or severe.
- Warn patient not to receive immunizations that contain live vaccines while taking ixekizumab.

J K L

ketorolac tromethamine

Sprix, Toradol (CAN)

≣ Class and Category

Pharmacologic class: NSAID
Therapeutic class: Analgesic

≣ Indications and Dosages

* *To provide short-term management of moderate to severe acute pain that requires analgesia at the opioid level, usually in a postoperative setting*

TABLETS

Adults ages 17 to 64 following parenteral therapy. *Initial:* 20 mg as single dose, followed by 10 mg every 4 to 6 hr, as needed, up to four times a day. *Maximum:* 40 mg daily for no more than 5 days including parenteral dosage.

±**DOSAGE ADJUSTMENT** For elderly patients (65 years or older), patients with impaired renal function, or patients weighing less than 50 kg (110 lb), initial dose reduced to 10 mg and given after receiving parenteral therapy followed by 10 mg every 4 to 6 hr, as needed, up to four times daily. *Maximum:* 40 mg daily for no more than 5 days including parenteral dosage.

I.M. INJECTION

Adults less than 65 years of age. *Initial:* 60 mg as single dose, followed by oral ketorolac, if needed; or 30 mg every 6 hr, as needed. *Maximum:* 120 mg daily for no more than 2 days or 5 days for combined oral and intramuscular therapy.

±**DOSAGE ADJUSTMENT** For elderly patients (65 years and older), patients with impaired renal function, or patients weighing less than 50 kg (110 lb), initial dose reduced to 30 mg as a single dose, followed by oral ketorolac if needed; or 15 mg every 6 hr as needed. *Maximum:* 60 mg daily for no more than 2 days or no more than 5 days for combined oral and intramuscular therapy.

I.V. INJECTION

Adults less than 65 years of age. *Initial:* 30 mg given as single dose, followed by oral ketorolac if needed; or 30 mg every 6 hr as needed. *Maximum:* 120 mg daily for no more than 2 days or no more than 5 days for combined oral and intravenous therapy.

±**DOSAGE ADJUSTMENT** For elderly patients (65 years and over), patients with impaired renal function, or patients weighing less than 50 kg (110 lb), initial dose reduced to 15 mg as a single dose, followed by oral ketorolac if needed; or 15 mg every 6 hr, as needed. *Maximum:* 60 mg daily for no more than 2 days or no more than 5 days for combined oral and intravenous therapy.

NASAL SPRAY (SPRIX)

Adults less than 65 years of age. 15.75 mg (1 spray) in each nostril every 6 to 8 hr. *Maximum:* 126 mg (four doses) daily for no more than 5 days.

±**DOSAGE ADJUSTMENT** For elderly patients (65 years and older), patients with impaired renal function, or patients weighing less than 50 kg (110 lb), 15.75 mg in only one nostril every 6 to 8 hr with maximum dose of 63 mg (four doses) daily for no more than 5 days.

≣ Drug Administration

P.O.

- Oral drug only given after a parenteral dose of drug has been administered first.
- Administer with an antacid, food, or milk to lessen GI upset, and give with a full glass of water.
- Patient should not lie down for at least 15 minutes after administration.

I.V.

- Administer as an I.V. injection over more than 15 seconds.
- Store at room temperature and protect from light.
- *Incompatibilities:* Hydroxyzine hydrochloride, meperidine hydrochloride, morphine sulfate, promethazine hydrochloride

I.M.

- Administer slowly and deeply into the muscle.
- Store at room temperature and protect from light.

J
K
L

INTRANASAL

- Have patient blow nose before administration and sit up straight or stand with head tilting slightly forward.
- Give container to patient and have patient insert tip of container into one nostril, pointing container away from the center of the nose.
- Tell patient to hold breath and spray once by pressing down evenly on both sides. Immediately after administration, patient should resume breathing through mouth to reduce expelling the product. The nose can also be pinched to help retain spray if it starts to drip.
- If two sprays are prescribed (one in each nostril), repeat procedure using other nostril.
- Replace clear plastic cover and store bottle in cool, dry place out of direct sunlight.
- After administering the first dose, discard after 24 hrs regardless of what is remaining in the bottle (each bottle contains dosage for 8 sprays).

Route	Onset	Peak	Duration
P.O.	30–60 min	1–2 hr	4–6 hr
I.M., I.V.	<30 min	1–2 hr	4–6 hr
Nasal	Unknown	45 min	Unknown

Half-life: 2–6 hr

▤ Mechanism of Action

Blocks cyclooxygenase, an enzyme needed to synthesize prostaglandins. Prostaglandins mediate inflammatory response and cause local vasodilation, pain, and swelling. They also promote pain transmission from periphery to spinal cord. By blocking cyclooxygenase and inhibiting prostaglandins, this NSAID reduces inflammation and relieves pain.

▤ Contraindications

Active peptic ulcer disease or recent GI bleeding or perforation; advanced renal impairment or risk of renal impairment due to volume depletion; cerebrovascular bleeding, hemorrhagic diathesis, incomplete hemostasis, or high risk of bleeding; history of asthma, urticaria, or other allergic-type reactions after taking aspirin or other NSAIDs; hypersensitivity to ketorolac tromethamine or its components; labor and delivery; postoperative pain after coronary artery bypass graft (CABG) surgery; use as a prophylactic analgesic before any major surgery

▤ Interactions

DRUGS

ACE inhibitors, angiotensin II receptor antagonists: Decreased antihypertensive effect of these drugs; increased risk of decreased renal function in patients who are elderly or volume depleted or have existing renal impairment

anticoagulants such as warfarin, platelet aggregation inhibitors such as aspirin, pentoxifylline, selective serotonin reuptake inhibitors, serotonin–norepinephrine reuptake inhibitors: Increased risk of serious bleeding

antiepileptic drugs such as carbamazepine, phenytoin: Increased risk of seizures

aspirin and other salicylates, other NSAIDs: Increased risk of GI adverse reactions and bleeding, including GI toxicity

cyclosporine: Increased risk of cyclosporine-induced nephrotoxicity

digoxin: Increased digoxin levels with risk of digoxin toxicity

diuretics: Reduced effects of loop and thiazide diuretics in some patients

lithium: Possibly increased blood lithium level and increased risk of lithium toxicity

methotrexate: Possibly methotrexate toxicity

pemetrexed: Increased risk of pemetrexed-associated myelosuppression and GI and renal toxicity

probenecid: Decreased elimination of ketorolac, increased risk of adverse effects

ACTIVITIES

alcohol use: Increased risk of adverse GI effects

▤ Adverse Reactions

CNS: Aseptic meningitis, cerebral hemorrhage, coma, CVA, dizziness, drowsiness, headache, psychosis, **seizures**

CV: Edema, hypertension

EENT: Laryngeal edema, stomatitis

ENDO: Hyperglycemia

GI: Abdominal pain; **acute pancreatitis;** bloating; constipation; diarrhea; diverticulitis; elevated liver enzymes; flatulence; **GI**

bleeding, **perforation**, or ulceration; **hepatitis; hepatic failure**; jaundice; indigestion; nausea; vomiting; worsening of inflammatory bowel disease

GU: Interstitial nephritis, **renal failure**, urine retention

HEME: Agranulocytosis, anemia, **aplastic or hemolytic anemia**, eosinophilia, **leukopenia, pancytopenia, thrombocytopenia**

RESP: Bronchospasm, pneumonia, **respiratory depression**

SKIN: Diaphoresis, **erythema multiforme, exfoliative dermatitis**, photosensitivity, pruritus, rash, **Stevens–Johnson syndrome, toxic epidermal necrolysis**, urticaria

Other: Anaphylaxis, angioedema, hyperkalemia, hyponatremia, injection-site pain, lymphadenopathy, **sepsis**, unusual weight gain

☰ Childbearing Considerations

PREGNANCY

- Drug increases risk of premature closure of the fetal ductus arteriosus if given during the third trimester of pregnancy and fetal renal dysfunction if given after 20 weeks' gestation.
- Drug should be avoided in pregnant women starting at 20 weeks of gestation and onward.

LABOR & DELIVERY

- Drug may affect fetal circulation and inhibit uterine contractions.
- Use of drug is contraindicated during labor and delivery.

LACTATION

- Drug is present in breast milk.
- Patient should check with prescriber before breastfeeding.

REPRODUCTION

- Drug may affect fertility by delaying or preventing rupture of ovarian follicles.
- Drug should not be given to women who are planning to conceive or who are having difficulty conceiving.

☰ Nursing Considerations

- Be aware that NSAIDs like ketorolac should be avoided in patients with a recent MI because risk of reinfarction increases with NSAID therapy. If therapy is unavoidable, monitor patient closely for signs of cardiac ischemia.

- Know that the risk of heart failure increases with ketorolac use because drug is a NSAID. This class of drugs should not be used in patients with severe heart failure but, if unavoidable, monitor patient for worsening of heart failure.
- Notify prescriber if pain relief is inadequate or if breakthrough pain occurs between doses because supplemental doses of an opioid analgesic may be required.

! **WARNING** Monitor liver enzymes, as ordered. If elevated levels persist or worsen, notify prescriber and expect to stop drug, as ordered, to prevent hepatic impairment.

! **WARNING** Monitor patients with a history of peripheral edema, heart failure, or hypertension for adequate fluid balance because drug can promote fluid retention and worsen these conditions. Assess patient for decreased activity tolerance, dyspnea, edema, and unexplained rapid weight gain. Notify prescriber if such symptoms develop.

- Use ketorolac with extreme caution in patients with history of GI bleeding or ulcer disease because NSAIDs like ketorolac increase risk of GI bleeding and ulceration. Use ketorolac in these patients for shortest length of time possible.
- Know that serious GI tract bleeding and ulceration and perforation of intestine or stomach can occur without warning or symptoms. Elderly patients are at greater risk. To minimize risk, give drug with food. If GI distress occurs, withhold drug and notify prescriber immediately.
- Monitor patient with history of inflammatory bowel disease, such as Crohn's disease or ulcerative colitis, because ketorolac may worsen these conditions.
- Use ketorolac cautiously in patients with hypertension, and monitor blood pressure closely throughout therapy because drug can lead to onset of hypertension or worsen existing hypertension.

! **WARNING** Monitor patient closely for thrombotic events, including MI and stroke, because NSAIDs such as ketorolac increase risk. These events may occur early in treatment and risk increases with duration of use. Be aware that these events have

J
K
L

occurred even in patients who do not have a history of or risk factors for cardiovascular disease. Monitor patient for warning signs such as chest pain, shortness of breath, slurring of speech, or weakness. If any signs and symptoms develop, withhold ketorolac, alert prescriber immediately, and provide supportive care, as prescribed.

- Monitor patient—especially if elderly—for less common but serious adverse GI reactions, including anorexia, constipation, diverticulitis, dysphagia, esophagitis, gastritis, gastroenteritis, gastroesophageal reflux disease, hemorrhoids, hiatal hernia, melena, stomatitis, and vomiting.
- Monitor BUN and serum creatinine levels in the elderly; patients with heart failure, hepatic impairment, or impaired renal function; and those who are taking ACE inhibitors or diuretics, because drug may cause renal failure.
- Monitor CBC for decreased hemoglobin and hematocrit because drug may worsen anemia.

! **WARNING** Know that in a patient who has bone marrow suppression or is receiving antineoplastic drug therapy, monitor laboratory results (including WBC) and assess for evidence of infection because ketorolac has anti-inflammatory and antipyretic actions that may mask signs and symptoms, such as fever and pain.

! **WARNING** Assess patient's skin routinely for rash or other evidence of hypersensitivity reactions because ketorolac is an NSAID and may cause serious skin reactions without warning, even in patients with no history of NSAID hypersensitivity. Stop drug at first sign of reaction, and notify prescriber.

PATIENT TEACHING

- Alert patient that tablets are not used as initial therapy but follow an intramuscular or intravenous injection. Instruct patient to take ketorolac tablets with an antacid, a meal, or a snack to prevent stomach upset. Advise him to take drug with a full glass of water and to stay upright for at least 15 minutes afterward.
- Teach patient how to prime bottle and administer nasal spray form, if prescribed. Remind patient that nasal spray form is not to be inhaled. Tell patient not to use any single nasal spray bottle for more than 1 day, as it will not deliver the intended dose after 24 hours.
- Advise patient not to take aspirin, other NSAIDs, or other salicylates while taking ketorolac without consulting prescriber. Urge patient to limit use of acetaminophen to only a few days during ketorolac therapy and to notify prescriber of use.
- Caution patient not to use ketorolac for more than 5 days, as serious adverse effects may occur.
- Instruct him to immediately report blood in urine, easy bruising, itching, rash, swelling, or yellow eyes or skin.
- Caution pregnant patient that NSAIDs like ketorolac shouldn't be taken from 20 weeks, gestation onward, because drug may cause premature closure of the ductus arteriosus and fetal renal dysfunction.
- Explain that ketorolac may increase risk of serious adverse cardiovascular reactions; urge patient to seek immediate medical attention if signs or symptoms arise, such as chest pain, edema, shortness of breath, slurring of speech, unexplained weight gain, or weakness.
- Tell patient that ketorolac also may increase risk of serious adverse GI reactions; stress importance of seeking immediate medical attention if signs or symptoms occur, such as abdominal or epigastric pain, black tarry stools, indigestion, and vomiting blood or coffee-ground material.

! **WARNING** Alert patient to the possibility of serious allergic and skin reactions, although rare, occurring with ketorolac therapy. Urge patient to seek immediate medical attention if signs or symptoms occur, such as blisters, fever, a rash, or other signs of hypersensitivity, such as itching.

- Caution patient to avoid hazardous activities until drug's CNS effects are known.
- Urge patient to avoid alcohol while taking ketorolac.
- Encourage patient to have dental procedures performed before starting drug therapy because of increased risk of bleeding.
- Teach patient proper oral hygiene measures, and encourage him to use a soft-bristled toothbrush while taking ketorolac.

labetalol hydrochloride

Class and Category

Pharmacologic class: Noncardioselective beta-blocker/alpha[1] blocker
Therapeutic class: Antihypertensive

Indications and Dosages

＊ *To manage hypertension*

TABLETS

Adults. *Initial:* 100 mg twice daily, increased by 100 mg twice daily as needed and tolerated semi-weekly or weekly. *Maintenance:* 200 to 400 mg twice daily. *Maximum:* 600 mg twice daily.

＊ *To manage severe hypertension*

TABLETS

Inpatient adults after receiving drug parenterally. *Initial:* 200 mg after supine blood pressure has begun to rise, followed by 200 to 400 mg in 6 to 12 hr. Subsequent titration may be made every 24 hr thereafter depending on blood pressure control as follows: 200 mg twice daily followed by 400 mg twice daily followed by 800 mg twice daily followed by 1,200 mg twice daily, as needed.

I.V. INFUSION

Adults. 2 mg/min continuously until desired response occurs.

I.V. INJECTION

Adults. 20 mg given over 2 min; additional doses given in increments of 40 to 80 mg every 10 min as indicated until desired response occurs. *Maximum:* 300 mg.

±**DOSAGE ADJUSTMENT** For elderly patients, patients with hepatic impairment, and patients receiving a diuretic or other antihypertensive drugs, lower dosages usually required.

Drug Administration

P.O.

- Administer tablets after food intake.

I.V.

- Keep patient in a supine position during I.V. administration and for 3 hours afterward.
- For I.V. injection, administer slowly over a 2-minute period. Immediately before injection and at 5 and 10 minutes after injection, take patient's blood pressure.
- For I.V. infusion, dilute by adding 200 mg of drug to 160 ml of 0.9% Sodium Chloride Injection or 5% Dextrose Injection (see manufacturer guidelines for other appropriate solutions) to make a concentration of 1 mg/ml, or add 200 mg of drug to 250 ml of any of the above diluents to make a concentration of 2 mg/3 ml. Both concentrations are administered continuously at 2 mg/min with rate of infusion adjusted according to blood pressure. Administer drug with an infusion control device.
- Monitor patient's blood pressure throughout administration and after infusion is discontinued according to facility protocol, which is usually every 5 minutes for 30 minutes, then every 30 minutes for 2 hours, and then every hour for 6 hours.
- *Incompatibilities:* Alkaline solutions such as 5% Sodium Bicarbonate Injection, alkaline drugs such as furosemide

Route	Onset	Peak	Duration
P.O.	20–120 min	1–2 hr	8–24 hr
I.V.	< 5 min	5–15 min	2–4 hr

Half-life: 5.5–8 hr

Mechanism of Action

Selectively blocks alpha[1] and beta[2] receptors in vascular smooth muscle and beta[1] receptors in heart to reduce blood pressure and peripheral vascular resistance. Potent beta-blockade prevents reflex tachycardia, which commonly occurs when alpha blockers reduce cardiac output, resting heart rate, or stroke volume.

Contraindications

Bronchial asthma, cardiogenic shock, hypersensitivity to labetalol or its components, obstructive airway disease, other conditions associated with severe and prolonged hypotension, overt heart failure, second- or third-degree heart block, severe bradycardia

Interactions

DRUGS

calcium antagonist of verapamil type: Increased risk of adverse reactions
cimetidine: Possibly increased labetalol concentration and effects

epinephrine: Possibly unresponsiveness to usual doses of epinephrine
halothane anesthesia: Increased risk of hypotension
nitroglycerin: Blunted reflex tachycardia
other beta-blocker agonists: Possibly blunted bronchodilator effect of these drugs in patients with bronchospasm
tricyclic antidepressants: Increased risk of tremor

Adverse Reactions

CNS: Anxiety, confusion, depression, dizziness, drowsiness, fatigue, paresthesia, syncope, vertigo, weakness, yawning
CV: Bradycardia, chest pain, edema, **heart block, heart failure, hypotension,** orthostatic hypotension, **ventricular arrhythmias**
EENT: Nasal congestion, taste perversion
GI: Elevated liver enzymes, **hepatic necrosis, hepatitis,** indigestion, jaundice, nausea, vomiting
GU: Ejaculation failure, impotence
RESP: Dyspnea, wheezing
SKIN: Pruritus, rash, scalp tingling

Childbearing Considerations

PREGNANCY

- It is not known if drug causes fetal harm. However, drug does cross the placental barrier and may cause bradycardia, hypoglycemia, hypotension, and respiratory depression in newborns of mothers who were treated with the drug for hypertension during late pregnancy.
- Use with caution only if benefit to mother outweighs potential risk to fetus.

LACTATION

- Drug is present in breast milk.
- Patient should check with prescriber before breastfeeding.

Nursing Considerations

! **WARNING** Be aware that labetalol masks common signs of shock.

- Monitor blood glucose level in diabetic patient because labetalol may conceal symptoms of hypoglycemia.
- Be aware that stopping labetalol tablets abruptly after long-term therapy could result in angina, MI, or ventricular arrhythmias. Expect to taper dosage over 2 weeks while monitoring response.

PATIENT TEACHING

- Inform patient receiving drug intravenously that he must remain lying down throughout administration and for 3 hours afterward.
- Advise patient to report confusion, difficulty breathing, rash, slow pulse, and swelling in arms or legs.
- Caution patient not to stop drug abruptly because doing so could cause angina and rebound hypertension.
- Suggest that patient minimize effects of orthostatic hypotension by avoiding sudden position changes, rising to a sitting or standing position slowly, and taking labetalol at bedtime, if approved by prescriber.
- Instruct diabetic patient to check blood glucose level often and to be alert for signs and symptoms of hypoglycemia.
- Inform patient that scalp tingling may occur early in treatment but is transient.
- Urge patient to avoid alcohol during labetalol therapy.
- Advise patient to inform eye healthcare provider if he needs cataract surgery because intraoperative floppy iris syndrome has occurred during cataract surgery in some patients treated with the class of drugs of which labetalol is a member.

lacosamide
Vimpat

Class and Category

Pharmacologic class: Functionalized amino acid
Therapeutic class: Anticonvulsant
Controlled substance schedule: V

Indications and Dosages

❋ *To treat partial-onset seizures as monotherapy or adjunctive therapy*

I.V. INFUSION, ORAL SOLUTION, TABLETS
Adults and adolescents age 17 and over.
Initial for monotherapy: 100 mg twice daily, increased by 50 mg twice daily every week to recommended maintenance dose. Alternatively, 200 mg given as single loading dose, followed 12 hr later by 100 mg twice daily for 1 wk. *Initial for adjunctive therapy:* 50 mg twice daily. Dosage increased for both monotherapy and adjunctive therapy

at weekly intervals by 50 mg twice daily, as needed, up to recommended maintenance dose. *Maintenance:* 150 to 200 mg twice daily for monotherapy; 100 to 200 mg twice daily for adjunctive therapy.

Infants 1 month and older and children weighing 50 kg (110 lb) or more. *Initial:* 50 mg twice daily, increased by 50 mg twice daily every week to recommended maintenance dose. *Maintenance:* 150 to 200 mg twice daily as monotherapy; 100 to 200 mg twice daily as adjunctive therapy.

Infants 1 month and older and children weighing 30 kg (66 lb) to less than 50 kg (110 lb). *Initial:* 1 mg/kg twice daily, increased by 1 mg/kg twice daily every week to recommended maintenance dose. *Maintenance:* 2 to 4 mg/kg twice daily.

Infants 1 month and older and children weighing 6 kg (13.2 lb) to less than 30 kg (66 lb). *Initial:* 1 mg/kg twice daily, increased by 1 mg/kg twice daily every week to recommended maintenance dose. *Maintenance:* 3 to 6 mg/kg twice daily.

ORAL SOLUTION

Infants weighing less than 6 kg (13.2 lb). *Initial:* 1 mg/kg twice daily, increased by 1 mg/kg twice daily every week to recommended maintenance dose. *Maintenance:* 3.75 to 7.5 mg/kg twice daily.

I.V. INFUSION

Infants weighing less than 6 kg (13.2 lb). *Initial:* 0.66 mg/kg three times daily, increased by 0.66 mg/kg three times daily every week to recommended maintenance dose. *Maintenance:* 2.5 to 5 mg/kg three times daily.

✳ *As adjunct to treat primary generalized tonic-clonic seizures*

I.V. INFUSION, ORAL SOLUTION, TABLETS

Adults and adolescents age 17 and over. *Initial:* 50 mg twice daily, increased by 50 mg twice daily at weekly intervals based on response and tolerance. Dosage increased at weekly intervals by 50 mg twice daily, as needed, up to recommended maintenance dose. *Maintenance:* 100 to 200 mg twice daily.

Children ages 4 to 17 weighing 50 kg (110 lb) or more. 50 mg twice daily, increased by 50 mg twice daily every week to recommended maintenance dose. *Maintenance:* 100 mg to 200 mg twice daily.

Children ages 4 to 17 weighing 30 kg (66 lb) to less than 50 kg (110 lb). 1 mg/kg twice daily, increased by 1 mg/kg twice daily every week to recommended maintenance dose. *Maintenance:* 2 mg/kg to 4 mg/kg twice daily.

Children ages 4 to 17 weighing 11 kg (24.2 lb) to less than 30 kg (66 lb). 1 mg/kg twice daily, increased by 1 mg/kg twice daily every week to recommended maintenance dose. *Maintenance:* 3 mg/kg to 6 mg/kg twice daily.

±**DOSAGE ADJUSTMENT** For patients with mild to moderate hepatic impairment or severe renal impairment (creatinine clearance less than 30 ml/min) including end-stage renal disease, dosage reduced by 25% of maximum dosage recommended. Following a 4-hr hemodialysis treatment, dosage supplementation of up to 50% may be required. For patients with hepatic or renal impairment taking strong CYP2C9 or CYP3A4 inhibitors concurrently, dosage may have to be reduced.

⬚ Drug Administration

P.O.

- Tablets should be swallowed whole with a beverage and not chewed, crushed, or split.
- Use a calibrated device to measure oral solution dosage. Discard after 6 months of first opening the bottle.
- Oral solution may be administered through a gastrostomy or nasogastric tube.

I.V.

- Drug may be administered without further dilution or may be mixed with 0.9% Sodium Chloride Injection, 5% Dextrose Injection, or Lactated Ringer's Injection. If diluted, do not store diluted solution for more than 4 hours at room temperature.
- Administer over 30 to 60 minutes, although more rapid infusion of 15 minutes may be used in adults, if needed, but not in children.
- *Incompatibilities:* None reported by manufacturer

Route	Onset	Peak	Duration
P.O.	Unknown	1–4 hr	Unknown
I.V.	Unknown	30–60 min	Unknown
Half-life: 13 hr			

⬚ Mechanism of Action

May selectively inactivate voltage-gated sodium channels, which prevents seizure

J
K
L

activity by inhibiting repetitive neuronal firing in the brain and stabilizing hyperexcitable neuronal membranes.

Contraindications

Hypersensitivity to lacosamide and its components

Interactions

DRUGS

beta-blockers, calcium channel blockers, potassium channel blockers, sodium channel blockers including those that prolong PR interval such as sodium channel blocking antiepileptic drugs: Increased risk of AV block, bradycardia, or ventricular tachyarrhythmias

strong CYP2C9 inhibitors or CYP3A4 inhibitors (in presence of hepatic or renal impairment): Possibly significant increase in lacosamide exposure and adverse effects

Adverse Reactions

CNS: Aggression, agitation, asthenia, ataxia, attention deficit, cerebellar syndrome, confusion, depression, dizziness, dyskinesia, fatigue, feeling drunk, fever, hallucinations, headache, hypoesthesia, impaired balance, insomnia, irritability, memory impairment, mood alteration, paresthesia, psychotic disorder, **seizures** (new or worsening), somnolence, **suicidal ideation**, tremor, vertigo
CV: Atrial fibrillation or flutter, AV block, bradycardia, conduction disturbances, palpitations, prolonged PR interval, **prolonged QT interval**
EENT: Blurred vision, diplopia, dry mouth, nystagmus, oral hypoesthesia, tinnitus
GI: Constipation, diarrhea, dyspepsia, nausea, vomiting
HEME: Agranulocytosis, anemia, **neutropenia**
MS: Dysarthria, muscle spasms
SKIN: Pruritus, rash, **Stevens–Johnson syndrome, toxic epidermal necrolysis**, urticaria
Other: Angioedema; delayed multiorgan hypersensitivity reaction; injection-site erythema, irritation, and pain

Childbearing Considerations

PREGNANCY

- Pregnancy exposure registry: 1-888-233-2334 or http://www. aedpregnancyregistry.org/.

- It is not known if drug may cause fetal harm.
- Use with caution only if benefit to mother outweighs potential risk to fetus.

LACTATION

- It is not known if drug is present in breast milk.
- Patient should check with prescriber before breastfeeding.

Nursing Considerations

- Use cautiously in patients with concomitant drug therapy with drugs that prolong the PR interval, conduction problems (such as AV block, sick sinus syndrome and no pacemaker in place), severe cardiac disease (such as heart failure, myocardial ischemia), or sodium channel disorders such as Brugada syndrome, because lacosamide may affect conduction. For these patients, ensure that an ECG has been done, as ordered, prior to starting therapy and after dosage titration.
- Use cautiously in patients with cardiovascular disease or diabetic neuropathy because drug may predispose them to atrial fibrillation or flutter.
- Know that in patients who are already taking a single antiepileptic and being converted to lacosamide monotherapy, the maintenance dose of lacosamide should be maintained for at least 3 days before beginning the withdrawal of the concomitant antiepileptic drug, as ordered. A gradual withdrawal of the concomitant antiepileptic drug over at least 6 weeks is recommended.
- Watch patient closely for suicidal tendencies, particularly when therapy starts and dosage changes, because depression may worsen temporarily during these times and lead to suicidal ideation.
- Be aware that lacosamide therapy should be discontinued gradually over at least 1 week to minimize seizure frequency.

! WARNING Monitor patient closely for hypersensitivity reactions to lacosamide, such as pruritus, rash, and more than one organ abnormality, such as elevated liver enzymes and myocarditis or pancreatitis. Be aware that drug reaction with eosinophilia and systemic symptoms (DRESS) has occurred with use of other antiepileptics and therefore may possibly occur with lacosamide use. Monitor patient closely and if signs and symptoms are present to suggest DRESS, notify prescriber immediately and expect that drug may be discontinued.

PATIENT TEACHING

- Tell patient that lacosamide tablet or oral solution may be taken with or without food. If using tablet form, instruct patient to swallow tablet whole with water and not chew, crush, or divide the tablets. If using oral solution, remind patient to measure and administer the dose using a calibrated measuring device because a household teaspoon or tablespoon may not deliver correct dose. The solution should be discarded if any remains after 6 months of first opening the bottle.
- Alert patient that the oral solution of lacosamide contains aspartame, a source of phenylalanine that could be harmful to patients with phenylketonuria (PKU).
- Urge family or caregiver to watch patient closely for suicidal tendencies, especially when therapy starts or dosage changes.

! **WARNING** Instruct patient to report any persistent, severe, or unusual signs and symptoms to prescriber immediately. If allergic reaction occurs, counsel patient to seek immediate emergency medical care.

- Caution patient to avoid hazardous activities until drug's CNS effects are known.
- Encourage patient to carry medical identification that indicates her diagnosis and drug therapy.

lactitol
Pizensy

☰ Class and Category
Pharmacologic class: Simple monosaccharide sugar alcohol
Therapeutic class: Osmotic laxative

☰ Indications and Dosages
✳ *To treat chronic idiopathic constipation*

POWDER FOR ORAL SOLUTION
Adults. 20 g once daily.

± **DOSAGE ADJUSTMENT** Dosage reduced to 10 grams once daily for persistent loose stools.

☰ Drug Administration
P.O.
- Administration with meals is preferable.
- To mix using multidose bottle: Bottle top is a measuring cap marked to contain 10 grams of powder. For a 20-gram dose, fill the measuring cap twice to the top of the white section in cap marked by the arrow. For a 10-gram dose, fill the measuring cap once to the top of the white section in cap marked by the arrow. Pour the measured dose into an empty 8-ounce glass. Add 4 to 8 ounces of common beverages (coffee, soda, tea), juice, or water and stir to dissolve. Have patient drink entire contents of the glass.
- To use unit-dose packets: Pour the contents of one or two unit-dose packets, as prescribed, into an empty 8-ounce glass. Add 4 to 8 ounces of common beverages (coffee, soda, tea), juice, or water and stir thoroughly to dissolve. Have patient drink entire contents of the glass.
- Administer other oral drugs at least 2 hours before or after administration of drug.

Route	Onset	Peak	Duration
P.O.	Unknown	2.4–4.8 hr	Unknown

Half-life: 2.4 hr

☰ Mechanism of Action
Exerts an osmotic effect, causing the influx of water into the small intestine leading to a laxative effect in the colon.

☰ Contraindications
Galactosemia, hypersensitivity to lactitol or its components, mechanical gastrointestinal obstruction

☰ Interactions
DRUGS
other oral drugs: Possibly decreased absorption

☰ Adverse Reactions
CV: Hypertension
EENT: Nasopharyngitis
GI: Abdominal distention or pain, diarrhea (may be severe), flatulence

GU: UTI
RESP: Upper respiratory infection
SKIN: Pruritus, rash
OTHER: Elevated blood creatinine phosphokinase, **hypersensitivity reactions**

Childbearing Considerations

PREGNANCY

- It is not known if drug can cause fetal harm.
- Although drug is minimally absorbed systemically, use with caution in pregnant women.

LACTATION

- It is not known if drug is present in breast milk.
- Patient should check with prescriber before breastfeeding.

Nursing Considerations

! **WARNING** Monitor patient for hypersensitivity reactions, such as pruritus and rash, after administration.

- Administer all other oral drugs 2 hours before or 2 hours after administration of lactitol to prevent interference with absorption.

PATIENT TEACHING

- Teach patient how to mix the powder to make an oral solution for the dose prescribed.
- Tell patient to take any other oral drugs 2 hours before or 2 hours after taking lactitol.

! **WARNING** Instruct patient to notify prescriber if itching or a rash appears after taking lactitol.

- Advise patient to stop drug and notify prescriber if persistent loose stools occur.

lactulose

Enulose, Generlac

Class and Category

Pharmacologic class: Disaccharide
Therapeutic: Colonic acidifier

Indications and Dosages

* *To treat constipation*

POWDER, ORAL SOLUTION

Adults. *Initial:* 10 to 20 g daily, increased as needed. *Maximum:* 40 g daily.

* *To treat portal-systemic (hepatic) encephalopathy*

POWDER, ORAL SOLUTION

Adults. *Initial:* 20 to 30 g three times daily or four times daily with dosage adjustment made every day or two, as needed, until two or three soft stools occur daily. *Usual:* 60 to 100 g daily in divided doses. *Rapid laxation:* 20 to 30 g every hr initially and then reduced to usual dosage.

RETENTION ENEMA

Adults. 200 g (300 ml); if evacuated too promptly, repeated immediately. Dosage given every 4 to 6 hr, as needed.

* *To prevent portal-systemic (hepatic) encephalopathy*

ORAL SOLUTION

Adults. 20 g (30 ml) to 30 g (45 ml) three or four times daily, adjusted every day or two to produce 2 to 3 soft stools daily.
Children age 1 and older. 26.7 g (40 ml) to 60 g (90 ml) daily in divided doses with dosage adjusted every day or two, as needed, to produce 2 to 3 soft stools daily.
Infants up to 1 year. 1.7 (2.5 ml) to 6.5 g (10 ml) daily in divided doses with dosage adjusted every day or two, as needed, to produce 2 to 3 soft stools daily.

Drug Administration

P.O.

- For powder form, dissolve contents of packet in 4 ounces of fruit juice, milk, or water. Shake well before using.
- Use calibrated device to measure dosage of oral solution.

P.R.

- Retention enema used for impending coma or when coma has already occurred.
- Dilute 300 ml of drug in 700 ml of water or normal saline solution and administer as an enema. Use a rectal tube with a balloon to help with retention.
- Patient should retain enema for 30 to 60 min. If retention is less than 30 min, enema repeated.

Route	Onset	Peak	Duration
P.O.	24–48 hr	Unknown	Unknown
P.R.	Unknown	Unknown	Unknown

Half-life: 1.7–2 hr

Mechanism of Action

Arrives unchanged in the colon, where it breaks down into lactic acid and small amounts of acetic and formic acids, acidifying fecal contents. Acidification leads to increased osmotic pressure in the colon, which, in turn, increases stool water content and softens stool.

Also, lactulose makes intestinal contents more acidic than blood. This prevents ammonia diffusion from intestine into blood, as occurs in hepatic encephalopathy. The trapped ammonia is converted into ammonia ions and, by lactulose's cathartic effect, is expelled in feces with other nitrogenous wastes.

Contraindications

Hypersensitivity to lactulose or its components, low-galactose diet

Interactions

DRUGS

antacids (nonabsorbable), antibiotics (especially oral neomycin): Decreased effectiveness of lactulose
other laxatives: Possibly falsely indicating adequate lactulose dosage when used to treat hepatic encephalopathy

Adverse Reactions

ENDO: Hyperglycemia
GI: Abdominal cramps and distention, diarrhea, flatulence
Other: Hypernatremia, hypokalemia, hypovolemia

Childbearing Considerations

PREGNANCY

- It is not known if drug causes fetal harm.
- Use with caution only if benefit to mother outweighs potential risk to fetus.

LACTATION

- It is not known if drug is present in breast milk.
- Patient should check with prescriber before breastfeeding.

Nursing Considerations

- Expect to periodically check serum electrolyte levels of debilitated or elderly patient who uses oral drug longer than 6 months.
- Monitor blood ammonia level in patient with hepatic encephalopathy. Also watch for dehydration, hypernatremia, and hypokalemia when giving higher lactulose doses to treat this condition.
- Monitor diabetic patient for hyperglycemia because lactulose contains galactose and lactose.
- Plan to replace fluids if frequent bowel movements cause hypovolemia.

PATIENT TEACHING

- Advise patient to take lactulose diluted with juice, milk, or water to reduce sweet taste.
- Direct patient not to use other laxatives while taking lactulose.
- Instruct patient to report abdominal distention or severe diarrhea.
- Advise diabetic patient to check blood glucose level often and to report hyperglycemia.
- Instruct patient to increase fluid intake if frequent bowel movements occur.
- Teach patient with chronic constipation the importance of exercising, increasing fiber in diet, and increasing fluid intake.
- Inform patient that because oral lactulose must reach the colon to work, bowel movement may not occur for 24 to 48 hours after taking drug.

lamivudine

Epivir, Epivir-HBV, Heptovir (CAN)

Class and Category

Pharmacologic class: Synthetic nucleoside analogue
Therapeutic class: Antiviral

Indications and Dosages

✳ *To treat chronic hepatitis B virus (HBV) infection associated with active liver inflammation and evidence of hepatitis B viral replication*

ORAL SOLUTION, TABLETS (EPIVIR-HBV)

Adults. 100 mg once daily.
Children ages 2 to 17. 3 mg/kg once daily. *Maximum:* 100 mg once daily.

✳ *As adjunct to treat human immunodeficiency virus type 1 (HIV-1) infection*

ORAL SOLUTION, TABLETS (EPIVIR)

Adults. 300 mg once daily or 150 mg twice daily.

TABLETS

Children weighing 25 kg (55 lb) or more. 300 mg once daily or 150 mg in a.m. and 150 mg in p.m. *Maximum:* 300 mg daily.

J
K
L

Children weighing 20 kg (44 lb) to less than 25 kg (55 lb). 225 mg once daily or 75 mg in a.m. and 150 mg in p.m. *Maximum:* 225 mg daily.

Children weighing 14 kg (30.8 lb) to less than 20 kg (44 lb). 150 mg once daily or 75 mg in a.m. and 75 mg in p.m. *Maximum:* 150 mg daily.

ORAL SOLUTION

Infants ages 3 months and over. 10 mg/kg once daily or 5 mg/kg twice daily. *Maximum:* 300 mg daily.

±**DOSAGE ADJUSTMENT** For adults receiving Epivir-HBV, dosage adjustment is as follows: Adults with creatinine clearance between 30 and 49 ml/min, 100 mg first dose, then reduced to 50 mg once daily thereafter. For adults with creatinine clearance between 15 and 29 ml/min, 100 mg first dose, then reduced to 25 mg once daily thereafter. For adults with creatinine clearance between 5 and 14 ml/min, first dose reduced to 35 mg, then reduced to 15 mg once daily thereafter. For adults with creatinine clearance less than 5 ml/min, first dose reduced to 35 mg, then reduced to 10 mg once daily thereafter. There is no recommendation for pediatric patients with renal impairment for Epivir-HBV. For adults receiving Epivir, dosage adjustment is as follows: Adults with creatinine clearance between 30 and 49 ml/min, dosage reduced to 150 mg once daily. For adults with creatinine clearance between 15 and 29 ml/min, 150 mg first dose, then reduced to 100 mg once daily thereafter. For adults with creatinine clearance between 5 and 14 ml/min, 150 mg first dose, then reduced to 50 mg once daily thereafter. For adults with creatinine clearance less than 5 ml/min, 50 mg first dose, then reduced to 25 mg once daily. For pediatric patients with renal impairment taking Epivir, dosage may be reduced or dosing interval increased.

≡ Drug Administration

P.O.

- Do not confuse Epivir with Epivir-HBV. They are not interchangeable.

Route	Onset	Peak	Duration
P.O.	Unknown	1–3 hr	Unknown

Half-life: 5–7 hr

≡ Mechanism of Action

After being phosphorylated to its active metabolite, lamivudine inhibits the DNA- and RNA-dependent polymerase activities of HBV and HIV-1 reverse transcriptases via DNA chain termination after incorporation of the nucleotide analogue into viral DNA. This destroys the activity of the hepatitis B and HIV-1 viruses.

≡ Contraindications

Hypersensitivity to lamivudine or its components

≡ Interactions

DRUGS

drugs inhibiting organic cation transporters such as trimethoprim: Possibly altered excretion of lamivudine
sorbitol: Reduced lamivudine exposure and effectiveness

≡ Adverse Reactions

CNS: Chills, depression, dizziness, fatigue, fever, headache, insomnia, malaise, neuropathy, paresthesia, peripheral neuropathy, sleep disorders, weakness
EENT: Ear, nose, throat infections; nasal congestion or discharge; sore throat; stomatitis
ENDO: Cushingoid appearance, fat redistribution, hyperglycemia
GI: Abdominal pain, anorexia, bilirubin increase, diarrhea, dyspepsia, elevated lipase and liver enzyme levels, **exacerbation of hepatitis posttreatment, hepatic decompensation in patient co-infected with HIV-1 and hepatitis C, hepatomegaly with steatosis,** nausea, **pancreatitis,** vomiting
HEME: Anemia, **severe anemias including pure red cell aplasia and neutropenia,** splenomegaly, **thrombocytopenia**
MS: Abdominal cramps, arthralgia, elevated CPK level, musculoskeletal pain, myalgia, **rhabdomyolysis**
RESP: Abnormal breath sounds, cough, wheezing
SKIN: Alopecia, pruritus, rash, urticaria
Other: **Anaphylaxis, emergence of resistant HBV infection or HIV-1 infection,** immune reconstitution syndrome, **lactic acidosis,** lymphadenopathy

≡ Childbearing Considerations

PREGNANCY

- Pregnancy exposure registry: 1-800-258-4263.

- It is not known if drug causes fetal harm.
- Use with caution only if benefit to mother outweighs potential risk to fetus.

LACTATION

- Drug is present in breast milk.
- The Centers for Disease Control and Prevention recommends that HIV-1 infected mothers not breastfeed to avoid risking postnatal transmission of HIV-1 infection to infants. They also do not recommend breastfeeding because of potential drug-induced adverse reactions in the infant.
- Mothers who are not HIV-1 positive should check with prescriber before breastfeeding.

Nursing Considerations

- Be aware that Epivir-HBV oral solution and tablets contain a lower dose of lamivudine than used to treat HIV-1 infection and should not be used to treat patients co-infected with HBV and HIV-1 infections. Patients with unrecognized or untreated HIV infection exposed to Epivir-HBV may develop a rapid emergence of HIV-1 resistance. Make sure appropriate HIV counseling and testing have been done before treatment and periodically during treatment with lamivudine to ensure this does not happen.
- Use extreme caution when administering lamivudine to patient with known risk factors for liver disease.
- Monitor patient throughout treatment for evidence of loss of therapeutic response. Indicators include increasing levels of HBV DNA over time after an initial decline below assay limit, progression of clinical signs or symptoms of hepatic disease and/or worsening of hepatic necroinflammatory findings, or return of persistently elevated ALT levels. These findings may require drug to be discontinued.
- Be aware that a switch to an alternative regimen may be needed for patients in whom serum HBV DNA remains detectable after 24 weeks of treatment, to reduce the risk of resistance in patients receiving monotherapy with Epivir-HBV.

! **WARNING** Know that lactic acidosis and severe hepatomegaly with steatosis have occurred with lamivudine therapy, and death has occurred in some patients. Risk factors include presence of obesity, prolonged nucleoside exposure, and being a woman. However, know that lactic acidosis and severe hepatomegaly with steatosis have also occurred in patients with no known risk factors. Expect lamivudine to be discontinued in any patient who develops clinical or laboratory findings suggestive of lactic acidosis or pronounced hepatotoxicity, even in the absence of marked transaminase elevations.

- Monitor patient's ALT and HBV DNA levels during treatment to determine treatment options if viral mutants emerge.
- Monitor patients co-infected with HIV-1 and hepatitis C closely for signs and symptoms of liver dysfunction, because hepatic decompensations, some of which resulted in death, have occurred in patients receiving combination antiretroviral therapy for HIV-1 that included interferon alfa.
- Be aware that immune reconstitution syndrome has occurred in patients treated with combination antiretroviral therapy, including lamivudine. The inflammatory response predisposes susceptible patients to opportunistic infections such as cytomegalovirus, *Mycobacterium avium* infection, *Pneumocystis jiroveci* pneumonia, or tuberculosis. Autoimmune disorders such as Graves' disease, Guillain–Barré syndrome, or polymyositis have also occurred. Report sudden or unusual adverse reactions to prescriber.
- Observe patient for redistribution of body fat, including breast enlargement, central obesity, development of buffalo hump, facial wasting, and peripheral wasting, which may produce a cushingoid-type appearance.
- Expect patient to be closely monitored for at least several months after lamivudine has been discontinued, because exacerbation of hepatitis may occur.

PATIENT TEACHING

- Instruct patient with hepatitis B on the importance of testing for HIV before therapy begins and then periodically throughout therapy to avoid development of resistance to HIV treatment.
- Instruct patient to take lamivudine once daily. If he misses a dose, tell him to take

it as soon as he remembers but not to double the next dose or take more than the prescribed dose.

- Advise patient that treatment with lamivudine does not reduce the risk of transmission of HBV or HIV to others through blood contamination or sexual contact.
- Inform diabetic patient using oral solution that each 15-ml dose of Epivir contains 3 g of sucrose; 20-ml dose of Epivir-HBV contains 4 g of sucrose.
- Tell patient being treated for hepatitis B to report immediately any new or worsening symptoms to prescriber, because emergence of resistant hepatitis B virus may occur or disease may worsen during treatment.

! **WARNING** Warn patient with hepatitis B that acute severe exacerbations of hepatitis B may occur following discontinuation of lamivudine. He should not discontinue drug without prescriber knowledge. Tell patient to report any reappearance of signs and symptoms of hepatitis B.

- Warn patient that fat distribution may occur with lamivudine therapy and may alter his appearance.
- Advise patient to alert all prescribers of lamivudine therapy and to tell the prescriber if patient is taking any other prescription or over-the-counter drugs. Instruct patient to avoid chronic use of sorbitol-containing drugs, when possible, as drug may become less effective.

! **WARNING** Alert patient that severe conditions may develop while taking lamivudine. Encourage him to stop taking drug and seek medical attention immediately if he experiences any persistent, severe, or unusual symptoms.

lamotrigine
Lamictal, Lamictal CD, Lamictal ODT, Lamictal XR

≣ Class and Category
Pharmacologic class: Phenyltriazine
Therapeutic class: Anticonvulsant

≣ Indications and Dosages
✱ *As adjunct to treat partial seizures; to treat generalized seizures of Lennox–Gastaut syndrome; to treat primary generalized tonic–clonic seizures*

CHEWABLE TABLETS, ORAL SUSPENSION, ORALLY DISINTEGRATING TABLETS, TABLETS

Adults and children over age 12 taking valproate. 25 mg every other day for 2 wk, followed by 25 mg once daily for 2 wk. Increased by 25 to 50 mg every 1 to 2 wk, if needed. *Maintenance:* 100 to 200 mg daily.
Children ages 2 to 12 taking valproate. 0.15 mg/kg/day (rounded down to nearest whole tablet) as a single dose or in divided doses twice daily for 2 wk and then 0.3 mg/kg/day (rounded down to nearest whole tablet) as single dose or in divided doses twice daily for next 2 wk. Increased by 0.3 mg/kg/day (rounded down to the nearest whole tablet and amount added to previously administered daily dose), every 1 to 2 wk, if needed, to reach maintenance dosage. *Maintenance:* 1 to 3 mg/kg/day as single dose or in divided doses twice daily. *Maximum:* 200 mg/day.
Adults and children over age 12 not taking carbamazepine, phenobarbital, phenytoin, primidone, or valproate. 25 mg once daily for 2 wk, followed by 50 mg once daily for 2 wk. Increased by 50 mg every 1 to 2 wk, if needed. *Maintenance:* 225 to 375 mg daily in 2 divided doses.
Children ages 2 to 12 not taking carbamazepine, phenobarbital, phenytoin, primidone, or valproate. 0.3 mg/kg/day (rounded down to the nearest whole tablet) in 1 or 2 divided doses for 2 wk; followed by 0.6 mg/kg/day (rounded down to the nearest whole tablet) in 2 divided doses for 2 wk. Increased by 0.6 mg/kg/day (rounded down to the nearest whole tablet and added to the previously administered daily dose) every 1 to 2 wk, if needed. *Maintenance:* 4.5 to 7.5 mg/kg/day in 2 divided doses. *Maximum:* 300 mg daily in two divided doses.
Adults and children over age 12 taking carbamazepine, phenobarbital, phenytoin, or primidone but NOT valproate. 50 mg once daily for 2 wk and then 100 mg daily in 2 divided doses for 2 wk. Increased by 100 mg/day every 1 to 2 wk, if needed.

Maintenance: 300 to 500 mg daily in 2 divided doses.

Children ages 2 to 12 taking carbamazepine, phenobarbital, phenytoin, or primidone but NOT valproate. 0.6 mg/kg/day (rounded down to the nearest whole tablet) in 2 divided doses for 2 wk and then 1.2 mg/kg/day (rounded down to the nearest whole tablet) in 2 divided doses for 2 wk. Increased by 1.2 mg/kg/day (rounded down to the nearest whole tablet and this amount added to the previously administered daily dose) every 1 to 2 wk, if needed to reach maintenance dosage. *Maintenance:* 5 to 15 mg/kg/day (rounded down to the nearest whole tablet) in 2 divided doses. *Maximum:* 400 mg daily in 2 divided doses.

±**DOSAGE ADJUSTMENT** For children ages 2 to 12 weighing less than 30 kg (66 lb), maintenance dosage, regardless of what drugs are or are not taken adjunctively, may have to be increased by 50%, based on clinical response.

✳ *To treat partial seizures as monotherapy with conversion from carbamazepine, phenobarbital, phenytoin, primidone, or valproate*

CHEWABLE TABLETS, ORAL SUSPENSION, ORALLY DISINTEGRATING TABLETS, TABLETS

Adults and adolescents age 16 and over converting from carbamazepine, phenytoin, phenobarbital, or primidone. 50 mg once daily for 2 wk, followed by 50 mg twice daily for next 2 wk. Increased by 100 mg daily every 1 to 2 wk (while continuing to take carbamazepine, phenobarbital, phenytoin, or primidone), until usual maintenance dosage—500 mg daily in 2 divided doses—is achieved. Then carbamazepine, phenobarbital, phenytoin, or primidone dosage tapered in 20% decrements weekly over 4 wk and then discontinued.

Adults and adolescents age 16 and over converting from valproate. 25 mg every other day for 2 wk followed by 25 mg once daily for 2 wk. Then increased by 25 to 50 mg daily every 1 to 2 wk until maintenance dosage of 200 mg daily is achieved. Then valproate dosage decreased to 500 mg daily by decrements no greater than 500 mg daily every wk and then maintained at 500 mg daily for 1 wk. After

valproate dosage has been at 500 mg for 1 wk, lamotrigine dosage increased to 300 mg daily while valproate dosage decreased to 250 mg daily for 1 wk. Then lamotrigine dosage increased by 100 mg daily every wk until maintenance dose of 500 mg daily is reached (given in 2 divided doses). Valproate therapy is then discontinued.

E.R. TABLETS

Adults and adolescents age 13 and over converting from carbamazepine, phenobarbital, phenytoin, or primidone. 50 mg once daily for first 2 wk, then increased as follows: 100 mg once daily for wk 3 and 4, then 200 mg once daily for wk 5, then 300 mg once daily for wk 6, then 400 mg once daily for wk 7, and 500 mg once daily for wk 8. Once maintenance dosage of 500 mg daily has been reached, carbamazepine, phenobarbital, phenytoin, or primidone dosage tapered in 20% decrements weekly over 4 wk and then discontinued. Two weeks after carbamazepine, phenobarbital, phenytoin, or primidone has been discontinued, lamotrigine dosage decreased no faster than 100 mg/day each week until monotherapy maintenance dosage of 250 to 300 mg daily has been reached.

Adults and adolescents age 13 and over converting from valproate. 25 mg every other day for 2 wk, then increased as follows: 25 mg once daily for wk 3 and 4, then 50 mg once daily for wk 5, then 100 mg once daily for wk 6, then 150 mg once daily for wk 7. Once lamotrigine dosage has reached 150 mg once daily, valproate dosage decreased by decrements no greater than 500 mg/day/wk to 500 mg/day and then maintained for 1 wk. Then lamotrigine dosage increased to 200 mg daily with valproate dosage decreased to 250 mg/day for 1 wk. This is followed by lamotrigine dosage increased to 250 to 300 mg daily and valproate discontinued.

✳ *To treat partial seizures with conversion from a single antiepileptic drug other than carbamazepine, phenobarbital, phenytoin, primidone, or valproate*

E.R. TABLETS

Adults and adolescents age 13 and over converting from an antiepileptic drug other than carbamazepine, phenobarbital, phenytoin, primidone, or valproate. 25 mg once daily for 2 wk, followed by 50 mg once

J
K
L

daily for next 2 wk. Increased to 100 mg once daily for wk 5, followed by 150 mg once daily for wk 6 and 200 mg once daily for wk 7. Further increased by 100 mg once daily at weekly intervals beginning at week 8 and onward until usual maintenance dosage—300 to 400 mg daily—is reached. Once dosage has reached 250 to 300 mg once daily, antiepileptic drug tapered in 20% decrements weekly over 4 wk and then discontinued.

* *As adjunct to treat primary generalized tonic-clonic seizures and partial-onset seizures*

E.R. TABLETS

Adults and children age 13 and over taking valproate. 25 mg every other day for 2 wk, followed by 25 mg once daily for 2 wk, followed by 50 mg once daily for 1 wk. Then 100 mg once daily for 1 wk, then 150 mg once daily. Dosage increased further, as needed, but increase not greater than 100 mg/day on a weekly basis. *Maintenance:* 200 to 250 mg once daily.

Adults and children age 13 and over NOT taking carbamazepine, phenobarbital, phenytoin, primidone, or valproate. 25 mg once daily for 2 wk, followed by 50 mg once daily for 2 wk, followed by 100 mg once daily for 1 wk. Then 150 mg once daily for 1 wk, followed by 200 mg once daily. Dosage increased further, as needed, but increase not greater than 100 mg/daily on a weekly basis. *Maintenance:* 300 to 400 mg once daily.

Adults and children age 13 and over taking carbamazepine, phenobarbital, phenytoin, or primidone and NOT taking valproate. 50 mg once daily for 2 wk, followed by 100 mg once daily for 2 wk, followed by 200 mg once daily for 1 wk. Then, 300 mg once daily for 1 wk, followed by 400 mg once daily. Dosage increased further, as needed, but increase not greater than 100 mg/daily on a weekly basis. *Maintenance:* 400 to 600 mg once daily.

* *As maintenance therapy for bipolar 1 disorder to delay occurrence of mood episodes (depression, mania, hypomania, mixed episodes) in patients being treated for acute mood episodes with standard therapy*

CHEWABLE TABLETS, ORAL SUSPENSION, ORALLY DISINTEGRATING TABLETS, TABLETS

Adults not taking carbamazepine, phenobarbital, phenytoin, primidone, rifampin, or valproate. 25 mg once daily for 2 wk, followed by 50 mg once daily for 2 wk, followed by 100 mg once daily for 1 wk, and then increased to 200 mg once daily as maintenance dose. *Maximum:* 200 mg daily.

Adults taking valproate. 25 mg every other day for 2 wk, followed by 25 mg once daily for 2 wk, followed by 50 mg once daily for 1 wk, and then increased to 100 mg once daily as maintenance dose.

Adults taking carbamazepine, lopinavir/ritonavir, phenobarbital, phenytoin, primidone, or rifampin, but not valproate. 50 mg once daily for 2 wk, followed by 100 mg once daily in divided doses for 2 wk, followed by 200 mg once daily in divided doses for 1 wk, then increased to 300 mg daily in divided doses for 1 wk, and then increased to 400 mg daily in divided doses as maintenance dose.

±**DOSAGE ADJUSTMENT** *For all indications:* For women taking estrogen-containing oral contraceptives and NOT taking carbamazepine, phenobarbital, phenytoin, primidone, or other drugs such as rifampin and protease inhibitors such as atazanavir/ritonavir or lopinavir/ritonavir, maintenance dose may have to be increased gradually by as much as twofold over recommended target maintenance dose. For women discontinuing estrogen-containing oral contraceptives who have been stabilized on lamotrigine prior to discontinuation and NOT taking carbamazepine, phenobarbital, phenytoin, primidone, or other drugs such as rifampin and protease inhibitors such as atazanavir/ritonavir or lopinavir/ritonavir, maintenance dose may have to be decreased gradually by as much as half. For patient with moderate to severe hepatic impairment without ascites, all dosages decreased by 25%, and for patient with severe hepatic impairment with ascites, all dosages decreased by 50%. For patient with significant renal impairment, maintenance dosage may have to be reduced on individual basis. Dosage may have to be increased during pregnancy.

Drug Administration

P.O.

- Starter and titration kits can be used for the first 5 weeks of treatment, based upon concomitant medications, for patients with epilepsy (older than 12 years) and bipolar I disorder (adults). The kits are recommended for use in appropriate patients who are starting or restarting drug.

- E.R. tablets should be swallowed whole and not chewed, crushed, or split.
- Tablets for oral suspension may be swallowed whole, chewed, or dispersed in water or diluted with fruit juice. If the tablets are chewed, administer a small amount of water or diluted fruit juice to aid in swallowing. To disperse tablets for oral suspension, add tablets to a small amount of liquid (1 teaspoon, or enough to cover drug). Wait 1 minute for dispersion to take place, swirl solution, and administer immediately. Never attempt to administer partial quantities of the dispersed tablets.
- Have patient place oral disintegrating tablets onto tongue and move around in mouth. The ODT tablets can be swallowed with or without water.

Route	Onset	Peak	Duration
P.O.	Unknown	1–5 hr	Unknown
P.O./E.R.	Unknown	4–11 hr	Unknown

Half-life: Variable

⸬ Mechanism of Action

May stabilize neuron membranes by blocking their sodium channels and inhibiting release of excitatory neurotransmitters, such as aspartate and glutamate, through these channels. By blocking the release of neurotransmitters, lamotrigine inhibits the spread of seizure activity in the brain, reduces seizure frequency, and diminishes mood swings.

⸬ Contraindications

Hypersensitivity to lamotrigine or its components

⸬ Interactions

DRUGS

atazanavir/ritonavir, carbamazepine, lopinavir/ritonavir, phenobarbital, phenytoin, primidone, rifampin: Decreased blood lamotrigine level
estrogen-containing oral contraceptive preparations containing 30 mcg ethinylestradiol and 150 mcg levonorgestrel: Decreased blood levels of both drugs
organic cationic transporter 2 (OCT2) substrates such as dofetilide: Possibly increased plasma levels of these drugs
valproic acid: Increased lamotrigine level

⸬ Adverse Reactions

CNS: Aggression, amnesia, anxiety, **aseptic meningitis**, ataxia, confusion, depression, dizziness, drowsiness, emotional lability, exacerbation of parkinsonian symptoms, fever, headache, **increased seizure activity**, lack of coordination, **suicidal ideation**, tics
CV: Chest pain, **conduction abnormalities, proarrhythmias**, vasculitis
EENT: Blurred vision, diplopia, dry mouth, nystagmus
GI: Abdominal pain, anorexia, constipation, diarrhea, esophagitis, **hepatic failure, pancreatitis**, vomiting
HEME: Agranulocytosis, anemia, **aplastic or hemolytic anemia, disseminated intravascular coagulation (DIC)**, eosinophilia, **hemophagocytic lymphohistiocytosis, leukopenia, neutropenia, pancytopenia, severe anemia such as pure red cell aplasia, thrombocytopenia**
MS: Rhabdomyolysis
RESP: Apnea
SKIN: Petechiae, photosensitivity, pruritus, rash, **Stevens–Johnson syndrome, toxic epidermal necrolysis**
Other: Angioedema, drug reaction with eosinophilia and systemic symptoms (DRESS), flu-like symptoms, hypogammaglobulinemia lupus-like reaction, lymphadenopathy, **progressive immunosuppression**

⸬ Childbearing Considerations

PREGNANCY

- Pregnancy exposure registry: 1-888-233-2334 or http://www. aedpregnancyregistry.org/.
- It is not known if drug causes fetal harm, but animal studies suggest developmental toxicity may occur.
- Use with caution only if benefit to mother outweighs potential risk to fetus.
- Dosage may have to be adjusted during pregnancy.

LACTATION

- Drug is present in breast milk.
- Patient should check with prescriber before breastfeeding.
- If breastfeeding occurs, infant should be monitored for lamotrigine toxicity; if present, breastfeeding should be discontinued.

J
K
L

REPRODUCTION

- Women taking estrogen-containing oral contraceptive preparations containing 30 mcg ethinyl estradiol and 150 mcg levonorgestrel should use a different contraceptive method because of decreased blood levels of both drugs.

Nursing Considerations

! WARNING Know that lamotrigine is not recommended for patients with functional or structural heart disease, because drug could widen QRS interval and induce proarrhythmias (severe enough to cause death). Also know that concomitant use of other sodium channel blockers may further increase the risk for proarrhythmias in these patients.

- Use cautiously in patients with illnesses that could affect elimination or metabolism of lamotrigine, such as cardiac, hepatic, or renal functional impairment.
- Be aware that the patient may be converted directly from immediate-release lamotrigine to extended-release lamotrigine with the initial dose of extended-release matching the total daily dose of immediate-release lamotrigine. However, monitor effects closely, especially for patient who is receiving an enzyme-inducing agent that may lower plasma levels of lamotrigine on conversion. If drug effectiveness appears to be altered, notify prescriber and expect a dosage adjustment.

! WARNING Be aware that lamotrigine may cause potentially life-threatening rash. Notify prescriber at first sign, and expect to discontinue drug. Lamotrigine therapy shouldn't be restarted after rash subsides.

- Monitor patient for adverse reactions, especially suicidal thoughts, at start of therapy and with each dosage increase.

! WARNING Monitor patient for hypersensitivity, such as fever, rash, or lymphadenopathy in association with other organ system dysfunction that may be suggestive of DRESS. Although rare, DRESS may be life-threatening. If suspected, notify prescriber immediately and expect lamotrigine to be discontinued.

! WARNING Monitor patient closely for signs and symptoms of aseptic meningitis such as fever, headache, nausea, nuchal rigidity, or vomiting. Additional signs and symptoms may include altered consciousness, chills, myalgia, photophobia, rash, and somnolence. These symptoms may occur within 1 day to 1.5 months following the initiation of lamotrigine therapy. Notify prescriber immediately, if suspected, and expect drug to be discontinued.

- Monitor patient for seizure activity during lamotrigine therapy.

! WARNING Monitor patient closely for signs and symptoms of hemophagocytic lymphohistiocytosis such as coagulation abnormalities, cytopenias, fever, hepatosplenomegaly, liver dysfunction, lymphadenopathy, neurologic symptoms, and rash that may occur within 8 to 24 days from start of lamotrigine therapy. Be aware that this is a life-threatening condition of extreme systemic inflammation.

- Expect to taper dosage over at least 2 weeks, even for treatment of bipolar disorder, to avoid stopping lamotrigine abruptly, which may increase seizure activity.

PATIENT TEACHING

- Advise patient to take lamotrigine exactly as prescribed and not to stop abruptly because seizure activity may increase.
- Instruct patient how to make oral suspension, if prescribed, from special tablets made just for oral suspension. Once tablets are dissolved, patient should take suspension immediately. Also, tell patient ordered orally disintegrating tablets how to take them.

! WARNING Instruct patient to seek immediate emergency help or call local poison control center if too much lamotrigine is taken.

! WARNING Advise patient to notify prescriber immediately if rash or other symptoms of hypersensitivity, such as a fever or swollen glands, occur.

- Instruct patient to report increased seizure activity, vision changes, and vomiting.

! WARNING Inform patient that excessive immune activation may occur with lamotrigine therapy and to immediately report fever, rash, or swollen lymph nodes.

- Caution patient to avoid hazardous activities until drug's CNS effects are known.
- Advise patient to avoid direct sunlight and to wear protective clothing to minimize risk of photosensitivity.
- Instruct patient to wear or carry medical identification stating that she takes lamotrigine.
- Caution patient or caregiver about possibility of suicidal thoughts, especially when therapy begins or dosage changes.

! WARNING Advise patient to notify prescriber immediately if she develops any combination of an abnormal sensitivity to light, chills, confusion, drowsiness, fever, headache, myalgia, nausea, rash, stiff neck, or vomiting while taking lamotrigine.

- Instruct patient to notify prescriber if an irregular pulse occurs.
- Advise patient that if syncope occurs, to lie down with legs raised and contact prescriber.
- Tell female patient to notify prescriber if she becomes pregnant, is considering pregnancy, or starts or stops an oral hormonal contraceptive or other female hormonal preparation.

lansoprazole
Prevacid, Prevacid-24 Hour, Prevacid SoluTab

dexlansoprazole
Dexilant

⬚ Class and Category
Pharmacologic class: Proton pump inhibitor
Therapeutic class: Antiulcer

⬚ Indications and Dosages
✳ *To treat duodenal ulcers short-term and maintain healed duodenal ulcers*

DELAYED-RELEASE CAPSULES, DELAYED-RELEASE SUSPENSION, DELAYED-RELEASE ORALLY DISINTEGRATING TABLETS (LANSOPRAZOLE)
Adults. 15 mg daily for 4 wk. *Maintenance: 15 mg daily.*
✳ *To treat benign gastric ulcers short-term*

DELAYED-RELEASE CAPSULES, DELAYED-RELEASE SUSPENSION, DELAYED-RELEASE ORALLY DISINTEGRATING TABLETS (LANSOPRAZOLE)
Adults. 30 mg daily for up to 8 wk.
✳ *To treat NSAID-associated gastric ulcer and risk reduction for NSAID-associated gastric ulcer in patients who need to continue NSAID therapy*

DELAYED-RELEASE CAPSULES, DELAYED-RELEASE SUSPENSION, DELAYED-RELEASE ORALLY DISINTEGRATING TABLETS (LANSOPRAZOLE)
Adults. 30 mg daily for 8 wk. *Risk reduction: 15 mg daily for up to 12 wk.*
✳ *To treat symptomatic gastroesophageal reflux disease (GERD) short-term*

DELAYED-RELEASE CAPSULES, DELAYED-RELEASE SUSPENSION, DELAYED-RELEASE ORALLY DISINTEGRATING TABLETS (LANSOPRAZOLE)
Adults and children ages 12 to 17. 15 mg daily for up to 8 wk.
Children ages 1 to 12 weighing more than 30 kg (66 lb). 30 mg once daily for up to 12 wk.
Children ages 1 to 12 weighing 30 kg (66 lb) or less. 15 mg once daily for up to 12 wk.
✳ *To treat symptomatic nonerosive gastroesophageal reflux disease*

DELAYED-RELEASE CAPSULES (DEXLANSOPRAZOLE)
Adults and children ages 12 and over. 30 mg once daily for 4 wk.
✳ *To heal all grades of erosive esophagitis*

DELAYED-RELEASE CAPSULES (DEXLANSOPRAZOLE)
Adults and children ages 12 and over. 60 mg once daily for up to 8 wk.

J
K
L

❋ *To treat erosive esophagitis short-term*

DELAYED-RELEASE CAPSULES, DELAYED-RELEASE SUSPENSION, DELAYED-RELEASE ORALLY DISINTEGRATING TABLETS (LANSOPRAZOLE)

Adults and children ages 12 and over.
30 mg once daily for up to 8 wk. Course may be repeated an additional 8 wk, if needed (adults).

Children ages 1 to 12 weighing more than 30 kg (66 lb). 30 mg once daily for up to 12 wk.

Children ages 1 to 12 weighing 30 kg (66 lb) or less. 15 mg once daily for up to 12 wk.

❋ *To maintain healed erosive esophagitis*

DELAYED-RELEASE CAPSULES, DELAYED-RELEASE SUSPENSION, DELAYED-RELEASE ORALLY DISINTEGRATING TABLETS (LANSOPRAZOLE)

Adults and children ages 12 and over. 15 mg once daily.

DELAYED-RELEASE CAPSULES (DEXLANSOPRAZOLE)

Adults and children ages 12 and over. 30 mg once daily.

❋ *To treat pathological hypersecretory conditions, such as Zollinger–Ellison syndrome*

DELAYED-RELEASE CAPSULES, DELAYED-RELEASE SUSPENSION, DELAYED-RELEASE ORALLY DISINTEGRATING TABLETS (LANSOPRAZOLE)

Adults. *Initial:* 60 mg daily, increased as needed according to patient's condition. Doses exceeding 120 mg/day administered in divided doses.

❋ *To eradicate* Helicobacter pylori *to reduce risk of duodenal ulcer recurrence*

DELAYED-RELEASE CAPSULES, DELAYED-RELEASE SUSPENSION, DELAYED-RELEASE ORALLY DISINTEGRATING TABLETS (LANSOPRAZOLE)

Adults. 30 mg plus 1 g amoxicillin and 500 mg clarithromycin every 12 hr for 10 to 14 days. Or, 30 mg plus 1 g amoxicillin three times daily for 14 days.

❋ *To treat frequent heartburn*

E.R. CAPSULES (PREVACID 24-HR)

Adults. 15 mg daily for 14 days. May repeat course every 4 months.

±**DOSAGE ADJUSTMENT** For patients with severe hepatic impairment prescribed lansoprazole, dosage not to exceed 15 mg daily regardless of condition being treated. For patients with moderate hepatic impairment prescribed dexlansoprazole for the healing of erosive esophagitis, dosage not to exceed 30 mg once daily.

Drug Administration

P.O.

- Antacids may be administered with drug.
- Drug should be administered at least 30 minutes before taking sucralfate, if prescribed.
- Delayed-release capsules (lansoprazole) should be administered before meals and not chewed or crushed. Delayed-release capsules (dexlansoprazole) may be administered with or without food but should be swallowed whole, without chewing.
- For patient who has difficulty swallowing capsules, lansoprazole delayed-release capsules may be opened and contents sprinkled on 60 ml of apple, orange, or tomato juice. Mix briefly and have patient swallow immediately. Rinse glass with 60 ml of juice and have patient swallow immediately to ensure entire contents have been given. If patient is taking dexlansoprazole brand, place one tablespoon of applesauce into a clean container and sprinkle capsule contents on applesauce. Administer immediately, making sure patient does not chew granules. Do not save mixture. Alternatively, dexlansoprazole granules may be mixed with 20 ml of water, gently swirled, withdrawn into a syringe, and administered. After administration, syringe should be refilled with 10 ml of water, swirled gently, and administered.
- Delayed-release capsules may be opened and administered through a nasogastric tube (16 French or greater) by opening and sprinkling contents into 40 ml of apple juice (lansoprazole) or mixed with 20 ml of water (dexlansoprazole). Mix briefly and draw up mixture using a catheter-tipped syringe. Inject drug mixture through the nasogastric tube. Flush with additional fluid used to mix drug to clear the tube.
- Delayed-release suspension should be administered before meals. Shake well

before use. Use the calibrated device that comes with drug to measure dose. May be given through feeding tubes; flush the tube afterward.

- To administer delayed-release orally disintegrating tablets, place tablet on patient's tongue with gloved hand without breaking or cutting it. Tablet should disintegrate in less than one minute.
- For patient who has difficulty using orally disintegrating tablets, place a 15-mg tablet in oral syringe and draw up 10 ml of water. Shake gently. After tablet has been dispersed, administer contents into patient's mouth within 15 minutes of mixing. Refill syringe with about 2 ml (for 15-mg tablet) or 5 ml (for 30-mg tablet) of water, shake gently, and administer any remaining contents.
- For patient with a nasogastric tube 8 French or greater who is prescribed orally disintegrating tablets, place tablet in catheter-tip syringe and draw up 4 ml of water (for 15-mg tablet) or 10 ml of water (for 30-mg tablet). Shake gently. After tablet has dispersed, shake syringe gently again to keep granules from settling and immediately inject mixture through the nasogastric tube within 15 minutes of mixing. Refill syringe with about 5 ml of water, shake gently, and flush tube.

Route	Onset	Peak	Duration
P.O./D.R.	1–3 hr	1.7 hr	>24 hr

Half-life: < 2 hr.

Mechanism of Action

Binds to and inactivates the hydrogen-potassium adenosine triphosphate enzyme system (also called the proton pump) in gastric parietal cells. This action blocks the final step of gastric acid production.

Contraindications

Concurrent therapy with rilpivirine-containing products, hypersensitivity to lansoprazole or its components

Interactions

DRUGS

antiretrovirals such as atazanavir, nelfinavir, rilpivirine: Possible decreased antiviral effect and increased risk of drug resistance to antiretroviral

dasatinib, erlotinib, iron salts, itraconazole, ketoconazole, mycophenolate mofetil, nilotinib, other drugs that depend on low gastric pH for bioavailability: Inhibited absorption of these drugs.

digoxin: Increased digoxin absorption with possible toxicity

methotrexate: Possibly elevated methotrexate levels, which may cause toxicity

rifampin, St. John's wort, and other strong CYP2C19 or CYP3A4 inducers: Decreased plasma levels of dexlansoprazole

saquinavir: Possibly increased toxicity of saquinavir

sucralfate: Decreased and delayed lansoprazole absorption

tacrolimus: Possibly increased blood tacrolimus levels

theophylline: Increased clearance of theophylline reducing effectiveness

voriconazole and other strong CYP2C19 or CYP3A4 inhibitors: Increased exposure of lansoprazole possibly causing toxicity

warfarin: Increased INR and PT with possibly increased risk of serious bleeding

Adverse Reactions

CNS: CVA, dizziness, headache, transient ischemic attack

EENT: Blurred vision, deafness, oral edema oropharyngeal pain, **pharyngeal edema, throat tightness**

GI: Abdominal pain, anorexia, *Clostridium difficile*-**associated diarrhea,** diarrhea, elevated liver enzymes, flatulence, fundic gland polyps, **hepatitis, hepatotoxicity,** increased appetite, nausea, **pancreatitis,** vomiting

GU: Acute renal failure, acute tubulointerstitial nephritis, urine retention

HEME: Agranulocytosis, aplastic anemia, decreased hemoglobin, **hemolytic anemia, idiopathic thrombocytopenic purpura, leukopenia, neutropenia, pancytopenia, thrombocytopenia, thrombotic thrombocytopenic purpura**

MS: Arthralgia, bone fracture, bursitis, myositis

RESP: Upper respiratory tract infection

SKIN: Cutaneous lupus erythematosus, **erythema multiforme, exfoliative dermatitis,** leukocytoclastic vasculitis, pruritus, rash, **Stevens–Johnson syndrome, toxic epidermal necrolysis**

Other: Hyperkalemia, drug reaction with eosinophilia and systemic symptoms (DRESS), hypersensitivity reactions (acute tubulointerstitial nephritis, anaphylaxis, angioedema, bronchospasm, urticaria), hypocalcemia, hypokalemia, hypomagnesemia, hyponatremia, injection-site reaction, systemic lupus erythematosus, vitamin B_{12} deficiency

Childbearing Considerations

PREGNANCY
- It is not known if drug causes fetal harm.
- Use with caution only if benefit to mother outweighs potential risk to fetus.

LACTATION
- It is not known if drug is present in breast milk.
- Patient should check with prescriber before breastfeeding.

Nursing Considerations
- Know that drug should not be given to children under 1 year of age because of the risk of heart valve thickening.

> ! **WARNING** Monitor patient closely for hypersensitivity reactions and serious skin reactions that may become life-threatening. If present, notify prescriber, expect drug to be discontinued, and appropriate supportive measures given as prescribed.

- Be aware that diarrhea from *C. difficile* infection can occur with or without concurrent antibiotics when lansoprazole is used. If *C. difficile*-associated diarrhea occurs, notify prescriber and expect to withhold drug and treat with an antibiotic effective against *C. difficile,* electrolytes, fluids, and protein.
- Monitor patient for bone fracture, especially in patients receiving multiple daily doses for more than a year, because proton pump inhibitors, such as lansoprazole, increase risk for osteoporosis-related fractures of the hip, spine, or wrist.
- Monitor patient, especially patient on long-term therapy for hypomagnesemia. If patient is to remain on lansoprazole long term, expect to monitor patient's serum magnesium level, as ordered, and if level becomes low, anticipate that magnesium replacement therapy will be started and lansoprazole will be discontinued.

- Monitor patient for renal dysfunction because drug may cause acute interstitial nephritis at any point during lansoprazole therapy. Expect drug to be discontinued if it occurs.
- Be aware that drug may cause false-positive results in diagnostic investigations for neuroendocrine tumors. Expect drug to be temporarily discontinued for at least 14 days before testing is done. Also know that drug can cause a hyper-response in gastrin secretion in response to secretin stimulation test. Expect lansoprazole to be temporarily withheld at least 30 days before assessment is done. Be aware that false-positive urine screening tests for tetrahydrocannabinol may occur during lansoprazole therapy.
- Monitor patient for cutaneous and systemic lupus erythematosus either as new onset or exacerbation of existing disorder. Know that cutaneous lupus erythematosus occurs more commonly. Expect lansoprazole to be discontinued if present.
- Be aware that long-term use (especially more than one year) of lansoprazole increases risk for the development of fundic gland polyps. Be aware that drug should be given for the shortest duration possible for the condition being treated.

PATIENT TEACHING
- Urge patient to take lansoprazole exactly as prescribed, usually before a meal to decrease gastric acid output. Tell patient taking dexlansoprazole that drug may be taken with or without food.
- Tell patient who is having trouble swallowing dexlansoprazole capsules to open them and sprinkle granules on 1 tablespoon of applesauce and swallow immediately. If patient has trouble swallowing lansoprazole capsules, tell her to open them and sprinkle granules on 2 ounces of apple, orange, or tomato juice, mix quickly, and swallow immediately. Tell her to refill glass with 2 or more ounces of juice and drink immediately to ensure a full dose.
- Tell patient prescribed delayed-release orally disintegrating tablets to place tablet on tongue, let it dissolve, and then swallow particles with or without water. Also tell her not to break, cut, or chew the tablets.

- Tell patient prescribed delayed-release oral suspension to shake container before each use and to use the calibrated device that comes with drug.
- Inform patient that she may take antacids with lansoprazole. But also tell patient to inform all prescribers of lansoprazole therapy.

! WARNING Instruct patient to seek immediate medical attention if a serious hypersensitivity reaction occurs. Also tell patient to notify prescriber immediately if a rash or other skin reactions occur.

- Tell patient to stop taking drug and report to prescriber blood in urine or decrease in urination, joint pain that is new or worsening, or a rash on arms or cheeks that gets worse in the sun.
- Advise patient to report severe headache or worsening of symptoms immediately to prescriber.
- Urge patient to tell prescriber about diarrhea that's severe or lasts longer than 3 days. Remind patient that bloody or watery stools can occur 2 or more months after antibiotic therapy and can be serious, requiring prompt treatment.

lanthanum carbonate
Fosrenol

Class and Category
Pharmacologic class: Rare earth element
Therapeutic class: Phosphate binder

Indications and Dosages
✽ *To reduce serum phosphate levels in patients with end-stage renal disease*

ORAL POWDER, TABLETS (CHEWABLE)
Adults. *Initial:* 500 mg three times daily, increased, as needed, by 750 mg daily every 2 to 3 wk until acceptable serum phosphate level is reached.

Drug Administration
P.O.
- Administer drug with or immediately after meals.
- Chewable tablets should be chewed thoroughly before swallowing or, if patient has trouble chewing tablets, they can be crushed.

- Sprinkle oral powder form on a small quantity of applesauce or other similar foods and administer immediately.
- Administer tetracyclines and drugs with a narrow therapeutic range at least 1 hour before or 3 hours after lanthanum administration; quinolone antibiotics at least 1 hour before or 4 hours after lanthanum administration; levothyroxine at least 2 hours before or 2 hours after lanthanum administration; and any other drugs known to bind to cationic antacids (aluminum-, magnesium-, or calcium-based) by several hours to prevent a reduction in bioavailability.

Route	Onset	Peak	Duration
P.O.	Unknown	0.5–3 hr	Unknown

Half-life: 53 hr

Contraindications
Bowel obstruction, fecal impaction, hypersensitivity to lanthanum carbonate or any of its components, hypophosphatemia, ileus

Interactions
DRUGS
ACE inhibitors; antibiotics such as ampicillin, fluoroquinolones or tetracyclines; antimalarials; drugs with narrow therapeutic range; statins; thyroid hormones: Possibly reduced bioavailability with these drugs

Adverse Reactions
CNS: Headache
CV: **Hypotension**
EENT: Rhinitis, tooth injury while chewing tablet
GI: Abdominal pain, constipation, diarrhea, dyspepsia, fecal impaction, **GI obstruction or perforation**, ileus, nausea, subileus, vomiting
GU: Dialysis graft occlusion
RESP: Bronchitis
SKIN: Pruritus, rash, urticaria
Other: **Hypercalcemia, hypocalcemia, hypophosphatemia**

Childbearing Considerations
PREGNANCY
- It is not known if drug causes fetal harm.
- Drug is not recommended for use during pregnancy.

☰ Mechanism of Action

During digestion, phosphate is released into the upper GI tract (below left) and absorbed into the bloodstream, increasing serum phosphate levels. In patients with end-stage renal disease, however, inefficient phosphate clearance from the blood leads to abnormally elevated levels.

Lanthanum dissociates in the upper GI tract, releasing ions that attach to unbound phosphate to form an insoluble complex (below right). Unabsorbed into the bloodstream, these altered phosphate molecules can't elevate the patient's serum phosphate level.

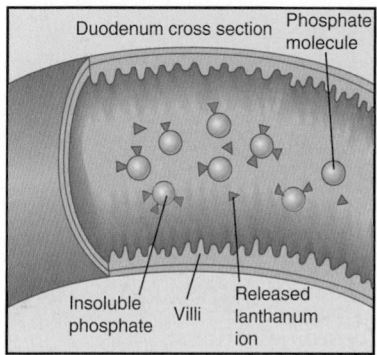

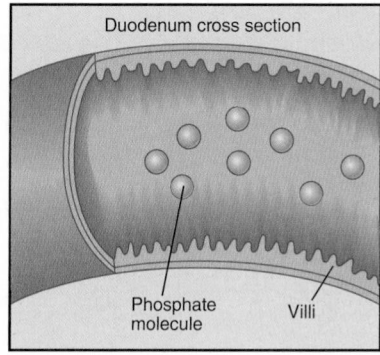

LACTATION

- It is not known if drug is present in breast milk.
- Drug is not recommended during breastfeeding.

☰ Nursing Considerations

- Use lanthanum carbonate cautiously in patients with acute peptic ulcer, bowel obstruction, Crohn's disease, or ulcerative colitis because drug effects are unknown in these patients.
- Monitor the patient's serum phosphate levels, as ordered, especially during dosage adjustment, to determine effectiveness of lanthanum carbonate therapy. Serum phosphate levels should fall below 6 mg/dl.
- Monitor patient closely for signs and symptoms of bowel obstruction, fecal impaction, or ileus, especially the patient with a history of colon cancer, gastrointestinal surgery, or hypomotility disorders, as well as patient receiving calcium channel blockers. Notify prescriber if present, because these gastrointestinal adverse effects may become serious enough to require hospitalization or surgery.

PATIENT TEACHING

- Instruct patient to take lanthanum carbonate with or immediately after meals.
- Advise patient to chew each tablet thoroughly before swallowing. If patient has trouble chewing tablets, tell her she may crush them.
- Tell patient to sprinkle the prescribed oral powder form on a small quantity of applesauce or other similar foods and consume immediately.
- Urge patient to take drug exactly as prescribed, and explain that it may take weeks to reach a desired serum phosphate level.
- Advise patient to notify prescriber if she experiences gastrointestinal discomfort that becomes prolonged or severe.

lefamulin
Xenleta

☰ Class and Category
Pharmacologic class: Pleuromutilin derivative
Therapeutic class: Antibacterial

☰ Indications and Dosages
* *To treat community-acquired bacterial pneumonia caused by* Chlamydophila pneumoniae, Haemophilus influenzae, Legionella pneumophila, Mycoplasma

pneumoniae, Staphylococcus aureus (*methicillin-susceptible isolates*), *or* Streptococcus pneumoniae

TABLETS
Adults. 600 mg every 12 hr for 5 days.

I.V. INFUSION
Adults. 150 mg every 12 hr for 5 to 7 days.

± **DOSAGE ADJUSTMENT** For patients with severe hepatic impairment, dosing interval increased to every 24 hours when administering drug intravenously. Oral dosage is not recommended for patients with moderate or severe hepatic impairment.

Drug Administration

P.O.
- Administer tablets at least 1 hour before a meal or 2 hours after a meal with 6 to 8 ounces of water.
- Tablets should be swallowed whole and not chewed, crushed, or split.

I.V.
- Dilute vial contents with 250-ml solution of 10-mM citrate buffered 0.9% Sodium Chloride for Injection supplied with drug. Mix thoroughly. Solution should be clear.
- After drug is diluted, it may be stored for up to 24 hours at room temperature or 48 hours if refrigerated.
- Do not use the diluent bag in series connections.
- Infuse over 60 minutes. Do not exceed the recommended rate of infusion of 60 minutes or increase the concentration of drug because the magnitude of QT prolongation may be increased.
- *Incompatibilities:* Other I.V. drugs or solutions

Route	Onset	Peak	Duration
P.O.	Unknown	0.88–2 hr	Unknown
I.V.	Unknown	Unknown	Unknown

Half-life: 8 hr

Mechanism of Action
Inhibits bacterial protein synthesis through interactions with the A- and P- sites of the peptidyl transferase center (PTC) in the V domain of the 23s rRNA of the 50s subunit.

Contraindications
Concurrent use with sensitive CYP3A4 substrates that prolong QT interval, such as pimozide; hypersensitivity to lefamulin, other pleuromutilin-class drugs, or their components

Interactions

DRUGS
drugs that prolong QT interval, such as Class IA antiarrhythmics (procainamide, quinidine), Class III antiarrhythmics (amiodarone, sotalol), antipsychotics, erythromycin, moxifloxacin, pimozide, tricyclic antidepressants: Increased risk of prolonged QT interval and life-threatening arrhythmias

moderate and strong CYP3A inducers, P-gp inducers: Decreased lefamulin concentration and effectiveness

moderate and strong CYP3A inhibitors, P-gp inhibitors: Increased lefamulin concentration and risk of adverse reactions

sensitive CYP3A4 substrates (alprazolam, diltiazem, pimozide, verapamil, simvastatin, vardenafil): Increased risk of cardiac conduction toxicities

Adverse Reactions
CNS: Anxiety, headache, insomnia, somnolence
CV: **Atrial fibrillation**, palpitations, **prolonged QT interval**
EENT: Oropharyngeal candidiasis
GI: Abdominal pain, *Clostridium difficile colitis*, constipation, diarrhea, dyspepsia, elevated liver enzymes, epigastric discomfort, erosive gastritis, nausea, vomiting
GU: Urine retention, vulvovaginal candidiasis
HEME: Anemia, **thrombocytopenia**
Other: Elevated alkaline phosphatase and creatine phosphokinase, **hypersensitivity reactions, hypokalemia,** injection-site reactions (pain, phlebitis, reactions)

Childbearing Considerations

PREGNANCY
- Pregnancy exposure registry: 1-855-5NABRIVA.
- Pregnancy status of females of childbearing age should be verified before drug therapy is initiated.
- Drug may cause fetal harm based on animal studies.
- Drug is not recommended for use during pregnancy and should be discontinued as soon as pregnancy is known.

LACTATION
- It is not known if drug is present in breast milk.

- Breastfeeding mothers should pump and discard breast milk for the duration of treatment with drug and for 2 days after final dose.

REPRODUCTION

- Females of childbearing age should use effective contraception during treatment with drug and for 2 days after final dose.
- Known or suspected pregnancy should be reported immediately.

Nursing Considerations

- Know that lefamulin should not be given to patients with known prolongation of the QT interval or ventricular arrhythmias (including torsades de pointes), or in patients receiving class IA or class III antiarrhythmics or other drugs that prolong the QT interval. Lefamulin should also not be given to patients with hepatic impairment or renal failure (if dialysis is required), because metabolic disturbances associated with these conditions may lead to QT prolongation.
- Expect ECG monitoring in patients who are predisposed to QT prolongation for whom use of lefamulin cannot be avoided.
- Be aware that patient may be switched to the oral form of lefamulin to complete the treatment.
- Assess patients for signs of secondary infection, such as profuse, watery diarrhea. If such diarrhea develops, contact prescriber and expect to obtain a stool specimen to rule out pseudomembranous colitis caused by *Clostridium difficile*. If confirmed, expect to discontinue lefamulin and treat with electrolytes, fluids, protein, and an antibiotic effective against *C. difficile*.
- Monitor patient with hepatic impairment for adverse reactions throughout lefamulin therapy.

PATIENT TEACHING

- Instruct patient to take oral form of lefamulin at least 1 hour before a meal or 2 hours after a meal by swallowing tablets whole with 6 to 8 ounces of water. Caution patient not to crush or divide tablets.
- Tell patient that if a dose is missed, he should take it as soon as possible any time up to 8 hours prior to the next scheduled dose. If less than 8 hours remains before the next scheduled dose, he should not take the missed dose, but take drug at the next scheduled dose.

- Urge patient to tell prescriber if diarrhea develops, even 2 months or more after lefamulin therapy ends.
- Inform patient that nausea and vomiting are common adverse reactions.
- Advise patient to tell prescriber of all drugs taken, including over-the-counter drugs and herbal products, because lefamulin can interact with other drugs.
- Inform patient that allergic reactions may occur and that serious allergic reactions require immediate treatment.

! **WARNING** Warn patient of risks to the fetus if taken during pregnancy. Tell women of childbearing age that a pregnancy test will be performed before lefamulin therapy is begun. Instruct these women to use effective contraception throughout drug therapy and for 2 days after the last dose.

- Instruct women who are breastfeeding to pump and discard breast milk throughout lefamulin therapy and for 2 days after the last dose.

leflunomide
Arava

Class and Category

Pharmacologic class: Pyrimidine synthesis inhibitor
Therapeutic class: Antirheumatic

Indications and Dosages

✳ *To treat active rheumatoid arthritis*

TABLETS

Adults who are at low risk for hepatotoxicity and myelosuppression.
Loading: 100 mg daily for 3 days, followed by 20 mg daily. *Maximum:* 20 mg/day.
Adults at high risk for hepatotoxicity or myelosuppression. 20 mg daily without a loading dose. *Maximum:* 20 mg/day.
±**DOSAGE ADJUSTMENT** Dosage reduced to 10 mg daily if poorly tolerated.

Drug Administration

P.O.

- Store at room temperature and protect from light.
- Be prepared to assist with an accelerated drug elimination procedure when drug is

discontinued; without such a procedure it may take up to 2 years for undetectable plasma concentrations to occur.

Route	Onset	Peak	Duration
P.O.	Unknown	6–12 hr	Unknown

Half-life: 2 wk

Mechanism of Action

Inhibits dihydroorotate dehydrogenase, the enzyme in autoimmune process that leads to rheumatoid arthritis. With this action, leflunomide relieves inflammation and prevents alteration of the autoimmune process.

Contraindications

Hypersensitivity to leflunomide, teriflunomide, or their components; pregnancy; severe hepatic impairment

Interactions

DRUGS

BCRP and organic anion transporting polypeptide B1 and B3 (AOTP1B1) substrates such as HMG-Co reductase inhibitors (atorvastatin, nateglinide, pravastatin, repaglinide, rosuvastatin, simvastatin), methotrexate, mitoxantrone, rifampin: Elevated blood levels of these drugs

CYP1A2 substrates such as alosetron, duloxetine, theophylline, tizanidine: Possibly decreased exposure with decreased effectiveness of these drugs

CYP2C8 substrates such as paclitaxel, pioglitazone, repaglinide, rosiglitazone: Possibly increased levels of these drugs with increased risk of adverse reactions

oral contraceptives, organic anion transporter 3 (OAT3) substrates such as cefaclor, cimetidine, ciprofloxacin, furosemide, ketoprofen, methotrexate, penicillin G, zidovudine: Possibly increased exposure of these drugs with increased risk of adverse reactions

rifampin: Increased blood leflunomide level

warfarin: Possibly decreased peak INR by about 25%

Adverse Reactions

CNS: Anxiety, dizziness, drowsiness, fatigue, fever, headache, paresthesia, peripheral neuropathy

CV: Chest pain, hypertension, palpitations, tachycardia, vasculitis

EENT: Blurred vision, conjunctivitis, dry mouth, epistaxis, mouth ulcers, pharyngitis, rhinitis, sinusitis

GI: Abdominal pain, **acute hepatic necrosis**, cholestasis, colitis, constipation, diarrhea, elevated liver enzymes, flatulence, gastritis, gastroenteritis, **hepatic injury or failure**, **hepatitis**, jaundice, nausea, **pancreatitis**, vomiting

GU: Hypophosphaturia, UTI

HEME: **Agranulocytosis**, anemia, **leukopenia, neutropenia, pancytopenia, thrombocytopenia**

MS: Back pain, synovitis, tendinitis

RESP: **Asthma**, bronchitis, dyspnea, **interstitial lung disease, pulmonary fibrosis or hypertension**, respiratory tract infection

SKIN: Alopecia (transient), cutaneous lupus erythematosus, cutaneous necrotizing vasculitis, **erythema multiforme**, erythematous rash, pruritus, pustular psoriasis, **Stevens–Johnson syndrome, toxic epidermal necrolysis**, urticaria, worsening psoriasis

Other: **Angioedema, drug reaction with eosinophilia and systemic symptoms (DRESS)**, opportunistic infections, **sepsis**, weight loss

Childbearing Considerations

PREGNANCY

- Pregnancy exposure registry: 1-877-311-8972 or http://www.pregnancystudies.org /participate-in-a-study/.
- Drug can cause fetal harm.
- Drug is contraindicated during pregnancy.
- A negative pregnancy test must be obtained before drug therapy is begun.
- If pregnancy occurs, drug must be discontinued immediately and an accelerated drug elimination procedure done in an effort to reduce the risk to the fetus.

LACTATION

- It is not known if drug is present in breast milk.
- Breastfeeding should be discontinued during drug therapy.

REPRODUCTION

- Women of childbearing age need to use an effective contraception during drug therapy and also when drug is discontinued while undergoing the drug elimination procedure until verification that the plasma teriflunomide concentration is less than 0.02 mg/L.
- Women of childbearing age should immediately report suspected or known pregnancy to prescriber.

≡ Nursing Considerations

- Know that leflunomide isn't recommended for patients with severe immunodeficiency, or severe, uncontrolled infections because of its immunosuppressant effect. It is also not recommended for patients with liver disease or those with a serum alanine aminotransferase level greater than two times the upper level normal prior to initiation of therapy, because drug may worsen liver dysfunction.
- Use cautiously in patients who are over 60 years of age, in patients taking concomitant neurotoxic drugs, or in patients with diabetes because of an increased risk of developing peripheral neuropathy. If peripheral neuropathy occurs during leflunomide therapy, notify prescriber and expect drug to be discontinued and possibly cholestyramine washout to be ordered.
- Test patient for latent tuberculosis before starting leflunomide, as ordered. If positive, expect standard medical treatment to be given before leflunomide therapy starts.
- Obtain baseline blood pressure before starting leflunomide, and monitor periodically thereafter because drug may cause hypertension.
- Know that patients at high risk for drug-associated hepatotoxicity are those who are taking concomitant methotrexate. Patients at high risk for drug-associated myelosuppression are those who are taking concomitant immunosuppressants.
- Assess liver enzyme (ALT and AST) levels at start of therapy, monthly during first 6 months, and if stable, every 6 to 8 weeks thereafter, as ordered. If levels become elevated greater than threefold upper-level normal, notify prescriber and expect leflunomide therapy to be withheld until underlying cause is determined. If the elevation is thought to be leflunomide-induced, expect to start cholestyramine washout, as ordered, and monitor liver test weekly until normalized. If another cause is found for the elevation, expect to resume leflunomide therapy.
- Obtain platelet count, hemoglobin or hematocrit, and WBC count at start of therapy and every 4 to 8 weeks thereafter, as ordered.
- Notify prescriber if patient develops serious infection, because drug may have to be interrupted and charcoal or cholestyramine given to eliminate drug rapidly.

! **WARNING** Monitor patient's respiratory function closely because drug may cause interstitial lung disease that could become life-threatening. If patient develops a cough and dyspnea, notify prescriber; drug will have to be stopped, and patient may need charcoal or cholestyramine to eliminate drug rapidly.

! **WARNING** Assess patient's skin regularly for evidence of serious skin reactions. If present, notify prescriber, as drug will have to be discontinued, and patient may need charcoal or cholestyramine to eliminate drug rapidly.

PATIENT TEACHING

- Advise patient that leflunomide doesn't cure arthritis but may relieve its symptoms and improve physical function.
- Inform patient that reversible hair loss may occur.
- Caution woman of childbearing potential not to become pregnant while taking drug, because of the high risk of birth defects. Also, tell patient that breastfeeding should be discontinued during drug therapy.
- Instruct patient to report signs of hepatotoxicity, such as mouth ulcers, unusual bleeding or bruising, and yellow skin or eyes.
- Tell patient to report signs of respiratory dysfunction, such as cough and dyspnea, and signs of persistent or serious skin reactions.
- Advise patient to avoid live vaccines during leflunomide therapy.
- Instruct patient to notify prescriber if she develops an infection.

leuprolide acetate

Eligard, Fensolvi, Lupron, Lupron Depot 3.75 mg, Lupron Depot-3 Month 11.25 mg, Lupron Depot-3 Month 22.5 mg, Lupron Depot-4 Month 30 mg, Lupron Depot-6 Month 45 mg, Lupron Depot-Ped-1 Month, Lupron Depot-Ped-3 Month

☰ Class and Category

Pharmacologic class: Gonadotropin-releasing hormone analogue
Therapeutic class: Antineoplastic, gonadotropin inhibitor

☰ Indications and Dosages

✳ *To provide palliative treatment of advanced prostate cancer*

SUBCUTANEOUS INJECTION (ELIGARD)

Adults. 7.5 mg/mo, 22.5 mg every 3 mo, 30 mg every 4 mo, or 45 mg every 6 mo.

SUBCUTANEOUS INJECTION (LUPRON)

Adults. 1 mg daily.

I.M. INJECTION (LUPRON DEPOT, LUPRON DEPOT-3 MONTH, LUPRON DEPOT-4 MONTH, LUPRON DEPOT-6 MONTH)

Adults. 7.5 mg/mo, 22.5 mg every 3 mo, 30 mg every 4 mo, or 45 mg every 6 mo.

✳ *To treat central precocious puberty*

I.M. INJECTION (LUPRON DEPOT-PED-1 MONTH)

Children weighing more than 37.5 kg (83 lb). 15 mg every 4 wk. *Maximum:* 15 mg every 4 wk.

Children weighing more than 25 kg (55 lb) to 37.5 kg (83 lb). *Initial:* 11.25 mg every 4 wk. Dosage increased to next available dose at next monthly injection, if needed. *Maximum:* 15 mg every 4 wk.

Children weighing 25 kg (55 lb) or less. *Initial:* 7.5 mg every 4 wk. Dosage increased to next available dose at next monthly injection, if needed. *Maximum:* 15 mg every 4 wk.

I.M. INJECTION (LUPRON DEPOT-PED-3 MONTH)

Children age 2 and over. 11.25 or 30 mg once every 3 mo (dose not based on weight).

SUBCUTANEOUS INJECTION (FENSOLVI)

Children age 2 years and older. 45 mg once every 6 months.

✳ *To treat endometriosis as monotherapy or as adjunctive therapy in combination with norethindrone acetate*

I.M. INJECTION (LUPRON DEPOT 3.75 MG, LUPRON DEPOT-3 MONTH)

Adults. 3.75 mg every mo for up to 6 mo or 11.25 mg every 3 mo for up to 6 mo.

✳ *As adjunct to treat anemia due to uterine leiomyomas in combination with iron therapy*

I.M. INJECTION (LUPRON DEPOT 3.75 MG, LUPRON DEPOT-3 MONTH)

Adults. 3.75 mg every consecutive mo up to 3 mo or 11.25 mg as a single dose. *Maximum:* 11.25 mg total dose.

☰ Drug Administration

- Never administer by I.V. route.
- Do not substitute one product for another. Be sure the product prescribed is the one to be administered.
- Do not substitute one strength for another by giving a lesser amount, administering more often in place of another product, or increasing dose to achieve dosage of another product.
- Do not administer longer than product indicates.

I.M.

- Let drug come to room temperature before using.
- Reconstitute leuprolide acetate depot suspension with diluent provided by manufacturer. Add diluent to powder for suspension and thoroughly shake vials to disperse particles into a uniform milky suspension.
- Administer within 30 minutes after mixing, and discard any unused portion.
- If using a prefilled dual-chamber syringe, follow manufacturer's instructions to release diluent into chamber containing powder. Shake gently after dilution to disperse particles evenly in solution.
- Rotate sites.

SUBCUTANEOUS

- No dilution or reconstitution is needed for leuprolide acetate injection (Lupron).
- Leuprolide acetate for injectable suspension (Eligard) is approved only for use in men for palliative treatment of prostate cancer. Use provided syringes and delivery system, and read and follow instructions carefully to ensure proper

J
K
L

mixing of product; shaking alone is inadequate to mix it.

- Leuprolide acetate for injectable suspension (Fensolvi) is approved only for use in children age 2 and older with central precocious puberty. Allow drug to reach room temperature before reconstitution. Drug comes packaged in a carton containing two trays (syringe A contains diluent in a prefilled syringe and syringe B contains 45 mg of drug powder in a single-dose prefilled syringe) and guidelines on how to prepare drug. Follow guidelines to obtain a concentration of 45 mg/0.375 ml. Administer within 30 minutes of reconstitution or discard.
- Rotate sites.

Route	Onset	Peak	Duration
I.M./SubQ	2–4 wk	1–2 mo	60–90 days

Half-life: 3 hr

Mechanism of Action

After stimulating follicle-stimulating hormone (FSH) and luteinizing hormone (LH), continuous leuprolide therapy suppresses secretion of gonadotropin-releasing hormone, decreasing estradiol and testosterone levels. In children with central precocious puberty, this stops menses and reproductive organ development.

In adult men, continuous suppression decreases testosterone levels and causes pharmacologic castration, which slows the activity of prostatic neoplastic cells. In women with endometriosis or uterine leiomyomas, leuprolide suppresses ovarian function, inactivating endometrial tissues and resulting in amenorrhea.

Contraindications

For all forms: Hypersensitivity to leuprolide, other gonadotropin-releasing hormone analogues, or their components; *For leuprolide acetate for depot:* Breastfeeding, pregnancy, undiagnosed abnormal uterine bleeding; *For injectable suspension (Fensolvi):* Pregnancy

Interactions

DRUGS

None reported by manufacturer

Adverse Reactions

CNS: Aggression, anger, anxiety, asthenia, CVA, delusions, depression, dizziness, emotional lability, fatigue, fever, headache including migraine, hyperkinesia, insomnia, irritability, lethargy, malaise, memory loss, mood changes, nervousness (adult women), paresthesia, paralysis (from spinal fracture), peripheral neuropathy, personality disorder, rigors, seizures, somnolence, suicidal ideation, syncope, thirst, transient ischemic attacks, vertigo, weakness

CV: Arrhythmias, bradycardia, chest pain, deep vein thrombosis, edema, elevated cholesterol and triglyceride levels, hypertension, hypotension, palpitations, peripheral vascular disorder, prolonged QT interval, tachycardia, vasodilation; angina, MI, thrombophlebitis (adult men), vasodilation

EENT: Blurred vision, conjunctivitis, decreased vision, dry mouth, epistaxis, gingivitis, hearing disorder, pharyngitis, rhinitis, sinusitis

ENDO: Amenorrhea, androgenic effects in women, breast tenderness or swelling, decreased testicle size, diabetes mellitus, goiter, growth retardation, gynecomastia, hot flashes, hyperglycemia, increased signs and symptoms of puberty (children), pituitary apoplexy

GI: Anorexia, colitis, constipation, diarrhea, dyspepsia, dysphagia, elevated liver enzymes, flatulence, gastroenteritis, hepatic dysfunction, increased appetite, nausea, vomiting

GU: Bladder spasm, cervix disorder, cervical neoplasm, decreased libido, decreased penis size, dysmenorrhea and other menstrual disorders, dysuria, endometriosis flare-up, impotence, incontinence, nocturia, prostate cancer flare-up, prostate pain, renal calculus, urinary incontinence, uterine bleeding, vaginal bleeding or discharge in girls, vaginitis

HEME: Leukopenia, purpura

MS: Arthralgia, bone density loss, bone or limb pain, epiphysiolysis, fibromyalgia, joint disorder, leg cramps, myalgia, myopathy, severe muscle pain (children), spinal fracture, tenosynovitis-like symptoms

RESP: Asthmatic attack, dyspnea, interstitial lung disease, pulmonary embolism

SKIN: Acne, alopecia, clamminess, ecchymosis, erythema multiforme, hirsutism, leukoderma, nail disorder, night sweats, photosensitivity, rash, seborrhea, skin hypertrophy, urticaria

Other: Aggravation of preexisting tumor; **anaphylaxis; angioedema (face);** body pain (children); elevated uric acid; flu-like symptoms; infection; injection-site abscess, burning, edema, induration, itching, pain, redness, or swelling; **tumor flare;** weight gain or loss

Childbearing Considerations

PREGNANCY

- Drug may cause fetal harm such as major fetal abnormalities and increases risk for pregnancy loss.
- Drug is contraindicated in pregnant women and in women who may become pregnant.
- Women of childbearing age should have a negative pregnancy test before starting drug therapy.

LACTATION

- It is not known if drug is present in breast milk.
- Patient should check with prescriber before breastfeeding. Drug may be contraindicated with breastfeeding for leuprolide acetate for depot.

REPRODUCTION

- Women of childbearing age should use a nonhormonal method of contraception throughout drug therapy.
- Women of childbearing age should notify prescriber immediately if pregnancy occurs.
- Drug may impair fertility.

Nursing Considerations

- Use cautiously in patients at risk for prolonged QT interval, such as in the presence of congenital long QT syndrome, congestive heart failure, or frequent electrolyte abnormalities, and in patients taking drugs that may prolong the QT interval. Know that electrolyte abnormalities should be corrected, as ordered, prior to therapy beginning. Monitor patient's electrocardiogram and electrolytes regularly throughout therapy, as ordered. Notify prescriber of any abnormalities.

! **WARNING** Be aware that life-threatening hypersensitivity reactions such as anaphylaxis and asthmatic attacks have occurred with leuprolide therapy. Patients at higher risk for an asthma attack include those with a preexisting history of asthma, drug and environmental allergies, and sinusitis. If present, alert prescriber and provide supportive emergency care, as prescribed. Also monitor patient for possible allergic reaction (erythema and induration) at injection site because leuprolide injections contain benzyl alcohol. Manufacturer recommends that injection be given by physician.

- Be aware that during first weeks of leuprolide therapy, patient being treated for prostate cancer should be monitored for initial worsening of symptoms, such as difficulty urinating, increased bone pain, and paralysis or paresthesia (in patients with vertebral metastasis). Also be aware that, following the first dose of leuprolide depot form used to treat endometriosis, an increase in symptoms may occur during the initial days of therapy because of a temporary rise in the hormone levels. These symptoms usually abate with time.
- Monitor patient's PSA and serum testosterone levels periodically, as ordered, to determine response to leuprolide therapy used to treat prostate cancer.
- Monitor patient's blood glucose level, as ordered, because leuprolide therapy may elevate blood glucose levels, leading to a diagnosis of diabetes mellitus, or may adversely affect glycemic control in patients with diabetes.
- Watch patient closely for signs and symptoms of cardiovascular disease because leuprolide therapy increases risk of myocardial infarction, stroke, and sudden cardiac death.
- Expect to stop drug before age 11 in female patients and age 12 in male patients treated for precocious central puberty.
- Monitor bone density test results, as ordered, of women at risk for osteoporosis who are receiving leuprolide because of possible drug-induced estrogen loss, which may result in decreased bone density.
- Be aware that therapeutic doses of leuprolide suppress the pituitary–gonadal system and that normal function doesn't return for 4 to 12 weeks after drug is stopped.

! **WARNING** Monitor patient for evidence of pituitary apoplexy, such as altered mental

J
K
L

status, and possibly cardiovascular collapse, ophthalmoplegia, sudden headache, visual changes, and vomiting. Although rare, it may occur within 2 weeks of first dose, sometimes within the first hour. Notify prescriber immediately and provide supportive care.

- Institute seizure precautions, especially in patients with a history of central nervous system dysfunction or tumors, cerebrovascular disorders, epilepsy, or history of seizures or in patients who are taking medications that may cause seizures.

PATIENT TEACHING

- Instruct patient who is self-administering leuprolide injection to use syringe provided by manufacturer. If manufacturer's syringe is unavailable, advise him to use only a 0.5-ml disposable, low-dose, U-100 insulin syringe to ensure accurate dosage. Substitution of syringes is not recommended for leuprolide acetate for injectable suspension.
- Stress importance of compliance with dosing schedule.
- Prepare patient for possible injection-site reactions and to notify prescriber, if present.
- Advise women to report monthly menses or breakthrough bleeding to prescriber immediately.
- Instruct female patient of childbearing age to use a nonhormonal form of contraception during leuprolide therapy. Advise her to stop taking drug and notify prescriber at once if she becomes pregnant. Be aware that patient should check with prescriber before breastfeeding because it may be contraindicated depending on product used.
- Inform patient with osteoporosis or at risk for developing it that drug may increase bone density loss.
- Inform parents of child being treated for central precocious puberty that they should expect normal gonadal-pituitary function to return 4 to 12 weeks after therapy ends. Also tell parents to notify prescriber if an increase in signs and symptoms of puberty, including vaginal bleeding, occurs during the first weeks of therapy or after subsequent doses.
- Advise patient to report symptoms of depression or memory problems.

- Caution patient being treated for prostate cancer that drug may initially worsen such symptoms as bone pain and that it may cause new signs or symptoms to occur during first few weeks of treatment. Also inform women receiving drug for treatment of endometriosis that an increase in symptoms may occur during the initial days of therapy. Reassure these patients that these reactions are transient.
- Instruct patient to report to prescriber any symptoms that are new, prolonged, or worsen.
- Advise patient with diabetes to monitor his blood glucose level closely.

! **WARNING** Emphasize importance of seeking immediate emergency care if patient develops symptoms suggestive of a heart attack or stroke, or symptoms of an allergic reaction.

- Inform caregivers to watch for emotional lability such as aggression, anger, crying, depression, impatience, or irritability. Also warn caregivers that although rare, suicidal behaviors and thoughts have occurred during leuprolide therapy. If present, tell caregiver to notify prescriber.
- Review seizure precautions with patient and family or caregiver.

levalbuterol hydrochloride
Xopenex

levalbuterol tartrate
Xopenex HFA

☰ Class and Category
Pharmacologic class: Beta^2 agonist
Therapeutic class: Bronchodilator

☰ Indications and Dosages
✳ *To prevent or treat bronchospasm in reversible obstructive airway disease*

INHALATION AEROSOL (XOPENEX HFA)
Adults and children age 4 and over. 45 or 90 mcg (1 or 2 inhalations) every 4 to 6 hr.

INHALATION SOLUTION (XOPENEX)
Adults and children age 12 and over.
Initial: 0.63 three times daily every 6 to 8 hr, increased to 1.25 mg three times daily every 6 to 8 hr, as needed. *Maximum:* 1.25 mg three times daily.

Children ages 6 to 11. *Initial:* 0.31 mg three times daily, increased to 0.63 mg three times daily, as needed. *Maximum:* 0.63 mg three times daily.

±**DOSAGE ADJUSTMENT** For elderly patients using Xopenex, dosage limited to 0.63 mg three times daily every 6 to 8 hr and only increased if needed.

▤ Drug Administration
INHALATION
Xopenex
- Administer solution by nebulization. Solution should be colorless; if not, discard.
- Monitor blood pressure and pulse rate before and after nebulizer treatment.
- Dilute with sterile 0.9% Sodium Chloride Injection before administration. Do not add any other drugs to reservoir.
- If dosage is less than 1.25 mg, use only the 3-ml inhalation solution vials.
- Use with a standard jet nebulizer (with a face mask or mouthpiece) connected to an air compressor (PARI Master Dura-Neb 2000 or Dura-Neb 3000).
- Do not exceed recommended dose. Monitor patients receiving the highest dose for adverse systemic effects.
- Store unused vials in the protective foil pouch at room temperature and protect from excessive heat and light.
- Once foil pouch is opened, use vial immediately.

Xopenex HFA
- Prime inhaler before using it for the first time or when it hasn't been used for more than 3 days by releasing 4 test sprays into the air, aiming inhaler away from face.
- Shake inhaler well before each use, including when priming.
- A spacer device may be used, if recommended.
- Clean inhaler at least weekly by washing actuator with warm water and let it air-dry. If it becomes clogged, wash the actuator to remove blockage.
- The inhaler will deliver 200 actuations. When nearing the end of the usable inhalations, the color behind the number in the dose indicator window will change to red. Discard when display window shows 0. Never immerse canister in water to determine how full the canister is.

Route	Onset	Peak	Duration
Inhalation	5–15 min	1 hr	3–4 hr

Half-life: 3–4 hr

▤ Mechanism of Action
Attaches to beta$_2$ receptors on bronchial cell membranes, which stimulates the intracellular enzyme adenyl cyclase to convert adenosine triphosphate to cAMP. Increased intracellular cAMP level relaxes bronchial smooth muscle and inhibits histamine release from mast cells.

▤ Contraindications
Hypersensitivity to levalbuterol, racemic albuterol, or their components

▤ Interactions
DRUGS
beta-blockers: Possibly block pulmonary effects of levalbuterol; may cause severe bronchospasms
digoxin: Decreased blood digoxin level and effectiveness
loop or thiazide diuretics: Increased risk of hypokalemia
MAO inhibitors, sympathomimetics, tricyclic antidepressants: Increased risk of adverse cardiovascular effects

▤ Adverse Reactions
CNS: Anxiety, chills, dizziness, dysphonia, hypertonia, insomnia, migraine headache, nervousness, paresthesia, syncope, tremor
CV: **Arrhythmias,** chest pain, hypertension, **hypotension,** tachycardia
EENT: Dry mouth and throat, rhinitis, sinusitis
GI: Diarrhea, gastroesophageal reflux disease (GERD), indigestion, nausea, vomiting
MS: Leg cramps, myalgia
RESP: **Asthma exacerbation,** cough, dyspnea, **paradoxical bronchospasm**
SKIN: Rash, urticaria
Other: **Anaphylaxis, angioedema,** flu-like symptoms, lymphadenopathy, **metabolic acidosis**

J
K
L

Childbearing Considerations

PREGNANCY

- Pregnancy exposure registry: 1-877-311-8972 or www.mothertobaby.org/ongoing-study/asthma
- It is not known if drug causes fetal harm.
- Use with caution only if benefit to mother outweighs potential risk to fetus.

LABOR & DELIVERY

- Drug should not be used during labor and delivery unless there are no other alternatives because drug may interfere with uterine contractility.
- Be aware drug has not been approved for management of preterm labor. Serious adverse reactions, including maternal pulmonary edema, have occurred during or following treatment of premature labor.

LACTATION

- It is not known if drug is present in breast milk.
- Patient should check with prescriber before breastfeeding.

Nursing Considerations

- Use levalbuterol cautiously in patients with arrhythmias, diabetes mellitus, hypertension, hyperthyroidism, or a history of seizures.
- Observe for dyspnea, increased coughing, and wheezing, because drug may provoke paradoxical bronchospasm.

PATIENT TEACHING

- Teach patient how to use levalbuterol nebulizer, if prescribed.
- Instruct patient how to use inhalation aerosol, if prescribed. Instruct patient to prime inhaler before using it for the first time or when it hasn't been used for more than 3 days by releasing 4 test sprays into the air, aiming it away from her face. Tell patient that inhaler canister must be shaken well before each use, including when priming.
- Inform patient that inhaler canister has a dose indicator display, which will change after every tenth actuation. When nearing the end of usable inhalations, the color behind the number in the dose indicator window will change to red. Tell patient to discard the inhaler when the display window shows zero.
- Show patient how to clean inhaler, and explain the need to do so at least once weekly.
- Instruct patient to notify prescriber if drug fails to work or if she needs more treatments because asthma is worsening.
- Inform patient that common side effects with levalbuterol use include chest pain, nervousness, palpitations, rapid heart rate, and tremor.
- Instruct patient not to increase dosage or frequency unless told by prescriber.
- Urge patient to stop drug and call prescriber if she has paradoxical bronchospasm.
- Urge patient to consult prescriber before using OTC or other drugs.

levamlodipine

Conjupri

Class and Category

Pharmacologic class: Dihydropyridine calcium channel blocker
Therapeutic class: Antihypertensive

Indications and Dosages

❋ *To treat hypertension*

TABLETS

Adults. *Initial:* 2.5 mg once daily increased after 7 to 14 days to 5 mg once daily, as needed. *Maximum:* 5 mg once daily.
Children ages 6 to 17. *Initial:* 1.25 to 2.5 mg once daily. *Maximum:* 2.5 mg once daily.
±**DOSAGE ADJUSTMENT** For elderly or frail patients and patients with hepatic insufficiency, initial dose decreased to 1.25 mg once daily and titrated slowly.

Drug Administration

P.O.

- Administer once daily keeping time of day consistent.
- Keep in tight, light-resistant containers.

Route	Onset	Peak	Duration
P.O.	Unknown	6 to 12 hr	Unknown
Half-life: 30–50 hr			

Mechanism of Action

Inhibits the transmembrane influx of calcium ions into vascular smooth muscle to produce peripheral vasodilation, which reduces peripheral vascular resistance and thus reduces blood pressure.

Contraindications

Hypersensitivity to levamlodipine, amlodipine, or their components

Interactions

DRUGS

immunosuppressants (cyclosporine, tacrolimus), simvastatin: Increased systemic exposure of these drugs with increased risk of adverse reactions
moderate and strong CYP3A inducers: Decreased concentration of levamlodipine
moderate and strong CYP3A inhibitors: Increased exposure of levamlodipine and risk of adverse reactions
sildenafil: Increased risk of hypotension

Adverse Reactions

CNS: Abnormal dreams, anxiety, asthenia, depersonalization, depression, dizziness, extrapyramidal disorder, fatigue, hypoesthesia, insomnia, malaise, nervousness, paresthesia, peripheral neuropathy, rigors, somnolence, syncope, thirst, tremor, vertigo
CV: **Arrhythmias (including atrial fibrillation, ventricular tachycardia), bradycardia,** chest pain, edema, palpitation, peripheral ischemia, tachycardia, vasculitis
EENT: Abnormal vision, conjunctivitis, diplopia, dry mouth, epistaxis, eye pain, gingival hyperplasia, tinnitus
ENDO: Hot flashes, hyperglycemia
GI: Abdominal pain, anorexia, cholestasis, constipation, diarrhea, dysphagia, elevated liver enzymes, flatulence, **hepatitis,** jaundice, nausea, **pancreatitis,** vomiting
GU: Female and male sexual dysfunction, nocturia, urinary frequency or other micturition disorders
HEME: Leukopenia, **purpura, thrombocytopenia**
MS: Arthralgia, arthrosis, back pain, muscle cramps, myalgia
RESP: Dyspnea
SKIN: Diaphoresis, **erythema multiforme,** flushing, pruritus, rash
Other: **Angioedema,** generalized pain, **hypersensitivity reactions,** weight gain or loss

Childbearing Considerations

PREGNANCY

- It is not known if drug causes fetal harm.
- Use with caution only if benefit to mother outweighs potential risk to fetus.

LACTATION

- Drug is present in breast milk.
- Patient should check with prescriber before breastfeeding.

Nursing Considerations

- Monitor patient's blood pressure to determine effectiveness. Know that symptomatic hypotension is possible, particularly in patients with severe aortic stenosis.

! WARNING Monitor patient closely after levamlodipine is initiated or dosage is increased, especially in patients with severe obstructive coronary artery disease, because drug may cause an acute myocardial infarction or worsen angina.

! WARNING Monitor patient for hypersensitivity reactions. Although uncommon, hypersensitivity reactions may become life-threatening. Notify prescriber; expect drug to be discontinued and appropriate supportive care given, as prescribed.

PATIENT TEACHING

- Instruct patient to inform prescriber of all medications taken, including over-the-counter and herbal products.
- Tell patient to keep levamlodipine out of the light.

! WARNING Urge patient to seek immediate emergency care if serious allergic reactions occur or heart disorders worsen.

levetiracetam

Elepsia XR, Keppra, Keppra XR, Spritam

Class and Category

Pharmacologic class: Pyrrolidine derivative
Therapeutic class: Anticonvulsant

Indications and Dosages

❋ *To treat partial seizures as monotherapy or adjunctive therapy*

I.V. INFUSION, ORAL SOLUTION

Adults and adolescents age 16 and over.
Initial: 500 mg twice daily, increased by
500 mg twice daily every 2 wk, if needed,
until the recommended daily dose of
3,000 mg given in two divided doses is
reached. *Maximum:* 3,000 mg daily in two
divided doses.

Children ages 4 to 16. *Initial:* 10 mg/kg twice
daily, increased by 10 mg/kg twice daily every
2 wk until recommended daily dose of
60 mg/kg given in 2 divided doses is reached.
Maximum: 3,000 mg daily in two divided
doses.

Children 6 months to 4 years. *Initial:* 10 mg/
kg twice daily, increased by 10 mg/kg twice
daily every 2 wk until the recommended
daily dose of 50 mg/kg given in 2 divided
doses is reached.

Infants 1 to 6 months of age. *Initial:* 7 mg/kg
twice daily, increased by 7 mg/kg twice
daily every 2 wk until recommended daily
dose of 42 mg/kg given in 2 divided doses is
reached.

TABLETS (KEPPRA)

Adults and adolescents ages 16 and over.
Initial: 500 mg twice daily, increased by
1,000 mg daily every 2 wk, if needed, until the
recommended daily dose of 3,000 mg given in
two divided doses is reached. *Maximum:*
3,000 mg daily in two divided doses.

**Children ages 4 to 16 weighing more than
40 kg (88 lb).** *Initial:* 500 mg twice daily,
increased by 1,000 mg daily every 2 wk
to a maximum recommended daily dose.
Maximum: 1,500 mg twice daily.

**Children ages 4 to 16 weighing 20 to
40 kg (44 to 88 lb):** *Initial:* 250 mg twice
daily, increased by 500 mg daily every 2 wk
to a maximum recommended daily dose.
Maximum: 750 mg twice daily. *Maximum:*
750 mg twice daily.

TABLETS (SPRITAM)

**Adults and children age 4 and over
weighing more than 40 kg (88 lb).**
Initial: 500 mg twice daily, increased by
1,000 mg daily every 2 wk to a maximum
recommended daily dose. *Maximum:*
3,000 mg daily given in 2 divided doses.

**Children age 4 and over weighing 20 to
40 kg (44 to 88 lb).** *Initial:* 250 mg twice
daily, increased by 500 mg every 2 wk until
maximum recommended daily dose is

reached. *Maximum:* 1,500 mg daily in
2 divided doses.

XR TABLETS (ELEPSIA XR, KEPPRA XR)

Adults and children age 12 and over. 1,000
mg once daily, increased by 1,000 mg daily
every 2 wk until maximum recommended
daily dose is reached. *Maximum:* 3,000 mg
once daily.

* *As adjunct to treat myoclonic seizures in
patients with juvenile myoclonic epilepsy*

I.V. INFUSION, ORAL SOLUTION, TABLETS

Adults and children age 12 and over. *Initial:*
500 mg twice daily, increased by
500 mg twice daily every 2 wk to maximum
recommended dose. *Maximum:* 3,000 mg
daily given in 2 divided doses.

* *As adjunct to treat primary generalized tonic-
clonic seizures in patients with idiopathic
generalized epilepsy*

I.V. INFUSION, ORAL SOLUTION, TABLETS

Adults and children age 16 and over.
Initial: 500 mg twice daily, increased by
500 mg twice daily every 2 wk to the
maximum recommended dose given in 2
divided doses. *Maximum:* 3,000 mg given in
2 divided doses.

Children ages 6 to 16. *Initial:* 10 mg/kg twice
daily, increased by 10 mg/kg twice daily every
2 wk to the maximum recommended daily
dose and given in 2 divided doses. *Maximum:*
60 mg/kg/day in 2 divided doses.

TABLETS (SPRITAM)

**Adults and children age 6 and over
weighing more than 40 kg (88 lb).** *Initial:*
500 mg twice daily, increased by 1,000 mg
daily every 2 wk to recommended daily dose
of 3,000 mg given in 2 divided doses.

**Children age 6 and over weighing 20 to
40 kg (44 to 88 lb).** *Initial:* 250 mg twice
daily, increased by 500 mg every 2 wk to the
recommended daily dose of 1,500 mg given
in 2 divided doses.

± **DOSAGE ADJUSTMENT** Maximum dosage
reduced to 2,000 mg daily for patients with
creatinine clearance of 50 to 80 ml/min; to
1,500 mg daily for clearance of 30 to 50 ml/
min; and to 1,000 mg daily for clearance less
than 30 ml/min. For patients with end-stage
renal disease who are having dialysis, expect
to give another 250 to 500 mg, as prescribed,
after each dialysis session. For children who
can't tolerate maximum daily dose, dosage
reduced to point of tolerance.

☰ Drug Administration

- Keep in mind that when switching patient from oral dosing to intravenous dosing and from intravenous dosing to oral dosing, no dosage or frequency changes are needed.

P.O.

- Tablets and X.R. tablets should be swallowed whole and not chewed, crushed, or split.
- Know that children weighing 20 kg (44 lb) or less should be given only the oral solution form.
- Do not push Spritam tablet through the foil; peel foil from blister.
- Administer Spritam tablets by having patient place tablet on tongue with a dry hand and immediately follow with a sip of water, as it is intended to disintegrate in the mouth. Alternatively, add whole tablet(s) to about 1 tablespoon of liquid to cover tablet(s) in a cup. Allow tablet(s) to disperse prior to administering the entire contents to patient immediately. After administration, resuspend any residue by adding an additional small volume of liquid to cup and have patient swallow the full amount. Do not administer partial quantities of the dispersed tablets.
- For solution administered orally, shake bottle well before using and use a calibrated measuring device to measure dose.

I.V.

- Intravenous form should be used only as an alternative for patients when oral administration is temporarily not possible.
- Do not dilute if drug is already premixed as a single-dose I.V. bag.
- For vials, dilute in 100 ml of compatible diluent, such as 0.9% Sodium Chloride Injection, 5% Dextrose Injection, or Lactated Ringer's solution. If a smaller volume is needed (fluid restriction or for children), the amount of diluent should be calculated to not exceed maximum concentration of 15 mg/ml of diluted solution.
- Use within 4 hours of dilution.
- Infuse each dose over 15 minutes.
- Store drug at room temperature.
- *Incompatibilities:* Other drugs except for diazepam, lorazepam, and valproate sodium; other solutions except for 0.9% Sodium Chloride Injection, 5% Dextrose Injection, and Lactated Ringer's solution.

Route	Onset	Peak	Duration
P.O.	1 hr	1 hr	12 hr
P.O./X.R.	Unknown	4 hr	Unknown
I.V.	Unknown	5–30 min	Unknown

Half-life: 6–8 hr

☰ Mechanism of Action

May protect against secondary generalized seizure activity by preventing coordination of epileptiform burst firing. Levetiracetam doesn't seem to involve inhibitory and excitatory neurotransmission.

☰ Contraindications

Hypersensitivity to levetiracetam or its components

☰ Interactions

DRUGS

None reported by manufacturer

☰ Adverse Reactions

CNS: Abnormal gait, affect lability, aggression, agitation, altered mood, amnesia, anger, anxiety, apathy, asthenia, ataxia, behavioral difficulties (children), choreoathetosis (movement disorder), confusion, coordination difficulties, depersonalization, depression, dizziness, dyskinesia, emotional lability, fatigue, hallucinations, headache, hostility, hypersomnia, increased reflexes, insomnia, involuntary movements, irritability, lethargy, mental or mood changes, nervousness, neurosis, panic attacks, paranoia, paresthesia, personality disorder, psychosis, **seizures** (worsening), somnolence, **suicidal ideation**, vertigo

CV: Elevated diastolic blood pressure (children up to 4 years of age), **hypotension**

EENT: Amblyopia, conjunctivitis, diplopia, ear pain, nasal congestion, nasopharyngitis, pharyngitis, rhinitis, sinusitis

GI: Abdominal pain (upper), anorexia, constipation, diarrhea, elevated liver enzymes, gastroenteritis, **hepatic failure**, **hepatitis**, **pancreatitis**, vomiting

GU: **Acute kidney injury**, albuminuria

HEME: **Agranulocytosis**; decreased hematocrit, hemoglobin, and red blood cell counts; elevated eosinophil count; **leukopenia**; **neutropenia**; **pancytopenia**; **thrombocytopenia**

J
K
L

MS: Arthralgia, joint sprain, muscle weakness, neck pain
RESP: **Asthma,** cough, dyspnea
SKIN: Alopecia, ecchymosis, **erythema multiforme,** pruritus, rash, skin discoloration, **Stevens–Johnson syndrome, toxic epidermal necrolysis,** vesiculobullous rash, urticaria
Other: **Anaphylaxis, angioedema,** dehydration, **drug reaction with eosinophilia and systemic symptoms (DRESS),** flu-like symptoms, **hyponatremia,** infection, weight loss

Childbearing Considerations

PREGNANCY

- Pregnancy exposure registry: 1-888-233-2334 or http://www.aedpregnancyregistry.org/.
- It is not known if drug causes fetal harm.
- Use with caution only if benefit to mother outweighs potential risk to fetus.
- Drug levels may decrease during pregnancy, requiring dosage adjustments.

LACTATION

- Drug is present in breast milk.
- Patient should check with prescriber before breastfeeding.

Nursing Considerations

! **WARNING** Monitor patient for hypersensitivity and skin reactions. Know that anaphylaxis or angioedema have occurred with levetiracetam therapy as early as after the first dose, but also at other times during treatment. Monitor patient for difficulty breathing, hives, hypotension, rash, and swelling. If present, withhold drug, notify prescriber immediately, and provide emergency supportive care, as ordered. Expect drug to be discontinued.

- Monitor patient for seizure activity during therapy. As appropriate, implement seizure precautions according to facility policy.
- Avoid stopping drug abruptly because doing so may increase seizure activity. Expect to taper dosage gradually.
- Monitor patient for bleeding, fever, recurrent infections, or significant weakness. If present, notify prescriber and expect to obtain a complete blood count to assess patient's hematological status.

- Assess compliance, especially during the first 4 weeks of therapy, when certain adverse effects, including abnormal behaviors, coordination problems, fatigue, and somnolence may be more likely to occur.
- Monitor blood pressure in children because increased diastolic blood pressure may occur in patients up to 4 years old.
- Monitor patient closely for evidence of suicidal thinking or behavior, especially when therapy starts or dosage changes.
- Monitor patient for a rash and other adverse skin reactions because serious dermatological reactions have occurred with levetiracetam therapy. Although these adverse reactions usually appear within 14 to 17 days after therapy has begun, some have occurred as late as 4 months later. Notify prescriber at the first sign of a rash and expect drug to be discontinued.

PATIENT TEACHING

- Instruct patient prescribed Spritam form of levetiracetam to peel foil from the blister by bending up and lifting the peel tab around the blister seal and not to just push tablet through the foil. Then instruct patient to place tablet on tongue with a dry hand and immediately follow with a sip of water, as it is intended to disintegrate in the mouth when taken with a sip of water. Alternatively, tell patient to add whole tablet(s) to about 1 tablespoon of liquid to cover tablet(s) in a cup. Allow tablet(s) to disperse prior to immediately taking the entire contents of the drug mixture. Tell patient after administration to resuspend any residue left in cup by adding an additional small volume of liquid and swallowing the full amount. Instruct patient not to take partial quantities of the dispersed tablets.
- Remind patient prescribed X.R. tablet form to swallow tablet whole. It should not be broken, chewed, or crushed. Reassure patient that they may occasionally notice something that looks like swollen pieces of the original tablet in stool but not to be concerned.

! **WARNING** Tell patient to seek immediate emergency care if an allergic or skin reaction occurs, especially if he experiences difficulty breathing, hives, low blood pressure, rash, or swelling.

- Caution patient that levetiracetam may cause dizziness and drowsiness, especially during first 4 weeks of therapy.
- Advise patient to avoid hazardous activities until drug's CNS effects are known.
- Caution patient not to stop taking levetiracetam abruptly; inform her that drug dosage should be tapered under prescriber's direction to reduce the risk of breakthrough seizures.
- Explain to patient and family that levetiracetam may cause mental and behavioral changes, such as aggression, depression, irritability, and rarely psychotic symptoms. The prescriber should be contacted about any bothersome changes.
- Advise patient to keep taking other anticonvulsants, as ordered, while taking levetiracetam.
- Instruct patient to see prescriber regularly so that her progress can be monitored.
- Urge caregivers to watch patient closely for evidence of suicidal tendencies, especially when therapy starts or dosage changes, and to report concerns immediately.

levocetirizine
Xyzal, Xyzal 24-HR

▤ Class and Category
Pharmacologic class: H_1-receptor antagonist
Therapeutic class: Antihistamine

▤ Indications and Dosages
✴ *To treat uncomplicated skin manifestations of chronic idiopathic urticaria*

TABLETS, ORAL SOLUTION
Adults and children age 12 and over. 2.5 or 5 mg once daily. *Maximum:* 5 mg daily.
Children ages 6 to 11. 2.5 mg once daily. *Maximum:* 2.5 mg daily.
Children 6 months to age 5. 1.25 mg once daily. *Maximum:* 1.25 mg daily.
✴ *To relieve symptoms associated with seasonal and perennial allergic rhinitis*

ORAL SOLUTION, TABLETS
Adults and children age 12 and over. 2.5 or 5 mg once daily. *Maximum:* 5 mg daily.

Children ages 6 to 11. 2.5 mg once daily. *Maximum:* 2.5 mg daily.
Children ages 2 to 5. 1.25 mg once daily. *Maximum:* 1.25 mg daily.
✴ *To relieve symptoms associated with pediatric perennial allergic rhinitis*

ORAL SOLUTION
Children 6 months of age to 2 years. 1.25 mg once daily. *Maximum:* 1.25 mg daily.
±**DOSAGE ADJUSTMENT** Maximum dosage should not be exceeded in children because systemic exposure in children is about twice that of adults. For adult patient or child 12 years of age and older with mild renal impairment (creatinine clearance 50 to 80 ml/min), dosage should not exceed 2.5 mg daily. For adult patient with moderate renal impairment (creatinine clearance 30 to 50 ml/min), dosage should not exceed 2.5 mg once every other day. For adult patient with severe renal impairment (creatinine clearance 10 to 30 ml/min), dosage should not exceed 2.5 mg once every 3 to 4 days. Drug should not be used in the presence of renal impairment in children.

▤ Drug Administration
P.O.
- Administer drug in evening.
- Use calibrated device to measure dosage of oral solution.

Route	Onset	Peak	Duration
P.O.	<1 hr	0.5–1 hr	24 hr

Half-life: 8–9 hr

▤ Mechanism of Action
Binds to central and peripheral H_1 receptors, competing with histamine for these sites and preventing it from reaching its site of action. By blocking histamine, levocetirizine produces antihistamine effects, inhibiting respiratory, vascular, and GI smooth-muscle contraction; decreasing capillary permeability, which reduces wheals, flares, and itching; and decreasing salivary and lacrimal gland secretions to relieve chronic urticaria and signs and symptoms of allergic rhinitis.

▤ Contraindications
Children ages 6 months to 11 years with impaired renal function; creatinine clearance less than 10 ml/min (end-stage renal disease):

J
K
L

hemodialysis; hypersensitivity to levocetirizine, cetirizine or their components

Interactions

DRUGS

CNS depressants: Possibly increased CNS depression
ritonavir: Possibly increased risk of adverse effects of levocetirizine
theophylline: Possibly decreased clearance of levocetirizine

ACTIVITIES

alcohol use: Possibly increased CNS depression

Adverse Reactions

CNS: Aggression, agitation, asthenia, depression, dizziness, fatigue, fever, hallucinations, insomnia, movement disorders, myoclonus and extrapyramidal symptoms, paresthesia, **seizures,** somnolence, **suicidal ideation,** syncope, tic, tremor, vertigo
CV: Edema, palpitations, tachycardia
EENT: Blurred vision, dry mouth, epistaxis, nasopharyngitis, pharyngitis, visual disturbances
GI: Hepatitis, increased appetite, nausea, vomiting
GU: Dysuria, urinary retention
MS: Arthralgia, myalgia
RESP: Cough, dyspnea
SKIN: Acute generalized exanthematous pustulosis, fixed drug eruption, pruritus, rash, urticaria
Other: Anaphylaxis, angioedema, weight gain

Childbearing Considerations

PREGNANCY

- It is not known if drug causes fetal harm.
- Use with caution only if benefit to mother outweighs potential risk to fetus.

LACTATION

- It is not known if levocetirizine is present in breast milk although cetirizine is present.
- Patient should check with prescriber before breastfeeding.

Nursing Considerations

- Use levocetirizine cautiously in patients with predisposing risk factors for urinary retention, such as prostatic hyperplasia or spinal cord lesion. Monitor patient's intake and output closely. If urinary retention is

suspected, notify prescriber and expect drug to be discontinued if confirmed.
- Monitor patient for abnormal thinking, such as desire to harm oneself. Notify prescriber immediately if present.
- Expect to stop drug at least 72 hours before skin tests for allergies because drug may inhibit cutaneous histamine response, thus producing false-negative results.

PATIENT TEACHING

- Instruct patient to take drug exactly as prescribed and to take drug in the evening. For oral solution, patient should use appropriate measuring device.
- Urge patient to avoid alcohol while taking levocetirizine.
- Advise patient to avoid hazardous activities until drug's CNS effects are known.
- Tell patient to notify prescriber if he is feeling bladder fullness or notices that his urine output is significantly less than his intake.
- Warn patient that if he develops abnormal thoughts, especially thoughts of harming himself, he should notify prescriber immediately.
- Alert patient taking levocetirizine long term that rebound itching may occur within days after drug is discontinued.

levofloxacin

Class and Category

Pharmacologic class: Fluoroquinolone
Therapeutic class: Antibiotic

Indications and Dosages

✴ *To reduce incidence or progression of inhalation anthrax after exposure to aerosolized* Bacillus anthracis; *to treat plague, including pneumonic and septicemic plague, caused by* Yersinia pestis; *to provide prophylaxis for plague*

I.V. INFUSION, ORAL SOLUTION

Adults and children weighing 50 kg (110 lb) or more. 500 mg daily for 60 days for treatment of inhalation anthrax and 10 to 14 days for treatment of plague.
Infants age 6 months and older and children weighing less than 50 kg (110 lb). 8 mg/kg every 12 hr for 60 days for treatment

of inhalation anthrax and 10 to 14 days for treatment of plague. *Maximum:* 250 mg/dose.

TABLETS

Children weighing more than 30 kg (66 lb) but less than 50 kg (110 lb). 250 mg every 12 hr for 60 days.

✱ *To treat acute bacterial sinusitis caused by* Haemophilus influenzae, Moraxella catarrhalis, *or* Streptococcus pneumoniae

TABLETS, I.V. INFUSION, ORAL SOLUTION

Adults. 500 mg daily for 10 to 14 days. Or 750 mg daily for 5 days.

✱ *To treat acute exacerbation of chronic bacterial bronchitis caused by* H. influenzae, H. parainfluenzae, M. catarrhalis, S. pneumoniae, *or* Staphylococcus aureus

TABLETS, I.V. INFUSION, ORAL SOLUTION

Adults. 500 mg daily for 7 days.

✱ *To treat community-acquired pneumonia caused by* Chlamydophila pneumoniae, H. influenzae, H. parainfluenzae, Klebsiella pneumoniae, Legionella pneumophila, M. catarrhalis, Mycoplasma pneumoniae, S. aureus, *or* S. pneumoniae

TABLETS, I.V. INFUSION, ORAL SOLUTION

Adults. 500 mg daily for 7 to 14 days. Alternatively, for infection caused by *C. pneumoniae, H. influenzae, H. parainfluenzae, M. pneumoniae,* or *S. pneumoniae,* 750 mg daily for 5 days.

✱ *To treat uncomplicated UTI caused by* Escherichia coli, K. pneumoniae, *or* Staphylococcus saprophyticus

TABLETS, I.V. INFUSION, ORAL SOLUTION

Adults. 250 mg daily for 3 days.

✱ *To treat complicated UTI caused by* Enterococcus faecalis, E. cloacae, E. coli, K. pneumoniae, Proteus mirabilis, *or* Pseudomonas aeruginosa; *acute pyelonephritis caused by* E. coli

TABLETS, I.V. INFUSION, ORAL SOLUTION

Adults. 250 mg daily for 10 days.

✱ *To treat complicated UTI caused by* E. coli, K. pneumoniae, *or* P. mirabilis *or acute pyelonephritis caused by* E. coli

TABLETS, I.V. INFUSION, ORAL SOLUTION

Adults. 750 mg daily for 5 days.

✱ *To treat mild to moderate skin and soft-tissue infections caused by* S. aureus *or* Streptococcus pyogenes

TABLETS, I.V. INFUSION, ORAL SOLUTION

Adults. 500 mg daily for 7 to 10 days.

✱ *To treat complicated skin and soft-tissue infections caused by methicillin-sensitive* E. faecalis, Proteus mirabilis, S. aureus, *or* S. pyogenes; *to treat nosocomial pneumonia caused by* E. coli, H. influenzae, K. pneumoniae, Pseudomonas aeruginosa, S. aureus, Serratia marcescens, *or* S. pneumoniae

TABLETS, I.V. INFUSION, ORAL SOLUTION

Adults. 750 mg daily for 7 to 14 days.

✱ *To treat chronic bacterial prostatitis caused by* E. coli, E. faecalis, *or* S. epidermidis

TABLETS, I.V. INFUSION, ORAL SOLUTION

Adults. 500 mg daily for 28 days.

±**DOSAGE ADJUSTMENT** For patients with creatinine clearance of 20 to 49 ml/min and normal dosage of 750 mg daily, dosage interval increased to every 48 hr; for normal dosage of 500 mg, initial dose of 500 mg given, followed by 250 mg every 24 hr. For patients with creatinine clearance of 10 to 19 ml/min or who are receiving dialysis, and normal dosage is 750 mg, initial dose of 750 mg given, followed by 500 mg every 48 hr; for normal dosage of 500 mg, initial dose of 500 mg given, followed by 250 mg every 48 hr; and for normal dosage of 250 mg (no information on dosing adjustment available for patient on dialysis at this dosage), dosage interval increased to every 48 hr unless the 250-mg dosage is used to treat uncomplicated UTI, then no dosage adjustment is required. Supplemental doses of levofloxacin are not required following continuous ambulatory peritoneal dialysis or hemodialysis because dialysis is not effective in removing levofloxacin from the body.

☰ Drug Administration

- Administer drug with plenty of fluid to prevent crystalluria.

P.O.

- Tablets should be swallowed whole and not chewed, crushed, or split.
- Administer oral solution 1 hour before or 2 hours after eating. Use a calibrated device to measure dosage.
- Administer antacid containing aluminum or magnesium, didanosine, iron, multivitamins with zinc, sucralfate, or zinc at least 2 hours before or after levofloxacin.

I.V.

- Drug is supplied as a premixed solution in single-use flexible container with a

J
K
L

concentration of 5 mg/ml. It comes with a foil overwrap. Do not dilute further. Discard any unused portion.

- To prepare the premixed solution, tear outer wrap at the notch and remove solution container. Check for minute leaks by squeezing the inner bag firmly. Discard if leaks are found or if seal is not intact. Also discard if solution is cloudy or a precipitate is present.
- Do not use flexible containers in series connections because an air embolism might result.
- Administer a dosage of 250 or 500 mg slowly as an I.V. infusion over 60 minutes; a dosage of 750 mg slowly over 90 minutes. Do not administer as a rapid or bolus I.V. injection because hypotension may occur.
- Do not administer by any other route.
- If the same intravenous line is used to administer other drugs, flush line before and after infusion of levofloxacin with a solution compatible with the drug and any other drugs administered via the common I.V. line.
- *Incompatibilities:* Other additives, drugs, or substances; solutions containing multivalent cations

Route	Onset	Peak	Duration
P.O./I.V.	Unknown	1–2 hr	Unknown

Half-life: 6–8 hr

Mechanism of Action

Interferes with bacterial cell replication by inhibiting the bacterial enzyme DNA gyrase, which is essential for repair and replication of bacterial DNA.

Contraindications

Hypersensitivity to levofloxacin, other fluoroquinolones, or their components; myasthenia gravis

Interactions

DRUGS

aluminum-, calcium-, or magnesium-containing antacids; didanosine; iron; sucralfate; zinc: Reduced GI absorption of levofloxacin
cyclosporine: Increased risk of nephrotoxicity
NSAIDs: Possibly increased CNS stimulation and risk of seizures
oral anticoagulants: Increased anticoagulant effect and risk of bleeding
oral antidiabetic drugs: Possibly hyperglycemia or hypoglycemia
theophylline: Increased blood theophylline level and risk of toxicity

Adverse Reactions

CNS: Agitation, anxiety, CNS stimulation, confusion, delirium, depression, disorientation, disturbance in attention, dizziness, electroencephalogram abnormalities, **encephalopathy** (rare), fever, hallucinations, headache, hoarse voice, **increased intracranial pressure**, insomnia, light-headedness, memory impairment, nervousness, nightmares, paranoia, peripheral neuropathy, **pseudotumor cerebri**, psychosis, restlessness, **seizures**, sleep disturbance, **suicidal ideation**, toxic psychoses, tremors

CV: Aortic dissection, **arrhythmias**, leukocytoclastic vasculitis, **prolonged QT interval**, **rupture of aortic aneurysm**, tachycardia, **torsades de pointes**, vasculitis, vasodilation

EENT: Blurred vision, decreased visual acuity, diplopia, dysphonia, scotoma, smell or taste perversion, tinnitus, uveitis

ENDO: Hyperglycemia, **hypoglycemia**

GI: Abdominal pain, **acute hepatic failure or necrosis**, anorexia, constipation, diarrhea, flatulence, **hepatitis**, **hepatotoxicity**, indigestion, jaundice, nausea, **pseudomembranous colitis**, vomiting

GU: **Acute renal failure or insufficiency**, crystalluria, interstitial nephritis, vaginal candidiasis

HEME: **Agranulocytosis**, **aplastic anemia**, eosinophilia, **hemolytic anemia**, **leukopenia**, **pancytopenia**, **prolonged international normalized ratio (INR) and prothrombin time**, **thrombocytopenia**

MS: Arthralgia, arthritis, back pain, elevated muscle enzymes, gait abnormality, myalgia, **rhabdomyolysis**, tendon or muscle rupture, tendinopathy

RESP: **Hypersensitivity pneumonitis**

SKIN: **Erythema multiforme**, photosensitivity, pruritus, rash, **Stevens–Johnson syndrome**, **toxic epidermal necrolysis**, urticaria

Other: Anaphylaxis, **angioedema**, exacerbation of myasthenia gravis, **multiorgan failure**, serum sickness

≡ Childbearing Considerations

PREGNANCY

- It is not known if drug causes fetal harm.
- Use with caution only if benefit to mother outweighs potential risk to fetus.

LACTATION

- Drug is present in breast milk.
- Breastfeeding is not recommended during drug therapy and for 2 days after last dose; mother may consider pumping and discarding breast milk during drug therapy and for 2 days after last dose.

≡ Nursing Considerations

- Use levofloxacin cautiously in patients with renal insufficiency. Monitor renal function as appropriate during treatment.
- Use drug cautiously in patients with CNS disorders, such as epilepsy or renal dysfunction, as well as certain drug therapies, that may lower the seizure threshold. Also use cautiously in patients taking corticosteroids, especially elderly patients, because of increased risk of tendon rupture.
- Expect to obtain culture and sensitivity tests before levofloxacin treatment begins.
- Know that levofloxacin therapy should begin as soon as possible after suspected or confirmed exposure to *Y. pestis*.

! **WARNING** Stop levofloxacin at first sign of hypersensitivity, including rash, because drug may lead to anaphylaxis. Reaction may occur after first dose. Expect to give epinephrine and provide supportive care.

- Monitor blood glucose level, especially in diabetic patient who takes an oral antidiabetic or uses insulin, because levofloxacin may alter blood glucose level. If so, notify prescriber, stop drug immediately if patient has hypoglycemia, and provide prescribed treatment.
- Monitor QT interval if needed. If it lengthens, notify prescriber at once and stop drug. Patients with cardiomyopathy, hypokalemia, or significant bradycardia and those receiving a class IA or III antiarrhythmic shouldn't receive levofloxacin.

! **WARNING** Be aware that levofloxacin increases risk of aortic aneurysm and dissection within 2 months following drug use, especially in elderly patients.

- Notify prescriber if patient has symptoms of peripheral neuropathy (altered sensations of light touch, pain, position sense, temperature, or vibration sense), which could be permanent; or CNS or psychiatric abnormalities (e.g., CNS stimulation, increased ICP, psychosis, or seizures), which may lead to more serious adverse reactions, such as suicidal ideation. In each case, expect to discontinue levofloxacin.
- Watch for evidence of tendon rupture (inflammation, pain, swelling) during and up to several months after therapy, especially in children, elderly patients, patients receiving corticosteroids, and patients with heart, kidney, and lung transplants. Notify prescriber about suspected tendon rupture, and have patient rest and refrain from exercise until tendon rupture has been ruled out. If present, expect to provide supportive care, as ordered.
- Be aware that children have a higher incidence of musculoskeletal adverse reactions, especially arthralgia, arthritis, gait abnormality, and tendinopathy. Report any complaint involving the musculoskeletal system promptly to prescriber.
- Monitor patient's bowel elimination. If diarrhea develops, obtain stool culture to check for pseudomembranous colitis. If confirmed, expect to stop drug and give antibiotics effective against *Clostridium difficile*, electrolytes, and fluids.
- Know that fluoroquinolones like levofloxacin have caused disabling and potentially irreversible serious adverse reactions from different body systems that can occur together in the same patient. These reactions can occur within hours to weeks after starting the drug and usually cause central nervous system effects, peripheral neuropathy, tendinitis, and tendon rupture. All ages of patients and patients without any preexisting risk factors have experienced these reactions. Notify prescriber and expect to discontinue levofloxacin immediately at the first signs or symptoms of any serious adverse reactions.

PATIENT TEACHING

- Tell patient prescribed oral solution to take it 1 hour before or 2 hours after eating.
- Advise patient to increase fluid intake during therapy to prevent crystalluria.

J
K
L

- Direct patient to take an antacid containing aluminum or magnesium, didanosine, iron, multivitamins containing sucralfate or zinc at least 2 hours before or after levofloxacin.
- Tell patient to complete the drug as prescribed, even if symptoms subside.
- Urge patient to avoid excessive sun exposure and to wear sunscreen because of increased risk of photosensitivity. Tell patient to notify prescriber at first sign of photosensitivity.
- Caution patient to avoid hazardous activities until drug's CNS effects are known.
- Tell patient to stop drug and notify prescriber if he develops abnormal changes in motor or sensory function, or if he experiences bruising right after an injury in a tendon area, hearing or feeling a pop or snap in a tendon area, or is unable to move the affected area or bear weight. Inform patient tendon problems may be permanent.

! **WARNING** Urge patient experiencing a rash or other allergic reactions to stop drug and tell prescriber.

- Urge patient to notify prescriber if patient experiences pain or tenderness in the upper right side of the abdomen.
- Advise diabetic patient to monitor blood glucose level and report changes.
- Urge patient to tell prescriber about severe diarrhea, even if it's more than 2 months after drug therapy ends. Additional treatment may be needed.
- Advise patient to notify prescriber about heart palpitations or loss of consciousness.
- Advise patient to stop taking levofloxacin immediately and notify prescriber if any persistent, serious, or worsening adverse effects occur.

levomilnacipran hydrochloride
Fetzima

Class and Category
Pharmacologic class: Selective norepinephrine and serotonin reuptake inhibitor (SSNRI)
Therapeutic class: Antidepressant

Indications and Dosages
✳ *To treat major depressive disorder*
E.R. CAPSULES
Adults. *Initial:* 20 mg once daily for 2 days then increased to 40 mg once daily. Dosage further increased in 40-mg increments at intervals of 2 or more days, as needed. *Maximum:* 120 mg once daily.
±**DOSAGE ADJUSTMENT** For patients with moderate renal impairment (creatinine clearance of 30 to 59 ml/min), maintenance dosage should not exceed 80 mg once daily. For patients with severe renal impairment (creatinine clearance of 15 to 29 ml/min), maintenance dosage should not exceed 40 mg once daily.

Drug Administration
P.O.
- E.R. capsules should be swallowed whole and not chewed, crushed, or opened.
- Administer at about the same time every day.

Route	Onset	Peak	Duration
P.O./E.R.	1–2 wk	6–8 hr	Unknown

Half-life: 12 hr

Mechanism of Action
Inhibits reuptake of norepinephrine and serotonin by CNS neurons without affecting uptake of dopamine or other neurotransmitters, thereby increasing amount of norepinephrine and serotonin available in nerve synapses in the central nervous system. Elevated norepinephrine and serotonin levels may relieve symptoms of depression and may improve symptoms of fibromyalgia, including central analgesic effect.

Contraindications
Hypersensitivity to levomilnacipran, milnacipran, or its components; use within 14 days of MAO inhibitor therapy, including reversible agents such as intravenous methylene blue or linezolid

Interactions
DRUGS
antipsychotics or other dopamine antagonists, MAO inhibitors, other serotonergic drugs (amphetamines, buspirone, fentanyl, lithium, St. John's wort, tramadol, tricyclic

antidepressants, triptans, tryptophan), selective serotonin reuptake inhibitors, serotonin–norepinephrine reuptake inhibitors: Possibly development of neuroleptic malignant syndrome-like reactions or serotonin syndrome

aspirin, NSAIDs, warfarin: Increased risk of bleeding

CNS-active drugs: Possibly increased CNS effects

strong CYP3A4 inhibitors such as clarithromycin, itraconazole, ketoconazole: Increased exposure of levomilnacipran resulting in increased risk of adverse reactions

ACTIVITIES

alcohol use: Increased risk of adverse reactions

Adverse Reactions

CNS: Activation of hypomania or mania, aggression, agitation, anger, anxiety, delirium, depression, dizziness, extrapyramidal disorder, fatigue, fever, hallucinations, headache, hypoesthesia, insomnia, irritability, loss of consciousness, migraine, panic attack, paresthesia, **seizures, serotonin syndrome, suicidal ideation,** syncope, thirst, tremor

CV: Chest pain, elevated cholesterol levels, **extrasystoles,** hypertension, **hypertensive crisis, hypotension,** increased heart rate, palpitations, peripheral edema, **supraventricular tachycardia,** tachycardia, **Takotsubo cardiomyopathy**

EENT: Angle-closure glaucoma, blurred vision, conjunctival hemorrhage, dry eye, epistaxis, mydriasis

ENDO: Hot flashes

GI: Abdominal distention or pain, anorexia, constipation, diarrhea, elevated liver enzymes, flatulence, nausea, vomiting

GU: Decreased libido, delayed or absent orgasm (females), dysuria, ejaculation disorder, erectile dysfunction, hematuria, prostatitis, proteinuria, scrotal or testicular pain, testicular swelling, urinary hesitation or retention

HEME: Bleeding risk including **hemorrhage,** hematoma

RESP: Dyspnea,

SKIN: Dry skin, ecchymosis, **erythema multiforme,** excessive sweating including night sweats, flushing, petechiae pruritus, rash, urticaria

Other: Hyponatremia

Childbearing Considerations

PREGNANCY

- Pregnancy exposure registry: 1-844-405-6185 or https://www.womens mentalhealth.org/clinical-and-research -programs/pregnancyregistry/ antidepressants/.
- Drug may cause fetal harm. Neonates exposed to drug late in the third trimester have developed complications requiring prolonged hospitalization, respiratory support, and tube feeding. Such complications can arise immediately upon delivery.
- Use with caution, especially late in the third trimester, only if benefit to mother outweighs potential risk to fetus.

LABOR & DELIVERY

- Drug use late in pregnancy increases risk of postpartum hemorrhage.

LACTATION

- It is not known if drug is present in breast milk.
- Patient should check with prescriber before breastfeeding.
- If breastfeeding occurs, infant should be monitored for agitation, irritability, or poor feeding or weight gain.

Nursing Considerations

- Use levomilnacipran cautiously in patients with cardiac disease or significant hypertension and in patients with renal impairment. Also use cautiously in patients with a history of dysuria, especially men with prostatic hypertrophy, prostatitis, and other lower urinary tract obstructive disorders.
- Know that at least 14 days should elapse between stopping an MAO inhibitor and starting levomilnacipran. At least 7 days should elapse between stopping levomilnacipran and starting an MAO inhibitor antidepressant.
- Measure patient's blood pressure and heart rate before starting and periodically during levomilnacipran therapy because drug can raise blood pressure and heart rate. If hypertension or tachycardia occurs and persists, notify prescriber and expect to reduce dosage or discontinue drug.
- Watch closely for suicidal tendencies, especially when therapy starts and after dosage changes.

J
K
L

! **WARNING** Monitor patient closely for serotonin syndrome, a rare but serious adverse effect of selective serotonin reuptake inhibitors such as levomilnacipran. Signs and symptoms include agitation, confusion, diaphoresis, diarrhea, fever, hyperactive reflexes, poor coordination, restlessness, shaking, talking or acting with uncontrolled excitement, tremor, and twitching. In its most severe form, it can resemble neuroleptic malignant syndrome with autonomic instability with possible rapid fluctuation of vital signs, mental status changes, and muscle rigidity. If symptoms occur, notify prescriber immediately, expect to discontinue drug, and provide supportive care.

- Assess effectiveness of levomilnacipran periodically, being aware that therapy may be required for several months or longer. Expect to taper drug when no longer needed, as ordered, to minimize adverse reactions.

PATIENT TEACHING

- Instruct patient to take levomilnacipran capsules whole and not to chew, crush, or open capsules.
- Advise patient that drug may cause mild pupillary dilation, which may lead to an episode of acute-closure glaucoma. Encourage patient to have an eye exam before starting therapy to see if he is at risk.
- Urge family or caregiver to watch patient closely for suicidal tendencies, especially when therapy starts or dosage changes.
- Caution patient against stopping drug abruptly because serious adverse effects may result.
- Instruct patient to alert all prescribers of levomilnacipran therapy.
- Tell patient to have his blood pressure monitored regularly throughout levomilnacipran therapy.
- Advise patient to avoid activities, such as driving, that require alertness until the CNS effects of levomilnacipran are known.
- Monitor patient to avoid aspirin and NSAIDs, if possible, while taking levomilnacipran and to take bleeding precautions.
- Instruct patient to report any persistent, severe, or unusual adverse effects to prescriber immediately.
- Advise patient to consult prescriber with concerns of sexual dysfunction.

levothyroxine sodium

(l-thyroxine sodium, T₄, thyroxine sodium)

Eltroxin (CAN), Euthyrox, Levo-T, Levoxyl, Synthroid, Tirosint, Tirosint-Sol, Unithroid

Class and Category

Pharmacologic class: Synthetic thyroxine (T_4)
Therapeutic class: Thyroid hormone replacement

Indications and Dosages

* *To treat primary, secondary, or tertiary hypothyroidism*

CAPSULES, ORAL SOLUTION (TIROSINT-SOL), TABLETS

Adults and adolescents in whom growth and puberty are complete. *Initial:* 1.6 mcg/kg once daily. Dosage adjusted by 12.5 to 25 mcg every 4 to 6 wk, as needed. Usual maintenance dose: 100 to 125 mcg daily.

Adults with severe long-standing hypothyroidism. *Initial:* 12.5 to 25 mcg daily with dosage adjusted in 12.5- to 25-mcg increments every 2 to 4 wk, as needed.

Elderly patients or patients with cardiac disease. *Initial:* 12.5 to 25 mcg daily, increased gradually every 6 to 8 wk, as needed.

Children age 12 and over in whom growth and puberty are incomplete. 2 to 3 mcg/kg daily.

Children ages 6 to 12. 4 to 5 mcg/kg daily.

ORAL SOLUTION (TIROSINT-SOL), TABLETS

Children ages 1 to 5. 5 to 6 mcg/kg daily.

Infants ages 6 to 12 months. 6 to 8 mcg/kg daily.

Infants ages 3 to 6 months. 8 to 10 mcg/kg daily.

Infants and neonates birth to age 3 months. 10 to 15 mcg/kg daily.

Infants and neonates birth to age 3 months at risk for cardiac failure. *Initial:* Highly individualized but less than 10 mcg/kg daily with dosage increased every 4 to 6 wk, as needed.

✷ *As adjunct to surgery and radioiodine therapy in the management of thyrotropin-dependent well-differentiated thyroid cancer*

ORAL SOLUTION, CAPSULES, TABLETS

Adults. Highly individualized. *Usual:* Greater than 2 mcg/kg daily but could be less.

✷ *To treat myxedema coma*

I.V. INJECTION

Adults. *Initial as loading dose:* 300 to 500 mcg, followed by 50 to 100 mcg once daily until patient able to tolerate drug orally.

±**DOSAGE ADJUSTMENT** Dosage adjustment highly individualized according to patient's response and tolerance as well as age, degree of hypothyroidism present, general physical condition, and presence and severity of cardiac risk factors. Dosage possibly increased during pregnancy. For children at risk for hyperactivity, initial dosage reduced by 75% of normal dosage with dosage increased by 25% of the full recommended replacement dosage weekly until the full replacement dosage is reached.

⦀ Drug Administration

P.O.

- Administer once daily, preferably on an empty stomach, one-half to one hour before first meal of the day.
- Administer capsules or tablets with a full glass of water. Have patient swallow drug whole and not chew or divide tablet, or open capsule.
- Administer oral solution by squeezing contents of single-dose unit ampule into a cup or glass containing only water. Stir mixture and give to patient to drink immediately. Add more water to cup or glass and have patient drink mixture to obtain the full dose. Alternatively, administer oral solution by squeezing contents into the patient's mouth or onto a spoon before administering without using water.
- Administer at least 4 hours before or after drugs known to interfere with absorption.
- For patient, infants, and children who cannot swallow capsules or tablets, obtain order for oral solution. Alternatively for tablet form, crush tablet, and mix in 5 to 10 ml of breast milk, formula

(except soy-based), or water. Administer immediately by dropper or spoon. Do not store mixture. Do not administer in foods that decrease absorption. Do not administer capsule form to children under 6 years of age.

I.V.

- Reconstitute drug by adding 5 ml of 0.9% Sodium Chloride Injection to drug vial.
- Shake vial to mix well.
- Administer immediately as an I.V. injection at a rate not to exceed 100 mcg/min.
- Discard any solution left in vial.
- *Incompatibilities:* I.V. solutions except for 0.9% Sodium Chloride Injection

Route	Onset	Peak	Duration
P.O.	3–5 days	2–4 hr	Unknown
I.V.	6–8 hr	Unknown	Unknown

Half-life: 3–10 days

⦀ Mechanism of Action

Replaces endogenous thyroid hormone, which may exert its physiologic effects by controlling DNA transcription and protein synthesis. Levothyroxine has all the following actions of endogenous thyroid hormone. The drug:

- increases energy expenditure
- accelerates the rate of cellular oxidation, which stimulates body tissue growth, maturation, and metabolism
- regulates differentiation and proliferation of stem cells
- aids in myelination of nerves and development of synaptic processes in the nervous system
- regulates growth
- decreases blood and hepatic cholesterol concentrations
- enhances carbohydrate and protein metabolism, increasing gluconeogenesis and protein synthesis.

⦀ Contraindications

Hypersensitivity to levothyroxine or its components, uncorrected adrenal insufficiency

⦀ Interactions

DRUGS

5-fluorouracil, clofibrate, estrogens (oral), estrogen-containing oral contraceptives, heroin, methadone, mitotane, tamoxifen: Possibly

J
K
L

increased serum thyroxine-binding globulin (TBG) concentration

aluminum- and magnesium-containing antacids, calcium carbonate, cholestyramine, colestipol, colesevelam, ferrous sulfate, kayexalate, lanthanum, orlistat, proton pump inhibitors, sevelamer, simethicone, sucralfate: Possibly decreased absorption and reduced effects of levothyroxine

amiodarone, glucocorticoids: Possibly hyperthyroidism from decreased peripheral conversion of T_4 to T_3, leading to decreased T_3 levels

anabolic steroids, androgens, asparaginase, glucocorticoids, slow-release nicotinic acid: Possibly decreased serum TBG concentration

beta-blockers: Possibly impaired action of beta-blockers and decreased conversion of T_4 to triiodothyronine (T_3)

carbamazepine, fenamates, furosemide (greater than 80 mg I.V.), heparin, hydantoins, NSAIDs, salicylates (greater than 2 g/ day): Transient increase in FT4 followed by decreased serum T_4 and normal FT4 and TSH concentrations with continued administration

digoxin: Reduced digoxin effects

insulin, oral antidiabetic drugs: Decreased effectiveness of these drugs

ketamine: Possibly marked hypertension and tachycardia

oral anticoagulants: Altered anticoagulant activity

phenobarbital: Reduces response to thyroxine decreasing effectiveness

rifampin: Accelerates metabolism of levothyroxine

sympathomimetics: Increased risk of coronary insufficiency in patients with coronary artery disease; increased effects of both drugs

tetracyclic and tricyclic antidepressants: Increased therapeutic and toxic effects of both drugs

tyrosine-kinase inhibitors: Possible decreased effectiveness of levothyroxine leading to hypothyroidism

FOODS

cottonseed meal, dietary fiber, soybean flour (infant formula), walnuts: Possibly decreased absorption of levothyroxine from GI tract

grapefruit juice: Possible delayed absorption of levothyroxine and reduced bioavailability

☰ Adverse Reactions

CNS: Anxiety, craniosynostosis (infants with overtreatment), emotional lability, fatigue, fever, headache, heat intolerance, hyperactivity, insomnia, irritability, nervousness, **pseudotumor cerebri** (children), **seizures** (rare), somnolence, tremors

CV: Angina, **arrhythmias, cardiac arrest, heart failure,** increased blood pressure and pulse, **MI,** palpitations, tachycardia

ENDO: Hyperthyroidism (with over-replacement), **myxedema coma (with undertreatment),** worsening of diabetic control

GI: Abdominal cramps or pain, diarrhea, dysphagia, elevated liver enzymes, increased appetite, nausea, vomiting

GU: Impaired fertility, menstrual irregularities

MS: Arthralgia, decreased bone mineral density (with over-replacement), muscle spasm or weakness, myalgia, premature closure of the epiphysis (children), slipped capital femoral epiphysis (children)

RESP: Dyspnea, wheezing

SKIN: Alopecia (transient), diaphoresis, flushing, pruritus, rash, urticaria

Other: **Angioedema,** serum sickness, weight gain or loss

☰ Childbearing Considerations

PREGNANCY

- Drug is not known to cause fetal harm and should not be stopped during pregnancy.
- Be aware that pregnancy may increase dosage requirements.

LACTATION

- Drug is present in breast milk.
- Patient should check with prescriber before breastfeeding.

☰ Nursing Considerations

- Be aware that levothyroxine therapy is not to be used for treatment of obesity or for weight loss.
- Use levothyroxine cautiously in the elderly and patients with underlying cardiovascular disease. Know that levothyroxine should be started at a lower dose in these patients because overtreatment can increase cardiac contractility, cardiac wall thickness, and heart rate, which can precipitate angina or arrhythmias. Also use caution in

patients with coronary artery disease undergoing surgery while receiving suppressive levothyroxine therapy and in patients receiving sympathomimetic drugs concurrently. Monitor for signs and symptoms of coronary insufficiency.

- Use caution when administering levothyroxine to children to avoid overtreatment or undertreatment. Be aware that overtreatment may cause craniosynostosis in infants, may adversely affect brain maturation, and may accelerate the bone age and result in premature epiphyseal closure, which will compromise stature for life. Undertreatment may cause adverse effects on intellectual development and linear growth of the child.
- Monitor PT of patient who is receiving anticoagulants, as a dosage adjustment may be required.
- Monitor blood glucose level of diabetic patient because drug may worsen glycemic control and result in increased antidiabetic agent or insulin requirement. Carefully monitor patient after starting, changing, or discontinuing levothyroxine.
- Expect patient to undergo thyroid function tests regularly during levothyroxine therapy. Monitor patient for signs and symptoms of over- or undertreatment with levothyroxine because drug has a narrow therapeutic index. Be aware that atrial fibrillation is the most common arrhythmia with levothyroxine overtreatment in the elderly.
- Keep in mind when interpreting TBG levels that many disorders and medications can decrease TBG concentration, causing a TBG deficiency.

PATIENT TEACHING

- Inform patient that levothyroxine replaces a hormone that is normally produced by the thyroid gland and that she'll probably need to take drug for life.
- Instruct patient to take drug at least 30 minutes before breakfast because drug absorption is increased on an empty stomach and evening doses may cause insomnia.
- Emphasize the need to take levothyroxine with a full glass of water to avoid choking, gagging, having tablet stick in throat, and developing heartburn afterward.

- Instruct patient to separate antacids and calcium or iron supplements by at least 4 hours from levothyroxine doses.
- Inform patient that drug may require a few weeks to take effect.
- Advise patient not to stop drug or change dosage unless instructed by prescriber.
- Instruct patient to report signs of hyperthyroidism, such as chest pain, diarrhea, excessive sweating, fever, headache, heat intolerance, insomnia, irritability, leg cramps, nervousness, palpitations, shortness of breath, tremors, vomiting, weight loss.
- Tell patient to notify prescriber if hives or rash develop during drug use.
- Inform patient that transient hair loss may occur during first few months of levothyroxine therapy.

lidocaine hydrochloride
Lidoderm, Xylocaine, Xylocard (CAN)

J
K
L

Class and Category
Pharmacologic class: Amide derivative
Therapeutic class: Class IB antiarrhythmic, local anesthetic

Indications and Dosages
* *To treat ventricular arrhythmias occurring during cardiac manipulations, such as cardiac surgery; to treat life-threatening ventricular arrhythmias, such as occurring during acute myocardial infarction*

I.V. INFUSION AND INJECTION
Adults. *Loading:* 50 to 100 mg (0.70 to 1.4 mg/kg). If desired response isn't achieved after 5 to 10 min, second dose of 25 to 50 mg (or 0.5 to 0.75 mg/kg) given every 5 min until desired response occurs or maximum dose (300 mg in 1 hr) has been reached. *Maintenance:* 20 to 50 mcg/kg/ min (1 to 4 mg/min) by continuous infusion (rarely longer than 24 hr). Smaller bolus dose repeated 15 to 20 min after start of infusion if needed to maintain therapeutic blood level. *Maximum:* 300 mg (or 3 mg/kg) over 1 hr.
Children. *Loading:* 1 mg/kg (not to exceed 100 mg). *Maintenance:* 20 to 50 mcg/kg/min by continuous infusion.

±**DOSAGE ADJUSTMENT** For patient receiving prolonged lidocaine therapy intravenously (24 hours), dosage reduced. For patients with decreased hepatic function or diminished hepatic blood flow as in heart failure or after cardiac surgery or elderly patients who are 70 years and older, loading dose reduced to one-half and maintenance dose lowered.

✳ *To provide topical anesthesia for mucous membranes or skin*

FILM-FORMING GEL, JELLY, OR OINTMENT

Adults. Thin layer applied to skin or mucous membranes, as needed, before procedure.

✳ *To provide pain relief of postherpetic neuralgia*

TRANSDERMAL PATCH (LIDODERM 5%)

Adults. 1 to 3 patches applied over most painful area only once for up to 12 hr within a 24-hr period.

≣ Drug Administration

I.V.

- Administer I.V. injection as a bolus at a rate of 25 to 50 mg/min.
- Follow manufacturer guidelines for diluting lidocaine in one liter of 5% Dextrose in Water.
- Check premixed solutions carefully to ensure correct solution is being used.
- Solution should be clear. If not, discard.
- Use an infusion pump for continuous infusion.
- Administer I.V. infusion at 20 to 50 mcg/kg/min (1 to 4 mg/min) at the specific rate prescribed. Do not exceed the maximum rate of 4 mg/min, as toxicity risk increases above this rate.
- Reduce continuous infusion dosage to one-half, as ordered, if infusion continues beyond 24 hours.
- Cardiac monitoring should be in place when administering lidocaine continuously.
- *Incompatibilities:* Blood transfusions, cefazolin, methohexital, phenytoin

TOPICAL

- Apply lidocaine jelly or ointment to gauze or bandage before applying to skin.

TRANSDERMAL

- Patches may be cut into smaller sizes with scissors prior to removal of the release liner, if needed.
- Apply immediately upon removal from the protective envelope to clean, dry skin. Patch may not stick if it gets wet.

- If patient complains of burning or irritation, remove the patch(es) and do not reapply until irritation is gone.
- Wash hands immediately after applying patch.
- Do not store patch outside of the sealed envelope.
- Fold used patches so that the adhesive side sticks to itself and safely discard.

Route	Onset	Peak	Duration
I.V.	45–90 sec	Unknown	10–20 min
Topical	2–5 min	3–5 min	0.5–1 hr
Transdermal	0.5–3 hr	Unknown	Unknown

Half-life: 1.5–2 hr

≣ Mechanism of Action

Combines with fast sodium channels in myocardial cell membranes, which inhibits sodium influx into cells and decreases ventricular depolarization, as well as automaticity and excitability during diastole. Lidocaine also blocks nerve impulses by decreasing the permeability of neuronal membranes to sodium, which produces local anesthesia.

≣ Contraindications

Adams–Stokes syndrome; hypersensitivity to lidocaine, amide anesthetics, or their components; severe heart block (without artificial pacemaker); Wolff–Parkinson–White syndrome

≣ Interactions

DRUGS

amiodarone, phenytoin, procainamide, propranolol, quinidine: Additive cardiac effects possibly resulting in toxicity; antagonistic cardiac effects
beta-blockers, CYP1A2 inhibitors such as fluvoxamine, CYP3A4 inhibitors such as propofol, cimetidine: Increased blood lidocaine level and risk of toxicity
CYP1A2 inducers, CYP3A4 inducers: Decreased blood lidocaine level with decreased effectiveness
digoxin: Increased toxicity

≣ Adverse Reactions

CNS: Agitation; anxiety; apprehension; confusion; difficulty speaking; disorientation; dizziness; drowsiness; euphoria; hallucinations; lethargy;

light-headedness; **malignant hyperthermia;** paresthesia; **seizures;** sensation of cold, heat, or numbness; tremors; twitching; unconsciousness
CV: Bradycardia, cardiac arrest, hypotension, new or worsening arrhythmias, tachycardia
EENT: Blurred vision, diplopia, oral hypoesthesia, tinnitus
GI: Nausea, vomiting
HEME: Methemoglobinemia
MS: Dysarthria, muscle weakness, myalgia
RESP: Respiratory arrest or depression
Other: Anaphylaxis; injection-site burning, irritation, petechiae, redness, stinging, swelling, and tenderness; other less severe hypersensitivity reactions; worsened pain

Childbearing Considerations
PREGNANCY
- It is not known if drug causes fetal harm.
- Use with caution only if benefit to mother outweighs potential risk to fetus.

LACTATION
- Drug is present in breast milk.
- Patient should check with prescriber before breastfeeding.

Nursing Considerations
- Use caution in patients with severe hepatic or renal disease because accumulation of lidocaine may occur and lead to toxicity. Also, use caution in patients with any form of AV block, including AV block caused by digitalis toxicity, as well as in patients with hypovolemia and shock.
- Use caution when administering lidocaine to patients with compromised myocardial function because of risk of electrolyte disturbances or fluid overload.
- Observe for respiratory depression after bolus injection and during I.V. infusion of lidocaine.

! **WARNING** Monitor patient for hypersensitivity reactions that can be as severe as anaphylaxis following lidocaine administration. Keep life-support equipment and vasopressors nearby during I.V. use in case of respiratory depression or other reactions. If anaphylaxis occurs, discontinue drug, notify prescriber, and provide supportive care.

- Check blood drug level, as ordered. Therapeutic level is 2 to 5 mcg/ml.

- If signs of toxicity, such as dizziness, occur, notify prescriber and expect to discontinue or slow infusion.

! **WARNING** Monitor for malignant hyperthermia. If present, stop lidocaine administration immediately, notify prescriber, and provide therapeutic countermeasures, as indicated and ordered.

- Monitor vital signs as well as BUN and serum creatinine and electrolyte levels during and after therapy.

PATIENT TEACHING
- Instruct patient how to administer topical form of lidocaine.
- Inform patient who receives lidocaine as an anesthetic that she'll feel numbness.

! **WARNING** Tell patient to immediately report any signs or symptoms of an allergic reaction.

- Advise patient to report difficulty speaking, dizziness, injection-site pain, nausea, numbness or tingling, and vision changes.
- Caution patient to keep lidocaine topical preparations and patches out of reach of children and pets.
- Tell patient to wash hands thoroughly after handling lidocaine topical forms or patch and to avoid getting drug in eyes.
- Remind patient using patches to store them in their sealed envelopes until needed and to apply immediately after removing from the envelope. Tell patient to remove patch if burning or irritation occurs at the site and not to reapply until irritation is gone.
- Tell patient to fold used patches so that the adhesive side sticks to itself and discard where children or pets cannot get to them.
- Warn patient prescribed a lidocaine patch not to place external heat sources, such as electric blanket or heating pad, on it while wearing it, because heat may cause the drug to be absorbed faster, increasing the risk of adverse effects.

linaclotide
Linzess

Class and Category
Pharmacologic class: Guanylate cyclase-C agonist

Therapeutic class: Bowel stimulator

Indications and Dosages

❋ *To treat irritable bowel syndrome with constipation*

CAPSULES

Adults. 290 mcg once daily.

❋ *To treat chronic, idiopathic constipation*

CAPSULES

Adults. 72 or 145 mcg once daily.

Drug Administration

P.O.

- Administer on an empty stomach, at least 30 minutes before the first meal of the day.
- Capsules should be swallowed whole and not chewed or crushed.
- If patient has difficulty swallowing, capsules can be opened and contents sprinkled on 1 teaspoon of room-temperature applesauce and administered immediately. Ensure that patient does not chew beads. Alternatively, capsule contents may be mixed with 30 ml of room-temperature water, gently swirled for at least 20 seconds, and administered immediately. Add another 30 ml of water to beads remaining in cup and repeat process. Do not store mixture for later use.
- Drug may be administered through a gastrostomy or nasogastric tube by mixing content of capsules with 30 ml of water in a cup; swirl gently for at least 20 seconds. Draw mixture up in a catheter-tipped syringe and apply rapid and steady pressure (10 ml/10 seconds) to dispense into the tube. Add another 30 ml of water to any beads remaining in cup and repeat process. After administering mixture, flush nasogastric/gastrostomy tube with a minimum of 10 ml of water.

Route	Onset	Peak	Duration
P.O.	1 wk	Unknown	Unknown

Half-life: 11–12 hr

Mechanism of Action

Acts locally on the luminal surface of the intestinal epithelium through activation of guanylate cyclase-C, which increases both extracellular and intracellular concentrations of cyclic guanosine monophosphate (cGMP). Elevation in intracellular cGMP stimulates secretion of bicarbonate and chloride into the intestinal lumen, which increases intestinal fluid and accelerates GI transit to relieve constipation. Increased extracellular cGMP decreases the activity of pain-sensing nerves, resulting in a reduction of intestinal pain present with constipation and irritable bowel syndrome.

Contraindications

Hypersensitivity to linaclotide or its components, known or suspected mechanical gastrointestinal obstruction, pediatric patients under 2 years of age

Interactions

DRUGS

None reported by manufacturer

Adverse Reactions

CNS: Fatigue, headache
EENT: Sinusitis
GI: Abdominal distention or pain, defecation urgency, diarrhea (may become severe), dyspepsia, fecal incontinence, flatulence, gastroesophageal reflux, hematochezia, **melena, rectal hemorrhage,** vomiting
RESP: Upper respiratory infection
SKIN: Urticaria
Other: **Hypersensitivity reactions** (**anaphylaxis, angioedema,** rash, urticaria)

Childbearing Considerations

PREGNANCY

- It is not known if drug can cause fetal harm but is not expected to harm fetus as drug is negligibly absorbed systemically.
- Use with caution only if benefit to mother outweighs potential risk to fetus.

LACTATION

- It is not known if drug is present in breast milk.
- Patient should check with prescriber before breastfeeding.

Nursing Considerations

- Be aware that although linaclotide is contraindicated in children under 2 years of age due to potential for serious dehydration, it also is not recommended to be given to children younger than 18 years.
- Monitor patient for diarrhea that may become severe. If severe diarrhea occurs, assess patient for dizziness, electrolyte abnormalities (hypokalemia and hyponatremia), hypotension, and

syncope. Notify prescriber if diarrhea occurs. Expect to withhold drug. Also know that if severe, patient may require hospitalization and intravenous fluid administration.

PATIENT TEACHING

- Instruct patient to swallow capsules whole and to avoid chewing or crushing the capsule. However, if patient has difficulty swallowing capsules, tell patient to open capsule and mix with either 1 teaspoon of room-temperature applesauce or 1 ounce of room-temperature water (swirl beads in the container for at least 20 seconds) immediately before ingesting. Tell patient using water method to add another 30 ml of water to beads remaining in cup and repeat process. Do not store mixture for later use.
- Tell patient that linaclotide is to be taken on an empty stomach 30 minutes before the first meal of the day.
- Advise patient to stop taking linaclotide if severe diarrhea occurs and to contact prescriber immediately because hospitalization and intravenous fluid replacement may be necessary.
- Instruct patient to store linaclotide out of the reach of children.

linagliptin
Tradjenta

Class and Category
Pharmacologic class: Dipeptidyl peptidase-4 (DDP-4) enzyme inhibitor
Therapeutic class: Antidiabetic

Indications and Dosages
✱ *As adjunct to improve glycemic control in type 2 diabetes mellitus*

TABLETS
Adults. 5 mg once daily.
±**DOSAGE ADJUSTMENT** For patients taking a supplemental oral hypoglycemic agent or insulin, dosage may have to be reduced.

Drug Administration
P.O.
- No special administration guidelines given by manufacturer.

Route	Onset	Peak	Duration
P.O.	Unknown	1.5 hr	Unknown

Half-life: 11–12 hr

Mechanism of Action
Inhibits the enzyme, dipeptidyl peptidase-4, that degrades incretin hormones responsible for glucose elevation. This allows levels of incretin hormones to rise, stimulating the release of insulin in a glucose-dependent manner while decreasing the glucagon level in the blood. In addition, glucagon secretion from pancreatic alpha cells is reduced, resulting in a reduction in the amount of glucose released by the liver. These combined actions reduce blood glucose levels, thereby improving glycemic control in type 2 diabetes.

Contraindications
Hypersensitivity to linagliptin or its components

Interactions
DRUGS
CYP3A4 or P-gp inducers (strong) such as rifampin: Decreased linagliptin effectiveness
insulin, sulfonylureas: Increased risk of hypoglycemia

Adverse Reactions
CNS: Headache
CV: Hyperlipidemia, hypertriglyceridemia
EENT: Mouth ulceration, nasopharyngitis, stomatitis
ENDO: Hypoglycemia
GI: Acute pancreatitis, constipation, diarrhea, elevated lipase level
GU: UTI
MS: Arthralgia (may be disabling and severe); back, extremity, or joint pain; myalgia; rhabdomyolysis
RESP: Bronchial hyperreactivity, cough
SKIN: Bullous pemphigoid, localized skin exfoliation, rash, urticaria
Other: Anaphylaxis, angioedema, elevated uric acid, weight gain

Childbearing Considerations
PREGNANCY
- It is not known if drug causes fetal harm.
- Use with caution only if benefit to mother outweighs potential risk to fetus.

- It is not known if drug is present in breast milk.
- Patient should check with prescriber before breastfeeding.

≡ Nursing Considerations

! **WARNING** Know that linagliptin's hypersensitivity may be exhibited through serious adverse reactions such as anaphylaxis, angioedema, bronchial hyperreactivity, exfoliative skin conditions, or urticaria. Monitor patient closely for hypersensitivity reactions. If present, withhold drug immediately, notify prescriber, and be prepared to administer emergency care, as ordered.

- Be aware that heart failure has been linked to two other drugs in the same class as linagliptin. Use caution when administering linagliptin, especially to patients with a prior history of heart failure or renal impairment. Monitor patient for signs and symptoms of heart failure and report any to prescriber immediately.

! **WARNING** Monitor patient closely for hypoglycemia, especially if another antidiabetic drug, such as insulin or a sulfonylurea, is used concomitantly. If signs and symptoms of hypoglycemia occur, check patient's blood glucose level. If confirmed, administer 15 g of an oral rapid-acting carbohydrate. After 15 minutes, repeat blood glucose and, if needed, administer 15 g of an oral rapid-acting carbohydrate again. (Administer glucagon 1 mg parenterally, as ordered, if patient is unresponsive, and repeat dose in 15 minutes, if needed.) Notify prescriber of incident, as dosage of the other antidiabetic drug may have to be reduced.

- Monitor patient's blood glucose level routinely to determine response to drug. Expect to check patient's glycosylated hemoglobin every 3 to 6 months or as ordered to evaluate long-term blood glucose control.
- Monitor patient for signs and symptoms of pancreatitis such as abdominal pain, fever, nausea, sweating, and vomiting. Notify prescriber if present, and expect drug to be discontinued, as acute pancreatitis may become life-threatening.

PATIENT TEACHING

- Advise patient that if a dose is missed he should not double up on the next dose.
- Urge patient to report evidence of hypoglycemia, such as anxiety, confusion, dizziness, excessive sweating, headache, and nausea.
- Encourage patient to carry hard candy or other simple sugars to treat mild hypoglycemia.
- Urge patient to carry identification indicating that he has diabetes.
- Teach patient how to monitor his blood glucose level.
- Instruct patient about diet, exercise, foot care, hygiene, signs of hyperglycemia and hypoglycemia, and ways to avoid infection.

! **WARNING** Tell patient to stop drug if he experiences signs and symptoms of an allergic reaction such as difficulty breathing, hives, rash, or swelling of face or skin or signs and symptoms of acute pancreatitis such as persistent severe abdominal pain radiating to the back, which may or may not be accompanied by vomiting, and to seek medical attention immediately.

- Review signs and symptoms of heart failure with patient such as difficulty breathing; swelling or fluid retention, especially in ankles, feet, or legs; unusual tiredness; or fast weight gain. Tell patient to report any such symptoms immediately.
- Inform patient that disabling and severe arthralgia may occur with linagliptin therapy beginning within a day of starting therapy or years later. Patient should notify prescriber if severe joint pain occurs.
- Advise patient to report blisters or erosions that occur on his skin to prescriber.

linezolid

Zyvox

≡ Class and Category
Pharmacologic class: Oxazolidinone
Therapeutic class: Antibiotic

⚏ Indications and Dosages

✳ *To treat vancomycin-resistant* Enterococcus faecium *infections, including concurrent bacteremia*

ORAL SUSPENSION, TABLETS, I.V. INFUSION

Adults and children 12 and older. 600 mg every 12 hr for 14 to 28 days.

Neonates age 7 days and over, infants, and children age 11 and younger. 10 mg/kg every 8 hr for 14 to 28 days.

Neonates younger than 7 days. 10 mg/kg every 12 hr, increased to every 8 hr when neonate is 7 days old. Given for 14 to 28 days.

✳ *To treat nosocomial pneumonia caused by* Staphylococcus aureus *(methicillin-susceptible and resistant strains) or* Streptococcus pneumoniae *(penicillin-susceptible strains only) and community-acquired pneumonia, including accompanying bacteremia, caused by* S. aureus *(methicillin-susceptible strains only) or* S. pneumoniae *(penicillin-susceptible strains only); to treat complicated skin and soft-tissue infections, including diabetic foot infections without concomitant osteomyelitis, caused by* S. aureus *(methicillin-susceptible and resistant strains),* Streptococcus agalactiae, *or* Streptococcus pyogenes

ORAL SUSPENSION, TABLETS, I.V. INFUSION

Adults and children age 12 and older. 600 mg every 12 hr for 10 to 14 days.

Neonates age 7 days or older, infants, and children age 11 and younger. 10 mg/kg every 8 hr for 10 to 14 days.

Neonates younger than 7 days. 10 mg/kg every 12 hr, increased to every 8 hr when neonate is 7 days old. Given for 10 to 14 days.

✳ *To treat uncomplicated skin and soft-tissue infections caused by* S. aureus *(methicillin-susceptible strains only) or* S. pyogenes

ORAL SUSPENSION, TABLETS

Adults. 400 mg every 12 hr for 10 to 14 days.

Children age 12 and older. 600 mg every 12 hr for 10 to 14 days.

Children age 5 to 11. 10 mg/kg every 12 hr for 10 to 14 days.

Neonates age 7 days and over, infants, and children to age 5. 10 mg/kg every 8 hr.

Neonates younger than 7 days. 10 mg/kg every 12 hr, increased to every 8 hr when neonate is 7 days old. Given for 10 to 14 days.

⚏ Drug Administration

P.O.

- Administer oral suspension to neonates, infants, and children who cannot swallow tablets.
- Prepare oral suspension by gently tapping bottle to loosen powder. Add about 63 ml distilled water, shake vigorously, then add 60 ml more of distilled water and shake vigorously again. Concentration will be 100 mg/5 ml.
- Before each use, gently invert bottle 3 to 5 times to mix. Do not shake. Use a calibrated device to measure dosage.
- Store oral suspension at room temperature and discard any unused portion after 21 days.
- Tablets should be swallowed whole and not chewed, crushed, or split.

I.V.

- Supplied in single-dose, ready-to-use infusion bags.
- Keep infusion bags in the overwrap until ready to use.
- Check for minute leaks by firmly squeezing the bag. If leaks are detected, discard the solution.
- Solution may exhibit a yellow color that can intensify over time but does not affect potency of drug.
- Do not use with series plastic connections.
- Don't add other drugs to linezolid solution.
- Infuse I.V. solution over 30 to 120 minutes.
- Flush intravenous line before and after infusion of drug if other drugs will be administered in same line.
- *Incompatibilities:* Amphotericin B, ceftriaxone, chlorpromazine hydrochloride, cotrimoxazole, diazepam, erythromycin lactobionate, pentamidine isethionate, phenytoin sodium, or trimethoprim-sulfamethoxazole; I.V. solutions other than 0.9% Sodium Chloride Injection, 5% Dextrose Injection, or Lactated Ringer's Injection

Route	Onset	Peak	Duration
P.O.	Unknown	1–2 hr	Unknown
I.V.	Unknown	30 min	Unknown

Half-life: 3.4–7 hr

▤ Mechanism of Action

Linezolid inhibits bacterial protein synthesis by interfering with translation of ribonucleic acid (RNA) to protein. In bacteria, protein synthesis begins with binding of a 30S ribosomal subunit and a 50S ribosomal subunit to a messenger RNA (mRNA) molecule to form a 70S initiation complex. The 50S ribosomal subunit consists of 23S ribosomal RNA (rRNA) and other ribosomal subunits. Then translation begins. Transfer RNA (tRNA) attaches to the 50S subunit and brings specific amino acids into place. As the tRNA and amino acids fall into place, they are joined together by peptide bonds and elongate to form a polypeptide chain,

as shown below left. This chain eventually combines with other polypeptide chains to form a complete protein molecule. After translation is complete, the ribosomal subunits fall away and are ready to combine with more mRNA to start the translation process over again.

Linezolid binds to a site on the bacterial 23S rRNA of the 50S subunit. This action prevents formation of a functional 70S initiation complex, an essential component of the bacterial translation. Without proper protein production, as shown below right, susceptible bacteria are unable to multiply. Linezolid is bactericidal against most streptococci and bacteriostatic against staphylococci and enterococci.

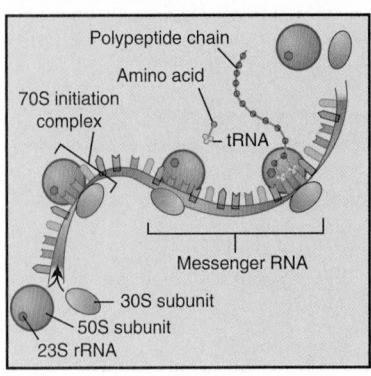

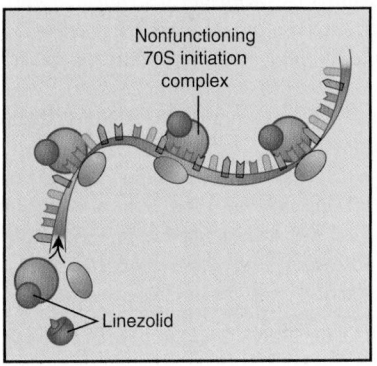

▤ Contraindications

Hypersensitivity to linezolid or its components, use within 14 days of an MAO inhibitor

▤ Interactions

DRUGS

bupropion, buspirone, meperidine, serotonergics, tricyclic antidepressants, triptans: Possibly serotonin syndrome
dopaminergic agents (dobutamine, dopamine), sympathomimetic agents (pseudoephedrine), vasopressive agents (epinephrine, norepinephrine): Increased risk of altered blood pressure
MAO inhibitors: Increased risk of life-threatening adverse effects

FOODS

tyramine-containing beverages and foods: Possibly hypertension

▤ Adverse Reactions

CNS: Dizziness, fever, headache, insomnia, peripheral neuropathy, **seizures, serotonin syndrome**, vertigo
CV: Hypertension
EENT: Optic neuropathy with possible loss of vision, oral candidiasis, taste alteration, tooth or tongue discoloration
ENDO: Syndrome of inappropriate antidiuretic hormone secretion (SIADH)
GI: Abdominal pain, constipation, diarrhea, elevated liver enzymes, indigestion, nausea, **pseudomembranous colitis**, vomiting
GU: Vaginal candidiasis
HEME: Anemia, eosinophilia, **leukopenia, pancytopenia, sideroblastic anemia, thrombocytopenia**
SKIN: Bullous dermatitis, pruritus, rash, **Stevens–Johnson syndrome, toxic epidermal necrolysis**

Other: **Anaphylaxis, angioedema,** fungal infections, **hyponatremia, lactic acidosis**

Childbearing Considerations

PREGNANCY

- It is not known if drug causes fetal harm.
- Use with caution only if benefit to mother outweighs potential risk to fetus.

LACTATION

- Drug is present in breast milk.
- Patient should check with prescriber before breastfeeding.
- If breastfeeding occurs, mother should monitor infant for diarrhea and vomiting.

REPRODUCTION

- May impair fertility in male patients that is reversible, based on animal studies.

Nursing Considerations

- Obtain body tissue and fluid specimens for culture and sensitivity tests, as ordered, before giving first dose of linezolid. Expect to start drug before test results are known.
- Be aware that linezolid shouldn't be used to treat catheter-related bloodstream infections, catheter-site infections, or infections caused by gram-negative bacteria because the risk of death is higher in these infections.

! **WARNING** Monitor CBC weekly, as ordered, to detect or track worsening myelosuppression in patients who need more than 2 weeks of therapy, who have preexisting myelosuppression and are receiving drugs that produce bone marrow suppression, or who have chronic infection and are receiving or have received antibiotic therapy.

- Notify prescriber if patient develops visual impairment that suggests optic neuropathy, such as blurred vision, changes in color vision or visual acuity, lost vision, or visual field defect. If optic or peripheral neuropathy develops, drug may have to be stopped.

! **WARNING** Monitor patient for signs and symptoms of hyponatremia and SIADH such as confusion, generalized weakness, and somnolence; if severe, respiratory failure and death may occur. Expect to monitor serum sodium levels regularly in patients at risk, such as the elderly, patients taking diuretics, and patients already at risk for hyponatremia or SIADH. If present, notify prescriber and expect drug to be discontinued.

- Know that if patient takes a dopaminergic agent, sympathomimetic agent, or vasopressive agent, monitor blood pressure closely; if monitoring isn't possible, know that linezolid shouldn't be prescribed.
- Be aware that while linezolid should not be given to patients receiving serotonergic drugs, there are some conditions that may be life-threatening and require the use of linezolid, such as the presence of vancomycin-resistant *Enterococcus faecium* (VRE) or infections such as nosocomial pneumonia and complicated skin and skin structure infections, including those caused by methicillin-resistant *Staphylococcus aureus* (MRSA). If patient takes buspirone, meperidine, or a serotonergic or tricyclic antidepressant, watch closely for signs and symptoms of serotonin syndrome; if monitoring isn't possible, know that linezolid shouldn't be prescribed.
- Assess bowel pattern daily. Also watch for secondary infection, including oral candidiasis and profuse, watery diarrhea.
- Monitor patient with diabetes who is also taking antidiabetic medication because hypoglycemia has been linked to linezolid use in these patients. If hypoglycemia occurs, treat appropriately and notify prescriber, as dosage of the antidiabetic medication may have to be decreased.
- Monitor patient with a seizure history closely for development of seizure activity.

PATIENT TEACHING

- Caution patient with phenylketonuria that oral suspension contains phenylalanine and that he should receive tablets instead.
- Instruct patient to take drug exactly as prescribed, including the length of time drug should be taken even if patient feels better. Inform patient that drug may be taken with or without food.
- Tell patient that tablets should be swallowed whole and not chewed, crushed, or split.

J
K
L

- Tell patient to invert bottle of oral suspension three to five times before measuring dose and to use a calibrated device to measure dosage of oral suspension. Tell patient to store oral suspension at room temperature and to discard any unused portion after 21 days.
- Advise patient not to take OTC cold remedies without consulting prescriber because medications that contain propanolamine or pseudoephedrine may cause or worsen hypertension.
- Instruct patient to avoid beverages and foods that contain large amounts of tyramine, including aged cheese, air-dried or fermented meats, protein-rich foods that have been stored for long periods or poorly refrigerated, red wines, soy sauce, and tap beers.
- Instruct patient to notify prescriber at once about severe diarrhea, even up to 2 months after linezolid therapy has ended, because additional treatment may be needed. Also, advise patient to report repeated episodes of nausea and vomiting as well as any other serious or unusual signs and symptoms that may occur during drug therapy.
- Alert patient that blood tests to check patient's sodium level may be ordered periodically. Review signs and symptoms of hyponatremia and SIADH with patient and family and advise to notify prescriber if present because drug will have to be discontinued if confirmed.
- Tell patient to report changes in limb sensation (such as numbness, pins and needles, or tingling) or vision changes because drug may have to be stopped. Also, tell patient to notify prescriber immediately if persistent, severe, or unusual signs and symptoms develop.
- Reassure patient with tooth discoloration that professional dental cleaning can restore tooth color.
- Advise diabetic patients prescribed antidiabetic medications to monitor their blood glucose closely and be prepared to treat hypoglycemia if it should occur. If present, tell patient to notify prescriber, as a dosage adjustment may be required in his antidiabetic medication.
- Alert male patients that drug may impair fertility but that it may be reversible.

liraglutide
Saxenda, Victoza

☰ Class and Category
Pharmacologic class: Glucagon-like peptide-1 receptor agonist
Therapeutic class: Antidiabetic

☰ Indications and Dosages
❋ *To improve glycemic control as an adjunct to diet and exercise in patients with type 2 diabetes mellitus*

SUBCUTANEOUS INJECTION (VICTOZA)
Adults and children age 10 and over. *Initial:* 0.6 mg daily for 1 wk, then increased to 1.2 mg daily. Dosage increased to 1.8 mg daily after 1 additional week. *Maximum:* 1.8 mg daily.

❋ *To reduce risk of major adverse cardiovascular events such as CVA or MI in patients with type 2 diabetes mellitus and established cardiovascular disease*

SUBCUTANEOUS INJECTION (VICTOZA)
Adults. *Initial:* 0.6 mg daily for 1 wk, then increased to 1.2 mg daily.

❋ *As adjunct for chronic weight management in patients with an initial body mass index of 30 kg/m² or greater, or 27 kg/m² or greater in the presence of at least one weight-related comorbid condition such as dyslipidemia, hypertension, or type 2 diabetes mellitus; as adjunct to reduced-calorie diet and increased physical activity for chronic weight management in children 12 years and older with a body weight above 60 kg and an initial BMI corresponding to 30 kg/m² for adults (obese) by international cut-offs*

SUBCUTANEOUS INJECTION (SAXENDA)
Adults and children age 12 years and older. *Initial:* 0.6 mg daily for wk 1, increased to 1.2 mg daily for wk 2, increased to 1.8 mg daily for wk 3, increased to 2.4 mg daily for wk 4, and increased to 3 mg daily for wk 5 and onward. *Maintenance:* 3 mg daily.
± **DOSAGE ADJUSTMENT** For children who do not tolerate an increased dose during dose escalation, dose reduced to the previous level with dose escalation taking up to 8 weeks. Also, for children who cannot tolerate a maintenance dose of 3 mg daily, dosage reduced to 2.4 mg daily.

Drug Administration
SUBCUTANEOUS

- Drug is supplied in a multidose prefilled syringe and kept in refrigerator until first use. Discard if pen freezes. Once used, pen may be stored at room temperature for 30 days but should be protected from excessive heat and sunlight.
- May be administered at any time of day, but keep administration time consistent.
- Solution should be clear, colorless, and contain no particles.
- Inject drug into abdomen, thigh, or upper arm.
- Rotate sites.
- When patient is also taking insulin, inject at separate injection sites, but can be in same anatomical area. Never mix the two drugs.
- If more than 3 days have elapsed without liraglutide administration, drug will have to be reinitiated.

Route	Onset	Peak	Duration
SubQ	Unknown	8–12 hr	Unknown

Half-life: 13 hr

Mechanism of Action

Activates the glucagon-like peptide-1 site on pancreatic beta cells, which increases intracellular cyclic AMP, which increases insulin release when blood glucose level is elevated. In addition, because glucagon and insulin levels occur in an inverse relationship to plasma glucose level, increased insulin level will decrease glucagon level, which inhibits glucagon stimulation of the liver that increases plasma glucose level. Although its exact mechanism is unclear, liraglutide also delays gastric emptying, which helps prevent a sudden rise in plasma glucose level after eating. Together these actions work to lower plasma glucose level.

Binds to the glucagon-like peptide-1 receptor and activates it to regulate appetite and calorie intake, resulting in weight loss.

Contraindications

Family or personal history of medullary thyroid cancer, hypersensitivity to liraglutide or its components, pregnancy (Saxenda), presence of multiple endocrine neoplasia syndrome type 2

Interactions
DRUGS

oral hypoglycemic agents such as sulfonylureas: Increased risk of hypoglycemia
orally administered drugs: Possibly decreased absorption of these drugs

Adverse Reactions

CNS: Anxiety, asthenia, dizziness, fatigue, fever, headache, insomnia, malaise, **suicidal ideation**
CV: Dyslipidemia, edema, hypertension, **hypotension**, palpitations
EENT: Dry mouth, nasopharyngitis, sinusitis, taste distortion
ENDO: Elevated calcitonin levels, **hypoglycemia, medullary thyroid cancer, thyroid C-cell hyperplasia**
GI: Abdominal distention or pain, **acute pancreatitis**, anorexia, cholecystitis, cholelithiasis, constipation, diarrhea, dyspepsia, elevated liver or pancreatic enzymes, eructation, flatulence, gastroenteritis, **hemorrhagic and necrotizing pancreatitis, hepatitis**, hyperbilirubinemia, jaundice, nausea, slowed gastric emptying, vomiting
GU: **Acute renal failure**, elevated serum creatinine level, UTI, **worsening of chronic renal failure**
MS: Back pain
RESP: Cough, dyspnea, upper respiratory tract infection
SKIN: Pruritus, rash, urticaria
Other: **Anaphylaxis; angioedema;** anti-liraglutide antibodies; dehydration; elevated creatine kinase levels; influenza-like symptoms; injection-site reaction including erythema, pruritus, rash; **malignancies such as breast and papillary thyroid cancer**

Childbearing Considerations
PREGNANCY

- It is not known if Victoza brand of drug causes fetal harm, but animal studies suggest it may.
- Saxenda brand of drug is contraindicated in pregnancy because weight loss offers no benefit to a pregnant woman and may result in fetal harm.
- Use Victoza with caution only if benefit to mother outweighs potential risk to fetus.

J
K
L

LACTATION

- It is not known if drug is present in breast milk.
- Patient should check with prescriber before breastfeeding.

Nursing Considerations

- Be aware that liraglutide isn't recommended as first-line therapy for patients with type 2 diabetes mellitus not well controlled with diet and exercise. It also isn't a substitute for insulin therapy. Saxenda brand shouldn't be given with insulin, nor should it be combined with other products intended for weight loss, including herbal preparations, over-the-counter products, or prescription drugs.
- Know that liraglutide shouldn't be given to a patient with a history of thyroid C-cell tumors, including medullary thyroid carcinoma, or to patients with multiple endocrine neoplasia syndrome type 2 because drug may stimulate tumor growth.
- Use liraglutide cautiously in patients with a history of pancreatitis because drug can cause pancreatitis, in patients with impaired hepatic function because drug effects in these patients are unknown, and in patients with renal dysfunction because liraglutide may adversely affect renal function.
- Be aware that dosage of liraglutide given during first week of therapy to lower blood glucose level isn't enough to provide glycemic control, but is given to minimize adverse effects when dosage is increased.

! **WARNING** Monitor patient closely for signs and symptoms of a hypersensitivity reaction that may become serious, especially in patients with a history of angioedema to other medications. If any hypersensitivity reaction occurs, discontinue liraglutide and notify the prescriber.

- Monitor patient's fluid intake, especially if gastrointestinal dysfunction occurs, because dehydration can lead to renal dysfunction that can become severe enough to require dialysis.
- Monitor patient's serum calcitonin levels, as indicated. Be aware that elevations occur more often when liraglutide dosage is 1.8 mg daily.
- Monitor patient for pancreatitis, especially when therapy starts or dosage increases.

Report persistent severe abdominal pain; it may radiate to the back and may be accompanied by vomiting. If pancreatitis is confirmed, expect to stop drug and know that it should not be restarted after episode has been resolved.
- Also monitor patient for acute gallbladder disease. Risk is increased in patients who experience a rapid or substantial weight loss, although it may also occur in patients who have lost weight more slowly or less significantly. Notify prescriber if signs and symptoms occur and expect diagnostic testing to be performed.

! **WARNING** Monitor patient for hypoglycemia, especially if he takes another antidiabetic, such as a sulfonylurea or insulin. Know that the risk of hypoglycemia is higher in children regardless of concomitant antidiabetic therapies. Report any episode of hypoglycemia because dosage of other antidiabetic may require adjustment. Treat hypoglycemia with a glucose-containing beverage or food, or give glucagon, as ordered, to raise blood glucose level.

- Monitor patient's blood glucose level and hemoglobin A_{1C} regularly, as ordered, to assess effectiveness of drug when used to treat diabetes mellitus.
- Monitor effectiveness of all other oral drugs because liraglutide slows gastric emptying and may impair their absorption. Alert prescriber to any concerns.
- Monitor patient closely for suicidal ideation such as depression, or unusual changes in behavior or mood. If patient becomes suicidal, take safety precautions immediately, discontinue liraglutide therapy, as ordered, and notify prescriber.
- Monitor patient's heart rate regularly. If patient develops a sustained increase in resting heart rate while taking Saxenda, notify prescriber, as drug will have to be discontinued.

PATIENT TEACHING
- Teach patient how to use prefilled multidose pen and how to give a subcutaneous injection. Explain that he'll need to inject drug daily but that he can do it at any time of day, independent of meals, but timing should be consistent when he gives it each day. Tell patient to inject drug into his

abdomen, thigh, or upper arm and to rotate sites to minimize injection-site reactions. Warn patient not to share his pen with anyone.

- Instruct patient to maintain an adequate fluid intake, as dehydration may cause kidney dysfunction.
- Advise patient of possible risk of medullary thyroid cancer or multiple endocrine neoplasia syndrome type 2 and the need to report any symptoms, such as dysphagia, dyspnea, a neck mass, or persistent hoarseness.
- Tell caregivers to monitor patient closely for depression or changes in behavior or mood. If suicidal, have them take safety precautions, stop the drug, and seek emergency medical help for patient.
- Emphasize that liraglutide therapy (Victoza brand) isn't a substitute for diet and exercise when used to treat diabetes mellitus but is used to enhance the effectiveness of these measures. However, alert patient that hypoglycemia can occur with drug use, especially if also taking other antidiabetic drugs and in children regardless of concomitant antidiabetic treatment. Review signs and symptoms of low blood sugar with patient and appropriate treatment.

! **WARNING** Instruct patient to discontinue drug immediately and seek emergency care if he experiences a serious hypersensitivity reaction, such as difficulty breathing, feeling acutely ill, or swelling of the face or throat area.

- Tell patient to alert prescriber if palpitations or feelings of a racing heartbeat while at rest occur during Saxenda therapy.
- Inform patient that drug may increase risk for gallbladder disease. If abdominal pain, nausea, and vomiting occur, instruct patient to notify prescriber. Also, tell patient to report yellowing of skin or white of the eye along with gastrointestinal signs and symptoms to prescriber.
- Inform patient that drug may increase risk for acute pancreatitis. Tell patient to report persistent severe abdominal pain that may radiate to the back and may be accompanied by vomiting and to stop taking drug.

- Instruct female patients prescribed Saxenda to notify prescriber immediately if pregnancy is suspected or occurs, as drug will have to be discontinued.
- Have patient monitor her weight to assess effectiveness of drug (Saxenda) when prescribed for weight management. Tell patient that Saxenda used for weight loss must be discontinued if she has not achieved a 4% weight loss by 16 weeks.
- Tell patient prescribed Saxenda brand of drug that it should not be given with insulin, nor should it be combined with other products intended for weight loss, including herbal preparations, over-the-counter products, and prescription drugs.
- Alert women that liraglutide does have an effect on preexisting breast neoplasia that may increase risk of breast cancer. In addition, inform all patients that there may be an increase in the development of colorectal neoplasms. Encourage all patients to have cancer screenings done as recommended by their doctor.

lisdexamfetamine dimesylate

Vyvanse

Class, Category, and Schedule

Pharmacologic class: Amphetamine
Therapeutic class: CNS stimulant
Controlled substance schedule: II

Indications and Dosages

* *To treat attention deficit hyperactivity disorder (ADHD)*

CAPSULES, CHEWABLE TABLETS

Adults, adolescents, and children age 6 and over. *Initial:* 30 mg once daily, increased, as needed, in increments of 10 or 20 mg daily every wk. *Maximum:* 70 mg daily.

* *To treat moderate to severe binge eating disorder*

CAPSULES, CHEWABLE TABLETS

Adults. *Initial:* 30 mg once daily, increased as needed in increments of 20 mg weekly to reach target dosage of 50 to 70 mg/day. *Maximum:* 70 mg daily.

±**DOSAGE ADJUSTMENT** For patients with severe renal impairment (GFR from 15 ml/min to less than 30 ml/min), maximum dose is limited to 50 mg daily. For patients with end-stage renal disease (GFR less than 15 ml/min), maximum dose is limited to 30 mg daily. For patients taking agents that alter urinary pH, dosage adjustments are individualized.

Drug Administration

P.O.

- Administer drug in the morning to avoid insomnia.
- Capsules should be swallowed whole and not chewed or crushed. For patient who cannot swallow the capsule, it may be opened and contents dissolved in a glass of orange juice or water. Administer immediately. Alternatively, the contents may be mixed with yogurt until completely dispersed and administered immediately.
- Chewable tablets should be chewed thoroughly before swallowing.
- Capsules and chewable tablets are interchangeable on a mg-per-mg basis.

Route	Onset	Peak	Duration
P.O.	2 hr	3.5 hr	10–12 hr

Half-life: < 1 hr

Mechanism of Action

Produces CNS stimulant effects, probably by facilitating release and blocking reuptake of norepinephrine at adrenergic nerve terminals and by stimulating alpha and beta receptors in peripheral nervous system. The drug also releases and blocks reuptake of dopamine in limbic regions of brain. These actions cause decreased motor restlessness and increased alertness. Lisdexamfetamine's action in the treatment of binge eating is unknown.

Contraindications

Hypersensitivity, or idiosyncratic reaction to lisdexamfetamine, other sympathomimetic amines, or their components; MAO inhibitor therapy including intravenous methylene blue and linezolid within 14 days

Interactions

DRUGS

acidifying agents (urinary) such as ammonium chloride, sodium acid phosphate: Decreased blood level and effects of lisdexamfetamine

alkalinizing agents (urinary) such as acetazolamide, some thiazides: Increased blood level and effects of lisdexamfetamine
buspirone, fentanyl, lithium, MAO inhibitors, selective serotonin reuptake inhibitors, serotonin–norepinephrine reuptake inhibitors, St. John's wort, tricyclic antidepressants, triptans, tryptophan: Increased risk of serotonin syndrome
CYP2D6 inhibitors such as fluoxetine, paroxetine, quinidine, ritonavir: Increased exposure to dextroamphetamine; increased risk of serotonin syndrome
MAO inhibitors: Potentiated effects of lisdexamfetamine, possibly hypertensive crisis
tricyclic antidepressants: Possibly increased antidepressant effects and cardiovascular effects can be potentiated

Adverse Reactions

CNS: Affect lability, aggression, agitation, anxiety, depression, dizziness, dyskinesia, dysphoria, energy increase, euphoria, fever, hallucinations, headache, insomnia, irritability, jittery feeling, mania, mood swings, nightmare, paranoia, paresthesia, psychomotor hyperactivity, psychotic episodes, restlessness, **seizures, serotonin syndrome,** somnolence, tics, tremor
CV: Cardiomyopathy, chest pain, hypertension, increased heart rate, palpitations, peripheral vasculopathy, including Raynaud's phenomenon, tachycardia, ventricular hypertrophy
EENT: Blurred vision, diplopia, dry mouth, mydriasis, oropharyngeal pain, taste alterations, teeth grinding, visual accommodation difficulties
ENDO: Long-term growth suppression
GI: Anorexia, constipation, diarrhea, gastroenteritis, **hepatitis,** intestinal ischemia, nausea, upper abdominal pain, vomiting
GU: Decreased libido, erectile dysfunction, frequent or prolonged erections, priapism, UTI
MS: Rhabdomyolysis
RESP: Dyspnea
SKIN: Alopecia, diaphoresis, pruritus, rash, **Stevens–Johnson syndrome, toxic epidermal necrolysis,** uncontrolled picking at skin, urticaria
Other: Anaphylaxis, angioedema, physical or psychological dependence, weight loss

Childbearing Considerations

PREGNANCY

- Pregnancy exposure registry: 1-866-961-2388 or https://womensmentalhealth.org/clinical-and-researchprograms/pregnancyregistry/adhd-medications/.
- Drug may cause fetal harm because as an amphetamine, vasoconstriction occurs, which may decrease placental perfusion. Prenatal or early postnatal exposure can result in long-term neurochemical and behavioral alterations according to animal studies.
- Use with caution only if benefit to mother outweighs potential risk to fetus.

LABOR & DELIVERY

- Be aware that drug can stimulate uterine contractions, increasing the risk of premature delivery.
- Infants born to mothers taking amphetamines should be monitored for symptoms of withdrawal upon birth, such as agitation, excessive drowsiness, feeding difficulties, and irritability.

LACTATION

- Drug is present in breast milk.
- Breastfeeding is not recommended during drug use.

Nursing Considerations

> ! **WARNING** Keep in mind lisdexamfetamine shouldn't be given to patients with cardiac abnormalities (structural), cardiomyopathy, or other serious heart problems or rhythm abnormalities because even usual CNS stimulant dosages increase risk of sudden death in patients with these conditions.

- Use lisdexamfetamine cautiously in patients with heart failure, hypertension, recent MI, or ventricular arrhythmia because drug may increase blood pressure and worsen these conditions.
- Know that patient should be screened for psychiatric risk factors such as a family or personal history of bipolar disorder, depression, or suicidal ideation because lisdexamfetamine may cause psychiatric adverse reactions. Monitor patients with bipolar disorder for mania.
- Monitor patient's blood pressure closely; stimulant drugs such as lisdexamfetamine may increase it.

> ! **WARNING** Monitor patient closely for serotonin syndrome, a rare but serious adverse effect of lisdexamfetamine. Signs and symptoms include agitation, confusion, diaphoresis, diarrhea, fever, hyperactive reflexes, poor coordination, restlessness, shaking, talking or acting with uncontrolled excitement, tremor, and twitching. If symptoms occur, notify prescriber immediately, expect drug to be discontinued, and provide supportive care.

- Know that chest pain or fainting should be reported to prescriber immediately.
- Monitor patients with bipolar illness, a history of aggression or hostility or psychosis; CNS stimulation may worsen symptoms.
- Assess growth pattern in pediatric patients because stimulants such as lisdexamfetamine may suppress growth. If so, notify prescriber and expect therapy to be halted.
- Know that if patient has a history of seizures or EEG abnormality, watch for seizure activity because stimulants may lower seizure threshold. Rarely, lisdexamfetamine may cause seizures in a patient with no history of them. Take seizure precautions in all patients, and notify prescriber if a seizure occurs. Expect to discontinue lisdexamfetamine, as prescribed.
- Take safety precautions because stimulants may alter accommodation and cause blurred vision. Although these effects haven't been reported with lisdexamfetamine, drug is a known stimulant.
- Be aware that therapy may be stopped temporarily to assess continued need for it, as evidenced by a return of attention deficit and hyperactivity.
- Know that lisdexamfetamine can cause a significant elevation in plasma corticosteroid levels, especially in the evening, which may interfere with urinary steroid determinations.

PATIENT TEACHING

- Warn patient or caregiver that drug must be taken exactly as prescribed and dosage increased only at prescriber's instruction because drug can be abused or lead to dependence.

- Instruct patient or caregiver that capsule must be swallowed whole and not chewed or crushed. However, it may be opened and contents dissolved in a glass of orange juice or water and drunk immediately. Alternatively, the contents of capsule may be mixed with yogurt until completely dispersed; the entire mixture must be consumed immediately.
- Inform patient that chewable tablets must be chewed thoroughly before swallowing.
- Tell patient or caregiver that drug should only be taken in the morning because taking it later in the day may cause insomnia.
- Tell patient with symptoms such as chest pain or fainting to contact prescriber immediately.

! **WARNING** Instruct patient to tell all prescribers about lisdexamfetamine therapy, as serious drug interactions can occur. Stress importance of seeking immediate medical care if persistent, severe, or unusual adverse reactions occur.

- Advise patient or caregiver to report any symptoms that suggest heart disease, such as exertional chest pain or unexplained syncope.
- Urge patient to avoid hazardous activities until drug effects are known.
- Warn male patients and parents of male children that painful or prolonged penile erections may occur while taking the drug, especially after a dose increase or during a period of drug withdrawal. In the event this happens, immediate medical attention should be sought.
- Instruct patient or parents to monitor fingers and toes for soft-tissue breakdown and/or ulceration. If noticed, prescriber should be notified. Reassure patient that signs and symptoms generally improve after the dose is reduced or drug is discontinued.
- Tell female patient of childbearing age to notify prescriber if pregnancy is suspected or occurs. Also inform women wanting to breastfeed that breastfeeding is not recommended during lisdexamfetamine therapy.

lisinopril
Prinivil, Qbrelis, Zestril

Class and Category
Pharmacologic class: Angiotensin-converting enzyme (ACE) inhibitor
Therapeutic class: Antihypertensive

Indications and Dosages
✳ *To treat hypertension*

ORAL SOLUTION OR SUSPENSION, TABLETS

Adults. *Initial:* 5 mg (if taking a diuretic) or 10 mg once daily (if no diuretic therapy), adjusted according to blood pressure. *Maintenance:* 20 to 40 mg once daily. *Maximum:* 80 mg once daily.

Children age 6 and over with a GFR of at least 30 ml/min. *Initial:* 0.07 mg/kg (maximum 5 mg) daily, adjusted according to blood pressure. *Maximum:* 0.61 mg/kg or 40 mg daily.

✳ *As adjunct with digitalis and diuretics to treat heart failure*

ORAL SOLUTION OR SUSPENSION, TABLETS

Adults. *Initial:* 5 mg once daily. *Maintenance:* 5 to 20 mg once daily. *Maximum:* 40 mg once daily.

±**DOSAGE ADJUSTMENT** For patients with hyponatremia or creatinine clearance of 30 ml/min or less, initial dosage reduced to 2.5 mg daily with maximum dosage not to exceed 40 mg once daily.

✳ *To improve survival in hemodynamically stable patient within 24 hours of an acute MI*

ORAL SOLUTION OR SUSPENSION, TABLETS

Adults. *Initial:* 5 mg within 24 hr after onset of symptoms, followed by 5 mg after 24 hr and 10 mg after 48 hr and daily thereafter. *Maintenance:* 10 mg daily for 6 wk.

±**DOSAGE ADJUSTMENT** For patients with baseline systolic blood pressure of 120 mm Hg or less, initial dosage decreased to 2.5 mg daily for first 3 days after MI. If systolic blood pressure falls to 100 mm Hg or less during therapy, maintenance dosage decreased to 2.5 or 5 mg as tolerated; if systolic blood pressure is 90 mm Hg or less for more than 1 hr, drug discontinued. For adult patients, regardless of indication, with impaired renal function (creatinine clearance of 10 to 30 ml/min), initial dosage reduced by half; for patients on hemodialysis or with a creatinine clearance of less than 10 ml/min, initial dose reduced to 2.5 mg once daily.

Drug Administration

P.O.

- Use a calibrated device when measuring dosage of oral solution or suspension.
- If oral solution is not available, request that an oral suspension form be prepared by pharmacist. Shake suspension before each use and discard after 4 weeks.

Route	Onset	Peak	Duration
P.O.	1 hr	6–8 hr	24 hr

Half-life: 12 hr

Mechanism of Action

May reduce blood pressure by inhibiting conversion of angiotensin I to angiotensin II. Angiotensin II is a potent vasoconstrictor that also stimulates adrenal cortex to secrete aldosterone. Lisinopril may also inhibit renal and vascular production of angiotensin II. Decreased release of aldosterone reduces sodium and water reabsorption and increases their excretion, thereby reducing blood pressure.

Contraindications

Concurrent aliskiren use in patients with diabetes; hereditary or idiopathic angioedema or history of angioedema related to previous treatment with an ACE inhibitor; hypersensitivity to lisinopril, other ACE inhibitors, or their components; use of a neprilysin inhibitor such as sacubitril within 36 hours of lisinopril initiation

Interactions

DRUGS

aliskiren (in presence of diabetes or renal impairment), other ACE inhibitors, angiotensin receptor blockers: Increased risk of hypotension, hyperkalemia, and renal impairment
diuretics, other antihypertensives: Increased hypotensive effect
gold (injectable form such as sodium aurothiomalate): Possibly nitroid reaction

(facial flushing, hypotension, nausea, vomiting)
insulin, oral antidiabetics: Increased risk of hypoglycemia
lithium: Increased blood lithium level and risk of lithium toxicity
mTOR inhibitors such as everolimus, sirolimus, temsirolimus; neprilysin inhibitors such as sacubitril: Increased risk for angioedema
NSAIDs: Possibly reduced antihypertensive effect; possibly reduced renal function in patients with preexisting renal dysfunction, the elderly and patients who are volume-depleted
potassium-sparing diuretics: Increased risk of hyperkalemia
thiazide diuretics: Increased risk of hypokalemia

FOODS

high-potassium diet, potassium-containing salt substitutes: Increased risk of hyperkalemia

Adverse Reactions

CNS: Ataxia, confusion, CVA, depression, dizziness, fatigue, hallucinations, headache, insomnia, irritability, memory impairment, mood alterations, nervousness, paresthesia, peripheral neuropathy, somnolence, syncope, transient ischemic attack, tremor, vertigo
CV: Arrhythmias, chest pain, fluid overload, hypotension, MI, orthostatic hypotension, palpitations, peripheral edema, vasculitis
ENDO: Hyperglycemia, syndrome of inappropriate ADH secretion
EENT: Blurred vision, diplopia, dry mouth, olfactory or taste disturbance, photophobia, tinnitus, visual loss
GI: Abdominal pain, anorexia, cholestatic jaundice, constipation, diarrhea, elevated liver enzymes, flatulence, fulminant hepatic necrosis, gastritis, hepatitis, indigestion, nausea, pancreatitis, vomiting
GU: Acute renal failure, decreased libido, impotence, pyelonephritis
HEME: Agranulocytosis, anemia, hemolytic anemia, neutropenia, thrombocytopenia
MS: Arthralgia, arthritis, bone or joint pain, muscle spasms, myalgia
RESP: Bronchospasm, cough, dyspnea, paroxysmal nocturnal dyspnea, pulmonary embolism and infarction, upper respiratory tract infection
SKIN: Alopecia, cutaneous pseudolymphoma, diaphoresis, erythema,

J
K
L

flushing, herpes zoster, infections, pemphigus, photosensitivity, pruritus, psoriasis, rash, **Stevens–Johnson syndrome, toxic epidermal necrolysis,** urticaria
Other: Anaphylaxis, angioedema, dehydration, gout, **hyperkalemia, hyponatremia,** weight gain or loss

Childbearing Considerations
PREGNANCY
- Drug can cause fetal harm. Drug given during the second or third trimester reduces fetal renal function and increases fetal and neonatal morbidity and death. Resulting oligohydramnios can cause fetal lung hypoplasia and skeletal malformations.
- Drug should be discontinued as soon as pregnancy is known.

LACTATION
- It is not known if drug is present in breast milk.
- A decision should be made to discontinue breastfeeding or the drug to avoid potential serious adverse reactions in the breastfed infant.

Nursing Considerations
- Be aware that lisinopril should not be given to a patient who is hemodynamically unstable after an acute MI.
- Use lisinopril cautiously in patients with fluid volume deficit, heart failure, impaired renal function, or sodium depletion.
- Also use cautiously in patients with severe aortic stenosis or hypertrophic cardiomyopathy because symptomatic hypotension may occur.
- Monitor blood pressure often, especially during the first 2 weeks of therapy and whenever the dose of lisinopril and/or prescribed diuretic is increased. If excessive hypotension develops, expect to withhold drug for several days.

! WARNING Keep in mind if angioedema, affects face, glottis, larynx, limbs, lips, mucous membranes, or tongue, notify prescriber immediately and expect to stop lisinopril and start appropriate therapy at once. If airway obstruction threatens, promptly give 0.3 to 0.5 ml of epinephrine 1:1000 solution subcutaneously, as prescribed.

! WARNING Monitor patient for anaphylaxis, especially patient being dialyzed with high-flux membranes. If anaphylaxis occurs, stop dialysis immediately and treat aggressively (antihistamines are ineffective in this situation), as ordered. Anaphylaxis has also occurred with some patients undergoing low-density lipoprotein apheresis with dextran sulfate absorption.

- Notify prescriber if patient has persistent, nonproductive cough, a common adverse effect of ACE inhibitors such as lisinopril.
- Monitor for dehydration, which can lead to hypotension especially if patient experiences diarrhea or vomiting.
- Monitor patient for hepatic dysfunction because lisinopril, an ACE inhibitor, may rarely cause a syndrome that starts with cholestatic jaundice or hepatitis and progresses to fulminant hepatic necrosis. If patient develops jaundice or a marked elevation in liver enzymes, withhold drug and notify prescriber.
- Monitor patient's serum creatinine, as ordered because changes in renal function can occur with lisinopril use. If renal function decreases, alert prescriber and expect drug to be withheld or discontinued.
- If patient takes insulin or an oral antidiabetic, monitor blood glucose level closely because risk of hypoglycemia increases, especially during first month of therapy.
- Monitor patient's serum potassium level, as ordered because drugs that inhibit the renin–angiotensin system such as lisinopril can cause hyperkalemia. Patients at increased risk for developing hyperkalemia include patients with diabetes or renal insufficiency or who are also taking potassium-sparing diuretics, potassium-containing salt substitutes, or potassium supplements.

PATIENT TEACHING
- Explain that lisinopril helps to control, but doesn't cure, hypertension and that patient may need lifelong therapy.

! WARNING Warn patient to seek immediate emergency treatment if she experiences difficulty breathing or swallowing or notices swelling of her eyes, extremities, face, lips, or tongue.

- Advise patient to take lisinopril at the same time every day.
- Emphasize need to take drug as ordered, even if patient feels well; caution her not to stop drug without consulting prescriber.
- Instruct patient to report dizziness, especially during first few days of therapy.
- Caution her to avoid hazardous activities such as driving until dizziness or other nervous system symptoms abates.
- Inform patient that persistent, nonproductive cough may develop during lisinopril therapy. Urge her to notify prescriber immediately if cough becomes difficult to tolerate.
- Advise patient to drink adequate fluids and avoid excessive sweating, which can lead to dehydration and hypotension. Make sure she understands that diarrhea, excessive perspiration, and vomiting can also cause hypotension.
- Caution patient not to use salt substitutes that contain potassium.
- Instruct patient to report signs of infection, such as fever and sore throat, which may indicate neutropenia.
- Advise patient to change position slowly to minimize orthostatic hypotension.
- If patient has diabetes and takes insulin or an oral antidiabetic, urge her to monitor her blood glucose level closely and watch for symptoms of hypoglycemia.
- Caution female patient to notify prescriber immediately if she is or could be pregnant because lisinopril must be discontinued. Also inform her that breastfeeding is not recommended during lisinopril therapy.
- Advise patient to inform all prescribers of lisinopril therapy.

lithium carbonate
Carbolith (CAN), Lithane (CAN), Lithobid

lithium citrate

≡ Class and Category
Pharmacologic class: Alkali metal
Therapeutic class: Antimanic

≡ Indications and Dosages

✳ *To treat acute mania episodes of bipolar disorder; to maintain patients with bipolar disorder*

CAPSULES, TABLETS

Adults and children age 7 and over weighing more than 30 kg (66 lb). *Initial:* 300 mg three times daily, increased every 3 days by 300 mg, as needed. *Acute goal:* 600 mg two to three times daily. *Maintenance:* 300 to 600 mg two to three times daily.
Children ages 7 and over weighing 20 (44 lb) to 30 kg (66 lb). *Initial:* 300 mg twice daily, increased 300 mg weekly. *Acute goal:* 600 mg to 1,500 mg in divided doses daily. *Maintenance:* 600 mg to 1,200 mg in divided doses daily.

ORAL SOLUTION

Adults and children age 7 and over weighing more than 30 kg (66 lb). *Initial:* 8 mEq (5 ml) three times daily, increased by 8 mEq (5 ml) every 3 days, as needed. *Acute goal:* 16 mEq (10 ml) two to three times daily. *Maintenance:* 8 to 16 mEq (5 to 10 ml) two to three times daily.
Children age 7 and over weighing 20 kg (44 lb) to 30 kg (66 lb). *Initial:* 8 mEq (5 ml) twice daily, increased by 8 mEq (5 ml) weekly, as needed. *Acute goal:* 16 to 40 mEq (10 to 25 ml) in divided doses daily. *Maintenance:* 16 to 32 mEq (10 to 20 ml) in divided doses daily.

E.R. TABLETS (LITHOBID)

Adults and children age 12 and over. *Initial:* 900 mg twice daily. *Maintenance:* 600 mg twice daily.

SYRUP (LITHIUM CITRATE)

Adults and children age 12 and over. Highly individualized. *Usual initial:* 16 mEq (10 ml) three times daily. *Usual maintenance:* 8 mEq (5 ml) three or four times daily.

±**DOSAGE ADJUSTMENT** For elderly patient and patient at risk for lithium toxicity, such as in the presence of severe debilitation or dehydration, or significant cardiovascular or renal disease or who is taking drugs that may affect kidney function such as angiotensin-converting enzyme inhibitors, angiotensin receptor blockers, diuretics, or NSAIDS, initial dosage may be reduced and titration done more slowly.

J
K
L

Drug Administration

P.O.

- Do not interchange one form of lithium with another.
- Administer drug in regularly spaced doses consistently.
- Administer drug with water after meals to slow absorption from GI tract and reduce adverse reactions.
- Use a calibrated device when measuring dose of liquid form of drug.
- Capsules and E.R. tablets should be swallowed whole and not chewed, crushed, or opened.

Route	Onset	Peak	Duration
P.O.	5–7 days	1–2 hr	Unknown
P.O./E.R.	5–7 days	4–5 hr	Unknown

Half-life: 18–36 hr

Mechanism of Action

May increase presynaptic degradation of the catecholamine neurotransmitters dopamine, norepinephrine, and serotonin; inhibit their release at neuronal synapses; and decrease postsynaptic receptor sensitivity. These actions may correct overactive catecholamine systems in patients with mania.

Contraindications

Hypersensitivity to lithium or its components

Interactions

DRUGS

ACE inhibitors, angiotensin receptor blockers, diuretics, metronidazole, NSAIDs: Possibly increased blood lithium level and increased risk of toxicity
acetazolamide, sodium bicarbonate, urea, xanthines: Decreased blood lithium level
buspirone, fentanyl, MAO inhibitors, norepinephrine reuptake inhibitors, selective serotonin reuptake inhibitors, St. John's wort, tramadol, tricyclic antidepressants, triptans, tryptophan: Increased risk of serotonin syndrome
calcium channel blockers: Increased risk of neurotoxicity from lithium
calcium iodide, iodinated glycerol, potassium iodide: Possibly increased hypothyroid effects of both drugs
carbamazepine, methyldopa, phenytoin: Possibly increased risk of adverse reactions with these drugs

haloperidol and other antipsychotics: Increased risk of neurotoxicity ranging from extrapyramidal symptoms to neuroleptic malignant syndrome
neuromuscular blockers: Risk of prolonged effects

Adverse Reactions

CNS: Ataxia, **coma**, confusion, depression, disorientation, dizziness, drowsiness, fatigue, headache, lethargy, **seizures**, **serotonin syndrome**, syncope, tremor (in hands), vertigo
CV: **Arrhythmias**, **bradycardia**, **ECG changes**, edema, **hypotension**, palpitations, **peripheral circulatory collapse**, tachycardia, unmasking of **Brugada syndrome**
EENT: Blurred vision, dental caries, dry mouth, exophthalmos
ENDO: Diabetes insipidus, euthyroid goiter, hypothyroidism, **myxedema**, polydipsia
GI: Abdominal distention and pain, anorexia, diarrhea, nausea, vomiting
GU: **Nephrotic syndrome**, polyuria, stress incontinence, urinary frequency
HEME: Leukocytosis
MS: Muscle twitching and weakness
RESP: Dyspnea
SKIN: Abnormally dry skin; acne; alopecia; chronic folliculitis; cutaneous ulcers; dermatitis; dry, thin hair; numbness of skin; pruritus; psoriasis (new onset or exacerbation); rash
Other: **Angioedema**, cold sensitivity, **drug reaction with eosinophilia and systemic symptoms (DRESS)**, weight gain or loss

Childbearing Considerations

PREGNANCY

- Drug may cause fetal harm in first trimester, such as cardiovascular and other anomalies, and especially Ebstein's anomaly.
- Drug may cause fetal harm late in pregnancy with increased risk of neonatal lithium toxicity at birth.
- Use with caution only if benefit to mother outweighs potential risk to fetus.

LACTATION

- Drug is present in breast milk.
- Breastfeeding is not recommended during drug therapy. However, if a woman chooses to breastfeed, infant should be monitored for signs of lithium toxicity. If present, breastfeeding must be discontinued.

⋮ Nursing Considerations

- Expect to monitor blood lithium level two or three times weekly during first month, and then weekly to monthly during maintenance therapy and when starting or stopping NSAID therapy. In uncomplicated cases, plan to monitor lithium level every 2 to 3 months.
- Be aware that lithium has a narrow therapeutic range. Even a slightly high blood level is dangerous, and some patients show signs of toxicity at normal levels. Be aware that risk of toxicity is increased in patients with electrolyte changes (especially potassium and sodium), recent onset of a concurrent febrile illness, severe debilitation or dehydration, or significant cardiovascular or renal disease, and in patients taking other drugs that affect kidney function, such as angiotensin-converting enzyme inhibitors, angiotensin receptor blockers, diuretics, and NSAIDs. Lithium toxicity signs and symptoms affect many areas of the body and can range from mild to severe and life-threatening symptoms. No antidote for lithium toxicity is available.
- Expect prescriber to decrease dosage after acute manic episode is controlled.

! **WARNING** Be aware that lithium affects extracellular and intracellular potassium ion shift, which can cause ECG changes, such as flattened or inverted T waves; it also can increase the risk of cardiac arrest.

- Monitor ECGs, renal and thyroid function test results, and serum electrolyte levels, as appropriate, during lithium treatment. Know that nephrotic syndrome has occurred with lithium use but has resulted in remission after lithium was discontinued.
- Be aware that lithium can cause reversible leukocytosis, which usually peaks within 7 to 10 days of starting therapy; WBC count typically returns to baseline within 10 days after therapy stops.
- Weigh patient daily to detect sudden weight changes.
- Monitor blood glucose level often in diabetic patient because lithium alters glucose tolerance.
- Palpate thyroid gland to detect enlargement because drug may cause goiter.

- Ensure that patient's fluid and sodium intake is adequate during treatment.

! **WARNING** Monitor patient closely for unexplained palpitations or syncope after starting lithium therapy, as these symptoms may be caused by the unmasking of Brugada syndrome by lithium. Know that Brugada syndrome is a disorder in which electrocardiographic abnormalities occur and can result in sudden death. Patients at risk include those with a family history of Brugada syndrome or a family history of sudden death before the age of 45 years. Notify prescriber if palpitations or syncope occur and expect to discontinue lithium therapy.

! **WARNING** Monitor patient closely for serotonin syndrome, a rare but serious adverse effect of lithium. Signs and symptoms include agitation, confusion, diaphoresis, diarrhea, fever, hyperactive reflexes, poor coordination, restlessness, shaking, talking or acting with uncontrolled excitement, tremor, and twitching. If symptoms occur, notify prescriber immediately, expect drug to be discontinued, and provide supportive care.

- Monitor patient's skin for abnormalities. Report any such findings to prescriber, as some can be serious.

PATIENT TEACHING

- Advise patient to take lithium after meals to minimize adverse reactions.
- Instruct patient to swallow capsules or E.R. form whole. Tell patient prescribed liquid form of drug to use a calibrated device to measure dosage.
- Inform patient that frequent urination, nausea, and thirst may occur during the first few days of treatment.
- Caution patient not to stop taking lithium or adjust dosage without first consulting prescriber.
- Instruct patient to report signs of toxicity, such as diarrhea, drowsiness, muscle weakness, tremor, uncoordinated body movements, and vomiting.
- Urge patient to avoid hazardous activities until drug's CNS effects are known.
- Advise patient to maintain normal fluid and sodium intake.

J
K
L

- Emphasize importance of complying with scheduled checkups and laboratory tests.

> **! WARNING** Instruct patient to seek immediate emergency care if he experiences abnormal heartbeats, fainting, light-headedness, or shortness of breath.

- Stress importance of alerting prescriber of pregnancy. Inform mothers that breastfeeding is not recommended during lithium therapy.

lixisenatide
Adlyxin

☰ Class and Category
Pharmacologic class: Glucagon-like peptide receptor agonist
Therapeutic class: Antidiabetic

☰ Indications and Dosages
✳ *Adjunct to diet and exercise to improve glycemic control in patients with type 2 diabetes mellitus*

SUBCUTANEOUS INJECTION
Adults. *Initial:* 10 mcg once daily for 14 days. Increased to 20 mcg once daily on day 15 and thereafter. *Maintenance:* 20 mcg once daily.

☰ Drug Administration
SUBCUTANEOUS
- Inspect solution before administration; it should be clear and colorless.
- Administer drug within 1 hour before patient's first meal of the day.
- Inject drug into patient's abdomen, thighs, or upper arm.
- If a dose is missed, give 1 hour before next meal.
- Rotate sites.
- Protect the pen device containing the drug from light by keeping it in its original packaging until ready for use.
- Do not store pen with needle attached. Unused pens should be stored in refrigerator.
- Write date that pen was first used, store pen at room temperature, and discard 14 days later.

Route	Onset	Peak	Duration
SubQ	Unknown	1–3.5 hr	Unknown

Half-life: 3 hr

☰ Mechanism of Action
As a glucagon-like peptide receptor agonist, lixisenatide decreases glucagon secretion, increases glucose-dependent insulin release, and slows gastric emptying. All of these actions work together to reduce blood glucose levels.

☰ Contraindications
Hypersensitivity to lixisenatide or its components

☰ Interactions
DRUGS
basal insulin, sulfonylureas: Increased risk of hypoglycemia
orally administered drugs: Possibly delayed absorption of orally administered drugs resulting in decreased effectiveness

☰ Adverse Reactions
CNS: Dizziness, headache
EENT: **Laryngeal edema**
GI: Abdominal distention or pain, **acute pancreatitis**, constipation, diarrhea, dyspepsia, nausea, vomiting
GU: **Acute kidney injury, worsening of chronic renal failure**
RESP: **Bronchospasms**
SKIN: Urticaria
Other: **Anaphylaxis; angioedema;** injection-site reactions such as erythema, pain, and pruritus; lixisenatide-induced antibodies

☰ Childbearing Considerations
PREGNANCY
- Drug may cause fetal harm based on animal studies.
- Use with caution only if benefit to mother outweighs potential risk to fetus.

LACTATION
- It is not known if drug is present in breast milk.
- Patient should check with prescriber before breastfeeding.

☰ Nursing Considerations

> **! WARNING** Monitor patient closely for hypersensitivity reactions that could become

serious, especially if patient has a history of hypersensitivity to other drugs in the same class.

- Monitor patient for signs and symptoms of pancreatitis, including persistent severe abdominal pain, sometimes radiating to the back, that may or may not be accompanied with vomiting. Know that risk increases in patients who have a history of alcohol abuse or cholelithiasis. If pancreatitis is suspected, notify prescriber, discontinue drug, and provide supportive care, as ordered.
- Monitor patient for hypoglycemia, especially in patients who also take basal insulin and/or a sulfonylurea. Be prepared to treat hypoglycemia should it occur. Notify prescriber of persistent or severe hypoglycemic episodes, as a dosage reduction in the insulin or sulfonylurea may be needed.
- Monitor patient's renal function before lixisenatide is initiated and during therapy, as ordered. Know that acute kidney injury can occur quickly even in patients who have no history of kidney disease. Patients are at increased risk when they experience dehydration, diarrhea, nausea, or vomiting. Notify prescriber immediately if patient's fluid balance is compromised.

PATIENT TEACHING

- Instruct patient or caregiver on how to administer drug subcutaneously, if self-administration is prescribed. Provide instructions on how to use the pen device correctly. Tell patient how to dispose of pen properly and to keep out of reach of children and pets.
- Tell patient to inspect solution in pen before administering. It should appear clear and colorless.
- Instruct patient to administer lixisenatide 1 hour before the first meal of the day by injecting into her abdomen, thigh, or upper arm. Stress importance of rotating sites. Tell her it is best to administer the drug before the same meal each day.
- Inform patient that if she forgets a dose, she should administer the drug within 1 hour prior to the next meal but never double the dose to make up for a missed dose.
- Tell patient to protect the pen from light by keeping it in the original packaging. She

should also write down the date the pen was first used, as pen must be discarded 14 days later. Unused pens should be refrigerated.

- Inform women who are taking oral contraceptives that lixisenatide may interfere with absorption and effectiveness of oral contraceptive. To avoid this, tell patient to take oral contraceptive 1 hour before or 11 hours after administering lixisenatide each day.
- Tell all patients taking oral medications to take them at least 1 hour before administering lixisenatide; if a prescribed drug requires food intake, take it with a meal or snack that does not coincide with lixisenatide administration.
- Warn patient never to share the pen used to inject lixisenatide even if the needle is changed, because of an increased risk for transmission of blood-borne diseases.
- Remind patient that lixisenatide does not take the place of dietary measures and exercise also used to control blood sugar.
- Advise patient to maintain adequate hydration. Emphasize importance of alerting prescriber immediately if she does become dehydrated or develops diarrhea, nausea, or vomiting.

! WARNING Instruct patient to seek immediate medical attention if she develops an allergic reaction to drug.

- Review signs and symptoms of pancreatitis with patient and urge her to stop taking drug and notify the prescriber, if present.
- Encourage patient to be on the alert for hypoglycemia, especially if she is taking basal insulin or sulfonylurea. Review the signs and symptoms and how to treat it. If episodes occur frequently or become severe, tell her to notify prescriber, as a dosage reduction may be needed for her basal insulin or sulfonylurea.

Iofexidine
Lucemyra

Class and Category
Pharmacologic class: Central alpha$_2$-agonist
Therapeutic class: Opioid withdrawal

☰ Indications and Dosages

* *To mitigate opioid withdrawal symptoms in order to facilitate abrupt opioid discontinuation*

TABLETS

Adults. 3 tablets (0.18 mg each) four times daily and continued during the period of peak withdrawal (usually first 5 to 7 days following last use of an opioid, although peak withdrawal may last up to 14 days). Then, dosage gradually reduced over 2 to 4 days by reducing 1 tablet per dose every 1 to 2 days. *Maximum:* 4 tablets (total 0.72 mg) for a single dose, 16 tablets (total 2.88 mg) daily.

±**DOSAGE ADJUSTMENT** For patients experiencing drug-related adverse reactions, dosage reduced, held, or drug discontinued depending on severity of reactions. Dosage may be reduced as opioid withdrawal symptoms wane. For patient with moderate hepatic or renal impairment, dosage reduced to 2 tablets four times daily; for patient with severe hepatic or renal impairment, dosage reduced to 1 tablet four times daily.

☰ Drug Administration

P.O.

- Administer drug with 5 to 6 hours between each dose.
- Do not remove desiccant pack from bottle.

Route	Onset	Peak	Duration
P.O.	Unknown	3–5 hr	Unknown

Half-life: 11–13 hr

☰ Mechanism of Action

Binds to receptors on adrenergic neurons to reduce the release of norepinephrine and decrease sympathetic tone, thereby reducing opioid withdrawal symptoms.

☰ Contraindications

Hypersensitivity to lofexidine or its components

☰ Interactions

DRUGS

CNS depressants such as barbiturates and other sedating drugs: Possibly potentiates effects of CNS depressants

CYP2D6 inhibitors such as paroxetine: Increased absorption of lofexidine, increasing risk for bradycardia and orthostatic hypotension

methadone: Increased risk of QT prolongation leading to life-threatening arrythmias

naltrexone (oral): Possibly reduced effectiveness of oral naltrexone if administered within 2 hours of lofexidine

ACTIVITIES

alcohol use: Possibly potentiates CNS depressant effect of alcohol

☰ Adverse Reactions

CNS: Dizziness, insomnia, sedation, somnolence, syncope

CV: Bradycardia, **hypotension**, orthostatic hypotension, **QT prolongation, torsades de pointes**

EENT: Dry mouth, tinnitus

Other: Discontinuation effects (anxiety, chills, diarrhea, elevation of blood pressure, extremity pain, hyperhidrosis, insomnia)

☰ Childbearing Considerations

PREGNANCY

- It is not known if drug causes fetal harm.
- Use with caution only if benefit to mother outweighs potential risk to fetus.

LACTATION

- It is not known if drug is present in breast milk.
- Patient should check with prescriber before breastfeeding.

☰ Nursing Considerations

- Be aware that lofexidine should not be used in patients with cerebrovascular disease, congenital long QT syndrome, marked bradycardia, recent myocardial infarction, or severe coronary insufficiency.
- Monitor vital signs before administering each dose of lofexidine, because drug may cause a decrease in blood pressure or pulse and cause syncope.

! **WARNING** Know that lofexidine prolongs the QT interval. Expect to monitor patient's ECG if he has a history of bradyarrhythmias, congestive heart failure, or hepatic or renal impairment; ECG should also be monitored in patients with electrolyte abnormalities such as hypokalemia or hypomagnesemia. Know that electrolyte imbalances should be corrected before lofexidine therapy begins.

- Be aware that lofexidine therapy should not be stopped abruptly but gradually withdrawn to reduce the risk of discontinuation symptoms such as a sudden rise in blood pressure along with anxiety, chills, diarrhea, excessive sweating, extremity pain, and insomnia. If patient stops drug use abruptly, symptoms can be managed by administering the previous lofexidine dose and then subsequently gradually tapering drug dosage downward.

PATIENT TEACHING

- Instruct patient to take lofexidine exactly as prescribed. Warn patient that stopping drug abruptly can result in a sudden rise in blood pressure along with anxiety, chills, diarrhea, excessive sweating, extremity pain, and insomnia. Caution him that drug must be gradually withdrawn.
- Tell patient that lofexidine therapy will help with opioid withdrawal symptoms but will not completely prevent them.
- Inform patient that lofexidine may cause a sudden drop in blood pressure or pulse. Instruct patient to rise slowly from a lying or sitting position and to maintain adequate hydration, as well as avoid becoming overheated, to help minimize these effects. Tell patient that if he experiences low blood pressure or decreased pulse rate to withhold drug and notify prescriber for guidance on how to adjust his dose.
- Tell patient to inform all prescribers of lofexidine therapy and not to take any over-the-counter preparations, including herbal products, without consulting prescriber, as the combination may cause an excessive drop in blood pressure or pulse rate.
- Instruct patient to avoid performing hazardous activities such as driving until the drug's effects on his nervous system are known.

! **WARNING** Alert patient that lofexidine is not a treatment for opioid use. Tell patient that upon complete opioid discontinuation, he is more likely to have a reduced tolerance to opioids and is at increased risk for a fatal overdose should he resume opioid use. Make sure both patient and caregivers are aware of the increased risk of overdose.

- Warn patient to avoid taking any CNS depressant drugs such as barbiturates, benzodiazepines, or other sedating drugs while taking lofexidine, because severe respiratory depression and sedation may occur. Also warn patient not to drink alcohol while taking drug, for the same reason.

lomitapide mesylate
Juxtapid

Class and Category

Pharmacologic class: Microsomal triglyceride transfer protein (MTP) inhibitor
Therapeutic class: Antilipemic

Indications and Dosages

✴ *To control lipid levels as adjunct to diet and other lipid-lowering treatments in homozygous familial hypercholesterolemia*

CAPSULES

Adults. *Initial:* 5 mg once daily with dosage increased to 10 mg once daily after 2 wk, as needed. Dosage further increased in 4 wk increments to 20 mg once daily, then to 40 mg once daily to 60 mg once daily, as needed. *Maximum:* 60 mg once daily.

±**DOSAGE ADJUSTMENT** For patients with mild hepatic impairment or with end-stage renal impairment requiring dialysis, dosage not to exceed 40 mg once daily. For patients receiving weak CYP3A4 inhibitors such as alprazolam, amiodarone, amlodipine, atorvastatin, bicalutamide, cilostazol, cimetidine, cyclosporine, fluoxetine, fluvoxamine, ginkgo, goldenseal, isoniazid, lapatinib, nilotinib, pazopanib, ranolazine, ticagrelor, or zileuton, dosage of 10 mg or more reduced by half and maximum dosage not to exceed 30 mg once daily. However, for patient taking oral contraceptives which are also weak CYP3A4 inhibitors, maximum daily dosage reduced to 40 mg daily. For patients who develop elevated transaminases three times or greater but less than five times upper normal limits during therapy, daily dosage reduced with degree of reduction individualized.

Drug Administration

P.O.

- Administer drug with a full glass of water 2 hours after the evening meal because taking drug with food may increase the risk of gastrointestinal adverse reactions.

J
K
L

- Capsules should be swallowed whole and not chewed, crushed, dissolved, or opened.

Route	Onset	Peak	Duration
P.O.	Unknown	6 hr	Unknown

Half-life: 39.7 hr

Mechanism of Action

Binds and inhibits microsomal triglyceride transfer protein, located in the lumen of the endoplasmic reticulum of cells which in turn prevents the assembly of apo B-containing lipoproteins in enterocytes and hepatocytes. This then prevents the synthesis of chylomicrons and very low-density lipoproteins (VLDL). Lower VLDL levels leads to reduced levels of plasma low-density lipoprotein-cholesterol.

Contraindications

Active liver disease, concurrent therapy with moderate or strong CYP3A4 inhibitors, hypersensitivity to lomitapide or its components, moderate or severe hepatic impairment, pregnancy, unexplained persistent elevations of serum transaminases

Interactions

DRUGS

bile acid sequestrants: Possibly decreased absorption of lomitapide
CYP3A inhibitors: Increased lomitapide exposure with possible increased risk of adverse reactions
lovastatin, simvastatin: Increased risk of myopathy, including rhabdomyolysis
P-glycoprotein substrates such as aliskiren, colchicine, dabigatran etexilate, digoxin, everolimus, fexofenadine, imatinib, lapatinib, maraviroc, nilotinib, posaconazole, ranolazine, saxagliptin, sirolimus, sitagliptin, talinolol, tolvaptan, topotecan: Increased absorption of these drugs resulting in higher drug levels
warfarin: Increased plasma warfarin levels with possible increased risk of bleeding events

FOODS

grapefruit juice: Increased lomitapide exposure and adverse reactions

ACTIVITIES

alcohol use: Possibly increased risk of hepatic steatosis

Adverse Reactions

CNS: Dizziness, fatigue, fever, headache

CV: Chest pain, palpitations
EENT: Nasal congestion, nasopharyngitis, pharyngolaryngeal pain
GI: Abdominal distention or pain, constipation, defecation urgency, diarrhea (may become severe), dyspepsia, elevated liver enzymes, flatulence, gastroenteritis, gastroesophageal reflux disease, hepatic steatosis, **hepatotoxicity**, nausea, rectal tenesmus, transaminase elevations, vomiting
MS: Back pain, myalgia
SKIN: Alopecia
Other: Fat-soluble vitamin deficiency, flu-like symptoms, serum fatty acid deficiency, weight loss

Childbearing Considerations

PREGNANCY

- Pregnancy Exposure Registry: 1-877-902-4099.
- Drug may cause fetal harm.
- Drug is contraindicated in pregnancy.
- Women of childbearing age should have a negative pregnancy test before starting drug.

LACTATION

- It is not known if drug is present in breast milk.
- A decision should be made to discontinue breastfeeding or the drug to avoid potential serious adverse reactions in the breastfed infant.

REPRODUCTION

- Advise women of childbearing age pregnancy should be avoided during drug therapy.
- Women of childbearing age must use effective contraception during drug therapy.

Nursing Considerations

- Be aware that lomitapide should not be given to patients with rare, hereditary problems of galactose intolerance, glucose–galactose malabsorption, or Lapp lactase deficiency because drug may cause diarrhea and malabsorption in these patients.
- Know that because lomitapide increases risk of hepatotoxicity, the drug can only be administered through the Juxtapid REMS program.
- Determine that patient has had ALT, AST, alkaline phosphatase and total bilirubin measured, has had a negative pregnancy

test if patient is female, and has initiated a low-fat diet supplying less than 20% of energy from fat prior to initiating lomitapide therapy.

■ Be aware that ALT and AST levels should be measured prior to potential dosage increase or monthly, whichever comes first, for first year of therapy and then before each actual dosage increase and every 3 months thereafter. If transaminase values are equal to or greater than three times upper limit normal but less than five times upper limit normal, expect to confirm elevation with a repeat measurement within 1 week. If confirmed, expect dosage to be decreased and additional liver-related tests done, such as measurement of alkaline phosphatase, total bilirubin, and patient's INR. Repeat tests weekly, as ordered, and expect to withhold drug if there are signs of abnormal liver function such as an elevation in patient's bilirubin or an increase in patient's INR. If transaminase levels are above five times upper limit normal, or if transaminase levels do not fall below three times upper limit normal within about 4 weeks, expect drug to be withheld or discontinued. Know that if drug therapy is resumed, dosage should be reduced and more frequent liver-related tests ordered.

■ Monitor patient closely for signs and symptoms of liver impairment, such as presence of abdominal pain, fever, flu-like symptoms, jaundice, or lethargy; a bilirubin result that is equal to or greater than two times upper limit normal, or active liver disease is suspected, because risk of hepatotoxicity increases with lomitapide therapy.

■ Monitor patient for fat-soluble vitamin and fatty acids deficiencies, especially patients with chronic bowel or pancreatic diseases that predispose to malabsorption, because lomitapide reduces the absorption of fat-soluble vitamins.

■ Monitor patient for adverse reactions, especially gastrointestinal reactions, which are the most common reactions associated with lomitapide therapy. Ensure patient is adhering to a low-fat diet that supplies less than 20% of energy needs from fat, to reduce the risk of adverse gastrointestinal reactions.

■ Know that lomitapide may cause severe diarrhea in some patients, requiring hospitalization because of diarrhea-induced volume depletion. Monitor patients closely, especially the elderly and those who are taking drugs that can lead to hypotension or volume depletion.

PATIENT TEACHING

■ Advise patient to take lomitapide with a full glass of water 2 hours after the evening meal because taking drug with food may increase the risk of gastrointestinal adverse reactions.

■ Caution patient to swallow capsule whole and not to chew, crush, dissolve, or open capsule.

■ Instruct patient to take daily supplements of 400 international units of vitamin E and at least 210 mg alpha-linolenic acid, 110 mg eicosapentaenoic acid, and 80 mg of docosahexaenoic acid to prevent deficiencies.

■ Remind patient of importance of adhering to the low-fat diet prescribed, as lomitapide therapy is not a replacement for dietary control of fat in her diet.

■ Tell patient to inform all prescribers about lomitapide therapy because of potential drug interactions.

■ Review signs and symptoms of liver impairment, and emphasize importance of reporting such to prescriber. Inform patient of need for blood tests to monitor her liver function and importance of compliance with test schedule.

■ Instruct patient to stop taking drug and notify prescriber if severe diarrhea occurs or if he experiences symptoms such as decreased urine output, light-headedness, or unexplainable tiredness that accompanies diarrhea.

! **WARNING** Instruct patient not to consume more than one alcoholic beverage daily.

! **WARNING** Caution women of childbearing age to notify prescriber immediately if pregnancy occurs or is suspected because drug will have to be discontinued. Also inform these women that breastfeeding is not recommended during drug therapy.

lorazepam
Ativan, Lorazepam Intensol

Class, Category, and Schedule
Pharmacologic class: Benzodiazepine
Therapeutic class: Anxiolytic
Controlled substance schedule: IV

Indications and Dosages
* *To treat anxiety*

ORAL CONCENTRATE, TABLETS
Adults. *Initial:* 2 to 3 mg twice daily or three times daily, increased as needed. *Maximum:* 10 mg daily.
±**DOSAGE ADJUSTMENT** For elderly or debilitated patients, initial dosage may be reduced to 1 to 2 mg daily in divided doses.

* *To treat insomnia caused by anxiety*

ORAL CONCENTRATE, TABLETS
Adults. 2 to 4 mg as a single daily dose, as needed.
±**DOSAGE ADJUSTMENT** Dosage possibly reduced for elderly or debilitated patients.

* *To provide preoperative sedation*

I.V. INJECTION
Adults. 0.044 mg/kg or 2 mg, whichever is less, 2 hr before procedure. Higher dosage may be required for some patients but not to exceed maximum dose. *Maximum:* 0.05 mg/kg or total of 4 mg.

I.M. INJECTION
Adults. 0.05 mg/kg up to maximum dosage 2 hr before procedure. *Maximum:* 4 mg.

* *To treat status epilepticus*

I.V. INJECTION, I.M. INJECTION
Adults. *Initial:* 4 mg I.V. at a rate of 2 mg/min. Repeated in 10 to 15 min if seizures don't subside. I.M. route used only if I.V. route is not accessible. *Maximum:* 8 mg/24 hr.
±**DOSAGE ADJUSTMENT** For patients receiving drug I.M. or I.V. and also taking probenecid or valproate, dosage reduced by 50%. Dosage may have to be increased in female patients who are concomitantly taking oral contraceptives.

Drug Administration
- Drug not FDA approved for use in children.
- Have emergency resuscitation equipment readily available when administering drug parenterally.

P.O.
- When administering oral concentrate, use calibrated dropper supplied with drug to measure dosage.
- Mix oral concentrate with a liquid (water, carbonated beverages, juices) or semisolid food (applesauce or pudding). Gently stir for a few seconds and administer immediately. Do not store mixture for future use.
- For anxiety, administer in divided doses with the largest dose given before bedtime.
- For insomnia caused by anxiety, administer at bedtime.

I.V.
- Preferred route for treatment of status epilepticus.
- Dilute lorazepam with equal amount of 0.9% Sodium Chloride Injection, 5% Dextrose Injection, or Sterile Water for Injection.
- Gently invert container repeatedly to mix. Do not shake vigorously, as this will result in air entrapment.
- Administer as an I.V. injection slowly, at no more than 2 mg/min.
- For preoperative sedation, administer 15 to 20 minutes before procedure.
- Monitor patient's respirations every 5 to 15 minutes and keep emergency resuscitation equipment readily available.
- Store unopened multidose vials in refrigerator and protect from light.
- Discard multidose vial after 28 days of initial use.
- *Incompatibilities:* None listed by manufacturer

I.M.
- For status epilepticus, I.M. route used only if I.V. route is not available.
- Inject undiluted deep into large muscle mass, such as gluteus maximus.
- For preoperative sedation, administer 2 hours before procedure.
- Store unopened multidose vials in refrigerator and protect from light.
- Discard multidose vial after 28 days of initial use.

Route	Onset	Peak	Duration
P.O.	1 hr	2 hr	12–24 hr
I.V.	1–3 min	1–1.5 hr	6–8 hr
I.M.	15–30 min	< 3 hr	6–8 hr
Half-life: 10–20 hr			

Mechanism of Action

May potentiate the effects of gamma-aminobutyric acid (GABA) and other inhibitory neurotransmitters by binding to specific benzodiazepine receptors in cortical and limbic areas of CNS. GABA inhibits excitatory stimulation, which helps control emotional behavior. Limbic system contains a highly dense area of benzodiazepine receptors, which may explain drug's antianxiety effects. Also, lorazepam hyperpolarizes neuronal cells, thereby interfering with their ability to generate seizures.

Contraindications

For all forms of lorazepam: Acute angle-closure glaucoma; hypersensitivity to lorazepam, other benzodiazepines, or their components; *For parenteral form:* intra-arterial delivery, severe respiratory insufficiency (except in patients requiring anxiety relief and/or diminished recall of events while being mechanically ventilated), sleep apnea syndrome

Interactions

DRUGS

aminophylline, theophylline: Possibly reduced sedative effects of lorazepam
clozapine: Increased risk of ataxia, delirium, excessive salivation, hypotension, marked sedation, and respiratory arrest
CNS depressants: Additive CNS depression, potentially fatal respiratory depression
fentanyl: Possibly decreased therapeutic effects of fentanyl
probenecid, valproate: Possibly increased therapeutic and adverse effects of lorazepam
other benzodiazepines, sedating antihistamines, opioids, tricyclic antidepressants: Increased risk of profound respiratory depression, sedation, and somnolence

ACTIVITIES

alcohol use: Increased CNS depression and severe respiratory depression

Adverse Reactions

CNS: Amnesia, anxiety, ataxia, **coma**, confusion, delusions, depression, dizziness, drowsiness, euphoria, extrapyramidal symptoms, fatigue, headache, hypokinesia, irritability, malaise, nervousness, **seizures**, slurred speech, **suicidal ideation**, tremor, unsteadiness, vertigo

CV: Chest pain, palpitations, tachycardia
EENT: Blurred vision, diplopia, dry mouth, increased salivation, photophobia
ENDO: Syndrome of inappropriate ADH
GI: Abdominal pain, constipation, diarrhea, elevated liver enzymes, jaundice, nausea, thirst, vomiting
GU: Libido changes
HEME: **Agranulocytosis, pancytopenia, thrombocytopenia**
RESP: **Apnea, respiratory depression,** worsening of obstructive pulmonary disease or sleep apnea
SKIN: Diaphoresis
Other: **Anaphylaxis**, injection-site pain (I.M.) or phlebitis (I.V.), physical and psychological dependence, withdrawal symptoms

Childbearing Considerations

PREGNANCY

- Drug may cause fetal harm such as congenital abnormalities, neurotoxicity, and neonatal withdrawal symptoms.
- Drug should not be used during pregnancy except in life-threatening situations.
- If mother ingests drug for several weeks or more prior to delivery, monitor infant closely for withdrawal symptoms.

LACTATION

- Drug is present in breast milk.
- Drug should not be given to breastfeeding mothers unless benefit to mother outweighs the potential risk to breastfed infant.
- Infants being breastfed should be observed for inability to suckle, irritability, and sedation.

Nursing Considerations

- Before starting lorazepam therapy in a patient with depression, make sure he already takes an antidepressant, because of the increased risk of suicide in patients with untreated depression.
- Use extreme caution when giving lorazepam to elderly patients, especially those with compromised respiratory function, because drug can cause hypoventilation, respiratory depression, sedation, and unsteadiness.
- Use drug cautiously in patients with a history of alcohol or drug abuse or a personality disorder because of an increased risk of physical and psychological

dependence. Also use cautiously in patients with encephalopathy or severe hepatic insufficiency because drug may worsen hepatic encephalopathy.

- Be aware that benzodiazepine therapy such as lorazepam should only be used concomitantly with opioids in patients for whom other treatment options are inadequate because adverse effects could be profound and possibly result in death. If prescribed together, expect dosing and duration of the opioid to be limited. Monitor patient closely for signs and symptoms of profound decrease in consciousness, including coma, sedation, and respiratory depression. Notify prescriber immediately and provide emergency supportive care.

! **WARNING** Monitor patient's respiratory status closely because drug may cause life-threatening respiratory depression.

- Know that stopping drug abruptly increases risk of withdrawal symptoms, which may last from weeks to more than 12 months and could be life-threatening. Dosage should be tapered gradually, especially in epileptic patients.

PATIENT TEACHING

- Instruct patient to take lorazepam exactly as prescribed and not to stop without consulting prescriber because of the risk of withdrawal symptoms. Inform patient that withdrawal symptoms could last for weeks to more than 12 months and could be life-threatening.

! **WARNING** Warn patient that drug use may become addictive and, if misused, could result in overdose or even death.

- Advise patient to avoid hazardous activities until drug's CNS effects are known.
- Urge patient to avoid alcohol while taking lorazepam because it increases drug's CNS depressant effects and can cause severe respiratory depression which may lead to death.
- Instruct patient to report excessive drowsiness and nausea.
- Advise patient to alert prescriber if pregnancy occurs, as drug will have to be discontinued.

! **WARNING** Warn patient about potentially fatal additive effects of combining lorazepam with an opioid, such as potentially fatal respiratory depression and sedation. Instruct him to inform all prescribers of lorazepam use, especially when pain medication may be prescribed.

losartan potassium
Cozaar

Class and Category
Pharmacologic class: Angiotensin II receptor blocker (ARB)
Therapeutic class: Antihypertensive

Indications and Dosages
✳ *To manage hypertension*

ORAL SUSPENSION, TABLETS

Adults. *Initial:* 50 mg daily. *Maintenance:* 25 to 100 mg as a single dose or in 2 divided doses.

Children age 6 and over with an estimated glomerular filtration rate 30 ml/min or greater. *Initial:* 0.7 mg/kg (up to 50 mg total) once daily, with dosage adjusted, as needed. *Maximum:* 1.4 mg/kg or 100 mg daily.

✳ *To treat nephropathy in patients with type 2 diabetes and hypertension*

ORAL SUSPENSION, TABLETS

Adults. *Initial:* 50 mg daily, increased to 100 mg daily, as needed.

✳ *To reduce stroke risk in patients with hypertension and left ventricular hypertrophy*

ORAL SUSPENSION, TABLETS

Adults. *Initial:* 50 mg daily. Hydrochlorothiazide 12.5 mg daily added and/or dosage increased to 100 mg daily, as needed, followed by hydrochlorothiazide increased to 25 mg, daily, as needed.

±**DOSAGE ADJUSTMENT** Initial losartan dosage reduced to 25 mg daily for patients with impaired hepatic function or volume depletion.

Drug Administration
P.O.

- Shake oral suspension before each use.
- Use a calibrated device to measure dosage of oral suspension.

- Store oral suspension in refrigerator for up to 4 weeks.

Route	Onset	Peak	Duration
P.O.	6 hr	1–1.5 hr	24 hr

Half-life: 2–6 hr

Mechanism of Action

Blocks binding of angiotensin II to receptor sites in many tissues, including adrenal glands and vascular smooth muscle. Angiotensin II is a potent vasoconstrictor that also stimulates the adrenal cortex to secrete aldosterone. The inhibiting effects of angiotensin II reduce blood pressure. Decreases left ventricular mass index in patients with left ventricular hypertrophy who also have hypertension. By targeting the renin–angiotensin system, a renoprotective action occurs through the lowering of the albumin excretion rate in patients with type 2 diabetes.

Contraindications

Concurrent aliskiren therapy (in patients with diabetes), hypersensitivity to losartan or its components

Interactions

DRUGS

ACE inhibitors, aliskiren (in patients with diabetes or renal impairment with a glomerular filtration rate less than 60 ml/min), other angiotensin receptor blockers: Increased risk of hyperkalemia, hypotension, and renal dysfunction
lithium: Increased serum lithium levels and risk of lithium toxicity
NSAIDs: Possibly decreased renal function in elderly patients or those with renal dysfunction or volume depletion; possibly decreased effectiveness of losartan
potassium-sparing diuretics, potassium supplements: Increased risk of hyperkalemia

FOODS

high-potassium diet, potassium-containing salt substitutes: Increased risk of hyperkalemia

Adverse Reactions

CNS: Dizziness, fatigue, headache, insomnia, malaise
CV: Hypotension
EENT: Nasal congestion
GI: Diarrhea, indigestion, nausea, vomiting

HEME: Thrombocytopenia
MS: Back pain, leg pain, muscle spasms
RESP: Cough, upper respiratory tract infection
SKIN: Erythroderma
Other: Angioedema, hyperkalemia, hyponatremia

Childbearing Considerations

PREGNANCY

- Drug can cause fetal harm and should be discontinued as soon as pregnancy is known.
- Drug given during the second or third trimester reduces fetal renal function and increases fetal and neonatal morbidity and death. Resulting oligohydramnios can cause fetal lung hypoplasia and skeletal malformations.

LACTATION

- It is not known if drug is present in breast milk.
- A decision should be made to discontinue breastfeeding or the drug to avoid potential serious adverse reactions in the breastfed infant.

Nursing Considerations

- Know that patients of African descent with hypertension and left ventricular hypertrophy may not benefit from losartan to reduce stroke risk.

! **WARNING** Be aware that patients who have renal artery stenosis or severe heart failure may experience acute renal failure from losartan therapy because losartan inhibits the angiotensin–aldosterone system, on which renal function depends.

- Monitor blood pressure and renal function studies, as ordered, to evaluate drug effectiveness.
- Periodically monitor patient's serum potassium level, as ordered, to detect hyperkalemia.
- Monitor patient for muscle pain; rarely, rhabdomyolysis has developed in patients taking other angiotensin II receptor blockers.

PATIENT TEACHING

- Instruct patient to avoid potassium-containing salt substitutes because they may increase risk of hyperkalemia.

J
K
L

- Advise patient to avoid exercising in hot weather and drinking excessive amounts of alcohol; instruct her to notify prescriber if she has prolonged diarrhea, nausea, or vomiting.
- Warn patient to tell all prescribers of losartan therapy.
- Instruct women to notify prescriber immediately if pregnancy occurs or is suspected as drug may cause fetal harm and will have to be discontinued. Breastfeeding should also not be undertaken.

lovastatin
(mevinolin)
Altoprev

≣ Class and Category
Pharmacologic class: HMG-CoA reductase inhibitor (statin)
Therapeutic class: Antilipemic

≣ Indications and Dosages
* *As adjunct to diet to reduce LDL and total cholesterol levels in patients with primary hypercholesterolemia; to reduce risk of coronary revascularization procedures, myocardial infarction, or unstable angina in patients without symptomatic cardiovascular disease and who have average to moderately elevated total-C and LDL-C, and below average HDL-C as primary prevention of coronary heart disease; to slow progression of coronary atherosclerosis in patients with coronary heart disease*

TABLETS
Adults. *Initial:* 20 mg once daily for LDL-C reduction of 20% or more, 10 mg daily for LDL-C reduction of less than 20%; dosage adjusted after at least 4 wk. *Maintenance:* 10 to 80 mg daily as a single dose or in 2 divided doses. *Maximum:* 80 mg daily.

* *To reduce apolipoprotein B, LDL, and total cholesterol levels in adolescents with heterozygous familial hypercholesterolemia*

TABLETS
Adolescent boys and girls who are at least 1 yr postmenarche and ages 10 to 17. *Initial:* 20 mg daily for LDL-C reduction of 20% or more, 10 mg daily for LDL-C reduction of less than 20%; dosage adjusted after at least 4 wk. *Maintenance:* 10 to 40 mg daily. *Maximum:* 40 mg daily.

±**DOSAGE ADJUSTMENT** For patients taking immediate-release form: concomitant therapy with amiodarone limits maximum dosage to 40 mg daily; concomitant therapy with danazol, diltiazem, dronedarone, or verapamil, initial therapy begun at 10 mg daily and maximum dosage limited to 20 mg daily; and for patients with creatinine clearance less than 30 ml/min, maximum dosage limited to 20 mg daily or increased, if needed, very carefully.

* *As adjunct to diet to reduce elevated total-C, LDL-C, Apo B, and TG, and to increase HDL-C in patients with primary hypercholesterolemia (heterozygous familial and nonfamilial) and mixed dyslipidemia (Fredrickson types IIa and IIb); to reduce risk of coronary revascularization procedures, myocardial infarction, or unstable angina in patients without symptomatic cardiovascular disease and who have average to moderately elevated total-C and LDL-C, and below average HDL-C as primary prevention of coronary heart disease; to slow progression of coronary atherosclerosis in patients with coronary heart disease*

E.R. TABLETS (ALTOPREV)
Adults. *Initial:* 20 to 60 mg daily as a single dose. *Maximum:* 60 mg daily.

±**DOSAGE ADJUSTMENT** For patients taking extended-release form: concomitant therapy with amiodarone limited to 40 mg daily; concomitant therapy with danazol, diltiazem, dronedarone, or verapamil, dosage limited to 20 mg daily; and for patients who are 65 years and older or who have a creatinine clearance less than 30 ml/min, initial dosage limited to 20 mg daily and dosage increased, if needed, very carefully.

≣ Drug Administration
P.O.
- Administer immediate-release tablet with evening meal; extended-release tablet at bedtime.
- Extended-release tablets should be swallowed whole and not chewed, crushed, or split.
- Give drug 1 hour before or 4 hours after bile acid sequestrant, cholestyramine, or colestipol.

Route	Onset	Peak	Duration
P.O.	Unknown	2–4 hr	Unknown
P.O./E.R.	3 days	14 hr	Unknown

Half-life: 1.1–1.7 hr

Mechanism of Action

Interferes with the hepatic enzyme hydroxymethylglutaryl-coenzyme A reductase. By doing so, lovastatin reduces formation of mevalonic acid (a cholesterol precursor), thus interrupting the pathway by which cholesterol is synthesized. When cholesterol level declines in hepatic cells, LDLs are consumed, which also reduces amount of circulating total cholesterol and serum triglycerides. The decrease in LDLs may result in decreased level of apolipoprotein B, which is found in each LDL particle.

Contraindications

Acute hepatic disease; breastfeeding; concomitant therapy with cobicistat-containing products or strong CYP3A4 inhibitors (such as boceprevir, clarithromycin, erythromycin, HIV protease inhibitors, itraconazole, ketoconazole, nefazodone, posaconazole, telaprevir, telithromycin, voriconazole); hypersensitivity to lovastatin or its components; pregnancy; unexplained elevated liver enzymes

Interactions

DRUGS

amiodarone, boceprevir, cobicistat-containing products, clarithromycin, colchicine, cyclosporine, danazol, diltiazem, dronedarone, erythromycin, fibric acid derivatives, gemfibrozil and other fibrates, HIV protease inhibitors, itraconazole, ketoconazole, nefazodone, niacin (1 g daily or more), posaconazole, ranolazine, telaprevir, telithromycin, verapamil, voriconazole: Increased risk of severe myopathy or rhabdomyolysis
oral anticoagulants: Increased anticoagulant effect and risk of bleeding

FOODS

grapefruit juice (more than 1 qt daily): Increased risk of myopathy or rhabdomyolysis

ACTIVITIES

alcohol use: Increased lovastatin blood level

Adverse Reactions

CNS: Anxiety, asthenia, cognitive impairment, chills, confusion, cranial nerve dysfunction, depression, dizziness, fatigue, fever, headache, insomnia, malaise, memory loss, paresthesia, peripheral nerve palsy, peripheral neuropathy, psychic disturbances, tremor, vertigo
CV: Vasculitis
EENT: Blurred vision, cataracts, ophthalmoplegia, pharyngitis, rhinitis, sinusitis
ENDO: Elevated glycosylated hemoglobin levels, gynecomastia, hyperglycemia, thyroid function abnormalities
GI: Abdominal cramps and pain, anorexia, cholestatic jaundice, **cirrhosis**, constipation, diarrhea, elevated liver enzymes, flatulence, **fulminant hepatic necrosis, hepatic failure** (rare), **hepatitis**, hyperbilirubinemia, indigestion, nausea, hepatoma, **pancreatitis**, vomiting
GU: Erectile dysfunction, loss of libido
HEME: Elevated erythrocyte sedimentation rate (ESR), eosinophilia, **hemolytic anemia, leukopenia**, positive antinuclear antibodies (ANA), purpura, **thrombocytopenia**
MS: Arthralgias, arthritis, back pain, immune-mediated necrotizing myopathy, muscle pain, myalgia, myopathy, myositis, polymyalgia rheumatica, **rhabdomyolysis**
RESP: Cough, dyspnea, **interstitial lung disease**, upper respiratory tract infection
SKIN: Alopecia, changes to hair and nails, dermatomyositis, discolored or dry skin, **erythema multiforme**, flushing, photosensitivity, pruritus, rash, **Stevens–Johnson syndrome, toxic epidermal necrolysis**, urticaria
Other: **Anaphylaxis, angioedema,** elevated alkaline phosphatase, lupus erythematosus-like syndrome

Childbearing Considerations

PREGNANCY

- Drug may cause fetal harm according to animal studies.
- Drug is contraindicated in pregnancy because there is no apparent benefit to drug therapy in pregnancy and it may cause fetal harm.

J
K
L

LACTATION

- It is not known if drug is present in breast milk.
- Drug is contraindicated in breastfeeding.

REPRODUCTION

- Women of childbearing age should be advised to use effective contraception during drug treatment.

Nursing Considerations

- Give lovastatin cautiously in patients who have a history of liver disease and patients who consume large amounts of alcohol.
- Expect patient to be prescribed a standard low-cholesterol diet during therapy.
- Be aware that drug affects mainly total cholesterol and LDL levels; it has only slight effects on HDL and triglyceride levels.
- Monitor liver enzymes before therapy begins, as ordered. If indicated, expect to measure them during therapy, as ordered. If ALT or AST level reaches or exceeds three times upper limit of normal and persists at that level, expect to discontinue lovastatin.
- Monitor patient closely for muscle pain, tenderness, or weakness suggestive of myopathy. Also monitor creatinine kinase, as ordered. If patient becomes symptomatic or creatine kinase becomes highly elevated, withhold drug, notify prescriber and expect drug to be discontinued. Be especially alert for myopathy that could become its more severe form, rhabdomyolysis, in patients with other disorders such as diabetes complicated with renal dysfunction.
- Expect to withhold drug temporarily in patients who develop an acute or serious condition predisposing patient to the development of renal failure secondary to rhabdomyolysis. Conditions to be watchful for include hypotension; major surgery or trauma; sepsis; or severe electrolyte, endocrine, or metabolic disorders; or uncontrolled epilepsy. Be mindful that the drug interactions may not be the same for the extended-release formulation of lovastatin as for those encountered with the immediate-release formulation.

PATIENT TEACHING

- Tell patient who takes immediate-release drug once daily to do so with evening meal to enhance absorption. For patient who takes extended-release tablets, advise to take once-daily dose at bedtime and to swallow tablets whole and not to chew, crush, or split tablets.
- Advise patient to report muscle aches, pains, tenderness, or weakness, being especially watchful of these symptoms when dosage is increased. If present, tell him to stop taking lovastatin immediately and notify prescriber.
- Instruct patient to report severe GI distress or vision changes, as well as the development of dark urine, fatigue, loss of appetite, right upper abdominal pain or yellowing of skin.
- Advise patient to avoid performing any hazardous activity, such as driving, if cognitive impairment develops and to notify prescriber.
- Tell patient to alert prescriber of any over-the-counter or prescription drugs being taken, because serious drug interactions could occur.
- Urge patient to avoid consuming alcohol or more than 1 quart of grapefruit juice daily while taking drug.
- Direct patient to follow a low-cholesterol diet during therapy. Recommend exercise and weight loss programs as appropriate.
- Emphasize the importance of periodic eye examinations during therapy.
- Teach female patients the need to report suspected pregnancy immediately.
- Tell mothers that breastfeeding is contraindicated while taking lovastatin.

lubiprostone
Amitiza

Class and Category
Pharmacologic class: Chloride channel activator
Therapeutic class: GI motility

Indications and Dosages
❋ *To treat chronic idiopathic constipation; to treat opioid-induced constipation in patients with chronic noncancer pain*

CAPSULES
Adults. 24 mcg twice daily.
❋ *To treat irritable bowel syndrome with constipation*

CAPSULES

Women at least 18 years of age. 8 mcg twice daily.

± **DOSAGE ADJUSTMENT** For patients with chronic idiopathic constipation or opioid-induced constipation who have moderate liver impairment, dosage reduced to 16 mcg twice daily. For patients being treated for any indication who have severe liver impairment, dosage reduced to 8 mcg once daily.

Drug Administration

P.O.

- Administer drug with food and water to reduce nausea.
- Capsules should be swallowed whole and not chewed, crushed, or opened.

Route	Onset	Peak	Duration
P.O.	Unknown	1 hr	Unknown

Half-life: 0.9–1.4 hr

Mechanism of Action

Enhances a chloride-rich intestinal fluid secretion specifically by activating CIC-2, which is a normal constituent of the apical membrane of the human intestine. By increasing intestinal fluid secretion, motility in the intestine is increased, which facilitates the passage of stool to alleviate the symptoms associated with chronic idiopathic constipation. In addition, activation of the apical CIC-2 channels in intestinal epithelial cells bypasses the antisecretory action of opiates through suppression of secretomotor neuron excitability.

Contraindications

Hypersensitivity to lubiprostone or its components, mechanical gastrointestinal obstruction

Interactions

DRUGS

diphenylheptane opioids such as methadone: Decreased effectiveness of lubiprostone

Adverse Reactions

CNS: Anxiety, asthenia, depression, dizziness, fatigue, headache, lethargy, malaise, syncope, tremor
CV: Chest discomfort or pain, **hypotension**, palpitations, peripheral edema, tachycardia

EENT: Distortion of sense of smell, dry mouth, pharyngolaryngeal pain, **throat tightness**
GI: Abdominal distention or pain, anorexia, constipation, defecation urgency, diarrhea, dyspepsia, elevated liver enzymes, eructation, fecal incontinence, flatulence, frequent bowel movements, gastritis, gastroesophageal reflux disease, intestinal functional disorder, **ischemic colitis**, nausea, **rectal hemorrhage**, vomiting
GU: Pollakiuria, UTI
MS: Fibromyalgia, joint swelling, muscle cramps or spasms, myalgia
RESP: Cough, dyspnea
SKIN: Cold sweat, erythema, excessive diaphoresis, rash
Other: Flu-like symptoms, generalized pain, **hypokalemia**, swelling, weight gain

Childbearing Considerations

PREGNANCY

- It is not known if drug causes fetal harm.
- Use with caution only if benefit to mother outweighs potential risk to fetus.

LACTATION

- It is not known if drug is present in breast milk.
- Patient should check with prescriber before breastfeeding.
- If breastfeeding occurs, infant should be monitored for diarrhea.

Nursing Considerations

- Be aware that lubiprostone should not be given to patients with severe diarrhea. If severe diarrhea occurs while patient is taking drug, notify prescriber and expect drug to be discontinued.
- Monitor patient's blood pressure for hypotension. Syncope and hypotension have occurred with lubiprostone therapy and sometimes within 1 hour after drug administration, including the first dose. Risk factors include the presence of diarrhea or vomiting or taking drugs known to lower blood pressure.
- Assess patient for dyspnea, which generally has occurred as an acute onset within 30 to 60 minutes after being given the first dose of lubiprostone. Although dyspnea usually resolves within 3 hours after taking drug, it may reoccur with subsequent doses. If it becomes severe or reoccurs, notify prescriber.

J
K
L

PATIENT TEACHING

- Instruct patient to swallow capsules whole and not to break apart or chew the capsules.
- Tell patient to take lubiprostone with food and water.
- Inform patient of the possibility of diarrhea occurring with lubiprostone therapy. If diarrhea becomes severe, tell patient to stop taking drug and notify prescriber.
- Tell patient that drug may lower his blood pressure to the point of fainting. Caution patient to avoid performing hazardous activities until the effects of drug are known.
- Instruct patient to inform all prescribers of lubiprostone therapy, because drugs known to lower blood pressure increase patient's risk of low blood pressure and possibly fainting.
- Alert patient that difficulty breathing may occur after the first dose of lubiprostone but generally resolves within 3 hours. Tell patient to notify prescriber if dyspnea occurs.
- Tell mothers who are breastfeeding while taking lubiprostone to monitor the infant for diarrhea.

lumateperone tosylate

Caplyta

≣ Class and Category

Pharmacologic class: Neuroleptic
Therapeutic class: Atypical antipsychotic

≣ Indications and Dosages

✳ *To treat schizophrenia; to treat depressive episodes associated with bipolar I or II disorder as monotherapy or as adjunctive therapy with lithium or valproate*

CAPSULES

Adults. 42 mg once daily.

≣ Drug Administration

P.O.

- Administer drug with food.

Route	Onset	Peak	Duration
P.O.	Unknown	1–2 hr	Unknown

Half-life: 13–18 hr

≣ Mechanism of Action

Although exact mechanism is unknown, drug may be mediated through a combination of antagonist activity of central serotonin 5-HT$_{2A}$ receptors and postsynaptic antagonist activity at central dopamine D$_2$ receptors.

≣ Contraindications

Hypersensitivity to lumateperone or its components

≣ Interactions

DRUGS

CYP3A4 inducers: Decreased exposure and effectiveness of lumateperone
Moderate to strong CYP3A4 inhibitors, UGT inhibitors: Increased exposure and risk of adverse reactions to lumateperone

≣ Adverse Reactions

CNS: Body temperature dysregulation, cognitive and motor impairment, dizziness, dystonia, extrapyramidal symptoms, fatigue, **neuroleptic malignant syndrome, seizures,** somnolence, **suicidal ideation,** syncope, tardive dyskinesia
CV: Dyslipidemia, orthostatic hypotension
EENT: Dry mouth
ENDO: Hyperglycemia
GI: Anorexia, dysphagia, nausea, vomiting
HEME: Agranulocytosis, leukopenia, neutropenia
MS: Elevated creatine phosphokinase levels

≣ Childbearing Considerations

PREGNANCY

- Pregnancy exposure registry: 1-866-961-2388 or http://womensmentalhealth.org/clinical-and-research-programs/pregnancyregistry.
- Drug may cause fetal harm if fetus is exposed to drug during the third trimester, as extrapyramidal and/or withdrawal symptoms may occur after delivery.
- Use with caution only if benefit to mother outweighs potential risk to fetus.

LACTATION

- It is not known if drug is present in breast milk.
- Breastfeeding is not recommended during drug therapy.

REPRODUCTION

- Drug may impair female and male fertility, based on animal studies.

☰ Nursing Considerations

! WARNING Know that lumateperone shouldn't be used in elderly patients with dementia-related psychosis because drug increases risk of death in these patients. Also, know that lumateperone should not be given to patients with moderate or severe hepatic impairment or to patients taking CYP3A4 inducers or moderate to strong CYP3A4 inhibitors.

- Use lumateperone cautiously in patients at risk for aspiration because drug may cause dysphagia.

! WARNING Monitor patient for signs and symptoms of neuroleptic malignant syndrome (autonomic instability, delirium, hyperpyrexia, muscle rigidity) and report any such effects to prescriber immediately. Expect lumateperone to be discontinued and appropriate intensive treatment instituted, as prescribed.

- Notify prescriber if patient develops tardive dyskinesia, as the risk it will become irreversible increases with duration of treatment and cumulative dose. Be aware that tardive dyskinesia can develop after only a relatively brief treatment period, even at low doses, and it may occur after drug has been discontinued.
- Monitor patient's blood glucose and lipid levels as well as weight because drug may cause metabolic changes such as hyperglycemia, dyslipidemia, and weight gain.

! WARNING Monitor patient with clinically significant neutropenia for fever or other signs of infection and report promptly. Expect to monitor patient's complete blood count during drug therapy. Know that lumateperone should be discontinued if patient's absolute neutrophil count falls to less than 1,000/mm³.

- Assess patient for orthostatic hypotension, especially elderly patients; patients with concomitant treatment with antihypertensive drugs, dehydration, or hypovolemia; patients with known cardiovascular disease; and patients with cerebrovascular disease.

- Institute fall precautions, because lumateperone may cause motor and sensory instability, postural hypotension, and somnolence, which may lead to falls.
- Institute seizure precautions, as lumateperone may cause seizures.

PATIENT TEACHING

- Instruct patient to take drug with food.
- Encourage patient to inform all prescribers of lumateperone therapy and any other drugs taken, including over-the-counter and herbal products.
- Instruct patient to rise from a lying or sitting position slowly, especially early in drug therapy and when drug is being reinitiated, to avoid a drop in blood pressure. Inform patient that hot tubs, prolonged hot showers, and saunas may worsen this effect.
- Review signs and symptoms of infection with patient and stress importance of reporting a suspected infection to prescriber.
- Encourage patient to monitor weight and report excessive weight gain. Also inform patient that drug may increase blood glucose and lipid levels. Review signs and symptoms of hyperglycemia with patient and stress importance of complying with laboratory testing for these metabolic alterations.
- Review signs and symptoms of tardive dyskinesia and tell patient to report these abnormal movements, if present.
- Tell family or caregiver to monitor patient for suicidal thought and behaviors, especially during the initial few months of drug therapy and with dosage changes. If present, prescriber should be alerted.

! WARNING Review signs and symptoms of neuroleptic malignant syndrome with patient and family. Urge patient to seek emergency care if present.

- Caution patient to avoid hazardous activities until drug's CNS effects are known.
- Advise women of childbearing age to notify prescriber if pregnancy is suspected or known. Also alert pregnant women that breastfeeding is not recommended during lumateperone therapy.
- Inform patient that drug may impair fertility.

J
K
L

lurasidone hydrochloride

Latuda

Class and Category

Pharmacologic class: Atypical antipsychotic
Therapeutic class: Antipsychotic

Indications and Dosages

✴ *To treat schizophrenia*

TABLETS

Adults. *Initial:* 40 mg once daily, increased as needed. *Maximum:* 160 mg once daily.
Adolescents ages 13 to 17. *Initial:* 40 mg once daily, increased as needed. *Maximum:* 80 mg daily.

✴ *To treat depressive episodes associated with bipolar I disorder as monotherapy or adjunctive therapy with either lithium or valproate*

TABLETS

Adults. *Initial:* 20 mg once daily, increased as needed. *Maximum:* 120 mg once daily.

✴ *To treat depressive episodes associated with bipolar I disorder as monotherapy*

TABLETS

Children age 10 to 17 years. *Initial:* 20 mg once daily, increased weekly, as needed. *Usual:* 20 to 40 mg once daily. *Maximum:* 80 mg daily.

±**DOSAGE ADJUSTMENT** For patients already taking a moderate CYP3A4 drug or who have moderate hepatic impairment or moderate (creatinine clearance 30 to less than 50 ml/min) or severe (creatinine clearance less than 30 ml/min) renal impairment, initial dosage not to exceed 20 mg daily and maximum dose should not exceed 80 mg once daily. For patient with severe hepatic impairment, initial dosage should not exceed 20 mg daily and maximum dose should not exceed 40 mg once daily. For patient newly prescribed a moderate CYP3A4 inhibitor, dosage reduced to half of the original dose of lurasidone prescribed. For patient receiving a moderate CYP3A4 inducer, dosage may have to be increased after CYP3A4 inducer therapy has been in place for at least 7 days.

Drug Administration

P.O.

▪ Administer drug with a meal consisting of at least 350 calories.

Route	Onset	Peak	Duration
P.O.	Unknown	1–3 hr	Unknown

Half-life: 18 hr

Mechanism of Action

Possibly mediated through a combination of central dopamine type 2 and serotonin type 2 receptor antagonism to suppress psychotic symptoms and elevate mood.

Contraindications

Concurrent therapy with strong CYP3A4 inducers such as avasimibe, carbamazepine, phenytoin, rifampin, or St. John's wort; concurrent therapy with strong CYP3A4 inhibitors such as clarithromycin, ketoconazole, mibefradil, ritonavir, or voriconazole; hypersensitivity to lurasidone or its components

Interactions

DRUGS

CYP3A4 inducers: Possibly decreased effect of lurasidone
CYP3A4 inhibitors: Possibly increased effect of lurasidone

Adverse Reactions

CNS: Agitation, akathisia, anxiety, **CVA**, dizziness, dystonia, extrapyramidal symptoms, fatigue, hypomania or mania activation, impaired cognitive and motor function, insomnia, **neuroleptic malignant syndrome**, parkinsonism, psychomotor hyperactivity, restlessness, **seizures**, somnolence, **suicidal ideation**, syncope, tardive dyskinesia, transient ischemic attacks
CV: Hypertension, orthostatic hypotension, tachycardia
EENT: Blurred vision, dry mouth, increased salivation, oropharyngeal pain, rhinitis, **throat swelling, tongue swelling**
ENDO: Hyperglycemia, hyperprolactinemia
GI: Abdominal pain, anorexia, diarrhea, dyspepsia, dysphagia, nausea, vomiting
GU: Elevated creatinine level
HEME: **Agranulocytosis, leukopenia, neutropenia**
MS: Back pain, **rhabdomyolysis**
RESP: Dyspnea
SKIN: Pruritus, rash, urticaria
Other: Elevated CPK level, **hyponatremia**, weight gain

☰ Childbearing Considerations

PREGNANCY

- Pregnancy exposure registry: 1-866-961-2388 or http:// womensmentalhealth.org/ clinical-and-research-programs/ pregnancyregistry/.
- Drug may cause fetal harm. Neonates exposed to the drug in the third trimester of pregnancy are at risk for extrapyramidal and/or withdrawal symptoms following delivery.
- Use with caution only if benefit to mother outweighs potential risk to fetus.

LACTATION

- It is not known if drug is present in breast milk.
- Patient should check with prescriber before breastfeeding.

☰ Nursing Considerations

! WARNING Be aware that lurasidone should not be used to treat dementia-related psychosis in the elderly because of an increased risk of death, nor in patients at risk for aspiration pneumonia because drug may cause esophageal dysmotility, resulting in dysphagia.

- Use lurasidone cautiously in patients with cardiovascular disease, cerebrovascular disease, or conditions that would predispose them to hypotension. Also, use cautiously in those with a history of seizures or with conditions that lower the seizure threshold, such as Alzheimer's disease.
- Also, use cautiously in elderly patients because of increased risk of serious adverse cerebrovascular effects, such as stroke and transient ischemic attack.

! WARNING Monitor patient closely for neuroleptic malignant syndrome, seizures, and tardive dyskinesia throughout therapy, and take safety precautions, as needed. Notify prescriber immediately of any occurrence.

- Monitor patient's blood glucose level routinely; risk of hyperglycemia may increase.

- Watch patients closely for suicidal tendencies, especially in children and young adults, and particularly when therapy starts and dosage changes, because depression may worsen temporarily during these times.
- Monitor patient's CBC, as ordered, because serious adverse hematologic reactions may occur, such as agranulocytosis, leukopenia, and neutropenia. Assess more often during first few months of therapy if patient has a history of drug-induced leukopenia or neutropenia or a significantly low WBC count. If abnormalities occur during therapy, watch for fever or other signs of infection, notify prescriber, and, if severe, expect drug to be discontinued.
- Know that extrapyramidal symptoms and withdrawal symptoms may occur in newborns following delivery to mothers taking lurasidone during the third trimester.
- Be aware that the occurrence of tardive dyskinesia and the chances of the dyskinesia being irreversible increase the longer therapy continues, as well as with the total cumulative dose. Although less common, tardive dyskinesia may also occur after relatively short periods of therapy at low doses and may even occur after therapy has been discontinued. Monitor patient closely and notify prescriber at once if present.
- Assess patient for fall risk and institute fall precautions.

PATIENT TEACHING

- Instruct patient or caregiver that lurasidone must be taken with a meal consisting of at least 350 calories.
- Urge patient to avoid alcohol during lurasidone therapy.
- Instruct patient to avoid hazardous activities until drug's effects are known. Warn patient that falls can also occur due to the effects of drug on the nervous system. Review fall precautions with patient.
- Caution patient to avoid dehydration, exercising strenuously, exposure to extreme heat or taking medication with anticholinergic activity because lurasidone therapy may interfere with being able to reduce the body's core body temperature.

M

magnesium chloride
Chloromag, Mag-L-100, Slow-Mag

magnesium citrate
(citrate of magnesia)
Citroma, Citro-Mag (CAN)

magnesium gluconate
Almora, Maglucate (CAN), Magonate, Magtrate

magnesium hydroxide
(milk of magnesia)
Phillips' Chewable Tablets, Phillips' Magnesia Tablets (CAN), Phillips' Milk of Magnesia, Phillips' Milk of Magnesia Concentrate

magnesium lactate
Mag-Tab SR Caplets

magnesium oxide
Mag-200, Mag-Ox 400, Maox, Uro-Mag

magnesium sulfate

⬚ Class and Category
Pharmacologic class: Mineral
Therapeutic class: Electrolyte replacement

⬚ Indications and Dosages
✴ *To correct magnesium deficiency caused by alcoholism, magnesium-depleting drugs, malnutrition, or restricted diet; to prevent magnesium deficiency based on recommended daily allowances according to the National Institutes of Health*

CAPSULES, CHEWABLE TABLETS, CRYSTALS, ENTERIC-COATED TABLETS, E.R. TABLETS, LIQUID, LIQUID CONCENTRATE, ORAL SOLUTION, TABLETS (MAGNESIUM CHLORIDE, CITRATE, GLUCONATE, HYDROXIDE, LACTATE [EXCEPT IN CHILDREN], OXIDE, SULFATE)

Dosage individualized based on severity of deficiency and normal recommended daily allowances listed below.
Adult men age 31 years and older. 420 mg daily.
Adult women age 31 years and older. 320 mg daily (360 mg daily during pregnancy, 320 mg daily during breastfeeding).
Adult men age 19 to 30 years. 400 mg daily.
Adult women age 19 to 30 years. 310 mg daily (350 mg daily during pregnancy, 310 mg daily during breastfeeding).
Adolescent boys age 14 to 18 years. 410 mg daily.
Adolescent girls age 14 to 18 years. 360 mg daily (400 mg daily during pregnancy, 360 mg daily during breastfeeding).
Boys age 9 to 13 years. 240 mg daily.
Girls age 9 to 13 years. 240 mg daily.
Children age 4 to 8 years. 130 mg daily.
Children age 1 to 3 years. 80 mg daily.
Infants age 7 to 12 months. 75 mg daily.
Infants age birth to 6 months. 30 mg daily.
✴ *To provide magnesium supplementation in total parenteral nutrition (TPN)*

I.V. INFUSION (MAGNESIUM SULFATE)
Adults. *Usual:* 8 to 24 mEq daily added to the TPN solution.
✴ *To treat mild magnesium deficiency*

I.M. INJECTION (MAGNESIUM SULFATE)
Adults and adolescents. 1 g every 6 hr for 4 doses.
✴ *To treat severe hypomagnesemia*

I.V. INFUSION (MAGNESIUM CHLORIDE)
Adults. 4 g diluted in 250 ml D_5W and infused at no more than 3 ml/min. Then, dosage adjusted according to patient's magnesium level. *Maximum:* 40 g daily.

I.V. INFUSION (MAGNESIUM SULFATE)
Adults and adolescents. 5 g diluted in 1 liter I.V. solution and infused over 3 hr.
✴ *To prevent and control seizures in preeclampsia or eclampsia*

M

I.M. INJECTION, I.V. INFUSION OR INJECTION (MAGNESIUM SULFATE)

Adults. *Loading:* 4 to 5 g of a 10% to 20% solution and given I.V. very slowly following manufacturer's guidelines for type of solution used. Simultaneously up to 10 g I.M. Alternatively, 4 g I.V. injected over 3 to 4 minutes and subsequent I.M. injection of 4 to 5 g every 4 hr, as needed. *Maintenance required for some patients:* 1 to 2 g/hr by continuous infusion. *Maximum:* 40 g/day and for no longer than 5 to 7 days.

✳ *To control seizures due to acute nephritis in children*

I.M. INJECTION (MAGNESIUM SULFATE)

Children. 20 to 40 mg/kg of a 20% solution, repeated as needed.

✳ *To treat torsades de pointes*

I.V. INFUSION

Adults. *For patient with pulse:* 1 to 2 g diluted in 50 to 100 ml D_5W and infused over 5 to 60 min, followed by 0.5 to 1 g/hr. *For patient in cardiac arrest:* 1 to 2 g diluted in 10 ml D_5W and infused over 5 to 20 min.

✳ *To relieve indigestion with hyperacidity*

CHEWABLE TABLETS, LIQUID, LIQUID CONCENTRATE, ORAL SOLUTION TABLETS (MAGNESIUM HYDROXIDE)

Adults and adolescents. 400 to 1,200 mg (5 to 15 ml liquid or 2.5 to 7.5 ml liquid concentrate) up to four times daily with water, or 622 to 1,244 mg (tablets or chewable tablets) up to four times daily.

CAPSULES, TABLETS (MAGNESIUM OXIDE)

Adults and adolescents. 140 mg (capsules) three times daily or four times daily with water or milk, or 400 to 800 mg (tablets) daily.

✳ *To relieve constipation, to evacuate colon for rectal or bowel examination*

LIQUID, LIQUID CONCENTRATE (MAGNESIUM HYDROXIDE)

Adults and children age 12 and over. 2.4 to 4.8 g (30 to 60 ml) daily as single dose at bedtime or divided doses.
Children ages 6 to 11. 1.2 to 2.4 g (15 to 30 ml)/day as a single dose or in divided doses.
Children ages 2 to 5. 0.4 to 1.2 g (5 to 15 ml) daily as single dose or divided doses.

ORAL SOLUTION (MAGNESIUM CITRATE)

Adults and children age 12 and over. Up to 10 ounces with 8 ounces of water as a single dose or in divided doses.
Children ages 6 to 11. Up to 5 ounces with 8 ounces of water.
Children ages 2 to 5. Highly individualized.

CRYSTALS (MAGNESIUM SULFATE)

Adults and children age 12 and over. 10 to 30 g daily with 8 ounces of water as single dose or divided doses. *Maximum: Two* times daily.
Children age 6 to 12. 5 to 10 g with 8 ounces of water as a single dose or divided doses.

±**DOSAGE ADJUSTMENT** Dosage limited to 20 g of magnesium sulfate/48 hr for patients with severe renal impairment.

☰ Drug Administration

P.O.

- Oral forms are not all interchangeable.
- Chewable tablets should be chewed thoroughly before swallowing, followed by a full glass of water.
- Avoid giving other oral drugs within 2 hours of magnesium-containing antacid.
- Before giving drug as laxative, shake oral solution, liquid, or liquid concentrate well and give with a large amount of water.
- Refrigerate magnesium citrate solution.

I.V.

- Magnesium chloride for injection contains the preservative benzyl alcohol, which may cause fatal toxic syndrome in neonates and premature infants.
- Prepare solution for administration according to manufacturer guidelines and administer according to condition being treated (see Indication and Dosage section).
- For I.V. injection, administer slowly, as a rapid injection may cause hypotension.
- For I.V. infusion, dilute to a concentration of 20% or less prior to administration. Commonly used diluents include 0.9% Sodium Chloride Injection and 5% Dextrose Injection. Infuse at a rate given under indication. Use an infusion pump for administration.
- *Incompatibilities:* Alkali carbonates and bicarbonates, alkali hydroxides, arsenates, calcium, clindamycin phosphate, dobutamine, fat emulsions, heavy metals, hydrocortisone sodium

succinate, phosphates, polymyxin B, procaine hydrochloride, salicylates, sodium bicarbonate, strontium, and tartrates

I.M.

- Administer as a deep I.M. injection undiluted (50%) solution in adults, but dilute to a 20% or less concentration prior to such injection in children.

Route	Onset	Peak	Duration
P.O.	0.5–6 hr	Unknown	Unknown
I.V.	Immediate	Unknown	30 min
I.M.	1 hr	Unknown	3–4 hr

Half-life: Unknown

Mechanism of Action

Assists all enzymes involved in phosphate transfer reactions that use adenosine triphosphate (ATP). Magnesium is required for normal function of the ATP-dependent sodium–potassium pump in muscle membranes. It may effectively treat digitalis glycoside–induced arrhythmias because correction of hypomagnesemia improves the sodium–potassium pump's ability to distribute potassium into intracellular spaces and because magnesium decreases calcium uptake and potassium outflow through myocardial cell membranes.

As a laxative, magnesium exerts a hyperosmotic effect in the small intestine. It causes water retention that distends the bowel and causes the duodenum to secrete cholecystokinin. This substance stimulates fluid secretion and intestinal motility.

As an antacid, magnesium reacts with water, converting magnesium oxide to magnesium hydroxide. Magnesium hydroxide rapidly reacts with gastric acid to form water and magnesium chloride, which increases gastric pH.

As an anticonvulsant, magnesium depresses the CNS and blocks peripheral neuromuscular impulse transmission by decreasing available acetylcholine.

Contraindications

Hypersensitivity to magnesium salts or any component of magnesium-containing preparations

For magnesium chloride: Coma, marked heart disease, renal impairment

For magnesium sulfate: Heart block, MI, preeclampsia 2 hours or less before delivery (I.V. form)

For use as laxative: Acute abdominal problem (as indicated by abdominal pain, nausea, or vomiting), diverticulitis, fecal impaction, intestinal obstruction or perforation, colostomy or ileostomy, severe renal impairment, ulcerative colitis

Interactions

DRUGS

calcium channel blockers: Possibly enhanced adverse/toxic effects of magnesium salts

calcium salts (I.V.): Possibly neutralization of magnesium sulfate's effects

CNS depressants: Increased CNS depression

digoxin: Possibly heart block and conduction changes

misoprostol: Increased misoprostol-induced diarrhea

neuromuscular blockers: Possibly increased neuromuscular blockade

oral drugs: Possibly decreased absorption of oral drugs when magnesium salts given orally

sodium polystyrene sulfonate resin: Possibly metabolic alkalosis

FOODS

high glucose intake: Increased urinary excretion of magnesium

ACTIVITIES

alcohol use: Increased urinary excretion of magnesium

Adverse Reactions

CNS: Confusion, decreased reflexes, dizziness, syncope

CV: Arrhythmias, hypotension

GI: Flatulence, vomiting

MS: Muscle cramps

RESP: Dyspnea, **respiratory depression or paralysis**

SKIN: Diaphoresis

Other: Hypermagnesemia, hypersensitivity reactions, injection-site pain or irritation (I.M. form), laxative dependence, **magnesium toxicity**

Childbearing Considerations

PREGNANCY

- It is not known if drug causes fetal harm for some forms of magnesium.

M

- Magnesium sulfate may cause fetal harm if administered continuously beyond 5 to 7 days to pregnant women, causing hypocalcemia and bone abnormalities in the developing fetus.
- Use with caution only if benefit to mother outweighs potential risk to fetus.

LABOR & DELIVERY

- Some authorities recommend magnesium chloride and magnesium sulfate not be administered within 2 hours prior to delivery because of the risk of hypermagnesemia-stimulated respiratory depression in the neonate.
- Magnesium sulfate is not approved to treat preterm labor.
- If magnesium sulfate is administered by continuous I.V. infusion, especially for more than 24 hours preceding delivery, to control seizures in a toxemic woman, monitor newborn for signs of magnesium toxicity, including neuromuscular or respiratory depression.

LACTATION

- Drug is present in breast milk.
- Patient should check with prescriber before breastfeeding.

Nursing Considerations

- Be aware that drug isn't metabolized. Drug remaining in the GI tract produces watery stool within 30 minutes to 3 hours.

! **WARNING** Observe for and report early evidence of hypermagnesemia: bradycardia, depressed deep tendon reflexes, diplopia, dyspnea, flushing, hypotension, nausea, slurred speech, vomiting, and weakness.

! **WARNING** Be aware that magnesium may precipitate myasthenic crisis by decreasing patient's sensitivity to acetylcholine.

- Frequently assess cardiac status of patient taking drugs that lower heart rate, such as beta-blockers because magnesium may aggravate symptoms of heart block.
- Provide adequate diet, exercise, and fluids for patient being treated for constipation.
- Monitor serum electrolyte levels in patients with renal insufficiency because they're at risk for magnesium toxicity.
- Be aware that magnesium salts aren't intended for long-term use. For example,

magnesium sulfate may cause fetal abnormalities if administered for more than 5 to 7 days to pregnant women. When magnesium sulfate is administered by continuous I.V. infusion (especially for more than 24 hours preceding delivery) to control convulsions in a toxemic woman, monitor newborn for signs of magnesium toxicity, such as neuromuscular or respiratory depression.

PATIENT TEACHING

- Advise patient to chew magnesium chewable tablets thoroughly before swallowing, and then drink a full glass of water. Mention that tablets have a chalky taste.
- Instruct patient to take magnesium-containing antacid between meals and at bedtime. Urge him not to take other drugs within 2 hours of the antacid.
- Tell patient to notify prescriber and avoid using magnesium-containing laxative if he has abdominal pain, nausea, or vomiting.
- Instruct patient to refrigerate magnesium citrate solution.
- Caution patient about risk of dependence with long-term laxative use.
- Teach patient to prevent constipation by increasing dietary fiber and fluid intake and exercising regularly.
- Inform patient that magnesium supplements used to replace electrolytes can cause diarrhea.

mannitol
Aridol, Bronchitol, Osmitrol

Class and Category
Pharmacologic class: Osmotic diuretic
Therapeutic class: Diuretic

Indications and Dosages

* *To reduce intracranial pressure and cerebral edema; to reduce intraocular pressure*

I.V. INFUSION (OSMITROL)

Adults and children. *Intracranial pressure:* 0.25 g/kg repeated every 6 to 8 hrs. *Intraocular pressure:* 1.5 to 2 g/kg of a 15% or 20% solution infused as a single dose.

* *Adjunct as add-on maintenance therapy to improve pulmonary function in patients with cystic fibrosis*

ORAL INHALATION (BRONCHITOL)

Adults. 400 mg (10 capsules) twice daily with second dose given 2 to 3 hr before bedtime.

* *To assess bronchial hyperresponsiveness in patients who do not have clinically apparent asthma*

ORAL INHALATION (ARIDOL)

Adults and children 6 years and older. Bronchial challenge testing started with 0 mg of mannitol dosage, increased to 5 mg with second dose, 10 mg with third dose, 20 mg with fourth dose, 40 mg with fifth dose, 80 mg with sixth dose, and 160 mg for 3 remaining doses. Doses spaced equally apart. Increased doses given until patient has a positive response or 635 mg of mannitol has been administered.

Drug Administration

I.V.

- Drug is supplied in single-dose containers.
- Crystals may form, especially if solution is chilled. To dissolve, warm the bottle in hot water at 80°C and periodically shake vigorously. Cool to body temperature or less before administering. Never administer solution with undissolved crystals.
- Do not place 25% strength in polyvinylchloride bags, as a white flocculent precipitate may form.
- Use an infusion pump and administer with a filter such as a blood filter set to prevent infusion of mannitol crystals.
- To prevent air embolism, use a nonvented infusion set, avoid multiple connections, do not connect flexible containers in series, fully evacuate residual gas in the container prior to administration, do not pressurize the flexible container to increase flow rates, and, if administration is controlled by a pumping device, turn off pump before container runs dry.
- Administer through a large central vein, if possible, because severe infusion-site reactions can occur if administered through a peripheral vein.
- For reduction of intracranial or intraocular pressure, infuse over 30 min.
- If used for eye surgery, infuse 60–90 minutes before procedure.
- Never administer as an I.V. injection.
- *Incompatibilities:* Blood products, other drugs

ORAL INHALATION

± BRONCHITOL

- Ensure patient has passed the Bronchitol Tolerance Test before first administration.
- Administer a short-acting bronchodilator by oral inhalation, as prescribed, 5 to 15 minutes before each dose.
- Use only with provided inhaler.
- Each capsule contains 40 mg of drug and each dose will require 10 capsules. Each of the 10 capsules must be inhaled individually once in the morning and once in the evening. Evening dose should be given 2 to 3 hours before bedtime.
- To use inhaler, remove cap and twist open inhaler by turning the mouthpiece.
- Take 1 capsule out of the package and put it in the chamber. (Do not put capsule into the mouthpiece.)
- Hold inhaler upright and turn the mouthpiece until it locks in place.
- Push both buttons at the same time while keeping inhaler upright. Then release both buttons at the same time. Never keep buttons pressed.
- Hand inhaler to patient; have patient close lips around mouthpiece and take a steady deep breath and then remove inhaler. The patient should then hold breath for 5 seconds before exhaling. Do not have patient inhale into inhaler.
- A rattling sound while breathing in should be heard. If it is not heard, have patient tap bottom of inhaler firmly and have patient repeat breathing administration again.
- Afterward, open inhaler, remove empty capsule and throw capsule away. If capsule is not empty, have patient repeat breathing administration again.
- Repeat procedure 9 more times for each dose.
- Inhaler should be discarded and replaced after 7 days of use.
- If inhaler has to be washed, the inhaler should be thoroughly air-dried before the next use.

± ARIDOL

- Use the Aridol Bronchial Challenge Test Kit, when administering test.
- A nose clip may be used, if needed. Once clip is in place, patient should breathe through the mouth.

M

- To start test, insert 0 mg capsule into inhalation device. Puncture capsule by depressing buttons on side of device slowly, and only once.
- Have patient exhale completely, before inhaling from device in a controlled deep inspiration. At the end of the deep inspiration, start 60-second timer, have patient hold breath for 5 seconds, and exhale through mouth before removal of nose clip.
- After 60 seconds, measure the patient's FEV_1 in duplicate (measurement after inhaling the 0 mg capsule is the baseline FEV_1).
- Repeat steps following the mannitol capsule dose instruction schedule that comes with the kit until patient has a positive response (a 15% reduction in FEV_1 from 0 mg baseline or a 10% incremental reduction in FEV_1 between consecutive doses) or 635 mg dose of mannitol has been reached, which indicates a negative test.

Route	Onset	Peak	Duration
I.V.*	1–3 hr	Unknown	Up to 8 hr
I.V.†	30–60 min	Unknown	4–8 hr
I.V.‡	0.5–3 hr	30–60 min	3–8 hr
Inhalation	Unknown	1.5 hr	Unknown

Half-life: 100 minutes (Osmitrol); 4.7 hr (Aridol, Bronchitol)

* To produce diuresis.
† To decrease intraocular pressure.
‡ To decrease intracranial pressure.

Mechanism of Action

FOR ARIDOL AND BRONCHITOL

Mechanism of action is unknown in inducing bronchial hyperresponsiveness (Aridol) or improving pulmonary function in cystic fibrosis patients (Bronchitol).

FOR OSMITROL

Elevates plasma osmolality, causing water to flow from tissues, such as brain and eyes, and from CSF, into extracellular fluid, thereby decreasing intracranial and intraocular pressure.

As an osmotic diuretic, mannitol increases the osmolarity of glomerular filtrate, which decreases water reabsorption. This leads to increased excretion of chloride, sodium, water, and toxic substances.

As an irrigant, mannitol minimizes the hemolytic effects of water used as an irrigant and reduces the movement of hemolyzed blood from the urethra to the systemic circulation, which prevents hemoglobinemia and serious renal complications.

Contraindications

FOR ARIDOL

Conditions that may be compromised by induced bronchospasm or repeated spirometry maneuvers such as aortic or cerebral aneurysm, CVA, recent MI, or uncontrolled hypertension; known hypersensitivity to mannitol or to the gelatin used to make capsules

FOR BRONCHITOL

Failure to pass the Bronchitol Tolerance Test, hypersensitivity to mannitol or any of the capsule components

FOR OSMITROL

Active intracranial bleeding (except during craniotomy), anuria, hypersensitivity to mannitol or its components, severe pulmonary vascular congestion or pulmonary edema, severe hypovolemia

Interactions

DRUGS

For Aridol and Bronchitol
None reported by manufacturer
For Osmitrol
digoxin, drugs that prolong the QT interval, neuromuscular blocking agents: Increased risk of electrolyte imbalances resulting in serious cardiac adverse reactions; increased risk of digitalis toxicity from hypokalemia
diuretics; nephrotoxic drugs such as aminoglycosides, cyclosporine: Increased risk of renal failure and toxicity
lithium: Initial increased elimination of lithium followed by increased risk of lithium toxicity in patients with hypovolemia or renal impairment
neurotoxic drugs such as aminoglycosides: Increased risk of CNS toxicity
renally eliminated drugs: Increased elimination and decreased effectiveness of these drugs

Adverse Reactions

FOR ARIDOL

CNS: Dizziness, headache

CV: Chest discomfort
EENT: Gagging, pharyngolaryngeal pain, rhinorrhea, throat irritation
GI: Nausea, vomiting
RESP: Bronchospasm, cough, decreased forced expiratory volume, dyspnea, **wheezing**

FOR BRONCHITOL

CNS: Fever
EENT: Oropharyngeal pain
GI: Vomiting
MS: Arthralgia
RESP: Bronchospasm, cough, hemoptysis

FOR OSMITROL

CNS: Asthenia, chills, **coma,** confusion, dizziness, fever, headache, lethargy, malaise, **rebound increased intracranial pressure, seizures**
CV: Angina-like chest pain, **cardiac arrest,** chest pain, **heart failure,** hypertension, **hypotension,** palpitations, peripheral edema, tachycardia, thrombophlebitis, **venous thrombosis**
EENT: Blurred vision, dry mouth, rhinitis
GI: Diarrhea, nausea, vomiting
GU: Acute kidney injury, anuria, azotemia, hematuria, oliguria, osmotic nephrosis, polyuria, urine retention
MS: Musculoskeletal stiffness, myalgia
RESP: Cough, dyspnea, **pulmonary edema**
SKIN: Diaphoresis, pruritus, rash, urticaria
Other: Anaphylaxis, dehydration, extravasation (with compartment syndrome, swelling, and tissue necrosis), generalized discomfort or pain, **hyperkalemia, hypernatremia, hyperosmolarity,** hypervolemia, **hypokalemia, hyponatremia** (dilutional), hypovolemia, infusion-site reactions (erythema, inflammation, pain, phlebitis, pruritus, or extravasation complications of compartment syndrome, tissue necrosis), **metabolic acidosis,** thirst

▤ Childbearing Considerations

PREGNANCY

- It is not known if drug causes fetal harm. However, use of Bronchitol may increase risk for preterm delivery.
- Use with caution only if benefit to mother outweighs potential risk to fetus.

LACTATION

- It is not known if drug is present in breast milk.

- Patient should check with prescriber before breastfeeding.

▤ Nursing Considerations

FOR BRONCHITOL

- Know that the Bronchitol Tolerance Test is administered before Bronchitol brand is prescribed to identify patients who are suitable candidates for Bronchitol therapy. The test must be administered by a health care practitioner skilled in managing acute bronchospasms. Only patients who experience bronchospasm, a decrease in FEV_1, or a decrease in oxygen saturation with administration of Bronchitol are candidates for drug use.
- Monitor patient for hemoptysis. If present, notify prescriber and expect Bronchitol to be discontinued.

FOR ARIDOL

- Be aware that the bronchial challenge test should not be performed in any patient with clinically apparent asthma or very low baseline pulmonary function tests (less than 70% of the predicted values).
- Administer with caution in patients with conditions that may increase sensitivity to the bronchoconstricting or other potential effects of the drug.
- Know that the bronchial challenge test is for diagnostic purposes only. It should only be conducted by trained professionals.

> **! WARNING** Monitor patient for bronchospasms that could become severe. Have emergency equipment on standby to treat severe bronchospasm that may occur during the test. Expect to administer a short-acting inhaled beta-agonist to treat bronchospasm.

FOR OSMITROL

- Know that elderly patients and patients with preexisting renal disease are at greater risk for developing adverse reactions. Expect to evaluate patient's cardiac, pulmonary, and renal status and correct any preexisting fluid and electrolyte imbalances before therapy begins, as ordered.
- Be aware that depending on dosage and duration of mannitol administration, acid–base and electrolyte imbalances may occur, which can be severe and potentially fatal. Monitor central venous pressure, fluid

M

intake and output, and vital signs every hour during I.V. infusion of mannitol. Measure urine output with indwelling urinary catheter, as appropriate. Notify prescriber if renal function worsens and expect mannitol to be discontinued.

! **WARNING** Assess patient for hypersensitivity reactions, including anaphylaxis, dyspnea, and hypotension; cardiac arrest and death have occurred. If hypersensitivity reactions present, stop infusion immediately, notify prescriber, and expect to provide supportive emergency care. Be aware that concomitant administration of nephrotoxic drugs or other diuretics should be avoided during mannitol therapy.

- Check weight and monitor BUN and serum creatinine electrolyte levels daily, as ordered.
- Expect to monitor patient's cardiac, pulmonary, and renal function as well as signs and symptoms of hyper- or hypovolemia for patient receiving mannitol therapy for reduction in intracranial pressure. Also expect to monitor this patient's acid–base balance, intracranial pressure, osmol gap, and serum electrolytes and osmolarity.

! **WARNING** Monitor patient, especially patient with impaired renal function, for CNS toxicity such as coma, confusion, or lethargy. This may occur as a result of high serum mannitol concentrations or disturbances of electrolyte and acid–base balance caused by mannitol administration. Patients with preexisting compromise of the blood–brain barrier are at increased risk for increasing cerebral edema with mannitol use. Monitor patient closely for a rebound increase in intracranial pressure for at least several hours after mannitol has been discontinued. Know that use of neurotoxic drugs should be avoided, if possible, during mannitol administration.

- Provide frequent mouth care to relieve dry mouth and thirst.
- Know that high concentrations of mannitol may produce false low results for inorganic phosphorus blood concentrations. Mannitol therapy may also produce false positive results in tests for blood ethylene glycol concentrations.

PATIENT TEACHING

For Bronchitol
- Tell patient that a test must be administered to see if he will benefit from Bronchitol therapy before drug is prescribed.
- Instruct patient how to use and clean inhaler.
- Inform patient that 10 capsules will have to be administered, one at a time, with the inhaler for each dose.
- Instruct patient to take each dose, once in the morning and once in the evening. For the evening dose, tell patient to take it at least 2 to 3 hours before bedtime.
- Tell patient to notify prescriber if he sees blood in his sputum, as drug will have to be discontinued.

For Aridol
- Review how test is to be done with patient beforehand.
- Reassure patient she will not be left alone during the test.
- Inform patient that if test is positive or patient develops significant respiratory symptoms, a short-acting inhaled beta-agonist will be given to the patient.

For Osmitrol
- Inform patient that he may experience dry mouth and thirst during mannitol therapy.
- Instruct patient to report chest pain, difficulty breathing, or pain at I.V. site, along with any other new, persistent, or severe adverse reactions.

maraviroc
Selzentry

Class and Category
Pharmacologic class: CCR5 co-receptor antagonist
Therapeutic class: Antiretroviral

Indications and Dosages
* As adjunct to treat CCR5-tropic human immunodeficiency virus type 1 (HIV-1) infection combined with potent CYP3A inhibitors (with or without a potent CYP3A inducer) such as boceprevir, delavirdine, clarithromycin, elvitegravir/ritonavir, itraconazole, ketoconazole, nefazodone, protease inhibitors except tipranavir/ritonavir, or telithromycin

ORAL SOLUTION, TABLETS

Adults and children age 2 and over weighing 40 kg (88 lb) or more. 150 mg twice daily.

Children age 2 and over weighing at least 30 kg (66 lb) to less than 40 kg (88 lb). 100 mg twice daily.

Children age 2 and over weighing at least 20 kg (44 lb) to less than 30 kg (66 lb). 75 mg (tablet) or 80 mg (oral solution) twice daily.

Children age 2 and over weighing at least 10 kg (22 lb) to less than 20 kg (44 lb). 50 mg twice daily.

✳ *To treat CCR5-tropic HIV-1 infection combined with potent CYP3A inducers (without a potent CYP3A inhibitor) such as carbamazepine, efavirenz, etravirine, phenobarbital, phenytoin, or rifampin*

ORAL SOLUTION, TABLETS

Adults. 600 mg twice daily.

✳ *To treat CCR5-tropic HIV-1 infection in combination with drugs that are not potent CYP3A inducers or inhibitors*

ORAL SOLUTION, TABLETS

Adults and children age 2 and over weighing at least 30 kg (66 lb). 300 mg twice daily.

Children age 2 and older weighing 14 kg (30.8 lb) to 30 kg (66 lb). 200 mg twice daily.

Children age 2 and older weighing 10 kg (22 lb) to 14 kg (30.8 lb). 150 mg twice daily.

ORAL SOLUTION

Infants and children age 2 and older weighing 6 kg (13.2 lb) to less than 10 kg (22 lb). 100 mg twice daily.

Neonates, infants, and children weighing 4 kg (8.8 lb) to less than 6 kg (13.2 lb). 40 mg twice daily.

Neonates and infants weighing 2 kg (4.4 lb) to less than 4 kg (8.8 lb). 30 mg twice daily.

≣ Drug Administration

P.O.

- Oral solution is available for patient who is unable to swallow tablets or for children weighing at least 2 kg (4.4 lb) but less than 10 kg (22 lb). Measure dosage using a dosing syringe.
- Discard oral solution 60 days after first opening the bottle.

Route	Onset	Peak	Duration
P.O.	Unknown	0.5–4 hr	Unknown

Half-life: 14–18 hr

≣ Mechanism of Action

Selectively binds to the human chemokine receptor CCR5 present on the cell membrane, preventing an interaction that would allow CCR5-tropic HIV-1 to enter the cell. This prevents replication of the CCR5-tropic human immunodeficiency virus type I.

≣ Contraindications

End-stage renal disease or severe renal impairment in patients receiving potent CYP3A inducers or inhibitors, hypersensitivity to maraviroc or its components

≣ Interactions

DRUGS

CYP3A and P-gp inducers: Decreased effectiveness of maraviroc

CYP3A and P-gp inhibitors: Increased plasma concentration of maraviroc with increased risk of adverse reactions

multidrug resistance-associated protein (MRP)2 and organic anion transporting polypeptide (OATP)1B1 inducers: Possibly decreased effectiveness of maraviroc

multidrug resistance-associated protein (MRP)2 and organic anion transporting polypeptide (OATP)1B1 inhibitors: Possibly increased plasma concentration of maraviroc with increased risk of adverse reactions

St. John's wort: Decreased plasma concentration of maraviroc with substantially decreased effectiveness; increased risk of development of resistance to maraviroc

≣ Adverse Reactions

CNS: Anxiety, changes in levels of consciousness including loss of consciousness, CVA, depression, dizziness, dysesthesias, facial palsy, fever, malaise, memory loss excluding dementia, paresthesias, peripheral neuropathies, seizures, sensory abnormalities, sleep disturbances, syncope, tremor

CV: Acute heart failure, coronary artery disease, coronary artery occlusion, endocarditis, hypertension, MI, myocardial ischemia, orthostatic hypotension, unstable angina

EENT: Conjunctivitis, ear disorders, hemianopia, nasal or ocular infections or inflammations, oral lesions, paranasal sinus disorders, visual field defects

GI: Abdominal distention, appetite disorders, bilirubin increase, bloating, cholestatic jaundice, constipation, elevated pancreatic and liver enzymes, flatulence, gastrointestinal atonic and hypomotility disorders, **hepatic cirrhosis or failure, hepatitis, hepatotoxicity,** jaundice, **portal vein thrombosis**

GU: Ejaculation and erection disorders, urinary tract signs and symptoms

HEME: Anemias, eosinophilia, **hypoplastic anemia, marrow depression, neutropenia**

MS: Elevated creatine kinase, joint or muscle aches or pains, myositis, osteonecrosis, **rhabdomyolysis**

RESP: Breathing difficulties, cough, respiratory infections

SKIN: Acne, alopecia, apocrine and eccrine gland disorders, benign skin neoplasms, blisters, erythemas, lipodystrophies, nail and nail bed disorders, pruritus, rash (could be severe), **Stevens–Johnson syndrome, toxic epidermal necrolysis**

Other: Angioedema; **drug reaction with eosinophilia and systemic symptoms (DRESS);** elevated IgE; generalized discomfort or pain; immune reconstitution syndrome; infections such as bacterial, herpes, *Neisseria,* respiratory, tinea, and viral

Childbearing Considerations

- Pregnancy exposure registry: 1-800-258-4263.
- It is not known if drug causes fetal harm.
- Use with caution only if benefit to mother outweighs potential risk to fetus.

LACTATION

- It is not known if drug is present in breast milk.
- The Centers for Disease Control and Prevention recommends that HIV-1 infected mothers not breastfeed to avoid risking postnatal transmission of HIV-1 infection to infants. They also do not recommend breastfeeding because of potential drug-induced adverse reactions in the infant.

Nursing Considerations

- Know that maraviroc is not recommended in patients with dual/mixed- or CXCR4-tropic HIV-1 infections.
- Be sure patient has been checked for CCR5 tropism before treatment with maraviroc is started, because it is only effective against this type of infection.

! WARNING Check patient's bilirubin and liver enzyme levels before maraviroc treatment is started and periodically throughout treatment, as ordered, because drug increases risk of hepatotoxicity. Know that patients with a history of liver dysfunction or patients with co-infection with hepatitis B and/or C virus may require additional monitoring. Severe rash or evidence of systemic allergic reactions (including DRESS, eosinophilia, elevated IgE, and other systemic symptoms) has occurred with hepatotoxicity about 1 month after maraviroc therapy was started in some patients. Know that cases of hepatitis have occurred in some patients in the absence of allergic manifestations or who have had no history of hepatic disease.

! WARNING Monitor patient closely for severe skin reactions. Notify prescriber and expect maraviroc to be discontinued immediately if patient develops a rash that is accompanied by blisters, conjunctivitis, eosinophilia, facial edema, fever, joint or muscle aches, lip swelling, malaise, or oral lesions. Be aware that a delay in discontinuing the drug may result in a life-threatening situation.

- Monitor patient's cardiovascular status throughout maraviroc therapy because, although uncommon, major events such as acute heart failure, endocarditis, hypertension, ischemia, myocardial infarction, and unstable angina have been reported with maraviroc therapy. Pay close attention to the patient's blood pressure if renal impairment is present, because of risk of orthostatic hypotension. Patients with severe renal impairment or end-stage renal disease experiencing orthostatic hypotension should be evaluated for a dosage reduction.
- Be aware that immune reconstitution syndrome has occurred in patients treated with combination antiretroviral therapy,

including maraviroc. The inflammatory response predisposes susceptible patients to opportunistic infections such as cytomegalovirus, *Mycobacterium avium* infection, *Pneumocystis jiroveci* pneumonia, or tuberculosis. Autoimmune disorders such as Graves' disease, Guillain–Barré syndrome, or polymyositis have also occurred. Report sudden or unusual adverse reactions to prescriber.

- Assess patient frequently for signs and symptoms of infection, because maraviroc affects some immune cells, placing patient at increased risk.
- Be aware that maraviroc may put patient at increased risk for malignant tumors because of its effect on the immune system.

PATIENT TEACHING

- Tell patient oral solution is available if patient is unable to swallow tablets. Dosage of oral solution should only be measured using a dosing syringe, not a household spoon.
- Instruct patient prescribed oral solution to throw away any unused solution 60 days after first opening the bottle.
- Advise patient to avoid missing doses of maraviroc, as it can result in the development of resistance to drug. If she misses a dose, she should take it as soon as she remembers, but should not double the next dose or take more than prescribed.

! **WARNING** Inform patient to seek immediate medical attention if signs and symptoms of hepatitis or an allergic or skin reaction occurs.

- Advise patients with a history of cardiovascular disease or postural hypotension to notify prescriber if signs and symptoms develop or increase, as such patients are at increased risk for cardiovascular events.
- Tell patient to avoid hazardous activities, such as driving, until drug's CNS effects are known. Urge her to take safety precautions to prevent falling if she has adverse reactions, such as dizziness.
- Instruct patient to alert all prescribers of maraviroc therapy and not to take any over-the-counter medication, including herbal products, without the consent of the prescriber. Inform her that St. John's wort

should not be taken while on maraviroc therapy.

- Inform mothers that breastfeeding is not recommended during maraviroc therapy.

meloxicam

Anjeso, Qmiiz ODT, Vivlodex

☰ Class and Category

Pharmacologic class: NSAID
Therapeutic class: Analgesic

☰ Indications and Dosages

✳ *To relieve signs and symptoms of osteoarthritis*

ORAL DISINTEGRATING TABLETS, ORAL SUSPENSION, TABLETS

Adults. 7.5 mg daily. *Maximum:* 15 mg daily.

CAPSULES (VIVLODEX)

Adults. 5 mg once daily. *Maximum:* 10 mg once daily.

✳ *To relieve signs and symptoms of rheumatoid arthritis*

ORAL DISINTEGRATING TABLETS, ORAL SUSPENSION, TABLETS

Adults. 7.5 mg daily. *Maximum:* 15 mg daily.

✳ *To relieve pauciarticular or polyarticular signs and symptoms of juvenile rheumatoid arthritis*

ORAL SUSPENSION, TABLETS

Children age 2 and over. 0.125 mg/kg daily. *Maximum:* 7.5 mg daily.

ORAL DISINTEGRATING TABLETS (QMIIZ ODT)

Children weighing 60 kg (132 lb) or more. *Initial:* 7.5 mg once daily increased, as needed. *Maximum:* 15 mg once daily.

±**DOSAGE ADJUSTMENT** For patient on hemodialysis, the maximum dosage of oral suspension of meloxicam not to exceed 7.5 mg daily and for Vivlodex brand not to exceed 5 mg daily.

✳ *To relieve moderate to severe pain, alone or in combination with non-NSAID analgesics*

I.V. INJECTION (ANJESO)

Adults. 30 mg once daily.

☰ Drug Administration

P.O.

- Do not interchange the various forms of drug even if milligram strength is the same.
- Administer with food if GI upset occurs.

M

- Shake oral suspension well before using. Use a calibrated device to measure dosage. Store at room temperature.
- Do not remove ODT tablet until ready for administration. Peel back foil to release tablet; do not push through the foil. Using a dry, gloved hand, place ODT tablet in patient's mouth or onto the tongue. Patient can swallow tablet with or without a beverage.

I.V.

- Patient must be well hydrated before administration.
- Administer over 15 seconds as an I.V. injection.
- Drug has a delayed onset of action. If rapid pain relief is needed, expect to administer another analgesic as well but not a NSAID or salicylate.

Route	Onset	Peak	Duration
P.O.	Unknown	2.5–11 hr	Unknown
I.V.	2–3 hr	Unknown	24 hr or less
Half-life: 15–24 hr			

Mechanism of Action

Blocks cyclooxygenase, the enzyme needed to synthesize prostaglandins, which mediate the inflammatory response and cause local pain, swelling, and vasodilation. By inhibiting prostaglandins, the NSAID meloxicam reduces inflammatory symptoms. It also relieves pain because prostaglandins promote pain transmission from the periphery to the spinal cord.

Contraindications

History of angioedema, asthma, bronchospasm, nasal polyps, rhinitis, or urticaria induced by hypersensitivity to aspirin or other NSAIDs; hypersensitivity to meloxicam or its components; moderate to severe renal insufficiency in patients at risk for renal failure (Anjeso only); setting of coronary artery bypass graft (CABG) surgery

Interactions

DRUGS

ACE inhibitors, angiotensin receptor blockers, beta-blockers: Decreased antihypertensive effect, increased risk of renal failure in patients who are elderly, volume-depleted, or have existing renal impairment

anticoagulants (warfarin), antiplatelets (aspirin), selective serotonin reuptake inhibitors (SSRIs), serotonin–norepinephrine reuptake inhibitors (SNRIs): Synergistic effect on bleeding.

aspirin: Increased risk of GI adverse reactions such as bleeding and ulceration

cyclosporine: Increased risk of nephrotoxicity

diuretics (loop and thiazide): Decreased diuretic effect; possibly renal impairment

lithium: Elevated blood lithium level, possibly lithium toxicity

methotrexate: Increased risk of methotrexate toxicity

NSAIDs, salicylates: Increased risk of GI toxicity

pemetrexed: Increased risk of GI toxicity, myelosuppression, and renal toxicity

ACTIVITIES

alcohol use, smoking: Increased risk of GI bleeding

Adverse Reactions

CNS: Confusion, **CVA**, dizziness, fever, headache, insomnia, masking of fever, mood alteration, **seizures**

CV: Chest pain, edema, **heart failure**, hypertension, **MI**, tachycardia, vasculitis

EENT: Laryngitis, pharyngitis, sinusitis

GI: Abdominal pain, anorexia, colitis, constipation, diarrhea, diverticulitis, dyspepsia, dysphagia, elevated liver enzymes, esophagitis, flatulence, gastritis, gastroenteritis, gastroesophageal reflux disease, **GI bleeding** and ulceration, **hepatic failure**, **hepatitis**, indigestion, **melena**, nausea, **pancreatitis**, **perforation of intestines or stomach**, stomatitis, vomiting

GU: **Acute renal failure**, acute urine retention (children), urinary frequency, UTI

HEME: **Agranulocytosis**, anemia, **hemolytic anemia**, **leukopenia**, **neutropenia**, **pancytopenia**, **thrombocytopenia**

MS: Arthralgia; back pain; joint crepitation, effusion, or swelling; muscle spasms; myalgia

RESP: **Asthma exacerbation**, **bronchospasm**, cough, dyspnea, **respiratory depression**, upper respiratory tract infection

SKIN: Easy bruising, **erythema multiforme**, **exfoliative dermatitis**, photosensitivity, pruritus, rash, **Stevens–Johnson syndrome**, **toxic epidermal necrolysis**

Other: **Anaphylaxis, angioedema, drug reaction with eosinophilia and systemic**

symptoms (**DRESS**), flu-like symptoms, hyperkalemia, masking of inflammation

Childbearing Considerations

PREGNANCY

- Drug increases risk of premature closure of the fetal ductus arteriosus if given during the third trimester of pregnancy. It may also damage kidneys in the fetus if given after 20 weeks of gestation, possibly leading to oligohydramnios and neonatal renal impairment.
- Drug should be avoided in pregnant women starting at 30 weeks of gestation and onward.
- Drug should only be given between 20 and 30 weeks gestation if absolutely necessary, with lowest dosage and shortest dosage interval possible used.

LACTATION

- It is not known if drug is present in breast milk.
- Patient should check with prescriber before breastfeeding.

REPRODUCTION

- Be aware that drug may delay or prevent rupture of ovarian follicles, which has been associated with reversible infertility in some women.
- Drug is not recommended for use in women having difficulty conceiving or who are undergoing investigation of infertility.

Nursing Considerations

- Be aware that NSAIDs like meloxicam should be avoided in patients with a recent MI because risk of reinfarction increases with NSAID therapy. If therapy is unavoidable, monitor patient closely for signs of cardiac ischemia.
- Know that the risk of heart failure increases with NSAID use. Meloxicam should not be used in patients with severe heart failure but, if unavoidable, monitor patient for worsening of heart failure.
- Use meloxicam with extreme caution in patients with history of GI bleeding or ulcer disease because NSAIDs, such as meloxicam, increase risk of GI bleeding and ulceration. Expect to use drug for shortest time possible in these patients.
- Be aware that serious GI tract bleeding, perforation, and ulceration may occur without warning symptoms. Elderly patients

are at greater risk. To minimize risk, give drug with food and a full glass of water. If GI distress occurs, withhold drug and notify prescriber immediately.

- Use meloxicam cautiously in patients with hypertension, and monitor blood pressure closely throughout therapy. Drug may cause hypertension or worsen it.

! WARNING Monitor patient closely for thrombotic events, including MI and stroke, because NSAIDs increase the risk. These events may occur early in treatment and risk increases with duration of use. Be aware that these events have occurred even in patients who do not have a history or risk factors for cardiovascular disease. Monitor patient for warning signs such as chest pain, slurring of speech, shortness of breath, or weakness. If any signs and symptoms develop, withhold meloxicam, alert prescriber immediately, and provide supportive care, as prescribed.

- Monitor patient—especially if elderly or taking meloxicam long-term—for less common but serious adverse GI reactions, including anorexia, constipation, diverticulitis, dysphagia, esophagitis, gastritis, gastroenteritis, gastroesophageal reflux disease, hemorrhoids, hiatal hernia, melena, stomatitis, and vomiting.
- Monitor liver enzymes because, rarely, elevations may progress to severe hepatic reactions, including fatal hepatitis, hepatic failure, or liver necrosis.
- Monitor BUN and serum creatinine levels in elderly patients; patients taking ACE inhibitors, angiotensin II receptor antagonists, or diuretics; and patients with heart failure, hepatic dysfunction, or impaired renal function. Drug may cause renal failure.
- Monitor CBC for decreased hemoglobin and hematocrit. Drug may worsen anemia.

! WARNING Keep in mind if patient has bone marrow suppression or is receiving an antineoplastic drug, monitor laboratory results (including WBC count), and watch for evidence of infection because anti-inflammatory and antipyretic actions of meloxicam may mask signs and symptoms, such as fever and pain.

M

> **! WARNING** Assess patient's skin regularly for rash or other hypersensitivity reaction because meloxicam is an NSAID and may cause serious skin reactions without warning, even in patients with no history of NSAID sensitivity. At first sign of reaction, stop drug and notify prescriber.

- Monitor patient for adequate hydration before beginning meloxicam therapy to decrease risk of renal dysfunction.

PATIENT TEACHING

- Instruct patient to take meloxicam with food or after meals if she has stomach upset.
- Instruct patient how to administer an oral disintegrating tablet. Stress importance of peeling back foil instead of pushing tablet through the foil to access tablet. Inform patient that tablet will disintegrate quickly in saliva and can be easily swallowed with or without drinking a beverage.
- Instruct patient using oral suspension to shake container before each use and to use a calibrated device to measure dosage, not a household spoon. Suspension may be stored at room temperature.
- Caution patient to avoid using other NSAIDs, aspirin, or products containing aspirin while taking meloxicam.
- Advise patient to refrain from alcohol use or smoking because these activities may increase risk of adverse GI reactions.
- Instruct patient to notify prescriber if she develops signs or symptoms of hepatic dysfunction, such as dark yellow or brown urine, fatigue, fever, itching, lethargy, nausea, or yellowing of eyes or skin.
- Advise patient, especially if she's taking an oral anticoagulant such as warfarin, to report immediately signs of bleeding, such as black or tarry stools, blood in urine, easy bruising, or stomach pain.
- Caution pregnant patient not to take NSAIDs, such as meloxicam, between 20 and 30 weeks gestation without prescriber knowledge because drug may cause neonatal renal impairment, and avoid use of drug from 30 weeks gestation onward because drug may cause premature closure of ductus arteriosus.
- Explain that meloxicam may increase risk of serious adverse cardiovascular reactions including heart failure; urge patient to seek

immediate medical attention if signs or symptoms arise, such as chest pain, edema, shortness of breath, slurring of speech, unexplained weight gain, or weakness.
- Explain that meloxicam may increase risk of serious adverse GI reactions; emphasize importance of seeking immediate medical attention for such signs and symptoms as abdominal or epigastric pain, black or tarry stools, indigestion, or vomiting blood or material that looks like coffee grounds.

> **! WARNING** Alert patient to rare but serious skin reactions. Urge her to seek immediate medical attention for blisters, fever, itching, rash, or other indications of hypersensitivity.

memantine hydrochloride
Namenda, Namenda XR

Class and Category
Pharmacologic class: N-methyl-D-aspartate (NMDA) receptor antagonist
Therapeutic class: Antidementia agent

Indications and Dosages
✳ *To treat moderate to severe dementia of the Alzheimer's type*

ORAL SOLUTION, TABLETS
Adults. *Initial:* 5 mg daily, increased by 5 mg/wk, as needed, to 10 mg daily in two divided doses; then 15 mg daily with one 5-mg and one 10-mg dose daily; then 20 mg daily in two divided doses. *Maintenance:* 20 mg daily.

E.R. CAPSULES
Adults. *Initial:* 7 mg once daily, increased by 7 mg/wk, as needed, to 28 mg once daily. *Maximum:* 28 mg once daily.

±**DOSAGE ADJUSTMENT** For patients with severe renal impairment, maintenance dosage reduced to 5 mg twice daily for oral solution and tablet form and 14 mg once daily for extended-release capsules.

Drug Administration
P.O.
- Tablets and capsules should be swallowed whole and not chewed or crushed. However if patient has difficulty swallowing capsules, open capsule, sprinkle contents on

applesauce, and immediately have patient consume entire amount of applesauce.

- For oral solution, use the calibrated device that comes with drug to measure dosage. Once measured, squirt into the corner of patient's mouth. Store at room temperature.
- If several days of drug therapy are missed, patient will need to begin titration of drug dosage again.

Route	Onset	Peak	Duration
P.O.	Unknown	3–7 hr	Unknown
P.O./E.R.	Unknown	9–12 hr	Unknown

Half-life: 15–24 hr

☰ Contraindications

Hypersensitivity to memantine, amantadine, or their components

☰ Interactions

DRUGS

amantadine, dextromethorphan, ketamine: Possibly additive effects
carbonic anhydrase inhibitors, sodium bicarbonate: Decreased memantine clearance, leading to increased blood drug levels and risk of adverse effects

☰ Adverse Reactions

CNS: Abnormal gait, agitation, akathisia, anxiety, confusion, **CVA**, delirium, delusions, depression, dizziness, drowsiness, dyskinesia, fatigue, hallucinations, headache, hyperexcitability, insomnia, **neuroleptic malignant syndrome**, psychosis, restlessness, **seizures**, somnolence, **suicidal ideation**, tardive dyskinesia
CV: **AV block**, chest pain, **congestive heart failure**, hypertension, peripheral edema,

☰ Mechanism of Action

Memantine blocks the excitatory amino acid glutamate on N-methyl-D-aspartate (NMDA) receptor cells in the CNS. In Alzheimer's disease, glutamate levels are abnormally high when brain cells are both active and at rest. Normally, when certain brain cells are resting, magnesium ions block NMDA receptors and prevent influx of calcium and sodium ions and outflow of potassium ions. When learning and memory cells in the brain are active, glutamate engages with NMDA receptors, magnesium ions are removed from NMDA receptors, and cells are depolarized. During depolarization, calcium and sodium ions enter brain cells, and potassium ions leave. In Alzheimer's disease, excessive circulating glutamate permanently removes magnesium ions and opens ion channels. Excessive influx of calcium may damage brain cells and play a major role in Alzheimer's disease. What's more, dying brain cells release additional glutamate, worsening the cycle of brain cell destruction.

Memantine replaces magnesium on NMDA receptors of brain cells, closing ion channels and preventing calcium influx and the resulting damage to brain cells. By preventing excessive brain cell death, memantine slows progression of Alzheimer's disease.

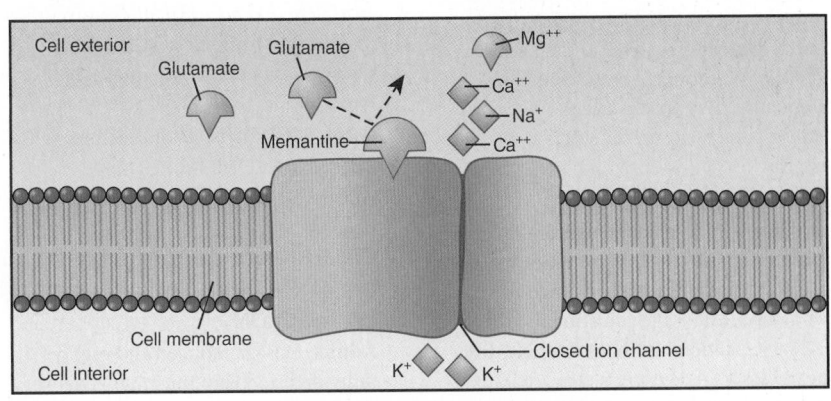

prolonged QT interval, supraventricular tachycardia, tachycardia
ENDO: Hypoglycemia
GI: Acute pancreatitis, anorexia, colitis, constipation, diarrhea, hepatic failure, hepatitis, ileus, nausea, pancreatitis, vomiting
GU: Acute renal failure, elevated creatinine levels, impotence, renal insufficiency, urinary incontinence, UTI
HEME: Agranulocytosis, leukopenia, neutropenia, pancytopenia, thrombocytopenia, thrombotic thrombocytopenic purpura
MS: Arthralgia, back pain
RESP: Bronchitis, cough, dyspnea, upper respiratory tract infection
SKIN: Stevens–Johnson syndrome
Other: Generalized pain, flu-like symptoms

Childbearing Considerations
PREGNANCY
- It is not known if drug causes fetal harm.
- Use with caution only if benefit to mother outweighs potential risk to fetus.

LACTATION
- It is not known if drug is present in breast milk.
- Patient should check with prescriber before breastfeeding.

Nursing Considerations
- Use memantine cautiously in patients with renal tubular acidosis or severe UTI because these conditions make urine alkaline, reducing memantine excretion and increasing the risk of adverse reactions.
- Use cautiously in patients with severe hepatic impairment, because drug undergoes partial hepatic metabolism, which may increase risk of adverse reactions.
- Monitor patient's response to memantine, and notify prescriber if bothersome or serious adverse reactions occur.
- Monitor patient closely for suicidal thoughts.

PATIENT TEACHING
- Instruct patient to take memantine exactly as prescribed. Inform him to notify the prescriber if he fails to take drug for several days, as dosage adjustments will be necessary. Caution him not to double dose if he misses a single dose. Instead, tell him to take the next dose as scheduled.

- Tell patient that capsule should be swallowed whole and not chewed or crushed. If patient has difficulty swallowing the capsule, instruct him to open capsule, sprinkle contents on applesauce, and immediately consume entire amount of applesauce.
- Instruct patient taking oral solution to measure dose using a calibrated device, not a household spoon. Tell him to store oral solution at room temperature.
- Advise patient to avoid a diet excessively high in fruits and vegetables because these foods contribute to alkaline urine, which can alter memantine clearance and increase adverse reactions.
- Caution patient to avoid hazardous activities until drug's CNS effects are known.
- Alert patient or caregiver that memantine has the potential to cause suicidal thoughts. If present, prescriber should be notified immediately.

meperidine hydrochloride
(pethidine hydrochloride)
Demerol

Class, Category, and Schedule
Pharmacologic class: Opioid
Therapeutic class: Opioid analgesic
Controlled substance schedule: II

Indications and Dosages
* *To relieve pain severe enough to require opioid treatment and for which alternative treatment options such as nonopioid analgesics or opioid combination products are inadequate or not tolerated*

ORAL SOLUTION, TABLETS, I.M. OR SUBCUTANEOUS INJECTION
Adults. 50 to 150 mg every 3 to 4 hr, as needed.
Children. 1.1 to 1.8 mg/kg every 3 to 4 hr, as needed. *Maximum:* Not to exceed adult dose.

I.V. INJECTION
Adults. Dosage reduced and highly individualized with injection given very slowly, preferably using a diluted solution.

✳ *To provide preoperative sedation*

I.M. OR SUBCUTANEOUS INJECTION

Adults. 50 to 100 mg 30 to 90 min before surgery.
Children. 1.1 to 2.2 mg/kg 30 to 90 min before surgery. *Maximum:* Not to exceed adult dose.

✳ *As adjunct to anesthesia*

I.V. INFUSION OR INJECTION

Adults. Individualized. Repeated slow injections of fractional doses such as 10 mg/ml solution or continuous infusion of dilute solution (1 mg/ml) titrated as needed.

✳ *To provide obstetric analgesia*

I.M. OR SUBCUTANEOUS INJECTION

Adults. 50 to 100 mg given with regular, painful contractions; repeated every 1 to 3 hr.

±**DOSAGE ADJUSTMENT** For elderly patients, total daily dosage decreased. For patients receiving CNS depressants, phenothiazines, and tranquilizers concurrently, dosage proportionately reduced by 25% to 50%.

Drug Administration

P.O.

- Dosing errors related to confusion between milligrams (mg) and milliliters (ml) and different concentrations of oral solutions can result in accidental overdose and death. Check dosage and concentration of oral solution very carefully before administering.
- Dilute oral solution in half a glass of water because undiluted solution may exert a slight topical anesthetic effect on mucous membranes.
- Use calibrated device when measuring dosage of oral solution.

I.V.

- Patient should be lying down during I.V. administration.
- For I.V. injection, administer diluted to a 10 mg/ml concentrate or use solution already containing 10 mg/ml that does not require further dilution (use with a compatible infusion device) and inject very slowly.
- For I.V. infusion, mix with 0.9% Sodium Chloride Injection, 5% Dextrose Injection, or Ringer's or Lactated Ringer's solution to a concentration of 1 mg/ml. Administer as a slow continuous infusion usually at 15 to 35 mg/hr.
- Keep naloxone available.

- *Incompatibilities:* Aminophylline, barbiturates, heparin, iodides, methicillin, morphine sulfate, phenytoin, sodium bicarbonate, sulfadiazine, or sulfisoxazole.

I.M.

- Inject into a large muscle mass.

SUBCUTANEOUS

- Subcutaneous injection is painful and isn't recommended unless no other route can be used.

Route	Onset	Peak	Duration
P.O.	15 min	1–1.5 hr	2–4 hr
I.V.	1 min	5–7 min	2–4 hr
I.M., SubQ	10–15 min	30–50 min	2–4 hr

Half-life: 2.5–4 hr

Mechanism of Action

Binds with opiate receptors in the spinal cord and higher levels of the CNS. In this way, meperidine stimulates kappa and mu receptors, which alters the perception of and emotional response to pain.

Contraindications

Acute or severe bronchial asthma in an unmonitored setting or in the absence of resuscitative equipment; hypersensitivity to meperidine or its components; known or suspected gastrointestinal obstruction, including paralytic ileus; significant respiratory depression; use within 14 days of MAO inhibitor therapy

Interactions

DRUGS

5-HT3 receptor antagonists, drugs that affect the serotonin neurotransmitter system (mirtazapine, tramadol, trazodone), MAO inhibitors including I.V. methylene blue and linezolid, selected muscle relaxants (cyclobenzaprine, metaxalone), selective serotonin reuptake inhibitors (SSRIs), serotonin and norepinephrine reuptake inhibitors (SNRIs), tricyclic antidepressants, triptans: Increased risk of serotonin syndrome
acyclovir: Possibly increased blood meperidine level
anticholinergics: Increased risk of severe constipation which may lead to paralytic ileus; increased risk of urinary retention
benzodiazepines, CNS depressants, muscle relaxants, other opioids, sedating

M

antihistamines, tricyclic antidepressants: Increased risk of significant respiratory depression and other life-threatening adverse effects

cimetidine: Reduced clearance and volume of distribution of meperidine

CYP3A4 inducers such as carbamazepine, phenytoin, rifampin: Increased clearance of meperidine with decreased effectiveness

CYP3A4 inhibitors such as azole-antifungals, macrolide antibiotics, protease inhibitors: Decreased clearance of meperidine resulting in increased or prolonged opioid effects

diuretics: Reduced effectiveness of diuretics

mixed agonist/antagonist and partial agonist opioid analgesics such as buprenorphine, butorphanol, nalbuphine, pentazocine: Decreased analgesic effect of meperidine; possibly precipitation of withdrawal symptoms

MAO inhibitors: Increased risk of coma, hypotension, or severe respiratory depression

muscle relaxants: Possibly enhanced neuromuscular blocking action of skeletal muscle relaxants; increased degree of respiratory depression

ACTIVITIES

alcohol use: Possibly increased CNS and respiratory depression and hypotension

Adverse Reactions

CNS: Agitation, confusion, delirium, depression, dizziness, drowsiness, headache, **increased intracranial pressure**, lack of coordination, malaise, mood changes, nervousness, nightmares, restlessness, **seizures**, syncope, transient hallucinations or disorientation, tremor, weakness

CV: **Hypotension**, orthostatic hypotension, tachycardia

EENT: Blurred vision, diplopia, dry mouth

ENDO: **Adrenal insufficiency**

GI: Abdominal cramps or pain, anorexia, constipation, ileus, nausea, vomiting

GU: Decreased libido, dysuria, erectile dysfunction, impotence, infertility, lack of menstruation, urinary frequency, urine retention

MS: Involuntary muscle movements

RESP: Dyspnea, **respiratory arrest or depression**, wheezing

SKIN: Diaphoresis, flushing, pruritus, rash, urticaria

Other: **Anaphylaxis**; injection-site pain, redness, or swelling; physical and psychological dependence

Childbearing Considerations

PREGNANCY

- Drug may cause fetal harm.
- Prolonged use of drug during pregnancy can result in neonatal opioid withdrawal syndrome (NOWS), which may be life-threatening if not recognized and treated.
- Avoid prolonged use during pregnancy. Use with caution only if benefit to mother outweighs potential risk to fetus.

LABOR & DELIVERY

- Drug is not recommended for use in pregnant women immediately before or during labor. Opioids may alter length of time of labor.
- Opioids cross the placental barrier and may produce respiratory depression and psycho-physiologic effects in the newborn. Monitor newborn closely for signs of excess sedation and respiratory depression.
- An opioid antagonist, such as naloxone, must be available at the time of delivery in the event it is needed to reverse opioid-induced respiratory depression in the neonate.

LACTATION

- Drug is present in breast milk.
- Patient should check with prescriber before breastfeeding.
- If breastfeeding occurs, monitor infant for excess sedation and respiratory depression and for withdrawal symptoms when breastfeeding is stopped.

REPRODUCTION

- Chronic use of opioids may reduce fertility.

Nursing Considerations

- Be aware that excessive use of opioids like meperidine may lead to abuse, addiction, misuse, overdose, and possibly death. Because of this, a Risk Evaluation and Mitigation Strategy (REMS) is required. Monitor patient's intake of drug closely and for evidence of physical dependence.
- Know that chronic maternal use of meperidine during pregnancy can result in neonatal opioid withdrawal syndrome (NOWS), which may be life-threatening if

not recognized and treated appropriately. NOWS occurs when a newborn has been exposed to opioid drugs like meperidine for a prolonged period while in utero.

- Use meperidine with extreme caution in patients with acute abdominal conditions, hepatic or renal disorders, hypothyroidism, prostatic hyperplasia, seizures, or supraventricular tachycardia.
- Use cautiously in debilitated patients or patients with adrenocortical insufficiency, pheochromocytoma, sickle cell anemia, toxic psychosis, and any other condition that might worsen with CNS depression, such as acute alcoholism.
- Be aware that meperidine should only be used concomitantly with benzodiazepine and other CNS depressants therapy in patients for whom other treatment options are inadequate. If prescribed together, expect dosing and duration of meperidine to be limited. Monitor patient closely for signs and symptoms of a decrease in consciousness, including coma, profound sedation, and significant respiratory depression. Notify prescriber immediately and provide emergency supportive care, as death may occur.

! WARNING Monitor patient's respiratory and cardiovascular status during treatment. Notify prescriber immediately and expect to discontinue drug if respiratory rate falls to less than 12 breaths/minute or if respiratory depth decreases because serious, life-threatening, or fatal respiratory depression may occur. Monitor patient especially during initiation or following a dose increase.

- Monitor patient's bowel function to detect constipation, and assess the need for stool softeners.
- Know that prolonged use may increase risk of toxicity exhibited by seizures from the accumulation of the meperidine metabolite, normeperidine.
- Expect withdrawal symptoms to occur if drug is abruptly withdrawn after long-term use.
- Be aware that concomitant use with CYP3A4 inhibitors or discontinuation of CYP3A4 inducers can result in fatal overdose of meperidine.

! WARNING Know that many drugs may interact with opioids like meperidine to cause serotonin syndrome. Monitor patient closely for signs and symptoms such as agitation, diaphoresis, diarrhea, fever, hallucinations, labile blood pressure, muscle twitching or stiffness, nausea, shakiness, shivering, tachycardia, trouble with coordination, or vomiting. Notify prescriber at once because serotonin syndrome may be life-threatening. Be prepared to discontinue drug, if possible and ordered, and provide supportive care.

- Monitor patient for adrenal insufficiency. Although rare, it can be life-threatening. Monitor patient for anorexia, dizziness, fatigue, hypotension, nausea, vomiting, or weakness. Notify prescriber if adrenal insufficiency is suspected and expect diagnostic testing to be done. If confirmed, expect to administer corticosteroids and wean patient off meperidine, if possible.

PATIENT TEACHING

- Inform patient that meperidine is a controlled substance.
- Instruct patient to use only a calibrated measuring device when measuring a dose of oral solution and never use a teaspoon or tablespoon, because a spoon is inexact and it is easy to use the wrong size spoon when measuring. Advise patient to dilute oral solution in half a glass of water before taking, because the undiluted solution may exert a slight topical anesthetic effect on mucous membranes.
- Advise patient to take drug exactly as prescribed. Warn patient that excessive or prolonged use can lead to abuse, addiction, misuse, overdose, and possibly death. If patient has been receiving meperidine for more than a few weeks and the drug is to be discontinued, advise patient to taper dosage off, as abrupt discontinuation could precipitate withdrawal symptoms.
- Encourage patient and family or caregiver to obtain naloxone for home use; if and when needed it will be readily available. Review signs and symptoms of an opioid overdose and how to administer naloxone. Stress importance of the need to call 911 if naloxone is administered.
- Instruct patient to report constipation, severe nausea, and shortness of breath.

- Advise patient to avoid hazardous activities until drug's CNS effects are known.
- Instruct patient to prevent postoperative atelectasis by turning, coughing, and deep breathing.
- Warn patient not to consume alcohol or take a benzodiazepine without prescriber knowledge, as severe respiratory depression can occur and may lead to death.
- Urge patient to avoid alcohol, sedatives, and tranquilizers during therapy.
- Inform patient that long-term use of opioids like meperidine may decrease sex hormone levels, causing decreased libido, erectile dysfunction, impotence, infertility, or lack of menstruation. Encourage patient to report any symptoms to prescriber.
- Caution pregnant patient not to increase dosage or take drug for a prolonged period, as adverse effects can cause infant to experience life-threatening withdrawal when born.
- Instruct patient to notify all prescribers of opioid use.
- Stress importance of keeping meperidine out of the reach of children, as ingestion may lead to a fatal overdose.

meropenem
Merrem I.V.

☰ Class and Category
Pharmacologic class: Carbapenem
Therapeutic class: Antibiotic

☰ Indications and Dosages
✳ *To treat complicated intra-abdominal infections caused by susceptible strains of alpha-hemolytic streptococci,* Bacteroides fragilis, B. thetaiotaomicron, Escherichia coli, Klebsiella pneumoniae, Peptostreptococcus species, *or* Pseudomonas aeruginosa

I.V. INFUSION OR INJECTION
Adults and children weighing more than 50 kg (110 lb). 1 g every 8 hr.
Children over age 3 months weighing less than 50 kg (110 lb). 20 mg/kg every 8 hr.
Maximum: 1 g every 8 hr.

I.V. INFUSION
Infants with gestational age of 32 weeks and over and postnatal age of 2 weeks and over. 30 mg/kg every 8 hr.

Infants with gestational age of 32 weeks and over but postnatal age less than 2 weeks or infants with gestational age less than 32 weeks but postnatal age of 2 weeks or over. 20 mg/kg every 8 hr.
Infants with gestational age less than 32 weeks and postnatal age less than 2 weeks. 20 mg/kg every 12 hr.

✳ *To treat complicated skin and skin structure infections caused by* B. fragilis, Enterococcus faecalis *(excluding vancomycin-resistant isolates),* E. coli, Peptostreptococcus *species,* Proteus mirabilis, P. aeruginosa, Staphylococcus aureus, Streptococcus agalactiae, S. pyogenes, *and viridans group streptococci*

I.V. INFUSION OR INJECTION
Adults and children weighing more than 50 kg (110 lb). 500 mg (1 g if caused by *Pseudomonas aeruginosa*) every 8 hr.
Children over age 3 months weighing 50 kg (110 lb) or less. 10 mg/kg (20 mg/kg if caused by *Pseudomonas aeruginosa*) every 8 hr. *Maximum:* 500 mg every 8 hr.

✳ *To treat bacterial meningitis caused by* Haemophilus influenzae, Neisseria meningitidis, *or* Streptococcus pneumoniae (penicillin-susceptible isolates)

I.V. INFUSION OR INJECTION
Children weighing more than 50 kg (110 lb). 2 g every 8 hr.
Children over age 3 months weighing less than 50 kg (110 lb). 40 mg/kg every 8 hr. *Maximum:* 2 g every 8 hr.

±**DOSAGE ADJUSTMENT** For adult patients with a creatinine clearance of 26 to 50 ml/min, dosage interval increased to every 12 hours. For adult patients with a creatinine clearance of 10 to 25 ml/min, dosage reduced by half and given every 12 hr. For adults with creatinine clearance less than 10 ml/min, dosage reduced by half and given every 24 hr. There is no experience for children with renal impairment.

☰ Drug Administration
I.V.
- For I.V. injection, add 10 ml Sterile Water for Injection to 500-mg vial, or 20 ml to 1-g vial of drug. Shake to dissolve. Administer over 3 to 5 minutes. Once reconstituted, drug may be stored for up to 3 hours at room temperature or for 13 hours if refrigerated.

- For I.V. infusion, drug vials may be directly reconstituted with 0.9% Sodium Chloride Injection or 5% Dextrose Injection. Alternatively, a drug vial may be reconstituted then the resulting solution added to 0.9% Sodium Chloride Injection or 5% Dextrose Injection container and further diluted. Solutions for infusion should have a concentration ranging from 1 mg/ml to 20 mg/ml. Infuse over 15 to 30 minutes. If mixed with 0.9% Sodium Chloride Injection, solution may be stored for 1 hour at room temperature and up to 15 hours if refrigerated. If mixed with 5% Dextrose Injection, solution must be used immediately.
- Follow manufacturer guidelines for preparing ADD-Vantage vials for administration.
- Do not use flexible container in series plastic connections.
- *Incompatibilities:* Other drugs, including solutions containing other drugs

Route	Onset	Peak	Duration
I.V.	Unknown	1 hr	Unknown

Half-life: 1–1.5 hr

Mechanism of Action

Penetrates cell walls of most gram-negative and gram-positive bacteria, inactivating penicillin-binding proteins. This action inhibits bacterial cell wall synthesis and causes cell death.

Contraindications

Hypersensitivity to meropenem, other carbapenem drugs, beta-lactams, or their components

Interactions

DRUGS

probenecid: Inhibited renal excretion of meropenem increasing meropenem plasma concentrations
valproic acid: Possibly reduced blood level of valproic acid to subtherapeutic level

Adverse Reactions

CNS: Headache, paresthesias, **seizures**
CV: **Shock**
EENT: Epistaxis, glossitis, oral candidiasis
GI: Anorexia, constipation, diarrhea, elevated liver enzymes, nausea, **pseudomembranous colitis**, vomiting

GU: Elevated BUN and serum creatinine levels, hematuria, **renal failure**
HEME: **Agranulocytosis, hemolytic anemia, leukopenia, neutropenia**, positive Coombs' test
RESP: **Apnea**, dyspnea
SKIN: Acute generalized exanthematous pustulosis, diaper rash from candidiasis (children), **erythema multiforme**, pruritus, rash, **Stevens–Johnson syndrome, toxic epidermal necrolysis**
Other: **Anaphylaxis; angioedema; drug reaction with eosinophilia and systemic symptoms (DRESS)**; injection-site inflammation, pain, phlebitis, or thrombophlebitis; **sepsis**

Childbearing Considerations

PREGNANCY

- It is not known if drug causes fetal harm.
- Use with caution only if benefit to mother outweighs potential risk to fetus.

LACTATION

- Drug is present in breast milk.
- Patient should check with prescriber before breastfeeding.

Nursing Considerations

- Obtain body fluid and tissue samples, as ordered, for culture and sensitivity testing. Expect to review test results, if possible, before giving first dose of meropenem.

! **WARNING** Be aware that fatal hypersensitivity reactions have occurred with meropenem use. Determine whether patient has had previous reactions to antibiotics or other allergens. Monitor patient closely and stop drug immediately if signs and symptoms of anaphylaxis occur. Notify prescriber, and expect to provide supportive emergency care that may include airway management, epinephrine and I.V. steroid administration, and oxygen.

- Monitor patient closely for diarrhea, which may indicate pseudomembranous colitis caused by *Clostridium difficile*. If diarrhea occurs, notify prescriber and expect to withhold meropenem and treat with an antibiotic effective against *C. difficile*, and electrolytes, fluids, and protein.
- Monitor patient for blister formation, rash, and other cutaneous abnormalities, because drug may cause severe cutaneous adverse

reactions that may become life-threatening. At first sign of skin abnormality, stop drug therapy immediately and notify prescriber.
- Take seizure precautions according to facility policy, especially for patients with bacterial meningitis or CNS or renal disorders because of an increased risk of seizures with meropenem.
- Monitor patient with creatinine clearance of 10 to 26 ml/min for signs and symptoms of heart failure, renal failure, seizures, or shock.

PATIENT TEACHING

! WARNING Tell patient to report immediately difficulty breathing, injection-site pain, skin changes (blister formation, rash), and sore mouth.

- Urge patient to tell prescriber about diarrhea that's severe or lasts longer than 3 days. Remind patient that bloody or watery stools can occur 2 or more months after antibiotic therapy and can be serious, requiring prompt treatment.
- Instruct patient to avoid hazardous activities until drug's CNS effects are known.

mesalamine

Apriso, Asacol HD, Canasa, Delzicol, Lialda, Rowasa, Salofalk (CAN), sfROWASA

☰ Class and Category

Pharmacologic class: Aminosalicylate
Therapeutic class: Anti-inflammatory

☰ Indications and Dosages

✴ *To treat actively mild to moderate ulcerative colitis*

DELAYED-RELEASE TABLETS (ASACOL HD)

Adults. 1,600 mg three times daily for 6 wk. *Maximum:* 4.8 g daily.

DELAYED-RELEASE CAPSULES (DELZICOL)

Adults. *Initial:* 800 mg three times daily for 6 wk.
Children age 5 years and older weighing 54 kg (118.8 lb) to 90 kg (198 lb). 27 to 44 mg/kg/day divided into two doses given in morning and evening for 6 wk. *Maximum:* 2.4 grams daily.

Children age 5 years and older weighing 33 kg (72.6 lb) to less than 54 kg (118.8 lb). 37 to 61 mg/kg/day divided into two doses given in morning and evening for 6 wk. *Maximum:* 2 grams daily.
Children age 5 years and older weighing 17 kg (37.4 lb) to less than 33 kg (72.6 lb). 36 to 71 mg/kg/day divided into two doses given in morning and evening for 6 wk. *Maximum:* 1.2 grams daily.

✴ *To induce remission in patients with actively mild to moderate ulcerative colitis.*

DELAYED-RELEASE TABLETS (LIALDA)

Adults. *Initial:* 2.4 or 4.8 g once daily with a meal.
Children weighing more than 50 kg (110 lb). 4.8 g once daily with a meal for 8 wk then reduced to 2.4 g once daily.
Children weighing more than 35 kg (77 lb) to and including 50 kg (110 lb). 3.6 g once daily with a meal for 8 wk then reduced *to* 2.4 g once daily after wk 8.
Children weighing 24 kg (52.8 lb) to 35 kg (77 lb). 2.4 g once daily with a meal for 8 wk then reduced to 1.2 g once daily after wk 8.

✴ *To maintain remission in patients with mild to moderate ulcerative colitis*

DELAYED-RELEASE CAPSULES (DELZICOL)

Maintenance: 1.6 g daily in 2 to 4 divided doses.

DELAYED-RELEASE TABLETS (LIALDA)

Adults. *Maintenance:* 2.4 g once daily.

E.R. CAPSULES (APRISO)

Adults. 1.5 g once daily.

✴ *To treat mild to moderate distal ulcerative colitis, proctitis, and proctosigmoiditis*

RECTAL SUSPENSION (ROWASA, SFROWASA)

Adults. 4 g (60 ml) daily at bedtime for 3 to 6 wk.

✴ *To treat active ulcerative proctitis*

SUPPOSITORIES (CANASA)

Adults. 1 g once daily for 3 to 6 wk.

☰ Drug Administration

P.O.

- Do not interchange or substitute one brand for another or the strength of the same brand for another.
- Capsules and tablets should be swallowed whole and not chewed, crushed, or split/opened. An exception is Delzicol capsules,

which can be opened and the inner tablets swallowed.

- Do not coadminister drug with antacids.
- Ensure that patient is well hydrated.
- Administer Lialda brand with food.
- Administer Asacol HD on an empty stomach, at least 1 hour before or 2 hours after a meal.

P.R.

- Administer suppository at bedtime. Ensure that suppository is firm before inserting it. If it's too soft, chill in refrigerator for 30 minutes or run under cold water before removing wrapper. Moisten with water-soluble lubricant or tap water before insertion. Have patient retain suppository for 1 to 3 hours. Avoid suppository touching surfaces to prevent staining.
- To administer rectal suspension, shake suspension bottle before each dose, then remove protective covering from applicator tip. Place patient on left side or in a knee-chest position. Insert applicator tip gently into the rectum pointing toward the umbilicus. Squeeze bottle in a steady manner. Give suspension at bedtime, and have patient retain for prescribed time of about 8 hours, if possible. Retention time ranges from 3.5 to 12 hours.
- Suspension may darken slightly over time but this change doesn't affect potency. Discard rectal suspension that turns dark brown.

Route	Onset	Peak	Duration
P.O.	1 wk–3 mo	3–12 hr	Unknown
P.R.	Unknown	4–7 hr	Unknown

Half-life: 7–12 hr

Mechanism of Action

May reduce inflammation by inhibiting the enzyme cyclooxygenase and decreasing production of arachidonic acid metabolites, which may be increased in patients with inflammatory bowel disease. Cyclooxygenase is needed to form prostaglandins from arachidonic acid. Prostaglandins mediate inflammatory activity and produce signs and symptoms of inflammation. Mesalamine also may reduce inflammation by interfering with leukotriene synthesis and inhibiting the enzyme lipoxygenase, both of which take part in inflammatory response.

Contraindications

Hypersensitivity to mesalamine, other salicylates including aminosalicylates, or their components

Interactions

DRUGS

azathioprine, 6-mercaptopurine: Possibly increased risk for blood disorders
nephrotoxic agents including NSAIDs: Possibly increased risk of nephrotoxicity

Adverse Reactions

CNS: Chills, confusion, depression, dizziness, drug fever, emotional lability, fatigue, fever, **Guillain–Barré syndrome**, headache (severe), **intracranial hypertension**, peripheral neuropathy, somnolence, transverse myelitis, tremor, vertigo, weakness
CV: Myocarditis, pericardial effusion, pericarditis
EENT: Blurred vision, dry mouth, pharyngitis, rhinitis, sinusitis, swelling of eye, taste perversion, tinnitus
GI: Abdominal cramps or pain (severe), anal pruritus, anorexia, bloody diarrhea, cholecystitis, colitis, constipation, diarrhea, discoloration of feces, distention (abdomen), elevated liver enzymes, feeling of incomplete defecation, flatulence, gastritis, **GI bleeding, hepatitis, hepatotoxicity**, indigestion, jaundice, Kawasaki-like syndrome, **liver failure or necrosis**, mucous stools, nausea, **pancreatitis, perforated peptic ulcer**, rectal discharge or pain, vomiting
GU: Acute or chronic renal failure, decreased libido, dysmenorrhea, dysuria, epididymitis, hematuria, interstitial nephritis, menorrhagia, minimal change disease, nephrogenic diabetes insipidus, nephrolithiasis, **nephrotoxicity**, reversible oligospermia, urinary frequency and urgency
HEME: Agranulocytosis, anemia, **aplastic anemia**, eosinophilia, **granulocytopenia, leukopenia**, lymphadenopathy, **neutropenia, pancytopenia, thrombocytopenia**
MS: Back pain, dysarthria, myalgia
RESP: Allergic alveolitis, pneumonitis, asthma exacerbation, bronchitis, **eosinophilic or interstitial pneumonitis, fibrosing alveolitis**, pleurisy/pleuritis
SKIN: Acne, acute generalized exanthematous pustulosis (AGEP), alopecia, diaphoresis, dryness, erythema including

M

erythema nodosum, photosensitivity, psoriasis, pruritus, pyoderma gangrenosum, rash, **Stevens–Johnson syndrome, toxic epidermal necrolysis (TEN),** urticaria
Other: Acute intolerance syndrome, anaphylaxis, angioedema, drug reaction with eosinophilia and systemic symptoms (DRESS), gout, systemic lupus erythematosus or lupus-like syndrome

Childbearing Considerations

PREGNANCY

- It is not known if drug causes fetal harm although it does cross the placental barrier.
- Use with caution only if benefit to mother outweighs potential risk to fetus.

LACTATION

- Drug is present in breast milk.
- Patient should check with prescriber before breastfeeding.
- If breastfeeding occurs, infant should be monitored for diarrhea.

Nursing Considerations

! WARNING Use mesalamine cautiously in patients with sulfite sensitivity. Some drug formulations contain sulfites, which may cause hypersensitivity reactions in these patients. Know that hypersensitivity reactions may affect internal organs such as the heart (myocarditis, pericarditis), kidneys (nephritis), liver (hepatitis), and lungs (pneumonitis), as well as cause hematologic adverse effects. If hypersensitivity is suspected, notify prescriber immediately, expect mesalamine to be discontinued, and provide supportive care, as ordered.

- Use mesalamine cautiously in patients with liver disease because hepatic dysfunction may occur. Monitor patient's liver enzymes, as ordered, for elevations.
- Expect to assess patient's renal function prior to the initiation of mesalamine therapy and then periodically throughout therapy, as ordered, because drug may cause renal impairment.
- Assess patient for evidence of acute intolerance similar to flare-up of inflammatory bowel disease: acute abdominal cramps and pain, bloody diarrhea, and, possibly, fever, headache, and rash. If present, notify prescriber.

- Monitor patient's CBC with differential for eosinophilia, which may indicate an allergic reaction, and other hematological adverse reactions. Know that patients age 65 and over are at increased risk for blood dyscrasias such as agranulocytosis, neutropenia, and pancytopenia.
- Be aware that mesalamine may interfere with the measurement of urinary normetanephrine, producing falsely elevated test results if the test is done by liquid chromatography with electrochemical detection.
- Monitor patient for signs and symptoms of acute intolerance syndrome, such as acute abdominal pain, bloody diarrhea, fever, headache, and rash. If suspected, expect to discontinue mesalamine therapy and provide supportive care, as ordered.
- Be aware that patients with preexisting skin conditions such as atopic dermatitis and atopic eczema are at higher risk for more severe photosensitivity reactions.

! WARNING Monitor patient for serious skin reactions. Expect drug to be discontinued at the first sign or symptom of severe cutaneous adverse reactions.

PATIENT TEACHING

- Instruct patient how to take the brand of mesalamine prescribed. Some may be taken with food and others not; some capsules may be opened and others not. If capsules are not to be opened or patient is taking a tablet form, tell patient to swallow drug whole and not to chew, crush, or split/open drug form.
- Teach patient how to use rectal suspension or suppositories correctly. Emphasize shaking suspension bottle well before using. Tell patient not to break or cut suppository. Remind him to retain the suppository for 1 to 3 hours or longer, if possible, and the suspension for 8 hours. Caution patient not to use two suppositories at the same time to make up for a missed dose. Make patient aware that suppository will cause staining if drug comes into direct contact with surfaces, such as clothing, floors, enamel, granite, marble, painted surfaces, and vinyl. Tell patient to take the rectal suspension or suppository at bedtime.

- Advise patient to notify prescriber immediately about abdominal cramps or pain, bloody diarrhea, fever, headache, or rash or any other adverse effects that are persistent, severe, or worsen during mesalamine therapy.
- Advise patient to take sun precautions such as using sunscreen and protective clothing while outdoors, as drug may cause photosensitivity reactions that could be severe, especially in patient with preexisting skin conditions.
- Tell patient to alert all prescribers of mesalamine therapy because of potential drug interactions, especially those drugs that increase sensitivity to sun and UV light.

! **WARNING** Advise patient to stop taking drug and to notify prescriber immediately if serious skin adverse reactions or an allergic reaction occurs.

metformin hydrochloride

Glucophage, Glucophage XR, Glumetza, Riomet

Class and Category

Pharmacologic class: Biguanide
Therapeutic class: Antidiabetic

Indications and Dosages

✴ *As adjunct to reduce blood glucose level in type 2 diabetes mellitus*

ORAL SOLUTION (RIOMET), TABLETS (GLUCOPHAGE)

Adults. *Initial:* 500 mg twice daily or 850 mg daily with meals, increased by 500 mg/wk or by 850 mg every 2 wk until desired response occurs. *Maximum:* 2,550 mg daily given in divided doses.

Children ages 10 and older. 500 mg twice daily with meals, increased as prescribed by 500 mg/wk until desired response occurs. *Maximum:* 2,000 mg daily in divided doses.

±**DOSAGE ADJUSTMENT** For patients not tolerating maximum dosage, total daily dose may be divided into 3 doses and given with meals.

E.R. TABLETS (GLUCOPHAGE XR, GLUMETZA)

Adults. *Initial:* 500 mg once daily with evening meal. Increased by 500 mg/wk (Glucophage XR) or 1 to 2 wk (Glumetza), as needed. *Maximum:* 2,000 mg daily.

±**DOSAGE ADJUSTMENT** For patient taking Glucophage XR but not achieving adequate glucose control at maximum dose of 2,000 mg once daily, dosage split to 1,000 mg twice daily. If that does not achieve adequate control, patient switched to immediate-release glucophage so dosage can be increased.

Drug Administration

P.O.

- Administer twice-daily dosages with meals, once in the morning and once in the evening.
- Administer once-daily dosages of immediate-release tablets with morning meal.
- Administer extended-release tablets with evening meal.
- Extended-release tablets should be swallowed whole and not chewed, crushed, or split.

Route	Onset	Peak	Duration
P.O.	3 hr	2–3 hr	Unknown
P.O./Solution	Unknown	3.5–6.5 hr	Unknown
P.O./E.R.	Unknown	4–8 hr	Unknown

Half-life: 4–9 hr

Mechanism of Action

May promote storage of excess glucose as glycogen in the liver, which reduces glucose production. Metformin also may improve glucose use by adipose tissue and skeletal muscle to increase glucose transport across cell membranes. This drug also may increase the number of insulin receptors on cell membranes and make them more sensitive to insulin. In addition, metformin modestly decreases blood total cholesterol and triglyceride levels.

Contraindications

Acute or chronic metabolic acidosis, including diabetic ketoacidosis with or without coma; hypersensitivity to metformin or its components; severe renal disease

M

(estimated glomerular filtration rate below 30 ml/min)

Interactions

DRUGS

calcium channel blockers, corticosteroids, estrogens, isoniazid, nicotinic acid, oral contraceptives, phenothiazines, phenytoin, sympathomimetics, thiazide and other diuretics, thyroid drugs: Possibly reduced effectiveness of metformin resulting in hyperglycemia

carbonic anhydrase inhibitors such as acetazolamide, dichlorphenamide, topiramate, zonisamide: Possibly increased risk of lactic acidosis

cimetidine, dolutegravir, ranolazine, vandetanib: Increased blood metformin level and possibly increased risk of lactic acidosis

insulin, sulfonylureas: Increased risk of hypoglycemia

ACTIVITIES

alcohol use: Increased risk of hypoglycemia and lactate formation

Adverse Reactions

CNS: Headache
EENT: Metallic taste
ENDO: **Hypoglycemia**
GI: Abdominal distention, anorexia, constipation, diarrhea, flatulence, **hepatic injury**, indigestion, nausea, vomiting
HEME: **Aplastic anemia**, megaloblastic anemia, **thrombocytopenia**
SKIN: Photosensitivity, rash
Other: **Lactic acidosis**, vitamin B$_{12}$ deficiency (with immediate-release formulation), weight loss

Childbearing Considerations

PREGNANCY

- It is not known if drug causes fetal harm although it does cross the placental barrier.
- Use with caution only if benefit to mother outweighs potential risk to fetus.

LACTATION

- Drug is present in breast milk.
- Patient should check with prescriber before breastfeeding.

REPRODUCTION

- Caution women of childbearing age of the potential for unintended pregnancy as drug may cause ovulation in some anovulatory women.
- Advise women of childbearing age not wishing to conceive to use effective contraception measures while taking drug.

Nursing Considerations

- Know that metformin should never be given to a patient with severe renal impairment (eGFR below 30 ml/min). Also be aware that metformin is not recommended for use in patients with hepatic impairment because of risk of lactic acidosis.
- Expect prescriber to alter dosage if patient has a condition that decreases or delays gastric emptying, such as diarrhea, gastroparesis, GI obstruction, ileus, or vomiting.
- Expect to assess patient's estimated glomerular filtration rate (eGFR) at least annually. Anticipate that the elderly and those at increased risk for renal impairment may be tested more frequently. Be aware that initiation of metformin is not recommended in patients who have an eGFR between 45 and 60 ml/min.

! WARNING Monitor patient closely for signs and symptoms of lactic acidosis that often are subtle and nonspecific, such as abdominal pain, increased somnolence, malaise, myalgias, and respiratory distress. Know that hypotension and resistant bradyarrhythmias have occurred with severe acidosis. Be aware that most cases of lactic acidosis have occurred in patients with significant renal impairment because metformin is substantially excreted by the kidneys. Other risk factors include being age 65 or older; certain drug interactions, such as carbonic anhydrase inhibitors; excessive alcohol intake; hepatic impairment; hypoxic states; radiologic studies with contrast; and withholding of fluids and food, which increases risk of volume depletion. If lactic acidosis is suspected, notify prescriber, expect metformin to be immediately discontinued, and provide appropriate supportive care. Know that prompt hemodialysis may be needed to correct the acidosis and remove the accumulated metformin.

- Monitor patient's blood glucose level to evaluate drug effectiveness. Assess for hyperglycemia and the need for insulin during times of increased stress, such as infection and surgery.

- Withhold drug, as ordered, if patient becomes dehydrated or develops hypoxemia or sepsis because these conditions increase the risk of lactic acidosis.
- Know that iodinated contrast media used in radiographic studies increase risk of renal failure and lactic acidosis during metformin therapy. Expect to withhold drug for 48 hours before and after testing.
- Expect yearly measurements of patient's hematologic status as well as vitamin B_{12} level. Be aware that vitamin B_{12} deficiency has occurred with use of the immediate-release formulation of metformin.

PATIENT TEACHING

- Instruct patient to take immediate-release metformin tablet at breakfast if taking drug once a day, or at breakfast and dinner if taking drug twice a day. Instruct him to take E.R. tablets once daily with evening meal and to swallow tablets whole without chewing or crushing.
- Direct patient to take drug exactly as prescribed and not to change the dosage or frequency unless instructed.
- Emphasize importance of checking blood glucose level regularly, controlling weight, exercising regularly, and following prescribed diet.
- Teach patient how to measure blood glucose level and recognize hyperglycemia and hypoglycemia. Urge him to notify prescriber of abnormal blood glucose level.
- Caution patient to avoid alcohol, which can increase the risk of hypoglycemia and lactic acidosis.

! WARNING Instruct patient to report early signs of lactic acidosis, including drowsiness, hyperventilation, malaise, and muscle pain.

- Advise patient to expect laboratory testing of glycosylated hemoglobin every 3 months until blood glucose is controlled.
- Alert women of childbearing age that metformin may cause ovulation in some premenopausal anovulatory women, which may lead to unintended pregnancy.

methadone hydrochloride
Dolophine, Metadol (CAN), Methadose

Class, Category, and Schedule
Pharmacologic class: Opioid
Therapeutic class: Opioid agonist
Controlled substance schedule: II

Indications and Dosages
* *To manage opioid detoxification and then maintenance of opioid abstinence*

DISPERSIBLE TABLETS, ORAL CONCENTRATE, ORAL SOLUTION, TABLETS

Adults. *Initial on day 1:* 20 to 30 mg as a single dose, followed by 5 to 10 mg 2 to 4 hr later, if needed. *Maximum for day 1:* 40 mg. *Maintenance:* Highly individualized with dosage adjustments made until opioid withdrawal symptoms have ceased for 24 hr. *Maximum:* 120 mg daily.

I.V., I.M., OR SUBCUTANEOUS INJECTION

Hospitalized adults unable to take drug orally. Highly individualized. If oral methadone had been used prior to hospitalization, dosage initially decreased by 50%.

* *To manage moderate to severe pain when a continuous, around-the-clock opioid analgesic is needed for an extended period of time and for which alternative treatment options are inadequate*

TABLETS

Adults. *Initial:* 2.5 mg every 8 to 12 hr increased slowly, as needed, every 3 to 5 days.

I.V., I.M., OR SUBCUTANEOUS INJECTION

Adults unable to take drug orally. *Initial:* 2.5 to 10 mg every 8 to 12 hr increased slowly, as needed, every 3 to 5 days.

±DOSAGE ADJUSTMENT For elderly patients and patients with hepatic or renal dysfunction, initial dose reduced.

Drug Administration
- Store all forms of drug at room temperature. Protect from light.
- Make sure opioid antagonist and equipment for administering oxygen and controlling

M

respiration are nearby before giving methadone.
- Protect parenteral forms from light.
- Have naloxone readily available to treat an emergency opioid overdose.

P.O.
- For liquid forms, dilute with at least 120 ml water or an acidic beverage such as orange juice and use a calibrated device to measure dosage.
- Dissolve dispersible tablets in 120 ml of water, orange juice, or other citrus-flavored non-alcoholic beverage before giving. Administer immediately. Dispersible tablet may not completely dissolve in water. If a residue remains in the cup after initial administration with water, add a small amount of liquid to the cup and give to patient to drink to ensure that all of the drug has been ingested. Do not store mixture.

I.V.
- Follow manufacturer guidelines for preparation and administration of drug, as it is highly individualized.
- *Incompatibilities:* None listed by manufacturer

I.M.
- Preferred parenteral route.
- Inject into a large muscle mass.
- Rotate sites.

SUBCUTANEOUS
- Rotate sites.

Route	Onset	Peak	Duration
P.O.	30–60 min	1–7 hr	4–8 hr
I.V.	Unknown	Unknown	4–8 hr
I.M./SubQ	10–20 min	Unknown	4–8 hr

Half-life: 8–59 hr.

Mechanism of Action

Binds with and activates opioid receptors (primarily mu receptors) in spinal cord and higher levels of CNS to produce analgesia and euphoric effects.

Contraindications

Acute or severe bronchial asthma in unmonitored setting or in absence of resuscitative equipment, hypersensitivity to methadone or its components, paralytic ileus, significant respiratory depression

Interactions

DRUGS

5-HT3 receptor antagonists, certain muscle relaxants (cyclobenzaprine, metaxalone), drugs that affect the serotonin neurotransmitter system (mirtazapine, tramadol, trazodone), I.V. methylene blue, linezolid, MAO inhibitors, selective serotonin reuptake inhibitors (SSRIs), serotonin and norepinephrine reuptake inhibitors (SNRIs), tricyclic antidepressants, triptans: Increased risk of serotonin syndrome
anticholinergics: Possibly severe constipation leading to ileus; urine retention
benzodiazepines, CNS depressants, other opioids, sedating antihistamines, tricyclic antidepressants: Increased risk of significant respiratory depression and other life-threatening adverse effects
CYP3A4, CYP2B6, CYP2C19, CYP2C9 inducers such as carbamazepine, phenobarbital, phenytoin, rifampin, St. John's wort: Decreased methadone concentration, resulting in decreased efficacy or onset of withdrawal symptoms in patients dependent on methadone
CYP3A4, CYP2B6, CYP2C19, CYP2C9, CYP2D6 inhibitors such as azole-antifungal agents, macrolide antibiotics, protease inhibitors, some selective serotonin reuptake inhibitors (fluvoxamine, sertraline): Increased methadone concentration, resulting in increased or prolonged opioid effects that may result in a fatal overdose
desipramine: Increased plasma desipramine levels
didanosine, stavudine: Decreased area under the concentration-time curve and peak levels of these drugs
diuretics: Decreased diuresis
diuretics, laxatives, mineralocorticoid hormones: Increased risk of electrolyte disturbances and prolonged QT interval
MAO inhibitors: Possibly increased risk of opioid toxicity or serotonin syndrome
mixed agonist-antagonist analgesics and partial agonist opioid analgesics such as buprenorphine, butorphanol, nalbuphine, pentazocine: Possibly reduced analgesic effect of methadone; possibly precipitation of withdrawal symptoms
muscle relaxants: Possibly enhanced neuromuscular blocking action of skeletal

muscle relaxants; increased degree of respiratory depression

zidovudine: Increased zidovudine levels possibly resulting in toxic effects

ACTIVITIES

alcohol use: Increased CNS and respiratory depression, possibly hypotension

Adverse Reactions

CNS: Agitation, amnesia, anxiety, asthenia, **coma**, confusion, decreased concentration, delirium, delusions, depression, dizziness, drowsiness, dysphoria, euphoria, fever, hallucinations, headache, insomnia, lethargy, light-headedness, malaise, psychosis, restlessness, sedation, **seizures**, syncope, tremor

CV: Bradycardia, cardiac arrest, cardiomyopathy, edema, **heart failure, hypotension**, orthostatic hypotension, palpitations, phlebitis, **prolonged QT interval, shock**, tachycardia, **torsades de pointes**, T-wave inversion on ECG, **ventricular fibrillation or tachycardia**

EENT: Blurred vision, diplopia, dry mouth, glossitis, **laryngeal edema or laryngospasm**, miosis, nystagmus, rhinitis, strabismus

ENDO: Adrenal insufficiency, hypoglycemia

GI: Abdominal cramps or pain, anorexia, biliary tract spasm, constipation, diarrhea, dysphagia, elevated liver enzymes, gastroesophageal reflux, hiccups, ileus and **toxic megacolon** (in patients with inflammatory bowel disease), indigestion, nausea, vomiting

GU: Amenorrhea, decreased ejaculate potency, decreased libido, difficult ejaculation, impotence, infertility, lack of menstruation, urinary hesitancy, urine retention

HEME: Anemia, **leukopenia, thrombocytopenia**

MS: Arthralgia

RESP: Apnea, asthma exacerbation, atelectasis, bronchospasm, depressed cough reflex, **hypoventilation, pulmonary edema, respiratory arrest or depression**, wheezing

SKIN: Diaphoresis, flushing

Other: Allergic reaction; angioedema; hypokalemia; hypomagnesemia; injection-site edema, pain, rash, or redness; physical and psychological dependence; weight gain; withdrawal symptoms

Childbearing Considerations

PREGNANCY

- Drug may cause fetal harm.
- Prolonged use of drug during pregnancy can result in neonatal opioid withdrawal syndrome (NOWS), which may be life-threatening if not recognized and treated.
- Use with extreme caution only if benefit to mother outweighs potential risk to fetus.
- Pregnancy can decrease the terminal half-life of drug during the second and third trimesters resulting in possible withdrawal symptoms in some pregnant women. To avoid this, dosage may have to be increased or the dosing interval decreased to achieve therapeutic effect.

LABOR & DELIVERY

- Opioid-dependent women on methadone maintenance therapy may need additional analgesia during labor.
- Opioids cross the placental barrier and may produce respiratory depression and psycho-physiologic effects in the newborn. Monitor newborn closely for signs of excess sedation and respiratory depression.
- An opioid antagonist, such as naloxone, must be available at the time of delivery in the event it is needed to reverse opioid-induced respiratory depression in the neonate.

LACTATION

- Drug is present in breast milk.
- Patient should check with prescriber before breastfeeding.
- If breastfeeding occurs, monitor infant for excess sedation and respiratory depression.

REPRODUCTION

- Chronic use of opioids may reduce fertility.

Nursing Considerations

- Assess patient's current drug use, including all prescription and OTC drugs before therapy begins. Be aware that excessive use of methadone may lead to abuse, addiction, misuse, overdose, and possibly death. Monitor patient's intake of drug closely.
- Be aware that use of methadone requires a Risk Evaluation and Mitigation Strategy (REMS) before drug can be dispensed, to ensure that the benefits outweigh the risks of abuse, addiction, and misuse.

M

- Know that benzodiazepine and other CNS depressant therapy should only be used concomitantly in patients for whom other treatment options are inadequate. If prescribed together, expect dosing and duration of methadone to be limited. Monitor patient closely for signs and symptoms of a decrease in consciousness, including coma, profound sedation, and significant respiratory depression. Notify prescriber immediately and provide emergency supportive care, as death may occur.
- Use extreme caution when administering methadone to patients with conditions accompanied by hypercapnia or hypoxia or decreased respiratory reserve such as asthma, chronic obstructive pulmonary disease or cor pulmonale, CNS depression or coma, kyphoscoliosis, myxedema, severe obesity, or sleep apnea syndrome. This is because methadone, even with usual therapeutic doses, may decrease respiratory drive while simultaneously increasing airway resistance to the point of apnea. Know that the peak respiratory depressant effect of methadone occurs later and persists longer than the peak analgesic effect. Monitor patient's respiratory status closely, especially when initiating drug or following a dosage increase.

! WARNING Give drug cautiously to patients at risk for a prolonged QT interval, such as those with cardiac hypertrophy, hypokalemia, or hypomagnesemia; those with a history of cardiac conduction abnormalities; and those taking diuretics or medications that affect cardiac conduction.

- Monitor patient for expected excessive confusion, drowsiness, or unsteadiness during first 3 to 5 days of therapy, and notify prescriber if effects continue to worsen or persist beyond this time.

! WARNING Monitor circulatory and respiratory status carefully and often during methadone therapy, especially when drug therapy is initiated and when patient is being converted to methadone, because cardiac arrest, circulatory or respiratory depression, hypotension, respiratory arrest, and shock can develop. Life-threatening respiratory depression can occur even when drug is being used as prescribed and is not abused or misused. Be especially vigilant with cachectic, debilitated, and elderly patients, who are at higher risk for developing respiratory depression. Assess patient for excessive or persistent sedation; dosage may have to be adjusted.

- Be aware that patients tolerant to other opioids may be incompletely tolerant to methadone. A high degree of "opioid tolerance" does not eliminate the possibility of methadone toxicity. Some patients have died during conversion from chronic high-dose therapy with other opioid agonists. Monitor patient closely during the conversion process.
- Watch for drug tolerance, especially in patients with a history of chronic drug abuse, because methadone can cause physical and psychological dependence.
- Monitor patient for pain because maintenance dosage doesn't provide pain relief; patients with tolerance to opiate agonists, including those with chronic cancer pain, may require a higher dosage.
- Know that chronic maternal use of methadone during pregnancy can result in NOWS, which may be life-threatening if not recognized and treated appropriately. Monitor patients who are pregnant or who have liver or renal impairment for increased adverse effects from methadone because drug may have a prolonged duration and cumulative effect in these patients. Methadone may prolong labor by reducing duration, frequency, or strength of uterine contractions, so expect dosage to be tapered before third trimester of pregnancy. Breastfeeding mothers on maintenance therapy put their infants at risk of withdrawal symptoms if they abruptly stop breastfeeding or discontinue methadone therapy. Methadone also accumulates in CNS tissue, increasing the risk of seizures in infants.
- Check plasma amylase and lipase levels in patients who develop biliary tract spasms because levels may increase up to 15 times normal. Notify prescriber immediately of any significant or sustained increase.

- Monitor patients who have head injuries or other conditions that may increase intracranial pressure (ICP) because methadone may further increase ICP.
- Assess patient for withdrawal symptoms and tolerance to therapy because physiologic dependence can occur with long-term methadone use. Avoid abrupt discontinuation because withdrawal symptoms will occur within 3 to 4 days after last dose.
- Monitor patients, especially the elderly, for cardiac arrhythmias, hypotension, hypovolemia, orthostatic hypotension, and vasovagal syncope because methadone may produce cholinergic effects in patients with cardiac disease, resulting in bradycardia and peripheral vasodilation; dosage decrease may be indicated.
- Monitor patients with prostatic hypertrophy, renal disease, or urethral stricture for urine retention and oliguria because methadone can increase tension of detrusor muscle.
- Be prepared to treat patient's symptoms of anxiety; be aware that anxiety may be confused with symptoms of opioid abstinence and that methadone doesn't have antianxiety effects.
- Monitor patients with seizure disorders because methadone may induce or aggravate seizure activity.

! **WARNING** Know that many drugs may interact with opioids like methadone to cause serotonin syndrome. Monitor patient closely for signs and symptoms such as agitation, diaphoresis, diarrhea, fever, hallucinations, labile blood pressure, muscle twitching or stiffness, nausea, shakiness, shivering, tachycardia, trouble with coordination, or vomiting. Notify prescriber at once because serotonin syndrome may be life-threatening. Be prepared to discontinue drug, if possible and ordered, and provide supportive care. Also be aware that concomitant use of methadone with CYP3A4, CYP2B6, CYP2C19, or CYP2D6 inhibitors or discontinuation of concomitantly used CYP3A4, CYP2B6, CYP2C19, or CYP2C9 inducers can result in a fatal overdose.

- Monitor patient for adrenal insufficiency. Although rare, it can be life-threatening.

Monitor patient for anorexia, dizziness, fatigue, hypotension, nausea, vomiting, or weakness. Notify prescriber if adrenal insufficiency is suspected and expect diagnostic testing to be done. If confirmed, expect to administer corticosteroids and wean patient off methadone, if possible.

PATIENT TEACHING

- Inform patient that misuse of drug either by taking excessive amounts or by taking drug for prolonged periods of time can lead to addiction, overdose, or even death. Therefore, tell patient to take drug exactly as prescribed and for the shortest time possible.
- Instruct patient taking liquid forms of drug to dilute in 120 ml of water or an acidic beverage, take immediately, and use a calibrated device to measure dosage (not a household spoon).
- Instruct patient to dissolve dispersible tablets in 120 ml of water, orange juice, or other citrus-flavored non-alcoholic liquid immediately before administration. Alert patient that if residue is left in the cup after ingesting, he should add a little more liquid to the cup and drink to ensure that all the drug was consumed.
- Advise patient to notify prescriber of all other drugs he's currently taking, including benzodiazepines, and to avoid alcohol and other depressants, such as sleeping pills and tranquilizers, because they may increase drug's CNS depressant effects and cause severe respiratory depression that could result in death.

! **WARNING** Warn patient and family that an opioid overdose can result in death. Instruct family or caregiver on the signs and symptoms of an overdose, including respiratory depression. Stress importance of having naloxone available for emergency use in the event patient experiences an opioid overdose. Instruct family or caregiver how to administer naloxone and stress the need to call 911 right away because naloxone effects are only temporary.

- Inform patient that abrupt cessation of methadone therapy can precipitate withdrawal symptoms. Urge him to notify prescriber if he develops any concerns over therapy.

- Urge patient to notify prescriber if he experiences dizziness, light-headedness, palpitations, or syncope, which may be caused by methadone-induced arrhythmias.
- Instruct patient to avoid potentially hazardous activities or those that require mental alertness because methadone therapy may cause drowsiness or sleepiness.
- Teach patient to change positions slowly to minimize the effects of orthostatic hypotension.
- Instruct patient to notify prescriber of worsening or breakthrough pain because dosage may have to be adjusted.
- Instruct female patient to notify prescriber immediately if she becomes pregnant.
- Instruct patient or parents to keep methadone out of the reach of children because accidental ingestion can be fatal.
- Inform patient that long-term use of opioids like methadone may decrease sex hormone levels, causing decreased libido, erectile dysfunction, impotence, infertility, or lack of menstruation. Encourage patient to report any symptoms.
- Advise patient that drug may cause severe constipation and to take measures to avoid constipation. If unresolved or severe, tell patient to seek medical attention.

methimazole

Tapazole

Class and Category

Pharmacologic class: Thyroid hormone antagonist
Therapeutic class: Antithyroid

Indications and Dosages

* *To treat hyperthyroidism in preparation for radioactive iodine therapy or thyroidectomy; to treat Graves' disease with hyperthyroidism or toxic multinodular goiter for whom radioactive iodine therapy or surgery is not an appropriate treatment option*

TABLETS

Adults. *Initial:* 15 mg daily for mild hyperthyroidism, 30 to 40 mg daily for moderate hyperthyroidism, and 60 mg daily for severe hyperthyroidism given in divided doses three times daily 8 hr apart for 6 to 8 wk or until euthyroid level is reached. *Maintenance:* 5 to 15 mg daily.
Children. *Initial:* 0.4 mg/kg daily in divided doses three times daily 8 hr apart. *Maintenance:* 0.2 mg/kg daily.

Drug Administration

P.O.

- Use gloves when administering tablets because it is classified as a hazardous drug.

Route	Onset	Peak	Duration
P.O.	12–18 hr	1–2 hr	36–72 hr

Half-life: 4–6 hr

Mechanism of Action

Directly interferes with thyroid hormone synthesis in the thyroid gland by inhibiting iodide incorporation into thyroglobulin. Iodination of thyroglobulin is an important step in synthesizing the thyroid hormones thyroxine and triiodothyronine. Eventually, thyroglobulin is depleted and the circulating thyroid hormone level drops.

Contraindications

Breastfeeding, hypersensitivity to methimazole or its components

Interactions

DRUGS

beta-blockers: Possibly increased blood levels of these drugs when patient becomes euthyroid
digoxin: Possibly increased blood digoxin level when patient becomes euthyroid
oral anticoagulants: Possibly action of oral anticoagulants may be potentiated
theophylline: Increased blood theophylline level when patient becomes euthyroid

Adverse Reactions

CNS: Drowsiness, headache, paresthesia, vertigo
CV: Edema
EENT: Loss of taste
ENDO: Hypothyroidism
GI: Diarrhea, indigestion, jaundice, nausea, vomiting
HEME: Agranulocytosis, aplastic anemia, leukopenia, thrombocytopenia
MS: Arthralgia, myalgia
SKIN: Alopecia, pruritus, rash, skin discoloration, urticaria

Other: Lupus-like symptoms, lymphadenopathy

Childbearing Considerations

PREGNANCY

- Drug may cause fetal harm as it crosses the placental barrier and can induce goiter and even cretinism in the developing fetus. In addition, rare cases of congenital defects have occurred in infants born to mothers who received the drug during pregnancy.
- If pregnancy occurs, it is recommended that drug be discontinued and an alternative drug substituted during the pregnancy.

LACTATION

- Drug is present in breast milk.
- Patient should check with prescriber before breastfeeding.

Nursing Considerations

- Closely monitor thyroid function test results during methimazole therapy.
- Check CBC results to detect abnormalities caused by inhibition of myelopoiesis.
- Watch for signs and symptoms of hypothyroidism, such as cold intolerance, depression, and edema.
- Be aware that hyperthyroidism may increase metabolic clearance of beta-blockers and theophylline and that dosages of these drugs may have to be reduced as the patient's thyroid condition becomes corrected.

PATIENT TEACHING

- Explain about possible hair loss or thinning during and for months after therapy.
- Instruct patient to notify prescriber immediately about cold intolerance, fever, sore throat, tiredness, and unusual bleeding or bruising.

methocarbamol

Class and Category

Pharmacologic class: Carbamate derivative
Therapeutic class: Skeletal muscle relaxant

Indications and Dosages

∗ *As adjunct to relieve discomfort caused by acute, painful musculoskeletal conditions*

TABLETS

Adults. *Initial:* 1,500 mg four times daily for 2 to 3 days; for severe discomfort 8,000 mg daily in divided doses.
Maintenance: 1,000 mg four times daily. Alternatively, 750 mg every 4 hr, or 1,500 mg three times daily.

I.M. INJECTION, I.V. INJECTION

Adults. *Initial:* 1 g followed by 1 g every 8 hours, if needed, for a total of 3 g in 24 hr. Then, 1 g every 8 hr for no longer than 2 more days, if needed. *Maximum:* 3 g daily for no longer than 3 days.

∗ *To provide supportive therapy for tetanus*

TABLETS

Adults and adolescents. Up to 24 g daily in divided doses given by nasogastric tube.

I.V. INFUSION OR INJECTION

Adults. *Initial:* 1 or 2 g followed by an additional 1 or 2 g for a total dose of up to 3 g. Dosing procedure repeated every 6 hr, as needed, until nasogastric tube can be inserted and oral therapy begun.
Children. *Initial:* 15 mg/kg and repeated every 6 hr, as needed. *Maximum:* $1.8 \text{ g/m}^2/$ day for 3 consecutive days only.

Drug Administration

P.O.

- Administer tablets with food or milk to minimize nausea.
- Crush tablets and mix with water or saline solution for administration by NG tube.

I.V.

- For I.V. injection, administer undiluted into the vein or give through infusion line at a maximum rate of 3 ml/min.
- For I.V. infusion, add 10 ml of drug to no more than 250 ml 0.9% Sodium Chloride Injection or 5% Dextrose in Water. Infuse at no more than 300 mg (3 ml)/min to avoid hypotension and seizures.
- Care should be taken to avoid extravasation because thrombophlebitis may occur.
- Keep patient recumbent during I.V. administration and for at least 15 minutes afterward. Then have him rise slowly.
- *Incompatibilities:* None listed by manufacturer

I.M.

- Inject deep into large muscle, such as the gluteus.
- Give no more than 5 ml/gluteal region.
- Don't give methocarbamol by subcutaneous route.

M

Route	Onset	Peak	Duration
P.O.	30 min	2 hr	Unknown
I.V.	Immediate	Unknown	Unknown
I.M.	Unknown	Unknown	Unknown

Half-life: 1–2 hr

Mechanism of Action

May depress CNS, which leads to sedation and reduced skeletal muscle spasms. Methocarbamol also alters perception of pain.

Contraindications

Hypersensitivity to methocarbamol or its components

Interactions

DRUGS

anticholinesterase drugs: Possibly inhibit the effect of these drugs such as pyridostigmine bromide.
CNS depressants: Increased CNS depression

ACTIVITIES

alcohol use: Increased CNS depression

Adverse Reactions

CNS: Dizziness, drowsiness, fever, headache, light-headedness, **seizures (I.V.)**, syncope, vertigo, weakness
CV: **Bradycardia**, **hypotension**, and thrombophlebitis (parenteral)
EENT: Blurred vision, conjunctivitis, diplopia, metallic taste, nasal congestion, nystagmus
GI: Nausea
GU: Black, brown, or green urine
SKIN: Flushing, pruritus, rash, urticaria
Other: **Anaphylaxis (parenteral)**, **angioedema**, injection-site irritation or pain (I.M.), injection-site sloughing (I.V.)

Childbearing Considerations

PREGNANCY

- Drug may cause fetal harm. Reports of congenital abnormalities following in utero exposure to drug have occurred.
- Drug should not be given to women who are or may become pregnant, especially early in pregnancy unless the benefit to mother outweighs potential risk to fetus.

LACTATION

- It is not known if drug is present in breast milk.

- Patient should check with prescriber before breastfeeding.

Nursing Considerations

- Keep antihistamines, corticosteroids, and epinephrine available in case patient experiences anaphylactic reaction.
- Be aware that the parenteral dosage form shouldn't be used in patients with renal dysfunction because the polyethylene glycol 300 vehicle is nephrotoxic.

PATIENT TEACHING

- Tell patient to take drug exactly as prescribed.
- Advise patient to take drug with food or milk to avoid nausea.
- Inform patient that urine may turn black, brown, or green until methocarbamol is discontinued.
- Advise patient to avoid hazardous activities until drug's CNS effects are known.
- Instruct patient to avoid alcohol and other CNS depressants during therapy.

methotrexate
(amethopterin)

Otrexup, Rasuvo, Reditrex, Xatmep

methotrexate sodium

Trexall

Class and Category

Pharmacologic class: Folate antagonist (antimetabolite)
Therapeutic class: Antineoplastic

Indications and Dosages

❋ *To treat severe psoriasis unresponsive to other therapy*

TABLETS (TREXALL)

Adults. 10 to 25 mg once weekly. *Maximum:* 30 mg/wk.

I.V. OR I.M. INJECTION (METHOTREXATE SODIUM), SUBCUTANEOUS INJECTION (OTREXUP, RASUVO, REDITREX)

Adults. 10 to 25 mg as a single dose weekly. *Maximum:* 25 to 30 mg weekly depending on product being used.

✳ *To treat severe rheumatoid arthritis unresponsive to other therapy*

TABLETS (TREXALL)

Adults. 7.5 mg once weekly. *Maximum:* 20 mg/wk.

SUBCUTANEOUS INJECTION (OTREXUP, RASUVO, REDITREX, TREXALL)

Adults. 7.5 mg once weekly, then gradually increased to achieve an optimal response. *Maximum:* 20 mg/wk.

✳ *To treat active polyarticular juvenile idiopathic arthritis unresponsive to other therapy*

ORAL SOLUTION (XATMEP), I.M. INJECTION (METHOTREXATE SODIUM), SUBCUTANEOUS INJECTION (OTREXUP, RASUVO, REDITREX), TABLETS (TREXALL)

Children ages 2 to 16. *Initial.* 10 mg/m^2 once weekly, increased gradually, as needed.

✳ *To treat neoplastic disease (acute lymphoblastic leukemia, breast cancer, gestational trophoblastic neoplasia, meningeal leukemia, non-Hodgkin lymphoma, osteosarcoma, squamous cell carcinoma of the head and neck)*

I.V. OR I.M. INJECTION (METHOTREXATE SODIUM), INTRATHECAL (METHOTREXATE), TABLETS (TREXALL)

Adults. Highly individualized depending on type of neoplasm present and product being used.

±**DOSAGE ADJUSTMENT** For patients with hepatic or renal failure, a reduced dose may be required.

☰ Drug Administration

P.O.

- Follow facility policy for handling and disposing drug because it is cytotoxic.
- Tablets should be swallowed whole and not chewed, crushed, or split.
- Administer at least 1 hour before or 2 hours after food or drink except for water.
- Use a calibrated device when measuring oral solution dosage.

I.V.

- Verify pregnancy status before initiating drug therapy in women of childbearing age.
- Follow facility policy for preparing and handling drug; parenteral form poses a risk of carcinogenicity, mutagenicity, and teratogenicity. Avoid skin contact.

- Use only preservative-free formulation of methotrexate when administering high-dose therapy or when drug is administered intrathecally to neonates or low-birth-weight infants..
- Follow manufacturer guidelines for preparation and administration, as guidelines vary between product and dosages.
- Liquid parenteral products can be further diluted with 0.9% Sodium Chloride Injection. Once diluted, drug should be used within 4 hours if stored at room temperature or 24 hours if stored in refrigerator.
- Expect to administer leucovorin rescue in patients receiving intermediate- or high-dose regimens for neoplastic disorders. Expect to administer folic acid or folinic acid to patients being treated for polyarticular juvenile idiopathic arthritis, psoriasis, or rheumatoid arthritis to reduce the risk of adverse reactions to the drug.
- *Incompatibilities:* None listed by manufacturers

I.M.

- Verify pregnancy status before initiating drug therapy in women of childbearing age.
- Follow facility policy for preparing and handling drug; parenteral form poses a risk of carcinogenicity, mutagenicity, and teratogenicity. Avoid skin contact.
- Rotate sites.

SUBCUTANEOUS

- Verify pregnancy status before initiating drug therapy in women of childbearing age.
- Follow facility policy for preparing and handling drug; subcutaneous form poses a risk of carcinogenicity, mutagenicity, and teratogenicity. Avoid skin contact.
- Administer Otrexup and Rasuvo injection using the single-dose auto-injector. If dosage not available with auto-injector, use a different formulation.
- Administer injection into patient's abdomen or thigh only.

INTRATHECAL

- Follow facility policy for preparing and handling drug; intrathecal form poses a risk of carcinogenicity, mutagenicity, and teratogenicity. Avoid skin contact.

M

- Use only preservative-free form.
- Administered only by person skilled in intrathecal injections.

Route	Onset	Peak	Duration
P.O.	Unknown	1–2 hr	Unknown
I.V.	Unknown	Unknown	Unknown
I.M.	Unknown	30–60 min	Unknown
SubQ	Unknown	1–2 hr	Unknown
Intrathecal	Unknown	Unknown	Unknown

Half-life: 3–15 hr

Mechanism of Action

May exert immunosuppressive effects by inhibiting replication and function of T and possibly B lymphocytes. Methotrexate also slows rapidly growing cells, such as epithelial skin cells in psoriasis. This action may result from the drug's inhibition of dihydrofolate reductase, the enzyme that reduces folic acid to tetrahydrofolic acid. Inhibition of tetrahydrofolic acid interferes with DNA synthesis and cell reproduction in rapidly proliferating cells. Methotrexate also interrupts the process that causes inflammation to prevent damage to joints.

Contraindications

For all conditions: Breastfeeding, hypersensitivity to methotrexate or its components; for treatment of psoriasis or rheumatoid arthritis: alcoholism; alcoholic liver disease; chronic liver disease; laboratory evidence or overt immunodeficiency syndromes; pregnancy; preexisting blood dyscrasias such as bone marrow hypoplasia, leukopenia, significant anemia, or thrombocytopenia

Interactions

DRUGS

bone marrow depressants: Possibly increased bone marrow depression
chloramphenicol, nonabsorbable broad spectrum antibiotics, tetracycline: Possibly decreased methotrexate absorption
co-trimoxazole: Possibly increased bone marrow suppression
folic acid: Possibly decreased effectiveness of methotrexate
hepatotoxic drugs: Increased risk of hepatotoxicity

NSAIDs, penicillins, phenylbutazone, phenytoin, probenecid, salicylates, sulfonamides: Increased risk of methotrexate toxicity
theophylline: Possibly increased risk of theophylline toxicity
vaccines: Risk of disseminated infection with live-virus vaccines, risk of suppressed response to killed-virus vaccines

ACTIVITIES

alcohol use: Increased risk of hepatotoxicity

Adverse Reactions

CNS: Aphasia, **cerebral thrombosis,** chills, dizziness, drowsiness, fatigue, fever, headache, hemiparesis, **leukoencephalopathy,** malaise, paresis, **seizures**
CV: Chest pain, **deep vein thrombosis, hypotension, pericardial effusion, pericarditis, thromboembolism**
ENDO: Gynecomastia
EENT: Blurred vision, conjunctivitis, gingivitis, glossitis, pharyngitis, stomatitis, transient blindness, tinnitus
GI: Abdominal pain, anorexia, **cirrhosis,** diarrhea, elevated liver enzymes, enteritis, **GI bleeding** and ulceration, **hepatitis, hepatotoxicity,** nausea, **pancreatitis,** vomiting
GU: Cystitis, hematuria, infertility, menstrual dysfunction, nephropathy, **renal failure, tubular necrosis,** vaginal discharge
HEME: Anemia, **aplastic anemia, leukopenia, neutropenia, pancytopenia, thrombocytopenia**
MS: Arthralgia, dysarthria, myalgia, stress fracture
RESP: Dry nonproductive cough, dyspnea, **interstitial pneumonitis,** pneumonia, **pulmonary fibrosis or failure, pulmonary infiltrates**
SKIN: Acne, alopecia, altered skin pigmentation, ecchymosis, **erythema multiforme, exfoliative dermatitis,** furunculosis, necrosis, photosensitivity, pruritus, psoriatic lesions, rash, **Stevens–Johnson syndrome,** telangiectasia, **toxic epidermal necrolysis,** ulceration, urticaria
Other: **Anaphylaxis,** increased risk of infection, lymphadenopathy, **lymphoproliferative disease**

⊟ Childbearing Considerations

PREGNANCY

- Drug can cause fetal harm such as embryotoxicity and fetal defects or death.
- Drug is contraindicated in pregnant women with psoriasis or rheumatoid arthritis and should be used in the treatment of neoplastic disease only if benefit to the mother outweighs the risk to the fetus.
- A negative pregnancy test should be obtained before drug therapy is started.

LACTATION

- Drug may be present in breast milk.
- Breastfeeding should not be undertaken during drug therapy and for 1 wk after final dose because it may cause myelosuppression in the breastfed infant.

REPRODUCTION

- Because of fetal harm, both partners should avoid conception during and after drug is discontinued for 3 months for male patients and 6 months for female patients.
- Drug may cause fertility impairment, menstrual dysfunction, and oligospermia during drug therapy. It is not known if infertility is reversible.

⊟ Nursing Considerations

- Monitor results of CBC, chest x-ray, liver and renal function tests, and urinalysis before and during treatment because drug can cause serious adverse reactions to many systems.
- Increase patient's fluid intake to 2 to 3 L daily, unless contraindicated, to reduce the risk of adverse GU reactions.
- Assess patient for bleeding and infection.

! WARNING Monitor patient for hypersensitivity reactions to drug because severe reactions such as anaphylaxis have occurred with drug use. Report any such reactions immediately and provide supportive care, as ordered.

- Be aware that high doses of methotrexate can impair renal elimination by forming crystals that obstruct urine flow. To prevent drug precipitation, alkalinize patient's urine with sodium bicarbonate tablets, as ordered.
- Follow standard precautions because drug can cause immunosuppression.

- Be aware that if patient becomes dehydrated from vomiting, prescriber should be notified, and expect to withhold drug until patient recovers.
- Be aware that methotrexate resistance may develop with prolonged use.

PATIENT TEACHING

- Prepare a calendar of treatment days for patient, and emphasize importance of following instructions exactly.
- Advise parents or caregivers administering oral solution form of methotrexate to use a calibrated measuring device and never to use a household measuring teaspoon because it is not an accurate measuring device.
- Teach patient prescribed weekly subcutaneous injections how to administer the injection using the single-dose auto-injector. Tell him to give the injection into his abdomen or thigh and to rotate injection sites.

! WARNING Alert patient to notify prescriber if an allergic reaction occurs; if severe, advise patient to seek immediate medical care.

- Instruct patient to avoid alcohol during methotrexate therapy. Tell patients being treated for cancer to also avoid folic acid or folinic acid unless they are directed to do so by the prescriber. However, tell patients being treated for polyarticular juvenile idiopathic arthritis, psoriasis, or rheumatoid arthritis that folic acid or folinic acid therapy may be needed to reduce the risk of adverse reactions to the drug.
- Tell patient to inform all prescribers of methotrexate therapy as well as any concomitant drugs they may be taking, including over-the-counter drugs, herbal products, and vitamins.
- Encourage frequent mouth care to reduce the risk of mouth sores.
- Instruct patient to use sunblock when exposed to sunlight.
- Instruct patient on infection control measures to take while receiving methotrexate.
- Advise patient to notify prescriber about bruising, chills, cough, dark or bloody urine, fever, mouth sores, shortness of

M

breath, sore throat, and yellow skin or eyes as well as any other serious or unusual adverse reaction.

- Urge women of childbearing age to use reliable contraception during methotrexate therapy and for 6 mo after last dose. Also tell women who are breastfeeding not to breastfeed during drug therapy and for 1 wk following final dose.

methoxypolyethylene glycol-epoetin beta
Mircera

Class and Category
Pharmacological class: Erythropoietin stimulating protein
Therapeutic class: Antianemic

Indications and Dosages
✴ *To treat anemia associated with chronic renal failure in dialysis-dependent and dialysis-independent patients*

I.V. INJECTION, SUBCUTANEOUS INJECTION

Adults not currently being treated with an erythropoiesis-stimulating agent.
Initial: 0.6 mcg/kg every 2 wk, increased or decreased by 25% monthly as needed.
Maintenance: Twice that of the every-two-week dose every 4 wk and subsequently titrated as necessary.

Adults stabilized on less than 8,000 units/wk of epoetin alfa or 40 mcg/wk of darbepoetin alfa. 60 mcg every 2 wk or 120 mcg every 4 wk.

Adults stabilized on 8,000 to 16,000 units/wk of epoetin alfa or 40 to 80 mcg/wk of darbepoetin alfa. 100 mcg every 2 wk or 200 mcg every 4 wk.

Adults stabilized on more than 16,000 units/wk of epoetin alfa or more than 80 mcg/wk of darbepoetin alfa. 180 mcg every 2 wk or 360 mcg every 4 wk.

I.V. INJECTION

Children ages 5 to 17 on hemodialysis who are converting from another erythropoiesis-stimulating agent (ESA) after hemoglobin level stabilized with an ESA. 4x previous weekly epoetin alfa

dose (units)/125 or 4x previous weekly darbepoetin alfa dose (mcg)/0.55.

±**DOSAGE ADJUSTMENT** If hemoglobin increase is greater than 1 g/dl during any 2-wk period or hemoglobin is approaching or exceeding 11 g/dl in adult patients on dialysis or exceeds 10 g/dl in adult patients not on dialysis, dosage reduced or interrupted. If hemoglobin continues to increase despite this reduction, drug discontinued until hemoglobin begins to decrease; then drug restarted at a dose 25% less than previously given. If hemoglobin doesn't increase by 1 g/dl after 4 wk of therapy in adult patients, dosage increased by 25%.

Drug Administration
I.V.
- Drug packaged as single-dose prefilled syringes.
- Drug contains no preservatives, so discard any unused portion.
- Do not pool unused portions from the prefilled syringes.
- Do not use the prefilled syringe more than once.
- Fully depress the plunger during injection in order for the needle guard to activate.
- Store in original cartons.
- Avoid vigorous shaking or prolonged exposure to light.
- Store in refrigerator or at room temperature (for no more than 30 days).
- *Incompatibilities:* Parenteral solutions, other drugs mixed in prefilled syringes

SUBCUTANEOUS
- Follow guidelines for I.V. administration.
- Administer in the abdomen, arm, or thigh.
- Rotate sites.

Route	Onset	Peak	Duration
I.V., SubQ	7–15 days	72 hr	Unknown

Half-life: 134 hours

Mechanism of Action
Stimulates release of reticulocytes from bone marrow into the bloodstream, where they develop into mature RBCs.

Contraindications
Hypersensitivity to methoxypolyethylene glycol-epoetin beta or its components, pure red cell aplasia, uncontrolled hypertension

☰ Interactions

DRUGS

None reported by manufacturer

☰ Adverse Reactions

CNS: CVA, headache, **seizures**
CV: Chest pain, **congestive heart failure, deep vein thrombosis,** hypertension, **hypotension, MI,** tachycardia, vascular access thrombosis
EENT: Nasopharyngitis
GI: Constipation, diarrhea, **GI bleeding,** vomiting
GU: UTI
HEME: Severe anemia including pure red cell aplasia
MS: Back or limb pain, muscle spasms
RESP: Bronchospasms, cough, upper respiratory tract infection
SKIN: Erythema, pruritus, rash, **Stevens–Johnson syndrome, toxic epidermal necrolysis,** urticaria
Other: Anaphylaxis, angioedema, antibody formation to drug

☰ Childbearing Considerations

PREGNANCY

- It is not known if drug causes fetal harm.
- Use with caution only if benefit to mother outweighs potential risk to fetus.

LACTATION

- It is not known if drug is present in breast milk.
- Patient should check with prescriber before breastfeeding.

☰ Nursing Considerations

- Use drug cautiously in patients who have conditions that could decrease or delay response to drug, such as aluminum intoxication, folic acid deficiency, hemolysis, infection, inflammation, iron deficiency, malignant neoplasm, osteitis (birrosa cystica), or vitamin B_{12} deficiency.
- Also use drug cautiously in patients with a cardiovascular disorder caused by a history of seizures, hypertension, vascular disease. Also use cautiously in patients with a hematologic disorder, such as hypercoagulation, myelodysplastic syndrome, or sickle cell disease.
- Be aware that if patient's blood pressure is difficult to control even with dietary measures or drug therapy, dose of

methoxypolyethylene glycol-epoetin beta should be reduced or drug withheld until blood pressure is controlled.

! WARNING Know that target hemoglobin shouldn't exceed 11 g/dl because it increases risk of life-threatening adverse cardiovascular effects.

- Monitor drug effectiveness by checking hemoglobin every 2 weeks until stabilized and maintenance dose has been established. Then expect hemoglobin to be monitored at least monthly unless dosage adjustment is needed.
- Expect to give an iron supplement because iron requirements rise when erythropoiesis consumes existing iron stores.
- Notify prescriber if patient has sudden loss of response to drug, evidenced by low reticulocyte count or severe anemia. Anti-erythropoietin antibody-related anemia may be present, which requires stopping drug and any other erythropoietic proteins.
- Take seizure precautions, especially during the first couple months of therapy.
- Keep in mind the risk of hypertensive or thrombotic complications increases if hemoglobin rises more than 1 g/dl over 2 weeks.

PATIENT TEACHING

- Teach patient how to administer drug and how to dispose of needles properly. Caution against reusing needles.
- Stress importance of complying with dosage regimen and keeping follow-up laboratory and medical appointments.
- Review possible adverse reactions, and urge patient to notify prescriber about chest pain, headache, hives, rapid heartbeat, rash, seizures, shortness of breath, or swelling.

! WARNING Warn patient to stop taking drug immediately if an allergic reaction occurs and notify prescriber. If serious, tell patient to seek emergency treatment.

- Advise patient that the risk of seizures is highest during the first couple of months of methoxypolyethylene glycol-epoetin beta therapy. Urge him to avoid hazardous activities during this time.
- Encourage patient to eat iron-rich foods.

M

methyldopa

Class and Category
Pharmacologic class: Central alpha agonist
Therapeutic class: Antihypertensive

Indications and Dosages
✳ *To manage hypertension*

TABLETS
Adults. *Initial:* 250 mg twice daily or three times daily for first 48 hr, decreased or increased as needed after 2 days with adjustments made no less than every 2 days. *Maintenance:* 500 to 2,000 mg daily in divided doses twice daily to four times daily. *Maximum:* 3,000 mg daily.
Children. *Initial:* 10 mg/kg daily in divided doses twice daily to four times daily for first 48 hr, decreased or increased as needed after 2 days with adjustments made no less than every 2 days. *Maximum:* 65 mg/kg or 3,000 mg daily, whichever is less.

Drug Administration

P.O.
- Drug should be administered consistently at same time each day.
- Store at room temperature.
- *Incompatibilities:* Barbiturates, sulfonamides

Route	Onset	Peak	Duration
P.O.	3–6 hr	2–4 hr	12–48 hr

Half-life: 1.5–2 hr

Mechanism of Action
Is decarboxylated in the body to produce alpha-methylnorepinephrine, a metabolite that stimulates central inhibitory alpha-adrenergic receptors. This action may reduce blood pressure by decreasing sympathetic stimulation of heart and peripheral vascular system.

Contraindications
Active hepatic disease, hypersensitivity to methyldopa or its components, impaired hepatic function from previous methyldopa therapy, use within 14 days of MAO inhibitor

Interactions

DRUGS
anesthetics: Possibly enhanced effect requiring reduced dosage of anesthetics
antihypertensives: Increased hypotension
CNS depressants: Possibly increased CNS depression
ferrous gluconate, ferrous sulfate: Decreased bioavailability of methyldopa
lithium: Increased risk of lithium toxicity
MAO inhibitors: Possibly hallucinations, headaches, hyperexcitability, and severe hypertension

ACTIVITIES
alcohol use: Possibly increased CNS depression

Adverse Reactions
CNS: Decreased concentration, depression, dizziness, drowsiness, fever, headache, involuntary motor activity, memory loss (transient), nightmares, paresthesia, Parkinsonism, sedation, vertigo, weakness
CV: Angina, **bradycardia**, edema, **heart failure, myocarditis**, orthostatic hypotension
EENT: Black or sore tongue, dry mouth, nasal congestion
ENDO: Gynecomastia
GI: Constipation, diarrhea, flatulence, **hepatic necrosis, hepatitis**, jaundice, nausea, **pancreatitis**, vomiting
GU: Decreased libido, impotence
HEME: **Agranulocytosis, hemolytic anemia, leukopenia**, positive Coombs' test, positive tests for ANA and rheumatoid factor, **thrombocytopenia**
SKIN: Eczema, rash, urticaria
Other: Weight gain

Childbearing Considerations

PREGNANCY
- It is not known if drug causes fetal harm.
- Use with caution only if benefit to mother outweighs potential risk to fetus.

LACTATION
- Drug is present in breast milk.
- Patient should check with prescriber before breastfeeding.

Nursing Considerations
- Expect to monitor CBC and differential results before and periodically during methyldopa therapy.
- Monitor blood pressure regularly during therapy.
- Monitor results of Coombs' test; a positive result after several months of treatment indicates that patient has hemolytic anemia. Expect to discontinue drug.

- Assess for edema and weight gain. If they develop, give a diuretic, as prescribed.
- Notify prescriber if patient has signs of heart failure (dyspnea, edema, hypertension) or involuntary, rapid, jerky movements.
- Be aware that hypertension may return within 48 hours after stopping drug.

PATIENT TEACHING

- Instruct patient to take methyldopa exactly as prescribed and not to skip a dose. Explain that hypertension can return within 48 hours after stopping drug.
- Instruct patient to weigh himself daily and to report a gain of more than 5 lb (2.3 kg) in 2 days.
- Advise patient to change position slowly to minimize orthostatic hypotension.
- Direct patient to notify prescriber about bruising, chest pain, fever, involuntary jerky movements, prolonged dizziness, rash, and yellow eyes or skin.
- Caution patient not to stop drug abruptly; doing so may cause withdrawal symptoms, such as headache, hypertension, increased sweating, nausea, and tremor.

methylnaltrexone bromide

Relistor

▤ Class and Category

Pharmacologic class: Peripheral mu-opioid receptor antagonist
Therapeutic class: GI effector

▤ Indications and Dosages

✶ *To treat opioid-induced constipation in patients receiving palliative care and not responsive to laxative therapy.*

SUBCUTANEOUS INJECTION

Adults weighing more than 114 kg (251 lb). 0.15 mg/kg every other day, as needed.
Adults weighing 62 to 114 kg (136 to 251 lb). 12 mg every other day, as needed.
Adults weighing 38 to less than 62 kg (84 to less than 136 lb). 8 mg every other day, as needed.
Adults weighing less than 38 kg (84 lb). 0.15 mg/kg every other day, as needed.

±**DOSAGE ADJUSTMENT** For patient with moderate to severe renal impairment, dosage reduced by half.

✶ *To treat opioid-induced constipation in patients with chronic noncancer pain*

SUBCUTANEOUS INJECTION

Adults. 12 mg once daily.

TABLETS

Adults. 450 mg once daily in the morning.

±**DOSAGE ADJUSTMENT** For patients receiving palliative care, with moderate to severe renal failure (creatinine clearance less than 60 ml/min), dosage reduced by half for subcutaneous injection. For patients with chronic noncancer pain with moderate to severe hepatic or renal impairment taking tablet form, daily dosage reduced to 150 mg daily.

▤ Drug Administration

P.O.

- Administer with water on an empty stomach at least 30 minutes before first meal of the day.

SUBCUTANEOUS

- To determine volume of drug to give to patients who weigh more than 114 kg (251 lb) or less than 38 kg (84 lb), multiply patient's weight in pounds by 0.0034 and round up to the nearest 0.1 ml. Or, multiply patient's weight in kilograms by 0.0075 and round up to the nearest 0.1 ml. For patients who weigh 62 to 114 kg (136 to 251 lb), injection volume administered should be 0.6 ml. For patients who weigh 38 to less than 62 kg (84 to less than 136 lb), injection volume administered should be 0.4 ml.
- Solution should be clear and colorless to pale yellow.
- Once drug is drawn into syringe, drug is stable for 24 hours at room temperature.
- Inject into abdomen, thigh, or upper arm.
- Rotate injection sites.

Route	Onset	Peak	Duration
P.O.	30–60 min	30 min	Unknown
SubQ	Unknown	0.5 hr	Unknown

Half-life: 8 hr

▤ Mechanism of Action

Binds to peripherally acting mu-opioid receptors in the GI tract, preventing opioid-induced slowing of GI motility and

M

transit time. When motility and transit time are restored to normal, constipation is relieved.

Contraindications

Hypersensitivity to methylnaltrexone bromide or its components, GI obstruction

Interactions

DRUGS

other opioid antagonists: Possible additive effects and increased risk of opioid withdrawal

Adverse Reactions

CNS: Anxiety, chills, dizziness, headache, malaise, tremor
EENT: Rhinorrhea
ENDO: Hot flashes
GI: Abdominal distention, pain, or tenderness; diarrhea; flatulence; GI cramping, **GI perforation**; nausea; vomiting
MS: Muscle spasms
SKIN: Excessive diaphoresis, piloerection

Childbearing Considerations

PREGNANCY

- Drug may cause fetal harm as drug may precipitate opioid withdrawal in a fetus at birth.
- Use with caution only if benefit to mother outweighs potential risk to fetus.

LACTATION

- It is not known if drug is present in breast milk.
- Breastfeeding should not be undertaken during drug therapy

Nursing Considerations

- Use methylnaltrexone cautiously in patients with known or suspected lesions of the gastrointestinal (GI) tract as well as conditions that may affect the structural integrity of the GI tract wall, such as diverticular disease, infiltrative GI tract malignancies, Ogilvie's syndrome, peptic ulcer disease, and peritoneal metastases, because of increased risk of GI perforation.
- Know that food affects absorption of tablet form of drug. Give on an empty stomach only with water 30 minutes before the first meal of the day.
- Notify prescriber about persistent or severe diarrhea, and expect drug to be discontinued. Be aware that elderly patients experience a higher incidence of diarrhea.

- Monitor patient for development of persistent, severe, or worsening abdominal pain because gastrointestinal perforation may occur with severe constipation that has not responded to methylnaltrexone therapy. Notify prescriber immediately and expect drug to be discontinued.
- Monitor patient for symptoms of opioid withdrawal such as abdominal pain, anxiety, chills, diaphoresis, diarrhea, or yawning that has occurred with methylnaltrexone therapy. Patients at greatest risk for opioid withdrawal are those who have disruptions to the blood–brain barrier with opioid administration.

PATIENT TEACHING

- Instruct patient prescribed tablet form to take it on an empty stomach with water 30 minutes before the first meal of the day.
- Teach patient or caregiver how to prepare and give methylnaltrexone subcutaneously. Stress need to rotate injection sites.
- Inform patient that a bowel movement may occur within 30 minutes after drug has been administered.
- Advise patient that if abdominal pain, nausea, persistent or severe diarrhea, or vomiting that is new or worsens occurs, prescriber should be notified and drug discontinued.
- Reassure patient that drug is not a controlled substance.
- Tell patient to stop taking methylnaltrexone if she stops taking opioid pain medication.

methylphenidate hydrochloride

Adhansia XR, Aptensio XR, Concerta, Cotempla XR-ODT, Daytrana, Jornay PM, Methylin, Methylin ER, QuilliChew ER, Quillivant XR, Ritalin, Ritalin SR

Class, Category, and Schedule

Pharmacologic class: Piperidine
Therapeutic class: CNS stimulant
Controlled substance schedule: II

Indications and Dosages

* *To treat attention-deficit hyperactivity disorder (ADHD)*

ORAL SOLUTION, S.R. TABLETS, TABLETS (METHYLIN, RITALIN)

Adults. *Initial:* 10 mg twice daily or three times daily 30 to 45 min before breakfast and lunch, and a third dose between 2 and 4 pm, if needed. Increased by 5 to 10 mg weekly, as needed. *Maximum:* 60 mg daily in two or three divided doses.

Children age 6 and over. *Initial:* 5 mg twice daily 30 to 45 min before breakfast and lunch; increased by 5 to 10 mg daily at 1-wk intervals. *Maximum:* 60 mg daily in two to three divided doses.

SUSTAINED-RELEASE TABLETS (RITALIN SR)

Adults and children age 6 and over who are switching from immediate-release to sustained-release form. *Initial:* If dosage same as immediate release and not taken more frequently than every 8 hr, sustained-release dosage taken once daily before breakfast and increased by 10 mg weekly, as needed. *Maximum:* 60 mg once daily before breakfast.

E.R. CAPSULES (RITALIN LA)

Adults and children ages 6 to 12 years. *Initial:* 10 or 20 mg once daily, increased weekly in increments of 10 mg, as needed. *Maximum:* 60 mg daily.

±**DOSAGE ADJUSTMENT** For children switching from Ritalin twice daily or Ritalin SR: if previous dose was 10 mg twice daily, dosage changed to 20 mg once daily; if previous dose was 15 mg twice daily, dosage changed to 30 mg once daily; if previous dose was 20 mg twice daily, dosage changed to 40 mg once daily; and if previous dose was 30 mg twice daily, dosage changed to 60 mg once daily.

E.R. ORAL SUSPENSION (QUILLIVANT XR)

Adults and children age 6 and over. *Initially:* 20 mg once daily in morning; increased weekly in increments of 10 to 20 mg, as needed. *Maximum:* 60 mg daily.

E.R. TABLETS (CONCERTA)

Adults age 18 to 65 years and children age 6 and over who are methylphenidate-naive. 18 mg daily before breakfast for children and adolescents and 18 mg to 36 mg once daily before breakfast for adults; increased in 18-mg increments at 1-wk intervals. *Maximum:* 72 mg daily (adults and children over age 12), 54 mg/day (children ages 6 to 12).

Adults and children age 6 and over who are currently taking immediate-release methylphenidate tablets. If previous dosage was 5 mg twice daily or three times daily, dosage switched to 18 mg once daily in morning; if previous dosage was 10 mg twice daily or three times daily, dosage switched to 36 mg once daily in morning; if previous dosage was 15 mg twice daily or three times daily, dosage switched to 54 mg in the morning; and for adults only if dosage was 20 mg twice daily or three times daily, dosage switched to 72 mg in the morning.

E.R. CAPSULES (ADHANSIA XR)

Adults and children age 6 and over. *Initial:* 25 mg once daily in morning increased in increments of 10 to 15 mg at intervals of at least 5 days. *Maximum:* 85 mg daily for adults; 70 mg daily or children.

E.R. CAPSULES (APTENSIO XR)

Adults and children age 6 and over. *Initial:* 10 mg once daily in morning, increased by 10 mg once daily weekly, as needed. *Maximum:* 60 mg once a day in the morning.

ORALLY DISINTEGRATING TABLET (COTEMPLA XR-ODT)

Children ages 6 to 17. *Initial:* 17.3 mg once daily in the morning, then titrated weekly in increments of 8.6 mg to 17.3 mg. *Maximum:* 51.8 mg daily.

E.R. CHEWABLE TABLETS (QUILLICHEW ER)

Adults and children ages 6 and over. *Initial:* 20 mg once daily in the morning, increased weekly in increments of 10 mg, 15 mg, or 20 mg daily, as needed. *Maximum:* 60 mg once daily in the morning.

E.R. CAPSULES (JORNAY PM)

Adults and children age 6 and over. 20 mg once daily in evening, increased weekly in increments of 20 mg, as needed. *Maximum:* 100 mg once daily.

TRANSDERMAL PATCH (DAYTRANA)

Adults and children age 6 and over. *Initial:* 10-mg (12.5-cm^2) patch worn 9 hr daily for wk 1; 15-mg (18.75-cm^2) patch worn 9 hr daily for wk 2; 20-mg (25-cm^2) patch worn 9 hr daily for wk 3; 30-mg (37.5-cm^2) patch worn 9 hr daily for wk 4 and thereafter.

M

Maximum: 30-mg (37.5-cm^2) patch worn 9 hr daily.

＊ *To treat narcolepsy*

ORAL SOLUTION, TABLETS (METHYLIN, RITALIN)

Adults. *Initial:* 10 mg twice daily or three times daily 30 to 45 min before meals, increased by 5 to 10 mg daily every wk, as needed. *Maximum:* 60 mg daily in two or three divided doses.

Children age 6 and over. *Initial:* 5 mg twice daily before breakfast and lunch, increased weekly in increments of 5 to 10 mg weekly. *Maximum:* 60 mg daily in divided doses.

SUSTAINED-RELEASE TABLETS (RITALIN SR)

Adults who are switching from immediate-release to sustained-release form. *Initial:* If dosage same as immediate release and not taken more frequently than every 8 hr, dosage same for sustained release taken once daily before breakfast, increased by 10 mg weekly, as needed. *Maximum:* 60 mg once daily before breakfast.

⬛ Drug Administration

P.O.

- Administer in relationship to meals or time of day according to product being administered. See Indications and Dosages section.
- Administer last dose of the day by 6 p.m., except for Jornay PM, which is administered in the evening.
- Chewable tablets should be thoroughly chewed before swallowing and administered with a full glass of water or another type of beverage.
- Tablets and capsules should be swallowed whole and not chewed, crushed, or split/opened, except for Adhansia, Aptensio XR, Jornay PM, or Ritalin LA, which may be opened and contents sprinkled onto a small amount of cool applesauce and ingested immediately. Follow with water.
- Vigorously shake oral suspension bottle for at least 10 seconds before each dose. If using the oral dosing dispenser, remove the bottle cap and confirm that the bottle adapter has been inserted into the top of the bottle. Insert the tip of the oral dosing dispenser provided into the bottle adapter, turn bottle

upside down, and withdraw prescribed amount of liquid into the oral dosing dispenser. Then remove the filled oral dosing dispenser from bottle and dispense drug directly into patient's mouth. Replace the bottle cap and wash the oral dosing dispenser after each use. Store at room temperature. Discard after 4 months.

- Use calibrated device to measure dosage of oral solution.
- Administer ODT tablets with dry, gloved hands by first peeling back the foil on the blister pack. Do not push tablet through the foil. Carefully remove tablet from blister pack and place on patient's tongue. There is no need for patient to take a drink following administration.

TRANSDERMAL

- After opening pouch and removing protective liner, apply patch to a clean, dry area on patient's hip. Press patch firmly in place for about 30 seconds.
- Avoid applying patch to skin that's damaged, irritated, or oily and avoid the waistline, where clothing may dislodge the patch.
- If a patch does fall off, a new patch may be applied, but the total exposure time for the day shouldn't exceed 9 hours.
- Rotate alternate sides of body for application.

Route	Onset	Peak	Duration
P.O. (tablets)	20–60 min	2–4 hr	3–6 hr
P.O./E.R.	20–60 min	8–12 hr	Unknown
P.O./S.R.	20–60 min	3–8 hr	Unknown
P.O. (E.R. once daily)	Unknown	Unknown	About 12 hr
Transdermal	2 hr	8–10 hr	10 hr

Half-life: 3–8 hr

⬛ Mechanism of Action

Blocks the reuptake mechanism of dopaminergic neurons in the cerebral cortex and subcortical structures of the brain, including the thalamus, decreasing motor restlessness, and improving concentration. Methylphenidate also may trigger sympathomimetic activity. This action produces decreased fatigue and increased alertness and motor activity in patients with narcolepsy.

☰ Contraindications

Agitation, marked anxiety, tension; glaucoma; hypersensitivity to methylphenidate or its components; tics or diagnosis or history of Tourette's syndrome; use within 14 days of an MAO inhibitor

☰ Interactions

DRUGS

anticonvulsants, oral anticoagulants, phenylbutazone, tricyclic antidepressants: Inhibited metabolism and increased blood levels of these drugs

antihypertensives: Decreased effectiveness of antihypertensives

buspirone, fentanyl, lithium, MAO inhibitors, selective serotonin reuptake inhibitors, serotonin–norepinephrine reuptake inhibitors, St. John's wort, tricyclic antidepressants, triptans, tryptophan: Increased risk of serotonin syndrome

gastric pH modulators: May interfere with the pharmacodynamics of ODT form

MAO inhibitors: Possibly increased adverse effects of methylphenidate, possibly severe hypertension

risperidone: Increased risk of extrapyramidal symptoms

FOODS

caffeine: Increased methylphenidate effects

ACTIVITIES

alcohol use: Possibly increased CNS effects; with long-acting forms, possible increased adverse effects

☰ Adverse Reactions

CNS: Aggressiveness, agitation, anger, anxiety, cerebral arteritis, **cerebral occlusion**, confusion, **CVA**, depression, disorientation, dizziness, drowsiness, dyskinesia, emotional lability, excessive talkativeness, fatigue, fever, hallucinations, headache, hyperactivity, hypomania, insomnia, irritability, ischemic neurologic defects (reversible), lability of affect, lethargy, mania, migraine, motor tics, nervousness, **neuroleptic malignant syndrome**, obsessive–compulsive disorder (rare), paresthesia, psychosis, restlessness, sedation, **seizures**, somnolence, **suicidal ideation**, transient mood depression, tension, tremor, Tourette's syndrome (rare), toxic psychosis, vertigo

CV: Angina, **arrhythmias, bradycardia, cardiac arrest**, chest discomfort or pain, **extrasystoles**, hypertension, **hypotension, MI**, necrotizing vasculitis, palpitations, peripheral vasculopathy including Raynaud's phenomenon, **sudden death, supraventricular tachycardia**, tachycardia, vasculitis

EENT: Accommodation abnormality, blurred vision, diplopia, dry mouth or throat, mydriasis, nasopharyngitis, pharyngitis, rhinitis, sinusitis, vision changes

ENDO: Dysmenorrhea, growth suppression in children with long-term use, gynecomastia

GI: Abdominal pain, anorexia, constipation, diarrhea, dyspepsia, elevated bilirubin and liver enzymes, **hepatotoxicity**, nausea, **severe hepatic failure or injury**, vomiting

GU: Decreased libido, hematuria, priapism

HEME: Anemia, **decreased platelet count, leukopenia, pancytopenia, thrombocytopenia, thrombocytopenic purpura**

MS: Arthralgia, myalgia, muscle tightness or twitching, **rhabdomyolysis**

RESP: Cough, dyspnea, upper respiratory tract infection

SKIN: Allergic contact dermatitis, alopecia, application-site reactions (transdermal patch), bullous skin conditions, chemical leukoderma (persistent loss of skin pigmentation with transdermal patch), excessive diaphoresis, erythema, **erythema multiforme**, exanthemas, **exfoliative dermatitis**, fixed drug eruption, pruritus, rash, urticaria

Other: **Anaphylaxis, angioedema**, elevated alkaline phosphatase, physical and psychological dependence, weight loss (prolonged use)

☰ Childbearing Considerations

PREGNANCY

- Pregnancy exposure registry: 1-866-961-2388 or https://womensmentalhealth.org/adhd-medications/.
- It is not known if drug causes fetal harm.
- Use with caution only if benefit to mother outweighs potential risk to fetus.

LACTATION

- Drug is present in breast milk.
- Patient should check with prescriber before breastfeeding.

M

- If breastfeeding occurs, infant should be monitored for agitation, anorexia, insomnia, and reduced weight gain.

Nursing Considerations

! WARNING Be aware that methylphenidate may induce CNS stimulation and psychosis and may worsen behavior disturbances and thought disorders in patients who already have psychosis. Use drug cautiously in patients with psychosis.

- Keep in mind that, when signs and symptoms of ADHD occur with acute stress reactions or with preexisting structural cardiac abnormalities or other serious heart problems, methylphenidate usually isn't indicated because of possible worsened reaction or sudden death.
- Monitor children and adolescents for first-time psychotic or manic symptoms. If present, notify prescriber and expect drug to be discontinued.

! WARNING Know that the E.R. tablet form (Concerta) shouldn't be given to patients with esophageal motility disorders; drug may cause GI obstruction because tablet doesn't change shape in GI tract.

- Monitor blood pressure and pulse rate to detect hypertension and excessive stimulation. Notify prescriber if present. For patient with hypertension, expect to increase antihypertensive dosage or add another antihypertensive to regimen.

! WARNING Watch for signs of physical or psychological dependence. Methylphenidate's abuse potential is similar to that of amphetamines; use cautiously in patients with a history of drug abuse.

- Stopping drug abruptly after long-term use may unmask dysphoria, paranoia, severe depression, or suicidal thoughts.
- Monitor growth in children. Report failure to grow or gain weight, and expect to stop drug.
- Watch closely (especially children, adolescents, and young adults), for suicidal tendencies, particularly when therapy starts and dosage changes, because depression may worsen temporarily during these times, possibly leading to suicidal ideation.

- Monitor transdermal patch application site for erythema. If more intense reactions occur with erythema, such as local edema or papule or vesicle formation that doesn't improve within 48 hours after patch is removed from irritated site or that spreads beyond the patch site, further diagnostic testing is required to determine presence of allergic contact dermatitis.
- Know that patients with allergic contact dermatitis from transdermal patch may develop systemic allergy reaction if methylphenidate is taken by another route, such as by mouth. Monitor patient closely if route of administration changes, and report any evidence of flare-up of previous dermatitis or positive patch-test sites, generalized skin eruptions in previously unaffected skin, or other symptoms such as arthralgia, diarrhea, fever, headache, malaise, or vomiting because drug may have to be discontinued.
- Observe patient for paradoxical aggravation of symptoms or other serious adverse reactions. If present, notify prescriber and expect dosage to be reduced or drug discontinued.

! WARNING Monitor patient closely for serotonin syndrome, a rare but serious adverse effect of methylphenidate when taken in combination with serotonergic drugs. Signs and symptoms include agitation, confusion, diaphoresis, diarrhea, fever, hyperactive reflexes, poor coordination, restlessness, shaking, talking or acting with uncontrolled excitement, tremor, and twitching. If symptoms occur, notify prescriber immediately, expect drug to be discontinued, and provide supportive care.

- Inspect patient's fingers and toes for signs of peripheral vasculopathy, such as digital ulceration and/or soft-tissue breakdown. Although usually mild and intermittent, more severe manifestation may occur. Notify prescriber if present, and expect dose to be reduced or drug discontinued.

PATIENT TEACHING

- Warn patient that methylphenidate is a controlled substance and can be abused and lead to dependence. Dosage should not be increased or dosage interval shortened without prescriber knowledge.

- For transdermal form, teach patient to apply patch to a clean, dry location in his hip area 2 hours before effect is needed and to remove it 9 hours after application. Caution patient to avoid applying patch to skin that's damaged, irritated, or oily and to avoid the waistline, where clothing may dislodge the patch. Tell patient to rotate application sites between hips.

- Instruct patient to apply patch immediately after opening pouch and removing protective liner. Tell him to press patch firmly in place with palm of his hand for about 30 seconds. Reassure patient that exposing site to water shouldn't cause patch to fall off. If a patch does fall off, explain that a new patch may be applied but that the total exposure time for the day shouldn't exceed 9 hours.

- Alert patient prescribed transdermal patch that a persistent loss of skin pigmentation, most commonly at and around the application site, may occur. Tell patient to notify prescriber if this occurs and expect this form of methylphenidate to be discontinued.

- Urge patient not to chew or crush E.R. tablets but swallow them whole.

- Tell patient to take tablets at least 6 hours before bedtime to avoid insomnia (unless prescribed Jornay PM) and to take E.R. once-daily tablets in the morning.

- Advise patient taking E.R. once-daily tablets (Concerta) that he may see intact tablet in stool. Explain that drug is slowly released from nonabsorbable tablet shell.

- Tell patient taking capsule form to swallow it whole or if using Adhansia, Aptensio XR, Jornay PM, or Ritalin LA, capsule may be opened and contents sprinkled onto a tablespoon of applesauce and taken immediately, followed by a liquid such as water.

- Instruct patient taking E.R. oral suspension form to vigorously shake the bottle for at least 10 seconds before measuring dose to ensure that the proper dose is being taken. If using the oral dosing dispenser, tell patient to remove the bottle cap and confirm that the bottle adapter has been inserted into the top of the bottle. Tell him to insert the tip of the oral dosing dispenser provided into the bottle adapter, turn bottle upside down, and withdraw prescribed amount of liquid into the oral dosing dispenser. Then have patient remove the filled oral dosing dispenser from bottle and dispense drug directly into his mouth. Tell him to then replace the bottle cap and wash the oral dosing dispenser after each use (components are dishwasher-safe).

- Tell patient taking ODT tablet not to remove the tablet from the blister pack until just prior to dosing and to take the tablet immediately after opening the blister pack. Tell him to use dry hands when opening the blister pack and remove tablet by peeling back the foil on the blister pack. Caution him not to push the tablet through the foil. Tell patient to place the whole tablet on his tongue and allow it to disintegrate without chewing or crushing it. Inform patient that no liquid is needed to take the tablet.

- Alert patient taking drug long term that prescriber may take patient off of drug periodically to determine continued need.

! WARNING Urge patient to seek immediate emergency attention if symptoms of a heart attack or stroke occur. Also teach patient how to take a blood pressure and pulse and to monitor both regularly.

- Direct patient to notify prescriber about excessive nervousness, fever, insomnia, palpitations, rash, or vomiting.

- Instruct patient to tell all prescribers about methylphenidate therapy, as serious drug interactions can occur. Stress importance of seeking immediate medical care if persistent, severe, or unusual adverse reactions occur.

- Warn patient with seizure disorder that drug may cause seizures.

- Inform parents of children on long-term therapy that drug may delay growth.

- Warn male patients and parents of male children that painful or prolonged penile erections may occur while taking the drug, especially after a dosage increase or during period of drug withdrawal. In the event that this happens, immediate medical attention should be sought.

- Instruct patient or parents to monitor fingers and toes for ulceration and/or soft-tissue breakdown. If noticed, prescriber should be called. Reassure patient that signs and symptoms generally improve after the dose is reduced or drug is discontinued.

- Urge family or caregiver to watch patient closely for suicidal tendencies, especially when therapy starts or dosage changes and particularly if patient is a child, teenager, or young adult.
- Alert patient and caregiver that psychotic or manic symptoms, even without a prior history, may occur and should be reported to prescriber.
- Advise patient to avoid alcohol while taking methylphenidate.

methylprednisolone
Medrol

methylprednisolone acetate
Depo-Medrol

methylprednisolone sodium succinate
Solu-Medrol

☰ Class and Category
Pharmacologic class: Glucocorticoid
Therapeutic class: Corticosteroid

☰ Indications and Dosages
∗ *To treat immune and inflammatory disorders*

TABLETS (METHYLPREDNISOLONE)
Adults. 4 to 48 mg daily as a single dose or in divided doses. Alternatively, twice the daily dose every other day.
Children. 0.11 to 1.66 mg/kg daily in divided doses three times daily or four times daily.

I.V. INFUSION, I.M. INJECTION, I.V. INJECTION (METHYLPREDNISOLONE SODIUM SUCCINATE)
Adults. *Initial:* 10 to 40 mg with subsequent doses dictated by patient's response and condition being treated.
Children. 0.11 to 1.66 mg/kg daily in divided doses three times daily or four times daily.

I.M. INJECTION (METHYLPREDNISOLONE ACETATE)
Adults. *Initial:* 4 to 120 mg daily according to clinical response.

INTRA-ARTICULAR, INTRALESIONAL, OR SOFT-TISSUE INJECTION (METHYLPREDNISOLONE ACETATE)
Adults. 4 to 10 mg for small joints; 10 to 40 mg for medium joints; and 20 to 80 mg for large joints every 1 to 5 wk, according to clinical response.

∗ *To treat acute exacerbations of multiple sclerosis*

TABLETS (METHYLPREDNISOLONE)
Adults. 200 mg daily for 7 days followed by 80 mg every other day for 1 mo.

I.M. INJECTION (METHYLPREDNISOLONE ACETATE), I.V. INFUSION (METHYLPREDNISOLONE SODIUM SUCCINATE)
Adults. 160 mg daily for 1 wk followed by 64 mg every other day for 1 mo.

☰ Drug Administration
P.O.
- Give drug with food to minimize GI irritation and indigestion.
- For once-daily dosing, give in the morning to coincide with normal cortisol secretion.

I.V.
- Store drug at room temperature. Protect from light.
- Never administer methylprednisolone acetate intravenously.
- Use only the accompanying diluent or Bacteriostatic Water for Injection with Benzyl Alcohol for reconstitution.
- Do not use formulations containing benzyl alcohol in neonates. Instead, use preservative-free formulations.
- Compatible diluents include 0.9% Sodium Chloride Injection, 5% Dextrose in Water, and 5% Dextrose in Water/0.9% Sodium Chloride Injection.
- Reconstitute and further dilute drug following manufacturer guidelines.
- When using the ACT-O-VIAL system, press down on plastic activator to force diluent into the lower compartment. Gently agitate to mix solution. After removing plastic tab covering center of stopper and sterilizing stopper, insert needle squarely

through center of stopper until tip is just visible. Invert vial and withdraw dose. Then continue to follow manufacturer guidelines.

- For I.V. injection, administer diluted drug directly into a vein or through a free-flowing compatible I.V. solution over at least 1 minute.
- For I.V. infusion, administer diluted drug over 30 minutes for doses less than 0.5 g and over at least 30 to 60 minutes for doses greater than 0.5 g or 30 mg/kg.
- Discard mixed solution after 48 hours.
- *Incompatibilities:* None listed by manufacturer

I.M.
- Inject slowly and deeply into gluteal muscle.
- Do not inject into deltoid muscle because of risk of subcutaneous atrophy.
- If a large dose is prescribed, divide dose into several small injections rather than administering as a single large dose.
- Rotate sites.

INTRA-ARTICULAR/INTRALESIONAL/ SOFT-TISSUE INJECTIONS
- Administered by health professional trained in these types of injections.

Route	Onset	Peak	Duration
P.O.	Rapid	1–2 hr	30–36 hr
I.V.	< 1 hr	0.8 hr	12 hr
I.M.	6–48 hr	4–8 days	1–4 wk
Intra-articular/ intralesional/ soft tissue	Rapid	7 days	1–5 wk

Half-life: 12–36 hr

Mechanism of Action

Binds to intracellular glucocorticoid receptors and suppresses inflammatory and immune responses by inhibiting accumulation of monocytes and neutrophils at inflammation sites, stabilizing lysosomal membranes, suppressing the antigen response of macrophages and helper T cells, and inhibiting the synthesis of inflammatory response mediators, such as cytokines, interleukins, and prostaglandins.

Contraindications

Hypersensitivity to cow's milk or other dairy products for Solu-Medrol 40-mg formulation, hypersensitivity to methylprednisolone or its components, idiopathic thrombocytopenic purpura (I.M.), intrathecal administration, premature infants (preparations containing benzyl alcohol), systemic fungal infections

Interactions
DRUGS
aminoglutethimide: Possibly loss of methylprednisolone-induced adrenal suppression
amphotericin B, potassium-depleting diuretics: Possibly severe hypokalemia
anticholinesterases: Possibly severe weakness in patients with myasthenia gravis
aspirin, NSAIDs: Increased risk of adverse GI effects and bleeding
barbiturates, carbamazepine, phenytoin, rifampin: Decreased blood methylprednisolone level
cholestyramine: Possibly increased methylprednisolone clearance
cyclosporine: Increased activity of both drugs
digoxin: Possibly hypokalemia-induced arrhythmias and digitalis toxicity
estrogens, oral contraceptives: Possibly increased therapeutic and toxic effects of methylprednisolone
insulin, oral antidiabetic drugs: Possibly increased blood glucose level
isoniazid: Possibly decreased therapeutic effects of isoniazid
ketoconazole, macrolide antibiotics such as erythromycin and troleandomycin: Decreased methylprednisolone clearance and increased risk of adverse effects
oral anticoagulants, thrombolytics: Increased risk of decreased therapeutic effects of these drugs
vaccines: Decreased antibody response and increased risk of neurologic complications

ACTIVITIES
alcohol use: Increased risk of adverse GI effects including bleeding

Adverse Reactions
CNS: Ataxia, behavioral changes, depression, dizziness, euphoria, fatigue, headache, **increased intracranial pressure with papilledema**, insomnia, malaise, mood changes, neuropathy, paresthesia, restlessness, **seizures**, steroid psychosis, syncope, vertigo
CV: Arrhythmias, cardiac arrest, edema, **fat embolism, heart failure**, hypertension, **hypertrophic cardiomyopathy** (premature

infants), **hypotension, myocardial rupture following recent MI**, tachycardia, **thromboembolism**, thrombophlebitis
EENT: Exophthalmos, glaucoma, increased intraocular pressure, nystagmus, posterior subcapsular cataracts
ENDO: Adrenal insufficiency, cushingoid symptoms (buffalo hump, central obesity, moon face, supraclavicular fat pad enlargement), diabetes mellitus, growth suppression in children, hyperglycemia
GI: Abdominal distention, **acute hepatitis**, elevated liver enzymes, hepatomegaly, hiccups, increased appetite, **melena**, nausea, **pancreatitis**, peptic ulcer, ulcerative esophagitis, vomiting
GU: Amenorrhea, glycosuria, menstrual irregularities, perineal burning or tingling
HEME: Easy bruising, leukocytosis
MS: Arthralgia; aseptic necrosis of femoral and humeral heads; Charcot-like arthropathy; compression fractures; muscle atrophy, twitching, or weakness; myalgia; osteoporosis; spontaneous fractures; steroid myopathy; tendon rupture
RESP: Pulmonary edema
SKIN: Acne; allergic dermatitis; altered skin pigmentation; diaphoresis; dry, scaly skin; erythema; hirsutism; necrotizing vasculitis; petechiae; purpura; rash; scarring; sterile abscess; striae; subcutaneous fat atrophy; thin, fragile skin; urticaria
Other: Activation of latent infections, **anaphylaxis, angioedema**, exacerbation of systemic fungal infections, **hypernatremia, hypocalcemia, hypokalemia, hypokalemic alkalosis**, impaired wound healing, masking of signs of infection, **metabolic alkalosis**, negative nitrogen balance from protein catabolism, suppressed skin test reaction, weight gain

Childbearing Considerations

PREGNANCY

- Drug may cause fetal harm. Some formulations contain benzyl alcohol, which can cross the placental barrier and cause "gasping syndrome" in premature infants when born.
- Use with caution only if benefit to mother outweighs potential risk to fetus.
- Infants born to mothers who have received corticosteroids during pregnancy should be observed for hypoadrenalism.

LACTATION

- Drug appears in breast milk and could suppress growth, interfere with endogenous corticosteroid production, or cause other adverse effects if infant is breastfed.
- A decision should be made to discontinue breastfeeding or the drug to avoid potential serious adverse reactions in the breastfed infant.

Nursing Considerations

- Know that high doses of systemic corticosteroids, including methylprednisolone, should not be used for the treatment of traumatic brain injury because of increased risk of death or in patients with active ocular herpes simplex because of risk of corneal perforation. Preparations containing benzyl alcohol should not be used to treat pediatric patients because of risk of "gasping syndrome."
- Administer methylprednisolone with extreme caution in patients with a recent myocardial infarction because corticosteroid use may increase risk of left ventricular free wall rupture.
- Use cautiously in patients with congestive heart failure or renal insufficiency because sodium retention and edema can occur in patients taking a corticosteroid. Also use cautiously in patients with diverticulitis, fresh intestinal anastomoses, nonspecific ulcerative colitis, or peptic ulcer; these conditions increase risk of perforation during corticosteroid therapy. In addition, use caution in patients with systemic sclerosis, because drug may increase risk of scleroderma renal crisis.
- Arrange for low-sodium diet with added potassium, as prescribed.
- Protect patient from falling, especially elderly patient at risk for fractures from osteoporosis.
- Closely monitor patient for signs of infection because drug may mask them or may worsen systemic fungal infections or active latent disease. Be aware that chickenpox and measles can become life-threatening in patients taking a corticosteroid.
- Assess for possible depression or psychotic episodes during therapy.

- Monitor blood glucose level; dosage of insulin or oral antidiabetic drug may have to be adjusted in diabetic patient.

! WARNING To avoid possibly fatal acute adrenocortical insufficiency, expect to taper long-term therapy when discontinuing drug, but expect dosage to be increased during times of stress.

- Be aware that changes in thyroid function, such as development of hyperthyroidism or hypothyroidism, may require dosage adjustment in chronic therapy because metabolic clearance of methylprednisolone is affected by thyroid activity.
- Know that skin testing should be avoided during methylprednisolone therapy because drug may suppress reaction.
- Monitor patient's liver enzymes, as ordered, especially in patients receiving high doses such as 1 g/day intravenously (usually for treatment of exacerbations of multiple sclerosis). This is important because, although rare, this can develop into a toxic form of acute hepatitis. The onset of liver dysfunction can occur several weeks or even longer after administration of methylprednisolone. Notify prescriber if liver dysfunction is suspected and expect drug to be discontinued, as condition can develop into acute liver failure and death.

PATIENT TEACHING

- Instruct patient to take drug with food or milk.
- Caution patient not to stop taking methylprednisolone abruptly or to change dosage without consulting prescriber.
- Tell patient to take a missed dose as soon as he remembers unless it's nearly time for the next dose. Caution against double-dosing.
- Urge patient to notify prescriber immediately about dark or tarry stools; signs of impending adrenocortical insufficiency, such as anorexia, dizziness, fainting, fatigue, fever, joint pain, muscle weakness, or nausea; and swelling or sudden weight gain.
- Instruct patient not to obtain vaccinations unless approved by prescriber.
- Urge patient to take calcium supplements, vitamin D, or both if recommended by prescriber.

- Inform patient that insomnia and restlessness usually resolve after 1 to 3 weeks.
- Caution patient to avoid people with contagious diseases.
- Explain the need for regular exercise or physical therapy to maintain muscle mass.
- Advise patient to carry medical identification that documents his need for long-term corticosteroid therapy.

metoclopramide
Gimoti

metoclopramide hydrochloride
Reglan

Class and Category
Pharmacologic class: Dopamine-2 receptor antagonist
Therapeutic class: Antiemetic, upper GI stimulant

Indications and Dosages
✳ *To treat diabetic gastroparesis*

ODT TABLETS, ORAL SOLUTION, TABLETS

Adults experiencing mild symptoms. 10 mg four times daily before each meal and at bedtime for 2 to 8 wk. *Maximum:* 40 mg daily in divided doses.

I.V. OR I.M. INJECTION

Adults experiencing severe symptoms. 10 mg four times a day for up to 10 days.

NASAL SPRAY (GIMOTI)

Adults less than 65 years of age. 15 mg (1 spray) in one nostril four times daily for 2 to 8 wk. *Maximum:* 60 mg (4 sprays) daily.

±**DOSAGE ADJUSTMENT** For patients age 65 and older, nasal spray not used for initial therapy. If patient is already stabilized on a dosage of 10 mg four times daily with another form of drug, patient may be switched to nasal spray with a dosage of 15 mg (1 spray) in one nostril four times daily for 2 to 8 wk.

✳ *To treat gastroesophageal reflux disease*

M

ODT TABLETS, ORAL SOLUTION, TABLETS

Adults. *Continuous dosing:* 10 to 15 mg four times a day for 4 to 12 wk. *Intermittent dosing:* Up to 20 mg as a single dose prior to provoking situation. *Maximum:* 60 mg daily in divided doses.

ODT TABLETS

Adults. 10 to 15 mg up to four times daily at least 30 min before eating and at bedtime for 4 to 12 weeks.

±**DOSAGE ADJUSTMENT** For patients with diabetic gastroparesis or gastroesophageal reflux disease who are taking tablet form (not ODT) and are elderly, dosage reduced to 5 mg four times daily; patients who are CYP2D6 poor metabolizers or have moderate to severe hepatic or renal impairment or are taking strong CYP2D6 inhibitors such as bupropion, fluoxetine, paroxetine, or quinidine, dosage reduced to 5 mg four times daily or 10 mg three times daily; and for patients with end-stage renal disease, including those treated with continuous ambulatory peritoneal dialysis or hemodialysis, dosage reduced to 5 mg four times daily or 10 mg twice daily. For patients who are taking ODT tablets or oral solution and have a creatinine clearance of less than 40 ml/min, dosage reduced by 50%.

✳ *To prevent or reduce nausea and vomiting from emetogenic cancer chemotherapy*

I.V. INFUSION

Adults receiving less emetogenic regimens. 1 mg/kg 30 min before chemotherapy and repeated every 2 hr for 2 additional doses, then every 3 hr for 3 doses.
Adults receiving highly emetogenic regimens with drugs such as cisplatin or dacarbazine. 2 mg/kg 30 min before chemotherapy and repeated every 2 hr for 2 additional doses, then every 3 hr for 3 doses.

✳ *To prevent postoperative nausea and vomiting*

I.M. INJECTION

Adults. 10 to 20 mg given at or near end of surgery.

✳ *To facilitate small bowel intubation; to aid in radiological examinations*

I.V. INJECTION

Adults and adolescents over age 14. 10 mg as a single dose.
Children ages 6 to 14 years. 2.5 to 5 mg as a single dose.

Children under 6 years. 0.1 mg/kg as a single dose.

±**DOSAGE ADJUSTMENT** Parenteral dosages given for any condition, reduced by half if creatinine clearance is less than 40 ml/min.

☰ Drug Administration

P.O.

- Give oral solution and tablets 30 minutes before meals and at bedtime when used to treat gastroparesis and GERD. A single dose may be given prior to provoking situation for GERD.
- Use a calibrated device to measure dosage of oral solution.
- Give ODT tablets 30 minutes before each meal and at bedtime. A single dose may be given prior to provoking situation for GERD. Remove ODT tablet from sealed blister (do not push tablet through covering) with dry, gloved hand and give to patient to place on her tongue. If ODT tablet breaks or crumbles, discard and obtain a new one.

I.V.

- I.V. injection is given for doses of 10 mg or less. Inject undiluted over 1 to 2 minutes.
- I.V. infusion is used for doses greater than 10 mg. Dilute in 50 ml 0.45% or 0.9% Sodium Chloride Injection, 5% Dextrose in Water, Lactated Ringer's, or Ringer's solution. Infuse over at least 15 minutes. Diluted drug can be stored for 48 hours if refrigerated and protected from light.
- Avoid rapid I.V. delivery because it may cause anxiety, restlessness, and drowsiness.
- *Incompatibilities:* Cephalothin sodium, chloramphenicol, sodium bicarbonate

I.M.

- Inject into a large muscle mass.
- Rotate sites.

INTRANASAL

- Administer 30 minutes before each meal and at bedtime.
- Prime spray bottle before first use by pressing down firmly and releasing 10 times on the finger flange (a spray should appear after the first few times of pressing down).
- Clear a nozzle that has become clogged by removing the spray nozzle and soaking it in warm water and then rinse. Do not insert a pin or other sharp object into nozzle

to clear clog. Dry spray nozzle at room temperature and when dry place back on the spray bottle.

Route	Onset	Peak	Duration
P.O.	30–60 min	1–2 hr	1–2 hr
I.V.	1–3 min	15 min	1–2 hr
I.M.	10–15 min	Unknown	1–2 hr
Intranasal	30–60 min	Unknown	Unknown

Half-life: 5–6 hr; 8 hr (nasal spray)

Mechanism of Action

Antagonizes the inhibitory effect of dopamine on GI smooth muscle. This causes gastric contraction, which promotes gastric emptying and peristalsis, and also reduces gastroesophageal reflux. Metoclopramide also blocks dopaminergic receptors in the chemoreceptor trigger zone, preventing nausea and vomiting.

Contraindications

Catecholamine-releasing paragangliomas; epilepsy; history of dystonic reaction or tardive dyskinesia to metoclopramide; hypersensitivity to metoclopramide or its components; pheochromocytoma; when stimulation of gastrointestinal motility might be dangerous, such as in the presence of gastrointestinal hemorrhage, mechanical obstruction, or perforation

Interactions

DRUGS

anticholinergics, antidiarrheals, antiperistaltics, antipsychotic drugs: Potential for additive effects, including increased frequency and severity of neuroleptic malignant syndrome, other extrapyramidal symptoms, and tardive dyskinesia
CNS depressants such as anxiolytics, hypnotics, opiates, sedatives: Increased risk of CNS depression
atovaquone, cimetidine, digoxin, posaconazole (oral suspension): Decreased absorption and reduced effectiveness of these drugs
CNS depressants: Possibly increased CNS depression
cyclosporine, sirolimus, tacrolimus: Increased absorption and risk of adverse effects
CYP2D6 inhibitors (strong) such as bupropion, fluoxetine, paroxetine, quinidine: Increased plasma concentrations of metoclopramide; risk of exacerbation of extrapyramidal symptoms
dopaminergic agonists and other drugs that increase dopamine concentrations such as apomorphine, bromocriptine, cabergoline, levodopa, pramipexole, ropinirole, rotigotine: Decreased effectiveness of metoclopramide; potential for exacerbation of symptoms such as Parkinsonian symptoms
MAO inhibitors: Increased risk of severe hypertension
mivacurium, succinylcholine: Enhanced neuromuscular blockade
serotonergic drugs: Possible development of serotonin syndrome

ACTIVITIES

alcohol use: Risk of increased CNS depression

Adverse Reactions

CNS: Agitation, anxiety, confusion, depression, dizziness, drowsiness, extrapyramidal reactions (motor restlessness, Parkinsonism, tardive dyskinesia), fatigue, hallucinations, headache, insomnia, irritability, lassitude, nervousness, **neuroleptic malignant syndrome**, panic reaction, restlessness, **seizures, suicidal ideation**
CV: **AV block, bradycardia,** fluid retention, **heart failure,** hypertension, **hypotension, supraventricular tachycardia**
EENT: Dry mouth, glossal edema, **laryngeal edema,** visual disturbances
ENDO: Galactorrhea, gynecomastia, hyperprolactinemia
GI: Constipation, diarrhea, nausea
GU: Impotence, menstrual irregularities, urinary frequency or incontinence
HEME: **Agranulocytosis, leukopenia, methemoglobinemia, neutropenia, sulfhemoglobinemia**
RESP: **Bronchospasm**
SKIN: Rash, urticaria
Other: **Angioedema,** porphyria, restless leg syndrome

Childbearing Considerations

PREGNANCY

- It is not known if drug causes fetal harm.
- Use with caution only if benefit to mother outweighs potential risk to fetus.

LABOR & DELIVERY

- Drug crosses the placental barrier and may cause extrapyramidal signs and

M

methemoglobinemia in the neonate if given to mother during delivery.

- Use with caution only if benefit to mother outweighs potential risk to fetus.

LACTATION

- Drug is present in breast milk and may cause gastrointestinal adverse effects in the breastfed infant such as intestinal discomfort and increased intestinal gas formation as well as extrapyramidal signs (dystonias) and methemoglobinemia.
- Patient should check with prescriber before breastfeeding.

Nursing Considerations

- Know that orally disintegrating tablets are not recommended for use in children because of increased risk of tardive dyskinesia and other extrapyramidal symptoms.
- Be aware that metoclopramide therapy should not be used in patients with depression because of increased risk of suicidal ideation. Also know that drug should not be given to patients with a history of hypertension or patients taking monoamine oxidase inhibitors, because of increased risk of hypertension that could lead to a hypertensive crisis.
- Use metoclopramide cautiously in patients with hypertension because it may increase catecholamine levels. Monitor blood pressure throughout therapy. Expect drug to be discontinued in any patient with a rapid rise in blood pressure.

! WARNING Watch closely for tardive dyskinesia, especially in the elderly, women, and patients with diabetes, because this serious adverse effect is often irreversible even after therapy stops. Therapy lasting longer than 12 weeks isn't recommended because risk of tardive dyskinesia increases the longer the patient takes metoclopramide. Risk also has been linked to total cumulative dose so prescriber must take this into account when setting dosage. Also be aware that drug can cause other extrapyramidal symptoms besides tardive dyskinesia. For example, though rare, drug may cause dystonic reactions such as dyspnea and stridor, possibly caused by laryngospasm. At first sign of involuntary movements of face, tongue, or limbs, or any other abnormal sign

---

or symptom, notify prescriber and expect to discontinue drug.

- Monitor patient with NADH-cytochrome b5 reductase deficiency because metoclopramide increases risk of methemoglobinemia and sulfhemoglobinemia. For patients with glucose-6-phosphate dehydrogenase (G6PD) deficiency, methylene blue treatment is not recommended if metoclopramide-induced methemoglobinemia occurs because the treatment may cause hemolytic anemia in these patients, which may be fatal.
- Assess patient for signs of intestinal obstruction, such as abnormal bowel sounds, diarrhea, nausea, and vomiting, before administering metoclopramide. Notify prescriber if you detect them.

! WARNING Notify prescriber if patient shows signs of toxicity, such as disorientation, drowsiness, and extrapyramidal reactions.

- Monitor patient, especially one with heart failure or cirrhosis, for possible fluid retention or volume overload due to transient increase in plasma aldosterone level. Expect metoclopramide to be discontinued if fluid retention occurs.

! WARNING Monitor patient closely for neuroleptic malignant syndrome, a rare but potentially fatal disorder characterized by altered level of consciousness, arrhythmias, diaphoresis, hyperthermia, irregular pulse or blood pressure, muscle rigidity, and tachycardia. Know that risk increases in patients experiencing a toxic reaction to metoclopramide as a result of overdosage or receiving concomitant treatment with another drug associated with neuroleptic malignant syndrome. Expect metoclopramide to be discontinued immediately, if present.

- Monitor patient for abnormal behaviors or thoughts suggestive of suicidal ideation because depression may occur while taking metoclopramide even in patients without a history of depression.

PATIENT TEACHING

- Instruct patient on how to take the form of metoclopramide prescribed.

- Advise against activities that require alertness.
- Urge patient to avoid alcohol and CNS depressants while taking metoclopramide. They may increase CNS depression.
- Tell patient to immediately report involuntary movements of face, eyes, tongue, or hands, including lip smacking, chewing, puckering of mouth, frowning, scowling, sticking out tongue, blinking, moving eyes, or shaking arms and legs.
- Explain that stopping metoclopramide may cause withdrawal symptoms that include dizziness, headache, and nervousness.
- Warn patient's family or caregiver to monitor patient for abnormal behavior or thoughts that may be suggestive of suicidal ideation. If concerns are raised, urge them to contact prescriber.
- Urge patient to tell all prescribers about metoclopramide therapy.
- Stress importance of reporting signs and symptoms that are persistent, severe, or unusual.

metolazone

Zaroxolyn

Class and Category

Pharmacologic class: Thiazide-like diuretic
Therapeutic class: Diuretic

Indications and Dosages

✴ *To manage mild to moderate hypertension*

TABLETS

Adults. 2.5 to 5 mg once daily.

✴ *To manage edema from heart failure or renal disease*

TABLETS

Adults. 5 to 10 mg once daily for edema of heart failure; 5 to 20 mg once daily for edema of renal disease.

Drug Administration

P.O.

- Administer at same time every day in the morning.

Route	Onset	Peak	Duration
P.O.	1 hr	8 hr	24 hr

Half-life: 6–14 hr

Mechanism of Action

Promotes renal excretion of sodium and water by inhibiting their reabsorption in distal convoluted tubules. The resulting reduction in extracellular fluid volume and plasma reduces blood pressure. Metolazone also helps reduce blood pressure by decreasing peripheral vascular resistance.

Contraindications

Anuria, hepatic coma or precoma, hypersensitivity to metolazone or its components

Interactions

DRUGS

ACTH or corticosteroids: Possible increased risk of hypokalemia and salt and water retention
antigout drugs: Increased blood uric acid level and risk of gout attack
barbiturates, narcotics, other antihypertensives: Increased risk of orthostatic hypotension
digoxin: Increased risk of electrolyte imbalances and digoxin-induced arrhythmias
diuretics: Additive effects of both drugs, possibly leading to electrolyte imbalances and severe hypovolemia
hydralazine: Possibly interference with the natriuretic action of metolazone
insulin, oral antidiabetic drugs: Decreased effectiveness of these drugs, increased risk of hyperglycemia
lithium: Increased risk of lithium toxicity
neuromuscular blockers: Increased risk of hypokalemia and neuromuscular blockade, increased risk of respiratory depression
NSAIDs, sympathomimetics: Possibly decreased metolazone effectiveness

ACTIVITIES

alcohol use: Increased risk of orthostatic hypotension

Adverse Reactions

CNS: Anxiety, chills, depression, dizziness, drowsiness, headache, insomnia, neuropathy, paresthesia, restlessness, syncope, weakness
CV: Chest pain, cold extremities, orthostatic hypotension, palpitations, peripheral edema, vasculitis, **venous thrombosis**
EENT: Bitter taste, blurred vision, dry mouth, epistaxis, pharyngitis, sinus congestion, tinnitus
ENDO: Hyperglycemia

GI: Abdominal pain, anorexia, cholecystitis, constipation, diarrhea, **hepatic dysfunction**, **hepatitis**, indigestion, nausea, **pancreatitis**, vomiting
GU: Decreased libido, glycosuria, impotence
HEME: **Agranulocytosis, aplastic anemia, leukopenia, thrombocytopenia**
MS: Arthralgia, gout, myalgia
RESP: Cough
SKIN: Dry skin, necrosis, petechiae, photosensitivity, pruritus, rash, urticaria
Other: Hypochloremia, **hypokalemia, hyponatremia**, hypovolemia, **metabolic alkalosis**

Childbearing Considerations
PREGNANCY
- Drug may cause fetal harm such as fetal or neonatal jaundice, thrombocytopenia, and possibly other adverse reactions that have occurred in adults.
- Use with caution only if benefit to mother outweighs potential risk to fetus.

LACTATION
- Drug is present in breast milk.
- Breastfeeding is not recommended during drug therapy.

Nursing Considerations
- Anticipate giving metolazone with a loop diuretic if patient responds poorly to loop diuretic alone.
- Measure patient's fluid intake and output and daily weight to monitor drug's diuretic effect.
- Monitor blood chemistry test results and assess for evidence of hypochloremia, hypokalemia, and, possibly, mild metabolic alkalosis.
- Monitor serum calcium and uric acid levels, especially if patient has a history of gout or renal calculi. Metolazone may slightly increase calcium reabsorption and decrease uric acid excretion.

PATIENT TEACHING
- Inform patient that metolazone controls but doesn't cure hypertension. Discuss possible need for lifelong therapy and consequences of uncontrolled hypertension.
- Instruct patient to take drug at the same time each day.
- Advise patient to change position slowly to minimize orthostatic hypotension.

- Urge patient to notify prescriber about persistent, severe diarrhea, nausea, or vomiting, which can cause dehydration and orthostatic hypotension.
- Emphasize the importance of diet control, especially limiting sodium intake, and maintaining a normal weight.
- Inform diabetic patient that metolazone may increase blood glucose level and that he should check his level often.

metoprolol succinate
Kapspargo Sprinkle, Toprol-XL

metoprolol tartrate
Lopresor (CAN), Lopresor SR (CAN), Lopressor

Class and Category
Pharmacologic class: Beta$_1$-adrenergic blocker
Therapeutic class: Antianginal, antihypertensive

Indications and Dosages
✳ *To manage hypertension, alone or with other antihypertensives*

E.R. CAPSULES (KAPSPARGO SPRINKLE), E.R. TABLETS (TOPROL-XL)
Adults. *Initial:* 25 to 100 mg once daily, adjusted weekly as prescribed. *Maximum:* 400 mg daily.
Children 6 years and over. *Initial:* 1 mg/kg once daily, not to exceed 50 mg once daily with initial dose, adjusted weekly as prescribed. *Maximum:* 2 mg/kg once daily, not to exceed 200 mg once daily.

TABLETS (LOPRESSOR)
Adults. *Initial:* 100 mg once daily or 50 mg twice daily increased weekly, if needed, to achieve optimum blood pressure control. *Usual effective dose:* 100 to 450 mg daily. *Maximum:* 450 mg daily as a single dose or in divided doses.

✳ *To provide early treatment of acute MI or evolving acute MI*

TABLETS (LOPRESSOR), I.V. INJECTION (LOPRESSOR)
Adults. *Initial:* 5 mg by I.V. bolus every 2 min for three doses followed by 25 to 50 mg P.O. every 6 hr for 48 hr, starting 15 min after

final I.V. dose. *Maintenance:* 100 mg P.O. twice daily for at least 3 mo.

✳ *To treat angina pectoris and chronic stable angina*

E.R. CAPSULES (KAPSPARGO SPRINKLE), E.R. TABLETS (TOPROL-XL)

Adults. 100 mg daily, increased weekly as needed. *Maximum:* 400 mg daily.

TABLETS (LOPRESSOR)

Adults. *Initial:* 50 mg twice daily, adjusted weekly in increments of 50 mg twice daily, if needed. *Maximum:* 400 mg daily.

✳ *To treat stable, symptomatic (New York Heart Association [NYHA] class II or III) heart failure of ischemic, hypertensive, or cardiomyopathic origin*

E.R. TABLETS (TOPROL-XL)

Adults. *Initial:* 25 mg once daily for class II heart failure or 12.5 mg once daily for more severe heart failure for 2 wk. Then dosage doubled every 2 wk as tolerated. *Maximum:* 200 mg daily.

E.R. CAPSULES (KAPSPARGO SPRINKLE)

Adults. *Initial:* 25 mg once daily for 2 wk. Then dosage doubled every 2 wk, as tolerated. *Maximum:* 200 mg daily.

±**DOSAGE ADJUSTMENT** For elderly patients or patients with hepatic impairment, initial dosage reduced with gradual dose titration.

☰ Drug Administration

P.O.

- Administer with or immediately after a meal.
- Tablets may be cut in half, but not chewed or crushed. E.R. tablets should be swallowed whole and not chewed, crushed, or split.
- For patient unable to swallow E.R. capsules, open capsule and sprinkle over soft food such as applesauce or pudding. Mixture must be swallowed within 60 minutes and never stored for later use.
- E.R. capsule form can be administered via a nasogastric tube by mixing contents of opened capsule with water and drawing mixture up into a syringe. Gently shake mixture for about 10 seconds, then flush it through the tube. Rinse the tube with water until all of drug is washed out.

I.V.

- Administer drug undiluted as an I.V. injection over 1 to 2 minutes.

- Drug should only be administered in a coronary care or intensive care setting.
- *Incompatibilities:* None listed by manufacturer

Route	Onset	Peak	Duration
P.O.	15 min	1 hr	3–6.5 hr
P.O. (E.R.)	15 min	6–12 hr	24 hr
I.V.	5 min	20 min	5–8 hr

Half-life: 3–7 hr

☰ Mechanism of Action

Inhibits stimulation of beta$_1$-receptor sites, located mainly in the heart, resulting in decreased cardiac excitability, cardiac output, and myocardial oxygen demand. These effects help relieve angina, minimize cardiac tissue damage from a myocardial infarction, and help relieve symptoms of heart failure. Metoprolol also helps reduce blood pressure by decreasing renal release of renin.

☰ Contraindications

For all indications: Hypersensitivity to metoprolol, other beta-blockers, or their components
For angina and hypertension: Cardiogenic shock, heart block greater than first degree, overt cardiac failure, sinus bradycardia
For myocardial infarction: Heart rate less than 45 beats/minute, moderate to severe cardiac failure, second- and third-degree heart block, significant first-degree heart block (P-R interval 0.24 seconds or greater), systolic blood pressure less than 100 mm Hg

☰ Interactions

DRUGS

alpha-adrenergic agents such as alpha-methyldopa, betanidine, guanethidine, reserpine: Possibly increased antihypertensive effects
calcium channel blockers: Increased risk of additive reduction in myocardial contractility
catecholamine-depleting drugs such as reserpine: Possibly additive effect resulting in hypotension or marked bradycardia
CYP2D6 inhibitors such as antiarrhythmics (propafenone, quinidine), antidepressants (bupropion, clomipramine, desipramine, fluoxetine, fluvoxamine, paroxetine, sertraline), antifungals (terbinafine), antihistamines (diphenhydramine), antimalarials (hydroxychloroquine, quinidine),

M

antipsychotics (chlorpromazine, fluphenazine, haloperidol, thioridazine), antiretrovirals (ritonavir): Increased plasma metoprolol level causing decrease in the cardioselectivity of metoprolol

clonidine: Increased risk of bradycardia and hypotension; increased risk of rebound hypertension when clonidine is discontinued

digoxin, other beta-blockers: Decreased heart rate and slowed atrioventricular conduction

dipyridamole: Possibly altered heart rate

ergot alkaloids: Possibly enhanced vasoconstrictive action of ergot alkaloids

hydralazine: Increased metoprolol concentration

MAO inhibitors: Possibly significant hypertension

other antihypertensives: Additive hypotensive effect

prazosin: Possibly increased postural hypotensive effect of first dose of prazosin

FOODS

all foods: Increased bioavailability of metoprolol

▤ Adverse Reactions

CNS: Anxiety, confusion, **CVA**, depression, dizziness, drowsiness, fatigue, hallucinations, headache, insomnia, nightmares, paresthesia, short-term memory loss, somnolence, syncope, tiredness, vertigo, weakness

CV: Angina, **arrhythmias (including AV block and bradycardia), arterial insufficiency, cardiac arrest, cardiogenic shock**, chest pain, decreased HDL level, increased triglyceride levels, gangrene of extremity, **heart failure**, hypertension, orthostatic hypotension, palpitations, peripheral edema

EENT: Blurred vision, dry eyes or mouth, nasal congestion, rhinitis, taste disturbance, tinnitus

GI: Constipation, diarrhea, flatulence, heartburn, **hepatitis**, nausea, vomiting

GU: Decreased libido, impotence

HEME: Agranulocytosis, leukopenia, thrombocytopenia

MS: Arthralgia, back pain, myalgia

RESP: Bronchospasm, dyspnea, shortness of breath

SKIN: Alopecia, diaphoresis, photosensitivity, pruritus, rash, urticaria, worsening of psoriasis

▤ Childbearing Considerations

PREGNANCY

- It is not known if drug causes fetal harm. However, drug crosses the placenta, placing the fetus at risk for bradycardia, hypoglycemia, hypotension, and respiratory depression at birth.
- Use with caution only if benefit to mother outweighs potential risk to fetus.

LACTATION

- Drug is present in breast milk.
- Patient should check with prescriber before breastfeeding.
- If breastfeeding occurs with a mother who is a slow metabolizer of drug, breastfed infant should be monitored for bradycardia and other symptoms of beta-blockade such as constipation, diarrhea, or dry eyes, mouth, or skin.

▤ Nursing Considerations

- Know that patients undergoing noncardiac major surgery should not begin a high-dose regimen using extended-release metoprolol because such use in patients with cardiovascular risk factors has been associated with bradycardia, hypotension, stroke, and death. However, also be aware that beta-blocker therapy such as metoprolol that is already in place should not be routinely discontinued prior to major surgery.
- Use metoprolol with extreme caution in patients with bronchospastic disease who don't respond to or can't tolerate other antihypertensives. Expect to give smaller doses more often to avoid the higher plasma levels in longer dosage intervals.
- Use cautiously in patients with angina or hypertension who have congestive heart failure because beta-blockers such as metoprolol can further depress myocardial contractility, worsening heart failure.
- Expect patients with acute MI who can't tolerate initial dosage or who delay treatment to start with maintenance dosage, as prescribed and tolerated.
- Before starting therapy for heart failure, expect to give an ACE inhibitor, digoxin, and a diuretic to stabilize patient.
- Be aware that if patient has pheochromocytoma, alpha blocker therapy should start first, followed by metoprolol

to prevent paradoxical increase in blood pressure from attenuation of beta-mediated vasodilation in skeletal muscle.

- Monitor patient for evidence of worsening heart failure during dosage increases. If heart failure worsens, expect to increase diuretic dosage and possibly decrease metoprolol dosage or temporarily discontinue drug, as prescribed. Metoprolol dosage shouldn't be increased until worsening heart failure has been stabilized.
- If patient with heart failure develops symptomatic bradycardia, expect to decrease the metoprolol dosage.

! **WARNING** Know that if dosage exceeds 400 mg daily, patient should be monitored for bronchospasm and dyspnea because metoprolol competitively blocks beta$_2$-adrenergic receptors in bronchial and vascular smooth muscles.

! **WARNING** When substituting metoprolol for clonidine, expect to gradually reduce clonidine and increase metoprolol dosage over several days. Given together, these drugs have additive hypotensive effects.

- Assess ECG of patients who take metoprolol, because they may be at risk for AV block. If AV block results from depressed AV node conduction, prepare to give appropriate drug, as ordered, or assist with insertion of temporary pacemaker.
- Check for signs of poor glucose control in patient with diabetes mellitus. Metoprolol may interfere with therapeutic effects of insulin and oral antidiabetic drugs. It also may mask evidence of hypoglycemia, such as palpitations, tachycardia, and tremor.
- Monitor patient with hyperthyroidism closely because beta-adrenergic blockers such as metoprolol may mask signs of hyperthyroidism, such as tachycardia. Also know that abrupt discontinuation of metoprolol should be avoided because thyroid storm could be precipitated.
- Monitor patient with peripheral vascular disease for evidence of arterial insufficiency (coldness, pain, and pallor in affected extremity). Metoprolol can precipitate or aggravate peripheral vascular disease.
- Be aware that patients with a history of severe anaphylactic reactions may be more reactive to repeated challenges of the allergen while taking beta-blocker therapy, such as metoprolol, and may be unresponsive to the usual doses of epinephrine used to treat an allergic reaction.

! **WARNING** Expect to taper dosage over 1 to 2 weeks when drug is discontinued; stopping abruptly can cause MI, myocardial ischemia, severe hypertension, or ventricular arrhythmias, especially in patients with cardiac disease.

PATIENT TEACHING

- Instruct patient to take metoprolol with or immediately after the same meal every day. Explain that he may halve tablets but not chew or crush them.
- Tell patient unable to swallow E.R. capsules that the capsule may be opened and sprinkled over soft food such as applesauce or pudding. Mixture must be swallowed within 60 minutes and never stored for later use.
- Advise patient to notify prescriber if pulse rate falls below 60 beats/minute or is significantly lower than usual.
- Urge diabetic patient to check blood glucose level often during therapy.
- Caution patient not to stop drug abruptly.

metronidazole
Flagyl, Flagyl ER, Flagyl I.V. RTU, Metro I.V.

☰ Class and Category
Pharmacologic class: Nitroimidazole
Therapeutic class: Antiprotozoal

☰ Indications and Dosages
✱ *To treat systemic anaerobic infections caused by* Bacteroides fragilis, Clostridium difficile, Clostridium perfringens, Eubacterium, Fusobacterium, Peptococcus, Peptostreptococcus, *and* Veillonella *species*

CAPSULES, TABLETS
Adults. 7.5 mg/kg up to 1,000 mg every 6 hr for 7 to 10 days or longer. *Maximum:* 4,000 mg daily.

I.V. INFUSION
Adults. *Initial:* 15 mg/kg as a single dose and then 7.5 mg/kg up to 1,000 mg every 6 hr for

7 to 10 days or longer. *Maximum:* 4,000 mg daily.

* *To treat amebiasis* (Entamoeba histolytica)

CAPSULES, TABLETS

Adults. *For acute amebic dysentery:* 750 mg three times daily for 5 to 10 days. *For amebic liver abscess:* 500 (tablets only) or 750 mg (tablets or capsules) three times daily for 5 to 10 days.

Children. 35 to 50 mg/kg/24 hr divided into three times daily for 10 days.

* *To treat trichomoniasis* (Trichomonas vaginalis)

TABLETS

Adults. 2,000 mg as a single dose, 1,000 mg twice daily for 1 day, or 250 mg three times daily for 7 days.

CAPSULES

Adults. 375 mg two times daily for 7 days.

* *To prevent postoperative bowel infection in elective colorectal surgery which is contaminated or potentially contaminated*

I.V. INFUSION

Adults. 15 mg/kg 1 hr before surgery and then 7.5 mg/kg 6 and 12 hr after initial dose. *Maximum:* 4,000 mg during a 24-hour period.

* *To treat bacterial vaginosis*

E.R. TABLETS

Adult nonpregnant women and postmenarchal adolescents. 750 mg once daily for 7 days.

±**DOSAGE ADJUSTMENT** For patients with severe hepatic impairment, dosage reduced by 50%. For patient with end-stage renal failure receiving hemodialysis and the administration of drug cannot be separated from the dialysis session, a supplemental dose of the drug is recommended to be given following hemodialysis.

* *Topical and vaginal forms presented in appendix.*

≡ Drug Administration

P.O.

- Administer immediate-release drug with food to minimize adverse GI reactions.
- Administer E.R. tablets 1 hour before or 2 hours after a meal.
- Capsules and tablets should be swallowed whole and not chewed, crushed, or split/opened.

I.V.

- Do not use aluminum equipment such as needles or cannulae that would come in contact with drug solution, as precipitates may form.
- Don't give drug by I.V. injection.
- Do not add any other additives or drug to solution.
- Do not use if solution is cloudy or precipitated or if the seal is not intact.
- Do not connect flexible plastic containers in series or pressurize intravenous solutions contained in flexible plastic containers to increase flow rate because an air embolism could result when administering drug in Viaflex plus plastic container. In addition, vented intravenous administration sets with the vent in the open position should not be used with flexible plastic containers.
- Discontinue primary I.V. infusion during metronidazole infusion.
- Using ready-to-use solutions, infuse over 30 to 60 minutes.
- Change intravenous administration equipment at least once every 24 hours.
- Store at room temperature. Refrigeration may cause precipitation to occur.
- *Incompatibilities:* Aztreonam, cefamandole nafate, cefoxitin, penicillin G

Route	Onset	Peak	Duration
P.O.	Unknown	1–2 hr	Unknown
P.O./E.R.	15 min	4.6–6.8 hr	Unknown
I.V.	Immediate	1 hr	Unknown

Half-life: 8 hr

≡ Mechanism of Action

Undergoes intracellular chemical reduction during anaerobic metabolism. After metronidazole is reduced, it damages DNA's helical structure and breaks its strands, which inhibits bacterial nucleic acid synthesis and causes cell death.

≡ Contraindications

Alcohol use, including products containing propylene glycol during and for at least 3 days after metronidazole therapy; Cockayne syndrome; hypersensitivity to metronidazole, other nitroimidazole derivatives, or their components; use of disulfiram within past 2 weeks

Interactions

DRUGS

5-fluorouracil: Decreased clearance of 5-fluorouracil and potential for 5-fluorouracil toxicity

amiodarone, carbamazepine, cyclosporine, phenytoin, quinidine, tacrolimus: Increased plasma levels of these drugs

busulfan: Increased risk of serious busulfan toxicity

cimetidine and other drugs that inhibit CYP450 enzymes: Possibly delayed elimination and increased blood level of metronidazole

disulfiram: Possibly combined toxicity, with confusion and psychotic reactions

drugs known to prolong QT interval: Increased risk of QT prolongation

lithium: Possible development of elevated lithium levels with potential for toxicity in patients on high doses

oral anticoagulants: Possibly increased anticoagulant effect

phenobarbital, phenytoin, and other drugs that induce microsomal liver enzyme activity: Possibly accelerated elimination of metronidazole and decreased effectiveness

ACTIVITIES

alcohol use: Possibly disulfiram-like effects

Adverse Reactions

CNS: **Aseptic meningitis (parenteral form),** asthenia, ataxia, chills, confusion, depression, dizziness, dysarthria, **encephalopathy,** fever, headache, hypoesthesia, incoordination, insomnia, irritability, jumpy eye movements, light-headedness, malaise, numbness, paresthesia, peripheral neuropathy, psychosis, **seizures** (high doses), somnolence, syncope, vertigo, weakness

CV: Chest pain, **hypotension,** palpitations, peripheral edema, **prolonged QT interval,** tachycardia

EENT: Dry mouth, furry tongue, glossitis, lacrimation (topical form), metallic taste, nasal congestion, nystagmus, optic neuropathy, pharyngitis, rhinitis, sinusitis, stomatitis

GI: Abdominal cramps or pain, anorexia, constipation, diarrhea, elevated liver enzymes, epigastric distress, **hepatic failure or hepatotoxicity** (patients with Cockayne syndrome), nausea, **pancreatitis,** vomiting

GU: Burning or irritation of sexual partner's penis, candidal cervicitis or vaginitis, chromaturia, dark urine, decreased libido, dryness of vagina or vulva, dysmenorrhea, dyspareunia, dysuria, genital pruritus, moniliasis, proctitis, urinary frequency, UTI

HEME: **Agranulocytosis,** eosinophilia, **leukopenia, neutropenia, thrombocytopenia**

MS: Arthralgia, back pain, dysarthria, muscle spasms, myalgia

RESP: Dyspnea, risk of upper respiratory infection

SKIN: Bullae, burning or stinging sensation, erythema, erythematous rash, flushing, hyperhidrosis, pruritus, rash, **Stevens–Johnson syndrome, toxic epidermal necrolysis,** urticaria

Other: **Anaphylaxis; angioedema;** bacterial infection; **drug reaction with eosinophilia and systemic symptoms (DRESS);** flu-like symptoms; infusion-site edema, pain, or tenderness

Childbearing Considerations

PREGNANCY

- It is not known if drug causes fetal harm.
- Use with caution only if benefit to mother outweighs potential risk to fetus.

LACTATION

- Drug is present in breast milk.
- A decision should be made to discontinue breastfeeding or the drug to avoid potential serious adverse reactions in the breastfed infant. Alternatively, a mother may choose to pump and discard breast milk for the duration of drug therapy and for 24 hours after therapy ends and feed her infant breast milk stored before therapy began or formula.

Nursing Considerations

- Use parenteral metronidazole with extreme caution in patients with Cockayne syndrome, because acute hepatic failure and severe hepatotoxicity have occurred as rapid as within 2 days, with some fatalities. If no other treatment is available, expect to obtain liver function studies before metronidazole is given parenterally, again within the first 2 to 3 days after treatment is initiated, frequently during therapy, and at the end of therapy. If liver enzymes become elevated, expect metronidazole to be discontinued

and liver enzymes monitored until they have returned to baseline values.
- Use cautiously in patients with CNS diseases.
- Use cautiously in patients with blood dyscrasias or a history of such because metronidazole therapy has caused agranulocytosis, leukopenia, and neutropenia in some patients.

> ! **WARNING** Know that if patient has adverse CNS reactions, such as peripheral neuropathy or seizures, prescriber must be told and drug stopped immediately.

- Monitor patient with severe liver disease because slowed metronidazole metabolism may cause drug to accumulate in body and increase the risk of adverse effects.
- Monitor patients with end-stage renal disease who are not on hemodialysis or patients with severe renal impairment for adverse reactions, because reduced urinary excretion may cause metronidazole and its metabolites to accumulate in the body.
- Monitor CBC and culture and sensitivity tests if therapy lasts longer than 10 days or if second course of treatment is needed.
- Monitor patient's neurologic status throughout metronidazole therapy. If abnormal neurologic signs and symptoms occur, notify prescriber and expect to discontinue drug. Be aware that prolonged oral administration of the drug may cause persistent peripheral neuropathy.
- Be aware that parenteral form of metronidazole contains 790 mg of sodium per 100 ml. Monitor patients predisposed to edema or who are receiving corticosteroids or a reduced-sodium diet.
- Assess patient for fungal superinfections. Candidiasis may occur and present with more serious symptoms during therapy with metronidazole and requires treatment with a candidacidal agent.
- Be aware that metronidazole may interfere with certain chemistry values, such as alanine aminotransferase (AST, SGOT), aspartate aminotransferase, glucose hexokinase, lactate dehydrogenase (LDH), and triglycerides.
- Monitor patient with Crohn's disease exposed to metronidazole at high doses for extended periods of time because

these patients have an increased risk of extraintestinal and gastrointestinal cancers such as breast and colon cancers.

PATIENT TEACHING
- Urge patient to take metronidazole at evenly spaced intervals during the day and with food to minimize adverse GI reactions, except for E.R. tablets, which should be taken 1 hour before or 2 hours after a meal.
- Urge patient to complete the entire course of therapy.
- Caution patient to avoid alcohol during therapy and for at least 3 days afterward.
- Advise patient to avoid hazardous activities until drug's CNS effects are known and to report any abnormal neurologic signs or symptoms, such as numbness, seizures, weakness, or vision changes.
- If patient reports dry mouth, suggest ice chips or sugarless hard candy or gum; suggest a dental visit if dryness lasts longer than 2 weeks.
- Instruct patient to notify prescriber if no improvement occurs within a few days of taking tablets or capsules.
- Inform patient with trichomoniasis that her male sexual partners should wear condoms during her treatment and that they may need treatment themselves to prevent reinfection.
- Urge patient to follow up with prescriber to make sure infection is gone.
- Tell patient with Cockayne syndrome who is receiving metronidazole to stop drug immediately if signs and symptoms of liver dysfunction occur, such as abdominal pain, change in skin or stool color, or nausea, and to notify prescriber.

micafungin sodium
Mycamine

≡ Class and Category
Pharmacologic class: Echinocandin
Therapeutic class: Antifungal

≡ Indications and Dosages
✱ *To treat esophageal candidiasis*

I.V. INFUSION
Adults. 150 mg once daily for 10 to 30 days (mean duration: 15 days).

Children age 4 months and over weighing more than 30 kg. 2.5 mg/kg once daily. *Maximum*: 150 mg once daily.

Children age 4 months and over weighing 30 kg or less. 3 mg/kg once daily.

✳ *To prevent* Candida *infection in patients undergoing hematopoietic stem cell transplantation*

I.V. INFUSION

Adults. 50 mg once daily for 6 to 51 days (mean duration: 19 days).

Children age 4 months and over. 1 mg/kg once daily. *Maximum:* 50 mg once daily.

✳ *To treat candidemia, acute disseminated candidiasis, and* Candida *peritonitis and abscesses*

I.V. INFUSION

Adults. 100 mg once daily for 10 to 47 days (mean duration: 15 days).

Children age 4 months and over. 2 mg/kg once daily. *Maximum*: 100 mg once daily.

✳ *To treat candidemia, acute disseminated candidiasis, and* Candida *peritonitis and abscesses without meningoencephalitis and/or ocular dissemination*

I.V. INFUSION

Children less than 4 months of age. 4 mg/kg once daily.

Drug Administration

I.V.

- Reconstitute by adding 5 ml of 0.9% Sodium Chloride Injection (without a bacteriostatic agent) or 5% Dextrose Injection to each 50-mg vial to yield 10 mg/ml and to each 100-mg vial to yield 20 mg/ml.
- Swirl vial gently to minimize excessive foaming.
- Reconstituted solution may be stored for up to 24 hours at room temperature. Protect from light.
- For adult patients, add reconstituted solution to 100 ml 0.9% Sodium Chloride Injection or 5% Dextrose Injection.
- For pediatric patients, follow manufacturer guidelines for calculating volume to use for dilution.
- Infuse over 1 hour for both adults and children after flushing an existing I.V. line with 0.9% Sodium Chloride Injection. Protect diluted solution from light, although

the infusion drip chamber or tubing need not be covered.

- Administer concentrations greater than 1.5 mg/ml through a central catheter to minimize risk of infusion reactions.
- Monitor infusion rate carefully because infusions that took less than 1 hour to infuse have been associated with more frequent hypersensitivity reactions.
- *Incompatibilities:* Other drugs

Route	Onset	Peak	Duration
I.V.	Unknown	Unknown	Unknown

Half-life: 11–21 hr

Mechanism of Action

Inhibits synthesis of 1,3-beta-D-glucan, which is an essential component of the *Candida* fungal cell wall. Without 1,3-beta-D-glucan, the fungal cell dies.

Contraindications

Hypersensitivity to micafungin, other echinocandins, or their components

Interactions

DRUGS

itraconazole, nifedipine, sirolimus: Increased plasma levels of these drugs

Adverse Reactions

CNS: Anxiety, delirium, dizziness, dysgeusia, fatigue, fever, headache, insomnia, **intracranial hemorrhage**, rigors, **seizures**, somnolence

CV: Arrhythmia, atrial fibrillation, bradycardia, cardiac arrest, deep vein thrombosis, hypertension, **hypotension,** MI, peripheral edema, phlebitis, tachycardia, **shock,** vasodilation

EENT: Epistaxis, mucosal inflammation

ENDO: Hyperglycemia, **hypoglycemia**

GI: Abdominal pain, anorexia, constipation, diarrhea, dyspepsia, elevated liver enzymes, **hepatic dysfunction, hepatitis,** hiccups, hyperbilirubinemia, jaundice, nausea, vomiting, **worsening hepatic failure**

GU: Acute renal failure, anuria, elevated blood urea and serum creatinine levels, oliguria, **renal tubular necrosis**

HEME: Anemia, **coagulopathy, disseminated intravascular coagulation (DIC),** eosinophilia, **hemolytic anemia,**

M

leukopenia, **lymphopenia, neutropenia, pancytopenia, thrombocytopenia**
RESP: Apnea, cough, **cyanosis,** dyspnea, **hypoxia,** pneumonia, **pulmonary embolism**
SKIN: Erythema, **erythema multiforme,** flushing, necrosis, pruritus, rash, **Stevens–Johnson syndrome, toxic epidermal necrolysis,** urticaria
Other: Acidosis, anaphylaxis, angioedema, bacteremia, **hyperkalemia, hypernatremia,** hypocalcemia, hypokalemia, **hypomagnesemia, hyponatremia, hypophosphatemia,** injection-site reactions including phlebitis and thrombophlebitis, **sepsis**

Childbearing Considerations
PREGNANCY
- It is not known if drug causes fetal harm although animal studies suggest a possibility.
- Use with caution only if benefit to mother outweighs potential risk to fetus.

LACTATION
- It is not known if drug is present in breast milk.
- Patient should check with prescriber before breastfeeding.

Nursing Considerations
- Use cautiously in patients with hepatic insufficiency.

! **WARNING** Monitor patient closely for hypersensitivity reactions, including anaphylaxis and angioedema. Stop infusion immediately if present, notify prescriber, and provide supportive care, as prescribed.

- Monitor patient's liver and renal function closely throughout therapy because liver and renal abnormalities may occur in patients receiving micafungin.
- Monitor hematologic status closely because hematologic abnormalities may occur. If they do, monitor patient closely. If patient's condition worsens, expect micafungin to be discontinued.

PATIENT TEACHING
- Instruct patient to report any infusion-site discomfort immediately.
- Tell patient to report any unusual or persistent signs and symptoms to prescriber.

- Stress importance of seeking emergency treatment if difficulty breathing or swallowing occurs or other signs of an allergic reaction occurs.
- Advise women of childbearing age to notify prescriber if pregnancy is known or suspected.

midazolam
Nayzilam

midazolam hydrochloride
Seizalam

Class, Category, and Schedule
Pharmacologic class: Benzodiazepine
Therapeutic class: Sedative-hypnotic
Controlled substance schedule: IV

Indications and Dosages
✳ *To induce preoperative sedation or amnesia, to control preoperative anxiety*

SYRUP
Children ages 6 to 16 years and cooperative children. 0.25 to 0.5 mg/kg as a single dose 30 to 45 min before surgery. *Usual:* 0.5 mg/kg. *Maximum:* 20 mg.
Children 6 months to 6 years of age and less cooperative children. 0.25 to 1 mg/kg as a single dose 30 to 45 min before surgery. *Maximum:* 20 mg.
±**DOSAGE ADJUSTMENT** For children with cardiac or respiratory compromise, high-risk children, and children who have received concomitant narcotics or other CNS depressants, dosage kept at 0.25 mg/kg. For obese children, dose should be calculated based on ideal body weight.

I.V. INJECTION
Adults age 60 and over and adults who are debilitated or chronically ill. *Initial:* 1 to 1.5 mg over 2 min immediately before procedure. After 2-minute waiting period, an additional 1-mg dose given, if needed. *Maintenance:* After another 2-min waiting period, dosage adjusted to desired level in 25% increments every 2 minutes, as needed. *Maximum:* 3.5 mg total initial dosage.

Adults under age 60 and adolescents. *Initial:* Up to 2.5 mg over 2 min immediately before procedure. After 2-min waiting period, dosage adjusted to desired level in 25% increments, as needed with smaller doses and 2 minutes between each dose. *Maximum:* 5 mg.

Children ages 6 to 12. *Initial:* 0.025 to 0.05 mg/kg, over 2 min up to 0.4 mg/kg, if needed immediately before procedure. *Maintenance:* After a 2- to 3-min waiting period, dosage adjusted as needed. *Maximum:* 10 mg.

Children ages 6 months to 5 years. *Initial:* 0.05 to 0.1 mg/kg, over 2 min up to 0.6 mg/kg, if needed immediately before procedure. *Maintenance:* After waiting 2 to 3 min, dosage adjusted, as needed. *Maximum:* 6 mg.

I.M. INJECTION

Adults age 60 and over. 0.02 to 0.05 mg/kg as a single dose 30 to 60 min before surgery.

Adults under age 60 and adolescents. 0.07 to 0.08 mg/kg as a single dose 30 to 60 min before surgery.

Children ages 6 months to 12 years. 0.1 to 0.15 mg/kg, up to 0.5 mg/kg for more anxious patients as a single dose 30 to 60 min before surgery. *Maximum:* 10 mg.

±**DOSAGE ADJUSTMENT** For elderly patients and patients who are chronically ill, maintenance dosage reduced by 50%. For adults who have been premedicated with an opiate, maintenance dosage reduced by 25%.

✳ *To induce general anesthesia*

I.V. INJECTION

Adults older than 55 years. 0.3 mg/kg over 20 to 30 seconds (if not premedicated) or 0.2 mg/kg over 20 to 30 seconds (if premedicated). After 2-minute waiting period, additional doses given, if needed, in increments of 25% of initial dose.

Adults under the age of 55 years. 0.3 to 0.35 mg/kg over 20 to 30 seconds (if not premedicated) or 0.25 mg/kg over 20 to 30 seconds (if premedicated). After 2-minute waiting period, additional doses given, if needed, in increments of 25% of initial dose.

✳ *To relieve agitation and anxiety in mechanically ventilated patients*

I.V. INFUSION

Adults. *Initial:* 0.01 to 0.05 mg/kg infused over several min, repeated at 10- to 15-min intervals until adequate sedation occurs. *Maintenance:* 0.02 to 0.1 mg/kg/hr initially, adjusted at intervals of 30 min to desired level in 25% to 50% increments, as ordered. After achieving desired level of sedation, infusion rate decreased by 10% to 25% every few hr, as ordered, until minimum effective infusion rate is determined.

Children. *Initial bolus:* 0.05 to 0.2 mg/kg. *Maintenance:* 0.06 to 0.12 mg/kg/hr by continuous infusion with dosage adjusted, as needed, to maintain effect.

Infants over age 32 weeks. 0.06 mg/kg/hr by continuous infusion with rate adjusted, as needed.

Infants under age 32 weeks. *Initial:* 0.03 mg/kg/hr by continuous infusion with rate adjusted, as needed.

±**DOSAGE ADJUSTMENT** For children who are hemodynamically compromised, the usual loading dose is titrated in small increments, separated by 2 to 3 min.

✳ *To treat acute, intermittent, stereotypic episodes of frequent seizure activity (i.e., seizure clusters, acute repetitive seizures) that are distinct from a patient's usual seizure pattern in patients with epilepsy*

NASAL SPRAY (NAYZILAM)

Adults and children age 12 and over. 5 mg (1 spray) into one nostril. After 10 min, an additional 5 mg (1 spray) into the opposite nostril, if needed. *Maximum:* 10 mg (2 sprays) to treat a single episode and used no more than one episode every three days and no more than 5 episodes a month.

✳ *To treat status epilepticus*

I.M. INJECTION

Adults. 10 mg as a single dose.

▤ Drug Administration

- Drug may cause respiratory depression and arrest. For all forms, have appropriate resuscitative drugs and equipment readily available during drug therapy, as well as staff knowledgeable and skilled in airway management.
- Drug forms other than nasal spray should only be administered in settings in which patient's cardiac and respiratory functions can be continuously monitored.

P.O.

- Syrup form can cause same severe respiratory symptoms as parenteral form.

- To use oral dispenser that comes with bottle, push plunger completely down toward the tip of the oral dispenser and insert tip firmly into opening of the bottle adapter.
- Turn entire bottle and oral dispenser upside down. Pull plunger out slowly until the desired dosage is withdrawn into the oral dispenser. Turn entire unit right side up and remove the oral dispenser slowly from the bottle. Cover tip with cap until ready to administer.
- Administer directly into patient's mouth. Do not dilute with any liquid.

I.V.

- Never administer excessive single doses or by rapid administration, because airway obstruction or respiratory arrest or depression may occur.
- Avoid administering by any other parenteral route, especially intra-arterially.
- Drug may be mixed in same syringe with atropine sulfate, meperidine hydrochloride, morphine sulfate, or scopolamine hydrobromide, if needed. The resulting solution is stable for 30 minutes.
- Follow manufacturer guidelines if using the Carpuject Syringe with the reusable Carpuject Holder.
- Administration rates determined by purpose of drug therapy. See Indications and Dosages section.
- Midazolam at a concentration of 0.5 mg/ml is compatible with 0.9% Sodium Chloride, or 5% Dextrose in Water for up to 24 hours and with Lactated Ringer's solution for up to 4 hours; 1 mg/ml or 5 mg/ml formulations are compatible with 0.9% Sodium Chloride Injection or 5% Dextrose in Water.
- For I.V. injection, administer slowly over at least 2 minutes and wait at least 2 minutes to evaluate therapeutic effects when initiating or titrating doses. For I.V. infusion, infuse at the rate specified (See Indications and Dosages section). Rate adjusted as needed.
- *Incompatibilities:* None listed by manufacturer

I.M.

- Administer deeply into a large muscle mass except for Seizalam, which should be injected only into the mid-outer thigh.

- Rotate sites for additional dosages.

INTRANASAL

- Drug available as a single-dose nasal spray unit. Do not open blister packaging until ready to use.
- Do not test or prime unit before use and discard if the nasal spray unit appears damaged.
- When ready to administer drug, remove nasal spray unit from blister package carefully. Hold the nasal spray unit with thumb on the plunger and middle and index fingers on each side of the nozzle. Place the tip of the nozzle into one nostril until fingers on either side of the nozzle touch the bottom of the nose. Press the plunger firmly to deliver the dose using only one motion. It is not necessary to have the patient breathe deeply when drug is administered. Discard the nasal spray unit and packaging.
- Do not administer a second dose if patient's breathing is compromised.
- Store at room temperature.

Route	Onset	Peak	Duration
P.O.	10–20 min	45–60 min	2–6 hr
I.V.	3–5 min	3–5 min	2–6 hr
I.M.	15 min	0.5–1 hr	2–6 hr
Intranasal	10 min	0.5–2 hr	4 hr

Half-life: 1.5–2.5 hr

Mechanism of Action

May exert sedating effect by increasing activity of gamma-aminobutyric acid, a major inhibitory neurotransmitter in the brain. As a result, midazolam produces a calming effect, relaxes skeletal muscles, and—at high doses—induces sleep.

Contraindications

Acute angle closure glaucoma; acute pulmonary insufficiency; debilitated or elderly patients outside the ICU setting; hypersensitivity to midazolam, other benzodiazepines, or their components; severe chronic obstructive pulmonary disease

Interactions

DRUGS

cimetidine, diltiazem, erythromycin, fluconazole, itraconazole, ketoconazole, ritonavir, saquinavir, verapamil: Intense and prolonged sedation caused by reduced midazolam metabolism

CNS depressants (secobarbital), droperidol-fentanyl combination, opioids (fentanyl, meperidine, morphine): Possibly increased CNS and respiratory depression and hypotension
halothane: Reduced minimum alveolar concentration of halothane required during maintenance of anesthesia
pancuronium: Potentiated effect of pancuronium
sodium valproate: Increased effect of midazolam
thiopental: Slight reduction in dosage requirement of thiopental following I.M. midazolam

Adverse Reactions

CNS: Agitation, delirium, or dreaming during emergence from anesthesia; anxiety; ataxia; chills; combativeness; confusion; dizziness; drowsiness; euphoria; excessive sedation; headache; impaired cognitive function; insomnia; lethargy; nervousness; nightmares; paresthesia; prolonged emergence from anesthesia; restlessness; retrograde amnesia; sleep disturbance; slurred speech; **suicidal ideation** (nasal spray form); weakness; yawning
CV: Cardiac arrest, hypotension, nodal rhythm, PVCs, tachycardia, **vasovagal episodes**
EENT: Blurred vision, diplopia, or other vision changes; increased salivation; **laryngospasm**; miosis; nystagmus; toothache
GI: Hiccups, nausea, retching, vomiting
RESP: Airway obstruction, bradypnea, bronchospasm, coughing, decreased tidal volume, dyspnea, hyperventilation, **respiratory arrest, shallow breathing,** tachypnea, wheezing
SKIN: Pruritus, rash, urticaria
Other: Injection-site burning, edema, induration, pain, redness, and tenderness; physical or psychological dependence, withdrawal reactions

Childbearing Considerations

PREGNANCY

- Pregnancy exposure registry for Nayzilam and Seizalam brands: 1-888-233-2334 or http://www.aedpregnancyregistry.org/.
- Drug may cause fetal harm based on benzodiazepines as a class such as an increased risk of congenital malformations if given in the first trimester.
- Drug is not recommended for obstetrical use because other benzodiazepines given in the last weeks of pregnancy have resulted in neonatal CNS depression. Withdrawal can occur in neonates when mother has used the nasal spray form during the later stages of pregnancy.

LABOR & DELIVERY

- Drug is not recommended for use during labor and delivery as administration may result in a floppy infant syndrome, which occurs mainly within the first hours after birth and may last up to 14 days.

LACTATION

- Drug is excreted in breast milk.
- Breastfeeding is not recommended during drug therapy. If nasal spray formulation is used with breastfeeding, infant should be monitored for lethargy, poor sucking, and somnolence.

Nursing Considerations

- Determine whether patient consumes alcohol or takes antibiotics, antihypertensives, or protease inhibitors because these substances can produce an intense and prolonged sedative effect when taken with midazolam.
- Assess patient's current drug use, including all prescription and OTC drugs, before nasal spray therapy begins. Be aware that excessive use of nasal spray may lead to abuse, addiction, misuse, overdose, and possibly death. Monitor patient's intake of drug closely.
- Know that repeated or lengthy use of sedation drugs such as midazolam and general anesthetics during procedures or surgeries should be avoided in children younger than 3 years of age or in pregnant women during their third trimester, because the combined use may affect the development of children's brains.
- Assess level of consciousness frequently because the range between sedation and unconsciousness or disorientation is narrow with midazolam.
- Be aware that recovery time for drug administered for surgery or procedures is usually 2 hours but may be up to 6 hours.

M

! WARNING Be aware that concomitant use of benzodiazepines such as midazolam with opioids may result in coma, profound sedation, respiratory depression, and death. Monitor patient closely.

! WARNING Know that even though nasal spray form is indicated only for intermittent use by the patient, if it is used more often than recommended, is stopped abruptly, or a rapid dosage reduction occurs, an acute withdrawal reaction may occur that could be life-threatening. In addition, a protracted withdrawal syndrome may occur that could last weeks to more than 12 months. Expect dosage to be tapered before being totally discontinued if patient has abused the use of the drug.

PATIENT TEACHING

- Inform patient that misuse of nasal spray, either by taking excessive amounts or by taking drug for prolonged periods of time, can lead to addiction, overdose, or even death. Stress importance of taking drug exactly as prescribed.
- Instruct patient how to administer nasal spray form, if prescribed for seizure activity. Stress importance of avoiding opioid use unless under supervision of a prescriber because of risk of severe respiratory depression and sedation.

! WARNING Stress importance of not taking a second dose of nasal spray if breathing difficulties occur and to seek immediate emergency attention.

- Inform patient that he may not remember procedure because midazolam produces amnesia.
- Advise patient to avoid hazardous activities until drug's adverse CNS effects, such as dizziness and drowsiness, have worn off.
- Instruct patient to avoid alcohol and other CNS depressants for 24 hours after receiving drug after surgery or a procedure, as directed by prescriber.
- Warn patient prescribed nasal spray form to avoid alcohol or other CNS depressants during midazolam nasal spray therapy to avoid risk of airway obstruction, apnea, or profound hypoventilation.

- Urge family or caregiver to watch patient taking nasal spray closely for suicidal tendencies, especially when therapy starts or dosage changes.

! WARNING Warn patient that if nasal spray is abused and abrupt cessation of drug therapy occurs, it can precipitate acute withdrawal symptoms, which could be life-threatening or last from a few weeks to over 12 months.

miglitol
Glyset

Class and Category
Pharmacologic class: Alpha glucosidase inhibitor
Therapeutic class: Antidiabetic

Indications and Dosages
* As adjunct to manage type 2 diabetes mellitus

TABLETS
Adults. *Initial:* 25 mg three times daily. Or, 25 mg daily increased gradually to 25 mg three times daily. After 4 to 8 wk, dosage increased to 50 mg three times daily for 3 months if needed, with a further increase to 100 mg three times daily, if needed. *Maximum:* 100 mg three times daily.

Drug Administration
P.O.
- Administer drug when patient takes first bite of each main meal.

Route	Onset	Peak	Duration
P.O.	Rapid	2–3 hr	Unknown

Half-life: 2 hr

Mechanism of Action
Inhibits intestinal glucoside hydrolase enzymes, which normally hydrolyze disaccharides and oligosaccharides to glucose and other monosaccharides. This action delays carbohydrate absorption and digestion and reduces postprandial blood glucose level.

Contraindications
Chronic intestinal diseases associated with marked disorders of absorption or digestion, colonic ulceration, conditions that may deteriorate as a result of increased

gas formation in the intestine, diabetic ketoacidosis, hypersensitivity to miglitol or its components, inflammatory bowel disease, partial intestinal obstruction, predisposition to intestinal obstruction

Interactions

DRUGS

digestive enzyme preparations, intestinal adsorbents (activated charcoal): Decreased miglitol effects
digoxin: Possibly decreased blood digoxin level
insulin, sulfonylureas: Increased risk and severity of hypoglycemia
propranolol: Decreased bioavailability of these drugs

Adverse Reactions

GI: Abdominal distention or pain, diarrhea, flatulence, **hepatotoxicity**, ileus including paralytic ileus, nausea, pneumatosis cystoides intestinalis (rare), subileus
HEME: Low serum iron level
SKIN: Rash (transient)

Childbearing Considerations

PREGNANCY

- It is not known if drug causes fetal harm.
- Use with caution only if benefit to mother outweighs potential risk to fetus.

LACTATION

- Drug is present in breast milk.
- Breastfeeding is not recommended during drug therapy.

Nursing Considerations

- Use miglitol cautiously in patient with serum creatinine level above 2 mg/dl.
- Be aware that some patients with type 2 diabetes also may receive insulin or a sulfonylurea as an adjunct to miglitol therapy. Monitor these patients closely for hypoglycemia because insulin and sulfonylureas may cause hypoglycemia, and miglitol therapy may make it more severe. If hypoglycemia occurs, use an oral glucose product such as dextrose to treat mild to moderate hypoglycemia rather than sucrose, whose hydrolysis to fructose and glucose is inhibited by miglitol.
- Review patient's HbA_{1C} level, as appropriate, to monitor long-term glucose control.
- Monitor patient for evidence of overdose, such as transient increases in abdominal

discomfort, diarrhea, and flatulence (but not hypoglycemia).
- Monitor patient for constipation, diarrhea, mucus discharge, or rectal bleeding suggestive of pneumatosis cystoides intestinalis. If suspected, notify prescriber and prepare patient for diagnostic imaging, as ordered. If confirmed, expect drug to be discontinued.

PATIENT TEACHING

- Explain that miglitol is an adjunct to diet, which is the primary treatment for type 2 diabetes mellitus.
- Instruct patient to take drug with first bite of each meal.
- Describe signs and symptoms of hypoglycemia and pathophysiology of diabetes to patient and family members.
- Alert patient that if miglitol is the only drug patient takes to control blood glucose level, it won't cause hypoglycemia.
- Instruct patient who takes insulin or a sulfonylurea with miglitol to keep a source of glucose readily available to reverse hypoglycemia.
- Explain importance of monitoring blood glucose levels.
- Explain that adverse GI reactions usually decrease in frequency and intensity over time.
- Teach obese patient about calorie restriction, diet, regular exercise, and weight loss, as indicated.
- Instruct patient to report to prescriber diarrhea, mucus discharge, persistent or severe constipation, or rectal bleeding.

milnacipran hydrochloride

Savella

Class and Category

Pharmacologic class: Selective norepinephrine and serotonin reuptake inhibitor (SSNRI)
Therapeutic class: Antifibromyalgia

Indications and Dosages

⁎ *To manage fibromyalgia*

TABLETS

Adults. *Initial:* 12.5 mg on day 1; 12.5 mg twice daily on days 2 and 3; 25 mg twice daily on days 4 through 7; and then 50 mg twice daily, increased if needed to 100 mg twice daily. *Maximum:* 100 mg twice daily.

±**DOSAGE ADJUSTMENT** For patients with severe renal impairment (creatinine clearance of 5 to 29 ml/min), maintenance dosage reduced by half.

Drug Administration

P.O.

- Administer with food to improve tolerability.

Route	Onset	Peak	Duration
P.O.	Unknown	2–4 hr	Unknown
Half-life: 6–8 hr			

Mechanism of Action

Inhibits reuptake of norepinephrine and serotonin by CNS neurons without affecting uptake of dopamine or other neurotransmitters, thereby increasing amount of norepinephrine and serotonin available in nerve synapses. Elevated norepinephrine and serotonin levels may improve symptoms of fibromyalgia, including central analgesic effect.

Contraindications

Hypersensitivity to milnacipran or its components, use within 14 days of MAO inhibitor, including I.V. methylene blue and linezolid

Interactions

DRUGS

amphetamines, buspirone, fentanyl, I.V. methylene blue, linezolid, lithium, MAO inhibitors, selective serotonin reuptake inhibitors, serotonin–norepinephrine reuptake inhibitors, St. John's wort, tramadol, tricyclic antidepressants, triptans: Increased risk of serotonin syndrome

clomipramine: Increased risk of euphoria and postural hypotension

clonidine: Possibly inhibited antihypertensive effect

CNS-active drugs: Possibly increased CNS effects

digoxin: Possibly increased risk of postural hypotension and tachycardia

epinephrine, norepinephrine: Increased risk of arrhythmias and paroxysmal hypertension

MAO inhibitors: Possibly hyperpyretic episodes, hypertensive crisis, serotonin syndrome, and severe seizures

ACTIVITIES

alcohol use: Increased risk of liver impairment

Adverse Reactions

CNS: Aggression, anger, anxiety, chills, delirium, depression, dizziness, fatigue, fever, hallucinations, headache, **homicidal ideation**, hypoesthesia, insomnia, irritability, loss of consciousness, migraine, **neuroleptic malignant syndrome**, Parkinsonism, paresthesia, **seizures**, **serotonin syndrome**, **suicidal ideation**, tremor

CV: Chest pain, hypercholesterolemia, hypertension, **hypertensive crisis**, increased heart rate, palpitations, peripheral edema, **supraventricular tachycardia**, tachycardia, **Takotsubo cardiomyopathy**

EENT: Accommodation abnormality, angle closure glaucoma, blurred vision, dry mouth, mydriasis

ENDO: Galactorrhea, hot flashes, hyperprolactinemia

GI: Abdominal distention or pain, **acute pancreatitis**, anorexia, constipation, diarrhea, dyspepsia, elevated liver enzymes, gastroesophageal reflux, flatulence, **hepatitis**, jaundice, liver dysfunction, nausea, vomiting

GU: **Acute renal failure**, cystitis, decreased libido, delayed or absent orgasm (females), dysuria, ejaculation disorder, erectile dysfunction, prostatitis, scrotal or testicular pain, testicular swelling, urinary hesitation, urine retention, urethral pain, UTI

HEME: **Leukopenia**, **neutropenia**, **thrombocytopenia**

MS: **Rhabdomyolysis**

RESP: Dyspnea, upper respiratory infection

SKIN: **Erythema multiforme**, flushing, hyperhidrosis, night sweats, pruritus, rash, **Stevens–Johnson syndrome**

Other: **Hyponatremia**, weight gain or loss

Childbearing Considerations

PREGNANCY

- Pregnancy exposure registry: 1-877-643-3010, email: pregnancyregistries@incresearch.com, or www.savellapregnancyregistry.com.
- Drug may cause fetal harm, especially if given during the third trimester. Neonate

may require prolonged hospitalization, respiratory support, and tube feeding immediately upon birth.

- Use with caution only if benefit to mother outweighs potential risk to fetus.

LACTATION

- Drug is present in breast milk.
- Patient should check with prescriber before breastfeeding.

≡ Nursing Considerations

- Keep in mind that because milnacipran may aggravate liver disease, it shouldn't be given to patients with alcohol addiction or chronic liver disease.
- Ensure patient has had an ophthalmic examination before milnacipran therapy is begun because pupillary dilation that occurs with drug use may trigger an angle closure attack in a patient with anatomically narrow angles who does not have a patent iridectomy.
- Use cautiously in patients with cardiac disease, mild to moderate renal impairment or significant hypertension. Also use cautiously in patients with a history of dysuria, especially men with prostatic hypertrophy, prostatitis, and other lower urinary tract obstructive disorders.
- Know that at least 14 days should elapse between stopping an MAO inhibitor and starting milnacipran. At least 5 days should elapse between stopping milnacipran and starting an MAO inhibitor.
- Measure patient's blood pressure and heart rate before starting and periodically during milnacipran therapy because drug can raise blood pressure and heart rate. If hypertension or tachycardia occurs and persists, notify prescriber and expect to reduce dosage or discontinue drug.
- Watch closely for suicidal tendencies, especially when therapy starts and dosage changes.

! WARNING Monitor patient closely for serotonin syndrome, a rare but serious adverse effect of selective serotonin reuptake inhibitors such as milnacipran. Signs and symptoms include agitation, confusion, diaphoresis, diarrhea, fever, hyperactive reflexes, poor coordination, restlessness, shaking, talking or acting with uncontrolled excitement, tremor, and twitching. In its most severe form, it can resemble neuroleptic malignant syndrome with autonomic instability with possible rapid fluctuation of vital signs, mental status changes, and muscle rigidity. If symptoms occur, notify prescriber immediately, expect to discontinue drug, and provide supportive care.

- Monitor patient's liver function. If jaundice or signs and symptoms of liver dysfunction occur, notify prescriber and expect drug to be discontinued.

! WARNING Watch for hypersensitivity reactions, especially in patients with aspirin sensitivity, because drug contains the yellow dye tartrazine.

- Check patient's serum sodium level, as ordered, because drug may cause hyponatremia, especially in elderly patients, patients taking diuretics, and patients who are volume-depleted.
- Expect to taper drug when no longer needed, as ordered, to minimize adverse reactions.

PATIENT TEACHING

- Advise patient to take drug with food to improve tolerability.
- Urge family or caregiver to watch patient closely for suicidal tendencies, especially when therapy starts or dosage changes.
- Caution patient against stopping drug abruptly because serious adverse effects may result.
- Instruct patient to alert all prescribers that he takes milnacipran.
- Tell patient to have his blood pressure monitored regularly throughout milnacipran therapy.
- Advise patient to avoid activities, such as driving, that require alertness until the CNS effects of milnacipran are known.
- Caution patient to avoid aspirin and NSAIDs, if possible, while taking milnacipran.
- Instruct patient to notify prescriber if any persistent, severe, or unusual signs or symptoms occur. Also, have patient speak with prescriber about sexual dysfunction concerns, if present.

M

milrinone lactate

Class and Category

Pharmacologic class: Phosphodiesterase 3 inhibitor

Therapeutic class: Inotropic

Indications and Dosages

* *To provide short-term treatment of acute heart failure*

I.V. INFUSION

Adults. *Loading:* 50 mcg/kg slowly over 10 minutes followed by 0.375 to 0.75 mcg/kg/min as a continuous infusion with infusion rate adjusted, as needed. *Maximum:* 1.13 mg/kg daily.

±**DOSAGE ADJUSTMENT** Dosage adjusted according to cardiac output, pulmonary artery wedge pressure (PAWP), and clinical response. If creatinine clearance is 50 ml/min, infusion rate reduced to 0.43 mcg/kg/min; if 40 ml/min, infusion rate reduced to 0.38 mcg/kg/min; if 30 ml/min, infusion rate reduced to 0.33 mcg/kg/min; if 20 ml/min, to 0.28 mcg/kg/min; if 10 ml/min, to 0.23 mcg/kg/min; and if 5 ml/min, to 0.2 mcg/kg/min.

Drug Administration

I.V.

- For I.V. infusion used for loading dose, infuse drug directly into I.V. line with compatible solution slowly over 10 minutes. Drug may be given undiluted but diluting to a rounded total volume of 10 or 20 ml may simplify controlling the rate of delivery. Use a controlled-rate infusion device for administration.
- For continuous I.V. infusion, dilute drug with 0.45% or 0.9% Sodium Chloride Injection or 5% Dextrose Injection to achieve a 200-mcg/ml concentration using 1-mg/ml vial as follows: Add 40 ml of above solution to 10 ml of drug to achieve a total volume of 50 ml or add 80 ml of above solution to 20 ml of drug to achieve a total volume of 100 ml. Using a calibrated electronic infusion device, infuse continuously at a rate between 0.375 mcg/kg/min up to 0.75 mcg/kg/min depending on patient's needs and response to drug but not

exceeding 1.13 mg/kg/day. Discard unused portion in vial.
- Be aware drug also comes premixed and does not require further dilution.
- Store unused vials at room temperature, avoiding excessive heat or cold.
- *Incompatibilities:* None listed by manufacturer

Route	Onset	Peak	Duration
I.V.	5–15 min	1–2 hr	3–6 hr

Half-life: 2.5 hr

Contraindications

Hypersensitivity to milrinone or its components

Interactions

DRUGS

None reported by manufacturer

Adverse Reactions

CNS: Headache, tremor

CV: Angina, **hypotension, supraventricular arrhythmias, torsades de pointes,** ventricular ectopic activity, **ventricular fibrillation and tachycardia, torsades de pointes**

GI: Liver function test abnormalities

HEME: Thrombocytopenia

RESP: Bronchospasm

SKIN: Rash

Other: **Anaphylactic shock, hypokalemia,** infusion-site reactions (pain, redness, swelling)

Childbearing Considerations

PREGNANCY

- It is not known if drug causes fetal harm.
- Use with caution only if benefit to mother outweighs potential risk to fetus.

LACTATION

- It is not known if drug is present in breast milk.
- Patient should check with prescriber before breastfeeding.

Nursing Considerations

- Make sure ECG equipment is available for continuous monitoring during milrinone therapy.
- Check platelet count before and periodically during infusion, as ordered. Expect to discontinue drug if platelet count falls below 150,000/mm^3.

☰ Mechanism of Action

An inotropic drug, milrinone increases the force of myocardial contraction—and cardiac output—by blocking the enzyme phosphodiesterase. Normally, this enzyme is activated by hormones binding to cell membrane receptors. As shown below left, phosphodiesterase normally degrades intracellular cAMP, which restricts calcium movement into myocardial cells. By inhibiting phosphodiesterase, as shown below right, milrinone slows the rate of cAMP degradation, increasing the intracellular cAMP level and the amount of calcium that enters myocardial cells. In blood vessels, increased cAMP causes smooth-muscle relaxation, which improves cardiac output by reducing preload and afterload.

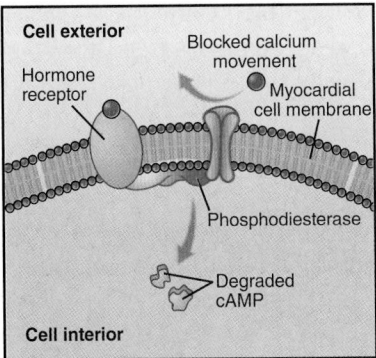
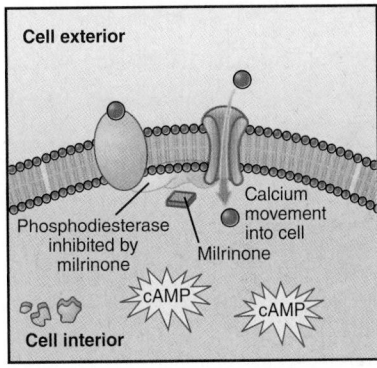

- Monitor blood pressure, cardiac output, fluid status, heart rate, pulmonary artery wedge pressure, and weight during therapy to determine drug effectiveness.
- Monitor liver and renal function test results and serum electrolyte levels. Notify prescriber of abnormalities.
- If severe hypotension develops, notify prescriber at once and expect to stop drug.
- Expect patient to receive digoxin before starting milrinone, which can increase ventricular response rate.

PATIENT TEACHING
- Reassure patient that he will be monitored constantly during therapy.

minocycline hydrochloride

CoreMino, Dynacin, Minocin, Minolira, Solodyn, Ximino

☰ Class and Category

Pharmacologic class: Tetracycline
Therapeutic class: Antibiotic

☰ Indications and Dosages

✳ *To treat infections as follows: bartonellosis due to* Bartonella bacilliformis; *brucellosis due to* Brucella *species;* Campylobacter fetus *infections caused by* Campylobacter fetus; *chancroid caused by* Haemophilus ducreyi; *cholera caused by* Vibrio cholerae; *granuloma inguinale caused by* Klebsiella granulomatis; *inclusion conjunctivitis caused by* Chlamydia trachomatis; *lymphogranuloma venereum caused by* Chlamydia trachomatis; *plague caused by* Yersinia pestis; *psittacosis due to* Chlamydophila psittaci; *relapsing fever due to* Borrelia recurrentis; *respiratory tract infections caused by* Mycoplasma pneumoniae; *Rocky Mountain spotted fever, typhus fever and the typhus group, q fever, rickettsialpox and tick fevers caused by* rickettsiae; *trachoma caused by* Chlamydia trachomatis; *or tularemia due to* Francisella tularensis; *other gram-negative infections caused by* Acinetobacter *species,* Enterobacter aerogenes, Escherichia coli, *respiratory tract infections caused by* Haemophilus influenzae, *or respiratory tract and urinary tract infections caused by* Klebsiella species; *other gram-positive infections such as skin and skin*

M

structure infections caused by Staphylococcus aureus *or upper respiratory tract infections caused by* Streptococcus pneumoniae; *and infections when penicillin is contraindicated such as actinomycosis caused by* Actinomyces israelii, *anthrax due to* Bacillus anthracis, *listeriosis due to* Listeria monocytogenes, *Vincent's infection caused by* Fusobacterium fusiforme, *or yaws caused by* Treponema pallidum *subspecies* pertenue

CAPSULES, ORAL SUSPENSION, TABLETS

Adults and adolescents. *Initial:* 200 mg. *Maintenance:* 100 mg every 12 hr. Or 100 to 200 mg initially, followed by 50 mg every 6 hr.

Children over age 8. *Initial:* 4 mg/kg. *Maintenance:* 2 mg/kg every 12 hr. *Maximum:* 200 mg as initial dose; 100 mg/dose for maintenance.

I.V. INFUSION

Adults and adolescents. *Initial:* 200 mg. *Maintenance:* 100 mg every 12 hr. *Maximum:* 200 mg daily.

Children over age 8. *Initial:* 4 mg/kg. *Maintenance:* 2 mg/kg every 12 hr. *Maximum:* 200 mg for initial dose; 100 mg/dose for maintenance dose; and 400 mg total daily dose.

± **DOSAGE ADJUSTMENT** For patient with renal impairment, dosage decreased or dosage interval increased; dosage not to exceed 200 mg daily.

✳ *To treat uncomplicated gonorrhea from* Neisseria gonorrhoeae *in nonpregnant patients allergic to penicillin*

CAPSULES, ORAL SUSPENSION, TABLETS

Adults and adolescents. *Initial:* 200 mg. *Maintenance:* 100 mg every 12 hr for at least 4 days.

✳ *To treat uncomplicated gonococcal urethritis in men allergic to penicillin*

CAPSULES, ORAL SUSPENSION, TABLETS

Adults. 100 mg every 12 hr for 5 days.

✳ *To treat asymptomatic meningococcal carriers with* Neisseria meningitidis *in nasopharynx*

CAPSULES, ORAL SUSPENSION, TABLETS

Adults and adolescents. 100 mg every 12 hr for 5 days.

Children over age 8. *Initial:* 4 mg/kg. *Maintenance:* 2 mg/kg every 12 hr for 5 days.

✳ *To treat infections caused by* Mycobacterium marinum

CAPSULES, ORAL SUSPENSION, TABLETS

Adults. 100 mg every 12 hr for 6 to 8 wk.

✳ *To treat uncomplicated nongonococcal endocervical, rectal, or urethral infection caused by* Chlamydia trachomatis *or* Ureaplasma urealyticum

CAPSULES, ORAL SUSPENSION, TABLETS

Adults. 100 mg every 12 hr for at least 7 days.

✳ *To treat syphilis caused by* Treponema pallidum *in patients allergic to penicillin*

CAPSULES, ORAL SUSPENSION, TABLETS

Adults. *Initial:* 200 mg, followed by 100 mg every 12 hr for 10 to 15 days.

✳ *To treat acne including inflammatory, nonnodular, moderate to severe*

CAPSULES, TABLETS

Adults and children 8 years and older. 50 to 100 mg twice daily for up to 12 wks.

E.R. CAPSULES (XIMINO)

Adults and children 12 years and older. 1 mg/kg/dose once daily for 12 wks.

E.R. TABLETS (MINOLIRA)

Adults weighing 126 to 136 kg (277 to 299 lb). 135 mg once daily.

Adults weighing 90 to 125 kg (198 to 275 lb). 105 mg once daily.

Adults weighing 60 to 89 kg (132 to 196 lb). 67.5 mg (one-half of the 135 mg-tablet) once daily.

Adults weighing 45 to 59 kg (99 to 130 lb). 52.5 mg (one-half of the 105-mg tablet) once daily.

E.R. TABLET (COREMINO, SOLODYN)

Adults weighing 126 to 136 kg (277 to 299 lb). 135 mg once daily.

Adults weighing 111 to 125 kg (244 to 275 lb). 115 mg once daily.

Adults weighing 97 to 110 kg (213 to 242 lb). 105 mg once daily.

Adults weighing 85 to 96 kg (187 to 211 lb). 90 mg once daily.

Adults weighing 72 to 84 kg (158 to 184 lb). 80 mg once daily.

Adults weighing 60 to 71 kg (132 to 156 lb). 65 mg once daily.

Adults weighing 50 to 59 kg (110 to 130 lb). 55 mg once daily.

Adults weighing 45 to 49 kg (99 to 108 lb). 45 mg once daily.

≡ Drug Administration

P.O.

- Shake oral suspension well before use.
- Use calibrated device to measure dosage of oral suspension.
- Administer drug with a full glass of water or milk, or with food.
- Capsules, E.R. tablets, and immediate-release tablets should be swallowed whole and not chewed, crushed, or split.
- Ensure that patient does not lie down immediately after administration, to minimize esophageal and GI irritation.
- Do not administer drug within 2 hours of an antacid or 3 hours of an iron preparation.

I.V.

- I.V. route used only when oral administration is not possible.
- Reconstitute each 100-mg vial with 5 to 10 ml Sterile Water for Injection.
- Further dilute in 100 to 1,000 ml 0.9% Sodium Chloride Injection, 5% Dextrose in Water, 5% Dextrose Injection with 0.9% Sodium Chloride Injection, or Lactated Ringer's solution.
- Flush I.V. line with any of the above diluents before and after administration if I.V. line is used for administration of other drugs.
- Infuse over 60 minutes.
- Store reconstituted drug at room temperature for up to 4 hours or refrigerated for up to 24 hours.
- *Incompatibilities:* Calcium-containing solutions, other drugs

Route	Onset	Peak	Duration
P.O.	Unknown	1–4 hr	Unknown
P.O./E.R.	Unknown	3.5–4 hr	Unknown
I.V.	Unknown	Unknown	Unknown

Half-life: 2.7–5.5 hr

≡ Mechanism of Action

Inhibits bacterial protein synthesis by competitively binding to the 30S ribosomal subunit of the mRNA–ribosome complex of certain organisms.

≡ Contraindications

U.S.: Hypersensitivity to minocycline, other tetracyclines, or their components; *Canada in addition to U.S.:* Breastfeeding children under age 12, complete renal failure, myasthenia gravis, pregnancy, severe liver disease

≡ Interactions

DRUGS

aluminum-, calcium-, or magnesium-containing antacids; calcium supplements; choline and magnesium salicylates; iron-containing preparations; magnesium-containing laxatives; sodium bicarbonate: Possibly formation of nonabsorbable complex, impaired minocycline absorption

atazanavir: Possibly decreased serum concentration of atazanavir

BCG (immunization or intravesical): Possibly decreased effectiveness of BCG

bile acid sequestrants, calcium salts: Decreased minocycline absorption

bismuth subsalicylate: Possibly decreased serum concentration of minocycline

cholera or typhoid vaccines: Possibly diminished effectiveness of vaccines

CNS depressants: Possibly enhanced CNS depressant effect

lactobacillus and estriol: Possibly diminished effectiveness of these products

lanthanum: Possible decreased effectiveness of minocycline

mecamylamine: Possibly enhanced neuromuscular blocking effect of mecamylamine

methoxyflurane: Increased risk of nephrotoxicity

mipomersen: Possibly enhanced hepatotoxicity of mipomersen

multivitamins/minerals: Possibly decreased concentration of minocycline

neuromuscular blocking agents: Enhanced neuromuscular blocking effect of these agents

penicillin: Interference with bactericidal action of penicillin

quinapril: Possibly decreased effectiveness of minocycline

retinoic acid derivatives: Possibly enhanced adverse effects of these drugs

sucralfate, zinc salts: Possibly decreased absorption of minocycline

sucroferric oxyhydroxide: Possibly decreased serum concentration of minocycline

vitamin K antagonists: Possibly enhanced anticoagulant effect of vitamin K antagonists

≡ Adverse Reactions

CNS: Dizziness, fever, headache, intracranial hypertension, light-headedness, unsteadiness, vertigo

CV: **Myocarditis, pericarditis**
EENT: Blurred vision, darkened or discolored tongue, glossitis, papilledema, tooth discoloration, vision changes
ENDO: Thyroid function abnormality, **thyroid cancer**
GI: Abdominal cramps or pain, anorexia, diarrhea, dysphagia, enterocolitis, esophageal irritation and ulceration, **hepatitis, hepatotoxicity, jaundice,** indigestion, nausea, **pancreatitis, pseudomembranous colitis,** vomiting
GU: Genital candidiasis, **nephritis, nephrotoxicity**
HEME: Eosinophilia, **hemolytic anemia, neutropenia, thrombocytopenia, thrombocytopenic purpura**
MS: Arthralgia, myopathy (transient)
RESP: **Pneumonitis, pulmonary infiltrates**
SKIN: **Erythema multiforme, exfoliative dermatitis,** brown pigmentation of skin and mucous membranes, **erythema multiforme,** erythematous and maculopapular rash, **exfoliative dermatitis,** onycholysis, photosensitivity, pruritus, purpura (anaphylactoid), rash, **Stevens–Johnson syndrome,** urticaria
Other: **Anaphylaxis, angioedema,** serum sickness-like reaction, systemic lupus erythematosus exacerbation

Childbearing Considerations

PREGNANCY

- Drug may cause fetal harm as it crosses the placental barrier and may discolor teeth.
- Like other tetracyclines, rare reports of congenital anomalies including limb reduction have been reported.
- Drug is not recommended for use during pregnancy.

LACTATION

- Drug is present in breast milk.
- A decision should be made to discontinue breastfeeding or the drug to avoid potential serious adverse reactions in the breastfed infant.

Nursing Considerations

- Use minocycline cautiously in patients with hepatic or renal dysfunction and in those taking other hepatotoxic drugs, because drug may cause nephrotoxicity or hepatotoxicity.

- Use minocycline cautiously in patients with a history of predisposition to oral candidiasis, because safety and effectiveness of drug have not been established for treatment of periodontitis in patients with coexistent oral candidiasis.
- Monitor blood, hepatic, and renal tests before and during long-term therapy.
- Assess patient for signs of superinfection; if signs appear, notify prescriber, discontinue minocycline, and start appropriate therapy, as ordered.
- Monitor patient for development of foul-smelling diarrhea, which suggests *Clostridium difficile.* If present, notify prescriber, obtain stool culture, and expect to withhold minocycline and provide supportive care, as indicated and ordered.
- Monitor PT in patient who also takes an anticoagulant during minocycline therapy.
- Monitor patient for signs and symptoms of thyroid cancer such as alteration in thyroid function or presence of nodule in patients receiving minocycline therapy over prolonged periods.

! WARNING Monitor patient for blurred vision or headache because benign intracranial hypertension has occurred with the use of minocycline. If present, notify prescriber and expect drug to be discontinued. Know that although intracranial hypertension usually resolves after drug is discontinued, permanent visual loss can occur. Expect patient with suspected intracranial hypertension to undergo a prompt ophthalmologic evaluation and be monitored until vision is stabilized, as intracranial pressure can remain elevated for weeks after drug is discontinued.

PATIENT TEACHING

- Instruct patient to shake oral suspension well and to use calibrated measuring device.
- Advise patient to take minocycline with a full glass of water, with food or milk, and to remain in an upright position to minimize esophageal and GI irritation.
- Direct patient to take a missed dose as soon as he remembers unless it's nearly time for the next dose. Caution against double-dosing.

- Instruct patient not to take minocycline within 2 hours of an antacid or 3 hours of an iron preparation.
- Urge patient to complete full course of treatment even if he feels better before finishing.
- Instruct patient to notify prescriber if no improvement occurs in a few days.
- Advise patient to avoid prolonged exposure to sun or sunlamps during therapy.
- Instruct patient to notify prescriber immediately about blurred vision, dizziness, headache, known or suspected pregnancy, and unsteadiness.
- Explain that diarrhea may occur up to 2 months after completing therapy; urge patient to notify prescriber if it occurs.

mirabegron
Myrbetriq, Myrbetriq Granules

☰ Class and Category
Pharmacologic class: Beta-3 adrenergic agonist
Therapeutic class: Bladder antispasmodic

☰ Indications and Dosages
✳ *To treat overactive bladder with symptoms of urge urinary incontinence, urgency, and urinary frequency as monotherapy or in combination with solifenacin succinate*

E.R. TABLETS
Adults. *Initially:* 25 mg once daily, increased as needed to 50 mg once daily after 4 to 8 wk.
±**DOSAGE ADJUSTMENT** For patients with severe hepatic or renal impairment, dosage should not exceed 25 mg once daily.

✳ *To treat pediatric neurogenic detrusor overactivity (NDO)*

E.R. TABLETS
Children age 3 years and older weighing 35 kg (77 lb) or more. 25 mg once daily, increased to 50 mg once daily after 4 to 8 wk, if needed.
±**DOSAGE ADJUSTMENT** For children weighing 35 kg (77 kb) or more with severe hepatic or renal impairment, dosage should not exceed 25 mg once daily.

E.R. ORAL SUSPENSION
Children age 3 years and older weighing 35 kg (77 lb) or more. 48 mg (6 ml) once daily, increased to 80 mg (10 ml) once daily after 4 to 8 wk, if needed. *Maximum:* 80 mg (10 ml) once daily.
Children age 3 years and older weighing 22 kg (48.4 lb) to less than 35 kg (77 lb). 32 mg (4 ml) once daily, increased to 64 mg (8 ml) once daily after 4 to 8 wk, if needed.
Children age 3 years and older weighing 11 kg (24.2 lb) to less than 22 kg (48.4 lb). 24 mg (3 ml) once daily, increased to 48 mg (6 ml) once daily after 4 to 8 wk, if needed.
±**DOSAGE ADJUSTMENT** For children with severe hepatic or renal dysfunction and weighing 35 kg (77 lb) or more, dosage should not exceed 48 mg (6 ml); for children weighing 22 kg (48.4 lb) to less than 35 kg (77 lb), dosage should not exceed 32 mg (4 ml); and for children weighing 11 kg (24.2 lb) to less than 22 kg (48.4 lb), dosage should not exceed 24 mg (3 ml).

☰ Drug Administration
P.O.
- Do not interchange E.R. tablets with E.R. oral suspension.
- A recommended adult dosage for E.R. oral suspension has not been determined.
- Do not combine E.R. tablets and E.R. oral suspension to achieve a total dose.
- Administer E.R. tablets with water. E.R. tablets should not be chewed, crushed, or divided. Adults may take tablets with or without food; children weighing more than 35 kg (77 lb) should take tablets with food.
- To make E.R. suspension, tap closed bottle several times to loosen granules, then add 100 ml of water to bottle and shake vigorously for 1 minute. Then let stand for 10 to 30 minutes followed by shaking bottle vigorously again for 1 minute (suspension will contain 8 mg/ml of drug). Measure dosage using a calibrated device. Administer with food. Store suspension at room temperature for up to 28 days.
- If a dose is missed and less than 12 hours has passed since missed dose, administer drug; if more than 12 hours has passed, skip missed dose.

Route	Onset	Peak	Duration
P.O.	Unknown	3.5 hr	Unknown

Half-life: 50 hr

Mechanism of Action

Relaxes the detrusor smooth muscle during the storage phase of the urinary bladder fill-void cycle by activating the beta-3 adrenergic receptor, which increases bladder capacity. With increased bladder capacity, urge sensation is decreased, which in turn decreases urinary frequency.

Contraindications

Hypersensitivity to mirabegron or its components

Interactions

DRUGS

CYP2D6 substrates such as desipramine, flecainide, metoprolol, propafenone, thioridazine: Increased blood levels of these drugs

digoxin: Increased risk of digoxin toxicity

warfarin: Possibly changes in INR and prothrombin time with multiple doses of warfarin

Adverse Reactions

CNS: Anxiety, confusion, dizziness, fatigue, hallucinations, headache, insomnia

CV: Atrial fibrillation, elevated LDH levels, hypertension, palpitations, tachycardia

EENT: Dry mouth, glaucoma, nasopharyngitis, rhinitis, sinusitis

GI: Abdominal distention or pain, constipation, diarrhea, dyspepsia, elevated liver enzymes, gastritis, nausea

GU: Bladder pain, cystitis, nephrolithiasis, **prostate cancer,** urinary retention, UTI, vaginal infections, vulvovaginal pruritis

MS: Arthralgia, back pain

RESP: Cough (children)

SKIN: Pruritis, rash, **Stevens–Johnson syndrome**

Other: Angioedema, flu-like symptoms

Childbearing Considerations

PREGNANCY

- It is not known if drug causes fetal harm.
- Use with caution only if benefit to mother outweighs potential risk to fetus.

LACTATION

- It is not known if drug is present in breast milk.
- Patient should check with prescriber before breastfeeding.

Nursing Considerations

- Know that mirabegron should not be given to patients with severe uncontrolled hypertension (defined as systolic blood pressure 180 mm Hg or higher and/or diastolic blood pressure 110 mm Hg or higher) because drug can increase blood pressure. Monitor patient's blood pressure regularly and report persistent or significant increases to prescriber.
- Be aware that mirabegron should not be given to patients with end-stage renal disease or to patients with severe hepatic impairment because drug has not been studied in these conditions, and adverse effects are unknown.
- Use mirabegron cautiously in patients with bladder outlet obstruction and in patients taking antimuscarinic drugs for the treatment of this condition, because drug may cause urinary retention.

! **WARNING** Monitor patient closely for angioedema of the face, larynx, lips, and tongue, which may occur as soon as the first dose or hours after the first dose or after multiple doses. Be prepared to administer emergency treatment for life-threatening upper airway swelling, as ordered, and maintain a patent airway. Notify prescriber and expect drug to be discontinued.

PATIENT TEACHING

- Instruct adult patient and children weighing more than 35 kg (77 lb) age 3 and older to take mirabegron tablets with water and to swallow tablet whole. Caution patient not to chew, crush, or divide tablets prior to ingesting. Tablets should be taken with food if administered to a child weighing 35 kg (77 lb) or more.
- Instruct family or caregiver how to mix granules. Advise the use of a calibrated device to measure dosage, not a household spoon, and to administer oral suspension with food. Tell family or caregiver to store oral suspension at room temperature and to discard after 28 days.

! **WARNING** Alert patient that serious allergic reactions can occur and to seek immediate medical care if serious swelling around face, neck, or tongue occurs.

- Warn patient that drug may increase blood pressure. Encourage patient to have his blood pressure checked regularly, especially if he has hypertension.
- Review common adverse effects of drug with patient. Tell patient to notify prescriber if he experiences a decrease in urinary output despite a normal intake. Also remind patient that drug may cause itching, rapid heartbeat, rash, or urinary tract infections and to alert prescriber if present.

mirtazapine

Remeron, Remeron SolTab

Class and Category

Pharmacologic class: Tetracyclic antidepressant
Therapeutic class: Antidepressant

Indications and Dosages

✴ *To treat major depression*

ORAL DISINTEGRATING TABLETS, TABLETS

Adults. *Initial:* 15 mg daily at bedtime. Increased as needed and tolerated at 1- to 2-wk intervals. *Maximum:* 45 mg daily.

±**DOSAGE ADJUSTMENT** For the elderly and patients with hepatic or renal impairment, dosage may have to be reduced.

Drug Administration

P.O.

- Administer dose preferably at bedtime with water.
- Tablets should be swallowed whole and not chewed, crushed, or split.
- Remove oral disintegrating tablets gently from blister pack with dry, gloved hands. Patient should hold tablet on tongue and let it dissolve, which will occur within 30 seconds. ODT tablets should not be swallowed whole and should not be chewed or crushed. Water may be taken once tablet has dissolved.

Route	Onset	Peak	Duration
P.O.	Unknown	2 hr	Unknown

Half-life: 20–40 hr

Mechanism of Action

May inhibit neuronal reuptake of norepinephrine and serotonin. By doing so, this tetracyclic antidepressant increases the action of these neurotransmitters in nerve cells. Increased neuronal serotonin and norepinephrine levels may elevate mood.

Contraindications

Hypersensitivity to mirtazapine or its components; use within 14 days of an MAO inhibitor, including I.V. methylene blue and linezolid

Interactions

DRUGS

anxiolytics, hypnotics, other CNS depressants (including sedatives): Increased CNS depression
CYP3A4 inducers such as carbamazepine, phenytoin, rifampicin: Decreased mirtazapine effects and effectiveness
CYP3A4 inhibitors such as azole-antifungals, cimetidine, CYP3A4 inhibitors, erythromycin, HIV protease inhibitors, ketoconazole, nefazodone: Increased serum mirtazapine effects and risk of adverse reactions
MAO inhibitors, including I.V. methylene blue and linezolid; other serotonergic drugs: Possibly hyperpyrexia, hypertension, seizures, and serotonin syndrome
QTc-prolonging drugs: Increased risk of QT prolongation and/or ventricular arrhythmias such as torsades de pointes
warfarin: Possible increase in INR

ACTIVITIES

alcohol use: Increased CNS depression

Adverse Reactions

CNS: Agitation, akathisia, amnesia, anxiety, apathy, asthenia, ataxia, **cerebral ischemia**, chills, confusion, delirium, delusions, depersonalization, depression, dizziness, dream disturbances, drowsiness, dyskinesia, dystonia, emotional lability, euphoria, extrapyramidal reactions, fever, hallucinations, hostility, hyperkinesia, hyperreflexia, hypoesthesia, hypokinesia, lack of coordination, malaise, mania, migraine headache, **neuroleptic malignant syndrome-like reactions**, neurosis, paranoia, paresthesia, psychomotor restlessness, **seizures**, **serotonin syndrome**, somnambulism (ambulation and other complex behaviors out of bed), somnolence, syncope, tremor, vertigo
CV: Angina, **bradycardia**, edema, hypercholesterolemia, hypertension,

M

hypertriglyceridemia, **hypotension**, **MI**, orthostatic hypotension, peripheral edema, **PVCs**, **torsades de pointes**, vasodilation, **ventricular arrhythmia**

EENT: Accommodation disturbances, conjunctivitis, dry mouth, earache, epistaxis, eye pain, gingival bleeding, glaucoma, glossitis, hearing loss, hyperacusis, keratoconjunctivitis, lacrimation, pharyngitis, sinusitis, stomatitis

ENDO: Breast pain, galactorrhea, gynecomastia, hyperprolactinemia

GI: Abdominal distention and pain, anorexia, cholecystitis, colitis, constipation, elevated ALT level, eructation, increased appetite, nausea, thirst, vomiting

GU: Amenorrhea, cystitis, dysmenorrhea, dysuria, hematuria, impotence, increased libido, leukorrhea, renal calculi, urinary frequency and incontinence, urine retention, UTI, vaginitis

HEME: **Agranulocytosis**, **neutropenia**

MS: Arthralgia, back pain, dysarthria, elevated creatine kinase blood level, muscle twitching, myalgia, myasthenia, neck pain and rigidity, **rhabdomyolysis**

RESP: **Asthma**, bronchitis, cough, dyspnea, pneumonia

SKIN: Acne, alopecia, bullous dermatitis, dry skin, **erythema multiforme**, **exfoliative dermatitis**, photosensitivity, pruritus, rash, **Stevens–Johnson syndrome**, **toxic epidermal necrolysis**

Other: **Angioedema**, dehydration, flu-like symptoms, herpes simplex, **hyponatremia**, weight change

Childbearing Considerations

PREGNANCY

- Pregnancy exposure registry: 1-844-405-6185 or https://womensmentalhealth.org/clinical-and-research-programs/pregnancyregistry/antidepressants/.
- It is not known if drug causes fetal harm.
- Use with caution only if benefit to mother outweighs potential risk to fetus.

LACTATION

- Drug may be present in breast milk.
- Patient should check with prescriber before breastfeeding.

Nursing Considerations

- Use mirtazapine cautiously in elderly patients and in those receiving concurrent medication known to cause hyponatremia, because drug may lower the serum sodium level in these patients.

! WARNING Don't give drug within 14 days of an MAO inhibitor or concurrent therapy with serotonin-precursors such as L-tryptophan and oxitriptan, to avoid serious, possibly fatal, serotonin syndrome reaction. Use drug cautiously in patients receiving other serotonergic drugs such as lithium, St. John's wort, tramadol, triptans, and most tricyclic antidepressants because of increased risk for serotonin syndrome. Know that both disorders can occur as an adverse drug reaction to mirtazapine therapy without the concomitant use of other drugs. Monitor patient closely for signs and symptoms of serotonin syndrome such as alteration in vital signs, gastrointestinal symptoms, mental status changes, or neuromuscular abnormalities. Its most severe form resembles neuroleptic malignant syndrome and presents with autonomic instability with possible rapid changes in vital signs, hyperthermia, mental status changes, and muscle rigidity. If any of these symptoms occur, notify prescriber immediately, provide supportive care, as ordered, and expect mirtazapine to be discontinued.

- Monitor patient closely, especially during the first few weeks of therapy, for the development of akathisia, an unpleasant or distressing restlessness and need to move, often accompanied by an inability to sit or stand still. Notify prescriber, if present, and know that increasing the dose may worsen patient's condition.

! WARNING Monitor patient for hypersensitivity, especially angioedema. If present, stop drug, notify prescriber, and provide supportive care, as ordered.

- Watch closely for suicidal tendencies, especially when therapy starts or dosage changes, because depression may briefly worsen.

- Monitor patient closely for infection (fever, pharyngitis, stomatitis), which may be linked to a low WBC count. If these signs occur, notify prescriber and expect to stop drug.
- Expect mirtazapine therapy to last 6 months or longer for acute depression.
- Be aware that mirtazapine therapy should not be discontinued abruptly because adverse reactions may occur.

PATIENT TEACHING

- Tell patient to take drug at bedtime.
- Instruct patient to remove oral disintegrating tablet from blister package gently with dry hands. Tell patient not to chew, crush, or swallow disintegrating tablet. Tell him to hold tablet on tongue and let it dissolve. Inform him that tablet will dissolve within 30 seconds and water may be taken afterward, if desired.
- Inform phenylketonuric patient that mirtazapine disintegrating tablets contain phenylalanine 2.6 mg per 15-mg tablet, 5.2 mg per 30-mg tablet, and 7.8 mg per 45-mg tablet.

> **! WARNING** Alert patient that drug may cause an allergic reaction. Tell patient to seek immediate medical attention if severe or if swelling of face, neck, or tongue occurs.

- Advise patient that drug may cause mild pupillary dilation, which may lead to an episode of acute closure glaucoma. Encourage patient to have an eye exam before starting therapy to see if he is at risk.
- Instruct patient to avoid alcohol and other CNS depressants during therapy and for up to 7 days after drug is discontinued.
- Advise patient to avoid hazardous activities until drug's CNS effects are known.
- Direct patient to change position slowly to minimize the effects of orthostatic hypotension.
- Instruct patient to notify prescriber at once about chills, fever, mouth irritation, sore throat, and other signs of infection.
- Encourage patient to visit prescriber regularly during therapy to monitor progress.
- Caution patient not to discontinue mirtazapine therapy abruptly.

mitoxantrone hydrochloride

Class and Category

Pharmacologic class: Anthracenedione
Therapeutic class: Antineoplastic

Indications and Dosages

✳ *To reduce neurologic disability and frequency of relapses in patients with secondary (chronic) progressive, progressive relapsing, or worsening relapsing-remitting multiple sclerosis (patients whose neurologic status is significantly abnormal between relapses)*

I.V. INFUSION

Adults. 12 mg/m^2 every 3 mo and dosage adjusted, as needed. *Maximum:* Cumulative lifetime dose of 140 mg/m^2.

✳ *As adjunct to treat pain related to advanced hormone-refractory prostate cancer*

I.V. INFUSION

Adults. 12 to 14 mg/m^2 every 21 days.

✳ *As adjunct to treat acute nonlymphocytic leukemia (ANLL)*

I.V. INFUSION

Adults. *Induction:* 12 mg/m^2 on days 1 to 3 with 100 mg/m^2 of cytarabine as a continuous 24-hr infusion on days 1 to 7. If patient's antileukemic response is inadequate or incomplete, second induction course is given at same dosage but only for 2 days with mitoxantrone and 5 days for cytarabine.

Drug Administration

I.V.

- Follow facility policy for handling antineoplastics. Be aware that manufacturer recommends goggles, gloves, and a gown during drug preparation and delivery.
- After penetration of multidose stopper, store undiluted drug concentrate for up to 7 days at room temperature or 14 days refrigerated. Avoid freezing drug.
- Before administering drug, dilute it in at least 50 ml of 0.9% Sodium Chloride Injection or 5% Dextrose in Water. Drug may be further diluted with 0.9% Sodium Chloride Injection, 5% Dextrose in Water, or 5% Dextrose in Water with 0.9% Sodium Chloride Injection. Use immediately.

M

- Administer diluted solution slowly into the tubing as a freely running intravenous infusion of 0.9% Sodium Chloride Injection or 5% Dextrose in Water over no less than 3 minutes. A short infusion should be administered over 5 to 15 minutes.
- Drug shouldn't be given intra-arterially, intramuscularly, intrathecally, or subcutaneously because of possible severe adverse reactions.
- If mitoxantrone solution contacts skin or mucosa, the area should be washed thoroughly with warm water. If it contacts eyes, irrigate them thoroughly with water or Normal Saline solution.
- Discard unused diluted solution immediately, because it contains no preservatives.
- If any signs of extravasation occur (bluish discoloration, burning, erythema, pain, swelling, or ulceration), stop infusion immediately and notify prescriber. Reinsert I.V. line in another large vein and resume administration slowly. Apply ice bags intermittently to affected site and elevate affected extremity. Extravasation reactions may progress so site should be assessed frequently. Be aware a surgical consult may be needed if there is any sign of a local reaction.
- *Incompatibilities:* Other drugs, including heparin

Route	Onset	Peak	Duration
I.V.	Unknown	Unknown	Unknown
Half-life: 23–215 hr			

Mechanism of Action

Binds to DNA, causing cross-linkage and strand breakage, interfering with RNA synthesis, and inhibiting topoisomerase II, an enzyme that uncoils and repairs damaged DNA. Mitoxantrone produces a cytocidal effect on proliferating and nonproliferating cells and doesn't appear to be cell-cycle specific. It's known to inhibit B-cell, T-cell, and macrophage proliferation and impair antigen function.

Contraindications

Hypersensitivity to mitoxantrone or its components

Interactions

DRUGS

vaccines, killed virus: Decreased antibody response to vaccine
vaccines, live virus: Increased risk of replication of and adverse effects of vaccine virus, decreased antibody response to vaccine

Adverse Reactions

CNS: Headache, **seizures**
CV: Arrhythmias, cardiotoxicity, chest pain, **congestive heart failure**, decreased left ventricular ejection fraction, **ECG changes**
EENT: Blue-colored cornea, conjunctivitis, mucositis, stomatitis
GI: Abdominal pain, diarrhea, elevated liver enzymes, **GI bleeding**, jaundice, nausea, vomiting
GU: Blue-green urine, **renal failure**
HEME: Acute myelogenous leukemia, leukopenia, other leukemias, thrombocytopenia
MS: Myelodysplasia
RESP: Cough, dyspnea
SKIN: Alopecia, extravasation
Other: Anaphylaxis, hypersensitivity reactions, hyperuricemia, infection, infusion-site pain or redness

Childbearing Considerations

PREGNANCY

- Drug may cause fetal harm.
- A negative pregnancy test must be obtained prior to each dose.
- Drug should not be given to pregnant women.

LACTATION

- Drug is present in breast milk.
- Breastfeeding should be discontinued prior to drug therapy.

REPRODUCTION

- Women of childbearing age should use an effective form of contraception during drug therapy.
- If pregnancy occurs while taking drug, patient should notify prescriber immediately.

Nursing Considerations

- Know that before mitoxantrone therapy and before each dose, expect patient to have an ECG and evaluation of left ventricular ejection fraction. Expect to obtain CBC with platelet count, and hematocrit and hemoglobin level(s). If patient's left ventricular ejection fraction drops below normal, expect drug to be discontinued.

- Be aware that drug shouldn't be given to patient with multiple sclerosis whose neutrophil count is less than 1,500/mm^3 or who has a below-normal left ventricular ejection fraction.
- Check liver enzymes, as ordered, before each course of therapy. Expect that drug won't be given to multiple sclerosis patient with abnormal liver function.

! WARNING Monitor I.V. site closely for extravasation, which may cause a severe reaction.

- Assess patient for cardiac dysfunction throughout therapy. Watch for evidence of cardiotoxicity, such as arrhythmias and chest pain, in patient with heart disease. Risk increases when cumulative dose reaches 140 mg/m^2 in cancer or 100 mg/m^2 in multiple sclerosis. Notify prescriber of any significant changes, and expect drug to be discontinued. Be aware that congestive heart failure may occur months or years after drug has been discontinued.
- Anticipate obtaining pregnancy test before each course of therapy for women of childbearing age with multiple sclerosis.
- Monitor patients with chickenpox or recent exposure and patients with herpes zoster for severe, generalized disease.
- Monitor blood uric acid level for hyperuricemia in patients with a history of gout or renal calculi. Expect to give allopurinol, as prescribed, to patients with leukemia or lymphoma and elevated blood uric acid level to prevent uric acid nephropathy.

! WARNING Be aware that if severe or life-threatening nonhematologic or hematologic toxicity occurs during first induction course, the second course will probably be withheld until it resolves.

- Know that if patient develops thrombocytopenia, precautions should be taken per facility policy.
- Assess patient for evidence of infection, such as fever, if leukopenia occurs. Expect to obtain appropriate specimens for culture and sensitivity testing.

- Be aware that patients receiving mitoxantrone in combination with other antineoplastics or radiation therapy or who have multiple sclerosis are at risk for developing secondary leukemia, including acute myelogenous leukemia.

PATIENT TEACHING

- Advise patient to complete dental work, if possible, before treatment begins or defer it until blood counts return to normal; drug may delay healing and cause gingival bleeding. Teach patient proper oral hygiene, and advise use of a toothbrush with soft bristles.

! WARNING Instruct patient to notify medical personnel immediately if a bluish discoloration, burning, pain, redness, swelling, or ulceration occurs at intravenous site used to administer drug.

- Urge patient to drink plenty of fluid to increase urine output and uric acid excretion.
- Advise patient to contact prescriber immediately if GI upset occurs, but to continue taking drug unless otherwise directed.
- Emphasize the importance of complying with the dosage regimen and keeping follow-up medical and laboratory appointments.
- Explain that urine may appear blue-green for 24 hours after treatment and that the whites of the eyes may appear blue. Emphasize that these effects are temporary and harmless. Explain that hair loss is possible, but that hair should return after therapy ends.
- Caution patient not to receive immunizations unless approved by prescriber. Also, advise persons who live in same household as patient to avoid receiving immunization with oral polio vaccine. Tell patient to avoid persons who recently received the oral polio vaccine or to wear a mask over his nose and mouth.
- Instruct patient to avoid persons with infections if bone marrow depression occurs. Advise patient to contact prescriber if chills, cough, fever, hoarseness, lower back or side pain, or difficult or painful urination occurs; these changes may signal an infection.

M

- Tell patient to contact prescriber immediately if he has black or tarry stools, unusual bleeding or bruising, blood in urine or stool, or pinpoint red spots on his skin.
- Urge patient not to touch his eyes or the inside of his nose unless he has just washed his hands.
- Emphasize the need to avoid accidental cuts, as from fingernail clippers or a razor, because of possible excessive bleeding or infection.
- Caution patient to avoid contact sports or activities that may cause bruising or injury.
- Urge patient to comply with yearly examinations after therapy ends to check for late-occurring drug-induced heart problems. Tell patient to report trouble breathing, swelling in ankles or legs, or a fast or uneven heartbeat even after drug has been discontinued.
- Warn women of childbearing age to avoid pregnancy but if pregnancy occurs to notify prescriber immediately.

modafinil
Provigil

Class, Category, and Schedule
Pharmacologic class: Analeptic
Therapeutic class: CNS stimulant
Controlled substance schedule: IV

Indications and Dosages

＊ *To improve daytime wakefulness in patients with narcolepsy, obstructive sleep apnea-hypopnea syndrome, and shift work sleep disorder*

TABLETS
Adults. 200 mg daily. *Maximum:* 400 mg daily.

±**DOSAGE ADJUSTMENT** For patients with severe hepatic impairment, dosage should be reduced by 50%.

Drug Administration

P.O.
- Administer daily dose in morning or 1 hr before starting work shift.
- Administer drug on an empty stomach, if possible, because food may delay drug's absorption and onset of action.

Route	Onset	Peak	Duration
P.O.	Unknown	2–4 hr	Unknown

Half-life: 15 hr

Mechanism of Action
May inhibit the release of gamma-aminobutyric acid (GABA), the most common inhibitory neurotransmitter, or CNS depressant, in the brain. Modafinil also increases the release of glutamate, an excitatory neurotransmitter, or CNS stimulant, in the hippocampus and thalamus. These two actions may improve wakefulness.

Contraindications
Hypersensitivity to modafinil, armodafinil, or their components

Interactions

DRUGS
CYP2C19 substrates such as clomipramine, diazepam, omeprazole, phenytoin, propranolol: Increased systemic exposure of these drugs
CYP3A4/5 substrates such as cyclosporine, midazolam, steroidal contraceptives, triazolam: Decreased systemic exposure of these drugs, with steroidal contraceptives continuing to have decreased effectiveness for one month after modafinil is discontinued
MAO inhibitors: Increased risk of adverse effects
warfarin: Possibly decreased warfarin metabolism and increased risk of bleeding

Adverse Reactions
CNS: Aggressiveness, agitation, anxiety, confusion, delusions, depression, hallucinations, headache, insomnia, mania, nervousness, psychomotor hyperactivity, psychosis, **suicidal ideation**
GI: Nausea
HEME: Agranulocytosis
SKIN: Rash, **Stevens–Johnson syndrome, toxic epidermal necrolysis**
Other: Anaphylaxis, angioedema, **drug reaction with eosinophilia and systemic symptoms (DRESS), infection, multiorgan hypersensitivity**

Childbearing Considerations

PREGNANCY
- Pregnancy exposure registry: 1-866-404-4106.

- Drug may cause fetal harm such as intrauterine growth restriction and spontaneous abortion based on animal studies.
- Use with caution only if benefit to mother outweighs potential risk to fetus.

LACTATION

- It is not known if drug is present in breast milk.
- Patient should check with prescriber before breastfeeding.

REPRODUCTION

- Women of childbearing age using steroidal contraceptives (including depot or implantable contraceptives) should be advised to use an alternative contraceptive method during drug therapy and for 1 month after drug is discontinued.

Nursing Considerations

- Keep in mind that modafinil shouldn't be given to patients with mitral valve prolapse syndrome or a history of left ventricular hypertrophy because drug may cause ischemic changes.
- Use cautiously in patients with recent MI or unstable angina because effect of drug is unknown in these disorders.
- Use cautiously in patients with a history of depression, mania, or psychosis because these conditions may worsen during therapy and may require modafinil to be stopped.

! **WARNING** Monitor patient with a history of alcoholism, stimulant abuse, or other substance abuse for compliance with modafinil therapy. Observe for signs of abuse or misuse, including drug-seeking behavior, frequent prescription refill requests, or increased frequency of dosing. Also watch for evidence of excessive modafinil dosage, including aggressiveness, anxiety, confusion, decreased prothrombin time, diarrhea, irritability, nausea, nervousness, palpitations, sleep disturbances, and tremor.

- Be aware that modafinil, like other CNS stimulants, may alter feelings, judgment, mood, motor skills, perception, thinking, and signs that patient needs sleep.
- Know that if giving drug to patient with emotional instability, a history of psychosis, or psychological illness with psychotic features, be prepared to perform baseline

behavioral assessments or frequent clinical observation.
- Stop drug at first sign of rash, and notify prescriber. Although rare, rash may indicate a potentially life-threatening event.

! **WARNING** Monitor patient for signs and symptoms of multisystem organ hypersensitivity, such as asthenia, fever, hematologic abnormalities, hepatitis, myocarditis, pruritus, rash, or any other serious abnormality, because multiorgan hypersensitivity may vary in its presentation. Notify prescriber if suspected, and expect to discontinue drug and provide supportive care, as ordered.

- Watch closely for suicidal tendencies, especially in patients with a psychiatric history.

PATIENT TEACHING

- Inform patient that modafinil can help, but not cure, narcolepsy and that drug's full effects may not be seen right away.
- Instruct patient to take drug in the morning or 1 hour before starting work shift.
- Advise patient to avoid taking modafinil within 1 hour of eating because food may delay drug's absorption and onset of action. If he drinks grapefruit juice, encourage him to drink a consistent amount daily.
- Instruct patient to stop taking modafinil and to notify prescriber if he develops a fever, rash, or other serious effect.
- Urge patient to report anxiety, chest pain, depression, or evidence of mania or psychosis to prescriber.

! **WARNING** Stress importance of stopping drug, seeking immediate medical care, and contacting prescriber if serious or unusual adverse reactions occur including the appearance of blisters, difficulty breathing or swallowing, hives, mouth sores, peeling skin, or a rash.

- Inform patient that drug can affect concentration and function and can hide signs of fatigue. Urge him not to drive or perform activities that require mental alertness until full CNS effects are known.
- Advise patient to avoid alcohol while taking modafinil.
- Encourage a regular sleeping pattern.

- Caution patient to avoid excessive intake of beverages, foods, and OTC drugs that contain caffeine because caffeine may lead to increased CNS stimulation.
- Inform female patient that modafinil can decrease the effectiveness of certain contraceptives, including birth control pills and implantable hormonal contraceptives. If she uses such contraceptives, urge her to use an alternate birth control method during modafinil therapy and for up to 1 month after she stops taking the drug.
- Advise patient to keep follow-up appointments with prescriber so that her progress can be monitored.
- Urge family or caregiver to watch patient closely for abnormal behaviors, including suicidal tendencies, especially if patient has a psychiatric history.

molnupiravir*

FDA Emergency Use Authorization

Class and Category
Pharmacologic class: Nucleoside analogue
Therapeutic class: Antiviral

Indications and Dosages
* *To treat mild to moderate coronavirus disease 2019 (COVID-19) in patients with a positive result of direct SARS-CoV-2 viral testing at high risk for progression to severe COVID-19, including hospitalization or death and for whom alternative COVID-19 treatment options approved or authorized by the FDA are not accessible or clinically appropriate.*

CAPSULES
Adults. 800 mg every 12 hr for 5 consecutive days and administered as soon as possible after a diagnosis of COVID-19 has been made, and within 5 days of symptom onset.

Drug Administration
TABLET
- Drug may be administered with or without food.
- Capsules should be swallowed whole and not broken, crushed, or opened.
- If a dose is missed within 10 hours of the administration time, administer the drug as soon as possible. If the dose is missed and it is longer than 10 hours since the last dose, do not administer drug until the next scheduled time. Dose should not be doubled to make up for missed dose.

Route	Onset	Peak	Duration
P.O.	Unknown	1–1.75 hr	Unknown

Half-life: 1 hr

Mechanism of Action
Metabolizes to cytidine nucleoside analogue (NHC), which distributes into cells where NHC is then phosphorylated to an active form. When the active form accumulates in the SARS-CoV-2 RNA, a number of errors in the viral genome occur, leading to inhibition of replication.

Contraindications
Hypersensitivity to molnupiravir or its components.

Interactions
DRUGS
None listed by manufacturer

Adverse Reactions
CNS: Dizziness
GI: Diarrhea, elevated lipase or liver enzymes, nausea
GU: Elevated creatinine levels
HEME: Abnormal hemoglobin, leukocytes, or platelet values
SKIN: Erythema, rash, urticaria
OTHER: Anaphylaxis, angioedema, other hypersensitivity reactions

Childbearing Considerations
PREGNANCY
- Pregnancy exposure registry: 1-877-888-4231 or pregnancyreporting .msd.com.
- Drug may cause fetal harm, including death, based on animal studies.
- Prescriber must document the known and potential benefits as well as the potential risks of use on the pregnant patient and that this information was communicated to the pregnant patient prior to administration. This documentation must then be submitted to the manufacturer, Merck Sharp & Dohme.
- Prior to administration of the drug, determine patient's pregnancy status. Expect to administer a pregnancy test in women of childbearing age who have irregular menstrual cycles, are unsure of the

first day of last menstrual period, or are not using effective contraception correctly and consistently.

- Drug is authorized for use in a pregnant patient only after prescriber has determined that the benefits outweigh the risks.

LACTATION

- It is not known if drug is present in breast milk.
- Breastfeeding is not recommended during drug therapy. Mother should discard breast milk during drug therapy and for 4 days after last dose.

REPRODUCTION

- Women of childbearing age should use an effective method of contraception during drug treatment and for 4 days after the final dose.

Nursing Considerations

- Know that molnupiravir is authorized only for the duration of the FDA declaration for emergency use.
- Be aware that molnupiravir is not authorized for use in patients who are less than 18 years old (affects bone and cartilage growth) and is not authorized to treat patients hospitalized due to COVID-19. It also is not authorized for use for longer than 5 consecutive days and is not authorized for preexposure or postexposure prophylaxis for prevention of COVID-19.
- Know that molnupiravir has not received full FDA approval to treat any indication, including the treatment of COVID-19.
- Ensure that prescriber has considered the benefit–risk ratio for the patient prior to administration of drug.
- Expect patient started on molnupiravir therapy and then requiring hospitalization to continue on to complete the full 5-day treatment course at the prescriber's discretion.
- Continue isolation protocols according to public health recommendations during drug therapy to minimize the transmission of SARS-CoV-2 virus.

! WARNING Monitor patient closely for adverse reactions, because serious and unexpected adverse reactions may occur that are still unknown because of the drug's emergency authorization with limited use.

! WARNING Monitor patient for hypersensitivity reaction to molnupiravir because hypersensitivity reactions, including anaphylaxis, have been reported with drug use. If signs and symptoms occur that are significant or anaphylaxis occurs, immediately stop drug therapy, notify prescriber, and provide supportive care, as needed and prescribed.

- Expect all serious adverse reactions and medication errors potentially related to molnupiravir to be reported within 7 calendar days from the time of the prescriber's awareness of the event, using FDA Form 3500. Once completed, form should be submitted to the FDA MedWatch online, mailed, or faxed. In addition, a copy of the form should be faxed or emailed to Merck Sharp & Dohme Corp. Be prepared to provide any information prescriber requests when form is completed.

PATIENT TEACHING

- Ensure that patient has received the "Fact Sheet for Patients and Caregivers."
- Instruct patient to take molnupiravir with or without food and to swallow capsules whole and not break, crush, or open the capsules.
- Advise patient on what to do if a drug dose is missed. Stress importance of never doubling the dose.
- Stress need for patient to complete the full 5-day treatment and to continue isolation as per public health recommendations.

! WARNING Inform patient that an allergic reaction may occur to molnupiravir. If present, advise patient or caregiver to notify prescriber and, if serious, to seek immediate emergency help.

! WARNING Alert women of childbearing age that drug is not recommended during pregnancy because of the risk of fetal toxicity. Stress importance of patient notifying prescriber before drug therapy begins if pregnancy is suspected or confirmed. Advise patient who becomes pregnant during molnupiravir therapy how to enroll in the pregnancy exposure registry and how to report pregnancy to manufacturer.

- Tell mothers who are breastfeeding that breastfeeding is not recommended during drug therapy. Instruct them to interrupt breastfeeding and discard the breast milk during drug therapy and for 4 days after the last dose.
- Instruct women of childbearing age to use an effective contraceptive during drug therapy and for 4 days after last dose. Also tell male patients with a partner of childrearing potential to use an effective contraceptive during drug therapy and for at least 3 months after the last dose because effects on offspring of treated males are not completely known.

mometasone furoate
Asmanex HFA, Asmanex Twisthaler, Sinuva

mometasone furoate monohydrate
Nasonex

Class and Category
Pharmacologic class: Glucocorticoid
Therapeutic class: Anti-inflammatory

Indications and Dosages
✷ *To manage symptoms of seasonal or allergic rhinitis*

NASAL SPRAY (NASONEX)
Adults and children 12 years and over. 100 mcg (2 sprays) in each nostril once daily.
Children ages 2 to 11. 50 mcg (1 spray) in each nostril once daily.

✷ *To prevent seasonal allergic rhinitis*

NASAL SPRAY (NASONEX)
Adults and adolescents 12 years and over. 100 mcg (2 sprays) in each nostril once daily, started 2 to 4 wk prior to anticipated start of pollen season, if known.

✷ *To treat nasal polyps*

NASAL SPRAY (NASONEX)
Adults. 100 mcg (2 sprays) in each nostril once or twice daily.

✷ *To treat patients with nasal polyps who have had ethmoid sinus surgery*

SINUS IMPLANT (SINUVA)
Adults. Implant placed under endoscopic visualization. Removed in 90 days or earlier, if needed, using standard surgical instruments.

✷ *To maintain asthma control*

ORAL INHALATION (ASMANEX TWISTHALER)
Adults and children age 12 and over who have been taking bronchodilators alone or inhaled corticosteroids. *Initial:* 220 mcg (1 inhalation) once daily, and increased, as needed. *Maximum:* 440 mcg once daily or in divided doses of 220 mcg and given twice daily.
Adults and children age 12 and over who have taken oral corticosteroids. 440 mcg (2 inhalations) twice daily. *Maximum:* 880 mcg daily.
Children ages 4 to 11 regardless of prior therapy. 110 mcg (1 inhalation) once daily. *Maximum:* 110 mcg daily.

ORAL INHALATION (ASMANEX HFA)
Adults and children age 12 and over not taking an inhaled corticosteroid. *Initial:* Using a 100-mcg inhaler, 2 inhalations twice daily, increased, as needed, after 2 wks. *Maximum:* Using a 200-mcg inhaler, two inhalations twice daily for maximum dosage of 800 mcg/day.
Adults and children age 12 and over taking oral corticosteroid therapy. *Initial:* Using a 200-mcg inhaler, 2 inhalations twice daily, increased, as needed after 2 wks. *Maximum:* Using a 200-mcg inhaler, two inhalations twice daily for maximum dosage of 800 mcg/day.
Children age 5 to less than 12 years. Using a 50-mcg inhaler, two inhalations twice daily. *Maximum:* 200 mcg daily.

Drug Administration
ORAL INHALATION
- Asmanex contains small amounts of lactose, which contains trace levels of milk proteins. Do not administer to patients with a milk protein allergy, because anaphylactic reactions have occurred.

Asmanex Twisthaler
- Administer once-daily dose for asthma control in the evening; twice daily in the morning and evening.

- Place inhaler in an upright position. Twist cap counterclockwise while holding colored base, making sure indented arrow (on white portion of the inhaler directly above the colored base) is pointing to the dose counter. Removing the cap loads inhaler with drug, and the dose counter on the base will count down by one.
- Have patient take a full breath in and out, and then place mouthpiece in patient's mouth. Have patient firmly close lips around mouthpiece, taking care not to cover ventilation holes on the inhaler. Then have patient take a fast, deep breath. Patient may not feel, smell, or taste anything with the inhalation. After taking the breath, patient should remove inhaler from mouth and hold breath for about 10 seconds. Patient should not exhale into the inhaler.
- Have patient rinse mouth with water and spit out contents afterward without swallowing the water.
- Wipe the mouthpiece dry, if needed, and replace the cap right away, turning it clockwise while pressing down. A click should be heard when the cap is fully closed.
- Write down the date inhaler is opened, and discard it 45 days from that date or when dose counter reads 00, whichever comes first.

Asmanex HFA
- Remove cap from the mouthpiece of the actuator. If using the inhaler for the first time, prime it by releasing 4 test sprays into the air, away from face, shaking well before each spray. If inhaler has not been used for more than 5 days, inhaler requires priming again.
- Use only the Asmanex HFA canister with the Asmanex HFA actuator.
- Shake inhaler before each use.
- Have patient breathe out as fully as possible through mouth.
- Holding the inhaler in an upright position, have patient insert the mouthpiece into mouth, and close lips around it.
- Patient should take a deep breath in slowly through mouth and while doing this press down firmly and fully on the top of the canister until it stops moving in the actuator. Then patient should take finger off the canister.

- When patient is finished breathing in, have patient hold breath as long as possible (10 seconds, if possible). Then inhaler is removed from mouth and patient should breathe out through nose, while keeping lips closed.
- Wait at least 30 seconds before administering second inhalation and then shake inhaler well again and repeat earlier steps.
- Replace cap over the mouthpiece right away after use.
- Do not wash inhaler in water, but wipe the mouthpiece clean using a dry wipe after every 7 days of use.
- Have patient rinse mouth after each use of oral inhaler to help prevent mouth and throat dryness, relieve throat irritation, and prevent oropharyngeal infection.

INTRANASAL

Nasonex
- Prime nasal spray bottle before using for the first time by pressing down and releasing pump 10 times or until a fine spray appears. If drug is not used for more than 1 week, container will have to be reprimed by spraying 2 times or until a fine spray appears.
- Shake container before each use.
- Have patient blow nose, tilt head slightly forward, and insert tube into a nostril, pointing toward inner corner of eye, away from nasal septum.
- Have patient hold the other nostril closed and spray while inhaling gently.
- Repeat the procedure in the other nostril.

Sinuva
- Implant inserted by physicians trained in otolaryngology.
- To prepare for insert, open package. Do not use if package is already opened, the package or product is damaged, or has evidence of gross contamination.
- Avoid bending, damaging, or twisting implant.
- Implant should not be compressed and loaded into the delivery system more than 2 times.
- Follow manufacturer guidelines when assisting physician in removal of the implant.

M

Route	Onset	Peak	Duration
Inhalation	Unknown	1–2.5 hr	Unknown
Intranasal including implant	Unknown	Unknown	Unknown

Half-life: 5–6 hr

Mechanism of Action

Inhibits the activity of cells and mediators active in the inflammatory response, possibly by decreasing influx of inflammatory cells into nasal passages and thereby decreasing nasal inflammation.

Inflammation is a key component in asthma pathophysiology. Decreasing the inflammatory response in lung tissue helps to relieve asthma symptoms.

Contraindications

For all forms: Hypersensitivity to mometasone or its components; *For Asmanex HFA:* Status asthmaticus or other asthma episodes that require emergency care; *For Asmanex Twisthaler:* Hypersensitivity to milk proteins, status asthmaticus or other asthma episodes that require emergency care; *For Sinuva Sinus Implant:* Hypersensitivity to mometasone, any of the copolymers of the implant, or their components

Interactions

DRUGS

strong CYP4503A4 inhibitors such as atazanavir, clarithromycin, cobicistat-containing products, indinavir, itraconazole, ketoconazole, nefazodone, nelfinavir, ritonavir, saquinavir, telithromycin: Increased plasma mometasone levels leading to possible increased adverse reactions

Adverse Reactions

CNS: Headache, presyncope (implant)
CV: Chest pain
EENT: Blurred vision, cataracts, conjunctivitis, dry mouth, earache, epistaxis, glaucoma, nasal irritation, nasopharyngitis, oral and pharyngeal candidiasis, otitis media, pharyngitis, rhinitis, sinusitis, **throat tightness**, unpleasant taste; *For implant:* Epistaxis; implant migration; nasal infection, irritation, pain, perforation
ENDO: Adrenal insufficiency, growth suppression

GI: Diarrhea, dyspepsia, nausea, vomiting
GU: Dysmenorrhea
MS: Arthralgia, decreased bone mineral density, myalgia, pain
RESP: Asthma aggravation, bronchitis, **bronchospasm**, increased cough, upper respiratory tract infection, wheezing
SKIN: Pruritus, rash, urticaria
Other: Anaphylaxis, angioedema, flu-like symptoms, immunosuppression, viral infection

Childbearing Considerations

PREGNANCY

- It is not known if drug causes fetal harm.
- Use with caution only if benefit to mother outweighs potential risk to fetus.

LACTATION

- It is not known if drug is present in breast milk, although other corticosteroids are.
- Patient should check with prescriber before breastfeeding.

Nursing Considerations

- Be aware that oral inhalation should not be used to treat bronchospasm or other acute episodes of asthma. Ensure that a short-acting beta$_2$-agonist, such as albuterol, is available, if needed, to treat acute asthma symptoms.
- Use mometasone cautiously if patient has ocular herpes simplex; tubercular infection; or untreated bacterial, fungal, or systemic viral infection.
- Be aware that a sinus implant is now available as a nonsurgical treatment for nasal polyps. It should not be used in patients with nasal ulcers or trauma.
- If patient takes an oral corticosteroid, expect to taper it slowly 1 week after changing to mometasone. If patient takes prednisone, expect to reduce it by no more than 2.5 mg daily at weekly intervals, beginning at least 1 week after mometasone therapy starts. Monitor patient for symptoms of systemically active corticosteroid withdrawal such as depression, joint and muscle pain, and lassitude, despite maintenance or even improvement of respiratory symptoms.

! **WARNING** Assess patient switched from systemic corticosteroid to mometasone for adrenal insufficiency (fatigue, hypotension, lassitude, nausea, vomiting, weakness) during initial treatment and during infection, stress, surgery, trauma, or an electrolyte-depleting condition. Notify prescriber immediately if signs or symptoms arise because adrenal insufficiency may be life-threatening. Hypothalamic-pituitary-adrenal axis function may take several months to recover after systemic corticosteroids are discontinued. Abrupt withdrawal of mometasone also may precipitate adrenal insufficiency.

! **WARNING** Monitor patient for allergic conditions that may have been masked by corticosteroid therapy when switching patient from systemic corticosteroid to mometasone. Also monitor these patients for corticosteroid withdrawal symptoms.

- Know that drug may cause adrenal suppression and hypercortisolism in susceptible patients or in patients who exceed the recommended dosages.
- Notify prescriber immediately if patient has bronchospasm after mometasone oral inhalation, and expect to give a fast-acting inhaled bronchodilator, discontinue mometasone, and use an alternate drug.
- Closely monitor a child's growth pattern; drug may stunt growth.
- Report oropharyngeal candidiasis, and expect patient to receive appropriate antifungal therapy while remaining on mometasone therapy. If candidiasis is severe, however, mometasone therapy may have to be temporarily halted.

! **WARNING** Monitor patient for infections, as drug causes immunosuppression, increasing risk for infections. Notify prescriber if an infection is present because it can become severe or even life-threatening. Be aware that if patient is exposed to chickenpox, prescriber may order varicella zoster immune globulin to be given or, if chickenpox develops, treatment with antiviral agents may be prescribed. In addition, if patient is exposed to measles, prophylaxis with pooled I.M. immunoglobulin may be prescribed.

PATIENT TEACHING

- Tell patient to take drug exactly as prescribed and not to change dosage without consulting with prescriber first.

- Instruct patient using nasal spray to shake container before each use. Instruct her to blow her nose, tilt her head slightly forward, and insert tube into a nostril, pointing toward inner corner of eye, away from nasal septum. Tell her to hold the other nostril closed and spray while inhaling gently. Then have her repeat the procedure in the other nostril.
- Review procedure for inserting implant. Tell patient it will stay in place for up to 90 days. Tell patient to report any adverse reactions, especially nasal bleeding or infection and signs of migration such as choking, throat irritation, or swallowing of the implant.
- Instruct patient using the Asmanex Twisthaler inhaler how to use inhaler: Remove cap only after placing inhaler in an upright position. Twist cap counterclockwise while holding colored base, making sure indented arrow (on white portion of the inhaler directly above the colored base) is pointing to the dose counter. Removing the cap loads inhaler with drug, and the dose counter on the base will count down by one. Tell her to take a full breath in and out, and then place mouthpiece in her mouth. Firmly close her lips around mouthpiece, taking care not to cover ventilation holes on the inhaler. Then take a fast, deep breath. Remind her she may not taste, smell, or feel anything with the inhalation. After taking the breath, she should remove inhaler from her mouth and hold her breath for about 10 seconds. She should not exhale into the inhaler. Then she should rinse mouth with water and spit out contents without swallowing. Afterward, she should wipe the mouthpiece dry, if needed, and replace cap, turning it clockwise while pressing down. A click should be heard when cap is fully closed.
- Tell her to write down the date inhaler is opened, and discard it 45 days from that date or when dose counter reads 00, whichever comes first.
- Instruct patient using Asmanex Twisthaler and prescribed one inhalation daily to take it in the evening.
- Instruct patient using Asmanex HFA inhaler to remove cap from the mouthpiece of the actuator. If using the inhaler for the first time, tell patient to prime it by

M

releasing 4 test sprays into the air, away from the face, shaking well before each spray. If inhaler has not been used for more than 5 days, inhaler requires priming again. Warn patient only to use the Asmanex HFA canister with the Asmanex HFA actuator. Instruct patient not to wash inhaler in water but to wipe the mouthpiece clean using a dry wipe after every 7 days.

- Instruct patient to rinse after each use of oral inhaler to help prevent mouth and throat dryness, relieve throat irritation, and prevent oropharyngeal infection.

! **WARNING** Caution patient not to use mometasone oral inhalation to relieve acute bronchospasm and to notify prescriber if rescue inhaler is required more often or doesn't seem to be as effective.

- Keep in mind that if patient switches from an oral corticosteroid to mometasone, she should be advised to carry or wear medical identification indicating the need for supplemental systemic corticosteroids during stress or severe asthma attack. Tell her to seek emergency care if either occurs.
- Instruct patient to contact prescriber if symptoms persist or worsen after 3 weeks.
- Caution patient about risk for infection and to avoid exposure to chickenpox and measles. If exposed, patient should contact prescriber immediately. Also alert patient of potential worsening of existing infections.

! **WARNING** Urge patient to seek emergency care if allergic reactions occur and to stop taking drug.

- Review adverse reactions with patient and family and to contact prescriber if bothersome or severe.

monomethyl fumarate

Bafiertam

Class and Category

Pharmacologic class: Nuclear factor erythroid-2 related factor 2 (Nrf2) activator
Therapeutic class: Immunomodulator

Indications and Dosages

* *To treat relapsing forms of multiple sclerosis, including active secondary progressive disease, clinically isolated syndrome, or relapsing-remitting disease*

D.R. CAPSULES

Adults. 95 mg twice daily for 7 days, then increased to 190 mg twice daily. *Maintenance:* 190 mg twice daily.

±**DOSAGE ADJUSTMENT** For patient unable to tolerate maintenance dose, dosage decreased to 95 mg twice daily for up to 4 weeks before resuming maintenance dosage of 190 mg twice daily.

Drug Administration

P.O.

- Expect to administer nonenteric-coated aspirin up to a dose of 325 mg 30 minutes before monomethyl fumarate administration to reduce severity of flushing.
- May be taken with or without food.
- Capsules should be swallowed whole without chewing, crushing, or opening capsule.

Route	Onset	Peak	Duration
P.O.	Unknown	4.03 hr	Unknown

Half-life: 0.5 hr

Mechanism of Action

Exact mechanism is unknown, but may work by decreasing inflammation and preventing nerve damage associated with multiple sclerosis.

Contraindications

Concurrent therapy with dimethyl fumarate or diroximel fumarate; hypersensitivity to dimethyl fumarate, diroximel fumarate, monomethyl fumarate, or their components

Interactions

DRUGS

dimethyl fumarate, diroximel fumarate: Increased serum monomethyl fumarate levels, increasing risk of adverse reactions

Adverse Reactions

CNS: Progressive multifocal leukoencephalopathy
GI: Abdominal pain, diarrhea, dyspepsia, elevated liver enzymes, liver injury, nausea, vomiting

GU: Albumin in urine
HEME: Eosinophilia (transient), lymphopenia
SKIN: Erythema, flushing, pruritus, rash
Other: Anaphylaxis, angioedema, herpes zoster and other serious opportunistic infections

Childbearing Considerations

PREGNANCY

- It is not known if drug can cause fetal harm, although animal studies suggest fetal harm may occur.
- Use with caution only if benefit to mother outweighs potential risk to fetus.

LACTATION

- It is not known if drug is present in breast milk.
- Patient should check with prescriber before breastfeeding.

Nursing Considerations

- Ensure that the following tests have been done prior to beginning monomethyl fumarate therapy: alkaline phosphatase, complete blood cell count (including lymphocyte count), serum aminotransferase, and total bilirubin levels. A baseline is needed because of drug's ability to cause liver damage and lymphopenia once therapy starts.

> **! WARNING** Monitor patient for anaphylaxis and angioedema after the first dose as well as any time during treatment. Report signs and symptoms such as difficulty breathing, swelling of the throat or tongue, and urticaria. If present, discontinue monomethyl fumarate, notify prescriber and provide supportive therapy, as prescribed.

- Monitor patient's complete blood cell count, including lymphocyte count, for 6 months after drug therapy starts and then every 6 to 12 months, as indicated, because monomethyl fumarate can decrease lymphocyte counts. Be aware that interruption of drug therapy may be needed if lymphocyte counts decrease to less than 0.5×10^9/L and persisting more than 6 months.
- Monitor patient's liver alkaline phosphatase, serum aminotransferase, and total bilirubin levels during treatment, because monomethyl fumarate can cause liver injury. Expect drug to be discontinued if liver injury is suspected.
- Monitor patient for signs and symptoms of herpes zoster and other serious opportunistic infections that can affect the patient's brain, ears, eyes, gastrointestinal tract, lungs, meninges, skin, or spinal cord. These infections can become serious. If present, notify prescriber and provide appropriate treatment, as ordered. If patient develops herpes zoster or other infections become serious, monomethyl fumarate may have to be discontinued.

> **! WARNING** Be aware that progressive multifocal leukoencephalopathy (PML) has occurred with the prodrug of monomethyl fumarate, especially in patients who develop lymphopenia. The majority of cases occurred in patients with lymphocyte counts less than 0.5×10^9/L. Notify prescriber at first sign of PML, withhold drug, and expect patient to undergo a diagnostic workup to confirm diagnosis. Signs and symptoms to be alert for include changes in thinking, memory, and orientation that lead to confusion; disturbances of vision; personality changes; and progressive clumsiness or weakness on one side of the body. Be aware that these changes can gradually occur over days to weeks.

PATIENT TEACHING

- Instruct patient to swallow D.R. capsules whole and not chew, crush, or open capsules. Also tell patient not to mix capsule content with food.
- Tell patient to keep unopened bottles of drug in refrigerator and opened bottle at room temperature.
- Alert patient that flushing and gastrointestinal adverse reactions (abdominal pain, diarrhea, and nausea) are the most common reactions to monomethyl fumarate therapy and may diminish over time. Tell patient to notify prescriber if flushing or gastrointestinal adverse reactions become persistent and/or severe. Let patient know that taking a nonenteric-coated aspirin, if not contraindicated, prior to taking drug may help reduce flushing.
- Review infection control measures and tell patient to alert prescriber if signs

M

and symptoms of herpes zoster or other infections develop.

- Inform patient that blood tests will be required before and during monomethyl fumarate therapy.
- Instruct patient to notify prescriber if anorexia, dark urine, fatigue, jaundice, or right upper abdominal discomfort occurs.

> **! WARNING** Warn patient that monomethyl fumarate may cause allergic reactions that could become life-threatening. Urge patient to seek immediate emergency care if patient develops difficulty breathing, hives, or swelling of throat or tongue.

montelukast sodium
Singulair

Class and Category

Pharmacologic class: Leukotriene receptor antagonist
Therapeutic class: Antiallergen, antiasthmatic

Indications and Dosages

✳ *To prevent or treat asthma*

TABLETS

Adults and adolescents age 15 and over. 10 mg daily in evening. *Maximum:* 10 mg daily.

CHEWABLE TABLETS

Children ages 6 to 14 years. 5 mg daily. *Maximum:* 5 mg daily.
Children ages 2 to 5 years. 4 mg daily in evening. *Maximum:* 4 mg daily.

ORAL GRANULES

Children ages 1 to 5 years. 4 mg daily in evening. *Maximum:* 4 mg daily.

✳ *To treat seasonal allergic rhinitis*

TABLETS

Adults and adolescents age 15 years and older. 10 mg daily.

CHEWABLE TABLETS

Children ages 6 to 14 years. 5 mg daily.
Children ages 2 to 5 years. 4 mg daily.

ORAL GRANULES

Children ages 2 to 5 years. 4 mg daily.

✳ *To treat perennial allergic rhinitis*

TABLETS

Adults and adolescents age 15 years and over. 10 mg daily.

CHEWABLE TABLETS

Children ages 6 to 14 years. 5 mg daily.
Children ages 2 to 5 years. 4 mg daily.

ORAL GRANULES

Children ages 6 months to 5 years. 4 mg daily.

✳ *To prevent exercise-induced bronchoconstriction*

TABLETS

Adults and adolescents age 15 and over. 10 mg at least 2 hr before exercise. *Maximum:* 10 mg in 24 hr.

CHEWABLE TABLETS

Children ages 6 to 14. 5 mg at least 2 hr before exercise. *Maximum:* 5 mg in 24 hr.

Drug Administration

P.O.

- Administer drug used to prevent or treat asthma in the evening.
- Administer drug to prevent exercise-induced bronchoconstriction at least 2 hours before exercise.
- Administer all forms of drug used to treat rhinitis at any time of day, but be consistent.
- Tablets should be swallowed whole and not chewed, crushed, or split.
- Chewable tablets should be thoroughly chewed before swallowing.
- To administer oral granules, pour contents directly into child's mouth or mix with 1 teaspoon of ice cream or cold or room-temperature applesauce, carrots, or rice—but not liquids (except for breast milk or baby formula) or other foods—just before administration. Liquids may be given after drug has been administered. Once packet is opened, the full dose must be administered within 15 minutes. Drug must not be stored for future use if mixed with food.

Route	Onset	Peak	Duration
P.O.	Unknown	3–4 hr	Unknown
P.O./Chewable	Unknown	1–2.5 hr	Unknown
P.O./Granules	Unknown	1–3 hr	Unknown
Half-life: 2.7–5.5 hr			

Mechanism of Action

Antagonizes receptors for cysteinyl leukotrienes, produced by arachidonic acid metabolism and released from eosinophils, mast cells, and other cells. When cysteinyl leukotrienes bind to receptors in bronchial airways, they increase endothelial membrane permeability, which leads to airway edema, smooth-muscle contraction, and altered activity of cells in asthma's inflammatory process. Also, antagonizes receptors for cysteinyl leukotrienes in nasal tissue that are responsible for producing rhinitis caused by allergens. Montelukast blocks these effects.

Contraindications

Hypersensitivity to montelukast or its components

Interactions

DRUGS

phenobarbital: Decreased amount of circulating montelukast

Adverse Reactions

CNS: Aggression, agitation, anxiousness, asthenia, attention disturbance, depression, disorientation, dizziness, dream abnormalities, drowsiness, fatigue, fever, hallucinations, headache, hostility, hypoesthesia, insomnia, irritability, memory impairment, obsessive–compulsive symptoms, paresthesia, restlessness, **seizures**, sleep walking, somnambulism, somnolence, stuttering, **suicidal ideation**, tic, tremor
CV: Palpitations, edema
EENT: Conjunctivitis, dental pain or tooth infection, epistaxis, laryngitis, myopia (children), nasal congestion, otitis media, pharyngitis, rhinorrhea, rhinitis (children), sinusitis, tonsillitis
GI: Abdominal pain, **cholestatic hepatitis**, diarrhea, dyspepsia, elevated liver enzymes, **hepatic eosinophilic infiltration**, **hepatotoxicity**, indigestion, infectious gastroenteritis, nausea, **pancreatitis**, vomiting
GU: Enuresis (children), pyuria
HEME: **Increased bleeding tendency**, systemic eosinophilia, **thrombocytopenia**
MS: Arthralgia, muscle cramps, myalgia
RESP: Acute bronchitis (children), cough, pneumonia (children), **pulmonary eosinophilia**, upper respiratory tract infection, wheezing (children)
SKIN: Atopic dermatitis (children), **bruising, eczema (children), erythema multiforme**, erythema nodosum, pruritus, rash, skin infection (children), **Stevens–Johnson syndrome, toxic epidermal necrolysis**, urticaria

Other: Anaphylaxis, angioedema; flu-like syndrome, varicella (children), viral-like infection (in children)

Childbearing Considerations

PREGNANCY

- It is not known if drug causes fetal harm.
- Use with caution only if benefit to mother outweighs potential risk to fetus.

LACTATION

- Drug is present in breast milk.
- Patient should check with prescriber before breastfeeding.

Nursing Considerations

> ! **WARNING** Know that montelukast isn't for acute asthma attack or status asthmaticus.

- Keep in mind that montelukast shouldn't be abruptly substituted for inhaled or oral corticosteroids; expect to taper corticosteroid dosage gradually, as directed.
- Monitor patient for adverse reactions, such as eosinophilia, cardiac and pulmonary symptoms, and vasculitis, in patient undergoing corticosteroid withdrawal. Notify prescriber if such reactions occur.
- Watch patient closely for suicidal tendencies during montelukast therapy, especially when therapy starts or dosage changes.
- Monitor patient for adverse neuropsychiatric effects that may become serious and may occur even after drug is discontinued. Notify prescriber if present. Drug may have to be discontinued.

PATIENT TEACHING

- Advise patient to take montelukast daily as prescribed, even when he feels well. Urge him not to decrease dosage or stop taking other prescribed allergy or asthma drugs unless instructed by prescriber.
- Instruct patient prescribed drug for asthma to take drug in the evening. If prescribed to prevent exercise-induced bronchospasms, patient should take drug 2 hours before anticipated exercise. If drug is prescribed for rhinitis, advise patient to take drug at any time of day but to be consistent.
- Caution patient prescribed drug for asthma not to use drug for acute asthma attack or status asthmaticus; make sure he

M

has appropriate short-acting rescue drug available.

- Tell parents administering oral granules to pour contents directly into child's mouth or mix with ice cream or cold or room-temperature applesauce, carrots, or rice—but not liquids or other foods—just before administration. Liquids may be given after drug has been administered. Once packet is opened, the full dose must be administered within 15 minutes. Drug must not be stored for future use if mixed with food.
- Instruct patient prescribed drug for asthma to notify prescriber if he needs a short-acting inhaled bronchodilator more often than usual, or more often than prescribed, to control symptoms.
- Teach patient prescribed drug for asthma to use a peak flow meter to determine his personal best expiratory volume.
- Caution patient with aspirin sensitivity to avoid aspirin and NSAIDs during montelukast therapy. Montelukast may not effectively reduce bronchospasm in such a patient.
- Inform patient (or parents of child) with phenylketonuria that chewable tablet contains phenylalanine.

! **WARNING** Urge family or caregiver to watch patient closely for abnormal behaviors, including depression, stuttering, or suicidal tendencies, during therapy, and urge them to notify prescriber if present and to stop taking drug.

- Instruct patient to report increased bleeding tendency or severe skin reaction that occurs without warning immediately to prescriber.

morphine sulfate
Arymo ER, Duramorph PF, Infumorph, Kadian, M-Eslon (CAN), Mitigo, MorphaBond ER, MS Contin, MS-IR (CAN), Statex (CAN)

≡ Class, Category, and Schedule
Pharmacologic class: Opioid
Therapeutic class: Opioid analgesic
Controlled substance schedule: II

≡ Indications and Dosages

✴ *To relieve pain severe enough to require opioid treatment and for which alternative treatment options such as nonopioid analgesics or opioid combination products are inadequate or not tolerated*

TABLETS
Adults. 15 to 30 mg every 4 hr, as needed.
Children weighing at least 50 kg (110 lb). *Initial:* 15 mg every 4 hr, as needed. *Maximum:* 30 mg for initial dose.

ORAL SOLUTION
Adults. 10 to 20 mg every 4 hr, as needed.
Children age 2 to 17 years. 0.15 to 0.3 mg/kg (acute pain only and only certain brands), as needed.

I.V. INFUSION
Adults. Highly individualized and dependent on product being used and patient's response.

I.V. INJECTION
Adults. 0.1 to 0.2 mg/kg every 4 hr, as needed.

I.M. INJECTION
Adults. 10 mg every 4 hr, as needed.

EPIDURAL INJECTION (MORPHINE SULFATE PRESERVATIVE FREE)
Adults. *Initial:* 5 mg as a single dose. If pain isn't relieved after 1 hr, 1- to 2-mg doses given at appropriate intervals to relieve pain. *Maximum:* 10 mg/24 hr.

EPIDURAL INJECTION (INFUMORPH)
Adults with no tolerance to opioids. *Initial:* 3.5 to 7.5 mg/day.
Adults with some tolerance to opioids. *Initial:* 4.5 to 10 mg/day.

INTRATHECAL INJECTION (MORPHINE SULFATE PRESERVATIVE FREE)
Adults. 0.2 to 1 mg as a single dose.

INTRATHECAL INJECTION (INFUMORPH)
Adults with no tolerance to opioids. *Initial:* 0.2 to 1 mg/day.
Adults with some tolerance to opioids. *Initial:* 1 to 10 mg/day.

SUPPOSITORIES
Adults. 10 to 20 mg every 4 hr, as needed.
Children. Individualized dosage based on patient's age, size, and need.

✴ *To manage moderate to severe pain when a continuous, around-the-clock opioid analgesic is needed for an extended period of time*

E.R. CAPSULES (KADIAN)

Adults who are not opioid tolerant. *Initial:* 30 mg every 24 hr, as needed.

Adults converting from other oral morphine formulations: Total previous daily dose every 24 hr. Alternatively, one-half total previous daily dose every 12 hr.

Adults converting from parenteral morphine. Highly individualized. *Usual:* Three times the previous daily parenteral morphine dosage.

Adults converting from other nonmorphine opioids (oral or parenteral). Highly individualized. *Usual:* Half of the estimated daily morphine requirements every 24 hr, and then increased as needed.

E.R. TABLETS (MORPHABOND, MS CONTIN)

Adults who are opioid-naive. 15 mg every 8 or 12 hr.

Adults who are not opioid tolerant. 15 mg every 12 hr (MS Contin) or 8 or 12 hr (Morphabond E.R.), as needed.

Adults converting from other oral morphine formulations. One-half of patient's previous 24-hr requirements every 12 hr. Alternatively for MS Contin, one-third of patient's previous 24-hr requirements every 8 hr.

Adults converting from parenteral morphine. Highly individualized. *Usual:* Three times the previous daily parenteral morphine dosage.

Adults converting from other parenteral or oral nonmorphine opioids. Highly individualized. *Usual:* Half of the estimated daily morphine requirements, and then increased as needed.

E.R. TABLETS (ARYMO ER)

Adults who are opioid-naive or are not opioid tolerant. 15 mg every 8 or 12 hr.

Adults converting from other oral morphine formulations. One-half of patient's previous 24-hr requirements every 12 hr. Alternatively, one-third of patient's previous 24-hr requirements every 8 hr.

Adults converting from parenteral morphine. Highly individualized. *Usual:* Three times the previous daily parenteral morphine dosage.

Adults converting from other opioids. 15 mg every 8 to 12 hr.

Drug Administration

- Ensure that before giving morphine, opioid antagonist and equipment for oxygen delivery and respiration are available.
- Store morphine at room temperature.
- Avoid medication errors by checking dosage (mg vs. ml), concentration, and product being used.
- Have naloxone readily available.

P.O.

- MorphaBond ER formulation has an added abuse deterrent property that makes it difficult to break, crush, or cut the tablet. It also resists extraction and forms a viscous liquid when physically compromised and placed in a liquid. This abuse deterrent helps prevent abuse when attempts are made to administer it intranasally or by injection.
- Give oral form with food or milk to minimize adverse GI reactions, if needed.
- Use dosing syringe or dosing cup that comes with product to measure dosage of oral solution. Use only 2 mg/ml or 4 mg/ml strengths for children. Never use the 20 mg/ml strength for children.
- Tablets should not be chewed, crushed, or dissolved (pellets) in mouth.
- Kadian E.R. capsules should be swallowed whole or capsules can be opened and contents sprinkled on applesauce (at room temperature or cooler). It can also be given through a gastrostomy tube (but not a nasogastric tube) by first flushing the tube with water; then sprinkle pellets into 10 ml of water. Using a funnel, swirl the pellets and water into the tube. Rinse container with another 10 ml and pour this into the funnel. Repeat rinsing until no pellets remain in the container.
- E.R. forms of morphine aren't interchangeable.

I.V.

- Discard injection solution that is discolored or darker than pale yellow or that contains precipitates that don't dissolve with shaking.
- Don't use highly concentrated solutions (such as 10 to 25 mg/ml) for single-dose administration. These solutions are intended for use in continuous, controlled microinfusion devices.

M

- For direct I.V. injection, dilute appropriate dose with 4 to 5 ml of Sterile Water for Injection. Inject directly into tubing of free-flowing I.V. solution slowly over 4 to 5 minutes. Rapid I.V. injection may increase adverse reactions.
- For continuous I.V. infusion, dilute drug in 5% Dextrose in Water to obtain a concentration of 0.1 to 1 mg/ml. Administer with infusion-control device. Adjust dose and rate based on patient response, as prescribed.
- *Incompatibilities:* None listed by manufacturer

I.M.

- Avoid I.M. route for long-term therapy because of injection-site irritation.
- Drug for I.M. injection comes either in a prefilled syringe or an auto-injector.
- To use the prefilled syringe, inject into a large muscle mass.
- To use the single-dose auto-injector system, remove red safety cap, place purple end on patient's outer thigh, and push the unit firmly against the patient until injector functions. Discard system after it has been activated.
- Rotate sites.

INTRATHECAL

- Drug administered intrathecally only by health care professional skilled in this type of injection.
- Administer no more than 2 ml of 0.5-mg/ml solution or 1 ml of 1-mg/ml solution.
- Intrathecal dosage is about one-tenth of epidural dosage.

EPIDURAL

- Drug administered epidurally only by health care professional skilled in this type of injection.
- Dosage must be individualized according to patient's age, body mass, physical status, previous experience with opioids, risk factors for respiratory depression, and drugs to be coadministered before or during surgery.

P.R.

- If rectal suppository is too soft to insert, refrigerate for 30 minutes or run wrapped suppository under cold tap water.
- Moisten suppository before inserting.

Route	Onset	Peak	Duration
P.O.	15–30 min	> 1 hr	3–5 hr
P.O. (E.R.)	1–2 hr	3–4 hr	8–24 hr
I.V.	>5 min	20 min	4–5 hr
I.M.	10–30 min	30–60 min	4–5 hr
Epidural	15–60 min	15–60 min	24 hr
Intrathecal	15–60 min	30–60 min	24 hr
P.R.	20–60 min	20–60 min	3–7 hr

Half-life: 1.5–4.5 hr

Mechanism of Action

Binds with and activates opioid receptors (mainly mu receptors) in brain and spinal cord to produce analgesia and euphoria.

Contraindications

For all forms: Acute or severe bronchial asthma in an unmonitored setting or in the absence of resuscitative equipment; gastrointestinal obstruction, including paralytic ileus; hypersensitivity to morphine sulfate or its components; significant respiratory depression; use of MAO inhibitors within past 14 days; *For neuraxial administration:* Concomitant anticoagulant therapy, infection at the injection microinfusion site, presence of any other concomitant therapy or medical condition which would render epidural or intrathecal administration of morphine especially hazardous

Interactions

DRUGS

5-HT3 receptor antagonists; cyclobenzaprine; linezolid; methylene blue; selected psychiatric drugs such as amoxapine, buspirone, lithium, mirtazapine, nefazodone, trazodone, vilazodone; selective serotonin reuptake inhibitors; serotonin–norepinephrine reuptake inhibitors; St. John's wort; tricyclic antidepressants; tramadol; triptans; tryptophan: Increased risk of serotonin syndrome
anticholinergics: Possibly severe constipation leading to ileus, urine retention
antipsychotics, anxiolytics, benzodiazepines, cimetidine, CNS depressants, general anesthetics, muscle relaxants other opioids, P-glycoprotein inhibitors, sedating antihistamines, tranquilizers, tricyclic

antidepressants: Increased additive effects increasing risk of coma, hypotension, profound sedation, respiratory depression, death

diuretics: Decreased diuretic efficacy

MAO inhibitors: Increased risk of opioid toxicity (coma, respiratory depression) or serotonin syndrome

mixed agonist-antagonist and partial agonist analgesics such as butorphanol, buprenorphine, nalbuphine, pentazocine: Possibly withdrawal symptoms or reduced analgesic effect

oral P2Y12 inhibitors: Decreased absorption and peak concentration of oral P2Y12 inhibitors and delayed onset of antiplatelet effect when given with intravenous morphine sulfate

ACTIVITIES

alcohol use: Increased morphine plasma levels and potentially fatal overdose of morphine from increased CNS and respiratory depression and hypotension

Adverse Reactions

CNS: Agitation, amnesia, anxiety, ataxia, chills, **coma**, confusion, decreased concentration, delirium, delusions, depression, dizziness, dream abnormalities, drowsiness, edema, euphoria, fever, gait disturbance, hallucinations, headache, **increased intracranial pressure**, insomnia, lethargy, light-headedness, malaise, mood alterations, psychosis, restlessness, rigidity, sedation, **seizures**, syncope, thinking disturbances, tremor, uncoordinated muscle movements, unresponsiveness, vertigo, weakness

CV: **Bradycardia, cardiac arrest**, edema, hypertension, **hypotension**, orthostatic hypotension, palpitations, **shock**, tachycardia, vasodilation

EENT: Amblyopia, blurred vision, diplopia, dry mouth, eye pain, hiccup, **laryngeal edema or laryngospasm** (allergic), miosis, nystagmus, rhinitis, taste or voice alteration

ENDO: **Adrenal insufficiency** (rare), hypogonadism

GI: Abdominal cramps or pain, anorexia, biliary tract spasm, constipation, diarrhea, dysphagia, elevated liver enzymes, flatulence, gastroenteritis, gastroesophageal reflux, hiccups, ileus (in patients with inflammatory bowel disease) indigestion, **intestinal obstruction**, nausea, **toxic megacolon** (in patients with inflammatory bowel disease), vomiting

GU: Decreased ejaculate potency, decreased libido, difficult ejaculation, dysuria, impotence, infertility, menstrual irregularities, oliguria, prolonged labor, urinary hesitancy, urine retention

HEME: Anemia, **leukopenia, thrombocytopenia**

MS: Arthralgia, decreased bone mineral density, skeletal muscle rigidity

RESP: **Apnea, asthma exacerbation, atelectasis, bronchospasm**, decreased oxygen saturation, depressed cough reflex, **hypoventilation, pulmonary edema, respiratory arrest and depression**, wheezing

SKIN: Diaphoresis, dryness, flushing, pallor, pruritus, rash, urticaria

Other: **Allergic reaction; anaphylaxis; angioedema**; injection-site edema, pain, rash, or redness; physical and psychological dependence; weight loss; withdrawal symptoms

Childbearing Considerations

PREGNANCY

- Drug may cause fetal harm.
- Prolonged use of drug during pregnancy can result in neonatal opioid withdrawal syndrome (NOWS), which may be life-threatening if not recognized and treated.
- Avoid prolonged use during pregnancy. Use with caution only if benefit to mother outweighs potential risk to fetus.

LABOR & DELIVERY

- Drug is not recommended for use in pregnant women immediately before or during labor. Opioids may alter length of time of labor.
- Opioids cross the placental barrier and may produce respiratory depression and psycho-physiologic effects in the neonate. Monitor neonate closely for signs of excess sedation and respiratory depression.
- An opioid antagonist, such as naloxone, must be available at the time of delivery in the event it is needed to reverse opioid-induced respiratory depression in the neonate.

M

LACTATION

- Drug is present in breast milk.
- Breastfeeding is not recommended during drug therapy.

REPRODUCTION

- Chronic use of opioids may reduce fertility.

Nursing Considerations

- Be aware that morphine can lead to abuse, addiction, and misuse. To ensure that benefits of morphine therapy outweigh risks, a Risk Evaluation and Mitigation Strategy (REMS) is required.

! **WARNING** Know that chronic maternal use of morphine during pregnancy can result in NOWS, which may be life-threatening if not recognized and treated appropriately. NOWS occurs when a newborn has been exposed to opioid drugs like morphine for a prolonged period while in utero.

! **WARNING** Use extreme caution when administering morphine to patients with conditions accompanied by hypercapnia, hypoxia, or decreased respiratory reserve such as asthma, chronic obstructive pulmonary disease (COPD), or cor pulmonale. This is because, even with usual therapeutic doses, morphine may decrease respiratory drive while simultaneously increasing airway resistance to the point of apnea. Monitor patient's respiratory status closely, especially during the initiation of therapy or following a dose increase.

! **WARNING** Use morphine with extreme caution in patients who may be at risk for carbon dioxide retention (e.g., those with brain tumors or increased intracranial pressure). Monitor for signs of sedation and respiratory depression, especially when initiating therapy. Morphine may reduce respiratory drive, and the resultant carbon dioxide retention can further increase intracranial pressure. Also know that opioids like morphine may obscure signs and symptoms in a patient with a head injury.

! **WARNING** Know that morphine should only be used concomitantly with benzodiazepine and other CNS depressant therapy in patients for whom other treatment options are inadequate. If prescribed together, expect dosing and duration of morphine to be limited. Monitor patient closely for signs and symptoms of a decrease in consciousness, including coma, profound sedation, and significant respiratory depression. Ensure that naloxone is readily available to treat significant respiratory depression and profound sedation. Notify prescriber immediately and provide additional emergency supportive care, as death may occur.

- Use cautiously in patients about to undergo surgery of the biliary tract and patients with acute pancreatitis secondary to biliary tract disease because morphine may cause spasm of the sphincter of Oddi.
- Use cautiously in patients with sleep-related breathing disorders because morphine increases the risk of central sleep apnea in a dose-dependent fashion. If patient has central sleep apnea, know that morphine dosage may have to be reduced.

! **WARNING** Monitor circulatory and respiratory status carefully and frequently during morphine therapy, especially when drug therapy is initiated and when patient is being converted to morphine because respiratory depression and severe hypotension can develop. Be especially vigilant with cachectic, debilitated, and elderly patients who are at higher risk. Know that life-threatening depression can occur even when morphine is taken as prescribed and is not misused or abused.

- Monitor patient with seizure disorder for increased seizure activity because morphine may worsen the disorder.
- Monitor patient for excessive or persistent sedation; dosage may have to be adjusted.
- Know that if patient is receiving a continuous morphine infusion, watch for and notify prescriber about new neurologic signs or symptoms. Inflammatory masses (such as granulomas) have caused serious neurologic reactions, including paralysis.
- Expect morphine to cause physical and psychological dependence; watch for drug tolerance and withdrawal, such as

body aches, diaphoresis, diarrhea, fever, piloerection, rhinorrhea, sneezing, and yawning.

- Keep in mind if tolerance to morphine develops, expect prescriber to increase dosage.
- Know that morphine may have a prolonged duration and cumulative effect in patients with impaired hepatic or renal function. It also may prolong labor.

! **WARNING** Know that many drugs may interact with opioids like morphine to cause serotonin syndrome. Monitor patient closely for signs and symptoms such as agitation, diaphoresis, diarrhea, fever, hallucinations, labile blood pressure, muscle twitching or stiffness, nausea, shakiness, shivering, tachycardia, trouble with coordination, or vomiting. Notify prescriber at once because serotonin syndrome may be life-threatening. Be prepared to discontinue drug, if possible and ordered, and provide supportive care.

- Monitor patient for adrenal insufficiency. Although rare, it can be life-threatening. Monitor patient for anorexia, dizziness, fatigue, hypotension, nausea, vomiting, and weakness. Notify prescriber if adrenal insufficiency is suspected and expect diagnostic testing to be done. If confirmed, expect to administer corticosteroids and wean patient off morphine, if possible.
- Keep in mind when discontinuing morphine in patients receiving more than 30 mg daily, expect prescriber to reduce daily dose by about one-half for 2 days and then by 25% every 2 days thereafter until total dose reaches initial amount recommended for patients who haven't received opioids (15 to 30 mg daily). This regimen minimizes the risk of withdrawal symptoms.

PATIENT TEACHING

- Instruct patient to take morphine exactly as prescribed and not to change dosage without consulting prescriber. Tell patient this is because excessive or prolonged use can lead to abuse, addiction, misuse, overdose, and possibly death.
- Encourage patient and family or caregiver to have naloxone in household to treat an emergency opioid overdose. Instruct on

how to recognize respiratory depression and how to give naloxone. Emphasize that even if naloxone is given, 911 should be called immediately with naloxone administration.

- Explain that patient may take tablets or capsules with food or milk to relieve GI distress.
- Urge patient not to break, chew, or crush tablets to avoid rapid release and, possibly, toxicity.
- Explain to patient who has difficulty swallowing capsules that he can open Kadian E.R. capsules and sprinkle contents on food or liquids. Urge him to take drug immediately and not let capsule contents dissolve in his mouth.
- Instruct patient taking oral solution to use the calibrated syringe that comes with the drug, never a household spoon, to measure dosage.
- Instruct patient to moisten rectal suppository before inserting it.
- Urge patient to avoid alcohol and other CNS depressants, including benzodiazepines, during therapy without prescriber knowledge, as severe respiratory depression can occur and may lead to death.
- Advise patient to avoid potentially hazardous activities during morphine therapy.
- Tell patient to change positions slowly to minimize orthostatic hypotension.
- Instruct patient to notify prescriber about worsening or breakthrough pain.
- Explain that morphine may be habit-forming. Urge patient to notify prescriber if he experiences anxiety, decreased appetite, excessive tearing, irritability, muscle aches or twitching, rapid heart rate, or yawning.
- Advise female patient to notify prescriber if she becomes pregnant. Regular morphine use during pregnancy may cause physical dependence in fetus and withdrawal in neonate.
- Inform breastfeeding mothers that breastfeeding is not recommended during morphine therapy.
- Tell patient to alert all prescribers of morphine use. This is important because a potentially fatal effect can occur when an

M

opioid like morphine is combined with a benzodiazepine.

- Warn patient not to discontinue morphine use abruptly if more than a few weeks of use has occurred, as withdrawal symptoms may develop.
- Caution patient to keep drug out of reach of children because accidental consumption by a child may be fatal.
- Inform patient that long-term use of opioids like morphine may decrease sex hormone levels, causing decreased libido, erectile dysfunction, impotence, infertility, or lack of menstruation. Encourage patient to report any symptoms.
- Instruct patient that when morphine is no longer needed, patient should dispose of drug promptly. Expired, unused, or unwanted drug can be disposed of by flushing the drug down the toilet if a drug-take back option is not available.

moxifloxacin hydrochloride

Avelox, Avelox I.V.

⦀ Class and Category

Pharmacologic class: Fluoroquinolone
Therapeutic class: Antibiotic

⦀ Indications and Dosages

✶ *To treat acute sinusitis caused by* Haemophilus influenzae, Moraxella catarrhalis, *or* Streptococcus pneumoniae; *to treat mild to moderate community-acquired pneumonia caused by* Chlamydia pneumoniae, H. influenzae, Klebsiella pneumoniae, M. catarrhalis, Mycoplasma pneumoniae, Staphylococcus aureus, *or* S. pneumoniae *(including penicillin- or multi-drug-resistant strains)*

TABLETS, I.V. INFUSION

Adults. 400 mg every 24 hr for 10 days for acute sinusitis and 7 to 14 days for community-acquired pneumonia.

✶ *To treat acute exacerbation of chronic bronchitis caused by* H. influenzae, H. parainfluenzae, Klebsiella pneumoniae, M. catarrhalis, S. pneumoniae, *or* Staphylococcus aureus

TABLETS, I.V. INFUSION

Adults. 400 mg every 24 hr for 5 days.

✶ *To treat uncomplicated skin and soft-tissue infections caused by* S. aureus *or* Streptococcus pyogenes

TABLETS, I.V. INFUSION

Adults. 400 mg every 24 hr for 7 days.

✶ *To treat complicated skin and skin structure infections caused by* Enterobacter cloacae, E. coli, K. pneumoniae, *or* S. aureus

TABLETS, I.V. INFUSION

Adults. 400 mg every 24 hr for 7 to 21 days.

✶ *To treat complicated intra-abdominal infections, including polymicrobial infections such as abscesses caused by* Bacteroides fragilis, B. thetaiotaomicron, Clostridium perfringens, Enterococcus faecalis, E. coli, Peptostreptococcus *species,* Proteus mirabilis, Streptococcus anginosus, *or* S. constellatus

TABLETS, I.V. INFUSION

Adults. 400 mg every 24 hr for 5 to 14 days with initial dosage given as I.V. infusion.

✶ *To prevent or treat plague, including pneumonic and septicemic plague, caused by* Yersinia pestis

I.V. INFUSION, TABLETS

Adults. 400 mg every 24 hr for 10 to 14 days after exposure confirmed or suspected.

⦀ Drug Administration

P.O.

- Administer drug at least 4 hours before and 8 hours after aluminum- or magnesium-containing antacids, didanosine chewable buffered tablets or oral solution prepared from powder, multivitamins containing iron or zinc, or sucralfate.

I.V.

- Flush I.V. line before and after infusion with a compatible solution, such as 0.9% Sodium Chloride Injection, 5% Dextrose Injection, Lactated Ringer's solution, or Sterile Water for Injection.
- Stop other solutions during moxifloxacin infusion.
- Infuse drug over 60 minutes using ready-to-use flexible bags with 400 mg of moxifloxacin in 250 ml of 0.9% Sodium Chloride Injection. Don't dilute further.
- Don't refrigerate drug, because precipitation will occur.

- Discard any unused portion; premixed bags are for single-use only.
- *Incompatibilities:* Other I.V. additives or drugs

Route	Onset	Peak	Duration
P.O./I.V.	Unknown	Unknown	Unknown

Half-life: 12 hr

Mechanism of Action

Inhibits synthesis of bacterial enzyme DNA gyrase by counteracting excessive supercoiling of DNA during replication or transcription. Inhibiting DNA gyrase causes rapid- and slow-growing bacterial cells to die.

Contraindications

Hypersensitivity to moxifloxacin, other fluoroquinolones, or their components; myasthenia gravis

Interactions

DRUGS

aluminum- or magnesium-containing antacids; drug formulations with divalent or trivalent cations, such as didanosine chewable buffered tablets or powder for oral solution; metal cations, such as iron; multivitamins containing iron or zinc; sucralfate: Possibly substantial interference with moxifloxacin absorption, causing low blood moxifloxacin level

antidiabetic agents: Increased risk of either hyperglycemia or hypoglycemia

class IA antiarrhythmics, such as quinidine; class III antiarrhythmics, such as sotalol; other drugs known to prolong QTc interval, such as antipsychotics, cisapride, disopyramide erythromycin, pentamidine and tricyclic antidepressants: Possibly prolonged QTc interval

corticosteroids: Increased risk of Achilles and other tendon ruptures

NSAIDs: Increased risk of CNS stimulation and seizures

warfarin: Possibly increased anticoagulation

Adverse Reactions

CNS: Abnormal gait, agitation, altered coordination, anxiety, confusion, delirium, depression, disorientation, disturbance in attention, dizziness, fever, hallucinations, headache, **increased intracranial pressure (including pseudotumor cerebri)**, insomnia, memory impairment, nervousness, paranoia, peripheral neuropathy, psychosis, psychotic reaction, **seizures, suicidal ideation**, syncope, **toxic psychosis**, tremors

CV: **Aortic dissection**, hypertension, **hypotension**, palpitations, peripheral edema, **prolonged QT interval, rupture of aortic aneurysm**, tachycardia, vasculitis, vasodilation, **ventricular tachyarrhythmias**

EENT: Altered taste, deafness or other hearing impairments, **laryngeal edema**, vision loss

ENDO: Hyperglycemia, **hypoglycemia**

GI: Abdominal pain, abnormal liver enzymes, **acute hepatic necrosis, cholestatic hepatitis**, diarrhea, dyspepsia, **hepatic failure, hepatitis**, jaundice, nausea, **pseudomembranous colitis**, vomiting

GU: **Acute renal insufficiency or failure**, interstitial nephritis

HEME: **Agranulocytosis, aplastic anemia**, eosinophilia, **hemolytic anemia, leukopenia, pancytopenia, prolonged prothrombin time, thrombocytopenia**

MS: Arthralgia; muscle weakness; myalgia; tendon inflammation, pain, or rupture

RESP: **Allergic pneumonitis**

SKIN: Photosensitivity, rash, **Stevens–Johnson syndrome, toxic epidermal necrolysis**

Other: **Anaphylaxis, anaphylactic shock, angioedema**, serum sickness, worsening of myasthenia gravis

Childbearing Considerations

PREGNANCY

- It is not known if drug causes fetal harm.
- Use with caution only if benefit to mother outweighs potential risk to fetus.

LACTATION

- Drug may be present in breast milk.
- Breastfeeding is not recommended during drug therapy.

Nursing Considerations

- Be aware that if patient has hypokalemia, expect to correct it before beginning moxifloxacin therapy to prevent arrhythmias.
- Determine if patient has a history of CNS disorder, such as cerebral arteriosclerosis or epilepsy, because drug may lower seizure threshold. Notify prescriber before starting drug, and take seizure precautions.

- Be aware that there is an increased risk of aortic aneurysm and dissection within 2 months following use of moxifloxacin as a fluroquinolone, especially in elderly patients. Moxifloxacin should be reserved for patients with a known aortic aneurysm or patients who are at greater risk for aortic aneurysms only when there are no alternative antibacterial therapies available.
- Use cautiously in patients with liver dysfunction, including cirrhosis, because drug may adversely affect liver function.
- Obtain a fluid or tissue specimen for culture and sensitivity, as ordered. Expect to begin therapy before results are available.

! **WARNING** Keep in mind before starting moxifloxacin therapy, determine if patient takes a class IA antiarrhythmic, such as quinidine; a class III antiarrhythmic, such as sotalol; or other drugs that prolong the QTc interval, such as antipsychotics, cisapride, erythromycin, or tricyclic antidepressants. These drugs should be avoided in patients taking moxifloxacin because they may prolong the QTc interval and lead to life-threatening ventricular tachycardia or torsades de pointes. Monitor patient closely throughout therapy, especially if he has significant acute myocardial ischemia or bradycardia, because these conditions increase risk of prolonging the QTc interval.

- Expect to obtain a 12-lead ECG to assess patient for prolonged QTc interval. Ask patient if he or a blood relative has a history of prolonged QTc interval. Monitor elderly patients closely; they may have increased risk of prolonged QT interval.
- Monitor patient for central nervous system (including psychiatric) adverse reactions such as confusion, depression, dizziness, hallucinations, peripheral neuropathy, psychosis, suicidal ideation, and tremors. If any occurs, notify prescriber and expect moxifloxacin to be discontinued.
- Monitor patient for diarrhea. If profuse, watery diarrhea develops, contact prescriber and expect to obtain a stool specimen to rule out pseudomembranous colitis caused by *Clostridium difficile*. If diarrhea occurs, notify prescriber and expect to withhold moxifloxacin and treat with fluids, an antibiotic effective against *C. difficile,* electrolytes, fluids, and protein, as ordered.
- Monitor serum potassium level, as ordered, during therapy to assess for hypokalemia.

! **WARNING** Keep emergency resuscitation equipment readily available, and observe for evidence of hypersensitivity, such as angioedema, dyspnea, and urticaria. If you suspect anaphylaxis, prepare to give epinephrine, corticosteroids, diphenhydramine, and epinephrine, as prescribed.

- Monitor patients who are prone to tendinitis, such as athletes, the elderly, and those taking corticosteroids, for complaints of tendon inflammation, pain, or rupture. If present, notify prescriber and expect to discontinue moxifloxacin, place patient on bedrest with no exercise of affected limb, and obtain diagnostic tests to confirm rupture.
- Monitor patient's blood glucose, especially in diabetic patients receiving concomitant treatment with insulin or an oral hypoglycemic agent, for changes in blood glucose levels that could become decreased or increased. If dysglycemia occurs, treat according to standard of care and expect that drug may have to be discontinued.
- Know that fluoroquinolones like moxifloxacin have caused disabling and potentially irreversible serious adverse reactions from different body systems that can occur together in the same patient. These reactions can occur within hours to weeks after starting the drug and usually cause central nervous system effects, peripheral neuropathy, tendinitis and tendon rupture. All ages of patients and patients without any preexisting risk factors have experienced these reactions. Notify prescriber and expect to discontinue moxifloxacin immediately at the first signs or symptoms of any serious adverse reactions.

PATIENT TEACHING

- Instruct patient that if a dose is missed, it can be taken anytime but not later than 8 hours prior to the next scheduled dose. If less than 8 hours, the dose should be missed and treatment continued with the next scheduled dose. Warn patient not to compensate for the missed dose by doubling next dose.
- Teach patient to take drug at least 4 hours before and 8 hours after aluminum- or magnesium-containing antacids, didanosine chewable buffered tablets or oral solution prepared from powder, multivitamins containing iron or zinc, or sucralfate.
- Urge patient to drink plenty of fluids while taking moxifloxacin.
- Urge patient to notify prescriber at once about fainting or palpitations because they may indicate a serious arrhythmia. Also, tell patient to seek emergency help immediately if patient develops sudden back, chest, or stomach pain.

! **WARNING** Caution patient to stop drug and notify prescriber if he has a rash, trouble breathing, or other signs of an allergic reaction. Also advise patient to stop taking moxifloxacin immediately and notify prescriber if any persistent, serious, or worsening adverse effects occur.

- Urge patient to stop any exercise and contact prescriber immediately if he develops tendon inflammation, pain, or rupture.
- Tell patient to notify prescriber if motor or sensory changes occur.
- Caution patient to avoid hazardous activities until adverse CNS effects are known.
- Urge patient to tell prescriber if diarrhea develops, even more than 2 months after moxifloxacin therapy ends.
- Caution patient to complete the prescribed course of therapy even if he feels better before it's completed.
- Tell patient to avoid excessive exposure to sunlight or artificial ultraviolet light because severe sunburn may result. Instruct patient to notify prescriber if sunburn develops because moxifloxacin may have to be discontinued.

- Warn patient, especially diabetics, that moxifloxacin may alter blood glucose levels. Review signs and symptoms of hyperglycemia and hypoglycemia. Tell patient to report symptomatic changes in blood glucose levels to prescriber and review how to treat hypoglycemia.

mycophenolate mofetil
CellCept

mycophenolate mofetil hydrochloride
CellCept, CellCept Intravenous

mycophenolic acid
Myfortic

Class and Category
Pharmacologic class: Mycophenolic acid
Therapeutic class: Immunosuppressant

Indications and Dosages
❋ *To prevent organ rejection in patients receiving allogenic kidney transplants*

CAPSULES, ORAL SUSPENSION, TABLETS, I.V. INFUSION
Adults. 1 g twice daily.

DELAYED-RELEASE TABLETS
Adults. 720 mg twice daily.

Children age 5 and older who are at least 6 months post kidney transplant. 400 mg/m^2 twice daily. Alternatively, 540 mg twice daily if body surface area is between 1.19 to 1.58 m^2 or 720 mg twice daily if body surface area is greater than 1.58 m^2.

ORAL SUSPENSION
Children age 3 months to 18 years. 600 mg/m^2 twice daily. *Maximum:* 2 g (10 ml) daily divided into 2 doses.

CAPSULES
Children with body surface area of 1.25 m^2 to less than 1.5 m^2. 750 mg twice daily.

CAPSULES, TABLETS

**Children with body surface area of 1.5 m²
or greater.** 1 g twice daily.

✱ *To prevent organ rejection in patients receiving
allogenic heart transplants*

**CAPSULES, ORAL SUSPENSION, TABLETS,
I.V. INFUSION**

Adults. 1.5 g twice daily.

✱ *To prevent organ rejection in patients receiving
allogenic liver transplants*

I.V. INFUSION

Adults. 1 g twice daily.

**CAPSULES, ORAL SUSPENSION,
TABLETS**

Adults. 1.5 g twice daily.

Drug Administration

- Handle drug similarly to a
  chemotherapeutic drug because
  mycophenolate mofetil is embryotoxic
  and genotoxic and may have mutagenic
  properties.
- Avoid inhalation or contact of skin or
  mucous membranes with the powder found
  in capsules or oral suspension. If contact
  occurs, wash area thoroughly with soap and
  water; rinse eyes with plain water.

P.O.

- Capsules, oral suspension, or tablets
  should not be used interchangeably with
  delayed-release tablets.
- Capsules and tablets should be swallowed
  whole and not chewed, crushed, or split/
  opened.
- Administer on an empty stomach 1 hour
  before or 2 hours after a meal. However,
  in stable transplant patients, drug may be
  taken with food, if needed.
- Wearing gloves, prepare oral suspension
  by tapping closed bottle several times to
  loosen powder and then measure 94 ml of
  water in a graduated cylinder. Add half of
  the water to the bottle and shake for about
  1 minute. Then add remainder of water
  and shake again for 1 minute. Remove
  child-resistant cap and push bottle adapter
  into neck of bottle. Close bottle tightly
  with child-resistant cap. Be aware that
  the suspension bottle may become cold
  immediately after reconstitution.
- When giving oral suspension, don't mix
  with any other drugs.

- Ask patient about history of
  phenylketonuria before initial
  administration, because oral suspension
  contains aspartame.
- Oral suspension can be administered
  through an 8 F or larger nasogastric tube.
- Store drug at room temperature. Oral
  suspension also may be stored in
  refrigerator. Discard oral suspension once
  mixed after 60 days.

I.V.

- Expect to give I.V. form within 24 hours of
  transplantation and for no longer than 14
  days. Expect to switch patient to oral form
  as soon as possible, as ordered.
- Reconstitute with 14 ml of 5% Dextrose in
  Water for each vial (2 vials will be needed
  for 1-g dose; 3 vials for 1.5-g dose), then
  shake gently.
- Further dilute 1-g dose with 140 ml of 5%
  Dextrose in Water and 210 ml for 1.5-g
  dose. Concentration should be 6 mg/ml.
- Administer within 4 hours once
  reconstituted and diluted.
- Administer infusion over no less than 2
  hours. Never administer by rapid or bolus
  I.V. injection.
- *Incompatibilities:* Other I.V. drugs and
  solutions

Route	Onset	Peak	Duration
P.O.	Unknown	0.5–2 hr	Unknown
P.O./D.R.	Unknown	1.5–2.7 hr	Unknown
I.V.	Unknown	Unknown	Unknown

Half-life: 8–18 hr

Mechanism of Action

Hydrolyzes to form mycophenolic acid
(MPA), which inhibits guanosine nucleotide
synthesis and proliferation of T and B
lymphocytes. MPA also suppresses antibody
formation by B lymphocytes and prevents
glycosylation of lymphocyte and monocyte
glycoproteins involved in adhesion to
endothelial cells. MPA also may inhibit
leukocytes from sites of inflammation and
graft rejection, which may explain how
mycophenolate mofetil prolongs allogeneic
transplant survival.

Contraindications

Hypersensitivity to mycophenolate mofetil,
mycophenolic acid, mycophenolate sodium,

or any of their components; hypersensitivity to polysorbate 80 (I.V. form)

Interactions

DRUGS

acyclovir, ganciclovir, probenecid, valacyclovir, valganciclovir: Increased plasma concentrations and/or adverse reactions of these drugs

aminoglycosides, bile acid sequestrants, cephalosporins, fluoroquinolones, penicillins, rifampin, sulfamethoxazole/trimethoprim: Decreased effectiveness of mycophenolate mofetil

antacids with aluminum and magnesium hydroxides, sevelamer: Decreased absorption of oral mycophenolate mofetil

isavuconazole: Increased risk of adverse reactions caused by mycophenolate mofetil

live vaccines: Decreased effectiveness of live vaccines

oral contraceptives (combination): Possibly decreased effectiveness of oral contraceptives

proton pump inhibitors such as lansoprazole, pantoprazole: Possibly decreased effectiveness of mycophenolate mofetil

telmisartan: Decreased mycophenolate mofetil system exposure reducing effectiveness

Adverse Reactions

CNS: Agitation, anxiety, chills, confusion, delirium, depression, dizziness, emotional lability, fever, hallucinations, headache, hypertonia, hypesthesia, insomnia, malaise, meningitis, nervousness, neuropathy, paresthesia, **progressive multifocal leukoencephalopathy**, psychosis, **seizures**, somnolence, syncope, thinking abnormality, tremor, vertigo

CV: Angina pectoris, **arrhythmias, arterial thrombosis, atrial fibrillation or flutter, bradycardia, cardiac arrest**, CV disorder, **congestive heart failure, extrasystoles**, generalized edema, **hemorrhage**, hypercholesterolemia, hyperlipemia, hypertension, **hypotension**, increased lactic dehydrogenase, increased SGOT and SGPT, increased venous pressure, **infectious endocarditis**, orthostatic hypotension, palpitations, **pericardial effusion**, peripheral edema, peripheral vascular disorder, **supraventricular tachycardia, thrombosis**, vasodilation, vasospasm, **ventricular extrasystole, ventricular tachycardia**

EENT: Amblyopia, cataract, conjunctivitis, deafness, dry mouth, ear disorder or pain, epistaxis, eye hemorrhage, gingivitis, gum hyperplasia, lacrimation disorder, mouth ulceration, oral candidiasis, pharyngitis, rhinitis, sinusitis, stomatitis, tinnitus, vision abnormality, voice alteration

ENDO: Cushing's syndrome, diabetes mellitus, hypercalcemia, **hypoglycemia**, hypothyroidism, parathyroid disorder

GI: Abdomen enlargement or pain, anorexia, ascites, cholangitis, cholestatic jaundice, colitis, constipation, diarrhea, dyspepsia, dysphagia, elevated liver enzymes, esophagitis, flatulence, gastritis, gastroenteritis, **GI hemorrhage or perforation**, GI infection, GI candidiasis, **hepatitis**, hernia, ileus, intestinal villous atrophy, jaundice, **liver damage, melena**, nausea, **pancreatitis, peritonitis**, rectal disorder, stomach ulcer, **ulceration of GI tract**, vomiting

GU: Albuminuria; bilirubinemia; BK virus-related nephropathy; dysuria; hematuria; hydronephrosis; impotence; increased BUN or creatinine levels; **kidney tubular necrosis**; nocturia; oliguria; pain; polyomavirus-associated nephropathy; prostatic disorder; **pyelonephritis; renal failure**; scrotal edema; urinary tract disorder or infection; urine abnormality, frequency, incontinence, or retention

HEME: Anemia, **bone marrow failure, coagulation disorder**, hypochromic anemia, hypogammaglobulinemia, **increased prothrombin time or thromboplastin time**, leukocytosis, **leukopenia, neutropenia, pancytopenia**, polycythemia, pure red cell aplasia, **thrombocytopenia**

MS: Arthralgia; back, neck or pelvic pain; joint disorder; leg cramps; myalgia; myasthenia; osteoporosis

RESP: **Apnea; asthma; atelectasis**; bronchiectasis; bronchitis; candidiasis; cough; dyspnea; **hemoptysis**; hyperventilation; **hypoxia**; interstitial lung disease; **neoplasm**; pleural effusion; pneumonia; **pneumothorax; pulmonary edema, fibrosis, or hypertension; respiratory acidosis**; sputum increase

M

SKIN: Abscess; acne; alopecia; benign neoplasm, **carcinoma**, hypertrophy, or ulcer; cellulite; ecchymosis; fungal dermatitis; hirsutism; pallor; petechia; pruritus; rash; sweating; vesiculobullous rash

Other: Abnormal healing; **acidosis**; activation of latent infections (such as tuberculosis) or **reactivation of hepatitis B or hepatitis C**; acute inflammatory syndrome; **alkalosis**; **angioedema**; bacterial, fungal, protozoal, and viral infections, including opportunistic infections; congenital defects; cyst; dehydration; flu-like syndrome; gout; hiccup; **hyperkalemia**; **hypersensitivity reactions**; hyperuricemia; hypervolemia; hypochloremia; **hypocalcemia**; **hypokalemia**; **hypomagnesemia**; **hyponatremia**; **hypophosphatemia**; hypoproteinemia; increased alkaline phosphatase; increased gamma glutamyl transpeptidase; lymphocele; **lymphoma**; **malignancies**; **sepsis**; thirst; weight gain or loss

Childbearing Considerations

PREGNANCY

- Pregnancy exposure registry: 1-800-617-8191 or www.mycophenolateREMS.com.
- Drug causes fetal harm such as an increased risk of first-trimester pregnancy loss and an increased risk of multiple congenital malformations in multiple organ systems.
- A negative pregnancy test should be performed and a second one done 8 to 10 days later before drug therapy is begun.
- Drug is not recommended for use during pregnancy.

LACTATION

- It is not known if drug is present in breast milk.
- Patient should check with prescriber before breastfeeding.

REPRODUCTION

- Know that female patients of childbearing age must receive contraceptive counseling and use at least two contraceptives simultaneously throughout drug therapy and for 6 weeks following drug discontinuation unless abstinence is practiced, an intrauterine device is in place, or tubal ligation or vasectomy has occurred.
- Know that male patients and their partner must also receive contraceptive counseling and use an effective contraceptive throughout drug therapy for male patient and for 90 days following drug discontinuation unless abstinence is practiced.
- Inform female patient that drug may make combination oral hormonal contraceptives ineffective.
- Female patient or female partner should be made aware that follow-up pregnancy testing will be done during drug use.
- Instruct male patients not to donate sperm during drug therapy and for at least 90 days following drug discontinuation.

Nursing Considerations

- Keep in mind, before starting mycophenolate therapy in a woman of childbearing potential, to make sure she has a negative pregnancy test within 1 week of starting therapy, using a test with a sensitivity of at least 25 mIU/ml. Therapy shouldn't start until results are confirmed.
- Know that mycophenolate mofetil therapy should be avoided in patients with hypoxanthine-guanine phosphoribosyl-transferase deficiency, because drug may exacerbate disease symptoms.
- Know that corticosteroids and cyclosporine should be used with mycophenolate mofetil therapy.
- Obtain CBC weekly during first month of therapy, twice monthly for the second and third months of therapy, and then monthly through the first year, as ordered. Notify prescriber of any abnormalities. If significant, anticipate dosage reduction if absolutely necessary because reduced immunosuppression increases the risk of organ rejection. Also provide supportive care. Monitor patient for signs and symptoms of infection and institute infection control measures.
- Monitor patient's serum creatinine levels, as ordered, to detect changes in kidney function because drug may cause polyomavirus-associated nephropathy. Notify prescriber if changes occur and expect dosage to be reduced, if needed.

! **WARNING** Monitor patient closely for adverse reactions because drug has many adverse effects, some of which can be serious or severe, such as the development of lymphoma and other malignancies, especially of the skin. Also know that patient may be at increased risk for bacterial, fungal, protozoal, and viral infections, including opportunistic infections and viral reactivation of hepatitis B and C, which may lead to hospitalization and possibly fatal outcome.

- Expect to stop drug or reduce the dose and provide supportive care, as ordered, if neutropenia develops.
- Monitor patient for acute inflammatory syndrome characterized by arthralgias, arthritis, elevated inflammatory markers, fever, and muscle pain. Symptoms may occur weeks to months after drug is initiated or after a dosage increase. If present, expect drug to be discontinued and patient to improve within 24 to 48 hours.

! **WARNING** Know that mycophenolate mofetil therapy has been associated with JC-virus-associated progressive multifocal leukoencephalopathy that can be life-threatening. Monitor patient for apathy, ataxia, cognitive deficiencies, and confusion. Report suspicions of disorder immediately to prescriber. Also, know that patient is at increased risk for other viral infections such as cytomegalovirus infections, COVID-19 infections, and polyomavirus-associated nephropathy. Expect dosage to be reduced or drug possibly discontinued in patients who develop new infections or reactivated viral infections.

PATIENT TEACHING
- Advise women of childbearing age that two forms of contraceptives should be used simultaneously before beginning mycophenolate mofetil therapy and for 6 weeks following discontinuation of therapy, because of potential for fetal harm. Tell male patients that they and their female partner should use effective contraception during therapy and for 90 days following discontinuation of therapy. Inform women who use combination oral contraceptives that drug may decrease effectiveness of oral contraceptives. Urge patient to notify prescriber immediately if pregnancy occurs because drug increases risk of first-trimester pregnancy loss and congenital malformations.
- Tell patient about increased risk of lymphomas or other malignancies, especially of the skin, before therapy starts. Tell patient to report any unusual signs or symptoms to prescriber.
- Tell patient to take oral form of drug on an empty stomach.
- Inform patient prescribed oral suspension that it contains aspartame, which is a source of phenylalanine.
- Instruct patient not to crush tablets or capsules or open capsules.
- Inform patient not to receive live vaccines during therapy. Urge him to avoid people who have received such vaccines or to wear a protective mask when he's around them.
- Tell patient to report any serious or ongoing adverse reactions, especially neurologic abnormalities, to prescriber immediately. Also alert patient that drug can cause an acute inflammatory syndrome. Review signs and symptoms and advise patient to notify prescriber, as drug may have to be discontinued.
- Caution patient not to engage in hazardous activities such as driving a car or using machines until the effects of the drug are known and patient is not experiencing confusion, dizziness, low blood pressure, somnolence, or tremors.
- Caution patient to avoid contact with people who have infections because drug causes immunosuppression, placing patient at increased risk for developing an infection.
- Urge patient to report any signs of infection, unexpected bleeding or bruising, or any other sign of bone marrow depression immediately.
- Tell patient that frequent laboratory tests may be needed during therapy. Emphasize that having these tests done is essential to continuing therapy.
- Advise patient to avoid exposure to direct sunlight and UV light and to wear sunscreen when outdoors because of increased risk for skin cancer.

M

- Advise patient not to take antacids at the same time as oral mycophenolate mofetil because some antacids can decrease drug's absorption.
- Tell patient to report dizziness, fainting, lack of energy, paleness, or unusual tiredness, because dosage may have to be reduced or drug discontinued.
- Emphasize importance of follow-up care to monitor the drug's effectiveness and possible adverse effects because of the increased risk for cancer and infections as a result of immunosuppression. Inform patient of the need for periodic laboratory tests.
- Caution patient not to donate blood during therapy and for at least 6 weeks following discontinuation of drug. Tell male patients not to donate semen during therapy and for 90 days following discontinuation of drug.

N O

nadolol
Corgard

⊟ Class and Category
Pharmacologic class: Nonselective beta-blocker
Therapeutic class: Antianginal, antihypertensive

⊟ Indications and Dosages
✽ *To manage hypertension, alone or with other antihypertensives*

TABLETS
Adults. *Initial:* 40 mg daily, increased by 40 to 80 mg as needed. *Maintenance:* 40 to 80 mg daily. *Maximum:* 320 mg daily.

✽ *To manage angina pectoris as long-term therapy*

TABLETS
Adults. *Initial:* 40 mg daily, increased by 40 to 80 mg daily every 3 to 7 days, as needed. *Maintenance:* 40 to 80 mg daily. *Maximum:* 240 mg daily.

±**DOSAGE ADJUSTMENT** Interval possibly increased to every 24 to 36 hr if creatinine clearance is 31 to 50 ml/min; to every 24 to 48 hr if it's 10 to 30 ml/min; or to every 40 to 60 hr if it's less than 10 ml/min.

⊟ Drug Administration
P.O.
- Check apical pulse before administering drug. If slower than 60 beats/minute, notify prescriber and withhold drug.
- Administer drug once daily at about the same time of day.
- Store at room temperature, avoiding excessive heat. Protect from light.

Route	Onset	Peak	Duration
P.O.	1 hr	3–4 hr	24 hr

Half-life: 10–24 hr

⊟ Mechanism of Action
Selectively blocks alpha$_1$ and beta$_2$ receptors in vascular smooth muscle and beta$_1$ receptors in the heart, thereby reducing peripheral vascular resistance and blood pressure. Potent beta blockade decreases cardiac excitability, cardiac output, and myocardial oxygen demand, thus reducing angina. It also prevents reflex tachycardia, which typically occurs with most alpha blockers.

⊟ Contraindications
Bronchial asthma; cardiogenic shock; heart failure; hypersensitivity to nadolol, other beta-blockers, or their components; second- or third-degree AV block; sinus bradycardia

⊟ Interactions
DRUGS
digoxin: Increased risk of bradycardia
epinephrine: Possibly unresponsive to usual doses of epinephrine used to treat allergic reaction
general anesthetics: Increased risk of hypotension and myocardial depression
insulin, oral antidiabetic drugs: Possibly increased risk of hyperglycemia and hypoglycemia
reserpine and other catecholamine-depleting drugs: Increased risk of bradycardia and hypotension

⊟ Adverse Reactions
CNS: Anxiety, depression, dizziness, drowsiness, fatigue, headache, paresthesia, syncope, vertigo, weakness, yawning
CV: **Bradycardia**, chest pain, edema, **heart block**, **heart failure**, **hypotension**, orthostatic hypotension, **ventricular arrhythmias**
EENT: Nasal congestion, taste perversion
GI: Dyspepsia, elevated liver enzymes, **hepatic necrosis**, **hepatitis**, jaundice, nausea, vomiting
GU: Ejaculation failure, impotence
RESP: Cough, dyspnea, wheezing
SKIN: Pruritus, scalp tingling

⊟ Childbearing Considerations
PREGNANCY
- It is not known if drug causes fetal harm.
- Use with caution only if benefit to mother outweighs potential risk to fetus.

LABOR & DELIVERY
- Monitor neonate whose mothers are receiving nadolol at parturition for bradycardia, hypoglycemia, or other associated symptoms.

N O

LACTATION

- Drug is present in breast milk.
- A decision should be made to discontinue breastfeeding or the drug to avoid potential serious adverse reactions in the breastfed infant.

Nursing Considerations

- Use nadolol cautiously in patients with diabetes mellitus because it may prolong or worsen hypoglycemia by interfering with glycogenolysis.
- Anticipate that drug may worsen psoriasis; in patients with myasthenia gravis, it may worsen muscle weakness and diplopia.
- Be aware that chronic beta-blocker therapy such as nadolol is not routinely withheld prior to major surgery because the benefits outweigh the risks associated with its use with general anesthesia and surgical procedures.

> ! **WARNING** Withdraw drug gradually over 2 weeks, or as ordered, to avoid MI caused by unopposed beta stimulation or thyroid storm caused by underlying hyperthyroidism. Expect drug to mask tachycardia caused by hyperthyroidism.

PATIENT TEACHING

- Teach patient how to take her radial pulse, and direct her to do so before each dose of nadolol.
- Instruct patient to notify prescriber if pulse rate falls below 60 beats/minute.
- Tell patient to take drug at about the same time every day.
- Caution patient not to stop taking nadolol abruptly or change dosage. Tell her to take a missed dose as soon as possible unless it's within 8 hours of the next scheduled dose.
- Advise patient with diabetes to check blood glucose level often because nadolol may mask signs of hypoglycemia, such as tachycardia.
- Review signs of impending heart failure, and urge patient to notify prescriber immediately if they occur.

nafcillin sodium

Class and Category

Pharmacologic class: Penicillin
Therapeutic class: Antibiotic

Indications and Dosages

✳ *To treat infections caused by penicillinase-producing* Staphylococcus aureus

I.V. INFUSION, I.V. INJECTION

Adults. 500 mg every 4 hr for mild to moderate infections; 1,000 mg every 4 hr for severe infections. Duration of therapy is continued for at least 48 hr after patient is afebrile, asymptomatic, and cultures are negative. Severe infections require at least 14 days of therapy although endocarditis and osteomyelitis may require a longer time of therapy.

I.M. INJECTION

Adults. 500 mg every 4 to 6 hr for mild to moderate infections; 1,000 mg every 4 hr for severe infections.

Infants and children weighing less than 40 kg (88 lb). 25 mg/kg twice daily
Neonates. 10 mg/kg twice daily. Duration of therapy for all ages is continued for at least 48 hr after patient is afebrile, asymptomatic, and cultures are negative. Severe infections require at least 14 days of therapy, although endocarditis and osteomyelitis may require a longer duration of therapy.

Drug Administration

I.V.

- For I.V. injection, reconstitute with 15 to 30 ml of Sterile Water for Injection or 0.9% Sodium Chloride Injection. Inject directly into a vein or through the tubing of an intravenous infusion. Administer over 5 to 10 minutes.
- For I.V. infusion, reconstitute with 15 to 30 ml of Sterile Water for Injection or 0.9% Sodium Chloride Injection. Further dilute following manufacturer guidelines prior to administration. Infuse over 30 to 60 minutes.
- *Incompatibilities:* Other drugs

I.M.

- Reconstitute with Sterile Water for Injection, 0.9% Sodium Chloride Injection, or Bacteriostatic Water for Injection by adding 3.4 ml to a 1-gram bottle and 6.6 ml to a 2-gram bottle to provide a concentration of 250 mg/ml.
- Inject the clear solution immediately by deep intragluteal injection.
- Rotate sites.
- Reconstituted solution is stable for 3 days at room temperature and 7 days refrigerated.

Route	Onset	Peak	Duration
I.V.	Immediate	Immediate	Unknown
I.M.	Unknown	30–60 min	Unknown

Half-life: 33–61 min

Mechanism of Action

Binds to certain penicillin-binding proteins in bacterial cell walls, thereby inhibiting the final stage of bacterial cell wall synthesis. The result is cell lysis. Nafcillin's action is bolstered by its chemical composition; its unique side chain resists destruction by beta-lactamases.

Contraindications

Hypersensitivity to nafcillin, other penicillins, or their components

Interactions

DRUGS

cyclosporine: Increased risk of subtherapeutic cyclosporine levels
tetracycline: Possible antagonized bactericidal effect of nafcillin
warfarin: Decreased effectiveness of warfarin

Adverse Reactions

CNS: Depression, fever, headache, **seizures**
CV: **Hypotension, vascular collapse**
EENT: Black or hairy tongue, **laryngospasm,** oral candidiasis, stomatitis
GI: Abdominal pain, cholestasis, diarrhea, elevated liver enzymes, nausea, **pseudomembranous colitis,** vomiting
GU: **Acute kidney injury,** hematuria, interstitial nephritis, proteinuria, **renal tubular damage,** vaginitis
HEME: **Agranulocytosis, bone marrow depression, leukopenia, neutropenia**
RESP: **Bronchospasm**
SKIN: **Exfoliative dermatitis,** pruritus, rash, urticaria
Other: **Anaphylaxis; angioedema; hypokalemia;** injection-site pain, redness, and swelling; phlebitis; serum sickness-like reaction; skin sloughing; thrombophlebitis; tissue necrosis (severe)

Childbearing Considerations

PREGNANCY

- It is not known if drug causes fetal harm.
- Use with caution only if benefit to mother outweighs potential risk to fetus.

LACTATION

- Drug is present in breast milk.

- Patient should check with prescriber before breastfeeding.

Nursing Considerations

- Obtain body fluid or tissue samples for culture and sensitivity testing, as prescribed, and obtain test results, if possible, before giving nafcillin, as ordered.
- Expect to have the following laboratory tests ordered before and then periodically during nafcillin therapy: alkaline phosphatase, bilirubin, blood urea nitrogen, creatinine, liver enzymes, and urinalysis; this provides a baseline and then allows monitoring for adverse effects stemming from nafcillin therapy.
- Know that when giving nafcillin to patient at risk for fluid overload or hypertension, each gram contains 2.5 mEq sodium.

! **WARNING** Monitor patient for hypersensitivity reactions, which could be serious. Stop drug, notify prescriber, and provide supportive care, as ordered.

- Watch for evidence of superinfection, such as oral candidiasis and pseudomembranous colitis, especially in elderly, immunocompromised, or debilitated patients who receive large doses of nafcillin. If profuse, watery diarrhea develops, contact prescriber and expect to obtain a stool specimen to rule out pseudomembranous colitis caused by *Clostridium difficile.* If diarrhea occurs, notify prescriber and expect to withhold nafcillin and treat with electrolytes, fluids, protein, and an antibiotic effective against *C. difficile.*

PATIENT TEACHING

! **WARNING** Advise patient to notify prescriber if she experiences chills, fever, GI distress, or rash.

- Urge patient to tell prescriber if diarrhea develops, even 2 or more months after nafcillin therapy ends.

nalbuphine hydrochloride
Nubain

Class and Category

Pharmacologic class: Opioid
Therapeutic class: Opioid analgesic

Indications and Dosages

＊ *To relieve pain severe enough to require an opioid analgesic and for which alternative treatment options such as nonopioid analgesics or opioid combination products are inadequate or not tolerated*

I.M., I.V., OR SUBCUTANEOUS INJECTION

Adults weighing 70 kg (154 lb). 10 mg every 3 to 6 hr and adjusted, as needed.

±**DOSAGE ADJUSTMENT** Dosage adjusted for patients weighing more or less than 70 kg, other medications that the patient may be receiving, severity of pain, and physical status of patient. For nontolerant adults, single maximum dose increased to 20 mg with a maximum total daily dose of 160 mg.

＊ *As adjunct to balanced anesthesia, for obstetrical analgesia during labor and delivery, and for preoperative and postoperative analgesia*

I.V. INJECTION

Adults. 0.3 to 3 mg/kg followed by 0.25 to 0.5 mg/kg, as needed.

Drug Administration

- Keep resuscitation equipment and naloxone readily available to reverse nalbuphine's effects, if needed.
- Store ampuls in carton and protect from light.

I.V.

- For direct I.V. injection used as an analgesic, inject through an I.V. line with a compatible infusing solution slowly—no more than 10 mg over at least 2 to 3 minutes.
- Inject into free-flowing 0.9% Sodium Chloride Injection, 5% Dextrose in Water, or Lactated Ringer's solution.
- For direct I.V. injection used as adjunct to balanced anesthesia, inject drug over 10 to 15 min.
- *Incompatibilities:* None listed by manufacturer

I.M.

- Rotate sites.

SUBCUTANEOUS

- Rotate sites.

Route	Onset	Peak	Duration
I.V.	2–3 min	2–3 min	3–6 hr
I.M.	15 min	30 min	3–6 hr
SubQ	15 min	Unknown	3–6 hr

Half-life: 5 hr

Mechanism of Action

Binds with and stimulates kappa and mu opiate receptors in the spinal cord and higher levels in the CNS. In this way, nalbuphine alters the perception of and emotional response to pain.

Contraindications

Acute or severe bronchial asthma in an unmonitored setting or in the absence of resuscitative equipment; gastrointestinal obstruction, including paralytic ileus; hypersensitivity to nalbuphine or any of its components; significant respiratory depression

Interactions

DRUGS

5-HT3 receptor antagonists, cyclobenzaprine; metaxalone; methylene blue (I.V.); selected psychiatric drugs such as buspirone, lithium, mirtazapine, nefazodone, trazodone, vilazodone; selective serotonin reuptake inhibitors; serotonin–norepinephrine reuptake inhibitors; St. John's wort; tramadol; tricyclic antidepressants; triptans; tryptophan: Increased risk of serotonin syndrome
anticholinergics: Increased risk of severe constipation and urine retention
antipsychotics, anxiolytics, benzodiazepines, CNS depressants, general anesthetics, muscle relaxants, other opioids, other sedative/hypnotics, sedating antihistamines, tranquilizers, tricyclic antidepressants: Increased risk of coma, severe respiratory depression, profound sedation, and death
diuretics: Reduced effectiveness of diuretics
MAO inhibitors: Risk of opioid toxicity or serotonin syndrome
neuromuscular blockers: Increased risk of respiratory depression severity

ACTIVITIES

alcohol use: Increased risk of coma, hypotension, profound sedation, and respiratory depression

Adverse Reactions

CNS: Confusion, depression, dizziness, euphoria, fatigue, hallucinations, headache, nervousness, restlessness, **seizures**, syncope, tiredness, weakness
CV: Hypertension, **hypotension**, tachycardia
EENT: Blurred vision, diplopia, dry mouth
ENDO: Adrenal insufficiency

GI: Abdominal cramps, anorexia, constipation, nausea, vomiting
GU: Decreased libido, decreased urine output, impotency, infertility, lack of menstruation, ureteral spasm
RESP: Dyspnea, **pulmonary edema**, **respiratory depression**, wheezing
SKIN: Diaphoresis, flushing, pruritus, rash, sensation of warmth, urticaria
Other: Injection-site burning, pain, redness, swelling, and warmth

Childbearing Considerations

PREGNANCY

- Drug may cause fetal harm.
- Prolonged use of drug during pregnancy can result in neonatal opioid withdrawal syndrome (NOWS), which may be life-threatening if not recognized and treated.
- Avoid prolonged use during pregnancy. Use with caution only if benefit to mother outweighs potential risk to fetus.

LABOR & DELIVERY

- Drug is not recommended for use in pregnant women immediately before or during labor as drug can cause severe fetal bradycardia. Opioids may alter length of time of labor.
- Opioids cross the placental barrier and may produce respiratory depression and psycho-physiologic effects in the newborn. Monitor neonate closely for signs of excess sedation and respiratory depression.
- An opioid antagonist, such as naloxone, must be available at the time of delivery in the event it is needed to reverse opioid-induced respiratory depression in the neonate.

LACTATION

- Drug is present in breast milk.
- Patient should check with prescriber before breastfeeding.
- If breastfeeding occurs, monitor infant for excess sedation and respiratory depression.

REPRODUCTION

- Chronic use of opioids may reduce fertility.

Nursing Considerations

- Be aware that excessive use of opioids like nalbuphine may lead to abuse, addiction, misuse, overdose, and possibly death. Monitor patient's intake of drug closely and for evidence of physical dependence.

- Know that chronic maternal use of nalbuphine during pregnancy can result in NOWS, which may be life-threatening if not recognized and treated appropriately. NOWS occurs when a newborn has been exposed to opioid drugs like nalbuphine for a prolonged period while in utero.
- Use nalbuphine cautiously in patients taking other drugs that can cause respiratory depression.

! WARNING Be aware that nalbuphine should only be used concomitantly with benzodiazepine therapy in patients for whom other treatment options are inadequate. If prescribed together, expect dosing and duration of nalbuphine to be limited. Monitor patient closely for signs and symptoms of a decrease in consciousness, including coma, profound sedation, and significant respiratory depression. Notify prescriber immediately and provide emergency supportive care, as death may occur.

- Be aware that during prolonged use, a stool softener may be given to minimize constipation.
- Know that if patient is opioid-dependent, drug will usually not be discontinued abruptly. Monitor patient for withdrawal symptoms, such as abdominal cramps, anorexia, anxiety, backache, bone or joint pain, confusion, depression, diaphoresis, dysphoria, erythema, fear, fever, irritability, labile blood pressure and pulse, lacrimation, muscle spasms, myalgia, mydriasis, nasal congestion, nausea, opioid craving, piloerection, restlessness, rhinorrhea, sensation of crawling skin, sleep disturbances, tremor, uneasiness, vomiting, and yawning.

! WARNING Know that many drugs may interact with opioids like nalbuphine to cause serotonin syndrome. Monitor patient closely for signs and symptoms such as agitation, diaphoresis, diarrhea, fever, hallucinations, labile blood pressure, muscle twitching or stiffness, nausea, shakiness, shivering, tachycardia, trouble with coordination, or vomiting. Notify prescriber at once because serotonin syndrome may be life-threatening. Be prepared to discontinue drug, if possible and ordered, and provide supportive care.

- Monitor patient for adrenal insufficiency. Although rare, it can be life-threatening. Monitor patient for anorexia, dizziness, fatigue, hypotension, nausea, vomiting, or weakness. Notify prescriber if adrenal insufficiency is suspected and expect to do diagnostic testing. If confirmed, expect to administer corticosteroids and wean patient off nalbuphine, if possible.

! **WARNING** Be aware that drug may obscure neurologic assessment findings if patient has a cerebral aneurysm, head injury, or increased intracranial pressure.

PATIENT TEACHING

- Warn patient not to take drug longer than absolutely needed because excessive or prolonged use can lead to abuse, addiction, misuse, overdose, and possibly death.
- Advise patient to avoid hazardous activities until nalbuphine's CNS effects are known.

! **WARNING** Warn patient not to consume alcohol or take a benzodiazepine without prescriber knowledge while taking nalbuphine, as severe respiratory depression can occur and may lead to death. Inform patient about potentially fatal additive effects of combining a benzodiazepine with an opioid. Instruct patient to inform all prescribers of nalbuphine use.

- Counsel patient against making important decisions while receiving drug because it may cloud her judgment.
- Inform patient that long-term use of opioids like nalbuphine may decrease sex hormone levels, causing decreased libido, erectile dysfunction, impotence, infertility, or lack of menstruation. Encourage patient to report any symptoms to prescriber.
- Instruct patient to notify all prescribers of opioid use.

naldemedine
Symproic

Class and Category
Pharmacologic class: Opioid receptor antagonist
Therapeutic class: Opioid antagonist of GI tract

Indications and Dosages
∗ *To treat opioid-induced constipation in patients with chronic noncancer pain*

TABLETS
Adults. 0.2 mg once daily.

Drug Administration
P.O.
- Keep in light-resistant container until ready to administer.

Route	Onset	Peak	Duration
P.O.	Unknown	45 min	Unknown

Half-life: 11 hr

Mechanism of Action
Functions as a peripherally acting mu-opioid receptor antagonist in the gastrointestinal tract to decrease the constipating effects of opioids.

Contraindications
Gastrointestinal obstruction or increased risk of recurrent obstruction due to the potential for gastrointestinal perforation, hypersensitivity to naldemedine or its components

Interactions
DRUGS
moderate CYP3A inhibitors such as aprepitant, atazanavir, diltiazem, erythromycin, fluconazole; P-glycoprotein inhibitors such as amiodarone, captopril, cyclosporine, quercetin, quinidine, verapamil; strong CYP3A inhibitors such as itraconazole: Increased plasma naldemedine concentrations increasing risk of adverse reactions
other opioid antagonists: Possible additive effect of opioid receptor antagonism and increased risk of opioid withdrawal
strong CYP3A inducers such as carbamazepine, phenytoin, rifampin, St. John's wort: Significant decrease in plasma naldemedine concentrations, which may decrease effectiveness

Adverse Reactions
GI: Abdominal pain, diarrhea, gastroenteritis, **GI perforation**, nausea, vomiting
RESP: Bronchospasm
SKIN: Rash
Other: Opioid withdrawal

Childbearing Considerations

PREGNANCY

- Drug may cause fetal harm.
- Prolonged use of drug during pregnancy can result in neonatal opioid withdrawal syndrome (NOWS), which may be life-threatening if not recognized and treated.
- Avoid prolonged use during pregnancy. Use with caution only if benefit to mother outweighs potential risk to fetus.

LACTATION

- It is not known if drug is present in breast milk.
- A decision should be made to discontinue breastfeeding or the drug to avoid potential serious adverse reactions in the breastfed infant.

Nursing Considerations

- Know that patients receiving opioids for less than a month may be less responsive to naldemedine therapy.
- Expect naldemedine to be discontinued if treatment with an opioid pain medication is discontinued.
- Monitor patient closely for abdominal pain. Know that gastrointestinal perforation has occurred with use of another peripherally acting opioid antagonist in patients with conditions that affect the gastrointestinal tract wall integrity, such as diverticular disease, infiltrative gastrointestinal tract malignancies, Ogilvie's syndrome, peptic ulcer disease, or peritoneal metastases. Patients with Crohn's disease may be at increased risk for gastrointestinal perforation. Notify prescriber immediately if abdominal pain becomes persistent, severe, or worsens. Expect drug to be discontinued.
- Monitor patient for signs and symptoms of opioid withdrawal such as abdominal pain, chills, diarrhea, feeling cold, fever, flushing, hyperhidrosis, increased lacrimation, nausea, and vomiting. Patients who develop disruptions to the blood–brain barrier may be at increased risk for opioid withdrawal or reduced analgesia.

PATIENT TEACHING

- Inform patient that naldemedine should be discontinued if treatment with the opioid pain medication is discontinued.
- Tell patient that the most common side effects of naldemedine include abdominal pain, diarrhea, nausea, and vomiting.
- Advise patient to seek immediate emergency care if persistent, severe, or worsening abdominal pain occurs.
- Review the signs and symptoms of withdrawal with patient and tell her to notify prescriber if these symptoms occur.
- Inform women of childbearing age to notify prescriber if pregnancy occurs.
- Inform mothers that breastfeeding is not recommended.

naloxegol oxalate
Movantik

Class and Category

Pharmacologic class: Opioid receptor antagonist
Therapeutic class: Opioid antagonist of gastrointestinal tract

Indications and Dosages

✻ *To treat opioid-induced constipation in patients with chronic noncancer pain*

TABLETS

Adults. 25 mg once daily.

±**DOSAGE ADJUSTMENT** For patients unable to tolerate naloxegol at the normal dose, patients with renal impairment (creatinine clearance less than 60 ml/min), and patients taking moderate CYP3A4 inhibitor drugs such as diltiazem, erythromycin, or verapamil, dosage reduced to 12.5 mg once daily. If dose is well tolerated in patients with renal impairment, dosage increased to 25 mg once daily.

Drug Administration

P.O.

- Administer drug on an empty stomach at least 1 hour prior to the first meal of the day or 2 hours after the meal.
- Do not administer with grapefruit juice.
- Tablet can be crushed to a powder and mixed with 4 ounces of water for patient who is unable to swallow tablet whole. Once mixed, patient must drink mixture immediately. Refill same glass with 4 ounces of water, stir, and have patient drink contents again.

N
O

- Drug may be administered through a nasogastric tube. Flush tube with 30 ml of water using a 60-ml syringe. Crush tablet to a powder in a container and mix with 60 ml of water. Draw up mixture using the 60-ml syringe and administer contents through the nasogastric tube. Add about 60 ml of water to same container used to prepare the dose. Draw up the water using the same 60-ml syringe and use all the water to flush the nasogastric tube and any remaining drug from the nasogastric tube into the stomach.

Route	Onset	Peak	Duration
P.O.	6–12 hr	2–3 hr	Unknown

Half-life: 6–11 hr

Mechanism of Action

Functions as a peripherally acting mu-opioid receptor antagonist in tissues such as the gastrointestinal tract, thereby decreasing the constipating effects of opioids.

Contraindications

Concomitant therapy with strong CYP3A4 inhibitors such as clarithromycin and ketoconazole, gastrointestinal obstruction or risk of recurrent obstruction due to potential for gastrointestinal perforation, hypersensitivity to naloxegol or its components

Interactions

DRUGS

CYP3A4 inducers such as carbamazepine, rifampin, St. John's wort: Decreased plasma naloxegol levels and effectiveness
CYP3A4 inhibitors such as clarithromycin, diltiazem, erythromycin, itraconazole, ketoconazole, verapamil: Increased plasma naloxegol levels, possibly increasing risk of adverse reactions including opioid withdrawal
other opioid antagonists: Potential for additive effects and increased risk of opioid withdrawal

FOOD

grapefruit, grapefruit juice: Increased plasma naloxegol levels

Adverse Reactions

CNS: Headache
GI: Abdominal pain (may become severe), diarrhea, flatulence, **GI perforation**, nausea, vomiting

SKIN: Diaphoresis, rash, urticaria
Other: **Angioedema**, opioid withdrawal

Childbearing Considerations

PREGNANCY

- Drug may cause fetal harm.
- Prolonged use of drug during pregnancy can result in neonatal opioid withdrawal syndrome (NOWS), which may be life-threatening if not recognized and treated.
- Avoid prolonged use during pregnancy. Use with caution only if benefit to mother outweighs potential risk to fetus.

LACTATION

- It is not known if drug is present in breast milk.
- Drug is not recommended for use in a mother who is breastfeeding.

Nursing Considerations

- Expect all maintenance laxative therapy to be discontinued prior to patient starting naloxegol therapy but know that laxatives may be given, as ordered and if needed, after 3 days of naloxegol therapy.
- Monitor patient for the development of persistent, severe, or worsening abdominal pain and/or diarrhea because gastrointestinal perforation has occurred with use of naloxegol. Symptoms generally occur within a few days of starting naloxegol therapy. If this type of abdominal pain occurs, withhold drug and notify prescriber. Know that drug may be restarted at a lower dose (12.5 mg daily), once symptoms have resolved and if drug is still needed.
- Monitor patient's reaction to naloxegol therapy, especially in patients who have taken opioids for at least 4 weeks prior to starting naloxegol, because sustained exposure to opioids may cause an increased response to naloxegol.
- Monitor patient for opioid withdrawal symptoms such as abdominal pain, anxiety, chills, diaphoresis, diarrhea, irritability, and yawning. Clusters of these symptoms may occur with naloxegol therapy, especially if patient is receiving methadone or has a disruption in opioid therapy.
- Know that if opioid therapy is discontinued, naloxegol therapy should be discontinued.

PATIENT TEACHING

- Tell patient to stop all maintenance laxative therapy prior to starting naloxegol therapy. Reassure him that laxatives may be used, if needed, after the first 3 days of therapy.
- Instruct patient to take naloxegol at least 1 hour prior to the first meal of the day or 2 hours after the meal.
- Tell patient who is unable to swallow tablet whole to crush it to a fine powder, mix it with 4 ounces of water and drink the mixture immediately. To ensure that all the drug has been ingested, have patient refill the same glass with 4 ounces of water again, stir, and drink entire content.
- Teach caregiver how to administer drug via a nasogastric tube, if necessary.
- Remind patient not to consume grapefruit or grapefruit juice while taking naloxegol.
- Tell patient to notify prescriber if opioid therapy is discontinued.
- Advise patient to inform prescriber of all medications being taken, including over-the-counter drugs and any new drug therapy begun once naloxegol therapy begins.
- Instruct patient to stop drug and seek medical attention promptly if he develops persistent, severe, or worsening abdominal pain and/or diarrhea. Tell patient symptoms may occur a few days after starting treatment.
- Warn patient that opioid withdrawal symptoms may occur while taking naloxegol and to notify prescriber.
- Caution female patients of childbearing age to notify prescriber immediately if pregnancy is suspected or has occurred.
- Advise females who might wish to breastfeed their infants not to do so.

naloxone hydrochloride

Kloxxado, Narcan, Zimhi

◢ Class and Category

Pharmacologic class: Opioid antagonist
Therapeutic class: Antidote

◢ Indications and Dosages

✳ *To treat known or suspected opioid overdose*

I.V., I.M., OR SUBCUTANEOUS INJECTION (NARCAN)

Adults. 0.4 to 2 mg repeated every 2 to 3 min, as needed. If no response after 10 mg, patient may not have opioid-induced respiratory depression.

Neonates and children. 0.01 mg/kg as a single dose I.V.; if no improvement, 0.1 mg/kg given I.V. as a second dose. If I.V. route is not available, drug may be given as an I.M. or subcutaneous injection in divided doses.

NASAL SPRAY (NARCAN)

Adults and children. 2 mg (1 spray) to 4 mg (2 sprays) repeated every 2 to 3 min, as needed, alternating nostrils with each dose.

NASAL SPRAY (KLOXXADO)

Adults and children. 8 mg (1 spray) repeated every 2 to 3 min, as needed, alternating nostrils with each dose.

I.M. OR SUBCUTANEOUS INJECTION (ZIMHI)

Adults and children. 5 mg/0.5 ml repeated every 2 to 3 min, as needed, until emergency medical assistance is available.

✳ *To treat postoperative opioid-induced respiratory depression*

I.V. INJECTION (NARCAN)

Adults. *Initial:* 0.1 to 0.2 mg every 2 to 3 min until desired response occurs. Additional doses given every 1 to 2 hr, if needed, based on patient response.

Children. *Initial:* 0.005 to 0.01 mg every 2 to 3 min until desired response occurs. Additional doses given every 1 to 2 hr, as needed, based on patient response.

✳ *To reverse opioid-induced depression*

I.V., I.M., OR SUBCUTANEOUS INJECTION (NARCAN)

Neonates. *Initial:* 0.01 mg/kg every 2 to 3 min until desired response occurs. Additional doses given every 1 to 2 hr, if needed, based on patient response.

✳ *As adjunct to treat hypotension caused by septic shock*

I.V. INFUSION OR INJECTION (NARCAN)

Adults. Highly individualized.

◢ Drug Administration

- Keep resuscitation equipment readily available during drug administration.
- Administer parenteral drug by I.V. route whenever possible.

N O

≣ Narcan

I.V.

- For I.V. infusion, dilute 2 mg of drug in 500 ml of 0.9% Sodium Chloride Injection or 5% Dextrose solution to provide a concentration of 0.004 mg/ml. Infuse at a rate titrated to patient's response.
- Discard any unused diluted solution after 24 hours.
- *Incompatibilities:* Preparations containing bisulfite, metabisulfite, long-chain or high molecular weight anions; solutions with an alkaline pH; other drugs

I.M.

- Inject undiluted into large muscle of arm, buttocks, or thigh.
- If more than one dose is needed, rotate sites.

SUBCUTANEOUS

- Inject undiluted into subcutaneous tissue.
- If more than one dose is needed, rotate sites.

≣ Zimhi

I.M. AND SUBCUTANEOUS

- Keep in outer case provided to protect from light until ready to use.
- Inspect solution in viewing window of device. If discolored yellow, brown color, cloudy, or contains particles, discard device and obtain a new one.
- Device is meant for single use only; do not attempt to reuse.
- Administer into anterolateral aspect of thigh after placing patient in the supine position. May be injected through clothing, if needed.
- Immediately after injection, using one hand slide the safety guard over the needle. Then place patient in the lateral recumbent position.

≣ Kloxxado, Narcan

NASAL SPRAY

- Each nasal spray contains a single dose and cannot be reused.
- Place patient in supine position to administer, making sure device nozzle is inserted in either of patient's nostrils. Provide support to the back of patient's neck to allow the head to tilt back.
- Do not prime or test the device prior to administration. Press firmly on the device plunger to administer the dose. Remove the device nozzle from patient's nostril after use and turn patient on side.

- If repeat doses are needed, alternate nostrils, using a new container each time.

Route	Onset	Peak	Duration
I.V.	1–2 min	5–15 min	45–60 min
I.M., SubQ	2–5 min	5–15 min	1–2 hr
Intranasal	8–13 min	20–30 min	30–120 min

Half-life: 30–90 min; 2 hr (intranasal)

≣ Mechanism of Action

Briefly and competitively antagonizes mu, kappa, and sigma receptors in the CNS, thus reversing analgesia, hypotension, respiratory depression, and sedation caused by most opioids. Mu receptors are responsible for analgesia, euphoria, miosis, and respiratory depression. Kappa receptors are responsible for analgesia and sedation. Sigma receptors control dysphoria and other delusional states.

≣ Contraindications

Hypersensitivity to naloxone or its components

≣ Interactions

DRUGS

naloxegol: Possibly increased risk of opioid withdrawal

≣ Adverse Reactions

CNS: Excitement, headache, irritability, nervousness, restlessness, **seizures**, tremor, violent behavior
CV: Cardiac arrest, hypotension, severe hypertension, ventricular fibrillation, ventricular tachycardia
EENT: Nasal congestion, dryness, edema, inflammation, or pain (spray form); toothache
GI: Constipation, nausea, vomiting
MS: Muscle spasms, musculoskeletal pain
RESP: Dyspnea, **pulmonary edema**
SKIN: Diaphoresis, xeroderma
Other: Withdrawal symptoms

≣ Childbearing Considerations

PREGNANCY

- Drug may cause fetal harm.
- Drug crosses the placental barrier and may precipitate withdrawal (maybe severe) in the fetus, as well as in the opioid-dependent mother.
- Monitor fetus for signs of distress after drug is given and until fetus and mother are stable.

LACTATION

- It is not known if drug is present in breast milk.
- Patient should check with prescriber before breastfeeding following drug administration.

≡ Nursing Considerations

- Anticipate that rapid reversal of opioid effects can cause diaphoresis, nausea, and vomiting in addition to serious adverse effects such as hypotension, pulmonary edema, seizures, and ventricular arrhythmias. Monitor patient closely, especially patients at risk because of the presence of preexisting cardiovascular disorders or who are receiving drugs that cause similar adverse cardiovascular effects.

! WARNING Watch for opioid withdrawal symptoms, especially when giving naloxone to opioid-dependent patient. Symptoms may include abdominal cramps, anorexia, anxiety, backache, bone or joint pain, confusion, depression, diaphoresis, dysphoria, erythema, fear, fever, irritability, labile blood pressure and pulse, lacrimation, muscle spasms, myalgia, mydriasis, nasal congestion, nausea, opioid craving, piloerection, restlessness, rhinorrhea, sensation of crawling skin, sleep disturbances, tremor, uneasiness, vomiting, and yawning.

- Monitor patients in postoperative setting who have received naloxone because abrupt postoperative reversal of opioid depression after using naloxone may cause serious adverse effects. Excessive doses of naloxone in the postoperative setting have also caused significant reversal of analgesia and have caused patient to become agitated.
- Expect patient with hepatic or renal dysfunction to have increased circulating blood naloxone level.

PATIENT TEACHING

- Inform patient or family that naloxone will reverse opioid-induced adverse reactions. Instruct them on the signs and symptoms of an opioid overdose such as inability to wake up and severe breathing problems.
- Instruct family or caregiver on how to administer naloxone by nasal spray (Kloxxado, Narcan) or via an injection (Zimhi). Alert family using Zimhi

injectable form that drug should only be administered by individuals who are 12 years and older.
- Stress importance of calling 911 immediately after administration. Instruct family/caregiver to repeat dosage every 2 to 3 minutes if patient does not respond until emergency medical personnel arrive. Remind family or caregiver that each dose requires the use of a new device.
- Urge opioid-dependent patient to seek drug rehabilitation.

naltrexone
Vivitrol

naltrexone hydrochloride
Revia (CAN)

≡ Class and Category

Pharmacologic class: Opioid antagonist
Therapeutic class: Opioid and alcohol blocker

≡ Indications and Dosages

✴ *To provide blockade of the effects of exogenously administered opioids*

TABLETS

Adults. *Initial:* 25 mg, and if no withdrawal symptoms occur, dosage increased following day to 50 mg and then 50 mg given once daily thereafter. Alternatively, 50 mg every weekday with 100-mg dose on Saturday, 100 mg every other day, or 150 mg every third day.

✴ *To prevent relapse to opioid dependence following opioid detoxification*

I.M. INJECTION (VIVITROL)

Adults. 380 mg every 4 wk or once monthly.

✴ *As adjunct to treat alcoholism*

TABLETS

Adults. 50 mg daily for 12 wk.

I.M. INJECTION (VIVITROL)

Adults. 380 mg every 4 wk or once monthly.

≡ Drug Administration

- Don't administer drug to patients who have not been free of opioids for at least 7 days.
- A naloxone challenge test may have to be done before drug therapy begins.

P.O.
- Give drug with antacids or food to decrease adverse GI reactions.

I.M.
- If drug is stored in refrigerator, allow it to warm up to room temperature before administering.
- Dilute using only diluent supplied in carton. Don't substitute any components for components in carton.
- Inject into the gluteal muscle using only needle supplied in carton.
- Rotate sites using other gluteal muscle for next injection.
- Store entire dose pack in refrigerator; unrefrigerated drug can be stored at room temperature for no more than 7 days.
- Avoid administering as a subcutaneous injection because of increased risk of severe injection-site reactions.
- Never give drug intravenously or subcutaneously.
- Inspect injection site for reactions. Report any such findings to prescriber because abscesses and site necrosis may occur and may require surgical intervention.

Route	Onset	Peak	Duration
P.O.	15–30 min	1 hr	24–72 hr
I.M.	Unknown	2 hr	Unknown

Half-life: 12–17 hr

Mechanism of Action

Displaces opioid agonists from—or blocks them from binding with—delta, kappa, and mu receptors. Opioid receptor blockade reverses the euphoric effect of opioids. Naltrexone also inhibits the effects of endogenous opioids, thus reducing alcohol craving.

Contraindications

Acute opioid withdrawal, concurrent therapy with opioid analgesics; dependency on opioids, including those currently maintained on opiate agonists (methadone) or partial agonists (buprenorphine); failure of the naloxone challenge test or has a positive urine screen for opioids; hypersensitivity to naltrexone or its components

Interactions

DRUGS
disulfiram: Increased risk of hepatoxicity

opioid analgesics: Reversal of analgesic and adverse effects of these drugs, possibly withdrawal symptoms in opioid-dependent patients
thioridazine: Increased lethargy and somnolence

Adverse Reactions

CNS: Abnormal thinking, agitation, anxiety, asthenia, chills, confusion, depression, dizziness, euphoria, fatigue, fever, hallucinations, headache, hyperkinesia, insomnia, irritability, malaise, nervousness, restlessness, somnolence, **suicidal ideation**, syncope, tremor
CV: Chest pain, edema, hypertension, palpitations, tachycardia
EENT: Blurred vision, burning eyes, conjunctivitis, dry mouth, eyelid swelling, hoarseness, pharyngitis, rhinitis, sneezing, tinnitus, vision abnormalities
ENDO: Hot flashes
GI: Abdominal cramps, anorexia, constipation, diarrhea, elevated liver enzymes, GI ulceration, **hepatotoxicity** (excessive doses), nausea, vomiting
GU: Difficult ejaculation, urinary frequency
HEME: **Idiopathic thrombocytopenic purpura**
MS: Arthralgia, back pain or stiffness, joint stiffness, muscle cramps, myalgia
RESP: Cough, dyspnea, **eosinophilic pneumonia**, upper respiratory tract infection
SKIN: Increased sweating, pruritus, rash
Other: **Anaphylaxis**; injection-site reactions, such as bruising, erythema, induration, pain, tenderness; thirst

Childbearing Considerations

PREGNANCY
- It is not known if drug causes fetal harm.
- Use with caution only if benefit to mother outweighs potential risk to fetus.

LACTATION
- Drug is present in breast milk.
- Patient should check with prescriber before breastfeeding.

Nursing Considerations

- Use naltrexone cautiously in patients with hemophilia, severe hepatic failure, severe renal impairment, or thrombocytopenia.
- Prepare patient for naloxone challenge test if there are any doubts about patient's abstinence of 7 to 10 days.

- Be aware that patients who receive naltrexone and need pain management are more likely to have longer, deeper respiratory depression and histamine-release reactions (such as bronchoconstriction, facial swelling, generalized erythema, and itching) if given an opioid analgesic. Expect alternative analgesics to be used, such as conscious sedation with a benzodiazepine, general anesthesia, nonopioid analgesics, or regional anesthesia. If an opioid analgesic must be used, monitor patient closely.
- Watch patient closely for suicidal tendencies throughout naltrexone therapy.
- Anticipate that some patients may need treatment for up to 1 year.
- Be aware that after opioid detoxification, patients may have lowered tolerance to opioids that could result in life-threatening circulatory collapse or respiratory compromise if patient uses previously tolerated doses of opioids.

PATIENT TEACHING

! **WARNING** Caution patient against taking opioids during naltrexone therapy or in the future because she'll be more sensitive to them. In fact, strongly warn patient that taking large doses of heroin or any other opioid (including LAAM or methadone) while taking naltrexone could lead to coma, serious injury, or death. Emphasize importance of having access to naloxone for emergency treatment of opioid overdose. Instruct family/caregiver when and how to administer naloxone, if needed.

- Explain that patient may have nausea after first injection but that it is usually mild and subsides within a few days. Most patients don't have nausea with repeat doses.
- Instruct patient to take oral drug with an antacid or food if stomach upset occurs.

! **WARNING** Urge patient to seek immediate emergency help if serious hypersensitivity reactions occur such as difficulty breathing or swallowing.

- Tell patient to report adverse reactions promptly, especially abdominal pain, coughing, dyspnea, jaundice, and wheezing. Also, tell patient to report any injection-site reactions to prescriber, especially if reaction does not improve in 1 month following the injection or worsens, as further treatment may be necessary.
- Caution patient to avoid performing hazardous activities, such as driving, until CNS effects of drug are known.
- Urge family or caregiver to watch patient closely for abnormal behaviors, including suicidal tendencies, even after patient stops taking naltrexone.
- Inform patient that naltrexone doesn't eliminate or diminish alcohol withdrawal symptoms.
- Urge patient to have comprehensive rehabilitation in addition to receiving naltrexone.
- Inform patient about nonopioid treatments for cough, diarrhea, and pain.
- Tell patient while taking drug she may not experience the expected effects from opioid-containing analgesic, antidiarrheal, or antitussive drugs.
- Warn patient that drug may cause liver damage. Tell her to report any signs of liver dysfunction, such as anorexia, digestive problems, or yellowing of skin or whites of her eyes.
- Instruct patient to carry medical identification that lists naltrexone therapy.

naproxen
EC-Naprosyn, Naprosyn

naproxen sodium
Aleve, Anaprox DS, Flanax, Mediproxen, Naprelan, Naprosyn-SR (CAN)

Class and Category
Pharmacologic class: NSAID
Therapeutic class: Analgesic

Indications and Dosages
* *To relieve mild to moderate musculoskeletal inflammation, including ankylosing spondylitis, osteoarthritis, and rheumatoid arthritis*

DELAYED-RELEASE TABLETS, ORAL SUSPENSION, TABLETS (NAPROXEN)
Adults. 250 to 500 mg twice daily. *Maximum:* 1,500 mg daily for limited periods, as prescribed.

DELAYED-RELEASE TABLETS (EC-NAPROSYN)

Adults. 375 or 500 mg twice daily. *Maximum: 1,500 mg daily.*

E.R. TABLETS (NAPROXEN)

Adults. 750 to 1,000 mg daily. *Maximum: 1,500 mg daily.*

TABLETS (NAPROXEN SODIUM)

Adults. 275 to 550 mg twice daily. *Maximum: 1,650 mg daily for limited periods, as prescribed.*

SUPPOSITORIES (NAPROXEN SODIUM)

Adults. 500 mg in addition to P.O. administration. *Maximum: 1,500 mg daily (P.O. and suppository combined).*

✳ *To relieve symptoms of juvenile rheumatoid arthritis and other inflammatory conditions in children*

ORAL SUSPENSION

Children age 2 and older. 10 mg/kg daily in divided doses twice daily.

✳ *To relieve symptoms of acute gouty arthritis*

ORAL SUSPENSION, TABLETS (NAPROXEN)

Adults. *Initial:* 750 mg, then 250 mg every 8 hr until symptoms subside.

TABLETS (NAPROXEN SODIUM)

Adults. *Initial:* 825 mg, then 275 mg every 8 hr until symptoms subside.

✳ *To relieve mild to moderate pain, including acute tendinitis and bursitis, arthralgia, dysmenorrhea, and myalgia*

ORAL SUSPENSION, TABLETS (NAPROXEN)

Adults. *Initial:* 500 mg, then 250 mg every 6 to 8 hr, as needed. *Maximum: 1,250 mg daily.*

TABLETS (NAPROXEN SODIUM)

Adults. *Initial:* 550 mg followed by 550 mg every 12 hr. Alternatively, 275 mg every 6 to 8 hr, as needed. *Maximum: 1,375 mg for initial total daily dose; subsequent days total daily dose should not exceed 1,100 mg.*

✳ *To relieve fever and mild to moderate musculoskeletal inflammation or pain*

CAPLET, CAPSULES, TABLETS (OTC NAPROXEN SODIUM)

Adults and adolescents. 220 mg every 8 to 12 hr; or 440 and 220 mg 12 hr later. *Maximum: 660 mg daily for 10 days unless directed otherwise.*

± **DOSAGE ADJUSTMENT** For patients over age 65, 220 mg every 12 hr. *Maximum: 440 mg for 10 days unless directed otherwise.*

☰ Drug Administration

P.O.

- Delayed-release, extended-release, and film-coated tablets should be swallowed whole and not broken, chewed, or crushed.
- Administer drug with food and a full glass of water to reduce GI distress.
- Have patient remain upright for 15 to 30 minutes after administration of tablet to prevent drug from lodging in esophagus and causing irritation.
- Shake suspension well before administering.
- Use a calibrated device to measure dosage.

P.R.

- If too soft to administer, place suppository in refrigerator for 30 minutes or run under cold water before removing wrap.
- Administer at bedtime in conjunction with daytime dosage.

Route	Onset	Peak	Duration
P.O.	30–60 min	2–4 hr	< 12 hr
P.O./D.R./ E.R.	30–60 min	2–12 hr	< 12 hr
P.R.	Unknown	Unknown	Unknown

Half-life: 12–17 hr

☰ Mechanism of Action

Blocks cyclooxygenase, the enzyme needed to synthesize prostaglandins, which mediate the inflammatory response and cause local pain, swelling, and vasodilation. Thus, naproxen, an NSAID, reduces symptoms of inflammation and relieves pain. Antipyretic action probably stems from effects on the hypothalamus, which increases peripheral blood flow, causing vasodilation and heat dissipation.

☰ Contraindications

History of asthma, urticaria, or other allergic-type reactions induced by aspirin or other NSAIDs; hypersensitivity to naproxen or its components; postoperatively for pain management after coronary artery bypass graft (CABG) surgery

☰ Interactions

DRUGS

angiotensin converting enzyme (ACE) inhibitors, angiotensin receptor blockers

(ARBs): Decreased antihypertensive effects; increased risk of renal dysfunction, especially in the elderly and those with impaired renal function or volume depletion

aluminum hydroxide or magnesium oxide antacids, cholestyramine, sucralfate: Possibly delayed absorption of naproxen

anticoagulants, antiplatelets, selective serotonin reuptake inhibitors, serotonin–norepinephrine reuptake inhibitors: Prolonged PT, increased risk of bleeding

aspirin: Decreased aspirin effectiveness with its antiplatelet effect taken to protect against CVA or MI; increased risk of GI adverse reactions compared to use of NSAID alone

beta-blockers: Decreased antihypertensive effects of these drugs

cyclosporine: Increased risk of nephrotoxicity

digoxin: Increased blood digoxin level and risk of digitalis toxicity

diuretics: Decreased diuretic effectiveness

lithium: Increased risk of lithium toxicity

methotrexate: Increased risk of methotrexate toxicity

other albumin-bound drugs: Increased risk of interference with binding requiring dosage changes of these drugs

other NSAIDs, salicylates: Increased risk of GI toxicity

pemetrexed: Increased risk of pemetrexed-associated GI and renal toxicity, myelosuppression

probenecid: Increased risk of naproxen toxicity

ACTIVITIES

alcohol use, smoking: Increased risk of naproxen-induced GI ulceration

Adverse Reactions

CNS: **Aseptic meningitis**, chills, cognitive impairment, **CVA**, decreased concentration, depression, dizziness, dream disturbances, drowsiness, fever, headache, insomnia, light-headedness, malaise, **seizures**, vertigo

CV: Edema, **heart failure**, hypertension, **MI**, palpitations, tachycardia, vasculitis

EENT: **Papilledema**, papillitis, retrobulbar optic neuritis, stomatitis, tinnitus, vision or hearing changes

ENDO: Hyperglycemia, **hypoglycemia**

GI: Abdominal pain, anorexia, colitis, constipation, diarrhea, diverticulitis, dyspepsia, dysphagia, elevated liver enzymes, esophagitis, flatulence, gastritis, gastroenteritis, gastroesophageal reflux disease, **GI bleeding** and ulceration, heartburn, hematemesis, **hepatitis**, indigestion, **melena**, nausea, **pancreatitis**, **perforation of intestines or stomach**, vomiting

GU: Elevated serum creatinine level, **glomerulonephritis**, hematuria, infertility (in women), interstitial nephritis, menstrual irregularities, **nephrotic syndrome**, **renal failure**, **renal papillary necrosis**

HEME: **Agranulocytosis**, anemia, **aplastic anemia**, eosinophilia, **granulocytopenia**, **hemolytic anemia**, **leukopenia**, **neutropenia**, **pancytopenia**, **thrombocytopenia**

MS: Muscle weakness, myalgia

RESP: Asthma, dyspnea, **eosinophilic pneumonitis**, **respiratory depression**

SKIN: Alopecia, diaphoresis, ecchymosis, **erythema multiforme**, photosensitivity, pruritus, pseudoporphyria, purpura, rash, **Stevens–Johnson syndrome**, **toxic epidermal necrolysis**, urticaria

Other: **Anaphylaxis**, angioedema, **drug reaction with eosinophilia and systemic symptoms (DRESS)**, hyperkalemia, systemic lupus erythematosus

Childbearing Considerations

PREGNANCY

- Drug increases risk of premature closure of the fetal ductus arteriosus if given during the third trimester of pregnancy.
- Drug can cause fetal renal dysfunction leading to oligohydramnios and possibly neonatal renal impairment if given at or after 20 weeks of gestation.
- Drug should be avoided in pregnant women starting at 30 weeks of gestation and onward.
- Drug should only be given, if absolutely needed, using lowest dose and shortest duration possible between 20 and 30 weeks of gestation.

LACTATION

- Drug is present in breast milk.
- Patient should check with prescriber before breastfeeding.

REPRODUCTION

- Drug may delay or prevent rupture of ovarian follicles, which may cause reversible infertility in some women.

N
O

- Drug should not be used in women who have difficulty conceiving or who are undergoing investigation of infertility.

Nursing Considerations

- Be aware that NSAIDs like naproxen should be avoided in patients with a recent MI because risk of reinfarction increases with NSAID therapy. If therapy is unavoidable, monitor patient closely for signs of cardiac ischemia.
- Know that the risk of heart failure increases with use of NSAIDs such as naproxen. NSAIDs should not be used in patients with severe heart failure but, if unavoidable, monitor patient for worsening of heart failure.
- Use naproxen with extreme caution in patients with a history of GI bleeding or ulcer disease because NSAIDs, such as naproxen, increase risk of GI bleeding and ulceration. Expect to use naproxen for the shortest time possible in these patients.
- Be aware that naproxen may decrease benefit of aspirin when taken for a heart attack or stroke.
- Use naproxen cautiously in patients with hypertension, and monitor blood pressure closely. Drug may cause hypertension or worsen it. Because of naproxen's sodium content, watch for fluid retention.
- Use naproxen cautiously in patients with heart failure, hypovolemia, liver dysfunction, renal dysfunction, salt depletion, or patients taking ACE inhibitors or ARBs and diuretics, and the elderly because of increased risk of renal decompensation. Be aware that naproxen is not recommended for patients with advanced renal disease.
- Monitor patient for serious GI tract bleeding, perforation, and ulceration, which may occur without warning symptoms. Elderly patients are at greater risk. To minimize risk, give drug with food. If GI distress occurs, withhold drug and notify prescriber immediately.
- Rehydrate a dehydrated patient before giving drug. If patient has renal disease, monitor renal function closely during therapy.

! **WARNING** Monitor patient closely for thrombotic events, including MI and stroke, because NSAIDs increase the risk, especially if used in higher doses than recommended or for extended periods of time. These events have occurred even in patients who do not have a history or risk factors for cardiovascular disease. Monitor patient for warning signs such as chest pain, slurring of speech, shortness of breath, or weakness. If present, withhold naproxen, alert prescriber immediately, and provide supportive care as prescribed.

- Monitor patient—especially if elderly or receiving long-term naproxen therapy— for less common but serious adverse GI reactions, including anorexia, constipation, diverticulitis, dysphagia, esophagitis, gastritis, gastroenteritis, gastroesophageal reflux disease, hemorrhoids, hiatal hernia, melena, stomatitis, and vomiting.
- Monitor liver enzymes because, in rare cases, elevations may progress to severe hepatic reactions, including fatal hepatitis, hepatic failure, or liver necrosis.
- Monitor BUN and serum creatinine levels in elderly patients, patients taking diuretics or ACE inhibitors, and patients with heart failure, hepatic dysfunction, or impaired renal function; naproxen may cause renal failure.
- Monitor CBC for decreased hemoglobin and hematocrit because drug may worsen anemia.

! **WARNING** Know that if patient has bone marrow suppression or is receiving treatment with an antineoplastic drug, laboratory results (including WBC count) must be monitored; watch for evidence of infection because anti-inflammatory and antipyretic actions of naproxen may mask signs and symptoms, such as fever and pain.

! **WARNING** Assess patient's skin regularly for signs of rash or other hypersensitivity reaction because naproxen is an NSAID and may cause serious skin reactions without warning, even in patients with no history of NSAID sensitivity. At first sign of reaction, stop drug and notify prescriber.

- Assess drug effectiveness in ankylosing spondylitis, as evidenced by decreased morning stiffness, night pain, and pain at rest; in osteoarthritis: decreased joint pain or tenderness and increased ability to perform daily activities, mobility, and range of motion; in rheumatoid arthritis: decreased joint swelling and morning stiffness and increased mobility; in acute gouty arthritis: decreased heat, pain, swelling, and tenderness in affected joints.

- Tell prescriber if patient complains of vision changes; patient may need ophthalmic exam.

PATIENT TEACHING

- Caution patient not to exceed recommended dosage, take for longer than directed, or take for more than 10 days without consulting prescriber because serious adverse reactions, such as a heart attack, heart failure, or stroke, may occur.
- Tell patient to swallow delayed-release or extended-release tablets whole and not to break, chew, or crush them.
- Advise patient to take drug with food to reduce GI distress.
- Tell patient to take drug with a full glass of water and to remain upright for 15 to 30 minutes after taking it to prevent drug from lodging in esophagus and causing irritation.
- Caution patient to avoid hazardous activities until drug's CNS effects are known.
- Urge patient to keep scheduled appointments with prescriber to monitor progress.
- Tell pregnant patient to avoid taking naproxen-containing products late in pregnancy.
- Explain that naproxen may increase risk of serious adverse cardiovascular reactions; urge patient to seek immediate medical attention if signs or symptoms arise, such as chest pain, edema, shortness of breath, slurring of speech, unexplained weight gain, and weakness.
- Inform patient that naproxen may increase risk of serious adverse GI reactions; stress the importance of seeking immediate medical attention for such signs and symptoms as abdominal or epigastric pain, black or tarry stools, indigestion, or vomiting blood or material that looks like coffee grounds.

! **WARNING** Alert patient to allergic reactions and rare but serious skin reactions. Urge her to seek immediate medical attention for blisters, fever, itching, rash, or other indications of hypersensitivity.

- Advise patient to consult prescriber before taking naproxen-containing OTC products if he has asthma, bleeding problems, heart or kidney disease, high blood pressure, or ulcers; a need for diuretic therapy; persistent stomach problems, such as heartburn, stomach pain, or upset stomach; or serious adverse effects from previous use of fever reducers or pain relievers.

naratriptan hydrochloride
Amerge

☰ Class and Category

Pharmacologic class: Selective serotonin 5-HT receptor agonist
Therapeutic class: Antimigraine

☰ Indications and Dosages

✴ *To relieve acute migraine with or without aura*

TABLETS

Adults. 1 or 2.5 mg as a single dose, repeated once in 4 hr, as needed, if headache returns or only partial relief obtained. *Maximum:* 5 mg daily.

±**DOSAGE ADJUSTMENT** For patients with mild to moderate hepatic or renal impairment, initial dose not to exceed 1 mg and maximum dosage reduced to 2.5 mg daily.

☰ Drug Administration

P.O.

- Administer drug as soon as symptoms of a migraine appear.
- Store away from heat and light.

Route	Onset	Peak	Duration
P.O.	1–2 hr	2–3 hr	Unknown

Half-life: 6 hr

☰ Mechanism of Action

Binds to receptors on intracranial blood vessels and sensory nerves in trigeminal-vascular system to stimulate negative feedback, which halts serotonin release. Thus, naratriptan selectively constricts dilated and inflamed cranial vessels in the carotid circulation and inhibits production of proinflammatory neuropeptides to relieve migrainal pain.

N
O

Contraindications

History of basilar or hemiplegic migraine, coronary artery disease, coronary artery vasospasm, stroke, or transient ischemic attack; hypersensitivity to naratriptan or its components; ischemic bowel disease; peripheral vascular disease; recent (within 24 hr) use of another 5-HT1 agonist or an ergotamine-containing drug; severe hepatic or renal impairment; uncontrolled hypertension; Wolff-Parkinson-White syndrome or other cardiac accessory conduction pathway disorders

Interactions

DRUGS

ergot-containing drugs: Possibly additive or prolonged vasospastic reactions
MAO inhibitors, selective serotonin reuptake inhibitors, serotonin–norepinephrine reuptake inhibitors, tricyclic antidepressants, triptans: Increased risk of serotonin syndrome
other selective serotonin 5-HT receptor agonists (including triptans): Possibly additive risk of vasospastic reactions

Adverse Reactions

CNS: Dizziness, drowsiness, fatigue, malaise, paresthesia
CV: Chest heaviness, pain, or pressure; hypertension; **hypertensive crisis**
EENT: Decreased salivation, otitis media, pharyngitis, photophobia, rhinitis, **throat tightness**
GI: Nausea, vomiting
Other: Anaphylaxis, angioedema

Childbearing Considerations

PREGNANCY

- It is not known if drug causes fetal harm.
- Use with caution only if benefit to mother outweighs potential risk to fetus.
- Women with migraine may be at increased risk of preeclampsia during pregnancy.

LACTATION

- It is not known if drug is present in breast milk.
- Patient should check with prescriber before breastfeeding.

Nursing Considerations

! WARNING Know that because naratriptan therapy can cause coronary artery vasospasm, monitor patient with coronary artery disease for signs or symptoms of angina while taking drug. Because naratriptan may also cause peripheral vasospastic reactions, such as ischemic bowel disease, monitor patient for abdominal pain and bloody diarrhea.

- Monitor patient for hypertension during naratriptan therapy even in patients with no history of hypertension because drug can cause significant elevation in blood pressure.
- Be prepared to perform complete neurovascular assessment in any patient who reports an unusual headache or who fails to respond to first dose of naratriptan.

! WARNING Monitor patient closely for serotonin syndrome if she is taking naratriptan along with a selective serotonin reuptake inhibitor or serotonin–norepinephrine reuptake inhibitor. Notify prescriber immediately if the patient exhibits agitation, coma, diarrhea, hallucinations, hyperreflexia, hyperthermia, incoordination, labile blood pressure, nausea, tachycardia, or vomiting because serotonin syndrome can be life-threatening. Provide supportive care.

PATIENT TEACHING

- Inform patient that naratriptan is used to treat acute migraine attacks and that it won't prevent or reduce the number of migraines.
- Instruct patient to take drug at first sign of migraine. Tell patient if she has no relief from initial dose of naratriptan, she should notify prescriber rather than taking another dose in 4 hours; she may need a different drug.
- Advise patient not to take more than maximum prescribed amount of naratriptan during any 24-hour period or to exceed 10 times or more instances of drug use each month. Overuse can cause headaches to become worse or increase frequency of migraine attacks. Tell patient that if she is using naratriptan 10 times or more in a 30-day period she should notify prescriber, as drug may have to be discontinued. Also tell patient that she may need to be treated for withdrawal symptoms upon discontinuation.
- Advise patient to seek reevaluation by prescriber if she has more than four headaches during any 30-day period while taking naratriptan.

- Urge patient to inform all prescribers that she is receiving naratriptan therapy because serious drug interactions may occur.

natalizumab
Tysabri

Class and Category
Pharmacologic class: Monoclonal antibody
Therapeutic class: Immunomodulator

Indications and Dosages
✴ *To treat relapsing forms of multiple sclerosis including active secondary progressive disease, clinically isolated syndrome, and relapsing-remitting disease; to induce and maintain remission in moderately to severely active Crohn's disease with evidence of inflammation in patients who had inadequate response to or are unable to tolerate conventional therapy and inhibitors of tumor necrosis factor alpha*

I.V. INFUSION
Adults. 300 mg every 4 wk.

Drug Administration
I.V.
- Dilute 300 mg/15 ml in 100 ml of 0.9% Sodium Chloride Injection.
- Gently invert solution to mix completely. Do not shake.
- Infuse drug over 1 hour.
- After infusion, flush line with 0.9% Sodium Chloride Injection.
- Do not give drug by I.V. push or bolus injection.
- Refrigerate drug and use within 8 hours if not used immediately.
- *Incompatibilities:* Other drugs, solutions other than 0.9% Sodium Chloride Injection

Route	Onset	Peak	Duration
I.V.	Unknown	Unknown	Unknown

Half-life: 12–20 days

Mechanism of Action
Inhibits migration of leukocytes from vascular space, increasing the number of circulating leukocytes. It does this by binding to integrins on the surface of leukocytes (except neutrophils) and inhibiting adhesion of leukocytes to their counter receptors to help relieve symptoms of Crohn's disease. In multiple sclerosis, lesions probably occur when activated inflammatory cells, including T-lymphocytes, cross the blood–brain barrier.

Contraindications
History of or presence of progressive multifocal leukoencephalopathy, hypersensitivity to natalizumab or its components

Interactions
DRUGS
antineoplastics, immunomodulating agents, immunosuppressants, inhibitors of TNF-α: Increased risk of life-threatening infection

Adverse Reactions
CNS: Depression, dizziness, **encephalitis**, fatigue, headache, **herpes encephalitis**, **meningitis**, **progressive multifocal leukoencephalopathy (PML)**, rigors, somnolence, **suicidal ideation**, vertigo
CV: Chest discomfort, peripheral edema
EENT: Acute retinal necrosis, sinusitis, tonsillitis, tooth infection
GI: Abdominal discomfort, cholelithiasis, diarrhea, elevated liver enzymes, gastroenteritis, **hepatotoxicity**, jaundice, nausea
GU: Amenorrhea; dysmenorrhea; irregular menstruation; ovarian cysts; UTI; urinary frequency, incontinence, or urgency; vaginitis
HEME: **Hemolytic anemia, immune thrombocytopenic purpura, thrombocytopenia**
MS: Arthralgia, back or limb pain, joint swelling, muscle cramp
RESP: Cough, pneumonia or other respiratory tract infection
SKIN: Dermatitis, night sweats, pruritus, rash, urticaria
Other: **Acute hypersensitivity reaction, anaphylaxis**, antibody formation, flu-like illness, herpes, immune reconstitution inflammatory syndrome, opportunistic infections, weight gain or loss

Childbearing Considerations
PREGNANCY
- It is not known if drug causes fetal harm.
- Use with caution only if benefit to mother outweighs potential risk to fetus.

N O

LACTATION

- Drug is present in breast milk.
- Patient should check with prescriber before breastfeeding.

☰ Nursing Considerations

- Make sure patient has enrolled in the TOUCH prescribing program before giving natalizumab. Once patient has signed and initialed the TOUCH program enrollment form, place original signed form in the patient's medical record, send a copy to Biogen Idec, and give a copy to patient.
- Be aware that all atypical and serious opportunistic infections must be reported to Biogen Idec at 1-800-456-2255 and the FDA's MedWatch Program at 1-800-FDA-1088.
- Make sure patient with multiple sclerosis has had an MRI of the brain before starting natalizumab therapy. It will help distinguish evidence of multiple sclerosis from PML symptoms if they occur after therapy starts. Also know that the following three factors increase the risk of PML in patients treated with natalizumab: longer treatment duration, especially beyond 2 years; prior treatment with an immunosuppressant; and the presence of anti-JCV antibodies.
- Observe patient during and for 1 hour after infusion for hypersensitivity reaction, evidenced by chest pain, dizziness, dyspnea, fever, flushing, hypotension, nausea, pruritis, rash, rigors, and urticaria. Reaction is more likely to occur if natalizumab therapy was interrupted. If hypersensitivity reaction occurs, notify prescriber; expect to withhold drug and provide supportive care.

! **WARNING** Monitor patient closely for evidence of PML, a viral brain infection that may be disabling or fatal, because natalizumab increases the risk. Patients at increased risk include those who have received natalizumab for longer than 2 years, have had prior treatment with an immunosuppressant, and who have anti-JCV antibodies. If patient has unexplained neurologic changes, notify prescriber, withhold natalizumab, and prepare patient for a gadolinium-enhanced brain MRI and possible cerebrospinal fluid analysis, as ordered. Be aware that immune reconstitution inflammatory syndrome may occur in patients who develop PML, even when drug has been discontinued. Monitor such patients for evidence of an overwhelming inflammatory response either to an opportunistic infection or the paradoxical symptomatic relapse of a prior infection despite it having been treated successfully in the past.

- Expect that patient will be reevaluated 3 months after first infusion, 6 months after first infusion, and every 6 months thereafter.
- Assess patient for evidence of infection because natalizumab may adversely affect immune system, increasing risk of infection. For example, drug increases the risk for encephalitis and meningitis as well as acute retinal necrosis caused by herpes simplex and varicella zoster viruses that could become life-threatening or result in blindness. Other infections that may occur but are uncommon may include aspergilloma, *Candida* pneumonia, cryptococcal fungemia, or pulmonary mycobacterium avium intracellulare. If infection occurs, expect to obtain appropriate specimens for culture and sensitivity and to treat accordingly. If infection is serious, expect drug to be discontinued.
- Be aware that if patient with Crohn's disease has no therapeutic response after 12 weeks, natalizumab should be discontinued. If patient is on chronic oral corticosteroid therapy, expect tapering of oral corticosteroid dose to begin. If patient can't be tapered off oral corticosteroids within 6 months of starting natalizumab therapy, expect natalizumab to be discontinued. Likewise, if patient needs additional steroid use that extends beyond 3 months in a calendar year to control signs and symptoms of Crohn's disease, expect natalizumab to be discontinued.
- Assess patient's liver function regularly, as ordered, because natalizumab may cause significant liver damage. Expect drug to be discontinued if patient becomes jaundiced or liver enzymes become elevated.
- Monitor patient's platelet counts for thrombocytopenia. If suspected, notify prescriber and expect drug to be discontinued.

- Ensure that when natalizumab is discontinued, patient completes the "Initial Discontinuation Questionnaire" and then has an appointment in 6 months to complete the "6-Month Discontinuation Questionnaire."

PATIENT TEACHING

- Instruct patient on benefits and risks of natalizumab therapy, and provide medication guide for patient to read before therapy begins.
- Encourage patient to ask questions before signing the enrollment form.
- Emphasize need to report any worsening symptoms that persist over several days.
- Tell patient to inform all healthcare providers that he is receiving natalizumab therapy.
- Stress the need to have follow-up visits 3 months after first infusion, 6 months after first infusion, and at least every 6 months thereafter.

! WARNING Instruct patient to report evidence of allergic reaction.

- Instruct patient to avoid people who have infections. Advise him or family members to report confusion, cough, fever, headache, lower-back or side pain, or other unexplained signs and symptoms because they may indicate infection. Also tell patient to report decreased visual acuity or eye pain or redness, as these may be early signs of acute retinal necrosis caused by a herpes virus.
- Alert patient that signs and symptoms suggestive of PML can occur up to 6 months after drug is discontinued and should be reported immediately.
- Advise patient to notify prescriber if any of the following adverse reactions occur: bleeding that is difficult to stop, including from gums, nose, or a cut; easy bruising; heavier menstrual periods than normal; and small, scattered, spots on skin that appear pink, purple, or red.

nateglinide
Starlix

Class and Category
Pharmacologic class: Meglitinide
Therapeutic class: Antidiabetic

Indications and Dosages
* *As adjunct to control blood glucose level in type 2 diabetes mellitus*

TABLETS
Adults. 120 mg three times daily.
± **DOSAGE ADJUSTMENT** Dosage reduced to 60 mg three times daily in patients with near-goal glycemic control.

Drug Administration
P.O.
- Administer within 30 minutes before meals to reduce risk of hypoglycemia.
- Do not administer if a meal is skipped.

Route	Onset	Peak	Duration
P.O.	20 min	1 hr	4 hr

Half-life: 1.5 hr

Contraindications
Hypersensitivity to nateglinide or its components

Interactions
DRUGS
beta-blockers, clonidine, guanethidine, reserpine: Possibly blunted signs and symptoms of hypoglycemia
corticosteroids, phenytoin, rifampin, somatostatin analogues (lanreotide, octreotide), somatropin, St. John's wort, sympathomimetics, thiazide diuretics, thyroid products: Possibly reduced hypoglycemic effects of nateglinide
CYP2C9 substrate poor metabolizers, CYP2C9 inhibitors (amiodarone, fluconazole, sulfinpyrazone), glucomannan, guanethidine, gymnema sylvestre, MAO inhibitors, methandrostenolone and other anabolic hormones, nonselective beta-adrenergic blockers, NSAIDs, salicylates, somatostatin analogues: Possibly additive hypoglycemic effects of nateglinide

ACTIVITIES
alcohol use: Increased risk of hypoglycemia

Adverse Reactions
CNS: Dizziness
ENDO: Hypoglycemia
GI: Cholestatic hepatitis, diarrhea, elevated liver enzymes, jaundice
MS: Arthropathy, back pain
RESP: Bronchitis, cough, upper respiratory tract infection

N
O

Mechanism of Action

Nateglinide stimulates the release of insulin from functioning beta cells of the pancreas. In patients with type 2 diabetes mellitus, a lack of functioning beta cells diminishes blood levels of insulin and causes glucose intolerance. By interacting with the adenosine triphosphatase (ATP)-potassium channel on the beta cell membrane, nateglinide prevents potassium (K^+) from leaving the cell. This causes the beta cell to depolarize and the cell membrane's calcium channel to open. Consequently, calcium (Ca^{++}) moves into the cell and insulin moves out of it. The extent of insulin release is glucose dependent; the lower the glucose level, the less insulin is secreted from the cell.

By promoting insulin secretion in patients with type 2 diabetes mellitus, nateglinide improves glucose tolerance.

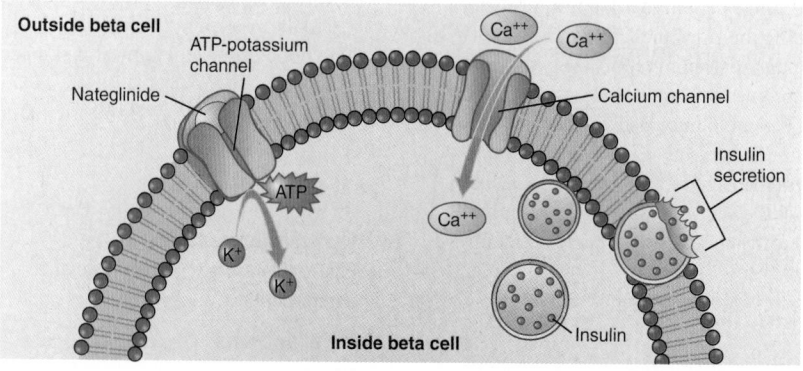

SKIN: Pruritus, rash, urticaria
Other: Flu-like symptoms

Childbearing Considerations

PREGNANCY

- It is not known if drug causes fetal harm.
- Use with caution only if benefit to mother outweighs potential risk to fetus.

LACTATION

- It is not known if drug is present in breast milk.
- A decision should be made to discontinue breastfeeding or the drug to avoid potential serious adverse reactions in the breastfed infant such as hypoglycemia.

Nursing Considerations

- Monitor fasting glucose and HbA_{1c} levels periodically, as ordered, to evaluate treatment effectiveness.
- Monitor patient often in event of fever, infection, surgery, or trauma because transient loss of glucose control may occur, requiring an alteration in therapy.
- Know that patients who are poor metabolizers of CYP2CP substrates are at increased risk of developing hypoglycemia because they may experience an additive hypoglycemic effect from nateglinide therapy.

PATIENT TEACHING

- Instruct patient to take nateglinide within 30 minutes before meals. Advise her to skip scheduled dose if she skips a meal, to reduce the risk of hypoglycemia.
- Teach patient how to measure blood glucose level and how to recognize hyperglycemia and hypoglycemia. Advise her to notify prescriber if blood glucose level is persistently abnormal. Review how to treat hypoglycemia.
- Inform patient that persistent consumption of alcohol, insufficient calorie intake, and strenuous exercise increase risk of hypoglycemia.
- Advise patient to monitor blood glucose level as prescribed and to keep follow-up appointments to monitor HbA_{1c} level because drug may become less effective over time.
- Tell patient to inform all prescribers of nateglinide therapy and not to take any over-the-counter drugs, including herbal preparations, without prescriber's knowledge.

nebivolol hydrochloride

Bystolic

Class and Category

Pharmacologic class: Beta-adrenergic blocker
Therapeutic class: Antihypertensive

Indications and Dosages

＊ *To treat hypertension*

TABLETS

Adults. *Initial:* 5 mg once daily, increased at 2-wk intervals, as needed. *Maximum:* 40 mg once daily.

±**DOSAGE ADJUSTMENT** For patients with moderate hepatic impairment (Child-Pugh Class B) or moderate renal impairment (creatinine clearance less than 30 ml/min), initial dose reduced to 2.5 mg.

Drug Administration

P.O.

- Protect from light.
- Administer at about the same time daily.

Route	Onset	Peak	Duration
P.O.	Unknown	1.5–4 hr	Unknown

Half-life: 12–19 hr

Mechanism of Action

May prevent arterial dilation and inhibit renin secretion, although precise mechanism of action isn't known. Negative chronotropic effects may slow resting heart rate, and negative inotropic effects may reduce cardiac output, myocardial contractility, and myocardial oxygen consumption during exercise or stress. All of these actions may work together to lower systolic and diastolic blood pressure.

Contraindications

Cardiogenic shock, decompensated cardiac failure, heart block greater than first degree, hypersensitivity to nebivolol or its components, sick sinus syndrome (unless permanent pacemaker is in place), severe bradycardia, severe hepatic impairment

Interactions

DRUGS

antiarrhythmics such as beta-blockers, digoxin, disopyramide, selected calcium antagonists such as diltiazem and verapamil: Increased effect on AV conduction and myocardial depression; increased risk of bradycardia
clonidine: Further decrease in blood pressure; possible life-threatening rebound hypertension when clonidine is discontinued
CYP2D6 inhibitors such as fluoxetine, paroxetine, propafenone, quinidine: Increased hypertensive effect of nebivolol
guanethidine, reserpine: Possibly excessive reduction of sympathetic activity with resulting bradycardia or severe hypotension

Adverse Reactions

CNS: Asthenia, dizziness, fatigue, headache, insomnia, paresthesia, somnolence, syncope, vertigo
CV: Allergic vasculitis, **AV block**, **bradycardia**, chest pain, hypercholesterolemia, hyperuricemia, **hypotension**, MI, peripheral edema, peripheral ischemia, Raynaud's phenomenon
ENDO: Hyperglycemia, mask symptoms of **hypoglycemia**
GI: Abdominal pain, diarrhea, elevated bilirubin and liver enzymes, nausea, vomiting
GU: **Acute renal failure**, elevated BUN level, erectile dysfunction
HEME: **Leukopenia, thrombocytopenia**
RESP: **Acute pulmonary edema, bronchospasms,** dyspnea
SKIN: Pruritus, psoriasis, rash, urticaria
Other: **Angioedema** (rare)

Childbearing Considerations

PREGNANCY

- It is not known if drug causes fetal harm.
- Use with caution only if benefit to mother outweighs potential risk to fetus.

LABOR & DELIVERY

- Monitor neonates of mothers who have been treated with drug during the third trimester of pregnancy for bradycardia, hypoglycemia, hypotension, and respiratory depression.

LACTATION

- It is not known if drug is present in breast milk.
- Drug is not recommended for mothers who are breastfeeding because of the potential for serious adverse reactions in breastfed infant, especially bradycardia.

N
O

Nursing Considerations

- Know that patients with bronchospastic disease usually shouldn't be treated with beta-blocker therapy such as nebivolol.
- Use nebivolol cautiously in patients with impaired hepatic or renal function.
- Expect to administer an alpha blocker, as ordered, before starting nebivolol therapy in patients with pheochromocytoma.
- Monitor blood pressure and pulse rate often, especially at start of nebivolol therapy and during dosage adjustments. Also monitor fluid intake and output and daily weight, and watch for evidence of heart failure, such as dyspnea, edema, fatigue, and jugular vein distention. If heart failure occurs or worsens, expect drug to be discontinued.
- Be aware that nebivolol shouldn't be stopped abruptly because MI, myocardial ischemia, severe hypertension, or ventricular arrhythmias may result.
- Expect nebivolol therapy to continue throughout the perioperative period of major surgery. However, monitor patient closely for protracted severe hypotension and difficulty restarting and keeping a heartbeat. Be prepared to administer a beta agonist such as dobutamine or isoproterenol, as ordered, to reverse the effects of nebivolol, if needed.
- Assess distal circulation and peripheral pulses in patient with peripheral vascular disease because drug can worsen it.
- Be aware that nebivolol may mask tachycardia from hyperthyroidism and that abrupt withdrawal can cause thyroid storm. Drug also can decrease blood glucose level, prolong or mask symptoms of hypoglycemia, promote hyperglycemia in patient with diabetes mellitus, or worsen psoriasis.

! **WARNING** Monitor patient closely for hypersensitivity reactions that may occur with beta-blockers, especially patients with a history of severe anaphylactic reactions who may not be responsive to usual doses of epinephrine used to treat allergic reactions.

- Monitor neonates born to mothers treated with beta-blockers such as nebivolol during the third trimester of pregnancy. Watch for bradycardia, hypoglycemia, hypotension, and respiratory depression.

PATIENT TEACHING

- Instruct patient to take nebivolol exactly as prescribed and not to stop using it abruptly.
- Tell patient to weigh herself daily during nebivolol therapy and to notify prescriber if she gains more than 2 lb (0.9 kg) in 1 day or 5 lb (2.3 kg) in 1 week.

! **WARNING** Tell patient that drug may cause an allergic reaction. If serious, tell patient to seek immediate emergency care.

- Advise patient to rise slowly from a lying or seated position to minimize effects of orthostatic hypotension.
- Advise patient to avoid hazardous activities until drug's CNS effects are known.
- Instruct patient to contact prescriber about bleeding or bruising, cough at night, dizziness, edema, rash, shortness of breath, or slow pulse rate.
- Advise diabetic patient to monitor her blood glucose level more often during nebivolol therapy because drug may mask symptoms of hypoglycemia.
- Inform patient with psoriasis that drug may aggravate this condition.

nelfinavir mesylate
Viracept

Class and Category

Pharmacologic class: Protease inhibitor
Therapeutic class: Antiretroviral

Indications and Dosages

* *As adjunct to treat human immunodeficiency virus-1 (HIV-1) infection*

ORAL POWDER, TABLETS

Adults and adolescents. 1,250 mg twice daily or 750 mg three times daily. *Maximum:* 2,500 mg daily.
Children ages 2 years and over. 45 to 55 mg/kg twice daily or 25 to 35 mg/kg three times daily. *Maximum:* 2,500 mg daily.

Drug Administration

P.O.

- Administer drug with food.
- For patients who cannot swallow tablets, tablets may be dissolved or oral solution made from powder may be given instead.

- To dissolve tablets, place in a small amount of water. Once dissolved, the mixture should be stirred well and consumed immediately. Add water to the container the tablets were mixed in and then have the patient swallow the rinse to ensure that the entire dose has been consumed.
- To mix oral powder, use a small amount of formula, milk, dietary supplements, or water. Do not mix with water in its original container. Do not mix with acidic food or juice because result will be a bitter taste. Stir well and administer immediately. If not administered immediately, it can be stored under refrigeration for up to 6 hours.

Route	Onset	Peak	Duration
P.O.	Unknown	2–4 hr	Unknown

Half-life: 3.5–5 hr

Mechanism of Action

Selectively inhibits the virus-specific processing of specific polyproteins in HIV-1-infected cells to prevent formation of mature virions.

Contraindications

Concomitant therapy with drugs highly dependent on CYP3A for clearance and for which elevated plasma concentrations are associated with serious and/or life-threatening events such as alfuzosin, amiodarone, cisapride, dihydroergotamine, ergotamine, lovastatin, lurasidone, methylergonovine, midazolam (oral), pimozide, quinidine, rifampin, St. John's wort, sildenafil (for treatment of pulmonary arterial hypertension), simvastatin, or triazolam; hypersensitivity to nelfinavir or its components

Interactions

DRUGS

atorvastatin, azithromycin, bosentan, colchicine, fluticasone, PDE-5 inhibitors (sildenafil, tadalafil, vardenafil), quetiapine, rosuvastatin: Increased concentration of these drugs, with possible increased effect and risk of adverse reactions
carbamazepine, ethinyl estradiol, norethindrone, phenobarbital, phenytoin: Decreased concentration of these drugs and nelfinavir, interfering with their effectiveness

cyclosporine, sirolimus, tacrolimus: Increased concentrations of these drugs and nelfinavir
delavirdine: Decreased concentrations of delavirdine and its effectiveness and increased concentration of nelfinavir, with possible increased effect and risk of adverse reactions
indinavir, saquinavir: Increased concentration of these drugs and nelfinavir, with possible increased effects and risk of adverse reactions
methadone, nevirapine, omeprazole, ritonavir: Decreased concentration of these drugs and possible reduced effectiveness
rifabutin: Decreased concentration of nelfinavir and effectiveness and increased concentration of rifabutin, with possible increased effects and risk of adverse reactions
salmeterol: Increased risk of cardiovascular adverse events such as palpitations, QT prolongation, and sinus tachycardia
trazodone: Increased concentration of trazodone, with possible increased effect and risk of dizziness, hypotension, nausea, and syncope
warfarin: Possible changes in international normalized ratio (INR) requiring dosage change of warfarin

Adverse Reactions

CNS: Anxiety, asthenia, depression, dizziness, emotional lability, fever, headache, hyperkinesia, insomnia, malaise, migraine, paresthesia, **seizures**, sleep disorder, somnolence, **suicidal ideation**
CV: Edema, hyperlipidemia, **prolonged QT interval, torsades de pointes**
EENT: Acute iritis, eye disorders, mouth ulcers, pharyngitis, rhinitis, sinusitis
ENDO: Fat redistribution, hyperglycemia, **hypoglycemia**
GI: Abdominal pain, anorexia, bilirubinemia, diarrhea, dyspepsia, elevated liver and pancreatic enzymes, epigastric pain, flatulence, **GI bleeding, hepatitis**, jaundice, nausea, **pancreatitis**, vomiting
GU: Kidney calculus, sexual dysfunction, urine abnormality
HEME: Anemia, **leukopenia, neutropenia, thrombocytopenia**
MS: Arthralgia, arthritis, back pain, cramps, elevated creatine kinase, myalgia, myasthenia, myopathy
RESP: **Bronchospasms**, dyspnea

SKIN: Dermatitis including fungal, diaphoresis, folliculitis, maculopapular rash, pruritus, rash, urticaria

Other: **Dehydration**, generalized pain, **hypersensitivity reactions**, hyperuricemia, immune reconstitution syndrome, **metabolic acidosis**

Childbearing Considerations

PREGNANCY

- Pregnancy exposure registry: 1-800-258-4263.
- It is not known if drug causes fetal harm but it is known to cause harm to pregnant women because of potential for hepatic adverse reactions that could lead to hepatic failure.
- Drug should not be used during pregnancy.

LACTATION

- Drug may be present in breast milk.
- The Centers for Disease Control and Prevention recommends that HIV-1 infected mothers not breastfeed to avoid risking postnatal transmission of HIV-1 infection to infants. They also do not recommend breastfeeding because of potential drug-induced adverse reactions in the infant.

REPRODUCTION

- Drug may reduce efficacy of estrogen-based oral contraceptives so women of childbearing age should use an additional or alternative contraceptive measure if taking oral contraceptives containing ethinyl estradiol or norethindrone.

Nursing Considerations

- Monitor patient's blood glucose level, because nelfinavir may cause changes in blood glucose levels. Other drugs in the same class as nelfinavir have caused exacerbation of preexisting diabetes mellitus and new-onset diabetes mellitus, including diabetic ketoacidosis.
- Assess patients who have hemophilia type A or B closely for bleeding, because spontaneous skin hematomas and hemarthrosis have occurred with other protease inhibitors. In some cases, treatment with factor VIII was required.
- Be aware that immune reconstitution syndrome has occurred in patients treated with combination antiretroviral therapy, including nelfinavir. The inflammatory

response predisposes susceptible patients to opportunistic infections such as cytomegalovirus, *Mycobacterium avium* infection, *Pneumocystis jiroveci* pneumonia, or tuberculosis. Autoimmune disorders such as Graves' disease, Guillain–Barré syndrome, or polymyositis have also occurred. Report sudden or unusual adverse reactions to prescriber.

PATIENT TEACHING

- Instruct patient to take drug with food. If patient is unable to swallow tablets, instruct how to dissolve tablet in water or how to mix oral powder form.
- Advise patient to avoid missing doses of nelfinavir. If she misses a dose, she should take it as soon as she remembers but should not double the next dose or take more than prescribed.
- Review signs and symptoms of hyperglycemia and hypoglycemia even if patient is not diabetic. Urge patient to report any such findings to prescriber.
- Warn patients with hemophilia that nelfinavir may increase the risk of bleeding and to seek immediate medical attention if bleeding occurs.
- Inform patient that nelfinavir therapy may cause changes in his body appearance because of fat redistribution. Prepare him for the possibility of developing breast enlargement, central obesity, dorsocervical fat enlargement (buffalo hump), facial wasting, and peripheral wasting.
- Instruct patient to report any persistent, severe, or unusual signs and symptoms.
- Inform women using oral contraceptives that an alternative or additional contraceptive should be used during nelfinavir therapy, because drug may make the oral contraceptive unreliable. Encourage women of childbearing age to report known or suspected pregnancy.
- Alert mothers that breastfeeding is not recommended during nelfinavir therapy.
- Tell patient to report all drugs being taken, including over-the-counter medications and herbals, as serious drug interactions may occur. Advise patient not to begin any new drug therapy without first checking with prescriber.
- Warn male patients who are taking a PDE-5 inhibitor to discuss use with prescriber

before continuing and, if used, to seek immediate medical attention for prolonged penile erection.

- Inform patient that the most common side effect of nelfinavir is diarrhea, which can be controlled with over-the-counter drugs such as loperamide if prescriber so advises.

nevirapine
Viramune, Viramune XR

Class and Category
Pharmacologic class: Non-nucleoside reverse transcriptase inhibitor (NNRTI)
Therapeutic class: Antiretroviral

Indications and Dosages
∗ *As adjunct to treat human immunodeficiency virus (HIV-1) infection*

ORAL SUSPENSION, TABLETS
Adults. 200 mg once a day for 14 days. Maintenance: 200 mg twice daily. Maximum: 200 mg/dose.
Adolescents, children, and infants 15 days old and over. 150 mg/m^2 once a day for 14 days. *Maintenance:* 150 mg/m^2 twice daily. *Maximum:* 200 mg/dose.

E.R. TABLETS
Adults. 400 mg once daily after an initial dose of 200 mg (immediate-release tablets) given for 14 days.
Children age 6 to less than 18 years with a body surface area (BSA) 1.17 m^2 or greater. 400 mg once a day after an initial dose of 150 mg/m^2 (immediate-release tablets) given once a day for 14 days.
Children age 6 to less than 18 years with a BSA 0.84 to 1.16 m^2. 300 mg once a day after an initial dose of 150 mg/m^2 (immediate-release tablets) given once a day for 14 days.
Children age 6 to less than 18 years with a BSA 0.58 to 0.83 m^2. 200 mg once a day after an initial dose of 150 mg/m^2 (immediate-release tablets) given once a day for 14 days.
±**DOSAGE ADJUSTMENT** For patient experiencing a mild to moderate rash without constitutional symptoms during the 14-day lead-in period of 200 mg/day for adults and 150 mg/m^2 for infants and children using immediate-release formulation, maintenance

dosage not increased to twice-daily or extended-release tablets administered until rash is resolved. If rash not resolved after 28 days of taking nevirapine once daily, drug discontinued. For adult patient with end-stage renal disease receiving dialysis, an additional dose of 200 mg immediate-release formulation given following each dialysis session.

Drug Administration
P.O.
- Shake oral suspension container gently prior to measuring dose. Use an oral syringe or dosing cup to measure dosage, especially if volume to be administered is 5 ml or less. If a dosing cup is used, thoroughly rinse the cup with water and have patient drink the rinse.
- Extended-release tablets should be swallowed whole and not chewed, crushed, or divided.

Route	Onset	Peak	Duration
P.O.	Unknown	4 hr	Unknown
P.O./E.R.	Unknown	24 hr	Unknown

Half-life: 25–30 hr

Mechanism of Action
Binds directly to reverse transcriptase and blocks the RNA-dependent and DNA-dependent DNA polymerase activities by causing a disruption of the enzymes' catalytic site.

Contraindications
Hypersensitivity to nevirapine or its components, moderate to severe hepatic impairment, use as part of nonoccupational and occupational postexposure prophylaxis regimens

Interactions
DRUGS
amiodarone, boceprevir, cisapride, clarithromycin, cyclophosphamide, cyclosporine, diltiazem, disopyramide, efavirenz, ergotamine, ethinyl estradiol, fentanyl, ketoconazole, indinavir, itraconazole, lidocaine, lopinavir/ritonavir, nelfinavir, nifedipine, norethindrone, saquinavir/ritonavir, sirolimus, tacrolimus, telaprevir, verapamil: Possible decreased concentration of these drugs with possible decreased effectiveness

N
O

atazanavir/ritonavir, fosamprenavir, fosamprenavir/ritonavir: Decreased concentration with these drugs with possible decreased effectiveness and increased nevirapine concentration with possible risk of prolonged action and adverse reactions
carbamazepine, clonazepam, ethosuximide: Decreased concentrations of these drugs and nevirapine with possible decreased effectiveness
fluconazole: Increased nevirapine concentration with possible increased risk of prolonged action and adverse reactions
methadone: Decreased concentration of methadone, increasing risk of opiate withdrawal
other NNRTI agents such as delavirdine, etravirine, rilpivirine: Possible plasma concentration alteration
rifabutin: Increased concentration of rifabutin with possible risk of prolonged action and adverse reactions
rifampin: Decreased concentration of nevirapine with possible decreased effectiveness
warfarin: Possible increased concentration of warfarin with possible alteration in anticoagulation

Adverse Reactions
CNS: Fatigue, fever, headache, **hepatic encephalopathy**, malaise, paresthesia, somnolence
EENT: Conjunctivitis, oral lesions, ulcerative stomatitis
ENDO: Cushingoid appearance, fat redistribution
GI: Abdominal pain, anorexia, **cholestatic and fulminant hepatitis**, diarrhea, elevated liver enzymes, **hepatic failure or necrosis, hepatotoxicity**, hyperbilirubinemia, jaundice, liver tenderness, nausea, vomiting
GU: Renal dysfunction
HEME: Anemia, **granulocytopenia, leukopenia, neutropenia, prolonged partial thromboplastin time, thrombocytopenia**
MS: Arthralgia, joint and muscle aches, myalgia, **rhabdomyolysis**
SKIN: Blisters, bullous eruptions, pruritus, rash, **Stevens–Johnson syndrome, toxic epidermal necrolysis**, urticaria
Other: **Anaphylaxis, angioedema, drug reaction with eosinophilia and systemic symptoms (DRESS),** drug withdrawal symptoms, flu-like symptoms, **hypophosphatemia,** immune reconstitution syndrome, lymphadenopathy, organ dysfunction

Childbearing Considerations
PREGNANCY
- Pregnancy exposure registry: 1-800-258-4263.
- It is not known if drug causes fetal harm.
- Chronic use of drug can cause severe hepatic dysfunction, including fatalities, in pregnant women receiving nevirapine therapy as part of combination treatment for HIV-1 infection.
- Pregnant women with CD4+ cell counts greater than 250 cells/mm^3 should not be started on the drug.
- Use with extreme caution only if benefit to mother outweighs potential risk to fetus.

LACTATION
- Drug is present in breast milk.
- The Centers for Disease Control and Prevention recommends that HIV-1 infected mothers not breastfeed to avoid risking postnatal transmission of HIV-1 infection to infants. They also do not recommend breastfeeding because of potential drug-induced adverse reactions in the infant.

REPRODUCTION
- Drug may reduce fertility in females of reproductive potential. It is not known if these effects on fertility are reversible.

Nursing Considerations
- Know that nevirapine should never be used as monotherapy, because a resistant virus emerges rapidly.
- Check patient's liver enzymes before initiating nevirapine therapy, as ordered and regularly thereafter.
- Expect to strictly follow the initial 14-day period of once-daily dosing to decrease the incidence of a rash. If a mild to moderate rash develops, know that the 14-day once-daily dosing period should be extended to as long as 28 days total. However, if rash continues to persist after 28 days of therapy, expect drug to be discontinued. Report a severe rash or any rash that is accompanied by other signs and symptoms to prescriber immediately and expect drug to be discontinued.

- Be aware that the oral suspension formulation is not recommended for use initially in adult female patients with a CD4+ cell count greater than 250 cells/mm³ or adult male patients with a CD4+ cell count greater than 400 cells/mm³, because of risk for serious or life-threatening hepatotoxicity.
- Know that if nevirapine therapy is interrupted for more than 7 days, the initial dosage regimen using the immediate-release formulation can be expected to be repeated for the first 14 days.

! **WARNING** Monitor patient closely during the first 18 weeks of therapy to detect potentially life-threatening hepatotoxicity or skin reactions. Know that the greatest risk occurs during the first 6 weeks of therapy; patients at greatest risk include females and those having higher CD4+ cell counts at the initiation of therapy. Women with CD4+ cell count greater than 250 cells/mm³ are at greatest risk. Patients coinfected with hepatitis B or C and/or who have increased transaminase levels at the start of therapy are at a greater risk of symptomatic events that may appear 6 weeks or more after starting nevirapine therapy. However, monitor all patients at all times, as these adverse reactions have also occurred in patients not considered at risk. Monitor patient closely for rash that may be combined with signs and symptoms of hepatitis that may progress to hepatic failure. If patient develops signs and symptoms of hepatitis or presents with increased transaminases accompanied with a rash or systemic symptoms such as blisters, conjunctivitis, facial edema, fatigue, fever, joint or muscle aches, malaise, oral lesions, or renal dysfunction, notify prescriber immediately; check transaminases levels, as ordered; and expect nevirapine to be discontinued.

- Be aware that immune reconstitution syndrome has occurred in patients treated with combination antiretroviral therapy, including nevirapine. The inflammatory response predisposes susceptible patients to opportunistic infections such as cytomegalovirus, *Mycobacterium avium* infection, *Pneumocystis jiroveci* pneumonia, or tuberculosis. Autoimmune disorders such as Graves' disease, Guillain–Barré syndrome, or polymyositis have also occurred. Report sudden or unusual adverse reactions to prescriber.

PATIENT TEACHING

- Advise patient to avoid missing doses of nevirapine. If she misses a dose, she should take it as soon as she remembers, but should not double the next dose or take more than prescribed.
- Tell patient prescribed oral suspension to shake oral suspension container gently prior to measuring dose. Use an oral syringe or dosing cup to measure dosage, especially if volume to be administered is 5 ml or less. If a dosing cup is used, tell patient to thoroughly rinse the cup with water and drink the rinse.

! **WARNING** Inform patient about severe liver disease that may occur with nevirapine. Tell her to report signs and symptoms of liver disease such as acholic stools, anorexia, fatigue, malaise, nausea, tenderness over liver area, or yellowing of skin or whites of the eyes, and to seek immediate medical attention.

- Stress importance of being compliant with tests ordered to screen for adverse effects of nevirapine therapy.

! **WARNING** Advise patient that nevirapine therapy may cause severe hypersensitivity or skin reactions. Tell her to report a rash, especially if it is accompanied by blisters, conjunctivitis, facial edema, fatigue, fever, joint or muscle aches, liver problems, or oral lesions, and to seek immediate medical attention.

- Inform patient that nevirapine therapy may cause changes in her body appearance because of fat redistribution. Prepare her for the possibility of developing breast enlargement, central obesity, dorsocervical fat enlargement (buffalo hump), facial wasting, and peripheral wasting.
- Instruct patient to report any persistent, severe, or unusual signs and symptoms.
- Inform female patients of childbearing age that nevirapine may impair fertility.
- Alert mothers that breastfeeding is not recommended during nevirapine therapy.

N
O

- Tell patient to report all drugs being taken, including over-the-counter medications and herbals, as serious drug interactions may occur. Advise patient not to begin any new drug therapy without first checking with prescriber.

nicardipine hydrochloride

⬚ Class and Category
Pharmacologic class: Calcium channel blocker
Therapeutic class: Antianginal, antihypertensive

⬚ Indications and Dosages
✳ *To manage chronic stable angina pectoris*
CAPSULES
Adults. 20 mg three times daily, increased every 3 days, as needed. *Maintenance:* 20 to 40 mg three times daily.
✳ *To manage hypertension*
CAPSULES
Adults. 20 mg three times daily, increased every 3 days, as needed. *Maintenance:* 20 to 40 mg three times daily.
✳ *To control hypertension when oral therapy is not desirable or feasible*
I.V. INFUSION
Adults. *Initial:* 5 mg/hr; increased by 2.5 mg/hr every 5 to 15 min, as prescribed. *Maximum:* 15 mg/hr.
±**DOSAGE ADJUSTMENT** For patients with impaired liver function, initial dose reduced to 20 mg twice daily with slow titration. For patients with impaired renal function, initial dosage of 20 mg three times daily kept but titration done slower.

⬚ Drug Administration
P.O.
- Capsules should be swallowed whole and not chewed, crushed, or opened.
- May be administered with food, but avoid giving with a high-fat meal or grapefruit juice.
I.V.
- Dilute each 25-mg ampule of nicardipine with 240 ml of 0.45% or 0.9% Sodium Chloride Injection, 5% Dextrose in Water, or 5% Dextrose Injection and either

0.45% or 0.9% Sodium Chloride Injection combined to yield 0.1 mg/ml.
- Mixture is stable at room temperature for 24 hours.
- If using premixed nicardipine, strength must be checked carefully because drug comes as single strength (20 mg nicardipine in 200 ml of solution, providing 0.1 mg/ml) or double strength (40 mg nicardipine in 200 ml of solution, providing 0.2 mg/ml).
- Administer drug through large peripheral veins or central veins.
- Administer continuous infusion with I.V. pump or controller, and adjust according to patient's blood pressure, as prescribed.
- Titrate infusion dosage slowly in patients receiving a beta-blocker and in patients with heart failure or significant left ventricular dysfunction, because of possible negative inotropic effects. Also, patients with renal impairment require a more gradual titration.
- Change peripheral I.V. site every 12 hours, if feasible.
- Give first dose of oral nicardipine 1 hour before stopping I.V. infusion, as ordered.
- Use solution within 24 hours if stored at room temperature.
- *Incompatibilities:* Lactated Ringer's or Sodium Bicarbonate solution through same I.V. line, other drugs

Route	Onset	Peak	Duration
P.O.	0.5–2 hr	0.5–2 hr	< 8 hr
I.V.	10–20 min	45 min	3 hr

Half-life: 8.5 hr

⬚ Mechanism of Action
May slow extracellular calcium movement into myocardial and vascular smooth-muscle cells by deforming calcium channels in cell membranes, inhibiting ion-controlled gating mechanisms, and interfering with calcium release from the sarcoplasmic reticulum. By decreasing the intracellular calcium level, nicardipine inhibits smooth-muscle cell contraction and dilates coronary and systemic arteries. As with other calcium channel blockers, these actions lead to decreased myocardial oxygen requirements and reduced afterload, blood pressure, and peripheral resistance.

Contraindications

Advanced aortic stenosis, hypersensitivity to nicardipine and its components

Interactions

DRUGS

cimetidine: Increased nicardipine bioavailability
cyclosporine: Increased plasma cyclosporine levels
digoxin: Transiently increased blood digoxin level, increased risk of digitalis toxicity
fentanyl: Possibly severe hypotension
tacrolimus: Increased plasma tacrolimus levels

FOODS

grapefruit, grapefruit juice: Possibly increased bioavailability of nicardipine
high-fat meals: Decreased blood nicardipine level

Adverse Reactions

CNS: Anxiety, asthenia, ataxia, confusion, dizziness, drowsiness, headache, nervousness, paresthesia, psychiatric disturbance, syncope, tremor, weakness
CV: **Bradycardia**, chest pain, exacerbation of angina (chronic therapy), **heart failure**, **hypotension**, orthostatic hypotension, palpitations, peripheral edema, tachycardia
EENT: Altered taste, blurred vision, dry mouth, epistaxis, gingival hyperplasia, pharyngitis, rhinitis, tinnitus
ENDO: Gynecomastia, hyperglycemia
GI: Anorexia, constipation, diarrhea, elevated liver enzymes, indigestion, nausea, thirst, vomiting
GU: Dysuria, nocturia, polyuria, sexual dysfunction, urinary frequency
HEME: Anemia, **leukopenia**, **thrombocytopenia**
MS: Joint stiffness, muscle spasms
RESP: Bronchitis, cough, **decreased oxygen saturation**, upper respiratory tract infection
SKIN: Dermatitis, diaphoresis, **erythema multiforme**, flushing, photosensitivity, pruritus, rash, **Stevens–Johnson syndrome**, urticaria
Other: **Hypokalemia**, injection-site irritation, weight gain

Childbearing Considerations

PREGNANCY

- Drug may cause fetal harm such as transient fetal heart rate decelerations and neonatal hypotension when drug is given intravenously.
- Drug may also cause maternal harm causing such adverse reactions as dizziness, flushing, headache, hypotension, nausea, and reflex tachycardia when administered intravenously.
- Use with caution only if benefit to mother outweighs potential risk to fetus.

LABOR & DELIVERY

- Drug may slow or halt labor when given intravenously.
- Drug increases risk for postpartum hemorrhage for mother when given intravenously.

LACTATION

- Drug is present in breast milk.
- Breastfeeding is not recommended by some manufacturers.

Nursing Considerations

- Check blood pressure and pulse rate before nicardipine therapy begins, during dosage changes, and periodically throughout therapy. During prolonged therapy, periodically assess ECG tracings for arrhythmias and other changes.
- Monitor fluid intake and output and daily weight for signs of fluid retention, which may precipitate heart failure. Also assess for signs of heart failure, such as crackles, dyspnea, jugular vein distention, peripheral edema, and weight gain.
- During prolonged therapy, expect to periodically monitor liver and renal function test results. Anticipate drug dosage to be titrated slowly in these patients. Expect elevated liver enzymes to return to normal after drug is discontinued.
- Monitor patient with angina for increases in duration, frequency, or severity of symptoms because with chronic use of oral nicardipine (rarely with I.V. administration), exacerbation of angina may occur.
- Monitor serum potassium level during prolonged therapy. Hypokalemia increases the risk of arrhythmias.
- Monitor patients who take a beta-blocker or have heart failure or significant left ventricular dysfunction because of drug's negative inotropic effect on some patients.

N
O

! **WARNING** Expect to taper dosage gradually before discontinuing drug. Otherwise, angina or dangerously high blood pressure could result.

PATIENT TEACHING

- Urge patient to take nicardipine as prescribed, even if she feels well.
- Advise patient not to take drug within 1 hour of eating a high-fat meal or grapefruit product. Urge her not to alter the amount of grapefruit products in her diet without consulting prescriber.
- Instruct patient to swallow capsules whole and not to chew, crush, or open.

! **WARNING** Caution patient against stopping nicardipine abruptly because angina or dangerously high blood pressure could result.

- Teach patient how to take her pulse, and urge her to notify prescriber immediately if it falls below 50 beats/minute.
- Teach patient how to measure blood pressure, and urge her to do so weekly if drug was prescribed for hypertension. Suggest that she keep a log of blood pressure readings and take it to follow-up visits.
- Advise patient to change position slowly to minimize orthostatic hypotension.
- Urge patient to avoid potentially hazardous activities until drug's CNS effects are known.
- Advise patient to notify prescriber immediately about chest pain that's not relieved by rest or nitroglycerin, constipation, irregular heartbeats, nausea, pronounced dizziness, severe or persistent headache, and swelling of hands or feet.
- Encourage patient to comply with suggested lifestyle changes, such as alcohol moderation, low-fat or low-sodium diet, regular exercise, smoking cessation, stress management, and weight reduction.
- Inform patient that hot tubs, prolonged hot showers, or saunas may cause dizziness or fainting.
- Instruct patient to avoid prolonged sun exposure and to use sunscreen when going outdoors.

nicotine for inhalation
Nicotrol Inhaler

nicotine nasal solution
Nicotrol NS

nicotine polacrilex
Nicorette, Nicorette Plus (CAN)

nicotine transdermal system
Habitrol, NicoDerm CQ, Nicotine Transdermal System Patch Kit, Nicotrol, ProStep

Class and Category
Pharmacologic class: Nicotinic agonist
Therapeutic class: Smoking cessation adjunct

Indications and Dosages
✴ *As adjunct to smoking cessation for the relief of nicotine withdrawal symptoms, including craving*

CHEWING GUM (NICORETTE, NICORETTE PLUS)

Adults. *Initial:* For patient who smokes first cigarette later than 30 min after waking up, 2 mg (1 piece) or for patient who smokes first cigarette within 30 minutes of waking up, 4 mg (1 piece) every 1 to 2 hr, for 1 to 6 wk; then 2 or 4 mg every 2 to 4 hr for 7 to 9 wk; and then 2 or 4 mg every 4 to 8 hr for 10 to 12 wk. *Maximum:* 24 pieces daily for no longer than 12 wk.

NASAL SPRAY (NICOTROL NS)

Adults. 1 to 2 sprays (1 to 2 mg) in each nostril/hr. *Maximum:* 5 mg/hr or 40 mg daily for up to 3 mo.

LOZENGES (NICORETTE)

Adults who smoke first cigarette more than 30 min after waking up. 2 mg (1 lozenge) when needed using at least 9 lozenges daily for 6 wk, then daily amount decreased for remaining 6 wk.

Adults who smoke first cigarette within 30 min after waking up. 4 mg (1 lozenge), when needed using at least 9 lozenges daily for 6 wk, then daily amount decreased for remaining 6 wk. *Maximum:* No more than 1 lozenge at a time, no use of lozenges continuously one after another, no more than 5 lozenges in 6 hr; no more than 20 lozenges daily. Not to be used longer than 12 wk.

ORAL INHALATION (NICOTROL INHALER)

Adults. 6 to 16 cartridges (24 to 64 mg) daily for up to 12 wk with dosage adjustment made according to signs and symptoms of nicotine excess or withdrawal; then dosage gradually reduced over 12 wk or less. *Maximum:* 16 cartridges (64 mg) daily for 6 mo.

TRANSDERMAL PATCH (NICOTROL)

Adults who smoke more than 10 cigarettes a day. 15 mg patch once daily for 6 wk, then 10-mg patch once daily for 2 wk, then 5-mg patch once daily for 2 wk.

Adults who smoke 10 or less cigarettes a day. 10-mg patch once daily for 6 wk, then 5-mg patch once daily for 2 wk.

TRANSDERMAL SYSTEM (HABITROL, NICODERM CQ, NICOTINE TRANSDERMAL SYSTEM PATCH KIT)

Adults who smoke more than 10 cigarettes a day. 21-mg patch daily for wk 1 through 4; 14-mg patch daily for wk 5 & 6; 7-mg patch daily for wk 7 & 8.

Adults who smoke 10 cigarettes or less a day. 14-mg daily for 6 wk followed by 7-mg daily for 2 additional wk.

TRANSDERMAL SYSTEM (PROSTEP)

Adults. *Initial:* 11 to 22 mg daily, adjusted to lower-dose systems over 6 to 12 wk.

±**DOSAGE ADJUSTMENT** For patients with moderate to severe hepatic or renal impairment, dosage may have to be reduced.

Drug Administration

P.O.

- For chewing gum or lozenges, patient must wait at least 15 minutes after drinking coffee, juice, soft drink, tea, or wine before using these forms of drug.
- Gum should be chewed until a tingling sensation or peppery taste occurs and then gum placed in cheek until sensation or taste subsides. Gum then should be moved to a different site until tingling or taste subsides, repeating until there is no longer

a sensation—usually about 30 minutes. Caution against swallowing the gum.
- For lozenges, tell patient to allow lozenge to slowly dissolve and minimize swallowing. The lozenge should not be chewed or swallowed but moved from one side of mouth to the other until it is completely dissolved. It will take about 20 to 30 minutes.

INTRANASAL

- Have patient tilt head back and spray into a nostril. Caution against inhaling, sniffing, or swallowing spray because nicotine is absorbed through nasal and oral mucosa.
- Prolonged use of nasal form may cause dependence.
- Patient should not blow nose for several minutes after administration.

INHALATION

- Direct patient to inhale through device like a cigarette, puffing often for 20 minutes. 6 to 16 cartridges will have to be used daily to prevent or relieve withdrawal symptoms and craving.
- Clean mouthpiece with soap and water, as needed.

TRANSDERMAL

- Open package immediately before use. Apply system to a clean, dry, hairless site on outer arm or upper body. Save pouch for disposal of patch after use.
- After removing backing, press on skin for 10 seconds.
- Don't apply patch to damaged skin.
- Do not apply lotions, moisturizers, or similar products on skin where patch will be applied.
- Change systems and rotate sites every 24 hours.
- Do not use same site for 7 days.
- After removing patch, fold sticky ends together, put in pouch, and discard.
- Wash hands.

Route	Onset	Peak	Duration
P.O.	Unknown	30 min	Unknown
Inhalation	Unknown	<15 min	Unknown
Intranasal	Rapid	10–20 min	Unknown
Transdermal	Unknown	2–8 hr	24 hr

Half-life: 1–4 hr

Mechanism of Action

Binds selectively to nicotinic-cholinergic receptors at autonomic ganglia, in the adrenal medulla, at neuromuscular junctions, and in the brain. By providing a lower dose of nicotine than cigarettes, this drug reduces nicotine craving and withdrawal symptoms.

Contraindications

Hypersensitivity to nicotine or its components, including menthol or soy

Interactions

DRUGS

acetaminophen, adrenergic antagonists (labetalol, prazosin), beta-blockers, imipramine, insulin, oxazepam, pentazocine, theophylline: Possibly increased therapeutic effects of these drugs (chewing gum, nasal spray, transdermal system)
adrenergic agonists (isoproterenol): Decreased effectiveness of these drugs
tricyclic antidepressants: Possibly altered pharmacologic actions of these drugs (oral inhalation)

FOODS

acidic beverages (citrus juices, coffee, soft drinks, tea, wine): Decreased nicotine absorption from gum if beverages consumed within 15 minutes before or while chewing gum
caffeine: Increased effects of caffeine (chewing gum, nasal spray, transdermal system)

Adverse Reactions

CNS: Dizziness, dream disturbances, drowsiness, headache, irritability, light-headedness, nervousness (chewing gum, transdermal system); amnesia, confusion, difficulty speaking, headache, migraine headache, paresthesia (nasal spray); chills, fever, headache, paresthesia (oral inhalation)
CV: Arrhythmias (all forms); hypertension (chewing gum, transdermal system); peripheral edema (nasal spray)
EENT: Increased salivation, injury to teeth or dental work, mouth injury, oral blistering, pharyngitis, stomatitis (chewing gum); altered taste, dry mouth (chewing gum, transdermal system); altered smell and taste, burning eyes, dry mouth, earache, epistaxis, gum disorders, hoarseness, lacrimation, mouth and tongue swelling, nasal blisters, nasal irritation or ulceration, pharyngitis,

rhinitis, sinus problems, sneezing, vision changes (nasal spray); altered taste, lacrimation, pharyngitis, rhinitis, sinusitis, stomatitis (oral inhalation)
GI: Eructation (chewing gum); abdominal pain, constipation, diarrhea, flatulence, increased appetite, indigestion, nausea, vomiting (chewing gum, transdermal system); abdominal pain, constipation, diarrhea, flatulence, hiccups, indigestion, nausea (nasal spray); diarrhea, flatulence, hiccups, indigestion, nausea, peptic ulcer (transdermal); vomiting (oral inhalation)
GU: Dysmenorrhea (chewing gum, transdermal system); menstrual irregularities (nasal spray)
MS: Jaw and neck pain (chewing gum); arthralgia, myalgia (chewing gum, transdermal system); arthralgia, back pain, myalgia (nasal spray); back pain (oral inhalation)
RESP: Cough (chewing gum, transdermal system); bronchitis, bronchospasm, chest tightness, cough, dyspnea, increased sputum production (nasal spray); chest tightness, cough, dyspnea, wheezing (oral inhalation)
SKIN: Diaphoresis, erythema, pruritus, rash, urticaria (chewing gum, transdermal system); acne, flushing of face, pruritus, purpura, rash (nasal spray); pruritus, rash, urticaria (oral inhalation)
Other: Anaphylaxis, delayed wound healing, flu-like symptoms, generalized pain, physical dependence, hypersensitivity reactions, withdrawal symptoms

Childbearing Considerations

PREGNANCY

- Drug may cause fetal harm.
- Drug use is not recommended during pregnancy.

LACTATION

- Drug is present in breast milk.
- Patient should check with prescriber before breastfeeding.

Nursing Considerations

- Know that drug should be used with caution in patients with hyperthyroidism, insulin-dependent diabetes, or pheochromocytoma because nicotine releases catecholamines from the adrenal medulla, which affects the drug dosing treatment of these disorders.

- Use caution when nicotine is given with patients with active gastric or peptic ulcers or who have esophagitis because nicotine delays healing in ulcer disease.
- Keep in mind to avoid possible burns, remove patch before patient has an MRI.

PATIENT TEACHING

- Instruct patient to read and follow package instructions to obtain best results with nicotine product.
- Advise patient to notify prescriber about other conditions or drugs she takes.
- Emphasize that patient must stop smoking as soon as nicotine treatment starts to avoid toxicity.

! **WARNING** Tell patient to stop taking drug and notify prescriber or seek emergency medical care if she develops an allergic reaction such as difficulty breathing or a rash or experiences an irregular heartbeat or palpitations, or signs of nicotine overdose.

- Instruct patient using chewing gum or lozenges to wait at least 15 minutes after drinking coffee, juice, soft drink, tea, or wine.
- Advise patient to chew gum until she detects a tingling sensation or peppery taste and then to place gum between her cheek and gum until tingling or peppery taste subsides. Then direct her to move gum to a different site until tingling or taste subsides, repeating until she no longer feels the sensation—usually about 30 minutes. Caution against swallowing the gum. Advise her to stop use and contact prescriber if she experiences oral blistering.
- Tell patient to allow lozenge to slowly dissolve. The lozenge should not be chewed or swallowed but moved from one side of mouth to the other until it is completely dissolved. It will take about 20 to 30 minutes.
- Tell patient using nasal spray to tilt her head back and spray into a nostril. Caution against inhaling, sniffing, or swallowing spray, because nicotine is absorbed through nasal and oral mucosa.
- Warn patient that prolonged use of nasal form may cause dependence.
- Tell patient using oral inhalation form to use 6 to 16 cartridges daily to prevent or relieve withdrawal symptoms and craving.

Starting with 1 or 2 cartridges daily yields poor success. Direct patient to inhale through device like a cigarette, puffing often for 20 minutes.

- Tell patient using transdermal system not to open package until just before use, because nicotine is lost in the air. Advise her to apply system to clean, dry, hairless site on upper outer arm or upper body. Instruct her to change systems and rotate sites every 24 hours and not to use the same site for 7 days. To avoid possible burns, advise patient to remove patch before undergoing any MRI procedure.

! **WARNING** Urge patient to keep all unused nicotine forms safely away from children and pets and to discard used forms carefully. (Enough nicotine may remain in used systems to poison children and pets.) Instruct her to contact a poison control center immediately if she suspects that a child has ingested nicotine.

- Explain to patient with asthma or COPD that nicotine may cause bronchospasm.
- Inform patient that it may take several attempts to stop smoking. Urge her to join a smoking cessation program.

nifedipine
Adalat CC, Adalat XL (CAN), Afeditab CR, Procardia, Procardia XL

Class and Category
Pharmacologic class: Calcium channel blocker
Therapeutic class: Antianginal, antihypertensive

Indications and Dosages
* *To manage chronic stable angina, vasospastic angina*

CAPSULES (PROCARDIA)

Adults. *Initial:* 10 mg three times daily, increased over 1 to 2 wk as needed. *Maintenance:* 10 to 20 mg three times daily. *Maximum:* 180 mg daily, 30 mg/dose.

E.R. TABLETS (PROCARDIA XL)

Adults. *Initial:* 30 or 60 mg daily, increased over 7 to 14 days, as needed. *Maximum:* 120 mg daily.

E.R. TABLETS (ADALAT XL)

Adults. *Initial:* 30 mg once daily, increased, as needed, over 7 to 14 days. *Maximum:* 90 mg daily.

✳ *To manage hypertension*

E.R. TABLETS (ADALAT CC, AFEDITAB CR)

Adults. *Initial:* 30 mg daily, increased, as needed, over 7 to 14 days. *Maintenance:* 30 to 60 mg daily. *Maximum:* 90 mg daily.

E.R. TABLETS (ADALAT XL)

Adults. *Initial:* 20 or 30 daily, increased over 7 to 14 days, as needed. *Maintenance:* 30 to 60 mg daily. *Maximum:* 90 mg daily.

E.R. TABLETS (PROCARDIA XL)

Adults. 30 or 60 mg daily, increased over 7 to 14 days, as needed. *Maximum:* 120 mg daily.

±**DOSAGE ADJUSTMENT** Dosage may be reduced for elderly patients and those with heart failure or impaired hepatic or renal function.

Drug Administration

P.O.

- Extended-release tablets should be swallowed whole and not chewed, crushed, or opened.
- Administer Adalat CC brand of extended-release tablets on an empty stomach; other brands should not be administered within 1 hour of a high-fat meal.
- Do not administer with grapefruit juice.

Route	Onset	Peak	Duration
P.O.	30–60 min	30–120 min	8 hr
P.O./E.R.	20 min	6 hr	24 hr
Half-life: 2–7 hr			

Mechanism of Action

May slow movement of calcium into myocardial and vascular smooth-muscle cells by deforming calcium channels in cell membranes, inhibiting ion-controlled gating mechanisms, and disrupting calcium release from sarcoplasmic reticulum. Decreasing intracellular calcium level inhibits smooth-muscle cell contraction and dilates arteries, which decreases myocardial oxygen demand, peripheral resistance, blood pressure, and afterload.

Contraindications

Hypersensitivity to nifedipine or its components

Interactions

DRUGS

cimetidine, clarithromycin, erythromycin, fentanyl, fluconazole, fluoxetine, indinavir, itraconazole, nefazodone, nelfinavir, saquinavir: Increased risk of hypotension
beta-blockers: Increased risk of profound hypotension, heart failure, and worsening of angina
digoxin: Transiently increased blood digoxin level, increased risk of digitalis toxicity
oral anticoagulants: Possibly increased prothrombin time
phenytoin: Decreased systemic exposure of nifedipine
quinidine: Possibly decreased plasma quinidine level

FOODS

grapefruit, grapefruit juice: Possibly increased bioavailability of nifedipine

Adverse Reactions

CNS: Anxiety, ataxia, confusion, dizziness, drowsiness, headache, nervousness (possibly extreme), nightmares, paresthesia, psychiatric disturbance, syncope, tremor, weakness
CV: **Bradycardia**, chest pain, **heart failure**, **hypotension**, palpitations, peripheral edema, tachycardia
EENT: Altered taste, blurred vision, dry mouth, epistaxis, gingival hyperplasia, nasal congestion, pharyngitis, sinusitis, tinnitus
ENDO: Gynecomastia, hyperglycemia
GI: Anorexia; constipation; diarrhea; dyspepsia; elevated liver enzymes; **GI bleeding**, irritation, or **obstruction**; **hepatitis**; nausea; vomiting
GU: Dysuria, nocturia, polyuria, sexual dysfunction, urinary frequency
HEME: Anemia, **leukopenia**, positive Coombs' test, **thrombocytopenia**
MS: Joint stiffness, muscle cramps
RESP: Chest congestion, cough, dyspnea, respiratory tract infection, wheezing
SKIN: Acute generalized exanthematous pustulosis, diaphoresis, **erythema multiforme**, **exfoliative dermatitis**, flushing, photosensitivity, pruritus, rash, **Stevens–Johnson syndrome**, **toxic epidermal necrolysis**, urticaria

Childbearing Considerations

PREGNANCY

- Drug may cause fetal harm, according to animal studies.

- Use with caution only if benefit to mother outweighs potential risk to fetus.

LACTATION

- Drug is present in breast milk.
- Patient should check with prescriber before breastfeeding.

Nursing Considerations

- Be aware that patients with galactose intolerance should not take nifedipine because drug contains lactose. The capsule form of nifedipine should not be used to treat hypertension because its effects on blood pressure are not known.
- Use cautiously in patients with cirrhosis because it is unknown how nifedipine exposure may be altered in these patients.
- Know that when starting and stopping nifedipine therapy, taper it, as prescribed, over 7 to 14 days.
- Keep in mind that because of drug's negative inotropic effect on some patients, frequently monitor heart rate and rhythm, as well as blood pressure, especially in patients who take a beta-blocker or have heart failure, significant left ventricular dysfunction, or tight aortic stenosis.
- Monitor fluid intake/output and daily weight; fluid retention may lead to heart failure. Also assess for signs of heart failure, such as crackles, dyspnea, jugular vein distention, peripheral edema, and weight gain.

PATIENT TEACHING

- Urge patient to take nifedipine exactly as prescribed, even when she's feeling well. Advise her to notify prescriber if she misses two or more doses.
- Urge patient not to take drug within 1 hour of a high-fat meal or grapefruit juice. Instruct patient taking Adalat CC brand of E.R. tablets to take tablets on an empty stomach.
- Instruct patient to swallow E.R. tablets whole and not to break, chew, or crush them. Inform patient that their empty shells may appear in stool.

! **WARNING** Caution patient against stopping nifedipine abruptly because angina or dangerously high blood pressure could result.

- Teach patient to measure blood pressure and pulse rate, and advise her to call prescriber if they drop below accepted levels. Suggest keeping a log of weekly measurements and taking it to follow-up visits.
- Instruct patient to notify prescriber immediately about chest pain, difficulty breathing, ringing in ears, and swollen gums.
- Advise patient to avoid hazardous activities until drug's CNS effects are known.
- Urge patient to avoid alcoholic beverages because they may worsen dizziness, drowsiness, and hypotension.
- Teach patient to minimize constipation by increasing her intake of fluids, if allowed, and dietary fiber.
- Emphasize the need to comply with prescribed lifestyle changes, such as alcohol moderation, low-fat or low-sodium diet, regular exercise, smoking cessation, stress reduction, and weight reduction.
- Emphasize the need for good oral hygiene and regular dental visits.
- Caution patient that hot tubs, prolonged hot showers, and saunas may cause dizziness and fainting.
- Advise patient to avoid prolonged sun exposure and to wear sunscreen outdoors.

nirmatrelvir*

FDA Emergency Use Authorization

Class and Category

Pharmacologic class: Protease inhibitor
Therapeutic class: Antiviral

Indications and Dosages

✳ *As adjunct to treat mild to moderate coronavirus disease 2019 (COVID-19) with positive results of direct severe acute respiratory syndrome coronavirus 2 (SARS-CoV-2) viral testing and who are at high risk for progression to severe COVID-19, including hospitalization or death.*

P.O.

Adults and children age 12 and older weighing at least 40 kg (88 lb). 300 mg with 100 mg ritonavir twice daily for 5 days.

± **DOSAGE ADJUSTMENT** For patients with impaired renal function (an estimated glomerular filtration rate of 30 to less than 60 ml/min), dosage reduced to 150 mg (no dosage change for ritonavir).

Drug Administration

TABLET

- Know that nirmatrelvir and ritonavir are copackaged for oral use and supplied under the trade name of Paxlovid even though the two drugs are not combined into one tablet but are administered as two different drugs.
- Administer both nirmatrelvir and ritonavir tablets together at the same time because failure to do so may result in insufficient plasma levels of nirmatrelvir to achieve desired results.
- Have patient swallow the tablet whole and not break, chew, or crush the tablet.

Route	Onset	Peak	Duration
P.O.	Unknown	Unknown	Unknown

Half-life: 6.05 hr

Mechanism of Action

Inhibits the activity of SARS-CoV-2 main protease (Mpro), rendering it incapable of processing polyprotein precursors. This prevents viral replication.

Contraindications

Concurrent therapy with drugs that are highly dependent on CYP3A for clearance and for which elevated concentrations are associated with serious and/or life-threatening reactions such as alpha$_1$-adrenoreceptor antagonist (alfuzosin), analgesics (pethidine, piroxicam, propoxyphene), antianginal (ranolazine), antiarrhythmics (amiodarone, dronedarone, flecainide, propafenone, quinidine), anti-gout (colchicine), antipsychotics (lurasidone, pimozide, clozapine), ergot derivatives (dihydroergotamine, ergotamine, methylergonovine), HMG-CoA reductase inhibitors (lovastatin, simvastatin), PDE-5 inhibitor when used for pulmonary arterial hypertension (sildenafil [Revatio]), and sedative/hypnotics (triazolam, oral midazolam); hypersensitivity to nirmatrelvir or ritonavir or any of their components; within recent discontinuation of potent CYP3A inducers where significantly reduced nirmatrelvir or ritonavir plasma concentrations may be associated with the potential for loss of virologic response and possible resistance such as anticancer drugs (apalutamide), anticonvulsants (carbamazepine, phenobarbital, phenytoin), antimycobacterials (rifampin) and herbal products (St. John's wort)

Interactions

DRUGS

antiarrhythmics (bepridil, systemic lidocaine): Increased risk of change in therapeutic concentration for antiarrhythmics

anticancer drugs (abemaciclib, ceritinib, dasatinib, encorafenib, ibrutinib, ivosidenib, neratinib, nilotinib, venetoclax, vinblastine, vincristine): Potential for significant adverse reactions

anticoagulants (rivaroxaban, warfarin): Increased risk of INR change (warfarin) or bleeding (rivaroxaban)

antidepressants (bupropion, trazodone): Change in therapeutic response (bupropion) or increased risk of adverse reactions of dizziness, hypotension, nausea, and syncope (trazodone)

antifungals (ketoconazole, isavuconazonium sulfate, itraconazole): Plasma concentration increased with increased risk of adverse reactions

anti-HIV drugs (bictegravir/emtricitabine/ tenofovir, didanosine, delavirdine, efavirenz, maraviroc, nevirapine, raltegravir, zidovudine): Change in plasma concentration either affecting effectiveness of the anti-HIV drug or increasing risk of adverse reactions

anti-infective (clarithromycin, erythromycin), anti-HIV protease inhibitors (amprenavir, atazanavir, darunavir, fosamprenavir, indinavir, nelfinavir, saquinavir, tipranavir), antimycobacterial (bedaquiline, rifabutin), bosentan, calcium channel blockers (amlodipine, diltiazem, felodipine, nicardipine, nifedipine), digoxin, fentanyl, hepatitis C direct-acting antivirals (elbasvir/grazoprevir, glecaprevir/pibrentasvir, ombitasvir, paritaprevir, ritonavir and dasabuvir, sofosbuvir/velpatasvir/voxilaprevir), HMG-CoA reductase inhibitors (atorvastatin, rosuvastatin), immunosuppressants (cyclosporine, sirolimus, tacrolimus), parenteral midazolam, quetiapine, salmeterol, systemic corticosteroids (betamethasone, budesonide, ciclesonide, dexamethasone, fluticasone, methylprednisolone, mometasone, prednisone, triamcinolone): Increased plasma concentrations of these drugs increasing risk of adverse reactions

hormonal contraceptive (ethinyl estradiol):
Decreased effectiveness of ethinyl estradiol
methadone, voriconazole: Decreased plasma
concentration of these drugs
* Refer to manufacturer guidelines for ritonavir
drug interactions.

Adverse Reactions
CV: Hypertension
EENT: Alteration in taste
GI: Diarrhea
MS: Myalgia

Childbearing Considerations
PREGNANCY
- It is not known if drug can cause fetal harm.
- Use with caution only if benefit to mother outweighs potential risk to fetus.

LACTATION
- It is not known if drug is present in breast milk.
- Patient should check with prescriber before breastfeeding.

REPRODUCTION
- Women of childbearing age using a combined hormonal contraceptive should use an effective alternative contraceptive method or an additional barrier method of contraception during drug therapy.

Nursing Considerations
- Know that nirmatrelvir is authorized only for the duration of the FDA declaration for emergency use.
- Be aware that drug is not authorized for use in patients who are less than 12 years old and it is not authorized to treat patients hospitalized due to COVID-19. It is also not authorized for use for longer than 5 consecutive days and it is not authorized for preexposure or postexposure to prevent COVID-19.
- Know that nirmatrelvir has not received full FDA approval to treat any indication, including the treatment of COVID-19.
- Ensure that prescriber has considered the benefit–risk balance for patient prior to administration of drug.
- Know that nirmatrelvir is not recommended for patients with severe hepatic or renal impairment.
- Expect patient who is started on nirmatrelvir therapy and then requires hospitalization to continue on to complete the full 5-day treatment course at the prescriber's discretion.
- Continue isolation protocols according to public health recommendations during drug therapy to minimize the transmission of SARS-CoV-2 virus.

> **! WARNING** Monitor patient for hypersensitivity reaction to nirmatrelvir because patient sensitivity to this drug is unknown.

- Expect all serious adverse reactions and medication errors potentially related to nirmatrelvir to be reported within 7 calendar days from the time of the prescriber's awareness of the event, using FDA Form 3500. Once completed, form should be submitted to the FDA MedWatch online, mailed, or faxed. In addition, a copy of the form should be faxed or emailed to the manufacturer, Pfizer. Be prepared to provide any information prescriber requests when form is completed.

PATIENT TEACHING
- Ensure that patient has received the "Fact Sheet for Patients, Parents, and Caregivers."
- Instruct patient to swallow tablet whole and not to break, chew, or crush it.
- Stress importance of completing the full 5-day treatment with nirmatrelvir in combination with ritonavir.
- Tell patient that if a dose is missed and it is within 8 hours of the time it is usually taken, drug should be taken and normal dosing schedule resumed. If it is more than 8 hours, the missed dose should not be taken and dosage schedule resumed at the regularly scheduled time. The dose should not be doubled to make up for a missed dose.
- Tell patient to alert prescriber of all drug therapies taken, as nirmatrelvir/ritonavir combination can cause many drug interactions, resulting in adverse reactions that could be severe.
- Monitor patient with preexisting liver disease, liver enzyme abnormalities, or hepatitis closely, as clinical hepatitis, jaundice, and transaminase elevations have occurred in patients receiving ritonavir.
- Be aware that because nirmatrelvir is given with ritonavir, a risk of HIV-1 resistance

to HIV protease inhibitors may develop in patients with uncontrolled or undiagnosed HIV-1 infection.

- Stress need for patient to continue isolation per public health recommendations.

! **WARNING** Inform patient that an allergic reaction may occur with nirmatrelvir. If present, advise patient or caregiver to notify prescriber and, if serious, patient should seek immediate emergency help.

---

nitrofurantoin
Furadantin, Macrobid, Macrodantin

Class and Category
Pharmacologic class: Nitrofuran
Therapeutic class: Antibiotic

Indications and Dosages
* *To treat acute cystitis due to* Enterococci, Escherichia coli, *or* Staphylococcus aureus; *certain strains of* Enterobacter *or* Klebsiella *species*

CAPSULES, ORAL SUSPENSION
Adults and adolescents. 50 to 100 mg four times daily and continued for 1 wk or at least 3 days after urine is negative for bacteria. Alternatively using Macrobid, 100 mg every 12 hr for 7 days.
Children over age 1 month. 5 to 7 mg/kg/day in four divided doses, continued for 1 wk or at least 3 days after urine is negative for bacteria.

* *To suppress chronic cystitis*

CAPSULES, ORAL SUSPENSION
Adults. 50 to 100 mg daily at bedtime.
Children over age 1 month. 1 to 2 mg/kg daily at bedtime or divided into two doses and given every 12 hr.

Drug Administration
P.O.
- Give drug with food or milk to avoid staining teeth.
- Capsules should be swallowed whole and not chewed, crushed, or opened.
- Shake suspension before pouring dose, and use a calibrated device to measure dose. Mix with food or milk, as needed.
- Administer drug used to suppress chronic cystitis once daily at bedtime.

Route	Onset	Peak	Duration
P.O.	Unknown	30 min	Unknown

Half-life: 20–60 min

Mechanism of Action
Alters or inactivates bacterial ribosomal proteins and other macromolecules. This action of nitrofurantoin inhibits aerobic energy metabolism, bacterial protein synthesis, cell wall synthesis, DNA synthesis, and RNA synthesis. Nitrofurantoin is bacteriostatic at low doses and bactericidal at higher doses.

Contraindications
Acute porphyria (Macrobid, Macrodantin); age under 1 month (Furadantin), under 3 months (Macrodantin), or 12 years and under (Macrobid); anuria; creatinine clearance less than 60 ml/min; G6PD (Macrobid, Macrodantin); history of cholestatic jaundice or hepatic dysfunction with previous nitrofurantoin therapy; hypersensitivity to nitrofurantoin, other nitrofurans, or their components; oliguria; pregnancy near term (38 to 42 weeks)

Interactions
DRUGS
antacids containing magnesium trisilicate: Decreased nitrofurantoin absorption
live vaccines: Possibly diminished therapeutic effect of the vaccines
uricosuric such as probenecid, sulfinpyrazone: Increased nitrofurantoin serum levels with increased risk of toxicity; decreased urinary levels with decreased effectiveness

FOODS
all foods: Delays gastric emptying, thus increasing absorption

Adverse Reactions
CNS: Chills, confusion, depression, headache, **neurotoxicity**, peripheral neuropathy
CV: Vasculitis
EENT: Optic neuritis, parotitis, tooth discoloration
GI: Abdominal pain, anorexia, cholestatic jaundice, diarrhea, **hepatic necrosis**, **hepatitis**, jaundice, nausea, **pancreatitis**, **pseudomembranous colitis**, vomiting
GU: Rust-colored to brown urine

HEME: Aplastic anemia, granulocytopenia, hemolytic anemia, leukopenia, megaloblastic anemia, methemoglobinemia, thrombocytopenia
MS: Arthralgia, myalgia
RESP: Asthma (in asthmatic patients), cyanosis, interstitial pneumonitis, pulmonary fibrosis
SKIN: Alopecia; eczematous, erythematous, or maculopapular eruptions; erythema multiforme; exfoliative dermatitis; pruritus; rash; Stevens–Johnson syndrome
Other: Anaphylaxis, angioedema, drug-induced fever, lupus-like syndrome

☰ Childbearing Considerations

PREGNANCY
- It is not known if drug causes fetal harm.
- Use with caution only if benefit to mother outweighs potential risk to fetus.

LABOR & DELIVERY
- Drug is contraindicated when labor is imminent, during labor and delivery, and in the neonate under 1 month of age because drug may cause hemolytic anemia in the fetus and neonate.

LACTATION
- Drug is present in breast milk.
- A decision should be made to discontinue breastfeeding or the drug to avoid potential serious adverse reactions in the breastfed infant.

☰ Nursing Considerations
- Obtain a specimen of patient's urine for culture and sensitivity tests, as ordered; review test results if possible before giving nitrofurantoin.
- Monitor patient for evidence of superinfection, such as abdominal pain, diarrhea, and fever. If patient develops diarrhea, it may indicate pseudomembranous colitis caused by *Clostridium difficile*. Notify prescriber and expect to withhold nitrofurantoin and treat with electrolytes, fluids, protein, and an antibiotic effective against *C. difficile*.
- Monitor patient for hepatic and pulmonary abnormalities because rare but severe reactions have occurred with nitrofurantoin use, especially in the elderly.
- Observe patient for changes in nervous function because peripheral neuropathy, although uncommon, may become severe

or irreversible. Patients with anemia, debilitating disease, diabetes mellitus, electrolyte imbalance, renal impairment, or vitamin B deficiency are at higher risk for peripheral neuropathy.

PATIENT TEACHING
- Instruct patient to shake nitrofurantoin oral suspension before measuring dose and to take drug with food or milk to avoid staining teeth. Also tell patient to measure dose with a calibrated device, not a household spoon.
- Instruct patient to swallow capsules whole and not chew, crush, or open capsules.
- Caution patient against taking any preparations that contain magnesium trisilicate during therapy.
- Explain that urine may turn brown, orange, or rust-colored during therapy.
- Instruct patient to complete prescribed course of therapy even if symptoms subside before course is completed.
- Urge patient to tell prescriber about diarrhea that's severe or lasts longer than 3 days. Explain that bloody or watery stools can occur 2 or more months after nitrofurantoin therapy and can be serious, requiring prompt treatment.

nitroglycerin
(glyceryl trinitrate)

N O

GoNitro, Minitran Patch, Nitro-Bid Ointment, Nitro-Dur Patch, Nitrolingual Pumpspray, NitroMist, Nitrostat, Rectiv, Trinipatch (CAN)

☰ Class and Category
Pharmacologic class: Nitrate
Therapeutic class: Antianginal, vasodilator

☰ Indications and Dosages
✱ *To prevent anginal attacks due to coronary artery disease*

TRANSDERMAL OINTMENT (NITRO-BID)
Adults. *Initial:* 1/2 inch of 2% ointment twice daily with first dose applied upon awakening and second dose 6 hr later. Dosage increased, in 1/2 inch increments and/or dosing frequency to three or four times daily, as needed.

TRANSDERMAL PATCH (MINITRAN, NITRO-DUR, TRINIPATCH)

Adults. *Initial:* 0.2 to 0.4 mg/hr worn 12 to 14 hr, with dosage increased or decreased, as needed.

* *To treat acute angina pectoris; to reduce or limit anginal attacks before exercise*

S.L. TABLETS (NITROSTAT)

Adults. 0.3 to 0.6 mg, repeated every 5 min for an acute attack or taken 5 to 10 min before exercise. *Maximum:* 3 tabs in 15 min.

S.L. POWDER (GONITRO)

Adults. 400 or 800 mcg (1 or 2 packets) sprinkled under tongue, repeated every 5 min as needed for an acute attack, or taken 5 to 10 min before exercise. *Maximum:* 1,200 mcg (3 packets) in 15 min.

TRANSLINGUAL SPRAY (NITROLINGUAL, NITROMIST)

Adults. 1 or 2 metered doses (400 or 800 mcg) onto or under tongue, repeated every 5 min, as needed, for an acute attack or taken 5 to 10 min before exercise. *Maximum:* 3 sprays within 15 min.

* *To treat acute angina when oral therapy has been ineffective; to manage hypertension related to surgery or heart failure following an acute myocardial infarction; to induce intraoperative hypotension*

I.V. INFUSION (NITROGLYCERIN)

Adults. Highly individualized. *Suggested initial:* 5 mcg/min, increased by 5 mcg/min every 3 to 5 min to 20 mcg/min, as needed, and then by 10 to 20 mcg/min every 3 to 5 min, if higher dosage is needed.

* *To treat moderate to severe pain associated with chronic anal fissure*

RECTAL OINTMENT (RECTIV)

Adults. 1 inch (375 mg of ointment equivalent to 1.5 mg of nitroglycerin) to intra-anal area every 12 hr for up to 3 wk.

☰ Drug Administration

- Time administration according to route of administration and condition being treated. See Indications and Dosages section.

SUBLINGUAL

- Place S.L. tablet under patient's tongue and make sure it dissolves completely.
- Place patient in sitting position, if possible, when administering S.L. powder. Have patient open mouth; sprinkle powder under tongue. Have patient close mouth and breathe normally. Allow powder to dissolve without patient swallowing. Do not allow patient to rinse mouth or spit for 5 minutes after administration.

TRANSLINGUAL

- Prime container when using for first time by spraying five times into the air. If container is not used for 6 weeks, it will have to be reprimed by spraying it once; if not used within 3 months, reprime with up to five sprays.
- Don't shake container before administering.
- Have patient assume a sitting position. Then have patient inhale and hold her breath, and then spray drug under or on the tongue.
- Do not allow patient to rinse mouth or spit for 5 to 10 minutes after administration.

I.V.

- Dilute only in 0.9% Sodium Chloride Injection or 5% Dextrose in Water. Do not mix with other infusions.
- Always mix in a glass bottle, not a container made of polyvinyl chloride. Use with the special nonabsorbent polyvinyl chloride tubing supplied by manufacturer.
- Don't use a filter because plastic absorbs drug.
- Administer with infusion pump.
- *Incompatibilities:* Other drugs

TRANSDERMAL

- For ointment, apply correct amount on dose-measuring paper. Then place paper on hairless area of body and spread in a thin, even layer over an area at least 2 inches by 3 inches. Don't place on cuts or irritated areas. Cover with plastic film. Wash hands after application. Rotate sites. Store at room temperature.
- Open transdermal patch package immediately before use. Apply patch to hairless area, and press edges to seal. Rotate sites. Store at room temperature. If patient needs cardioversion or defibrillation, remove transdermal patch before procedure.

P.R.

- Cover finger with a finger cot or hand with a disposable surgical glove. Apply 1 inch of ointment onto a covered finger. Insert gently into the anal canal no further than the first finger joint. Remove finger and covering. Wash hands.

Route	Onset	Peak	Duration
I.V.	Immediate	1–2 min	3–5 min
S.L.	1–3 min	5–7 min	25 min
Translingual	1–3 min	4–15 min	25 min
Transdermal†	15–30 min	1 hr	7 hr
Transdermal‡	In 30 min	2 hr	10–12 hr
Topical	15–30 min	1 hr	7 hr
P.R.	Unknown	Unknown	Unknown

Half-life: 1–4 min

† Ointment.
‡ Patch.

☰ Mechanism of Action

May interact with nitrate receptors in vascular smooth-muscle cell membranes. This interaction reduces nitroglycerin to nitric oxide, which activates the enzyme guanylate cyclase, increasing intracellular formation of cGMP. Increased cGMP level may relax vascular smooth muscle by forcing calcium out of muscle cells, causing vasodilation. Venous dilation decreases venous return to the heart, reducing left ventricular end-diastolic pressure and pulmonary artery wedge pressure. Arterial dilation decreases systemic arterial pressure, systemic vascular resistance, and mean arterial pressure. Thus, nitroglycerin reduces preload and afterload, decreasing myocardial workload and oxygen demand. It also dilates coronary arteries, increasing blood flow to ischemic myocardial tissue and provides analgesic effects in anal tissue.

☰ Contraindications

Acute MI (S.L.), angle-closure glaucoma, cerebral hemorrhage, circulatory failure and shock, concurrent use of phosphodiesterase inhibitors (avanafil, sildenafil, tadalafil, vardenafil) or riociguat, constrictive pericarditis (I.V.), head trauma, hypersensitivity to adhesive in transdermal form, hypersensitivity to nitrates, or their components, hypotension (I.V.), hypovolemia (I.V.), inadequate cerebral circulation (I.V.), increased intracranial pressure, orthostatic hypotension, pericardial tamponade (I.V.), restrictive cardiomyopathy (I.V.), severe anemia

☰ Interactions

DRUGS

antihypertensives, beta-adrenergic blockers, calcium channel blockers: Increased risk of additive hypotensive effects.

aspirin: Increased nitroglycerin concentrations enhancing vasodilatory and hemodynamic effects of nitroglycerin
ergotamine and related drugs: Possibly precipitate angina (oral nitroglycerin)
heparin: Possibly decreased anticoagulant effect of heparin
phosphodiesterase inhibitors (such as avanafil, sildenafil, tadalafil, vardenafil), riociguat: Possibly severe hypotensive effect of nitroglycerin
tissue-type plasminogen activator (t-PA): Decreases thrombolytic effect of t-PA.

ACTIVITIES

alcohol use: Possibly increased orthostatic hypotension

☰ Adverse Reactions

CNS: Agitation, anxiety, dizziness, drowsiness, headache, insomnia, restlessness, syncope, weakness
CV: **Arrhythmias**, edema, **hypotension**, orthostatic hypotension, palpitations, tachycardia
EENT: Blurred vision, burning or tingling in mouth (S.L. forms), dry mouth
GI: Abdominal pain, diarrhea, indigestion, nausea, vomiting
GU: Dysuria, impotence, urinary frequency
HEME: **Methemoglobinemia**
MS: Arthralgia
RESP: Bronchitis, pneumonia, transient hypoxemia
SKIN: Contact dermatitis (transdermal forms), **exfoliative dermatitis**, flushing of face and neck, rash
OTHER: **Hypersensitivity reactions**

☰ Childbearing Considerations

PREGNANCY

- It is not known if drug causes fetal harm.
- Use with caution only if benefit to mother outweighs potential risk to fetus.

LACTATION

- It is not known if drug is present in breast milk.
- Patient should check with prescriber before breastfeeding.

☰ Nursing Considerations

- Use nitroglycerin cautiously in elderly patients, especially those who are volume-depleted or taking several medications, because of the increased risk of falls and hypotension. Hypotension may

N
O

be accompanied by angina and paradoxical slowing of the heart rate. Hypotension may become severe, especially in patients in an upright position, even with small doses, particularly in patients with aortic or mitral stenosis, constrictive pericarditis, or who are already experiencing hypotension. Symptoms of severe hypotension include collapse, nausea, pallor, perspiration, syncope, vomiting, and weakness. Notify prescriber immediately if these occur, and provide appropriate treatment, as ordered.

- Use nitroglycerin cautiously in patients with hypertrophic obstructive cardiomyopathy because nitrate therapy may aggravate angina in this condition.
- Plan a nitroglycerin-free period of about 10 hours each day, as prescribed, to maintain therapeutic effects and avoid tolerance.
- Check vital signs before every dosage adjustment and often during therapy.
- Monitor frequently heart and breath sounds, level of consciousness, fluid intake and output, and pulmonary artery wedge pressure, if possible.

! **WARNING** Assess patient for evidence of overdose, such as confusion, diaphoresis, dyspnea, flushing, headache, hypotension, nausea, palpitations, tachycardia, vertigo, vision changes, and vomiting. Treat as prescribed by removing nitroglycerin source, if possible; elevating legs above heart level; and administering an alpha-adrenergic agonist, as prescribed, to treat severe hypotension.

PATIENT TEACHING

- Teach patient to recognize signs and symptoms of angina pectoris, including chest fullness, pain, and pressure, possibly with sweating and nausea. Pain may radiate down left arm or into neck or jaw. Inform women and those with diabetes mellitus or hypertension that they may feel only fatigue and shortness of breath.
- Instruct patient to read and follow package instructions to obtain full benefits of drug.
- Inform patient that prescriber may order a 10- to 12-hour drug-free period at night (or at another time if she has chest pain at night or in the morning) to prevent drug tolerance. Also inform patient that drug should be taken as prescribed, as excessive use may lead to tolerance as well.

- For sublingual use, advise patient to place 1 or 2 packets of powder or 1 tablet under her tongue or in buccal pouch (tablet form only) when angina starts and then to sit or lie down. Instruct her not to swallow drug, but to let it dissolve. Explain that moisture in her mouth helps drug absorption. Remind patient not to rinse mouth or spit for 5 minutes after using drug. If angina doesn't subside, instruct patient to place another packet of powder or tablet under her tongue or in buccal pouch (tablet form only) after 5 minutes and to repeat, if needed, for three doses total. If pain doesn't subside after 15 minutes, urge patient to call 911 or another emergency service.
- Advise patient to carry S.L. packets of powder or tablets in their original brown bottle in a purse or jacket pocket, but not a place that will be affected by body heat. Instruct her to store drug in a dry place at room temperature and to discard cotton from container. Advise her to discard and replace S.L. tablets after 6 months. Tell her to note date on packets of powder and not to use beyond the expiration date printed.
- Instruct patient prescribed transdermal ointment or patch how to apply. Advise patient using transdermal ointment or patch to rotate sites to avoid skin sensitization.
- Inform patient that swimming or bathing doesn't affect transdermal forms but that electric blankets, hot tubs, magnetic therapy, prolonged hot showers, and saunas over the site may increase drug absorption and cause dizziness and hypotension.
- Caution against inhaling translingual spray. Before first use, tell patient to press actuator button 5 times to prime container and then hold container upright with forefinger on top of actuator button. Tell her to open her mouth, bring container as close as possible, press actuator button firmly to release spray onto or under tongue, and release button and immediately close her mouth. Remind her to replace plastic cover on container and to not spit out the drug or rinse her mouth for 5 to 10 minutes. Tell her to reprime container by pressing actuator button once if container hasn't been used for more than 6 weeks. Remind patient to periodically check level of fluid in container. If it reaches the top or middle hole on side

of container, more should be obtained. Caution patient not to let level of liquid get to bottom of hole.

- Inform patient that nitroglycerin commonly causes headache, which typically resolves after a few days of continuous therapy. Suggest taking acetaminophen, as needed, and not contraindicated.
- Advise patient to notify prescriber immediately about blurred vision, dizziness, and severe headache.
- Suggest that patient change positions slowly to minimize orthostatic hypotension.
- Advise patient to avoid hazardous activities until drug's CNS effects are known.
- Urge patient to avoid alcohol and erectile dysfunction drugs during therapy.
- Advise patient to alert all prescribers of nitroglycerin use because of potential drug interactions.
- Advise patient to alert all prescribers of nitroglycerin use because of potential drug interactions.

nitroprusside sodium
Nipride (CAN), Nitropress

☰ Class and Category
Pharmacologic class: Vasodilator
Therapeutic class: Antihypertensive, vasodilator

☰ Indications and Dosages
* *To treat hypertensive crisis and acute heart failure; to produce controlled hypotension in order to reduce bleeding during surgery*

I.V. INFUSION
Adults and children. *Initial:* 0.3 mcg/kg/min, increased gradually, waiting at least 5 minutes between titrations as needed, until desired level is reached. *Maximum:* 10 mcg/kg/min.
±**DOSAGE ADJUSTMENT** For children weighing less than 10 kg (22 lb), infusion rate may be reduced.

☰ Drug Administration
I.V.
- Obtain baseline vital signs before administering nitroprusside.
- Reconstitute 50 mg of drug with 2 or 3 ml 5% Dextrose in Water or, if using ADD-Vantage vials, reconstitute according to manufacturer guidelines.

- Further dilute reconstituted solution with 250 to 1000 ml 5% Dextrose in Water to produce concentrations of 50 to 200 mcg/ml.
- Don't use solution if it contains particles or is blue, green, red, or darker than faint brown.
- Diluted solution is stable at room temperature for 24 hours when protected from light.
- Use an infusion pump for administration. Never administer undiluted or as an I.V. injection.
- Place opaque cover over infusion container because drug is metabolized by light. I.V. tubing need not be covered.
- Keep patient supine when starting drug or titrating dose up or down.
- Infuse piggybacked into a peripheral vein through a main I.V. line with no other drug being infused at the same time. Do not change rate of main I.V. solution while nitroprusside is being infused.
- Monitor blood pressure continuously with intra-arterial pressure monitor. Record blood pressure every 5 minutes at start of infusion and every 15 minutes thereafter.
- If severe hypotension occurs, stop infusion immediately and notify prescriber. Because of drug's short half-life, drug effects on blood pressure are quickly reversed.
- *Incompatibilities:* Other drugs

Route	Onset	Peak	Duration
I.V.	Immediate	1–2 min	1–10 min

Half-life: 2 min

☰ Mechanism of Action
May interact with nitrate receptors in vascular smooth-muscle cell membranes. This action reduces nitroprusside to nitric oxide and then activates intracellular guanylate cyclase, which increases the cGMP level. Increased cGMP level may relax vascular smooth muscle by forcing calcium out of muscle cells. Smooth-muscle relaxation causes arteries and veins to dilate, which reduces peripheral vascular resistance and blood pressure.

☰ Contraindications
Acute heart failure associated with decreased peripheral vascular resistance, concomitant use of riociguat, compensatory hypertension

when primary hemodynamic lesion is aortic coarctation or arteriovenous shunting, congenital optic atrophy, decreased cerebral perfusion, hypersensitivity to nitroprusside or its components, tobacco-induced amblyopia, use of PDE-5 inhibitors, used to produce hypotension during surgery in patients with inadequate circulation or moribund patients (A.S.A. Class 5E) requiring emergency surgery

Interactions

DRUGS

ganglionic blockers, inhaled anesthetics, negative inotropic agents: Increased hypotensive effect
PDE-5 inhibitors, riociguat: Increased risk of hypotension

Adverse Reactions

CNS: Anxiety, dizziness, headache, **increased intracranial pressure,** nervousness, restlessness
CV: Hypotension, tachycardia
ENDO: Hypothyroidism
GI: Abdominal pain, ileus, nausea, vomiting
HEME: Methemoglobinemia
MS: Muscle twitching
SKIN: Diaphoresis, flushing, rash
Other: Infusion-site phlebitis

Childbearing Considerations

PREGNANCY

- It is not known if drug causes fetal harm.
- Use with caution only if benefit to mother outweighs potential risk to fetus.

LACTATION

- It is not known if drug is present in breast milk.
- A decision should be made to discontinue breastfeeding or the drug to avoid potential serious adverse reactions in the breastfed infant.

Nursing Considerations

- Obtain baseline vital signs before administering nitroprusside.
- Monitor blood pressure continuously with intra-arterial pressure monitor. Record blood pressure every 5 minutes at start of infusion and every 15 minutes thereafter.
- Be aware that if patient has severe heart failure, expect to administer an inotropic drug, such as dopamine or dobutamine, as prescribed.

! **WARNING** Know that patient who receives prolonged nitroprusside therapy or short-term high-dose therapy should be watched for evidence of thiocyanate toxicity (ataxia, blurred vision, delirium, dizziness, dyspnea, headache, hyperreflexia, loss of consciousness, nausea, tinnitus, and vomiting). Toxicity can cause arrhythmias, metabolic acidosis, severe hypotension, and death.

- Monitor serum thiocyanate level at least every 72 hours; levels above 100 mcg/ml are associated with toxicity.

! **WARNING** Assess patient for evidence of cyanide toxicity (absence of reflexes, coma, distant heart sounds, hypotension, metabolic acidosis, mydriasis, pink skin, shallow respirations, and weak pulse). If detected, discontinue nitroprusside, as ordered, and give 4 to 6 mg/kg sodium nitrite over 2 to 4 minutes to convert hemoglobin to methemoglobin. Follow with 150 to 200 mg/kg sodium thiosulfate. Repeat this regimen at half the original doses after 2 hours, as ordered.

PATIENT TEACHING

- Advise patient to change position slowly to minimize dizziness from sudden, severe hypotension.

norepinephrine bitartrate
(levarterenol bitartrate)
Levophed

Class and Category

Pharmacologic class: Sympathomimetic
Therapeutic class: Vasopressor

Indications and Dosages

＊ *To manage blood pressure in acute hypotensive states such as blood transfusion, drug adverse effect, myocardial infarction, pheochromocytomectomy, poliomyelitis, spinal anesthesia, and sympathectomy reactions; adjunct in treatment of cardiac arrest and profound hypotension*

I.V. INFUSION

Adults. *Initial average dose:* 8 to 12 mcg/min. Then titrated to maintain systolic blood pressure between 80 to 100 mm Hg in patients previously not hypertensive and 40 mm Hg below preexisting systolic blood pressure in patients previously hypertensive. *Maintenance:* 2 to 4 mcg/min.

Drug Administration

I.V.

- Dilute by adding 4 mg of drug to 1,000 ml of 5% Dextrose Injection or 5% Dextrose Injection with 0.9% Sodium Chloride solution to yield a concentration of 4 mcg/ml. Do not use 0.9% Sodium Chloride Injection alone. Never administer undiluted.
- Solution should be colorless. Do not use if it contains particles or is discolored such as a pinkish or darker than a slightly yellow color.
- Give drug using a flow-control device.
- Infuse through a central line or large peripheral vein to avoid extravasation. Do not infuse into leg veins in the elderly or in patients with occlusive vascular disease of the legs.
- Avoid using a catheter tie-in technique, if possible.
- Check blood pressure every 2 to 3 minutes, preferably by direct intra-arterial monitoring, until stabilized and then every 5 minutes.
- If extravasation occurs, it can cause severe tissue damage and necrosis. Notify prescriber and expect prescriber to give multiple subcutaneous injections of phentolamine (5 to 10 mg diluted in 10 to 15 ml of 0.9% Sodium Chloride Injection) around extravasated peripheral infusion site.
- If blanching occurs along vein, change infusion site and notify prescriber at once.
- When discontinuing infusion, reduce the flow rate gradually. Avoid abrupt withdrawal.
- *Incompatibilities:* Alkalis, iron salts, or oxidizing agents; whole blood or plasma

Route	Onset	Peak	Duration
I.V.	Immediate	1–2 min	1–10 min

Half-life: 1–2.5 min

Mechanism of Action

Inhibits adenyl cyclase and directly stimulates alpha-adrenergic receptors, which inhibits cAMP production. Inhibition of cAMP constricts arteries and veins and increases peripheral vascular resistance and systolic blood pressure.

Contraindications

Concurrent use of cyclopropane and hydrocarbon inhalation anesthetics, hypersensitivity to norepinephrine or its components, hypovolemia (except as an emergency measure), mesenteric or peripheral vascular thrombosis (except as an emergency measure), profound hypercarbia or hypoxia

Interactions

DRUGS

cyclopropane and halothane anesthetics: Increased cardiac autonomic irritability, sensitizing the myocardium to the action of norepinephrine
MAO inhibitors of the imipramine or triptyline types: May cause prolonged, severe hypertension

Adverse Reactions

CNS: Anxiety, dizziness, headache, insomnia, nervousness, tremor, weakness
CV: Angina, **bradycardia**, **ECG changes**, edema, hypertension, **hypotension**, palpitations, peripheral vascular insufficiency (including gangrene), **PVCs**, sinus tachycardia
GI: Nausea, vomiting
GU: Decreased renal perfusion
RESP: Apnea, dyspnea
SKIN: Pallor
Other: Infusion-site sloughing and tissue necrosis, **metabolic acidosis**

Childbearing Considerations

PREGNANCY

- It is not known if drug causes fetal harm.
- Use with caution only if benefit to mother outweighs potential risk to fetus.

LACTATION

- It is not known if drug is present in breast milk.
- Patient should check with prescriber before breastfeeding.

Nursing Considerations

- Check blood pressure every 2 to 3 minutes, preferably by direct intra-arterial monitoring, until stabilized and then every 5 minutes.
- Monitor continuous ECG during therapy.

PATIENT TEACHING

- Urge patient to immediately report burning, leaking, or tingling around I.V. site.

N O

nortriptyline hydrochloride
Aventyl (CAN), Pamelor

Class and Category
Pharmacologic class: Tricyclic antidepressant (TCA)
Therapeutic class: Antidepressant

Indications and Dosages
* *To treat depression*

CAPSULES, ORAL SOLUTION

Adults. *Initial:* 25 mg three times a day or four times a day. Alternatively, total daily dose once daily. *Maximum:* 150 mg daily.
Adolescents and the elderly. 30 to 50 mg daily in divided doses. Alternatively, total daily dose once daily.

Drug Administration
P.O.
- Capsules should be swallowed whole and not chewed, crushed, or opened.
- Use a calibrated device when measuring dosage for oral solution.

Route	Onset	Peak	Duration
P.O.	Unknown	7–8.5 hr	Unknown

Half-life: 16–38 hr

Mechanism of Action
May interfere with reuptake of serotonin (and possibly other neurotransmitters) at presynaptic neurons, thus enhancing serotonin's effects at postsynaptic receptors. By restoring normal neurotransmitter levels at nerve synapses, this tricyclic antidepressant may elevate mood.

Contraindications
Acute recovery phase of MI; hypersensitivity to nortriptyline, other dibenzazepines, tricyclic antidepressants, or their components; use within 14 days of MAO inhibitor therapy including intravenous methylene blue or linezolid

Interactions
DRUGS

barbiturates, CNS depressants: Possibly increased CNS depression
chlorpropamide: Possibly significant hypoglycemia
cimetidine: Increased plasma concentrations of nortriptyline
MAO inhibitors (including I.V. methylene blue, linezolid), serotonergic drugs (buspirone, fentanyl, lithium, St. John's wort, tramadol, tricyclic antidepressants, triptans, tryptophan): Increased risk of serotonin syndrome
P4502D6 inhibitors such as cimetidine, fluoxetine and other antidepressants, phenothiazines, quinidine, selective serotonin reuptake inhibitors, type IC antiarrhythmics (flecainide, propafenone): Possibly increased plasma concentration of these drugs with possible increase in adverse reactions
other anticholinergics, sympathomimetic drugs: Increased risk of profound hypertension
reserpine: Possibly produce a stimulating effect

ACTIVITIES

alcohol use: Increased alcohol effects, CNS and respiratory depression, hypertension

Adverse Reactions
CNS: Ataxia, confusion, **CVA**, delirium, dizziness, drowsiness, excitation, hallucinations, headache, insomnia, nervousness, nightmares, Parkinsonism, **serotonin syndrome**, **suicidal ideation**, tremor
CV: **Arrhythmias**, orthostatic hypotension, **unmasking of Brugada syndrome**
EENT: Angle-closure glaucoma, blurred vision, dry mouth, increased intraocular pressure, taste perversion
GI: Constipation, diarrhea, heartburn, ileus, increased appetite, nausea, vomiting
GU: Sexual dysfunction, urine retention
HEME: **Bone marrow depression**
RESP: Wheezing
SKIN: Diaphoresis, urticaria
Other: Weight gain

Childbearing Considerations
PREGNANCY
- It is not known if drug causes fetal harm.
- Use with caution only if benefit to mother outweighs potential risk to fetus.

LACTATION
- Drug is present in breast milk.
- Patient should check with prescriber before breastfeeding.

Nursing Considerations
- Expect to stop MAO inhibitor therapy, including intravenous methylene blue and

linezolid, 10 to 14 days before starting nortriptyline.

- Know that nortriptyline should be avoided in patients with Brugada syndrome or those suspected of having the disorder, because Brugada syndrome can cause abnormal ECG findings and syncope as well as increasing the risk of sudden death.
- Watch patient closely (especially adolescents and young adults), for suicidal tendencies, particularly when therapy starts and dosage changes because depression may worsen temporarily during these times, possibly leading to suicidal ideation.
- Be aware that oral solution (10 mg/5 ml) is 4% alcohol.

! **WARNING** Monitor patient for possible serotonin syndrome, characterized by agitation, chills, confusion, diaphoresis, diarrhea, fever, hyperactive reflexes, poor coordination, restlessness, shaking, talking or acting with uncontrolled excitement, tremor, and twitching. Notify prescriber immediately if serotonin syndrome is suspected because it can become life-threatening and expect to discontinue nortriptyline therapy.

- Monitor blood nortriptyline level; therapeutic range is 50 to 150 ng/ml.
- Monitor ECG tracing to detect arrhythmias.

PATIENT TEACHING

- Advise patient to use a calibrated device to measure oral solution, not a household spoon. Tell patient that oral solution contains alcohol.
- Discourage alcohol consumption during therapy.
- Explain that improvement may take weeks.
- Advise patient that drug may cause mild pupillary dilation, which may lead to an episode of acute angle-closure glaucoma. Encourage patient to have an eye exam before starting therapy to see if he is at risk.
- Advise patient to avoid hazardous activities until drug's CNS effects are known.
- Urge family or caregiver to watch patient closely for suicidal tendencies, especially when therapy starts or dosage changes and particularly if patient is a teenager or young adult.
- Instruct patient to change position slowly to minimize orthostatic hypotension.

- Encourage patient to inform prescriber if there is a family history of sudden unexplained death before the age of 45 before nortriptyline is begun or if abnormal heartbeat or unexplained fainting occurs during nortriptyline therapy.
- Suggest that patient minimize constipation by drinking plenty of fluids (if allowed), exercising regularly, and eating high-fiber foods.

nystatin

Class and Category
Pharmacologic class: Polyene macrolide
Therapeutic class: Antifungal

Indications and Dosages
* *To treat oral candidiasis (thrush)*

ORAL SUSPENSION

Adults and children. 400,000 to 600,000 units (4 to 6 ml) swished and swallowed four times a day until at least 48 hr after symptoms subside.

Infants. 200,000 units (2 ml) applied to each side of mouth four times a day until at least 48 hr after symptoms subside.

* *To treat intestinal candidiasis*

TABLETS

Adults. 500,000 to 1,000,000 units (1 to 2 tablets) every 8 hr.

* Topical use found in Appendix.

Drug Administration
P.O.

- Shake oral suspension well before measuring dose.
- Use supplied dropper or a calibrated syringe to measure dosage.
- Oral suspension should be swished and retained in mouth for several minutes before patient swallows it.
- When using powder form, prepare only a single dose at a time, because it does not contain preservatives. Add prescribed dosage to about 4 ounces of water. Stir well and divide into smaller portions. Administer immediately using one portion at a time until entire volume is used.
- Swab oral suspension on both sides of mouth or drop one-half the dose on each side of tongue when administering to infants.

N
O

Route	Onset	Peak	Duration
P.O.	24–72 hr	Unknown	Unknown

Half-life: 16–38 hr

Mechanism of Action

Binds to sterols in fungal cell membranes, impairing membrane integrity. Cells lose intracellular potassium and other cellular contents and, eventually, die.

Contraindications

Hypersensitivity to nystatin or its components

Interactions

DRUGS

None reported by manufacturer

Adverse Reactions

ENDO: Hyperglycemia (oral suspension)
GI: Abdominal pain, diarrhea, nausea, vomiting (oral forms)

Childbearing Considerations

PREGNANCY

- It is not known if drug causes fetal harm.
- Use with caution only if benefit to mother outweighs potential risk to fetus.

LACTATION

- It is not known if drug is present in breast milk.
- Patient should check with prescriber before breastfeeding.

Nursing Considerations

- Monitor patient for adverse reactions.

PATIENT TEACHING

- Instruct patient using oral suspension to use the dropper that comes with product or a calibrated device to measure dosage. Tell patient to shake suspension well before using.
- Tell patient using powder form to prepare only a single dose at a time, because it does not contain preservatives. Add prescribed dosage to about 4 ounces of water. Stir well and divide into smaller portions. Patient should take immediately, using one portion at a time, until entire volume is used.
- Teach parents or caregiver to swab oral suspension on both sides of mouth or drop one-half the dose on each side of tongue when administering to infants.
- Tell patient to swish oral suspension in her mouth as long as possible before swallowing.

- Review adverse reactions with patient and to report them to prescriber if prolonged or severe.

obiltoxaximab
Anthim

Class and Category

Pharmacologic class: Monoclonal antibody
Therapeutic class: Antianthrax agent

Indications and Dosages

* *To prevent inhalational anthrax due to* Bacillus anthracis *when alternative therapies are not appropriate or available; to treat inhalational anthrax due to* B. anthracis *in combination with appropriate antibacterial drugs*

I.V. INFUSION

Adults and children weighing more than 40 kg (88 lb). 16 mg/kg as a single dose.
Adults and children weighing more than 15 kg (33 lb) to 40 kg (88 lb). 24 mg/kg as a single dose.
Children weighing 15 kg (33 lb) or less. 32 mg/kg as a single dose.

Drug Administration

I.V.

- Do not shake drug vial.
- Expect to premedicate patient with diphenhydramine because drug can cause serious hypersensitivity reactions, including anaphylaxis.
- There are two ways to prepare and dilute the drug for infusion.
Using infusion-bag method
- First, calculate the required dosage and volume according to manufacturer guidelines. Each single vial allows delivery of 6 ml of obiltoxaximab.
- Select an appropriate-size bag of 0.9% Sodium Chloride Injection.
- Withdraw a volume of solution from the bag equal to the calculated volume in milliliters of drug to be administered and discard. Then withdraw the required volume of drug from the drug vial(s) and discard any unused portion remaining in the vial(s).
- Transfer the required volume of drug into the selected infusion bag.

- Gently invert bag to mix the solution. Do not shake.
- The prepared solution is stable for 8 hours stored in the refrigerator or at room temperature.

Using syringe method

- First calculate the required dosage and volume of drug according to manufacturer guidelines.
- Select an appropriate-size syringe for the total volume of infusion to be administered.
- Using the selected syringe, withdraw the required volume of drug. Discard any unused portion remaining in the vial(s).
- Withdraw an appropriate amount of 0.9% Sodium Chloride Injection, using the syringe containing drug, to prepare the total infusion volume specified in manufacturer guidelines.
- Gently mix solution. Do not shake.
- Once diluted in the syringe, administer immediately. Do not store solution in syringe.
- Administer as an infusion using either of the stated methods of dilution.
- Use a 0.22-micron in-line filter and infuse at the rate specified in the manufacturer guidelines in order for drug to be administered over 90 minutes.
- Flush the intravenous line with 0.9% Sodium Chloride Injection at the end of the infusion.
- *Incompatibilities:* Other drugs, other solutions except for 0.9% Sodium Chloride Injection

Route	Onset	Peak	Duration
I.V.	Unknown	Unknown	Unknown

Half-life: 15–23 days

Mechanism of Action

Binds to the PA component of the *B. anthracis* toxin to inactivate it.

Contraindications

Hypersensitivity to obiltoxaximab or its components

Interactions

DRUGS

None reported by manufacturer

Adverse Reactions

CNS: Dizziness, dysphonia, fatigue, fever, headache
CV: Chest discomfort or pain, palpitations

EENT: Dry mouth, nasal congestion, oropharyngeal pain, rhinorrhea, sinus congestion
GI: Vomiting
HEME: Leukopenia, lymphopenia, neutropenia
MS: Extremity pain, myalgia, musculoskeletal pain
RESP: Cough, cyanosis, dyspnea, upper respiratory infections
SKIN: Pruritus, urticaria
Other: Anaphylaxis; antibody formation against obiltoxaximab; increased creatine phosphokinase; infusion-site reactions of bruising, discoloration, pain, swelling, or urticaria

Childbearing Considerations

PREGNANCY

- It is not known if drug causes fetal harm.
- Use with caution only if benefit to mother outweighs potential risk to fetus.

LACTATION

- It is not known if drug is present in breast milk.
- Patient should check with prescriber before breastfeeding.

Nursing Considerations

- Know that obiltoxaximab should only be used for prophylaxis when its benefit for prevention of inhalational anthrax outweighs the risk of anaphylaxis and other hypersensitivity reactions.
- Be aware that because obiltoxaximab does not have antibacterial activity, it must be used in combination with appropriate antibacterial drugs.

! WARNING Be aware that because of the risk for serious hypersensitivity reactions, including anaphylaxis, drug should be administered in an environment conducive to treating anaphylaxis. Monitor patient closely for signs and symptoms of hypersensitivity that may progress rapidly to anaphylaxis. Know that hypersensitivity reactions were the most common adverse reactions that occurred in the safety trials for obiltoxaximab. Observe the patient throughout the infusion and for a period of time after administration. Stop infusion immediately if hypersensitivity or anaphylaxis occurs, notify prescribe and provide supportive care, as ordered.

N
O

PATIENT TEACHING

! WARNING Inform patient of the possibility of an allergic reaction that could become severe with obiltoxaximab administration. Reassure him that he will be given a drug to help prevent this before obiltoxaximab is given. Review the signs and symptoms of an allergic reaction with the patient and stress importance of alerting the healthcare staff administering drug if any should occur. Tell him that if he experiences any reactions after going home, he should seek immediate medical attention.

- Tell patient that he will only need to receive drug one time.

ocrelizumab
Ocrevus

Class and Category
Pharmacologic class: Monoclonal antibody
Therapeutic class: Antimultiple sclerotic

Indications and Dosages
✳ *To treat primary progressive multiple sclerosis; to treat relapsing forms of multiple sclerosis, including active secondary progressive disease, clinically isolated syndrome, or relapsing-remitting disease*

I.V. INFUSION
Adults. *Initial:* 300 mg, followed 2 wk later by a second 300-mg infusion. *Maintenance:* Single infusion of 600 mg every 6 months beginning 6 months after first 300-mg dose.

Drug Administration
- Expect to premedicate patient with 100 mg of methylprednisolone (or an equivalent corticosteroid) intravenously about 30 minutes before each ocrelizumab infusion, to reduce the frequency and severity of infusion reactions. Also expect to premedicate patient with an antihistamine such as diphenhydramine about 30 to 60 minutes prior to each ocrelizumab infusion to further reduce infusion reactions. Know that the administration of an antipyretic such as acetaminophen may also be ordered.

I.V.
- Do not shake drug vial.

- Withdraw prescribed dose and dilute in an infusion bag containing 0.9% Sodium Chloride Injection to a final drug concentration of approximately 1.2 mg/ml. For example, withdraw 10 ml (300 mg) from vial and inject into a 250-ml infusion bag or withdraw 20 ml (600 mg) from vial and inject into a 500-ml infusion bag. Do not use any other diluents to dilute ocrelizumab.
- Prepared solution can be stored for up to 24 hours in the refrigerator or 8 hours at room temperature, which must include the infusion time.
- Administer the diluted solution through a dedicated line using an infusion set with a 0.2- or 0.22-micron in-line filter.
- If prepared solution was refrigerated, allow solution to warm to room temperature before administering.
- Infuse initial two doses starting at 30 ml per hour, then increased by 30 ml per hour every 30 min to maximum infusion rate of 180 ml per hour with an infusion duration of 2.5 hours or longer.
- Infuse maintenance dose starting at 40 ml per hour, increased by 40 ml per hour every 30 min with maximum infusion of 200 ml per hour and duration of infusion 3.5 hours or longer. Alternatively, if patient has had no prior serious infusion reaction with any previous infusion, begin infusing drug at 100 ml per hour for the first 15 minutes, increase to 200 ml per hour for the next 15 minutes, then increase to 250 ml per hour for the next 30 minutes followed by an increase to 300 ml per hour for the remaining 60 minutes with an infusion duration of 2 hours or longer.
- Monitor patient for infusion reactions for at least 1 hour after completion of the infusion.
- Expect to administer a planned infusion that is missed as soon as possible. It should not be withheld until the next scheduled dose. Reset the dose schedule to administer the next sequential dose 6 months after the missed dose is administered, because doses must be separated by at least 5 months.
- *Incompatibilities:* Solutions other than 0.9% Sodium Chloride Injection

Route	Onset	Peak	Duration
I.V.	14 days	Unknown	72 wk

Half-life: 26 days

⧉ Mechanism of Action

Although precise mechanism is unknown, ocrelizumab binds to CD20, a cell surface antigen on pre-B and mature B lymphocytes, which results in antibody-dependent cellular cytolysis and complement-mediated lysis to help relieve symptoms of multiple sclerosis.

⧉ Contraindications

Active hepatitis B virus infection, hypersensitivity to ocrelizumab or its components

⧉ Interactions

DRUGS

other immune-modulating or immunosuppressants: Increased risk of immunosuppression

vaccines (live or live-attenuated): Possibly decreased effectiveness or increased risk of infection

⧉ Adverse Reactions

CNS: Depression, dizziness, fatigue, fever, headache

CV: Hypotension, peripheral edema, tachycardia

EENT: Laryngeal or pharyngeal edema, oropharyngeal pain, throat irritation

GI: Diarrhea, nausea

HEME: Neutropenia

MS: Back or extremity pain

RESP: Bronchospasms, cough, dyspnea, respiratory infections

SKIN: Erythema, flushing, pruritus, rash, skin infections, urticaria

Other: Anaphylaxis, anti-ocrelizumab antibody formation, decreased immunoglobulins, herpes virus-associated infections, infusion reactions (may become severe), reactivation of hepatitis B

⧉ Childbearing Considerations

PREGNANCY

- Pregnancy exposure registry: 1-833-872-4370 or www.ocrevuspregnancyregistry.com.
- It is not known if drug causes fetal harm. However, as a humanized monoclonal antibody, it may cross the placental barrier. This may increase the potential for transient peripheral B-cell depletion and lymphocytopenia in the neonate.
- The safety and effectiveness of vaccine administration in these infants are unknown. Live or live-attenuated vaccines should not be administered to infant exposed to the drug in utero before confirming the recovery of B-cell counts.
- Use with caution only if benefit to mother outweighs potential risk to fetus.

LACTATION

- It is not known if drug is present in breast milk. This makes B-cell depletion in the breast-fed infant unknown.
- Patient should check with prescriber before breastfeeding.

REPRODUCTION

- Instruct women of childbearing age to use effective contraception during drug therapy and for 6 months after the last drug dose.

⧉ Nursing Considerations

- Expect to perform hepatitis B virus (HBV) screening, as ordered, prior to initiating ocrelizumab therapy because drug is contraindicated in patients with active HBV that has been confirmed by positive test results.
- Administer all necessary immunizations, as ordered, according to guidelines at least 4 weeks prior to initiation of ocrelizumab therapy for live or live-attenuated vaccines and, whenever possible, at least 2 weeks before initiation of ocrelizumab therapy for nonlive vaccines. This is because drug may interfere with effectiveness of nonlive vaccines, and safety of immunization with live or live-attenuated vaccines following ocrelizumab therapy is unknown.
- Assess patient for evidence of an active infection prior to every infusion of ocrelizumab. Serious infections caused by herpes simplex virus and *varicella zoster* may occur at any time during drug therapy with ocrelizumab and may become life-threatening. Infections may include central nervous system infections such as encephalitis or meningitis, disseminated skin and soft-tissue infections, and intraocular infections. If present, know that the infusion must be delayed until the infection is resolved.

N
O

! WARNING Monitor patient for life-threatening infusion reactions. If present, stop infusion immediately, provide supportive care, as ordered, and know that drug will be permanently discontinued. If infusion reaction is not life-threatening but severe, expect to immediately interrupt the infusion and provide supportive treatment, as ordered and needed. Expect to restart the infusion only after all symptoms have resolved. When restarting, expect to restart at half the infusion rate at the time of onset of the infusion reaction. If this rate is tolerated, increase the rate per the standard protocol. If patient is experiencing a mild to moderate infusion reaction, expect to reduce the infusion rate to half the rate at the onset of the infusion reaction and maintain the reduced rate for at least 30 minutes. If this rate is tolerated, expect to increase the rate per the standard protocol.

! WARNING Know that progressive multifocal leukoencephalopathy (PML) has occurred in patients treated with other anti-CD20 antibodies and other multiple sclerosis therapies. Patients at risk included patients who were immunocompromised or received polytherapy with immunosuppressants. Monitor patient for PML, which may include changes in memory, orientation, or thinking that could lead to confusion and personality changes. Other symptoms include clumsiness of limbs, disturbance of vision, and progressive weakness on one side of the body. If present, notify prescriber immediately, because PML usually leads to death or severe disability.

PATIENT TEACHING

- Explain the importance of as well as the risks associated with ocrelizumab therapy.

! WARNING Tell patient she will receive medication before the infusion to lessen or prevent infusion reactions. However, inform patient that infusion reactions may occur up to 24 hours after the infusion and include allergic types of signs and symptoms. If adverse reactions occur in this time frame, patient should notify prescriber and if reactions are severe, seek immediate emergency medical care.

- Review signs and symptoms of herpes infection, including change in vision, cold or genital sores, confusion, eye redness or pain, persistent or severe headache, or shingles. If present, tell patient to notify prescriber.
- Instruct patient to report changes in memory, orientation, or thinking that could lead to confusion and personality changes. Other symptoms to report include clumsiness of limbs, disturbance of vision, and progressive weakness on one side of the body. If present, urge patient to notify prescriber immediately.
- Inform patient that live or live-attenuated vaccines should not be given within 4 weeks of starting drug therapy and for 2 weeks prior to starting drug therapy for nonlive vaccines. Also tell mothers of infants exposed to drug during pregnancy to inform pediatrician of exposure before any live or live-attenuated vaccines are administered to the infant.
- Inform patient that ocrelizumab may increase risk of breast cancer. Stress importance of following standard breast cancer screening guidelines.

ofatumumab
Kesimpta

Class and Category
Pharmacologic class: CD20-directed cytolytic antibody
Therapeutic class: Immunosuppressant

Indications and Dosages
* *To treat relapsing forms of multiple sclerosis, including clinically isolated syndrome, relapsing-remitting disease, and active secondary progressive disease*

SUBCUTANEOUS INJECTION
Adults. *Initial:* 20 mg, repeated at wks 2 and 3. *Maintenance:* 20 mg monthly starting at wk 4.

Drug Administration
SUBCUTANEOUS

- Remove pen or prefilled syringe from refrigerator and allow drug to reach room temperature (15–30 min).
- Inspect drug solution. Discard if particles are visible or solution appears cloudy.

- Administer in the abdomen, thigh, or outer upper arm.
- Do not inject into abnormal areas or where skin is bruised, hard, red, scaly, or tender.
- Pens and prefilled syringes are for one-time use.
- Store in refrigerator until ready to use.

Route	Onset	Peak	Duration
SubQ	Unknown	Unknown	Unknown

Half-life: 16 days

Mechanism of Action

Precise mechanism of action is unknown, but is thought to involve binding to CD20, a cell surface antigen present on pre-B and mature B lymphocytes. This binding results in antibody-dependent cellular cytolysis and complement-mediated lysis.

Contraindications

Active hepatitis B viral infection, hypersensitivity to ofatumumab or its components

Interactions

DRUGS

immunosuppressive drugs such as systemic corticosteroids: Increased risk of infection
live-attenuated or live vaccines: Increased risk of adverse effects

Adverse Reactions

CNS: Headache, **progressive multifocal leukoencephalopathy (PML)**
GU: UTI
MS: Back pain
RESP: Upper respiratory infections
Other: Anti-ofatumumab antibody formation, decreased blood immunoglobulin M, infections (bacterial, fungal, new or reactivated viral infections), injection-related systemic reactions (chills, fatigue, fever, headache, myalgia), injection-site local reactions (erythema, pain, pruritus, swelling)

Childbearing Considerations

PREGNANCY

- It is not known if drug causes fetal harm, but animal studies suggest that fetal harm can occur due to fetal B-cell lymphopenia and reduced antibody response.
- Use with caution only if benefit to mother outweighs potential risk to fetus.

- If infant was exposed to drug in utero, live or live-attenuated vaccines should be withheld until B-cell counts have recovered.

LACTATION

- It is not known if drug is present in breast milk.
- Patient should check with prescriber before breastfeeding.

REPRODUCTION

- Females of childbearing age should use effective contraception during drug therapy and for 6 months after drug is discontinued.

Nursing Considerations

- Determine that screenings for hepatitis B virus (HBV) and quantitative serum immunoglobulins have been done before first dose is given. Therapy with ofatumumab is contraindicated in the presence of HBV. Therapy may have to be withheld in patients with low serum immunoglobulins until levels are higher.
- Ensure that all immunizations according to immunization guidelines have been administered to patient at least 4 weeks prior to starting ofatumumab for live or live-attenuated vaccines, and whenever possible, at least 2 weeks before for inactivated vaccines.
- Expect to delay initiation of therapy if patient has an active infection until infection is resolved. Be aware patient is at risk for infections, including serious bacterial, fungal, and new or reactivated viral infections, during therapy. Some infections may become life-threatening. Monitor patient for infections and institute infection control measures. Notify prescriber if an infection is suspected.

! **WARNING** Be aware that progressive multifocal leukoencephalopathy (PML) has the potential to occur with ofatumumab therapy. Notify prescriber at the first sign of PML, withhold drug, and expect patient to undergo a diagnostic workup to confirm diagnosis. Signs and symptoms to be alert for include changes in thinking, memory, and orientation that lead to confusion; disturbances of vision; personality changes; and progressive clumsiness or weakness on one side of the body. Be aware that these changes can gradually occur over days to weeks. Expect drug to be discontinued if PML is confirmed.

N
O

PATIENT TEACHING

- Teach patient or caregiver how to administer a subcutaneous injection.
- Instruct patient or caregiver to remove pen or prefilled syringe from refrigerator and allow drug to reach room temperature (15–30 minutes).
- Tell patient to inspect drug solution. Discard if solution contains visible particles or is cloudy.
- Instruct patient to inject drug into the abdomen, thigh, or outer upper arm and not to inject into moles, scars, stretch marks, or areas where skin is bruised, hard, red, scaly, or tender.
- Remind patient or caregiver that pen or prefilled syringe is for one use only and that drug should be refrigerated until ready to use.
- Tell patient that if a dose is missed, it should be given as soon as possible without waiting until the next scheduled dose. Subsequent doses should be administered at the recommended intervals.
- Review signs and symptoms of infection and infection control measures. Stress importance of notifying prescriber if an infection occurs, as it can become quite serious.
- Inform patient that vaccines should not be received during ofatumumab therapy. Inform mothers who were treated with drug during pregnancy not to have their infants receive live or live-attenuated vaccines until prescriber indicates it is safe to do so.
- Tell patient that injection-site reactions may occur, usually within 24 hours and predominantly after the first injection. If present, tell patient to notify prescriber.
- Advise women of childbearing age to use effective contraception during drug therapy and for 6 months after drug has been discontinued.

ofloxacin

▤ Class and Category

Pharmacologic class: Fluoroquinolone
Therapeutic class: Antibiotic

▤ Indications and Dosages

✴ *To treat acute, uncomplicated cystitis caused by* Escherichia coli *or* Klebsiella pneumoniae

TABLETS

Adults. 200 mg every 12 hr for 3 days.

✴ *To treat uncomplicated cystitis caused by* Citrobacter diversus, Enterobacter aerogenes, Proteus mirabilis, *or* Pseudomonas aeruginosa

TABLETS

Adults. 200 mg every 12 hr for 7 days.

✴ *To treat complicated UTI caused by* C. diversus, E. coli, K. pneumoniae, P. mirabilis, *or* P. aeruginosa

Adults. 200 mg every 12 hr for 10 days.

✴ *To treat pelvic inflammatory disease caused by susceptible organisms only if standard cephalosporin therapy is not feasible and community prevalence of quinolone-resistant gonococcal organisms is low*

TABLETS

Adults. 400 mg every 12 hr with metronidazole P.O. for 10 to 14 days.

✴ *To treat prostatitis caused by* E. coli

TABLETS

Adults. 300 mg every 12 hr for 6 wk.

✴ *To treat acute exacerbation of chronic bronchitis or community-acquired pneumonia caused by* Haemophilus influenzae *or* Streptococcus pneumoniae *and uncomplicated skin and soft-tissue infections caused by* Proteus mirabilis, Staphylococcus aureus *or* Streptococcus pyogenes

TABLETS

Adults. 400 mg every 12 hr for 10 to 14 days.

±**DOSAGE ADJUSTMENT** If creatinine clearance is 20 to 50 ml/min, dosing interval possibly reduced to every 24 hr; if clearance is less than 10 ml/min, dosage possibly reduced by 50% and given every 24 hr. For patients with severe liver dysfunction, maximum dose limited to 400 mg daily.

▤ Drug Administration

P.O.

- Administer each dose with a full glass of water.
- Do not administer antacids, iron or zinc preparations, or other drugs (such as didanosine and sucralfate) within 2 hours of drug, to prevent decreased or delayed drug absorption.

Route	Onset	Peak	Duration
P.O.	Unknown	0.5–2 hr	Unknown

Half-life: 4–8 hr

Mechanism of Action

Inhibits synthesis of the bacterial enzyme DNA gyrase by counteracting excessive supercoiling of DNA during replication or transcription. Inhibition of DNA gyrase causes rapid- and slow-growing bacterial cells to die.

Contraindications

Hypersensitivity to ofloxacin, other fluoroquinolones, or their components

Interactions

DRUGS

aluminum-, calcium-, or magnesium-containing antacids; didanosine; ferrous sulfate; magnesium-containing laxatives; multivitamins; sevelamer; sucralfate; zinc: Decreased absorption of ofloxacin
insulin, oral antidiabetic drugs: Possibly disturbance in blood glucose control with these agents
NSAIDs: Possibly increased risk of CNS stimulation and seizures
theophylline: Increased risk of theophylline-related adverse reactions
procainamide: Decreased renal clearance of procainamide
warfarin: Possibly increased anticoagulant activity and risk of bleeding

Adverse Reactions

CNS: Aggressiveness, agitation, ataxia, **CVA**, delirium, disorientation, disturbance in attention, dizziness, drowsiness, emotional lability, exacerbation of extrapyramidal disorders and myasthenia gravis, fever, headache, incoordination, insomnia, light-headedness, mania, memory impairment, nervousness, peripheral neuropathy, psychotic reactions, restlessness, **suicidal ideation**, syncope
CV: Arrhythmias, prolonged QT interval, severe hypotension, torsades de pointes, vasculitis
EENT: Blurred vision; diplopia; disturbances in equilibrium, hearing, smell, and taste
ENDO: Hyperglycemia, **hypoglycemia**
GI: Abdominal cramps or pain, **acute hepatic necrosis or failure,** diarrhea, **hepatitis,** jaundice, nausea, **pseudomembranous colitis,** vomiting
GU: Acute renal insufficiency or failure, interstitial nephritis, renal calculi, vaginal candidiasis

HEME: Agranulocytosis, aplastic or hemolytic anemia, leukopenia, pancytopenia, thrombocytopenia
MS: Arthralgia; myalgia; **rhabdomyolysis;** tendinitis; tendon inflammation, pain, or rupture
RESP: Hypersensitivity pneumonitis, pulmonary edema
SKIN: Blisters, diaphoresis, erythema, **erythema multiforme, exfoliative dermatitis,** photosensitivity, pruritus, rash, **Stevens–Johnson syndrome, toxic epidermal necrolysis,** urticaria
Other: Acidosis, anaphylaxis, infusion-site phlebitis, serum sickness

Childbearing Considerations

PREGNANCY

- It is not known if drug causes fetal harm.
- Use with caution only if benefit to mother outweighs potential risk to fetus.

LACTATION

- Drug is present in breast milk.
- A decision should be made to discontinue breastfeeding or the drug to avoid potential serious adverse reactions in the breastfed infant.

Nursing Considerations

- Know that because of increased risk of prolonged QT interval, ofloxacin shouldn't be used if patient has had a prolonged QT interval, has an uncorrected electrolyte disorder, or takes a Class IA or III antiarrhythmic. Monitor elderly patients closely because risk of prolonged QT interval may be increased in this group.

! **WARNING** Monitor patient closely for hypersensitivity, which may occur as early as first dose. Reaction may include angioedema, bronchospasm, dyspnea, itching, jaundice, rash, shortness of breath, and urticaria. If these signs or symptoms appear, notify prescriber immediately and expect to discontinue drug.

- Know that fluoroquinolones like ofloxacin have caused disabling and potentially irreversible serious adverse reactions from different body systems that can occur together in the same patient. These reactions can occur within hours to weeks after starting the drug and usually cause central nervous system effects, peripheral neuropathy, tendinitis, and tendon rupture. All ages of patients and patients without any preexisting risk factors have experienced these reactions. Notify prescriber and expect to discontinue ofloxacin immediately at the first signs or symptoms of any serious adverse reactions.

- Notify prescriber if patient has symptoms of peripheral neuropathy (burning, numbness, pain, tingling, weakness, or altered sensations of light touch, pain, position sense, temperature, or vibration sense), which could be permanent; tendon rupture (inflammation and pain), which may occur more often in patients (especially elderly ones) taking corticosteroids and requires immediate rest; or a severe photosensitivity reaction. In each case, expect to stop ofloxacin.
- Maintain adequate hydration to prevent development of highly concentrated urine and crystalluria.
- Expect an increased risk of toxicity in severe hepatic disease, including cirrhosis.
- Be aware that ofloxacin may stimulate the CNS and aggravate seizure disorders. Also know that the drug may cause many psychiatric adverse reactions. Monitor patient closely.
- If diarrhea develops, notify prescriber because it may indicate pseudomembranous colitis. Ofloxacin may have to be discontinued and additional therapy started.
- Be alert for secondary fungal infection.
- Monitor patient closely for hypoglycemia, especially if patient is elderly, has diabetes or renal insufficiency, or is taking hypoglycemic drugs such as sulfonylureas. Hypoglycemia can become severe and result in coma. Treat hypoglycemia quickly and effectively. Notify prescriber of incident and expect that drug may be replaced with a different antibiotic for this patient.

PATIENT TEACHING
- Encourage patient to take each dose with a full glass of water.
- Tell patient to complete full course of ofloxacin therapy exactly as prescribed, even if he feels better before it's complete.
- Urge patient not to take antacids, iron or zinc preparations, or other drugs (such as didanosine and sucralfate), within 2 hours of ofloxacin to prevent decreased or delayed drug absorption.

- Advise patient to avoid hazardous activities until CNS effects of drug are known.
- Tell patient to limit exposure to sun and ultraviolet light to prevent phototoxicity.
- Advise patient to notify prescriber immediately about abnormal motor or sensory function, burning skin, hives, itching, rapid heart rate, rash, and tendon pain. Also advise patient to stop taking ofloxacin immediately and notify prescriber if any other persistent, serious, or worsening adverse effects occur.

! **WARNING** Urge patient to seek medical care immediately for trouble breathing or swallowing, which may signal an allergic reaction.

- Instruct diabetic patient who takes an antidiabetic agent or insulin to notify prescriber immediately if he develops a hypoglycemic reaction.
- Advise patient to notify prescriber if diarrhea develops, even up to 2 months after ofloxacin therapy ends. Additional therapy may be needed.

olanzapine
Zyprexa, Zyprexa IntraMuscular, Zyprexa Zydis

olanzapine pamoate monohydrate
Zyprexa Relprevv

Class and Category
Pharmacologic class: Thienobenzodiazepine derivative
Therapeutic class: Antipsychotic

Indications and Dosages
✱ *To treat schizophrenia*
ORALLY DISINTEGRATING TABLETS, TABLETS
Adults. *Initial:* 5 to 10 mg daily. Once 10 mg daily dosage reached, additional dosage adjustment made in 5-mg increments every wk, as needed. *Maintenance:* 10 mg daily. *Maximum:* 20 mg daily.

Adolescents age 13 and over. *Initial:* 2.5 to 5 mg daily, increased in increments of 2.5 mg or 5 mg, as needed. *Maintenance:* 10 mg daily. *Maximum:* 20 mg daily.

I.M. INJECTION-ER (ZYPREXA RELPREVV)

Adults who have been taking 10 mg daily orally. *Initial:* 210 mg every 2 wk for first 8 wk, then decreased to 150 mg every 2 wk. Alternatively, 405 mg every 4 wk for first 8 wk, then decreased to 300 mg every 4 wk. **Adults who have been taking 15 mg daily orally.** *Initial:* 300 mg every 2 wk for 8 wk, then decreased to 210 mg every 2 wk or 405 mg every 4 wk. **Adults who have been taking 20 mg daily orally.** 300 mg every 2 wk.

* *To treat manic phase of bipolar I disorder (manic or mixed episodes)*

ORALLY DISINTEGRATING TABLETS, TABLETS

Adults. *Initial:* 10 to 15 mg daily decreased or increased in 5-mg increments no less than every 24 hr, as needed. *Maintenance:* 5 to 20 mg daily. *Maximum:* 20 mg daily. **Adolescents age 13 and over.** *Initial:* 2.5 to 5 mg daily, increased, as needed, in 2.5- or 5-mg increments. *Maintenance:* 10 mg daily. *Maximum:* 20 mg daily.

* *As adjunct to lithium or valproate therapy to treat bipolar I disorder*

ORALLY DISINTEGRATING TABLETS, TABLETS

Adults. *Initial:* 10 mg daily with lithium or valproate sodium, increased or decreased by 5 mg no less than every 24 hr, as needed. *Maintenance:* 5 to 20 mg/day. *Maximum:* 20 mg daily.

* *To treat agitation associated with schizophrenia and bipolar I mania*

I.M. INJECTION (ZYPREXA INTRAMUSCULAR)

Adults. 5 to 10 mg, as needed. Repeat as needed every 2 to 4 hr for total of 3 doses. *Maximum:* Three doses of 10 mg administered with second dose given after 2 hr and third dose given 2 hr after second dose providing patient is not exhibiting orthostatic hypotension.

±**DOSAGE ADJUSTMENT** For short-acting oral form, initial dosage possibly reduced to 5 mg for debilitated patients, those prone to hypotension, and female nonsmokers over age 65. For short-acting I.M. form, dosage decreased to 5 mg for elderly patients and 2.5 mg for debilitated patients, female nonsmokers over age 65, and those prone to hypotension. For extended-release I.M. form, dosage decreased to 150 mg every 4 weeks for patients who are debilitated, female nonsmokers over 65, or those prone to hypotension.

Drug Administration

P.O.

- For oral disintegrating tablets, open sachet and peel back foil on blister. Do not push tablet through foil. Immediately upon opening the blister, remove tablet with dry, gloved hands. Place tablet on patient's tongue. It can be swallowed after it dissolves with or without liquid.

I.M.

- Keep patient recumbent after I.M. injection of olanzapine if bradycardia, dizziness, drowsiness, or hypoventilation occurs. Don't let patient sit or stand up until blood pressure and heart rate have returned to baseline.
- There are two formulations for I.M. injection. One is an immediate-release formulation and one is an extended release. They are not interchangeable. When administering drug intramuscularly, make sure the right formulation is being administered.

Immediate-release formulation

- Reconstitute by dissolving contents of vial in 2.1 ml Sterile Water to yield 5 mg/ml.
- Solution should be clear yellow.
- Administer within 1 hour.
- Inject I.M. slowly, deep into muscle mass.

Extended-release formulation

- Reconstitute using only the diluent provided as follows: for 150- or 210-mg dose, use 1.3 ml of diluent; for 300-mg dose, use 1.8 ml of diluent; and for 405-mg dose, use 2.3 ml of diluent.
- Loosen the powder in the vial by lightly tapping the vial.
- Withdraw predetermined diluent into syringe. Inject into powder vial and withdraw air to equalize pressure. Remove needle and hold vial upright.
- Pad a hard surface, then tap vial firmly and repeatedly on the surface until no powder is visible. Shake vial vigorously until

suspension appears smooth and consistent in color and texture (yellow and opaque). If foam has formed, let vial stand until it has dissipated.

- Administer immediately or, if stored for up to 24 hr, remember that drug vial must be vigorously shaken to resuspend solution prior to administration.
- Attach new needle to syringe and slowly withdraw desired amount into the syringe. Remove needle from syringe.
- Administer by first attaching a 19-gauge (1.5-inch) needle or larger to syringe to prevent clogging. Obese patients may need a 2-inch needle. Inject deeply into the gluteal muscle. Withdraw needle. Do not massage injection site.
- Following the injection of extended-release olanzapine, patient may experience a syndrome similar to an olanzapine overdose, with delirium and sedation being the primary symptoms. Patient must be observed for 3 hours following each injection for this syndrome. Notify prescriber immediately if it should occur.

Route	Onset	Peak	Duration
P.O.	Unknown	6 hr	Unknown
I.M.	Unknown	15–45 min	Unknown
I.M./E.R.	Unknown	7 days	Unknown

Half-life: 21–54 hr (P.O.); 30 days (I.M.)

Mechanism of Action

May achieve antipsychotic effects by antagonizing dopamine and serotonin receptors. Anticholinergic effects may result from competitive binding to and antagonism of the muscarinic receptors M_1 through M_5.

Contraindications

Hypersensitivity to olanzapine or its components

Interactions

DRUGS

anticholinergic drugs: May increase risk for severe GI adverse reactions related to hypomotility
antihypertensives: Increased effects of antihypertensives, increased risk of hypotension
carbamazepine, rifampin: Increased olanzapine clearance

charcoal: Reduced olanzapine level by about 60%; interferes with olanzapine effectiveness
CNS depressants: Additive CNS depression, potentiated orthostatic hypotension
diazepam: Potentiated orthostatic hypotension
dopamine agonists, levodopa: Antagonized effects of these drugs
fluoxetine, fluvoxamine: Decreased olanzapine clearance
lorazepam (parenteral): Possibly increased somnolence with I.M. olanzapine injection

ACTIVITIES

alcohol use: Potentiated orthostatic hypotension
smoking: Decreased blood olanzapine level

Adverse Reactions

CNS: Abnormal gait, agitation, akathisia, altered thermoregulation, amnesia, anxiety, asthenia, dizziness, euphoria, fatigue, fever, headache, hypertonia, insomnia, motor and sensory instability, nervousness, **neuroleptic malignant syndrome**, restless leg syndrome, restlessness, somnolence, stuttering, **suicidal ideation**, syncope, tardive dyskinesia, thirst, tremor

CV: Bradycardia, chest pain, elevated triglyceride levels, hyperlipidemia, hypertension, **hypotension**, orthostatic hypotension, peripheral edema, tachycardia, **venous thromboembolic events**

EENT: Amblyopia, dry mouth, increased salivation, pharyngitis, rhinitis

ENDO: Diabetic coma, diabetic ketoacidosis, hyperglycemia, **hyperprolactinemia**

GI: Abdominal pain, **cholestatic** or **mixed liver injury**, constipation, dysphagia, elevated liver enzymes, **hepatitis**, increased appetite, jaundice, nausea, **pancreatitis**, vomiting

GU: Priapism, urinary incontinence, UTI

HEME: Agranulocytosis, leukopenia, neutropenia

MS: Arthralgia; back, joint, or limb pain; muscle spasms and twitching; **rhabdomyolysis**

RESP: Cough, **pulmonary embolism**

SKIN: Ecchymosis, photosensitivity, pruritus, rash, urticaria

Other: Anaphylaxis, angioedema, discontinuation reaction, **drug reaction with eosinophilia and systemic symptoms (DRESS)**, flu-like symptoms, injection-site abscess, weight gain

Childbearing Considerations

PREGNANCY

- Pregnancy exposure registry: 1-866-961-2388 or http://womensmentalhealth.org/clinical-and-research-programs/pregnancyregistry/.
- Drug may cause fetal harm, as exposure to drug during the third trimester of pregnancy increases the risk for extrapyramidal and/or withdrawal symptoms following delivery.
- Use with caution only if benefit to mother outweighs potential risk to fetus.

LACTATION

- Drug is present in breast milk.
- Patient should check with prescriber before breastfeeding. However, if breastfeeding occurs, infant should be monitored for excess sedation, extrapyramidal symptoms, poor feeding, and irritability.

REPRODUCTION

- Drug may cause an increase in serum prolactin levels, which may lead to a reversible reduction in fertility in females of childbearing age.

Nursing Considerations

! **WARNING** Olanzapine shouldn't be used for elderly patients with dementia-related psychosis because drug increases risk of death in these patients.

- Use cautiously in patients with hepatic impairment or conditions associated with limited hepatic functional reserve and in patients who are being treated with potentially hepatotoxic drugs. Also use cautiously in patients with known cardiovascular or cerebrovascular disease and conditions that would predispose patient to hypotension, such as presence of dehydration, hypovolemia, or treatment with antihypertensive medications because of the increased risk for bradycardia, hypotension, and syncope.
- Use cautiously in patients with a current diagnosis or prior history of constipation, paralytic ileus or related conditions, significant prostatic hypertrophy, or urinary retention, because of drug's cholinergic antagonism.
- Be aware that olanzapine may worsen such conditions as angle-closure glaucoma, benign prostatic hyperplasia, and seizures. Monitor patient closely.

- Monitor patient's blood pressure routinely during therapy because olanzapine may cause orthostatic hypotension.
- Assess daily weight to detect fluid retention or metabolic changes.
- Notify prescriber if patient develops tardive dyskinesia or urinary incontinence.
- Be alert for and immediately report signs of neuroleptic malignant syndrome.
- Watch patient closely (especially adolescent and young adults), for suicidal tendencies, particularly when therapy starts and dosage changes, because depression may worsen temporarily during these times, possibly leading to suicidal ideation.
- Monitor patient's lipid levels throughout therapy, as ordered, because olanzapine may cause significant elevations.
- Monitor patient's blood glucose level routinely because olanzapine may increase risk of hyperglycemia.
- Monitor CBC often during first few months of therapy, especially if patient has low WBC count or history of drug-induced leukopenia or neutropenia. If WBC count declines, and especially if neutrophil count drops below 1,000/mm^3, expect olanzapine to be discontinued. If neutropenia is significant, also monitor patient for fever or other evidence of infection and provide appropriate treatment, as prescribed.
- Be aware that drug may cause hyperprolactinemia, which, in turn, may reduce pituitary gonadotropin secretion. This then inhibits reproductive function by impairing gonadal steroidogenesis in both female and male patients. In addition, longstanding hyperprolactinemia may decrease bone density in patient when it is associated with hypogonadism.

! **WARNING** Know that olanzapine may cause a drug reaction with eosinophilia and systemic symptoms called DRESS. Although uncommon, it can become fatal. Assess patient regularly for a cutaneous reaction exhibited by eosinophilia, exfoliative dermatitis, fever, lymphadenopathy, or rash. Know that systemic complications such as hepatitis, myocarditis and/or pericarditis, nephritis, or pneumonitis also may occur. If suspected, stop olanzapine and notify prescriber immediately. Expect to provide supportive care, as ordered.

- Institute fall precautions, especially in patients with conditions, diseases, or concurrent drug therapy that could exacerbate effects of motor and sensory instability, postural hypotension, and somnolence.

PATIENT TEACHING

- Teach patient to open orally disintegrating tablet sachet by peeling back foil on the blister, not by pushing tablet through the foil. Immediately after opening blister, tell him to use dry hands to remove tablet and place it in his mouth. Explain that tablet will disintegrate rapidly in saliva so he can easily swallow it without liquid.
- Caution patient with phenylketonuria that disintegrating olanzapine tablets contain phenylalanine.
- Tell patient receiving the extended-release parenteral form of olanzapine that she will need to be monitored for at least 3 hours following the injection. Stress importance of reporting any unusual symptoms, including altered thoughts and lethargy, immediately to healthcare professional.
- Advise patient to avoid alcohol and smoking during olanzapine therapy.
- Urge patient to avoid hazardous activities until drug's CNS effects are known. Also inform patient of increased risk for falls because of potential CNS effects. Review fall precautions with patient.
- Instruct patient to change position slowly to minimize effects of orthostatic hypotension.
- Encourage patient to weigh self frequently to detect weight gain. If diabetes is present, also instruct patient to monitor blood glucose level closely.
- Urge family or caregiver to watch patient closely for suicidal tendencies, especially when therapy starts or dosage changes and particularly if patient is a teenager or young adult.
- Warn patient that chronic olanzapine therapy may alter reproductive function through olanzapine-induced hyperprolactinemia causing amenorrhea and impotence. If reproductive adverse effects occur, patient should notify prescriber.

! **WARNING** Instruct patient to notify prescriber of any persistent, severe, or worsening adverse reactions, including fever, rash, or swollen glands or change in body function.

oliceridine
Olinvyk

☰ Class and Category

Pharmacologic class: Opioid agonist
Therapeutic class: Analgesic
Controlled substance schedule: II

☰ Indications and Dosages

✱ *To manage acute pain severe enough to require an intravenous opioid analgesic for patient for whom alternative treatments are inadequate*

I.V. INJECTION

Adults. *Initial:* 1.5 mg followed by 0.35-mg to 0.5-mg demand dose with a 6-minute lockout. Supplemental doses of 0.75 mg may be given by healthcare provider beginning 1 hr after initial dose and hourly thereafter, as needed. *Maximum:* 27 mg daily for no longer than 48 hr.

±**DOSAGE ADJUSTMENT** For patients experiencing unacceptable opioid-related adverse reaction, dosage may be reduced. Dosage adjustment is made to obtain an appropriate balance between management of pain and opioid-related adverse reactions.

☰ Drug Administration

I.V.

- Initiation of oliceridine dosing regimen should take into account patient's severity of pain, patient response, prior analgesic treatment experience, and risk factors for addiction, abuse, and misuse.
- Use of oliceridine (30 mg/30 ml) vial is intended for patient-controlled analgesia (PCA) only. Set demand dose with a 6-minute lockout.
- Draw oliceridine directly from vial into PCA syringe or I.V. bag without diluting.
- Know that drug solution should be clear and colorless.
- Individual single doses greater than 3 mg and use beyond 48 hours have not been evaluated.
- Know that if analgesia is still required with a 27-mg cumulative daily dose before 24 hours are up, an alternative analgesic regimen should be administered, as prescribed, until oliceridine can be resumed

the next day. Alternative analgesia may include multimodal therapies.

- Have naloxone readily available.
- *Incompatibilities:* None listed by manufacturer

Route	Onset	Peak	Duration
I.V.	2–5 min	Unknown	Unknown

Half-life: 1.3–3 hr

Mechanism of Action

The precise mechanism of the analgesic action is unknown. However, specific CNS opioid receptors with opioid-like activity have been identified throughout the brain and spinal cord and are thought to play a role in the analgesic effects of oliceridine.

Contraindications

Acute or severe bronchial asthma in an unmonitored setting or in the absence of resuscitative equipment; gastrointestinal obstruction, including paralytic ileus; hypersensitivity to oliceridine or its components; significant respiratory depression

Interactions

DRUGS

anticholinergic drugs: Possibly increased risk of urinary retention and/or severe constipation, which may lead to paralytic ileus

benzodiazepines and other CNS depressants (antipsychotics, anxiolytics, general anesthetics, muscle relaxants, other opioids, tranquilizers): Increased risk of coma, hypotension, profound sedation, respiratory depression, death

CYP2D6 moderate to strong inhibitors (bupropion, fluoxetine, paroxetine, quinidine), CYP3A4 moderate to strong inhibitors (antiretroviral agents, azole antifungal agents such as ketoconazole, macrolide antibiotics such as erythromycin, NS3/4A inhibitors, protease inhibitors such as ritonavir, selective serotonin reuptake inhibitors): Possibly increased plasma concentration of oliceridine, causing increased or prolonged opioid effects

CYP3A4 inducers (carbamazepine, phenytoin, rifampin): Possibly reduced plasma concentration of oliceridine, causing decreased effectiveness

diuretics: Possibly reduced effectiveness of diuretics

mixed agonist/antagonist, partial agonist opioid analgesics such as buprenorphine, butorphanol, nalbuphine, pentazocine: Possibly reduced analgesic effect of oliceridine and/or precipitation of withdrawal symptoms

muscle relaxants: Possibly enhanced neuromuscular blocking action of skeletal muscle relaxants and increased degree of respiratory depression

serotonergic drugs (5-HT$_3$ receptor antagonists; certain muscle relaxants such as cyclobenzaprine and metaxalone; drugs that affect the serotonin neurotransmitter system, such as mirtazapine, tramadol, trazodone; MAO inhibitors such as drugs used to treat psychiatric disorders and I.V. methylene blue, linezolid; norepinephrine reuptake inhibitors; selective serotonin reuptake inhibitors): Possibly development of serotonin syndrome

ACTIVITIES

alcohol: Increased risk of coma, hypotension, profound sedation, respiratory depression, and death

Adverse Reactions

CNS: Anxiety, dizziness, fever, headache, insomnia, restlessness, sedation, **seizures,** somnolence

CV: Increased blood pressure, **QT prolongation, severe hypotension,** tachycardia

EENT: Dry mouth

ENDO: **Adrenal insufficiency**

GI: Constipation, diarrhea, dyspepsia, elevated amylase or liver enzymes, flatulence, nausea, spasm of sphincter of Oddi, vomiting

HEME: Anemia

MS: Back pain, muscle spasms

RESP: Cough, decreased oxygen saturation, dyspnea, **hypoxia, respiratory depression**

SKIN: Excessive diaphoresis, flushing, hot flush, pruritus, urticaria

Other: **Hypocalcemia, hypokalemia, hypomagnesemia, hypophosphatemia,** physical and psychological dependence, withdrawal

Childbearing Considerations

PREGNANCY

- Drug may cause fetal harm.
- Prolonged use of drug during pregnancy can result in neonatal opioid withdrawal

syndrome (NOWS), which may be life-threatening if not recognized and treated.

- Avoid prolonged use during pregnancy. Use with caution only if benefit to mother outweighs potential risk to fetus.

LABOR AND DELIVERY

- Drug is not recommended for use in pregnant women immediately before or during labor. Opioids may alter length of time of labor.
- Opioids cross the placental barrier and may produce respiratory depression and psychological effects in the neonate. Monitor neonate closely for signs of excess sedation and respiratory depression.
- An opioid antagonist, such as naloxone, must be available at the time of delivery in case it is needed to reverse opioid-induced respiratory depression in the neonate.

LACTATION

- It is not known if drug is present in breast milk.
- Patient should check with prescriber before breastfeeding.
- If breastfeeding occurs, monitor infant for excess sedation and respiratory depression.
- Withdrawal symptoms can occur in breastfed infants when maternal administration of an opioid analgesic is stopped or when breastfeeding is stopped.

REPRODUCTION

- Chronic use of opioids may reduce fertility.

Nursing Considerations

- Be aware that use of opioids like oliceridine may lead to abuse, addiction, misuse, overdose, and possibly death. Addiction can occur even with appropriately prescribed dosages. Monitor patient's intake of drug closely and for evidence of physical dependence.
- Know that cumulative total daily dose of oliceridine should not exceed 27 mg daily because of risk of QT prolongation. Also monitor patient using PCA for signs of excessive sedation, respiratory depression, or other adverse effects, because PCA administration has resulted in adverse outcomes and episodes of respiratory depression.
- Use of oliceridine should be avoided in patients who are in a coma or have impaired consciousness, because drug can obscure their clinical course. Also know that patients susceptible to the intracranial

effects of carbon dioxide retention, such as patients with brain tumors or head injury, may develop further increased intracranial pressure because of oliceridine's ability to reduce respiratory drive, which causes carbon dioxide retention.

! **WARNING** Use extreme caution when administering oliceridine to patients with conditions accompanied by hypoxia or decreased respiratory reserve, such as asthma, COPD, or cor pulmonale. This is because even with usual therapeutic dosages, oliceridine may decrease respiratory drive while simultaneously increasing airway resistance to the point of apnea. Monitor patient's respiratory status closely, especially in cachectic, debilitated, and elderly patients and in patients with chronic pulmonary disease. Respiratory depression may occur at any time, but is most likely to occur during initiation of therapy or following a dosage increase. Have resuscitative equipment nearby and be prepared to administer supportive measures and use of opioid antagonists, as ordered.

! **WARNING** Be aware that overestimating the oliceridine dosage when converting patients from another opioid product can result in a fatal overdose with the first dose.

- Attempt to identify source of increased pain, if level of pain increases after dosage stabilization, before increasing oliceridine dosage, as prescribed.
- Evaluate patient continually to assess maintenance of pain control and relative incidence of adverse reactions.
- Know that an initial 1-mg dose of oliceridine is approximately equipotent to morphine 5 mg.
- Monitor patients with biliary tract disease for worsening symptoms, because oliceridine may cause spasm of the sphincter of Oddi.

! **WARNING** Know that chronic maternal use of oliceridine during pregnancy can result in neonatal opioid withdrawal syndrome (NOWS), which may be life-threatening if not recognized and treated appropriately. NOWS occurs when a newborn has been exposed to opioid drugs like oliceridine for a prolonged period while in utero.

! **WARNING** Be aware that oliceridine should only be used concomitantly with benzodiazepine or other CNS depressant therapy in patients for whom other treatment options are inadequate. If prescribed together, expect dosing and duration of oliceridine and/or benzodiazepine or other CNS depressant to be limited. Monitor patient closely for signs and symptoms of a decrease in consciousness, including coma, profound sedation, and significant respiratory depression. Notify prescriber immediately and provide emergency supportive care, as death may occur.

- Know that opioids such as oliceridine can cause sleep-related breathing disorders such as central sleep apnea and sleep-related hypoxemia. Risk for central sleep apnea increases in a dose-dependent fashion. If central sleep apnea occurs, notify prescriber, as dosage may have to be reduced.

! **WARNING** Know that many drugs may interact with opioids such as oliceridine to cause serotonin syndrome. Monitor patient closely for signs and symptoms such as agitation, diaphoresis, diarrhea, fever, hallucinations, labile blood pressure, muscle twitching or stiffness, nausea, shakiness, shivering, tachycardia, trouble with coordination, or vomiting. Notify prescriber at once, because serotonin syndrome may be life-threatening. Be prepared to discontinue drug, if possible and ordered, and provide supportive care.

- Monitor patient for adrenal insufficiency. Although rare, it can be life-threatening. Monitor patient for anorexia, dizziness, fatigue, hypotension, nausea, vomiting, or weakness. Notify prescriber if adrenal insufficiency is suspected and expect diagnostic testing to be done. If confirmed, expect to administer corticosteroids and wean patient off oliceridine, if possible.
- Monitor patients with seizure disorders closely because oliceridine may induce or aggravate seizures.
- Monitor patient's blood pressure closely, especially when initiating oliceridine therapy and when titrating dose, because drug may cause severe hypotension and syncope in ambulatory patients due to its vasodilatory effects.

- Be aware that risk of hypotension is greater in patients who have already been compromised by a reduced blood volume or concurrent administration of certain CNS depressant drugs, such as general anesthetics and phenothiazines.
- Know that oliceridine therapy should not be abruptly discontinued in a physically dependent patient. Instead, taper dose gradually while monitoring for withdrawal. If patient exhibits withdrawal signs and symptoms, be aware that dose should be raised to the previous level and then tapered more slowly, either by increasing the interval between decreases, decreasing the amount of dosage change, or both, as prescribed.

PATIENT TEACHING

- Explain to patient how PCA works, including the use of a 6-minute lockout for oliceridine. Tell patient to notify staff if pain is not controlled.
- Inform patient that drug can cause severe constipation and to notify prescriber if present.
- Alert patient to the possibility of addiction even with prescribed dosages.

olmesartan medoxomil

Benicar

N O

☰ Class and Category

Pharmacologic class: Angiotensin II receptor blocker (ARB)
Therapeutic class: Antihypertensive

☰ Indications and Dosages

✳ *To manage or as adjunct to manage hypertension*

SUSPENSION, TABLETS

Adults, adolescents, and children age 6 and over who weigh 35 kg (77 lb) or more. *Initial:* 20 mg daily, increased in 2 wk to 40 mg daily, as needed. *Maximum:* 40 mg daily.

Adolescents and children age 6 and over who weigh 20 kg (44 lb) to less than 35 kg (77 lb). *Initial:* 10 mg daily, increased in 2 wk to 20 mg daily, as needed. *Maximum:* 20 mg daily.

±DOSAGE ADJUSTMENT Lower starting dosage is recommended for patients with possible depletion of intravascular volume, such as those treated with diuretics, especially if impaired renal function is present.

Drug Administration

P.O.

- For patient who cannot swallow tablets, have pharmacist make a suspension form.
- Shake the suspension well before each use.
- Use a calibrated device to measure dosage of oral suspension.
- Refrigerate the suspension for up to 4 weeks. Return promptly to the refrigerator after each use.

Route	Onset	Peak	Duration
P.O.	<2 wk	1–2 hr	24 hr

Half-life: 13 hr

Contraindications

Aliskiren therapy in patients with diabetes or renal impairment (GFR less than 60 ml/min), hypersensitivity to olmesartan medoxomil or its components

Interactions

DRUGS

ACE inhibitors, aliskiren (in patients with diabetes or renal impairment), other angiotensin receptor blockers: Increased risk of hyperkalemia, hypotension, and renal dysfunction

colesevelam: Reduced effectiveness of olmesartan

drugs that may increase potassium levels such as heparin, potassium-sparing diuretics, potassium supplements: Increased risk of hyperkalemia

lithium: Increased serum lithium level with possible toxicity

NSAIDs: Increased risk of renal dysfunction in elderly patients and patients who are volume-depleted or have preexisting renal dysfunction; increased antihypertensive effect of olmesartan

FOOD

salt substitutes containing potassium: Increased risk of hyperkalemia

Adverse Reactions

CNS: Asthenia, dizziness, fatigue, headache, insomnia, vertigo
CV: Chest pain, hypercholesterolemia, hyperlipidemia, hypertriglyceridemia, peripheral edema, tachycardia

Mechanism of Action

Olmesartan medoxomil blocks angiotensin II from binding to receptor sites in many tissues, including adrenal glands and vascular smooth muscle.

Angiotensin II, a potent vasoconstrictor, is then free to stimulate the adrenal cortex to secrete aldosterone, and the inhibiting effects of angiotensin II reduce blood pressure.

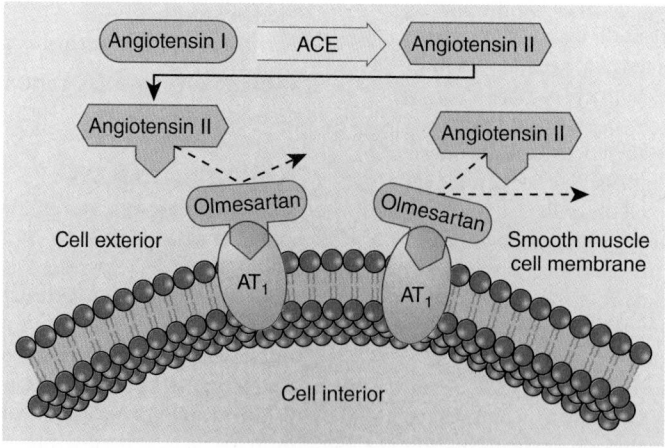

EENT: Pharyngitis, rhinitis, sinusitis
ENDO: Hyperglycemia
GI: Abdominal pain, diarrhea, gastroenteritis, indigestion, nausea, sprue-like enteropathy, vomiting
GU: **Acute renal failure**, elevated BUN and serum creatinine levels, hematuria, UTI
MS: Arthralgia, arthritis, back pain, myalgia, **rhabdomyolysis**, skeletal pain
RESP: Bronchitis, cough, upper respiratory tract infection
SKIN: Alopecia, pruritus, rash, urticaria
Other: **Anaphylaxis, angioedema, hyperkalemia**, hyperuricemia, increased CK level, flu-like symptoms, pain

Childbearing Considerations
PREGNANCY
- Drug causes fetal harm.
- Drug given during the second or third trimester reduces fetal renal function and increases fetal and neonatal morbidity and death. Resulting oligohydramnios can cause fetal lung hypoplasia and skeletal malformations.
- Drug should be discontinued as soon as pregnancy is known.

LACTATION
- It is not known if drug is present in breast milk.
- A decision should be made to discontinue breastfeeding or the drug to avoid potential adverse reactions in the breastfed infant.

Nursing Considerations
- Be aware that olmesartan should not be given to children under the age of 1 year because the drug can have adverse effects on the development of immature kidneys.
- Expect to provide treatment such as 0.9% Sodium Chloride Injection I.V., as prescribed, to correct known or suspected hypovolemia, before beginning olmesartan therapy.
- Monitor patient for increased BUN and serum creatinine levels, especially in a patient with impaired renal function, because drug may cause acute renal failure. If increased levels are significant or persist, notify prescriber immediately.
- Monitor blood pressure frequently to assess effectiveness of therapy. If blood pressure isn't controlled with olmesartan alone, expect to administer a diuretic, such as hydrochlorothiazide, as prescribed, but know that use of diuretics or other antihypertensive drugs during olmesartan therapy increases the risk of hypotension.
- Expect to discontinue drug temporarily if patient experiences hypotension. Place patient in supine position immediately and prepare to administer normal saline solution I.V., as prescribed. Expect to resume drug therapy after blood pressure stabilizes.
- Know that if patient also receives a diuretic, adequate hydration should be provided, as appropriate, to help prevent hypovolemia. Watch for evidence of hypovolemia, such as hypotension with dizziness and fainting.
- Monitor patient's electrolytes regularly, as ordered, and observe patient for signs and symptoms of electrolyte imbalances, especially hyperkalemia, because drug inhibits the renin–angiotensin system and may cause hyperkalemia. Risks for hyperkalemia include concomitant use of potassium-sparing diuretics, potassium supplements and/or potassium containing salt substitutes; and patients with diabetes mellitus or renal insufficiency.
- Monitor patient for chronic severe diarrhea and substantial weight loss, as drug may cause these symptoms even months to years after drug initiation.

PATIENT TEACHING
- Alert patient or caregiver that drug can be made into a suspension by the pharmacist if tablets cannot be swallowed. If using suspension, instruct patient or caregiver to shake bottle before each dose, use a calibrated device to measure dosage (not a household spoon), and keep suspension refrigerated. It should be discarded after 28 days.
- Advise patient to avoid exercise in hot weather and excessive alcohol use to reduce the risk of dehydration and hypotension. Also instruct him to notify prescriber if he has prolonged diarrhea, nausea, or vomiting.
- Caution patient to avoid hazardous activities until drug's CNS effects are known.
- Explain the importance of proper diet, regular exercise, and other lifestyle changes in controlling hypertension.
- Advise female patient to notify prescriber immediately about known or suspected pregnancy.

olodaterol
Striverdi Respimat

Class and Category
Pharmacologic class: Long-acting beta$_2$-adrenergic agonist
Therapeutic class: Bronchodilator

Indications and Dosages
✳ *To provide long-term maintenance for airflow obstruction in patients with chronic obstructive pulmonary disease (COPD), including chronic bronchitis and/or emphysema*

ORAL INHALATION
Adults. 5 mcg (2 inhalations) once daily at same time each day.

Drug Administration
INHALATION
- Load cartridge into the inhaler. Prime before first use by actuating inhaler toward the ground until an aerosol cloud is visible, and then repeat the process three more times. If not used for more than 7 days, actuate inhaler once before use; if not used for more than 21 days, reprime the same way as if using inhaler for the first time.
- Use inhalation spray only with the Striverdi Respimat inhaler. Do not use to administer other drugs.
- Administer by first pressing the safety catch while firmly pulling off the clear base with other hand. Do not touch the piercing element. Insert the narrow end of the cartridge into the inhaler. Place inhaler on a firm surface and push down firmly until it clicks. Replace the clear base. Then turn the clear base in the direction of the arrows on the label until it clicks. Open the cap until it snaps fully open. Device is ready for use.
- Have patient breathe out slowly and fully, then have patient close lips around the mouthpiece without covering the air vents. Have patient breathe in slowly through the mouth while pressing the dose release button. Patient should continue to finish the slow breath and then hold breath for 10 seconds, if able.
- Repeat for second inhalation. Close cap when finished.
- Inhaler will lock after 60 actuations (30-day supply), signifying it is empty.
- Discard after 3 months or when locking mechanism is engaged, whichever comes first.

Route	Onset	Peak	Duration
Inhalation	5 min	10–20 min	24 hr

Half-life: 7.5 hr

Mechanism of Action
By binding and activating beta$_2$-adrenoceptors in the airways, intracellular adenyl cyclase (an enzyme that mediates the synthesis of cyclic-3′ 5′-adenosine monophosphate [cAMP]) is stimulated. Elevated levels of cAMP cause bronchodilation by relaxing airway smooth-muscle cells.

Contraindications
Asthma without use of a long-term asthma control drug, hypersensitivity to olodaterol or its components

Interactions
DRUGS
adrenergic agents: Potentiated sympathetic effects
beta-blockers: Decreased effectiveness of olodaterol and beta-blockers; possibly severe bronchospasm
diuretics, steroids, xanthine derivatives: Increased risk of hypokalemia
drugs known to prolong QT interval, MAO inhibitors, tricyclic antidepressants: Possibly adverse cardiovascular effects
ketoconazole: Possibly increased serum olodaterol level
non-potassium-sparing diuretics: Possibly increased risk of ECG changes and hypokalemia

Adverse Reactions
CNS: Dizziness, fever
CV: Atrial fibrillation, chest pain, ECG changes, palpitations, tachycardia
EENT: Nasopharyngitis
ENDO: Hyperglycemia
GI: Constipation, diarrhea
GU: UTI
MS: Arthralgia, back pain
RESP: Bronchitis, COPD exacerbation, cough, paradoxical bronchospasms, pneumonia, upper respiratory infection
SKIN: Rash

Other: Anaphylaxis, angioedema, hypokalemia, immediate hypersensitivity reactions

Childbearing Considerations

PREGNANCY

- It is not known if drug causes fetal harm.
- Use with caution only if benefit to mother outweighs potential risk to fetus.

LABOR & DELIVERY

- Drug may inhibit labor due to a relaxant effect on uterine smooth muscle.

LACTATION

- It is not known if drug is present in breast milk.
- Patient should check with prescriber before breastfeeding.

Nursing Considerations

- Know that olodaterol therapy should not be used in patients with acutely deteriorating COPD, which may be a life-threatening condition. It should also not be used for relief of acute episodes of bronchospasm.
- Use caution when administering olodaterol to patients with cardiovascular disorders, such as arrhythmias, coronary insufficiency, hypertension, or hypertrophic obstructive cardiomyopathy; to patients with seizure disorders or thyrotoxicosis; and to patients who are unusually responsive to sympathomimetic amines or are at risk for developing prolonged QT interval.

! **WARNING** Watch patient closely for paradoxical bronchospasm. If present, discontinue olodaterol therapy immediately, notify prescriber, and implement treatment according to standard of care.

! **WARNING** Monitor patient for worsening or deteriorating asthma because asthma-related deaths have increased in patients receiving salmeterol, a drug in the same class as olodaterol. Be aware that use of long-acting beta$_2$-adrenergic agonists such as olodaterol is contraindicated in patients with asthma without the use of a long-term asthma control medication, such as an inhaled corticosteroid. Monitor patient closely and notify prescriber immediately of any changes in patient's respiratory status.

- Monitor patients with a history of cardiovascular disorders. Notify prescriber

of any significant increases in blood pressure or pulse rate or worsening of chronic conditions. Olodaterol may also cause ECG changes such as flattening of the T wave, prolonged QT interval, and ST-segment depression. Drug may have to be discontinued if such reactions occur.

! **WARNING** Watch patient closely for hypersensitivity reactions. If present, stop olodaterol therapy immediately, notify prescriber, and provide emergency treatment according to standard of care.

- Monitor patient's serum potassium level and assess for signs and symptoms of hypokalemia, especially if patient has severe COPD, because hypokalemia may be made worse by hypoxia and concomitant treatment.

PATIENT TEACHING

- Advise patient, especially if she has a significant cardiac history, to inform prescriber of any other drugs she is taking before beginning olodaterol therapy and to keep prescriber informed of any new drug therapies while taking olodaterol.
- Caution patient not to increase olodaterol dosage or frequency without consulting prescriber because serious adverse reactions may occur.
- Instruct patient on how to load the cartridge into the inhaler. Remind patient that after insertion, the unit must be primed before first use by actuating the inhaler toward the ground until an aerosol cloud is visible and then repeating the process three more times. If not used for more than 7 days, remind patient to actuate inhaler once before use; if not used for more than 21 days, tell patient to prime inhaler as if using for the first time.
- Teach patient how to use inhaler. Stress importance of using inhalation spray only with the Striverdi Respimat inhaler and that the inhaler should not be used for administering other drugs.

! **WARNING** Caution patient that immediate hypersensitivity reactions, including swelling of face or throat, may occur after administration of olodaterol. If present, patient should stop taking drug, seek immediate medical treatment, and notify prescriber.

- Urge patient to notify prescriber if her symptoms worsen, if olodaterol becomes less effective, or if she needs more inhalations of her prescribed short-acting beta$_2$-agonist than usual. This may indicate that her condition is worsening.

! **WARNING** Instruct patient to notify prescriber immediately if she experiences chest pain, palpitations, rapid heart rate, or other troublesome effects while taking olodaterol, because dosage may have to be adjusted.

! **WARNING** Tell patient that olodaterol may cause paradoxical bronchospasms. If present, tell patient to discontinue drug and notify prescriber. If severe or unrelieved, stress importance of seeking emergency treatment to relieve bronchospasms.

olsalazine sodium
Dipentum

Class and Category
Pharmacologic class: Salicylate
Therapeutic class: Anti-inflammatory

Indications and Dosages
✳ *To maintain remission of ulcerative colitis in patients who are intolerant of sulfasalazine*

CAPSULES
Adults and adolescents. 500 mg twice daily.

Drug Administration
P.O.
- Give drug with food to decrease adverse GI reactions and have patient drink plenty of water during therapy.

Route	Onset	Peak	Duration
P.O.	Unknown	1 hr	Unknown
Half-life: 0.9 hr			

Mechanism of Action
Exerts anti-inflammatory action in GI tract after being converted by colonic bacteria to mesalamine (5-aminosalicylic acid), which inhibits cyclooxygenase. Inhibition of cyclooxygenase reduces prostaglandin production in intestinal mucosa. This in turn reduces production of arachidonic acid metabolites, which may be increased in patients with inflammatory bowel disease. Olsalazine also exerts an anti-inflammatory effect by indirectly inhibiting leukotriene synthesis, which normally catalyzes production of arachidonic acid.

Contraindications
Hypersensitivity to olsalazine, aminosalicylates, other salicylates, or their components

Interactions
DRUGS
azathioprine, 6-mercaptopurine, thioguanine: Increased risk of myelosuppression
low-molecular-weight heparins or heparinoids: Increased risk of bleeding after neuraxial anesthesia
nephrotoxic agents, including NSAIDs: Increased risk of nephrotoxicity
oral anticoagulants: Possibly prolonged PT
varicella vaccine: Increased risk of Reye's syndrome

Adverse Reactions
CNS: Anxiety, depression, dizziness, drowsiness, fatigue, fever, headache, insomnia, lethargy, paresthesia, peripheral neuropathy, vertigo
CV: **Cardiac arrest, hypotension, myocarditis, pericarditis, prolonged QT interval, second-degree AV block**
ENDO: Hot flashes
EENT: Dry eyes and mouth, lacrimation, **laryngeal edema, stridor,** stomatitis, tinnitus
GI: Abdominal pain, anorexia, cholestatic jaundice, **cirrhosis,** diarrhea, dyspepsia, elevated bilirubin or liver enzymes, **hepatic failure or necrosis, hepatitis, hepatotoxicity,** nausea, vomiting
GU: Dysuria, hematuria, interstitial nephritis, nephrolithiasis, **nephrotic syndrome,** urinary frequency
HEME: **Aplastic or hemolytic anemia, lymphopenia, neutropenia, pancytopenia**
MS: Arthralgia, joint pain, muscle spasms, myalgia
RESP: **Bronchospasms,** dyspnea, **interstitial lung disease,** pleurisy/pleuritis, shortness of breath
SKIN: Acne, acute generalized exanthematous pustulosis, alopecia, angioneurotic edema, erythema nodosum,

flushing, photosensitivity, pruritus, rash, **Stevens–Johnson syndrome, toxic epidermal necrolysis**

Other: Anaphylaxis, angioedema, dehydration, **drug reaction with eosinophilia and systemic symptoms (DRESS),** mesalamine-induced acute intolerance syndrome

Childbearing Considerations

PREGNANCY

- It is not known if drug causes fetal harm.
- Use with caution only if benefit to mother outweighs potential risk to fetus.

LACTATION

- Drug may be present in breast milk.
- A decision should be made to discontinue breastfeeding or the drug to avoid potential adverse reactions in the breastfed infant.

Nursing Considerations

- Use olsalazine cautiously in patient with preexisting liver disease because hepatic failure may occur during olsalazine therapy, since drug is converted to mesalamine.
- Assess patient for aspirin allergy before giving olsalazine.

! **WARNING** Monitor patient for hypersensitivity reactions that may become serious. Also monitor patient for signs or symptoms of severe cutaneous adverse reaction. Notify prescriber at the first sign or symptom that appears.

- Know that if patient has severe allergies or asthma, he should be watched closely for worsening symptoms during olsalazine therapy; notify prescriber immediately if they occur.
- Assess consistency and quantity of stools and frequency of bowel movements before, during, and after therapy.
- Maintain adequate hydration, because kidney stones may develop.
- Assess patient for abdominal pain and hyperactive bowel sounds.
- Monitor hepatic and renal status in patient with underlying hepatic or renal dysfunction because drug may further impair these functions.
- Monitor patient for signs and symptoms of mesalamine-induced acute intolerance syndrome such as acute abdominal pain or

cramping, bloody diarrhea, fever, headache, and rash. This may occur because olsalazine is converted to mesalamine.

PATIENT TEACHING

- Instruct patient to take olsalazine with food and to drink plenty of water while taking drug.
- Urge patient to continue taking drug as prescribed, even if symptoms improve.

! **WARNING** Alert patient that drug may cause allergic reactions or serious skin conditions. Tell patient to stop drug, notify prescriber, and seek medical attention at the first sign of an allergic or skin reaction.

- Advise patient to watch for signs of dehydration.
- Tell patient to report unusual, persistent, or severe adverse effects to prescriber.
- Instruct patient to avoid sun exposure, wear protective clothing, and use a broad-spectrum sunscreen when outdoors, especially if patient has atopic dermatitis or atopic eczema.
- Tell patient and caregivers that salicylates, such as olsalazine, should not be given for 6 weeks after the varicella vaccine.

omadacycline

Nuzyra

Class and Category

Pharmacologic class: Aminomethylcycline of the tetracycline class
Therapeutic class: Antibacterial

Indications and Dosages

* *To treat community-acquired bacterial pneumonia caused by* Chlamydophila pneumoniae, Haemophilus influenzae, H. parainfluenzae, Klebsiella pneumoniae, Legionella pneumophilia, Mycoplasma pneumoniae, Staphylococcus aureus *(methicillin-susceptible isolates), or* Streptococcus pneumoniae

I.V. INFUSION, TABLETS

Adults. *Loading:* 200 mg I.V. once on day 1. Alternatively, 100 mg I.V. twice on day 1. *Maintenance:* 100 mg I.V. once daily for 7 to 14 days. Alternatively, 300 mg P.O. once daily for 7 to 14 days.

✱ *To treat acute bacterial skin structure and skin infections caused by* Enterobacter cloacae, Enterococcus faecalis, K. pneumoniae, S. anginosus group, S. aureus *(methicillin-susceptible and-resistant isolates),* S. lugdunensis, *or* S. pyogenes

I.V. INFUSION, TABLETS

Adults. *Loading:* 200 mg I.V. once on day 1. Alternatively, 100 mg I.V. twice on day 1 or 450 mg P.O. once daily on day 1 and day 2. *Maintenance:* 100 mg I.V. once daily for 7 to 14 days if loading dose was 200 mg administered I.V. once on day 1. Alternatively, 300 mg P.O. once daily for 7 to 14 days if loading dose was 100 mg administered I.V. twice on day 1 or 450 mg P.O. once on day 1 and day 2.

⬚ Drug Administration

P.O.

- Administer oral tablets with water after patient has fasted for at least 4 hours.
- After administration, patient should not drink (except water) or eat for 2 hours and not ingest any antacids, dairy products, iron preparations, or multivitamins for 4 hours after administration.

I.V.

- Reconstitute each 100-mg vial with 5 ml of 0.9% Sodium Chloride Injection, 5% Dextrose Injection, or Sterile Water for Injection.
- Gently swirl contents and let vial stand until the cake has completely dissolved and any foam disperses. Do not shake vial. If needed, invert vial to dissolve any remaining powder and swirl gently, to prevent foaming. Reconstituted solution should be yellow to dark orange in color; if not, discard solution.
- Dilute further within 1 hour by withdrawing reconstituted solution from vial and adding it to 100 ml or more of 0.9% Sodium Chloride Injection or 5% Dextrose Injection in an intravenous bag. Concentration of the final diluted infusion solution will be either 1 mg/ml or 2 mg/ml depending on number of vials reconstituted.
- Use within 24 hours if diluted drug is left at room temperature or within 7 days, if refrigerated.
- If refrigerated, remove infusion bag from refrigerator and place in a vertical position at room temperature 60 minutes before use.

- Administer total infusion over 60 minutes for a 200-mg dose or a total infusion time of 30 minutes for a 100-mg dose.
- Infuse through a dedicated line or through a Y-site.
- If the same intravenous line is used for sequential infusion of several drugs, flush with 0.9% Sodium Chloride Injection or 5% Dextrose Injection before and after infusion.
- *Incompatibilities:* Other drugs, solutions other than 0.9% Sodium Chloride Injection or 5% Dextrose Injection, solutions containing multivalent cations such as calcium and magnesium

Route	Onset	Peak	Duration
P.O.	Unknown	2.5 hr	Unknown
I.V.	Unknown	0.5 hr	Unknown

Half-life: 15.5–16.8 hr

⬚ Mechanism of Action

Binds to the 30S ribosomal subunit and blocks protein synthesis, exerting a bacteriostatic effect as well as a bactericidal effect against some isolates of S. pneumoniae and H. influenzae.

⬚ Contraindications

Hypersensitivity to omadacycline, other tetracycline-class antibacterial drugs or their components

⬚ Interactions

DRUGS

antacids containing aluminum, calcium, or magnesium; bismuth subsalicylate; iron preparations: Decreased absorption of oral omadacycline
anticoagulant drugs: Depressed plasma prothrombin activity

FOODS

all foods, especially dairy products: Decreased absorption of oral omadacycline

⬚ Adverse Reactions

CNS: Fatigue, headache, insomnia, lethargy, vertigo
CV: Atrial fibrillation, hypertension, tachycardia
EENT: Oral candidiasis, oropharyngeal pain, taste distortion
GI: Abdominal pain, *Clostridium difficile*-associated diarrhea (CDAD),

constipation, diarrhea, dyspepsia, elevated bilirubin and liver enzymes, elevated lipase levels, nausea, vomiting

GU: Vulvovaginal mycotic infection

HEME: Anemia, thrombocytosis

SKIN: Excessive diaphoresis, erythema, pruritus, urticaria

Other: Elevated alkaline phosphatase or creatinine phosphokinase, **hypersensitivity reactions**, infusion-site reactions (erythema, induration, inflammation, irritation, pain, swelling)

Childbearing Considerations

PREGNANCY

- Drug causes fetal harm such as adverse effects on skeleton growth and tooth development when given during the second and third trimester.
- The use of drug during last half of pregnancy may cause permanent discoloration of the child's teeth.
- Drug should not be used during pregnancy unless there is no alternative and benefit to mother outweighs potential risk to fetus.

LACTATION

- It is not known if drug is present in breast milk.
- Breastfeeding is not recommended during drug therapy and for 4 days following the last dose.

REPRODUCTION

- Patients should use effective contraception during drug therapy.
- Drug may reduce ovulation and increased embryonic loss in female patients, according to animal studies.
- Drug may cause injury to the testis and reduced motility and reduced sperm counts in male patients, according to animal studies.

Nursing Considerations

! WARNING Be aware that patients treated for community-acquired bacterial pneumonia with omadacycline may have a higher risk of death, especially patients over the age of 65 and patients with multiple disorders. Monitor patients with pneumonia closely for worsening and/or complications of infection and underlying conditions.

- Know that omadacycline, as a tetracycline, may cause permanent discoloration of the teeth, enamel hypoplasia, and inhibition of bone growth in the neonate if administered during the last half of pregnancy.

! WARNING Monitor patient for hypersensitivity reactions, because other tetracyclines have caused reactions, including anaphylaxis. If patient develops a reaction, notify prescriber and expect drug to be discontinued. Provide supportive care, as ordered and required.

- Assess patient for signs of secondary infection, such as profuse, watery diarrhea. If such diarrhea develops, contact prescriber and expect to obtain a stool specimen to rule out pseudomembranous colitis caused by *Clostridium difficile*. If diarrhea occurs, notify prescriber and expect to withhold omadacycline and treat with electrolytes, fluids, protein, and an antibiotic effective against *C. difficile*.
- Monitor patient for tetracycline-class effects such as abnormal liver function tests, acidosis, azotemia, hyperphosphatemia, increased BUN, pancreatitis, photosensitivity, and pseudotumor cerebri. Expect omadacycline to be discontinued if any of these adverse reactions occurs.

PATIENT TEACHING

- Instruct patient taking oral tablets of omadacycline to take drug with water after patient has fasted for at least 4 hours. After administration, patient should not drink (except water) or eat for 2 hours. Also tell patient not to ingest any antacids, dairy products, iron preparations, or multivitamins for 4 hours after administration.
- Inform patient that nausea and vomiting may occur with omadacycline use, especially if patient received the oral loading dose for treatment of acute bacterial skin and skin structure infections.
- Alert patient that diarrhea is a common problem with antibacterial drugs. Tell patient that bloody or watery stools can occur even after omadacycline therapy has been discontinued. Stress importance of reporting diarrhea to prescriber.

! WARNING Instruct patient to stop taking drug and seek medical attention if an allergic reaction occurs.

- Advise mothers not to breastfeed their infant during omadacycline therapy and for 4 days after the last dose of drug.

omalizumab
Xolair

Class and Category
Pharmacologic class: Monoclonal antibody
Therapeutic class: Antiallergenic, antiasthmatic

Indications and Dosages
❋ *To treat moderate to severe persistent asthma in patients with positive skin test or in vitro reactivity to a perennial aeroallergen and symptoms have been inadequately controlled with inhaled corticosteroids*

SUBCUTANEOUS INJECTION
Adults and adolescents age 6 and over. 75 to 375 mg every 2 or 4 wk. Dose and frequency determined by body weight and blood IgE levels.
±**DOSAGE ADJUSTMENT** Dosage adjusted for significant changes in body weight.

❋ *As add-on maintenance treatment for nasal polyps for patients with inadequate response to nasal corticosteroids*

SUBCUTANEOUS INJECTION
Adults. 75 mg to 600 mg every 2 to 4 wk. Dose and frequency determined by body weight and blood IgE levels.
±**DOSAGE ADJUSTMENT** Dosage adjusted for significant changes in body weight.

❋ *To treat chronic idiopathic urticaria in patients who remain symptomatic despite H$_1$ antihistamine treatment*

SUBCUTANEOUS INJECTION
Adults and adolescents age 12 and over. 150 or 300 mg every 4 wk.

Drug Administration
SUBCUTANEOUS
- Reconstitute by adding 1.4 ml Sterile Water for Injection into a 3-ml syringe with a 1-in 18G needle. Place drug vial upright and inject Sterile Water for Injection into vial.
- Gently swirl upright vial for about 1 minute to evenly wet powder. Don't shake. Every 5 minutes, gently swirl for 5 to 10 seconds until solution contains no gel-like particles, which usually takes 15 to 20 minutes.

Discard if powder takes longer than 40 minutes to dissolve, and start with a new vial. Solution should be clear or slightly opalescent and may have a few small bubbles or foam around edge of vial.
- Use omalizumab within 8 hours if refrigerated or 4 hours if stored at room temperature. Protect from sunlight.
- Remove reconstituted omalizumab from vial by inverting vial for 15 seconds to let solution drain toward stopper. Using a new 3-ml syringe with a 1-in 18G needle, insert needle into inverted vial and position needle tip at the very bottom of solution in the vial stopper. Then pull plunger all the way back to end of syringe barrel to remove all solution from inverted vial. To obtain full 150-mg dose (1 vial containing 1.2 ml of reconstituted omalizumab), all product must be withdrawn from vial before expelling any air or excess solution from syringe. Replace needle with a 25G needle for administration.
- Drug is also available as a prefilled syringe. The needle cover on the prefilled syringe contains dry natural rubber, which is a derivative of latex and may cause allergic reactions in individuals sensitive to latex. Do not remove from sealed outer carton until ready for use. Do not use syringe if it has been dropped or damaged or if packaging is damaged or appears to have been tampered with. Remove carton from refrigerator and allow syringe to warm up to room temperature on its own (at least 15 to 30 minutes), because drug when cold can cause discomfort for patient and make it hard to push the plunger. Leave syringe in carton to protect it from light during warming process. Do not warm in any other way and do not put syringe in a microwave or warm water. When removing syringe from carton, do not flip blister pack upside down to take out the syringe and do not touch the back of the syringe, as damage may occur. After peeling back blister pack cover, take syringe out by holding the middle part of the syringe. When administering, press plunger all the way down to give full dose. Allow needle to be covered by the needle shield.
- Don't give more than 150 mg of drug per injection site.

- Inject over 5 to 10 seconds because solution is slightly viscous. Do not rub injection site afterward. If needed, site may be covered with a small bandage.
- If skin contact occurred while preparing or administering drug, wash area with water.
- Reconstituted vials and prefilled syringes should be stored in refrigerator until ready for use.

Route	Onset	Peak	Duration
SubQ	Unknown	7–8 days	Unknown

Half-life: 24–26 days

Mechanism of Action

Helps reduce inflammation by binding to circulating IgE and keeping it from binding to mast cells. This action inhibits degranulation and blocks release of histamine and other chemical mediators. In asthma, inflammation results when antigen reexposure causes mast cells to degranulate and release histamine and chemical mediators. By blocking these responses, asthma and nasal polyp symptoms and urticaria are less likely to develop.

Contraindications

Hypersensitivity to omalizumab or its components

Interactions

DRUGS

None reported by manufacturer

Adverse Reactions

CNS: Dizziness, fatigue, fever, headache, vertigo
EENT: Earache, epistaxis, nasopharyngitis, otitis media, pharyngitis, sinusitis
GI: Gastroenteritis, nausea, upper abdominal pain
HEME: Eosinophilic conditions, **thrombocytopenia (severe)**
MS: Arm or leg pain, arthralgia, fractures
RESP: Bronchitis, cough, upper respiratory tract infection
SKIN: Alopecia, dermatitis, pruritus, rash, urticaria
Other: **Anaphylaxis**; antibodies to omalizumab; generalized pain; injection-site bruising, burning, hive or mass formation, induration, inflammation, itching, pain, redness, stinging, and warmth; lymphadenopathy; **malignancies**

Childbearing Considerations

PREGNANCY

- It is not known if drug causes fetal harm but drug crosses the placental barrier.
- Use with caution only if benefit to mother outweighs potential risk to fetus.

LACTATION

- It is not known if drug is present in breast milk.
- Patient should check with prescriber before breastfeeding.

Nursing Considerations

- Record patient's weight, and obtain blood IgE levels, as ordered, before starting omalizumab prescribed to treat asthma; dosage and dosing frequency are based on these factors.

! **WARNING** Monitor patient closely for hypersensitivity reactions, particularly for first 2 hours after administration. Although rare, anaphylaxis has occurred as early as first dose and more than 1 year after starting regular treatment. Monitor patient closely and keep emergency medication and equipment readily available.

! **WARNING** Monitor patient closely for signs of cancer. Report any abnormal findings to prescriber.

- Be aware that inhaled or systemic corticosteroids should not be discontinued abruptly upon initiation of omalizumab therapy for asthma or nasal polyps. Instead, dosage should be discontinued gradually.
- Know that serum total IgE levels obtained less than 1 year following omalizumab discontinuation should not be used to reassess dosing regimen because these levels may not reflect steady-state free IgE levels. Elevated IgE levels may persist for up to 1 year following discontinuation of drug.

PATIENT TEACHING

! **WARNING** Instruct patient to notify prescriber immediately about possible hypersensitivity, such as difficulty breathing, hives, or rash, and if severe to seek immediate medical care.

- Alert patient that prefilled syringe needle cover contains latex and should not be

N
O

used if allergic to latex. Have patient notify prescriber of latex allergy.

- Instruct patient or caregiver how to administer drug and a subcutaneous injection. If more than 1 injection is required for dose, tell patient all injections should be administered consecutively and at one sitting.
- Caution patient that any improvement in his condition may take time.
- Encourage patient to comply with regularly scheduled prescriber visits.
- Inform patient of risk of malignancy and suggest routine cancer screening.
- Explain that omalizumab prescribed for the treatment of asthma isn't used to treat acute bronchospasm or status asthmaticus. Tell patient to notify prescriber if asthma remains uncontrolled or worsens after initiation of omalizumab therapy.
- Tell patient not to abruptly stop any prescribed systemic or inhaled corticosteroid when starting omalizumab therapy for asthma treatment because steroid dosage must be tapered gradually under prescriber's supervision.
- If female patient becomes pregnant within 8 weeks before or during omalizumab therapy, urge her to enroll in the Xolair Pregnancy Exposure Registry at 1-866-496-5247. Also, tell her to notify prescriber because drug may have to be changed.

omega-3-acid ethyl esters
Lovaza

Class and Category
Pharmacologic class: Ethyl esters
Therapeutic class: Antilipemic

Indications and Dosages
* *As adjunct to diet to reduce severe triglyceride level that is equal to or exceeds 500 mg/dl*

CAPSULES
Adults. 4 g once daily or 2 g twice daily.

Drug Administration
P.O.
- Capsules should be swallowed whole and not chewed, crushed, or opened.

Route	Onset	Peak	Duration
P.O.	Unknown	5 hr	Unknown

Half-life: 89 hr

Mechanism of Action
Omega-3-acid ethyl esters are essential fatty acids that may inhibit very-low-density lipoprotein and triglyceride synthesis in the liver. With less triglyceride synthesis, plasma triglyceride levels decrease.

Contraindications
Hypersensitivity to omega-3-acid ethyl esters or their components

Interactions
DRUGS
anticoagulants, antiplatelets: Possibly increased bleeding time

Adverse Reactions
CV: Angina pectoris
EENT: Halitosis, nosebleeds, taste perversion
GI: Diarrhea, dyspepsia, eructation, nausea, vomiting
HEME: Prolonged bleeding time, hemorrhagic diathesis
MS: Back pain
SKIN: Bruising, rash, urticaria
Other: Anaphylaxis, flu-like symptoms

Childbearing Considerations
PREGNANCY
- It is not known if drug causes fetal harm.
- Use with caution only if benefit to mother outweighs potential risk to fetus.

LACTATION
- Drug is present in breast milk.
- Patient should check with prescriber before breastfeeding.

Nursing Considerations
- Be aware that drugs known to increase triglyceride levels—such as beta-blockers, thiazide diuretics, and estrogens—should be discontinued or changed, if possible, before omega-3 ethyl ester therapy starts.
- Expect to check patient's triglyceride level before starting and periodically throughout omega-3-acid ethyl ester therapy to determine effectiveness.
- Expect to stop omega-3-acid ethyl ester therapy after 2 months if patient's triglyceride level doesn't decrease as expected.

- Monitor patient with history of paroxysmal or persistent atrial fibrillation for recurrences of symptomatic atrial fibrillation or flutter, especially within the first 2 to 3 months of initiating omega-3 ethyl ester therapy.

PATIENT TEACHING

- Explain to patient the importance of dietary measures, an exercise program, and controlling other factors—such as blood glucose level—that may contribute to elevated triglyceride levels.
- Advise patient to take drug with meals. Tell patient to swallow capsule whole and not chew, crush, or open capsule.
- Explain that patient will need periodic laboratory tests to evaluate therapy.
- Instruct patient to seek immediate medical attention if an allergic reaction or chest pain occurs.

omega 3-carboxylic acids

Epanova

☰ Class and Category

Pharmacologic class: Fish oil derivative
Therapeutic class: Antilipemic

☰ Indications and Dosages

* *As adjunct to diet to reduce triglyceride levels in patients with severe (equal to or greater than 500 mg/dl) hypertriglyceridemia*

CAPSULES

Adults. 2 or 4 g once daily.

☰ Drug Administration

P.O.

- Capsules should be swallowed whole and not chewed, crushed, or opened.

Route	Onset	Peak	Duration
P.O.	Unknown	5–9 hr	Unknown

Half-life: 37–46 hr

☰ Mechanism of Action

Possibly reduces synthesis of triglycerides in the liver by inhibiting acyl-CoA-1,2 diacylglycerol acyltransferase, increasing mitochondrial and peroxisomal beta oxidation in the liver, decreasing lipogenesis in the liver, and increasing plasma lipoprotein lipase activity.

☰ Contraindications

Hypersensitivity to omega 3-carboxylic acids or its components

☰ Interactions

DRUGS

anticoagulants, antiplatelet agents: Possibly increased risk of bleeding

☰ Adverse Reactions

CNS: Fatigue
CV: Elevated LDL-C levels
EENT: Difficulty swallowing, nasopharyngitis
GI: Abdominal discomfort, distention, or pain; constipation; diarrhea; eructation; flatulence; nausea; vomiting
MS: Arthralgia

☰ Childbearing Considerations

PREGNANCY

- It is not known if drug causes fetal harm.
- Use with caution only if benefit to mother outweighs potential risk to fetus.

LACTATION

- It is not known if drug is present in breast milk.
- Patient should check with prescriber before breastfeeding.

☰ Nursing Considerations

! WARNING Monitor patient for signs and symptoms of a hypersensitivity reaction, because omega 3-carboxylic acids contain polyunsaturated free fatty acids derived from fish oils and it is not known if cross-sensitivity exists.

- Monitor LDL-C levels, as ordered, periodically during therapy with omega 3-carboxylic acids because drug may increase these levels in some patients.

PATIENT TEACHING

- Instruct patient to swallow capsules whole and not to break open, chew, crush, or dissolve the capsules.
- Advise patient that if a dose is missed, take it as soon as it is remembered, but never to double the next dose to make up for the missed dose.

N
O

- Inform patient that drug therapy is not a substitution for dietary measures. Adherence to dietary restrictions must be continued.

! **WARNING** Tell patient to notify prescriber if any signs or symptoms of an allergic reaction occur and to seek immediate emergency care, if severe.

omeprazole
Losec (CAN), Prilosec

omeprazole magnesium
Prilosec, Prilosec OTC

Class and Category
Pharmacologic class: Proton pump inhibitor
Therapeutic class: Antiulcer

Indications and Dosages
✳ *To treat symptomatic gastroesophageal reflux disease (GERD)*

DELAYED-RELEASE CAPSULES, DELAYED-RELEASE TABLETS, DELAYED-RELEASE ORAL SUSPENSION
Adults and adolescents 16 years and over. 20 mg daily for 4 wk.
Children age 1 to 16 years of age weighing 20 kg (44 lb) or more. 20 mg once daily for up to 4 wk.
Children age 1 to 16 weighing 10 kg (22 lb) to less than 20 kg (44 lb). 10 mg once daily for up to 4 wk.
Children age 1 to 16 weighing 5 kg (11 lb) to less than 10 kg (22 lb). 5 mg once daily for up to 4 wk.
✳ *To treat erosive esophagitis due to acid-mediated GERD*

DELAYED-RELEASE CAPSULES, DELAYED-RELEASE ORAL SUSPENSION
Adults and adolescents age 16 and over. 20 mg daily for 4 to 8 wk.
Children age 1 to 16 years of age weighing 20 kg (44 lb) or more. 20 mg daily for 4 to 8 wk.
Children age 1 to 16 weighing 10 kg (22 lb) to less than 20 kg (44 lb). 10 mg daily for 4 to 8 wk.

Children age 1 to 16 weighing 5 kg (11 lb) to less than 10 kg (22 lb). 5 mg daily for 4 to 8 wk.
Children ages 1 month to less than 1 year weighing 10 kg (22 lb) or more. 10 mg once daily up to 6 wk.
Children ages 1 month to less than 1 year weighing 5 kg (11 b) to less than 10 kg (22 lb). 5 mg once daily up to 6 wk.
Children ages 1 month to less than 1 year weighing 3 kg (6.6 lb) to less than 5 kg (11 lb). 2.5 mg once daily up to 6 wk.
✳ *To provide maintenance of healing of erosive esophagitis due to acid-mediated GERD*

DELAYED-RELEASE CAPSULES, DELAYED-RELEASE ORAL SUSPENSION
Adults and adolescents age 16 and over. 20 mg once daily up to 12 mo.
Children age 1 to 16 years of age weighing 20 kg (44 lb) or more. 20 mg once daily up to 12 mo.
Children age 1 to 16 weighing 10 kg (22 lb) to less than 20 kg (44 lb). 10 mg once daily up to 12 mo.
Children age 1 to 16 weighing 5 kg (11 lb) to less than 10 kg (22 lb). 5 mg once daily for up to 12 mo.
± **DOSAGE ADJUSTMENT** For adult patients with hepatic impairment and Asian patients, dosage reduced to 10 mg once daily.
✳ *To provide short-term treatment of active benign gastric ulcer*

DELAYED-RELEASE CAPSULES, DELAYED-RELEASE ORAL SUSPENSION
Adults. 40 mg daily for 4 to 8 wk.
✳ *To treat active duodenal ulcer short-term*

DELAYED-RELEASE CAPSULES, DELAYED-RELEASE ORAL SUSPENSION
Adults. 20 mg once daily for 4 wk, with an additional 4 wk of therapy, as needed.
✳ *To eradicate* Helicobacter pylori *in order to reduce risk of duodenal ulcer recurrence*

DELAYED-RELEASE CAPSULES, DELAYED-RELEASE ORAL SUSPENSION
Adults. 40 mg once daily with clarithromycin 500 mg three times daily for 14 days. If ulcer present at start of therapy, 20 mg once daily for an additional 14 days. Alternatively, 20 mg twice daily with amoxicillin 1,000 mg twice daily, and clarithromycin 500 mg twice daily for 10 days. If ulcer present at start of therapy, 20 mg once daily for an additional 18 days.

✳ *To provide long-term treatment of gastric hypersecretory conditions, such as multiple endocrine adenoma syndrome, systemic mastocytosis, and Zollinger–Ellison syndrome*

DELAYED-RELEASE CAPSULES, DELAYED-RELEASE ORAL SUSPENSION

Adults. 60 mg once daily or in divided doses for doses greater than 80 mg. *Maximum:* 120 mg three times daily.

Drug Administration

P.O.

- Give omeprazole before meals, preferably in the morning for once-daily dosing and before breakfast and dinner for twice-daily dosing. An antacid may also be given, as prescribed.
- Tablets and capsules should be swallowed whole and not chewed, crushed, or split/ opened. If patient has difficulty swallowing tablets or capsules, oral suspension form should be used.
- To prepare oral suspension form, empty contents into a container with 5 ml of water (2.5-mg packet) or 15 ml of water (10-mg packet). Stir. Let thicken for 2 to 3 minutes. Stir and administer within 30 minutes. If any material remains after patient drinks solution, add more water, stir, and have patient drink residual solution.
- To administer via a gastric or nasogastric tube, add 5 ml of water to a catheter-tipped syringe and then add contents of 2.5-mg packet (or 15 ml of water for 10-mg packet). Immediately shake the syringe and allow to thicken for 2 to 3 minutes. Shake syringe again and inject through tubing within 30 minutes. Refill syringe with equal amount of water, shake, and flush any remaining contents into tube.

Route	Onset	Peak	Duration
P.O.	1 hr	0.5–3.5 hr	72–96 hr

Half-life: 0.5–1 hr

Contraindications

Concurrent therapy with rilpivirine-containing products; hypersensitivity to omeprazole, substituted benzimidazoles, or their components

Interactions

DRUGS

atazanavir, nelfinavir, rilpivirine: Decreased plasma levels of these agents; promote drug resistance to these drugs

cilostazol diazepam, digoxin, phenytoin, tacrolimus: Increased exposure of these drugs

citalopram: Increased exposure of citalopram leading to increased risk of QT prolongation

clopidogrel: Reduced effectiveness of clopidogrel

CYP2C19 or CYP3A4 inducers such as rifampin, St. John's wort: Decreased exposure of omeprazole

CYP2C19 or CYP3A4 inhibitors such as voriconazole: Increased exposure of omeprazole

dasatinib, erlotinib, iron salts, itraconazole, ketoconazole, mycophenolate mofetil, nilotinib: Reduced absorption of these drugs

methotrexate: Possibly delayed methotrexate elimination and increased risk of toxicity

saquinavir: Increased plasma saquinavir level and risk of toxicity

St. John's wort, rifampin: Decreased plasma omeprazole level

warfarin: Possibly increased risk of abnormal bleeding

Adverse Reactions

CNS: Agitation, asthenia, dizziness, drowsiness, fatigue, fever, headache, malaise, psychic disturbance, somnolence

CV: Chest pain, hypertension, peripheral edema

EENT: Anterior ischemic optic neuropathy, optic atrophy or neuritis, otitis media, stomatitis

ENDO: Hypoglycemia

GI: Abdominal pain, acid regurgitation, constipation, diarrhea, *Clostridium difficile*-associated diarrhea, dyspepsia, elevated liver enzymes, flatulence, fundic gland polyps (long-term use), hepatic dysfunction or failure, indigestion, nausea, pancreatitis, vomiting

GU: Acute tubulointerstitial nephritis

HEME: Agranulocytosis, anemia, hemolytic anemia, leukopenia, leukocytosis, neutropenia, pancytopenia, thrombocytopenia

MS: Back pain, bone fracture, joint pain

RESP: Bronchospasms, cough, upper respiratory infection

N
O

☰ Mechanism of Action

Omeprazole interferes with gastric acid secretion by inhibiting the hydrogen potassium adenosine triphosphatase (H+ K+ -ATPase) enzyme system, or proton pump, in gastric parietal cells. Normally, the proton pump uses energy from hydrolysis of adenosine triphosphate to drive hydrogen (H^+) and chloride (Cl^-) out of parietal cells and into the stomach lumen in exchange for potassium (K^+), which leaves the stomach lumen and enters parietal cells. After this exchange, H^+ and Cl^- combine in the stomach to form hydrochloric acid (HCl), as shown below left. Omeprazole irreversibly blocks the exchange of intracellular H^+ and extracellular K^+, as shown below right. By preventing H^+ from entering the stomach lumen, omeprazole keeps additional HCl from forming.

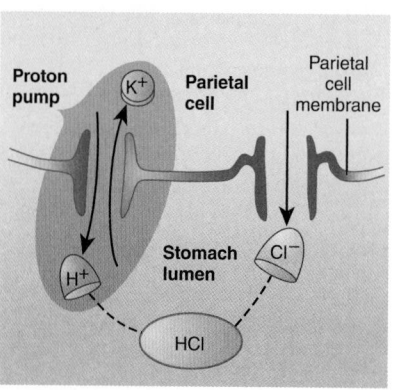
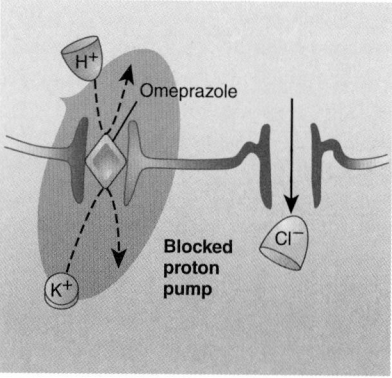

SKIN: Acute generalized exanthematous pustulosis, cutaneous lupus erythematosus, **erythema multiforme,** photosensitivity, pruritus, rash, **Stevens–Johnson syndrome, toxic epidermal necrolysis,** urticaria
Other: Anaphylaxis, angioedema, **drug reaction with eosinophilia and systemic symptoms (DRESS), hypocalcemia, hypokalemia, hypomagnesemia,** hyponatremia, systemic lupus erythematosus, vitamin B_{12} deficiency (long-term use), weight gain

☰ Childbearing Considerations

PREGNANCY

- It is not known if drug causes fetal harm.
- Use with caution only if benefit to mother outweighs potential risk to fetus.

LACTATION

- Drug may be present in breast milk.
- Patient should check with prescriber before breastfeeding.

☰ Nursing Considerations

! WARNING Monitor patient for hypersensitivity reactions such as acute tubulointerstitial nephritis, anaphylactic shock, anaphylaxis, angioedema, bronchospasm, and urticaria. Also, monitor patient for severe cutaneous adverse reactions. Be aware omeprazole should not be given to patients who have developed a hypersensitivity reaction with these symptoms in the past.

- Monitor patient's renal function closely because drug may cause acute tubulointerstitial nephritis at any time during therapy. Varying degrees of symptoms may occur or no symptoms at all. If renal function deteriorates, notify prescriber and expect drug to be discontinued.
- Know that because drug can interfere with absorption of vitamin B_{12}, monitor patient for macrocytic anemia.
- Monitor patient for bone fracture, especially in patients receiving multiple daily doses for more than a year, because proton pump inhibitors, such as omeprazole, increase risk for osteoporosis-related fractures of the hip, spine, or wrist.

- Be aware that long-term use of omeprazole may increase the risk of gastric carcinoma and symptomatic response to omeprazole therapy does not rule out the presence of gastric tumors.
- Know that omeprazole therapy may produce false elevations of serum chromogranin levels, used to help diagnosis presence of neuroendocrine tumors. If test results are high, withhold omeprazole therapy temporarily and repeat test, as ordered.
- Keep in mind that if omeprazole is given with antibiotics, watch for diarrhea from *C. difficile*. If diarrhea occurs, notify prescriber and expect to withhold drug and treat with electrolytes, fluids, protein, and an antibiotic effective against *C. difficile*.
- Monitor the patient, especially the patient on long-term therapy, for hypomagnesemia. If patient is to remain on omeprazole long term, expect to monitor the patient's serum magnesium level, as ordered, and if level becomes low, anticipate magnesium replacement therapy and omeprazole to be discontinued.
- Know that both cutaneous and systemic lupus erythematosus have occurred within days to years after proton pump therapy such as omeprazole was initiated. The most common symptoms presented were arthralgia, cytopenia, and rash. Report such findings to prescriber.
- Know that proton pump inhibitors such as omeprazole should not be prescribed longer than medically necessary.

PATIENT TEACHING

- Tell patient to take capsules or tablets whole and not to chew, crush, or split/open them. Tell patient taking once-daily dose to take drug before breakfast; if twice-daily dosing, tell patient to take drug before breakfast and dinner. If patient is unable to swallow tablets or capsules, advise patient that drug comes in a powder form to make an oral suspension.
- Instruct patient how to mix oral suspension form, if prescribed. Tell patient to take once-daily dose before breakfast and twice-daily dosing before breakfast and dinner. Tell patient to stir well, drink mixture within 30 minutes of mixing, and to refill cup with water and drink again.

> **! WARNING** Alert patient that drug may cause serious allergic and skin reactions that could be severe. At first sign of a rash or reaction, tell patient to stop drug and notify prescriber.

- Encourage patient to avoid alcohol, aspirin products, ibuprofen, and foods that may increase gastric secretions during therapy. Tell him to notify all prescribers about prescription drug use.
- Advise patient to notify prescriber immediately about abdominal pain or diarrhea. Also, tell patient to stop taking omeprazole and notify prescriber if serious or unusual reactions occur.
- Instruct patient to inform all prescribers of omeprazole therapy.
- Advise patient to notify prescriber if patient notices he is experiencing a decrease in the amount of urine voided or there is blood in his urine. Also tell him to notify prescriber if he experiences new or worsening joint pain or a rash on his arms or cheeks that gets worse in the sun.

ondansetron
Zofran ODT, Zuplenz

ondansetron hydrochloride
Zofran

⬚ Class and Category
Pharmacologic class: Selective serotonin (5-HT$_3$) receptor antagonist
Therapeutic class: Antiemetic

⬚ Indications and Dosages
✶ *To prevent nausea and vomiting associated with highly emetogenic cancer chemotherapy*

DISINTEGRATING TABLETS, ORAL SOLUTION, ORAL SOLUBLE FILM (ZUPLENZ), TABLETS

Adults. 24 mg 30 min before chemotherapy. Films and disintegrating tablets given as three 8-mg doses (allowing each 8-mg film or disintegrating tablet to dissolve completely before another given).

I.V. INFUSION

Adults and children ages 6 months to 18 years. Three 0.15-mg/kg doses, starting with first dose given 30 min before chemotherapy and second and third doses given 4 and 8 hr after first dose. *Maximum:* 16 mg per dose.

✴ *To prevent nausea and vomiting associated with moderately emetogenic cancer chemotherapy*

DISINTEGRATING TABLETS, ORAL SOLUTION, ORAL SOLUBLE FILM (ZUPLENZ), TABLETS

Adults and adolescents age 12 and over. *Initial:* One 8-mg dose given 30 min before chemotherapy and one 8-mg dose given 8 hr after the first dose. Then, one 8-mg dose given every 12 hr for 1 to 2 days after completion of chemotherapy.

Children ages 4 to 11. *Initial:* One 4-mg dose given 30 min before chemotherapy with one 4-mg dose given 4 and 8 hr after the first dose. Then, one 4-mg dose given every 8 hr for 1 to 2 days after completion of chemotherapy.

✴ *To prevent nausea and vomiting associated with initial and repeat courses of emetogenic chemotherapy*

I.V. INFUSION

Adults and children ages 6 months to 18 years. Three 0.15-mg/kg doses, starting with first dose given 30 min before chemotherapy and second and third doses given 4 and 8 hr after first dose. *Maximum:* 16 mg per dose.

✴ *To prevent nausea and vomiting associated with radiotherapy in patients receiving either total body irradiation, single high-dose fraction to the abdomen, or daily fractions to the abdomen*

DISINTEGRATING TABLETS, ORAL SOLUTION, ORAL SOLUBLE FILM (ZUPLENZ), TABLETS

Adults receiving total body irradiation. 8-mg dose given 1 to 2 hr before each fraction of radiotherapy administered each day.

Adults receiving single high-dose fraction radiotherapy to the abdomen. 8-mg dose given 1 to 2 hr before radiotherapy, with subsequent 8-mg doses given every 8 hr after the first dose for 1 to 2 days after completion of radiotherapy.

Adults receiving daily fractionated radiotherapy to the abdomen. 8-mg dose given 1 to 2 hr before radiotherapy with subsequent 8-mg doses given every 8 hr after the first dose for each day radiotherapy is given.

✴ *To prevent postoperative nausea and vomiting*

DISINTEGRATING TABLETS, ORAL SOLUTION, TABLETS

Adults. 16 mg as a single dose 1 hr before anesthesia induction.

ORAL SOLUBLE FILM (ZUPLENZ)

Adults. 16 mg given as two 8-mg films (first 8-mg film allowed to dissolve completely before second 8-mg film given) 1 hr before induction of anesthesia.

I.V. INJECTION

Adults and children age 12 and over. 4 mg undiluted as a single dose just before anesthesia induction or if nausea or vomiting develops within 2 hr after surgery, providing no prophylactic antiemetics had been given preoperatively.

Children ages 2 to 12 weighing more than 40 kg (88 lb). 4 mg as a single dose just before anesthesia induction or if nausea or vomiting develops within 2 hr after surgery, providing no prophylactic antiemetics had been given preoperatively.

Children ages 1 month to 12 years weighing 40 kg (88 lb) or less. 0.1 mg/kg as a single dose just before or immediately after anesthesia induction or if nausea or vomiting develops within 2 hr after surgery, providing no prophylactic antiemetics had been given preoperatively.

I.M. INJECTION

Adults and children age 12 and over. 4 mg undiluted as a single dose just before anesthesia induction or if nausea within 2 hr after surgery, providing no prophylactic antiemetics had been given preoperatively.

± **DOSAGE ADJUSTMENT** For patients with severe hepatic impairment, maximum dosage limited to 8 mg daily I.V. or P.O.

Drug Administration

P.O.

▪ For ODT tablet administration: With dry, gloved hands, open blister containing ODT tablet by peeling backing off. Don't push tablet through foil blister. Place on top of patient's tongue. It will dissolve in seconds. Then have patient swallow with saliva. A drink afterward is not needed.

- For oral film administration: With dry, gloved hands, open film pouch and immediately place film on top of patient's tongue. It will dissolve in 4 to 20 seconds. Then have patient swallow with or without a beverage. If using more than 1 film, allow each film to dissolve completely before administering the next film.
- For oral solution administration: Use calibrated container or oral syringe to measure dose of oral solution. Store at room temperature and protect from light. Oral solution container should also be stored upright.

I.V.

- Drug may precipitate at the stopper/vial interface in vials stored upright. If this happens, resolubilize by shaking the vial vigorously.
- For I.V. infusion used to prevent nausea and vomiting related to chemotherapy: Dilute drug for adults in 50 ml of 0.9% Sodium Chloride Injection or 5% Dextrose in Water. In children, dilute drug in 10 to 50 ml of 0.9% Sodium Chloride Injection or 5% Dextrose in Water depending on fluid needs. Infuse over 15 minutes.
- For I.V. injection used to prevent postoperative nausea and vomiting: Inject undiluted over more than 30 seconds but preferably over 2 to 5 minutes.
- After dilution, solution is stable at room temperature under normal lighting conditions for 48 hours if diluted with 0.9% Sodium Chloride Injection, 5% Dextrose Injection, 0.45% or 0.9% Sodium Chloride Injection, or 3% Sodium Chloride Injection.
- *Incompatibilities:* Alkaline solutions

I.M.

- Administer undiluted into a large muscle mass.

Route	Onset	Peak	Duration
P.O.	30 min	1–2 hr	Unknown
I.V.	5 min	10 min	Unknown
I.M.	Unknown	30 min	Unknown

Half-life: 3.1–5.8 hr

Mechanism of Action

Blocks serotonin receptors centrally in the chemoreceptor trigger zone and peripherally at vagal nerve terminals in the intestine. This action reduces nausea and vomiting by preventing serotonin release in the small intestine (probable cause of chemotherapy- and radiation-induced nausea and vomiting) and by blocking signals to the CNS. Ondansetron may also bind to other serotonin receptors and to mu-opioid receptors.

Contraindications

Concomitant use of apomorphine, hypersensitivity to ondansetron or its components

Interactions

DRUGS

5-HT3 receptor antagonists, selective serotonin reuptake inhibitors, serotonin and noradrenaline reuptake inhibitors: Increased risk of serotonin syndrome
carbamazepine, phenytoin, rifampin: Possibly decreased ondansetron blood concentrations
tramadol: Possibly interference with pain control from tramadol

Adverse Reactions

CNS: Agitation, akathisia, anxiety, ataxia, dizziness, drowsiness, dystonia, fever, headache, **hypotension**, restlessness, seizures, **serotonin syndrome**, syncope, somnolence, thirst, weakness
CV: Arrhythmias, cardiopulmonary arrest (parenteral form), chest pain, **hypotension, myocardial ischemia,** palpitations, **prolonged QT interval, shock,** tachycardia, **torsades de pointes**
EENT: Accommodation disturbances, altered taste, blurred vision, dry mouth, **laryngeal edema, laryngospasm, stridor,** transient blindness
GI: Abdominal pain, anorexia, constipation, diarrhea, elevated liver enzymes, flatulence, indigestion, **intestinal obstruction,** masking of progressive gastric and ileus distention
RESP: Bronchospasms, pulmonary embolism, shortness of breath
SKIN: Flushing, hyperpigmentation, maculopapular rash, pruritus, **Stevens–Johnson syndrome, toxic epidermal necrolysis,** urticaria
Other: Anaphylaxis; angioedema; hiccups; injection-site burning, pain, and redness

Childbearing Considerations

PREGNANCY

- It is not known if drug causes fetal harm.
- Use with caution only if benefit to mother outweighs potential risk to fetus.

LACTATION

- Drug may be present in breast milk.
- Patient should check with prescriber before breastfeeding.

Nursing Considerations

! WARNING Be aware that oral disintegrating tablets may contain aspartame, which is metabolized to phenylalanine and must be avoided in patients with phenylketonuria.

- Know that if hypokalemia or hypomagnesemia is present, these electrolyte imbalances should be corrected before ondansetron is administered because of increased risk for QT-interval prolongation, which could predispose the patient to develop torsades de pointes.

! WARNING Monitor patient closely for signs and symptoms of hypersensitivity to ondansetron because hypersensitivity reactions, including anaphylaxis and bronchospasm, may occur. If present, discontinue drug, notify prescriber, and provide supportive care.

! WARNING Monitor patient closely for serotonin syndrome, which may include agitation, chills, confusion, diaphoresis, diarrhea, fever, hyperactive reflexes, poor coordination, restlessness, shaking, talking or acting with uncontrolled excitement, tremor, and twitching.

- Monitor patient's electrocardiogram, as ordered, and especially in patients with bradyarrhythmias, congestive heart failure, hypokalemia, or hypomagnesemia or in patients taking other medications known to prolong the QT interval because ondansetron therapy can prolong the QT interval resulting in life-threatening arrhythmias such as torsades de pointes. Be aware that no dosage greater than 16 mg should be given intravenously at any one time due to increased risk of prolonged QT interval. Also, monitor patient for chest pain that may be caused by myocardial ischemia, which may appear immediately after administration.

! WARNING Be aware that ondansetron may mask symptoms of adynamic progressive ileus or gastric distention after abdominal surgery. Monitor patient for decreased bowel activity, especially if patient has risk factors for gastrointestinal obstruction.

PATIENT TEACHING

- Advise patient to use calibrated container or oral syringe to measure oral solution.

! WARNING Tell patient that oral disintegrating tablets may contain aspartame, which is metabolized to phenylalanine and must be used cautiously in patients with phenylketonuria. Tell patient each 4- and 8-mg orally disintegrating tablet contains less than 0.03 mg phenylalanine.

- Instruct patient to place ondansetron disintegrating tablet or oral soluble film on his tongue immediately after opening package and to let it dissolve on his tongue before swallowing. Advise patient not to push disintegrating tablet through foil blister but to open by peeling backing off.

! WARNING Advise patient to immediately report signs of hypersensitivity, such as rash or development of sudden chest pain or tightness. Also, advise patient to seek immediate medical attention if patient experiences persistent, severe, unusual, or worsening symptoms.

- Reassure patient with transient blindness that it will resolve within a few minutes to 48 hours.

opicapone
Ongentys

Class and Category

Pharmacologic class: Catechol-O-methyltransferase (COMT) inhibitor
Therapeutic class: Antiparkinsonian

Indications and Dosages

* *Adjunct treatment to levodopa/carbidopa in patients with Parkinson's disease experiencing "off" episodes*

CAPSULES

Adults. 50 mg once daily.

± **DOSAGE ADJUSTMENT** For patients with moderate hepatic impairment, dosage reduced to 25 mg once daily.

Drug Administration

P.O.

- Administer drug at bedtime.
- Patient should not eat food for 1 hour before and for at least 1 hour after taking drug.

Route	Onset	Peak	Duration
P.O.	Unknown	Unknown	<24 hr

Half-life: 1–2 hr

Mechanism of Action

Prevents the breakdown of levodopa where it turns into dopamine in the brain. Dopamine helps to maintain normal movement in Parkinson's disease.

Contraindications

Concomitant use of nonselective MAO inhibitors; hypersensitivity to opicapone or its components; presence of paraganglioma, pheochromocytoma, or other catecholamine-secreting neoplasms

Interactions

DRUGS

drugs metabolized by COMT such as dobutamine, dopamine, epinephrine, isoproterenol, norepinephrine; nonselective MAO inhibitors such as isocarboxazid, phenelzine, tranylcypromine: Increased levels of catecholamines, possibly leading to arrhythmias, excessive changes in blood pressure, and increased heart rate

Adverse Reactions

CNS: Agitation, aggressiveness, delusions, dizziness, dyskinesia, falling asleep during daytime, hallucinations, lack of impulse control, insomnia, somnolence, syncope
CV: Hypertension, **hypotension**
EENT: Dry mouth
GI: Constipation
Other: Elevated creatine kinase levels, weight loss

Childbearing Considerations

PREGNANCY

- It is not known if drug can cause fetal harm. However, animal studies suggest the possibility of fetal abnormalities.

- Use with caution only if benefit to mother outweighs potential risk to fetus.

LACTATION

- It is not known if drug is present in breast milk.
- Patient should check with prescriber before breastfeeding.

Nursing Considerations

- Know that opicapone is used in patients with dopamine dysregulation syndrome.
- Know that opicapone should not be given to patients with severe hepatic impairment.
- Provide safety measures for patients receiving opicapone, because drug may cause patient to fall asleep during activities of daily living. Monitor patient for excessive drowsiness, but know that patient may feel alert immediately prior to falling asleep. Notify prescriber of such problems, as drug may have to be discontinued. Also, if other drugs are being taken, such as other dopaminergic or sedating drugs, dosage of any of these drugs may have to be reduced.
- Monitor patient's blood pressure, because opicapone may cause both orthostatic and nonorthostatic hypotension. If hypotension occurs, notify prescriber, as drug may have to be discontinued or a dosage reduction in a concomitantly administered antihypertensive drug may be needed.
- Monitor patient for the development of dyskinesia or exacerbation of preexisting dyskinesia, as this was the most common adverse reaction associated with drug. Notify prescriber if present.
- Monitor patient for hallucinations and psychotic-like behavior. If present, notify prescriber, as drug may have to be discontinued.

! **WARNING** Be aware that a symptom complex resembling neuroleptic malignant syndrome (altered consciousness, autonomic instability, elevated temperature, and muscular rigidity) has occurred when opicapone dosage has been rapidly reduced, drug is withdrawn, or changes are made in dosages of other drugs that increase central dopaminergic tone. When drug is discontinued, monitor patient closely for adverse effects and expect prescriber to make adjustment of other dopaminergic therapies, as needed.

N
O

PATIENT TEACHING

- Instruct patient and caregiver that opicapone should be taken at bedtime and patient should not eat for 1 hour before and for at least 1 hour after taking drug.
- Tell patient and caregiver that if a dose is missed, the next dose should be taken at the scheduled time the next day.
- Alert patient and caregiver that falling asleep during activities of daily living may occur without warning. Caution patient to avoid driving, operating machinery, and other hazardous activity until effect of drug is known.
- Tell patient to rise from a lying or sitting position slowly to avoid fainting or light-headedness.
- Review adverse reactions with patient and caregiver, especially abnormal movement of body parts, hallucinations, and psychotic-like behaviors; falling asleep suddenly; and/or experiencing intense urges to binge-eat, gamble, have sex, or spend money. If present, instruct patient to notify prescriber.

! **WARNING** Urge patient not to discontinue opicapone suddenly. Tell patient to call prescriber if symptoms of confusion, fever, or severe muscle stiffness occur.

- Inform patient and caregiver to tell all prescribers that opicapone is being taken as well as any other drugs, including dietary supplements, herbal products, and over-the-counter drugs.

oritavancin diphosphate

Kimyrsa, Orbactiv

Class and Category

Pharmacologic class: Lipoglycopeptide
Therapeutic class: Antibiotic

Indications and Dosages

* *To treat acute bacterial skin and skin structure infections caused by gram-positive microorganisms such as* Enterococcus faecalis *(vancomycin-susceptible isolates only),* Staphylococcus aureus *(including methicillin-susceptible and methicillin-resistant isolates),* Streptococcus agalactiae, S. dysgalactiae, S. anginosus *group (S. anginosus, S. constellatus, S. intermedius), and* S. pyogenes

I.V. INFUSION

Adults. 1,200 mg as a one-time dose.

Drug Administration

- Be aware that there are two oritavancin products that are different in the following ways: dose strengths, duration of infusion, reconstitution and dilution instructions, and compatible diluents. Be sure the correct product is being prepared and administered properly.

I.V. (KIMYRSA)

- Reconstitute drug by adding 40 ml of Sterile Water for Injection to one vial to provide a 30 mg/ml solution.
- Gently swirl contents to avoid foaming and ensure that all powder is completely dissolved. Solution should appear clear and colorless to pink.
- Dilute further by withdrawing and discarding 40 ml from a 250-ml intravenous bag of either 0.9% Sodium Chloride Injection or 5% Dextrose in Water. Withdraw 40 ml of drug from vial and add to intravenous bag to bring volume back to 250 ml yielding 4.8 mg/ml.
- The combined storage time (reconstituted solution in the vial and diluted solution in the bag) and 1 hour infusion time should not exceed 4 hours at room temperature or 12 hours if refrigerated.
- Flush intravenous line with 0.9% Sodium Chloride Injection or 5% Dextrose in Water solution before and after administering drug.
- Infuse drug over 1 hour. If patient develops an infusion-related reaction such as flushing, pruritus, or urticaria, slow or stop the infusion and notify prescriber.
- *Incompatibilities for Kimyrsa:* Drugs formulated at a basic or neutral pH or solutions other than 0.9% Sodium Chloride Injection or 5% Dextrose in Water

I.V. (ORBACTIV)

- Reconstitute drug by adding 40 ml of Sterile Water for Injection to each vial (three vials are needed) to provide a 10-mg/ml solution per vial. Gently swirl to avoid foaming and to completely dissolve the powder.

Solution should appear clear, colorless to pale yellow.

- Withdraw and discard 120 ml from a 1,000-ml intravenous bag of 5% Dextrose in Water (never use 0.9% Sodium Chloride Injection). Then withdraw 40 ml from each of the three reconstituted vials and add to 5% Dextrose in Water intravenous bag to bring bag volume back to 1,000 ml. This will yield a concentration of 1.2 mg/ml.
- Once mixed in infusion bag, use within 6 hours when stored at room temperature or within 12 hours when refrigerated. These times include the additional 3 hours needed for administration.
- Flush intravenous line with 5% Dextrose in Water solution before and after administering drug.
- Infuse drug over 3 hours. If patient develops an infusion-related reaction such as flushing, pruritus, or urticaria, slow or stop the infusion and notify prescriber.
- *Incompatibilities for Orbactiv:* 0.9% Sodium Chloride Injection solution, other solutions containing 0.9% Sodium Chloride Injection, other additives or drugs mixed in 0.9% Sodium Chloride Injection, drugs formulated with a basic or neutral pH (possibly)

Route	Onset	Peak	Duration
I.V.	Unknown	Unknown	Unknown

Half-life: 245 hr

Mechanism of Action

Kills bacteria by inhibiting cell wall synthesis.

Contraindications

Hypersensitivity to oritavancin and its components, intravenous unfractionated heparin sodium administration used within 5 days following oritavancin administration

Interactions

DRUGS

drugs with a narrow therapeutic window that are predominantly metabolized by CYP450 enzymes: Possibly decreased or increased concentration of these drugs
warfarin: Increased risk of bleeding

Adverse Reactions

CNS: Dizziness, headache
CV: Peripheral edema, tachycardia

ENDO: Hypoglycemia
GI: Clostridium difficile-associated diarrhea, diarrhea, elevated liver enzymes, nausea, vomiting
HEME: Anemia, eosinophilia
MS: Myalgia, osteomyelitis, tenosynovitis
RESP: Bronchospasm, wheezing
SKIN: Erythema multiforme, leukocytoclastic vasculitis, pruritus, rash, urticaria
Other: Anaphylaxis; angioedema; antibodies to oritavancin; hyperuricemia; infusion reactions such as back or chest pain, chills, erythema, flushing of the upper body, pruritus, tremor, or urticaria; infusion-site extravasation, induration, or phlebitis

Childbearing Considerations

PREGNANCY

- It is not known if drug causes fetal harm.
- Use with caution only if benefit to mother outweighs potential risk to fetus.

LACTATION

- Drug may be present in breast milk.
- Patient should check with prescriber before breastfeeding.

Nursing Considerations

- Use oritavancin cautiously in patients with a history of hypersensitivity to glycopeptides because of the possibility of cross-sensitivity.
- Monitor patient closely for signs of bleeding, especially if patient is taking warfarin therapy, because drug may artificially prolong prothrombin time (PT) and INR for up to 12 hours, making monitoring of the effectiveness of warfarin unreliable for at least 12 hours after the administration of oritavancin. Drug may also artificially prolong activated partial thromboplastin time (aPTT) for up to 120 hours and activated clotting time (ACT) for up to 24 hours after a single 1,200-mg dose of oritavancin.

! **WARNING** Monitor patient closely for signs of hypersensitivity reactions because some reactions may be serious. If present, discontinue infusion immediately, notify prescriber, and implement appropriate standard of care.

- Assess patient for signs of secondary infection, such as profuse, watery diarrhea. If such diarrhea develops, contact prescriber and expect to obtain a stool specimen to rule out pseudomembranous colitis caused by *C. difficile*. If confirmed, expect to withhold drug and treat with electrolytes, fluids, protein, and an antibiotic effective against C. *difficile*.

- Monitor patient for osteomyelitis, as drug has been shown to produce more cases of osteomyelitis than vancomycin used to treat similar infections. If present, be prepared to institute appropriate alternative antibacterial therapy.
- Be aware that drug may artificially prolong certain coagulation test results. If patient requires monitoring of anticoagulation effects, a nonphospholipid-dependent coagulation test such as Factor Xa assay or an alternative anticoagulant not requiring aPTT monitoring may be required.

PATIENT TEACHING

! **WARNING** Alert patient that an allergic reaction can occur up to a day after oritavancin has been administered. Instruct him to notify prescriber of any signs of an allergic reaction and seek immediate medical attention if signs are severe or prolonged.

- Urge patient to tell prescriber if diarrhea develops, even 2 months or more after oritavancin ends.
- Advise patient to contact prescriber if serious or unusual adverse effects occur after receiving drug.

oseltamivir phosphate
Tamiflu

☰ Class and Category

Pharmacologic class: Selective neuraminidase inhibitor
Therapeutic class: Antiviral

☰ Indications and Dosages

＊ *To treat acute uncomplicated illness due to influenza A and B infection in patients who have been symptomatic for no more than 48 hours*

CAPSULES, ORAL SUSPENSION

Adults and adolescents. 75 mg twice daily for 5 days.
Children ages 1 to 12 years weighing more than 40 kg (88 lb). 75 mg twice daily.

Children ages 1 to 12 years weighing 23.1 kg (50.82 lb) to 40 kg (88 lb). 60 mg twice daily.
Children ages 1 to 12 years weighing 15.1 kg (33.22 lb) to 23 kg (50.6 lb). 45 mg twice daily.
Children ages 1 to 12 years weighing 15 kg (33 lb) or less. 30 mg twice daily.
Infants 2 weeks to less than 1 year at any weight. 3 mg/kg twice daily.

＊ *To prevent influenza A and B infection*

CAPSULES, ORAL SUSPENSION

Adults and adolescents. 75 mg once daily for at least 10 days following close contact with an infected individual, up to 6 wk during a community outbreak, and up to 12 wk for immunocompromised patients.
Children ages 1 to 12 years weighing more than 40.1 kg (88 lb). 75 mg once daily for at least 10 days following close contact with an infected individual, up to 6 wk during a community outbreak, and up to 12 wk for immunocompromised patients.
Children ages 1 to 12 years weighing 23.1 kg (50.82 lb) to 40 kg (88 lb). 60 mg once daily for at least 10 days following close contact with an infected individual, up to 6 wk during a community outbreak, and up to 12 wk for immunocompromised patients.
Children ages 1 to 12 years weighing 15.1 (33.22 lb) to 23 kg (50.6 lb). 45 mg once daily for at least 10 days following close contact with an infected individual, up to 6 wk during a community outbreak, and up to 12 wk for immunocompromised patients.
Children ages 1 to 12 years weighing 15 kg (33 lb) or less. 30 mg once daily for at least 10 days following close contact with an infected individual, up to 6 wk during a community outbreak, and up to 12 wk for immunocompromised patients.

±**DOSAGE ADJUSTMENT** For adult patients with a creatinine clearance between 30 and 60 ml/min, dosage reduced to 30 mg twice daily for 5 days to treat influenza A and B infection and 30 mg once daily to prevent influenza A and B infection for 10 days. For adult patients with a creatinine clearance of between 10 to 30 ml/min, dosage reduced to 30 mg once daily for 5 days to treat influenza A and B infection and 30 mg every other day to prevent influenza A and B infection for 10 days. For adult patients with end-stage renal disease on hemodialysis, dosage reduced to 30 mg given immediately and then 30 mg after each hemodialysis cycle (treatment duration not to exceed 5 days) to treat influenza A and B infection and 30 mg given immediately and then 30 mg after each hemodialysis cycles to prevent influenza A and B infection for 10 days. For patients with end-stage renal disease on continuous ambulatory peritoneal dialysis, dosage reduced to a single 30-mg dose administered immediately to treat influenza A and B infection and 30 mg given immediately and then 30 mg once weekly to prevent influenza A and B infection for 10 days.

▤ Drug Administration

P.O.

- Administer with or without food, but patient may tolerate drug better if given with food.
- Capsules should be swallowed whole and not chewed or crushed. However, for the patient who cannot swallow capsules, the capsules may be opened and mixed with sweetened liquids such as regular or sugar-free chocolate syrup, corn syrup, caramel topping, or light brown sugar (dissolved in water).
- To make oral suspension, tap closed bottle several times to loosen powder. Add 55 ml of water to drug bottle and shake closed bottle well for 15 seconds.
- During an emergency and when oral suspension is not available or the age-appropriate strengths of oseltamivir capsules to mix with sweetened liquids are not available, the pharmacist can make an emergency suspension preparation that contains 6 mg/ml using capsules. It is only stable for 5 days at room temperature or 5 weeks when stored in a refrigerator.
- Shake oral suspension well before using. Use the oral dispenser device that comes with the product to measure dosage.
- Manufactured oral suspension can be stored in the refrigerator for up to 17 days or 10 days if stored at room temperature; then discard. Avoid freezing.

Route	Onset	Peak	Duration
P.O.	Unknown	2.5–6 hr	Unknown

Half-life: 1–3 hr

▤ Mechanism of Action

After conversion to its active form, oseltamivir inhibits influenza virus neuraminidase, affecting release of viral particles.

▤ Contraindications

Hypersensitivity to oseltamivir phosphate or its components

▤ Interactions

DRUGS

live-attenuated influenza vaccine (intranasal): Possibly decreased effectiveness

▤ Adverse Reactions

CNS: Abnormal behavior, agitation, altered level of consciousness, anxiety, delirium, delusions, headache, **hypothermia,** nightmares, **seizures**
CV: Arrhythmia
ENDO: Aggravation of diabetes mellitus
GI: Diaper rash, diarrhea, elevated liver enzymes, **GI bleeding, hemorrhagic colitis, hepatitis,** nausea, vomiting
SKIN: Dermatitis, eczema, **erythema multiforme,** rash, **Stevens–Johnson syndrome, toxic epidermal necrolysis,** urticaria
Other: Anaphylaxis, angioedema, generalized pain

▤ Childbearing Considerations

PREGNANCY

- It is not known if drug causes fetal harm.
- Use with caution only if benefit to mother outweighs potential risk to fetus.

LACTATION

- Drug is present in breast milk.
- Patient should check with prescriber before breastfeeding.

▤ Nursing Considerations

! **WARNING** Monitor patient for serious hypersensitivity and skin reactions when administering oseltamivir. Know that anaphylaxis and skin reactions such as erythema multiforme, Stevens–Johnson syndrome, and toxic epidermal necrolysis have occurred. If present, discontinue oseltamivir therapy immediately, notify prescriber, and be prepared to provide emergency supportive care as ordered.

- Be aware that although uncommon, abnormal behavior and delirium have occurred after administration of oseltamivir, especially in children. While the onset is abrupt, rapid resolution usually occurs once oseltamivir is discontinued.

PATIENT TEACHING

- Instruct patient that for oseltamivir to be most effective, therapy should begin as soon as possible with the first appearance of flu symptoms: no later than 48 hours of onset of symptoms and as soon as possible after exposure.
- Tell patient to take a missed dose as soon as he remembers it, except if it is within 2 hours of the next scheduled dose.
- Warn patient that oral suspension contains above-normal maximum daily limits of sorbitol and may cause dyspepsia and diarrhea, especially in patients with hereditary fructose intolerance.
- Inform patient who cannot swallow capsules, when oral suspension is not available, that capsules may be opened and mixed with sweetened liquids such as caramel topping, corn syrup, light brown sugar dissolved in water, or regular or sugar-free chocolate syrup.
- Instruct patient, parent, or caregiver to use the oral dispenser device that comes with manufactured oral suspension.
- Instruct patient that oral suspension can be stored at room temperature for up to 10 days or in the refrigerator for up to 17 days before discarding. Caution against freezing.

! **WARNING** Advise patient to seek immediate medical attention if he experiences an allergic reaction or unusual or severe skin reactions.

- Alert patient and parents that, although uncommon, abnormal behavior and delirium have occurred, especially in children. Notify prescriber if present and expect drug to be discontinued.
- Inform patient that oseltamivir is not a substitute for receiving an annual flu vaccination.

oxandrolone

Oxandrin

≡ Class, Category, and Schedule

Pharmacologic class: Androgen
Therapeutic class: Appetite stimulant
Controlled substance schedule: III

≡ Indications and Dosages

✳ *As adjunct to offset protein catabolism from prolonged use of corticosteroids; to provide relief of bone pain from osteoporosis*

TABLETS

Adults. 2.5 to 20 mg in divided doses given twice daily to four times a day for 2 to 4 wk; intermittent therapy repeated as prescribed. *Maximum:* 20 mg daily.
Children. 0.1 mg/kg or less daily; intermittent therapy repeated as prescribed.

± **DOSAGE ADJUSTMENT** For elderly patients, dosage not to exceed 5 mg twice daily.

≡ Drug Administration

P.O.

- No specific administration guidelines given by manufacturer.

Route	Onset	Peak	Duration
P.O.	Unknown	1 hr	Unknown

Half-life: 10–13 hr`

≡ Mechanism of Action

Promotes tissue-building processes and reverses catabolic or tissue-depleting processes by promoting protein anabolism.

≡ Contraindications

Breast cancer (males); breast cancer with hypercalcemia (females); hypercalcemia; hypersensitivity to oxandrolone, anabolic steroids, or their components; nephrosis; pregnancy; prostate cancer

≡ Interactions

DRUGS

ACTH, adrenal steroids: Increased risk of edema
oral hypoglycemic agents: Inhibited metabolism of these drugs
warfarin: Increased risk anticoagulant effect

Adverse Reactions

CNS: Depression, excitement, insomnia

CV: Decreased serum HDL level, edema, hyperlipidemia, hypertension

ENDO: Feminization in postpubertal males (epididymitis, gynecomastia, impotence, oligospermia, priapism, testicular atrophy), glucose intolerance, virilism in females (acne, clitoral enlargement, decreased breast size, deepened voice, diaphoresis, emotional lability, flushing, hirsutism, hoarseness, libido changes, male-pattern baldness, menstrual irregularities, nervousness, oily skin or hair, vaginal bleeding, vaginitis, weight gain), virilism in prepubertal males (acne, decreased ejaculatory volume, penis enlargement, prepubertal closure of epiphyseal plates, unnatural growth of body and facial hair)

GI: Diarrhea, elevated liver enzymes, **hepatocellular carcinoma**, jaundice, nausea, vomiting

GU: Benign prostatic hyperplasia, **prostate cancer**, urinary frequency, urine retention (elderly men)

HEME: Iron deficiency anemia, **leukemia, prolonged bleeding time**

Other: Fluid retention, **hypercalcemia** (females), physical and psychological dependence, sodium retention

Childbearing Considerations

PREGNANCY

- Drug may cause fetal harm.
- Drug is contraindicated during pregnancy.

LACTATION

- It is not known if drug is present in breast milk.
- A decision should be made to discontinue breastfeeding or the drug to avoid potential adverse reactions in the breastfed infant.

REPRODUCTION

- Women of childbearing age should use an effective contraceptive throughout drug therapy.

Nursing Considerations

- Use oxandrolone cautiously in patients with heart disease because drug has hypercholesterolemic effects.
- Provide adequate calories and protein, as ordered, to maintain a positive nitrogen balance during oxandrolone therapy.
- Anticipate an increased risk of fluid and sodium retention in patients with cardiac, hepatic, or renal dysfunction.
- Weigh patient daily to detect fluid retention. If patient has fluid retention, expect a sodium-restricted diet or diuretics.
- Monitor blood glucose level frequently in patient with diabetes mellitus.
- Know that if patient takes an oral anticoagulant, check INR or PT should be checked as ordered.

PATIENT TEACHING

- Advise patient to consume a diet high in calories and protein to achieve maximum therapeutic effect of oxandrolone.
- Urge patient to weigh himself daily during therapy and to report swelling or unexplained weight gain at once.
- Explain that drug may alter libido.
- Inform woman that drug may cause permanent physical changes, such as clitoral enlargement, deepened voice, and hair growth.
- Advise female patient of childbearing age that she must use contraception during oxandrolone therapy and should notify prescriber immediately about suspected or known pregnancy.
- Instruct diabetic patient to monitor blood glucose level frequently.
- Advise bleeding precautions (such as an electric shaver and soft toothbrush) if patient takes warfarin. Tell patient to notify prescriber immediately if bleeding occurs.

N
O

oxaprozin
Daypro

oxaprozin potassium
Daypro Alta

Class and Category

Pharmacologic class: NSAID

Therapeutic class: Anti-inflammatory, antirheumatic

Indications and Dosages

✳ *To treat osteoarthritis and rheumatoid arthritis*

TABLETS

Adults. *Initial:* 1,200 mg once daily. Dosage adjusted based on response. *Maximum:*

1,200 mg daily (Daypro Alta) or 1,800 mg daily or 26 mg/kg daily (whichever is less) in divided doses (Daypro).

±**DOSAGE ADJUSTMENT** Initial dose limited to 600 mg daily for patients with low body weight or severe renal impairment.

✻ *To treat juvenile rheumatoid arthritis*

TABLETS (DAYPRO)

Children ages 6 to 16 years weighing 55 kg (121 lb) or more. 1,200 mg once daily. *Maximum:* 1,200 mg daily.

Children ages 6 to 16 weighing 32 to 54 kg (70.4 to 118.8 lb). 900 mg once daily.

Children ages 6 to 16 weighing 22 to 31 kg (48.4 to 68.2). 600 mg once daily.

±**DOSAGE ADJUSTMENT** For patient taking Daypro with low body weight or patient with severe renal impairment or on dialysis, initial dosage reduced to 600 mg once daily. In adults taking Daypro who require a quick onset of action, a one-time loading dose of 1,200 to 1,800 mg (not to exceed 25 mg/kg) may be given. For adult patients taking Daypro who require chronic dosage, weighing more than 50 kg (110 lb), have a normal renal and hepatic function, are at low risk of peptic ulcer, and whose severity of disease justifies maximal therapy, dosage larger than 1,200 mg/day may be given. For patients taking Daypro Alta who have a low body weight or milder disease, initial dose reduced to 600 mg. For patient taking Daypro Alta who has renal impairment or is elderly, reduced dosage may be needed.

☰ Drug Administration

P.O.

- Administer with food to minimize GI adverse effects and with a full glass of water.
- Have patient stay upright for 15 to 30 minutes after administration to keep drug from lodging in esophagus and causing irritation.

Route	Onset	Peak	Duration
P.O.	Unknown	2–4 hr	Unknown

Half-life: 22–55 hr

☰ Mechanism of Action

Blocks cyclooxygenase, the enzyme needed to synthesize prostaglandins, which mediate the inflammatory response and cause local vasodilation, pain, and swelling. By blocking cyclooxygenase and prostaglandins, the NSAID oxaprozin relieves pain.

☰ Contraindications

History of asthma, urticaria, or other allergic-type reactions after taking aspirin or other NSAIDs, hypersensitivity to oxaprozin or its components; postoperatively after coronary artery bypass graft (CABG) surgery

☰ Interactions

DRUGS

ACE inhibitors, angiotensin receptor blockers, beta-blockers: Diminished antihypertensive effect of these drugs; possibly impaired renal function especially in the elderly and patients with existing renal impairment or volume depletion

anticoagulants, antiplatelets, selective serotonin reuptake inhibitors, serotonin–norepinephrine reuptake inhibitors: Increased risk of bleeding

aspirin: Increased significant risk of GI bleeding reactions

corticosteroids: Increased risk of adverse GI effects

cyclosporine: Increased risk of nephrotoxicity

digoxin: Increased blood digoxin level and risk of digitalis toxicity

diuretics: Possibly decreased diuretic effect

glyburide: Possibly altered blood glucose level

lithium: Increased blood lithium level and increased risk of lithium toxicity

methotrexate: Increased blood methotrexate level and risk of methotrexate toxicity

other NSAIDs, salicylates: Increased GI irritability and bleeding

pemetrexed: Increased risk of pemetrexed-associated GI and renal toxicity, myelosuppression

ACTIVITIES

alcohol use, smoking: Increased risk of adverse GI effects

☰ Adverse Reactions

CNS: **Aseptic meningitis**, confusion, **CVA**, dizziness, drowsiness, fatigue, headache, insomnia, nervousness, sedation, transient ischemic attacks, vertigo, weakness

CV: **Deep vein thrombosis**, hypertension, **hypotension**, **MI**, peripheral edema

EENT: Tinnitus

ENDO: **Hypoglycemia**

GI: Abdominal pain, constipation, diarrhea, dyspepsia, elevated liver enzymes, **GI bleeding** or ulceration, **hepatitis**, jaundice, **liver failure**, nausea, **perforation of intestine or stomach**, vomiting

GU: **Acute renal failure,** dysuria, interstitial nephritis, urinary frequency

HEME: **Agranulocytosis,** anemia, **aplastic anemia, leukopenia, pancytopenia, thrombocytopenia**

SKIN: Alopecia, **erythema multiforme, exfoliative dermatitis,** maculopapular rash, photosensitivity, **Stevens–Johnson syndrome, toxic epidermal necrolysis**

Other: **Anaphylaxis, angioedema, drug reaction with eosinophilia and systemic symptoms (DRESS)**

Childbearing Considerations

PREGNANCY

- Drug increases risk of premature closure of the fetal ductus arteriosus if given at or beyond 30 weeks gestation.
- Drug may cause fetal renal dysfunction leading to oligohydramnios and possibly neonatal renal impairment if given at 20 weeks gestation or beyond.
- Drug should be avoided in pregnant women starting at 30 weeks of gestation and onward.
- Drug should only be given if absolutely necessary and no alternative is available, at lowest dose and shortest duration possible between 20 and 30 weeks gestation.

LACTATION

- It is not known if drug is present in breast milk.
- Patient should check with prescriber before breastfeeding.

REPRODUCTION

- Drug may delay or prevent rupture of ovarian follicles in females, causing reversible infertility and a reversible delay in ovulation.
- Drug should not be used in women of childbearing age who have difficulty conceiving or who are undergoing investigation of infertility.

Nursing Considerations

- Be aware that NSAIDs like oxaprozin should be avoided in patients with a recent MI because risk of reinfarction increases with NSAID therapy. If therapy is unavoidable, monitor patient closely for signs of cardiac ischemia.
- Know that the risk of heart failure increases with use of NSAIDs such as oxaprozin. NSAIDs should not be used in patients

with severe heart failure, but if unavoidable, monitor patient for worsening of heart failure.

- Use oxaprozin with extreme caution in patients with a history of GI bleeding or ulcer disease because NSAIDs, such as oxaprozin, increase risk of GI bleeding and ulceration. Expect to use oxaprozin for the shortest time possible in these patients. Also know that other risk factors for GI bleeding in patients taking oxaprozin include advanced liver disease and/or coagulopathy; concomitant use of antiplatelets, anticoagulants, oral corticosteroids, or selective serotonin reuptake inhibitors; older age; poor general health; smoking; and use of alcohol.
- Be aware that serious GI tract bleeding, perforation, and ulceration may occur without warning symptoms. Elderly patients are at greater risk. To minimize risk, give drug with food. If GI distress occurs, withhold drug and notify prescriber at once.
- Use oxaprozin cautiously in patients with hypertension, and monitor blood pressure closely throughout therapy. Drug may cause hypertension or worsen it.

! **WARNING** Monitor patient closely for thrombotic events, including MI and stroke, because NSAIDs increase the risk. These events have occurred even in patients who do not have a history or risk factors for cardiovascular disease. Monitor patient for warning signs such as chest pain, shortness of breath, slurring of speech, or weakness. If present, withhold oxaprozin, alert prescriber immediately, and provide supportive care as prescribed.

! **WARNING** If patient has bone marrow suppression or is receiving antineoplastic drug therapy, monitor laboratory results (including WBC count), and watch for evidence of infection because anti-inflammatory and antipyretic actions of oxaprozin may mask signs and symptoms, such as fever and pain.

- Watch for less common but serious adverse GI reactions, including anorexia, constipation, diverticulitis, dysphagia, esophagitis, gastritis, gastroenteritis, gastroesophageal reflux disease, hemorrhoids, hiatal hernia, melena, stomatitis, and vomiting. The risk is higher if patient is elderly or taking oxaprozin long term.

- Monitor liver enzymes because, in rare cases, elevated levels may progress to severe hepatic reactions, including fatal hepatitis, hepatic failure, and liver necrosis.
- Monitor BUN and serum creatinine levels in patients with heart failure, hepatic dysfunction, or impaired; those taking ACE inhibitors or diuretics; and elderly patients because drug may cause renal failure.
- Monitor CBC for decreased hemoglobin level and hematocrit because drug may worsen anemia.

! **WARNING** Assess patient's skin routinely for rash or other signs of hypersensitivity reaction because oxaprozin and other NSAIDs may cause serious skin reactions without warning, even in patients with no history of NSAID hypersensitivity. Stop drug at first sign of reaction, and notify prescriber.

PATIENT TEACHING
- Instruct patient to take oxaprozin exactly as prescribed.
- Advise patient to take drug with food and a full glass of water and to stay upright for 15 to 30 minutes afterward to keep drug from lodging in esophagus and causing irritation.
- Urge patient to avoid alcohol as well as aspirin and other NSAIDs during oxaprozin therapy, to avoid bleeding complications.
- Advise patient to avoid excessive sun exposure to reduce the risk of photosensitivity.
- Caution patient to avoid hazardous activities until drug's CNS effects are known.
- Inform patient that risk of bleeding may continue up to 2 weeks after stopping drug.
- Explain that oxaprozin may increase the risk of serious adverse cardiovascular reactions; urge patient to seek immediate medical attention if signs or symptoms arise, such as chest pain, edema, shortness of breath, slurring of speech, unexplained weight gain, or weakness.
- Inform patient that oxaprozin also may increase the risk of serious adverse GI reactions; stress need to seek immediate medical attention for such signs and

symptoms as abdominal or epigastric pain, black or tarry stools, indigestion or vomiting blood, or material that looks like coffee grounds.

! **WARNING** Alert patient to allergic and rare but serious skin reactions. Urge him to seek immediate medical attention for blisters, fever, itching, rash, or other indications of hypersensitivity.

oxazepam

≣ Class, Category, and Schedule
Pharmacologic class: Benzodiazepine
Therapeutic class: Anxiolytic
Controlled substance schedule: IV

≣ Indications and Dosages
✳ *To treat anxiety*

CAPSULES
Adults and adolescents. 10 to 15 mg three times a day or four times a day for mild to moderate anxiety; up to 30 mg three times a day or four times a day for severe anxiety.

✳ *To help manage acute alcohol withdrawal symptoms*

CAPSULES
Adults. 15 to 30 mg three times a day or four times a day.

±**DOSAGE ADJUSTMENT** For elderly or debilitated patients, initial dose reduced to 10 mg three times a day increased cautiously to 15 mg three times a day or four times a day.

≣ Drug Administration
P.O.
- Store at room temperature in a tight, light-resistant container.

Route	Onset	Peak	Duration
P.O.	30–60 min	2–3 hr	6–8 hr
Half-life: 6–15 hr			

≣ Mechanism of Action
May potentiate the effects of gamma-aminobutyric acid (GABA) and other inhibitory neurotransmitters by binding to specific benzodiazepine receptors in limbic and cortical areas of the CNS. GABA inhibits excitatory stimulation,

which helps control emotional behavior. The limbic system contains highly dense areas of benzodiazepine receptors, which may explain oxazepam's antianxiety and alcohol withdrawal effects.

Contraindications

Hypersensitivity to oxazepam or its components

Interactions

DRUGS

CNS depressants, opioids, other benzodiazepines: Increased risk of severe CNS and respiratory depression

ACTIVITIES

alcohol use: Increased risk of severe CNS and respiratory depression

Adverse Reactions

CNS: Anxiety (in daytime), ataxia, confusion, depression, dizziness, drowsiness, fatigue, headache, insomnia, nightmares, sleep disturbance, slurred speech, syncope, talkativeness, tremor, vertigo
GI: Nausea
Other: Drug tolerance, physical and psychological dependence, withdrawal symptoms

Childbearing Considerations

PREGNANCY

- It is not known if drug causes fetal harm. However, use of other minor tranquilizers during the first trimester of pregnancy has shown an increased risk for congenital malformations.
- Maternal use of drug shortly before delivery may result in floppy infant syndrome.
- Drug should be avoided during pregnancy, if possible.

LACTATION

- Drug is present in breast milk.
- Breastfeeding is not recommended during drug therapy.

Nursing Considerations

! **WARNING** Oxazepam may cause physical and psychological dependence.

- Be aware that drug shouldn't be stopped abruptly after prolonged use; doing so may cause seizures or withdrawal symptoms, such as insomnia, irritability, and nervousness.

- Be aware that withdrawal symptoms can occur when therapy lasts only 1 or 2 weeks.

! **WARNING** Be aware that oxazepam should only be used concomitantly with benzodiazepine therapy in patients for whom other treatment options are inadequate. If prescribed together, expect dosing and duration of oxazepam to be limited. Monitor patient closely for signs and symptoms of a decrease in consciousness, including coma, profound sedation, and significant respiratory depression. Notify prescriber immediately and provide emergency supportive care, as death may occur. Monitor respiratory status in patients with pulmonary disease (such as severe COPD), respiratory depression, or sleep apnea; drug may worsen ventilatory failure.

- Expect an increased risk of falls among elderly patients from impaired cognition and motor function. Take safety precautions.
- Be aware that drug may worsen acute intermittent porphyria, myasthenia gravis, and severe renal impairment.
- Expect patient with late-stage Parkinson's disease to experience decreased cognition or coordination and, possibly, increased psychosis.

PATIENT TEACHING

- Instruct patient to take oxazepam exactly as prescribed and not to stop taking it without consulting prescriber.
- Caution patient about possible drowsiness and reduced coordination.
- Urge patient to avoid alcohol, which increases oxazepam's sedative effects.

! **WARNING** Alert patient to the drug interaction between oxazepam and opioids and not to combine the two unless directed to do so by a prescriber and only after prescriber has been informed of oxazepam therapy.

oxcarbazepine

Oxtellar XR, Trileptal

Class and Category

Pharmacologic class: Carboxamide derivative
Therapeutic class: Anticonvulsant

≡ Indications and Dosages

* *As adjunct to treat partial seizures*

ORAL SUSPENSION, TABLETS (TRILEPTAL)

Adults and adolescents over age 16. *Initial:* 300 mg twice daily. Dosage increased by 600 mg/day every wk. *Usual:* 1,200 mg daily. *Maximum:* 2,400 mg daily.

Children ages 4 to 16. *Initial:* 4 to 5 mg/kg twice daily to maximum initial dose of 600 mg daily. *Usual:* 900 mg daily for children weighing 20 to 29 kg (44 to 64 lb); 1,200 mg daily for those weighing 29.1 to 39 kg (65 to 86 lb); 1,800 mg daily for those weighing more than 39 kg. *Maximum:* 1,800 mg daily.

Children ages 2 to 4. *Initial:* 8 to 10 mg/kg in two divided doses not to exceed 600 mg daily.

Children ages 2 to 4 weighing less than 20 kg (44 lb). *Initial:* 16 to 20 mg/kg daily in two divided doses, increased, as needed, over 2 to 4 wk to achieve maximum maintenance dose. *Maximum:* 60 mg/kg/day in two divided doses.

* *As monotherapy to treat partial seizures*

ORAL SUSPENSION, TABLETS (TRILEPTAL)

Adults and adolescents over age 16. *Initial:* 300 mg twice daily. Dosage increased by 300 mg/day every 3 days, as needed. *Usual:* 1,200 mg daily. *Maximum:* 2,400 mg daily.

Children ages 4 to 16. *Initial:* 4 to 5 mg/kg twice daily, increased by 5 mg/kg daily every third day, as needed. *Maintenance:* Based on weight as follows: 70 kg (154 lb)–1,500 to 2,100 mg/day; 60 to 65 kg (132 to 143 lb)–1,200 to 2,100 mg/day; 50 to 55 kg (110 to 121 lb)–1,200 to 1,800 mg/day; 45 kg (99 lb)–1,200 to 1,500 mg/day; 35 to 40 kg (77 to 88 lb)–900 to 1,500 mg/day; 25 to 30 kg (55 to 66 lb)–900 to 1,200 mg/day; and 20 kg (44 lb): 600 to 900 mg/day.

* *To convert to monotherapy in treating partial seizures*

ORAL SUSPENSION, TABLETS (TRILEPTAL)

Adults and adolescents over age 16. *Initial:* 300 mg twice daily while reducing dose of concomitant anticonvulsant drug. Dosage increased by up to 600 mg daily every wk over 2 to 4 wk, as needed, while dosage of other anticonvulsant reduced to complete withdrawal over 3 to 6 wk. *Usual:* 1,200 mg daily. *Maximum:* 2,400 mg daily.

Children ages 4 to 16. *Initial:* 4 to 5 mg/kg twice daily while reducing dose of concomitant anticonvulsant drug. Dosage increased by up to 10 mg/kg daily weekly as needed to maximum maintenance dosage while dosage of other anticonvulsant is reduced over 3 to 6 wk to complete withdrawal.

Maintenance: Based on weight as follows: 70 kg (154 lb)–1,500 to 2,100 mg/day; 60 to 65 kg (132 to 143 lb)–1,200 to 2,100 mg/day; 50 to 55 kg (110 to 121 lb)–1,200 to 1,800 mg/day; 45 kg (99 lb)–1,200 to 1,500 mg/day; 35 to 40 kg (77 to 88 lb)–900 to 1,500 mg/day; 25 to 30 kg (55 to 66 lb)–900 to 1,200 mg/day; and 20 kg (44 lb): 600 to 900 mg/day.

±**DOSAGE ADJUSTMENT** Dosage adjustment may be required with concomitant use of strong CYP3A4 enzyme inducers or UGT inducers. For patients with creatinine clearance less than 30 ml/min, usual initial dosage reduced by 50%.

* *To treat partial seizures*

XR TABLETS (OXTELLAR XR)

Adults and adolescents over age 16. *Initial:* 600 mg once daily for 1 wk, increased in 600 mg/day increments weekly to reach target dose. *Maintenance:* 1,200 to 2,400 mg once daily. *Maximum:* 2,400 mg once daily.

Children ages 6 to 17. *Initial:* 8 to 10 mg/kg once daily, not to exceed initial dose of 600 mg in first wk, then increased by 8 to 10 mg/kg in once-daily increments weekly, not to exceed dose of 600 mg daily. *Usual:* 1,800 mg daily for those weighing more than 39 kg (more than 86 lb); 1,200 mg daily for those weighing 29.1 to 39 kg (65 to 86 lb); 900 mg daily for children weighing 20 to 29 kg (44 to 64 lb). *Maximum:* 1,800 mg daily.

±**DOSAGE ADJUSTMENT** For patients taking concurrent strong CYP3A4 enzyme inducers or UGT enzyme inducers, initial dosage increased to 900 mg once daily for adults and 12 to 15 mg/kg (not to exceed 900 mg) once daily for pediatric patients. For adults with a creatinine clearance less than 30 ml/min, initial dosage decreased by 50% with subsequent dosage increases made weekly in increments of 300 to 450 mg/day to achieve desired response. For elderly patients, initial dosage reduced to 300 to 450 mg/day with subsequent dosage increases made weekly in increments of 300 to 450 mg/day to achieve desired response.

Drug Administration

P.O.

- Administer XR tablets 1 hour before or 2 hours after a meal, because adverse reactions are more likely to occur when taken with food. If patient has difficulty swallowing XR tablets, daily dosages can be achieved by using lower-strength tablets such as 150 mg.
- Be aware that in conversion of immediate-release form to extended-release form, higher dosages of extended-release form maybe necessary.
- Immediate-release tablets should be swallowed whole and not chewed, crushed, or split.
- Shake suspension well before using. Withdraw prescribed amount using supplied oral dosing syringe. Mix dose in a small glass of water just before administering it, or patient can swallow drug directly from syringe. Rinse syringe with warm water and let it dry thoroughly. Discard any unused oral suspension after 7 weeks of first opening the bottle.
- Oral immediate-release tablets and oral suspension may be interchanged at equal doses.

Route	Onset	Peak	Duration
P.O.	Unknown	3–13 hr	Unknown
P.O./E.R.	Unknown	7 hr	Unknown

Half-life: 2–11 hr

Mechanism of Action

May prevent or halt seizures by blocking or closing sodium channels in neuronal cell membrane. By preventing sodium from entering the cell, oxcarbazepine may slow nerve impulse transmission, thus decreasing the rate at which neurons fire.

Contraindications

Hypersensitivity to oxcarbazepine, eslicarbazepine acetate, or their components

Interactions

DRUGS

hormonal contraceptives: Rendered less effective by immediate-release oxcarbazepine
phenytoin: Possibly increased phenytoin levels with increased risk of adverse reactions

strong CYP3A4 or UGT inducers (carbamazepine, phenobarbital, phenytoin, rifampin): Decreased oxcarbazepine levels with decreased effectiveness

FOODS

all food (XR tablets): Increased risk of adverse effects

ACTIVITIES

alcohol use: Possibly additive CNS depressant effects

Adverse Reactions

CNS: Abnormal coordination or gait, agitation, amnesia, asthenia, ataxia, confusion, difficulty concentrating, dizziness, EEG abnormalities, emotional lability, fatigue, fever, headache, hypoesthesia, insomnia, language or speech problems, nervousness, psychomotor slowing, **seizures**, somnolence, **status epilepticus, suicidal ideation**, tremor, vertigo
CV: **AV block**, chest pain, **hypotension**, peripheral edema
EENT: Abnormal vision, diplopia, earache, ear infection, epistaxis, nystagmus, pharyngitis, rhinitis, sinusitis, taste perversion
ENDO: Hot flashes, hypothyroidism, syndrome of inappropriate antidiuretic hormone secretion
GI: Abdominal pain, anorexia, constipation, diarrhea, elevated liver or pancreatic enzymes, gastritis, indigestion, nausea, **pancreatitis**, vomiting
GU: Frequent urination, UTI, vaginitis
HEME: **Agranulocytosis, aplastic anemia,** eosinophilia, **leukopenia, pancytopenia,** purpura
MS: Arthralgia, back pain, decreased bone mineral density, dysarthria, fractures, muscle weakness, osteoporosis (long-term therapy with immediate-release form)
RESP: Bronchitis, cough, respiratory tract infection
SKIN: Acne, acute generalized exanthematous pustulosis, diaphoresis, **erythema multiforme**, maculopapular rash, rash, **Stevens–Johnson syndrome, toxic epidermal necrolysis**
Other: **Anaphylaxis, drug reaction with eosinophilia and systemic symptoms (DRESS), hyponatremia,** lymphadenopathy, **multiorgan hypersensitivity**

N
O

Childbearing Considerations

PREGNANCY

- Pregnancy exposure registry: 1-888-233-2334 or http://www.aedpregnancyregistry.org.
- Drug may cause fetal harm such as an increased risk of congenital malformations such as oral clefts and ventricular septal defects.
- An increase in seizure activity may occur during pregnancy.
- Use with caution only if benefit to mother outweighs potential risk to fetus.

LACTATION

- Drug is present in breast milk.
- Patient should check with prescriber before breastfeeding. If breastfeeding occurs, infant should be monitored for adverse effects.

REPRODUCTION

- Women using hormonal contraceptives should use an additional or alternative nonhormonal contraceptive during drug therapy.

Nursing Considerations

! WARNING Know that patient with allergic reaction to carbamazepine may have hypersensitivity to oxcarbazepine. Monitor patient closely.

- Monitor serum sodium level for signs of hyponatremia, especially during first 3 months. Know that elderly patients may be at higher risk for hyponatremia because of age-related reductions in creatinine clearance.
- Monitor therapeutic oxcarbazepine levels during initiation and titration, and expect to adjust dosage accordingly.
- Implement seizure precautions as needed. If seizures occur, expect oxcarbazepine to be discontinued.

! WARNING Monitor patient's skin closely. If a reaction develops, notify prescriber at once because skin reactions caused by oxcarbazepine may be serious or life-threatening. Be aware that patients carrying the HLA-B*1502 allele may be at increased risk for Stevens–Johnson syndrome or toxic epidermal necrolysis.

! WARNING Watch closely for evidence of multiorgan hypersensitivity, such as arthralgia, asthenia, fever, hematologic abnormalities, hepatitis, hepatorenal syndrome, liver function abnormalities, lymphadenopathy, nephritis, oliguria, organ dysfunction, pruritus, and rash. If suspected, notify prescriber and expect to stop drug. Provide supportive care, as prescribed.

- Monitor patient closely for evidence of suicidal thinking or behavior, especially when therapy starts or dosage changes.
- Monitor patient for CNS adverse reactions that may involve cognitive symptoms, coordination abnormalities, fatigue, and somnolence.
- Expect to discontinue oxcarbazepine gradually, as abrupt withdrawal may increase risk of seizure frequency and development of status epilepticus.

PATIENT TEACHING

- Teach patient to shake suspension well and measure dose immediately afterward. Tell him to then withdraw prescribed amount using supplied oral dosing syringe. Instruct him to mix dose in a small glass of water just before taking it, or tell him that he can swallow drug directly from syringe. Instruct him to close bottle and rinse syringe with warm water and let it dry thoroughly. Instruct patient to discard any unused oral suspension after 7 weeks of first opening the bottle.
- Instruct patient prescribed XR tablets not to break, chew, or crush tablets but to swallow them whole. Also tell patient to take XR tablets on an empty stomach.
- Inform patient that he may experience dizziness, double vision, and unsteady gait as well as other adverse CNS signs and symptoms. Caution him not to drive or perform any other hazardous activity if these effects occur.
- Instruct patient not to drink alcohol during oxcarbazepine therapy.
- Review signs and symptoms of low sodium level with patient. Tell him to report signs and symptoms such as confusion, increase in severity of seizures, lack of energy, nausea, or tiredness to prescriber.

! WARNING Warn patient to notify prescriber immediately if he develops difficulty breathing or swallowing; fever; rash; swelling of face, eyes, lips, tongue; or other evidence of hypersensitivity, such as a serious skin reaction, because drug may have to be stopped and emergency medical care given.

- Alert woman of childbearing age that oxcarbazepine may render hormonal contraceptives ineffective. Urge patient to use an additional or a different contraceptive during oxcarbazepine therapy. Also tell patient to alert prescriber if pregnancy is suspected or occurs. Breastfeeding should not occur during drug therapy.
- Urge caregivers to watch patient closely for evidence of suicidal tendencies, especially when therapy starts or dosage changes, and to report concerns to prescriber at once.
- Warn patient not to stop taking oxcarbazepine abruptly, as an increase in seizure activity may occur and possibly lead to status epilepticus.

oxybutynin
Oxytrol, Oxytrol for Women

oxybutynin chloride
Ditropan XL, Gelnique 10%

Class and Category
Pharmacologic class: Anticholinergic
Therapeutic class: Antispasmodic (urinary)

Indications and Dosages
✶ *To provide relief of symptoms of bladder instability associated with voiding in patients with uninhibited neurogenic or reflex neurogenic bladder (dysuria, frequency, urge incontinence, urgency, or urinary leakage)*

SYRUP, TABLETS (OXYBUTYNIN)
Adults. 2.5 to 5 mg twice or three times daily. *Maximum:* 5 mg four times daily.
Children over age 5. 5 mg twice daily. *Maximum:* 5 mg three times daily.

✶ *To treat overactive bladder with symptoms of frequency, urge urinary incontinence, or urgency*

E.R. TABLETS (DITROPAN XL)
Adults. *Initial:* 5 or 10 mg daily, adjusted by 5 mg/wk, as prescribed. *Maximum:* 30 mg daily.

TRANSDERMAL SYSTEM (OXYTROL)
Adults. System supplying 3.9 mg daily, applied twice weekly.

TOPICAL GEL (GELNIQUE 10%)
Adults. 1 sachet or one actuation of the metered dose pump applied once daily.

✶ *To treat symptoms of detrusor muscle overactivity of bladder associated with a neurological condition such as spina bifida*

E.R. TABLETS (DITROPAN XL)
Children age 6 and over. *Initial:* 5 mg once daily, increased in 5 mg increments weekly, as needed. *Maximum:* 20 mg once daily.

Drug Administration
P.O.
- E.R. tablets should be swallowed whole and not chewed, crushed, or divided.
- Use a calibrated device when measuring dosage. Store syrup at room temperature.

TRANSDERMAL
- Apply transdermal system to dry, intact, fold-free skin of abdomen, buttock, or hip immediately after removing from pouch. Do not store patch outside of sealed pouch.
- Avoid areas that are irritated or scraped.
- Apply by removing the first piece of the protective liner, placing the patch, adhesive side face down, and pressing firmly onto the skin. Bend the patch in half and gently roll the remaining part onto patient's skin using your fingertips. As patch is rolled in place, the second piece of protective liner should move off the patch. Apply firm pressure over the patch. Avoid touching the sticky adhesive side when putting on the patch, as this may cause the patch to fall off early.
- If patch partly or completely falls off, press it back in place. If it does not stay, replace with a new patch, but remove at scheduled time.
- Do not use same site for at least 7 days.
- Rotate sites.
- Remove old patch slowly and carefully to avoid damaging the skin. Once off, fold the patch in half with sticky sides together and discard.
- Store patches at room temperature, avoiding exposure to sunlight.

TOPICAL
- Put on gloves, then apply gel to dry, intact skin on patient's abdomen, shoulders, thighs, or upper arms immediately after sachet is opened.
- Avoid applying to recently shaved skin surfaces.
- Have patient cover area if close skin-to-skin contact at application site is anticipated.

- Make sure patient does not bathe or shower for 1 hour after application.
- Rotate application sites.

Route	Onset	Peak	Duration
P.O./E.R.	Unknown	4–6 hr	24 hr
Topical	Unknown	Unknown	Unknown
Transdermal	Unknown	24–48 hr	96 hr

Half-life: 2–13 hr (P.O.); Unknown (topical/transdermal)

Mechanism of Action

Exerts antimuscarinic (atropine-like) and potent direct antispasmodic (papaverine-like) actions on smooth muscle in the bladder and decreases detrusor muscle contractions. The result is increased bladder capacity and a decreased urge to void.

Contraindications

Angle-closure glaucoma, gastric retention, hypersensitivity to oxybutynin or its components, urine retention

Interactions

DRUGS

anticholinergics: Increased anticholinergic effects; possibly decreased absorption of some concomitantly administered drugs with major concern for those drugs with a narrow therapeutic index
antimycotic agents (itraconazole, miconazole), ketoconazole, macrolide antibiotics (erythromycin, clarithromycin): Increased plasma oxybutynin concentrations with increased risk of adverse reactions
carbamazepine concurrently with dantrolene: Increased risk of confusion, drowsiness, nystagmus, slurred speech, unsteadiness, and vomiting suggestive of carbamazepine toxicity

ACTIVITIES

alcohol use: Increased CNS effects

Adverse Reactions

CNS: **Abnormal behaviors**, **agitation**, asthenia, confusion, delirium, depression, dizziness, drowsiness, fatigue, hallucinations, headache, insomnia, memory impairment, nervousness, psychosis, restlessness, **seizures**, somnolence, thirst
CV: **Arrhythmias**, chest discomfort, edema, hypertension, **hypotension**, palpitations, peripheral edema, **QT-interval prolongation**, tachycardia, vasodilation
EENT: Abnormal or blurred vision; cycloplegia; dry eyes, mouth, nose, and throat; eye irritation; glaucoma; keratoconjunctivitis sicca; mydriasis; nasal congestion; nasopharyngitis; rhinitis; sinusitis
ENDO: Hot flashes, hyperglycemia, suppression of lactation
GI: Abdominal pain, anorexia, constipation, decreased GI motility, diarrhea, dysphagia, esophagitis, flatulence, gastroesophageal reflux, indigestion, nausea, vomiting
GU: Cystitis, dysuria, impotence, urinary hesitancy, urine retention, UTI
MS: Arthralgia, arthritis, back pain
RESP: **Asthma**, bronchitis, cough, dysphonia, upper respiratory tract infection
SKIN: Decreased sweating, dry skin, flushing, pruritus, rash, urticaria
Other: **Anaphylaxis**, **angioedema**, application-site reactions (anesthesia, dermatitis, erythema, irritation, papules, pruritus), flu-like symptoms, fungal infections, **heatstroke**

Childbearing Considerations

PREGNANCY

- It is not known if drug causes fetal harm.
- Use with caution only if benefit to mother outweighs potential risk to fetus.

LACTATION

- It is not known if drug is present in breast milk.
- Patient should check with prescriber before breastfeeding.

Nursing Considerations

- Use oxybutynin cautiously in patients with diarrhea because it may signal incomplete GI obstruction, especially in patients with colostomy or ileostomy. Also use cautiously in patients with dementia treated with cholinesterase inhibitors because drug may aggravate symptoms.
- Use cautiously in patients with GI disorders such as autonomic neuropathy, myasthenia gravis, or Parkinson's disease because drug may adversely affect these conditions. If exacerbation of symptoms occurs, notify prescriber and expect drug to be discontinued.
- Assess urinary symptoms before and after treatment.

! **WARNING** Monitor patient for angioedema of the face, lips, tongue, and/or larynx, even after just the first dose. If present, notify prescriber, stop oxybutynin therapy, as ordered, and provide emergency supportive care.

! **WARNING** Watch for adverse cardiovascular reactions in patients with arrhythmias, coronary artery disease, heart failure, or hypertension, because drug's antimuscarinic effects may increase their risk.

- Keep in mind that decreased GI motility can cause adynamic ileus; assess for abdominal pain and ileus. Also use with caution in patients who have intestinal atony or ulcerative colitis, because of decreased gastrointestinal motility.
- Be aware that drug may aggravate benign prostatic hyperplasia, gastroesophageal reflux disease, and hyperthyroidism.
- Monitor patient for anticholinergic CNS effects, such as agitation, confusion, hallucinations, and somnolence, especially in the first few months of therapy or when dosage is increased. If such effects occur, notify prescriber and expect dosage to be reduced or drug discontinued.

PATIENT TEACHING

- Advise patient to swallow E.R. tablets whole and not to break, chew, or crush tablets.
- Instruct patient how to apply transdermal system and how to remove it. Tell her to apply to clean, dry skin, avoiding areas that have open sores or rashes. Remind patient to wash hands after handling product. Inform patient not to reapply patch in same site within 7 days and not to expose patch to sunlight.
- Instruct patient how to and where to apply gel form. Warn patient that gel is flammable and that she should avoid open fire or smoking until gel has dried. Also tell patient to avoid bathing, exercising, showering, swimming, or immersing application site in water for 1 hour after application and to cover site with clothing once gel has dried. Remind patient not to apply to recently shaved skin.
- Warn of possible decreased alertness, and advise patient against performing hazardous activities until drug's CNS effects are known.

- Caution patient to avoid excessive sun exposure and strenuous exercise because of increased risk of heatstroke.
- Urge patient to avoid alcohol during therapy.

! **WARNING** Instruct patient to seek immediate emergency care if he experiences swelling of his face, lips, throat, or tongue, or if he has difficulty breathing.

oxycodone
Xtampza ER

oxycodone hydrochloride
Oxaydo, OxyContin, Roxicodone, Supeudol (CAN)

☰ Class, Category, and Schedule
Pharmacologic class: Opioid
Therapeutic class: Opioid analgesic
Controlled substance schedule: II

☰ Indications and Dosages
✱ *To relieve pain severe enough to require opioid treatment and for which alternative treatment options such as nonopioid analgesics or opioid combination products are inadequate or not tolerated*

CAPSULES (OXYCODONE), ORAL SOLUTION (ROXICODONE), TABLETS (OXAYDO, ROXICODONE)
Adults. 5 to 15 mg every 4 to 6 hr.

SUPPOSITORY (SUPEUDOL)
Adults. 1 suppository three to four times daily.

TABLETS (SUPEUDOL)
Adults. 5 to 10 mg every 6 hr.

✱ *To manage moderate to severe pain when a continuous around-the-clock opioid analgesic is needed for an extended period of time*

E.R. TABLETS (OXYCONTIN)
Adults who haven't received opioids before; adults converting from other opioids.
Initial: 10 mg every 12 hr, increased every 1 to 2 days, as needed to achieve desired pain control.

N
O

Adults converting from other oral oxycodone formulations. Half the 24-hr oxycodone dose every 12 hr.

Adults converting from methadone. Highly individualized.

Adults. Highly individualized. *Usual:* 10 mg oxycodone for each 25 mcg/hr of fentanyl patch dosage every 12 hr, beginning 18 hr after removing patch.

Children age 11 and over who are already receiving opioids for at least 5 consecutive days and requiring at least 20 mg of oxycodone daily. *Initial:* Highly individualized and based on the type of opioid taken prior to oxycodone dosing. For example, using the conversion factor of 0.9 for oral hydrocodone in manufacturer guidelines, a total daily hydrocodone dosage of 50 mg is converted to 45 mg of oxycodone daily or 22.5 mg every 12 hours. After rounding down to the nearest available strength, the dosage would be 20 mg every 12 hr, increased every 1 to 2 days, as needed.

E.R. CAPSULES (XTAMPZA ER)

Adults who are opioid-naïve, not opioid tolerant, or converting from other opioids. 9 mg every 12 hr, increased as needed, with dose adjusted to obtain balance between management of pain and opioid-related adverse reactions. *Maximum:* 288 mg daily in divided doses.

Adults converting from fentanyl transdermal patch. Highly individualized. *Usual:* 9 mg oxycodone for each 25 mcg/hr of fentanyl patch dosage every 12 hr, beginning 18 hr after removing patch.

Adults converting from other oral oxycodone formulations. Highly individualized. *Usual:* Half the 24-hr oxycodone dose every 12 hr.

Adults converting from methadone. Highly individualized.

±**DOSAGE ADJUSTMENT** For elderly patients, patients with hepatic impairment, or patients currently taking a CNS depressant, one-third to one-half the usual starting dose and then adjusted, as needed.

Drug Administration

P.O.

- Administer with food. Have patient consume about the same amount of food for every dose in order to maintain consistent blood levels of drug.

- Tablet should be swallowed whole and not broken, chewed, or crushed because of rapid release possibly causing a fatal overdose.

- Have patient swallow one E.R. tablet (OxyContin) at a time, with enough water to ensure complete swallowing immediately after patient places tablet in his mouth; otherwise, choking on tablets or difficulty swallowing tablets may occur due to the swelling and hydrogelling property of tablet if left in the mouth too long.

- Capsules should be swallowed whole without chewing or crushing. However for patient who has difficulty swallowing E.R. capsules, capsule can be opened and contents sprinkled on soft foods or sprinkled into a cup and then administered directly into patient's mouth. Give patient water to rinse mouth to ensure that all capsule contents have been swallowed.

- For patient with a gastrostomy or nasogastric tube, Xtampza ER capsules can be opened and carefully poured directly into the tube after the tube has been flushed with water. Do not pre-mix the capsule contents with the liquid used to flush them through the tube. After instilling capsule content into tube, draw up 15 ml of water into a syringe, insert syringe into the tube and flush the capsule content through the tube. Repeat flushing two more times, each with 10 ml of water, to ensure that no content is left in the tube. Milk or liquid nutritional supplement may be used in place of water to flush tube.

- E.R. tablets and capsules are not interchangeable.

- Check to be sure the right oral solution strength is being used before measuring dose. It comes in 5 mg per 5 ml and 100 mg per 5 ml. The 100 mg per 5 ml concentration should only be used in patients who are opioid tolerant.

- Use a calibrated device when measuring oral solution dosage. The 100 mg per 5 ml oral solution comes with an oral syringe that should always be used to measure the dose.

P.R.

- If suppository is soft, place in refrigerator for 30 minutes or run it under cold water while wrapped.

Route	Onset	Peak	Duration
P.O.	10–30 min	0.5–1 hr	3–6 hr
P.O./E.R.	Unknown	4–5 hr	12 hr
P.R.	Unknown	Unknown	Unknown

Half-life: 3–5 hr

Mechanism of Action

Alters perception of and emotional response to pain at spinal cord and higher levels of CNS by blocking release of inhibitory neurotransmitters, such as acetylcholine and gamma-aminobutyric acid.

Contraindications

Acute or severe bronchial asthma or hypercarbia in an unmonitored setting or in the absence of resuscitative equipment, gastrointestinal obstruction, hypersensitivity to oxycodone or its components, paralytic ileus, significant respiratory depression

Interactions

DRUGS

5-HT3 receptor antagonists, certain muscle relaxants (cyclobenzaprine, metaxalone), drugs that affect the serotonin neurotransmitter system (mirtazapine, tramadol, trazodone), MAO inhibitors including I.V. methylene blue and linezolid, selective serotonin reuptake inhibitors, serotonin and norepinephrine reuptake inhibitors, tricyclic antidepressants, triptans: Increased risk of serotonin syndrome

anticholinergics: Possibly severe constipation and ileus; increased risk of urinary retention

anxiolytics, antipsychotics, benzodiazepines, generalized anesthetics, muscle relaxants, other CNS depressants, other opioids, sedating antihistamines, tranquilizers, tricyclic antidepressants: Increased risk of severe respiratory depression and significant sedation and somnolence

CYP3A4 inducers such as carbamazepine, phenytoin, rifampin: Possibly decreased oxycodone levels making it less effective

CYP3A4 inhibitors such as azole antifungal drugs, macrolide antibiotics, and protease inhibitors: Possibly increased plasma oxycodone levels and prolonged opioid effects with possible overdose effects

diuretics: Reduced effectiveness of diuretics

MAO inhibitors such as linezolid, phenelzine, tranylcypromine: Increased risk of serotonin syndrome; increased risk of opioid toxicity

mixed agonist/antagonist and partial agonist opioid analgesics such as buprenorphine, butorphanol, nalbuphine, pentazocine: Decreased analgesic effect of oxycodone and/or precipitation of withdrawal symptoms

muscle relaxants such as cyclobenzaprine, metaxalone: Enhanced neuromuscular blocking action increasing degree of respiratory depression; increased risk of serotonin syndrome

ACTIVITIES

alcohol use: Additive CNS and respiratory depressive effects that may become severe

Adverse Reactions

CNS: Abnormal dreams, anxiety, asthenia, chills, dizziness, drowsiness, euphoria, excitation, headache, insomnia, nervousness, sedation, seizures, somnolence, syncope, twitching

CV: Bradycardia, chest pain, hypotension, orthostatic hypotension, palpitations

EENT: Blurred vision, choking or difficulty swallowing tablets (OxyContin), dry eyes or mouth, lens opacities, miosis

ENDO: Adrenal insufficiency (rare), syndrome of inappropriate antidiuretic hormone secretion

GI: Abdominal pain, anorexia, constipation, diarrhea, dyspepsia, dysphagia, elevated liver enzymes, gastritis, hiccups, ileus, nausea, vomiting

GU: Amenorrhea, decreased libido, erectile dysfunction, impotence, infertility, lack of menstruation, oliguria, urinary hesitancy, urine retention

RESP: Dyspnea, respiratory depression

SKIN: Diaphoresis, pruritus, rash

Other: Anaphylaxis, drug tolerance, hyponatremia, physical and psychological dependence, withdrawal symptoms

Childbearing Considerations

PREGNANCY

- Drug may cause fetal harm.
- Prolonged use of drug during pregnancy can result in neonatal opioid withdrawal syndrome (NOWS), which may be life-threatening if not recognized and treated.

- Avoid prolonged use during pregnancy. Use with caution only if benefit to mother outweighs potential risk to fetus.

LABOR & DELIVERY

- Drug is not recommended for use in pregnant women immediately before or during labor. Opioids may alter length of time of labor.
- Opioids cross the placental barrier and may produce respiratory depression and psycho-physiologic effects in the neonate. Monitor neonate closely for signs of excess sedation and respiratory depression.
- An opioid antagonist, such as naloxone, must be available at the time of delivery in the event it is needed to reverse opioid-induced respiratory depression in the neonate.

LACTATION

- Drug is present in breast milk.
- Patient should check with prescriber before breastfeeding.
- If breastfeeding occurs, monitor infant for excess sedation and respiratory depression.

REPRODUCTION

- Chronic use of opioids may reduce fertility.

Nursing Considerations

- Be aware that excessive use of opioids like oxycodone may lead to abuse, addiction, misuse, overdose, and possibly death. For this reason, a Risk Evaluation and Mitigation Strategy (REMS) is required for oxycodone to be prescribed. Monitor patient's intake of drug closely and for evidence of physical dependence. Also, have naloxone readily available for emergency treatment of opioid overdose.
- Know that chronic maternal use of oxycodone during pregnancy can result in NOWS, which may be life-threatening if not recognized and treated appropriately. NOWS occurs when a newborn has been exposed to opioid drugs like oxycodone for a prolonged period while in utero.
- Use extreme caution when administering oxycodone to patients with conditions accompanied by hypoxia or decreased respiratory reserve such as asthma, COPD, or cor pulmonale. This is because even with usual therapeutic dosages, oxycodone may decrease respiratory drive while simultaneously increasing airway resistance

to the point of apnea. Monitor patient's respiratory status closely, especially in cachectic, debilitated, and elderly patients and in patients with chronic pulmonary disease. Respiratory depression may occur at any time, but it is most likely to occur during the initiation of therapy or following a dose increase. Have resuscitative equipment nearby.

- Use oxycodone with extreme caution in patients who may be at risk for carbon dioxide retention (e.g., those with increased intracranial pressure or brain tumors). Monitor for signs of sedation and respiratory depression, especially when initiating therapy. Oxycodone may reduce respiratory drive, and the resultant carbon dioxide retention can further increase intracranial pressure. Also know that opioids like oxycodone may obscure signs and symptoms in a patient with a head injury.
- Know that oxycodone can cause sleep-related breathing disorders such as central sleep apnea (CSA) or sleep-related hypoxemia. Use of drug increases the risk of CSA in a dose-dependent way. Let prescriber know if patient experiences CSA and expect oxycodone dosage to possibly be reduced.

! WARNING Be aware that oxycodone should only be used concomitantly with benzodiazepine therapy in patients for whom other treatment options are inadequate. If prescribed together, expect dosing and duration of oxycodone to be limited. Monitor patient closely for signs and symptoms of a decrease in consciousness, including coma, profound sedation, and significant respiratory depression. Notify prescriber immediately and provide emergency supportive care, as death may occur.

- Assess patient's pain level regularly, and give drug as prescribed before pain becomes severe.
- Monitor patient's blood pressure closely, especially when initiating oxycodone therapy and when titrating the dose, because oxycodone may cause severe hypotension and syncope in ambulatory patients due to its vasodilatory effects.

Risk of hypotension is greater in patients who already have been compromised by a reduced blood volume or concurrent administration of certain CNS depressant drugs, such as general anesthetics and phenothiazines.

- Assess patient for possible paradoxical excitation during dosage titration.
- Assess patient for abdominal pain because oxycodone may mask underlying GI disorders.

! **WARNING** Know that many drugs may interact with opioids like oxycodone to cause serotonin syndrome. Monitor patient closely for signs and symptoms such as agitation, diaphoresis, diarrhea, fever, hallucinations, labile blood pressure, muscle twitching or stiffness, nausea, shakiness, shivering, tachycardia, trouble with coordination, or vomiting. Notify prescriber at once because serotonin syndrome may be life-threatening. Be prepared to discontinue drug, if possible and ordered, and provide supportive care.

- Monitor patient for adrenal insufficiency. Although rare, it can be life-threatening. Monitor patient for anorexia, dizziness, fatigue, hypotension, nausea, vomiting, or weakness. Notify prescriber if adrenal insufficiency is suspected and expect diagnostic testing to be done. If confirmed, expect to administer corticosteroids and wean patient off oxycodone, if possible.
- Monitor patients with seizure disorders closely because oxycodone may induce or aggravate seizures.

! **WARNING** Be aware that oxycodone given concomitantly with CYP3A4 inhibitors (or if CYP3A4 inducers are discontinued) can result in a fatal overdose of oxycodone.

! **WARNING** Be aware that abuse of crushed controlled-release tablets poses a hazard of overdose and death. If you suspect abuse and determine that patient also is abusing alcohol or illicit substances, notify prescriber immediately, because risk of overdose and death is increased. If you suspect parenteral abuse, be aware that tablet excipients, especially talc, may result in endocarditis, infection, local tissue necrosis, pulmonary granulomas, and valvular heart injury.

- Know that oxycodone therapy should not be stopped abruptly in a physically dependent patient.

PATIENT TEACHING

! **WARNING** Strongly warn patient to swallow oxycodone tablets whole and not to break, chew, or crush them because taking broken, chewed, or crushed tablets leads to rapid release and absorption of a potentially fatal dose.

- Remind patient that drug must be taken with food. Tell patient to consume about the same amount of food for every dose in order to maintain consistent blood levels of the drug.
- Instruct patient not to take oxycodone more often than prescribed and not to take it longer than absolutely needed because excessive or prolonged use can lead to abuse, addiction, misuse, overdose, and possibly death. Encourage patient and family to have naloxone available in the home in the event of an opioid overdose. Instruct family or caregiver how to recognize an opioid overdose such as severe respiratory depression and profound sedation and how to administer naloxone. Stress importance of immediately calling 911 when administering naloxone.
- Warn patient not to stop abruptly after long-term use.
- Caution patient prescribed extended-release tablets to take one tablet at a time; not to presoak, lick, or otherwise wet the tablet prior to placing in his mouth; and to take each tablet with enough water to ensure complete swallowing of tablet.
- Advise patient prescribed suppository form to store drug in refrigerator for 30 minutes or run under cold water if it is too soft to administer.

! **WARNING** Warn patient not to consume alcohol or take a benzodiazepine without prescriber knowledge, as severe respiratory depression can occur and may lead to death.

- Caution patient to avoid hazardous activities such as driving during oxycodone therapy.
- Tell patient to notify prescriber about signs of possible toxicity or hypersensitivity, such

N
O

as excessive light-headedness, extreme dizziness, itching, swelling, and trouble breathing.

- Warn patient to keep drug out of reach of children because ingestion of the drug by a child can be fatal.
- Inform patient that long-term use of opioids like oxycodone may decrease sex hormone levels, causing decreased libido, erectile dysfunction, impotence, infertility, or lack of menstruation. Encourage patient to report any symptoms to prescriber.
- Caution pregnant patient not to increase dosage or take drug for a prolonged period, as adverse effects can cause infant to experience life-threatening withdrawal when born.
- Instruct patient to notify all prescribers of opioid use.
- Instruct patient to dispose of unused drug by flushing down the toilet, if a drug take-back option is not readily available.

oxymorphone hydrochloride

Class, Category, and Schedule

Pharmacologic class: Opioid
Therapeutic class: Opioid analgesic
Controlled substance schedule: II

Indications and Dosages

∗ *To relieve pain severe enough to require opioid treatment and for which alternative treatment options such as nonopioid analgesics or opioid combination products are inadequate or not tolerated.*

TABLETS

Adults receiving an opioid for first time.
Initial: 10 to 20 mg every 4 to 6 hr, as needed with dosage adjusted based on patient response. *Maximum initial dose:* 20 mg.
Adults converting from parenteral oxymorphone. *Initial:* 10 times the patient's total daily parenteral oxymorphone dose divided by 4 or 6 to provide four or six equally divided doses every 4 to 6 hr.
Adults converting from other oral opioids. Highly individualized.

±**DOSAGE ADJUSTMENT** For patients with mild hepatic impairment or renal

impairment (a creatinine clearance less than 50 ml/min), or who are elderly, initial dose reduced to 5 mg and titrated slowly. For patient receiving a CNS depressant, dosage begun at one-third to one-half usual initial dose.

E.R. TABLETS

Adults who are opioid-naïve or opioid nontolerant. *Initial:* 5 mg every 12 hr and increased every 3 or 7 days, using increments of 5 to 10 every 12 hr.

±**DOSAGE ADJUSTMENT** For patients who are opioid-naïve with mild hepatic impairment or renal impairment or who are elderly, initial dose kept at 5 mg and dosage titrated slowly. For patient on prior opioid therapy with mild hepatic impairment or renal impairment, initial dosage reduced by 50% and titration done slowly. For patient receiving a CNS depressant, dosage begun at one-third to one-half the usual initial dose.

I.V. INJECTION

Adults. *Initial:* 0.5 mg with dosage adjusted based on patient response.
Adults converting from oral oxymorphone. *Initial:* One-tenth of oral oxymorphone daily dose divided into 4 or 6 equally divided doses.

I.M. OR SUBCUTANEOUS INJECTION

Adults. *Initial:* 1 to 1.5 mg every 4 to 6 hr, as needed.
Adults converting from oral oxymorphone. *Initial:* One-tenth of oral oxymorphone daily dose and divided into 4 or 6 equally divided doses.

±**DOSAGE ADJUSTMENT** For patient receiving parenteral oxymorphone and has mild hepatic impairment or for patients over the age of 65, initial dosage started with lowest dose and titration done slowly. For patient with renal impairment (a creatinine clearance of less than 50 ml/min), initial dosage reduced and titration done slowly. For patient receiving a CNS depressant, dosage begun at one-third to one-half the usual initial dose.

∗ *To provide support for anesthesia and use as preoperative medication; to relieve anxiety in patients with dyspnea from pulmonary edema caused by acute left ventricular dysfunction*

I.V. INJECTION

Adults. *Initial:* 0.5 mg and then dosage adjusted, as needed.

I.M. OR SUBCUTANEOUS INJECTION

Adults. *Initial:* 1 to 1.5 mg, repeated every 4 to 6 hr, as needed.

±**DOSAGE ADJUSTMENT** For patient receiving parenteral oxymorphone and has mild hepatic impairment or for patients over the age of 65, initial dosage started with lowest dose and titration done slowly. For patient with renal impairment (a creatinine clearance of less than 50 ml/min), initial dosage reduced and titration done slowly. For patient receiving a CNS depressant, dosage begun at one-third to one-half the usual initial dose.

SUPPOSITORIES

Adults. 5 mg every 4 to 6 hr, as needed.

✳ *To relieve obstetric pain during labor*

I.M. INJECTION

Adults. 0.5 to 1 mg as a single dose.

±**DOSAGE ADJUSTMENT** For patient with mild hepatic impairment, initial dosage started with lowest dose and titration done slowly. For patient with renal impairment (a creatinine clearance of less than 50 ml/min), initial dosage reduced and titration done slowly. For patient receiving a CNS depressant, dosage begun at one-third to one-half the usual initial dose.

Drug Administration

P.O.

- Administer tablets on an empty stomach at least 1 hour before or 2 hours after a meal.
- Tablets should be swallowed whole and not broken, chewed, crushed, or divided.

I.V.

- Manufacturer does not give specific guidelines for administering I.V.
- Store at room temperature and protect from light.
- Have naloxone readily available.
- *Incompatibilities:* None listed by manufacturer

I.M., SUBCUTANEOUS

- More than 1 ampul (1 mg/ml) may be needed for prescribed dosage.
- Rotate injection sites.
- Store at room temperature and protect from light.

P.R.

- If suppository is too soft, place it in refrigerator for 30 minutes or run wrapped suppository under cold water until firm.
- Store suppositories under refrigeration.

Route	Onset	Peak	Duration
P.O.	10–30 min	1–2 hr	3–6 hr
I.V.	5–10 min	15–30 min	3–6 hr
I.M.	10–30 min	30–60 min	3–6 hr
SubQ	10–30 min	30–90 min	3–6 hr
P.R.	15–30 min	20–60 min	3–6 hr

Half-life: 7–10 hr

Mechanism of Action

Alters perception of and emotional response to pain at spinal cord and higher levels of CNS by blocking release of inhibitory neurotransmitters, such as acetylcholine and gamma-aminobutyric acid.

Contraindications

Acute or severe bronchial asthma in an unmonitored setting or in the absence of resuscitative equipment; gastrointestinal obstruction, including paralytic ileus; hypersensitivity to oxymorphone or its components; moderate or severe hepatic impairment; significant respiratory depression

Interactions

DRUGS

5-HT3 receptor antagonists, certain muscle relaxants (cyclobenzaprine, metaxalone), drugs that affect the serotonin neurotransmitter system (mirtazapine, tramadol, trazodone), MAO inhibitors such as I.V. methylene blue or linezolid, selective serotonin reuptake inhibitors, serotonin and norepinephrine reuptake inhibitors, tricyclic antidepressants, triptans: Increased risk of serotonin syndrome

anticholinergics: Increased risk of urine retention, severe constipation

anxiolytics, antipsychotics, benzodiazepines, general anesthetics, muscle relaxants, other CNS depressants, other opioids, sedating antihistamines, tranquilizers: Increased risk of severe respiratory depression and significant sedation and somnolence

diuretics: Decreased effectiveness of diuretics

MAO inhibitors: Increased risk of serotonin syndrome; increased risk of opioid toxicity

mixed agonist/antagonist and partial agonist opioid analgesics such as buprenorphine, butorphanol, nalbuphine, pentazocine: Possibly reduced analgesic effect of oxymorphone

muscle relaxants: Enhanced neuromuscular blocking action increasing degree of respiratory depression

ACTIVITIES

alcohol use: Additive CNS and respiratory depressant effects which could be severe

Adverse Reactions

CNS: Agitation, asthenia, CNS depression, confusion, delusions, depersonalization, dizziness, drowsiness, euphoria, fatigue, hallucinations, headache, insomnia, light-headedness, nervousness, nightmares, restlessness, seizures, somnolence, tiredness, tremor, weakness

CV: Bradycardia, hypertension, hypotension, palpitations, tachycardia

EENT: Blurred vision, diplopia, dry mouth, laryngeal edema, laryngospasm, miosis, tinnitus

ENDO: Adrenal insufficiency

GI: Abdominal cramps or pain, anorexia, biliary colic, constipation, elevated serum amylase level, hepatotoxicity, ileus, nausea, vomiting

GU: Decreased urine output, decreased libido, dysuria, erectile dysfunction, impotence, infertility, lack of menstruation, urinary frequency and hesitancy, urine retention

MS: Muscle rigidity (with large doses), uncontrolled muscle movements

RESP: Apnea, atelectasis, bradypnea, bronchospasm, dyspnea, irregular breathing, respiratory depression, wheezing

SKIN: Dermatitis, diaphoresis, erythema, flushing of face, pruritus, urticaria

Other: Angioedema; injection-site burning, pain, redness, and swelling; psychological and physical dependence

Childbearing Considerations

PREGNANCY

- Drug may cause fetal harm.
- Prolonged use of drug during pregnancy can result in neonatal opioid withdrawal syndrome (NOWS), which may be life-threatening if not recognized and treated.
- Avoid prolonged use during pregnancy. Use with caution only if benefit to mother outweighs potential risk to fetus.

LABOR & DELIVERY

- Drug is not recommended for use in pregnant women immediately before or during labor. Opioids may alter length of time of labor.
- Opioids cross the placental barrier and may produce respiratory depression and psycho-physiologic effects in the neonate. Monitor neonate closely for signs of excess sedation and respiratory depression.
- An opioid antagonist, such as naloxone, must be available at the time of delivery in the event it is needed to reverse opioid-induced respiratory depression in the neonate.

LACTATION

- It is not known if drug is present in breast milk.
- Patient should check with prescriber before breastfeeding.
- If breastfeeding occurs, monitor infant for excess sedation and respiratory depression.

REPRODUCTION

- Chronic use of opioids may reduce fertility.

Nursing Considerations

- Be aware that excessive use of opioids like oxymorphone may lead to abuse, addiction, misuse, overdose, and possibly death. Monitor patient's intake of drug closely and watch for evidence of physical dependence. Know that drug use now requires a Risk Evaluation and Mitigation Strategy (REMS) for a prescription.
- Know that chronic maternal use of oxymorphone during pregnancy can result in NOWS, which may be life-threatening if not recognized and treated appropriately. NOWS occurs when a newborn has been exposed to opioid drugs like oxymorphone for a prolonged period while in utero.
- Use extreme caution when administering oxymorphone to patients with conditions accompanied by decreased respiratory reserve or hypoxia, such as asthma, COPD, or cor pulmonale. This is because oxymorphone, even with usual therapeutic dosages, may decrease respiratory drive while simultaneously increasing airway resistance to the point of apnea. Have naloxone readily available.
- Use oxymorphone with extreme caution in patients who may be at risk for carbon dioxide retention (e.g., those with brain tumors or increased intracranial pressure). Monitor for signs of respiratory depression

and sedation, especially when initiating therapy. Oxymorphone may reduce respiratory drive, and the resultant carbon dioxide retention can further increase intracranial pressure. Also know that opioids like oxymorphone may obscure signs and symptoms in a patient with a head injury.

- Use cautiously in patients with biliary tract disease because drug may cause spasm of sphincter of Oddi; mild hepatic impairment because drug is metabolized in liver; and impaired renal function because drug is excreted by kidneys.
- Use cautiously in patients receiving mixed agonist-antagonist opioid analgesics because these drugs may reduce analgesic effect of oxymorphone or may cause withdrawal symptoms.
- Use cautiously in elderly patients because plasma oxymorphone levels in the elderly are higher than in younger patients.
- Know that oral hydromorphone shouldn't be used "as needed" or for first 24 hours after surgery in patients not already taking opioids because of the risk of oversedation and respiratory depression.
- Taper dosage, as ordered, before stopping therapy, to prevent withdrawal in physically dependent patients.

! WARNING Monitor patient's respiratory status closely for respiratory depression, especially in cachectic, debilitated, or elderly patients; when initiating or titrating dosages; or when other drugs that depress respiration are given together. Have resuscitative equipment nearby. Report respiratory depression immediately, because severe respiratory depression may occur. Be prepared to provide supportive care.

- Monitor patient's blood pressure closely, especially when initiating oxymorphone therapy and when titrating the dose because oxymorphone may cause severe hypotension and syncope in ambulatory patients due to its vasodilatory effects. Risk of hypotension is greatest in patients who already have been compromised by a reduced blood volume or concurrent administration of certain CNS depressant drugs, such as general anesthetics and phenothiazines.

! WARNING Know that many drugs may interact with opioids like oxymorphone to cause serotonin syndrome. Monitor patient closely for signs and symptoms such as agitation, diaphoresis, diarrhea, fever, hallucinations, labile blood pressure, muscle twitching or stiffness, nausea, shakiness, shivering, tachycardia, trouble with coordination, or vomiting. Notify prescriber at once because serotonin syndrome may be life-threatening. Be prepared to discontinue drug, if possible and ordered, and provide supportive care.

- Monitor patient for adrenal insufficiency. Although rare, it can be life-threatening. Monitor patient for anorexia, dizziness, fatigue, hypotension, nausea, vomiting, or weakness. Notify prescriber if adrenal insufficiency is suspected and expect diagnostic testing to be done. If confirmed, expect to administer corticosteroids and wean patient off oxymorphone, if possible.
- Monitor patient for signs of excessive opioid-related adverse reactions. If present, notify prescriber and expect next dose to be reduced.
- Monitor bowel and urinary status; constipation may be so severe it causes ileus.
- Offer fluids to relieve dry mouth.

! WARNING Be aware that oxymorphone should only be used concomitantly with benzodiazepine therapy in patients for whom other treatment options are inadequate. If prescribed together, expect dosing and duration of oxymorphone to be limited. Monitor patient closely for signs and symptoms of a decrease in consciousness, including coma, profound sedation, and significant respiratory depression. Notify prescriber immediately and provide emergency supportive care, as death may occur.

PATIENT TEACHING

- Instruct patient to take oxymorphone exactly as prescribed and not to stop abruptly; warn that drug can cause abuse, misuse, overdose, physical dependence, and possibly death. Encourage patient and family/caregiver to have naloxone on hand. Instruct family/caregiver on recognizing signs and symptoms of an opioid overdose such as severe respiratory depression and profound sedation and instruct on how to administer naloxone. Stress importance of calling 911 immediately if naloxone is administered.

- Emphasize importance of taking drug before pain becomes severe.
- Instruct patient to take drug on an empty stomach.
- Instruct patient to store suppositories in refrigerator.
- Encourage patient to increase fluid and fiber intake during therapy to prevent constipation.
- Emphasize need to avoid alcohol, benzodiazepine therapy, and CNS depressants during therapy because of risk of severe life-threatening adverse reactions.
- Caution patient to avoid potentially hazardous activities until drug's CNS effects are known.
- Warn patient to keep drug out of the reach of children, as accidental ingestion may be fatal.
- Inform patient that long-term use of opioids like oxymorphone may decrease sex hormone levels, causing decreased libido, erectile dysfunction, impotence, infertility, or lack of menstruation. Encourage patient to report any symptoms to prescriber.
- Instruct patient to notify all prescribers of opioid use.
- Instruct patient to dispose of unused drug by flushing down the toilet, if a drug take-back option is not readily available.

ozanimod hydrochloride
Zeposia

Class and Category
Pharmacologic class: Sphingosine 1-phosphate receptor modulator
Therapeutic class: Immunosuppressant

Indications and Dosages
* *To treat relapsing forms of multiple sclerosis, including active secondary progressive disease, clinically isolated syndrome, and relapsing-remitting disease; to treat moderate to severe active ulcerative colitis*

CAPSULES

Adults. *Initial:* 0.23 mg once daily for days 1 through 4; increased to 0.46 mg once daily for days 5 through 7; increased to 0.92 mg once daily for day 8. *Maintenance:* 0.92 mg once daily.

±**DOSAGE ADJUSTMENT** For patients who miss a dose during the first 2 weeks of treatment, titration regimen must be reinitiated. For patients who miss a dose after the first 2 weeks of treatment, no retitration is necessary.

Drug Administration
P.O.
- Capsules should be swallowed whole and not chewed, crushed, or opened.
- Can be given with or without meals.

Route	Onset	Peak	Duration
P.O.	Unknown	6–8 hr	Unknown

Half-life: 21 hr

Mechanism of Action
Binds to sphingosine 1-phosphate receptors 1 and 2 to block the capability of lymphocytes to leave lymph nodes. This action reduces the number of lymphocytes in the bloodstream. This is thought to possibly reduce the lymphocyte migration into the central nervous system, which may help to reduce signs and symptoms of relapsing multiple sclerosis.

Contraindications
Experienced within the past 6 months class III or IV heart failure, decompensated heart failure requiring hospitalization, myocardial infarction, stroke, transient ischemic attack, or unstable angina; hypersensitivity to ozanimod or its components; presence of Mobitz type II second-degree or third-degree atrioventricular block, sick sinus syndrome, or sinoatrial block, unless a pacemaker is in place; severe, untreated sleep apnea; use within 14 days of MAO inhibitor therapy

Interactions
DRUGS

adrenergic and serotonergic drugs such as nonselective MAO inhibitors, opioids (meperidine and its derivatives, methadone, tramadol), selective norepinephrine reuptake inhibitors, selective serotonin reuptake inhibitors, tricyclics, tyramine: Increased risk of serious adverse reactions such as hypertensive crisis

antineoplastic, immune-modulating, or immunosuppressive drugs: Increased risk of additive immune effects

breast cancer resistance protein inhibitors: Increased exposure of active metabolites of ozanimod, which may increase risk of ozanimod adverse reactions

class Ia antiarrhythmics such as procainamide, quinidine; class III antiarrhythmics such as amiodarone, sotalol; QT-prolonging drugs with known arrhythmogenic properties: Possibly increased risk for torsades de pointes in patients with bradycardia

combined beta-blocker and calcium channel blocker: Possible additive effects on heart rate

CYP2C8 inducers (strong) such as rifampin: Reduced exposure of ozanimod active metabolites leading to reduced effectiveness

CYP2C8 inhibitors (strong) such as gemfibrozil: Increased risk of ozanimod adverse effects

live-attenuated vaccines: Increased risk of infection

MAO inhibitors: Possibly decreased exposure of ozanimod; possibly inhibition of MAO inhibitor effects

vaccinations: Possibly less effective

FOODS

tyramine-rich foods such as foods that are aged, cured, fermented, pickled, or smoked: Increased risk of hypertensive crisis

Adverse Reactions

CNS: Posterior reversible encephalopathy syndrome, progressive multifocal leukoencephalopathy

CV: Atrioventricular conduction delays, bradyarrhythmia, bradycardia (transient), hypertension, hypertensive crisis, orthostatic hypotension, peripheral edema

EENT: Macular edema

GI: Abdominal pain, elevated liver enzymes, hepatic dysfunction, rectal adenocarcinoma

GU: Cervical cancer, UTI

MS: Back pain

RESP: Decreased absolute forced expiratory volume over 1 second (FEV_1), dyspnea, upper respiratory infections

SKIN: Basal cell carcinoma, melanoma, rash, urticaria

Other: Immunosuppression; infections (maybe serious or life-threatening);

malignancies such as adenocarcinomas, breast cancer, or seminoma

Childbearing Considerations

PREGNANCY

- It is not known if drug can cause fetal harm. However, animal studies suggest that a serious risk may exist.
- Use with caution only if benefit to mother outweighs potential risk to fetus.

LACTATION

- It is not known if drug is present in breast milk.
- Patient should check with prescriber before breastfeeding.

REPRODUCTION

- Women of childbearing age should use an effective contraceptive method during treatment and for 3 months after treatment is discontinued.

Nursing Considerations

- Know that ozanimod should not be administered to patients who have received alemtuzumab, because of risk of additive immunosuppression. Also use ozanimod cautiously in patients receiving other antineoplastic, immune-modulating, or immunosuppressive drugs.
- Expect to obtain results of the following tests and evaluations prior to starting ozanimod therapy: cardiac evaluation, complete blood count, liver function tests, and an ophthalmic evaluation. In addition, determine if patient is taking or has taken antineoplastic, immune-modulating, or immunosuppressive therapies or drugs that could slow atrioventricular conduction or slow heart rate, because of increased risk for adverse reactions.
- Ensure that patient who has no history of having had chickenpox has been tested for antibodies to varicella zoster virus before ozanimod therapy begins. Expect to administer varicella zoster virus vaccine to antibody-negative patients. Know that live-attenuated vaccine immunizations should be administered at least 1 month prior to initiation of ozanimod.
- Plan to reinitiate ozanimod therapy using the titration regimen, as prescribed, if patient has missed a dose during the first 2 weeks of treatment. If a dose is missed after the first 2 weeks of therapy, continue treatment as prescribed.

N
O

! WARNING Monitor patient for signs and symptoms of infection, because serious, life-threatening, or even fatal (rare) infections have occurred with ozanimod therapy. Know that therapy should be delayed in patients with an active infection until the infection is resolved. Ozanimod particularly increases the risk of herpes zoster, urinary tract, and viral upper respiratory tract infections. Be aware that therapy may have to be interrupted if a serious infection occurs. Continue monitoring patient for infection for at least 3 months after ozanimod therapy is discontinued.

- Assess patient's heart rate regularly, because initiation of ozanimod may result in a transient decrease in heart rate or cause delays in atrioventricular conduction. If patient develops any of the following, expect prescriber to consult with a cardiologist: arrhythmias requiring treatment with Class 1a or Class III antiarrhythmic drugs; heart failure or ischemic heart disease; history of cardiac arrest, cerebrovascular disease, myocardial infarction, second-degree Mobitz type II or higher AV block, sick sinus syndrome, sinoatrial heart block, or uncontrolled hypotension; or significant QT prolongation.
- Monitor patient's liver enzymes, as ordered, because elevations may occur with ozanimod therapy. Notify prescriber if patient develops signs and symptoms of liver dysfunction such as unexplained abdominal pain, anorexia, fatigue, jaundice, nausea, or vomiting as well as an AST or ALT value greater than 1.5 times upper-level normal. If present, expect drug to be discontinued if significant liver injury is confirmed.
- Monitor elderly patients for cardiac and hepatic adverse drug reactions because of decreased cardiac and hepatic function in this population.

! WARNING Monitor patient for posterior reversible encephalopathy syndrome or progressive multifocal leukoencephalopathy and report suspicions immediately to prescriber. Expect ozanimod to be withheld until such disorder has been excluded. If confirmed, expect ozanimod to be discontinued and appropriate supportive care given, as prescribed.

- Assess patient's blood pressure regularly, as an increase may occur. Although uncommon, a hypertensive crisis may also occur as a result of ozanimod therapy. Do not give patient foods containing very large amounts (i.e., more than 150 mg) of tyramine because of an increased sensitivity to tyramine as a result of ozanimod therapy.
- Monitor patient's respiratory status and notify prescriber if patient develops dyspnea, because dose-dependent reductions in absolute forced expiratory volume over 1 second may occur with ozanimod therapy.
- Assess patient for changes in vision, as ozanimod may cause macular edema. Patients at increased risk are those who have a history of uveitis or diabetes mellitus.
- Be aware that a severe increase in disability may occur when ozanimod is discontinued, though this is rare. If present, notify prescriber and expect appropriate treatment to be given, as prescribed.
- Know that immunosuppression may continue for at least 30 days after ozanimod has been discontinued and therefore infection control measures should continue during this time.

PATIENT TEACHING

- Instruct patient to swallow capsules whole and not to chew, crush, or open capsule.
- Tell patient that if a dose is missed during the first 2 weeks of therapy, prescriber must be notified because therapy dosage must begin at the beginning again. If a dose is missed after the first 2 weeks of therapy, tell patient to continue same schedule and dosage as prescribed.

! WARNING Review with patient foods that are rich in tyramine, such as foods that are aged, cured, fermented, pickled, or smoked, and stress importance of avoiding these foods while taking ozanimod.

! WARNING Warn women of childbearing age to use effective contraception during ozanimod therapy and for 3 months following discontinuation of drug, because of potential fetal risk.

- Caution patient to notify prescriber if changes in breathing or vision occur.

> **! WARNING** Review signs and symptoms of infection and infection control measures to take while receiving ozanimod and for 3 months following drug discontinuation. Stress importance of notifying prescriber if an infection occurs.

- Inform patient that vaccines containing live virus should be avoided during ozanimod therapy and for 3 months after drug is discontinued, or given at least 1 month prior to start of therapy.
- Instruct patient to notify prescriber of any abnormal, serious, or unusual signs and symptoms.
- Tell patient to report any significant increase in disability after ozanimod is discontinued.

P

paliperidone
Invega

paliperidone palmitate
Invega Hafyera, Invega Sustenna, Invega Trinza

Class and Category
Pharmacologic class: Benzisoxazole derivative
Therapeutic class: Antipsychotic (atypical)

Indications and Dosages
∗ *To treat schizophrenia*

E.R. TABLETS (INVEGA)
Adults. *Initial:* 3 to 6 mg once daily; then increased or decreased in increments of 3 mg daily every 5 or more days, as needed. *Maximum:* 12 mg daily.
Adolescents 12 to 17. *Initial:* 3 mg once daily; then increased in increments of 3 mg daily every 6 or more days, as needed. *Maximum:* 12 mg once daily for adolescents weighing 51 kg (112.2 lb) or more; 6 mg for adolescents weighing less than 51 kg (112.2 lb).

I.M. INJECTION (INVEGA SUSTENNA)
Adults. *Initial:* 234 mg on day 1 and 156 mg on day 8. *Maintenance:* 39 to 234 mg monthly. Maintenance dosage decreased or increased monthly according to patient's response and tolerance. *Maximum:* 234 mg monthly.

I.M. INJECTION (INVEGA TRINZA)
Adults who have been adequately treated with Invega Sustenna for at least 4 mo. *Initial:* 273 mg if last monthly Sustenna dose was 78 mg; 410 mg if last monthly Sustenna dose was 117 mg; 546 mg if last monthly Sustenna dose was 156 mg; or 819 mg if last monthly Sustenna dose was 234 mg, administered within 7 days before or after next monthly Sustenna dose would have been given with dosage adjustment made thereafter every 3 mo, as needed.

Maintenance: 273 to 819 mg every 3 mo.
Maximum: 819 mg every 3 mo.

I.M. INJECTION (INVEGA HAFYERA)
Adults who have been adequately treated with Invega Sustenna for at least 4 months. *Initial:* 1,092 mg if last paliperidone palmitate extended-release injectable suspension dose was 156 mg or 1,560 mg if last paliperidone palmitate extended-release injectable suspension dose was 234 mg, administered within 7 days before or after next monthly Sustenna dose would have been given with dosage adjustment made every 6 months thereafter, as needed.
Adults who have been adequately treated with Invega Trinza for at least one 3-month injection cycle. *Initial:* 1,092 mg if last every 3-month paliperidone palmitate extended-release injectable suspension dose was 546 mg or 1,560 mg if last every-3-month paliperidone palmitate extended-release injectable suspension dose was 819 mg, administered within 14 days before or after next monthly Trinza dose would have been given with dosage adjustment made every 6 months thereafter, as needed.

∗ *To treat schizoaffective disorder*

E.R. TABLETS (INVEGA)
Adults. *Initial:* 6 mg once daily; then increased or decreased in increments of 3 mg daily every 4 or more days, as needed. *Maximum:* 12 mg daily.

I.M. INJECTION (INVEGA SUSTENNA)
Adults. *Initial:* 234 mg on day 1 and 156 mg on day 8. *Maintenance:* 78 to 234 mg monthly. Maintenance dosage decreased or increased monthly according to patient's response and tolerance. *Maximum:* 234 mg monthly.

±**DOSAGE ADJUSTMENT** For patients taking E.R. tablets with mild renal impairment (creatinine clearance 50 to 79 ml/min), initial dosage decreased to 3 mg daily then increased to maximum dosage 6 mg daily; moderate to severe renal impairment (creatinine clearance 10 ml/min to less than 50 ml/min), initial dose decreased to 1.5 mg daily, then increased to maximum dosage of 3 mg daily. For patient receiving Invega Sustenna with mild renal impairment (creatinine clearance equal to or greater than 50 ml/min but less than 80 ml/min),

P

initial dosage decreased to 156 mg on day 1 and second dose given 1 wk later decreased to 117 mg, followed by 78 mg monthly. For patient receiving Invega Trinza with mild renal impairment (creatine clearance greater than 50 ml/min to less than 80 ml/min), patient stabilized using Invega Sustenna then transitioned to Invega Trinza. Invega Trinza is not recommended in patients with moderate or severe renal impairment (creatinine clearance less than 50 ml/min). For elderly patient with any degree of renal impairment, Invega Hafyera should not be used. For patient receiving a strong CYP3A4 inducer such as carbamazepine, rifampin, or St. John's wort, these drugs should be avoided if patient is to receive an injectable form of paliperidone. If use of these drugs must continue, extended-release tablets (Invega) should be used instead of an injectable form.

Drug Administration

P.O.

- Administer with a liquid beverage.
- E.R. tablets must be swallowed whole and not chewed, crushed, or divided.

I.M.

- Do not administer by any other route.
- Drug is supplied in a prefilled syringe along with two different-size needles. Use only the needles provided with the product.
- Administer dose as a single injection.
- Do not mix with any product or diluent.
- When a patient who has been taking a long-acting injectable antipsychotic consistently is now switching to the long-lasting 1-month preparation of paliperidone, the first dose of paliperidone is given in place of the next scheduled injection of the other medication. Parenteral long-acting 1-month preparation of paliperidone therapy is then continued at monthly intervals. The 1-week initiation dosing is not required.
- For patient being switched from the 3-month long-acting paliperidone preparation to the 1-month preparation or to E.R. tablets, the new preparation is begun 3 months after the last dose of the long-acting 3-month preparation. Dosage adjustment is made according to the new preparation guidelines.
- A patient must not receive an every-6-month injection preparation unless patient

has already been adequately treated with a once-a-month form for at least 4 months or an every-3-month form has been administered for at least one 3-month cycle.
- Rotate sites.

Invega Sustenna
- When initiating drug, inject the first two doses into the deltoid muscle.
- For injection into the deltoid muscle for patient weighing less than 90 kg (198 lb), use the 1-inch, 23G needle; for patient weighing 90 kg (198 lb) or more, use the 1½-inch, 22G needle.
- When injecting into the gluteal muscle (upper outer quadrant), use the 1½-in, 22G needle regardless of patient weight and after two doses have been given in the deltoid muscle.
- Shake syringe vigorously for a minimum of 10 seconds before administration.
- Inject slowly, deep into muscle.

Invega Trinza
- Shake syringe vigorously for at least 15 seconds to ensure a homogeneous suspension and that the needle does not get clogged during injection, which would deliver an incomplete dose. Once syringe has been shaken, inject drug within 5 minutes.
- Use only the thin-wall needles provided with the 3-month product for the injection. Do not use needles from the 1-month product or other commercially available needles, to reduce risk of blockage.
- When injecting into the deltoid muscle for patient weighing less than 90 kg (198 lb), use the 1-inch, 22G needle; for patient weighing 90 kg (198 lb) or more, use the 1½-inch, 22G needle.
- Administer a deltoid injection into the center of the deltoid muscle.
- When injecting into the gluteal muscle (upper outer quadrant), use the 1½-inch, 22G needle regardless of patient weight.
- If an incomplete dose is administered, do not reinject the dose remaining in the syringe and do not administer another dose. Notify prescriber.
- May administer drug up to 2 weeks before or after the 3-month scheduled time.
- If 4 months or more have elapsed since last dose, do not give scheduled dose; instead obtain an order to follow manufacturer guidelines for reinitiation.

Invega Hafyera

- Shake syringe vigorously for at least 15 seconds, rest briefly, and then shake again for 15 seconds. Administer within 5 minutes. If more than a 5-minute lapse occurs, the syringe will have to be shaken vigorously again for at least 30 seconds.
- Use only the needle provided with the drug. Do not interchange needles from other dosage forms or use any other commercially available needle.
- Administer deeply into the gluteal muscle only. Inject slowly (will take about 30 seconds) and take care to avoid injection into a blood vessel. Resistance may be felt while administering drug but this is normal. Confirm that the entire content of syringe has been injected before removing needle from muscle. After injection, hold pressure over the site; do not rub the injection site.
- If an incomplete dose is administered, do not reinject the dose remaining in the syringe and do not administer another dose. Notify prescriber.
- Follow manufacturer guidelines if a dose is missed.

Route	Onset	Peak	Duration
P.O.	Unknown	24 hr	Unknown
I.M.	1 day	13 days	126 days

Half-life: 23 hr (P.O.); 25–49 hr (I.M.)

Mechanism of Action

The main active metabolite of risperidone, paliperidone selectively blocks serotonin and dopamine receptors in mesocortical tract of CNS to suppress psychotic symptoms.

Contraindications

For all forms: History of cardiac arrhythmias, congenital heart disease, or congenital long-QT syndrome; hypersensitivity to paliperidone, risperidone, or its components
For oral form: Preexisting severe gastrointestinal narrowing

Interactions

DRUGS

alpha agonists, alpha blockers, angiotensin-converting enzyme (ACE) inhibitors, angiotensin II receptor blockers (ARBs), beta-blockers, calcium channel blockers, diuretics including thiazide, nitrates, vasodilators: Increased risk of hypotension, including orthostatic

antiarrhythmics of class IA (such as quinidine, procainamide) and class III (such as amiodarone, sotalol), antibiotics (such as gatifloxacin, moxifloxacin), antipsychotics (such as chlorpromazine, thioridazine): Increased risk of QT-interval prolongation
CNS depressants: Additive CNS depression
CYP3A4 and P-gp strong inducers (carbamazepine, rifampin, St. John's wort): Decreased plasma paliperidone level and effectiveness
dopamine agonist including levodopa: Possibly antagonized effects of dopamine agonist and other dopamine agonists

ACTIVITIES

alcohol use: CNS depression

Adverse Reactions

CNS: Agitation, akathisia, anxiety, asthenia, bradykinesia, catatonia, cogwheel rigidity, **CVA**, depression, disruption of body temperature regulation, dizziness, drooling, dyskinesia, dystonia, extrapyramidal disorder, fatigue, fever, headache, hyperkinesia, hypertonia, insomnia, lethargy, **neuroleptic malignant syndrome**, nightmares, nuchal rigidity, Parkinsonism, psychomotor hyperactivity, psychosis, restlessness, **seizures**, sleep disorder, somnambulism, somnolence, syncope, tardive dyskinesia, transient ischemic attack, tremor, vertigo
CV: **Bradycardia**, bundle branch block, elevated cholesterol and triglyceride level, first-degree heart block, hypertension, ischemia, orthostatic hypotension, palpitations, peripheral edema, **prolonged QT interval**, tachycardia, vascular ischemia, **venous thrombosis**
EENT: Blurred vision, dry mouth, eye movement disorder, inability to open mouth or jaw (trismus), nasal congestion, nasopharyngitis, oromandibular dystonia, pharyngolaryngeal pain, rhinitis, salivary hypersecretion, **swollen tongue**, tonsillitis, toothache
ENDO: Breast discharge, engorgement, pain, or tenderness; gynecomastia; hyperglycemia; hyperinsulinemia; hyperprolactinemia
GI: Abdominal discomfort or pain, change in appetite, constipation, diarrhea, dyspepsia, dysphagia, elevated liver enzymes, flatulence, ileus, nausea, **small intestinal obstruction**, upper abdominal pain, vomiting

GU: Cystitis, erectile dysfunction, menstrual abnormalities, priapism, retrograde ejaculation, urinary incontinence or retention, UTI

HEME: Agranulocytosis, anemia, leukopenia, neutropenia, thrombocytopenia, thrombotic thrombocytopenic purpura

MS: Arthralgia; back or limb pain; dysarthria; joint stiffness; muscle rigidity, spasms, tightness, or twitching; myalgia; torticollis

RESP: Cough, dyspnea, upper respiratory tract infection

SKIN: Drug eruption, eczema, pruritus, rash, urticaria

Other: Anaphylaxis, angioedema, generalized chest discomfort, injection-site reactions, weight gain or loss

Childbearing Considerations

PREGNANCY

- Pregnancy exposure registry: 1-866-961-2388 or http://womensmentalhealth.org/clinical-and-research-programs/pregnancyregistry/.
- Drug may cause fetal harm.
- Exposure to drug during the third trimester of pregnancy increases the risk for extrapyramidal and/or withdrawal symptoms following delivery.
- Use with caution only if benefit to mother outweighs potential risk to fetus.

LACTATION

- Drug is present in breast milk.
- Patient should check with prescriber before breastfeeding.
- If breastfeeding occurs, advise mothers to monitor their infants for excess sedation, extrapyramidal symptoms (tremors and abnormal muscle movements), failure to thrive, and jitteriness.

REPRODUCTION

- Know that women of childbearing age may experience a decrease in fertility during drug therapy that is reversible when drug is discontinued.

Nursing Considerations

- Keep in mind paliperidone shouldn't be used to treat dementia-related psychosis in the elderly because of an increased mortality risk. Parenteral paliperidone

is not recommended for patients with moderate to severe renal impairment.

- Know that drug shouldn't be given if patient has a condition that severely narrows GI tract because tablet doesn't change shape as it passes and could cause blockage.
- Use paliperidone cautiously in patients with cardiovascular disease, because drug may cause orthostatic hypotension. Also use cautiously in patients with Lewy bodies, because these patients are more sensitive to antipsychotic drugs. Monitor patient for increased sensitivity manifested as confusion, extrapyramidal symptoms, neuroleptic malignant syndrome clinical features, postural instability with frequent falls, and obtundation.

! **WARNING** Notify prescriber immediately and expect to stop drug if patient shows signs of neuroleptic malignant syndrome (altered mental status, autonomic instability, hyperpyrexia, muscle rigidity). Patients at risk for developing neuroleptic malignant syndrome are patients with dementia with Lewy bodies or Parkinson's disease because these patients can experience increased sensitivity to paliperidone.

- Monitor patient for involuntary, dyskinetic movements that may occur during therapy or after drug is discontinued. Notify prescriber if present, and expect to stop therapy. In some cases, therapy may have to continue despite tardive dyskinesia.
- Monitor blood glucose level because drug increases risk of hyperglycemia and possible hyperosmolar coma or ketoacidosis.
- Keep in mind dosage adjustments of paliperidone may be needed when carbamazepine therapy is started or discontinued because of carbamazepine's interaction with paliperidone.
- Check CBC often during first few months of therapy, especially if patient has low WBC count or history of drug-induced leukopenia or neutropenia. If WBC count declines, and especially if neutrophil count goes below 1,000/mm^3, expect to stop drug. If neutropenia is significant, also watch for evidence of infection and provide appropriate treatment, as prescribed.
- Institute fall measures because of potential for adverse CNS effects.

PATIENT TEACHING

- Instruct patient to take tablet whole with liquid beverage. Caution against chewing, crushing, or splitting it because it's designed to release drug at a controlled rate.
- Explain that shell of tablet will be eliminated in stool and that patient need not worry if he sees tablet in stool.
- Stress importance of compliance with appointments for administration of injectable form and routine blood tests, if ordered.
- Advise patient to avoid alcohol while taking paliperidone.
- Urge patient to rise slowly from sitting or lying position to minimize orthostatic hypotension.
- Caution patient to avoid hazardous activities until CNS effects of drug are known. Review fall precautions with patient as well.
- Advise patient to avoid activities that may cause overheating, such as becoming dehydrated, being exposed to extreme heat, or exercising strenuously.
- Advise female patient of childbearing age to notify prescriber if she intends to become or suspects that she is pregnant during therapy.
- Inform a breastfeeding mother to monitor her infant for abnormal muscle movements, excess sedation, failure to thrive, jitteriness, or tremors.
- Alert the patient who experiences hyperprolactinemia as a result of paliperidone therapy that reproductive function may become impaired. Also, review signs and symptoms of amenorrhea or galactorrhea in females and erectile dysfunction or gynecomastia in males. If this is a concern for the patient, patient should consult prescriber.
- Tell male patients that painful or prolonged penile erections can occur while taking paliperidone. Instruct him to seek immediate emergency medical attention if this occurs.
- Instruct patient to alert prescriber immediately if he experiences any persistent, severe, or unusual signs and symptoms.
- Tell patient to contact prescriber if abnormal movements occur.
- Instruct patient with diabetes to monitor her blood glucose level closely, as drug can affect glycemic control. Also review signs and symptoms of hyperglycemia with all patients and tell them to notify prescriber if present.
- Advise patient to notify all prescribers of paliperidone therapy and not to take over-the-counter preparations, including herbal products, without consulting prescriber.

palonosetron hydrochloride
Aloxi

≣ Class and Category

Pharmacologic class: Selective serotonin subtype 3 (5-HT$_3$) receptor antagonist
Therapeutic class: Antiemetic

≣ Indications and Dosages

✳ *To prevent acute and delayed nausea and vomiting from chemotherapy*

I.V. INJECTION

Adults. 0.25 mg about 30 min before start of chemotherapy.

I.V. INFUSION

Infants 1 month of age and over to less than 17 years. 20 mcg/kg about 30 min before start of chemotherapy. *Maximum:* 1.5 mg.

✳ *To prevent postoperative nausea and vomiting for up to 24 hr after surgery*

I.V. INJECTION

Adults. 0.075 mg immediately before induction of anesthesia.

≣ Drug Administration

I.V.

- Flush I.V. line with 0.9% Sodium Chloride Injection before and after giving drug.
- Use either the single-dose vial or the prefilled syringe to administer a 0.25-mg dose. Do not use the prefilled syringe to administer a dose other than 0.25 mg.
- For I.V. injection, administer a 0.25-mg dose over 30 seconds and a 0.075-mg dose over 10 seconds.
- For I.V. infusion, administer over 15 minutes.
- Store at room temperature and protect from light.
- *Incompatibilities:* Other I.V. drugs

P

Route	Onset	Peak	Duration
I.V.	Unknown	Unknown	3–5 days

Half-life: 40 hr

Contraindications

Hypersensitivity to palonosetron or its components

Interactions

DRUGS

5-HT3 receptor antagonists, selective serotonin reuptake inhibitors, serotonin and noradrenaline reuptake inhibitors: Increased risk of serotonin syndrome

Adverse Reactions

CNS: Anxiety, dizziness, drowsiness, dyskinesia, fatigue, headache, insomnia, serotonin syndrome, weakness
CV: Bradycardia, hypotension, prolonged QT interval, tachycardia
GI: Abdominal pain, constipation, diarrhea
SKIN: Dermatitis, pruritus, rash

Other: Hyperkalemia, hypersensitivity reactions (anaphylaxis, angioedema, bronchospasm, dyspnea, erythema, pruritus, rash, swelling), injection-site reaction (burning, discomfort, induration, pain)

Childbearing Considerations

PREGNANCY

- It is not known if drug can cause fetal harm.
- Use with caution only if benefit to mother outweighs potential risk to fetus.

LACTATION

- It is not known if drug is present in breast milk.
- A decision should be made to discontinue breastfeeding or to discontinue the drug if breastfeeding occurs.

Nursing Considerations

- Use palonosetron cautiously in patients who have or may develop prolonged cardiac conduction intervals—especially QT interval—such as those with congenital QT syndrome, hypokalemia,

Mechanism of Action

Chemotherapy may induce nausea and vomiting by irritating the small intestine's mucosa, causing mucosal enterochromaffin cells to release serotonin (5-HT$_3$). 5-HT$_3$ stimulates sympathetic receptors on afferent vagal nerve endings causing the vomiting reflex.

Palonosetron selectively blocks 5-HT$_3$ receptors. By keeping the vagus nerve from inducing the vomiting reflex, drug reduces or prevents nausea and vomiting. It also may block 5-HT$_3$ receptors centrally, in the brain's chemoreceptor trigger zone.

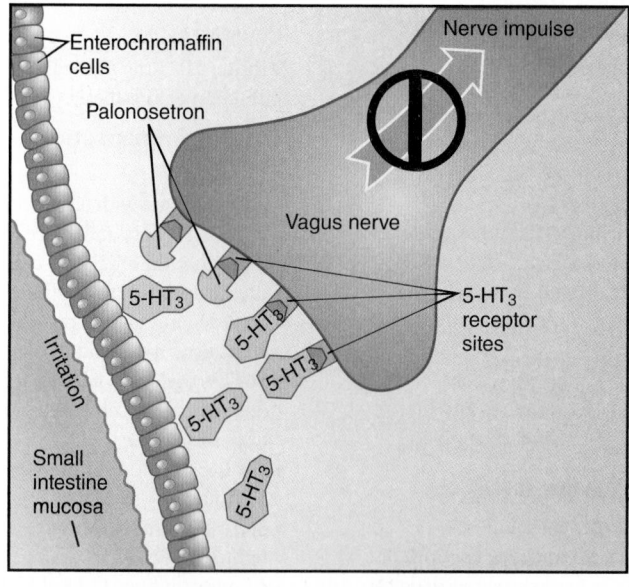

or hypomagnesemia; those taking an antiarrhythmic, a diuretic known to induce electrolyte abnormalities, or another drug that may prolong QT interval; and those who have received cumulative high-dose anthracycline therapy. With these patients, obtain a baseline ECG before giving palonosetron; repeat the ECG 15 minutes or 24 hours after giving drug, as ordered. Notify prescriber of any delayed conduction.

! **WARNING** Closely monitor any patient hypersensitive to other selective serotonin receptor antagonists for a similar reaction. If a reaction occurs, notify prescriber immediately. Expect drug to be discontinued and administer appropriate supportive care, as ordered.

! **WARNING** Monitor patient closely for serotonin syndrome, which is characterized by agitation, coma, diarrhea, hallucinations, hyperreflexia, hyperthermia, incoordination, labile blood pressure, nausea, tachycardia, or vomiting. Notify prescriber immediately because serotonin syndrome may be life-threatening, and provide supportive care.

PATIENT TEACHING
- Advise patient to avoid hazardous activities until drug's CNS effects are known.

! **WARNING** Instruct patient to notify prescriber of any hypersensitivity reaction, such as allergic dermatitis or rash.

- Also instruct patient to immediately report any persistent, severe, or unusual signs and symptoms.

pamidronate disodium

⌇ Class and Category
Pharmacologic class: Bisphosphonate
Therapeutic class: Antiosteoporotic

⌇ Indications and Dosages
＊ *To treat moderate or severe cancer-induced hypercalcemia*

I.V. INFUSION
Adults. 60 to 90 mg over 2 to 24 hr as a single dose when corrected serum calcium level is

12 to 13.5 mg/dl; 90 mg over 2 to 24 hr when corrected serum calcium level is greater than 13.5 mg/dl. May be repeated as prescribed after 7 days if hypercalcemia recurs.

＊ *To treat moderate to severe Paget's disease of bone*

I.V. INFUSION
Adults. 30 mg daily over 4 hr on 3 consecutive days for a total dose of 90 mg. Repeated as needed and tolerated.

＊ *To treat osteolytic bone metastases of breast cancer*

I.V. INFUSION
Adults. 90 mg over 2 hr every 3 to 4 wk.

＊ *To treat osteolytic bone lesions of multiple myeloma*

I.V. INFUSION
Adults. 90 mg over 4 hr every mo.

±**DOSAGE ADJUSTMENT** For patients with renal deterioration (normal baseline creatinine but an increase of 0.5 mg/dl or more or an abnormal baseline creatinine with an increase of 1 mg/dl or more) being treated for osteolytic bone metastases of breast cancer or osteolytic bone lesions of multiple myeloma, retreatment given only after creatinine has returned to within 10% of the baseline value.

⌇ Drug Administration
I.V.
- No more than 90 mg should be given at any one time because of increased risk of serious adverse effect on kidneys.
- For treatment of hypercalcemia of malignancy, dilute drug in 1,000 ml of 0.45% or 0.9% Sodium Chloride Injection or 5% Dextrose Injection and administer over at least 2 hours and up to 24 hours for the 60- and 90-mg doses.
- For treatment of Paget's disease, dilute drug in 500 ml of 0.45% or 0.9% Sodium Chloride Injection or 5% Dextrose Injection and infuse over 4 hours.
- For treatment of osteolytic bone metastases of breast cancer, dilute drug in 250 ml of 0.45% or 0.9% Sodium Chloride Injection or 5% Dextrose Injection and infuse over 2 hours.
- For treatment of osteolytic bone lesions of multiple myeloma, dilute 90 mg in 500 ml of 0.45% or 0.9% Sodium Chloride Injection or 5% Dextrose Injection and infuse over 4 hours.

P

- *Incompatibilities:* Calcium-containing solutions such as Ringer's solution, other drugs

Route	Onset	Peak	Duration
I.V.	24 hr	1 mo	Unknown
Half-life: 21–35 hr			

Mechanism of Action

Inhibits bone resorption, possibly by impairing attachment of osteoclast precursors to mineralized bone matrix, thus reducing the rate of bone turnover in Paget's disease and osteolytic metastases. Pamidronate also reduces the flow of calcium from resorbing bone into bloodstream.

Contraindications

Hypersensitivity to pamidronate, other bisphosphonates, or their components

Interactions

DRUGS

nephrotoxic drugs: Increased risk of nephrotoxicity
thalidomide: Increased risk of renal dysfunction in patients with multiple myeloma

Adverse Reactions

CNS: Confusion, fever, psychosis, visual hallucinations
CV: Hypotension
EENT: Conjunctivitis, ocular inflammation
GI: Abdominal cramps, anorexia, GI bleeding, indigestion, nausea, vomiting
GU: Azotemia, focal segmental glomerulosclerosis, glomerulonephropathies, hematuria, nephritis, nephrotic syndrome, renal toxicity leading to failure, renal tubular disorders
HEME: Leukopenia, lymphopenia
MS: Atypical fractures of femur; muscle spasms or stiffness; osteonecrosis (mainly of jaw); severe bone, joint, or muscle pain
RESP: Adult respiratory distress syndrome, dyspnea, interstitial lung disease
SKIN: Pruritus, rash
Other: Anaphylaxis, angioedema, flu-like symptoms, hyperkalemia, hypernatremia, hypocalcemia, hypokalemia, hypomagnesemia, hypophosphatemia, injection-site pain and swelling, reactivation of herpes simplex and zoster infections

Childbearing Considerations

PREGNANCY

- Drug may cause fetal harm such as skeletal and other abnormalities. This risk includes posttreatment if a woman becomes pregnant.
- Drug is not recommended for use during pregnancy.

LACTATION

- It is not known if drug is present in breast milk.
- A decision should be made to discontinue breastfeeding or the drug to avoid potential serious adverse reactions in the breastfed infant.

Nursing Considerations

- Make sure patient has had a dental checkup before invasive dental procedures during pamidronate therapy, especially if he has cancer; is receiving chemotherapy, a corticosteroid, or head or neck radiation; or has poor oral hygiene. Risk of osteonecrosis is increased in these patients.
- Obtain serum creatinine level before each treatment, as ordered. Notify prescriber of abnormal results because drug may have to be withheld or dosage adjusted until creatinine level returns to normal.
- Monitor patient's CBC differential; hematocrit and hemoglobin; and serum electrolytes including calcium, magnesium, and phosphate levels, as ordered throughout therapy because abnormalities may occur.
- Monitor patient for hypocalcemia, especially if patient has had thyroid surgery. Expect to administer calcium and vitamin D supplementation in the absence of hypercalcemia in patients with multiple myeloma or predominantly lytic bone metastases, who are at risk of calcium or vitamin D deficiency, and for patients with Paget's disease of the bone.
- Stay alert for fever during first 3 days of therapy, especially in patients receiving high doses. If fever develops, obtain patient's CBC with differential, as ordered.
- Assess patient with anemia, leukopenia, or thrombocytopenia for worsening of the condition during first 2 weeks of therapy.

PATIENT TEACHING

- Emphasize need to comply with prescribed administration schedule for pamidronate.

- Review if calcium and vitamin D supplementation should be or not be used, which is dependent on patient's calcium level and indication being treated.
- Instruct patient on proper oral hygiene and on need to notify prescriber about upcoming invasive dental procedures.
- Advise women of childbearing age to alert prescriber if she suspects or knows she is pregnant.
- Instruct patient to report to prescriber any new or unusual pain in hip or thigh in the absence of trauma.

pantoprazole sodium
Pantoloc (CAN), Protonix, Protonix I.V.

Class and Category
Pharmacologic class: Proton pump inhibitor
Therapeutic class: Antiulcer

Indications and Dosages
✶ *To treat erosive esophagitis associated with gastroesophageal reflux disease (GERD) short-term*

DELAYED-RELEASE ORAL SUSPENSION, DELAYED-RELEASE TABLETS
Adults. 40 mg daily for up to 8 wk. Repeated for another 4 to 8 wk if healing doesn't occur.
Children age 5 years and older weighing 40 kg (88 lb) or more. 40 mg once daily for up to 8 wk.
Children age 5 years and older weighing 15 kg (33 lb) up to 40 kg (88 lb). 20 mg once daily for up to 8 wks.

I.V. INFUSION
Adults. 40 mg once daily for 7 to 10 days, followed by oral doses.

✶ *To maintain healing of erosive esophagitis and reduce relapse of daytime and nighttime symptoms in patients with GERD*

DELAYED-RELEASE ORAL SUSPENSION, DELAYED-RELEASE TABLETS
Adults. 40 mg daily for up to 12 mo.

✶ *To treat pathological hypersecretion conditions, including Zollinger–Ellison*

DELAYED-RELEASE TABLETS
Adults. 40 mg twice daily. *Maximum:* 240 mg daily.

I.V. INFUSION
Adults. 80 mg every 12 hr adjusted based on patient's acid output measurements up to 80 mg every 8 hr. *Maximum:* 240 mg daily; no more than 6 days of therapy.

Drug Administration
P.O.
- Delayed-release tablets should be swallowed whole and not broken, chewed, or crushed.
- Mix delayed-release oral suspension in apple juice or applesauce only or, if given through a nasogastric tube, mix in apple juice only, because proper pH is necessary for stability.
- Administer oral suspension 30 minutes before a meal. When mixing with applesauce, administer within 10 minutes and encourage patient to take repeated sips of water to make sure granules are washed down into the stomach. When mixing with apple juice, use only 1 teaspoon of apple juice to mix granules in, stir for 5 seconds (granules will not dissolve) and give immediately to patient to drink. After administration, rinse container once or twice with more apple juice and give to patient to drink to ensure that full dose has been given.

I.V.
- Flush I.V. line with 0.9% Sodium Chloride Injection, 5% Dextrose in Water, or Lactated Ringer's Injection before and after giving drug.
- Administer through a dedicated line or through a Y-site.
- When giving I.V. infusion over 2 minutes, reconstitute with 10 ml of 0.9% Sodium Chloride Injection. Reconstituted solution may be stored up to 24 hours at room temperature.
- When giving I.V. infusion over 15 minutes at a rate of 7 ml/min, reconstitute with 10 ml 0.9% Sodium Chloride Injection. Then, further dilute with 100 ml (for GERD for final concentration of 0.4 mg/ml) or 80 ml (for pathological hypersecretion in Zollinger–Ellison syndrome for final concentration of 0.8 mg/ml) of 0.9% Sodium Chloride Injection, 5% Dextrose in Water, or Lactated Ringer's Injection.
- When giving through a Y-site, immediately stop administration if discoloration or precipitation occurs.

P

- Solution may be stored up to 6 hours before further dilution and up to 24 hours before use. Before reconstitution, store at room temperature and protect from light.
- *Incompatibilities:* Midazolam (Y-site administration), solutions other than 0.9% Sodium Chloride Injection, 5% Dextrose Injection, or Lactated Ringer's Injection, zinc-containing products

Route	Onset	Peak	Duration
P.O.	2.5 hr	2.5 hr	24 hr
I.V.	15–30 min	Unknown	24 hr
Half-life: 1 hr			

Mechanism of Action

Interferes with gastric acid secretion by inhibiting the hydrogen-potassium-adenosine triphosphatase (H^+-K^+-ATPase) enzyme system, or proton pump, in gastric parietal cells. Normally, the proton pump uses energy from hydrolysis of ATPase to drive H^+ and chloride (Cl^-) out of parietal cells and into the stomach lumen in exchange for potassium (K^+), which leaves the stomach lumen and enters parietal cells. After this exchange, H^+ and Cl^- combine in the stomach to form hydrochloric acid (HCl). Pantoprazole irreversibly inhibits the final step in gastric acid production by blocking the exchange of intracellular H^+ and extracellular K^+, thus preventing H^+ from entering the stomach and additional HCl from forming.

Contraindications

Concurrent therapy with rilpivirine-containing products, hypersensitivity to pantoprazole, substituted benzimidazoles, or their components

Interactions

DRUGS

atazanavir, nelfinavir, rilpivirine: Significantly decreased plasma levels of these drugs reducing antiviral effect; possible increased risk of drug resistance
dasatinib, erlotinib, iron salts, itraconazole, ketoconazole, mycophenolate mofetil, nilotinib: Possible decreased absorption of these drugs and decreased effectiveness
methotrexate: Increased risk of methotrexate toxicities

saquinavir: Possibly increased risk of antiretroviral toxicity
warfarin: Increased INR, PT, and bleeding risk

Adverse Reactions

CNS: Anxiety, asthenia, confusion, depression, dizziness, fatigue, fever, hallucinations, headache, hypertonia, hypokinesia, insomnia, malaise, migraine, somnolence, speech disorder, vertigo
CV: Chest pain, elevated triglycerides, hypercholesterolemia, hyperlipidemia
EENT: Anterior ischemic optic neuropathy, blurred vision, dry mouth, increased salivation, pharyngitis, rhinitis, sinusitis, taste disorder, tinnitus
ENDO: Hyperglycemia
GI: Abdominal pain, atrophic gastritis, *Clostridium difficile*-associated diarrhea, constipation, diarrhea, elevated liver enzymes, flatulence, fundic gland polyps (long-term use), gastroenteritis, hepatic failure, hepatitis, hepatotoxicity, indigestion, jaundice, nausea, pancreatitis, vomiting
GU: Elevated serum creatinine level, tubulointerstitial nephritis
HEME: Agranulocytosis, leukopenia, pancytopenia, thrombocytopenia
MS: Arthralgia, back or neck pain, bone fracture, myalgia, rhabdomyolysis
RESP: Bronchitis, dyspnea, increased cough, upper respiratory tract infection
SKIN: Acute generalized exanthematous pustulosis, cutaneous lupus erythematosus, erythema multiforme, photosensitivity, pruritus, rash, Stevens–Johnson syndrome, toxic epidermal necrolysis
Other: Anaphylaxis, angioedema, drug reaction with eosinophilia and systemic symptoms (DRESS), elevated creatine kinase and phosphokinase levels, flu-like symptoms, generalized pain, hyperuricemia, hypomagnesemia, hyponatremia, infection, injection-site reaction, systemic lupus erythematosus, vitamin B_{12} deficiency, weight changes

Childbearing Considerations

PREGNANCY

- It is not known if drug can cause fetal harm.
- Use with caution only if benefit to mother outweighs potential risk to fetus.

LACTATION

- Drug is present in breast milk.
- Patient should check with prescriber before breastfeeding.

Nursing Considerations

- Ensure the continuity of gastric acid suppression during transition from oral to I.V. pantoprazole (or vice versa) because even a brief interruption of effective suppression can lead to serious complications.
- Don't give pantoprazole within 4 weeks of testing for *Helicobacter pylori* because antibiotics, bismuth preparations, and proton pump inhibitors suppress *H. pylori* and may lead to false-negative results. Drug also may cause false-positive results in urine screening tests for tetrahydrocannabinol. Consult guidelines for pantoprazole use before testing.
- Expect to monitor PT or INR during therapy if patient takes an oral anticoagulant.
- Be aware that if therapy lasts more than 3 years, patient may not be able to absorb vitamin B_{12} because of achlorhydria or hypochlorhydria. Treatment for cyanocobalamin deficiency may be needed.

! WARNING Monitor patient for severe cutaneous and hypersensitivity adverse reactions. At the first sign of a rash or other hypersensitivity reactions, notify prescriber and expect drug to be discontinued.

- Monitor patient's urine output because pantoprazole may cause acute tubulointerstitial nephritis. Notify prescriber if urine output decreases or there is blood in the patient's urine.
- Monitor patient for bone fracture, especially in patients receiving multiple daily doses for more than a year because proton pump inhibitors, such as pantoprazole, increase risk of osteoporosis-related fractures of the hip, spine, or wrist.
- Monitor patient for diarrhea from *C. difficile*, which can occur with or without antibiotics in patients taking pantoprazole. If severe diarrhea occurs, notify prescriber and expect to withhold drug and treat with electrolytes, fluids, protein, and an antibiotic effective against *C. difficile*.

- Be aware that a symptomatic response to the drug does not rule out the presence of a gastric tumor.
- Monitor the patient, especially the patient on long-term therapy for hypomagnesemia. If patient is to remain on pantoprazole long-term, expect to monitor the patient's serum magnesium level, as ordered, and if level becomes low, anticipate magnesium replacement therapy to be given and pantoprazole to be discontinued.
- Know that both cutaneous and systemic lupus erythematosus have occurred within days to years after proton pump therapy such as pantoprazole was initiated. The most common symptoms presented were arthralgia, cytopenia, and rash. Report such findings to prescriber.
- Know that proton pump inhibitors such as pantoprazole should not be given longer than medically necessary.
- Expect drug to be withheld for at least 14 days before assessment of serum chromogranin A levels is performed, because levels increase when gastric acidity is decreased and thus interfere with diagnostic investigations for neuroendocrine tumors.
- Be aware that pantoprazole may result in false-positive urine screening tests for tetrahydrocannabinol.

PATIENT TEACHING

- Instruct patient to swallow delayed-release tablets whole and not to break, chew, or crush them. Warn patient not to exceed dosage or take for longer than prescribed, as long-term use increases risk of serious adverse reactions.
- Tell patient to take delayed-release oral suspension 30 minutes before a meal mixed in apple juice or applesauce; no other liquid or food should be used. When mixing with applesauce, tell patient to take mixture within 10 minutes and then to take repeated sips of water to make sure granules are washed down into the stomach. When mixing with apple juice, tell patient to use only 1 teaspoon of apple juice to mix granules in, stir for 5 seconds (granules will not dissolve) and drink immediately. After drinking, tell patient to rinse the container once or twice with more apple juice and then drink to ensure full dose has been given.

P

- Advise patient to expect relief of symptoms within 2 weeks of starting therapy. Tell patient to notify prescriber if he has a suboptimal response to drug or an early symptomatic relapse.
- Advise patient who takes warfarin to follow bleeding precautions and to notify prescriber immediately if bleeding occurs.

! **WARNING** Alert patient that drug may cause severe adverse skin and hypersensitivity reactions. Tell patient to stop drug immediately at the first sign of a rash or allergic reaction and contact prescriber.

- Instruct patient to notify prescriber if diarrhea occurs and becomes prolonged or severe.
- Advise patient to notify prescriber if patient notices he is experiencing a decrease in the amount of urine voided or there is blood in his urine. Also tell him to notify prescriber if he experiences new or worsening joint pain or a rash on his arms or cheeks that gets worse in the sun.
- Remind patient to notify all prescribers of pantoprazole use and not to take any over-the-counter medication, including herbal supplements, without discussing with prescriber.
- Advise patient taking pantoprazole for longer than 3 years to alert prescriber if he experiences signs and symptoms of vitamin B12 deficiency such as constipation or diarrhea, heart palpitations, mental problems such as depression or memory loss, pale skin, or feeling light-headed, tired, or weak. Also advise him to report any persistent, severe, or unusual signs or symptoms that may be suggestive of other adverse effects such as hypomagnesemia.

paroxetine hydrochloride

Paxil, Paxil CR

paroxetine mesylate

Brisdelle, Pexeva

☰ Class and Category

Pharmacologic class: Selective serotonin reuptake inhibitor (SSRI)

Therapeutic class: Antianxiety, antidepressant, antiobsessional, antipanic, premenstrual analgesic

☰ Indications and Dosages

✴ *To treat major depression*

C.R. TABLETS (PAXIL CR)

Adults. *Initial:* 25 mg daily, increased as tolerated by 12.5 mg daily every wk. *Maximum:* 62.5 mg daily.

ORAL SUSPENSION (PAXIL), TABLETS (PAXIL, PEXEVA)

Adults. *Initial:* 20 mg daily, increased as tolerated by 10 mg daily every wk. *Maximum:* 50 mg daily.

✴ *To treat obsessive–compulsive disorder*

ORAL SUSPENSION (PAXIL), TABLETS (PAXIL, PEXEVA)

Adults. *Initial:* 20 mg daily, increased as tolerated by 10 mg daily every wk. *Usual:* 20 to 60 mg daily. *Maximum:* 60 mg daily.

✴ *To treat panic disorder*

C.R. TABLETS (PAXIL CR)

Adults. *Initial:* 12.5 mg daily, increased by 12.5 mg daily every wk as needed. *Maximum:* **75** mg daily.

ORAL SUSPENSION (PAXIL), TABLETS (PAXIL, PEXEVA)

Adults. *Initial:* 10 mg daily, increased as tolerated by 10 mg daily every wk. *Usual:* 10 to 60 mg daily. *Maximum:* 60 mg daily.

✴ *To treat social anxiety disorder*

C.R. TABLETS (PAXIL CR)

Adults. *Initial:* 12.5 mg daily, increased by 12.5 mg daily every wk as needed. *Maximum:* 37.5 mg daily.

ORAL SUSPENSION (PAXIL), TABLETS (PAXIL)

Adults. *Initial:* 20 mg daily, increased as tolerated by 10 mg daily every wk. *Usual:* 20 to 60 mg daily. *Maximum:* 60 mg daily.

✴ *To treat generalized anxiety disorder*

ORAL SUSPENSION (PAXIL), TABLETS (PAXIL, PEXEVA)

Adults. *Initial:* 20 mg daily, increased as tolerated by 10 mg daily every wk. *Usual:* 20 to 50 mg daily. *Maximum:* 50 mg daily.

✴ *To treat posttraumatic stress disorder*

ORAL SUSPENSION, TABLETS (PAXIL)

Adults. *Initial:* 20 mg daily, increased as tolerated by 10 mg daily every wk. *Usual:* 20 to 50 mg daily. *Maximum:* 50 mg daily.

✳ *To treat premenstrual dysphoric disorder*

C.R. TABLETS (PAXIL CR)

Adults. *Initial:* 12.5 mg daily, increased as needed after 1 wk to 25 mg daily. Alternatively, 12.5 mg daily in the morning only during luteal phase of menstrual cycle (2-wk period before onset of menstrual cycle), increased as needed after 1 wk to 25 mg daily in the morning during luteal phase of menstrual cycle.

±**DOSAGE ADJUSTMENT** For patients who are debilitated, elderly, or have severe hepatic or renal dysfunction, initially 10 mg daily; maximum 40 mg daily. For these same patients who are taking C.R. tablets, initial dose is 12.5 mg but dosage may have to be reduced and titration intervals increased, if needed. If these patients are being treated for major depressive disorder or panic disorder, dosage should not exceed 50 mg daily and for social anxiety disorder dosage should not exceed 37.5 mg daily.

✳ *To treat moderate to severe vasomotor symptoms associated with menopause*

CAPSULES (BRISDELLE)

Adults. 7.5 mg once daily at bedtime.

▤ Drug Administration

P.O.

- Capsules and tablets should be swallowed whole and not broken, chewed, crushed, or opened.
- Shake oral suspension well before administration.
- Use a calibrated device or oral syringe to measure oral suspension dosage.
- Give immediate-release tablets and oral suspension in the morning.
- Give capsules at bedtime.

Route	Onset	Peak	Duration
P.O.	1–2 wk	3–8 hr	Unknown
P.O./E.R.	Unknown	6–10 hr	Unknown

Half-life: 15–33.2 hr

▤ Mechanism of Action

Exerts antianxiety, antidepressant, antiobsessional, and antipanic effects as well as relieving symptoms associated with premenstrual dysphoric disorder and hot flashes associated with menopause by potentiating serotonin activity in CNS and inhibiting serotonin reuptake at presynaptic neuronal membrane. Blocked serotonin reuptake increases levels and prolongs activity of serotonin at synaptic receptor sites.

▤ Contraindications

Hypersensitivity to paroxetine or its components, pimozide or thioridazine therapy, pregnancy (Brisdelle), use within 14 days of an MAO inhibitor including linezolid or methylene blue I.V.

▤ Interactions

DRUGS

amphetamines, buspirone, cisapride, fentanyl, isoniazid, linezolid, lithium, MAO inhibitors, methylene blue (I.V.), other selective serotonin reuptake inhibitors, other serotonin norepinephrine reuptake inhibitors, procarbazine, St. John's wort, tramadol, tricyclic antidepressants, triptans, tryptophan: Possibly increased risk of serotonin syndrome

aspirin, NSAIDs, warfarin: Increased anticoagulant activity and risk of bleeding

atomoxetine; risperidone; other drugs metabolized by CYP2D6, such as amitriptyline, desipramine, fluoxetine, imipramine, phenothiazines, type IC antiarrhythmics: Increased plasma levels of these drugs

cimetidine: Possibly increased blood paroxetine level

digoxin: Possibly decreased digoxin effects

drugs highly protein bound: Increased adverse reactions of these drugs and paroxetine

fosamprenavir/ritonavir: Significantly decreased plasma levels of paroxetine

phenytoin: Possibly altered levels of both drugs

pimozide: Increased risk of prolonged QT interval

procyclidine: Increased blood procyclidine level and anticholinergic effects

tamoxifen: Decreased tamoxifen effectiveness

theophylline: Possibly increased blood theophylline level and risk of toxicity

thioridazine: Increased thioridazine level, possibly leading to prolonged QT interval and life-threatening ventricular arrhythmias

tricyclic antidepressants: Increased blood antidepressant levels; increased risk of toxicity, including seizures

ACTIVITIES

alcohol use: Possibly altered psychomotor function

P

⊟ Adverse Reactions

CNS: Agitation, akathisia, asthenia, confusion, decreased concentration, dizziness, drowsiness, emotional lability, hallucinations, headache, hypomania, insomnia, mania, **neuroleptic malignant syndrome**, psychomotor agitation, restlessness, **seizures**, **serotonin syndrome**, somnolence, **suicidal ideation**, tremor

CV: Palpitations, tachycardia, **torsades de pointes**, **ventricular fibrillation or tachycardia**

EENT: Angle-closure glaucoma, blurred vision, dry mouth, rhinitis, taste perversion

GI: Abdominal cramps or pain, anorexia, constipation, diarrhea, flatulence, nausea, vomiting

GU: Decreased libido, absence or delayed orgasm (females), delayed or failed ejaculation, erectile dysfunction, impotence, sexual dysfunction, urine retention

HEME: **Bleeding events**

MS: Back pain, bone fracture, myalgia, myasthenia, myopathy

SKIN: Diaphoresis, rash, **Stevens–Johnson syndrome**

Other: **Hyponatremia**, weight gain or loss

⊟ Childbearing Considerations

PREGNANCY

- Drug causes fetal harm with congenital malformations, particularly cardiovascular malformations with exposure in first trimester.
- When drug is used late in the third trimester, the neonate may develop complications requiring prolonged hospitalization, respiratory support, and tube feeding.
- Drug is not recommended for use in pregnant women and is contraindicated for treatment of vasomotor symptoms during pregnancy.

LACTATION

- Drug is present in breast milk.
- Patient should check with prescriber before breastfeeding.

REPRODUCTION

- Drug may affect sperm quality, which may affect fertility in some men.

⊟ Nursing Considerations

- Be aware that Brisdelle is not used to treat any psychiatric condition because it contains a lower dose of paroxetine.

- Don't give enteric-coated form with antacids.
- Watch for akathisia (inner sense of restlessness) and psychomotor agitation, especially during the first few weeks of therapy.
- Watch patient closely (especially young adults), for suicidal tendencies, particularly when therapy starts and dosage changes, because depression may worsen temporarily during these times, possibly leading to suicidal ideation.
- Watch for mania, which may result from any antidepressant in a susceptible patient.
- Monitor patient closely for evidence of GI bleeding, especially if patient also takes a drug known to cause GI bleeding, such as aspirin, an NSAID, or warfarin.

> **! WARNING** Monitor patient closely for serotonin syndrome exhibited by agitation, coma, diarrhea, hallucinations, hyperreflexia, hyperthermia, incoordination, labile blood pressure, nausea, tachycardia, or vomiting. Notify prescriber immediately because serotonin syndrome may be life-threatening, and provide supportive care.

> **! WARNING** Be aware that serotonin syndrome in its most severe form may resemble neuroleptic malignant syndrome, which includes autonomic instability with possibly rapid changes in mental status and vital signs, hyperthermia, and muscle rigidity. Stop drug immediately, and provide supportive care.

- To minimize adverse reactions, expect to taper drug rather than stop it abruptly.
- Be aware that pathological fractures have been associated with antidepressant therapy. Monitor patient for unexplained bone pain, bruising, joint tenderness, or swelling.

PATIENT TEACHING

- Advise patient to take immediate-release form in the morning to minimize insomnia and to take it with food if adverse GI reactions develop.
- Instruct patient to avoid taking C.R. paroxetine within 2 hours of an antacid.
- Tell patient to swallow C.R. tablets whole and not to chew, crush, or cut them.
- Instruct patient prescribed Brisdelle to take drug at bedtime.

- Advise patient that drug may cause mild pupillary dilation, which may lead to an episode of acute angle-closure glaucoma. Encourage patient to have eye exam before starting therapy to see if he is at risk.
- Suggest that patient avoid hazardous activities until drug's CNS effects are known.
- Tell family or caregiver to observe patient closely for suicidal tendencies, especially when therapy starts or dosage changes and especially if patient is a young adult.
- Explain that full effect may take 4 weeks.
- Urge patient to avoid alcohol during therapy; effects with paroxetine are unknown.
- Tell patient not to take aspirin or NSAIDs during therapy because they increase the risk of bleeding. If patient takes warfarin, tell her to use bleeding precautions and to notify prescriber at once if bleeding occurs.
- Inform patient that episodes of acute depression may persist for months or longer and that they require continued follow-up.
- Instruct patient not to stop drug abruptly but to taper dosage as instructed.
- Alert female patients of childbearing age to use effective contraception and to notify prescriber if pregnancy occurs or is suspected.
- Caution patient to alert all prescribers about paroxetine therapy because of potentially serious drug interactions.
- Tell patient to notify prescriber if she develops unexplained bone pain, bruising, joint tenderness, or swelling. Also advise patient to report any persistent, severe, or unusual signs and symptoms to prescriber. Instruct patient to speak with prescriber with concerns about sexual dysfunction.

pegfilgrastim
Lapelga (CAN), Neulasta

pegfilgrastim-apgf
Nyvepria

pegfilgrastim-bmez
Ziextenzo

pegfilgrastim-cbqv
Udenyca

pegfilgrastim-jmdb
Fulphila

Class and Category
Pharmacologic class: Colony-stimulating factor
Therapeutic class: Hematopoietic

Indications and Dosages
* *To increase survival in patients acutely exposed to myelosuppressive doses of radiation.*

SUBCUTANEOUS INJECTION (NEULASTA)

Adults and children weighing 45 kg (99 lb) or more. 6 mg as soon as possible after exposure, followed by 6 mg 1 wk later.
Children weighing between 31 and 44 kg (68.2–96.8 lb). 4 mg as soon as possible after exposure, followed by 4 mg 1 wk later.
Children weighing between 21 and 30 kg (46.2–66 lb). 2.5 mg as soon as possible after exposure, followed by 2.5 mg 1 wk later.
Children weighing between 10 and 20 kg (22–44 lb). 1.5 mg as soon as possible after exposure, followed by 2.5 mg 1 wk later.
Children weighing less than 10 kg (22 lb). 0.1 mg/kg as soon as possible after exposure, followed by 0.1 mg/kg 1 wk later.

* *To reduce the risk of infection, as manifested by febrile neutropenia, in patients with nonmyeloid malignancies receiving myelosuppressive chemotherapy*

SUBCUTANEOUS INJECTION (FULPHILA, NEULASTA, NYVEPRIA, UDENYCA, ZIEXTENZO)

Adults and children weighing more than 45 kg (99 lb). 6 mg once with each chemotherapy cycle but not administered between 14 days before and 24 hours after administration of cytotoxic chemotherapy.
Children weighing between 31 and 44 kg (68.2–96.8 lb). 4 mg once with each chemotherapy cycle but not administered between 14 days before and 24 hours after administration of cytotoxic chemotherapy.
Children weighing between 21 and 30 kg (46.2–66 lb). 2.5 mg once with each chemotherapy cycle but not administered

P

between 14 days before and 24 hours after administration of cytotoxic chemotherapy. **Children weighing between 10 and 20 kg (22–44 lb).** 1.5 mg once with each chemotherapy cycle but not administered between 14 days before and 24 hours after administration of cytotoxic chemotherapy. **Children weighing less than 10 kg (22 lb).** 0.1 mg/kg once with each chemotherapy cycle but not administered between 14 days before and 24 hours after administration of cytotoxic chemotherapy.

SUBCUTANEOUS INJECTION (LAPELGA)
Adults. 6 mg once with each chemotherapy cycle and not administered sooner than 24 hours after the administration of cytotoxic chemotherapy.

Drug Administration
SUBCUTANEOUS
- Store drug in refrigerator and protect from freezing and light. If Fulphila or Lapelga become frozen, drug may be allowed to thaw one time in refrigerator before injection. Discard if either drug becomes frozen more than once.
- Needle cover for Lapelga, Neulasta, and Ziextenzo contains dry natural rubber and should not be handled by persons with a latex allergy.
- Don't use prefilled syringe for doses less than 0.6 ml (6 mg) because syringe does not bear graduation marks for doses that small.
- Let drug warm to room temperature for 30 minutes before injection and protect from light.
- Don't shake solution.
- Do not use prefilled syringe if it has been dropped on a hard surface.
- Discard drug that contains particles, is discolored, or was stored more than 48 hours at room temperature for Neulasta or Udenyca; 72 hours for Fulphila; 120 hours for Ziextenzo; or 15 days for Lapelga and Nyvepria.
- Administer via a single-dose prefilled syringe for manual administration or use an on-body injector for Neulasta, which is co-packaged with a single-dose prefilled syringe. The on-body injector form of Neulasta is not recommended for patients with hematopoietic subsyndrome or acute radiation syndrome.

- If using the on-body injector for Neulasta, fill it with drug using the prefilled syringe accompanying it and then apply the on-body injector to patient's intact, nonirritated skin (abdomen or back of arm). About 27 hours after it is applied, the device will deliver dose over 45 minutes. The prefilled syringe that comes with device can only be used for device. If given as a subcutaneous injection, patient will be given an overdose of the drug. If the single-dose prefilled syringe for manual use is used with the device, the patient will be underdosed.
- If using a prefilled syringe, inject drug into intact, nonirritated areas of the abdomen, back of arm, thigh, or upper outer area of buttocks.
- Rotate sites.

Route	Onset	Peak	Duration
SubQ	Unknown	16–120 hr	14 days

Half-life: 15–80 hr

Mechanism of Action
Induces formation of neutrophil progenitor cells by binding to receptors on granulocytes, which then divide. Pegfilgrastim also potentiates the effects of mature neutrophils, thus reducing fever and the risk of infection from severe neutropenia. It is pharmacologically identical to human granulocyte colony-stimulating factor.

Contraindications
Hypersensitivity to filgrastim, pegfilgrastim, or their components

Interactions
DRUGS
lithium: Increased neutrophil production

Adverse Reactions
CNS: Fever
CV: Aortitis, edema, hypotension
GI: Elevated liver enzymes, splenic rupture, splenomegaly
GU: Glomerulonephritis
HEME: Acute myeloid leukemia (patients with breast or lung cancer), capillary leak syndrome, hemoconcentration, leukocytosis, sickle cell crisis, thrombocytopenia
MS: Bone or extremity pain, myelodysplastic syndrome (patients with breast or lung cancer)

RESP: Acute respiratory distress syndrome, alveolar hemorrhage, dyspnea, hypoxia, pulmonary infiltrates

SKIN: Acute febrile neutrophilic dermatosis (Sweet's syndrome), contact dermatitis (on-body injector), cutaneous vasculitis, erythema, flushing, pruritus, rash, urticaria

Other: Anaphylaxis, angioedema, antibody formation to pegfilgrastim, application-site reactions with on-body injector (bruising, discomfort, erythema, hemorrhage, pain), elevated uric acid level, hypoalbuminemia, injection-site reactions (erythema, induration, pain)

Childbearing Considerations

PREGNANCY

- It is not known if drug can cause fetal harm.
- Use with caution only if benefit to mother outweighs potential risk to fetus.

LACTATION

- It is not known if drug is present in breast milk.
- Patient should check with prescriber before breastfeeding.

Nursing Considerations

- Check CBC, hematocrit, and platelet count before and periodically during therapy.

! WARNING Monitor patient for signs of hypersensitivity. If signs of allergy occur, notify prescriber at once. If anaphylaxis occurs, give antihistamine, bronchodilator, corticosteroid, and epinephrine, as ordered. Be aware that the on-body injector of Neulasta may cause application-site and local skin reactions, including contact dermatitis.

! WARNING Be aware that patients receiving filgrastim (parent drug) have had splenic rupture and acute respiratory distress syndrome, which may be life-threatening. Assess patient for fever, respiratory distress, and upper abdominal or shoulder tip pain and notify prescriber immediately, if present.

- Monitor patient's renal function, as ordered, because drug may cause glomerulonephritis. If renal dysfunction is suspected, notify prescriber and, if confirmed, expect drug to be withheld or dosage reduced.
- Monitor patient's platelet counts because of risk for thrombocytopenia.

- Monitor patient for signs and symptoms of aortitis such as abdominal pain, back pain, fever, increased inflammatory markers (C-reactive protein, white blood cell count), or malaise, as drug will have to be discontinued. Know that aortitis may occur as early as the first week after therapy is begun.
- Be aware that transient positive bone imaging changes may occur because of increased hematopoietic activity of the bone marrow in response to pegfilgrastim therapy.
- Assess patients with sickle cell disease for signs of sickle cell crisis; urge hydration. Know that drug should be discontinued if sickle cell crisis occurs.
- Give nonopioid and opioid analgesics, as ordered, if patient experiences bone pain.

! WARNING Monitor patient for edema and hypotension that may indicate development of capillary leak syndrome. If present, notify prescriber and be prepared to provide supportive care, as ordered. Be aware that the on-body injector of Neulasta may cause application-site and local skin reactions, including contact dermatitis.

PATIENT TEACHING

- Teach patient who will self-administer drug how to prepare, give, and store drug. However, alert patient that the on-body injector for drug uses acrylic adhesive, which can cause a significant reaction to those allergic to acrylic adhesive.
- Alert patient that needle cover contains dry natural rubber (Lapelga, Neulasta, and Ziextenzo) and should not be handled if she has a latex allergy.
- Tell patient to rotate injection sites among abdomen (except for 2 inches around navel), buttocks, outer upper arms, and thighs. Caution her to avoid bruised, hard, red, or tender areas.
- Urge patient to discard used needles and syringes in a puncture-resistant container and not to reuse them.
- Alert patient that missed or partial doses have been reported with the on-body injector Neulasta due to potential device failure. Also tell patient not to reapply the on-body injector Neulasta if it comes off before the full dose is delivered. Instruct

P

patient to notify prescriber immediately if the on-body injector Neulasta has come off or she suspects that the device may not have performed as intended, to get instructions on a possible replacement dose. Warn patient to avoid bumping the on-body injector Neulasta or knocking it off her body. Tell her she should not use additional materials to hold the on-body injector Neulasta in place, as this could dislodge the cannula and lead to a missed or incomplete dose.

- Tell patient to call prescriber immediately if the status light on the on-body injector Neulasta is flashing red. Also tell her not to remove the on-body injector Neulasta until the green light shines continuously. Tell patient to inform all healthcare workers of the presence of the on-body injector Neulasta, as it should not be exposed to medical imaging studies (CT scan, MRI, ultrasound, or X-ray), oxygen-rich environments, or radiation treatment.
- Remind patient not to use on-body injector Neulasta in the bathtub, hot tubs, saunas, or whirlpools and not to expose it to direct sunlight, as these may affect drug. Tell patient to avoid sleeping on the on-body injector Neulasta or getting cleaning agents, creams, lotions, or oils near the injector, as these products may loosen the adhesive.
- Advise patient to have a caregiver nearby when he administers the first dose and to avoid driving or operating heavy machinery during hours 26 to 29 following application of the on-body injector Neulasta.
- Warn patient to keep the on-body injector Neulasta at least 4 inches away from electrical equipment such as cell phones, cordless telephones, microwaves, and other common appliances, because of possible interference with its function.

! **WARNING** Alert patient that drug may cause serious allergic reactions. Tell patient to notify prescriber, if present, and to seek immediate emergency medical care, if severe.

- Urge patient to report promptly any potentially serious reactions (breathing difficulty, chest tightness, left upper abdominal pain, rash, shoulder tip pain) and evidence of infection (chills, fever).
- Emphasize the importance of follow-up tests.

- Advise patient to store pegfilgrastim in refrigerator and not to freeze it. Tell her to discard drug if left unrefrigerated for time frame specified for product being used.

penicillin G benzathine
Bicillin L-A

penicillin G potassium
Pfizerpen

penicillin G procaine

penicillin G sodium

penicillin V potassium
Penicillin-VK

≣ Class and Category
Pharmacologic class: Penicillin
Therapeutic class: Antibiotic

≣ Indications and Dosages
* *To treat systemic infections caused by gram-positive organisms (including* Bacillus anthracis, Corynebacterium diphtheriae, *enterococci,* Listeria monocytogenes, Staphylococcus aureus, *and* S. epidermidis), *gram-negative organisms (including* Neisseria gonorrhoeae, N. meningitidis, Pasteurella multocida, *and* Streptobacillus moniliformis [*rat-bite fever*]), *and gram-positive anaerobes (including* Actinomyces israelii [*actinomycosis*], Clostridium perfringens, C. tetani, Peptococcus *species,* Peptostreptococcus *species, and spirochetes, especially* Treponema carateum [*pinta*], T. pallidum, *and* T. pertenue [*yaws*])*

I.V. INFUSION, I.M. INJECTION (PENICILLIN G POTASSIUM, PENICILLIN G SODIUM)
Adults and children. Highly individualized based on type and severity of infection.

Dosage ranges from 1 to 24 million units daily in divided doses usually every 4 to 6 hr, although some infections may require divided dosing every 2 hr.

I.M. INJECTION (PENICILLIN G PROCAINE)

Adults and adolescents. Highly individualized based on severity and type of infection. Dosages range from 300,000 to 1,200,000 units daily and may be given in divided doses every 12 hr in some infections.

✱ *To treat Group A streptococcal respiratory infections*

I.M. INJECTION (PENICILLIN G BENZATHINE)

Adults and children weighing more than 45 kg (100 lb). 1.2 million units as a single injection.
Children weighing 27 to 45 kg (59 to 100 lb). 900,000 units as a single injection.
Infants and children weighing less than 27 kg (59 lb). 300,000 to 600,000 units as single injection.

✱ *To treat congenital syphilis*

I.M. INJECTION (PENICILLIN G BENZATHINE)

Children ages 2 to 12. Dosage adjusted based on adult dosing schedule.
Children under age 2. 50,000 units/kg as a single injection. *Maximum:* 2.4 million units/dose.

✱ *To treat primary, secondary, or latent syphilis*

I.M. INJECTION (PENICILLIN G BENZATHINE)

Adults. 2.4 million units as a single injection.

✱ *To treat late (neurosyphilis or tertiary) syphilis*

I.M. INJECTION (PENICILLIN G BENZATHINE)

Adults. 2.4 million units every wk for 3 wk.

✱ *To provide prophylaxis for glomerulonephritis and rheumatic fever*

I.M. INJECTION (PENICILLIN G BENZATHINE)

Adults. 1.2 million units once a month or 600,000 units every 2 wk following an acute attack.

✱ *To treat bejel, pinta, and yaws caused by susceptible organisms*

I.M. INJECTION (PENICILLIN G BENZATHINE)

Adults. 1.2 million units as a single injection.

✱ *To treat mild to moderate severe upper respiratory tract streptococcal infections, including erysipelas and scarlet fever*

ORAL SOLUTION, TABLETS (PENICILLIN V POTASSIUM)

Adults and adolescents. 125 to 250 mg (200,000 to 400,000 units) every 6 to 8 hr for 10 days.

✱ *To treat mild to moderate pneumococcal infections, mild skin and soft tissue staphylococcal infections, mild to moderate staphylococcal (Vincent's) infection of the oropharynx*

ORAL SOLUTION, TABLETS (PENICILLIN V POTASSIUM)

Adults and adolescents. 250 to 500 mg (400,000 to 800,000 units) every 6 to 8 hr.

✱ *To prevent recurrence following chorea and/or rheumatic fever*

ORAL SOLUTION, TABLETS (PENICILLIN V POTASSIUM)

Adults. 125 mg to 250 mg (200,000 to 400,000 units) twice daily on a continuing basis.

±**DOSAGE ADJUSTMENT** For uremic patient receiving penicillin G potassium or penicillin G sodium with creatinine clearance greater than 10 ml/min, full loading dose given followed by one-half of the loading dose every 4 to 5 hr. For patient receiving penicillin G potassium or penicillin G sodium with creatinine clearance of less than 10 ml/min, full loading dose given followed by one-half of the loading dose every 8 to 10 hr.

Drug Administration

P.O.

- Administer with a full glass of water on an empty stomach at least an hour before or 2 hours after eating.
- Reconstitute oral solution by tapping bottle until all powder flows freely. Slowly add 75 ml for 100-ml bottle size or 150 ml for a 200-ml bottle size by first partially filling bottle; replace cap and shake vigorously. Then add remaining water and shake again. Solution will be red in color.
- Shake oral solution container well before using.
- Use calibrated device to measure dosage when using oral solution.
- Store oral solution in refrigerator. Discard after 14 days.

P

I.V.

- Only penicillin G potassium or penicillin G sodium is administered intravenously.
- Do not administer penicillin G potassium to children requiring less than 1 million units per dose.
- Drug may come as a premixed solution or in powder form requiring reconstitution and further dilution.
- If reconstituting drug, use 0.9% Sodium Chloride Injection, 5% Dextrose in Water (penicillin G sodium only), or Sterile Water for Injection.
- Dilute by first loosening powder in vial. Then hold vial horizontally and rotate it while slowly directing the stream of diluent (amount of diluent to use is dependent on dose; see manufacturer guidelines) against the wall of vial. Shake vial vigorously after all the diluent has been added.
- To make a continuous intravenous drip using penicillin G potassium, determine the volume of fluid and rate of its administration required by patient in a 24-hour period in the usual manner for fluid therapy. Then add the appropriate daily dosage of diluted penicillin to this fluid. For example, if adult patient requires 2 liters of fluid over 24 hours and a daily dosage of 10 million units of penicillin, add 5 million units to each liter and adjust flow rate to infuse each liter over 12 hours.
- Administer penicillin at least 1 hour before other antibiotics.
- Administer intermittent I.V. infusion over 1 to 2 hr in adults and over 15 to 30 min in children or as a continuous infusion using penicillin G potassium, as ordered.
- Store penicillin G sodium in refrigerator for 7 days and penicillin G potassium for 3 days.
- *Incompatibilities:* Carbohydrate solutions at alkaline pH for penicillin G potassium; none listed by manufacturer for penicillin G sodium

I.M.

- Reconstitute using same technique as for intravenous solution except volume of diluent will be small; see manufacturer guidelines.
- Inject deep into large muscle mass such as the upper, outer quadrant of the dorsogluteal or the ventrogluteal site. In neonates, infants, and small children, the midlateral aspect of the thigh is usually preferred.
- Apply ice to relieve pain.
- Give penicillin G benzathine and penicillin G procaine only by deep I.M. injection; I.V. injection may be fatal, and intra-arterial injection may cause extensive organ and tissue necrosis. Also, injection of any penicillin into or near a nerve may result in permanent neurological damage.

Route	Onset	Peak	Duration
P.O.	Unknown	30–60 min	Unknown
I.V.	Unknown	Unknown	Unknown
I.M.	Unknown	Varies	Varies

Half-life: <1.4 hr

☰ Mechanism of Action

Inhibits final stage of bacterial cell wall synthesis by competitively binding to penicillin-binding proteins inside the cell wall. Penicillin-binding proteins are responsible for various steps in bacterial cell wall synthesis. By binding to these proteins, penicillin leads to cell wall lysis.

☰ Contraindications

Hypersensitivity to penicillin or its components

☰ Interactions

DRUGS

aspirin, ethacrynic acid, furosemide, indomethacin, phenylbutazone, probenecid, sulfonamides, thiazide diuretics: Possibly prolonged blood penicillin level
chloramphenicol, erythromycin, sulfonamides, tetracycline: Possibly interference with penicillin's bactericidal effect

☰ Adverse Reactions

CNS: Confusion, dizziness, dysphasia, hallucinations, headache, lethargy, permanent neurological damage (inadvertent intravascular administration), sciatic nerve irritation (I.M. injection), seizures
CV: Labile blood pressure, palpitations
EENT: Black "hairy" tongue, oral candidiasis, stomatitis, taste perversion
GI: Abdominal pain, diarrhea, elevated liver enzymes (transient), indigestion, nausea, pseudomembranous colitis

GU: Acute interstitial nephritis, vaginal candidiasis
MS: Muscle twitching
SKIN: Acute generalized exanthematous pustulosis, Nicolau syndrome, rash, **Stevens–Johnson syndrome, toxic epidermal necrolysis**
Other: Drug reaction with eosinophilia and systemic symptoms (DRESS); electrolyte imbalances; hypersensitivity reactions; injection-site necrosis, pain, or redness

Childbearing Considerations
PREGNANCY
- It is not known if drug causes fetal harm.
- Use with caution only if benefit to mother outweighs potential risk to fetus.

LACTATION
- Drug is present in breast milk.
- Patient should check with prescriber before breastfeeding.

Nursing Considerations
- Obtain body tissue and fluid samples for culture and sensitivity tests as ordered before giving first dose. Expect to begin drug therapy before test results are known.

! **WARNING** Monitor patient for hypersensitivity reactions that may be quite serious. If present, notify prescriber, expect drug to be discontinued, and provide appropriate supportive care.

- Assess patient for signs of secondary infection, such as profuse, watery diarrhea. If such diarrhea develops, contact prescriber and expect to obtain a stool specimen to rule out pseudomembranous colitis caused by *Clostridium difficile*. If diarrhea occurs, notify prescriber and expect to withhold penicillin and treat with electrolytes, fluids, protein, and an antibiotic effective against *C. difficile*.
- Monitor serum sodium level and assess for early signs of heart failure in patients receiving high doses of penicillin G sodium.
- When giving penicillin G potassium to patient at risk for fluid overload or hypertension, be aware that each gram of penicillin G potassium also contains 1.02 mEq of sodium.
- Monitor patient for severe cutaneous adverse reactions. If suspected, notify prescriber, and expect drug to be discontinued.

PATIENT TEACHING

! **WARNING** Instruct patient to report previous allergies to penicillins and to notify prescriber immediately about an allergic reaction.

- Tell patient to notify prescriber of any persistent, severe, or unusual adverse effects.
- Urge patient to tell prescriber if diarrhea develops, even 2 months or more after penicillin therapy ends.
- Inform patient taking penicillin V potassium oral solution that it contains phenylalanine.

phenazopyridine hydrochloride
Azo-Standard, Baridium, Phenazo (CAN), Pyridium

Class and Category
Pharmacologic class: Alpha$_1$ agonist
Therapeutic class: Urinary analgesic

Indications and Dosages
✴ *To relieve burning and pain on urination, and urinary frequency and urgency*

TABLETS
Adults. 190 to 200 mg three times after meals.

Drug Administration
P.O.
- Administer after a meal with a full glass of water.
- Drug therapy limited to 2 days when used concomitantly with an antibacterial agent for the treatment of a UTI.

Route	Onset	Peak	Duration
P.O.	55 min	112 min	Unknown

Half-life: Unknown

Mechanism of Action
Exerts a local anesthetic effect on urinary tract mucosa as drug is excreted in urine. Phenazopyridine's exact mechanism is unknown.

Contraindications
Hypersensitivity to phenazopyridine or its components, renal insufficiency

P

Interactions

DRUGS
None reported by manufacturer

Adverse Reactions
CNS: Headache
GI: Indigestion, nausea, vomiting
GU: Reddish-orange urine
SKIN: Pruritus, rash
Other: Discoloration of body fluids

Childbearing Considerations

PREGNANCY
- It is not known if drug can cause fetal harm.
- Use with caution only if benefit to mother outweighs potential risk to fetus.

LACTATION
- It is not known if drug is present in breast milk.
- Patient should check with prescriber before breastfeeding.

Nursing Considerations
- Notify prescriber if yellowish skin or sclerae develop in patient taking phenazopyridine because this may indicate drug accumulation from impaired renal excretion. Expect prescriber to discontinue drug.
- Be aware that phenazopyridine treatment should be limited to 2 days.

PATIENT TEACHING
- Instruct patient not to take drug for longer than 2 days and to notify prescriber if symptoms persist beyond that time.
- Advise patient to take drug after meals with a full glass of water.
- Inform patient that drug turns urine orange to red and may discolor other body fluids, such as tears.
- Advise patient not to wear contact lenses during therapy because they may become stained.

phentermine hydrochloride
Adipex-P, Lomaira

Class, Category, and Schedule
Chemical class: Sympathomimetic amine
Therapeutic class: Anorectic
Controlled substance schedule: IV

Indications and Dosages
✱ *Adjunct for short-term weight reduction in conjunction with behavioral modification, caloric restriction, and exercise in management of exogenous obesity in patients with an initial body mass index greater than or equal to 30 kg/m², or greater than or equal to 27 kg/m² in the presence of other risk factors such as controlled hypertension, diabetes, or hyperlipidemia*

CAPSULES, TABLETS (ADIPEX-P)
Adults. *Initial:* 18.75 to 37.5 mg once daily and then dosage adjusted to patient's need.
±**DOSAGE ADJUSTMENT** For patient with severe renal impairment (creatinine clearance between 15 to 29 ml/min), dosage reduced to 15 mg daily.

TABLETS (LOMAIRA)
Adults and adolescents age 17 and older. 8 mg three times daily.

Drug Administration

P.O.
- Adipex-P tablet may be halved as needed but should be swallowed without chewing or crushing.
- Capsules should be swallowed whole and not chewed, crushed, or opened.
- Administer Lomaira half an hour before meals. Adipex-P may be taken with or without food.
- Avoid administering in late evening, to prevent insomnia.

Route	Onset	Peak	Duration
P.O.	Unknown	3–4.4 hr	Unknown

Half-life: 20 hr

Mechanism of Action
Unknown, although thought to be related to its ability to suppress appetite.

Contraindications
Agitated states; breastfeeding; during or 14 days after MAO inhibitor therapy; glaucoma; history of cardiovascular disease such as arrhythmias, congestive heart failure, coronary artery disease, stroke, or uncontrolled hypertension; history of drug abuse; hypersensitivity to phentermine, other sympathomimetic amines, or their components; hyperthyroidism; pregnancy

Interactions

DRUGS

adrenergic neuron blocking drugs: Possibly decreased hypotensive effect of these drugs
insulin, oral hypoglycemic drugs: Possibly increased risk of hypoglycemia
MAO inhibitors: Increased risk of hypertensive crisis

ACTIVITIES

alcohol use: Possibly increased incidence of serious adverse reactions

Adverse Reactions

CNS: Dizziness, dysphoria, euphoria, headache, insomnia, overstimulation, psychosis, restlessness, tremor
CV: Hypertension, ischemic events, palpitations, **regurgitant cardiac valvular disease**, tachycardia
EENT: Dry mouth, unpleasant taste
GI: Constipation, diarrhea, other gastrointestinal disturbances
GU: Changes in libido, impotence
RESP: **Primary pulmonary hypertension**
SKIN: Urticaria
Other: Physical and psychological dependence

Childbearing Considerations

PREGNANCY

- Drug may cause fetal harm.
- Drug is contraindicated in pregnancy.

LACTATION

- It is not known if drug is present in breast milk.
- Drug is contraindicated during breastfeeding.

Nursing Considerations

- Use cautiously in patients with even mild hypertension, because drug can raise blood pressure; and in patients with diabetes who are taking insulin or oral hypoglycemic agents, as drug may enhance hypoglycemic effects.
- Use cautiously in patients with impaired renal function, especially the elderly, as phentermine is substantially excreted by the kidneys and can cause toxic effects in the presence of renal impairment.

! **WARNING** Monitor patient for anginal pain, dyspnea (most common), lower extremity edema, or syncope because a life-threatening disorder, primary pulmonary hypertension, has occurred in patients taking phentermine alone or concomitantly with dexfenfluramine or fenfluramine. If signs or symptoms develop, notify prescriber, expect drug to be discontinued, and assist with diagnostic testing to confirm presence of disorder.

- Know that serious regurgitant cardiac valvular disease has occurred in otherwise healthy patients taking phentermine alone or in combination with dexfenfluramine or fenfluramine. Regularly evaluate patient's heart sounds for presence of murmurs, especially those associated with aortic, mitral, or tricuspid valvular disease.
- Monitor patient's blood pressure regularly, as phentermine therapy may cause hypertension.
- Assess patients with diabetes who are taking insulin or oral hypoglycemic agents for signs and symptoms of hypoglycemia. If persistent or serious hypoglycemia occurs, notify prescriber and expect to adjust the antidiabetic medication dosage, as ordered.

PATIENT TEACHING

- Caution patient to take phentermine exactly as prescribed and not to increase dosage or dosage interval if tolerance to drug develops. Instead, instruct patient to notify prescriber, as drug will have to be discontinued.
- Tell patient that tablets may be halved as needed but should be swallowed without chewing or crushing. Capsules should be swallowed whole and not chewed, crushed, or opened.
- Tell patient to take drug half an hour to an hour before breakfast or 1 to 2 hours after breakfast; avoid taking in late evening, to prevent insomnia.
- Warn patient that drug is for short-term use only, as the drug may cause physical and/ or psychological dependence and can be abused for these effects.
- Inform patient that phentermine therapy is not a substitute for behavioral changes, caloric restriction, and exercise.
- Warn patient not to combine phentermine therapy with other drug products for weight loss, including herbal products, over-the-counter drugs, and prescription

P

drugs. Tell patient to inform all prescribers of phentermine use.

- Caution patient to avoid hazardous activities such as driving or operating machinery until the nervous system effects of the drug are known.
- Tell patient to keep drug out of reach of children and anyone who has a drug addiction and to take measures to prevent drug theft.
- Instruct patient to avoid drinking alcoholic beverages while taking phentermine, as serious adverse reactions may occur.
- Advise patients with diabetes who are taking medication to control their blood glucose levels to watch for low blood glucose reactions. If persistent or severe hypoglycemia occurs, instruct patient to notify prescriber, as dosage of the diabetic medication may have to be reduced. Also advise patient with high blood pressure to monitor blood pressure regularly.

! **WARNING** Instruct patient to discontinue phentermine therapy and notify prescriber if chest pain, decrease in exercise tolerance, difficulty breathing, lower extremity swelling, or shortness of breath develop during phentermine therapy.

- Warn women of childbearing age to notify prescriber immediately if pregnancy occurs or is suspected, as drug will have to be discontinued immediately. Also inform women who are breastfeeding that breastfeeding must be avoided during phentermine therapy.

phenytoin
Dilantin-125, Dilantin Infatabs

phenytoin sodium
Dilantin, Phenytek

Class and Category
Pharmacologic class: Hydantoin derivative
Therapeutic class: Anticonvulsant

Indications and Dosages
✳ *To treat tonic–clonic or psychomotor (temporal) seizures*

CHEWABLE TABLETS, ORAL SUSPENSION (PHENYTOIN)
Adults who have received no previous treatment. *Initial:* 125 mg suspension or 100 to 125 mg tablet three times a day, adjusted every 7 to 10 days as needed and tolerated.
Children. *Initial:* 5 mg/kg daily in divided doses twice daily or three times a day, adjusted as needed and tolerated. *Maintenance:* 4 to 8 mg/kg daily in divided doses twice daily or three times daily. *Maximum for children over the age of 6:* 300 mg daily.
✳ *To treat tonic–clonic or psychomotor (temporal) seizures; to prevent and treat seizures occurring during or following neurosurgery*

EXTENDED-RELEASE CAPSULES (PHENYTOIN SODIUM)
Adults who have received no previous treatment. *Initial:* 100 mg three times daily, adjusted every 7 to 10 days as needed and tolerated by adding fourth daily dose of 100 mg or increasing to 200 mg three times daily. Alternatively, once patient is stabilized on 100 mg three times daily, dosage regimen may be changed to 300 mg once daily. *Maintenance:* 100 mg three or four times daily, 200 mg three times daily, or 300 mg once daily.
± **DOSAGE ADJUSTMENT** For hospitalized patients without hepatic or renal disease, oral loading dose of 400 mg followed in 2 hr by 300 mg, and then followed in 2 more hr by another 300 mg, for a total of 1 g.
Children. *Initial:* 5 mg/kg daily in divided doses twice daily or three times a day, adjusted as needed and tolerated. *Maintenance:* 4 to 8 mg/kg daily in divided doses twice daily or three times a day. *Maximum for children over the age of 6:* 300 mg daily.
✳ *To treat status epilepticus; to prevent or treat seizures during neurosurgery*

I.V. INFUSION (PHENYTOIN SODIUM)
Adults and adolescents. *Loading dose:* 10 to 15 mg/kg not to exceed 50 mg/min. *Maintenance:* 100 mg I.V. or P.O. every 6 to 8 hr.
Children. *Loading dose:* 15 to 20 mg/kg not to exceed 3 mg/kg/min or 50 mg/min, whichever is slower. *Maintenance:* Highly individualized I.V. or P.O. every 6 to 8 hr.

± **DOSAGE ADJUSTMENT** For elderly patients dosage reduced. For patients who are known to be intermediate or poor metabolizers of CYP2C9 substrates, dosage reduced.

Drug Administration
P.O.
- Administer with meals to minimize GI upset.
- Capsules should be swallowed whole with a glass of water and not chewed, crushed, or opened.
- Shake oral suspension container before use.
- Use a calibrated device to measure oral suspension dosage.
- Store oral suspension at room temperature.
- Chewable tablets may be chewed thoroughly before swallowing or tablet can be swallowed whole.
- Dosage adjustment will be needed if patient switches to a different oral preparation. Oral preparations are not interchangeable mg per mg.

I.V.
- Can be initiated with either a loading dose or an infusion.
- If undiluted drug is refrigerated or becomes frozen, a precipitate might form; this will dissolve again after solution is allowed to stand at room temperature. A faint yellow coloration may develop but does not alter potency of drug.
- Check patency of I.V. catheter by testing with a flush of 0.9% Sodium Chloride Injection before administration. Repeat flush after administration.
- Administer directly into a central vein or large peripheral vein through a large-gauge catheter.
- For adult loading dose, infuse undiluted slowly at no more than 50 mg/min for adults (will take about 20 minutes for a 70-kg [150-lb] patient); for pediatric loading dose, infuse undiluted slowly at a rate not exceeding 3 mg/kg/min or 50 mg/min, whichever is slower.
- To prepare infusion, dilute drug in 0.9% Sodium Chloride Injection to a final concentration of no less than 5 mg/ml. Do not refrigerate diluted solution but administer immediately. Use an in-line filter (0.22 to 0.55 microns). Complete infusion within 1 to 4 hours.
- *Incompatibilities:* Dextrose and dextrose-containing solutions, other drugs

I.M.
- Although I.M. injection is a FDA-approved route of administration for phenytoin sodium, it is not recommended due to erratic absorption, pain on injection, and serious injection-site reactions that may occur, such as necrosis.
- A different anticonvulsant should be used in place of using I.M. phenytoin sodium.

Route	Onset	Peak	Duration
P.O.	Unknown	1.5–3 hr	Unknown
P.O./E.R.	Unknown	4–12 hr	Unknown
I.V.	10–60 min	1–2 hr	Unknown

Half-life: 7–42 hr

Mechanism of Action
Limits the spread of seizure activity and the start of new seizures by regulating voltage-dependent calcium and sodium channels in neurons, inhibiting calcium movement across neuronal membranes, and enhancing sodium-potassium ATP activity in neurons and glial cells. These actions all help stabilize the neurons.

Contraindications
For all forms: Concurrent use with delavirdine or nonnucleoside reverse transcriptase inhibitors; history of prior acute hepatoxicity attributed to phenytoin; hypersensitivity to phenytoin, other hydantoins, or their components; *For I.V. form:* Adams–Stokes syndrome, second- and third-degree A-V block, sinoatrial block, sinus bradycardia

Interactions
DRUGS
albendazole, anticoagulants (apixaban, dabigatran, edoxaban, rivaroxaban), antiepileptics (carbamazepine, felbamate, lamotrigine, oxcarbazepine, topiramate), antilipidemic agents (atorvastatin, fluvastatin, simvastatin), antiplatelets (ticagrelor), antiviral agents (efavirenz, fosamprenavir when given alone, indinavir, lopinavir/ ritonavir, nelfinavir, ritonavir, saquinavir), calcium channel blockers (nifedipine, nimodipine, verapamil), chlorpropamide, clozapine, cyclosporine, digoxin, disopyramide, folic acid, methadone, mexiletine, praziquantel, quetiapine: Decreased blood levels of these drugs by phenytoin

P

amiodarone, antidepressants (fluoxetine, fluvoxamine, sertraline), antiepileptic drugs (ethosuximide, felbamate, oxcarbazepine, topiramate), antineoplastic agents (capecitabine, fluorouracil), azoles (fluconazole, ketoconazole, itraconazole, miconazole, voriconazole), chloramphenicol, chlordiazepoxide, disulfiram, estrogen, fluvastatin, gastric acid reducing agents (H2 antagonist such as cimetidine, omeprazole), isoniazid, methylphenidate, phenothiazines, salicylates, sulfonamides (sulfadiazine, sulfamethizole, sulfamethoxazole-trimethoprim, sulfaphenazole), ticlopidine, tolbutamide, trazodone, warfarin: Possibly increased phenytoin serum levels
antiepileptics (carbamazepine, vigabatrin), antineoplastic agents usually in combination (bleomycin, carboplatin, cisplatin, doxorubicin, methotrexate), antiviral agents (fosamprenavir, nelfinavir, ritonavir), diazepam, diazoxide, folic acid, reserpine, rifampin, St. John's wort, theophylline: Possibly decreased phenytoin serum levels
antiepileptics (phenobarbital, valproate sodium, valproic acid): Possibly decreased or increased phenytoin serum levels
azoles (fluconazole, ketoconazole, itraconazole, posaconazole, voriconazole), antineoplastic agents (irinotecan, paclitaxel, teniposide), corticosteroids, delavirdine, doxycycline, estrogens, furosemide, neuromuscular blocking agents (cisatracurium, pancuronium, rocuronium, vecuronium), oral contraceptives, paroxetine, quinidine, rifampin, sertraline, theophylline, vitamin D, warfarin: Decreased effectiveness of these drugs by phenytoin
valproate: Increased risk of valproate-associated hyperammonemia

ACTIVITIES

alcohol use: Additive CNS depression, increased blood phenytoin levels with acute alcohol use; decreased blood phenytoin levels with chronic alcohol use

Adverse Reactions

CNS: Ataxia, cerebellar atrophy, confusion, depression, dizziness, drowsiness, excitement, fever, headache, involuntary motor activity, lethargy, nervousness, peripheral neuropathy, phenytoin-induced dyskinesias, restlessness, slurred speech, **suicidal ideation**, tremor, vertigo, weakness

CV: Bradycardia, **cardiac arrest**, **hypotension**, periarteritis nodosa, polyarteritis, vasculitis
EENT: Amblyopia, conjunctivitis, diplopia, earache, epistaxis, eye pain, gingival hyperplasia, hearing loss, loss of taste, nystagmus, pharyngitis, photophobia, rhinitis, sinusitis, taste perversion, tinnitus
ENDO: Gynecomastia, hyperglycemia
GI: Abdominal pain, **acute hepatic failure**, anorexia, constipation, diarrhea, epigastric pain, jaundice, hepatic dysfunction, **hepatic necrosis**, **hepatitis**, nausea, vomiting
GU: Glycosuria, Peyronie's disease, priapism, **renal failure**
HEME: Acute intermittent porphyria (exacerbation), **agranulocytosis**, anemia, eosinophilia, **granulocytopenia**, **leukopenia**, **pancytopenia**, **thrombocytopenia**
MS: Arthralgia, arthropathy, bone fractures, decreased bone mineral density, muscle twitching, osteomalacia, polymyositis
RESP: **Apnea**, **asthma**, bronchitis, cough, dyspnea, **hypoxia**, increased sputum production, pneumonia, **pneumothorax**, **pulmonary fibrosis**
SKIN: Acute generalized exanthematous pustulosis, bullous dermatitis, **exfoliative dermatitis**, maculopapular or morbilliform rash, purpuric dermatitis, **Stevens–Johnson syndrome**, **toxic epidermal necrolysis**, unusual hair growth, urticaria
Other: **Angioedema**, **drug reaction with eosinophilia and systemic symptoms (DRESS)**, facial feature coarsening or enlargement, immunoglobulin abnormalities, injection-site pain, lupus-like symptoms, lymphadenopathy, porphyria, weight gain or loss

Childbearing Considerations

PREGNANCY

- Pregnancy exposure registry: 1-888-233-2334 or http://www.aedpregnancyregistry.org/.

- Drug may cause fetal harm such as congenital malformations, adverse developmental outcomes, and less common malignancies, including neuroblastoma in children whose mothers received phenytoin during pregnancy.

- Be aware that a potentially life-threatening bleeding disorder may occur in newborns exposed to drug in utero but can be prevented with vitamin K administration to the mother before delivery and to the neonate after birth.

- Use with caution only if absolutely necessary and benefit to mother outweighs potential risk to fetus.
- Be aware that decreased serum concentrations of drug may occur during pregnancy requiring frequent monitoring of drug levels in mother throughout the pregnancy.

LACTATION

- Drug is present in breast milk.
- Patient should check with prescriber before breastfeeding.

REPRODUCTION

- Women of childbearing age using an oral contraceptive should use an additional or alternative nonhormonal contraceptive during drug therapy.

Nursing Considerations

! **WARNING** Know that patients of Asian ancestry who have the genetic allelic variant HLA-B 1502 or are CYP2C9*3 carriers can develop serious and sometimes fatal dermatologic reactions 10 times more often than people without these genetic variants. Phenytoin shouldn't be used as a substitute for carbamazepine in these patients.

- Continuously monitor blood pressure and ECG tracings when administering I.V. phenytoin. Be aware that bradycardia and cardiac arrest have occurred in patients receiving recommended dosages, in addition to patients experiencing phenytoin toxicity. Most cases of cardiac arrest occurred in patients with underlying cardiac disease.
- Frequently assess I.V. site for signs of extravasation because drug can cause tissue necrosis.

! **WARNING** Monitor patient closely for hypersensitivity to phenytoin therapy. Know that angioedema may occur. If patient develops facial, perioral, or upper airway swelling, drug should be discontinued immediately and supportive emergency care provided.

- Expect continuous enteral feedings to disrupt phenytoin absorption and,

possibly, reduce blood phenytoin level. Discontinue tube feedings 1 to 2 hours before and after phenytoin administration, as prescribed. Anticipate giving increased phenytoin doses to compensate for reduced bioavailability during continuous tube feedings.

- Monitor phenytoin level. Therapeutic level ranges from 10 to 20 mcg/L. Expect to monitor phenytoin serum levels based on the unbound fraction in patients with hepatic or renal disease or those with hypoalbuminemia because the fraction of unbound phenytoin is increased in these patients.
- Monitor patient closely for above therapeutic levels because high serum levels that are sustained may cause cerebellar atrophy (rare), delirium, encephalopathy, irreversible cerebellar dysfunction, or psychosis. Expect to obtain serum levels if early signs of dose-related CNS toxicity develops in any patient because some patients may be slow metabolizers of phenytoin. If above therapeutic range levels are found, expect phenytoin dosage to be reduced. If symptoms persist, expect drug to be discontinued.

! **WARNING** Monitor patient's hematologic status during therapy because phenytoin can cause blood dyscrasias. A patient with a history of agranulocytosis, leukopenia, or pancytopenia may have an increased risk of infection because phenytoin can cause myelosuppression.

- Anticipate that drug may worsen intermittent porphyria.

! **WARNING** Monitor patient for serious skin reactions. Onset usually occurs within 28 days but can occur later. Notify prescriber at the first sign of rash and expect phenytoin to be discontinued, unless rash is clearly not drug related. Also, expect patient with rash to be evaluated for severe cutaneous adverse reactions, which can be fatal.

- Frequently monitor blood glucose level of patient with diabetes mellitus because drug can stimulate glucagon secretion and impair insulin secretion, either of which can raise blood glucose level.
- Monitor thyroid hormone levels in patient receiving thyroid replacement

therapy because phenytoin may decrease circulating thyroid hormone levels and increase thyroid-stimulating hormone level. Also know that drug may decrease dexamethasone or metyrapone test results or increase serum levels of alkaline phosphatase, gamma glutamyl transpeptidase (GGT), or glucose.

- Be aware that long-term phenytoin therapy may increase patient's requirements for folic acid or vitamin D supplements. However, keep in mind that a diet high in folic acid may decrease seizure control.
- Monitor patient closely for evidence of suicidal thinking or behavior, especially when therapy starts or dosage changes.
- Know that phenytoin should not be stopped abruptly, as status epilepticus may occur. Instead, expect drug to be discontinued gradually.

PATIENT TEACHING

- Advise patient to take drug exactly as prescribed; she should not change brands, dosage, or stop taking drug unless instructed by prescriber.
- Instruct patients to use an accurately calibrated measuring device when using suspension form. Remind patient that a household teaspoon or tablespoon is not such a device.
- Tell patient to shake suspension bottle well before measuring dose. Suspension may be stored at room temperature.
- Tell patient chewable tablets may be chewed thoroughly before swallowing or may be swallowed whole.
- Instruct patient that capsules should be swallowed whole with a glass of water and not chewed, crushed, or opened.
- Advise patient to take drug with meals to minimize stomach upset.
- Tell patient to report any signs of heart dysfunction such as dizziness, feeling heart skipping beats, slow pulse, or tiredness.

! **WARNING** Instruct patient to stop taking phenytoin immediately and seek emergency help if signs of facial, perioral, or upper airway swelling occurs.

- Urge patient to avoid alcohol during therapy.
- Caution patient to avoid hazardous activities until drug's CNS effects are known.

- Inform patient with diabetes mellitus about the increased risk of hyperglycemia and the possible need for increased antidiabetic drug dosage during therapy. Advise her to check blood glucose level often.
- Emphasize the importance of good oral hygiene, and encourage patient to inform her dentist that she's taking phenytoin.
- Encourage patient to wear medical identification that indicates her diagnosis and drug therapy.
- Urge caregivers to watch patient closely for evidence of suicidal tendencies, especially when therapy starts or dosage changes, and to report concerns at once to prescriber.

! **WARNING** Instruct patient to notify prescriber at the first sign of a rash or if persistent, severe, or other unusual skin reactions occur.

- Inform women of childbearing age to notify prescriber immediately if pregnancy is suspected or occurs, as phenytoin may cause fetal harm. Instruct patients using a hormonal contraceptive to use an additional or alternative nonhormonal contraceptive during drug therapy.

pimavanserin
Nuplazid

☰ Class and Category
Pharmacologic class: Serotonin 5-HT receptor inverse agonist and antagonist
Therapeutic class: Atypical antipsychotic

☰ Indications and Dosages
✳ *To treat delusions and hallucinations associated with Parkinson's disease psychosis*

CAPSULES, TABLETS
Adults. 34 mg (two 17-mg tablets) once daily.
±**DOSAGE ADJUSTMENT** For patients taking strong CYP3A4 inhibitors such as ketoconazole concurrently, dosage reduced to 10 mg once daily.

☰ Drug Administration
P.O.
- Capsules may be swallowed whole or opened and contents sprinkled over

a tablespoon of applesauce, pudding, yogurt, or a liquid nutritional supplement. Administer immediately and warn patient not to chew it before swallowing.

Route	Onset	Peak	Duration
P.O.	Unknown	6 hr	Unknown

Half-life: 57 hr

Mechanism of Action

Precise mechanism is unknown, but possibly mediates through a combination of inverse agonist and antagonist activity at serotonin 5-HT2A receptors and to a lesser extent at serotonin 5-HT2C receptors to eradicate delusions and hallucinations associated with Parkinson's disease psychosis.

Contraindications

Hypersensitivity to pimavanserin or its components

Interactions

DRUGS

antibiotics such as gatifloxacin, moxifloxacin; antipsychotics such as chlorpromazine, thioridazine, ziprasidone; class 1A antiarrhythmics such as disopyramide, procainamide, quinidine; class 3 antiarrhythmics such as amiodarone, sotalol: Possible prolonged QT interval, increasing risk of cardiac arrhythmias
carbamazepine, efavirenz, modafinil, nafcillin, phenytoin, rifampin, St. John's wort, thioridazine: Possibly reduced pimavanserin exposure, resulting in decreased effectiveness
clarithromycin, itraconazole, ketoconazole, indinavir: Increased pimavanserin exposure, leading to possible adverse reactions

Adverse Reactions

CNS: Aggression, agitation, confusion, fatigue, gait disturbance, hallucination, somnolence
CV: Peripheral edema, **QT prolongation interval**
EENT: Circumoral edema, **throat tightness, tongue swelling**
GI: Constipation, nausea
GU: UTI
RESP: Dyspnea
SKIN: Rash, urticaria
Other: Angioedema

Childbearing Considerations

PREGNANCY

- It is not known if drug can cause fetal harm.
- Use with caution only if benefit to mother outweighs potential risk to fetus.

LACTATION

- It is not known if drug is present in breast milk.
- Patient should check with prescriber before breastfeeding.

Nursing Considerations

- Keep in mind that pimavanserin shouldn't be used to treat dementia-related psychosis in the elderly, because of an increased mortality risk.
- Know that pimavanserin therapy should be avoided in patients with a history of cardiac arrhythmias, known QT prolongation, or in combination with other drugs known to prolong the QT interval. Drug should also not be used in patients who are at risk for hypokalemia or hypomagnesemia or in the presence of congenital prolongation of the QT interval or symptomatic bradycardia. Monitor patient's EKG regularly for evidence of QT prolongation.
- Use cautiously in patients with renal impairment, including severe impairment and end-stage renal disease.

! WARNING Monitor patient for evidence of a hypersensitivity reaction that could include angioedema, rash, or urticaria. If present, notify prescriber, expect drug to be discontinued, and provide supportive care, as needed and prescribed.

PATIENT TEACHING

- Tell patient capsules may be swallowed whole or opened and contents sprinkled over a tablespoon of applesauce, pudding, yogurt, or a liquid nutritional supplement. Swallow immediately without chewing.

! WARNING Tell patient or family to stop pimavanserin therapy and notify prescriber if an allergic reaction occurs. If reaction is severe, urge patient to seek immediate emergency medical care.

- Instruct patient or family to alert all prescribers to pimavanserin therapy and not to take any over-the-counter drugs (including herbal preparations) without prescriber knowledge.

P

pioglitazone hydrochloride

Actos

Class and Category

Pharmacologic class: Thiazolidinedione
Therapeutic class: Antidiabetic

Indications and Dosages

* To achieve glucose control in type 2 diabetes
mellitus as monotherapy or in combination
with insulin, metformin, or a sulfonylurea

TABLETS

Adults. *Initial:* 15 or 30 mg daily, increased as
needed to maximum dose.
Maximum: 45 mg daily.

± DOSAGE ADJUSTMENT For patients with
congestive heart failure, starting dose is
15 mg once daily. For patients receiving
concomitant gemfibrozil or other strong
CYP2C8 inhibitors, maximum dose should
not exceed 15 mg once daily. For patients
taking insulin, insulin dosage decreased by
10% to 25%, as prescribed, once glucose level
reaches 100 mg/dl or less. If hypoglycemia
occurs, dosage of any concurrent antidiabetic
reduced, as prescribed.

Drug Administration

P.O.

- Drug may be given at any time of day but
consistently at the same time of day.

Route	Onset	Peak	Duration
P.O.	30 min	2 hr	24 hr

Half-life: 3–7 hr

Mechanism of Action

Decreases insulin resistance by enhancing
the sensitivity of insulin-dependent tissues,
such as adipose tissue, the liver, and skeletal
muscle, and reduces glucose output from the
liver. Drug activates peroxisome proliferator-
activated receptor-gamma (PPARg)
receptors, which modulate transcription
of insulin-responsive genes involved in
glucose control and lipid metabolism. In this
way, pioglitazone reduces hyperglycemia,
hyperinsulinemia, and hypertriglyceridemia
in patients with type 2 diabetes mellitus
and insulin resistance. However, to work

effectively, pioglitazone needs endogenous
insulin. Unlike sulfonylureas, it doesn't
increase pancreatic insulin secretion.

Contraindications

Hypersensitivity to pioglitazone or its
components, New York Heart Association
(NYHA) Class III or IV heart failure

Interactions

DRUGS

*gemfibrozil and other strong CYP2C8
inhibitors:* Increased pioglitazone effect
insulin, oral antidiabetic agents: Possibly
increased risk of hypoglycemia
ketoconazole: Possibly decreased metabolism
of pioglitazone
rifampin or other CYP2C8 inducers: Possibly
altered glucose control
topiramate: Decreased exposure of
pioglitazone and its active metabolites

Adverse Reactions

CNS: Headache
CV: Congestive heart failure, edema
EENT: Blurred vision, decreased visual
acuity, macular edema, pharyngitis, sinusitis,
tooth disorders
GI: Elevated liver enzymes, jaundice
HEME: Decreased hemoglobin level and
hematocrit
MS: Fractures, myalgia
RESP: Upper respiratory tract infection
Other: Weight gain

Childbearing Considerations

PREGNANCY

- It is not known if drug can cause fetal harm.
- Use with caution only if benefit to mother
outweighs potential risk to fetus.

LACTATION

- It is not known if drug is present in breast
milk.
- Patient should check with prescriber before
breastfeeding.

REPRODUCTION

- Be aware that drug may result in ovulation
in some anovulatory women, which
increases the risk of an unintended
pregnancy.

Nursing Considerations

- Be aware that pioglitazone isn't
recommended for patients with
symptomatic heart failure. It is also not

recommended in patients with active bladder cancer because there is insufficient information regarding the drug's role in promoting bladder tumors and should only be used with extreme caution in patients with a history of bladder cancer.

- Be prepared to monitor liver enzymes before therapy begins, every 2 months during first year, and annually thereafter, as ordered, because drug is extensively metabolized in the liver. Expect to stop drug if jaundice develops or ALT values exceed 2.5 times normal.

! WARNING Monitor patient for signs and symptoms of congestive heart failure—such as edema, rapid weight gain, or shortness of breath—because pioglitazone can cause fluid retention that may lead to or worsen heart failure. Notify prescriber immediately of any deterioration in the patient's cardiac status, and expect to discontinue drug, as ordered.

- Assess for signs and symptoms of hypoglycemia, especially if patient is also taking another antidiabetic drug.
- Monitor fasting glucose level, as ordered, to evaluate effectiveness of therapy.
- Monitor glycosylated hemoglobin level to assess drug's long-term effectiveness.

PATIENT TEACHING

- Emphasize the need for patient to continue, diet control, exercise program, and weight management during pioglitazone therapy.
- Advise patient to notify prescriber immediately if she experiences fluid retention, shortness of breath, or sudden weight gain, because drug may have to be discontinued.
- Urge patient to report vision changes promptly and expect to have an eye examination by an ophthalmologist, regardless of when the last examination occurred.
- Instruct patient to keep laboratory appointments for liver enzymes, as ordered, typically every 2 months during first year of therapy and annually thereafter.
- Inform female patient that she may be at risk for fractures during pioglitazone therapy, and urge her to take safety precautions to prevent falls and other injuries.

pitavastatin calcium
Livalo

pitavastatin magnesium
Zypitamag

Class and Category

Pharmacologic class: HMG-CoA reductase inhibitor (statin)
Therapeutic class: Antilipemic

Indications and Dosages

✳ *As adjunct to diet in patients with primary hyperlipidemia or mixed dyslipidemia*

TABLETS (LIVALO, ZYPITAMAG)

Adults. *Initial:* 2 mg once daily, increased as needed. *Maximum:* 4 mg once daily

±**DOSAGE ADJUSTMENT** For patients with moderate to severe renal impairment (glomerular filtration rate 30 to 59 ml/min) or patients receiving dialysis, initial dosage reduced to 1 mg once daily, with maximum of 2 mg once daily. For patients taking erythromycin, dosage shouldn't exceed 1 mg daily; for patients taking rifampin, dosage shouldn't exceed 2 mg daily.

✳ *To treat heterozygous familial hypercholesterolemia to reduce total cholesterol, low-density lipoprotein cholesterol, and apolipoprotein B*

TABLETS (LIVALO)

Children age 8 years and older. *Initial:* 2 mg once daily. *Maximum:* 4 mg once daily.

Drug Administration

P.O.

- Administer drug at any time of day but be consistent.

Route	Onset	Peak	Duration
P.O.	Unknown	1 hr	Unknown
Half-life: 12 hr			

Mechanism of Action

Reduces plasma cholesterol and lipoprotein levels by inhibiting cholesterol and HMG-CoA reductase synthesis in the liver. Consequently, number of LDL receptors on liver cells

P

increases, and LDL uptake and breakdown are enhanced. With sustained inhibition of cholesterol synthesis in the liver, levels of very low-density lipoproteins are decreased.

Contraindications

Active liver disease (including unexplained persistent hepatic transaminase elevation), breastfeeding, concurrent cyclosporine therapy, hypersensitivity to pitavastatin or its components, pregnancy

Interactions

DRUGS

colchicine, fibrates such as gemfibrozil: Increased risk of myopathy, including rhabdomyolysis

cyclosporine, erythromycin, rifampin: Increased pitavastatin exposure; increased risk of myopathy and rhabdomyolysis

niacin (1 gram or greater/day): Increased risk of adverse skeletal muscle effects

ACTIVITIES

alcohol: Increased risk of liver injury with heavy use

Adverse Reactions

CNS: Asthenia, cognitive impairment, confusion, depression, dizziness, fatigue, headache, hypoesthesia, insomnia, malaise, memory loss, peripheral neuropathy

EENT: Nasopharyngitis

ENDO: Elevated glycosylated hemoglobin level, hyperglycemia

GI: Abdominal discomfort or pain, constipation, diarrhea, dyspepsia, elevated liver enzymes, **hepatic failure, hepatitis,** jaundice, nausea

GU: **Acute renal failure,** erectile dysfunction, **myoglobinuria**

MS: Arthralgia, back or extremity pain, immune-mediated necrotizing myopathy (rare), muscle spasms, myalgia, myopathy, myositis, **rhabdomyolysis**

RESP: **Interstitial lung disease**

SKIN: Pruritus, rash, urticaria

Other: **Angioedema,** elevated creatine phosphokinase level, flu-like symptoms

Childbearing Considerations

PREGNANCY

- Drug may cause fetal harm.
- Drug is contraindicated in pregnant women and should be discontinued as soon as pregnancy is known.

LACTATION

- It is not known if drug is present in breast milk.
- Drug is contraindicated for use in women who are breastfeeding.

REPRODUCTION

- Advise females of childbearing age to use effective contraception during drug therapy.

Nursing Considerations

- Note that pravastatin, another HMG-CoA reductase inhibitor, sounds similar to pitavastatin and could be confusing. Make sure of correct drug before giving.
- Monitor liver enzymes, as ordered, before pravastatin therapy starts and as indicated during therapy. Know that patients who drink alcohol heavily and/or have a history of liver disease may be at increased risk for liver injury.
- Use pitavastatin cautiously in patients with risk factors for myopathy, such as concurrent use of colchicine, niacin-containing products (greater than 1 g daily), or fibrates and that cyclosporine is a contraindication and gemfibrozil not recommended during pitavastatin therapy. Additional risk factors include the elderly (over age 65), presence of renal impairment, or in patients who are being inadequately treated for hypothyroidism. Monitor patient throughout therapy for muscular complaints and an elevated blood creatine kinase level. Drug should be discontinued if patient's creatine kinase level becomes markedly elevated, or if myopathy is suspected or confirmed.
- Know that, although rare, immune-mediated necrotizing myopathy has been associated with statin therapy. Monitor patient for elevated serum creatine kinase levels and proximal muscle weakness, which persists despite discontinuation of the statin. Patient may need immunosuppressive therapy.
- Expect to monitor patient's lipid levels after 4 weeks of therapy to determine drug effectiveness and periodically thereafter, as ordered. Expect dosage to be adjusted if lipid levels remain elevated.
- Monitor patient's blood glucose levels and HbA1c in patients with diabetes because pitavastatin as a statin may increase blood glucose levels and alter control.

PATIENT TEACHING

- Emphasize that pitavastatin is an adjunct to, not a substitute for, a low-cholesterol diet.
- Tell patient to take drug at the same time each day to maintain its effects.
- Instruct patient to report unexplained muscle pain, tenderness, or weakness, especially if accompanied by fever or malaise.
- Advise patient to limit alcohol ingestion while taking pitavastatin because alcohol-induced liver dysfunction may be difficult to differentiate from pitavastatin-induced liver dysfunction.
- Instruct patient to consult prescriber before taking OTC niacin products because of increased risk of adverse muscle effects.
- Caution women of childbearing age that drug is contraindicated in pregnancy. If pregnancy is suspected, patient should notify prescriber immediately.
- Advise women not to breastfeed during pitavastatin therapy.
- Inform patient, especially diabetics, that pitavastatin may increase blood glucose levels and alter their control. Encourage patient to monitor their blood glucose levels closely throughout pitavastatin therapy.

plazomicin

Zemdri

≡ Class and Category

Pharmacologic class: Aminoglycoside
Therapeutic class: Antibiotic

≡ Indications and Dosages

∗ *To treat complicated urinary tract infections, including pyelonephritis, caused by* Enterobacter cloacae, Escherichia coli, Klebsiella pneumoniae, *or* Proteus mirabilis

I.V. INFUSION

Adults and adolescents age 18 and over who have a creatinine clearance greater than or equal to 90 ml/min. 15 mg/kg every 24 hr for 4 to 7 days.

±**DOSAGE ADJUSTMENT** For patient with a creatinine clearance less than 90 ml/min but equal to or greater than 60 ml/min, dosage remains at 15 mg/kg every 24 hr. For patient with a creatinine clearance less than 60 ml/min but greater than or equal to 30 ml/min, dosage reduced to 10 mg/kg every 24 hr. For

patient with a creatinine clearance less than 30 ml/min but greater than or equal to 15 ml/min, dosage reduced to 10 mg/kg and dosage interval increased to every 48 hr.

≡ Drug Administration

I.V.

- Each drug vial contains 500 mg plazomicin freebase in 10 ml Water for Injection, giving a concentration of 50 mg/ml.
- Dilute drug vial solution in 0.9% Sodium Chloride Injection or Lactated Ringer's Injection to achieve a final volume of 50 ml for intravenous infusion.
- After dilution, drug solution is stable for 24 hours at room temperature and up to 7 days if refrigerated.
- Infuse each dose over 30 minutes.
- *Incompatibilities:* Other I.V. drugs

Route	Onset	Peak	Duration
I.V.	Unknown	Unknown	Unknown

Half-life: 3.5 hr

≡ Mechanism of Action

Binds to bacterial 30S ribosomal subunit to inhibit protein synthesis, which exerts a bactericidal effect.

≡ Contraindications

Hypersensitivity to plazomicin, other aminoglycosides, or their components

≡ Interactions

DRUGS

None reported by manufacturer

≡ Adverse Reactions

CNS: Dizziness, headache, vertigo
CV: Hypertension, **hypotension**
EENT: Hearing loss, ototoxicity, tinnitus
GI: *Clostridium difficile*-associated diarrhea, constipation, diarrhea, elevated liver enzymes, gastritis, nausea, vomiting
GU: Elevated serum creatinine, hematuria, impaired renal function, **nephrotoxicity**
RESP: Dyspnea
Other: Hypersensitivity reactions, hypokalemia

≡ Childbearing Considerations

PREGNANCY

- Drug may cause fetal harm.
- Drug is not recommended during pregnancy.

P

LACTATION

- It is not known if drug is present in breast milk.
- Patient should check with prescriber before breastfeeding.

⬚ Nursing Considerations

- Expect to assess creatinine clearance in all patients prior to first dose of plazomicin and daily during therapy. For patients with renal impairment with a creatinine clearance of 15 ml/min or greater but less than 90 ml/min, expect plasma trough concentrations to be below 3 mcg/ml. Plasma trough level should be measured about 30 min before administration of second dose. If level is greater than or equal to 3 mcg/ml, expect a dosage adjustment to be made by extending the dosing interval by 1.5-fold; for example, from every 24 hours to every 36 hours or from every 48 hours to every 72 hours. Know that patients at greater risk for nephrotoxicity are the elderly, patients with existing impaired renal function, and those who are receiving concomitant nephrotoxic drugs.
- Monitor patient for hearing loss, tinnitus, and/or vertigo, because plazomicin may cause ototoxicity that may be irreversible and may not show up until after drug has been discontinued. Patients at higher risk include those with a family history of hearing loss, already have renal impairment, or are receiving higher doses and/or longer durations of therapy than recommended.

! **WARNING** Monitor patient for adverse reactions associated with neuromuscular blockade, because aminoglycosides such as plazomicin have been associated with neuromuscular blockade. Patients at high risk include patients with underlying neuromuscular disorders (including myasthenia gravis) or patients who are receiving concomitantly neuromuscular blocking drugs.

! **WARNING** Monitor patient for hypersensitivity reactions. Aminoglycosides have occasionally caused serious allergic reactions. Notify prescriber immediately and expect plazomicin to be discontinued. Provide supportive care, as ordered and needed.

- Assess patient for signs of secondary infection, such as profuse, watery diarrhea. If such diarrhea develops, contact prescriber and expect to obtain a stool specimen to rule out pseudomembranous colitis caused by *Clostridium difficile*. If diarrhea occurs, notify prescriber and expect to withhold plazomicin and treat with electrolytes, fluids, protein, and an antibiotic effective against *C. difficile*.

PATIENT TEACHING

- Tell patient that it is important to keep hydrated during plazomicin therapy, because dehydration increases the risk of kidney impairment.
- Alert patient that diarrhea is a common problem with antibacterial drugs. Tell patient that bloody or watery stools can occur even after plazomicin therapy has been discontinued. Stress importance of reporting diarrhea to prescriber.

! **WARNING** Instruct patient to report any adverse reactions that might indicate an allergic reaction (such as hives, itching, and rash), because an allergic reaction can become serious.

- Tell patient to report any changes in balance or hearing or if she experiences new onset or changes in preexisting buzzing or roaring in the ears, even after the course of plazomicin therapy has finished.
- Warn women of childbearing age to notify prescriber immediately if pregnancy is suspected or known, because aminoglycosides such as plazomicin can cause fetal harm.
- Inform patient with an underlying neuromuscular disease or patient who is receiving neuromuscular blocking agents that aggravation of muscle weakness has been reported with other aminoglycosides. Tell patient to report any muscle weakness that is abnormal for him to prescriber.

plecanatide
Trulance

⬚ Class and Category
Pharmacologic class: Guanylate cyclase-C agonist
Therapeutic class: Intestinal mobility agent

⋮ Indications and Dosages

✱ *To treat chronic idiopathic constipation or irritable bowel syndrome with constipation*

TABLETS

Adults. 3 mg once daily.

⋮ Drug Administration

P.O.

- Tablet should be swallowed whole.
- For patient who has difficulty swallowing tablets, crush tablet to a powder and mix with 1 teaspoon of room-temperature applesauce. Administer immediately. Do not store mixture for later use.
- Alternatively, drug may be administered in water by placing tablet in cup, adding 30 ml of room-temperature water, and gently swirling tablet/water mixture for at least 10 seconds. Have patient swallow entire contents of tablet/water mixture immediately. If any portion of tablet is left in the cup, add another 30 ml of room-temperature water to the cup, swirl for at least 10 seconds, and have patient swallow mixture immediately. Do not store the tablet/water mixture for later use.
- To administer drug through a gastric or nasogastric feeding tube, begin by placing tablet in a cup; then add 30 ml of room-temperature water. Gently swirl the tablet/water mixture for at least 15 seconds. Flush the feeding tube with 30 ml of water. Draw up drug mixture using the same syringe and immediately administer via the feeding tube. Do not reserve for future use. If any portion of tablet is left in the cup, add another 30 ml of room-temperature water, swirl for at least 15 seconds. Using the same syringe, administer via the feeding tube. Follow by flushing the feeding tube with at least 10 ml of water.
- Store in a dry place at room temperature, keeping desiccant in bottle.

Route	Onset	Peak	Duration
P.O.	Unknown	Unknown	Unknown

Half-life: Unknown

⋮ Mechanism of Action

Acts locally on the luminal surface of the intestinal epithelium, resulting in an increase in both extracellular and intracellular concentrations of cyclic guanosine monophosphate (cGMP). Elevation of intracellular cGMP stimulates secretion of bicarbonate and chloride into the intestinal lumen. This increases intestinal fluid and accelerates transit time, which relieves constipation.

⋮ Contraindications

Children less than 6 years of age, hypersensitivity to plecanatide or its components, known or suspected mechanical gastrointestinal obstruction.

⋮ Interactions

DRUGS

None reported by manufacturer

⋮ Adverse Reactions

CNS: Dizziness
EENT: Nasopharyngitis, sinusitis
GI: Abdominal distention or tenderness, diarrhea, flatulence, elevated liver enzymes, nausea
GU: UTI
RESP: Upper respiratory tract infection
Other: Dehydration

⋮ Childbearing Considerations

PREGNANCY

- Drug is negligibly absorbed systemically following oral administration so drug exposure to fetus is minimal. However, it is not known if drug causes fetal harm.
- Use with caution only if benefit to mother outweighs potential risk to fetus.

LACTATION

- It is not known if drug is present in breast milk.
- Patient should check with prescriber before breastfeeding.

⋮ Nursing Considerations

- Be aware that plecanatide therapy should be avoided in patients 6 years to less than 18 years of age and is contraindicated in patients who are less than 6 years of age because of the potential for serious dehydration from plecanatide use.
- Monitor patient for diarrhea, which can become severe. If severe diarrhea occurs, withhold drug. Notify prescriber and expect to follow measures to rehydrate patient, as ordered.

PATIENT TEACHING

- Caution patient not to exceed dosage, as severe dehydration may occur.

P

- Instruct patient to swallow tablet whole. If patient is unable to swallow tablet, tell patient how to mix in applesauce or room-temperature water. Warn patient to take mixture immediately and not to store for later use.
- Tell patient to store plecanatide in a dry place and protect from moisture. Also remind patient to keep drug in original bottle, with desiccant in the bottle, and not subdivide or repackage drug in any way. Instruct patient to keep bottle tightly closed when not in use.
- Tell patient to stop taking drug and notify prescriber if severe diarrhea occurs.
- Warn patient to keep plecanatide out of the reach of children, especially those who are less than 6 years of age.
- Tell patient if she misses a dose, she should skip the missed dose and take the next dose at the regular time. She should never double the dose.

ponesimod
Ponvory

⦀ Class and Category
Pharmacologic class: Sphingosine 1-phosphate receptor modulator
Therapeutic class: Immunomodulator

⦀ Indications and Dosages
✳ *To treat relapsing forms of multiple sclerosis (MS), to include active secondary progressive disease, clinically isolated syndrome, and relapsing-remitting disease*

TABLETS
Adults. *Initial:* 2 mg on days 1 and 2; 3 mg on days 3 and 4; 4 mg on days 5 and 6; 5 mg on day 7; 6 mg on day 8; 7 mg on day 9; 8 mg on day 10; 9 mg on day 11; 10 mg on days 12, 13, and 14 followed by 20 mg on day 15 and thereafter. *Maintenance:* 20 mg once a day.

⦀ Drug Administration
P.O.
- Expect to monitor patient with the following conditions for 4 hours or more after administering the first dose: presence of first- or second-degree Mobitz II AV block or sinus bradycardia with a heart rate less than 55 beats per minute or history of

heart failure or MI that has occurred more than 6 months prior to initiating drug therapy and patient is in stable condition.
- Ensure that resources are readily available to treat symptomatic bradycardia before administering first dose.
- Check that an EKG has been done before administering drug and then repeated 4 hours after first dose is administered.
- Administer tablet whole.
- Use starter pack when initiating drug therapy and follow titration schedule exactly, which helps reduce adverse cardiac reactions.
- Monitor patient for signs and symptoms of bradycardia. Assess patient's blood pressure and pulse at least hourly. Be aware that pulse rate may begin to decrease within an hour of administration but typically recovers to baseline levels 4–5 hours later.
- Additional monitoring of these patients is required if patient's heart rate postdose is less than 45 beats per minute, it is at the lowest value postdose, or the patient's 4-hour postdose EKG shows new onset of second-degree or higher AV block. If abnormalities are present, initiate continuous EKG monitoring and other appropriate treatment (may include need to monitor patient overnight or need for cardiologist consult), as ordered, until abnormalities are resolved.
- If fewer than 4 consecutive doses are missed during titration, resume treatment with the first missed titration dose and resume the titration schedule at that dose and titration day.
- If fewer than 4 consecutive doses are missed during maintenance, resume treatment with maintenance dosage.
- If 4 or more consecutive doses are missed during titration or maintenance, treatment should be reinitiated with day 1 of the titration regimen.

Route	Onset	Peak	Duration
P.O.	Unknown	2–4 hr	Unknown

Half-life: 33 hr

⦀ Mechanism of Action
Binds to sphingosine 1-phosphate (S1P) receptors to block the release of lymphocytes from lymph nodes. This action reduces the

number of lymphocytes in peripheral blood, which may involve reduction of lymphocyte migration into the central nervous system.

Contraindications

Class III or IV heart failure, decompensated heart failure requiring hospitalization, MI, transient ischemic attack (TIA), or unstable angina within the last 6 months; hypersensitivity to ponesimod or its components; presence of Mobitz type II second-degree, third-degree atrioventricular (AV) block, sick sinus syndrome, or sinoatrial block, unless a functioning pacemaker is in place

Interactions

DRUGS

antineoplastic, immune-modulating, or immunosuppressive drugs: Increased risk of additive immune effects during ponesimod therapy and for weeks following administration

beta-blockers: Additive effects on lowering heart rate

CYP3A4 (strong) and UGT1A1 inducers such as carbamazepine, phenytoin, rifampin: Possibly decreased systemic ponesimod levels, making drug less effective

live attenuated vaccines: Increased risk of infection during and for up to 2 weeks after ponesimod is discontinued

vaccinations: Decreased effectiveness of vaccinations during and for up to 2 weeks after ponesimod is discontinued

Adverse Reactions

CNS: Depression, dizziness, fatigue, fever, insomnia, migraine, **posterior reversible encephalopathy syndrome, seizures,** vertigo
CV: Atrioventricular conduction delays, bradycardia, chest discomfort, hypercholesterolemia, hypertension, peripheral edema
EENT: Dry mouth, macular edema, rhinitis, sinusitis
GI: Dyspepsia, elevated liver enzymes, **hepatic injury**
GU: UTI
MS: Back or extremity pain, joint swelling
RESP: Cough, dyspnea, increased risk of upper respiratory infection
SKIN: Cutaneous malignancies
OTHER: Immunosuppression, hyperkalemia, increased C-reactive

protein, infections (herpes zoster, viral), **lymphopenia**

Childbearing Considerations

PREGNANCY

- Drug may cause fetal harm based on animal studies.
- Use with caution only if benefit to mother outweighs potential risk to fetus.

LACTATION

- It is not known if drug is present in breast milk.
- Patient should check with prescriber before breastfeeding.

REPRODUCTION

- Women of childbearing age should use an effective contraception during drug therapy and for 1 week after drug is discontinued.

Nursing Considerations

- Ensure that the following has been assessed prior to administering the first dose of ponesimod: Cardiac evaluation (ECG and possible cardiologist consultation), complete blood count including lymphocyte count within past 6 months, liver function tests within last 6 months, drug therapy review (current or prior history of antineoplastic, immunosuppressive, or immune-modulating therapies and drugs that may slow atrioventricular conduction or heart rate), ophthalmic evaluation including the macula, presence of antibodies to varicella zoster virus if history or full course of vaccination against virus cannot be confirmed, and a detailed vaccination history.
- Be aware that live attenuated vaccine immunizations should be administered at least 1 month prior to the patient starting ponesimod therapy.
- Know that ponesimod therapy is not recommended in patients with a history of cardiac arrest, cerebrovascular disease, severe untreated sleep apnea, or uncontrolled hypertension because a serious reduction in heart rate may not be well tolerated in these patients. Also, know that ponesimod should not be initiated after treatment with alemtuzumab.
- Administer ponesimod with caution to patients who are or have received antineoplastic, immune-modulating, or immunosuppressive therapies including

P

corticosteroids, because additive immune system effects may occur predisposing patient to infection.

- Use caution when administering ponesimod to patients with severe respiratory disease such as asthma, chronic obstructive pulmonary disease, or pulmonary fibrosis because drug can adversely affect respiratory function, especially in the first month of drug therapy.
- Know that drug therapy should not be initiated in a patient with an infection until it is resolved because drug decreases peripheral lymphocyte counts by as much as 40% of baseline values.

! WARNING Monitor patient for infections throughout ponesimod therapy, as life-threatening infections such as cryptococcal meningitis, herpes simplex encephalitis, and varicella zoster meningitis have occurred with other drugs in the same class as ponesimod. Notify prescriber if signs and symptoms of an infection occur, as drug may have to be withheld until infection is resolved.

! WARNING Monitor patient for progressive multifocal leukoencephalopathy (PML), an opportunistic viral infection of the brain, which has occurred with other drugs in the same class. Notify prescriber immediately if signs and symptoms occur during drug therapy (sudden onset of altered mental status, seizures, severe headache, or visual disturbances) because delayed treatment could lead to permanent neurological damage. If confirmed, expect drug to be discontinued.

- Monitor patient for signs and symptoms of liver dysfunction such as unexplained abdominal pain, anorexia, fatigue, nausea, vomiting, or yellowing of skin or dark urine. This is because ponesimod may cause liver injury. If signs and symptoms of liver dysfunction are present, notify prescriber, expect liver function studies to be done, and, if significant liver injury is present, for drug to be discontinued.
- Assess patient's blood pressure regularly during ponesimod therapy because drug may cause hypertensive events, which could become serious.

- Assess patient's skin periodically for abnormalities because ponesimod may cause skin cancer, including melanoma, especially in patients with risk factors for skin cancer.
- Monitor patient's vision throughout drug therapy because ponesimod may cause macular edema, especially in patients with a history of diabetes mellitus or uveitis. If a change in vision occurs, notify the prescriber and expect an ophthalmic evaluation to be done.
- Expect to monitor patient even after ponesimod is discontinued. This is because severe exacerbation of MS resulting in a significant increase in disability may occur, although rarely, after the drug is discontinued.
- Be aware that ponesimod remains in the blood for up to 1 week after it is discontinued. Treatment with immunosuppressants during this time may cause additive effect on the immune system.

PATIENT TEACHING

- Instruct patient that tablet must be swallowed whole.
- Stress importance of patient following the titration schedule to reach maintenance dosing, as drug dosage may have to be reevaluated if more than 3 doses are missed.

! WARNING Alert patient that ponesimod increases risk of an infection during therapy and for up to 2 weeks after therapy is discontinued. Inform patient the most common infection is an upper respiratory infection, although other less common but more serious and possibly life-threatening infections could also occur. Know that taking immunosuppressants may increase patient's risk of infection. Review signs and symptoms of infection and tell patient to notify prescriber immediately, if present.

! WARNING Advise patient or family/caregiver to immediately notify the prescriber if patient develops a sudden onset of altered mental status, severe headache, seizure, or visual disturbances. Stress that a delay in reporting these symptoms could cause permanent neurologic deficits.

- Advise patient to avoid live, attenuated vaccines while taking ponesimod. If necessary, tell patient to alert prescriber, as ponesimod therapy will have to be withheld 1 week prior and for 4 weeks after the vaccination.

- Inform patients with first- or second-degree Mobitz type II AV block, history of a heart attack or heart failure that has occurred more than 6 months prior to initiating treatment with ponesimod, or sinus bradycardia less than 55 beats per minute that at first dose 4-hour monitoring will be required. If abnormalities develop, the monitoring may be extended and possibly include an overnight stay in a healthcare facility.
- Tell patient to notify prescriber if they experience new onset or worsening of dyspnea.
- Review signs and symptoms of hepatic dysfunction with patient and stress importance of notifying prescriber if present.
- Advise patient to assess the skin regularly. If any suspicious skin lesions appear, patient should have it assessed. Encourage patient to wear protective clothing and use a sunscreen with a high protection factor when outdoors and to avoid sunlight and ultraviolet light as much as possible.
- Alert patient that ponesimod may cause visual changes. If changes occur, patient should notify prescriber and expect to have an ophthalmic examination.
- Warn patient that severe disability, although rare, may occur when ponesimod therapy is discontinued. Tell them to report to the prescriber worsening symptoms of MS after drug has been discontinued.
- Tell patient that drug continues to have effects for up to 2 weeks after the last dose.
- Advise women of childbearing age to use an effective contraceptive during ponesimod therapy and for 1 week after drug has been discontinued. If pregnancy occurs, stress importance of notifying prescriber, as drug should not be taken during pregnancy.

posaconazole
Noxafil

▤ Class and Category
Pharmacologic class: Triazole
Therapeutic class: Antifungal

▤ Indications and Dosages

✱ *To prevent invasive Aspergillus and candida infections in patients at high risk because of severe immunocompromise from such conditions as graft-versus-host disease with hematopoietic stem-cell transplant or hematologic malignancies with prolonged neutropenia from chemotherapy*

ORAL SUSPENSION

Adults and adolescents. 200 mg (5 ml) three times a day until recovery from immunosuppression or neutropenia.

DELAYED-RELEASE ORAL SUSPENSION

Children age 2 and older who weigh between 36 kg (79.2 lb) and 40 kg (88 lb). *Loading dose:* 240 mg (8 ml) twice daily on first day. *Maintenance:* 240 mg (8 ml) once daily starting on second day.
Children age 2 and older who weigh 26 kg (57.2 lb) but less than 36 kg (79.2 lb). *Loading dose:* 210 mg (7 ml) twice daily on first day. *Maintenance:* 210 mg (7 ml) once daily starting on second day.
Children age 2 and older who weigh 21 kg (46.2 lb) but less than 26 kg (57.2 lb). *Loading dose:* 180 mg (6 ml) twice daily on first day. *Maintenance:* 180 mg (6 ml) once daily starting on second day.
Children age 2 and older who weigh 17 kg (37.4 lb) but less than 21 kg (46.2 lb). *Loading dose:* 150 mg (5 ml) twice daily on first day. *Maintenance:* 150 mg (5 ml) once daily starting on second day.
Children age 2 and older who weigh 12 kg (26.4 lb) but less than 17 kg (37.4 lb). *Loading dose:* 120 mg (4 ml) twice daily on the first day. *Maintenance:* 120 mg (4 ml) once daily starting on second day.
Children age 2 and older who weigh 10 kg (22 lb) but less than 12 kg (25.4 lb). *Loading dose:* 90 mg (3 ml) twice daily on the first day. *Maintenance:* 90 mg (3 ml) once daily starting on second day.

DELAYED-RELEASE TABLETS

Adults and children age 2 and older weighing more than 40 kg (88 lb). *Loading dose:* 300 mg twice daily on first day. *Maintenance:* 300 mg once daily starting on second day until recovery from immunosuppression or neutropenia.

I.V. INFUSION

Adults. *Loading dose:* 300 mg twice daily on first day. *Maintenance:* 300 mg once daily starting on second day until recovery from neutropenia or immunosuppression.

Children age 2 and older. *Loading dose:* 6 mg/kg up to maximum of 300 mg twice daily on first day. *Maintenance:* 6 mg/kg up to a maximum of 300 mg once daily starting on second day until recovery from immunosuppression or neutropenia.

✷ *To treat invasive aspergillosis*

DELAYED-RELEASE TABLETS, I.V. INFUSION

Adults and adolescents. *Loading dose:* 300 mg twice daily on first day. *Maintenance dose:* 300 mg once daily starting on second day for 6 to 12 wks.

✷ *To treat oropharyngeal candidiasis*

ORAL SUSPENSION

Adults and adolescents. *Initial:* 100 mg (2.5 ml) twice daily on first day, followed by 100 mg (2.5 ml) once daily for 13 days.

✷ *To treat oropharyngeal candidiasis refractory to fluconazole and/or itraconazole*

ORAL SUSPENSION

Adults and adolescents. 400 mg (10 ml) twice daily until underlying condition improves.

±**DOSAGE ADJUSTMENT** No adjustment need for oral dosing in patients with renal dysfunction. Injectable form should be avoided in patients with a creatinine clearance of less than 50 ml/min unless absolutely necessary. If serum creatinine levels increase, injectable form should be switched to oral form.

☰ Drug Administration

P.O.

- Do not interchange delayed-release tablet or oral suspension with immediate-release oral suspension because of differences in the dosing of each formulation.
- Shake immediate-release oral suspension well before administering. Use only the spoon provided in the package to measure dosage. Each dose should be administered during or immediately following (within 20 minutes) a full meal to enhance absorption. If patient cannot eat a full meal, administer drug with an acidic carbonated beverage or a liquid nutritional supplement. Rinse dosing spoon with water after each use. Store at room temperature.

- Administer delayed-release tablets with or without food. D.R. tablets should be swallowed whole and not chewed, crushed, or divided.
- Open packet of delayed-release oral suspension immediately before preparation. Remove cap from mixing liquid and push bottle adapter into the neck of bottle. Once in place, leave bottle adapter there. Remove 9 ml of mixing liquid using the provided blue syringe. Put cap back on bottle. Do not use any other solution to mix drug. Use the provided mixing cup to combine the 9 ml of liquid and entire contents of one packet of drug and mix, which will provide a final concentration of about 30 mg/ml. Stir the mixing cup vigorously for 45 seconds to mix powder and mixing liquid. The mixture should look cloudy and free of clumps when fully mixed. Administer delayed-release oral suspension with food within 1 hour. Using only the provided notched tip syringes provided by manufacturer, use the green one if dose is 3 ml or less and blue one if dose is more than 3 ml. Discard any remaining suspension. Hand wash mixing cup and reuse or use a similar mixing cup with a lid for subsequent doses. Store at room temperature.

I.V.

- Prepare drug by first removing vial from refrigerator and allowing it to warm to room temperature.
- Transfer 16.7 ml of the drug solution to an intravenous bag or bottle containing 0.45% or 0.9% Sodium Chloride Injection, 5% Dextrose in Water, 5% Dextrose Injection and 0.45% or 0.9% Sodium Chloride Injection, or 5% Dextrose Injection and 20 mEq Potassium Chloride to achieve a concentration between 1 mg/ml and 2 mg/ml. Solution should appear colorless to yellow. Variations of color within this range do not affect the quality of the drug.
- Once mixed, use immediately, or refrigerate for up to 24 hours. Discard any unused solution.
- Administer through a 0.22-micron polyethersulfone (PES) or polyvinylidene difluoride (PVD) filter using a central venous line.
- If a central venous line is not available, drug may be administered through a peripheral

venous catheter only as a single dose in advance of a central venous line being placed or to bridge the period during which a central venous line is replaced or is in use for other treatment.

- Infuse slowly over 90 minutes through a central venous line or 30 minutes through a peripheral line.
- Never administer drug by bolus injection.
- *Incompatibilities:* 4.2% Sodium Bicarbonate solution, 5% Dextrose with Lactated Ringer's solution, or Lactated Ringer's solution; drugs other than amikacin sulfate, caspofungin, ciprofloxacin, daptomycin, dobutamine hydrochloride, famotidine, filgrastim, gentamicin sulfate, hydromorphone hydrochloride, levofloxacin, lorazepam, meropenem, micafungin, morphine sulfate, norepinephrine bitartrate, potassium chloride, vancomycin hydrochloride

Route	Onset	Peak	Duration
P.O.	Unknown	3–5 hr	Unknown
I.V.	Unknown	1.5 hr	Unknown

Half-life: 24.5–35 hr

≣ Mechanism of Action

Blocks synthesis of ergosterol, an essential component of fungal cell membrane, by inhibiting 14 alpha-demethylase, an enzyme needed for conversion of lanosterol to ergosterol. Lack of ergosterol increases cellular permeability with cell contents leaking leak, making cells ineffective.

≣ Contraindications

Concurrent therapy with atorvastatin, lovastatin, simvastatin, sirolimus; concurrent therapy with venetoclax in patients with chronic lymphocytic leukemia or small lymphocytic lymphoma; hypersensitivity to posaconazole, its components, or other azole antifungals; use with ergot alkaloids or CYP3A4 substrates such as pimozide and quinidine; use of delayed-release oral suspension in patients with hereditary fructose intolerance

≣ Interactions

DRUGS

alprazolam, midazolam, triazolam: Increased plasma levels of these drugs which could potentiate and prolong hypnotic and sedative effects

calcium channel blockers (diltiazem, felodipine, nicardipine, nifedipine, verapamil): Increased plasma concentrations of these drugs with increased risk of adverse reactions

cimetidine (oral suspension only), efavirenz, esomeprazole (oral suspension only), fosamprenavir, metoclopramide (oral suspension only), phenytoin, rifabutin: Possibly decreased plasma level of posaconazole

cyclosporine, tacrolimus: Increased plasma levels of these drugs, with increased risk of adverse reactions

digoxin: Increased risk of digitalis toxicity

ergot alkaloids: Increased plasma ergot alkaloid level and increased risk of ergotism

HMG-CoA reductase inhibitors: Increased plasma statin level and increased risk of rhabdomyolysis

midazolam: Increased midazolam plasma concentrations by about 5-fold

pimozide, quinidine: Increased plasma concentrations of these drugs, leading to QT prolongation and torsades de pointes

sirolimus: Increased sirolimus blood concentration with possible sirolimus toxicity

vinca alkaloids: Increased plasma vinca alkaloid level and increased risk of neurotoxicity

ACTIVITIES

alcohol: Faster release for oral delayed-release suspension

≣ Adverse Reactions

CNS: Anxiety, asthenia, dizziness, fatigue, fever, headache, insomnia, rigors, tremor, weakness

CV: Edema, hypertension, **hypotension, QT-interval prolongation**, tachycardia

EENT: Blurred vision, epistaxis, herpes simplex, mucositis, pharyngitis, stomatitis, taste perversion

ENDO: Hyperglycemia, pseudoaldosteronism

GI: Abdominal pain, anorexia, bilirubinemia, constipation, diarrhea, dyspepsia, elevated liver enzymes, hepatomegaly, jaundice, nausea, **pancreatitis**, vomiting

GU: **Acute renal failure**, elevated blood creatinine level, **vaginal hemorrhage**

HEME: Anemia, **neutropenia (febrile), thrombocytopenia**

MS: Arthralgia, back or musculoskeletal pain

RESP: Cough, dyspnea, pneumonia, **respiratory failure**, upper respiratory tract infection
SKIN: Diaphoresis, petechiae, pruritus, rash
Other: **Bacteremia**, cytomegalovirus infection, dehydration, **hypocalcemia**, **hypokalemia**, **hypomagnesemia**, **septic shock**, weight loss

Childbearing Considerations
PREGNANCY
- Drug may cause fetal harm, based on animal studies.
- Use with caution only if benefit to mother outweighs potential risk to fetus.

LACTATION
- It is not known if drug is present in breast milk.
- Patient should check with prescriber before breastfeeding.

Nursing Considerations

! **WARNING** Determine sorbitol/fructose/sucrose exposure prior to administrating delayed-release oral suspension because life-threatening hypoglycemia, hypophosphatemia, lactic acidosis, and hepatic failure may occur in patients with hereditary fructose intolerance (HFI). Keep in mind the diagnosis of HFI may not yet be established in pediatric patients.

- Use cautiously in patients who have had a hypersensitivity reaction to other azoles because of risk for cross-sensitivity.
- Use cautiously in patients with hepatic or renal dysfunction. Know that posaconazole injection should be avoided, if possible, in patients with moderate or severe renal impairment (GFR less than 50 ml/min). If not possible, expect to monitor serum creatinine levels, as ordered, and if increases occur, anticipate patient being switched to oral posaconazole therapy.
- Use cautiously in patients with potentially proarrhythmic conditions because posaconazole may prolong QT interval.
- Expect to obtain electrolytes and correct any disturbances, as prescribed before and routinely during posaconazole therapy.
- Obtain baseline assessment of liver function and check periodically during therapy, as ordered. If elevations occur or patient has evidence of elevated liver enzymes, notify prescriber.

- Monitor patient experiencing severe diarrhea or vomiting for breakthrough fungal infections.

PATIENT TEACHING
- Advise patient prescribed oral suspension form to use the measuring spoon supplied by manufacturer and to rinse it with water after each use. Tell patient to shake bottle well before measuring dose and to store bottle at room temperature.
- Instruct patient to take posaconazole immediate-release oral suspension with or within 20 minutes after a full meal or liquid nutritional supplement to increase drug absorption. Tell patient that he also may take posaconazole immediate-release oral suspension with an acidic carbonated beverage such as ginger ale.
- Teach patient how to mix and administer delayed-release oral suspension for children. Stress importance of using only the notched-tip syringes that come with product and not opening packet until ready to mix. Tell patient to take drug with food and discard any remaining amount of suspension. Advise patient to store drug at room temperature.
- Advise patient prescribed delayed-release tablets to take with or without food; to swallow tablets whole; and to not chew, crush, or divide tablets.
- Tell patient to report severe diarrhea or vomiting because these conditions may interfere with drug effectiveness.

! **WARNING** Alert patient or family/caregiver before administering delayed-release oral suspension that a life-threatening condition can occur with patients with hereditary fructose intolerance (HFI). If patient has HFI, tell patient or family/caregiver to notify prescriber.

potassium acetate

potassium bicarbonate
K+Care ET, K-Electrolyte, K-Ide, Klor-Con/EF, K-Lyte

potassium bicarbonate and potassium chloride

Klorvess Effervescent Granules, Neo-K (CAN), Potassium Sandoz (CAN)

potassium bicarbonate and potassium citrate

Effer-K, K-Lyte DS

potassium chloride

Apo-K (CAN), K-10 (CAN), Kalium Durules (CAN), Kaochlor 10%, Kaochlor S-F 10%, Kaon-Cl, KCl 5% (CAN), K-Long (CAN), K-Lor, Klor-Con 10, Klor-Con Powder, Klor-Con/25 Powder, Klorvess 10% Liquid, Klotrix, K-Med 900 (CAN), K-Norm, K-Sol, K-Tab, Micro-K, Micro-K 10, Potasalan, Roychlor 10% (CAN), Ten-K

potassium citrate

Urocit-K

potassium gluconate

Glu-K, Kaon, Kaylixir, K-G Elixir, Potassium-Rougier (CAN)

potassium gluconate and potassium chloride

Kolyum

potassium gluconate and potassium citrate

Twin-K

trikates

Tri-K

▤ Class and Category

Pharmacologic class: Electrolyte cation
Therapeutic class: Electrolyte replacement

▤ Indications and Dosages

＊ *To prevent or treat hypokalemia in patients who can't ingest sufficient dietary potassium or who are losing potassium because of a condition (such as hepatic cirrhosis or prolonged vomiting) or drug (such as potassium-wasting diuretics or certain antibiotics)*

EFFERVESCENT TABLETS (POTASSIUM BICARBONATE)

Adults and adolescents. 25 to 50 mEq/g once or twice daily, as needed and tolerated. *Maximum:* 100 mEq daily.

EFFERVESCENT TABLETS (POTASSIUM BICARBONATE AND POTASSIUM CHLORIDE)

Adults and adolescents. 20, 25, or 50 mEq once or twice daily, as needed and tolerated. *Maximum:* 100 mEq daily.

EFFERVESCENT TABLETS (POTASSIUM BICARBONATE AND POTASSIUM CITRATE)

Adults and adolescents. 25 or 50 mEq once or twice daily, as needed and tolerated. *Maximum:* 100 mEq daily.

ELIXIR (POTASSIUM GLUCONATE)

Adults and adolescents. 20 mEq twice daily to four times daily, as needed and tolerated. *Maximum:* 100 mEq daily.
Children. 2 to 3 mEq/kg daily in divided doses.

E.R. CAPSULES (POTASSIUM CHLORIDE)

Adults and adolescents. 40 to 100 mEq daily in divided doses twice daily or three times a day for treatment; 16 to 24 mEq daily in divided doses twice daily or three times a day for prevention. *Maximum:* 100 mEq daily.

E.R. TABLETS (POTASSIUM CHLORIDE)

Adults and adolescents. 6.7 to 20 mEq three times a day. *Maximum:* 100 mEq daily.

GRANULE PACKETS (POTASSIUM BICARBONATE AND POTASSIUM CHLORIDE)

Adults and adolescents. 20 mEq once or twice daily, as needed and tolerated.

P

Maximum: 100 mEq daily.

GRANULES FOR ORAL SUSPENSION (POTASSIUM CHLORIDE)

Adults and adolescents. 20 mEq 1 to 5 times/day, as needed. *Maximum:* 100 mEq daily.

ORAL SOLUTION (POTASSIUM CHLORIDE)

Adults and adolescents. 20 mEq once daily to four times a day, as needed and tolerated. *Maximum:* 100 mEq daily.

Children. 1 to 3 mEq/kg daily in divided doses.

ORAL SOLUTION (POTASSIUM GLUCONATE AND POTASSIUM CHLORIDE, POTASSIUM GLUCONATE AND POTASSIUM CITRATE)

Adults and adolescents. 20 mEq twice daily to four times a day, as needed and tolerated. *Maximum:* 100 mEq daily.

Children. 2 to 3 mEq/kg daily in divided doses.

POWDER PACKET FOR ORAL SOLUTION (POTASSIUM CHLORIDE)

Adults. 15 to 25 mEq twice daily to four times a day, as needed and tolerated. *Maximum:* 100 mEq daily.

Children. 1 to 3 mEq/kg daily in divided doses, as needed and tolerated.

POWDER PACKET FOR ORAL SOLUTION (POTASSIUM GLUCONATE AND POTASSIUM CHLORIDE)

Adults and adolescents. 20 mEq twice daily to four times a day, as needed and tolerated. *Maximum:* 100 mEq daily.

Children. 2 to 3 mEq/kg daily in divided doses.

ORAL TRIKATES SOLUTION (POTASSIUM ACETATE, POTASSIUM BICARBONATE, AND POTASSIUM CITRATE)

Adults and adolescents. 15 mEq three times a day to four times a day, as needed and tolerated. *Maximum:* 100 mEq daily.

Children. 2 to 3 mEq/kg daily in divided doses.

TABLETS (POTASSIUM GLUCONATE)

Adults and adolescents. 5 to 10 mEq twice daily to four times a day, as needed and tolerated. *Maximum:* 100 mEq daily.

I.V. INFUSION (POTASSIUM ACETATE AND POTASSIUM CHLORIDE)

Adults and adolescents with serum potassium level above 2.5 mEq/L. Up to 10 mEq/hr. *Maximum:* 200 mEq daily.

Adults and adolescents with serum potassium level below 2 mEq/L, ECG changes, or paralysis. Up to 20 mEq/hr. *Maximum:* 400 mEq daily.

Children. 3 mEq/kg daily.

± **DOSAGE ADJUSTMENT** Dosage adjusted as prescribed based on patient's ECG patterns and serum potassium level.

✳ *To treat renal tubular acidosis with calcium stones, hypocitraturic calcium oxalate nephrolithiasis of any etiology, and uric acid lithiasis with or without calcium stones*

TABLETS (POTASSIUM CITRATE)

Adults. For patients with severe hypocitraturia, 15 mEq four times a day or 20 mEq three times a day. For patients with mild to moderate hypocitraturia, 10 mEq three times a day with meals.

± **DOSAGE ADJUSTMENT** For patients with cirrhosis or renal impairment, dosage should be started at the lower end of the dosing range for all formulations of potassium.

☰ Drug Administration

P.O.

- Administer with or immediately after meals.
- Mix potassium chloride for oral solution or potassium gluconate elixir in cold water, orange juice, tomato juice (if patient isn't sodium restricted), or apple juice, and stir for 1 full minute before administering.
- Mix potassium bicarbonate, potassium bicarbonate and potassium chloride, and potassium bicarbonate and potassium citrate effervescent tablets with cold water and allow to dissolve completely.
- Administer tablet forms of potassium with food to help prevent gastric irritation.

I.V.

- Use only when oral replacement is not feasible or life-threatening hypokalemia is present.
- Never directly inject undiluted potassium concentrate because it may be immediately fatal.
- Don't connect flexible plastic containers in series because of increased risk of residual air contained in the primary container that could cause an air embolism.
- Dilute potassium concentrate for injection with an adequate volume of solution before I.V. use following manufacturer guidelines.
- Infuse potassium slowly at a controlled rate using a calibrated infusion device.

Rate of infusion for an adult is dependent upon patient's needs. For example, if serum potassium level is greater than 2.5 mEq/liter, potassium chloride may be given at a rate not to exceed 10 mEq/hour in a concentration of up to 40 mEq/liter. However, if serum potassium level is less than 2.0 mEq/liter with ECG changes or paralysis present, drug may be infused very cautiously at a rate of up to 40 mEq/hour. Rate of infusion for children should be no greater than 0.5 mEq/kg/hr.

- In critical situations, potassium chloride should be administered in 0.9% Sodium Chloride Injection (unless contraindicated) rather than a dextrose-containing solution, as dextrose may lower serum potassium levels.
- If possible, administer via a central intravenous route.
- High concentrations of potassium should only should be given through a central line.
- *Incompatibilities:* None listed by manufacturer

Route	Onset	Peak	Duration
P.O.	Unknown	1–2 hr	Unknown
P.O./E.R.	Unknown	4 hr	8 hr
I.V.	Immediate	Unknown	Unknown

Half-life: Unknown

Mechanism of Action

Acts as the major cation in intracellular fluid, activating many enzymatic reactions essential for physiologic processes, including nerve impulse transmission and cardiac and skeletal muscle contraction. Potassium also helps maintain electroneutrality in cells by controlling exchange of intracellular and extracellular ions. It also helps maintain normal renal function and acid–base balance.

Contraindications

Acute dehydration, Addison's disease (untreated), concurrent use with amiloride or triamterene (potassium chloride), or potassium-sparing diuretics (all forms of potassium), crush syndrome, disorders that may delay drug passing through GI tract (potassium citrate), heat cramps, hyperkalemia, hypersensitivity to potassium salts or their components, peptic ulcer disease (potassium citrate), renal impairment with azotemia or oliguria, severe hemolytic anemia, UTI (potassium citrate)

Interactions

DRUGS

ACE inhibitors, aliskiren, amiloride, angiotensin II receptor antagonists, beta-blockers, blood products, corticosteroids, cyclosporine, eplerenone, heparin, NSAIDs, potassium-containing drugs, potassium-sparing diuretics, spironolactone, tacrolimus, triamterene: Increased risk of hyperkalemia that can become severe

amphotericin B, corticosteroids (glucocorticoids, mineralocorticoids), gentamicin, penicillins, polymyxin B: Possibly hypokalemia

anticholinergics, drugs with anticholinergic activity: Increased risk of GI ulceration, stricture, and perforation

antiepileptics, diuretics: Increased risk of hyponatremia when used with high concentration of potassium chloride

calcium salts (parenteral): Possibly arrhythmias

digoxin: Increased risk of digitalis toxicity

insulin, laxatives, sodium bicarbonate: Decreased serum potassium level

sodium polystyrene sulfonate: Possibly decreased serum potassium level and fluid retention

thiazide diuretics: Possibly hyperkalemia when diuretic is discontinued

FOODS

low-salt milk, salt substitutes: Increased risk of hyperkalemia

Adverse Reactions

CNS: Chills, confusion, fever, **hyponatremic encephalopathy (with use of high concentration of potassium chloride)**, paralysis, paresthesia, weakness

CV: Arrhythmias, **asystole, bradycardia, cardiac arrest**, chest pain, **ECG changes**, peripheral edema, **ventricular fibrillation**

EENT: Throat pain when swallowing

GI: Abdominal pain; **bloody stools**; diarrhea; flatulence; **GI bleeding, obstruction, perforation,** or ulceration; nausea; vomiting

RESP: Dyspnea, **pulmonary edema (with high concentration of potassium chloride)**

SKIN: Rash

Other: **Anaphylaxis; angioedema;** extravasation reactions such as necrosis,

P

nerve or tendon injury, ulcers, or vascular injury; **hyperkalemia**; hypervolemia (with high concentration of potassium chloride); **hypokalemia; hyponatremia (with use of high concentration of potassium chloride)**; infusion-site reactions such as burning sensation, erythema, irritation, pain, phlebitis, pruritus, rash, or **thrombosis**

Childbearing Considerations

PREGNANCY

- It is not known if drug causes fetal harm but may if hyperkalemia occurs.
- Use with caution only if benefit to mother outweighs potential risk to fetus.

LACTATION

- Potassium is normally present in breast milk.
- Patient should check with prescriber before breastfeeding.

Nursing Considerations

- Review patient's medical history before administering potassium chloride, because there are many conditions that may predispose patient to develop hyperkalemia and increased sensitivity to potassium.
- Be aware that liquid form of oral potassium is prescribed for patients with delayed gastric emptying, esophageal compression, or intestinal obstruction or stricture, as well as patients with dysphagia or swallowing disorders, to decrease the risk of tissue damage from solid forms of potassium that may remain in contact with the gastrointestinal mucosa for a prolonged period of time.
- Monitor patient receiving tablet forms of potassium for abdominal pain or distention, gastrointestinal bleeding, or severe vomiting, as this may indicate GI obstruction, perforation, or ulceration and should be reported immediately.
- Be aware that potassium chloride injection should be given with extreme caution, if at all, to patients with conditions that increase patient sensitivity to potassium or predispose patient to hyperkalemia, such as acute dehydration, congestive heart failure, extensive burns or tissue injury, or severe renal impairment. Also be aware that high concentration of potassium chloride for injection should be avoided in patients at risk for hyponatremia. If use cannot be avoided, monitor patient closely.

- Monitor serum potassium level before and during administration of I.V. potassium. Be aware that mild or moderate hyperkalemia is asymptomatic and may be manifested only by increased serum potassium concentrations, and possibly by characteristic ECG changes. Arrhythmias can develop at any time during hyperkalemia.

> **! WARNING** Be aware that some forms of potassium contain tartrazine, which may cause an allergic reaction, such as asthma. Some forms may also contain aluminum, which may become toxic in a patient with impaired renal function.

- Regularly assess patient for signs of hypokalemia, such as arrhythmias, fatigue, and weakness, and for signs of hyperkalemia, such as arrhythmias, confusion, dyspnea, and paresthesia.
- Monitor serum creatinine level and urine output during administration, because adequate renal function is needed for potassium supplementation. Notify prescriber about signs of decreased renal function, because renal impairment may predispose patient to fluid overload and/or hyperkalemia.

PATIENT TEACHING

- Inform patient that potassium is part of a normal diet and that most meats, seafoods, fruits, and vegetables contain sufficient potassium to meet recommended daily intake. Also advise her not to exceed recommended daily amount of potassium.
- Teach patient the correct way to take prescribed potassium. This can vary from swallowing a tablet with a full glass of water to mixing certain preparations with half to full glass of cold water or juice.
- Caution patient not to crush or chew E.R. forms unless instructed otherwise.
- Instruct patient to take drug with or right after food.
- Teach patient how to take her radial pulse, and advise her to notify prescriber about significant changes in heart rate or rhythm.
- Advise patient to watch stools for changes in color and consistency and to notify prescriber if they become black, tarry, or red.

- Inform patient that although she may see waxy form of E.R. tablet in stools, she has received all of the potassium.
- Urge patient to keep follow-up laboratory appointments as directed by prescriber to determine serum potassium level.

pramipexole dihydrochloride
Mirapex, Mirapex ER

Class and Category
Pharmacologic class: Nonergoline dopamine agonist
Therapeutic class: Antiparkinsonian

Indications and Dosages
✳ *To treat Parkinson's disease*

TABLETS
Adults. *Initial:* 0.125 mg three times a day for 1 wk, gradually increased every 5 to 7 days, as needed. Alternatively, can be increased weekly thereafter as follows: for wk 2, 0.25 mg three times a day; for wk 3, 0.5 mg three times a day; for wk 4, 0.75 mg three times a day; for wk 5, 1 mg three times day; for wk 6, 1.25 mg three times a day; and for wk 7, 1.5 mg three times a day. *Maintenance:* 1.5 to 4.5 mg daily in divided doses three times a day. *Maximum:* 4.5 mg daily.
±**DOSAGE ADJUSTMENT** For patients with renal impairment, dosage reduced as follows: for creatinine clearance greater than 50 ml/min, maximum dose limited to 1.5 mg three times a day; for creatinine clearance of 30 to 50 ml/min, maximum dose limited to 0.75 mg three times a day; for creatinine clearance of 15 to less than 30 ml/min, maximum dose limited to 1.5 mg once a day. Drug shouldn't be given to patients with creatinine clearance of less than 15 ml/min.

E.R. TABLETS
Adults. *Initial:* 0.375 mg once daily, increased every 5 to 7 days, first to 0.75 mg and then by 0.75-mg increments, as needed. *Maximum:* 4.5 mg daily.
±**DOSAGE ADJUSTMENT** For patients with moderate renal impairment (creatinine clearance between 30 and 50 ml/min), initial dosage taken every other day with dosage adjustment done after 1 wk in increments of 0.375 mg only, as needed, to maximum dosage of 2.25 mg daily.

✳ *To treat restless legs syndrome*

TABLETS
Adults. *Initial:* 0.125 mg once daily. Increased in 4 to 7 days to 0.25 mg once daily. Further increased in 4 to 7 days to 0.5 mg once daily.
±**DOSAGE ADJUSTMENT** For patients with moderate to severe renal impairment (creatinine clearance 20 to 60 ml/min) dosage interval for titration, if needed, increased to 14 days.

Drug Administration
P.O.
- Administer with food if GI upset occurs.
- Tablets should be swallowed whole and not chewed, crushed, or divided.
- Give drug used to treat restless leg syndrome 2 to 3 hours before bedtime.
- Patient may be switched overnight from immediate-release tablets to extended-release tablets at the same daily dose, but dosage adjustment may be needed after monitoring effectiveness of switch.
- A retitration of therapy may be required if a significant interruption in therapy occurs.
- Store drug at room temperature.

Route	Onset	Peak	Duration
P.O.	Rapid	2 hr	8–12 hr
P.O./E.R.	Unknown	6 hr	Unknown
Half-life: 8–12 hr			

Mechanism of Action
May stimulate dopamine receptors in the brain, thereby easing symptoms of Parkinson's disease, which is thought to be caused by a dopamine deficiency.

Contraindications
Hypersensitivity to pramipexole or its components

Interactions
DRUGS
butyrophenones, metoclopramide, phenothiazines, thioxanthenes: Decreased pramipexole effectiveness

Adverse Reactions
CNS: Abnormal behavior or thinking, amnesia, anxiety, asthenia, compulsive behaviors such as pathological gambling

or uncontrollable shopping or sexual activity, confusion, dream disturbances, drowsiness, dyskinesia, dystonia, fatigue, fever, hallucinations, headache, insomnia, malaise, paranoia, psychotic-like behavior, restlessness, syncope

CV: **Cardiac failure**, edema, orthostatic hypotension

EENT: Diplopia, dry mouth, rhinitis, vision changes

ENDO: Inappropriate antidiuretic hormone secretion (SIADH)

GI: Anorexia, constipation, dysphagia, eating disorders, nausea, vomiting

GU: Altered libido, hypersexuality, impotence, urinary frequency, urinary incontinence

MS: Arthralgia, myalgia, myasthenia, postural deformity, **rhabdomyolysis**

RESP: Pneumonia

SKIN: Diaphoresis, erythema, pruritis, rash, urticaria

Other: Weight gain or loss, withdrawal symptoms

Childbearing Considerations

PREGNANCY

- It is not known if drug can cause fetal harm.
- Use with caution only if benefit to mother outweighs potential risk to fetus.

LACTATION

- It is not known if drug is present in breast milk. However, lactation inhibition is likely to occur because drug inhibits prolactin secretion.
- Patient should check with prescriber before breastfeeding.

Nursing Considerations

- Use pramipexole cautiously in patients with hallucinations, hypotension, or retinal problems (such as macular degeneration). Drug may worsen these conditions.
- Also use cautiously in patients with renal impairment because pramipexole elimination may be decreased.
- Monitor patient for postural deformity (antecollis, bent spine syndrome, Pisa syndrome) that may occur several months after pramipexole therapy has been initiated or after increasing dose. If present, notify prescriber and expect dosage to be decreased or drug discontinued, which may improve condition.

- Take safety precautions per facility policy until drug's CNS effects are known.
- Avoid stopping pramipexole abruptly because doing so may cause a symptom complex resembling neuroleptic malignant syndrome and consisting of altered level of consciousness, autonomic instability, hyperpyrexia, and muscle rigidity. Also, be aware that withdrawal symptoms may occur during tapering or after drug is discontinued. Monitor patient for altered consciousness, fever, and muscular rigidity. If present, notify prescriber and expect to administer a low-dose dopamine agonist, if severe.
- Assess patient for skin changes regularly because melanomas may occur at a higher rate in patients with Parkinson's disease. It isn't clear if this is a result of the disease or drugs used to treat it.
- Know that some patients have reported worsening of their Parkinson's disease symptoms when tablet residue was visible in their stool. If this occurs, notify prescriber, as pramipexole therapy may have to be reevaluated.
- Monitor patient for hallucinations and psychotic-like behavior. Risk for hallucinations is higher if patient is older than 65 years. Changes in behavior or thinking may include aggressive behavior, agitation, confusion, delirium, delusions, disorientation, hallucinations, mania-like symptoms, paranoid ideation, and psychotic-like behavior.

PATIENT TEACHING

- Advise patient to take pramipexole with meals if nausea occurs.
- Inform patient that tablets should be swallowed whole and not chewed, crushed, or divided.
- Instruct patient taking drug for restless legs syndrome to take it 2 to 3 hours before bedtime.
- Inform patient that if drug is not taken for a period of time, the dosage may have to be retitrated when started again.
- Caution patient about possible dizziness, drowsiness, or light-headedness, which may result from orthostatic hypotension. Advise her not to rise quickly from a lying or sitting position to minimize these effects.

- Instruct patient to notify prescriber immediately about vision problems or urinary frequency or incontinence.
- Inform patient that improvement in motor performance and activities of daily living may take 2 to 3 weeks.
- Urge patient to have regular skin examinations by a dermatologist or other qualified health professional.
- Advise patient and his family to notify prescriber about onset of compulsive and intense urges, such as eating binges, compulsive shopping, hypersexuality, or pathological gambling. Dosage may have to be reduced or drug discontinued.
- Inform patient or caregivers that hallucinations and other psychotic-like behavior may occur, with elderly patients over age 65 more at risk. If present, notify prescriber.
- Caution patient not to stop taking pramipexole abruptly.
- Tell patient to alert prescriber if posture changes that cannot be controlled occur, such as neck bending forward; bending forward at the waist; or tilting sideways when sitting, standing, or walking.
- Advise patient to contact prescriber if he observes residue in his stool, which may resemble a swollen original E.R. tablet or swollen pieces of the original tablet.
- Advise patient to report unexplained muscle pain, tenderness, or weakness to prescriber.
- Inform patient that withdrawal symptoms may occur during or after drug is discontinued or dosage reduced. Review withdrawal symptoms with patient and tell patient to notify prescriber if present.
- Advise women of childbearing age to notify prescriber if pregnancy occurs or a pregnancy is being planned. Also, tell patient who plans to breastfeed their infant or are breastfeeding to alert prescriber before taking drug.

pramlintide acetate
Symlin-Pen 60, Symlin-Pen 120

☰ Class and Category

Pharmacologic class: Human amylin analogue
Therapeutic class: Antidiabetic

☰ Indications and Dosages

✶ *As adjunct to achieve euglycemia in patients with type 1 diabetes who use mealtime insulin therapy but have not achieved desired glucose control*

SUBCUTANEOUS INJECTION

Adults. *Initial:* 15 mcg just before major meals with 50% reduced dosage of preprandial rapid-acting or short-acting insulin, including fixed-mix insulins. Dosage increased in increments of 15 mcg, as tolerated, but no less than every 3 days to minimize nausea. *Maintenance:* 30 to 60 mcg before major meals.

±**DOSAGE ADJUSTMENT** Dosage decreased to 30 mcg if nausea occurs and persists at higher dosages.

✶ *As adjunct to achieve euglycemia in patients with type 2 diabetes who use mealtime insulin, with or without a sulfonylurea and/or metformin, and have not achieved desired glucose control*

SUBCUTANEOUS INJECTION

Adults. *Initial:* 60 mcg immediately before major meals combined with dosage reduction of preprandial rapid-acting or short-acting insulin, including fixed-mix insulins, by 50%. Dosage increased to 120 mcg before major meals if no significant nausea has occurred after at least 3 days.

±**DOSAGE ADJUSTMENT** Dosage decreased to 60 mcg before major meals if nausea occurs and persists with 120-mcg dosage.

☰ Drug Administration

SUBCUTANEOUS

- Ensure that mealtime insulin dose has been reduced by 50% upon initiation of drug therapy.
- Administer immediately prior to each major meal that contains 250 calories or more or 30 or more grams of carbohydrates.
- Allow drug to warm to room temperature before administering, to avoid injection-site adverse reactions.
- Inject drug into the abdomen or thigh. Do not inject into arm because absorption is variable from this site.
- Do not inject into same site as insulin.
- Rotate sites.
- Pramlintide and insulin should be administered in separate syringes, as drug should not be mixed with any type of insulin.

P

- Wait at least 3 days between dose titrations to minimize nausea.
- If drug is discontinued for illnesses or surgery, initiation protocol will have to be followed when drug is reinstituted.
- Store pens in refrigerator or at room temperature. Discard pens after 30 days regardless of how they were stored.

Route	Onset	Peak	Duration
SubQ	Unknown	19–21 min	3 hr

Half-life: 8 min

Mechanism of Action

Slows the rate at which food is released from stomach to small intestine, thus reducing initial postprandial rise in serum glucose level. Pramlintide also suppresses glucagon secretion and promotes satiety, thus furthering weight loss, which also lowers serum glucose level. Pramlintide is a synthetic analogue of amylin, a naturally occurring neuroendocrine hormone secreted with insulin by pancreatic beta cells. In diabetes, secretion of insulin and amylin is reduced or absent.

Contraindications

Gastroparesis, hypersensitivity to pramlintide or its components; hypoglycemia unawareness

Interactions

DRUGS

drugs that alter GI motility (such as anticholinergics) or slow intestinal absorption of nutrients (such as alpha-glucosidase inhibitors): Altered effects of these drugs
insulin: Alters pharmacokinetic parameters of pramlintide if mixed in the same syringe. Pramlintide and insulin must not be mixed together and must be administered as separate injections.
oral drugs: Delayed absorption

Adverse Reactions

CNS: Dizziness, fatigue, headache
EENT: Blurred vision, pharyngitis
GI: Abdominal pain, anorexia, nausea, **pancreatitis**, vomiting
MS: Arthralgia
RESP: Coughing
SKIN: Diaphoresis
Other: **Hypersensitivity reactions**; local injection-site reaction, such as redness, swelling, or pruritus

Childbearing Considerations

PREGNANCY

- It is not known if drug can cause fetal harm.
- Use with caution only if benefit to mother outweighs potential risk to fetus.

LACTATION

- It is not known if drug is present in breast milk.
- Patient should check with prescriber before breastfeeding.

Nursing Considerations

- Know that because of the risks involved with pramlintide therapy, insulin-using patients with type 1 or 2 diabetes must have failed to achieve adequate glycemic control despite individualized insulin management and must be receiving ongoing care with guidance of insulin prescriber and a diabetes educator before pramlintide is prescribed.
- Expect that certain patients won't be prescribed pramlintide because its risks may outweigh its benefits. These include patients with poor compliance with current insulin regimen, poor compliance with monitoring blood glucose level, a glycosylated hemoglobin greater than 9%, recurrent severe hypoglycemia that required assistance during past 6 months, hypoglycemia unawareness, gastroparesis, concurrent therapy with drugs that stimulate GI motility, and pediatric patients.
- Monitor patient's premeal and postmeal blood glucose levels regularly to determine effectiveness of pramlintide and insulin therapy and to detect hypoglycemia.
- Monitor patient for 3 hours after each dose of pramlintide, for hypoglycemia, which may be severe, especially in patients with type 1 diabetes. Effects may include hunger, headache, sweating, tremor, irritability, and trouble concentrating. They may occur with a rapid decrease in blood glucose level regardless of glucose values.
- Be aware that although pramlintide doesn't cause hypoglycemia, its use with insulin increases the risk of insulin-induced severe hypoglycemia, which can result in loss of consciousness, coma, or seizures. If hypoglycemia occurs, provide supportive care, including glucagon if prescribed, and notify prescriber. Expect insulin dosage accompanying pramlintide to be reduced.

- Know that early warning symptoms of hypoglycemia may be different or less severe if patient has had diabetes for a long time; has diabetic nerve disease; takes a beta blocker, clonidine, guanethidine, or reserpine; or is under intensified diabetes control.
- Closely monitor patients taking oral antidiabetics, ACE inhibitors, disopyramide, fibrates, fluoxetine, MAO inhibitors, pentoxifylline, propoxyphene, salicylates, or sulfonamide antibiotics, because of an increased risk of hypoglycemia.
- Expect pramlintide to be stopped if patient develops recurrent hypoglycemia that requires medical assistance, develops persistent nausea, or becomes noncompliant with therapy or follow-up visits.

PATIENT TEACHING

- Alert patient that insulin-induced hypoglycemia may occur within 3 hours of injecting pramlintide. Review signs and symptoms and appropriate treatment. Tell patient to notify prescriber if hypoglycemia occurs because insulin dosage will have to be reduced.
- Emphasize need to monitor blood glucose level often, especially before and after eating.
- Tell patient to inject drug subcutaneously immediately before major meals (contains 250 calories or more or contains 30 grams of carbohydrates or more) using the Symlin-Pen injector. Teach patient how to use the Symlin-Pen. Advise patient to inject drug into her abdomen or thigh and not to use her arm as an injection site because absorption may be too variable.
- Warn patient not to mix pramlintide and insulin together in the same syringe.
- Warn patient that nausea is common with pramlintide; urge her to notify prescriber because dosage may have to be decreased.
- Caution patient that if she misses a dose, she should skip the missed dose and continue with the next scheduled dose.
- Caution patient to avoid hazardous activities that require mental alertness until effects of pramlintide are known.
- Reassure patient that pramlintide won't alter her awareness of or her body's response to insulin-induced hypoglycemia.
- Alert patient that she'll need close follow-up care, at least weekly until a target dose

of pramlintide has been reached, she's tolerating the drug well, and her blood glucose level is stable.
- Explain that local injection-site reactions, such as itching, redness, or swelling, may occur but usually resolve in a few weeks.
- Instruct patient to never share the Symlin-Pen with anyone else, even if the needle has been changed, because of a risk for transmission of bloodborne pathogens.

prasugrel hydrochloride
Effient

Class and Category
Pharmacologic class: P2Y$_{12}$ platelet inhibitor (thienopyridine)
Therapeutic class: Antiplatelet

Indications and Dosages
✴ *To reduce rate of thrombotic cardiovascular events (including stent thrombosis) in patients with acute coronary syndrome who will be managed with percutaneous coronary intervention because of non-ST-elevation MI, ST-elevation MI, or unstable angina*

TABLETS
Adults. *Initial:* 60 mg as a loading dose and then 10 mg once daily. *Maintenance:* 10 mg once daily.
±**DOSAGE ADJUSTMENT** For patients weighing less than 60 kg (132 lb), daily maintenance dosage may be reduced to 5 mg once daily.

Drug Administration
P.O.
- Tablet should be swallowed whole and not broken, chewed, or crushed.
- Store at room temperature, keeping desiccant in bottle at all times.
- Drug should be taken with aspirin 75 mg to 325 mg daily.

Route	Onset	Peak	Duration
P.O.	< 30 min	30 min	5–9 days

Half-life: 2–15 hr

Mechanism of Action
After forming active metabolite, irreversibly binds to ADP receptors on platelets to inhibit

platelet activation and aggregation for the lifetime of the platelet, which is 7 to 10 days. Without platelet activation and aggregation, thrombus cannot form.

Contraindications

Active bleeding, history of transient ischemic attack or stroke, hypersensitivity to prasugrel or its components

Interactions

DRUGS

fibrinolytic agents, NSAIDs (chronic use), warfarin: Increased risk of bleeding
opioids: Decreased or delayed prasugrel absorption

Adverse Reactions

CNS: Dizziness, fatigue, fever, headache, **intracranial hemorrhage**
CV: Atrial fibrillation, bradycardia, hypercholesterolemia, hyperlipidemia, hypertension, **hypotension,** peripheral edema
EENT: Epistaxis, retinal hemorrhage
GI: Diarrhea, **GI or retroperitoneal hemorrhage,** hepatic dysfunction, nausea
HEME: Anemia, **bleeding, leukopenia, severe thrombocytopenia, thrombotic thrombocytopenia purpura**
MS: Back or limb pain
RESP: Cough, dyspnea, **hemoptysis**
SKIN: Subcutaneous hematoma, rash
Other: Anaphylaxis, angioedema, hypersensitivity reactions, malignancies, noncardiac chest pain

Childbearing Considerations

PREGNANCY

- Drug may cause fetal harm due to risk of bleeding.
- Use with caution only if benefit to mother outweighs potential risk to fetus.

LACTATION

- It is not known if drug is present in breast milk.
- Patient should check with prescriber once condition has stabilized before breastfeeding.

Nursing Considerations

- Be aware that patient should be receiving daily aspirin therapy (75 or 325 mg) throughout prasugrel therapy.
- Be aware that drug isn't recommended for patients age 75 or older (except in high-risk

situations such as history of previous MI or presence of diabetes) or in patients who have active bleeding or a history of a transient ischemic attack or stroke. Monitor patients closely who have other risk factors for bleeding, which include a body weight less than 60 kg or a history of bleeding. Also monitor patients who are also taking drugs that increase risk of bleeding, such as chronic use of NSAIDs, fibrinolytic therapy, heparin, or warfarin.

- Know that prasugrel shouldn't be given to patients likely to undergo emergency coronary artery bypass graft (CABG) surgery because of increased bleeding risk. Drug should be discontinued at least 7 days before any surgery.

! **WARNING** Monitor patient closely for bleeding because prasugrel can cause life-threatening hemorrhage. Report hypotension in patients who have recently undergone CABG surgery or other surgical procedures, coronary angiography, or percutaneous coronary intervention while taking drug. In this setting, expect therapy to continue because stopping prasugrel, especially in first few weeks after acute coronary syndrome, increases the risk of adverse cardiovascular effects.

- Be aware that because prasugrel inhibits platelet aggregation for the lifetime of the platelet, which is 7 to 10 days, withholding a dose is unlikely help in managing a bleeding event or the risk of bleeding associated with an invasive procedure. Expect to administer exogenous platelets but only 6 hours after prasugrel loading dose or 4 hours after maintenance dose was given.
- Monitor patient's CBC regularly, as ordered, watching for evidence of thrombotic thrombocytopenic purpura, such as abnormal blood counts, fever, neurologic abnormalities, or renal dysfunction. Notify prescriber immediately because condition can be fatal. Expect to implement emergency treatment, such as plasmapheresis.

! **WARNING** Monitor patient for serious allergic reactions, especially if patient has had a serious allergic reaction to thienopyridines such as clopidogrel or ticlopidine. Notify prescriber if present and provide supportive care per institution protocol.

PATIENT TEACHING

- Emphasize importance of taking prasugrel exactly as prescribed, without lapses in therapy, for drug to be effective and adverse reactions to be reduced.
- Advise patient to swallow tablets whole and not to break, chew, or crush the tablets. Also tell patient to keep drug in the container it comes in and to keep the container closed tightly with the gray cylinder (desiccant) inside.
- Instruct patient to take daily dose of aspirin as prescribed.
- Discourage use of NSAIDs, including OTC products, during prasugrel therapy because of risk of bleeding.
- Caution patient that bleeding may last longer than usual. Instruct him to report unusual bleeding or bruising.
- Instruct patient to inform healthcare providers that he takes prasugrel.
- Urge patient to take precautions against bleeding, such as using an electric shaver and a soft-bristled toothbrush.
- Advise patient to avoid activities that could cause traumatic injury and bleeding.

! **WARNING** Advise patient to seek immediate medical care if swelling of his face or throat occurs or if any signs of an allergic reaction develops that is persistent or becomes worse.

pravastatin sodium
Pravachol

≣ Class and Category
Pharmacologic class: HMG-CoA reductase inhibitor (statin)
Therapeutic class: Antilipemic

≣ Indications and Dosages
✳ *To prevent cardiovascular and coronary events in patients at risk; to treat hyperlipidemia*

TABLETS
Adults. *Initial:* 40 mg daily, increased in 4 wk to 80 mg daily if needed.
±**DOSAGE ADJUSTMENT** For patients with significant renal impairment, those taking immunosuppressants, and elderly patients,

initial dosage reduced to 10 mg daily at bedtime. For elderly patients and those taking immunosuppressants, maintenance dosage usually limited to 20 mg daily. For patients taking clarithromycin, dosage limited to 40 mg once daily.

✳ *To treat pediatric heterozygous familial hypercholesterolemia*

TABLETS
Adolescents ages 14 to 18. 40 mg daily.
Children ages 8 to 14. 20 mg daily.

≣ Drug Administration
P.O.
- Administer drug consistently at about the same time every day.
- Give drug 1 hour before or 4 hours after giving cholestyramine or colestipol.

Route	Onset	Peak	Duration
P.O.	Unknown	60–90 min	Unknown

Half-life: 2.6–3.2 hr

≣ Mechanism of Action
Inhibits cholesterol synthesis in liver by blocking the enzyme needed to convert hydroxymethylglutaryl-CoA (HMG-CoA) to mevalonate, a cholesterol precursor. When cholesterol synthesis is blocked, the liver also increases breakdown of LDL cholesterol.

≣ Contraindications
Active hepatic disease or unexplained, persistent elevated liver enzymes; breastfeeding; hypersensitivity to pravastatin or its components; pregnancy

≣ Interactions
DRUGS
clarithromycin and other macrolide antibiotics, colchicine, cyclosporine, gemfibrozil, other fibrates: Increased risk of rhabdomyolysis and acute renal failure
niacin: Increased risk of skeletal muscle effects

≣ Adverse Reactions
CNS: Anxiety, asthenia, chills, confusion, cognitive impairment, cranial nerve dysfunction, depression, dizziness, fatigue, headache, malaise, memory loss, nervousness, nightmare, peripheral nerve palsy, sleep disturbance
CV: Angina pectoris, chest pain, vasculitis

P

EENT: Blurred vision, diplopia, rhinitis
ENDO: Abnormal thyroid function, elevated glycosylated hemoglobin levels, gynecomastia, hyperglycemia
GI: Abdominal pain, cholestatic jaundice, cirrhosis, constipation, diarrhea, elevated liver enzymes, flatulence, **fulminant hepatic necrosis**, heartburn, hepatoma, **hepatic failure, hepatitis,** indigestion, nausea, **pancreatitis,** vomiting
GU: Dysuria, nocturia, urinary frequency
HEME: Hemolytic anemia, positive ANA, ESR elevation, purpura
MS: Arthralgia, immune-mediated necrotizing myopathy, musculoskeletal cramps or pain, myalgia, myopathy, polymyalgia rheumatica, **rhabdomyolysis,** tendon disorder
RESP: Cough, dyspnea, **interstitial lung disease,** upper respiratory tract infection
SKIN: Dermatomyositis, **erythema multiforme,** photosensitivity, rash, **Stevens–Johnson syndrome, toxic epidermal necrolysis**
Other: Anaphylaxis, angioedema, lupus-like syndrome

Childbearing Considerations

PREGNANCY
- Drug may cause fetal harm.
- Drug is contraindicated in pregnant women.
- Drug should be discontinued immediately when pregnancy is known.

LACTATION
- Drug is present in breast milk.
- Drug is contraindicated with breastfeeding,

REPRODUCTION
- Women of childbearing age should use a reliable contraceptive throughout pravastatin therapy.

Nursing Considerations

- Use pravastatin cautiously in patients with hepatic or renal impairment and in elderly patients.
- Monitor liver enzymes before pravastatin therapy starts and as indicated during therapy.
- Report unexplained muscle aches or weakness and significant increases in creatine kinase level to prescriber because in rare instances drug causes rhabdomyolysis with acute renal failure caused by

myoglobinuria. Expect to stop drug and provide supportive care.
- Monitor patient's BUN and serum creatinine levels periodically for abnormal elevations.
- Monitor blood lipoprotein level, as indicated, to evaluate response to therapy.

PATIENT TEACHING
- Instruct patient to take drug without regard to meals but to be consistent with timing of daily dose.
- Caution patient not to perform hazardous activities such as driving until effects of drug is known.
- Advise patient to notify prescriber at once about muscle pain, tenderness, weakness, and other evidence of myopathy.
- Urge woman of childbearing age to use a reliable method of contraception during pravastatin therapy and to notify prescriber at once if she becomes pregnant or thinks she may be pregnant.
- Advise women not to breastfeed while on pravastatin therapy.
- Instruct patient not to stop taking pravastatin without consulting prescriber, even when cholesterol level returns to normal.

prazosin hydrochloride
Minipress

Class and Category
Pharmacologic class: Alpha blocker
Therapeutic class: Antihypertensive

Indications and Dosages
✴ *To manage hypertension*

CAPSULES
Adults. *Initial:* 1 mg twice daily or three times a day. *Maintenance:* 6 to 15 mg daily in divided doses twice daily or three times a day. *Maximum:* 40 mg daily.
±**DOSAGE ADJUSTMENT** For patient taking a diuretic or other antihypertensive agent, dosage reduced to 1 or 2 mg three times a day and retitration done.

Drug Administration
P.O.
- Give drug at same times daily.

Route	Onset	Peak	Duration
P.O.	0.5–1.5 hr	2–4 hr	10–24 hr

Half-life: 2 to 3 hr

Mechanism of Action

Selectively and competitively inhibits alpha$_1$-adrenergic receptors. This action promotes peripheral arterial and venous dilation and reduces peripheral vascular resistance, thereby lowering blood pressure.

Contraindications

Hypersensitivity to prazosin, other quinazolines, or their components

Interactions

DRUGS

antihypertensives, beta-blockers, diuretics, phosphodiesterase-5 inhibitors: Increased risk of hypotension and syncope

Adverse Reactions

CNS: Asthenia, dizziness, drowsiness, fatigue, headache, insomnia, malaise, nervousness, syncope
CV: Angina, **bradycardia**, edema, orthostatic hypotension, palpitations, vasculitis
EENT: Dry mouth, eye pain
ENDO: Gynecomastia
GI: Nausea
GU: Priapism, urinary frequency or incontinence
SKIN: Urticaria
Other: Hypersensitivity reactions

Childbearing Considerations

PREGNANCY

- It is not known if drug can cause fetal harm.
- Use with caution only if benefit to mother outweighs potential risk to fetus.

LACTATION

- Drug is present in breast milk.
- Patient should check with prescriber before breastfeeding.

Nursing Considerations

- Use prazosin cautiously in patients with renal impairment because of increased sensitivity to prazosin's effects; in those with angina pectoris because drug may induce or aggravate angina; in those with narcolepsy because prazosin may worsen cataplexy; and in elderly patients because they're at increased risk for drug-induced hypotension.

- Monitor blood pressure regularly to evaluate effectiveness of therapy.

PATIENT TEACHING

- Emphasize need to take drug even if feeling well.
- Advise patient to avoid drinking alcohol, exercising in hot weather, or standing for long periods because these activities increase risk of orthostatic hypotension.
- Suggest rising slowly from lying or sitting position to minimize orthostatic hypotension.
- Urge patient to avoid hazardous activities until drug's CNS effects are known.
- Advise patient to notify prescriber immediately about adverse reactions, especially dizziness and fainting.
- Instruct patient not to take any drugs, including OTC forms, without consulting prescriber, to avoid serious interactions.
- Instruct male patient that a prolonged erection may occur with prazosin therapy. If it lasts longer than 4 hours, stress importance of seeking immediate medical assistance.

prednisolone
Delta-Cortef, Millipred

prednisolone sodium phosphate
Orapred ODT, Pediapred

Class and Category

Pharmacologic class: Glucocorticoid
Therapeutic class: Immunosuppressant

Indications and Dosages

✳ *To treat acute and chronic inflammatory and immunosuppressive disorders*

SYRUP, TABLETS (PREDNISOLONE); DISINTEGRATING TABLETS, ORAL SOLUTION (PREDNISOLONE SODIUM PHOSPHATE)

Adults. Highly individualized. *Dosage range:* 5 to 60 mg daily or in divided doses.
Children. *Initial:* 0.14 to 2 mg/kg/day divided and given 3 or 4 times daily. Then dosage adjusted, as needed. *Maintenance:* Gradual decrease in small decrements to lowest dose that maintains an adequate clinical response.

P

✳ *To treat acute exacerbations of multiple sclerosis*

SYRUP, TABLETS (PREDNISOLONE); DISINTEGRATING TABLETS, ORAL SOLUTION (PREDNISOLONE SODIUM PHOSPHATE)

Adults. 200 mg once daily for 1 wk, followed by 80 mg every other day for 1 mo.

✳ *To treat uncontrolled asthma in children taking inhaled corticosteroids and long-acting bronchodilators*

DISINTEGRATING TABLETS, ORAL SOLUTION (PREDNISOLONE SODIUM PHOSPHATE)

Children. 1 to 2 mg/kg once a day or in divided doses continued for 3 to 10 days but may be used longer, if needed.

✳ *To treat pediatric nephrotic syndrome*

DISINTEGRATING TABLETS, ORAL SOLUTION (PREDNISOLONE SODIUM PHOSPHATE)

Children. *Initial:* 60 mg/m^2/day divided into three doses for 4 wk, followed by 40 mg/m^2/day once every other day for 4 wks.

☰ Drug Administration

P.O.

- Administer once-daily dose in morning.
- Give with food to minimize GI upset.
- For oral solution, use the calibrated syringe that comes with it for measuring dosage. For syrup, use a calibrated device to measure dosage.
- For orally disintegrating tablets, do not remove tablet from blister pack until ready to administer. With dry, gloved hands, peel back the foil on the blister pack and carefully remove tablet. Do not push tablet through the foil because it can break easily. Place tablet on patient's tongue to dissolve completely. Patient may swallow after dissolution with saliva or with water. Tablet should not be broken, chewed, or crushed.

Route	Onset	Peak	Duration
P.O.	Rapid	1–2 hr	3–36 hr

Half-life: 2–3 hr

☰ Mechanism of Action

Binds to intracellular glucocorticoid receptors and suppresses inflammatory and immune responses by:

- inhibiting neutrophil and monocyte accumulation at inflammation site and suppressing their phagocytic and bactericidal activity
- stabilizing lysosomal membranes
- suppressing antigen response of macrophages and helper T cells
- inhibiting synthesis of inflammatory response mediators, such as cytokines, interleukins, and prostaglandins.

☰ Contraindications

Hypersensitivity to prednisolone or its components, idiopathic thrombocytopenic purpura (I.M. form), systemic fungal infection

☰ Interactions

DRUGS

aminoglutethimide: Possibly loss of induced adrenal suppression

amphotericin B, diuretics: Possibly severe hypokalemia

antacids, cholestyramine, colestipol: Decreased prednisolone absorption

anticholinesterase agents: Possibly severe weakness in patients with myasthenia gravis.

barbiturates, phenytoin, rifampin: Decreased prednisolone effects

cyclosporine: Increased risk of seizures

digoxin: Possibly arrhythmias and digitalis toxicity from hypokalemia

estrogens, oral contraceptives: Decreased clearance, increased elimination half-life, and increased therapeutic and toxic effects of prednisolone

insulin, oral antidiabetics: Increased risk of hyperglycemia

isoniazid, salicylates: Decreased blood level of these drugs

ketoconazole, macrolide antibiotics: Possibly decreased prednisolone metabolism

live or inactivated vaccines, toxoids: Possibly diminished response to vaccines or toxoids

NSAIDs: Increased risk of GI ulceration and bleeding, possibly added therapeutic effect when NSAIDs are used to treat arthritis

warfarin: Possibly inhibition of warfarin effect

FOODS

sodium-containing foods: Increased risk of edema and hypertension

ACTIVITIES

alcohol use: Increased risk of GI ulceration and bleeding

Adverse Reactions

CNS: Euphoria, headache, insomnia, nervousness, psychosis, restlessness, **seizures**, vertigo
CV: Edema, **heart failure**, hypertension
EENT: Cataracts, exophthalmos, glaucoma, increased ocular pressure
ENDO: Adrenal insufficiency, Cushing's syndrome, growth suppression in children, hyperglycemia
GI: Anorexia, **GI bleeding** and ulceration, increased appetite, indigestion, **intestinal perforation**, nausea, **pancreatitis**, vomiting
GU: Menstrual irregularities
MS: Avascular necrosis of joints, bone fractures, muscle atrophy or weakness, myalgia, osteoporosis
SKIN: Acne; diaphoresis; ecchymosis; flushing; petechiae; striae; thin, fragile skin
Other: Delayed wound healing, **hypernatremia, hypokalemia,** injection-site scarring, negative nitrogen balance

Childbearing Considerations

PREGNANCY

- Drug can cause fetal harm such as orofacial clefts when used in first trimester.
- Drug should be used with caution during pregnancy only if benefit to mother outweighs potential risk to fetus.
- Monitor infant for hypoadrenalism if mother has received large doses of drug during pregnancy.

LACTATION

- Drug is present in breast milk and, in high doses, could interfere with endogenous corticosteroid production, suppress growth, or cause other adverse effects in the breastfed infant.
- The lowest dose possible is recommended to minimize exposure to breastfed infant.

Nursing Considerations

! WARNING Avoid using prednisolone in patients with a history of active tuberculosis, because drug can reactivate the disease.

- Assess patient regularly for evidence of adverse reactions, including heart failure and hypertension. Also monitor patient's intake, output, and daily weight.
- Monitor growth pattern in children; prednisolone may retard bone growth.

- Be aware that prolonged use may cause hypothalamic-pituitary-adrenal suppression.

! WARNING Withdraw drug gradually, as ordered, if therapy lasts longer than 2 weeks. Stopping abruptly may cause acute adrenal insufficiency or, possibly, death.

- Be aware that patient may be at risk for emotional instability or psychic disturbance while taking prednisolone, especially if predisposed to them or taking high doses.

PATIENT TEACHING

- Instruct patient to take oral prednisolone with food to decrease stomach upset and to take once-daily dose in the morning.
- Emphasize need to take drug exactly as prescribed; taking too much increases risk of serious adverse reactions.
- Instruct patient taking orally disintegrating tablets to remove tablet from blister pack only when ready to take drug. With dry hands she should peel back foil on blister pack and remove tablet gently. Advise never to push tablet through the foil. Then patient should place tablet on tongue. Warn her not to break, cut, or split tablets.
- Advise patient taking oral solution to use the calibrated device packaged with the drug; if taking syrup, tell patient to measure dose with a calibrated device, not a household spoon.
- Caution patient not to discontinue drug abruptly.
- Urge patient to avoid alcohol during therapy because of increased risk of GI ulcers and bleeding.
- Urge patient to avoid hazardous activities until drug's CNS effects are known.
- Advise patient to avoid people with contagious infections because drug has an immunosuppressant effect. Urge her to notify prescriber immediately about exposure to measles or chickenpox.
- Caution against receiving vaccinations or other immunizations and coming in contact with people who have recently received oral poliovirus vaccine.
- Teach patient about potential side effects of prednisolone therapy, including restlessness, mood swings, nervousness, and delayed wound healing.

P

- Instruct patient to notify prescriber immediately about joint pain, swelling, tarry stools, and visual disturbances. Also instruct her to report signs of infection or injury for up to 12 months after therapy.
- Instruct diabetic patient to check her blood glucose level often because prednisolone may cause hyperglycemia.
- Advise patient to comply with follow-up visits to assess drug's effectiveness and detect adverse reactions.
- Urge patient to carry medical identification revealing prednisolone therapy.
- Advise female patients of childbearing age to notify prescriber immediately of suspected or known pregnancy.

prednisone
Prednisone Intensol, Rayos, Winpred (CAN)

Class and Category
Pharmacologic class: Glucocorticoid
Therapeutic class: Immunosuppressant

Indications and Dosages
✳ *To treat adrenal insufficiency and acute and chronic inflammatory and immunosuppressive disorders*

DELAYED-RELEASE TABLETS, ORAL SOLUTION, TABLETS
Adults and children. Highly individualized. *Range:* 5 to 60 mg daily as a single dose or in divided doses.

✳ *To treat acute exacerbations of multiple sclerosis*

DELAYED-RELEASE TABLETS, ORAL SOLUTION, TABLETS
Adults. 200 mg daily for 1 wk, then 80 mg every other day for 1 mo.

Drug Administration
P.O.
- Administer once-daily doses in the morning to match body's normal cortisol secretion schedule.
- Administer drug with food or milk to minimize GI upset.
- Delayed-release tablets should be swallowed whole and not broken, chewed, or crushed.
- For oral solution, use a calibrated device to measure dosage. Store at room temperature,

protected from light. Discard 90 days after opening container of oral solution.

Route	Onset	Peak	Duration
P.O.	Unknown	2 hr	Unknown
P.O./E.R.	4 hr	6–6.5 hr	Unknown

Half-life: 2–3 hr

Mechanism of Action
Binds to intracellular glucocorticoid receptors and suppresses inflammatory and immune responses by:
- inhibiting neutrophil and monocyte accumulation at inflammation site and suppressing their phagocytic and bactericidal activity
- stabilizing lysosomal membranes
- suppressing antigen response of macrophages and helper T cells
- inhibiting synthesis of inflammatory response mediators, such as cytokines, interleukins, and prostaglandins.

Contraindications
Hypersensitivity to prednisone or its components, systemic fungal infection

Interactions
DRUGS
aminoglutethimide: Possibly loss of corticosteroid-induced adrenal suppression
amphotericin B (parenteral): Possibly development of cardiac enlargement and congestive heart failure
anticholinesterase agents: Possibly severe weakness in patients with myasthenia gravis
cholestyramine: Increased clearance of prednisone
cyclosporine: Increased risk of seizures
CYP3A4 inducers (barbiturates, phenytoin, carbamazepine, rifampin): Increased metabolism of prednisone
CYP3A4 inhibitors (ketoconazole, macrolide antibiotics): Decreased prednisone metabolism
digoxin: Possibly arrhythmias and digitalis toxicity from hypokalemia
diuretics: Possibly decreased natriuretic and diuretic effects of diuretics, severe hypokalemia (with potassium-depleting diuretics)
estrogens, oral contraceptives: Decreased clearance, increased elimination half-life,

and increased therapeutic and toxic effects of prednisone

insulin, oral antidiabetic agents: Possibly less effective, causing increased blood glucose levels

isoniazid: Decreased blood isoniazid level

NSAIDs: Increased risk of GI ulceration and bleeding, possibly added therapeutic effect when NSAIDs are used to treat arthritis

toxoids, vaccines: Possibly loss of antibody response, increased risk of neurologic complications

warfarin: Increased risk of reduced effectiveness of warfarin

FOODS

sodium-containing foods: Increased risk of edema and hypertension

ACTIVITIES

alcohol use: Increased risk of GI ulceration and bleeding

Adverse Reactions

CNS: Euphoria, headache, insomnia, nervousness, psychosis, restlessness, **seizures**, vertigo

CV: Edema, **heart failure**, hypertension

EENT: Cataracts, exophthalmos, glaucoma, increased ocular pressure

ENDO: Adrenal insufficiency, Cushing's syndrome, growth suppression in children, hyperglycemia

GI: Anorexia, **GI bleeding** and ulceration, increased appetite, indigestion, **intestinal perforation**, nausea, **pancreatitis**, vomiting

GU: Menstrual irregularities

MS: Avascular necrosis of joints, bone fractures, muscle atrophy or weakness, myalgia, osteoporosis

SKIN: Acne; diaphoresis; ecchymosis; flushing; petechiae; striae; thin, fragile skin

Other: Delayed wound healing, **hypernatremia, hypokalemia,** negative nitrogen balance

Childbearing Considerations

PREGNANCY

- It is not known if drug can cause fetal harm, although animal studies suggest a higher risk for cleft palate.
- Drug should be used with caution during pregnancy only if benefit to mother outweighs potential risk to fetus.
- Monitor infant for hypoadrenalism if mother has received large doses of drug during pregnancy.

LACTATION

- Drug is present in breast milk and high doses could interfere with endogenous corticosteroid production, suppress growth, or cause other adverse effects in the breastfed infant.
- Lowest dose of drug used to minimize exposure to breastfed infant.

Nursing Considerations

- Assess patient for adverse reactions, especially signs and symptoms of such reactions as heart failure and hypertension. Also monitor fluid intake and output and daily weight.
- Monitor growth pattern in children. Prednisone may retard bone growth.
- Be aware that prolonged use of prednisone may cause hypothalamic-pituitary-adrenal suppression.

! **WARNING** Withdraw prednisone gradually, as ordered, if therapy lasts longer than 2 weeks. Stopping abruptly may cause acute adrenal insufficiency and, possibly, death.

PATIENT TEACHING

- Instruct patient to take prednisone with food to decrease GI distress and to take once-daily dose in the morning.
- Emphasize importance of taking drug exactly as prescribed; taking more than prescribed increases risk of serious adverse reactions.
- Tell patient prescribed delayed-release tablet form not to break, divide, or chew tablet because the delayed-release action is dependent on an intact coating.
- Caution patient not to stop drug abruptly.
- Urge patient to avoid alcohol during therapy because of increased risk of GI ulcers and bleeding.
- Urge patient to avoid hazardous activities until drug's CNS effects are known.
- Advise patient to avoid people with contagious infections because drug has an immunosuppressant effect. Urge her to notify prescriber immediately about possible exposure to measles or chickenpox.
- Caution against receiving vaccinations or other immunizations and coming in contact with people who have recently received oral poliovirus vaccine.

P

- Instruct patient to notify prescriber immediately about joint pain, swelling, tarry stools, and visual disturbances. Also instruct her to report signs of infection or injury for up to 12 months after therapy.
- Instruct diabetic patient to check blood glucose level often because prednisone may cause hyperglycemia.
- Advise patient to comply with follow-up visits to assess drug effectiveness and detect adverse reactions.
- Urge patient to carry medical identification revealing prednisone therapy.
- Advise patient to notify prescriber if pregnancy is suspected or known.

pregabalin
Lyrica, Lyrica CR

Class, Category, and Schedule
Pharmacologic class: Gamma-aminobutyric acid (GABA) analogue
Therapeutic class: Analgesic, anticonvulsant
Controlled substance schedule: V

Indications and Dosages
✷ *To relieve neuropathic pain associated with diabetic peripheral neuropathy*

CAPSULES, ORAL SOLUTION

Adults. *Initial:* 50 mg three times a day, increased to 100 mg three times a day, within 1 wk as needed. *Maximum:* 300 mg daily.

E.R. TABLETS

Adults. *Initial:* 165 mg once daily, then increased to 330 mg once daily within 1 wk, as needed and tolerated. *Maximum:* 330 mg once daily.

✷ *To relieve postherpetic neuralgia*

CAPSULES, ORAL SOLUTION

Adults. *Initial:* 75 mg twice daily or 50 mg three times a day, increased to 150 mg twice daily or 100 mg three times a day within 1 wk as needed. Then increased to 300 mg twice daily or 200 mg three times a day in 2 to 4 wk as needed.

E.R. TABLETS

Adults. *Initial* 165 mg once daily, then increased to 330 mg once daily within 1 wk, as needed and tolerated. Dosage further increased to 660 mg once daily after 2 to 4 wk, if needed and tolerated. Maximum: 660 mg once daily.

✷ *As adjunct therapy to manage partial-onset seizures*

CAPSULES, ORAL SOLUTION

Adults and adolescents 17 years and older. *Initial:* 150 mg daily in two or three divided doses, then increased as needed. *Maximum:* 600 mg daily in two or three divided doses.
Children weighing 30 kg (66 lb) or more. *Initial:* 2.5 mg/kg/day in two or three divided doses, then increased as needed. *Maximum:* 10 mg/kg/day in two or three divided doses, not to exceed 600 mg/day.
Children age 4 and over weighing less than 30 kg (66 lb). *Initial:* 3.5 mg/kg/day in two or three divided doses. *Maximum:* 14 mg/kg/day in two or three divided doses.
Infants and children age 1 month and over weighing less than 30 kg (66 lb). *Initial:* 3.5 mg/kg/day in three divided doses. *Maximum:* 14 mg/kg/day in three divided doses.

✷ *To manage fibromyalgia*

CAPSULES, ORAL SOLUTION

Adults. *Initial:* 75 mg twice daily, increased to 150 mg twice daily in 1 wk, as needed, and then to 225 mg twice daily in 1 wk as needed. *Maximum:* 450 mg daily.

✷ *To manage neuropathic pain associated with spinal cord injury*

CAPSULES, ORAL SOLUTION

Adults. *Initial:* 75 mg twice daily, increased to 150 mg twice daily in 1 wk, as needed, and then to 300 mg twice daily after 2 to 3 wk, as needed.

±**DOSAGE ADJUSTMENT** For adult patient with renal impairment with a creatinine clearance of 30 to 60 ml/min, daily dosage reduced by 50%. Extended-release pregabalin should not be given to patients with creatinine clearance less than 30 ml/min. If clearance is 15 to 30 ml/min, daily dosage of immediate-release form reduced by 75% and frequency reduced to once or twice daily. If clearance is less than 15 ml/min, daily dosage of immediate-release form reduced to as low as 25 mg daily. If patient is having hemodialysis, daily dosage of immediate-release form is reduced and supplemental dose given immediately after every 4-hour hemodialysis session as follows: If reduced daily dosage is 25 mg daily, give supplemental dose of 25 or 50 mg. If reduced daily dosage is 25 to 50 mg daily, give supplemental dose of 50 or 75 mg. If

reduced daily dosage is 50 to 75 mg daily,
give supplemental dose of 75 or 100 mg.
If reduced daily dosage is 75 mg,
give supplemental dose of 100 or 150 mg.

Drug Administration

P.O.

- Use calibrated device to measure dosage of oral solution.
- Extended-release tablets and capsules should be swallowed whole and not chewed, crushed, or split.
- Administer extended-release tablets after evening meal.
- When converting patient from immediate-release formulation to extended-release formulation, administer morning dose of immediate-release pregabalin and then administer first dose of extended-release form in the evening on the day of the switch following manufacturer guidelines for dosage conversion.
- Do not stop drug therapy abruptly; taper gradually over a minimum of 1 week, as ordered.

Route	Onset	Peak	Duration
P.O.	Unknown	1.5–3 hr	Unknown
P.O./E.R.	Unknown	8–12 hr	Unknown

Half-life: 6.3 hr

Mechanism of Action

Binds to alpha$_2$-delta site, an auxiliary subunit of voltage calcium channels, in CNS tissue where it may reduce calcium-dependent release of several neurotransmitters, possibly by modulating calcium channel function. With fewer neurotransmitters, pain sensation and seizure activity decline.

Contraindications

Hypersensitivity to pregabalin or its components

Interactions

DRUGS

CNS depressants: Increased risk of additive CNS adverse reactions such as dizziness, respiratory depression, or somnolence
lorazepam, oxycodone: Additive effects on cognitive and gross motor function
opioid analgesics: Increased risk of constipation, intestinal obstruction, or paralytic ileus

ACTIVITIES

alcohol use: Additive effects on cognitive and gross motor function

Adverse Reactions

CNS: Abnormal gait, amnesia, anxiety, asthenia, ataxia, balance disorder, confusion, depression, difficulty concentrating, dizziness, euphoria, extrapyramidal syndrome, fatigue, fever, headache, hypertonia, hypesthesia, incoordination, **intracranial hypertension**, myoclonus, nervousness, neuropathy, paresthesia, psychotic depression, schizophrenic reaction, somnolence, stupor, **suicidal ideation**, tremor, twitching, vertigo
CV: Chest pain, **heart failure**, peripheral edema, **ventricular fibrillation**
EENT: Amblyopia, blurred vision, conjunctivitis, decreased visual acuity, diplopia, dry mouth, nystagmus, otitis media, sinusitis, tinnitus, visual field defect
ENDO: Gynecomastia, **hypoglycemia**
GI: Abdominal distention or pain, constipation, diarrhea, flatulence, gastroenteritis, **GI hemorrhage**, increased appetite, nausea, vomiting
GU: **Acute renal failure**, anorgasmia, decreased libido, impotence, **nephritis**, urinary frequency, urinary incontinence, urine retention
HEME: **Leukopenia, thrombocytopenia**
MS: Arthralgia, back pain, elevated creatine kinase level, leg or muscle cramps, myalgia, myasthenia
RESP: Apnea, dyspnea, pneumonia, **respiratory depression (could be severe)**
SKIN: Bullous pemphigoid, ecchymosis, **exfoliative dermatitis**, pruritus, **Stevens–Johnson syndrome**
Other: **Anaphylaxis, angioedema, hypersensitivity reactions**, increased risk of viral infection, weight gain

Childbearing Considerations

PREGNANCY

- Pregnancy exposure registry: 1-888-233-2334 or http://www.aedpregnancyregistry.org/.
- Drug can cause fetal harm based on animal studies.
- Use with caution only if benefit to mother outweighs potential risk to fetus.

LACTATION

- Drug is present in breast milk.

P

- Breastfeeding is not recommended because of the potential risk of tumorigenicity in the breastfed infant.

REPRODUCTION

- Drug may cause a reduction in sperm concentration by 50% or more.

⬛ Nursing Considerations

- Know that pregabalin therapy should be stopped gradually over at least 1 week to decrease risk of seizure activity and avoid unpleasant symptoms such as diarrhea, headache, insomnia, and nausea.

! WARNING Be aware that if patient has evidence of hypersensitivity (dyspnea, facial swelling, rash, red skin, urticaria, wheezing) drug should be stopped at once; notify prescriber, and give supportive care.

- Monitor patient closely for adverse reactions. Notify prescriber if significant adverse reactions persist. Be aware that children younger than 4 years have a higher change of experiencing pneumonia, somnolence, or viral infection.
- Monitor patient closely for evidence of suicidal behavior or thinking, especially when therapy starts or dosage changes.

PATIENT TEACHING

- Instruct patient prescribed extended-release tablets not to chew, crush, or split tablets but to swallow tablets whole. Tell patient to take tablets after evening meal.
- Tell patient that if dose of extended-release formulation is missed, patient should take the missed dose prior to bedtime following a snack.
- Tell patient converting from immediate-release formulation to extended release to take morning dose of immediate-release pregabalin and take first dose of extended-release form in the evening on the day of the switch.
- Warn against stopping pregabalin abruptly. Tell patient that when pregabalin is no longer needed, the dosage should be tapered gradually over a minimum of one week before it is discontinued.

! WARNING Instruct patient to seek immediate emergency care if a serious allergic reaction occurs.

! WARNING Monitor patient's respiratory status closely, because respiratory depression that can become life-threatening has occurred with drug administration. Increased risk includes patients who are also taking other central nervous system depressants, including opioids, or patient who has an existing respiratory impairment disorder. If patient shows signs of respiratory depression and sedation, notify prescriber and expect dosage to be decreased or drug discontinued.

- Urge patient to avoid hazardous activities until she knows how drug affects her.
- Instruct patient to notify prescriber if she has changes in vision or unexplained muscle pain, tenderness, or weakness, especially if these muscle symptoms are accompanied by fever or malaise.
- Alert patient that drug may cause edema and weight gain.
- Tell patient who also takes a thiazolidinedione antidiabetic that these effects may be intensified. If significant, tell patient to notify prescriber.
- Inform male patient who plans to father a child that drug could impair his fertility.
- Instruct diabetic patients to inspect their skin while taking pregabalin.
- Urge caregivers to watch patient closely for evidence of suicidal tendencies, especially when therapy starts or dosage changes and to report concerns at once to prescriber.

probenecid
Benuryl (CAN), Probalan

⬛ Class and Category
Pharmacologic class: Sulfonamide derivative
Therapeutic class: Uricosuric

⬛ Indications and Dosages
✳ *To treat hyperuricemia due to chronic gout or gouty arthritis*

TABLETS

Adults and adolescents. *Initial:* 250 mg twice daily for 1 wk; then increased to 500 mg twice daily. Further increases may be made in 500-mg increments every 4 weeks if symptoms are not controlled or the 24-hour uric acid excretion is not above 700 mg. If no acute attacks of gout occur over next 6 mo

and serum uric acid level is within normal limits, dosage decreased by 500 mg every 6 mo until lowest effective maintenance dose is reached.
Maximum: 2 g daily.

* *As adjunct to antibiotic therapy with ampicillin, cloxacillin, methicillin, nafcillin, oxacillin, or penicillin*

TABLETS
Adults, adolescents age 14 and over, and children weighing more than 50 kg (110 lb). 500 mg four times a day.
Children ages 2 to 14 weighing up to 50 kg. 25 mg/kg as single dose, then 10 mg/kg four times a day.

Drug Administration
P.O.
- Administer drug with meals, if patient develops an upset stomach.
- Ensure patient is drinking plenty of water.
- Administer at least 30 minutes before antibiotic therapy if antibiotic is given I.M. or I.V.

Route	Onset	Peak	Duration
P.O.	0.5–2 hr	2–4 hr	8 hr

Half-life: 4–12 hr

Mechanism of Action
Increases urinary excretion of uric acid and lowers serum uric acid level, which may prevent or resolve urate deposits, tophus formation, and joint changes. Eventually, incidence of acute gout attacks decreases. Probenecid also inhibits renal excretion of penicillins and some cephalosporins, thereby increasing their serum concentration and prolonging their duration of action.

Contraindications
Acute gouty attacks (therapy not initiated), age less than 2 years, blood dyscrasias, hypersensitivity to probenecid or its components, renal calculi (urate)

Interactions
DRUGS
acetaminophen, indomethacin, ketoprofen, lorazepam, meclofenamate, methotrexate, naproxen, penicillin or other beta-lactams, rifampin, sulindac, sulfonamides: Possibly increased concentrations and adverse effects of these drugs

salicylates: Antagonized the uricosuric action of probenecid
thiopental: Increased plasma concentration of thiopental, which significantly requires reduced dosage for induction of anesthesia
theophylline: Possibly falsely high readings for theophylline using the Schack and Waxler technique

Adverse Reactions
CNS: Dizziness, headache
EENT: Sore gums
GI: Anorexia, nausea, vomiting
GU: Hematuria, renal calculi (urate), renal colic, urinary frequency
MS: Costovertebral pain; joint pain, redness, and swelling
SKIN: Facial flushing, pruritus, rash, urticaria

Childbearing Considerations
PREGNANCY
- It is not known if drug can cause fetal harm, although it does cross the placental barrier.
- Use with caution only if benefit to mother outweighs potential risk to fetus.

LACTATION
- Drug is present in breast milk.
- Patient should check with prescriber before breastfeeding.

Nursing Considerations
- Be aware that probenecid therapy shouldn't start until acute gout attack has subsided. If acute attack starts during therapy, continue therapy as prescribed.
- Use drug cautiously in patients with peptic ulcer disease.
- Expect to give sodium bicarbonate (3 to 7.5 g daily) or potassium citrate (7.5 g daily), as prescribed, to keep urine alkaline and prevent renal calculus formation.
- Monitor CBC, serum uric acid level, and liver and renal function test results during therapy.
- Closely monitor patients receiving intermittent therapy because they're more likely to develop allergic reactions.

PATIENT TEACHING
- Advise patient to take probenecid with meals to minimize GI distress.
- Encourage patient to increase fluid intake (up to 3 L daily, if not contraindicated) to help prevent renal calculus formation.

- Instruct patient to notify prescriber immediately if she has signs of an acute gout attack (joint pain, swelling, and redness) or of renal calculi (flank pain and blood in urine).
- Caution patient against taking salicylates while taking probenecid. Instead, advise acetaminophen to treat mild pain or fever.

procainamide hydrochloride

Class and Category
Pharmacologic class: Sodium channel blocker of cardiomyocytes
Therapeutic class: Antiarrhythmic (Class 1a)

Indications and Dosages
✱ *To treat life-threatening ventricular arrhythmias*

I.V. INFUSION OR INJECTION
Adults. *Initial loading dose:* 100 mg every 5 min until arrhythmia is controlled or maximum total dose of 500 mg is reached and given at a rate not to exceed 50 mg/min. Dosing should not be resumed for at least 10 minutes or longer at this point. Alternatively, 20 mg and given at a constant rate of 1 ml/min for 25 to 30 min. *Maintenance:* 2 to 6 mg/min by continuous infusion. *Maximum:* 1 gram.

✱ *To treat ventricular extrasystoles and arrhythmias associated with anesthesia and surgery*

I.M. INJECTION
Adults. 100 to 500 mg.

✱ *To treat less life-threatening arrhythmias in patients who are nauseated or vomiting, who are receiving nothing by mouth preoperatively, or who may have malabsorptive problems*

I.M. INJECTION
Adults. *Initial:* 50 mg/kg daily and divided into fractional doses of one-eighth to one-fourth given every 3 to 6 hr.

±**DOSAGE ADJUSTMENT** For elderly patients or those with hepatic or renal insufficiency, dosage possibly reduced or dosing intervals increased.

Drug Administration
- Place patient in a supine position before giving procainamide I.M. or I.V., to minimize hypotensive effects. Monitor

blood pressure often and ECG tracings continuously during administration and for 30 minutes afterward.
- Inspect parenteral solution for particles and discoloration before giving drug; discard if particles are present or solution is darker than light amber.

I.V.
- For I.V. injection as a loading dose, dilute procainamide with 5% Dextrose Injection according to manufacturer's instructions and inject into a vein or tubing of an established I.V. line slowly at a rate not to exceed 50 mg/minute.
- For I.V. infusion as a loading dose, dilute 1 gram with 50 ml 5% Dextrose Injection to a concentration of 20 mg/ml. Administer at a constant rate of 1 ml/min for 25 to 30 minutes.
- Administer I.V. infusion with an infusion pump or other controlled-delivery device.
- For I.V. infusion as a maintenance dose, dilute 1,000 mg of drug in 500 ml of 5% Dextrose Injection, which will produce a concentration of 2 mg/ml. Administer at a rate of 1 to 3 ml/min. However, if fluid intake must be limited, a 4 mg/ml concentration may be used by diluting 1 gram of drug in 250 ml of 5% Dextrose Injection and administering at 0.5 to 1.5 ml/min, which will deliver 2 to 6 mg/min.
- Don't infuse or inject more than recommended amount per minute because heart block or cardiac arrest may occur.
- *Incompatibilities:* None listed by manufacturer

I.M.
- Use I.M. route only if I.V. route is not feasible, because injection is painful.
- Inject deeply into a large muscle mass.
- Rotate injection sites.

Route	Onset	Peak	Duration
I.V.	Immediate	Immediate	Unknown
I.M.	10–30 min	15–60 min	Unknown

Half-life: 2.5–4.7 hr

Mechanism of Action
Prolongs recovery period after myocardial repolarization by inhibiting sodium influx through myocardial cell membranes. This action prolongs refractory period, causing

myocardial automaticity, excitability, and conduction velocity to decline.

Contraindications

Complete heart block, hypersensitivity to procainamide or its components, systemic lupus erythematosus, torsades de pointes

Interactions

DRUGS

antiarrhythmics: Additive cardiac effects
anticholinergics: Additive antivagal effects on A-V nodal conduction
neuromuscular blockers: Possibly increased or prolonged neuromuscular blockade

Adverse Reactions

CNS: Chills, disorientation, dizziness, light-headedness
CV: Heart block (second-degree), hypotension, pericarditis, prolonged QT interval, tachycardia
EENT: Bitter taste
GI: Abdominal distress, anorexia, diarrhea, nausea, vomiting
HEME: Agranulocytosis, neutropenia, thrombocytopenia
MS: Arthralgia, myalgia
RESP: Pleural effusion
SKIN: Pruritus, rash
Other: Drug-induced fever

Childbearing Considerations

PREGNANCY

- It is not known if drug can cause fetal harm.
- Use with caution only if benefit to mother outweighs potential risk to fetus.

LACTATION

- Drug is present in breast milk.
- A decision may have to be made to discontinue breastfeeding or the drug to avoid potential serious adverse reactions in the breastfed infant.

Nursing Considerations

- Know that if drug is to be given I.M. and patient's platelet count is below 50,000/mm³, notify prescriber at once because patient may develop bleeding, bruising, or hematomas from procainamide-induced bone marrow suppression and thrombocytopenia. Expect to give procainamide I.V.
- Anticipate that patient has reached maximum clinical response when ventricular tachycardia resolves,

hypotension develops, or QRS complex is 50% wider than original width.
- Monitor patient's CBC because drug can cause serious hematologic adverse effects such as agranulocytosis, neutropenia, and thrombocytopenia. Maintain infection control measures.

PATIENT TEACHING

- Advise patient to notify prescriber immediately about bruising, chills, diarrhea, fever, or rash.

prochlorperazine
Compro

prochlorperazine edisylate

prochlorperazine maleate

Class and Category

Pharmacologic class: Piperazine phenothiazine
Therapeutic class: Antiemetic

Indications and Dosages

✷ *To control nausea and vomiting related to surgery*

I.V. INFUSION OR INJECTION (PROCHLORPERAZINE EDISYLATE)

Adults. 5 to 10 mg at a rate not to exceed 5 mg/ml 15 to 30 min before anesthesia as needed. Dosage repeated once, if necessary. *Maximum:* 10 mg/dose, 40 mg daily.

I.M. INJECTION (PROCHLORPERAZINE EDISYLATE)

Adults. 5 to 10 mg 1 to 2 hr before anesthesia as needed. Repeated once in 30 min, if needed. *Maximum:* 10 mg/dose, 40 mg daily.

✷ *To control severe nausea and vomiting*

TABLETS (PROCHLORPERAZINE MALEATE)

Adults and adolescents. 5 to 10 mg three times a day or four times a day. *Maximum:* 40 mg daily.
Children age 2 and over weighing 18 kg (40 lb) to 38.5 kg (85 lb). 2.5 mg three times

P

a day or 5 mg two times a day. *Maximum:* 15 mg daily.

Children age 2 and over weighing 13.5 kg (30 lb) to 17 kg (39 lb). 2.5 mg two or three times daily. *Maximum:* 10 mg daily.

Children age 2 and over weighing 9 kg (20 lb) to 13 kg (29 lb). 2.5 mg once or twice daily. *Maximum:* 7.5 mg daily.

I.V. INFUSION OR INJECTION (PROCHLORPERAZINE EDISYLATE)

Adults. 2.5 to 10 mg at a rate not to exceed 5 mg/min. *Maximum:* 10 mg/dose; 40 mg daily.

I.M. INJECTION (PROCHLORPERAZINE EDISYLATE)

Adults and adolescents. 5 to 10 mg every 3 to 4 hr, as needed. *Maximum:* 40 mg daily.

Children ages 2 to 12. 0.132 mg/kg (0.06 mg/lb), then switched to oral form as soon as possible, usually after one dose.

SUPPOSITORIES (PROCHLORPERAZINE)

Adults. 25 mg twice daily.

✳ *To manage schizophrenia*

TABLETS (PROCHLORPERAZINE MALEATE)

Adults and adolescents. 5 to 10 mg three times a day or four times a day, increased gradually every 2 to 3 days, as needed and tolerated. *Maximum:* 150 mg daily.

Children age 2 to 12 years. *Initial:* 2.5 mg two or three times daily (maximum 10 mg first day), then increased, as needed. *Maximum:* For children 6 to 12, total daily dose of 25 mg beginning day 2 and onward, for children age 2 to 6, total daily dose of 20 mg beginning day 2 and onward.

I.M. INJECTION (PROCHLORPERAZINE EDISYLATE)

Adults and adolescents. *Initial:* 10 to 20 mg, repeated every 2 to 4 hr (or in resistant cases every hr), as needed, to bring symptoms under control (usually 3 to 4 doses). Then switched to oral dosing as soon as possible. *Maintenance:* If unable to switch to oral form, continue with 10 to 20 mg every 4 to 6 hr.

Children ages 2 to 12. 0.132 mg/kg (0.06 mg/lb) then switched to oral form as soon as possible, usually after one dose.

✳ *To treat non-psychotic anxiety*

TABLETS (PROCHLORPERAZINE MALEATE)

Adults. 5 mg three times daily or four times daily. *Maximum:* 20 mg daily for no longer than 12 wk.

±**DOSAGE ADJUSTMENT** Initial dose usually reduced and subsequent dosage increased more gradually for elderly, emaciated, and debilitated patients.

Drug Administration

P.O.
- Can be administered with or without food.

I.V.
- May be given undiluted as injection or diluted in 0.9% Sodium Chloride Injection when administered as an infusion.
- Administer slowly at no more than 5 mg/min as an injection or infusion.
- Never give as a I.V. bolus.
- Monitor patient for hypotension, as risk is higher with I.V. administration.
- Avoid contact between skin and solution because contact dermatitis could result.
- Protect drug from light.
- Parenteral solution may develop slight yellowing that won't affect potency. Don't use if discoloration is pronounced or precipitate is present.
- *Incompatibilities:* Other I.V. drugs

I.M.
- Inject slowly, deep into upper outer quadrant of buttocks.
- Rotate I.M. injection sites to prevent irritation and sterile abscesses.
- Avoid contact between skin and solution, because contact dermatitis could result.

P.R.
- If too soft, refrigerate drug for 30 minutes or run under cold water while still wrapped.
- Moisten suppository with water before insertion.

Route	Onset	Peak	Duration
P.O.	30–40 min	Unknown	3–4 hr
I.V.	Unknown	30–60 min	Unknown
I.M.	1–20 min	Unknown	3–4 hr
P.R.	1 hr	Unknown	3–12 hr

Half-life: 6–10 hr

Mechanism of Action

Alleviates psychotic symptoms by blocking dopamine receptors, depressing release of selected hormones, and producing alpha-adrenergic blocking effect in the brain.

Prochlorperazine also alleviates nausea and vomiting by centrally blocking dopamine receptors in the medullary chemoreceptor trigger zone and by peripherally blocking the vagus nerve in the GI tract.

Anticholinergic effects and alpha-adrenergic blockade reduce anxiety by decreasing arousal and filtering internal stimuli to the brain stem reticular activating system.

Contraindications

Age less than 2 years; coma, hypersensitivity to prochlorperazine, other phenothiazines or their components; pediatric surgery; severe CNS depression; use of large quantities of CNS depressants; weight less than 9 kg (20 lb)

Interactions

DRUGS

anticonvulsants: Possibly lowered seizure threshold by prochlorperazine
antihypertensives such as guanethidine and related compounds: Possibly action of these drugs may be counteracted by prochlorperazine
CNS depressants: Possibly intensify or prolong action of these drugs
oral anticoagulants: Possibly diminished effects of oral anticoagulants
phenytoin: Possible interference with phenytoin metabolism leading to phenytoin toxicity
propranolol: Increased plasma levels of both drugs
thiazide diuretics: Possibly accentuate orthostatic hypotension

ACTIVITIES

alcohol use: Additive CNS depression

Adverse Reactions

CNS: Akathisia, altered temperature regulation, dizziness, drowsiness, extrapyramidal reactions (such as dystonia, pseudoparkinsonism, tardive dyskinesia)
CV: **Hypotension,** orthostatic hypotension, tachycardia
EENT: Blurred vision, dry mouth, nasal congestion, ocular changes, pigmentary retinopathy
ENDO: Galactorrhea, gynecomastia

GI: Constipation, epigastric pain, nausea, vomiting
GU: Dysuria, ejaculation disorders, menstrual irregularities, urine retention
SKIN: Decreased sweating, photosensitivity, pruritus, rash
Other: Weight gain

Childbearing Considerations

PREGNANCY

- Drug may cause fetal harm.
- Neonates exposed to drug during the third trimester of pregnancy are at risk for extrapyramidal and withdrawal symptoms after birth.
- Use with caution only if benefit to mother outweighs potential risk to fetus.

LACTATION

- Drug may be present in breast milk.
- Patient should check with prescriber before breastfeeding.

Nursing Considerations

- Be aware that prochlorperazine shouldn't be used to treat dementia-related psychosis in the elderly because of increased mortality risk.

> **! WARNING** Monitor closely for numerous adverse reactions that may be serious.

PATIENT TEACHING

- Instruct patient using suppository to refrigerate it for 30 minutes or hold it under running cold water before removing the wrapper if it softens during storage.
- Teach patient correct administration technique for suppository.
- Caution patient on long-term therapy not to stop prochlorperazine abruptly; doing so may lead to such adverse reactions as nausea, trembling, and vomiting.
- Urge patient to avoid alcohol and OTC drugs that may contain CNS depressants.
- Advise patient to rise slowly from lying and sitting positions to minimize effects of orthostatic hypotension.
- Urge patient to avoid hazardous activities because of the risk of drowsiness and impaired judgment and coordination.
- Instruct patient to avoid excessive sun exposure and to wear sunscreen outdoors.
- Urge patient to notify prescriber about involuntary movements and restlessness.

P

progestins
levonorgestrel

medroxyprogester-
one acetate
Alti-MPA (CAN), Provera

megestrol acetate
Megace OS (CAN)

norethindrone
acetate
Aygestin, Norlutate (CAN)

progesterone
Crinone, PMS-Progesterone (CAN), Prometrium

▤ Class and Category
Pharmacologic class: Progesterone hormone
Therapeutic class: Ovarian hormone replacement

▤ Indications and Dosages
✳ *As adjunct to treat metastatic renal cancer*

I.M. INJECTION (MEDROXYPROGESTERONE)
Adults. *Initial:* 400 mg to 1 g every wk until improvement and stabilization. *Maintenance:* 400 mg or more every mo.

✳ *To treat metastatic breast cancer*

TABLETS (MEGESTROL)
Adults. 40 mg four times daily.

✳ *As adjunct to treat metastatic endometrial cancer*

TABLETS (MEGESTROL)
Adult women. 40 to 320 mg daily in divided doses.

I.M. INJECTION (MEDROXYPROGESTERONE)
Adults. *Initial:* 400 mg to 1 g every wk until improvement and stabilization. *Maintenance:* 400 mg or more every mo.

✳ *To treat anorexia, cachexia, or significant weight loss in patients who have AIDS*

SUSPENSION (MEGESTROL)
Adults. 800 mg daily for the first mo, and then 400 or 800 mg daily for the next 3 mo.

✳ *To treat endometriosis*

TABLETS (NORETHINDRONE ACETATE)
Adult women. *Initial:* 5 mg daily for 2 wk, increased by 2.5 mg daily at 2-wk intervals to total dose of 15 mg daily. *Maintenance:* 15 mg daily for 6 to 9 mo unless temporarily discontinued because of breakthrough menstrual bleeding.

✳ *To treat secondary amenorrhea*

TABLETS (MEDROXYPROGESTERONE)
Adult women. 5 to 10 mg daily for 5 to 10 days, starting anytime during menstrual cycle.

TABLETS (NORETHINDRONE ACETATE)
Adult women. 2.5 to 10 mg daily for 5 to 10 days during last half of menstrual cycle.

CAPSULES, TABLETS (PROGESTERONE)
Adult women. 400 mg daily at bedtime for 10 days.

I.M. INJECTION (PROGESTERONE)
Adult women. 5 to 10 mg daily for 6 to 8 days.

VAGINAL GEL (PROGESTERONE)
Adult women. 45 mg (1 applicatorful of 4% vaginal gel) every other day for up to 6 doses. Dosage increased, as needed, to 90 mg (1 applicatorful of 8% vaginal gel) every other day for up to 6 doses.

✳ *To treat dysfunctional uterine bleeding*

TABLETS (MEDROXYPROGESTERONE)
Adult women. 5 to 10 mg daily for 5 to 10 days, starting on day 16 or 21 of menstrual cycle.

TABLETS (NORETHINDRONE ACETATE)
Adult women. 2.5 to 10 mg daily for 5 to 10 days during last half of menstrual cycle.

I.M. INJECTION (PROGESTERONE)
Adult women. 5 to 10 mg daily for 6 consecutive days.

✳ *To reduce endometrial hyperplasia in nonhysterectomized postmenopausal women receiving daily oral conjugated estrogen therapy,*

TABLETS (MEDROXYPROGESTERONE)
Postmenopausal women with intact uterus. 5 to 10 mg for 12 to 14 consecutive days each

month, either beginning on the 1st day of the cycle or the 16th day of the cycle.

CAPSULES, TABLETS (PROGESTERONE)

Postmenopausal women with intact uterus. 200 mg once day at bedtime for 12 consecutive days per 28-day cycle.

* *To prevent pregnancy (postcoital)*

TABLETS (LEVONORGESTREL)

Adult and adolescent women. 0.75 mg as soon as possible within 72 hr of intercourse. Second dose given 12 hr later.

Drug Administration

- Drug is a hazardous drug requiring safe handling and disposal precautions.
- Pregnant women should avoid exposure to drug.

P.O.

- Administer tablets and capsules with a full glass of water.
- Administer progesterone at night because it can make patient dizzy or drowsy.
- Give medroxyprogesterone immediately before or after a meal to increase its bioavailability.
- Shake container vigorously for at least 1 minute for oral suspension form. Use a calibrated device to measure dose. Store at room temperature.

I.M.

- Shake suspension container vigorously for at least 1 minute before withdrawing dose.
- Use a 1½-inch, 22G needle for injection.
- Inject slowly, over 5 to 7 seconds, into deltoid or gluteal muscle. Pat site lightly after injection; don't rub it for medroxyprogesterone administration; massage area in a circular motion after progesterone administration.
- Rotate sites.

VAGINAL

- Remove applicator from sealed wrapper. Grip applicator firmly by thick end and shake it down like a thermometer to ensure that the contents are at the thin end.
- Twist tab off and discard.
- Insert thin end of applicator gently into the vagina while patient is in a sitting position or lying on her back with knees bent.
- Press thick end of applicator firmly to deposit gel.
- Remove applicator and discard.

Route	Onset	Peak	Duration
P.O.	Unknown	3 hr	Unknown
I.M.	Rapid	Unknown	3–4 hr
Vaginal	Unknown	Unknown	Unknown

Half-life: 5–20 min

Mechanism of Action

Progestins may diminish response to endogenous hormones in tumor cells by decreasing the number of steroid hormone receptors, causing a direct antiproliferative or cytotoxic effect on cell cycle growth and increased terminal cell differentiation. At higher doses, some progestins decrease adrenal production of androstenedione and estradiol, which may decrease estrogen- or testosterone-sensitive tumors. Megestrol stimulates appetite and metabolic effects, which promotes weight gain. Progestins also bind to cytosolic receptors that are loosely bound in cell nucleus, increasing protein synthesis and improving cachexia.

Progestins affect other hormones, especially estrogen, by reducing availability or stability of hormone receptor complex, shutting off estrogen-responsive genes, or causing negative feedback mechanism that decreases number of functioning estrogen receptors. These actions allow menstrual cycle to function normally, alleviating amenorrhea and dysfunctional uterine bleeding and inducing menses. Progestins also act to transform proliferative uterine endometrium into a more differentiated, secretory one, which is the basis for using medroxyprogesterone to treat some types of amenorrhea. In a normal ovulatory cycle not resulting in pregnancy, decline in progesterone secretion caused by degeneration of corpus luteum in late luteal phase results in endometrial sloughing. A similar sloughing occurs after 5 to 10 days of medroxyprogesterone, provided that adequate estrogen-stimulated proliferation has occurred during follicular phase.

The progestin, levonorgestrel, also inhibits secretion of gonadotropins from the pituitary gland, which creates an atrophic endometrium, resulting in contraceptive effect.

Contraindications

Active thromboembolic disorder; disease; hypersensitivity to sesame oil/seeds

P

(progesterone), progestins, or their components; known or suspected breast or genital cancer; missed abortion (progesterone); pregnancy; significant hepatic disease; thrombophlebitis; undiagnosed vaginal bleeding

Interactions

DRUGS

aminoglutethimide: Possibly decreased blood level of medroxyprogesterone
atazanavir, clarithromycin, indinavir, itraconazole, ketoconazole, nefazodone, nelfinavir, ritonavir, saquinavir, telithromycin, voriconazole: Possibly increased progestin level leading to potential for increased adverse reactions
barbiturates including bosentan, carbamazepine, felbamate, griseofulvin, oxcarbazepine, phenytoin, primidone, rifampin, St. John's wort, topiramate: Possibly decreased effectiveness of progestin
CYP3A4 inhibitors such as ketoconazole: Possibly increased bioavailability of progesterone
thyroid hormone: Decreased thyroid hormone effectiveness; increased thyroid hormonal levels
warfarin: Possibly increased INR

Adverse Reactions

CNS: Altered or reduced coordination or speech, depression, dizziness, drowsiness, fatigue, headache, irritability, migraine, mood changes, nervousness, postmenopausal dementia, syncope, unusual tiredness or weakness
CV: Fluid retention, **hypotension, thromboembolism**
ENDO: Adrenal insufficiency or suppression, breast pain or tenderness, Cushing's syndrome, decreased T$_3$ resin uptake, delayed return of fertility in women, elevated thyroid-binding globulin, galactorrhea, hyperglycemia
EENT: Gingival bleeding, swelling, or tenderness; vision changes or loss
GI: Abdominal cramps or pain, cholestatic jaundice, diarrhea, nausea, vomiting
GU: Amenorrhea, breakthrough bleeding or metromenorrhagia, changes in cervical erosion and secretions, decreased libido, hypermenorrhea, ovarian enlargement or cysts

HEME: Clotting and bleeding abnormalities
MS: Back pain, decreased bone density, osteoporosis, osteoporotic fractures
RESP: Acute eosinophilic pneumonia (progesterone in sesame oil), dyspnea
SKIN: Acne, alopecia, dermal edema, hirsutism, melasma, pruritus, rash, urticaria
Other: Anaphylaxis; angioedema; hot flashes; injection-site irritation, pain, or redness; numbness or pain in arm, chest, or leg; weight gain or loss

Childbearing Considerations

PREGNANCY

- Drug may cause fetal harm.
- Drug is contraindicated in pregnancy. If pregnancy occurs, drug should be discontinued immediately.

LACTATION

- Drug is present in breast milk in small amounts.
- A decision may have to be made to discontinue breastfeeding or the drug to avoid potential serious adverse reactions in the breastfed infant.

Nursing Considerations

- Be aware that progestin/estrogen therapy shouldn't be used to prevent cardiovascular disease or dementia.
- Use progestins cautiously in patients with risk factors for arterial vascular disease, such as diabetes mellitus, hypercholesterolemia, hypertension, obesity, systemic lupus erythematosus, tobacco use, or a family or personal history of venous thromboembolism. Drug worsens these conditions.
- Use progestins cautiously in patients who have CNS disorders, such as depression or seizures, because progestins may worsen these conditions.

! **WARNING** Notify prescriber immediately if patient develops signs of thrombotic events. Expect to discontinue progestin if such signs occur and provide emergency care, as ordered.

- Monitor patient for adrenal suppression, especially with megestrol therapy. If suspected, notify prescriber.
- Expect to stop progestin therapy in any woman who develops evidence of cancer;

cardiovascular disease such as CVA, MI, pulmonary embolism, or venous thrombosis; or dementia.

- Be aware that acute eosinophilic pneumonia may occur in patients receiving progesterone in sesame oil. Monitor patient for dyspnea with hypoxic respiratory insufficiency and fever that may occur 2 to 4 weeks after patient starts progesterone in sesame oil therapy. If this reaction is suspected, notify prescriber and expect drug to be discontinued immediately.

PATIENT TEACHING

- Explain risks of progestin therapy, including breast, endometrial, or ovarian cancer; cardiovascular disease; dementia; and gallbladder disease, especially in postmenopausal women.
- Instruct woman to notify prescriber if uterine bleeding continues longer than 3 months or if menstruation is delayed by 45 days.
- Warn patient taking progestin for noncontraceptive purposes to use a contraceptive method to prevent pregnancy, because drug may harm fetus.
- Advise female patient to contact prescriber immediately if she suspects pregnancy or misses a menstrual period.
- Advise patient that some products may contain peanut oil or sesame oil. If she is allergic to these, tell her to contact pharmacist to find out if prescribed progestin product contains peanut or sesame oil. Also tell patient to report difficulty breathing and fever to prescriber.
- Caution female patient who vomits within 1 hour of taking progestin for emergency contraception to contact prescriber about whether to repeat dose.
- Teach woman how to use vaginal gel, if prescribed. Tell her to avoid using other vaginal products for 6 hours before and after to ensure gel's complete absorption.
- Direct patient to alert all prescribers about progestin therapy, because certain blood tests may be affected.
- Emphasize importance of good dental hygiene and regular dental checkups because elevated progestin level increases growth of normal oral flora, which may lead to gum tenderness, bleeding, or swelling.

promethazine hydrochloride
Promethegan

Class and Category
Pharmacologic class: Phenothiazine
Therapeutic class: Antiemetic, antihistamine, antivertigo, sedative-hypnotic

Indications and Dosages
* *To prevent or treat motion sickness*

SUPPOSITORIES, SYRUP, TABLETS

Adults. 25 mg 30 to 60 min before travel and repeated 8 to 12 hr later, if needed. Then on succeeding days, 25 mg twice daily, once upon arising and again before evening meal, as needed.

Children age 2 and over. 12.5 to 25 mg every 12 hr, as needed.

* *To prevent or treat nausea and vomiting in certain types of anesthesia and surgery*

SYRUP, TABLETS

Adults. *Initial:* 12.5 to 25 mg every 4 to 6 hr, as needed. *Maximum:* 150 mg daily.

Children age 2 and over. 1.1 mg/kg/dose (maximum 25 mg/dose) every 4 to 6 hr as needed.

I.V. OR I.M. INJECTION

Adults. 12.5 to 25 mg every 4 to 6 hr, as needed. *Maximum:* 150 mg daily.

I.M. INJECTION

Children age 2 and over. 6.25 to 12.5 mg/dose every 4 to 6 hr, as needed.

SUPPOSITORIES

Adults. 12.5 to 25 mg every 4 to 6 hr, as needed. *Maximum:* 150 mg daily.

Children age 2 and over. 1.1 mg/kg/dose (maximum 25 mg/dose) every 4 to 6 hr, as needed.

* *To treat signs and symptoms of allergic response*

SUPPOSITORIES, SYRUP, TABLETS

Adults and adolescents. 12.5 mg four times a day before meals and at bedtime, as needed. Or, 25 mg at bedtime, as needed.

Children age 2 and over. 6.25 to 12.5 mg three times a day, as needed. Or, 25 mg at bedtime, as needed.

I.M. OR I.V. INJECTION

Adults. 25 mg repeated within 2 hr, as needed.

✱ As an adjunct to analgesics for preoperative or postoperative sedation

I.M. OR I.V. INJECTION, SUPPOSITORIES, SYRUP, TABLETS

Adults. 25 to 50 mg as a single dose.

SUPPOSITORIES, SYRUP, TABLETS

Children age 2 and over. 1.1 mg/kg as a single dose. *Maximum:* 25 mg/dose.

I.M. INJECTION

Children age 2 and over. 0.25 to 1.1 mg/kg as a single dose. Maximum: 25 mg/dose.

✱ To relieve apprehension and promote nighttime sleep

I.M. INJECTION, SYRUP, TABLETS, SUPPOSITORIES

Adults. 25 to 50 mg at bedtime.

±**DOSAGE ADJUSTMENT** Dosage usually decreased for elderly patients.

✱ To provide obstetric sedation

I.V. OR I.M. INJECTION

Adults and adolescents. 25 to 50 mg for early stages of labor; 25 to 75 mg after labor is established, repeated once or twice every 4 hr, as needed.

Drug Administration

P.O.

- Administer with food if GI irritation occurs.
- Use calibrated device to measure dosage of syrup.

I.V.

- Concentration should not exceed 25 mg/ml.
- Avoid inadvertent intra-arterial injection because it can cause arteriospasm.
- Inject through a running I.V. line at the port that is farthest from the patient's vein. Do not administer through a hand or wrist I.V.
- Inject over 10 to 15 minutes at no more than 25 mg/min; rapid I.V. administration may produce a transient drop in blood pressure.
- *Incompatibilities:* None listed by manufacturer

I.M.

- Parenteral route is preferred.
- Inject deep into large muscle mass.
- Rotate sites.
- Avoid injecting drug subcutaneously; severe tissue damage and gangrene may develop.

P.R.

- If suppository is too soft for administration, place in refrigerator for 30 minutes or run suppository under cold water before removing wrapper.
- Store in refrigerator.

Route	Onset	Peak	Duration
P.O.	15–60 min	Unknown	4–8 hr
I.V.	3–5 min	Unknown	4–8 hr
I.M., P.R.	20 min	Unknown	4–8 hr

Half-life: 10–19 hr

Mechanism of Action

Competes with histamine for H_1-receptor sites, thereby antagonizing many histamine effects and reducing allergy signs and symptoms. Promethazine also prevents motion sickness, nausea, and vertigo by acting centrally on medullary chemoreceptive trigger zone and by decreasing vestibular stimulation and labyrinthine function in the inner ear. It also promotes sedation and relieves anxiety by blocking receptor sites in CNS, directly reducing stimuli to the brain.

Contraindications

Children under the age of 2; comatose state; hypersensitivity to promethazine, other phenothiazines, or their components; intra-arterial or subcutaneous injection (parenteral)

Interactions

DRUGS

anticholinergics: Possibly intensified anticholinergic adverse effects
CNS depressants: Additive CNS depression
epinephrine: Reversed vasopressor effect of epinephrine; increased risk of hypotension
MAO inhibitors: Increased risk of extrapyramidal effects

ACTIVITIES

alcohol use: Additive CNS depression

Adverse Reactions

CNS: Akathisia, CNS stimulation, confusion, dizziness, drowsiness, dystonia, euphoria, excitation, fatigue, hallucinations, hysteria, incoordination, insomnia, irritability, nervousness, **neuroleptic malignant syndrome**, paradoxical stimulation, pseudoparkinsonism, restlessness, sedation, **seizures**, syncope, tardive dyskinesia, tremor
CV: Bradycardia, hypertension, **hypotension**, tachycardia

EENT: Blurred vision; diplopia; dry mouth, nose, and throat; nasal congestion; tinnitus; vision changes
ENDO: Hyperglycemia
GI: Anorexia, cholestatic jaundice, ileus, nausea, rectal burning or stinging (suppository form), vomiting
GU: Dysuria
HEME: Agranulocytosis, leukopenia, thrombocytopenia, thrombocytopenic purpura
RESP: Apnea, respiratory depression, tenacious bronchial secretions
SKIN: Dermatitis, diaphoresis, photosensitivity, rash, urticaria
Other: Angioedema, paradoxical reactions

Childbearing Considerations
PREGNANCY
- It is not known if drug can cause fetal harm. However, drug should not be used within 2 weeks of delivery due to potential inhibition of platelet aggregation in the newborn.
- Use with caution only if benefit to mother outweighs potential risk to fetus.

LACTATION
- It is not known if drug is present in breast milk.
- A decision may have to be made to discontinue breastfeeding or the drug to avoid potential serious adverse reactions in the breastfed infant.

Nursing Considerations
- Use promethazine cautiously in children and elderly patients because they may be more sensitive to its effects, patients with cardiovascular disease or hepatic dysfunction because of potential adverse effects, patients with asthma because of anticholinergic effects, and patients with seizure disorders or those who take drugs that may affect seizure threshold because drug may lower seizure threshold.

! **WARNING** Monitor respiratory function because drug may suppress cough reflex and cause thickening of bronchial secretions, aggravating such conditions as asthma and COPD. Rarely, it may depress respirations and induce apnea.

- Monitor patient's hematologic status as ordered because promethazine may cause

bone marrow depression, especially when used with other known marrow-toxic agents. Assess patient for signs and symptoms of infection or bleeding.

! **WARNING** Monitor patient for evidence of neuroleptic malignant syndrome, such as fever, hypertension or hypotension, involuntary motor activity, mental changes, muscle rigidity, tachycardia, and tachypnea. Be prepared to provide supportive treatment and drug therapy, as prescribed.

- Be aware that patient shouldn't have intradermal allergen tests within 72 hours of receiving promethazine because drug may significantly alter flare response.

PATIENT TEACHING
- Tell patient to use a calibrated device to ensure accurate doses of promethazine syrup.
- Teach patient correct administration technique for suppository, if needed.
- Advise patient to avoid OTC drugs unless approved by prescriber.
- Instruct patient to notify prescriber immediately if she has involuntary movements and restlessness.
- Urge patient to avoid alcohol and other CNS depressants during therapy.
- Instruct patient to avoid hazardous activities until drug's CNS effects are known.
- Suggest rinsing and use of sugarless gum or hard candy to relieve dry mouth.
- Urge patient to avoid excessive sun exposure and to use sunscreen when outdoors.

propafenone hydrochloride
Rythmol SR

Class and Category
Pharmacologic class: Sodium channel antagonist
Therapeutic class: Class IC antiarrhythmic

Indications and Dosages
* *To treat life-threatening ventricular arrhythmias; to prolong time of recurrence of paroxysmal supraventricular tachycardia*

associated with disabling symptoms in patients without structural heart disease

TABLETS

Adults. *Initial:* 150 mg every 8 hr; after 3 or 4 days, increased to 225 mg every 8 hr (U.S.) or 300 mg every 12 hr (Canada), as needed; after an additional 3 or 4 days, further increased to 300 mg every 8 hr, as needed. *Maximum:* 900 mg daily.

✳ *To prolong time of recurrence of symptomatic atrial fibrillation/flutter in patients with episodic (paroxysmal or persistent) atrial fibrillation who do not have structural heart disease*

TABLETS

Adults. Initial: 150 mg every 8 hr; after 3 or 4 days, increased to 225 mg every 8 hr (U.S.) or 300 mg every 12 hr (Canada), as needed; after an additional 3 or 4 days, further increased to 300 mg every 8 hr, as needed. *Maximum:* 900 mg daily.

E.R. CAPSULES

Adults. *Initial:* 225 mg every 12 hr, increased after 5 or more days to 325 mg every 12 hr, as needed, and further increased to 425 mg every 12 hr, as needed.

±**DOSAGE ADJUSTMENT** For patient with hepatic impairment, second- or third-degree AV block, or significant widening of the QRS complex, dosage may have to be reduced.

☰ Drug Administration

P.O.

- E.R. capsules should be swallowed whole and not chewed, crushed, or opened.

Route	Onset	Peak	Duration
P.O.	Unknown	2–3.5 hr	Unknown
P.O./E.R.	Unknown	3–8 hr	Unknown

Half-life: 2–10 hr

☰ Mechanism of Action

Prolongs recovery period after myocardial repolarization by inhibiting sodium influx through myocardial cell membranes. This action prolongs the refractory period, causing myocardial automaticity, excitability, and conduction velocity to decline.

☰ Contraindications

Bronchospastic disorders, such as asthma; Brugada syndrome; cardiogenic shock; concurrent use of both a CYP2D6 inhibitor and a CYP3A4 inhibitor (Rythmol SR); electrolyte imbalances; heart failure (uncontrolled); hypersensitivity to propafenone or its components; severe hypotension or obstructive pulmonary disease; sinus bradycardia or AV conduction disturbances (without artificial pacemaker)

☰ Interactions

DRUGS

amiodarone: Possibly altered cardiac conduction and repolarization
cimetidine, fluoxetine: Possibly increased blood propafenone level
CYP2D6 inhibitors and CYP3A4 inhibitors combined: Significantly increased concentration of propafenone, increasing risk of proarrhythmias and other adverse reactions
digoxin: Increased risk of digitalis toxicity
haloperidol, imipramine, venlafaxine: Possibly increased levels of these drugs
lidocaine: Possibly increased CNS adverse effects of lidocaine
metoprolol, propranolol: Increased blood level and half-life of these drugs
orlistat: Possibly decreased absorption of propafenone
quinidine: Decreased propafenone metabolism
rifampin: Possibly decreased propafenone level
warfarin: Increased blood warfarin level and risk of bleeding

FOODS

grapefruit juice: Possibly increased blood propafenone level

☰ Adverse Reactions

CNS: Anxiety, depression, dizziness, fatigue, headache, somnolence, tremor, weakness
CV: Angina, **atrial flutter, AV block, bradycardia,** chest pain, edema, **heart failure, hypotension, irregular heartbeat,** palpitations, **prolonged QT interval,** tachycardia, **ventricular arrhythmias, worsened supraventricular arrhythmias**
EENT: Altered taste, blurred vision, dry mouth
GI: Constipation, diarrhea, flatulence, nausea, vomiting
GU: Decreased sperm count, hematuria
HEME: Agranulocytosis
MS: Muscle weakness

RESP: Dyspnea, rales, upper respiratory tract infection, wheezes
SKIN: Ecchymosis, rash
Other: Elevated blood alkaline phosphatase, exacerbation of myasthenia gravis, flu-like symptoms, positive ANA titers

Childbearing Considerations

PREGNANCY

- It is not known if drug can cause fetal harm. However, other antiarrhythmic agents have caused fetal/neonatal arrhythmias when given during pregnancy.
- Fetal/neonatal monitoring for arrhythmia is recommended during and after drug therapy in pregnant women.
- Use with caution only if benefit to mother outweighs potential risk to fetus.

LABOR & DELIVERY

- Increased risk of arrhythmias during labor and delivery.

LACTATION

- Drug is present in breast milk.
- Patient should check with prescriber before breastfeeding.

REPRODUCTION

- Drug may transiently impair spermatogenesis in male patients.

Nursing Considerations

- Assess patient for electrolyte imbalances, such as hyperkalemia, before starting propafenone or any antiarrhythmic, to reduce risk of adverse cardiac reactions.
- Use propafenone cautiously in patients with heart failure or myocardial dysfunction because beta-blocking activity may further depress myocardial contractility.
- Use cautiously in patients with renal impairment because about 50% of the drug's metabolites are excreted in the urine, increasing risk of propafenone overdose.
- Monitor ECG tracings, blood pressure, and pulse rate, particularly at start of therapy and with dosage increases. Expect propafenone to be discontinued if Brugada syndrome is confirmed with ECG changes.
- Monitor patient for signs of infection such as chills, fever, or sore throat, because propafenone may cause agranulocytosis, particularly during the initial 3 months of therapy. If present, notify prescriber.

PATIENT TEACHING

- Instruct patient to take a missed dose if she remembers within 4 hours; otherwise, tell her to skip missed dose and to resume the regular dosing schedule.
- Tell patient to swallow E.R. capsules whole and not to chew, crush, or open capsules.
- Advise patient not to stop propafenone or change dosage without asking prescriber.
- Urge patient to carry medical identification showing that she takes propafenone.
- Advise patient to avoid hazardous activities until drug's CNS effects are known.
- Urge patient to increase fluid intake and dietary fiber if she becomes constipated.
- Explain that drug may cause an unusual taste. Advise patient to notify prescriber if taste interferes with compliance.
- Tell patient to notify prescriber promptly of any signs of infection such as fever, sore throat, or chills.

propofol
(disoprofol)
Diprivan

Class and Category
Pharmacologic class: Phenol derivative
Therapeutic class: Sedative-hypnotic

Indications and Dosages
* *To provide sedation for critically ill patients in intensive care*

I.V. INFUSION
Adults. *Initial:* 5 mcg/kg/min (0.3 mg/kg/h), increased in increments of 5 to 10 mcg/kg/min greater than every 5 min until desired level of sedation vis achieved. *Maintenance:* 5 to 50 mcg/kg/min or higher. *Maximum:* 4 mg/kg/hr.
±**DOSAGE ADJUSTMENT** For elderly, debilitated, or American Society of Anesthesiologists Physical Status (ASA-PS) III or IV patients, induction dose decreased and maintenance rate slower.

Drug Administration
I.V.
- Consult prescriber about pretreating injection site with 1 ml of 1% lidocaine to minimize pain, burning, or stinging that may occur. If ordered, lidocaine shouldn't be added to propofol solution in quantities

greater than 20 mg/200 mg because emulsion may become unstable.

- Don't use if emulsion appears to be separated.
- Give drug through a larger vein in forearm or antecubital fossa to minimize injection-site discomfort.
- Drug is provided as a ready-to-use formulation. However, if dilution is necessary, it should only be diluted with 5% Dextrose Injection and not diluted to a concentration less than 2 mg/ml, because it is an emulsion. In diluted form, drug is more stable when in contact with glass rather than with plastic.
- Shake container well before using and administer drug promptly after opening. Use prefilled syringes within 6 hours of opening.
- Use a drop counter syringe pump, or volumetric pump to safely control infusion rate.
- Don't infuse drug through filter with a pore size of less than 5 microns; doing so could cause emulsion to break down.
- A sterile vent spike must be used. Discard unused portion of propofol solution immediately after use or within 12 hours of administration (6 hours if propofol was transferred from original container) to prevent bacterial growth in stagnant solution. Also, protect solution from light.
- *Incompatibilities:* Blood and plasma, other I.V. drugs

Route	Onset	Peak	Duration
I.V.	15–30 sec	Unknown	3–10 min
Half-life: 2–10 min			

Mechanism of Action

Decreases cerebral blood flow, cerebral metabolic oxygen consumption, and intracranial pressure and increases cerebrovascular resistance, which may play a role in propofol's hypnotic effects.

Contraindications

Hypersensitivity to propofol or its components, to eggs or egg products, or to soybeans or soy products

Interactions
DRUGS

CNS depressants such as barbiturates, benzodiazepines, chloral hydrate, droperidol, *fentanyl, meperidine, morphine:* Additive CNS depressant, respiratory depressant, and hypotensive effects; possibly decreased emetic effects of opioids
nitrous oxide, opioids, potent inhalational agents (enflurane, halothane, isoflurane): Increased anesthetic, cardiorespiratory, or sedative effects of propofol
valproate: Increased blood levels of propofol increasing risk of cardiorespiratory depression and sedation

ACTIVITIES

alcohol use: Additive CNS depressant, respiratory depressant, and hypotensive effects

Adverse Reactions

CV: Bradycardia, hypotension
GI: Nausea, vomiting
MS: Involuntary muscle movement (transient)
RESP: Apnea
Other: Anaphylaxis, injection-site burning, pain, or stinging

Childbearing Considerations
PREGNANCY

- It is not known if drug can cause fetal harm.
- Use with caution only if benefit to mother outweighs potential risk to fetus.

LABOR & DELIVERY

- Drug is not recommended for obstetrics, including cesarean section deliveries, because drug crosses the placental barrier and may cause neonatal nervous and respiratory system depression.

LACTATION

- Drug is present in breast milk.
- Drug is not recommended during breastfeeding.

Nursing Considerations

- Know that repeated or lengthy (greater than 3 hours) use of sedation drugs such as propofol and general anesthetics during procedures or surgeries should be avoided, if possible, in children younger than 3 years of age or in pregnant women during their third trimester, because the combined use may affect the development of children's brains.
- Use propofol cautiously in patients with cardiac disease, peripheral vascular disease, impaired cerebral circulation, or increased

intracranial pressure, because drug may aggravate these disorders.

- Know that dosage must be tapered before stopping therapy. Stopping abruptly will cause rapid awakening, anxiety, agitation, and resistance to mechanical ventilation.
- Expect patient to recover from sedation within 8 minutes.

> ! **WARNING** Monitor patient for propofol infusion syndrome, especially with prolonged high-dose infusions. It may cause severe metabolic acidosis, hyperkalemia, lipemia, rhabdomyolysis, hepatomegaly and cardiac and renal failure. Alert prescriber at once and be prepared to provide emergency supportive care as ordered.

PATIENT TEACHING

- Urge patient and family to voice concerns and ask questions before administration.
- Reassure patient that she'll be monitored closely during administration and that vital functions will be supported as needed.
- Inform patient and family that caution is required when performing activities requiring mental alertness, such as driving, because mental alertness may be impaired for some time after general anesthesia or sedation such as propofol has been given.

propranolol hydrochloride

Hemangeol, Inderal LA, Inderal XL, InnoPran XL

☰ Class and Category

Pharmacologic class: Beta-adrenergic blocker
Therapeutic class: Antianginal, antiarrhythmic, antihypertensive, anti-MI, antimigraine, antitremor, hypertrophic cardiomyopathy, and pheochromocytoma therapy adjunct

☰ Indications and Dosages

✳ *To manage hypertension*

E.R. CAPSULES (INDERAL LA)

Adults. *Initial:* 80 mg once daily, increased to 120 mg or higher until blood pressure is adequately controlled. *Maintenance:* 120 to 160 mg once daily. *Maximum:* 640 mg once daily.

XL CAPSULES (INDERAL XL, INNOPRAN XL)

Adults. *Initial:* 80 mg once daily, increased, as needed, to 120 mg once daily.

ORAL SOLUTION, TABLETS

Adults. *Initial:* 40 mg twice daily, increased every 3 to 7 days, as needed. *Maintenance:* 80–240 mg every 8 to 12 hr. *Maximum:* 640 mg daily.

✳ *To treat chronic angina*

E.R. CAPSULES (INDERAL LA)

Adults. *Initial:* 80 mg once daily, increased at 3- to 7-day intervals, as needed. *Usual:* 160 mg once daily. *Maximum:* 320 mg once daily.

ORAL SOLUTION, TABLETS

Adults. 80 to 320 mg daily in divided doses twice daily, three times a day, or four times a day. *Maximum:* 320 mg/day in divided doses.

✳ *To treat supraventricular arrhythmia*

ORAL SOLUTION, TABLETS

Adults. 10 to 30 mg three times a day or four times a day, adjusted as needed.

✳ *To treat life-threatening cardiac arrhythmias*

I.V. INJECTION

Adults. 1 to 3 mg administered no greater than 1 mg/ml; repeated after 2 min and again after 4 hr, as needed.

✳ *To control tremor*

ORAL SOLUTION, TABLETS

Adults. *Initial:* 40 mg twice daily, adjusted as needed. *Maintenance:* 120 to 320 mg/day in 2 to 3 divided doses. *Maximum:* 320 mg daily.

✳ *To prevent vascular migraine headaches*

E.R. CAPSULES (INDERAL LA)

Adults. *Initial:* 80 mg once daily, increased gradually to achieve optimal migraine prophylaxis. *Usual:* 160 to 240 mg once daily.

ORAL SOLUTION, TABLETS

Adults. *Initial:* 20 mg four times a day, increased gradually, as needed. *Maximum:* 240 mg daily.

✳ *As adjunct to treat hypertrophic subaortic stenosis*

ORAL SOLUTION, TABLETS

Adults. 20 to 40 mg three or four times daily before meals and at bedtime.

E.R. CAPSULES (INDERAL LA)

Adults. 80 to 160 mg once daily.

✳ *As adjunct to manage pheochromocytoma*

P

ORAL SOLUTION, TABLETS

Adults. For operable tumors, 60 mg in divided doses for 3 days before surgery, concurrently with an alpha blocker. For inoperable tumors, 30 mg daily in divided doses concurrently with an alpha blocker.

✳ *To prevent MI*

ORAL SOLUTION, TABLETS

Adults. *Initial:* 40 mg three times a day for 1 mo, then increased to 60–80 mg three times a day, as tolerated. *Maintenance:* 180 to 240 mg daily in 2 to 4 divided doses. *Maximum:* 240 mg daily.

✳ *To treat proliferating infantile hemangioma requiring systemic therapy*

ORAL SOLUTION (HEMANGEOL)

Infants 5 weeks of age to 5 months. *Initial:* 0.6 mg/kg twice daily for 1 wk followed by 1.1 mg/kg twice daily for 1 wk followed by 1.7 mg/kg twice daily for 6 months.

±**DOSAGE ADJUSTMENT** Dosage increased or decreased for elderly patients, depending on sensitivity to propranolol.

☰ Drug Administration

- Obtain apical pulse and blood pressure before administering. If abnormal, withhold drug and notify prescriber.

P.O.

- Administer tablets with or without food.
- Administer oral solution used to treat hypertrophic subaortic stenosis before meals and at bedtime.
- Administer oral solution doses used to treat proliferating infantile hemangioma at least 9 hours apart during or after feeding.
- Administer extended-release capsules with or without food, but be consistent. Administer at bedtime.
- Use a calibrated device to measure dosage of oral solution.
- Store drug at room temperature.

I.V.

- Give I.V. injection at no more than 1 mg/min.
- Monitor ECG continuously, as ordered, when giving I.V. injection. Have emergency drugs and equipment available in case of hypotension or cardiac arrest.
- Protect injection solution from light.
- *Incompatibilities:* None listed by manufacturer

Route	Onset	Peak	Duration
P.O.	30 min	1–4 hr	6–12 hr
P.O./E.X.	Unknown	6–14 hr	24–27 hr
I.V.	Immediate	1 min	2–4 hr

Half-life: 3–6 hr

☰ Mechanism of Action

Through beta-blocking action, propranolol:

- prevents arterial dilation and inhibits renin secretion, resulting in decreased blood pressure (in hypertension and pheochromocytoma) and relief of migraine headaches
- decreases heart rate, which helps resolve tachyarrhythmias
- improves myocardial contractility, which helps ease symptoms of hypertrophic cardiomyopathy
- decreases myocardial oxygen demand, which helps prevent anginal pain and death of myocardial tissue.

In addition, peripheral beta-adrenergic blockade may play a role in propranolol's ability to alleviate tremor.

☰ Contraindications

Bronchial asthma; cardiogenic shock; decompensated heart failure; greater than first-degree block, sick sinus syndrome, or sinus bradycardia unless a permanent pacemaker is in place; hypersensitivity to propranolol or any of its components

☰ Interactions

DRUGS

alpha blockers (prazosin): May cause prolongation of first dose hypotension and syncope

cholestyramine, colestipol: Significantly reduces plasma concentrations of propranolol, which may result in loss of effectiveness

clonidine: Possibly antagonized antihypertensive effects of clonidine

corticosteroids: Possibly increased risk of hypoglycemia

CYP1A2 inducers (montelukast, phenytoin), CYP2C19 inducers (rifampin): Decreased plasma levels of propranolol resulting in loss of effectiveness

CYP1A2 inhibitors (ciprofloxacin, enoxamone, fluvoxamine), CYP2D6 inhibitors (bupropion, fluoxetine, paroxetine, quinidine): Increased exposure to propranolol increasing risks of adverse reactions such as bradycardia and hypotension

dobutamine: Reduced sensitivity to dobutamine stress echocardiography in patients undergoing evaluation for myocardial ischemia

MAO inhibitors, tricyclic antidepressants: Increased risk of significant hypertension

NSAIDs: Possibly decreased hypotensive effects

propafenone: Increased blood level and adverse reactions such as bradycardia and postural hypotension

warfarin: Increased risk of bleeding

ACTIVITIES

alcohol: Possibly decreased or increased plasma propranolol level

nicotine chewing gum, smoking cessation, smoking deterrents: Possibly decreased therapeutic effects of propranolol

▤ Adverse Reactions

CNS: Anxiety, depression, dizziness, drowsiness, fatigue, fever, insomnia, lethargy, nervousness, weakness

CV: AV conduction disorders, bradycardia, cold limbs, **heart failure, hypotension**

EENT: Dry eyes, **laryngospasm**, nasal congestion, pharyngitis

ENDO: Hypoglycemia

GI: Abdominal pain, constipation, diarrhea, nausea, vomiting

GU: Impotence, Peyronie's disease, sexual dysfunction

HEME: Agranulocytosis, nonthrombocytopenic purpura, **thrombocytopenic purpura**

MS: Muscle weakness, myopathy, myotonia

RESP: Bronchospasm, dyspnea, **respiratory distress,** wheezing

SKIN: Alopecia, **erythema multiforme,** erythematous rash, **exfoliative dermatitis,** psoriasiform rash, **Stevens–Johnson syndrome, toxic epidermal necrolysis,** urticaria

Other: Anaphylaxis, flu-like symptoms, systemic lupus-like reaction

▤ Childbearing Considerations

PREGNANCY

- Drug may have the potential to cause fetal harm such as congenital anomalies and intrauterine growth retardation.

- Use with caution only if benefit to mother outweighs potential risk to fetus.

LABOR & DELIVERY

- Neonates born to mothers who received drug at parturition may exhibit bradycardia, hypoglycemia, and/or respiratory depression.
- Neonates need to be monitored closely for adverse effects.

LACTATION

- Drug is present in breast milk.
- Patient should check with prescriber before breastfeeding.
- If breastfeeding occurs, mother should monitor infant for low pulse rate or signs and symptoms of low blood glucose level as well as respiratory depression.

REPRODUCTION

- Drug may cause erectile dysfunction.

▤ Nursing Considerations

- Use propranolol cautiously in patients with bronchospastic lung disease because it may induce asthmatic attack, and in patients with underlying skeletal muscle disease; isolated reports of myopathy and myotonia have occurred with propranolol use.
- Monitor blood pressure, apical and radial pulses, fluid intake and output, daily weight, respiration, and circulation in extremities before and during therapy.
- Know that because drug's negative inotropic effect can depress cardiac output, cardiac output should be monitored in patients with heart failure, particularly those with severely compromised left ventricular dysfunction.
- Be aware that propranolol can mask tachycardia in hyperthyroidism and that abrupt withdrawal in patients with hyperthyroidism or thyrotoxicosis can cause thyroid storm.
- Monitor diabetic patient taking an antidiabetic because propranolol can prolong hypoglycemia or promote hyperglycemia. It also can mask signs of hypoglycemia, especially tachycardia, palpitations, and tremor, but it doesn't suppress diaphoresis or hypertensive response to hypoglycemia.

! WARNING Be aware that stopping drug abruptly, even for surgery, may cause MI,

P

myocardial ischemia, severe hypertension, or ventricular arrhythmias, especially in patients with cardiac disease. However, be aware that the heart may not be able to respond to reflex adrenergic stimuli normally during surgery, which increases the risks of general anesthesia and surgical procedures. It also may cause increased intraocular pressure to return. Dosage should be reduced gradually.

PATIENT TEACHING

- Instruct patient to take propranolol at the same time every day.
- Tell patient to take tablets on an empty stomach and extended-release capsules with or without food but to be consistent.
- Instruct patient to take extended-release capsules at bedtime.
- Instruct patient to use a calibrated device to measure dosage of oral solution, never a household spoon.
- Instruct parents/caregiver to administer drug to infant at least 9 hours apart.
- Caution patient not to change dosage without consulting prescriber and not to stop taking drug abruptly.
- Advise patient to notify prescriber immediately if she has shortness of breath, weight gain, or signs and symptoms of worsening heart failure.

! WARNING Instruct diabetic patient to check blood glucose level regularly because drug may mask signs and symptoms of hypoglycemia. Instruct parents administering Hemangeol form to infant to monitor for signs and symptoms of hypoglycemia, which can occur at any time during treatment. Warn parents that risk is increased during poor oral food intake, infection, or vomiting or when glucose demands are increased such as during a cold, infection, or time of stress. If any of these situations occur, parents should be told to withhold drug and notify prescriber. Instruct parents on how to treat hypoglycemia.

- Advise patient to consult prescriber before taking OTC drugs, especially cold products.
- Urge patient to avoid hazardous activities until CNS effects of drug are known.
- Advise smoker to notify prescriber immediately if she stops smoking because cessation may decrease drug metabolism, calling for dosage adjustments.
- Tell patient to notify prescriber if she is or could be pregnant because drug may have to be discontinued.

protamine sulfate

⊟ Class and Category
Pharmacologic class: Heparin antagonist
Therapeutic class: Heparin antidote

⊟ Indications and Dosages
⁎ *To treat heparin toxicity or hemorrhage associated with heparin therapy*

I.V. INJECTION
Adults. Dosage dependent on lapse of time from when severe bleeding begins in relationship to when heparin dosage was given. *For severe bleeding occurring a few minutes after I.V. injection of heparin:* 1 mg for every 100 units of heparin administered. *For severe bleeding occurring 30 to 60 min after I.V. injection of heparin:* 0.5 to 0.75 mg for every 100 units of heparin given. *For severe bleeding occurring 2 hr or more after I.V. injection of heparin:* 0.25 to 0.375 mg for every 100 units of heparin given. *For severe bleeding after subcutaneous injection of heparin:* 1 to 1.5 mg for every 100 units of heparin given.

⊟ Drug Administration
I.V.
- Have fluids—epinephrine 1:1,000, dobutamine, or dopamine—available for allergic or hypotensive reactions.
- Expect to administer I.V. protamine undiluted. However, if dilution is ordered, dilute with 0.9% Sodium Chloride Injection or 5% Dextrose Injection. Do not store diluted solutions.
- Inject drug slowly at 5 mg/min; administer no more than 50 mg in 10 minutes.
- *Incompatibilities:* Other drugs, especially cephalosporin and penicillin antibiotics

Route	Onset	Peak	Duration
I.V.	5 min	Unknown	2 hr

Half-life: 5 to 7 min

Mechanism of Action

Neutralizes anticoagulant activity. A strong basic polypeptide, protamine combines with strongly acidic heparin complex to form an inactive stable salt, thereby neutralizing anticoagulant activity of both drugs.

Contraindications

Allergy to fish, hypersensitivity to protamine or its components

Interactions

DRUGS

heparin: Neutralized anticoagulant effect of heparin
insulin: Prolongs absorption of insulin
low molecular weight heparins: Incomplete neutralization of anticoagulant activity of low molecular weight heparin

Adverse Reactions

CNS: Weakness
CV: Bradycardia, hypertension, hypotension, shock
GI: Nausea, vomiting
HEME: Unusual bleeding or bruising
RESP: Dyspnea, pulmonary edema (noncardiogenic), pulmonary hypertension
SKIN: Flushing, sensation of warmth
Other: Anaphylaxis

Childbearing Considerations

PREGNANCY

- It is not known if drug may cause fetal harm.
- Use with caution only if benefit to mother outweighs potential risk to fetus.

LACTATION

- It is not known if drug is present in breast milk.
- Patient should check with prescriber before breastfeeding.

Nursing Considerations

- Be prepared to obtain coagulation studies (APTT, activated clotting time) 5 to 15 minutes after giving drug and to repeat them in 2 to 8 hours to detect heparin-rebound hypotension, shock, and bleeding.
- Monitor vital signs, hemodynamic parameters, and fluid intake and output, and assess for flushing sensation.
- Be aware that men with vasectomy have an increased risk of hypersensitivity reaction because of possible accumulation of antiprotamine antibodies.

PATIENT TEACHING

- Instruct patient to report adverse reactions immediately.

protriptyline hydrochloride

Triptil (CAN), Vivactil

Class and Category

Pharmacologic class: Tricyclic antidepressant
Therapeutic class: Antidepressant

Indications and Dosages

* *To treat depression*

TABLETS

Adults. *Initial:* 5 to 10 mg three times a day or four times a day, increased every wk by 10 mg daily, as needed. *Maximum:* 60 mg daily.
±**DOSAGE ADJUSTMENT** For adolescents and elderly patients, initial dosage limited to 5 mg three times a day, then adjusted, as needed.

Drug Administration

P.O.

- Any dosage increase made in morning dose.

Route	Onset	Peak	Duration
P.O.	1–2 wk	6–12 hr	24–48 hr

Half-life: 54–92 hr

Mechanism of Action

May block reuptake of norepinephrine and serotonin (and possibly other neurotransmitters) at neuronal membranes, thus enhancing their effects at postsynaptic receptors. These neurotransmitters may play a role in relieving depression symptoms.

Contraindications

Acute recovery phase after MI, concurrent therapy with cisapride, hypersensitivity to protriptyline or its components, use within 14 days of MAO inhibitor therapy

Interactions

DRUGS

anticholinergic agents, neuroleptic drugs: Increased risk of hyperpyrexia, especially in hot weather
anticholinergics, sympathomimetic drugs (epinephrine) combined with local anesthetics: Altered dosage requirements

cimetidine: Possible reduced metabolism of protriptyline with increased blood levels

CNS depressants: Possible increased CNS depressant effects

CYP2D6 substrates such as other antidepressants, phenothiazines, selective serotonin reuptake inhibitors, type I C antiarrhythmics: Possibly increased blood protriptyline levels leading to toxicity unexpectedly

tramadol: Increased seizure risk

ACTIVITIES

alcohol use: Possibly increased CNS depression alcohol

Adverse Reactions

CNS: Agitation, ataxia, confusion, **CVA**, dizziness, drowsiness, exacerbation of psychosis, extrapyramidal reactions, fatigue, lack of coordination, paresthesia, peripheral neuropathy, **suicidal ideation**, tremor, weakness

CV: Arrhythmias, including heart block; hypertension; **hypotension; MI**; orthostatic hypotension; palpitations; tachycardia

EENT: Angle-closure glaucoma, black tongue, blurred vision, dry mouth, increased intraocular pressure, lacrimation, stomatitis, tongue swelling

ENDO: Hyperglycemia, **hypoglycemia**

GI: Abdominal cramps, anorexia, constipation, diarrhea, epigastric discomfort, hepatic dysfunction, nausea, vomiting

GU: Impotence, libido changes, nocturia, urinary frequency and hesitancy, urine retention

SKIN: Diaphoresis, petechiae, photosensitivity, rash, urticaria

Other: Angioedema, weight gain or loss

Childbearing Considerations

PREGNANCY

- It is not known if drug may cause fetal harm.
- Use with caution only if benefit to mother outweighs potential risk to fetus.

LACTATION

- It is not known if drug is present in breast milk.
- Patient should check with prescriber before breastfeeding.

Nursing Considerations

- Use protriptyline cautiously in patients with a history of seizures, because drug can lower seizure threshold.

- Use cautiously in patients with a history of urine retention or increased intraocular pressure because of drug's autonomic activity.

! WARNING Avoid giving protriptyline with an MAO inhibitor. If patient is being switched from an MAO inhibitor to protriptyline, make sure MAO inhibitor has been discontinued for 14 days before starting protriptyline.

- Watch patients closely (especially children, adolescents, and young adults) for suicidal tendencies, particularly when therapy starts or dosage changes, because depression may worsen temporarily during these times, possibly leading to suicidal ideation.

PATIENT TEACHING

- Inform patient that protriptyline therapy may take several weeks to reach full effect.
- Advise patient that drug may cause mild pupillary dilation, which may lead to an episode of acute angle-closure glaucoma. Encourage patient to have an eye exam before starting therapy to see if he is at risk.
- Instruct patient to avoid hazardous activities until drug's CNS effects are known.
- Advise patient to change position slowly to minimize orthostatic hypotension.
- Urge patient to avoid alcohol while taking drug.
- Suggest drinking water and using sugarless gum or hard candy to relieve dry mouth.
- Advise patient to avoid sunlight and tanning booths and to wear protective clothing, a hat, and sunscreen when outdoors.
- Instruct diabetic patient to check blood glucose level frequently during first few weeks of protriptyline therapy.
- Urge family or caregiver to watch patient for suicidal tendencies, especially when therapy starts or dosage changes and particularly if patient is a child, teenager, or young adult.

prucalopride succinate
Motegrity

Class and Category

Pharmacologic class: Serotonin-4 (5-HT$_4$) receptor agonist

Therapeutic class: Intestinal mobility agent

Indications and Dosages

* *To treat chronic idiopathic constipation*

TABLETS

Adults. 2 mg once daily.

±**DOSAGE ADJUSTMENT** For patients with severe renal impairment (creatinine clearance less than 30 ml/min), dosage reduced to 1 mg once daily.

Drug Administration

P.O.

- Administered with or without food.

Route	Onset	Peak	Duration
P.O.	Unknown	2–3 hr	Unknown
Half-life: 24 hr			

Mechanism of Action

Stimulates colonic peristalsis, which increases bowel motility to relieve constipation.

Contraindications

Hypersensitivity to prucalopride or its components; intestinal obstruction or perforation due to functional or structural disorder of the gut wall, obstructive ileus, or severe inflammatory conditions of the intestinal tract such as Crohn's disease, toxic megacolon/megarectum, and ulcerative colitis

Interactions

DRUGS

None reported by manufacturer

Adverse Reactions

CNS: Dizziness, fatigue, headache, migraine, **suicidal ideation**
GI: Abdominal discomfort, distension, pain, or tenderness; abnormal gastrointestinal sounds; anorexia; diarrhea; epigastric discomfort; flatulence; nausea; vomiting
GU: Abnormal frequent urination during the day
RESP: Dyspnea
SKIN: Pruritus, rash, urticaria
Other: Hypersensitivity reactions, including facial angioedema

Childbearing Considerations

PREGNANCY

- Pregnancy exposure registry: 1-877-311-8972 or https://mothertobaby. org/pregnancy-studies/.
- It is not known if drug can cause fetal harm.

- Use with caution only if benefit to mother outweighs potential risk to fetus.

LACTATION

- Drug is present in breast milk.
- Patient should check with prescriber before breastfeeding.

Nursing Considerations

- Assess effectiveness of prucalopride therapy regularly.
- Monitor patient for persistent worsening of depression and emergence of suicidal thoughts and behavior, because prucalopride may cause suicidal ideation.

! **WARNING** Monitor patient for hypersensitivity reactions such as dyspnea, facial swelling, pruritus, rash, or urticaria. If present, stop drug therapy, notify prescriber, and provide supportive care, as prescribed.

PATIENT TEACHING

- Inform patient that prucalopride tablets may be taken without regard to food intake. Tell patient to store drug in original container to protect from moisture.
- Advise patient and caregiver that prucalopride may cause unusual changes in behavior or mood, persistent worsening of symptoms of depression, or emergence of suicidal thoughts or behavior. Instruct patient or caregiver to discontinue prucalopride therapy if any of these symptoms are present, and notify prescriber.

! **WARNING** Alert patient that prucalopride may cause an allergic reaction. If present, advise patient to stop taking drug, seek immediate emergency attention if serious, and notify prescriber.

pyridostigmine bromide

Mestinon, Mestinon-SR (CAN), Mestinon Timespans, Regonol

Class and Category

Pharmacologic class: Cholinesterase inhibitor
Therapeutic class: Muscle stimulant

≣ Indications and Dosages

✳ *To treat symptoms of myasthenia gravis*

SYRUP, TABLETS

Adults and adolescents. Highly individualized. *Average dose:* 600 mg daily spaced to provide maximum relief when maximum strength is needed. *For mild symptoms:* 60 mg to 360 mg daily, spaced to provide maximum relief. *For severe symptoms:* As high as 1,500 mg daily, spaced to provide maximum relief.

E.R. TABLETS

Adults and adolescents. 180 to 540 mg once or twice daily (at least 6 hr between doses).

✳ *To reverse the effects of neuromuscular blockers*

I.V. INJECTION

Adults. 0.1 to 0.25 mg/kg no faster than 1 mg/min immediately before or with 0.6 to 1.2 mg of I.V. atropine.

±**DOSAGE ADJUSTMENT** Dosage possibly reduced for patients with renal impairment.

≣ Drug Administration

P.O.

- Administer with a full glass of water or with food or milk if GI distress occurs.
- E.R. tablets should be swallowed whole and not chewed, crushed, or split.
- Use a calibrated device to measure dosage of syrup.

I.V.

- Administer as an I. V. injection no faster than 1 mg/min.
- *Incompatibilities:* None listed by manufacturer

Route	Onset	Peak	Duration
P.O.	20–30 min	1–2 hr	3–4 hr
P.O. (E.R.)	30–60 min	1–2 hr	6–12 hr
I.V.	2–5 min	Unknown	2–4 hr

Half-life: 1–3 hr

≣ Mechanism of Action

Improves muscle strength compromised by myasthenia gravis or neuromuscular blockade by competing with acetylcholine for its binding site on acetylcholinesterase. This action potentiates the effects of acetylcholine on skeletal muscle and the GI tract. Inhibited destruction of acetylcholine allows freer transmission of nerve impulses across the neuromuscular junction.

≣ Contraindications

Hypersensitivity to pyridostigmine or its components, mechanical obstruction of GI or urinary tract

≣ Interactions

DRUGS

4-aminopyridine: Delayed onset of action of pyridostigmine

aminoglycosides, bacitracin, colistin, magnesium salts, polymyxin B, sodium colistimethate, tetracyclines: Possible antagonized effects of pyridostigmine

quinidine: Possibly recurrent paralysis

≣ Adverse Reactions

EENT: Increased salivation, lacrimation, miosis

GI: Abdominal cramps, diarrhea, increased peristalsis, nausea, vomiting

GU: Urinary frequency, incontinence, or urgency

MS: Fasciculations, muscle spasms or weakness

RESP: Increased tracheobronchial secretions

SKIN: Diaphoresis

≣ Childbearing Considerations

PREGNANCY

- It is not known if drug may cause fetal harm.
- Use with caution only if benefit to mother outweighs potential risk to fetus.

LACTATION

- Drug may be present in breast milk.
- Patient should check with prescriber before breastfeeding.

≣ Nursing Considerations

- Use pyridostigmine cautiously in patients with renal disease because drug is mainly excreted unchanged by kidneys. Monitor BUN and serum creatinine levels.

! **WARNING** Maintain a rigid dosing schedule because a missed or late dose can precipitate myasthenic crisis.

- Observe for cholinergic reactions when administering drug I.V.

! **WARNING** Pyridostigmine overdose may obscure diagnosis of myasthenic crisis because main symptom in both is muscle weakness. Treat cholinergic crisis by stopping anticholinesterase, giving atropine as prescribed, and helping with endotracheal intubation and mechanical ventilation, if needed.

- Be aware that reversal of neuromuscular blockade usually occurs in 15 to 30 minutes. Be prepared to maintain patent airway and ventilation until normal voluntary respiration returns completely. Assess respiratory measurements and muscle tone with peripheral nerve stimulator device, as indicated.

PATIENT TEACHING

- Instruct patient to take pyridostigmine as directed and on schedule. Explain that a late or missed dose can precipitate a crisis. Suggest the use of a battery-operated alarm clock as a reminder.
- Tell patient to take drug with a full glass of water or with food or milk if GI distress occurs.
- Warn patient not to crush or chew E.R. tablets.
- Ask patient to record pyridostigmine dosage, times taken, and drug effects to help determine optimal dosage and schedule.
- Urge patient to carry medical identification describing her condition and drug regimen.

Q R S

quetiapine fumarate
Seroquel, Seroquel XR

☰ Class and Category
Pharmacologic class: Dibenzothiazepine derivative
Therapeutic class: Antipsychotic

☰ Indications and Dosages
✽ *To treat schizophrenia*

TABLETS
Adults. *Initial:* 25 mg twice daily on day 1. Increased by 25 to 50 twice daily or three times a day on days 2 and 3, then to 300 to 400 mg daily by day 4, in divided doses twice daily or three times a day. Increased every 2 days or more in increments of 25 to 50 mg twice daily, as needed. *Maximum:* 750 mg daily.

Adolescents ages 13 to 17 years. *Initial:* 25 mg twice daily on day 1; 50 mg twice daily on day 2; 100 mg twice daily on day 3; 150 mg twice daily on day 4; and 200 mg twice daily on day 5. Increased further in increments no greater than 100 mg/day. *Maximum:* 800 mg daily.

E.R. TABLETS
Adults. *Initial:* 300 mg once daily in evening. Dosage increased daily in increments up to 300 mg, as needed. *Maximum:* 800 mg daily.

Adolescents age 13 to 17 years. *Initial:* 50 mg daily on day 1; 100 mg daily on day 2; 200 mg daily on day 3; 300 mg daily on day 4; 400 mg daily on day 5. Increased further in increments no greater than 100 mg/day, as needed. *Maximum:* 800 mg daily.

✽ *To maintain schizophrenia therapy with monotherapy*

E.R. TABLETS, TABLETS
Adults. 400 to 800 mg daily after dosage has been titrated to usual dosage. Maximum: 800 mg daily.

✽ *To treat bipolar mania as monotherapy or as an adjunct to lithium or divalproex*

TABLETS
Adults. Initial: 50 mg twice daily on day 1; 100 mg twice daily on day 2; 150 mg twice

daily on day 3; and 200 mg twice daily on day 4. Increased in increments of no greater than 200 mg/day, as needed by day 6. Usual: 400 to 800 mg/day. Maximum: 800 mg/day.

E.R. TABLETS
Adults. Initial: 300 mg once daily on day 1; 600 mg once daily on day 2; and between 400 and 800 mg once daily on day 3 and beyond. Usual: 400 to 800 mg once daily. Maximum: 800 mg/day.

✽ *To treat mixed bipolar I disorder as monotherapy or adjunct to lithium or divalproex*

E.R. TABLETS
Adults. Initial: 300 mg once daily on day 1; 600 mg once daily on day 2; and between 400 and 800 mg once daily on day 3 and beyond. Usual: 400 to 800 mg once daily. Maximum: 800 mg/day.

✽ *To treat pediatric bipolar mania as monotherapy*

TABLETS
Children and adolescents age 10 to 17. *Initial:* 25 mg twice daily on day 1; 50 mg twice daily on day 2; 100 mg twice daily on day 3; 150 mg twice daily on day 4, and 200 mg twice daily on day 5. Increased in no greater increments than 100 mg/day, as needed. *Usual:* 400 to 600 mg/day. *Maximum:* 600 mg/day.

E.R. TABLETS
Children and adolescents age 10 to 17. *Initial:* 50 mg once daily on day 1; 100 mg once daily on day 2; 200 mg once daily on day 3; 300 mg once daily on day 4; and 400 mg once daily on day 5. *Usual:* 400 to 600 mg daily. *Maximum:* 600 mg/day.

✽ *To treat bipolar depression*

TABLETS
Adults. *Initial:* 50 mg at bedtime on day 1; 100 mg at bedtime on day 2; 200 mg at bedtime on day 3; and 300 mg at bedtime on day 4. *Maximum:* 300 mg/day.

E.R. TABLETS
Adults. *Initial:* 50 mg once daily on day 1; 100 mg once daily on day 2; 200 mg once daily on day 3; and 300 mg once daily on day 4. *Usual:* 300 mg daily. *Maximum:* 300 mg/day.

✽ *As adjunct to divalproex or lithium therapy as part of maintenance therapy for bipolar I disorder*

Q
R
S

E.R. TABLETS

Adults. Continued on same dosage stabilized on with doses given twice daily totaling 400 to 800/day. *Maximum:* 800 mg/day.

* *As adjunctive therapy with antidepressants to treat major depressive disorder*

E.R. TABLETS

Adults. *Initial:* 50 mg once daily on days 1 and 2 and 150 mg once daily on day 3. *Usual:* 150 to 300 mg once daily. *Maximum:* 300 mg once daily.

±**DOSAGE ADJUSTMENT** For patients with hepatic impairment, initial dosage no higher than 25 mg once daily for immediate-release form and 50 mg once daily for extended-release form and increased in increments of 25 mg/day for immediate-release form and 50 mg/day for extended-release form depending on response and tolerance. For elderly patients, initial dosage of either form reduced to 50 mg/day and dose increased in increments of 50 mg/day, as needed. For patients receiving CYP3A4 inducers (avasimibe, carbamazepine, phenytoin, rifampin, St. John's wort), dosage increased up to fivefold of the original dose. When CYP3A4 inducer is discontinued, dosage reduced to original level within 7 to 14 days. For patients receiving CYP3A4 inhibitors (ketoconazole, itraconazole, indinavir, nefazodone, ritonavir), dosage reduced to one-sixth of original dose. When CYP3A4 drug is discontinued, dosage increased sixfold.

Drug Administration

P.O.

- Administer immediate-release tablets without regard to food intake; administer extended-release tablets without food or with a light meal of about 300 calories.
- E.R. tablets should be swallowed whole and not chewed, crushed, or divided.
- E.R. tablets are administered at different times of the day depending on condition being treated (see Indications and Dosages section).

Route	Onset	Peak	Duration
P.O.	Unknown	1.5 hr	Unknown
P.O./E.R.	Unknown	6 hr	Unknown

Half-life: 6–7 hr

Mechanism of Action

May produce antipsychotic effects by interfering with dopamine binding to dopamine type 2 (D_2)-receptor sites in the brain and by antagonizing serotonin 5-HT_2, dopamine type 1 (D_1), histamine H_1, and adrenergic alpha$_1$ and alpha$_2$ receptors.

Contraindications

Hypersensitivity to quetiapine or its components

Interactions

DRUGS

anticholinergic drugs: Increased risk of severe gastrointestinal adverse reactions related to hypomotility
antihypertensives: Increased risk of hypotension
CNS depressants: Possibly increased CNS depression
CYP3A4 inducers (avasimibe, carbamazepine, phenytoin, rifampin, St. John's wort): Decreased exposure of quetiapine with decreased effectiveness
CYP3A4 inhibitors (ketoconazole, indinavir, itraconazole, nefazodone, ritonavir): Increased exposure of quetiapine increasing risk of adverse reactions
dopamine agonists, levodopa: Possibly antagonized effects of these drugs

ACTIVITIES

alcohol use: Possibly enhanced CNS depression

Adverse Reactions

CNS: Abnormal dreams, akathisia, anxiety, attention disturbance, confusion, depression, disorientation, dizziness, drowsiness, dystonia, extrapyramidal reactions, fatigue, hypertonia, **hypothermia**, irritability, lethargy, mental impairment, migraine, **neuroleptic malignant syndrome**, restless leg syndrome, motor and sensory instability, paresthesia, retrograde amnesia, somnolence, **suicidal ideation**, tardive dyskinesia, tremor
CV: **Cardiomyopathy**, dyslipidemia, hypercholesterolemia, **hypotension**, increased heart rate, **myocarditis**, orthostatic hypotension, palpitations, **prolongation of QT interval**, tachycardia
EENT: Blurred vision, cataracts, dry mouth, ear pain, nasal congestion, pharyngitis, rhinitis, sinusitis

ENDO: Galactorrhea, hyperglycemia, **hyperosmolar coma,** hyperprolactinemia, hypothyroidism, **ketoacidosis,** syndrome of inappropriate ADH secretion

GI: Anorexia, constipation, dysphagia, **hepatitis,** ileus, indigestion, **intestinal obstruction, ischemic colon, liver necrosis or failure, pancreatitis,** vomiting

GU: Decreased libido, nocturnal enuresis, pollakiuria, UTI, urinary retention

HEME: Agranulocytosis, leukopenia, neutropenia, thrombocytopenia

MS: Back or neck pain, dysarthria, muscle spasms or weakness, myalgia, **rhabdomyolysis**

RESP: Cough, dyspnea, **sleep apnea**

SKIN: Acute generalized exanthematous pustulosis, cutaneous vasculitis, diaphoresis, **Stevens–Johnson syndrome, toxic epidermal necrolysis**

Other: Anaphylaxis, drug reaction with eosinophilia and systemic symptoms (DRESS), flu-like symptoms, **hyponatremia,** weight gain

Childbearing Considerations

PREGNANCY
- Pregnancy exposure registry: 1-866-961-2388 or http://womensmentalhealth.org/clinical-and-research-programs/pregnancyregistry/.
- Drug may cause fetal harm if exposed in the third trimester increasing risk for extrapyramidal and/or withdrawal symptoms following delivery.

LACTATION
- Drug is present in breast milk.
- Patient should check with prescriber before breastfeeding.

REPRODUCTION
- Drug may increase prolactin levels, which may lead to a reversible reduction in fertility in female patients.

Nursing Considerations

! WARNING Know that quetiapine shouldn't be used for elderly patients with dementia-related psychosis because drug increases the risk of death in these patients.

- Know that quetiapine should not be given to patients who have a history of cardiac arrhythmias, such as bradycardia, or who experience hypokalemia or hypomagnesemia. The drug also should not be used with other drugs that prolong the QT interval or in a patient who has a congenital prolongation of the QT interval because quetiapine may increase the QT interval, which may increase the risk of torsades de pointes and/or sudden death.
- Use quetiapine cautiously in patients who have a history of cardiovascular disease, a family history of QT prolongation, or in patients who are elderly or take medications that may cause an electrolyte imbalance, such as diuretics, or who have congestive heart failure or heart hypertrophy, because these factors may increase the risk of a prolonged QT interval. Also use cautiously in cardiac patients because quetiapine may cause orthostatic hypotension.
- Monitor patients (particularly children and young adults) closely for suicidal tendencies, especially when therapy starts or dosage changes, because depression may worsen temporarily during these times.

! WARNING Monitor patient taking quetiapine for predisposing factors for neuroleptic malignant syndrome, such as dehydration, heat stress, organic brain disease, and physical exhaustion. Neuroleptic malignant syndrome includes altered mental status, autonomic instability (which may include arrhythmias, blood pressure abnormalities, diaphoresis, irregular pulse, or tachycardia), hyperpyrexia, and muscle rigidity.

- Monitor patient for signs of tardive dyskinesia, a potentially irreversible complication characterized by involuntary, dyskinetic movements of eyelids, face, jaw, mouth, or tongue. Notify prescriber if such signs develop, because quetiapine therapy may have to be stopped.
- Monitor patient for orthostatic hypotension, especially during initial dosage titration period. Be prepared to correct underlying conditions, such as dehydration and hypovolemia, before starting quetiapine therapy, as prescribed. Also monitor patient for an increase in blood pressure. Check blood pressure, especially in adolescents

Q
R
S

and children, at the beginning of and periodically during treatment.

- Monitor patient for prolonged abnormal muscle contractions, especially during the first few days of quetiapine therapy, in male patients and in younger patients.
- Assess patient for hypothyroidism because drug can cause dose-dependent decreases in total and free thyroxine (T_4) levels.
- Monitor laboratory results during first 3 weeks of therapy for transient elevations in hepatic enzyme levels. Notify prescriber if they persist or worsen.
- Monitor patient's blood glucose and lipid levels routinely, as ordered, because drug increases the risk of hyperglycemia and hypercholesterolemia.
- Check CBC often during the first few months of therapy, as ordered, in patients with a low white blood cell count or a history of drug-induced hematologic problems. If counts drop or patient develops a fever or other signs of infection, notify prescriber and expect to discontinue drug and provide supportive care.
- Institute fall precautions, because patients receiving quetiapine have a greater risk of falling.
- Expect to gradually taper off quetiapine therapy when discontinued, as ordered, to avoid acute withdrawal symptoms such as insomnia, nausea, and vomiting.

PATIENT TEACHING

- Instruct patient that quetiapine may be taken without regard to food, although extended-release form may be taken with a light meal of about 300 calories.
- Caution patient not to chew, crush, or divide extended-release tablets.
- Instruct patient to take extended-release tablets at the time of day prescribed.
- Advise patient not to stop taking quetiapine suddenly because doing so may exacerbate his symptoms or produce withdrawal symptoms.
- Inform patient that quetiapine therapy may cause dizziness or drowsiness. Advise him not to drive or perform other activities that require alertness until drug's full CNS effects are known. Also, review fall precautions with patient.
- Instruct patient to rise slowly from a lying or seated position to reduce the risk of dizziness or fainting.

- Caution patient to avoid consuming alcoholic beverages, because they can increase dizziness and drowsiness.
- Urge family or caregiver to watch patient closely for suicidal tendencies, especially when therapy starts or dosage changes and particularly if patient is a child or young adult.
- Encourage patient on long-term therapy to have regular eye examinations so that cataracts can be detected.
- Advise patient to contact prescriber if his pulse rate becomes abnormally slow or irregular.
- Alert patient that a false-positive drug test for methadone or tricyclic antidepressants may occur with quetiapine use.
- Urge patient to notify prescriber if a fever, flu-like symptoms, sore throat, or any other infection occurs, as drug may have to be discontinued and an evaluation for a potential infection be done.
- Caution patient to avoid dehydration, exposure to extreme heat, or exercising strenuously, because drug may disrupt body's ability to reduce body temperature.

quinapril hydrochloride
Accupril

Class and Category

Pharmacologic class: Angiotensin-converting enzyme (ACE) inhibitor
Therapeutic class: Antihypertensive

Indications and Dosages

* *To treat hypertension*

TABLETS

Adults not on diuretics. *Initial:* 10 or 20 mg daily, adjusted every 2 wk based on clinical response. *Maintenance:* 20 to 80 mg daily or in divided doses twice daily.

* *As adjunct to manage heart failure*

TABLETS

Adults. *Initial:* 5 mg twice daily, increased, weekly as needed and tolerated. *Maintenance:* 20 to 40 mg twice daily given in two equally divided doses.

±**DOSAGE ADJUSTMENT** For patients who are dehydrated from previous diuretic therapy, those who are still receiving diuretic therapy, and those with creatinine clearance of 30 to 60 ml/min, initial dosage reduced to 5 mg daily. For patients with creatinine clearance of 10 to 30 ml/min, initial dosage reduced to 2.5 mg daily. For elderly patients, initial dosage reduced to 10 mg once daily, then titrated slowly to optimal response.

Drug Administration

P.O.

- Administer with or without food but avoid giving with a high-fat meal because of decreased absorption.

Route	Onset	Peak	Duration
P.O.	1 hr	1–2 hr	24 hr

Half-life: 0.8–3 hr

Mechanism of Action

Blocks conversion of angiotensin I to angiotensin II, leading to vasodilation, and reduces aldosterone secretion, which prevents water retention. Quinapril also reduces peripheral arterial resistance. These combined actions lead to a reduction in blood pressure. The reduction of aldosterone secretion also helps to relieve fluid buildup in heart failure.

Contraindications

Aliskiren therapy in patients with diabetes, history of angioedema related to previous treatment with ACE inhibitor, hypersensitivity to quinapril or its components, use of a neprilysin inhibitor such as sacubitril within 36 hours

Interactions

DRUGS

aliskiren (patients with diabetes and/or renal impairment), angiotensin receptor blockers, other ACE inhibitors: Increased risk of hyperkalemia, hypotension, and renal dysfunction
diuretics: Increased risk of hypotension
lithium: Possibly increased blood lithium level and risk of toxicity
mTOR inhibitors such as temsirolimus, neprilysin inhibitors such as sacubitril: Increased risk of angioedema
NSAIDs: Decreased antihypertensive effect of quinapril; increased risk of renal dysfunction in the elderly or patients who have preexisting renal dysfunction or are volume depleted
potassium preparations, potassium-sparing diuretics, potassium supplements: Increased risk of hyperkalemia
sodium aurothiomalate: Possibly nitritoid reactions such as facial flushing, hypotension, nausea, vomiting
tetracyclines: Reduced tetracycline absorption

FOODS

foods high in potassium such as milk or potatoes, potassium-containing salt substitutes: Increased risk of hyperkalemia

Adverse Reactions

CNS: CVA, depression, dizziness, drowsiness, fatigue, fever, headache, insomnia, light-headedness, malaise, nervousness, paresthesia, sleep disturbance, somnolence, syncope, vertigo
CV: Angina pectoris, **arrhythmias, cardiogenic shock,** chest pain, edema, **heart failure, hypertensive crisis, hypotension,** orthostatic hypotension, **MI,** palpitations, tachycardia, vasodilation
EENT: Amblyopia, dry mouth or throat, loss of taste, pharyngitis
GI: Abdominal pain, constipation, diarrhea, dyspepsia, elevated liver enzymes, flatulence, **GI hemorrhage, hepatitis,** indigestion, nausea, **pancreatitis,** vomiting
GU: **Acute renal failure,** elevated blood urea nitrogen and creatinine, impotence, UTI, **worsening renal failure**
HEME: **Agranulocytosis, hemolytic anemia, thrombocytopenia**
MS: Arthralgia, back pain, myalgia
RESP: Cough, dyspnea, **eosinophilic pneumonitis**
SKIN: Alopecia, dermatopolymyositis, diaphoresis, **exfoliative dermatitis,** flushing, pemphigus, photosensitivity, pruritus, rash, urticaria
Other: Anaphylaxis, **angioedema, hyperkalemia,** hyponatremia

Childbearing Considerations

PREGNANCY

- Drug can cause fetal harm, especially if exposure occurs during the second or third trimester.
- Drug reduces fetal renal function, leading to anuria and renal failure, and increases fetal and neonatal morbidity and death.

Q
R
S

It can also cause fetal lung hypoplasia, hypotension, and skeletal deformations such as skull hypoplasia.

- Drug is contradicated in pregnant women and should be discontinued as soon as possible if pregnancy occurs.

LACTATION
- Drug is present in breast milk.
- Patient should check with prescriber before breastfeeding.

≣ Nursing Considerations
- Use quinapril cautiously in patients with diabetes mellitus, renal impairment, or patients taking concomitant therapy with drugs that raise potassium levels. Monitor serum potassium levels, as ordered, in these patients and assess patient often for signs and symptoms of hyperkalemia.

! **WARNING** Keep in mind patients with heart failure, hyponatremia, or severe salt or volume depletion; those who've recently received intensive diuresis or an increase in diuretic dosage; and those undergoing dialysis may be at risk for excessive hypotension. Monitor blood pressure often for first 2 weeks of therapy and whenever quinapril or diuretic dosage increases. If excessive hypotension occurs, notify prescriber immediately, place patient in a supine position, and, if prescribed, infuse normal saline solution.

! **WARNING** Know that because of the risk of angioedema, be prepared to discontinue drug and administer emergency measures, including subcutaneous epinephrine 1:1,000 (0.3 to 0.5 ml), if swelling of glottis, larynx, or tongue causes airway obstruction. Know that patients with a history of angioedema unrelated to ACE inhibitor therapy may be at increased risk of angioedema while receiving quinapril.

- Monitor patient's vital signs and cardiopulmonary status often to assess drug's effectiveness.

PATIENT TEACHING
- Advise patient to avoid taking drug with a high-fat meal because drug absorption may be affected.

! **WARNING** Instruct patient to notify prescriber immediately and stop taking

quinapril if he has difficulty breathing or swallowing or he experiences swelling of the eyes, face, lips, or tongue.

- Explain that drug may cause dizziness and light-headedness, especially for first few days of therapy. Advise patient to avoid hazardous activities until drug's CNS effects are known and to notify prescriber if he faints.
- Inform women of childbearing age of risks of taking quinapril during pregnancy. Caution her to use effective contraception and to notify prescriber immediately of known or suspected pregnancy.
- Advise patient having surgery or receiving anesthesia to tell specialist that he takes quinapril.
- Instruct patient to consult prescriber before using potassium supplements or salt substitutes that contain potassium.

quinidine gluconate

quinidine sulfate

≣ Class and Category
Pharmacologic class: Cinchona alkaloid
Therapeutic class: Class IA antiarrhythmic

≣ Indications and Dosages
* *To restore normal sinus rhythm in patients with symptomatic atrial fibrillation or atrial flutter*

E.R. TABLETS (QUINIDINE GLUCONATE)
Adults. 648 mg every 8 hr, increased cautiously after 3 to 4 doses, if needed.

E.R. TABLETS (QUINIDINE SULFATE)
Adults. 300 every 8 to 12 hr with dosage cautiously increased if conversion not attained.

TABLETS (QUINIDINE SULFATE)
Adults. *Initial:* 400 mg every 6 hr with dosage cautiously increased if conversion not attained after 4 or 5 doses.

* *To reduce frequency of relapse into atrial fibrillation or atrial flutter*

E.R. TABLETS (QUINIDINE GLUCONATE)
Adults. 324 mg every 8 to 12 hr, then dosage cautiously increased if serum quinidine levels

are within therapeutic range and average time between arrhythmic episodes has not been satisfactorily increased.

E.R. TABLETS (QUINIDINE SULFATE)

Adults. 300 mg every 8 to 12 hr with dosage cautiously increased if serum quinidine levels are within therapeutic range and average time between arrhythmic episodes has not been satisfactorily increased.

TABLETS (QUINIDINE SULFATE)

Adults. 200 mg every 6 hr with dosage cautiously increased if serum quinidine levels are within therapeutic range and average time between arrhythmic episodes has not been satisfactorily increased.

✳ *To suppress ventricular arrhythmias*

E.R. TABLETS (QUINIDINE SULFATE), E.R. TABLETS (QUINIDINE GLUCONATE), TABLETS (QUINIDINE SULFATE)

Adults. Highly individualized based on the results of programmed electrical stimulation and/or Holter monitoring with exercise.

☰ Drug Administration

P.O.

- Administer drug at the same time every day and at evenly spaced intervals with a full glass of water.
- E.R. tablets should be swallowed whole and not chewed, crushed, or opened.
- Administer drug with food if GI upset occurs, but not with grapefruit juice.

Route	Onset	Peak	Duration
P.O.	1–3 hr	2–5 hr	6–8 hr
P.O. (E.R.)	Unknown	Unknown	12 hr

Half-life: 6–8 hr

☰ Mechanism of Action

Depresses conduction velocity, contractility, and excitability of the myocardium and increases the effective refractory period, thus suppressing arrhythmic activity in the atria, ventricles, and His-Purkinje system.

☰ Contraindications

History of quinidine- or quinine-associated thrombocytopenic purpura; hypersensitivity to quinidine or its components; myasthenia gravis or other conditions that might be adversely affected by anticholinergic effects; presence of AV junctional or idioventricular pacemaker, including those in complete AV block

☰ Interactions

DRUGS

antacids: Possibly delayed oral absorption of quinidine

antiarrhythmics, phenothiazines: Additive cardiac effects

anticholinergics: Possibly intensified atropine-like adverse effects

anticonvulsants: Possible accelerated clearance of quinidine reducing effectiveness

antihypertensives: Increased risk of hypotension

cimetidine: Increased elimination half-life, possibly leading to quinidine toxicity

cholinergic agents: Antagonized effects of cholinergic agents

clarithromycin: Possible but rarely torsades de pointes occurrence

dextromethorphan: Substantial increase in bioavailability of dextromethorphan

digoxin: Possibly digitalis toxicity

diltiazem: Decreased clearance and increased half-life of quinidine

felodipine: Possibly decreased metabolism of felodipine

haloperidol: Increased serum haloperidol concentrations

ketoconazole: Increased plasma quinidine levels

nifedipine: Decreased serum quinidine concentrations and decreased rate of nifedipine metabolism

neuromuscular blockers: Possibly potentiated neuromuscular blockade

reserpine: Possible additive cardiac depressant effects

rifampin: Possible accelerated quinidine elimination

quinine: Increased risk of quinidine toxicity

verapamil: Possibly decreased clearance of quinidine, additive effects, and hypotension in patients with an arrhythmia or hypertrophic cardiomyopathy

warfarin: Potentiates anticoagulant effect of warfarin

FOOD

grapefruit juice: Possibly delay GI absorption of oral quinidine

☰ Adverse Reactions

CNS: Anxiety, asthenia, ataxia, confusion, delirium, difficulty speaking, dizziness, drowsiness, extrapyramidal reactions, fever, headache, hypertonia, syncope, vertigo

Q
R
S

CV: **Complete heart block,** orthostatic hypotension, palpitations, peripheral edema, **prolonged QT interval, torsades de pointes,** vasculitis, **ventricular arrhythmias, widening QRS complex**
EENT: Blurred vision, change in color perception, diplopia, dry mouth, hearing loss (high-frequency), pharyngitis, photophobia, rhinitis, tinnitus
GI: Abdominal pain, anorexia, constipation, diarrhea, indigestion, nausea, vomiting
HEME: **Agranulocytosis, hemolytic anemia, leukopenia, neutropenia, thrombocytopenia, thrombocytopenic purpura**
MS: Arthralgia, myalgia
RESP: Dyspnea
SKIN: Diaphoresis, eczema, **exfoliative dermatitis,** flushing, hyperpigmentation, photosensitivity, pruritus, psoriasis, purpura, rash, urticaria
Other: **Angioedema,** flu-like symptoms, weight gain

Childbearing Considerations
PREGNANCY
- It is not known if drug causes fetal harm.
- Use with caution only if benefit to mother outweighs potential risk to fetus.

LACTATION
- Drug is present in breast milk.
- Breastfeeding is not recommended during breastfeeding.

Nursing Considerations
- Monitor therapeutic blood level of quinidine, as ordered.
- Monitor heart rate and rhythm closely because quinidine may cause serious adverse reactions and can be cardiotoxic, especially at dosages exceeding 2.4 g daily. Implement continuous cardiac monitoring, as ordered.
- Assess for early signs and symptoms of cinchonism, including blurred vision, change in color perception, confusion, diplopia, headache, and tinnitus, which may indicate quinidine toxicity.

PATIENT TEACHING
- Advise patient to take quinidine at the same times every day and at evenly spaced intervals.
- Instruct patient to swallow E.R. tablets whole, with a full glass of water and not chew, crush, or divide tablets.

- Advise patient to take drug with food if GI upset occurs, but not to take with grapefruit juice.
- Urge patient to inform prescriber immediately of blurred or double vision, change in color perception, confusion, diarrhea, fever, headache, loss of hearing, or tinnitus.

rabeprazole sodium
AcipHex, AcipHex Sprinkle

Class and Category
Pharmacologic class: Proton pump inhibitor
Therapeutic class: Antiulcer

Indications and Dosages
✱ *To provide short-term treatment of erosive esophagitis or ulcerative gastroesophageal reflux disease (GERD)*

DELAYED-RELEASE TABLETS
Adults. 20 mg once daily for 4 to 8 wk; course may be repeated if healing has not occurred at the end of 8 wk.

✱ *To treat symptomatic GERD*

DELAYED-RELEASE TABLETS
Adults and adolescents age 12 and over. 20 mg daily for 4 wk (adults) and 8 weeks (adolescents). Course may be repeated if symptoms aren't completely resolved (adults).

DELAYED-RELEASE CAPSULES (ACIPHEX SPRINKLE)
Children ages 1 to 11 weighing 15 kg (33 lb) or more. 10 mg once daily for up to 12 wk.
Children ages 1 to 11 weighing less than 15 kg (33 lb). 5 mg once daily up to 12 wk. Increased to 10 mg once daily, as needed.

✱ *To provide maintenance treatment of erosive esophagitis or GERD*

DELAYED-RELEASE TABLETS
Adults. 20 mg once daily for no longer than 12 months.

✱ *To promote healing of duodenal ulcer*

DELAYED-RELEASE TABLETS
Adults. 20 mg once daily after the morning meal for up to 4 wk. Course may be repeated if symptoms aren't completely resolved.

✱ *As adjunct to reduce the risk of duodenal ulcer recurrence by eradicating* Helicobacter pylori

DELAYED-RELEASE TABLETS
Adults. 20 mg twice daily with morning and evening meals in conjunction with

amoxicillin 1,000 mg and clarithromycin 500 mg twice daily for 7 days.

✳ *To treat hypersecretory conditions, such as Zollinger–Ellison syndrome*

DELAYED-RELEASE TABLETS

Adults. *Initial:* 60 mg once daily; may be increased, if needed, to 100 mg daily or 60 mg twice daily.

⊟ Drug Administration

P.O.

- Delayed-release tablets are to be swallowed whole and not chewed, crushed, or divided; they can be administered with or without food. If used to heal a duodenal ulcer, D.R. tablets should be administered after morning meal; if used to eradicate *Helicobacter pylori*, administer before morning and evening meals.
- Delayed-release capsules should be administered 30 minutes before a meal. Be aware that the if patient cannot swallow capsule whole; open and pour content onto a small amount of soft food (applesauce, vegetable-based baby food, or yogurt) or into a small amount of liquid (apple juice, infant formula, or pediatric electrolyte solution). Food or liquid should be at or below room temperature. Administer within 15 minutes. Discard leftover mixture.

Route	Onset	Peak	Duration
P.O./D.R.	< 1 hr	1–6.5 hr	24 hr

Half-life: 1–2 hr

⊟ Mechanism of Action

Decreases gastric acid secretion by suppressing its release at the secretory surface of gastric parietal cells. Rabeprazole also increases gastric pH and decreases basal acid output, which helps to heal ulcerated areas. In gastric parietal cells, it's transformed to an active sulfonamide, which increases the clearance rate of *H. pylori*.

⊟ Contraindications

Concurrent therapy with rilpivirine-containing products; hypersensitivity to rabeprazole, other substituted benzimidazoles (lansoprazole, omeprazole), or their components

⊟ Interactions

DRUGS

atazanavir, nelfinavir, rilpivirine: Decreased exposure of these antiretrovirals with possible decreased antiviral effect and increased development of drug resistance

clarithromycin: Increased risk of serious adverse reactions, including possibly fatal arrhythmias

dasatinib, erlotinib, iron salts, itraconazole, ketoconazole, mycophenolate mofetil, nilotinib: Reduced absorption of these drugs decreasing effectiveness

digoxin: Increased risk of digitalis toxicity

methotrexate: Increased risk of methotrexate toxicities

saquinavir: Increased exposure resulting in possible increased toxicity

tacrolimus: Possibly increased exposure of tacrolimus, especially in transplant patients who are intermediate or poor metabolizers of CYP2C19

warfarin: Possibly increased prothrombin time (PT), international normalized ratio (INR)

⊟ Adverse Reactions

CNS: **Coma**, delirium, disorientation, dizziness, headache, malaise, vertigo

EENT: Blurred vision

ENDO: Elevated TSH levels

GI: Abdominal pain, *Clostridium difficile-associated diarrhea*, diarrhea, fundic gland polyps, jaundice, nausea, vomiting

GU: Acute tubulointerstitial nephritis

HEME: **Agranulocytosis, hemolytic anemia, leukopenia, pancytopenia, thrombocytopenia**

MS: Bone fracture, **rhabdomyolysis**

RESP: **Bronchospasm, interstitial pneumonia**

SKIN: Cutaneous lupus erythematosus, bullous and other drug skin eruptions, **erythema multiforme**, rash, **Stevens–Johnson syndrome, toxic epidermal necrolysis**, urticaria

Other: **Anaphylaxis, angioedema, hyperammonemia, hypomagnesemia**, systemic lupus erythematosus, vitamin B_{12} deficiency (long-term use)

⊟ Childbearing Considerations

PREGNANCY

- It is not known if drug can cause fetal harm.
- Use with caution only if benefit to mother outweighs potential risk to fetus.

LACTATION

- It is not known if drug is present in breast milk.

- Patient should check with prescriber before breastfeeding.

Nursing Considerations

- Use rabeprazole cautiously in patients with hepatic dysfunction.
- Obtain a serum magnesium level, as ordered, prior to starting rabeprazole therapy for those patients expected to be on prolonged therapy or who also take digoxin or drugs that may cause hypomagnesemia such as diuretics when taken with rabeprazole.
- Expect to monitor serum gastrin level in long-term therapy to detect elevation.
- Closely monitor Japanese men receiving rabeprazole for adverse reactions because they're more likely than other patients to have increased blood drug levels.

> **! WARNING** Monitor patient closely for hypersensitivity reactions such as acute tubulointerstitial nephritis (may or may not have symptoms), anaphylaxis, angioedema, bronchospasm, and urticaria. Notify prescriber, if suspected, and expect drug to be discontinued. Provide supportive care, as needed and prescribed.

- Be aware that symptomatic response to rabeprazole therapy does not preclude the presence of a gastric tumor. Expect patients who have a suboptimal response or an early symptomatic relapse after completing rabeprazole therapy to have further diagnostic testing done.
- Monitor patient for bone fracture, especially in patient receiving multiple daily doses for more than a year, because proton pump inhibitors like rabeprazole increase risk of osteoporosis-related fractures of the hip, wrist, and spine.
- Monitor patient for diarrhea because diarrhea including *C. difficile*-associated diarrhea may occur with rabeprazole therapy. Notify prescriber if persistent or severe diarrhea develops.
- Monitor patient's magnesium level, as ordered during therapy, because hypomagnesemia may occur with rabeprazole therapy that has lasted longer than 3 months, although most cases have occurred after therapy had been given for more than a year. Notify prescriber if magnesium level drops below normal, as hypomagnesemia may cause arrhythmias, seizures, and tetany. Expect patient to receive magnesium replacement and drug to be discontinued.
- Monitor patient for arthralgia and rash, as rabeprazole may cause either cutaneous or systemic lupus erythematosus in patients as a new onset or an exacerbation of the existing autoimmune disease. Know that proton pump inhibitors like rabeprazole should not be given longer than necessary. If patient becomes symptomatic, notify prescriber. If confirmed, expect drug to be discontinued. Know that most patients improve within 12 weeks after drug is discontinued.
- Be aware that rabeprazole may produce false readings on the following tests: secretin stimulation test assessing for gastrinoma and serum chromogranin levels assessing for neuroendocrine tumors; these require rabeprazole to be withheld for at least 14 days before tests are performed. Urine tests for tetrahydrocannabinol may result in a false-positive result.

PATIENT TEACHING

- Instruct patient to swallow delayed-release tablets whole and not to chew, crush, or divide and take with or without food.
- Instruct patient receiving delayed-release capsules to take capsules 30 minutes before a meal. Tell patient if capsule cannot be swallowed whole, to open and pour content onto a small amount of soft food (applesauce, vegetable-based baby food, or yogurt) or into a small amount of liquid (apple juice, infant formula, or pediatric electrolyte solution). Food or liquid should be at or below room temperature. Tell patient to take within 15 minutes and to discard leftover mixture.

> **! WARNING** Alert patient that drug may cause an allergic reaction. If an allergic reaction occurs, tell patient to stop drug, notify prescriber, and, if severe, to seek emergency medical care.

- Instruct patient to notify prescriber immediately if he develops new or worsening joint pain or a rash on his arms or cheeks that gets worse in the sun.
- Inform patients with hypersecretory conditions, such as Zollinger–Ellison

syndrome, that treatment can last for a year or longer.

- Tell patient to notify prescriber immediately if he experiences a decrease in the amount of urine voided or if urine has blood in it.
- Advise patient to contact prescriber if he develops persistent or severe diarrhea that is accompanied by abdominal pain and fever.
- Instruct patient to notify prescriber of any persistent, severe, or unusual adverse reactions.
- Tell patient to inform all prescribers of rabeprazole therapy.
- Inform patient that vitamin B$_{12}$ deficiency may occur if drug is taken longer than 3 years.

raloxifene hydrochloride
Evista

Class and Category
Pharmacologic class: Selective estrogen receptor modulator (SERM)
Therapeutic class: Antiosteoporotic

Indications and Dosages
∗ *To prevent osteoporosis in postmenopausal women; to reduce risk of invasive breast cancer in postmenopausal women with osteoporosis; to reduce risk of invasive breast cancer in postmenopausal women at high risk*

TABLETS
Adults. 60 mg daily.

Drug Administration
P.O.
- Do not administer drug for at least 72 hours before and during prolonged immobilization. Expect to resume therapy after patient is fully mobile again.

Route	Onset	Peak	Duration
P.O.	Unknown	0.5–6 hr	24 hr

Half-life: 1–2 hr

Mechanism of Action
Prevents osteoporosis by binding to estrogen receptors, which decreases bone resorption and increases bone mineral density in postmenopausal women. May reduce risk of invasive breast cancer because of its binding effects on estrogen receptors.

Contraindications
Active or past history of thromboembolic disease, hypersensitivity to raloxifene or its components, pregnancy

Interactions
DRUGS
cholestyramine: Decreased raloxifene absorption
diazepam, diazoxide, lidocaine, other highly protein-bound drugs: Possibly interference with binding sites
systemic estrogens: Safety not known
warfarin: Possibly decreased PT

Adverse Reactions
CNS: CVA, depression, fever, insomnia, migraine
CV: Chest pain, hot flashes, peripheral edema, **thromboembolism**, thrombophlebitis
EENT: Laryngitis, pharyngitis, sinusitis
ENDO: Hot flashes
GI: Abdominal pain, cholelithiasis, flatulence, indigestion, nausea, vomiting
GU: Cystitis, infertility, leukorrhea, UTI, vaginitis
MS: Arthralgia, arthritis, leg cramps or spasms, myalgia
RESP: Cough, pneumonia, **pulmonary embolism**
SKIN: Diaphoresis, rash
Other: Flu-like symptoms, weight gain

Childbearing Considerations
PREGNANCY
- Drug is not for use in females of childbearing age.
- Drug is contraindicated in pregnant women.

LACTATION
- It is not known if drug is present in breast milk.
- Drug is not for use in females of childbearing age.

Nursing Considerations
- Be aware that raloxifene should not be used in premenopausal women.
- Use cautiously in patients who smoke or have a history of atrial fibrillation, hypertension stroke, or TIA, because raloxifene may increase the risk of stroke.

Q
R
S

- Use cautiously in patients with renal impairment because effects of raloxifene on renal system are unknown.

> **! WARNING** Monitor patient's limbs for impaired circulation and pain (possible thromboembolism).

- Expect prescriber to stop drug at least 72 hours before and during periods of prolonged immobilization. Resume raloxifene therapy as prescribed after patient is fully ambulatory.

PATIENT TEACHING

- Advise patient to avoid lengthy immobility during travel while taking raloxifene because of the increased risk of thromboembolism.
- Instruct patient to report adverse reactions to prescriber immediately, especially coughing up blood, leg pain or swelling, shortness of breath, a sudden change in vision, or sudden chest pain.
- Emphasize the importance of compliance with long-term raloxifene therapy.
- Advise patient that postmenopausal women require an average of 1,500 mg of elemental calcium and 400 to 800 international units of vitamin D daily. Vitamin D requirement is increased in women who are chronically ill or nursing-home bound, women with GI malabsorption syndromes, and women over age 70. Review dietary sources of calcium and vitamin D, and have patient discuss supplements with prescriber, as needed.

raltegravir potassium

Isentress, Isentress HD

▤ Class and Category

Pharmacologic class: HIV integrase strand transfer inhibitor
Therapeutic class: Antiretroviral

▤ Indications and Dosages

✱ *As adjunct to treat human immunodeficiency virus (HIV-1) infection*

CHEWABLE TABLETS, TABLETS

Adults who are treatment-naïve or who are virologically suppressed on an initial regimen of raltegravir of 400 mg twice daily. 1,200 mg once daily if using 600-mg film-coated tablets or 400 mg twice daily if using 400-mg film-coated tablets.

Adults who are treatment-experienced. 400 mg twice daily using 400-mg film-coated tablets.

Adults who are treatment-experienced or treatment-naïve and taking rifampin concomitantly. 800 mg twice daily using 400-mg film-coated tablets.

Children weighing at least 40 kg (88 lb) and are treatment-naïve or virologically suppressed on an initial regimen of raltegravir 400 mg twice daily. 1,200 mg once daily using 600-mg film-coated tablets, 400 mg twice daily using 400-mg film-coated tablets, or 300 mg twice daily using chewable tablets.

Children who weigh at least 28 kg (61.6 lb) but less than 40 kg (88 lb). 400 mg twice daily using 400-mg film-coated tablets or 200 mg twice daily using chewable tablets.

Children who weigh at least 25 kg (55 lb) but less than 28 kg (61.6 lb). 400 mg twice daily using 400-mg film-coated tablets or 150 mg twice daily using chewable tablets.

CHEWABLE TABLETS

Children who weigh 20 kg (44 lb) to less than 25 kg (55 lb) and are 4 weeks of age and over. 150 mg twice daily.

CHEWABLE TABLETS, ORAL SUSPENSION

Children who are 4 weeks of age and older and weigh 14 kg (30.8 lb) to less than 20 kg (44 lb). 100 mg twice daily.

Children who are 4 weeks of age and older and weigh 11 kg (24.2 lb) to less than 20 kg (44 lb). 75 mg twice daily using chewable tablets or 80 mg twice daily using oral suspension.

ORAL SUSPENSION

Children who are at least 4 weeks of age and who weigh 8 kg (17.6 lb) to less than 11 (24.2 lb). 60 mg twice daily.

Children who are at least 4 weeks of age and who weigh 6 kg (13.2 lb) to less than 8 kg (17.6 lb). 40 mg twice daily.

Children who are at least 4 weeks of age and who weigh 4 kg (8.8 lb) to less than 6 kg (13.2 lb). 30 mg twice daily.

Children who are at least 4 weeks of age and who weigh 3 kg (6.6 lb) to less than 4 kg (8.8 lb). 25 mg twice daily.

Neonates age 1 to 4 weeks weighing 4 kg (8.8 lb) to less than 5 kg (11 lb). 15 mg twice daily.
Neonates age 1 to 4 weeks weighing 3 kg (6.6 lb) to less than 4 kg (8.8 lb). 10 mg twice daily.
Neonates age 1 to 4 weeks weighing 2 kg (4.4 lb) to less than 3 kg (6.6 lb). 8 mg twice daily.
Neonates age birth to 1 week weighing 4 kg (8.8 lb) to less than 5 kg (11 lb). 7 mg once daily.
Neonates age birth to 1 week weighing 3 kg (6.6 lb) to less than 4 kg (8.8 lb). 5 mg once daily.
Neonates age birth to 1 week weighing 2 kg (4.4 lb) to less than 3 kg (6.6 lb). 4 mg once daily.

±**DOSAGE ADJUSTMENT** If the mother has taken raltegravir 2 to 24 hours before delivery, then the neonate, age birth to 4 weeks, should be given the first dose, regardless of weight, between 24 and 48 hr after birth.

Drug Administration

P.O.

- Chewable tablets and oral suspension cannot be substituted for the 400-mg or 800-mg film-coated tablets, because the formulations have different pharmacokinetic profiles.
- Do not administer drug before dialysis, because the extent to which the drug is dialyzable is unknown.
- Film-coated tablets must be swallowed whole and not chewed, crushed, or divided.
- Chewable tablets may be chewed or swallowed whole. Maximum dose is 300 mg twice daily. Chewable tablets can be crushed and added to 5 ml of breast milk, juice, or water. After 2 minutes, crush any remaining pieces of the tablet(s) with a spoon and administer immediately. Add 5 ml of liquid to cup again, swirl and administer immediately to ensure that entire dose has been given.
- Mix oral suspension form using the provided mixing cup by pouring packet contents into 10 ml of water in the cup and mixing. Gently swirl the cup for 45 seconds in a circular motion to mix powder. Do not shake. Once mixed, measure the recommended dose with a syringe and administer within 30 minutes of mixing. Discard any remaining suspension. Maximum daily dose is 100 mg twice daily.

Route	Onset	Peak	Duration
P.O.	Unknown	1.5–3 hr	24 hr

Half-life: 9 hr

Mechanism of Action

Inhibits HIV integrase by binding to the integrase active site and blocking the strand transfer step of retroviral DNA integration, which is needed for the HIV replication cycle.

Contraindications

Hypersensitivity to raltegravir or its components

Interactions

DRUGS

aluminum- and/or magnesium-containing antacids, calcium carbonate antacid, carbamazepine, etravirine, phenobarbital, phenytoin, rifampin: Decrease in plasma concentration of raltegravir and its effectiveness

Adverse Reactions

CNS: Abnormal dreams, asthenia, cerebellar ataxia, depression, dizziness, fatigue, fever, headaches, insomnia, malaise, nightmares, paranoia, **suicidal ideation**
CV: Elevated cholesterol and triglycerides
EENT: Conjunctivitis
ENDO: Hyperglycemia
GI: Abdominal pain, anorexia, bilirubin increase, diarrhea, dyspepsia, elevated liver and pancreatic enzymes, flatulence, gastritis, **hepatic failure**, **hepatitis**, nausea, vomiting
GU: Genital herpes, nephrolithiasis, **renal failure**
HEME: Decreased hemoglobin count, **neutropenia**, **thrombocytopenia**
MS: Elevated creatine kinase, myopathy, **rhabdomyolysis**
SKIN: Blisters, rash, **Stevens–Johnson syndrome**, **toxic epidermal necrolysis**
Other: **Angioedema**, herpes zoster, **hypersensitivity reactions**, immune reconstitution syndrome

Childbearing Considerations

PREGNANCY

- Pregnancy exposure registry: 1-800-258-4263.
- It is not known if drug can cause fetal harm.

Q
R
S

- Use with caution only if benefit to mother outweighs potential risk to fetus.

LACTATION

- It is not known if drug is present in breast milk.
- The Centers for Disease Control and Prevention recommends that HIV-1 infected mothers not breastfeed to avoid risking postnatal transmission of HIV-1 infection to infants. They also do not recommend breastfeeding because of potential drug-induced adverse reactions in the infant.

☰ Nursing Considerations

- Ask patient before starting raltegravir therapy if he has ever experienced an elevated creatine kinase level, myopathy, or rhabdomyolysis or is taking any drugs known to cause these conditions (such as fenofibrate, gemfibrozil, statins, or zidovudine), because drug may increase risk of developing these conditions.

! WARNING Monitor patient closely for severe skin reactions. Notify prescriber and expect raltegravir to be discontinued immediately if patient develops a rash that is accompanied by angioedema, blisters, conjunctivitis, eosinophilia, facial edema, fatigue, fever, joint or muscle aches, lip swelling, malaise, or oral lesions. Be aware that a delay in discontinuing drug may result in a life-threatening situation.

- Be aware that immune reconstitution syndrome has occurred in patients treated with combination antiretroviral therapy, including raltegravir. The inflammatory response predisposes susceptible patients to opportunistic infections such as cytomegalovirus, *Mycobacterium avium* infection, *Pneumocystis jiroveci* pneumonia, or tuberculosis. Autoimmune disorders such as Graves' disease, Guillain–Barré syndrome, or polymyositis have also occurred. Report sudden or unusual adverse reactions to prescriber.

PATIENT TEACHING

- Advise patient to avoid missing doses of raltegravir, as it can result in the development of resistance to the drug. If he misses a dose, he should take it as soon as he remembers, but should not double the next dose or take more than prescribed.

- Instruct patient to swallow film-coated tablets whole; chewable tablets may be swallowed whole, chewed, or dissolved in 5 ml of breast milk, juice, or water.
- Tell patient or parents, if patient is prescribed oral suspension form, to pour packet into 10 ml of water in the provided mixing cup and mix. Dosage of drug should be measured with a syringe and administered within 30 minutes of mixing. Any leftover suspension should be discarded.
- Alert patient or parents that chewable tablet form contains phenylalanine and can be harmful to patients with phenylketonuria.

! WARNING Inform patient to seek immediate medical attention if a rash develops or other signs and symptoms that are new, persistent, or severe appear, including evidence of an infection.

- Advise female patient to alert prescriber if pregnancy is suspected or has occurred.
- Inform mothers that breastfeeding is not recommended during raltegravir therapy.
- Instruct patient to immediately report any unexplained muscle pain, tenderness, or weakness.

ramelteon
Rozerem

☰ Class and Category

Pharmacologic class: Melatonin receptor agonist
Therapeutic class: Hypnotic

☰ Indications and Dosages

✳ *To treat insomnia in patients having difficulty falling asleep*

TABLETS

Adults. 8 mg once nightly.

☰ Drug Administration

P.O.

- Administer drug 30 minutes before bedtime.
- Tablets should be swallowed whole and not chewed, crushed, or divided.
- Avoid giving with or after a high-fat meal.

Route	Onset	Peak	Duration
P.O.	30 min	0.5–1.5 hr	Unknown

Half-life: 1–2.6 hr

Mechanism of Action

Binds to melatonin receptors MT1 and MT2 in the suprachiasmatic nucleus (SCN) of the hypothalamus. The SCN regulates the sleep–wake cycle, and endogenous melatonin probably is involved in maintaining the circadian rhythm underlying that cycle.

Contraindications

Concurrent therapy with fluvoxamine, history of angioedema with previous ramelteon treatment, hypersensitivity to ramelteon or its components

Interactions

DRUGS

benzodiazepines, melatonin, other sedative-hypnotics: Possible additive sedative effects

donepezil, doxepin, fluconazole, fluvoxamine, ketoconazole: Increased plasma ramelteon levels

rifampin: Decreased ramelteon effectiveness

ACTIVITIES

alcohol use: Possibly additive CNS effect

Adverse Reactions

CNS: Agitation, amnesia, anxiety, bizarre behavior, complex behaviors such as sleep driving, depression, dizziness, fatigue, hallucinations, headache, insomnia exacerbation, mania, somnolence, **suicidal ideation**

EENT: Throat tightness

ENDO: Decreased testosterone level, increased prolactin level

GI: Diarrhea, dysgeusia, nausea, vomiting

MS: Arthralgia, myalgia

RESP: Dyspnea, upper respiratory tract infection

Other: **Anaphylaxis, angioedema**

Childbearing Considerations

PREGNANCY

- It is not known if drug can cause fetal harm.
- Use with caution only if benefit to mother outweighs potential risk to fetus.

LACTATION

- It is not known if drug is present in breast milk.

- Patient should check with prescriber before breastfeeding.
- If breastfeeding occurs, advise mother to monitor breastfed infant for feeding difficulties and somnolence.

Nursing Considerations

- Be aware that ramelteon therapy is not recommended for patients with COPD or severe sleep apnea because its effects have not been studied in these patient populations.
- Use cautiously in patients with mild-to-moderate hepatic dysfunction. Drug is contraindicated in severe hepatic dysfunction.
- Ramelteon is the first approved hypnotic not classified as a controlled substance.

! WARNING Monitor patient closely for hypersensitivity reactions such as dyspnea, nausea, swelling, throat tightness, and vomiting. If present, discontinue ramelteon immediately, notify prescriber, and provide supportive care.

- Watch patient closely for suicidal tendencies, particularly when therapy starts and dosage changes, because depression may worsen temporarily during these times, possibly leading to suicidal ideation.

PATIENT TEACHING

- Instruct patient to take drug 30 minutes before bedtime and not to take ramelteon with or immediately after eating a high-fat meal.

! WARNING Alert patient that drug may cause an allergic reaction. If present, tell patient to notify prescriber and, if severe, to seek emergency medical care.

- Caution patient to avoid potentially hazardous activities after taking ramelteon; drug's intended effect is to decrease alertness.
- Advise patient that drug may cause abnormal behaviors during sleep, such as driving a car, eating, having sex, or talking on the phone without any recall of the event. If family members notice any such behavior or patient sees evidence of such behavior upon awakening, prescriber should be notified.
- Advise limiting alcohol during therapy.

- Tell patient to notify prescriber if insomnia worsens or new signs or symptoms occur.
- Inform patient that drug may affect reproductive hormones; urge patient to report cessation of menses, galactorrhea (females), decreased libido, or problems with infertility.
- Urge family or caregiver to watch patient closely for suicidal tendencies, especially when therapy starts or dosage changes.

ramipril
Altace

Class and Category
Pharmacologic class: Angiotensin-converting enzyme (ACE) inhibitor
Therapeutic class: Antihypertensive

Indications and Dosages
* *To treat heart failure after MI*

CAPSULES
Adults. *Initial:* 2.5 mg twice daily with dose decreased to 1.25 mg twice daily if hypotension occurs. Dosage increased after 1 week, if tolerated. Dosage further increased about every 3 wk to achieve maintenance dose. *Maintenance:* 5 mg twice daily.

±**DOSAGE ADJUSTMENT** For patients with renal impairment (creatinine clearance less than 40 ml/min), initial dose reduced to 1.25 mg once daily and then increased to 1.25 mg twice daily, and up to maximum dose of 2.5 mg twice daily, as needed.

* *To reduce risk of MI or stroke and death from cardiovascular causes*

CAPSULES
Adults age 55 and over. *Initial:* 2.5 mg once daily for 1 wk, followed by 5 mg once daily for 3 wk, and then increased, as tolerated to 10 mg once daily.

±**DOSAGE ADJUSTMENT** For patient who is also hypertensive or recently post-myocardial infarction, daily dosage may also be divided.

* *To treat hypertension*

CAPSULES
Adults not taking a diuretic. *Initial:* 2.5 mg daily with dosage adjusted according to blood pressure response. *Maintenance:* 2.5 to 20 mg once daily or in divided doses twice daily.

±**DOSAGE ADJUSTMENT** For patients who have hypertension with renal impairment (creatinine clearance less than 40 ml/min), initial dose reduced to 1.25 mg once daily and then titrated upward till blood pressure is controlled or maximum total daily dose (not to exceed 5 mg) is reached. For patients with hypertension who experience a diminished drug effect toward end of dosing interval, dosage increased or dosage divided into 2 daily doses. For all patients regardless of indication being treated, if dehydrated from past or present diuretic use or who have renal artery stenosis, initial dosage reduced to 1.25 mg daily.

Drug Administration
P.O.
- Capsules should be swallowed whole and not chewed or crushed.
- If patient cannot swallow capsule, open and sprinkle contents onto about 4 ounces of applesauce or mix with 4 ounces of apple juice or water. If not administered immediately, mixture may be stored for 24 hours at room temperature or 48 hours in refrigerator.

Route	Onset	Peak	Duration
P.O.	1–2 hr	1–4 hr	24 hr
Half-life: 13–17 hr			

Mechanism of Action
Blocks conversion of angiotensin I to angiotensin II, causing vasodilation, and reduces aldosterone secretion, which prevents water retention. Ramipril also reduces peripheral arterial resistance. Combined, these actions reduce blood pressure.

Contraindications
Aliskiren therapy in patients with diabetes; hypersensitivity to ramipril, other ACE inhibitors or their components; use of neprilysin inhibitor such as sacubitril within 36 hours

Interactions
DRUGS
aliskiren (patients with diabetes and/or renal impairment), angiotensin receptor blockers, other ACE inhibitors: Increased risk of hyperkalemia, hypotension, and renal dysfunction
diuretics: Possibly hypotension

lithium: Increased risk of lithium toxicity
mTOR inhibitors such as temsirolimus,
neprilysin inhibitor such as sacubitril:
Increased risk of angioedema
NSAIDs: Decreased antihypertensive
effect of ramipril; increased risk of renal
dysfunction in the elderly and patients with
preexisting renal dysfunction or volume
depletion
potassium preparations, potassium-sparing
diuretics: Risk of hyperkalemia
sodium aurothiomalate: Increased risk
of nitritoid reaction (facial flushing,
hypotension, nausea, vomiting)

FOODS

potassium-rich foods such as milk and
potatoes, potassium-containing salt substitutes:
Increased risk of hyperkalemia

Adverse Reactions

CNS: Depression, dizziness, drowsiness,
fatigue, fever, headache, insomnia,
light-headedness, malaise, paresthesia, sleep
disturbance, syncope, vertigo
CV: Chest pain, **hypotension,** orthostatic
hypotension, palpitations, tachycardia
EENT: Amblyopia, dry mouth, loss of taste,
pharyngitis
GI: Abdominal pain, constipation, diarrhea,
elevated liver enzymes, jaundice, **hepatic**
failure, hepatitis, nausea, vomiting
GU: Acute renal failure, elevated BUN and
serum creatinine levels, impotence, oliguria,
progressive azotemia
HEME: Agranulocytosis, anemia, **bone**
marrow depression, pancytopenia
MS: Arthralgia, back pain, myalgia
RESP: Cough, dyspnea
SKIN: Alopecia, diaphoresis, flushing,
onycholysis, pemphigoid, photosensitivity,
pruritus, rash, **Stevens–Johnson syndrome,**
toxic epidermal necrolysis, urticaria
Other: Anaphylaxis, angioedema,
hyperkalemia

Childbearing Considerations

PREGNANCY

- Drug can cause fetal harm, especially if
  exposure occurs during the second or third
  trimester.
- Drug reduces fetal renal function leading
  to anuria and renal failure and increases
  fetal and neonatal morbidity and death.
  It can also cause fetal lung hypoplasia,

hypotension, and skeletal deformations
such as skull hypoplasia.
- Drug is not recommended in pregnant
  women and should be discontinued as soon
  as possible if pregnancy occurs.

LACTATION

- It is not known if drug is present in breast
  milk.
- Drug is not recommended for use during
  breastfeeding.

Nursing Considerations

- Use ramipril cautiously in patients with
  renal or hepatic impairment.
- Monitor patient's serum potassium level,
  as ordered, and assess often for signs and
  symptoms of hyperkalemia, especially
  in patients with diabetes mellitus or
  renal insufficiency and those taking
  concomitantly other drugs that raise serum
  potassium levels.

! **WARNING** Keep in mind patients with
dehydration, heart failure, or hyponatremia;
those who've recently received intensive diuresis
or an increase in diuretic dosage; and those
having dialysis may risk excessive hypotension.
Monitor such patients closely the first 2 weeks
of therapy and whenever ramipril or diuretic
dosage increases. If excessive hypotension
occurs, notify prescriber immediately, place
patient in a supine position, and, if prescribed,
infuse normal saline solution.

! **WARNING** Know that because of the risk of
angioedema, be prepared to stop drug and
provide emergency measures, including
subcutaneous epinephrine 1:1,000 (0.3 to
0.5 ml), if swelling of glottis, larynx, or
tongue causes airway obstruction.

- Monitor blood pressure frequently during
  therapy to assess drug's effectiveness.
- Monitor patient's hepatic and renal function
  closely during therapy. If patient develops
  jaundice or marked elevations of hepatic
  enzymes, notify prescriber and expect
  ramipril to be discontinued.

PATIENT TEACHING

- Advise patient to swallow capsules whole
  and not to chew or crush capsules.
- Tell patient who cannot swallow capsules to
  open and sprinkle contents onto about
  4 ounces of applesauce or mix with 4 ounces

of apple juice or water. If not administered immediately, tell patient that mixture may be stored for 24 hours at room temperature or 48 hours in refrigerator.

! **WARNING** Advise patient to stop taking ramipril and inform prescriber immediately if she experiences difficulty breathing or swallowing or develops swelling of the eyes, face, lips, or tongue.

- Explain that drug may cause dizziness and light-headedness, especially during first few days of therapy. Instruct patient to notify prescriber immediately if she has fainting episode.
- Inform female patient of childbearing age of the risks of taking ramipril during pregnancy and to report known or suspected pregnancy immediately.
- Urge patient to tell providers that she takes ramipril before having surgery or receiving anesthesia.
- Tell patient to ask prescriber before using supplements or salt substitutes that contain potassium.

ranolazine

Ranexa

Class and Category

Pharmacologic class: Cardiac agent
Therapeutic class: Antianginal

Indications and Dosages

✴ *To treat chronic angina*

E.R. TABLETS

Adults. *Initial:* 500 mg twice daily, increased to 1,000 mg twice daily, as needed. *Maximum:* 1,000 mg twice daily.

± **DOSAGE ADJUSTMENT** For patients taking a moderate CYP3A inhibitor, such as diltiazem, erythromycin, or verapamil, maximum dosage reduced to 500 mg twice daily. For patients taking P-gp inhibitors, such as cyclosporine, dosage may have to be reduced.

Drug Administration

P.O.

- Tablets should be swallowed whole and not chewed, crushed, or divided.
- Avoid administering drug with grapefruit juice.

Route	Onset	Peak	Duration
P.O.	Unknown	2–5 hr	Unknown

Half-life: 7 hr

Mechanism of Action

Exerts antianginal and anti-ischemic effects by an unknown mechanism not dependent on reductions in blood pressure or heart rate. Ranolazine inhibits cardiac late sodium current, but how this action inhibits angina symptoms is also unknown.

Contraindications

Hypersensitivity to ranolazine or its components, liver cirrhosis, use of CYP3A inducers or strong inhibitors

Interactions

DRUGS

CYP2D6 substrates such as antipsychotics, tricyclic antidepressants: Increased plasma levels of these drugs
CYP3A inducers, such as carbamazepine, phenobarbital, phenytoin, rifabutin, rifampin, rifapentine, St. John's wort: Decreased blood ranolazine level and decreased effectiveness
CYP3A substrates, such as cyclosporine, lovastatin, simvastatin, sirolimus, tacrolimus: Possibly increased blood levels of these drugs
CYP3A inhibitors, such as clarithromycin, diltiazem, erythromycin, fluconazole, indinavir, itraconazole, ketoconazole, nefazodone, nelfinavir, ritonavir, saquinavir, verapamil: Increased blood ranolazine level and increased risk of adverse reactions
digoxin: Increased blood digoxin level
metformin: Increased metformin levels when ranolazine dosage reaches 1,000 mg twice daily

ACTIVITIES

grapefruit juice, grapefruit containing products: Increased blood ranolazine level and increased risk of adverse reactions

Adverse Reactions

CNS: Abnormal coordination, asthenia, confusion, dizziness, hallucination, headache, hypoesthesia, myoclonus, paresthesia, syncope, tremor, vertigo
CV: Bradycardia, hypotension, orthostatic hypotension, palpitations, peripheral edema, QT-interval prolongation
EENT: Blurred vision, dry mouth, tinnitus
ENDO: Hypoglycemia

GI: Abdominal pain, anorexia, constipation, dyspepsia, nausea, vomiting
GU: Dysuria, elevated blood urea and creatinine levels, hematuria, **renal failure,** urinary retention
HEME: Eosinophilia, **leukopenia, pancytopenia, thrombocytopenia**
RESP: Dyspnea, **pulmonary fibrosis**
SKIN: Diaphoresis, pruritus, rash
Other: Angioedema

☰ Childbearing Considerations

PREGNANCY

- It is not known if drug can cause fetal harm.
- Use with caution only if benefit to mother outweighs potential risk to fetus.

LACTATION

- It is not known if drug is present in breast milk.
- The drug should be discontinued during breastfeeding or breastfeeding should be discontinued during drug therapy.

☰ Nursing Considerations

- Monitor patient's QT interval, as ordered, because ranolazine prolongs it in a dose-related manner.
- Assess effectiveness of ranolazine at preventing anginal pain.
- Know that acute renal failure may occur in some patients with severe renal impairment (creatinine clearance less than 30 ml/min) while taking drug. Monitor patient's serum creatinine levels and blood urea nitrogen after drug therapy begins and then periodically, as ordered. If elevations occur, notify prescriber and expect drug to be discontinued.
- Monitor patient's serum magnesium, potassium, and liver enzyme levels.

PATIENT TEACHING

- Instruct patient to take ranolazine exactly as prescribed.
- Inform patient that drug may be taken with or without food.
- Caution patient to swallow tablets whole and not to break, chew, or crush them.
- Advise patient to limit the amount of grapefruit and grapefruit juice consumed while taking this drug. Advise patient not to use grapefruit juice to take drug.
- Advise patient to notify prescriber if persistent or severe adverse reactions occur.
- Instruct patient to notify all prescribers of ranolazine use.

rasagiline
Azilect

☰ Class and Category

Pharmacologic class: Irreversible monoamine oxidase inhibitor (MAOI)
Therapeutic class: Antiparkinsonian

☰ Indications and Dosages

✳ *To treat Parkinson's disease as monotherapy*

TABLETS

Adults. 1 mg once daily.

✳ *As adjunct with levodopa in treatment of Parkinson's disease*

TABLETS

Adults. 0.5 mg once daily increased to 1 mg once daily, as needed.

±**DOSAGE ADJUSTMENT** For patients with mild hepatic failure or taking ciprofloxacin or other CYP1A2 inhibitors, dosage shouldn't exceed 0.5 mg daily.

☰ Drug Administration

P.O.

- Administer at about the same time each day.

Route	Onset	Peak	Duration
P.O.	Unknown	1 hr	1 wk

Half-life: 1.5–3.5 hr

☰ Mechanism of Action

Inhibits metabolic degradation of catecholamines and serotonin in the CNS and peripheral tissues, increasing extracellular dopamine level in the striatum. The increased dopamine level helps control alterations in voluntary muscle movement (such as rigidity and tremors) in Parkinson's disease because dopamine, a neurotransmitter, is essential for normal motor function. By stimulating central and peripheral dopaminergic 2 (D_2) receptors on postsynaptic cells, dopamine inhibits firing of striatal neurons (such as cholinergic neurons), improving motor function.

☰ Contraindications

Concurrent therapy with cyclobenzaprine, dextromethorphan, or St. John's wort; hypersensitivity to rasagiline or its components; use within 14 days of MAO inhibitors, meperidine, methadone, other

Q
R
S

selective MAO-B inhibitors, propoxyphene, or tramadol

Interactions

DRUGS

antipsychotics, metoclopramide: Possible diminished effectiveness of rasagiline
CYP1A2 inhibitors such as ciprofloxacin: Increased plasma rasagiline concentrations
dextromethorphan: Increased risk of bizarre behavior or episodes of psychosis
MAO inhibitors, meperidine, selective MAO-B inhibitors: Increased risk of serious, sometimes fatal, adverse reactions
MAO inhibitors, sympathomimetics: Increased risk of hypertensive crisis
selective serotonin reuptake inhibitors; serotonin–norepinephrine reuptake inhibitors; tetracyclic, triazolopyridine, or tricyclic antidepressants: Increased risk of serotonin syndrome

Activities

FOOD

foods high in tyramine: Possibly significant increase in blood pressure

Adverse Reactions

CNS: Abnormal dreams, amnesia, anxiety, asthenia, ataxia, **cerebral ischemia, coma,** compulsive behaviors (binge eating, increased sexual urges, intense urges to spend money), confusion, **CVA,** daytime sleepiness, depression, difficulty thinking, dizziness, dyskinesia, dystonia, fever, hallucinations, headache, malaise, manic-depressive reaction, nightmares, paresthesia, psychotic-like behavior, **seizures, serotonin syndrome,** somnolence, stupor, syncope, vertigo
CV: Angina, bundle branch heart block, chest pain, **heart failure, MI, hypertensive crisis,** postural hypotension, thrombophlebitis, **ventricular fibrillation or tachycardia**
EENT: Blurred vision, conjunctivitis, dry mouth, epistaxis, gingivitis, **hemorrhage, laryngeal edema,** retinal detachment or hemorrhage, rhinitis
GI: Abdominal pain, anorexia, constipation, diarrhea, dyspepsia, dysphagia, elevated liver enzymes, gastroenteritis, **GI hemorrhage, intestinal obstruction or perforation,** nausea, vomiting
GU: **Acute renal failure,** albuminuria, decreased libido, hematuria, impotence, incontinence, priapism

HEME: Anemia, **leukopenia, thrombocytopenia**
MS: Arthralgia, arthritis, bone necrosis, bursitis, leg cramps, myasthenia, neck pain or stiffness, tenosynovitis
RESP: **Apnea, asthma,** cough, dyspnea, pleural effusion, **pneumothorax, interstitial pneumonia**
SKIN: Alopecia, **carcinoma,** diaphoresis, ecchymosis, **exfoliative dermatitis, melanoma,** pruritus, ulcer, vesiculobullous rash
Other: **Angioedema,** flu-like symptoms, **hypersensitivity reactions, hypocalcemia,** weight loss

Childbearing Considerations

PREGNANCY

- It is not known if drug can cause fetal harm.
- Use with caution only if benefit to mother outweighs potential risk to fetus.

LACTATION

- It is not known if drug is present in breast milk.
- Patient should check with prescriber before breastfeeding.

Nursing Considerations

! WARNING Monitor patient's blood pressure closely throughout therapy. Notify prescriber immediately if patient has evidence of hypertensive crisis or signs and symptoms suggesting a stroke. Expect to stop drug immediately if these occur.

- Keep phentolamine readily available to treat hypertensive crisis. Give 5 mg by slow I.V. infusion, as prescribed, to reduce blood pressure without causing excessive hypotension. Use external cooling measures, as prescribed, to manage fever.
- Monitor patient receiving rasagiline with levodopa for worsening of preexisting dyskinesia. If it occurs, notify prescriber and expect levodopa dosage to be decreased.
- Be aware that patient may experience orthostatic hypotension, especially in the first 2 months of rasagiline therapy and that it may also occur while patient is supine.

PATIENT TEACHING

! WARNING Inform patient taking recommended dosage of rasagiline that dietary tyramine restriction is no longer needed except for avoidance of very tyramine-rich foods such as aged cheese (e.g., Stilton), which may increase blood pressure greatly. If patient doesn't feel well soon after eating a suspected high-tyramine meal, he should contact prescriber immediately.

- Remind patient not to exceed the recommended dose because of risk of hypertension.

! WARNING Advise patient to stop taking rasagiline and to notify prescriber immediately if he develops blurred vision, chest pain, coma, nausea, palpitations, seizures, severe headache, stiff neck, stupor, trouble thinking, vomiting, or evidence of stroke.

! WARNING Monitor patient closely for serotonin syndrome, a rare but serious adverse effect of rasagiline. Signs and symptoms include agitation, confusion, diaphoresis, diarrhea, fever, hyperactive reflexes, poor coordination, restlessness, shaking, talking or acting with uncontrolled excitement, tremor, and twitching. If symptoms occur, notify prescriber immediately, expect to discontinue drug, and provide supportive care.

- Suggest that patient change position slowly to minimize orthostatic hypotension.
- Alert patient that drug may cause changes in behavior that may be severe or hallucinations, especially at the initiation of drug therapy or when an increase in dosage occurs. If they occur, tell patient to notify prescriber promptly.
- Alert patient and caregivers that drug may cause compulsive or impulsive behaviors such as binge eating, gambling, increased sexual activities, or spending money inappropriately. If any questionable behavior occurs, instruct patient or caregiver to notify prescriber, as dosage may have to be adjusted or drug discontinued.
- Instruct patient to notify all prescribers of rasagiline therapy, especially if antidepressants or antibiotics such as ciprofloxacin or a similar drug are being considered, and to avoid taking any over-the-counter cold medications.

- Caution patient not to perform hazardous activities until CNS effects of drug are known. Some patients have fallen asleep without warning while engaged in activities of daily living, including driving.

remdesivir
Veklury

☰ Class and Category
Pharmacologic class: SARS-CoV-2 nucleotide analog RNA polymerase inhibitor
Therapeutic class: Antiretroviral

☰ Indications and Dosages
✳ *To treat coronavirus disease 2019 (COVID-19) in patients with positive results of direct severe acute respiratory syndrome coronavirus 2 (SARS-CoV-2) viral testing and requiring hospitalization*

I.V. INFUSION
Adults and children weighing at least 40 kg (88 lb). *Loading dose*: 200 mg as a single dose on day 1. *Maintenance:* 100 mg once daily beginning on day 2 for 4 additional days for patients not requiring invasive mechanical ventilation and/or extracorporeal membrane oxygenation (ECMO) and who show signs of improvement or 9 additional days if patient does not demonstrate clinical improvement or patient requires invasive mechanical ventilation and/or ECMO.

I.V. INFUSION (USING ONLY INJECTION FORM SUPPLIED AS 100-MG LYOPHILIZED POWDER IN VIAL)
Infants 28 days of age and older weighing at least 3 kg (6.6 lb) to children weighing less than 40 kg (88 lb). *Loading dose*: 5 mg/kg as a single dose on day 1. *Maintenance:* 2.5 mg/kg once daily beginning on day 2 for 4 additional days for patients not requiring invasive mechanical ventilation and/or extracorporeal membrane oxygenation (ECMO) and who show signs of improvement or 9 additional days if patient does not demonstrate clinical improvement or patient requires invasive mechanical ventilation and/or ECMO.

✳ *To treat symptomatic coronavirus disease 2019 (COVID-19) within 7 days of symptom onset in nonhospitalized patients who have mild-to-moderate COVID-19, and are at high risk for progression to severe COVID-19, including hospitalization or death*

I.V. INFUSION

Adults and children weighing at least 40 kg (88 lb). *Loading dose:* 200 mg as a single dose on day 1. *Maintenance:* 100 mg once daily given on days 2 and 3.

I.V. INFUSION (USING ONLY INJECTION FORM SUPPLIED AS 100-MG LYOPHILIZED POWDER IN VIAL)

Infants 28 days of age and older at least weighing 3 kg (6.6 lb) to children weighing less than 40 kg (88 lb). *Loading dose:* 100 mg as a single dose on day 1. *Maintenance:* 2.5 mg/kg once daily on days 2 and 3.

Drug Administration

I.V.

- Drug is available in two dosage forms: as a 100-mg lyophilized powder in a vial, which must be reconstituted, and as a 100-mg/20-ml solution.
- Solution or powder (when reconstituted), should appear clear, colorless to yellow, and free of visible particles.
- Do not exceed infusion rate, to help prevent hypersensitivity reactions. Slower infusion rates, with a maximum infusion time of up to 120 minutes, can potentially prevent infusion-related hypersensitivity reactions.
- *Incompatibilities:* Other drugs or solutions other than 0.9% Sodium Chloride Injection

Lyophilized powder form

- Only use the 100-mg lyophilized powder in vial for pediatric patients 28 days of age and older and weighing at least 3 kg (6.6 lb) to children weighing less than 40 kg (88 lb).
- First, reconstitute with 19 ml of Sterile Water for Injection. Do not use any other solution to reconstitute drug. Discard vial if a vacuum does not pull the Sterile Water for Injection into the vial. Immediately shake vial for 30 seconds. Allow contents to settle for 2 to 3 minutes. Solution should be clear after 3 minutes. If not, shake vial again for 30 seconds and allow contents to settle for 2 to 3 minutes. Repeat as needed until contents of vial are completely dissolved. Discard vial if contents do not completely dissolve. Following reconstitution, each vial contains 100 mg/20 ml (5 mg/ml) of drug solution. Follow with dilution immediately.

- For pediatric patients 28 days of age and older and weighing at least 3 kg to children weighing less than 40 kg, dilute reconstituted powder in 0.9% Sodium Chloride Injection to achieve a concentration of 1.25 mg/ml. Small 0.9% Sodium Chloride Injection infusion bags (e.g., 25, 50, or 100 ml) or an appropriately sized syringe should be used for pediatric dosing. After withdrawing the required volume of reconstituted solution from the vial into the bag or syringe, gently invert the bag or syringe 20 times to mix the solution. Do not shake. Infuse the prepared diluted solution immediately. A syringe and syringe pump may be used for infusion volumes less than 50 ml.
- For adults and pediatric patient weighing 40 kg or more, dilute reconstituted powder in either a 100-ml or 250-ml 0.9% Sodium Chloride Injection infusion bag as follows: Withdraw and discard from infusion bag the volume of 0.9% Sodium Chloride Injection solution to be replaced by drug solution. Withdraw the required volume of drug from vial and transfer to the selected infusion bag. Gently invert bag 20 times to mix solution. Do not shake. The prepared infusion solution is stable for 24 hours at room temperature or 48 hours if refrigerated.
- Infuse over 30 to 120 min. If using a 250-ml infusion bag volume, rate should be 8.33 ml/min to deliver drug in 30 minutes; 4.17 ml/min to deliver drug in 60 minutes; and 2.08 ml/min to deliver drug in 120 min. If using a 100-ml infusion bag volume, rate should be 3.33 ml/min to deliver drug in 30 minutes; 1.67 ml/min to deliver drug in 60 minutes; and 0.83 ml/min to deliver drug in 120 minutes.

Solution form

- Do not use this form in pediatric patients weighing 3 kg (6.6 lb) to children weighing less than 40 kg (88 lb).
- Withdraw and discard volume of 0.9% Sodium Chloride Injection solution to be replaced by drug solution from a 250-ml infusion bag. Do not use a 100-ml infusion bag. Withdraw the required volume of drug from vial by first pulling syringe plunger rod back to fill syringe with about 10 ml of air. Inject air into drug vial above the level of the solution. Invert vial and withdraw the

required volume of drug solution into the syringe. The last 5 ml of solution requires more force to withdraw. Transfer the required volume of drug solution into the 250-ml infusion bag.

- Gently invert bag 20 times to mix solution in the bag. Do not shake. The prepared infusion solution is stable for 24 hr at room temperature or 48 hr if refrigerated.
- Infuse over 30 to 120 min. Rate should be 8.33 ml/min to deliver drug in 30 minutes; 4.17 ml/min to deliver drug in 60 minutes; and 2.08 ml/min to deliver drug in 120 min.

Route	Onset	Peak	Duration
I.V.	Unknown	Unknown	Unknown

Half-life: 1 hr

Mechanism of Action

Blocks the COVID-19 virus from copying itself, although how it does this is not known.

Contraindications

Hypersensitivity to remdesivir or its components

Interactions

DRUGS

chloroquine phosphate, hydroxychloroquine sulfate: Potential antagonism to remdesivir interfering with drug's effectiveness against COVID-19

Adverse Reactions

CNS: Seizures
CV: Decreased heart rate
ENDO: Increased blood glucose level
GI: Elevated bilirubin and liver enzymes, nausea
GU: Acute kidney injury, decreased creatinine clearance and eGFR, elevated creatinine
HEME: Decreased hemoglobin or lymphocytes, elevated prothrombin time
SKIN: Rash
Other: Anaphylaxis, angioedema, hypersensitivity reactions, infusion reactions

Childbearing Considerations

PREGNANCY

- Pregnancy exposure registry: 1-800-616-3791 or https://covid-pr. pregistry.com
- Drug may cause fetal harm.

- Use with caution only if benefit to mother outweighs potential risk to fetus.

LACTATION

- It is not known if drug is present in breast milk.
- Patient should check with prescriber before breastfeeding.

Nursing Considerations

- Determine patient's eGFR, liver enzymes, and prothrombin time before starting remdesivir therapy and continue to monitor during therapy, as ordered, because drug may adversely alter these values.
- Expect not to administer remdesivir to patients with an eGFR less than 30 ml/min.

! WARNING Monitor patient closely during and after drug administration for hypersensitivity reactions that could include anaphylactic reactions or are infusion related. Assess patient for angioedema, bradycardia, diaphoresis, dyspnea, fever, hypertension, hypotension, hypoxia, nausea, rash, shivering, tachycardia, or wheezing. Slower infusion rates, with a maximum infusion time of up to 120 minutes, can potentially prevent these signs and symptoms. If signs and symptoms are serious, immediately discontinue infusion, notify prescriber, and institute appropriate care, as ordered.

- Notify prescriber if patient's ALT levels increase to greater than 10 times the upper limit of normal, as drug may have to be discontinued. However, if patient exhibits signs or symptoms of liver inflammation that are accompanied by an ALT elevation, drug will have to be discontinued.
- Be aware that chloroquine phosphate or hydroxychloroquine sulfate should not be coadministered with remdesivir because remdesivir becomes less effective.

PATIENT TEACHING

- Caution patient to notify prescriber if adverse reactions occur.

! WARNING Review signs and symptoms of an allergic reaction and urge patient to report symptoms immediately.

- Instruct patient to notify remdesivir prescriber of all drugs taken, including

Q
R
S

nonprescription drugs and herbal products, because of potential drug interactions.

- Tell women of childbearing age to alert prescriber of a suspected or known pregnancy, because drug effects on fetus are unknown.

- If a meal is skipped, also skip the scheduled dose for that meal.

Route	Onset	Peak	Duration
P.O.	15–60 min	1 hr	4–6 hr

Half-life: 1 hr

repaglinide
Prandin

Class and Category
Pharmacologic class: Meglitinide
Therapeutic class: Antidiabetic

Indications and Dosages
＊ *As adjunct to achieve glucose control in type 2 diabetes mellitus as monotherapy in patients whose glycosylated hemoglobin (HbA1c) level is less than 8%*

TABLETS
Adults. *Initial:* 0.5 mg daily 30 minutes before each meal. Dosage doubled, as needed, every wk until adequate glucose response obtained. *Maintenance:* 0.5 to 4 mg/dose up to four times a day. *Maximum:* 16 mg daily in divided doses of not more than 4 mg/dose.

＊ *As adjunct to achieve glucose control in type 2 diabetes mellitus as monotherapy in patients whose HbA1c is 8% or greater*

TABLETS
Adults. *Initial:* 1 or 2 mg daily 30 minutes before each meal. Dosage doubled, as needed, every wk until adequate glucose response obtained. *Maintenance:* 0.5 to 4 mg/dose up to four times a day. *Maximum:* 16 mg daily in divided doses of not more than 4 mg/dose.

±**DOSAGE ADJUSTMENT** For patients with severe renal impairment, dosage initiated at 0.5 mg before each meal and then titrated gradually, as needed. Concomitant use with clopidogrel should be avoided but if not possible, dosage initiated at 0.5 mg and total daily dose not to exceed 4 mg. Individualized dosing adjustments needed for patients taking concomitant strong CYP2C8 or CYP3A4 inducers or CYP2C8 or CYP3A4 inhibitors. Total daily dose of 6 mg should not be exceeded in patients receiving cyclosporine.

Drug Administration
P.O.
- Administer drug within 30 minutes of each meal.

Mechanism of Action
Stimulates release of insulin from functioning pancreatic beta cells. In patients with type 2 diabetes mellitus, a shortage of these cells decreases blood insulin levels and causes glucose intolerance. By interacting with the adenosine triphosphatase (ATP)–potassium channel on the beta cell membrane, repaglinide prevents potassium from leaving the cell. This causes the beta cell to depolarize and the cell membrane's calcium channel to open. As a result, calcium moves into the cell and insulin moves out. The extent of insulin release is glucose dependent; the lower the glucose level, the less insulin is secreted from the cell.

Contraindications
Concurrent therapy with gemfibrozil, hypersensitivity to repaglinide or its components

Interactions
DRUGS
ACE inhibitors, angiotensin II receptor blocking agents, disopyramide, fibrates, fluoxetine, monoamine oxidase inhibitors, nonsteroidal anti-inflammatory agents (NSAIDs), pentoxifylline, pramlintide, propoxyphene, salicylates, somatostatin analogues (e.g., octreotide), and sulfonamide antibiotics: Increased risk of hypoglycemia
atypical antipsychotics (clozapine, olanzapine), calcium channel blockers, corticosteroids, danazol, diuretics, estrogens, glucagon, isoniazid, niacin, oral contraceptives, phenothiazines, progestogens (in oral contraceptives), protease inhibitors, somatropin, sympathomimetics (albuterol, epinephrine, terbutaline), thyroid hormones: Possibly decreased effectiveness of repaglinide; loss of glucose control
beta-blockers, clonidine, guanethidine, reserpine: Possibly blunt signs and symptoms of hypoglycemia
cyclosporine, CYP2C8 inhibitors (clopidogrel, deferasirox, gemfibrozil, montelukast,

trimethoprim), *CYP3A4 inhibitors (clarithromycin, erythromycin, ketoconazole, itraconazole):* Increased blood repaglinide level, resulting in enhanced and prolonged blood glucose–lowering effects

CYP2C8 and CYP3A4 inducers: Decreased blood repaglinide level, resulting in decreased effectiveness

Adverse Reactions

CNS: Headache
CV: Angina
EENT: Rhinitis, sinusitis
ENDO: Hypoglycemia
GI: Diarrhea, elevated liver enzymes, hepatitis, nausea, pancreatitis
HEME: Hemolytic anemia, leukopenia, thrombocytopenia
MS: Arthralgia, back pain
RESP: Bronchitis, upper respiratory tract infection
SKIN: Alopecia, Stevens–Johnson syndrome
Other: Anaphylaxis

Childbearing Considerations

PREGNANCY
- It is not known if drug can cause fetal harm.
- Use with caution only if benefit to mother outweighs potential risk to fetus.

LACTATION
- It is not known if drug is present in breast milk.
- Drug is not recommended during breastfeeding because of the potential for hypoglycemia in the breastfed infant.

Nursing Considerations

- Be aware that repaglinide shouldn't be used with NPH insulin because the combination may increase the risk of angina.
- Expect to check HbA$_{1c}$ level every 3 months, as ordered, to assess patient's long-term control of blood glucose level.
- During times of increased stress, such as from infection, surgery, or trauma, monitor blood glucose level often and assess need for additional insulin.

PATIENT TEACHING
- Instruct patient to take repaglinide within 30 minutes before meals and to skip dose whenever she skips a meal.
- Explain that repaglinide is an adjunct to diet in managing type 2 diabetes mellitus.
- Inform patient that changes in blood glucose level may cause blurred vision

or visual disturbances, especially when repaglinide therapy starts. Reassure him that these changes are usually transient.
- Teach patient how to monitor her blood glucose level and when to notify prescriber about changes.
- Review signs and symptoms of hyperglycemia and hypoglycemia with patient and family. Instruct patient to notify prescriber immediately if she experiences anxiety, confusion, dizziness, excessive sweating, headache, increased thirst, increased urination, or nausea.
- Advise patient to wear or carry identification indicating that she has diabetes. Encourage her to carry candy or other simple carbohydrates with her to treat mild episodes of hypoglycemia.
- Inform patient that her HbA$_{1c}$ level will be tested every 3 to 6 months until her blood glucose level is controlled.

reslizumab

Cinqair

Class and Category

Pharmacologic class: Interleukin-5 antagonist monoclonal antibody
Therapeutic class: Immunomodulator

Indications and Dosages

* *Adjunct for add-on maintenance treatment in patients with severe asthma who have an eosinophilic phenotype*

I.V. INFUSION
Adults. 3 mg/kg every 4 wk.

Drug Administration

I.V.
- Remove drug from refrigerator and allow to come to room temperature.
- To minimize foaming, do not shake vial.
- Inspect for particulate matter and discoloration. Solution should be clear to slightly hazy/opalescent, colorless to slightly yellow. Know that because reslizumab is a protein, particles may be present that appear translucent to white and amorphous. Do not use if discolored or other foreign particulate matter is present.
- Withdraw proper volume and discard any unused portion.

- Inject drug slowly into an infusion bag containing 50 ml of 0.9% Sodium Chloride Injection to minimize foaming. Drug is compatible with polyvinylchloride (PVC) or polyolefin infusion bags.
- Gently invert the bag to mix the solution. Do not shake.
- If not administered immediately, diluted solution may be stored in refrigerator or at room temperature, protected from light, for up to 16 hours, which must include the time for administration.
- Use an infusion set with an in-line, low-protein-binding filter (pore size of 0.2 micron).
- Infuse drug over 20 to 50 minutes according to total volume to be infused and patient's weight. Do not infuse in the same intravenous line with other agents.
- Never administer drug by I.V. push.
- After infusion is complete, flush the intravenous line with 0.9% Sodium Chloride Injection.
- *Incompatibilities:* Other I.V. drugs or solution other than 0.9% Sodium Chloride Injection

Route	Onset	Peak	Duration
I.V.	Unknown	Unknown	Unknown

Half-life: 24 days

Mechanism of Action

Inhibits IL-5 activity (the major cytokine responsible for activation and survival, differentiation, growth, and recruitment of eosinophils) by blocking its binding to the IL-5 receptor complex found on the eosinophil cell surface. Eosinophils are among many cell types involved in inflammation. By inhibiting IL-5 signaling, the production and survival of eosinophils are reduced, which then reduces inflammation present in asthma.

Contraindications

Hypersensitivity to reslizumab or its components

Interactions

DRUGS

None reported by manufacturer

Adverse Reactions

EENT: Oropharyngeal pain
GI: Vomiting

MS: Elevated CPK levels; chest, extremity, or neck musculoskeletal pain; muscle fatigue or spasms; myalgia
RESP: Decreased oxygen saturation, dyspnea, wheezing
SKIN: Urticaria
Other: Anaphylaxis, antibodies to reslizumab, malignancy

Childbearing Considerations

PREGNANCY

- It is not known if drug can cause fetal harm although monoclonal antibodies are transported across the placental barrier in a linear fashion as pregnancy progresses; therefore, potential effects on a fetus increases as the pregnancy progresses.
- Use with caution only if benefit to mother outweighs potential risk to fetus.

LACTATION

- It is not known if drug is present in breast milk, although human IgG is present in breast milk.
- Patient should check with prescriber before breastfeeding.

Nursing Considerations

- Know that reslizumab should not be used to treat acute asthma symptoms or acute exacerbations, including acute bronchospasm or status asthmaticus.
- Check to see that patient with an existing parasitic (helminth) infection has received treatment prior to starting reslizumab therapy because drug may interfere with resolving the infection. If patient becomes infected while receiving reslizumab and does not respond to antihelminth treatment, notify prescriber, as reslizumab will have to be discontinued until infection is resolved.
- Be aware that concurrent inhaled or systemic corticosteroid therapy should not be abruptly discontinued when reslizumab therapy is initiated, as systemic withdrawal symptoms may occur. Expect reductions to be done gradually, as ordered.

! **WARNING** Monitor patient closely for allergic reactions to reslizumab, including anaphylaxis exhibited by decreased oxygen saturation, dyspnea, urticaria, vomiting, or wheezing. These reactions most often occur during or within 20 minutes after completion of the infusion, although reactions have occurred before the second dose 4 weeks later. If severe symptoms, such as anaphylaxis, occur, stop infusion at once, notify prescriber, and provide supportive care, as ordered. Know that if anaphylaxis occurs, drug should be permanently discontinued. Be aware that reslizumab-specific IgE antibodies may not be detected in patients who have had a past experience of anaphylactic reactions to the drug.

- Be aware that, infrequently, malignancies of many different types have occurred within six months after patient's exposure to reslizumab. Report any persistent, severe, or unusual symptoms immediately to the prescriber.

PATIENT TEACHING

- Remind patient that reslizumab is not used to treat acute asthma symptoms or acute exacerbations. If asthma symptoms worsen or become acute, instruct patient to seek immediate emergency care.

! WARNING Inform patient that drug may cause an allergic reaction that could become life-threatening. Review signs and symptoms with patient and instruct her to seek immediate emergency care, if any occurs.

- Instruct patient to have any persistent, severe, or unusual symptoms checked out by prescriber.
- Tell patient not to change any concurrent inhaled or systemic corticosteroid dosage when starting reslizumab until instructed to do so by prescriber. Inform patient that if a dosage reduction is done, it will be done gradually to avoid withdrawal symptoms. Remind her that corticosteroids should never be abruptly stopped.

revefenacin
Yupelri

▤ Class and Category
Pharmacologic class: Anticholinergic
Therapeutic class: Bronchodilator

▤ Indications and Dosages
✱ *To provide maintenance therapy for patients with chronic obstructive pulmonary disease (COPD)*

INHALATION SOLUTION
Adults. 175-mcg once daily by nebulizer.

▤ Drug Administration
INHALATION
- Remove unit-dose vial from foil pouch and open immediately before use.
- Administer by the orally inhaled route via a standard jet nebulizer connected to an air compressor and using a mouthpiece.
- Do not mix any other drugs in the nebulizer with revefenacin, as drug compatibility is unknown.

Route	Onset	Peak	Duration
Inhalation	45 min	14–41 min	24 hr

Half-life: 22–70 hr

▤ Mechanism of Action
Inhibits muscarinic receptor M3 in smooth muscles of the airways to produce bronchodilation

▤ Contraindications
Hypersensitivity to revefenacin or its components

▤ Interactions
DRUGS
OATP1B1 and OATP1B3 inhibitors such as cyclosporine, rifampicin: Possibly increased systemic exposure of revefenacin leading to increased adverse reactions
other anticholinergics: Possible additive anticholinergic effects leading to increased adverse reactions

▤ Adverse Reactions
CNS: Dizziness, headache
CV: Hypertension
EENT: Nasopharyngitis, oropharyngeal pain
MS: Back pain
RESP: Bronchitis, cough, **paradoxical bronchospasms**, upper respiratory infection
Other: Immediate hypersensitivity reactions

▤ Childbearing Considerations
PREGNANCY
- It is not known if drug can cause fetal harm.
- Use with caution only if benefit to mother outweighs potential risk to fetus.

LACTATION
- It is not known if drug is present in breast milk.

Q
R
S

- Patient should check with prescriber before breastfeeding.

Nursing Considerations

- Be aware that revefenacin should not be initiated in patients during acutely deteriorating or potentially life-threatening episodes of COPD. It should also not be used to relieve acute bronchospasms; know that acute symptoms should be treated with an inhaled, short-acting beta₂-agonist.
- Use cautiously in patients with narrow-angle glaucoma, because revefenacin may worsen the condition. Question patient frequently about presence of blurred vision, colored images, eye discomfort or pain, or visual halos in association with red eyes from conjunctival congestion and corneal edema. Notify prescriber immediately, if present.
- Use cautiously in patients with urinary retention, because revefenacin may worsen condition. Monitor patient for signs and symptoms of urinary retention such as difficulty passing urine or painful urination, especially in patients with bladder-neck obstruction or prostatic hyperplasia.
- Notify prescriber if revefenacin no longer controls symptoms of bronchoconstriction, because this may indicate that patient's condition is deteriorating and other forms of therapy may be required. The dosage or frequency of revefenacin should not be increased in this situation.

! **WARNING** Monitor patient for paradoxical bronchospasm that may become life-threatening. If this should occur following a nebulizer treatment with revefenacin, notify prescriber immediately; expect to administer an inhaled, short-acting bronchodilator, as prescribed; and know that revefenacin should be discontinued immediately and alternative therapy substituted.

PATIENT TEACHING

- Inform patient that revefenacin therapy is not meant to relieve acute symptoms of COPD and extra doses should never be used for that purpose. Instead, acute symptoms should be treated with an inhaled short-acting beta₂ agonist such as albuterol.
- Teach patient how to administer drug using a standard jet nebulizer. Tell patient drug should only be administered via this device. Warn him not to inject or swallow the solution and not to mix it with other medications.
- Warn patient not to inhale more than one dose at any given time. Remind him the daily dosage should not exceed one unit-dose vial. Tell him to inhale the dosage via nebulization daily at the same time every day. He should throw the plastic dispensing vials away immediately after use.
- Stress importance of keeping plastic vials out of the reach of children, because the vials' small size poses a choking danger if swallowed.
- Instruct patient to notify prescriber immediately if he experiences decreased effectiveness or needs more of his inhaled short-acting beta₂ agonist or experiences a decrease in lung function. Warn him not to stop taking revefenacin without consulting prescriber, as symptoms may reoccur or become worse.

! **WARNING** Tell patient drug may cause allergic reactions that may occur after revefenacin has been administered. Instruct patient to notify prescriber, as drug will have to be discontinued, and to seek emergency care if reaction is severe.

- Instruct patient to report the presence of blurred vision, colored images, eye discomfort or pain, or visual halos in association with red eyes from conjunctival congestion and corneal edema.
- Tell patient, especially if he has bladder-neck obstruction or prostatic hyperplasia, to report difficulty passing urine or painful urination.

! **WARNING** Inform patient that drug may cause paradoxical bronchospasm. If present, patient should use an inhaled, short-acting bronchodilator immediately, stop taking revefenacin, and notify prescriber.

ribavirin
Rebetol, Ribasphere, Virazole

Class and Category
Pharmacologic class: Nucleoside analogue
Therapeutic class: Antiviral

Indications and Dosages
＊ *As adjunct to treat chronic hepatitis C (CHC) infection in combination with interferon alfa-2 b (pegylated and nonpegylated) in patients with compensated liver disease*

CAPSULES (REBETOL, RIBASPHERE), ORAL SOLUTION (REBETOL)
Adults weighing more than 105 kg (231 lb). 600 mg in morning and 800 mg in evening for 24 to 48 wks depending on genotype.
Adults weighing between 81 and 105 kg (178 to 231 lb) and children ages 3 to 18 weighing more than 73 kg (162 lb). 600 mg in morning and 600 mg in evening for 24 to 48 wks depending on genotype.
Adults weighing between 66 and 80 kg (145 to 177 lb) and children ages 3 to 18 weighing 60 to 73 kg (132 to 162 lb). 400 mg in morning and 600 mg in evening for 24 to 48 wks depending on genotype.
Adults weighing less than 66 kg (144 lb) and children ages 3 to 18 weighing between 47 and 59 kg (103 to 131 lb). 400 mg in morning and 400 mg in evening for 24 to 48 wks depending on genotype.

ORAL SOLUTION (REBETOL)
Children ages 3 to 18 weighing less than 47 kg (103 lb). 15 mg/kg/day divided and given in 2 doses for 24 to 48 wk depending on genotype.

＊ *As adjunct to treat chronic hepatitis C (CHC) infection in combination with peginterferon alfa-2a in patients with compensated liver disease who have not been previously treated with interferon alpha*

TABLETS
Adults with genotypes 1 or 4 weighing 75 kg (165 lb) or more. 600 mg in morning and 600 mg in evening for 48 wks.
Adults with genotypes 1 or 4 weighing less than 75 kg (165 lb). 400 mg in morning and 600 mg in evening for 48 wks.
Adults with genotypes 2 or 3. 400 mg in morning and 400 mg in evening for 24 wks.

Children ages 5 to 18 weighing 75 kg (165 lb) or more. 600 mg in morning and 600 mg in evening for 24 to 48 wks depending on genotype.
Children ages 5 to 18 weighing 60 to 74 kg (132 to 162.8 lb). 400 mg in morning and 600 mg in evening for 24 to 48 wks depending on genotype.
Children ages 5 to 18 weighing 47 to 59 kg (103.4 to 129.8. lb). 400 mg in morning and 400 mg in evening for 24 to 48 wks depending on genotype.
Children ages 5 to 18 weighing 34 to 46 kg (74.8 to 101.2 lb). 200 mg in morning and 400 mg in evening for 24 to 48 wks depending on genotype.
Children ages 5 to 18 weighing 23 to 33 kg (50.6 to 72.6 lb). 200 mg in morning and 200 mg in evening for 24 to 48 wks depending on genotype.

＊ *To treat hospitalized infants and young children with severe lower respiratory tract infections due to respiratory syncytial virus (RSV)*

INHALATION SOLUTION (VIRAZOLE)
Hospitalized infants and young children. 20 mg/ml administered by SPAG-2 unit with continuous aerosol for 12 to 18 hr daily for 3 to 7 days.

± **DOSAGE ADJUSTMENT** Dosage adjustment individualized for patients with renal dysfunction and severe adverse reactions.

Drug Administration
P.O.
- Administer with food.
- Administer consistently at the same times daily, morning and evening.
- Capsules should be swallowed whole and not chewed, crushed, or opened.
- Use a calibrated device to measure oral solution.

INHALATION
- Use in children only.
- Do not mix with or simultaneously give with other aerosolized medications.
- Prepare powder for administration as a solution by reconstituting drug with a minimum of 75 ml of Sterile Water for Injection or Inhalation in the original 100-ml glass vial. Do not use Bacteriostatic Water. Shake well.
- Transfer solution to the clean, sterilized 500-ml SPAG-2 reservoir.

Q.
R
S

- Further dilute to a final volume of 300 ml with Sterile Water for Injection or Inhalation. Do not use Bacteriostatic Water. The final concentration should be 20 mg/ml.
- Discard solutions in the SPAG-2 unit at least every 24 hours and when the liquid level is low before adding newly reconstituted solution.

Route	Onset	Peak	Duration
P.O.	Unknown	1–2 hr	Unknown
Inhalation	Unknown	Unknown	Unknown

Half-life: 12 days

Mechanism of Action

Precise action unknown, but may inhibit HCV polymerase or respiratory syncytial virus in a selective biochemical reaction.

Contraindications

Autoimmune hepatitis, coadministration with didanosine, creatinine clearance less than 50 ml/min, hemoglobinopathies (i.e., sickle cell anemia, thalassemia major), hypersensitivity to ribavirin or its components, men whose female partners are pregnant, pregnancy

Interactions

DRUGS

azathioprine: Increased risk of azathioprine-related myelotoxicity and severe pancytopenia

didanosine: Increased risk of didanosine-induced toxicities such as hepatic failure, pancreatitis, peripheral neuropathy, and symptomatic hyperlactatemia/lactic acidosis

lamivudine, stavudine, zidovudine: Possibly decreased effectiveness of these drugs; increased risk of hepatic toxicity, anemia, and hepatic decompensation

Adverse Reactions

CNS: Aggression, agitation, anger, anxiety, asthenia, chills, **CVA**, depression, dizziness, emotional swings in mood, fatigue, fever, hallucinations, headache, impaired concentration, insomnia, irritability, lethargy, malaise, memory impairment, nervousness, peripheral neuropathy, psychosis, rigors, **suicidal ideation**, vertigo

CV: Angina, **bigeminy, bradycardia** (inhalation solution), **cardiac arrest**, chest pain, **hypotension** (inhalation solution)

EENT: Blurred vision, conjunctivitis, dry mouth, hearing impairment or loss, pharyngitis, retinal detachment or exudates, rhinitis, significant ophthalmologic disorders, sinusitis, taste perversion, transient blindness

ENDO: Hyperglycemia, hypothyroidism, growth retardation (children)

GI: Abdominal pain, anorexia, cholangitis, colitis, constipation, diarrhea, dyspepsia, elevated liver enzymes, fatty liver, **GI bleeding, hepatic decompensation,** hepatomegaly, hyperbilirubinemia, nausea, **pancreatitis,** peptic ulcer, vomiting

GU: Menstrual disorder

HEME: Anemia, **hemolytic anemia, leukopenia, neutropenia, pure red cell aplasia,** reticulocytosis (inhalation solution), **thrombocytopenia, thrombotic thrombocytopenic purpura**

MS: Arthralgia, back pain, extremity pain, musculoskeletal pain, myalgia, myositis

RESP: Cough, dyspnea, **pulmonary embolism or hypertension** (inhalation solution in children); **apnea, atelectasis,** bacterial pneumonia, **bronchospasm, cyanosis,** dyspnea, **hypoventilation, pneumothorax, pulmonary edema, ventilator dependence, worsening of respiratory status** (inhalation solution)

SKIN: Alopecia, dermatitis, diaphoresis, dry skin, eczema, erythroderma, flushing, pruritus, rash, **Stevens–Johnson syndrome, toxic epidermal necrolysis,** urticaria

Other: Anaphylaxis; angioedema; autoimmune disorders; bacterial, fungal, or viral infections; dehydration; flu-like symptoms; graft rejection (liver or renal); hyperuricemia; weight loss

Childbearing Considerations

PREGNANCY

- Pregnancy exposure registry: 1-800-593-2214.
- Drug can cause fetal harm as significant embryocidal and teratogenic effects.
- A negative pregnancy must be obtained immediately before drug therapy is begun and periodic pregnancy tests done during treatment and for 9 months following discontinuation of drug.
- Drug is contraindicated in women who are pregnant and in male partners of women who are pregnant. If pregnancy occurs, drug must be discontinued immediately.

LACTATION

- It is not known if drug is present in breast milk.
- Patient should check with prescriber before breastfeeding.

REPRODUCTION

- Females of childbearing age should use effective contraception during drug therapy and for 9 months after drug has been discontinued; male patients and their female partners of childbearing age should use effective contraception during drug therapy and for 6 months after drug has been discontinued.
- Drug may impair male fertility.

Nursing Considerations

- Know that patient requires the following tests to be performed before ribavirin therapy is started and then periodically thereafter, as ordered, to establish a baseline before treatment starts and allow early detection of adverse effects during treatment: ECG, standard hematologic tests including hemoglobin, liver function tests, monthly pregnancy tests for women of childbearing potential or partners of male patients, and TSH levels. Expect dosage to be temporarily withheld or discontinued, as ordered, if patient experiences severe adverse reactions or test abnormalities and drug to be discontinued immediately with confirmation of pregnancy.
- Be aware that ribavirin therapy should not be given to patients with a creatinine clearance less than 50 ml/min, because of risk of severe renal dysfunction. Ribavirin should not be given until a negative pregnancy test is obtained from women of childbearing age or the female partner of childbearing age of male patient. Also know that ribavirin should not be given to patient with a history of significant or unstable cardiac disease, because drug may cause a deterioration of cardiovascular status.
- Use caution when administering ribavirin to patient with preexisting but stable cardiac disease. Monitor these patients closely and expect that if there is any deterioration in cardiovascular status, ribavirin therapy will be discontinued.
- Monitor patients with impaired renal function and those over the age of 50 during therapy for anemia. Because anemia usually occurs early in treatment, expect to obtain a baseline of patient's hemoglobin and then assess at 2 and 4 weeks after therapy begins. Know that any patient who develops a decreased hemoglobin level below 10 g/dl should have dosage modified or drug discontinued, as ordered, because potentially fatal myocardial infarctions have occurred from anemia induced by ribavirin therapy. For patients with a history of stable cardiovascular disease, expect a permanent dosage reduction to occur if the hemoglobin decreases by more than or equal to 2 g/dl during any 4-week period. If the hemoglobin remains less than 12 g/dl after 4 weeks of therapy on a reduced dose, expect drug to be discontinued. Also monitor patient taking azathioprine concomitantly for pancytopenia and bone marrow suppression, which usually occurs within 3 to 7 weeks after concomitant administration of pegylated interferon/ribavirin and azathioprine. Expect drug to be discontinued if pancytopenia develops.
- Monitor patient for signs and symptoms of pancreatitis (abdominal pain and tenderness, anorexia, fever, nausea, vomiting). If present, notify prescriber and expect drug to be discontinued.

! **WARNING** Expect patient's lungs to be assessed regularly for evidence of pulmonary function impairment or pulmonary infiltrates, because drug can cause serious or even life-threatening pulmonary adverse reactions. If either develops, expect ribavirin therapy to be discontinued.

- Know that because ribavirin is used in conjunction with alpha interferons, serious and severe visual changes may occur. Know that patient should have a baseline ophthalmologic exam before therapy begins. Patients with preexisting ophthalmologic disorders such as diabetic or hypertensive retinopathy should receive periodic eye examinations throughout therapy or at any time ocular symptoms appear. Expect drug to be discontinued in patients who develop new or worsening ophthalmologic disorders.

! **WARNING** Monitor patient closely for suicidal ideation. Suicidal ideation or attempts occur more frequently among pediatric patients, primarily adolescents, when compared to adult patients during treatment and off-therapy follow-up.

PATIENT TEACHING

- Tell patient to take oral ribavirin with food.
- Instruct patient to take ribavirin exactly as prescribed. If a dose is missed, tell patient to take the missed dose as soon as possible during the same day but not to double the next dose.
- Warn patient not to chew, crush, or open capsules but to swallow them whole.
- Instruct patient to use a calibrated device to measure dosage of oral solution, not a household spoon.

! **WARNING** Instruct patients to use reliable form of contraception throughout treatment and for 6 months after drug has been discontinued. A pregnancy test must be performed monthly during ribavirin therapy and for 6 months after therapy is finished. Stress importance of notifying prescriber immediately if pregnancy occurs or is suspected.

- Instruct patient to comply with dental checkups and to brush teeth thoroughly twice daily. If vomiting should occur, stress importance of rinsing out mouth thoroughly afterward.
- Inform patients that growth retardation often occurs with combination therapy that includes ribavirin. Reassure parents that following treatment, rebound growth and weight gain occur in most children.
- Stress importance of complying with scheduled laboratory tests.
- Tell patient to maintain adequate hydration throughout ribavirin therapy.
- Caution patient not to perform hazardous activities such as driving until effects of ribavirin on his nervous system are known and resolved.

! **WARNING** Caution patient or parents to watch for changes in behavior or mood as ribavirin may cause suicidal ideation, especially in adolescent patients. If changes are noted, stress importance of contacting prescriber.

rifampin
(rifampicin)
Rifadin, Rifadin I.V. Rimactane, Rofact (CAN)

⦀ Class and Category
Pharmacologic class: Semisynthetic rifamycin
Therapeutic class: Antimycobacterial antitubercular

⦀ Indications and Dosages
✴ *As adjunct to treat tuberculosis caused by all strains of* Mycobacterium tuberculosis

CAPSULES, ORAL SUSPENSION, I.V. INFUSION
Adults. 10 mg/kg once daily with other antitubercular drugs for 2 mo. *Maximum:* 600 mg daily.
Children. 10 to 20 mg/kg once daily in combination with other antitubercular drugs for 2 mo. *Maximum:* 600 mg daily.

✴ *To eliminate meningococci from nasopharynx of asymptomatic carriers of* Neisseria meningitidis

CAPSULES, ORAL SUSPENSION, I.V. INFUSION
Adults. 600 mg every 12 hr for 2 days (total of 4 doses).
Infants age 1 month and over and children. 10 mg/kg every 12 hr for 2 days (total of 4 doses). *Maximum:* 600 mg/dose.
Infants under age 1 month. 5 mg/kg every 12 hr for 2 days (total of 4 doses).

⦀ Drug Administration
P.O.
- Administer 1 hour before or 2 hours after a meal with a full glass of water.
- If patient is unable to swallow a capsule, have pharmacist prepare an oral suspension.
- Shake oral suspension well before measuring dose. Use a calibrated device when measuring dose of oral suspension.
- Store oral suspension at room temperature or in refrigerator for 4 weeks, then discard.

I.V.
- Reconstitute by adding 10 ml Sterile Water for Injection to 600-mg vial. Swirl gently to dissolve to yield a concentration of 60 mg/ml.

- Reconstituted solution is stable at room temperature for up to 30 hours.
- Withdraw appropriate dose and add to 500 ml of 0.9% Sodium Chloride Injection or 5% Dextrose in Water (preferred solution) and infuse within 3 hours. Or, withdraw appropriate dose and add to 100 ml of 0.9% Sodium Chloride Injection or 5% Dextrose in Water (preferred solution) and infuse over 30 minutes.
- Dilutions using 5% Dextrose Injection are stable at room temperature for up to 8 hours; after 8 hours precipitation of rifampin may occur. Dilutions using 0.9% Sodium Chloride Injection are stable at room temperature for up to 6 hours.
- *Incompatibilities:* Diltiazem hydrochloride with Y-site administration

Route	Onset	Peak	Duration
P.O.	Unknown	2–4 hr	Unknown
I.V.	Unknown	0.5 to 3 hr	Unknown

Half-life: 2–3 hr

Mechanism of Action

Inhibits bacterial and mycobacterial RNA synthesis by binding to DNA-dependent RNA polymerase, thereby blocking RNA transcription. Exhibits dose-dependent bactericidal or bacteriostatic action. Rifampin is highly effective against rapidly dividing bacilli in extracellular cavitary lesions, such as those found in the nasopharynx.

Contraindications

Concurrent use of atazanavir, darunavir, fosamprenavir, praziquantel, ritonavir/saquinavir, saquinavir, or tipranavir; hypersensitivity to rifampin, other rifamycins or their components

Interactions

DRUGS

antacids: Possibly reduced rifampin absorption

antiarrhythmics (disopyramide, mexiletine, quinidine, propafenone, tocainide), anticonvulsants (phenytoin), antiestrogens (tamoxifen, toremifene), antifungals (fluconazole, itraconazole, ketoconazole), antipsychotics (haloperidol), antiretrovirals (atazanavir, darunavir, efavirenz, fosamprenavir, indinavir, saquinavir,
tipranavir, zidovudine), benzodiazepines (diazepam), benzodiazepine-related drugs (zopiclone, zolpidem), beta-blockers (metoprolol, propranolol), calcium channel blockers (diltiazem, nifedipine, verapamil), chloramphenicol, clarithromycin, corticosteroids (prednisolone), dapsone, digoxin, doxycycline, enalapril, fluoroquinolones (moxifloxacin, pefloxacin), hepatitis C antiviral (daclatasvir, simeprevir, sofosbuvir, telaprevir), hypoglycemic agents oral (glipizide, glyburide), immunosuppressive agents (cyclosporine, tacrolimus), irinotecan, levothyroxine, losartan, methadone, narcotic analgesics (morphine, oxycodone), praziquantel, quinine, selective 5-HT3 receptor antagonists (ondansetron), statins (simvastatin), systemic hormonal contraceptives (estrogens, progestins), telithromycin, theophylline, thiazolidinediones (rosiglitazone), ticagrelor, tricyclic antidepressants (nortriptyline), warfarin: Decreased exposure and effectiveness of these drugs

antihypertensives: Possibly interference of antihypertensive action of these drugs

atovaquone: Decreased concentration of atovaquone and increased concentration of rifampin, which may increase risk of toxicities

clopidogrel: Increased risk of bleeding

cotrimoxazole, probenecid: Increased rifampin concentration

halothane, isoniazid: Possibly hepatotoxicity

ritonavir/saquinavir: Increased risk of severe hepatotoxicity

ACTIVITIES

alcohol use: Increased risk of hepatotoxicity

Adverse Reactions

CNS: Ataxia, behavioral changes, chills, confusion, difficulty concentrating, dizziness, drowsiness, fatigue, fever, generalized numbness, headache, paresthesia, psychoses

CV: **Chest pain, hypotension, myopathy,** vasculitis

EENT: Conjunctivitis; discolored saliva, sputum, tears, and teeth; mouth or tongue soreness; periorbital edema; visual disturbances

ENDO: **Adrenal insufficiency** (rare), hyperglycemia or **hypoglycemia** (in patients with diabetes)

GI: Abdominal cramps, anorexia, cholestasis, diarrhea, discolored feces, elevated liver

Q
R
S

enzymes, epigastric discomfort, flatulence, heartburn, **hepatitis, hepatotoxicity,** jaundice, nausea, **pseudomembranous colitis, shock-like syndrome with hepatic involvement,** vomiting

GU: Acute renal failure or tubular necrosis, discolored urine, elevated BUN and serum uric acid, hematuria, interstitial nephritis, menstrual disturbances, **renal insufficiency**

HEME: Agranulocytosis (rare), decreased hemoglobin, **disseminated intravascular coagulation (DIC),** eosinophilia, **hemolytic anemia, leukopenia, neutropenia,** purpura, **thrombocytopenia** (rare)

MS: Arthralgia, extremity pain, muscle weakness, myalgia (rare)

RESP: Acute bronchospasm, cough, **pulmonary toxicity (interstitial lung disease),** shortness of breath, wheezing

SKIN: Acute generalized exanthematous pustulosis, discolored skin and sweat, **erythema multiforme,** flushing, pemphigoid reaction, pruritus, rash, **Stevens–Johnson syndrome, toxic epidermal necrolysis,** urticaria

Other: Anaphylaxis, angioedema, drug reaction with eosinophilia and systemic symptoms (DRESS), flu-like symptoms, lymphadenopathy, paradoxical drug reaction

Childbearing Considerations

PREGNANCY

- It is not known if drug causes fetal harm, but animal studies suggest it may as drug does cross the placental barrier. When given during the last few weeks of pregnancy drug can cause postnatal hemorrhages in both mother and infant.
- Use with caution only if benefit to mother outweighs potential risk to fetus.

LACTATION

- Drug is present in breast milk.
- A decision should be made to discontinue breastfeeding or the drug to avoid potential serious adverse reactions.

REPRODUCTION

- Female patient using an oral contraceptive should use an additional contraceptive throughout therapy.

Nursing Considerations

- Obtain blood samples or other specimens for culture and sensitivity testing, as ordered, before giving rifampin and

throughout therapy to monitor response to drug.

- Be aware that rifampin should not be used to treat meningococcal infection, because of the possibility of rapid emergence of resistant organisms.

! **WARNING** Monitor patient for acute respiratory distress syndrome or respiratory failure because rifampin may cause pulmonary toxicity. If present, drug will have to be discontinued immediately and emergency supportive care given, as ordered.

! **WARNING** Expect to monitor liver enzymes before and every 2 to 4 weeks during therapy. Immediately report abnormalities. Also monitor patient for liver dysfunction such as abdominal pain, darkened urine, loss of appetite, and yellowish discoloration of the eyes and skin. Know that drug can cause serious liver dysfunction that could become life-threatening.

- Use rifampin cautiously in patients with diabetes mellitus because rifampin therapy may make diabetes management more difficult because of its effect on blood glucose levels.
- Expect drug to discolor body fluids, skin, and teeth reddish orange to reddish brown.
- Be aware that rifampin can cause myelosuppression and increase risk of infection. Notify prescriber immediately if signs of infection, such as fever, develop.

! **WARNING** Monitor patient for signs and symptoms of hypersensitivity reactions. Notify prescriber if present, expect drug to be discontinued, and provide supportive care, as ordered.

- Monitor patient for rash or other skin abnormalities, as rifampin may cause severe skin reactions that could be life-threatening.
- Be aware that paradoxical drug reaction (recurrence or appearance of new symptoms) may occur in patients who have shown improvement to drug therapy. It is usually transient and should not be misunderstood as treatment failure.

PATIENT TEACHING

- Instruct patient to take rifampin 1 hour before or 2 hours after a meal with a full glass of water. Tell patient to swallow capsules whole and not to chew, crush, or open capsules.

- Inform patient unable to swallow capsules that pharmacist can make an oral suspension. If used, tell patient to shake suspension before using and measure dose with a calibrated device, not a household spoon. Also tell patient suspension can be stored in refrigerator or at room temperature for 4 weeks and then must be discarded.
- Emphasize the need to take drug exactly as prescribed. Explain that not completing the full course of therapy or skipping doses may decrease the effectiveness of the treatment and increase the chance that resistance to drug may develop, making it ineffective to treat an infection patient might develop in the future. Emphasize importance of compliance with the full course of therapy.
- Explain that drug may discolor feces, saliva, skin, sputum, sweat, tears, teeth, and urine reddish brown to reddish orange or yellow. Discoloration of teeth and soft contact lenses may be permanent.

! WARNING Alert patient that an allergic reaction may occur with rifampin therapy. Review signs and symptoms with patient. Advise patient to alert prescriber if an allergic reaction occurs; if severe, stress importance of seeking immediate medical care.

- Advise patient who takes an oral contraceptive to use an additional form of birth control during rifampin therapy.
- Urge patient to notify prescriber about anorexia, cough, darkened urine, fever, flu-like symptoms, joint pain or swelling, malaise, nausea, rash, shortness of breath, swollen lymph nodes, vomiting, wheezing, and yellowish eyes or skin. Also, advise patient to seek medical care immediately if symptoms worsen.
- Advise patient to avoid alcohol, herbal products, or any drug that adversely affects the liver (without prescriber consent) during rifampin therapy.
- Instruct patient to notify prescriber if no improvement occurs within 2 to 3 weeks.
- Inform patient with diabetes mellitus that rifampin therapy may affect his blood

glucose levels and to monitor his blood glucose levels closely.

- Tell patient to inform all prescribers of rifampin therapy.
- Instruct patient to notify prescriber immediately if rash or other skin abnormalities occur, as reaction may become severe.

rifamycin
Aemcolo

Class and Category
Pharmacologic class: Rifamycin antibacterial
Therapeutic class: Antibiotic

Indications and Dosages
* *To treat travelers' diarrhea caused by noninvasive strains of* Escherichia coli

DELAYED-RELEASE TABLETS

Adults. 388 mg twice daily for 3 days.

Drug Administration
P.O.
- Administer drug with 6 to 8 ounces of liquid.
- D.R. tablets should be swallowed whole and not chewed, crushed, or divided.

Route	Onset	Peak	Duration
P.O./D.R.	Unknown	2 hr	Unknown

Half-life: 1.5–5 hr

Mechanism of Action
As a semisynthetic derivative of rifampin, drug inhibits bacterial RNA synthesis by binding to DNA-dependent RNA polymerase, thereby blocking RNA transcription. This results in bacterial cell impairment or death.

Contraindications
Hypersensitivity to rifamycin, other rifamycin-class antimicrobial agents such as rifaximin, or their components

Interactions
DRUGS
None reported by manufacturer

Adverse Reactions
CNS: Fever, headache
GI: Abdominal pain, *Clostridium difficile-associated diarrhea*, constipation, dyspepsia

Childbearing Considerations
PREGNANCY
- It is not known if drug causes fetal harm. However, because systemic absorption is negligible, it not expected to affect the fetus.
- Use with caution only if benefit to mother outweighs potential risk to fetus.

LACTATION
- It is not known if drug is present in breast milk.
- Patient should check with prescriber before breastfeeding.

Nursing Considerations
- Be aware that rifamycin is not to be used in patients with diarrhea complicated by bloody stool or fever or due to pathogens other than noninvasive strains of *E. coli*.
- Know that drug should be discontinued if diarrhea gets worse or persists more than 48 hours.
- Assess patient for signs of secondary infection, such as profuse, watery diarrhea. If such diarrhea develops, contact prescriber and expect to obtain a stool specimen to rule out pseudomembranous colitis caused by *Clostridium difficile*. If diarrhea occurs, notify prescriber and expect to withhold rifamycin and treat with electrolytes, fluids, protein, and an antibiotic effective against *C. difficile*.

PATIENT TEACHING
- Tell patient to take rifamycin twice daily (once in morning and once in evening) with 6 to 8 ounces of liquid but not with alcohol.
- Caution patient not to break, chew, or crush tablets. Instead, tablets must be swallowed whole.
- Instruct patient to notify prescriber if diarrhea gets worse or persists for more than 48 hours, because drug will have to be discontinued and a different antibiotic prescribed.

rifaximin
Xifaxan

Class and Category
Pharmacologic class: Rifamycin
Therapeutic class: Antibiotic

Indications and Dosages
✴ *To treat irritable bowel syndrome with diarrhea (IBS-D)*

TABLETS
Adults. 550 mg three times daily for 14 days. May be repeated up to two times for reoccurrence.

✴ *To treat travelers' diarrhea caused by noninvasive strains of* Escherichia coli

TABLETS
Adults and children age 12 and over. 200 mg three times daily for 3 days.

✴ *To reduce risk of overt hepatic encephalopathy*

TABLETS
Adults. 550 mg twice daily.

Drug Administration
P.O.
- Administer drug without regard to food.

Route	Onset	Peak	Duration
P.O.	Unknown	1 hr	Unknown

Half-life: 2–5 hr

Mechanism of Action
As a semisynthetic derivative of rifampin, it inhibits bacterial RNA synthesis by binding to DNA-dependent RNA polymerase, thereby blocking RNA transcription. This results in bacterial cell impairment or death.

Contraindications
Hypersensitivity to rifaximin, any of the rifamycin antimicrobial agents, or their components

Interactions
DRUGS
P-glycoprotein inhibitors such as cyclosporine: Increased exposure to rifaximin leading to possible risk of increased adverse reactions
warfarin: Altered INR levels possibly requiring warfarin dosage adjustment

Adverse Reactions
CNS: Depression, dizziness, fatigue, fever, headache
CV: Peripheral edema
EENT: Nasal passage irritation, nasopharyngitis, taste loss
GI: Abdominal pain, anorexia, ascites, *Clostridium difficile*-associated colitis, dysentery, elevated ALT liver enzyme, nausea
HEME: Anemia

MS: Arthralgia, muscle spasms, myalgia, **rhabdomyolysis**
RESP: Dyspnea
SKIN: **Exfoliative dermatitis,** flushing, pruritus, rash, urticaria
Other: **Anaphylaxis, angioedema,** elevated blood creatine phosphokinase, weight loss

Childbearing Considerations

PREGNANCY
- It is not known if drug can cause fetal harm, although some animal studies suggest it may cause fetal harm.
- Use with caution only if benefit to mother outweighs potential risk to fetus.

LACTATION
- It is not known if drug is present in breast milk.
- Patient should check with prescriber before breastfeeding.

Nursing Considerations
- Be aware that rifaximin should not be used in patients with travelers' diarrhea complicated by blood in the stool, diarrhea due to pathogens other than *E. coli*, or in the presence of fever.
- Use extreme caution in patients with severe hepatic impairment because of increased rifaximin exposure leading to possible increased risk of adverse reactions.
- Notify prescriber if diarrhea gets worse or persists for more than 48 hours in patients being treated for diarrhea or for a new onset of diarrhea in patients being treated for hepatic encephalopathy. The patient may be experiencing *C. difficile* colitis associated with antibiotic use, requiring rifaximin to be discontinued and an antibiotic effective against *C. difficile* along with electrolytes, fluids, and protein replacement therapy, to be administered, as ordered.

PATIENT TEACHING
- Instruct patient to take drug for length of time prescribed, even when feeling better.
- Tell patient to report diarrhea that gets worse or persists for more than 48 hours or new onset or reoccurrence of diarrhea, as *C. difficile*-associated diarrhea may occur even after rifaximin has been discontinued, requiring additional treatment.

rilpivirine
Edurant

Class and Category
Pharmacologic class: Nonnucleoside reverse transcriptase inhibitor (NNRTI)
Therapeutic class: Antiretroviral

Indications and Dosages
＊ *As adjunct to treat human immunodeficiency virus type 1 (HIV-1) infection in antiretroviral treatment-naïve patients with NIV-1 RNA equal to or less than 100,000 copies/ml at the start of therapy*

TABLETS
Adults and children age 12 years and over weighing at least 35 kg (77 lb). 25 mg once daily with a meal.
± **DOSAGE ADJUSTMENT** For patient taking rifabutin concomitantly, dosage increased to 50 mg once daily.
＊ *To provide short-term treatment of HIV-1 infection in combination with cabotegravir in patients who are virologically suppressed (HIV-1 RNA less than 50 copies/ml) and on a stable antiretroviral regimen with no history of treatment failure and with no known or suspected resistance to either cabotegravir or rilpivirine as either an oral lead-in to assess the tolerability of rilpivirine prior to administration of the combination product Cabenuva (cabotegravir, rilpivirine E.R. injectable suspension) or to provide oral therapy for patients who will miss planned injection dosing with Cabenuva E.R. injectable suspension*

TABLETS
Adults requiring lead-in dosing. 25 mg rilpivirine with 30 mg cabotegravir once daily for at least 28 days with last oral dose given on the same day injections with Cabenuva are started.
Adults replacing planned missed Cabenuva injections. 25 mg rilpivirine with 30 mg cabotegravir once daily for up to 2 consecutive months of missed Cabenuva injections and started 1 month after last injection dose of Cabenuva and continued until the day injection dosing is restarted.

Drug Administration

P.O.
- Administer drug with a meal; a protein drink is not adequate to count as a meal.

Q
R
S

- Store drug protected from light.
- If administering drug with cabotegravir, administer both drugs at the same time each day with a meal.
- The last oral dose of drug administered with cabotegravir should be given on the same day injections with Cabenuva are started or restarted.

Route	Onset	Peak	Duration
P.O.	Unknown	4–5 hr	Unknown

Half-life: 50 hr

Mechanism of Action

Inhibits HIV-1 replication by noncompetitive inhibition of HIV-1 reverse transcriptase.

Contraindications

Concomitant therapy with carbamazepine, dexamethasone (more than a single dose), esomeprazole, lansoprazole, omeprazole, oxcarbazepine, pantoprazole, phenobarbital, phenytoin, rabeprazole, rifampin, rifapentine, or St. John's wort; hypersensitivity to rilpivirine or its components

Interactions

DRUGS

aluminum- or magnesium-containing antacids, calcium carbonate, cimetidine, famotidine: Decreased rilpivirine concentration and significantly decreased effectiveness

atazanavir, atazanavir/ritonavir, clarithromycin, darunavir/ritonavir, delavirdine, erythromycin, fluconazole, fosamprenavir, fosamprenavir/ritonavir, indinavir, itraconazole, lopinavir/ritonavir, nelfinavir, posaconazole, saquinavir/ritonavir, telithromycin, tipranavir, voriconazole: Increased concentration of rilpivirine with possible prolonged action and risk of adverse reactions

carbamazepine, dexamethasone (more than a single dose), phenobarbital, phenytoin, proton pump inhibitors, rifampin, rifapentine, St. John's wort: Possibly significant decrease in rilpivirine plasma concentrations, resulting in loss of virologic response

drugs that prolong QT interval: Increased risk of torsades de pointes

ketoconazole: Decreased ketoconazole concentration and effectiveness and increased rilpivirine concentration with possible prolonged action and risk of adverse reactions

methadone: Possible decreased methadone concentration with increased risk of opiate withdrawal

other NNRTIs (efavirenz, etravirine, nevirapine), rifabutin: Decreased concentration of rilpivirine with possible decreased effectiveness

Adverse Reactions

CNS: Abnormal dreams, anxiety, depression, dizziness, dysphoria, fatigue, fever, headache, insomnia, mood changes, sleep disorders, somnolence, suicidal ideation

CV: Elevated cholesterol and triglycerides

EENT: Conjunctivitis, oral ulceration

ENDO: Cushingoid appearance, fat redistribution

GI: Abdominal discomfort or pain, anorexia, bilirubin increase, cholecystitis, cholelithiasis, diarrhea, elevated liver enzymes, hepatitis, hepatotoxicity, nausea, vomiting

GU: Elevated creatinine, glomerulonephritis, nephrolithiasis, nephrotic syndrome

HEME: Eosinophilia

SKIN: Blisters, rash

Other: Angioedema, drug reaction with eosinophilia and systemic symptoms (DRESS), immune reconstitution syndrome

Childbearing Considerations

PREGNANCY

- Pregnancy exposure registry: 1-800-258-4263.
- Drug can be administered during pregnancy.

LACTATION

- It is not known if drug is present in breast milk.
- The Centers for Disease Control and Prevention recommends that HIV-1 infected mothers not breastfeed to avoid risking postnatal transmission of HIV-1 infection to infants. They also do not recommend breastfeeding because of potential drug-induced adverse reactions in the infant.

Nursing Considerations

- Know that drug should not be used in patients taking other medications with a known risk of torsades de pointes or in patients at higher risk of torsades de pointes, because rilpivirine may cause QT prolongation.

! WARNING Obtain liver enzymes before therapy begins, as ordered, in patients with marked transaminase elevations, patients treated with other medications associated with liver toxicity, and patients with underlying hepatic disease, including hepatitis B or C viral infections. Also monitor liver enzymes throughout therapy, as ordered, on all patients, because rilpivirine may cause hepatotoxicity. Know that persistent elevations of serum transaminase levels may require rilpivirine therapy to be discontinued.

- Obtain cholesterol and triglyceride levels before rilpivirine is begun and periodically throughout therapy, because drug may cause an increase in total cholesterol and triglycerides.

! WARNING Assess patient's skin regularly for rash or other abnormalities. Notify prescriber and expect rilpivirine to be discontinued immediately if a severe rash occurs and is accompanied by blisters, conjunctivitis, eosinophilia, facial edema, fever, joint or muscle aches, lip swelling, malaise, or oral lesions. Be aware that a delay in discontinuing drug may result in a life-threatening situation.

- Monitor patient's mood and emotional status, as rilpivirine may cause significant depression, mood changes, and suicidal ideation. Report any changes to prescriber.
- Be aware that immune reconstitution syndrome has occurred in patients treated with combination antiretroviral therapy, including rilpivirine. The inflammatory response predisposes susceptible patients to opportunistic infections such as cytomegalovirus, *Mycobacterium avium* infection, *Pneumocystis jiroveci* pneumonia, or tuberculosis. Autoimmune disorders such as Graves' disease, Guillain–Barré syndrome, or polymyositis have also occurred. Report sudden or unusual adverse reactions to prescriber.

PATIENT TEACHING

- Advise patient to avoid missing doses of rilpivirine. If she misses a dose, and it is less than 12 hours from the time of the missed dose, she should take it as soon as she remembers. However, if more than 12 hours has elapsed since missing dose, dose should not be taken and usual dosing schedule resumed. Stress importance of not doubling the next dose or taking more than prescribed.
- Inform patient that rilpivirine must be taken with a meal. Remind patient that a protein drink does not replace a meal.

! WARNING Inform patient about severe liver disease that may occur with rilpivirine. Tell her to report signs and symptoms of liver disease such as acholic stools, anorexia, fatigue, malaise, nausea, tenderness over liver area, or yellowing of skin or whites of the eyes and to seek immediate medical attention.

- Stress importance of being compliant with tests ordered to screen for adverse effects of rilpivirine therapy.

! WARNING Advise patient that rilpivirine therapy may cause severe hypersensitivity or skin reactions. Tell her to report a rash, especially if it is accompanied by blisters, conjunctivitis, facial edema, fatigue, fever, joint or muscle aches, liver problems, or oral lesions and to seek immediate medical attention.

- Inform patient that rilpivirine therapy may cause changes in her body appearance because of fat redistribution. Prepare her for the possibility of developing breast enlargement, central obesity, dorsocervical fat enlargement (buffalo hump), facial wasting, and peripheral wasting.
- Instruct patient to report any persistent, severe, or unusual signs and symptoms.
- Alert mothers that breastfeeding is not recommended during rilpivirine therapy.
- Tell patient to report all drugs being taken, including over-the-counter medications and herbals, as serious drug interactions may occur. Advise patient not to begin any new drug therapy without first checking with prescriber.
- Tell patient or caregiver to report any signs of depression, mood changes, sleep disorders, or suicidal thoughts to prescriber.

Q
R
S

rimegepant
Nurtec ODT

Class and Category
Pharmacologic class: Calcitonin gene-related peptide (CGRP) receptor antagonist
Therapeutic class: Antimigraine

Indications and Dosages
✴ *To treat acute migraine*

ORALLY DISINTEGRATING TABLETS
Adults. 75 mg. *Maximum:* 75 mg in a 24-hr period and no more than 18 doses in a 30-day period.

±**DOSAGE ADJUSTMENT** For patient taking a moderate inhibitor of CYP3A4 or potent inhibitors of P-gp, length of time a second dose may be taken increased to every 48 hours.

✴ *To prevent episodic migraines*

ORALLY DISINTEGRATING TABLETS
Adults. 75 mg every other day.

Drug Administration
P.O.
- Using dry gloved hands, peel back foil covering of one blister and gently remove tablet. Do not push tablet through the foil.
- Administer immediately, without additional liquid, by placing tablet on or under patient's tongue.
- Do not store tablet outside the blister pack for future use.

Route	Onset	Peak	Duration
P.O.	Unknown	1.5 hr	Unknown
Half-life: 11 hr			

Mechanism of Action
Blocks CGRP receptors to help stop inflammation, pain signals, and swelling of blood vessels that occur in the brain during a migraine headache.

Contraindications
Hypersensitivity to rimegepant or its components

Interactions
DRUGS
BCRP or P-gp inhibitors: Possibly increased exposure to rimegepant with possibly increased risk of adverse reactions

CYP3A4 moderate or strong inducers: Decreased rimegepant exposure with possible loss of effectiveness
CYP3A4 moderate or strong inhibitors: Increased (strong) or possible increased (moderate) rimegepant exposure with possibly increased risk of adverse reactions

Adverse Reactions
GI: Abdominal pain, dyspepsia, nausea
MS: Dyspnea
SKIN: Severe rash
Other: Hypersensitivity reactions

Childbearing Considerations
PREGNANCY
- Pregnancy exposure registry: 1-877-366-0324, web address: nurtecpregnancyregistry.com, or email: nurtecpregnancyregistry@ppd.com.
- It is not known if drug can cause fetal harm.
- Use with caution only if benefit to mother outweighs potential risk to fetus.
- Know that pregnant women with migraine may be at increased risk of gestational hypertension and preeclampsia.

LACTATION
- It is not known if drug is present in breast milk.
- Patient should check with prescriber before breastfeeding.

Nursing Considerations
- Know that rimegepant should not be administered to patients taking BCRP or P-gp inhibitors and moderate or strong CYP3A inducers, because these drugs interfere with the effectiveness of rimegepant.
- Know that rimegepant should not be administered to patients taking strong CYP3A inhibitors, because these drugs increase exposure of rimegepant and increase the risk of adverse reactions.
- Be aware that the safety of taking rimegepant more than 15 times in a 30-day period is unknown.

! **WARNING** Monitor patient for hypersensitivity reactions, including dyspnea and rash. Hypersensitivity has been known to occur days after administration and could be serious.

PATIENT TEACHING

- Instruct patient on how to handle, administer, and store rimegepant as an orally disintegrating tablet.

! **WARNING** Review signs and symptoms of an allergic reaction to rimegepant and remind patient that such a reaction may occur days after taking drug. If an allergic reaction occurs, urge patient to contact prescriber.

risankizumab-rzaa
Skyrizi

⊟ Class and Category

Pharmacologic class: Monoclonal antibody
Therapeutic class: Anti-inflammatory, immunosuppressant

⊟ Indications and Dosages

✳ *To treat moderate to severe plaque psoriasis in patients who are candidates for systemic therapy or phototherapy; to treat active psoriatic arthritis as monotherapy or in combination with nonbiologic disease-modifying antirheumatic drugs (DMARDs)*

SUBCUTANEOUS INJECTION

Adults. *Initial:* 150 mg (two consecutive 75-mg injections) followed by 150 mg (two consecutive 75-mg injections) 4 wk later and then 150 mg (two consecutive 75-mg injections) every 12 wk thereafter.

⊟ Drug Administration

SUBCUTANEOUS

- Take drug carton out of refrigerator and allow it to warm to room temperature keeping it out of direct sunlight (15 to 30 minutes) without removing the prefilled syringes from carton.
- Visually inspect syringes for particulate matter and discoloration (solution should be colorless to slightly yellow and clear to slightly opalescent).
- If using two separate 75-mg single-dose prefilled syringes for the full 150-mg dose, inject in two different anatomical sites.
- Inject into the abdomen, thigh, or upper outer arm. Do not inject into an area that is affected by psoriasis, bruised, indurated, red, or tender.

- If dose is missed, administer as soon as possible and then resume dosing at the regular scheduled time.

Route	Onset	Peak	Duration
SubQ	Unknown	Unknown	Unknown

Half-life: 28 days

⊟ Mechanism of Action

Unknown but thought to block interleukin-23, which causes inflammation and swelling, reducing the signs and symptoms of plaque psoriasis

⊟ Contraindications

Hypersensitivity to risankizumab-rzaa or its components

⊟ Interactions

DRUGS

immunosuppressants: enhanced immunosuppressive effect
live vaccines: Possibly increased risk of infection

⊟ Adverse Reactions

CNS: Fatigue, headache
MS: Asthenia, osteomyelitis
RESP: Pneumonia, upper respiratory infections
SKIN: Cellulitis, eczema, rash
Other: Anaphylaxis, antibody formation to risankizumab-rzaa; infections, including herpes zoster and tinea; injection-site reactions such as bruising, erythema, extravasation, hematoma, hemorrhage, infection, inflammation, irritation, pain, pruritus, swelling, warmth; sepsis

⊟ Childbearing Considerations

PREGNANCY

- Pregnancy exposure registry: 1-877-302-2161.
- It is not known if drug can cause fetal harm, but drug does cross the placental barrier and may be transmitted from mother to fetus.
- Use with caution only if benefit to mother outweighs potential risk to fetus.

LACTATION

- It is not known if drug is present in breast milk.
- Patient should check with prescriber before breastfeeding.

☱ Nursing Considerations

- Know that risankizumab-rzaa should not be given to patient with an active infection until infection resolves or is adequately treated.
- Use risankizumab-rzaa cautiously in patients with chronic infection or a history of recurrent infection.
- Be sure patient has been evaluated for tuberculosis prior to initiating treatment with risankizumab-rzaa. Expect tuberculosis treatment to be initiated in patients with a past history of active or latent TB in whom an adequate course of treatment cannot be confirmed. Monitor patient for signs and symptoms of active TB during and after drug therapy. Know that risankizumab-rzaa should not be given to patients with active TB.
- Check to determine that patient is up to date on immunizations before initiating treatment with risankizumab-rzaa.

! WARNING Monitor patient for hypersensitivity reactions, which could be severe. If present, stop drug therapy, notify prescriber, and expect to provide emergency supportive care, as ordered.

- Institute infection control measures and monitor patient for signs and symptoms of infection throughout therapy. Notify prescriber if an infection is suspected or known and expect drug to be withheld until infection is resolved.

PATIENT TEACHING

- Tell patient that the first dose of drug must be given under the supervision of a healthcare professional.
- Teach patient or caregiver how to administer a subcutaneous injection. Instruct patient or caregiver to first take drug carton out of the refrigerator and allow it to warm at room temperature out of direct sunlight (15 to 30 minutes) without removing the prefilled syringes from the carton. After visually inspecting syringes for particulate matter and discoloration (solution should be colorless to slightly yellow and clear to slightly opalescent), tell patient or caregiver to administer two separate 75-mg single-dose prefilled syringes for the full 150-mg dose by injecting into the abdomen or thigh and not into an area that is bruised, indurated, red, tender, or affected by psoriasis. Caregiver may inject drug into patient's upper, outer arm. Remind patient or caregiver to inject the two injections at different anatomic locations. Instruct patient or caregiver how to dispose of needle and syringe properly.

- Instruct patient or caregiver that if a dose is missed, to administer it as soon as possible and then resume dosing at the regular time.

! WARNING Alert patient to possibility of an allergic reaction. Advise patient, if an allergic reaction occurs, to stop drug, notify prescriber, and seek immediate emergency care if serious or severe symptoms occur.

- Review infection control measures with patient and family. Urge patient to notify prescriber immediately if an infection is suspected or known.
- Advise patient to avoid vaccination with live vaccines and immediately prior to or after drug therapy. Tell them to alert all prescribers about risankizumab-rzaa therapy prior to any potential vaccination.
- Encourage females of childbearing age who become pregnant during drug therapy to register their pregnancy.

risedronate sodium
Actonel, Atelvia

☱ Class and Category
Pharmacologic class: Bisphosphonate
Therapeutic class: Antiosteoporotic

☱ Indications and Dosages
✱ *To treat Paget's disease of bone*
TABLETS (ACTONEL)
Adults. 30 mg daily for 2 mo. Repeated after 2 mo if relapse occurs or if serum alkaline phosphatase level fails to normalize.
✱ *To prevent or treat glucocorticoid-induced osteoporosis in patients taking a dose of 7.5 mg or more of prednisone or equivalent daily*
TABLETS (ACTONEL)
Adults. 5 mg daily.
✱ *To prevent or treat postmenopausal osteoporosis*

TABLETS (ACTONEL)

Postmenopausal women. 5 mg daily. 35 mg once weekly, 75 mg taken on 2 consecutive days once a month, or 150 mg once a month.

✶ *To treat postmenopausal osteoporosis*

E.R. TABLETS (ATELVIA)

Adults. 35 mg once weekly.

✶ *To treat osteoporosis in men*

TABLETS (ACTONEL)

Adult men. 35 mg once weekly.

⬛ Drug Administration

P.O.

- Administer immediate-release tablet with 6 to 8 ounces of plain water (no supplements should be present in the water such as found in mineral water). Administer at least 30 minutes before the first beverage, food, or medication of the day. Tablet should be swallowed whole and not chewed or sucked on.
- E.R. tablets should be swallowed whole and not chewed, crushed, or divided. Administer in the morning following breakfast with at least 4 ounces of plain water (no supplements added such as found in mineral water).
- Ensure that patient is in an upright position when drug is administered and does not lie down for 30 minutes afterward.

Route	Onset	Peak	Duration
P.O.	1 hr	1 hr	Unknown
P.O./E.R.	Unknown	3 hr	Unknown

Half-life: 1.5 hr, initial; terminal exponential, 480 hr

⬛ Mechanism of Action

Hinders excessive bone remodeling characteristic of Paget's disease by binding to bone and reducing the rate at which osteoclasts are resorbed by bone. Also, decreases elevated rate of bone turnover that is typically seen in osteoporosis.

⬛ Contraindications

Esophageal abnormalities that delay esophageal emptying, such as achalasia or stricture; hypersensitivity to risedronate or its components; hypocalcemia; inability to sit or stand upright for at least 30 minutes

⬛ Interactions

DRUGS

angiogenesis inhibitors, chemotherapy, corticosteroids: Possibly increased risk of osteonecrosis of the jaw
aspirin, NSAIDs: Increased risk of GI irritation
calcium-containing preparations, including antacids: Impaired absorption of risedronate
histamine 2 blockers, proton pump inhibitors: Faster drug release of delayed-release form of drug increasing drug exposure and possible adverse reactions

FOODS

all foods: Decreased risedronate bioavailability when taking Actonel form of drug

⬛ Adverse Reactions

CNS: Anxiety, asthenia, depression, dizziness, fatigue, headache, insomnia, sciatica, syncope, vertigo, weakness
CV: Chest pain, hypercholesterolemia, hypertension, peripheral edema, vasodilation
EENT: Amblyopia, cataract, dry eyes, eye inflammation, nasopharyngitis, painful swallowing, pharyngitis, rhinitis, sinusitis, tinnitus
GI: Abdominal pain, colitis, constipation, diarrhea, dyspepsia, dysphagia, eructation, esophagitis, esophageal or gastric ulcers, flatulence, gastritis, nausea, vomiting
GU: UTI
MS: Arthralgia; atypical femur fractures; back, limb, neck, or shoulder pain; jaw osteonecrosis; leg cramps or spasms; myasthenia; myalgia; osteoarthritis; retrosternal pain; severe incapacitating bone, joint, or muscle pain
RESP: Asthma exacerbation; bronchitis, cough, pneumonia, upper respiratory tract infection
SKIN: Bullous reaction, pruritus, rash, Stevens–Johnson syndrome, toxic epidermal necrolysis
Other: Anaphylaxis, angioedema, flu-like symptoms, hypersensitivity reactions, hypocalcemia

⬛ Childbearing Considerations

PREGNANCY

- It is not known if drug can cause fetal harm.
- Know that there is a theoretical risk of fetal harm, especially skeletal, if a woman

becomes pregnant after completing a course of bisphosphonate therapy. Time between cessation of drug therapy to conception, the particular bisphosphonate used, and route of administration that may cause fetal harm are unknown.

- Use with caution only if benefit to mother outweighs potential risk to fetus.

LACTATION

- It is not known if drug is present in breast milk.
- A decision should be made to discontinue breastfeeding or the drug to avoid potential serious adverse reactions in the infant.

Nursing Considerations

- Be aware that risedronate isn't recommended for patients with severe renal impairment.
- Make sure patient has had a dental checkup before having invasive dental procedures during risedronate therapy, especially if patient has cancer; is receiving angiogenesis inhibitors, chemotherapy, corticosteroids, or head or neck radiation; or has poor oral hygiene, because risk of jaw osteonecrosis is increased in these patients.
- Give supplemental calcium and vitamin D, as prescribed, during risedronate therapy if patient's dietary intake is inadequate.
- Give calcium supplements and antacids at different time of day than risedronate administration to avoid impaired drug absorption and altered effectiveness.

! **WARNING** Watch for rare, but possibly severe hypersensitivity reactions such as angioedema, bullous skin reactions, or rash.

PATIENT TEACHING

- Instruct patient to take immediate-release risedronate at least 1 hour before first food or drink of day (except water) while in an upright position and with 6 to 8 oz of plain water (contains no supplements). Instruct patient taking extended-release form to take immediately after breakfast with at least 4 ounces of plain water (contains no supplements). Caution against lying down for at least 30 minutes after taking drug to keep it from lodging in esophagus and causing irritation. Also instruct patient not to chew or suck

on tablet because doing so may irritate mouth or throat.

- Advise patient to stop taking risedronate and to notify prescriber if she develops dysphagia, new or worsening heartburn, or pain while swallowing, retrosternal pain. Also alert patient that drug may cause severe bone, joint, or muscle pain and to notify prescriber if present occurs.
- Alert patient that drugs in the same class as risedronate have caused severe bone, joint, or muscle pain. If such symptoms appear while taking risedronate, advise patient to contact prescriber.
- Advise patient that if she takes 35 mg once weekly and misses a dose, tell her to take it the morning after she remembers and then to take the next dose on its usual day. If patient takes 75 mg on 2 consecutive days once monthly and she misses both doses with more than 7 days until the next scheduled dose, tell her to take the first missed dose on the morning after she remembers and the second dose the following day. If she misses only 1 of the 2 doses, tell her to take it the morning after she remembers and then resume her normal schedule. If patient takes 150 mg once monthly and misses a dose, urge her to contact prescriber for instructions. Caution patient not to take more than 150 mg within a 7-day period and not to take 2 tablets of any strength on the same day.
- Tell patient to take antacids or calcium supplements at different times than risedronate.
- Urge women of childbearing age to tell prescriber about planned, suspected, or known pregnancy because of risk to fetal skeleton.

! **WARNING** Tell patient to stop risedronate and contact prescriber if allergic reaction occurs. Stress importance of seeking immediate emergency care if she notices swelling or skin abnormalities.

- Instruct patient about proper oral hygiene and about the need to notify prescriber about invasive dental procedures.
- Instruct patient to notify prescriber immediately of any new groin or thigh pain that might be reflective of an atypical femur fracture.

risperidone

Perseris, Risperdal, Risperdal Consta

Class and Category

Pharmacologic class: Benzisoxazole derivative
Therapeutic class: Antipsychotic

Indications and Dosages

* *To treat schizophrenia*

ORAL SOLUTION, ORALLY DISINTEGRATING TABLETS, TABLETS

Adults. *Initial:* 2 mg once daily or divided and given as 1 mg twice daily, increased at intervals of 24 hr or longer in increments of 1 to 2 mg daily to target dose of 4 to 8 mg once daily or divided and given twice daily. *Effective dose range:* 4 to 16 mg once daily or divided and given twice daily. *Maximum:* 16 mg daily.

Adolescents ages 13 to 17. *Initial:* 0.5 mg once daily, increased as needed every 24 hr or longer in 0.5- to 1-mg increments to target dose of 3 mg daily. *Effective dose range:* 1 to 6 mg once daily. *Maximum:* 6 mg once daily.

I.M. INJECTION (RISPERDAL CONSTA)

Adults. *Initial:* After tolerability established with oral risperidone, 25 mg every 2 wk, increased as needed every 4 wk to 37.5 or 50 mg. *Maximum:* 50 mg every 2 wk.

SUBCUTANEOUS INJECTION (PERSERIS)

Adults. 90 mg or 120 mg injected into abdomen only once monthly. Tolerability should be established first with oral risperidone for patient who has never received drug before.

* *To treat bipolar mania as monotherapy*

ORAL SOLUTION, ORALLY DISINTEGRATING TABLETS, TABLETS

Adults. *Initial:* 2 or 3 mg daily, increased as needed by 1 mg every 24 hr or longer up to 6 mg. *Maximum:* 6 mg daily for no more than 3 wk.

Children and adolescents ages 10 to 17. *Initial:* 0.5 mg once daily, increased as needed every 24 hr or longer in 0.5- to 1-mg increments to recommended dose of 1 to 2.5 mg daily. *Maximum:* 2.5 mg once daily.

I.M. INJECTION (RISPERDAL CONSTA)

Adults. After tolerability established with oral risperidone, 25 mg every 2 wk, increased, as needed every 4 wk to 37.5 or 50 mg. *Maximum:* 50 mg every 2 wk.

* *As adjunct to treat bipolar mania with lithium or valproate therapy*

ORAL SOLUTION, ORALLY DISINTEGRATING TABLETS, TABLETS

Adults. *Initial:* 2 to 3 mg daily, increased as needed by 1 mg every 24 hr or longer up to 6 mg. *Maximum:* 6 mg daily for no more than 3 wk.

I.M. INJECTION (RISPERDAL CONSTA)

Adults. After tolerability established with oral risperidone, 25 mg every 2 wk, increased, as needed, every 4 wk to 37.5 or 50 mg. *Maximum:* 50 mg every 2 wk.

* *To treat irritability associated with autistic disorder*

ORAL SOLUTION, ORALLY DISINTEGRATING TABLETS, TABLETS

Children age 5 and over and adolescents weighing 20 kg (44 lb) or more. *Initial:* 0.5 mg daily, increased after 4 days to 1 mg daily. Dosage further increased, as needed, in 2-wk intervals in 0.5-mg increments.

Children age 5 and over and adolescents weighing less than 20 kg (44 lb). *Initial:* 0.25 mg daily, increased after 4 days to 0.5 mg daily. Dosage further increased, as needed, in 2-wk intervals in 0.25-mg increments.

±**DOSAGE ADJUSTMENT** *For oral dosage:* For elderly patients and patients with severe hepatic or renal impairment or who are taking CYP2D6 inhibitors, starting doses reduced to 0.5 mg twice daily, increased in increments of 0.5 mg or less twice daily. For doses above 1.5 mg twice daily, dosage increased in intervals of one week or greater. For patients taking CYP3A4 inducers such as carbamazepine, phenobarbital, phenytoin, or rifampin, dosage may have to be increased up to double the patient's usual dose. *For I.M. doses:* For patients with hepatic or renal impairment, initial dose may have to be reduced to 12.5 mg. For patients starting a CYP3A4 inducer during risperidone therapy, a dosage increase of risperidone may be needed. For patients starting a CYP2D6 inhibitor, a dosage decrease of risperidone may be needed. *For subcutaneous doses:* For patients with hepatic or renal impairment, the lower dose of 90 mg recommended for the initial dose. For patient receiving a CYP2D6 inhibitor, lowest dose of drug

Q
R
S

should be used with possible interruption of drug therapy, if needed. For patients receiving strong CYP3A4 inducers and a 90-mg dose, dosage may have to be increased to 120 mg; for patient already receiving a 120-mg dose, additional oral risperidone may be needed.

Drug Administration

P.O.

- Administer oral solution directly from the calibrated pipette or mix with water, coffee, orange juice, or low-fat milk, but not with cola or tea. Use a calibrated device to measure dosage.
- For orally disintegrating tablets, break open the blister unit with dry gloved hands by peeling the foil back to expose the tablet. Do not push tablet through the foil because this could damage tablet. Have patient place tablet immediately on the tongue, where it will dissolve within seconds. Orally disintegrating tablet should not be chewed or spit out of mouth.
- Continue oral therapy for 3 weeks after I.M. injection therapy is begun (not needed for subcutaneous injection therapy), then expect oral therapy to be discontinued.

I.M.

- Remove Risperdal Consta from refrigerator and allow it to come to room temperature for at least 30 minutes before reconstitution.
- Follow manufacturer's guidelines for reconstitution, following the illustrations closely, and use only the diluent supplied in the dose pack. After dilution, shake the vial vigorously while holding the plunger rod down for a minimum of 10 seconds to ensure a homogeneous suspension. Suspension should appear milky, thick, and uniform.
- Give using only the needle supplied in the dose pack. Within 2 minutes of reconstitution, inject entire contents of syringe into the upper outer quadrant of gluteal area using the 2-inch 20G needle (longer needle with yellow colored hub) or into the deltoid muscle using the 1-inch 21G needle (shorter needle with green colored hub).
- Never combine the two different dose strengths into a single injection.
- If drug can't be given right after reconstitution, shake the upright vial vigorously back and forth again

until particles are resuspended before administration.

- Discard reconstituted drug if not used within 6 hours.
- Never administer I.M. form intravenously.

SUBCUTANEOUS

- Drug by this route should only be given by a health professional.
- Neither a loading dose nor supplemental oral risperidone doses are needed when giving drug as a subcutaneous injection. Tolerance to drug should be established first in patients who have never received risperidone.
- Remove Perseris from refrigerator and allow it to come to room temperature for at least 15 minutes before preparing drug for administration. Only prepare drug when ready to administer the dose, not before.
- Wear gloves when preparing drug for administration.
- Follow manufacturer's guidelines for reconstitution, following the illustrations closely, and use only the diluent supplied in the dose pack.
- When fully mixed, drug should be a cloudy suspension that is uniform in color. It can vary from white to yellow-green. If any clear areas occur in the mixture, continue to mix it until the distribution of the color is uniform.
- Inject into the abdomen only after removing excess air from syringe; inject drug slowly and steadily.
- Do not rub the injection site after the injection. If there is bleeding, apply a bandage but use minimal pressure.
- Can be stored in refrigerator; if stored at room temperature, drug will have to be discarded after 7 days.

Route	Onset	Peak	Duration
P.O.	Unknown	1 hr	Unknown
I.M.	3 wk	4–6 wk	7 wk
SubQ	Unknown	4–6 hr	Unknown

Half-life: 3–20 hr (P.O.); 3–6 days (I.M.); 9–11 days (SubQ)

Mechanism of Action

Selectively blocks serotonin and dopamine receptors in the mesocortical tract of the CNS to suppress psychotic symptoms.

Contraindications

Hypersensitivity to risperidone, paliperidone, or its components

Interactions

DRUGS

antihypertensives: Increased antihypertensive effects

carbamazepine, phenobarbital, phenytoin, rifampin: Increased risperidone clearance with decreased effectiveness

clozapine: Decreased risperidone clearance with long-term concurrent use

CNS depressants: Additive CNS depression

fluoxetine, paroxetine: Increased plasma risperidone level

dopamine agonists, levodopa: Possibly antagonized effects of these drugs

methylphenidate: Increased risk of extrapyramidal symptoms

ACTIVITIES

alcohol use: Additive CNS depression

Adverse Reactions

CNS: Abnormal coordination, aggressiveness, agitation, akathisia, anxiety, asthenia, confusion, decreased concentration, depression, dizziness, dream disturbances, drooling, drowsiness, dyskinesia, dystonia, fatigue, fever, headache, **hypothermia,** insomnia, lassitude, malaise, mania, memory loss, nervousness, **neuroleptic malignant syndrome,** paresthesia, Parkinsonism, restlessness, **seizures,** shaking of head repeatedly, sleepwalking, somnambulism, somnolence, tardive dyskinesia, tremor, vertigo

CV: Atrial fibrillation, **bradycardia,** bundle branch block, **cardiopulmonary arrest,** chest pain, elevated triglyceride levels, first-degree AV block, hypercholesterolemia, orthostatic hypotension, palpitations, **QT-interval prolongation,** tachycardia

EENT: Conjunctivitis, decreased or increased salivation, dry mouth, ear pain, epistaxis, nasal congestion, pharyngitis, retinal artery occlusion, rhinitis, sinusitis, taste alteration, vision changes

ENDO: **Diabetic ketoacidosis** (patients with diabetes), elevated prolactin level, galactorrhea, hyperglycemia, hyperprolactinemia, **hypoglycemia,** inappropriate antidiuretic hormone secretion (SIADH), pituitary adenoma, precocious puberty, water intoxication

GI: Abdominal pain, anorexia, constipation, diarrhea, gastritis, ileus, indigestion, **intestinal obstruction,** jaundice, nausea, **pancreatitis,** vomiting

GU: Amenorrhea, decreased libido, delayed ejaculation, dysmenorrhea, dysuria, glucosuria, hypermenorrhea, incontinence, increased appetite, polyuria, priapism, sexual dysfunction, urinary incontinence or retention, UTI

HEME: Agranulocytosis, anemia, **leukopenia, neutropenia, thrombocytopenia, thrombotic thrombocytopenic purpura**

MS: Arthralgia; back, buttock, or neck pain; dysarthria; muscle weakness; myalgia

RESP: Cough, dyspnea, **pulmonary embolism, sleep apnea,** upper respiratory tract infection

SKIN: Alopecia, diaphoresis, dry skin, eczema, hyperpigmentation, photosensitivity, pruritus, rash, seborrhea, **Stevens–Johnson syndrome, toxic epidermal necrolysis**

Other: Anaphylaxis; angioedema; flu-like symptoms; infections; injection-site induration, pain, redness, or swelling; weight gain or loss

Childbearing Considerations

PREGNANCY

- Pregnancy exposure registry: 1-866-961-2388 or http://womensmentalhealth.org/clinical-and-research-programs/pregnancyregistry/.
- Drug may cause fetal harm.
- Neonates exposed to drug during the third trimester of pregnancy are at risk for extrapyramidal and withdrawal symptoms.
- Use with caution only if benefit to mother outweighs potential risk to fetus.

LACTATION

- Drug is present in human milk.
- Patient should check with prescriber before breastfeeding.
- If breastfeeding occurs, mother should monitor infant for signs of abnormal muscle movements, excess sedation, failure to thrive, jitteriness, and tremors.

REPRODUCTION

- Infertility may occur because of hyperprolactinemia but is reversible.

Q
R
S

Nursing Considerations

- Use risperidone cautiously in debilitated patients, elderly patients, and patients with hepatic or renal dysfunction or hypotension because of their increased sensitivity to the drug. Also use risperidone cautiously in patients with a history of seizures; although rare, seizures may occur in those with schizophrenia.

! **WARNING** Be aware that risperidone should not be used to treat elderly patients with dementia-related psychosis because it increases risk of death in these patients.

- Monitor for orthostatic hypotension, especially in patients with cardiac or cerebrovascular disease.

! **WARNING** Immediately notify prescriber and expect to stop giving risperidone if patient shows evidence of neuroleptic malignant syndrome (altered mental status, autonomic instability, hyperpyrexia, muscle rigidity), which can be fatal.

- Monitor patient's blood glucose and lipid levels as ordered because drug increases the risk of hyperglycemia and hypercholesterolemia.
- Assess patients with Parkinson's disease or Lewy body dementia for increased sensitivity to the drug, exhibited by confusion, extrapyramidal symptoms, frequent falls, obtundation, postural instability, and features of neuroleptic malignant syndrome.
- Monitor patient's CBC, as ordered, because serious adverse hematologic reactions may occur, such as agranulocytosis, leukopenia, or neutropenia. More frequent monitoring during the first few months of risperidone therapy is recommended for patients with a history of drug-induced leukopenia or neutropenia, or those who have had a significantly low WBC count in the past. If abnormalities occur during therapy, monitor patient for fever or other signs of infection, notify prescriber, and expect drug to be discontinued if severe.
- Monitor patient for tardive dyskinesia, especially in the elderly and particularly elderly women. Be aware it may occur even at low doses and after discontinuation of treatment. Alert prescriber, if present, as drug may have to be discontinued.
- Institute fall precautions.

PATIENT TEACHING

- Instruct patient to take oral solution directly from the calibrated pipette used to measure drug. Drug can be diluted with water, coffee, orange juice, or low-fat milk, but not with cola or tea, before administration.
- Tell patient prescribed orally disintegrating tablets to break open the blister unit with dry hands by peeling the foil back to expose the tablet. Emphasize the importance of not pushing tablet through the foil because this could damage the tablet. Once patient has removed tablet, she should place immediately on her tongue, where it will dissolve within seconds. Tell patient not to chew orally disintegrating tablet or attempt to spit it out of her mouth.
- Inform patient receiving parenteral risperidone that injections must be administered by a healthcare professional. Alert patient receiving drug by subcutaneous injection that a lump may be felt for several weeks at injection site. Caution patient not to rub or massage the injection site and to be careful in the placement of any belts or clothing waistbands.
- Urge patient to avoid alcohol because of its additive CNS effects.
- Inform patient with a preexisting hematologic condition of the need to comply with ordered laboratory tests done to monitor for adverse effects.
- Warn patient that drug may cause amenorrhea or galactorrhea in females or erectile dysfunction or gynecomastia in men and for patient to alert prescriber if present. Stress importance with male patient to seek emergency care if an erection becomes painful or lasts longer than usual.
- Tell patient to notify prescriber of any adverse reactions, especially if serious or unusual.
- Instruct patient that dizziness upon standing can be minimized by rising slowly from a sitting or lying position and to avoid sudden position changes.
- Caution diabetic patient to monitor blood glucose level closely, because risperidone may increase it.

- Caution patient that risperidone may cause sleepwalking.
- Alert patient that drug may cause involuntary movements that may not be reversible. If present, stress importance of notifying prescriber immediately.
- Inform patient or parents/caregivers that orally disintegrating tablets contain phenylalanine and should not be used if patient has been diagnosed with PKU.
- Instruct patient to inform all prescribers of risperidone therapy and not to take any new medication, including over-the-counter preparation, without discussing use with prescriber first.
- Caution patient to avoid performing hazardous activities such as driving until CNS effects are known and subside. Review fall precautions with patient.
- Instruct patient to avoid overheating and becoming dehydrated during drug therapy.
- Instruct mothers who are breastfeeding while taking risperidone to monitor the infant for abnormal muscle movements, excess sedation, failure to thrive, jitteriness, or tremors.

ritonavir
Norvir

☰ Class and Category
Pharmacologic class: Protease inhibitor
Therapeutic class: Antiretroviral

☰ Indications and Dosages
＊ *As adjunct to treat human immunodeficiency viral type 1 (HIV-1) infection*

ORAL POWDER, TABLETS
Adults. *Initial:* 300 mg twice daily, increased by 100 mg twice daily every 2 to 3 days until maximum dose reached. *Maximum:* 600 mg twice daily.
Children old enough to swallow tablets. *Initial:* 250 mg/m^2 twice daily, increased by 50 mg/m^2 twice daily every 2 to 3 days until a maintenance dosage is reached. *Maintenance:* 350 to 400 mg/m^2 twice daily. *Maximum:* 600 mg twice daily.

ORAL POWDER
Children. *Initial:* 250 mg/m^2 twice daily, increased by 50 mg/m^2 twice daily every 2 to 3 days until a maintenance dosage is reached.

Maintenance: 350 to 400 mg/m^2 twice daily. *Maximum:* 600 mg twice daily.

ORAL SOLUTION
Adults. *Initial:* 300 mg twice daily, increased by 100 mg twice daily every 2 to 3 days until maximum dose is reached. *Maximum:* 600 mg twice daily.
Infants at least 44 weeks old (calculated from first day of mother's last menstrual period to birth plus the time elapsed after birth) and children. *Initial:* 250 mg/m^2 twice daily, increased by 50 mg/m^2 twice daily every 2 to 3 days until a maintenance dosage is reached. *Maintenance:* 350 to 400 mg/m^2 twice daily. *Maximum:* 600 mg twice daily.
±**DOSAGE ADJUSTMENT** For patient taking other protease inhibitors such as atazanavir, darunavir, fosamprenavir, saquinavir, and tipranavir, dosage reduced.

☰ Drug Administration
P.O.
- Administer drug with meals.
- Tablets should be swallowed whole and not chewed, crushed, or divided.
- Use a calibrated device to measure dosage of oral solution. Mix oral solution with Advera, chocolate milk, or Ensure within 1 hour of administration to help improve the taste. Shake well after mixing.
- Be aware that oral powder form of ritonavir should only be used for dosing increments of 100 mg. If the dose is less than 100 mg or the dose falls between 100-mg intervals, other forms should be used instead of the powder.
- Mix oral powder form with soft food such as applesauce or vanilla pudding or mix with liquids such as chocolate milk or 4 ounces of infant formula, or water. Use a calibrated dosing syringe to measure dosage, especially for infants and children. Once mixed, use within 2 hours or discard.
- Know that the oral powder (mixed with water) or solution form may be given via a feeding tube.
- Do not use oral solution with polyurethane feeding tubes, because the presence of ethanol in the solution may be incompatible. Also know that oral solution should not be given to pregnant women because of the ethanol content. Be aware that the total amounts of ethanol and

Q
R
S

propylene glycol from all drugs given to infants 1 to 6 months of age should be taken into account to avoid toxicity.

Route	Onset	Peak	Duration
P.O.	Unknown	2–4 hr	Unknown

Half-life: 3–5 hr

Mechanism of Action

Inhibits HIV protease to render the enzyme incapable of processing the Gag-Pol polyprotein precursor, which leads to the production of noninfectious immature HIV particles.

Contraindications

Concomitant therapy with other protease inhibitors, potent CYP3A inducers, or therapy that is highly dependent on CYP3A for drug clearance and for which elevated plasma concentrations have resulted in serious and/or life-threatening reactions (alfuzosin, amiodarone, cisapride, colchicine, dihydroergotamine, dronedarone, ergotamine, flecainide, lomitapide, lovastatin, lurasidone, methylergonovine, midazolam [oral], pimozide, propafenone, quinidine, ranolazine, St. John's wort, sildenafil [when used for treatment of pulmonary arterial hypertension], simvastatin, triazolam, voriconazole); hypersensitivity to ritonavir or its components; use of potent CYP3A inducers where significantly reduced ritonavir plasma concentrations may be associated with the potential loss of virologic response and possible resistance and cross-resistance such as anticancer agents (apalutamide) or herbal products (St. John's wort)

Interactions

DRUGS

amprenavir, atazanavir, atorvastatin, bedaquiline, bosentan, buspirone, carbamazepine, clarithromycin, clonazepam, clorazepate, colchicine, corticosteroids, cyclosporine, darunavir, dasatinib, desipramine, diazepam, diltiazem, disopyramide, dronabinol, estazolam, ethinyl estradiol, ethosuximide, fentanyl, fluoxetine, flurazepam, ibrutinib, indinavir, itraconazole, ketoconazole, lidocaine, lomitapide, maraviroc, methamphetamine, metoprolol, mexiletine, midazolam (parenteral), nefazodone,

nifedipine, nilotinib, paroxetine, perphenazine, propoxyphene, quetiapine, quinine, rifabutin, risperidone, rosuvastatin, salmeterol, saquinavir, simeprevir, sirolimus, tacrolimus, thioridazine, timolol, tipranavir, trazodone, tricyclic antidepressants, venetoclax, verapamil, zolpidem: Increased concentration of these drugs with possible risk of prolonged action and adverse reactions

atovaquone, bupropion, divalproex, lamotrigine, phenytoin, raltegravir, rifampin, theophylline, voriconazole: Decreased concentration of these drugs with possible decreased efficacy

avanafil, sildenafil, tadalafil, vardenafil: Increased concentration of PDE5 inhibitors with possible increased risk of adverse reactions, including hypotension, prolonged erection, syncope, visual changes

delavirdine: Increased concentration of ritonavir with possible risk of prolonged action and adverse reactions

digoxin: Increased concentration of digoxin with possible increased risk of digitalis toxicity

disulfiram, metronidazole: Increased risk of adverse reactions, especially "hangover" symptoms, because ritonavir contains ethanol

methadone: Decreased concentration of methadone with increased risk of opiate withdrawal symptoms

meperidine: Increased concentrations of the metabolite of meperidine with possible risk of prolonged action and adverse reactions

rivaroxaban: Increased concentration of rivaroxaban with possible increased risk of bleeding

vinblastine, vincristine: Increased concentration of these drugs with increased risk of significant gastrointestinal or hematologic adverse reactions

warfarin: Altered INR in either direction requiring possible dosage adjustments

Adverse Reactions

CNS: Asthenia, attention disturbance, confusion, dizziness, fatigue, paresthesia, peripheral neuropathy, **seizures**, syncope

CV: **AV block**, elevated cholesterol and triglycerides, hypertension, **hypotension**, orthostatic hypotension, peripheral edema, right bundle branch block

EENT: Blurred vision, oral paresthesia, oropharyngeal pain

ENDO: Cushingoid appearance, fat redistribution, hot flashes

GI: Abdominal pain, bilirubin increase, diarrhea, dysgeusia, dyspepsia, elevated liver and pancreatic enzymes, flatulence, gastroesophageal reflux disease, **GI hemorrhage, hepatitis, hepatotoxicity,** jaundice, nausea, **pancreatitis,** vomiting

GU: Increased urination, nephrolithiasis, **renal insufficiency**

HEME: Anemia, decreased red blood cells, **leukopenia, neutropenia, thrombocytopenia**

MS: Arthralgia, back pain, elevated creatine phosphokinase, myalgia, myopathy, peripheral coldness

RESP: Bronchospasm, coughing

SKIN: Acne, facial edema, flushing, pruritus, rash, skin eruptions, **Stevens–Johnson syndrome, toxic epidermal necrolysis,** urticaria

Other: Anaphylaxis, angioedema, dehydration, **electrolyte imbalances,** gout, immune reconstitution syndrome, lipodystrophy (acquired)

Childbearing Considerations
PREGNANCY
- Pregnancy exposure registry: 1-800-258-4263.
- It is not known if drug can cause fetal harm.
- Be aware that the oral solution form is not recommended during pregnancy because there is no known safe level of ethanol exposure during pregnancy.
- Use other forms with caution only if benefit to mother outweighs potential risk to fetus.

LACTATION
- Drug is present in breast milk.
- The Centers for Disease Control and Prevention recommends that HIV-1 infected mothers not breastfeed to avoid risking postnatal transmission of HIV-1 infection to infants. They also do not recommend breastfeeding because of potential drug-induced adverse reactions in the infant.

REPRODUCTION
- Women of childbearing age using a hormonal form of contraception should use an additional or alternative form during drug therapy.

Nursing Considerations
- Use cautiously in patients with cardiomyopathies, ischemic heart disease, preexisting conduction system abnormalities, or structural heart disease, because ritonavir may prolong patient's PR interval.
- Use cautiously in patients with hepatitis (especially B and C), liver enzyme abnormalities, or preexisting liver disease, because of the increased risk of hepatotoxicity during ritonavir therapy. Expect to monitor liver enzymes, as ordered, in these patients more frequently during the first 3 months of ritonavir therapy.
- Expect to check patient's cholesterol and triglyceride levels prior to starting ritonavir therapy and then periodically throughout therapy. Notify prescriber if elevated, and expect patient to be treated for the lipid disorder.
- Know that dihydroergotamine or ergotamine should not be coadministered with ritonavir because acute ergot toxicity may occur, exhibited by ischemia of the extremities and other tissues including the central nervous system and vasospasm.
- Be aware that adrenal suppression and Cushing's syndrome may occur when ritonavir is coadministered with budesonide or fluticasone propionate.

! **WARNING** Assess patient's skin regularly for signs of a hypersensitivity reaction. Know that angioedema, mild skin eruptions, and urticaria have occurred with ritonavir therapy. Cases of anaphylaxis, Stevens–Johnson syndrome, and toxic epidermal necrolysis have also occurred with ritonavir therapy. Report any abnormal findings and expect ritonavir to be discontinued if reaction is severe.

- Monitor patient's liver enzymes, as ordered, and patient for signs and symptoms of liver dysfunction.
- Monitor patient for pancreatitis such as the presence of abdominal pain, abnormal serum amylase or lipase values, nausea, or vomiting. If suspected, notify prescriber and expect ritonavir to be discontinued if confirmed.
- Monitor patient's blood glucose levels throughout ritonavir therapy, because some

patients have experienced an exacerbation of diabetes mellitus or have developed hyperglycemia or new-onset diabetes mellitus with protease inhibitor therapy.

- Be aware that immune reconstitution syndrome has occurred in patients treated with combination antiretroviral therapy, including ritonavir. The inflammatory response predisposes susceptible patients to opportunistic infections such as cytomegalovirus, *Mycobacterium avium* infection, *Pneumocystis jiroveci* pneumonia, or tuberculosis. Autoimmune disorders such as Graves' disease, Guillain–Barré syndrome, or polymyositis have also occurred. Report sudden or unusual adverse reactions to prescriber.
- Observe patient for redistribution of body fat, including breast enlargement, central obesity, development of buffalo hump, facial wasting, and peripheral wasting, which may produce a cushingoid-type appearance.
- Monitor patients with hemophilia for increased bleeding, because spontaneous skin hemarthrosis and hematomas have occurred in these patients while taking ritonavir. Provide supportive care, as prescribed.

PATIENT TEACHING

- Instruct patient to swallow tablets whole and not to break, chew, or crush them.
- Tell patient prescribed the oral solution that the taste may be improved by mixing with Advera, chocolate milk, or Ensure within 1 hour of dosing.
- Instruct parents to mix oral powder with soft food such as applesauce or vanilla pudding or mix with liquid such as chocolate milk or water. The bitter aftertaste may be lessened if given with food.
- Instruct mothers not to breastfeed while receiving ritonavir therapy.
- Warn patient that fat distribution may occur with ritonavir therapy, altering appearance.
- Alert female patients using oral contraceptives or patch contraceptives containing ethinyl estradiol that alternative methods of contraception should be used.
- Tell women of childbearing age to report a known or suspected pregnancy.
- Inform patients with hemophilia of increased risk of bleeding and the need to seek immediate medical attention if bleeding occurs.

! **WARNING** Instruct patient to report any signs of an allergic reaction or skin abnormalities, especially a skin rash, immediately to the prescriber.

- Warn patient to alert all prescribers of ritonavir therapy, because serious drug interactions can occur.

rituximab
Rituxan

rituximab-abbs
Truxima

rituximab-pvvr
Ruxience

Class and Category
Pharmacologic class: Monoclonal antibody
Therapeutic class: Anti-inflammatory, immunosuppressant

Indications and Dosages
❊ *To treat rheumatoid arthritis*

I.V. INFUSION (RITUXAN, RUXIENCE, TRUXIMA)

Adults. Two 1,000-mg infusions separated by 2 wk. Subsequent courses administered every 24 wk or based on clinical evaluation, but no sooner than every 16 wk.

❊ *To treat moderate to severe pemphigus*

I.V. INFUSION (RITUXIMAB)

Adults. *Induction:* Two 1,000-mg infusions separated by 2 wk. *Maintenance:* 500-mg infusion at month 12 and every 6 months thereafter or based on clinical evaluation. **Adults who have relapsed.** 1,000-mg infusion on relapse. Subsequent infusions given no sooner than 16 wk following previous infusion.

❊ *To treat non-Hodgkin's lymphoma (NHL)*

I.V. INFUSION (RITUXIMAB, RUXIENCE, TRUXIMA)

Adults with relapsed or who have refractory, low-grade, or follicular CD20-positive, B-cell NHL. 375 mg/m² once a wk for 4 to 8 doses.

Adults receiving retreatment for relapsed or refractory, low-grade, or follicular CD20-positive, B-cell NHL. 375 mg/m^2 once a wk for 4 doses.

Adults with previously untreated follicular, CD20-positive, B-cell NHL. 375 mg/m^2 administered on day 1 of each cycle of chemotherapy for up to 8 doses. *Maintenance:* If complete or partial response occurs after chemotherapy, 375 mg/m^2 every 8 wk for 12 doses.

Adults with nonprogressing, low-grade, CD20-positive, B-cell NHL after first-line CVP chemotherapy. Following completion of 6 to 8 cycles of CVP chemotherapy, 375 mg/m^2 once weekly for 4 doses at 6-month intervals to a maximum of 16 doses.

Adults with diffuse large B-cell NHL. 375 mg/m^2 on day 1 of each cycle of chemotherapy for up to 8 infusions.

I.V. INFUSION (RITUXAN)

Children age 6 months and older with previously untreated, advanced stage, CD20-positive diffuse large B-cell lymphoma, Burkitt lymphoma, or Burkitt-like lymphoma. 375 mg/m^2 for six infusions (two doses during each of the induction courses, COPDAM1 and COPDAM2, and one dose during each of the two consolidation courses of CYM/CYVE). Infusion initiated at a rate of 0.5 mg/kg/hr (maximum 50 mg/hr) and if no infusion toxicity, infusion rate increased by 0.5 mg/kg/hr every 30 min to a maximum of 400 mg/hr. For subsequent infusions in the absence of infusion toxicity, infused at 1 mg/kg/hr (maximum 50 mg/hr) and if no infusion toxicity develops, infusion rate increased by 1 mg/kg/hr every 30 min to a maximum of 400 mg/hr.

✳ *To treat chronic lymphocytic leukemia (CLL)*

I.V. INFUSION (RITUXAN, RUXIENCE, TRUXIMA)

Adults. 375 mg/m^2 on day prior to initiation of FC chemotherapy, then 500 mg/m^2 on day 1 of cycles 2–6 (every 28 days).

✳ *To treat granulomatosis with polyangiitis (Wegener's granulomatosis) and microscopic polyangiitis*

I.V. INFUSION (RITUXAN, RUXIENCE, TRUXIMA)

Adults. *Induction:* 375 mg/m^2 once a wk for 4 wk. *Maintenance:* Two 500-mg infusions

separated by 2 wk, followed by a 500-mg infusion every 6 months based on clinical evaluation.

I.V. INFUSION (RITUXAN)

Children age 2 years and older. *Induction:* 375 mg/m^2 once a wk for 4 wk. *Maintenance:* Two 250-mg/m^2 infusions separated by 2 wk, followed by a 250-mg/m^2 infusion every 6 months based on clinical evaluation.

✳ *To treat mature B-cell acute leukemia in children*

I.V. INFUSION (RITUXAN)

Children 6 months of age and older with previously untreated mature B-cell acute leukemia. *Induction:* 375 mg/m^2 once a wk for 4 wk. *Maintenance:* Two 250-mg/m^2 infusions separated by 2 wk, followed by a 250-mg/m^2 infusion every 6 months based on clinical evaluation.

±**DOSAGE ADJUSTMENT** Follow manufacturer guidelines for each indication and the additional drugs given concomitantly that may have to be adjusted with rituximab therapy.

Drug Administration

I.V.

- Premedicate patient with acetaminophen and an antihistamine prior to each infusion, as ordered, to prevent or lessen severity of an infusion reaction. If glucocorticoid therapy is part of patient's regimen, it should also be administered about 30 minutes prior to infusion, as ordered.
- Prepare infusion by withdrawing the necessary amount of drug and dilute to a final concentration of 1 mg/ml to 4 mg/ml in an infusion containing either 0.9% Sodium Chloride Injection or 5% Dextrose Injection. Gently invert bag to mix the solution. Do not mix or dilute with other drugs. Discard any unused portion left in vial.
- Diluted solutions may be stored refrigerated for 24 hours.
- For adults, unless otherwise specified in manufacturer guidelines, infuse first infusion at 50 mg/hr. If no infusion toxicity noted, infusion rate increased by 50-mg/hr increments every 30 minutes to a maximum of 400 mg/hr. For subsequent infusions, initiate infusion rate at 100 mg/hr, and if no infusion toxicity noted, rate increased by 100-mg/hr increments at 30-minute intervals to a maximum of 400 mg/hr.

- For children, unless otherwise specified in manufacturer guidelines, initiate infusion at a rate of 0.5 mg/kg/hr (maximum 50 mg/hr) and if no infusion toxicity, infusion rate increased by 0.5 mg/kg/hr every 30 min to a maximum of 400 mg/hr. For subsequent infusions in the absence of infusion toxicity, infused at 1 mg/kg/hr (maximum 50 mg/hr) and if no infusion toxicity develops, infusion rate increased by 1 mg/kg/hr every 30 min to a maximum of 400 mg/hr.
- Most infusion reactions occur within 30 to 120 minutes of beginning the first infusion. Patients at higher risk include patients with preexisting cardiac or pulmonary conditions, those who experienced prior cardiopulmonary adverse reactions, and those with high numbers of circulating malignant cells (25,000/mm³ or greater). Stop infusion or slow infusion rate for infusion-related reactions, some of which could be life-threatening, such as angioedema, bronchospasms, and hypotension. Know that reaction may resolve with slowing or interruption of the infusion and with supportive care (acetaminophen, diphenhydramine, and intravenous saline). Expect to resume infusion upon improvement of symptoms by continuing infusion at one-half the previous rate.
- Never administer drug as an I.V. bolus or give as an intravenous push.
- *Incompatibilities:* Other drugs; other solutions except for 0.9% Sodium Chloride Injection or 5% Dextrose Injection

Route	Onset	Peak	Duration
I.V.	7–56 days	Unknown	Unknown

Half-life: 14–62 days

⦀ Mechanism of Action

Targets the CD20 antigen expressed on the surface of pre-B and mature B lymphocytes. Upon binding to CD20, drug-mediated B-cell lysis occurs. B cells are also believed to play a role in the pathogenesis of rheumatoid arthritis and associated chronic synovitis. In rheumatoid arthritis, B cells may be acting at multiple sites in the autoimmune/inflammatory process, including through production of rheumatoid factor and other auto-antibodies, antigen presentation, T-cell activation, and/or proinflammatory cytokine production. Improvement of rheumatoid arthritis signs and symptoms may occur when B-cell lysis occurs.

⦀ Contraindications

Hypersensitivity to rituximab or its components

⦀ Interactions

DRUGS

immunosuppressants: Enhanced immunosuppressive effects
vaccines (live): Possibly increased risk of infection

⦀ Adverse Reactions

CNS: Anxiety, asthenia, chills, depression, dizziness, fatigue, fever, headache, insomnia, irritability, migraine, paresthesia, peripheral sensory neuropathy, **progressive multifocal leukoencephalopathy (PML), posterior reversible encephalopathy syndrome, reversible posterior leukoencephalopathy syndrome**
CV: Cardiogenic shock, fatal cardiac failure, hypertension, **hypotension,** increased LDH, **MI,** peripheral edema, systemic vasculitis, tachycardia, **ventricular fibrillation**
EENT: Conjunctivitis, epistaxis, optic neuritis, rhinitis, sinusitis, throat irritation, uveitis
ENDO: Hyperglycemia, hypophosphatemia, weight gain
GI: Abdominal pain, **bowel obstruction and perforation,** diarrhea, dyspepsia, elevated liver enzymes, nausea, vomiting
GU: UTI
HEME: Anemia, bone marrow hypoplasia, febrile neutropenia, hyperviscosity syndrome in Waldenstrom's macroglobulinemia, leukopenia, lymphopenia, neutropenia, prolonged hypogammaglobulinemia, prolonged pancytopenia, thrombocytopenia
MS: Arthralgia, back pain, muscle spasms, musculoskeletal pain, myalgia, polyarticular arthritis
RESP: Bronchospasm, dyspnea, **fatal bronchiolitis obliterans and interstitial lung disease,** increased cough, pleuritis, upper respiratory infections
SKIN: Alopecia, flushing, lichenoid or vesiculobullous dermatitis, night sweats, **paraneoplastic pemphigus (blistering of**

mucous membranes and skin), pruritus, pyoderma gangrenosum (large, painful sores), rash, skin papilloma, **Stevens–Johnson syndrome, toxic epidermal necrolysis,** urticaria

Other: Angioedema, antibody formation to rituximab, **disease progression of Kaposi's sarcoma,** generalized pain, herpes simplex or zoster, **HIV-associated lymphoma (fatal),** infections (bacterial, fungal, viral), infusion reactions (**angioedema, bronchospasm,** chills/rigors, dizziness, fever, headache, myalgia, nausea, pruritus, rash, urticaria, vomiting), lupus-like syndrome, serum sickness, **tumor lysis (acute renal failure, hyperkalemia, hyperphosphatemia, hyperuricemia, hypocalcemia),** vasculitis with rash

Childbearing Considerations

PREGNANCY

- Drug can cause fetal harm such as B-cell lymphocytopenia.
- Use with caution only if benefit to mother outweighs potential risk to fetus.
- If drug used during pregnancy, neonate should be observed for signs of infection.

LACTATION

- It is not known if drug is present in breast milk.
- Breastfeeding is not recommended during drug therapy and for 6 months following last dose.

REPRODUCTION

- Advise women of childbearing age to use effective contraception during drug treatment and for at least 12 months after last dose.

Nursing Considerations

- Screen all patients for HBV by measuring HbsAg and anti-HBc before initiating rituximab, as ordered, because HBV reactivation can occur and can result in severe liver dysfunction or even death. Patient will need to be monitored for up to 24 months after completion of rituximab therapy. Also obtain complete blood count (CBC), including platelets, prior to first dose. Once treatment is begun, obtain CBC with differential and platelet counts prior to each drug course in patients with lymphoid malignancies. During treatment with chemotherapy, obtain CBC with differential and platelet counts at weekly to monthly

intervals and more frequently in patients who develop cytopenias.

- Ensure that patient is up to date on immunizations before rituximab is begun because immunization with live-virus vaccines is not recommended before or during rituximab therapy. Nonlive vaccines should be administered at least 4 weeks before a course of rituximab is given.
- Be prepared to perform cardiac monitoring during and after all infusions of rituximab for patients who develop clinically significant arrhythmias or who have a history of angina or arrhythmia. This is because life-threatening cardiac adverse reactions, such as cardiogenic shock, MI, or ventricular fibrillation, may occur with rituximab therapy.

! WARNING Monitor patient being treated for non-Hodgkin's lymphoma for tumor lysis syndrome (acute renal failure, hyperkalemia, hyperphosphatemia, and hypocalcemia), which can sometimes be fatal and usually occurs within 12 to 24 hours after the first infusion. Patients at higher risk include patients with high number of circulating malignant cells (25,000/mm^3 or greater) or high tumor burden. If present, expect to provide aggressive intravenous hydration and antihyperuricemic therapy in patients at high risk, as ordered. Expect electrolyte abnormalities to be corrected and renal function and fluid balance monitored, as ordered. Also, provide supportive care that may include dialysis, as ordered.

- Know that prophylaxis treatment for *Pneumocystis jirovecii* pneumonia and herpes virus infections may be given during treatment with rituximab and in some cases up to 6 or 12 months following last infusion.
- Obtain CBC with differential and platelet counts at 2- to 4-month intervals for patients with granulomatosis with polyangiitis, microscopic polyangiitis, and rheumatoid arthritis. Continue to monitor all patients throughout rituximab therapy for cytopenias and after final dose and until resolution, if present.

! WARNING Monitor patient for severe mucocutaneous reactions. If present, notify prescriber and expect drug to be discontinued.

Q
R
S

! **WARNING** Monitor patient for new-onset neurological manifestations that may be suggestive of progressive multifocal leukoencephalopathy (PML), which can occur with rituximab therapy. Know that most cases are diagnosed within 12 months of the last infusion of drug. If suspected, expect an MRI and lumbar puncture to be obtained. If confirmed, expect rituximab to be discontinued.

- Institute infection control measures and monitor patient for signs and symptoms of infection, as serious infections, including fatal bacterial, fungal, and new or reactivated viral infections, can occur. If infection is serious, expect rituximab to be discontinued and appropriate anti-infective therapy instituted.
- Monitor patient's serum creatinine level and patient for oliguria if being treated for NHL with rituximab because renal toxicity may occur. Renal toxicity may occur with tumor lysis syndrome but also in patients receiving cisplatin. Be aware that concomitant administration of cisplatin and rituximab is not an approved treatment regimen. In addition, patient treated for NHL is also at risk for bowel obstruction and perforation. If patient develops abdominal pain or repeated vomiting, notify prescriber at once.

PATIENT TEACHING

! **WARNING** Instruct patient on the signs and symptoms of an infusion reaction. Urge patient to report immediately if present.

- Tell patient or parents/caregivers to monitor the skin for abnormal effects. If blisters, painful sores, or ulcers appear in the mouth, or if peeling skin, pustules, or rash develops, tell patient to contact prescriber immediately.
- Review other signs and symptoms that should be reported to prescriber, including prolonged, severe, or unusual reactions that may warrant immediate attention, such as those that may occur with the cardiovascular system, hepatitis B virus reaction, progressive multifocal leukoencephalopathy, and tumor lysis syndrome.

- Instruct patient or parents/caregivers on infection control measures, including avoiding people who are ill.

! **WARNING** Advise women of childbearing age to use effective contraception while receiving rituximab and for 12 months after last dose.

- Instruct women not to breastfeed during treatment with rituximab and for at least 6 months after last dose.

rivaroxaban
Xarelto

Class and Category
Pharmacologic class: Factor Xa inhibitor
Therapeutic class: Anticoagulant

Indications and Dosages
✴ *To reduce the risk of stroke and systemic embolism in patients with nonvalvular atrial fibrillation*

TABLETS

Adults with creatinine clearance greater than 50 ml/min. 20 mg once daily with evening meal.
Adults with creatinine clearance between 15 and 50 ml/min. 15 mg once daily with evening meal.

✴ *To prevent deep vein thrombosis, which may lead to pulmonary embolism following knee or hip replacement surgery*

TABLETS

Adults with creatinine clearance of 15 ml/min or greater. 10 mg once daily begun 6 to 10 hr after surgery once hemostasis has been established and given for 12 days after knee replacement surgery and given 35 days after hip replacement surgery.

✴ *To treat deep vein thrombosis or pulmonary embolism*

TABLETS

Adults with creatinine clearance of 15 ml/min or greater. 15 mg twice daily for 21 days, followed by 20 mg once daily.

✴ *To reduce risk of recurrence of deep vein thrombosis or pulmonary embolism in patients at continued risk*

TABLETS

Adults with a creatinine clearance of 15 ml/min or greater. 10 mg once daily after at least 6 months of standard anticoagulant therapy.

* *To prevent venous thromboembolism in acutely ill medical patients at risk for thromboembolic complications not at high risk of bleeding*

TABLETS

Adults with a creatinine clearance of 15 mg/ml or greater. 10 mg once daily, for a total of 31 to 39 days.

* *To reduce risk of major cardiovascular events in patients with chronic coronary artery disease or peripheral artery disease*

TABLETS

Adults regardless of creatinine clearance level. 2.5 mg twice daily with 75 or 100 mg aspirin once daily.

* *To reduce risk of major thrombotic vascular events in patients with peripheral artery disease (PAD), including patients after lower extremity revascularization due to symptomatic PAD*

TABLETS

Adults regardless of creatinine clearance level. 2.5 mg twice daily with 75 or 100 mg aspirin once daily. For lower extremity revascularization, therapy started once hemostasis has been established.

* *To treat venous thromboembolism and reduce risk of recurrent venous thromboembolism in pediatric patients*

ORAL SUSPENSION, TABLETS

Children less than 18 years weighing 50 kg (110 lb) or greater. 20 mg once daily with food about 24 hr apart following at least 5 days of parenteral anticoagulation therapy.

Children less than 18 years weighing between 30 kg (66 lb) and 49.9 kg (109.78 lb). 15 mg once daily with food about 24 hr apart following at least 5 days of parenteral anticoagulation therapy.

ORAL SUSPENSION

Children less than 18 years of age weighing 12 kg (26.4 lb) to 29.9 kg (65.78 lb). 5 mg twice daily about 12 hr apart with food following at least 5 days of parenteral anticoagulation therapy. *Maximum: 10 mg daily.*

Children less than 18 years of age weighing 10 kg (22 lb) to 11.9 kg (26.18 lb). 3 mg three times daily about 8 hr apart with food following at least 5 days of parenteral

anticoagulation therapy. *Maximum: 9 mg daily.*

Children less than 18 years of age weighing 9 kg (19.8 lb) to 9.9 kg (21.78 lb). 2.8 mg three times daily about 8 hr apart with food following at least 5 days of parenteral anticoagulation therapy. *Maximum: 8.4 mg daily.*

Children weighing 8 kg (17.6 lb) to 8.9 kg (19.58 lb). 2.4 mg three times daily about 8 hr apart with food following at least 5 days of parenteral anticoagulation therapy. *Maximum: 7.2 mg daily.*

Infants from birth who were at least 37 weeks gestation at birth and have had at least 10 days of oral feeding and children weighing 7 kg (15.4 lb) to 7.9 kg (17.38 lb). 1.8 mg three times daily about 8 hr apart with feeding following at least 5 days of parenteral anticoagulation therapy. *Maximum: 5.4 mg daily.*

Infants from birth who were at least 37 weeks gestation at birth and have had at least 10 days of oral feeding and children weighing 5 kg (11 lb) to 6.9 kg (15.18 lb). 1.6 mg three times daily about 8 hr apart with feeding following at least 5 days of parenteral anticoagulation therapy. *Maximum: 4.8 mg daily.*

Infants from birth who were at least 37 weeks gestation at birth, have had at least 10 days of oral feeding, and weigh 4 kg (8.8 lb) to 4.9 kg (10.78 lb). 1.4 mg three times daily about 8 hr apart with feeding following at least 5 days of parenteral anticoagulation therapy. *Maximum: 4.2 mg daily.*

Infants from birth who were at least 37 weeks gestation at birth, have had at least 10 days of oral feeding, and weigh 3 kg (6.6 lb) to 3.9 kg (8.58 lb). 0.9 mg three times daily about 8 hr apart with feeding following at least 5 days of parenteral anticoagulation therapy. *Maximum: 2.7 mg daily.*

Infants from birth who were at least 37 weeks gestation at birth, have had at least 10 days of oral feeding, and weigh 2.6 kg (5.72 lb) to 2.9 g (6.38 lb). 0.8 mg three times daily about 8 hr apart with feeding following at least 5 days of parenteral anticoagulation therapy. *Maximum: 2.4 mg daily.*

±**DOSAGE ADJUSTMENT** Therapy continued for at least 3 months in children with thrombosis but may be extended up to 12 months except for children less than

Q
R
S

2 years old with catheter-related thrombosis. In these children, therapy continued for at least 1 month but may be extended up to 3 months, if needed. For patients 1 year of age and older with mild renal impairment (creatinine 50 to 80 ml/min), no dosage adjustment necessary. Drug should not be used if renal impairment is more severe. For patient less than 1 year, drug should be avoided in patients with serum creatinine results above 97.5 percentile (see manufacturer guidelines for chart).

＊ *To prevent thromboembolism in children with congenital heart disease after the Fontan procedure*

ORAL SUSPENSION, TABLETS

Children age 2 and older weighing 50 kg (110 lb) or more. 10 mg once daily about 24 hr apart. *Maximum:* 10 mg daily.

ORAL SUSPENSION

Children age 2 and older weighing 30 kg (66 lb) to 49.9 kg (109.78 lb). 7.5 mg once daily about 24 hr apart. *Maximum:* 7.5 mg daily.

Children age 2 and older weighing 20 kg (44 lb) to 29.9 kg (65.78 lb). 2.5 mg two times daily about 12 hr apart. *Maximum:* 5 mg.

Children age 2 and older weighing 12 kg (26.4 lb) to 19.9 kg (43.78 lb). 2 mg twice daily about 12 hr apart. *Maximum:* 4 mg.

Children age 2 and older weighing 10 kg (22 lb) and 11.9 kg (26.18 lb). 1.7 mg twice daily about 12 hr apart. *Maximum:* 3.4 mg daily.

Children age 2 and older weighing 8 kg (17.6 lb) to 9.9 kg (21.78 lb). 1.6 mg twice daily about 12 hr apart. *Maximum:* 3.2 mg daily.

Children age 2 and older weighing 7 kg (15.4 lb) to 7.9 kg (17.38 lb). 1.1 mg twice daily about 12 hr apart. *Maximum:* 2.2 mg daily.

Drug Administration

P.O.

- Follow manufacturer guidelines when patient is being switched to and from rivaroxaban and when a dose is missed.
- Be aware that oral suspension can be used with PVC, polyurethane, or silicone NG tubing.

Adults

- Give 15- or 20-mg tablets with food; 2.5- or 10-mg tablets need not be taken with food.

- For nonvalvular atrial fibrillation, give drug with the evening meal.
- For adults unable to swallow tablets, crush tablets and mix with applesauce immediately prior to administration and if dose is 15 mg or 20 mg then follow with food.
- Administering drug via a nasogastric tube or gastric feeding tube requires tablets to be crushed and suspended in 50 ml of water. Following administration, flush tube with water and give enteral feeding immediately if dose is 15 mg or 20 mg.
- Drug is stable in water or in applesauce for up to 4 hours.

Children

- For treatment of venous thromboembolism or reduction of recurrent venous thromboembolism, all doses should be given with food or a feeding to enhance absorption. Food or feedings are not necessary for thromboprophylaxis in children with congenital heart disease after the Fontan procedure.
- Measure child's weight routinely, especially children weighing less than 12 kg, because dosage is based upon weight.
- Oral suspension is prepared by a pharmacist and can be stored at room temperature. Use the calibrated syringe provided with drug to measure dosage.
- If infant or child vomits or spits up the dose within 30 minutes after administration, give a new dose. If it is more than 30 minutes, do not administer another dose and give the next dose as scheduled.
- Tablets must be swallowed whole and not chewed, crushed, or split.
- Administering drug via a nasogastric tube or gastric feeding tube requires tablets to be crushed and suspended in 50 ml of water or oral suspension to be used. After administration, flush the tube with water. Also following administration, enteral feeding should be given immediately if child is being treated for venous thromboembolism or reduction of recurrent venous thromboembolism.

Route	Onset	Peak	Duration
P.O.	Unknown	2–4 hr	Unknown

Half-life: 5–9 hr

Mechanism of Action

Selectively blocks the active site of factor Xa, which plays a central role in the cascade of blood coagulation. Without the action of factor Xa, blood clotting is impaired.

Contraindications

Active pathological bleeding, hypersensitivity to rivaroxaban or its components

Interactions

DRUGS

anticoagulants, aspirin, clopidogrel, dual antiplatelet therapy, fibrinolytic therapy, heparin, NSAIDs, other antithrombotic agents or platelet aggregation inhibitors, selective serotonin reuptake inhibitors, serotonin–norepinephrine reuptake inhibitors, warfarin: Possibly increased bleeding risk
combined strong CYP3A and P-glycoprotein (P-gp) inducers such as carbamazepine, phenytoin, rifampin, St. John's wort: Decreased effectiveness of rivaroxaban
combined CYP3A4 and P-gp inhibitors such as conivaptan, diltiazem, dronedarone, erythromycin, fluconazole, indinavir/ritonavir, itraconazole, ketoconazole, lopinavir/ritonavir, ritonavir, verapamil: Increased rivaroxaban exposure resulting in increased bleeding risk

Adverse Reactions

CNS: Anxiety, **cerebral hemorrhage**, depression, dizziness, epidural hematoma, fatigue, hemiparesis, insomnia, **subdural hematoma**, syncope
GI: Abdominal pain, cholestasis, **cytolytic hepatitis, GI bleeding**, jaundice, **retroperitoneal hemorrhage**
HEME: Agranulocytosis, excessive bleeding, hemorrhage, thrombocytopenia
MS: Back or extremity pain, muscle spasm
RESP: Pulmonary hemorrhage with or without bronchiectasis
SKIN: Pruritus, **Stevens–Johnson syndrome**
Other: Anaphylactic shock, anaphylaxis, angioedema, drug reaction with eosinophilia and systemic symptoms (DRESS)

Childbearing Considerations

PREGNANCY

- Drug has the potential to cause fetal harm as a result of bleeding at any site in the fetus and/or neonate from drug use during pregnancy.

- Use with caution only if benefit to mother outweighs potential risk to fetus.

LABOR & DELIVERY

- Drug may increase the risk of bleeding for both mother and fetus/neonate during labor and delivery.

LACTATION

- Drug is present in breast milk.
- Patient should check with prescriber before breastfeeding.

REPRODUCTION

- Women of childbearing age should discuss pregnancy planning with prescriber because of potential for significant uterine bleeding that may require surgery to stop bleeding.

Nursing Considerations

- Know that rivaroxaban should not be given to patients with moderate or severe hepatic impairment, to patients with any hepatic disease associated with coagulopathy, and to patients with a creatinine clearance that is less than 15 ml/min. Monitor patient's hepatic and renal function, as ordered, throughout rivaroxaban therapy.
- Know that rivaroxaban should not be given to acutely ill medical patients at high risk of bleeding to prevent a venous thrombosis event. High-srisk conditions include active cancer; gastroduodenal ulcer in the three months prior to treatment; or a history of bronchiectasis, bleeding in the three months prior to treatment, dual antiplatelet therapy, or pulmonary cavitation or hemorrhage.
- Do not expect to give rivaroxaban to patients with triple-positive antiphospholipid syndrome, because of increased rates of recurrent thrombotic events.
- Be aware that rivaroxaban should not be given to patients with prosthetic heart valves or as an alternative to unfractionated heparin in patients with pulmonary embolism who are hemodynamically unstable or who may receive pulmonary embolectomy or thrombolysis.
- Be aware that rivaroxaban should be used cautiously during pregnancy because drug has the potential to cross the placenta, causing bleeding at any site in the fetus and/or neonate.

Q
R
S

> **! WARNING** Monitor patient closely for signs and symptoms of a hypersensitivity reaction because severe hypersensitivity reactions have occurred following rivaroxaban therapy.

- Be aware that manufacturer guidelines should be followed when patient is switching from or to other anticoagulants. For example, when patient is switching from warfarin to rivaroxaban therapy, expect warfarin to be discontinued and rivaroxaban started when the international normalized ratio (INR) is below 3. For patients currently receiving an anticoagulant other than warfarin, such as low-molecular-weight heparin or nonwarfarin oral anticoagulant, expect to start rivaroxaban therapy within 2 hours of the next scheduled evening administration of the drug, and plan to omit administration of the other anticoagulant, as ordered. For unfractionated heparin being administered by continuous infusion, expect to stop the infusion and start rivaroxaban therapy at the same time. For patients currently taking rivaroxaban and transitioning to an anticoagulant with rapid onset, expect rivaroxaban to be discontinued and the first dose of the other anticoagulant given at the time the next rivaroxaban would have been given.
- Expect rivaroxaban to be discontinued if acute renal failure occurs.

> **! WARNING** Monitor patient closely for bleeding, as rivaroxaban therapy may cause life-threatening bleeding. Expect to administer the antidote available to reverse the anti-factor Xa activity of rivaroxaban if bleeding is significant. Be aware that bleeding risks are higher in elderly patients.

- Expect rivaroxaban to be discontinued 24 hours before an invasive procedure or surgery, if possible and restarted after adequate hemostasis has been established after the invasive surgery or procedure.
- Know that if patient has an epidural catheter inserted, it should not be removed any earlier than 18 hours for younger patients (less than 45 years) and 26 hours for older patients (60 years and over) after the last rivaroxaban dose was administered. Obtain specific guidelines for catheter removal from prescriber for patients between 45 and 60 years of age. The next rivaroxaban dose should not be administered any earlier than 6 hours after removal of the catheter because an epidural or spinal hematoma can occur and can result in long-term or permanent paralysis. If traumatic puncture occurs, know that rivaroxaban should be withheld for 24 hours.
- Be aware that if rivaroxaban is discontinued and adequate alternative anticoagulation is not present, the risk for thrombosis increases. Monitor patient closely.

PATIENT TEACHING

- Emphasize the importance of taking rivaroxaban exactly as prescribed.
- Instruct adults taking 15- or 20-mg tablets or parents/caregivers of children being treated for venous thromboembolism or reduction of the risk of recurrent venous thromboembolism to take tablets with food (or feeding); 2.5- or 10-mg tablets for children being treated for thromboprophylaxis after the Fontan procedure need not be taken with food. For adults unable to swallow tablets, tell patient to crush tablets and mix with applesauce immediately prior to taking and then follow with food. Alert patient and parents/caregiver that oral suspension is available.
- Tell patient not to stop taking rivaroxaban without first consulting prescriber.
- Instruct patient with atrial fibrillation to take drug with the evening meal.
- Advise patient to report any unusual bleeding or bruising to prescriber. Inform patient that it may take longer for him to stop bleeding and to take bleeding precautions, such as avoiding the use of a razor and using a soft-bristle toothbrush.
- Tell patient to alert all prescribers to use of rivaroxaban therapy before any invasive procedure, including dental work, is scheduled.
- Instruct patient who has had spinal anesthesia or puncture to watch for back pain, muscle weakness, numbness (especially in the lower limbs), stool or urine incontinence, or tingling. If present, stress importance of notifying prescriber immediately.
- Caution patient not to take any prescription or nonprescription medication, including

over-the-counter and herbal medicines, without first consulting with prescriber.

- Advise female patient to notify prescriber immediately if pregnancy is suspected or known.
- Alert women of childbearing age to discuss pregnancy planning because of the potential risk of significant bleeding with the drug that may require gynecological surgical intervention.

rivastigmine
Exelon Patch

rivastigmine tartrate
Exelon

Class and Category
Pharmacologic class: Cholinesterase inhibitor
Therapeutic class: Antidementia

Indications and Dosages
❋ *To treat mild-to-moderate Alzheimer's-type dementia*

CAPSULES, ORAL SOLUTION
Adults. *Initial:* 1.5 mg twice daily. Dosage increased after 2 wk to 3 mg twice daily followed by an increase to 4.5 mg twice daily after another 2 weeks and then increased to 6 mg twice daily after another 2 wk, as needed. *Maximum:* 6 mg twice daily.

❋ *To treat mild, moderate, and severe Alzheimer's disease*

TRANSDERMAL
Adults. *Initial:* 4.6 mg/24 hr. After 4 wk, increased to 9.5 mg/24 hr. When therapeutic effect begins to decrease and with at least 4 wk from last dosage increase, dosage increased to 13.3 mg/24 hr. *Maximum:* 13.3 mg/24 hr.

❋ *To treat mild-to-moderate dementia in Parkinson's disease*

CAPSULES, ORAL SOLUTION
Adults. *Initial:* 1.5 mg twice daily. Dosage increased after 4 wk to 3 mg twice daily followed by an increase to 4.5 mg twice daily after another 4 weeks and then increased to 6 mg twice daily after another 4 wk, as needed. *Maximum:* 6 mg twice daily.

TRANSDERMAL
Adults. *Initial:* 4.6 mg/24 hr. After 4 wk, increased to 9.5 mg/24 hr. When therapeutic effect begins to decrease, dosage increased to 13.3 mg/24 hr. *Maximum:* 13.3 mg/24 hr.

❋ *To convert patient from oral to transdermal rivastigmine therapy*

TRANSDERMAL
Adults. If total oral dosage was less than 6 mg daily, 4.6 mg/24 hr used, with first transdermal patch applied the day after the last oral dose. If total oral dosage was 6 to 12 mg daily, 9.5 mg/24 hr used, with first transdermal patch applied the day after the last oral dose.

±**DOSAGE ADJUSTMENT** If patient develops adverse effects (such as nausea or vomiting), oral treatment should be stopped for several doses, as prescribed and restarted at the same or next lower dose level if 3 days or less have passed; if more than 3 days has passed, treatment started with initial dose and retitrated. For patients with mild-to-moderate hepatic impairment or moderate to severe renal impairment, oral dosage may have to be reduced. For patient with mild-to-moderate hepatic impairment, 4.6 mg/24 hr patch used for both initial and maintenance dose. For patients with low body weight of less than 50 kg (110 lb) and experiencing excessive nausea and vomiting, maintenance dose of patch reduced to 4.6 mg/24 hr or oral dosage reduced.

Drug Administration
P.O.
- Measure oral solution with the calibrated syringe provided. Administer dose directly from the syringe or mix into a small glass of cold fruit juice, soda, or water; stir; and then administer.
- Capsules should be swallowed whole and not chewed, crushed, or opened.
- Administer with morning and evening meals.
- Capsules and oral solution are interchangeable at equal doses.

TRANSDERMAL
- Do not use patch if pouch seal is broken or the patch is cut, damaged, or changed in any way.
- Apply patch to clean, dry, hairless, intact skin in a location, such as the back, that

won't be rubbed by tight clothing and won't be affected by cream, lotion, or powder. However, if back is not possible, upper arm or chest may be used. Do not apply to skin that is cut, irritated, or red or skin where cream, lotion, or powder has recently been applied.

- Press firmly into place for about 30 seconds until the edges are adhered to skin.
- Remove the old patch before applying a new one and use a new application site daily. Do not reuse the same site for 14 days.
- If patch falls off or a dose is missed, apply a new patch immediately, and then replace this patch the following day at the usual application time.
- Wash hands with soap and water after removing patch. Place used patches in previously saved pouch and discard.

Route	Onset	Peak	Duration
P.O.	Unknown	1 hr	8–10 hr
Transdermal	Unknown	8–16 hr	24 hr

Half-life: 1.5–3 hr

Mechanism of Action

May slow the decline of cognitive function by increasing acetylcholine concentration at cholinergic transmission sites. This action prolongs and exaggerates the effects of acetylcholine that are otherwise blocked by toxic levels of anticholinergics. Cognitive decline is partially related to cholinergic deficits along neuronal pathways projecting from the basal forebrain to the cerebral cortex and hippocampus that are involved in attention, cognition, learning, and memory.

Contraindications

History of application-site reactions suggestive of allergic contact dermatitis (for patch form); hypersensitivity to carbamate derivatives, rivastigmine, or their components

Interactions

DRUGS

anticholinergics: Possibly decreased effectiveness of anticholinergics
beta-blockers: Possible additive bradycardic effects resulting in syncope
metoclopramide: Increased risk of additive extrapyramidal adverse reactions

other cholinomimetic drugs: Possibly increased cholinergic effects

Adverse Reactions

CNS: Aggression, anxiety, asthenia, confusion, depression, dizziness, extrapyramidal movements, fatigue, fever, hallucinations, headache, insomnia, malaise, nightmares, **seizures**, somnolence, tremor, worsening of parkinsonism
CV: Hypertension, tachycardia
EENT: Rhinitis
GI: Abdominal pain, anorexia, constipation, diarrhea, duodenal ulcers, elevated liver enzymes, flatulence, **hepatitis**, indigestion, nausea, vomiting
GU: UTI
SKIN: Allergic or disseminated dermatitis, increased sweating, reaction at patch application site (papule or vesicle formation, pruritus, redness, swelling), **Stevens–Johnson syndrome**, urticaria
Other: Dehydration, flu-like symptoms, weight loss

Childbearing Considerations

PREGNANCY

- It is not known if drug can cause fetal harm.
- Use with caution only if benefit to mother outweighs potential risk to fetus.

LACTATION

- It is not known if drug is present in breast milk.
- Patient should check with prescriber before breastfeeding.

Nursing Considerations

! WARNING Be aware that rivastigmine should be started at lowest recommended dosage and adjusted to effective maintenance dosage because initial therapy at high dosage can cause serious adverse GI reactions, including anorexia, nausea, and weight loss. Also, a higher than recommended starting dosage may cause severe vomiting and possibly esophageal rupture. If treatment is interrupted for longer than several days, expect to restart at lowest recommended dosage.

- Be aware that drug shouldn't be stopped abruptly because doing so may increase behavioral disturbances and precipitate a further decline in cognitive function.

- Monitor respiratory status of patients with pulmonary disease, including asthma, chronic bronchitis, and emphysema, because rivastigmine has a weak affinity for peripheral cholinesterase, which may increase bronchoconstriction and bronchial secretions.
- Monitor patient for adequate urine output because cholinomimetics, such as rivastigmine, may induce or exacerbate bladder or urinary tract obstruction.
- Monitor patients with Parkinson's disease for exaggerated parkinsonian symptoms, which may result from drug's increased cholinergic effects on CNS.

! **WARNING** Monitor patient closely for hypersensitivity skin reactions regardless of route of administration. If suspected, notify prescriber, and expect drug to be discontinued.

PATIENT TEACHING

- Explain to patient and family that rivastigmine can't cure Alzheimer's or Parkinson's disease but may slow the progressive deterioration of memory and improve patient's ability to perform activities of daily living.
- Teach patient and family how to administer oral solution, if prescribed, emphasizing need to use the oral dosing syringe provided. Explain that dose may be swallowed directly from the syringe or mixed into a small glass of cold fruit juice, soda, or water; stirred; and then drunk.
- Tell patient that capsules must be swallowed whole and not chewed, crushed, or opened.
- Explain that oral drug should be taken at morning and evening meals to reduce adverse GI effects.
- Instruct patient or caregiver to apply transdermal patch to clean, dry, hairless, intact skin in a location, such as the back, that won't be rubbed by tight clothing and won't be affected by cream, lotion, or powder. Tell patient to remove the old patch before applying a new one and to use a new application site daily. Caution against using the same site within 14 days.
- Tell patient applying transdermal patch to press patch firmly against skin for at least 30 seconds until the edges stick well. Reassure patient that patch may be worn while bathing or swimming.
- Instruct a family member to supervise patient's use of rivastigmine.
- Urge caregiver to contact prescriber and to withhold drug if patient stops taking it for more than several days.

! **WARNING** Emphasize importance of inspecting skin for signs of an allergic reaction, such as presence of hives, itching, rash, or redness. If present, instruct patient or family to notify prescriber, as drug will have to be discontinued.

rizatriptan benzoate
Maxalt, Maxalt-MLT

☰ Class and Category
Pharmacologic class: Selective serotonin receptor agonist
Therapeutic class: Antimigraine

☰ Indications and Dosages
✳ *To relieve acute migraine headache*

DISINTEGRATING TABLETS, TABLETS

Adults. 5 or 10 mg when migraine headache starts; repeated 2 hr later, as needed. Additional doses spaced at least 2 hr apart, if needed. *Maximum:* 30 mg daily and treating more than 4 headaches in a 30-day period.
Children age 6 to 17 years weighing 40 kg (88 lb) or more. 10 mg as a single dose when migraine headache starts.
Children age 6 to 17 years weighing less than 40 kg (88 lb). 5 mg as a single dose when migraine headache starts.

±**DOSAGE ADJUSTMENT** For adults taking propranolol, initial dosage should not exceed 5 mg, and maximum dosage limited to three 5-mg doses in any 24-hour period. For pediatric patients weighing 40 kg (88 lb) or more taking propranolol, dosage reduced to 5 mg as a single dose. For pediatric patients weighing less than 40 kg (88 lb) taking propranolol, rizatriptan should not be used.

☰ Drug Administration
P.O.
- Remove disintegrating tablets from blister pack with dry, gloved hands just before administering by peeling foil back from blister. Do not force tablet through foil.

- Place disintegrating tablet on patient's tongue and allow it to dissolve and be swallowed with saliva. Liquids are not needed.
- Immediate-release tablets should be swallowed whole and administered with a liquid.

Route	Onset	Peak	Duration
P.O.	0.5–2 hr	1–1.5 hr	Unknown
P.O./MLT	0.5–2 hr	1.6–2.5 hr	Unknown

Half-life: 2–3 hr

Mechanism of Action

Binds to selective 5-hydroxytryptamine receptor sites on cerebral blood vessels, causing vessels to constrict. This may decrease the characteristic pulsing sensation and thus relieve the pain of migraine headaches. Rizatriptan may also relieve pain by inhibiting the release of proinflammatory neuropeptides and reducing transmission of trigeminal nerve impulses from sensory nerve endings during a migraine attack.

Contraindications

Basilar or hemiplegic migraine, coronary artery vasospasm including Prinzmetal angina, history of stroke or transient ischemic attack, hypersensitivity to rizatriptan or its components, ischemic bowel disease, ischemic coronary artery disease or other significant underlying cardiovascular disease, uncontrolled hypertension, use within 14 days of MAO inhibitor therapy, use within 24 hours of ergotamine-containing or ergot-type drugs or other serotonin receptor agonists

Interactions

DRUGS

ergot-containing drugs: Prolonged vasospastic reactions
MAO inhibitors, propranolol: Increased blood rizatriptan level
selective serotonin reuptake inhibitors, serotonin–norepinephrine reuptake inhibitors, other triptans: Increased risk of serotonin syndrome
serotonin receptor agonists: Additive vasospastic effects

Adverse Reactions

CNS: Altered temperature sensation, anxiety, asthenia, ataxia, chills, confusion, depression, disorientation, dizziness, dream disturbances, drowsiness, euphoria, fatigue, hangover, headache, hypoesthesia, insomnia, mental impairment, nervousness, paresthesia, somnolence, tremor, vertigo
CV: Bradycardia, chest pain, hot flashes, hypertension, palpitations, tachycardia
EENT: Blurred vision; burning eyes; dry eyes, mouth, and throat; earache; eye irritation; lacrimation; nasal congestion and irritation or pain; pharyngeal edema; pharyngitis; tinnitus; tongue swelling
GI: Abdominal distention, constipation, diarrhea, dysphagia, flatulence, heartburn, indigestion, nausea, thirst, vomiting
GU: Menstrual irregularities, polyuria, urinary frequency
MS: Arthralgia; dysarthria; muscle spasms, stiffness, or weakness; myalgia
RESP: Dyspnea, upper respiratory tract infection, wheezing
SKIN: Diaphoresis, flushing, pruritus, rash, urticaria
Other: Angioedema, dehydration

Childbearing Considerations

PREGNANCY

- Pregnancy exposure registry: 1-800-986-8999 or http://www.merckpregnancyregistries.com/maxalt.html.
- It is not known if drug can cause fetal harm.
- Use with caution only if benefit to mother outweighs potential risk to fetus.
- Women with migraines are at increased risk of experiencing pre-eclampsia and gestational hypertension.

LACTATION

- It is not known if drug is present in breast milk.
- Patient should check with prescriber before breastfeeding.

Nursing Considerations

- Use rizatriptan cautiously in patients with hepatic or renal dysfunction because of impaired drug excretion or metabolism. Monitor patient's BUN and serum creatinine levels and liver enzymes, as appropriate.
- Also use cautiously in patients with peripheral vascular disease because drug may cause vasospastic reactions, leading to colonic and vascular ischemia with abdominal pain and bloody diarrhea. Assess bowel sounds and peripheral circulation frequently during therapy.
- Assess patient's cardiovascular status and institute continuous ECG monitoring,

as ordered, immediately after giving rizatriptan in patients with cardiovascular risk factors, because of possible asymptomatic cardiac ischemia.
- Monitor blood pressure regularly in patients with hypertension because rizatriptan may increase blood pressure.

! **WARNING** Monitor patient closely for serotonin syndrome if she is taking rizatriptan along with a selective serotonin reuptake inhibitor or serotonin–norepinephrine reuptake inhibitor. Notify prescriber immediately if the patient exhibits agitation, coma, diarrhea, hallucinations, hyperreflexia, hyperthermia, incoordination, labile blood pressure, nausea, tachycardia, or vomiting, as serotonin syndrome can be life-threatening. Provide supportive care.

PATIENT TEACHING
- Instruct patient taking rizatriptan-disintegrating tablets to remove tablet from blister pack with dry hands by peeling back foil and just before taking tablet. Tell patient to place tablet on tongue and allow it to dissolve and be swallowed with saliva. Tell patient to swallow immediate-release tablets whole and take with a liquid.
- Advise phenylketonuric patient not to use disintegrating tablet form because it contains phenylalanine.
- Instruct patient to seek emergency care immediately if cardiac symptoms, such as chest pain, occur after administration.
- Caution patient about possible adverse CNS reactions, and advise her to avoid potentially hazardous activities until drug's CNS effects are known.
- Urge patient to inform all prescribers of rizatriptan therapy because serious drug interactions may occur.

roflumilast
Daliresp

Class and Category
Pharmacologic class: Selective phosphodiesterase 4 inhibitor
Therapeutic class: Antipulmonic obstructive agent

Indications and Dosages
✽ *To reduce the risk of COPD exacerbations in patients with severe COPD associated with chronic bronchitis and a history of exacerbations*

TABLETS
Adults. *Initial:* 250 mcg once daily for 4 wk, then increased to maintenance dose of 500 mcg daily.

Drug Administration
P.O.
- Administer at same time daily.

Route	Onset	Peak	Duration
P.O.	Unknown	0.5–2 hr	Unknown
Half-life: 17–30 hr			

Mechanism of Action
Increases intracellular cyclic AMP in lung cells by inhibiting a major cyclic AMP-metabolizing enzyme in lung tissue to improve pulmonary function

Contraindications
Hypersensitivity to roflumilast or its components, moderate to severe liver impairment

Interactions
DRUGS
CYP450 inducers such as carbamazepine, phenobarbital, phenytoin, rifampicin: Decreased effectiveness of roflumilast
CYP450 inhibitors or dual inhibitors (both CYP1A2 and CYP3A4), such as cimetidine, enoxacin, erythromycin, fluvoxamine, ketoconazole; oral contraceptives containing gestodene and ethinyl estradiol: Increased roflumilast exposure with increased risk of adverse effects

Adverse Reactions
CNS: Anxiety, depression, dizziness, headache, insomnia, **suicidal ideation**, tremor
CV: **Atrial fibrillation**
EENT: Rhinitis, sinusitis
ENDO: Gynecomastia
GI: Abdominal pain, **acute pancreatitis**, anorexia, diarrhea, dyspepsia, gastritis, nausea, vomiting
GU: **Acute renal failure**, UTI
MS: Back pain, muscle spasms
SKIN: Rash, urticaria

Q
R
S

Other: Angioedema, flu-like symptoms, weight loss

Childbearing Considerations

PREGNANCY
- It is not known if drug can cause fetal harm.
- Use with caution only if benefit to mother outweighs potential risk to fetus.

LABOR & DELIVERY
- Drug should not be used during labor and delivery, as animal studies showed drug disrupts the labor and delivery process.

LACTATION
- It is not known if drug is present in breast milk.
- Breastfeeding is not recommended during drug therapy.

Nursing Considerations
- Monitor effectiveness of roflumilast to reduce COPD exacerbations.

! **WARNING** Be aware that drug is not to be used for relief of acute bronchospasm.

- Watch patient closely for suicidal tendencies because roflumilast has been associated with an increase in psychiatric adverse reactions, such as depression and insomnia, as well as suicidal ideation.
- Monitor patient's weight and notify prescriber if significant weight loss occurs.

PATIENT TEACHING
- Tell family or caregiver to monitor patient for suicidal tendencies because drug may worsen depression during roflumilast therapy and increase suicidal thinking.

! **WARNING** Warn patient that roflumilast is not a bronchodilator and should not be used to relieve acute bronchospasm.

- Inform mothers wishing to breastfeed to notify prescriber because drug will have to be discontinued.

rolapitant hydrochloride
Varubi

Class and Category
Pharmacologic class: Substance P and neurokinin-1 receptor antagonist
Therapeutic class: Antiemetic

Indications and Dosages
✳ *Adjunct to prevent delayed nausea and vomiting associated with initial and repeat courses of emetogenic cancer chemotherapy*

TABLETS
Adults receiving cisplatin-based highly emetogenic cancer chemotherapy; adults receiving moderately emetogenic cancer chemotherapy and combinations of anthracycline and cyclophosphamide.
180 mg in combination with dexamethasone and a 5-HT3 receptor antagonist within 2 hours prior to chemotherapy.

Drug Administration
P.O.
- Administer within 2 hours prior to chemotherapy.
- Administer again only after at least 2 weeks have passed.

Route	Onset	Peak	Duration
P.O.	30 min	4 hr	Unknown

Half-life: 169–183 hr

Mechanism of Action
Crosses the blood–brain barrier to occupy brain P/NK1 receptors, which prevents nerve transmission of signals that cause nausea and vomiting.

Contraindications
Children less than 2 years of age, concurrent therapy with CYP2D6 substrates with a narrow therapeutic index such as pimozide and thioridazine, hypersensitivity to rolapitant or its components

Interactions
DRUGS
dextromethorphan and other CYP2D6 substrates: May increase plasma concentrations of these drugs
digoxin and other P-gp substrates with a narrow therapeutic index; irinotecan, methotrexate, topotecan, and other BCRP substrates with a narrow therapeutic index: Increased plasma concentrations of these drugs, which increases risk of adverse reactions
pimozide, thioridazine, and other CYP2D6 substrates with a narrow therapeutic index: Increased plasma concentrations of these drugs, which can result in QT prolongation and torsades de pointes

rifampin and other strong CYP3A4 inducers: Decreased plasma concentrations and effectiveness of rolapitant

Adverse Reactions
CNS: Dizziness
EENT: Stomatitis
GI: Abdominal pain, anorexia, dyspepsia, hiccups
GU: UTI
HEME: Anemia, **neutropenia**

Childbearing Considerations
PREGNANCY
- It is not known if drug can cause fetal harm.
- Use with caution only if benefit to mother outweighs potential risk to fetus.

LACTATION
- It is not known if drug is present in breast milk.
- Patient should check with prescriber before breastfeeding.

REPRODUCTION
- Drug may impair fertility in females in a reversible fashion, according to animal studies.

Nursing Considerations
- Know that rolapitant should not be given to patients with severe hepatic impairment but in the event its use cannot be avoided, monitor patient closely for rolapitant-related adverse reactions.
- Make sure dexamethasone and a 5-HT3 receptor antagonist have also been prescribed and are on hand ready to be given, as directed.

PATIENT TEACHING
- Review with patient when rolapitant is to be administered in conjunction with the patient's chemotherapy. Also, instruct patient when to take dexamethasone if it is prescribed after his chemotherapy.
- Tell patient to inform all prescribers of rolapitant therapy.
- Advise women of childbearing age that rolapitant may impair fertility.

romosozumab-aqqg
Evenity

Class and Category
Pharmacologic class: Monoclonal antibody
Therapeutic class: Anti-osteoporotic

Indications and Dosages
* *To treat osteoporosis in postmenopausal women at risk for fracture or who have failed or are intolerant to other available osteoporosis therapy.*

SUBCUTANEOUS INJECTION
Postmenopausal women. 210 mg once a month for 12 months.

Drug Administration
SUBCUTANEOUS
- Administer by injecting two consecutive 105-mg injections to complete the 210-mg dose.
- Remove two prefilled syringes from carton by grasping the syringe barrel when removing from the tray. Do not grasp the plunger or gray needle cap and do not remove gray needle cap until ready to give injection.
- Visually inspect the solution in each syringe. It should be clear to opalescent, colorless to light yellow.
- Allow solution to sit at room temperature for at least 30 minutes before injecting. Do not warm in any other way.
- Inject each injection for the monthly dose in two separate locations such as abdomen, outer area of upper arm, or thigh. Do not inject where skin is bruised, hard, red, or tender, and avoid injecting into areas with scars or stretch marks. Repeat steps with second syringe.
- Administer a missed dose as soon as possible and reschedule remaining monthly doses from date of last dose.

Route	Onset	Peak	Duration
SubQ	2 wk	5 days	Unknown
Half-life: 12.8 days			

Mechanism of Action
Inhibits the action of sclerostin, a regulatory factor in bone metabolism, which increases bone formation and, to a lesser extent, decreases bone resorption.

Contraindications
Hypersensitivity to romosozumab or its components, uncorrected hypocalcemia

Interactions
DRUGS
None reported by manufacturer

Q
R
S

≡ Adverse Reactions

CNS: Asthenia, **CVA**, headache, insomnia, paresthesia
CV: MI, peripheral edema
MS: Arthralgia, atypical subtrochanteric and diaphyseal femoral fractures, muscle spasms, neck pain, osteonecrosis of the jaw
SKIN: Dermatitis, **erythema multiforme**, rash, urticaria
Other: Angioedema, antibody formation to romosozumab, **hypocalcemia**, injection-site reactions (erythema, pain)

≡ Childbearing Considerations

PREGNANCY

Drug is not indicated for use in women of childbearing age.

LACTATION

- Drug is not indicated for use in women of childbearing age.

≡ Nursing Considerations

- Know that romosozumab should not be administered to patients who have had an MI or CVA within the preceding year. Additionally, romosozumab should be discontinued if MI or stroke occurs during therapy.
- Ensure that preexisting hypocalcemia is corrected prior to initiating romosozumab therapy.
- Check to see if patient has had a routine oral exam and any abnormalities taken care of before starting romosozumab therapy because drug can cause osteonecrosis of the jaw, which could occur spontaneously with tooth extraction and/or local dental infection with delayed healing. Patients should be counseled to maintain good oral hygiene.

! **WARNING** Monitor patient for hypersensitivity reactions that could be life-threatening, such as angioedema or erythema multiforme. If signs and symptoms occur, stop romosozumab therapy and notify prescriber. Expect to provide supportive care, as ordered.

- Monitor patient's cardiac status throughout romosozumab therapy because drug increases the risk of major adverse cardiac events. If patient develops any abnormality, notify prescriber immediately. If confirmed, expect drug to be discontinued.

- Monitor patient's calcium level throughout therapy because drug may cause hypocalcemia. Patients at greater risk are those with severe renal impairment or who are receiving dialysis. Ensure that patient is taking adequate amounts of calcium and vitamin D supplements.

PATIENT TEACHING

- Inform patient that romosozumab therapy will be given monthly for 12 months and requires 2 consecutive subcutaneous injections each month.
- Instruct patient to take a calcium and vitamin supplement while taking romosozumab.
- Tell patient to alert prescriber if dull, aching thigh pain occurs or if new or unusual groin, hip, or thigh pain is present.

! **WARNING** Instruct patient on the signs and symptoms of a heart attack or stroke. Urge patient to seek immediate medical attention if present.

! **WARNING** Review signs and symptoms of an allergic reaction, such as hives, rash, swelling or difficulty swallowing, or unusual skin condition. Tell patient to seek emergency care if severe.

- Tell patient to inform dentist of romosozumab therapy before any dental work is done, especially invasive dental procedures.

ropinirole hydrochloride
Requip, Requip XL

≡ Class and Category

Pharmacologic class: Nonergot alkaloid dopamine agonist
Therapeutic class: Antiparkinsonian

≡ Indications and Dosages

✷ *To treat signs and symptoms of Parkinson's disease*

TABLETS

Adults. *Initial:* 0.25 mg three times a day. Dosage titrated upward every wk according to the following schedule: 0.25 mg three times a day in wk 1; 0.5 mg three times a day in wk 2; 0.75 mg three times a day in wk 3;

1 mg three times a day in wk 4. After wk 4, if needed, dosage increased by 1.5 mg daily every wk up to 9 mg daily, then by 3 mg/day up to 24 mg daily. *Maximum:* 24 mg/day in three divided doses.

E.R. TABLETS

Adults. *Initial:* 2 mg once daily for 1 to 2 wk, increased, as needed, in increments of 2 mg/day at 1 wk or longer intervals. *Maintenance:* For patients with early Parkinson's disease, 12 mg daily or lower; for patients with advanced Parkinson's disease, 8 mg daily or lower.

* *To treat moderate to severe primary restless legs syndrome*

TABLETS

Adults. *Initial:* 0.25 mg daily. Dosage increased, as needed, on day 3 to 0.5 mg and then to 1 mg at beginning of week 2 (day 8). If needed, dosage further increased in 0.5-mg increments every wk for 4 wk, followed by a 1-mg increase for wk 7, if needed. *Maximum:* 4 mg daily.

± **DOSAGE ADJUSTMENT** For patients with end-stage renal disease on hemodialysis, dosage titration of immediate-release tablets is based on tolerability and need for efficacy, with recommended maximum total daily dose reduced to 18 mg/day for treatment of Parkinson's disease and 3 mg daily for patients with restless legs syndrome receiving regular dialysis. For patients with end-stage renal disease on hemodialysis and taking extended-release tablets, initial dose is 2 mg daily with dosage titration based on tolerability and need for efficacy, with recommended maximum total daily dose limited to 18 mg/day in patients receiving regular dialysis.

Drug Administration

P.O.

- Administer drug with food if adverse GI effects occur.
- Extended-release tablets should be swallowed whole and not chewed, crushed, or divided.
- Administer drug to treat restless legs syndrome 1 to 3 hours before bedtime.

Route	Onset	Peak	Duration
P.O.	Unknown	1–2 hr	6 hr
P.O./E.R.	Unknown	6–10 hr	Unknown

Half-life: 6 hr

Mechanism of Action

Directly stimulates postsynaptic dopamine type 2 (D_2) receptors within the brain and acts as an agonist at peripheral D_2 receptors. These actions inhibit the firing of striatal cholinergic neurons, thus helping to control alterations in voluntary muscle movement (such as rigidity and tremors) associated with Parkinson's disease and restless legs syndrome.

Contraindications

Hypersensitivity to ropinirole or its components

Interactions

DRUGS

ciprofloxacin, other CYP1A2 inhibitors: Altered drug clearance and increased blood level of immediate-release ropinirole tablets
CYP1A2 inducers; dopamine antagonists such as butyrophenones, metoclopramide, phenothiazines, thioxanthenes: Possibly decreased effectiveness of ropinirole
ethinyl estradiol (higher doses associated with hormone replacement therapy): Possibly reduced clearance of ropinirole

ACTIVITIES

smoking: Increased clearance of ropinirole with decreased effectiveness

Adverse Reactions

CNS: Abnormal dreaming, aggression, agitation, amnesia, anxiety, asthenia, compulsive behaviors, confusion, delirium, delusions, disorientation, dizziness, dyskinesia, falling asleep during activities of daily living, fatigue, hallucinations, headache, hypoesthesia, hypokinesia, insomnia, malaise, mania, nervousness, neuralgia, paranoid ideation, paresis, paresthesia, psychotic-like behaviors, rigors, somnolence, syncope, transient ischemic attack, tremor, vertigo

CV: Acute coronary syndrome, angina, bradycardia, cardiac failure, chest pain, hypertension, MI, orthostatic hypotension, palpitations, peripheral edema, sick sinus syndrome, tachycardia

EENT: Abnormal vision, diplopia, dry mouth, increased salivation, nasal congestion, nasopharyngitis, rhinitis, toothache

GI: Abdominal pain, constipation, diarrhea, dyspepsia, dysphagia, flatulence, gastric hemorrhage, gastroenteritis, indigestion,

intestinal obstruction, ischemic hepatitis, nausea, **pancreatitis**, vomiting
GU: Elevated BUN level, erectile dysfunction, pyuria, urinary incontinence, UTI
HEME: Anemia
MS: Arthralgia; arthritis; back pain; exacerbation of limb pain (restless legs syndrome); muscle cramps, spasms, or stiffness; myalgia; neck pain; osteoarthritis; tendinitis
RESP: Asthma, bronchitis, cough, dyspnea, upper respiratory tract infection
SKIN: Diaphoresis, flushing, hot flashes, **melanoma**, night sweats, pruritus, rash, urticaria
Other: Angioedema, elevation of serum creatine phosphokinase (CPK), flu-like symptoms, viral infection, weight loss, withdrawal symptoms

Childbearing Considerations
PREGNANCY
- It is not known if drug can cause fetal harm, but animal studies suggest harm may occur.
- Use with caution only if benefit to mother outweighs potential risk to fetus.

LACTATION
- It is not known if drug is present in breast milk.
- Inhibition of lactation is likely because drug inhibits the secretion of prolactin.
- Patient should check with prescriber before breastfeeding.

Nursing Considerations

! **WARNING** Expect to reassess patient for excessive sedation periodically during therapy. Excessive, acute drowsiness may arise as late as 1 year after starting therapy.

- Know that when ropinirole is given as adjunct to levodopa, expect concurrent dosage of levodopa to be gradually decreased as tolerated.

! **WARNING** Monitor patient for hypersensitivity reaction such as angioedema, pruritus, rash, and urticaria. If present, notify prescriber immediately. Expect to provide supportive care.

! **WARNING** Expect to stop ropinirole gradually over 7 days, as follows: over first 4 days, reduce from three times a day to

twice daily; during last 3 days, reduce to once daily, followed by complete withdrawal of drug. Watch for withdrawal symptoms (anxiety, apathy, depression, fatigue, pain, and sweating) during and after drug is discontinued. Be aware that these symptoms do not usually respond to levodopa. Instead, in cases of severe withdrawal symptoms, expect a trial of readministration of a dopamine agonist at the lowest effective dose.

! **WARNING** Watch for altered mental status during drug withdrawal. Rapid dose reduction may lead to a symptom complex resembling neuroleptic malignant syndrome that includes altered level of consciousness, autonomic instability, fever, and muscle rigidity.

- Watch for orthostatic hypotension, especially in patient with early Parkinson's disease. Orthostatic hypotension can occur more than 4 weeks after start of therapy or after a dosage reduction because ropinirole may impair systemic regulation of blood pressure.
- Monitor patient for hallucinations or other psychotic-like behavior, especially if patient has Parkinson's disease, is elderly, or takes levodopa.
- Monitor patient for worsening of preexisting dyskinesia; ropinirole may potentiate dopaminergic adverse effects of levodopa.
- Avoid giving CNS depressants, other CNS-interacting drugs, and sleep aids during ropinirole therapy because they increase the risk of somnolence.
- Assess patient for skin changes regularly because risk of melanoma is higher in patients with Parkinson's disease. It isn't clear whether this results from disease or from the drugs used to treat it.

PATIENT TEACHING
- Inform patient with Parkinson's disease that ropinirole helps to improve muscle control and movement but doesn't cure Parkinson's disease.
- Encourage patient to take ropinirole with food to decrease risk of adverse GI effects. Tell her not to chew, crush, or divide extended-release tablets but to swallow them whole. If a dose is missed, instruct patient not to double their next dose.

! **WARNING** Caution patient not to stop taking ropinirole abruptly. If concerns arise over ropinirole therapy, encourage her to speak with prescriber. Remind patient that withdrawal symptoms (anxiety, apathy, depression, fatigue, pain, and sweating) can occur during dosage reduction or after discontinuation of drug or if dosage decreased rapidly (altered consciousness, fever, and muscular rigidity). In either case, instruct patient to notify prescriber immediately.

! **WARNING** Instruct patient to notify prescriber if allergic reactions occur, such as hives, itching, or rash. If facial swelling or difficulty breathing occurs, tell patient to seek immediate emergency treatment.

- Caution patient to avoid hazardous activities until CNS effects of drug—including sedation—are known.
- Tell the patient that if she falls asleep during normal activities, she should notify prescriber.
- Urge patient to avoid consuming alcohol and other sedating drugs (such as sleep aids) during therapy because they may increase drug's CNS depressant effects.
- Urge patient to stand up slowly from a lying or sitting position to avoid feeling dizzy, faint, nauseated, or sweaty.
- Alert patient and family/caregiver that drug may cause hallucinations and other psychotic-like behavior. Also, warn patient that drug may cause involuntary movements. Tell patient to notify prescriber right away, if present.
- Explain to patient with restless legs syndrome that symptoms might appear in early morning or have an earlier onset in the evening or even the afternoon during ropinirole therapy and could be worse or spread to other limbs. Urge patient to notify prescriber if this occurs.
- Urge patient to have regular skin examinations by a dermatologist or other qualified health professional.
- Advise patient to notify prescriber about intense urges (as for gambling or sex) because dosage may have to be reduced or drug discontinued.
- Tell patient to inform all prescribers of ropinirole therapy.

- Inform patient that smoking may decrease effectiveness of ropinirole. If smoking is started or stopped during therapy, patient should notify prescriber.
- Advise patients who are planning a pregnancy or do become pregnant or wish to breastfeed after infant is born, to discuss their wishes with prescriber.

rosiglitazone maleate
Avandia

Class and Category
Pharmacologic class: Thiazolidinedione
Therapeutic class: Antidiabetic

Indications and Dosages
* *As adjunct to diet and exercise to achieve glucose control in type 2 diabetes mellitus*

TABLETS
Adults. *Initial:* 4 mg once daily or 2 mg twice daily, increased to 8 mg once daily or 4 mg twice daily if glucose control is inadequate after 8 to 12 wk. *Maximum:* 8 mg daily.

Drug Administration
P.O.
- Administer once-daily dose in morning and twice-daily doses in morning and in evening.

Route	Onset	Peak	Duration
P.O.	Unknown	1 hr	Unknown

Half-life: 3–4 hr

Mechanism of Action
Increases tissue sensitivity to insulin. This peroxisome proliferator-activated receptor agonist regulates the transcription of insulin-responsive genes found in key target tissues, such as adipose tissue, the liver, and skeletal muscle. Enhanced tissue sensitivity to insulin lowers the blood glucose level.

Contraindications
Hypersensitivity to rosiglitazone or its components, New York Heart Association (NYHA) class III or IV heart failure

Interactions
DRUGS
CYP2C8 inducers, such as rifampin: Possibly decreased effects of rosiglitazone

Q
R
S

CYP2C8 inhibitors, such as gemfibrozil:
Possibly increased effects of rosiglitazone

Adverse Reactions

CNS: CVA, fatigue, headache
CV: Angina, **congestive heart failure,**
edema, hypertension, **myocardial ischemia
or infarction**
EENT: Blurred vision, decreased visual
acuity, macular edema, nasopharyngitis,
sinusitis
ENDO: Hyperglycemia, **hypoglycemia**
GI: Diarrhea, elevated liver enzymes,
hepatotoxicity
HEME: Anemia
MS: Arthralgia, back pain, bone fracture
(especially upper arm, foot, hand)
RESP: Dyspnea, upper respiratory tract
infection
SKIN: Pruritus, rash, **Stevens–Johnson
syndrome,** urticaria
Other: **Anaphylaxis, angioedema,** weight
gain

Childbearing Considerations

PREGNANCY

- It is not known if drug can cause fetal harm.
- Use with caution only if benefit to mother
  outweighs potential risk to fetus.

LACTATION

- It is not known if drug is present in breast
  milk.
- Patient should check with prescriber before
  breastfeeding.

REPRODUCTION

- Drug may result in unintended pregnancy
  in women of childbearing age who are
  anovulatory because drug may cause
  ovulation.

Nursing Considerations

- Give rosiglitazone cautiously in patients
  with edema, heart failure, or hepatic
  impairment because of potential adverse
  reactions.
- Be aware that drug isn't recommended for
  patients with symptomatic heart failure.
- Evaluate patient's liver function before
  starting drug and periodically throughout
  therapy, as ordered. Notify prescriber
  about abnormalities, such as abdominal
  pain, anorexia, dark urine fatigue, nausea,
  and vomiting. Drug may have to be
  stopped.

! WARNING Monitor patient for evidence of
congestive heart failure—such as edema,
rapid weight gain, or shortness of breath—
because rosiglitazone can cause fluid
retention that may lead to or worsen heart
failure. Notify prescriber immediately if
the patient's cardiac status deteriorates, and
expect to stop drug, as ordered.

- Monitor fasting glucose and glycosylated
  hemoglobin A_{1c} levels periodically,
  as ordered, to evaluate rosiglitazone
  effectiveness.
- Be aware that drug is effective only in the
  presence of endogenous insulin.

PATIENT TEACHING

- Advise patient to take once-daily dose in
  morning and twice-daily doses in morning
  and evening.
- Emphasize the need to follow an exercise
  program and a diet control program during
  rosiglitazone therapy.
- Advise patient to notify prescriber
  immediately if she has fluid retention,
  shortness of breath, or sudden weight gain,
  because drug may have to be discontinued.
- Instruct patient to have liver enzymes
  checked, as ordered, about every 2 months
  for first year and then annually.
- Inform anovulatory premenopausal patient
  that drug may induce ovulation, increasing
  risk of pregnancy.
- Urge patient, especially women, to take
  precautions against falling or experiencing
  trauma; drug increases risk of fractures,
  particularly of the foot, hand, and upper
  arm.
- Instruct patient to notify all prescribers
  of rosiglitazone therapy and not to take
  any medication such as over-the-counter
  medicines, including herbal supplements
  and vitamins, without consulting prescriber
  first.

rosuvastatin calcium

Crestor, Ezallor Sprinkle

Class and Category

Pharmacologic class: HMG-CoA reductase
inhibitor
Therapeutic class: Antilipemic

Indications and Dosages

* As adjunct to treat hyperlipidemia, mixed dyslipidemia, hypertriglyceridemia, and primary dysbetalipoproteinemia (type III hyperlipoproteinemia); to slow the progression of atherosclerosis; to prevent primary cardiovascular disease (reduce the risk of myocardial infarction, stroke, or need for arterial revascularization procedures) in patients without clinically evident CAD but with increased risk factors of cardiovascular disease such as age (men 50 years and over; women 60 years and over), hsCRP of 2 mg/l or greater, and the presence of at least one additional cardiovascular disease risk factor such as hypertension, low HDL-C, smoking, or a family history of premature CAD

TABLETS (CRESTOR)

Adults. *Initial:* 10 to 20 mg daily, increased every 2 to 4 wk, as needed. *Maximum:* 40 mg daily.

* To treat homozygous familial hypercholesterolemia

TABLETS (CRESTOR)

Adults. *Initial:* 20 mg daily, increased every 2 to 4 wk, as needed. *Maximum:* 40 mg daily.
Children ages 7 to 17. 20 mg once daily.

* To treat pediatric heterozygous familial hypercholesterolemia

TABLETS (CRESTOR)

Children ages 10 to 17. 5 to 20 mg daily. *Maximum:* 20 mg daily.
Children ages 8 to less than 10. 5 to 10 mg daily. *Maximum:* 10 mg daily.

* As adjunct to treat hypertriglyceridemia; as adjunct to treat primary dysbetalipoproteinemia (type III hyperlipoproteinemia)

CAPSULES (EZALLOR SPRINKLE)

Adults. *Initial:* 10 to 20 mg once daily, increased as needed. *Maximum:* 40 mg once daily.

* As adjunct to treat homozygous familial hypercholesterolemia

CAPSULES (EZALLOR SPRINKLE)

Adults. *Initial:* 20 mg once daily, increased as needed. Maximum: 40 mg once daily.

±**DOSAGE ADJUSTMENT** For patients taking cyclosporine or darolutamide, dosage shouldn't exceed 5 mg daily. For Asian patients, initial dosage limited to 5 mg daily. For patients taking regorafenib or a combination of dasabuvir/ombitasvir/paritaprevir/ritonavir, elbasvir/grazoprevir, sofosbuvir/velpatasvir, or glecaprevir/pibrentasvir, dosage should not exceed 10 mg daily. For patients taking combined atazanavir and ritonavir, lopinavir and ritonavir, gemfibrozil, or simeprevir or for patients with severe renal impairment (creatinine clearance less than 30 ml/min) not on hemodialysis, initial dosage reduced to 5 mg daily, with maintenance dose not to exceed 10 mg daily.

Drug Administration

P.O.

- Capsules should be swallowed whole and not chewed or crushed. However, capsules can be opened for patients who cannot swallow capsules and contents sprinkled on soft food such as applesauce or pudding. Drug mixture should be swallowed within 1 hour and not stored for future use.
- Capsules can be used to administer drug via a nasogastric tube (16-French or greater). Open capsule and empty content into a 60-ml catheter-tipped syringe, add 40 ml of water, replace plunger, and shake syringe vigorously for 15 seconds. Insert syringe into nasogastric tube and administer drug. Afterward, flush nasogastric tube with 20 ml of additional water. Do not use any other liquid except water. Once mixed in syringe, use immediately and do not store for future use.
- Space drug administration at least 2 hours apart when antacids are also administered.

Route	Onset	Peak	Duration
P.O.	1 wk	3–5 hr	Unknown

Half-life: 19 hr

Mechanism of Action

Cholesterol and triglycerides circulate in the blood as part of lipoprotein complexes. Rosuvastatin inhibits the enzyme 3-hydroxy-3-methylglutaryl-coenzyme A (HMG-CoA) reductase. This inhibition reduces lipid levels by increasing the number of hepatic low-density lipoprotein (LDL) receptors on the cell surface to increase uptake and catabolism of LDL. It also inhibits hepatic synthesis of very-low-density lipoprotein

Q
R
S

(VLDL), which decreases the total number of VLDL and LDL particles.

Contraindications

Active liver disease, breastfeeding, hypersensitivity to rosuvastatin or its components, pregnancy, unexplained persistent elevations of serum transaminase levels

Interactions

DRUGS

antacids: Decreased blood rosuvastatin level if given within 2 hours of rosuvastatin
atazanavir/ritonavir, cyclosporine, darolutamide, dasabuvir/ombitasvir/ paritaprevir/ritonavir, elbasvir/grazoprevir, gemfibrozil, glecaprevir/pibrentasvir, ledipasvir/sofosbuvir, lopinavir/ritonavir, other lipid-lowering drugs, regorafenib, simeprevir, sofosbuvir/velpatasvir, sofosbuvir/velpatasvir/ voxilaprevir: Increased rosuvastatin level and risk of myopathy
colchicine: Increased risk of myopathy, including rhabdomyolysis
fenofibrates: Possibly increased risk of myopathy
niacin (equal to or greater than 1 g/day): Increased risk of skeletal muscle effects
warfarin: Increased INR

Adverse Reactions

CNS: Asthenia, cognitive impairment, confusion, depression, dizziness, headache, hypertonia, insomnia, memory loss, nightmares, paresthesia, peripheral neuropathy
CV: Chest pain, hypertension, peripheral edema
EENT: Pharyngitis, rhinitis, sinusitis
ENDO: Elevated glycosylated hemoglobin levels, gynecomastia, hyperglycemia, thyroid function abnormalities
GI: Abdominal pain, constipation, diarrhea, elevated liver enzymes, gastroenteritis, **hepatic failure, hepatitis,** jaundice, nausea, **pancreatitis**
GU: **Acute renal failure,** proteinuria, UTI
HEME: Thrombocytopenia
MS: Arthralgia, arthritis, back pain, immune-mediated necrotizing myopathy, myalgia, myopathy, **rhabdomyolysis**
RESP: Bronchitis, increased cough, **interstitial lung disease**
SKIN: Rash, urticaria

Other: Angioedema, flu-like symptoms, generalized pain, infection

Childbearing Considerations

PREGNANCY

- Drug may cause fetal harm.
- Drug is contraindicated in pregnant women. Drug should be discontinued as soon as pregnancy is known.

LACTATION

- Drug is present in breast milk.
- Drug is contraindicated in women who are breastfeeding.

REPRODUCTION

- Advise women of childbearing age to use effective contraception during drug therapy.

Nursing Considerations

- Use rosuvastatin cautiously in patients who consume large quantities of alcohol or who have a history of liver disease, because drug is contraindicated in patients with active liver disease or unexplained persistent elevations of transaminase levels.
- Administer cautiously in patients with risk factors for myopathy, such as advanced age, hypothyroidism, or renal impairment.
- Know that if ALT or AST levels increase to more than three times the normal range, expect dosage to be reduced or drug discontinued.
- Monitor serum lipoprotein level, as ordered, to evaluate response to therapy.
- Expect rosuvastatin to be discontinued if patient develops markedly elevated creatinine kinase levels, or if myopathy is diagnosed or suspected. Drug may be temporarily withheld if patient develops any condition that may be related to myopathy or that predisposes her to renal failure, such as hypotension; major surgery; sepsis; severe electrolyte, endocrine, or metabolic disorders; trauma, or uncontrolled seizures.
- Obtain baseline liver enzymes and expect to monitor them thereafter, as indicated. Notify prescriber if proteinuria or hematuria appears in patient's routine urinalysis, because rosuvastatin dosage may have to be reduced.

PATIENT TEACHING

- Encourage patient to follow a low-fat, low-cholesterol diet.
- Tell patient who takes antacids to wait at least 2 hours after taking rosuvastatin.

- Instruct patient prescribed capsule form not to chew or crush capsules. If patient cannot swallow the capsule, it can be opened and the granules carefully emptied onto one teaspoon of applesauce. Patient should swallow mixture immediately, without chewing.
- Instruct patient to notify prescriber immediately about muscle pain, tenderness, or weakness, especially if accompanied by fever or malaise. He should also tell prescriber if these symptoms occur even after drug is discontinued.
- Encourage patient or family to notify prescriber if patient begins to notice new onset or worsening of confusion, forgetfulness, or memory loss.
- Tell woman of childbearing age about the need to use reliable contraceptive method while taking drug. Instruct her to notify prescriber at once if she suspects she may be pregnant.
- Instruct patient with diabetes to test his blood glucose regularly and have a HbA_{1c} level checked routinely.

safinamide mesylate
Xadago

Class and Category
Pharmacologic class: Monoamine oxidase type B (MAO-B) inhibitor
Therapeutic class: Antiparkinsonian

Indications and Dosages
∗ *As adjunct to levodopa/carbidopa treatment in patients with Parkinson's disease experiencing "off" episodes*

TABLETS
Adults. *Initial:* 50 mg once daily at the same time of day, increased after 2 wk to 100 mg once daily, if needed and tolerated.
±**DOSAGE ADJUSTMENT** For patient with moderate hepatic impairment, maximum dosage kept at 50 mg once daily.

Drug Administration
P.O.
- Administer drug consistently at about the same time each day.
- If a dose is missed, administer the next dose at the same time it's due the next day.
- Store at room temperature.

Route	Onset	Peak	Duration
P.O.	Unknown	1.8–2.8 hr	Unknown

Half-life: 20–26 hr

Mechanism of Action
Precise mechanism unknown, but by inhibiting monoamine oxidase B activity through blocking the catabolism of dopamine, it is thought this action increases dopamine levels, which in turn increase dopaminergic activity in the brain to improve Parkinson symptoms.

Contraindications
Concurrent use with amphetamine and their derivatives; cyclobenzaprine; dextromethorphan; linezolid; methylphenidate; opioid drugs *(meperidine and its derivatives, methadone, propoxyphene, or tramadol)*; other MAO inhibitors or other drugs that are potent inhibitors of MAOs; serotonin–norepinephrine reuptake inhibitors; St. John's wort; *tetracyclic, triazolopyridine, or tricyclic antidepressants;* hypersensitivity to safinamide or its components; severe hepatic impairment

Interactions
DRUGS
amphetamine, antidepressants (tetracyclic, triazolopyridine, tricyclic), cyclobenzaprine, methylphenidate, opioid drugs, serotonin–norepinephrine reuptake inhibitors, St. John's wort: Increased risk of life-threatening serotonin syndrome
antipsychotics, metoclopramide: Possibly decreased effectiveness of safinamide; exacerbation of Parkinson's disease symptoms
dextromethorphan: Increased risk of abnormal behavior or psychosis
isoniazid, other MAO inhibitors, other drugs that are potent inhibitors of MAO, sympathomimetics, tyramine: Increased risk of hypertensive crisis

Adverse Reactions
CNS: Anxiety, compulsive behaviors, confusion, dyskinesia, falling asleep during activities of daily living, fever, hallucinations, headache, insomnia, lack of impulse control, serotonin syndrome
CV: Hypertension, orthostatic hypotension
EENT: Gingival swelling, retinal pathology, tongue swelling

GI: Dyspepsia, elevated liver enzymes, nausea
RESP: Cough, dyspnea
SKIN: Rash
Other: Hypersensitivity reactions

Childbearing Considerations

PREGNANCY

- It is not known if drug may cause fetal harm, but animal studies suggest harm may occur.
- Use with caution only if benefit to mother outweighs potential risk to fetus.

LACTATION

- It is not known if drug is present in breast milk.
- Patient should check with prescriber before breastfeeding.

Nursing Considerations

- Be aware that safinamide therapy should not be used in patients with a major psychotic disorder because drug may exacerbate the psychosis.

! **WARNING** Monitor patient for hypersensitivity reactions such as dyspnea, rash, or swelling of tongue and gingiva. Notify prescriber immediately and be prepared to provide supportive emergency care.

- Monitor patient's blood pressure closely because safinamide may cause hypertension or exacerbate existing hypertension. Be aware that although dietary restriction is not necessary during treatment with recommended doses, certain foods that are very high in tyramine (more than 150 mg) could cause severe hypertension.

! **WARNING** Monitor patient closely for serotonin syndrome, a rare but serious adverse effect of MAO inhibitors such as safinamide. Signs and symptoms include agitation, confusion, diaphoresis, diarrhea, fever, hyperactive reflexes, poor coordination, restlessness, shaking, talking or acting with uncontrolled excitement, tremor, and twitching. If symptoms occur, notify prescriber immediately, expect to discontinue drug, and provide supportive care.

- Monitor patient for dyskinesia because safinamide may cause dyskinesia or exacerbate preexisting dyskinesia. Notify prescriber, because reducing the patient's daily levodopa dosage or the dosage of another dopaminergic drug may lessen the dyskinesia.
- Monitor patient for hallucinations or psychotic behavior. If present, expect dosage to be reduced or drug discontinued.
- Monitor patient for visual changes, especially in patients with a history of certain eye disorders such as active retinopathy, albinism, family history of hereditary retinal disease, inherited retinal conditions, macular or retinal degeneration, retinitis pigmentosa, or uveitis. This is because retinal degeneration and loss of photoreceptor cells may occur with safinamide therapy.

! **WARNING** Be aware that 100-mg dose should be tapered to 50 mg for 1 week before safinamide is discontinued. This is because a symptom complex resembling neuroleptic malignant syndrome, exhibited by altered consciousness, autonomic instability, elevated temperature, and muscular rigidity, has occurred with rapid dose reduction, withdrawal of, or changes in drugs that increase central dopaminergic tone.

PATIENT TEACHING

- Instruct patient to take daily dose at about the same time every day.
- Tell patient that if a dose is missed, he should take the next dose at the same time the next day.
- Instruct patient to avoid foods very high in tyramine, because consuming such may cause very high blood pressure.

! **WARNING** Alert patient that allergic reactions such as difficulty breathing, rash, or swelling of tongue and gingiva may occur. If present, instruct patient to seek immediate medical care.

- Advise patient to avoid performing hazardous activities, as drug may cause daytime sleepiness or episodes of falling asleep during activities that require full attention, such as driving. Tell patient to notify prescriber of any such occurrence.

- Tell patient drug may cause him to experience intense urges to perform compulsive behaviors such as binge eating, gambling excessively, having sex very frequently, or spending money uncontrollably. If present, tell him to notify prescriber, as dosage may have to be reduced or drug discontinued.
- Advise patient to inform all prescribers of safinamide therapy.
- Instruct patient and family to notify prescriber if persistent, severe, or unusual adverse effects occur, including dyskinesia, hallucinations, or psychotic behavior.
- Stress importance of not stopping drug abruptly. If patient has concerns about safinamide therapy, advise him to speak with prescriber.

salmeterol xinafoate

Serevent Diskus

Class and Category

Pharmacologic class: Long-acting beta$_2$ agonist (LABA)
Therapeutic class: Bronchodilator

Indications and Dosages

∗ *To treat asthma and prevent bronchospasm in patients with reversible obstructive airway disease, including symptoms of nocturnal asthma, who are currently using an inhaled corticosteroid*

ORAL INHALATION POWDER

Adults and children age 4 and over.
1 inhalation (50 mcg) every 12 hr in the morning and evening.

∗ *To provide maintenance treatment of bronchospasm associated with chronic obstructive pulmonary disease (COPD)*

ORAL INHALATION POWDER

Adults. 1 inhalation (50 mcg) every 12 hr in the morning and evening.

∗ *To prevent exercise-induced bronchospasm in patients who do not have persistent asthma or, if persistent asthma present, used in conjunction with an inhaled corticosteroid*

ORAL INHALATION POWDER

Adults and children age 4 and over.
1 inhalation (50 mcg) at least 30 min before exercise. *Maximum:* No more than 1 inhalation (50 mcg) every 12 hr.

Drug Administration

INHALATION

- Administer twice-daily doses 12 hours apart, morning and evening.
- Administer at least 30 minutes before exercise if used to prevent exercise-induced bronchospasm.
- Do not use a spacer device when administering drug.
- Remove diskus from foil pouch when administering for the first time and write date on label. Hold the diskus in left hand and place thumb of right hand in thumb grip. Push the thumb grip as far as it will go until the mouthpiece shows and snaps into place. Have patient hold the diskus in a level, flat position with the mouthpiece toward patient. Have patient slide the lever away from the mouthpiece as far as it will go until a click is heard. Then patient should exhale and then place mouthpiece to his lips and inhale through his mouth, not his nose. After removing mouthpiece from his mouth, patient should hold his breath for at least 10 seconds, and exhale slowly. To close diskus, place thumb in the thumb grip and slide it back as far as it will go.
- Have patient rinse mouth with water after each dose to minimize dry mouth.
- Store drug in a dry place away from heat and sunlight in the unopened foil pouch until ready for use.
- Discard diskus 6 weeks after removing it from overwrap or when dose indicator reads zero.

Route	Onset	Peak	Duration
Inhalation	0.5–2 hr	20 min	12 hr

Half-life: 5.5 hr

Mechanism of Action

Attaches to beta$_2$ receptors on bronchial cell membranes, stimulating the intracellular enzyme adenylate cyclase to convert adenosine triphosphate to cAMP. The resulting increase in intracellular cAMP level inhibits histamine release, relaxes bronchial smooth-muscle cells, and stabilizes mast cells.

Q
R
S

Contraindications

Hypersensitivity to salmeterol, its components, or to milk proteins (severe); primary treatment of status asthmaticus or other acute episodes of asthma or COPD where intensive measures are required; treatment of asthma without use of an inhaled corticosteroid

Interactions

DRUGS

atazanavir, clarithromycin, indinavir, itraconazole, ketoconazole, nefazodone, nelfinavir, ritonavir, saquinavir, telithromycin: Possibly increased risk of adverse cardiovascular effects

beta-blockers: Blocked pulmonary effect of salmeterol; possibly produce severe bronchospasms

loop or thiazide diuretics: Increased risk of hypokalemia and potentially life-threatening arrhythmias

MAO inhibitors, tricyclic antidepressants: Potentiated adverse vascular effects, such as hypertensive crisis

Adverse Reactions

CNS: Dizziness, fever, headache, nervousness, paresthesia, tremor
CV: Palpitations, tachycardia
EENT: Dry mouth, nose, and throat; sinus problems
GI: Nausea
MS: Arthralgia
RESP: Cough, **paradoxical bronchospasm**
SKIN: Contact dermatitis, eczema, rash, urticaria
Other: **Angioedema**, generalized aches and pains

Childbearing Considerations

PREGNANCY

- It is not known if drug can cause fetal harm.
- Use with caution only if benefit to mother outweighs potential risk to fetus.

LABOR & DELIVERY

- Drug use should be restricted to patients only if the benefit clearly outweighs the risk because drug may interfere with uterine contractions.

LACTATION

- It is not known if drug is present in breast milk.
- Patient should check with prescriber before breastfeeding.

Nursing Considerations

- Be aware that salmeterol shouldn't be used to relieve bronchospasm quickly because of its prolonged onset of action and that patients already taking drug twice daily shouldn't take additional doses for exercise-induced bronchospasm.

! WARNING Be aware that a recent study suggests that asthma-related deaths may increase in asthmatics receiving salmeterol. Know that salmeterol should not be used in patients whose asthma is adequately controlled on low- or medium-dose inhaled corticosteroids and it should only be used as additional therapy for patients with asthma who are currently taking but are not adequately controlled on an inhaled corticosteroid. Salmeterol should never be used as monotherapy in the treatment of asthma. Monitor this patient population closely throughout salmeterol therapy, and notify prescriber immediately of any changes in patient's respiratory status. Expect to discontinue use as soon as possible.

- Watch for arrhythmias and changes in blood pressure after use in patients with cardiovascular disorders, including arrhythmias, hypertension, and ischemic cardiac disease, because of drug's beta-adrenergic effects.
- Monitor patient's compliance. Expect adults with poor compliance and children and adolescents who require the addition of a long-acting beta agonist such as salmeterol to be prescribed a combination product containing both an inhaled corticosteroid and a long-acting beta agonist to increase compliance.

! WARNING Stop salmeterol immediately and notify prescriber if patient develops paradoxical bronchospasm. Risk is greatest with first use of a new canister or vial used as an inhalant.

PATIENT TEACHING

- Instruct patient to use salmeterol exactly as prescribed and not to increase dosage or frequency of use.
- Advise patient with asthma or COPD to take doses 12 hours apart for optimum

effect. Caution against using drug more than every 12 hours. Also, inform patients with asthma that salmeterol must be taken with an inhaled corticosteroid because a life-threatening reaction may occur if drug is taken alone. Tell patient using salmeterol to prevent exercise-induced bronchospasm to take drug at least 30 min before exercise.

- Teach patient how to use the diskus by instructing him to slide the lever only once when preparing dose, to avoid wasting doses. Advise him to exhale immediately before using the diskus and then to place mouthpiece to his lips and inhale through his mouth, not his nose. Then he should remove mouthpiece from his mouth, hold his breath for at least 10 seconds, and exhale slowly.
- Advise patient to rinse mouth with water after each dose to minimize dry mouth.
- Advise patient to store drug in a dry place away from heat and sunlight in the unopened foil pouch until ready for use. Also tell patient to discard diskus 6 weeks after removing it from overwrap or when dose indicator reads zero.

! WARNING Instruct patient to seek immediate medical attention if after taking salmeterol he develops breathing problems, a fast or irregular heartbeat, high blood glucose level, or any persistent, severe, or unusual side effects. Tell him that if he develops a low potassium level, that should also be reported to the prescriber.

- Instruct patient to notify prescriber if he needs four or more oral inhalations of rapid-acting inhaled bronchodilator a day for 2 or more consecutive days, or if he uses more than one canister of rapid-acting bronchodilator in an 8-week period.
- Caution patient not to use other drugs to treat his underlying respiratory condition without consulting prescriber and to let all prescribers know that he takes salmeterol.
- Caution patient to keep salmeterol diskus out of the reach of children. Also tell patient not to give the diskus to other people, even if they have the same symptoms, because it may harm them.

saquinavir mesylate
Invirase

Class and Category
Pharmacologic class: Protease inhibitor
Therapeutic class: Antiretroviral

Indications and Dosages
＊ *As adjunct to treat human immunodeficiency viral (HIV) infection in combination with ritonavir and other antiretroviral agents*

TABLETS
Adults and adolescents over the age of 16 who are treatment-naïve or are switching from a regimen containing delavirdine. *Initial:* 500 mg twice daily in combination with ritonavir 100 mg twice daily for 7 days, then increased to 1,000 mg twice daily in combination with ritonavir 100 mg twice daily.

Adults and adolescents over the age of 16 who are not treatment-naïve or are switching from another ritonavir-containing regimen or from a nonnucleoside reverse transcriptase inhibitor-based regimen not containing delavirdine or rilpivirine. 1,000 mg twice daily in combination with ritonavir 100 mg twice daily.

Drug Administration
P.O.
- Tablets should be swallowed whole and not chewed, crushed, or divided.
- Administer ritonavir at the same time as saquinavir.
- Administer within 2 hours after a meal.

Route	Onset	Peak	Duration
P.O.	Unknown	Unknown	Unknown

Half-life: 7–12 hr

Mechanism of Action
Inhibits HIV protease to render the enzyme incapable of processing the Gag-Pol polyprotein precursor, which leads to the production of noninfectious immature HIV particles.

Contraindications
Combination with drugs that both increase saquinavir plasma concentrations

and prolong the QT interval or CYP3A substrates that increase saquinavir levels resulting in serious or life-threatening adverse reactions; complete atrioventricular (AV) block without implanted pacemaker or at risk for complete AV block; concomitant therapy with alfuzosin, amiodarone, atazanavir, bepridil, clarithromycin, clozapine, dasatinib, dofetilide, disopyramide, ergot derivatives, erythromycin, flecainide, halofantrine, haloperidol, lidocaine, lovastatin, lurasidone, midazolam (oral), pentamidine, phenothiazines, pimozide, propafenone, quinidine, quinine, rifampin, rilpivirine (without a washout period of at least 2 weeks), sertindole, sildenafil (for treatment of pulmonary arterial hypertension), simvastatin, sunitinib, tacrolimus, trazodone, triazolam, ziprasidone; congenital long QT syndrome; high risk for complete AV block; hypersensitivity to saquinavir or its components; refractory hypokalemia or hypomagnesemia; severe hepatic impairment

Interactions

DRUGS

alfentanil, alfuzosin, amiodarone, amitriptyline, atorvastatin, benzodiazepines, bepridil, bosentan, calcium channel blockers, chlorpromazine, clarithromycin, clomipramine, clozapine, colchicine, dapsone, dasatinib, digoxin, disopyramide, dofetilide, ergot derivatives, erythromycin, fentanyl, flecainide, halofantrine, haloperidol, imipramine, immunosuppressants, ketoconazole, lidocaine (systemic), lovastatin, lurasidone, maraviroc, mesoridazine, midazolam, omeprazole, pimozide, propafenone, quetiapine, quinidine, quinine, rifabutin, rifampin, rilpivirine, salmeterol, sertindole, sildenafil, simvastatin, sunitinib, tacrolimus, tadalafil, thioridazine, trazodone, triazolam, vardenafil, vincamine, warfarin, ziprasidone: Increased concentration of these drugs

antiarrhythmics class 1A and class III, antidepressants, antihistaminics, antimicrobials, neuroleptics, PDE5 inhibitors (used for pulmonary arterial hypertension): Increased risk of prolonged PR and/or QT interval resulting in increased risk of ventricular arrhythmias, especially torsades de pointes

atazanavir: Increased concentration of atazanavir, ritonavir, and saquinavir
carbamazepine, efavirenz, garlic capsules, nevirapine, phenobarbital, phenytoin, St. John's wort, tipranavir/ritonavir: Decreased saquinavir concentration
corticosteroids: Decreased concentration of saquinavir and increased concentrations of corticosteroids
dalfopristin, quinupristin: Possibly increased saquinavir concentration
delavirdine, nefazodone, nelfinavir: Increased saquinavir concentration
ethinyl estradiol, methadone: Decreased concentration of these drugs
fusidic acid: Increased concentrations of fusidic acid, ritonavir, saquinavir
indinavir, itraconazole: Increased concentration of both drugs

Adverse Reactions

CNS: Abnormal coordination, anxiety, asthenia, confusion, depression, dizziness, fatigue, fever, headache, hypoesthesia, insomnia, **intracranial hemorrhage**, lethargy, loss of consciousness, paresthesia, peripheral neuropathy, psychotic disorder, **seizures**, somnolence, **suicidal ideation**, syncope, tremor
CV: Chest pain, edema, elevated LDH levels, hypertension, hypertriglyceridemia, heart murmur, **hypotension**, peripheral vasoconstriction, PR or **QT-interval prolongation, thrombophlebitis**
EENT: Sinusitis, taste distortion, tinnitus, visual impairment
ENDO: Diabetes mellitus (new-onset or worsening of existing condition), hyperglycemia
GI: Abdominal discomfort or pain, anorexia, ascites, constipation, diarrhea, dyspepsia, dysphagia, elevated liver and pancreatic enzymes, eructation, flatulence, gastritis, **gastrointestinal hemorrhage or obstruction, hepatitis**, hepatomegaly, hyperbilirubinemia, increased appetite, jaundice, nausea, **pancreatitis, portal hypertension**, vomiting
GU: Libido disorder, nephrolithiasis
HEME: Anemia including **hemolytic, leukopenia**, lymphadenopathy, **neutropenia, pancytopenia, thrombocytopenia**
MS: Arthralgia, back pain, muscle spasms, myalgia, polyarthritis

RESP: Bronchitis, cough, dyspnea, pneumonia

SKIN: Acne, alopecia, bullous dermatitis, diaphoresis, drug eruption, dry lips or skin, eczema, erythema, papillomatosis, pruritus, rash, **severe cutaneous reaction, Stevens–Johnson syndrome**, urticaria

Other: **Acute myeloid leukemia**, dehydration, elevated alkaline phosphatase, creatine phosphokinase, flu-like symptoms, **hypersensitivity reactions**, lipodystrophy, wasting syndrome, weight gain

▤ Childbearing Considerations

PREGNANCY

- Pregnancy exposure registry: 1-800-258-4263.
- It is not known if drug can cause fetal harm.
- Use with caution only if benefit to mother outweighs potential risk to fetus.

LACTATION

- It is not known if drug is present in breast milk.
- The Centers for Disease Control and Prevention recommends that HIV-1 infected mothers not breastfeed to avoid risking postnatal transmission of HIV-1 infection to infants. They also do not recommend breastfeeding because of potential drug-induced adverse reactions in the infant.

▤ Nursing Considerations

- Be aware that saquinavir must be used in combination with ritonavir because ritonavir significantly inhibits metabolism of saquinavir to provide increased plasma saquinavir levels. However, saquinavir is not recommended for use in combination with cobicistat because dosing recommendations for this combination have not been established.
- Be aware that tablets contain lactose and should not be taken by patients with rare hereditary problems of galactose intolerance, glucose-galactose malabsorption, or Lapp lactase deficiency.
- Monitor patient closely because saquinavir interacts with many drugs. These interactions may cause serious adverse reactions that could be life-threatening or increase adverse reactions from greater exposure to saquinavir. In addition, some drug interactions can lower the therapeutic effect of saquinavir and possibly cause resistance

to develop. Alert prescriber if a serious or severe toxicity occurs during treatment, as saquinavir will have to be discontinued.

- Obtain an ECG reading on all patients before starting saquinavir therapy, because of risk of PR or QT prolongation.
- Monitor patient's ECG for PR interval prolongation during therapy. Prolonged PR intervals can lead to conduction abnormalities including second- or third-degree atrioventricular block. Use caution with administering atazanavir, beta-adrenergic blockers, calcium channel blockers, or digoxin with saquinavir, because of the combined effect on the PR interval.
- Know that patients should also have ECG monitoring for QT-interval prolongation during therapy. Patients with long QT syndrome should not receive saquinavir, because of its effect on the QT interval. Risk factors for QT prolongation include presence of bradyarrhythmias, congestive heart failure, electrolyte abnormalities, or hepatic impairment. Know that hypokalemia or hypomagnesemia must be corrected before saquinavir therapy is begun. Expect to monitor patient's electrolyte levels throughout therapy. Know that saquinavir should be discontinued in any patient who develops a QT-interval prolongation greater than 20 msec over pretreatment measurement.
- Monitor patient's blood glucose levels, as new onset of diabetes mellitus, exacerbation of preexisting diabetes mellitus, and hyperglycemia have occurred with protease inhibitor therapy such as saquinavir.
- Monitor patient with underlying chronic alcoholism, cirrhosis, hepatitis B or C, or other liver abnormalities, because portal hypertension has occurred after saquinavir therapy has been initiated. If severe hepatic dysfunction occurs, expect drug to be discontinued.
- Know that spontaneous bleeding in patients with hemophilia A and B has occurred during treatment with protease inhibitors such as saquinavir. Additional factor VIII may be required.
- Monitor patient's lipid profile, as ordered, because elevated cholesterol and/or triglyceride levels have occurred with the combination therapy of saquinavir and ritonavir.

Q
R
S

- Be aware that immune reconstitution syndrome has occurred in patients treated with combination antiretroviral therapy, including saquinavir. The inflammatory response predisposes susceptible patients to opportunistic infections such as cytomegalovirus, *Mycobacterium avium* infection, *Pneumocystis jiroveci* pneumonia, or tuberculosis. Autoimmune disorders such as Graves' disease, Guillain–Barré syndrome, or polymyositis have also occurred. Report sudden or unusual adverse reactions to prescriber.

PATIENT TEACHING

- Instruct patient to swallow tablets whole and never chew, crush, or divide the tablets.
- Tell patient to take ritonavir at the same time as saquinavir and 2 hours after a meal.
- Tell patient with diabetes to monitor his blood glucose levels closely, as saquinavir may cause blood glucose levels to rise.
- Inform patient that saquinavir therapy may cause changes in her body appearance because of fat redistribution. Prepare her for the possibility of developing breast enlargement, central obesity, dorsocervical fat enlargement (buffalo hump), facial wasting, and peripheral wasting.
- Instruct patient to report any persistent, severe, or unusual signs and symptoms, such as dizziness, light-headedness, or palpitations.
- Inform patients with hemophilia that saquinavir may cause spontaneous bleeding and instruct them to seek immediate medical attention if bleeding occurs.
- Stress importance of compliance with ordered laboratory studies such as lipid profile to monitor for adverse reactions.
- Advise patient to notify all prescribers of saquinavir therapy, because of potential drug interactions, and advise patient not to take over-the-counter preparations (including herbal drugs and preparations) without consulting prescriber first.

sarecycline
Seysara

Class and Category

Pharmacologic class: Tetracycline
Therapeutic class: Antibacterial

Indications and Dosages

* *To treat inflammatory lesions of non-nodular moderate to severe acne vulgaris*

TABLETS

Adults and children age 9 and over weighing 85 kg (187 lb) to 136 kg (299.2 lb). 150 mg once daily.
Adults and children age 9 and over weighing 55 kg (121 lb) to 84 kg (184.8 lb). 100 mg once daily.
Adults and children age 9 and over weighing 33 kg (72.6 lb) to 54 kg (118.8 lb). 60 mg once daily.

Drug Administration

P.O.

- Administer drug with liberal amounts of fluid to reduce risk of esophageal irritation and ulceration.

Route	Onset	Peak	Duration
P.O.	Unknown	1.5–2 hr	Unknown

Half-life: 21–22 hr

Mechanism of Action

Although the exact mechanism of action is unknown for the treatment of acne vulgaris, the tetracycline class of antibiotics exerts a bacteriostatic effect by passing through the bacterial lipid bilayer, where it binds reversibly to 30S ribosomal subunits. This blocks the binding of aminoacyl transfer RNA to messenger RNA, thus inhibiting bacterial protein synthesis, which may relieve the inflammation of acne vulgaris.

Contraindications

Hypersensitivity to sarecycline, other tetracyclines, or their components

Interactions

DRUGS

aluminum-, calcium-, or magnesium-containing antacids, bismuth subsalicylate, iron-containing preparations: Possibly altered absorption of sarecycline
anticoagulants: Possibly depressed plasma prothrombin activity, which may increase risk of bleeding
oral retinoids: Possibly additive increased risk of intracranial pressure
penicillin: Possible interference with bactericidal action of penicillin

P-glycoprotein substrates such as digoxin: Possibly increased concentrations of P-gp substrates

Adverse Reactions

GI: *Clostridium difficile*-associated diarrhea, nausea

GU: Vulvovaginal candidiasis, vulvovaginal mycotic infection

Childbearing Considerations

PREGNANCY

- Drug can cause fetal harm such as adverse effects on skeletal and tooth development.
- The use of drug during last half of pregnancy may cause permanent discoloration of the child's teeth.
- Drug should not be used during pregnancy and should be discontinued as soon as pregnancy is known.

LACTATION

- Drug is present in breast milk.
- Breastfeeding is not recommended during drug therapy.

REPRODUCTION

- Know that drug should not be used in male patients attempting to conceive a child because animal studies have shown drug adversely affects spermatogenesis.

Nursing Considerations

- Assess patient for signs of secondary infection, such as profuse, watery diarrhea that has occurred with nearly all antibacterial agents. If such diarrhea develops, contact prescriber and expect to obtain a stool specimen to rule out pseudomembranous colitis caused by *C. difficile*. If diarrhea occurs, notify prescriber and expect to withhold penicillin and treat with electrolytes, fluids, protein, and an antibiotic effective against *C. difficile*.
- Monitor patient for central nervous system adverse reaction such as dizziness, light-headedness, and vertigo, because although sarecycline has not been known to cause such reactions, other tetracyclines have.

! **WARNING** Be aware that intracranial hypertension has occurred with the use of other tetracyclines. Monitor patient for blurred vision, headache, and papilledema.

If present, notify prescriber immediately, because even though intracranial hypertension usually resolves with discontinuation of the tetracycline, vision loss may become severe or even permanent. Women of childbearing age who are overweight are at higher risk for developing intracranial hypertension.

- Monitor patient for superinfection such as mycotic or vulvovaginal candidiasis infections. If present, notify prescriber and expect sarecycline therapy to be discontinued.

PATIENT TEACHING

- Tell patient to take sarecycline therapy exactly as directed. Also stress importance of completing the full course of therapy and not skipping doses, because not doing so may decrease the effectiveness of current therapy and increase the likelihood that bacteria may develop resistance to other antibacterial drugs in the future.
- Instruct patient to take tablets with liberal amounts of fluid, to reduce risk of esophageal irritation and ulceration.
- Advise women of childbearing age to notify prescriber of suspected or known pregnancy. Inform mothers that breastfeeding is not recommended during sarecycline therapy.
- Urge patient to tell prescriber if diarrhea develops, even 2 months or more after sarecycline therapy ends.
- Caution patient not to perform hazardous activities such as driving until possible adverse reactions are known.
- Warn patient to avoid exposure to artificial or natural sunlight because photosensitivity, manifested as an exaggerated sunburn reaction, has occurred in patients taking other tetracycline products. Instruct patient to wear protective clothing and use sunscreen if natural sunlight cannot be avoided. If skin redness occurs, tell patient to report this to prescriber, as drug should be discontinued at the first sign of skin redness.

! **WARNING** Instruct patient to report blurred vision or headaches immediately to prescriber.

Q
R
S

sarilumab

Kevzara

Class and Category

Pharmacologic class: Monoclonal antibody
Therapeutic class: Antiarthritic

Indications and Dosages

* *To treat moderate to severe active rheumatoid arthritis in patients who have had an inadequate response or intolerance to one or more disease-modifying antirheumatic drugs (DMARDs)*

SUBCUTANEOUS INJECTION

Adults. 200 mg once every 2 wk.

±**DOSAGE ADJUSTMENT** For patients who experience an absolute neutrophil count (ANC) between 500 to 1,000 cells/mm³, sarilumab withheld until ANC becomes greater than 1,000 cells/mm³. Dosage restarted at 150 mg every 2 wk and then dosage increased to 200 mg and given every 2 wk, when clinically appropriate. For patients experiencing an ANC less than 500 cells/mm³, drug discontinued. For patients who experience a low platelet count between 50,000 to 100,000 cells/mm³, drug withheld until platelets become greater than 100,000 cells/mm³. Dosage restarted at 150 mg every 2 wk and then dosage increased to 200 mg every 2 wk, when clinically appropriate. For patients experiencing a platelet count less than 50,000 cells/mm³ and confirmed with repeat testing, drug discontinued. For patients experiencing an elevated (ALT) greater than upper level normal (ULN) to three times ULN or less, dosage may have to be modified on an individual basis. For patients who experience an ALT greater than three times ULN to five times ULN or less, drug withheld until ALT is less than three times ULN. Dosage restarted at 150 mg every 2 wk and then dosage increased to 200 mg every 2 wk, as clinically appropriate. For patient experiencing an ALT greater than five times ULN, drug discontinued.

Drug Administration

SUBCUTANEOUS

- Remove drug from refrigerator and allow prefilled syringe to sit at room temperature for 30 minutes and the prefilled pen for 60 minutes prior to administering the injection. Do not warm drug any other way.
- Inspect the solution in the syringe. Solution should be clear and colorless to pale yellow. If solution is cloudy, discolored, or contains particles, discard it and use a new prefilled syringe or pen.
- Do not inject drug into areas of skin that appear bruised, damaged, tender, or has scars. Administer full amount in the syringe or pen.
- Rotate sites.
- Store drug in refrigerator in original carton and protect from light. However, if stored at room temperature, discard after 14 days.

Route	Onset	Peak	Duration
SubQ	Unknown	2–4 days	28–43 days

Half-life: 8–10 days

Mechanism of Action

Binds to IL-6 receptors to inhibit IL-6 mediated signaling of inflammatory processes, which occurs in rheumatoid arthritis. Without IL-6 mediated signaling, IL-6, as a proinflammatory cytokine, cannot be produced by endothelial and synovial cells in joints. This helps relieve inflammation present in rheumatoid arthritis.

Contraindications

Hypersensitivity to sarilumab or its components

Interactions

DRUGS

atorvastatin, lovastatin, oral contraceptives: Possibly decreased effectiveness of these drugs
CYP450 substrates with narrow therapeutic index, such as theophylline, warfarin: Possibly altered dosage requirements
live vaccines: Increased risk of vaccine-related infection

Adverse Reactions

CV: Elevated cholesterol and triglyceride levels
EENT: Nasopharyngitis
GI: Elevated liver enzymes, **GI perforation**
GU: UTI
HEME: **Neutropenia, thrombocytopenia**
RESP: Upper respiratory infections
SKIN: Rash, urticaria

Other: Anaphylaxis; anti-sarilumab antibody formation; herpes zoster reactivation; **immunosuppression**; infections such as bacterial, invasive fungal, mycobacterial, tuberculosis, viral, or other opportunistic infections; injection-site erythema, pruritis, rash; **malignancies**

Childbearing Considerations

PREGNANCY

- Pregnancy exposure registry: 1-877-311-8972.
- Drug may affect immune system of fetus/neonate in mothers exposed to drug during pregnancy because monoclonal antibodies cross the placental barrier.
- Use with caution only if benefit to mother outweighs potential risk to fetus.
- Be aware that administration of live vaccines may decrease response in infants exposed to the drug during pregnancy.

LACTATION

- It is not known if drug is present in breast milk.
- Patient should check with prescriber before breastfeeding.

Nursing Considerations

- Be aware that sarilumab therapy should not be started in patients who have an elevated ALT or AST above 1.5 times the upper limit of normal, an absolute neutrophil count (ANC) less than 2,000/mm^3, or platelet count less than 150,000/mm^3.
- Expect patient to be tested for latent tuberculosis before sarilumab therapy is started. If result is positive, patient will need to be treated before sarilumab is initiated. In patient who has a history of active or latent tuberculosis and for whom an adequate course of treatment cannot be confirmed or results are negative, but patient has risk factors for tuberculosis infection, patient may need to be treated before beginning sarilumab therapy.
- Know that sarilumab should not be used with biological DMARDs because of increased immunosuppression and increased risk of infection.
- Be aware that sarilumab should be avoided in patients with active infections.
- Know that patients with active hepatic disease or hepatic impairment are not candidates for sarilumab therapy, because drug can have adverse effects on liver, as evidenced by elevation in liver enzymes.

! **WARNING** Monitor patient for signs and symptoms of infection because of sarilumab's immunosuppressant action. Serious and sometimes fatal infections due to bacterial, invasive fungal, mycobacterial, viral, or other opportunistic pathogens have occurred with sarilumab therapy. If infection occurs, notify prescriber, expect drug to be withheld for serious infections until infection is eradicated, and administer prescribed treatment for the infection.

- Expect to monitor patient's ALT, ANC, and platelet counts regularly. Expect dosage modifications or drug withholding until target levels are met.

! **WARNING** Monitor patient for hypersensitivity reactions, If present, notify prescriber, expect drug to be withheld or discontinued based upon severity of the reaction, and provide supportive care.

PATIENT TEACHING

- Teach patient or caregiver how to administer a subcutaneous injection. Tell patient to rotate injection sites with each injection and not to inject into skin that is bruised, damaged, scarred, or tender.
- Instruct patient to allow prefilled syringe to sit at room temperature for 30 minutes and the prefilled pen for 60 minutes prior to administering the injection. Warn patient not to warm syringe any other way. Have patient inspect the solution in the syringe before administering the injection. Solution should be clear and colorless to pale yellow. If solution is cloudy, discolored, or contains particles, instruct patient to discard it and use a new prefilled syringe. Also tell patient to discard the prefilled syringe or pen if not used within 14 days after being taken out of the refrigerator.
- Tell patient to inject the full amount in syringe to receive the prescribed dose.
- Instruct patient on infection precautions. Warn patient to avoid people with an active infection. Review signs and symptoms of an infection with patient and tell him to report any such evidence to prescriber immediately.

Q
R
S

> **! WARNING** Warn patient that allergic reactions can occur with sarilumab therapy. Tell patient to alert prescriber if present, as drug may have to be discontinued if reaction is serious.

- Inform patient that frequent blood tests will have to be performed to monitor for adverse effects. Stress importance of patient compliance with these appointments.
- Warn patient not to receive any live vaccines while taking sarilumab.
- Instruct patient to notify prescriber and seek immediate emergency medical attention if abdominal signs and symptoms such as pain occur.

saxagliptin hydrochloride
Onglyza

Class and Category
Pharmacologic class: Dipeptidyl peptidase-4 (DPP-4) inhibitor
Therapeutic class: Antidiabetic

Indications and Dosages
* As adjunct to diet and exercise to improve blood glucose control in type 2 diabetes mellitus*

TABLETS
Adults. 2.5 or 5 mg once daily.

± **DOSAGE ADJUSTMENT** For patients with moderate or severe renal impairment (creatinine clearance 45 ml/min or less), patients with end-stage renal disease, patients having hemodialysis, and patients receiving strong CYP3A4/5 inhibitors (i.e., atazanavir, clarithromycin, indinavir, itraconazole, ketoconazole, nefazodone, nelfinavir, ritonavir, saquinavir, telithromycin), dosage shouldn't exceed 2.5 mg once daily.

Drug Administration
P.O.
- Tablets should be swallowed whole and not chewed, crushed, or divided.
- Tablets may be taken at any time of day regardless of meals but consistently.

Route	Onset	Peak	Duration
P.O.	Unknown	2 hr	24 hr

Half-life: 2.5 hr

Mechanism of Action
Incretin hormones, such as glucose-dependent insulinotropic polypeptide (GIP) and glucagon-like peptide-1 (GLP-1), are released into bloodstream from small intestine in response to meals. Upon arrival at the pancreas, they stimulate pancreatic beta cells to release insulin. GLP-1 also reduces glucagon secretion from pancreatic alpha cells, which reduces hepatic glucose production. Incretin hormones become inactivated within minutes of release by the enzyme, dipeptidyl peptidase-4. Saxagliptin inhibits this enzyme, thereby slowing inactivation of incretin hormones, which provides more time for them to increase insulin levels and blunt glucagon secretion. More insulin and less hepatic glucose production work together to lower blood glucose levels.

Contraindications
Hypersensitivity to saxagliptin or its components

Interactions
DRUGS
insulin, sulfonylureas: Increased risk of hypoglycemia
strong CYP3A4/5 inhibitors such as atazanavir, clarithromycin, indinavir, itraconazole, ketoconazole, nefazodone, nelfinavir, ritonavir, saquinavir, telithromycin: Increased plasma saxagliptin level
insulin, sulfonylureas: Increased risk of hypoglycemia

Adverse Reactions
CNS: Headache
CV: Heart failure, peripheral edema
EENT: Sinusitis, nasopharyngitis
ENDO: Hypoglycemia
GI: Abdominal pain, **acute pancreatitis**, gastroenteritis, vomiting
GU: Elevated plasma creatinine level, UTI
HEME: Lymphopenia
MS: Arthralgia (disabling, severe), **rhabdomyolysis**

RESP: Upper respiratory tract infection
SKIN: Bullous pemphigoid, **exfoliative skin conditions**, rash, urticaria
Other: **Anaphylaxis, angioedema**

Childbearing Considerations

PREGNANCY

- It is not known if drug can cause fetal harm.
- Use with caution only if benefit to mother outweighs potential risk to fetus.

LACTATION

- It is not known if drug is present in breast milk.
- Patient should check with prescriber before breastfeeding.

Nursing Considerations

- Know that saxagliptin shouldn't be used to treat type 1 diabetes mellitus or diabetic ketoacidosis.
- Use cautiously in patients who have experienced angioedema with another dipeptidyl peptidase-4 inhibitor, because it is not known if a cross-sensitivity reaction may occur with saxagliptin.
- Obtain a serum creatinine level, as ordered, before starting saxagliptin therapy and then periodically thereafter to monitor patient's renal function.

! WARNING Monitor patient closely for hypersensitivity to saxagliptin, especially within the first 3 months of therapy beginning with first dose. These reactions can be serious and life-threatening and may include anaphylaxis, angioedema, and exfoliative skin conditions. Discontinue saxagliptin immediately if hypersensitivity occurs, and notify prescriber.

- Monitor patient's blood glucose level and hemoglobin A_{1c} to assess effectiveness of saxagliptin therapy.
- Monitor patient for signs and symptoms of heart failure during saxagliptin therapy, because drug may increase risk. If present, notify prescriber, expect drug to be discontinued, and provide supportive care, as ordered.
- Watch for hypoglycemia in patients taking insulin or other antidiabetics, such as sulfonylureas. Expect dosage of insulin or other antidiabetics, such as sulfonylureas,

to be decreased to reduce risk of hypoglycemia.

! WARNING Monitor patient for signs and symptoms of acute pancreatitis such as severe, sharp pain in the upper abdominal accompanied by fever, nausea, and vomiting. If present, notify prescriber, expect to stop saxagliptin, as ordered, and provide supportive care, as indicated and ordered.

PATIENT TEACHING

- Inform patient that drug may be taken at any time of day regardless of meals but should be taken consistently at the same time.
- Emphasize that saxagliptin isn't a replacement for diet and exercise therapy.
- Explain importance of self-monitoring glucose levels during saxagliptin therapy.
- Teach patient to recognize hypoglycemia and how to treat it if it should occur. Urge him to carry glucose with him at all times in case hypoglycemia occurs.
- Review signs and symptoms of heart failure with patient, such as difficulty breathing; swelling of feet, hands, or legs; or unexplained weight gain. Tell patient to notify prescriber immediately, if present.
- Instruct patient to notify prescriber if fever, illness, infection, surgery, trauma, or other stress occurs because blood glucose control may be altered, requiring temporary insulin therapy.
- Tell patient to watch for the development of blisters or breakdown of the outer layer of his skin. If present, he should notify prescriber, as drug may have to be discontinued.

! WARNING Instruct patient to seek immediate medical attention if he experiences persistent, acute abdominal pain, fever, nausea, and vomiting, as well as any sign of hypersensitivity, such as difficulty breathing or swallowing, hives, rash, skin flaking or peeling, or swelling of any area on face or skin.

- Advise patient to seek medical attention if severe joint pain occurs. Tell patient that joint pain may develop within a day of taking saxagliptin or may develop years later.

Q
R
S

scopolamine transdermal system
Transderm-V (CAN)

Route	Onset	Peak	Duration
Transdermal	4 hr	24 hr	72 hr

Half-life: 9.5 hr

Class and Category
Pharmacologic class: Belladonna alkaloid
Therapeutic class: Antiemetic

Indications and Dosages
* *To prevent nausea and vomiting associated with motion sickness or recovery from anesthesia and/or opiate analgesia and surgery*

TRANSDERMAL SYSTEM
Adults and adolescents. 1 U.S. transdermal system (1 mg) applied behind ear before antiemetic effect is required as follows: 4 hr before event known to cause motion sickness, evening before surgery, or 1 hr before caesarian section. Patch removed 24 hr postsurgical procedure. Patch may remain in place up to 3 days for prevention of motion sickness and may be replaced, as needed. Or, 1 Canadian transdermal system (1 mg) applied behind ear for 3-day period, beginning at least 12 hr before antiemetic effect is required and no more than 2 patches worn for a total of 6 days.
± **DOSAGE ADJUSTMENT** Dosage reduction possible for elderly patients because of increased sensitivity to scopolamine.

Drug Administration
TRANSDERMAL
- Apply patch on hairless area behind ear and wash hands thoroughly with soap and water before and after applying.
- Do not apply more than 1 patch.
- Do not cut patch.
- If patch becomes displaced, remove it and apply a new one.
- When removing the old patch, fold the used patch in half with the sticky side together and discard.
- Remove patch before patient undergoes an MRI, as skin burns may occur if left in place.
- Store pouches at room temperature in an upright position and do not bend or roll the pouches.

Mechanism of Action
Blocks neural pathways in the inner ear to relieve motion sickness.

Contraindications
Angle-closure glaucoma; hypersensitivity to scopolamine, other belladonna alkaloids, or their components

Interactions
DRUGS
anticholinergics (other): Possibly intensified anticholinergic effects including CNS adverse reactions, intestinal obstruction, and/or urinary retention
CNS depressants: Possibly potentiated effects of either drug, resulting in additive sedation
oral drugs absorbed in stomach: Possibly delayed absorption of oral drugs

ACTIVITIES
alcohol use: Additive CNS effects

Adverse Reactions
CNS: Agitation, amnesia, attention disturbance, confusion, coordination abnormalities, delusions, dizziness, drowsiness, euphoria, exacerbation of psychosis, hallucinations, headache, insomnia, memory loss, paradoxical stimulation, paranoia, restlessness, speech disorder, **seizures**, somnolence, vertigo
CV: Palpitations, tachycardia
EENT: Acute angle-closure glaucoma; amblyopia; blurred vision; dry eyes, mouth, nose, and throat; eyelid irritation; increased intraocular pressure; itchy eyes; mydriasis; pharyngitis
GI: Constipation, decreased gastrointestinal motility, dysphagia
GU: Dysuria, urinary hesitancy, urine retention
SKIN: Decreased sweating, dry skin, erythema, flushing, rash, skin irritation
Other: Application site burning, withdrawal symptoms upon removal of patch

Childbearing Considerations
PREGNANCY
- It is not known if drug can cause fetal harm.

- Drug should be avoided in pregnant women experiencing severe preeclampsia because of increased risk for eclamptic seizures.
- Use with caution only if benefit to mother outweighs potential risk to fetus in other circumstances.

LACTATION

- Drug is present in breast milk.
- Patient should check with prescriber before breastfeeding.

Nursing Considerations

- Assess for bladder distention and monitor urine output because drug's antimuscarinic effects can cause urine retention. Also, monitor bowel sounds as drug may decrease gastrointestinal motility. Know that patch should be removed in patients experiencing difficulty in urination.
- Monitor patient who has worn the patch for several days for withdrawal symptoms, which usually occur 24 hours or more after the patch has been removed.
- Monitor for pain. In presence of pain, drug may act as a stimulant and produce delirium if used without meperidine or morphine.
- Monitor heart rate for transient tachycardia, which may occur with high doses of drug. Rate should return to normal within 30 minutes.
- Monitor patient for visual adverse effects; nervous system adverse reactions including cognitive, psychiatric reactions, and seizures; decreased gastrointestinal motility; urinary retention; and withdrawal symptoms.

PATIENT TEACHING

- Instruct patient to apply scopolamine transdermal patch on hairless area behind ear and to wash hands thoroughly with soap and water before and after applying. Remind patient that only one transdermal patch should be worn at one time. Patch should not be cut. If patch becomes displaced, tell patient to remove it and apply a new one. When removing the old patch, instruct patient to fold the used patch in half with the sticky side together and discard in a manner that prevents accidental contact or ingestion by children or pets.
- Advise patient to avoid hazardous activities until drug's CNS effects are known.
- Instruct patient to avoid alcohol while wearing the scopolamine patch.
- Suggest to patient who complains of dry eyes to use lubricating drops.
- Advise patient to immediately remove the transdermal system and contact prescriber if experiencing blurred vision, eye pain or discomfort, or halos or colored images in association with red eyes from conjunctival congestion and corneal edema.
- Review adverse reactions associated with drug and advise patient to alert prescriber if prolonged, severe, or unusual. Tell patient wearing patch for more than a couple of days to be alert for signs of withdrawal when patch is removed. If severe, patient should contact prescriber.
- Instruct patient to remove patch if undergoing an MRI, as skin burns can occur if left in place.

selegiline hydrochloride
Zelapar

selegiline transdermal system
Emsam

Class and Category

Pharmacologic class: Monoamine oxidase inhibitor (MAOI)
Therapeutic class: Antidepressant (Emsam), antidyskinetic

Indications and Dosages

⁎ *As adjunct to carbidopa-levodopa therapy to treat Parkinson's disease in patients whose response to therapy has deteriorated*

ORALLY DISINTEGRATING TABLETS (ZELAPAR)

Adults. *Initial:* 1.25 mg once daily for at least 6 wk; then increased to 2.5 mg once daily, as needed.

±**DOSAGE ADJUSTMENT** For patients with mild-to-moderate hepatic dysfunction, dosage kept at 1.25 mg once daily.

⁎ *To treat depression*

TRANSDERMAL SYSTEM (EMSAM)

Adults. *Initial:* 6 mg/24 hr daily. Increased every 2 wk in increments of 3 mg/24 hr, as needed. *Maximum:* 12 mg/24 hr.

± **DOSAGE ADJUSTMENT** For elderly patients (65 years and older), dosage not to exceed 6 mg/24 hr daily.

⬚ Drug Administration

P.O.

- Administer before breakfast without any liquid.
- Do not push tablet through the foil on the blister pack but instead peel back the foil with dry gloved hands and gently remove tablet.
- Immediately place tablet on top of patient's tongue and let it disintegrate.
- Do not have patient drink or ingest any food for 5 minutes before and after drug administration.
- Store blister tablets in sachet pouch at room temperature. Discard unused tablets 3 months after opening pouch.

TRANSDERMAL

- Apply patch at about the same time daily.
- Wash area gently and thoroughly with soap and warm water, then rinse until all soap is removed. After drying area, patch is ready to be applied.
- Apply patch to outer surface of upper arm, upper torso below the neck and above the waist, or upper thigh. Do not apply patch to broken, calloused, hairy, irritated, oily, or scarred skin. Also, patch should not be placed where clothing may rub patch off of site.
- Do not cut patch.
- Wash hands well after application.
- Only one patch may be worn at a time.
- If a patch falls off, apply a new patch to a new site and resume previous schedule.

Route	Onset	Peak	Duration
P.O.	5 min	15–40 min	Unknown
Transdermal	Unknown	Unknown	24 hr

Half-life: 1.3–10 hr

⬚ Mechanism of Action

Reduces dopamine metabolism by noncompetitively inhibiting the brain enzyme monoamine oxidase type B. This increases the amount of dopamine available to relieve symptoms of parkinsonism. Selegiline's metabolites may also enhance dopamine transmission by inhibiting its reuptake at synapses.

⬚ Contraindications

For all forms: Hypersensitivity to selegiline or its components; *For oral form:* Concurrent therapy with cyclobenzaprine, dextromethorphan, or St. John's wort; use of MAO inhibitors or meperidine or other opioids within 14 days of therapy; *For transdermal form:* Children less than 12 years, concomitant therapy within 2 weeks with carbamazepine, dextromethorphan, dual serotonin and norepinephrine reuptake inhibitors (duloxetine, venlafaxine), opiate analgesics (meperidine, methadone, pentazocine, propoxyphene, tramadol), oxcarbazepine, selective serotonin reuptake inhibitors (fluoxetine [use within 5 weeks], paroxetine, sertraline), tricyclic antidepressants (clomipramine, imipramine); pheochromocytoma

⬚ Interactions

DRUGS

amphetamines, buspirone, sympathomimetic amines: Increased risk of severe hypertension
carbamazepine: Increased risk of hypertensive crisis
dextromethorphan: Increased risk of brief episodes of bizarre behavior or psychosis, increased risk of serotonin syndrome
dopamine antagonists such as antipsychotics, metoclopramide: Possibly decreased effectiveness of selegiline
MAO inhibitors including linezolid: Increased risk for hypertensive crisis
serotonergic drugs such as opiate analgesics (meperidine, methadone, pentazocine, propoxyphene, tramadol), selective serotonin reuptake inhibitors (fluoxetine, paroxetine, sertraline), serotonin and norepinephrine reuptake inhibitors (duloxetine, venlafaxine), tricyclic antidepressants (clomipramine, imipramine): Increased risk of serotonin syndrome

FOODS

foods that contain tyramine or other high-pressor amines: Increased risk of sudden and severe hypertension

ACTIVITIES

alcohol use such as tap beer and beers not pasteurized: Increased risk of hypertension

Adverse Reactions

CNS: Anxiety, ataxia, chills, compulsive behaviors such as intense urges to perform certain activities (such as gambling or sex), confusion, depression, dizziness, drowsiness, dyskinesia, euphoria, extrapyramidal reactions, falling asleep during activities of daily living, fatigue, hallucinations, headache, insomnia, irritability, lethargy, memory loss, mood changes, nervousness, paresthesia, precipitation of manic/mixed episodes, restlessness, **serotonin syndrome**, somnolence, **suicidal ideation**, syncope, tremor, weakness

CV: Arrhythmias, chest pain, hypertension, orthostatic hypotension, palpitations, peripheral edema

EENT: Altered taste, blepharospasm, blurred vision, burning lips or mouth, diplopia, dry mouth, pharyngitis, rhinitis, sinusitis, stomatitis, tinnitus, tooth disorder

GI: Abdominal pain, anorexia, constipation, diarrhea, dyspepsia, dysphagia, flatulence, **GI bleeding**, heartburn, nausea, vomiting

GU: Dysuria, urinary hesitancy, urinary urgency, urine retention

MS: Arthralgia, back and leg pain, leg cramps, muscle fatigue and spasms, myalgia, neck stiffness

RESP: Asthma, dyspnea

SKIN: Dermatitis, diaphoresis, dry skin, ecchymosis, hypertrophy, photosensitivity, pruritus, rash, ulcers, urticaria

Other: Application site reactions (Emsam), **hypokalemia**

Childbearing Considerations

PREGNANCY

- It is not known if drug can cause fetal harm.
- Use with caution only if benefit to mother outweighs potential risk to fetus.

LACTATION

- It is not known if drug is present in breast milk.
- Patient should check with prescriber before breastfeeding if using oral form.
- Breastfeeding not recommended during treatment with transdermal form and for 5 days after the final dose.

Nursing Considerations

- Expect to screen patient for a family or personal history of bipolar disorder, hypomania, or mania before selegiline

therapy is begun, because drug may precipitate manic/mixed episodes.
- Be aware oral form contains phenylalanine and should not be given to patients with phenylketonuria (PKU).
- Assess patient for mental status and mood changes because selegiline can worsen such conditions as dementia, severe psychosis, tardive dyskinesia, and tremor. Be especially alert for suicidal tendencies, particularly when therapy starts or dosage changes.
- Monitor for decreased symptoms of Parkinson's disease to evaluate drug's effectiveness.

! **WARNING** Monitor patient for serotonin syndrome, which can be life-threatening. Signs and symptoms to watch for include autonomic instability, gastrointestinal symptoms, mental status changes, neuromuscular changes, and seizures. If present, stop selegiline therapy immediately (remove transdermal system, if present), notify prescriber, and provide supportive care, as ordered.

- Be aware that drug can reactivate gastric ulcers because it prevents breakdown of gastric histamine. Assess for related signs and symptoms, such as abdominal pain.
- Assess patient for skin changes regularly because risk of melanoma is increased in patients with Parkinson's disease. It isn't clear whether increase results from disease or drugs used to treat it.

PATIENT TEACHING

- Caution patient to take only prescribed amount because increased dosage may cause severe adverse reactions.
- Advise patient to avoid taking oral selegiline in the late afternoon or evening because it may interfere with sleep.
- For orally disintegrating tablets, tell patient to take it before breakfast without any liquid. Caution him not to push tablet through the foil on the blister pack but instead to peel back the foil with dry hands and gently remove the tablet. He should then immediately place the tablet on top of his tongue and let it disintegrate. Advise him not to drink or ingest any food for 5 minutes before and after taking the drug.
- Instruct patient taking oral form to store blister tablets in sachet pouch at all

Q
R
S

times and to keep pouch inside a clear child-resistant pouch provided. Unused tablets should be discarded 3 months after opening pouch. Store pouch at room temperature.

- For transdermal form, explain how and where (outer surface of upper arm, upper torso below the neck and above the waist, or upper thigh) to apply patch, stressing need to rotate sites. Remind patient to apply patch at about the same time of day. Tell patient not to apply patch to broken, calloused, hairy, irritated, oily, or scarred skin. Also, patch should not be placed where clothing is tight. Have patient wash the area gently and thoroughly with soap and warm water, then rinse until all soap is removed. After drying area, patch is ready to be applied. Tell patient to wash hands well after application and to dispose of removed patch immediately.
- Emphasize that only one patch may be worn at a time. If a patch falls off, tell patient to apply a new patch to a new site and to resume previous schedule.
- Caution patient to avoid exposing transdermal patch to sources of direct heat, such as electric blankets, heat lamps, heating pads, hot tubs, prolonged sunlight exposure, or saunas.
- Tell patient not to cut transdermal patch into smaller pieces.
- Alert patient that oral form contains phenylalanine and tell patient to alert prescriber if patient has phenylketonuria (PKU).
- Urge caregiver to monitor patient closely for suicidal tendencies, especially when therapy starts or dosage changes.

! WARNING Urge patient to avoid tyramine-rich foods and beverages during and for 2 weeks after stopping selegiline therapy unless patient is prescribed the lowest dosage of transdermal system (6 mg/24 hours), which doesn't require diet modification. Review which foods are considered tyramine-rich. Stress importance of seeking immediate medical attention if the following acute symptoms occur: heart racing or palpitations, neck stiffness, severe headache, or other sudden or unusual symptoms.

- Urge patient to avoid hazardous activities until drug's CNS effects are known.
- Instruct patient to immediately report neck stiffness, palpitations, racing heart, severe headache, or other sudden or unusual symptoms.
- Advise patient to change positions slowly to minimize the effects of orthostatic hypotension.
- Suggest that patient elevate his legs when sitting to reduce ankle swelling.
- Urge patient to avoid excessive sun exposure.
- Instruct patient to notify prescriber if symptoms develop that could indicate overdose, including muscle twitching and eye spasms.
- Urge patient to notify prescriber if dry mouth lasts longer than 2 weeks. Advise him to have routine dental checkups.
- Urge patient to have regular skin examinations done by a dermatologist or other qualified health professional.
- Tell patient to inform prescriber of any new medications, including prescription drugs, over-the-counter drugs, and also including herbal preparations.
- Advise patient to notify prescriber about intense urges (as for gambling or sex), because dosage may have to be reduced or drug discontinued.
- Inform mothers wishing to breastfeed their infants that breastfeeding is not recommended during treatment with selegiline and for 5 days after final dose.

semaglutide
Ozempic, Rybelsus, Wegovy

Class and Category
Pharmacologic class: Glucagon-like peptide-1 (GLP-1) receptor agonist
Therapeutic class: Antidiabetic

Indications and Dosages
∗ *As adjunct to diet and exercise to improve glycemic control in type 2 diabetes mellitus disease*

TABLETS (RYBELSUS)
Adults. 3 mg once daily for 30 days, then increased to 7 mg once daily for 30 days, and then further increased to 14 mg once daily, as needed.

SUBCUTANEOUS INJECTION (OZEMPIC)

Adults. *Initial:* 0.25 mg once a wk for 4 wk, then increased to 0.5 mg once a wk. Dosage further increased to 1 mg once a wk, if needed, after another 4 wk. *Maximum:* 1 mg once a wk.

✳ *To reduce risk of major adverse cardiovascular events (cardiovascular death, nonfatal MI or stroke) in patients with type 2 diabetes mellitus and established cardiovascular disease*

SUBCUTANEOUS INJECTION (OZEMPIC)

Adults. *Initial:* 0.25 mg once a wk for 4 wk, then increased to 0.5 mg once a wk. Dosage further increased to 1 mg once a wk, if needed, after another 4 wk. *Maximum:* 1 mg once a wk.

✳ *As adjunct to diet and exercise for chronic weight management in patients with an initial body mass index of 30 kg/m² or greater or 27 kg/m² in the presence of at least one weight-related comorbid condition such as dyslipidemia, hypertension, or type 2 diabetes mellitus*

SUBCUTANEOUS INJECTION (WEGOVY)

Adults. *Initial:* 0.25 mg once weekly for 4 wk. Dosage then increased as follows: 0.5 mg once weekly for wks 5–8, 1 mg once weekly for wks 9–12, 1.7 mg once weekly for wks 13–16 and 2.4 mg once weekly for wk 17 and onward. *Maintenance:* 2.4 mg once weekly.

⊟ Drug Administration

- Expect possible reduction in concomitantly administered insulin secretagogue or insulin to reduce the risk of hypoglycemia.

P.O.

- Administer tablet at least 30 minutes before first food, beverage, or other drug administration of the day and give with no more than 4 ounces of plain water.
- Tablets should be swallowed whole and not chewed, crushed, or divided.
- Use only 14-mg tablet to administer a 14-mg dose; do not use two 7-mg tablets to achieve a 14-mg dose.

SUBCUTANEOUS

- Inspect solution. It should be clear and colorless. Do not use if particles are present or solution is colored.
- Administer once weekly on the same day each week, without regard to meals. However, when administering Ozempic, day of weekly administration may be changed as long as the time between the two doses is at least 48 hours apart.
- Inject into patient's abdomen, thigh, or upper arm.
- Rotate sites.
- If Ozempic dose is missed, administer as soon as possible within 5 days of missed dose.
- Store unused pen in refrigerator with cap on, avoiding excessive heat and sunlight. Once first dose is given for Ozempic, pen can be stored at room temperature for up to 56 days. Store Wegovy pens in refrigerator or for 28 days if kept at room temperature.
- When administering with insulin, administer as separate injections; never mix the two drugs. Insulin can be injected into the same area as semaglutide but not adjacent to each other.

Route	Onset	Peak	Duration
P.O.	Unknown	1 hr	Unknown
SubQ	Unknown	1–3 days	Unknown

Half-life: 1 wk

≣ Mechanism of Action

Selectively binds to and activates the GLP-1 receptor to regulate appetite, thereby lowering body weight through decreased caloric intake. The binding of GLP-1 receptors also reduces blood glucose through a mechanism that stimulates insulin secretion and lowers glucagon secretion, both in a glucose-dependent manner. Thus, when blood glucose is high, insulin secretion is stimulated and glucagon secretion is inhibited, to lower blood glucose levels. A minor delay in gastric emptying in the early postprandial phase may also cause a minor glucose-lowering action.

≣ Contraindications

Family or personal history of medullary thyroid carcinoma, hypersensitivity to semaglutide or its components, multiple endocrine neoplasia syndrome type 2 (MEN 2)

≣ Interactions

DRUGS

insulin, insulin secretagogues such as sulfonylureas: Increased risk of hypoglycemia
oral drugs: Delayed absorption of these drugs

Adverse Reactions

CNS: Dizziness, fatigue, headache
EENT: Distortion of taste
ENDO: Hypoglycemia
GI: Abdominal distention or pain, cholelithiasis, constipation, diarrhea, dyspepsia, elevated pancreatic enzymes, flatulence, gastroesophageal reflux disease, gastritis, nausea, **pancreatitis**, vomiting
GU: Acute kidney injury, worsening of chronic renal failure
SKIN: Alopecia, rash, urticaria
Other: Anaphylaxis, angioedema, anti-semaglutide antibodies, injection-site reactions (discomfort, erythema)

Childbearing Considerations

PREGNANCY

- Pregnancy exposure registry: 1-800-727-6500 (for Wegovy exposure)
- Drug may cause fetal harm, based on animal studies.
- Use not recommended in pregnancy when using Wegovy and drug should be discontinued if pregnancy occurs; use with caution for other brands only if benefit to mother outweighs potential risk to fetus.

LACTATION

- It is not known if drug is present in breast milk.
- Breastfeeding is not recommended.

REPRODUCTION

- Women of childbearing age should be advised to consult prescriber for an alternative drug at least 2 months before a planned pregnancy.

Nursing Considerations

- Be aware that semaglutide is not recommended as a first-line therapy for patients who have inadequate glycemic control using diet and exercise, because of the uncertain relevance of possible tumor findings in animals.
- Know that semaglutide should not be given to patients with a history of pancreatitis, because effects are unknown. Monitor all patients for signs and symptoms of pancreatitis such as persistent severe abdominal pain which sometimes may radiate to the back and which may or may not be accompanied by vomiting. If pancreatitis is suspected, expect drug to be discontinued.

- Monitor patient with a history of diabetic retinopathy for progression of the disorder.
- Monitor patient for hypoglycemia, especially if patient is also taking insulin or an insulin secretagogue such as a sulfonylurea.
- Monitor patient closely for renal dysfunction, especially when initiating or escalating the dose of semaglutide or if patient develops severe adverse gastrointestinal reactions.

! **WARNING** Monitor patient for serious hypersensitivity reactions such as anaphylaxis and angioedema. If present, stop drug therapy immediately and provide supportive care, as needed and prescribed.

PATIENT TEACHING

- Instruct patient taking oral form to take tablet at least 30 minutes before the first food, beverage, or other drugs are taken for the day and to take with no more than 4 ounces of water. Stress importance of swallowing tablets whole and not chewing, crushing, or dividing tablets. Warn patient to use only the 14-mg tablet for the 14-mg dose; not to use two 7-mg tablets to make up the 14-mg dose.
- Teach patient or caregiver how to administer a subcutaneous injection. Tell her to administer drug into the abdomen, thigh, or upper arm using a different injection site each time. Review how to store drug and when to discard depending on brand of drug being used.
- Instruct patient to administer the once-weekly dosage subcutaneously at the same day each week at any time of the day and without regard to meals. However, let patient who is taking Ozempic brand know that the day of weekly subcutaneous administration can be changed, if needed, as long as the time between two doses is more than 48 hours.
- Inform patient that if a subcutaneous dose of Ozempic is missed, she should take the drug as soon as possible if within 5 days after the missed dose. If more than 5 days have passed, she should skip the missed dose and administer the next dose on the regularly scheduled day.
- Tell patient who is also administering insulin to administer the two drugs as

separate injections and never to mix them. The two injections can be administered in the same body region, but injections should not be adjacent to each other.

- Remind patient never to share the semaglutide pen with anyone else, even if the needle has been changed, because of an increased risk of transmitting bloodborne pathogens.
- Review signs and symptoms of hypoglycemia with patient and how to treat if it should occur. This is especially important in patients at increased risk, such as patients taking concurrent insulin or a sulfonylurea.
- Tell patient to report acute gastrointestinal adverse reactions, severe abdominal pain that may or may not radiate to the back and possibly be accompanied by vomiting. Tell patient to report any visual changes to prescriber.
- Advise women of childbearing age to alert prescriber if pregnancy occurs or 2 months in advance if pregnancy is being planned.

! **WARNING** Warn patient to seek immediate emergency care if severe or persistent signs and symptoms of an allergic reaction occur.

sertraline hydrochloride
Zoloft

Class and Category
Pharmacologic class: Selective serotonin reuptake inhibitor (SSRI)
Therapeutic class: Antianxiety, antidepressant, antiobessive-compulsant, antipanic, antiposttraumatic stress, antipremenstrual dysphoric

Indications and Dosages
✳ *To treat major depression*
ORAL SOLUTION, TABLETS
Adults. *Initial:* 50 mg daily, increased in increments of 25 to 50 mg daily every wk, as needed. *Maximum:* 200 mg daily.
✳ *To treat obsessive–compulsive disorder*
ORAL SOLUTION, TABLETS
Adults and adolescents. *Initial:* 50 mg daily, increased in increments of 25 to 50 mg daily every wk, as needed. *Maximum:* 200 mg daily.

Children ages 6 to 12. *Initial:* 25 mg daily, increased in increments of 25 mg every wk, as needed. *Maximum:* 200 mg daily.
✳ *To treat panic disorder, with or without agoraphobia; to treat posttraumatic stress disorder; to treat social anxiety disorder*
ORAL SOLUTION, TABLETS
Adults. *Initial:* 25 mg daily, increased by 25 to 50 mg daily every wk, as needed. *Maximum:* 200 mg daily.
✳ *To treat premenstrual dysphoric disorder (PMDD)*
ORAL SOLUTION, TABLETS
Adult women. *Initial:* 50 mg daily throughout menstrual cycle; or, 50 mg daily during luteal phase of menstrual cycle only (starting 14 days prior to menses and continuing through onset of menses). Dosage increased each menstrual cycle in 50-mg increments up to 150 mg daily, or each luteal phase up to 100 mg daily, as needed. If 100-mg daily dosage given, dosage regimen given as 50 mg daily for first 3 days followed by 100 mg daily during remaining dosage cycle. *Maximum:* 150 mg daily for dosing throughout menstrual cycle, or 100 mg daily for dosing during luteal phase only.
±**DOSAGE ADJUSTMENT** For patients with mild hepatic dysfunction, all dosages reduced by 50%.

Drug Administration
P.O.
- Use the supplied calibrated dropper to measure oral solution dose. However, don't use if allergic to latex, as dropper contains dry natural rubber.
- Mix oral solution with 4 ounces of ginger ale, lemon/lime soda, lemonade, orange juice, or water. Do not mix with any other solutions. Stir. A slight haze may appear but is normal.
- Administer oral solution immediately after mixing.
- Store oral solution and tablets at room temperature.

Route	Onset	Peak	Duration
P.O.	1–2 wk	4.5–8.8 hr	Unknown

Half-life: 26 hr

Mechanism of Action
Inhibits reuptake of the neurotransmitter serotonin by CNS neurons, thereby increasing the amount of serotonin available

Q
R
S

in nerve synapses. An elevated serotonin level may result in elevated mood and reduced depression. This action may also relieve symptoms of other psychiatric conditions attributed to serotonin deficiency and premenstrual dysphoric disorder.

Contraindications

Concurrent use of disulfiram (oral solution) or pimozide; hypersensitivity to sertraline or its components; use within 14 days of an MAO inhibitor, including intravenous methylene blue and linezolid.

Interactions

DRUGS

antibiotics (erythromycin, gatifloxacin, moxifloxacin, sparfloxacin), antipsychotics (chlorpromazine, droperidol, iloperidone, mesoridazine, ziprasidone), Class 1A antiarrhythmics (procainamide, quinidine), Class III antiarrhythmics (amiodarone, sotalol), dolasetron, halofantrine, levomethadyl, mefloquine, methadone, pentamidine, pimozide, probucol, tacrolimus: Increased risk of QT-interval prolongation and/or ventricular arrhythmias

aspirin, clopidogrel, heparin, NSAIDs, warfarin: Increased anticoagulant activity and risk of bleeding

atomoxetine, desipramine, dextromethorphan, flecainide, metoprolol, nebivolol, perphenazine, phenytoin, propafenone, thioridazine, tolterodine, venlafaxine: Possibly increased blood levels of these drugs, leading to increased risk of arrhythmias

buspirone, fentanyl, lithium, MAO inhibitors (I.V. methylene blue, linezolid, selegiline, tranylcypromine), other selected serotonin reuptake inhibitors, serotonin–norepinephrine reuptake inhibitors, St. John's wort, tricyclic antidepressants, triptans, tryptophan: Increased risk of potentially fatal serotonin syndrome

disulfiram: May interact with oral solution that contains alcohol

highly bound drugs to plasma protein: Increased free concentrations of sertraline, increasing risk of adverse reactions

Adverse Reactions

CNS: Abnormal dreams, aggressiveness, agitation, amnesia, anxiety, apathy, ataxia, **cerebrovascular spasm, coma,** confusion, delusions, depression, dizziness, drowsiness, emotional lability, euphoria, extrapyramidal symptoms, fatigue, fever, hallucination, headache, hyperkinesia, hypoesthesia, insomnia, lethargy, malaise, nervousness, **neuroleptic malignant syndrome-like reaction,** paranoid reaction, paresthesia, psychomotor hyperactivity, psychosis, **seizures, serotonin syndrome,** somnolence, **suicidal ideation,** syncope, tremor, weakness, yawning

CV: Atrial arrhythmias, **AV block, bradycardia,** hypertension, palpitations, **prolonged QT interval, torsades de pointes,** vasculitis, vasodilation, **ventricular tachycardia**

EENT: Abnormal accommodation, acute angle-closure glaucoma, blindness, cataract, conjunctivitis, dry mouth, earache, epistaxis, eye pain, optic neuritis, rhinitis, sinusitis, teeth grinding, tinnitus, vision changes

ENDO: Galactorrhea, hyperglycemia, hyperprolactinemia, hypothyroidism, syndrome of inappropriate ADH secretion

GI: Abdominal cramps or pain, anorexia, constipation, diarrhea, elevated liver enzymes, flatulence, hepatic dysfunction, **hepatic failure, hepatitis,** increased appetite, indigestion, jaundice, nausea, **pancreatitis,** vomiting

GU: **Acute renal failure;** anorgasmia (females); decreased libido; ejaculation disorders; erectile dysfunction; enuresis; hematuria; impotence; leucorrhea; menstrual disorders; priapism; polyuria; urinary frequency, incontinence, or retention; vaginal hemorrhage

HEME: Agranulocytosis, altered platelet function, aplastic anemia, hemorrhage, leukopenia, pancytopenia, thrombocytopenia

MS: Arthralgia, dystonia, lockjaw, muscle cramps or weakness, myalgia, **rhabdomyolysis**

RESP: Bronchospasm, coughing, dyspnea, **pulmonary hypertension**

SKIN: Alopecia, dermatitis including bullous, diaphoresis, flushing, photosensitivity, pruritus, purpura, rash, severe cutaneous disorders, **Stevens–Johnson syndrome, toxic epidermal necrolysis,** urticaria

Other: Anaphylaxis, angioedema, hyponatremia, lupus-like syndrome, serum sickness, weight loss

Childbearing Considerations

PREGNANCY

- Drug may cause fetal harm, especially if given in late pregnancy, as drug exposure increases risk of multiple neonatal complications after birth including feeding difficulties, respiratory complications, seizures, and persistent pulmonary hypertension of the newborn.
- Use with caution only if benefit to mother outweighs potential risk to fetus.
- Oral solution contains 12% alcohol and is not recommended during pregnancy.

LACTATION

- Drug is present in breast milk.
- Patient should check with prescriber before breastfeeding.

Nursing Considerations

- Be aware that sertraline should not be given to patients with bradycardia, congenital long QT syndrome, hypokalemia or hypomagnesemia, recent acute myocardial infarction, or uncompensated heart failure because of increased risk of prolonged QT interval and torsades de pointes. It should also not be given to patients who are taking other drugs that prolong the QT interval. Expect hypokalemia and hypomagnesemia to be corrected before sertraline therapy is begun.
- Monitor liver enzymes and BUN and serum creatinine levels, as appropriate, in patients with hepatic or renal dysfunction.

! **WARNING** Monitor patient closely for evidence of serotonin syndrome, such as agitation, coma, diarrhea, hallucinations, hyperthermia, hyperreflexia, incoordination, labile blood pressure, nausea, tachycardia, and vomiting. Serotonin syndrome in its most severe form can resemble neuroleptic malignant syndrome, which includes autonomic instability, hyperthermia, mental status changes, muscle rigidity, and possibly rapid changes in vital signs. Notify prescriber immediately because serotonin syndrome reactions that resemble neuroleptic malignant syndrome may be life-threatening. Be prepared to provide supportive care.

- Monitor patient for hypo-osmolarity of serum and urine and for hyponatremia, which may indicate sertraline-induced syndrome of inappropriate ADH secretion.

- Be aware that effective antidepressant therapy can promote development of mania in predisposed people. If mania develops, notify prescriber immediately and expect to withhold sertraline.
- Watch closely for suicidal tendencies, especially when therapy starts and dosage changes and especially in children and adolescents.
- Monitor patient closely for evidence of GI bleeding, especially if patient takes a drug known to cause it, such as aspirin, an NSAID, or warfarin.
- When therapy stops, expect to taper dosage to minimize adverse effects rather than stopping drug abruptly.

PATIENT TEACHING

- Advise patient that drug may cause mild pupillary dilation, which may lead to an episode of acute angle-closure glaucoma. Encourage patient to have an eye exam before starting therapy to see if he is at risk.
- Inform patient that oral solution contains alcohol and should not be taken with disulfiram.
- Teach patient to dilute oral solution before taking it. Tell him to use supplied dropper to remove prescribed amount and mix it with 4 oz (one-half cup) of ginger ale, lemon or lime soda, lemonade, orange juice, or water. Warn him not to mix oral solution with anything else. Explain that it's normal for mixture to be slightly hazy.
- Tell patient to take dose immediately after mixing it.
- Advise patient with a latex sensitivity to use an alternate dispenser because the supplied dropper dispenser contains dry natural rubber.
- Advise patient to avoid hazardous activities until drug's CNS effects are known.
- Inform patient that use of certain drugs, such as aspirin, NSAIDs, other antiplatelet drugs, warfarin, or other anticoagulants, with sertraline may increase his risk for bleeding.

! **WARNING** Tell patient that sertraline increases the risk of serotonin syndrome and reactions that resemble neuroleptic malignant syndrome, rare but serious complications, when taken with some other

Q
R
S

drugs. Teach patient how to recognize signs and symptoms of these disorders and advise him to notify prescriber immediately if they occur.

- Warn family or caregiver to watch patient closely for evidence of suicidal thinking or behavior, especially when therapy starts or dosage changes, and especially if patient is a child or adolescent.
- Caution patient not to stop taking drug abruptly. Explain that gradual tapering helps to avoid withdrawal symptoms.
- Advise patient to consult prescriber before taking any OTC product, especially aspirin products or NSAIDs.
- Alert patient that false-positive urine testing for benzodiazepines may occur while taking sertraline, requiring a more sensitive test to be performed.
- Encourage patient to discuss concerns about sexual dysfunction, if present.

sevelamer hydrochloride
Renagel

sevelamer carbonate
Renvela

⊒ Class and Category
Pharmacologic class: Polymeric phosphate binder
Therapeutic class: Phosphate binder

⊒ Indications and Dosages
✳ *To control serum phosphate level in patients with chronic kidney disease on dialysis*

TABLETS (RENAGEL)
Adults not taking a phosphate binder.
Initial: 800 mg three times a day with meals if serum phosphorus level is greater than 5.5 to less than 7.5 mg/dl; 1,600 mg three times a day with meals if serum phosphorus level is 7.5 mg/dl or greater.
±**DOSAGE ADJUSTMENT** Dosage adjusted based on the serum phosphorus concentration with goal of lowering serum phosphorus to 5.5 mg/dl or less and increased or decreased by 800 mg/meal

at 2-week intervals, as needed. If serum phosphorus level is greater than 5.5 mg/dl, dosage increased by 800 mg/meal at 2-week intervals; if serum phosphorus level is between 3.5 and 5.5 mg/dl, dosage remains unchanged; and if serum phosphorus level is less than 3.5 mg/dl, dosage decreased by 800 mg/meal at 2-week intervals. *Maximum average dose:* 13 g daily. For adult patients being switched from calcium acetate to sevelamer carbonate, 800 mg of sevelamer can be substituted for every 667 mg of calcium acetate being taken.

POWDER FOR ORAL SUSPENSION (RENVELA), TABLETS (RENVELA)
Adults not taking a phosphate binder.
800 mg three times a day with meals if serum phosphorus level is greater than 5.5 to less than 7.5 mg/dl; 1,600 mg three times a day with meals if serum phosphorus level is 7.5 mg/dl or greater. Dosage increased or decreased by 800 mg/meal at 2-wk intervals, as needed. *Maximum:* 14 g daily.
Children age 6 years and over not taking a phosphate binder. 800 mg three times a day with meals if body surface area is 0.75 m^2 or greater to less than 1.2 m^2, with dosage titrated every 2 weeks by 400 mg/meal, as needed; 1,600 mg three times a day with meals if body surface area is 1.2 m^2 or greater, with dosage titrated every 2 weeks by 800 mg/meal, as needed.
±**DOSAGE ADJUSTMENT** For adult patients being switched from calcium acetate to sevelamer carbonate, 800 mg of sevelamer can be substituted for every 667 mg of calcium being taken.

⊒ Drug Administration
P.O.
- Administer with meals.
- Tablets should be swallowed whole with water and not broken, chewed, or crushed.
- When using powder to make oral suspension for dose increments of 0.4 g, use one-half of a 0.8-g packet.
- Mix with 1 ounce of water for a 0.4-g or 0.8-g dose; 2 ounces for a 2.4-g dose. More than one packet can be mixed together.
- Stir mixture vigorously, even though it does not dissolve, and have patient drink entire preparation immediately or restir prior to administration if taken up to 30 minutes after being mixed.

- As an alternative to water, packet may be pre-mixed with a small amount of food or beverage and administered within 30 min as part of the meal.
- Do not heat powder mixture or add to heated foods or liquids.
- Do not administer other drugs 1 hour before or 3 hours after sevelamer.

Route	Onset	Peak	Duration
P.O.	1–2 wk	Unknown	Unknown

Half-life: Unknown

▤ Mechanism of Action

Inhibits phosphate absorption in the intestine by binding dietary phosphate, thereby lowering serum phosphorus level.

▤ Contraindications

Bowel obstruction; hypersensitivity to sevelamer carbonate, sevelamer hydrochloride, or their components

▤ Interactions

DRUGS

oral drugs such as ciprofloxacin, cyclosporine, levothyroxine, mycophenolate mofetil, tacrolimus: Possible decreased bioavailability of oral drugs requiring separate administration times

▤ Adverse Reactions

CNS: Headache, fever
CV: Hypertension, **hypotension, thrombosis**
EENT: Nasopharyngitis
GI: Abdominal pain, **bleeding gastrointestinal ulcers**, colitis, constipation (severe), diarrhea, dysphagia, fecal impaction, flatulence, **gastrointestinal necrosis**, ileus, indigestion, **intestinal obstruction or perforation**, nausea, vomiting
RESP: Bronchitis, dyspnea, increased cough, upper respiratory tract infection
MS: Arthralgia, back or limb pain
SKIN: Pruritus, rash
Other: **Hypersensitivity reactions**, infection

▤ Childbearing Considerations

PREGNANCY

- Drug is not absorbed systemically and is not expected to result in fetal exposure.
- Drug may decrease serum levels of fat-soluble vitamins and folic acid in pregnant women.

- Use with caution only if benefit to mother outweighs potential risk to fetus.

LACTATION

- Drug is not absorbed systemically.
- Drug is not expected to be in breast milk.

▤ Nursing Considerations

- Suggest suspension form be used in patients with swallowing disorders because tablet may get stuck in the esophagus in these individuals, and they may require hospitalization and emergency intervention to remove it.
- Be aware that severe hypophosphatemia may occur in patient with dysphagia, major GI tract surgery, or severe GI motility disorder (including severe constipation) because drug prevents phosphate absorption.
- Monitor blood pressure frequently.
- Monitor serum phosphorus level to determine drug's effectiveness; monitor other serum electrolyte levels, especially bicarbonate and chloride, to detect imbalances.

PATIENT TEACHING

- Tell patient to take drug with meals and to swallow tablets whole with water and not to break, chew, or crush them.
- Instruct patient taking suspension form to mix entire contents of each packet of powder thoroughly with the amount of water indicated on packet. More than one packet can be mixed together. He should stir the mixture vigorously, even though it does not dissolve, and drink entire preparation immediately or up to 30 minutes later (but he will need to stir the mixture again vigorously right before drinking if it was not consumed immediately). Warn patient not to heat mixture in microwave or add to heated foods or beverages.
- Caution patient to take other drugs 1 hour before or 3 hours after sevelamer.
- Review symptoms of thrombosis, and advise patient to report them immediately.
- Instruct patient to report new onset or worsening of existing constipation to prescriber, because additional treatment may be needed to prevent serious complications. Also, advise patient to report new onset of bloody stools.
- Inform patient of potential need for fat-soluble vitamins and folic acid supplements, especially if patient is pregnant.

Q
R
S

sildenafil citrate
Revatio, Viagra

Class and Category
Pharmacologic class: Phosphodiesterase 5 (PDE5) inhibitor
Therapeutic class: Antihypertensive (pulmonary arterial), erectile dysfunction agent

Indications and Dosages
✳ *To treat erectile dysfunction*

TABLETS (VIAGRA)
Men younger than 65. *Initial:* 50 mg taken 30 min to 4 hr before sexual activity although best if taken 1 hr before sexual activity; decreased or increased as needed based upon response. *Usual range:* 25 to 100 mg. *Maximum:* Once per day with dosage not exceeding 100 mg.

±**DOSAGE ADJUSTMENT** Initially, 25 mg for men over 65 years of age, those with hepatic dysfunction or severe renal insufficiency (creatinine clearance less than 30 ml/min), and those taking an alpha blocker or potent CYP3A4 inhibitors (erythromycin, itraconazole, ketoconazole, saquinavir) or ritonavir. Maximum dosage for patient taking ritonavir is 25 mg within a 48-hr period.

✳ *To treat pulmonary arterial hypertension in order to improve exercise ability and delay clinical worsening of condition in patients classified as group 1 by the World Health Organization*

ORAL SUSPENSION, TABLETS (REVATIO)
Adults. 5 or 20 mg three times a day 4 to 6 hr apart.

I.V. INJECTION (REVATIO)
Adults. 2.5 or 10 mg three times a day.

Drug Administration
P.O.
- Reconstitute powder for oral suspension by tapping bottle to release the powder; then remove the cap. Accurately measure out 60 ml of water and pour the water into bottle, replace cap, and shake bottle vigorously for a minimum of 30 seconds. Then add another 30 ml of water to bottle. Replace cap and shake bottle vigorously again for a minimum of 30 seconds. Solution should be clear and colorless and contain 10 mg sildenafil per ml.

Press bottle adaptor into the neck of the bottle. The adaptor should be used so the oral syringe can be filled with the drug from the bottle. Replace cap on the bottle.
- Do not mix with any other drug or additional flavoring agent.
- Store reconstituted oral suspension at room temperature or in refrigerator.
- Discard any remaining oral suspension 60 days after reconstitution.

I.V.
- Used for patients unable to take oral medication.
- Drug supplied as a ready-to-use solution in a single-use glass vial.
- Inspect solution before administering. It should be clear and colorless.
- Administer as an I.V. bolus.
- *Incompatibilities:* None listed by manufacturer

Route	Onset	Peak	Duration
P.O.	30–60 min	30–120 min	4 hr

Half-life: 4 hr

Mechanism of Action
Enhances the effect of nitric oxide released in the penis by stimulation. Nitric oxide increases cGMP level, relaxes smooth muscle, and increases blood flow to the corpus cavernosum, thus producing an erection. By preventing breakdown of cyclic guanosine monophosphate by phosphodiesterase, levels increase, leading to smooth-muscle relaxation of the pulmonary vasculature and subsequently, vasodilation. Vasodilation causes the pressure within the pulmonary vasculature to decrease, which improves tolerance to exercise and delays worsening of pulmonary arterial hypertension.

Contraindications
Concomitant riociguat, a guanylate cyclase stimulator, continuous or intermittent nitrate therapy, hypersensitivity to sildenafil or its components

Interactions
DRUGS
alpha-blockers, amlodipine, nitrates: Possible additive blood pressure-lowering effects
erythromycin, itraconazole, ketoconazole, ritonavir, saquinavir, and other CYP3A4 inhibitors: Significantly increased systemic

exposure of sildenafil, increasing risk of adverse reactions

Adverse Reactions

CNS: CVA, dizziness, headache, migraine, seizures, syncope, transient global amnesia, transient ischemic attack

CV: Heart failure, hypertension, hypotension, myocardial infarction or ischemia, orthostatic hypotension, palpitations, sudden cardiac death, tachycardia, vaso-occlusive crisis (presence of sickle cell disease), ventricular arrhythmias

EENT: Blurred vision; change in color perception; diplopia; epistaxis; hearing loss; increased intraocular pressure; nasal congestion; nonarteritic anterior ischemic optic neuropathy (NAION); ocular burning, pressure, redness, or swelling; paramacular edema; photophobia; retinal vascular bleeding or disease; tinnitus; visual decrease or temporary vision loss; vitreous detachment

ENDO: Uncontrolled diabetes mellitus

GI: Diarrhea, indigestion

GU: Cystitis, dysuria, painful erection, priapism, UTI

MS: Arthralgia, back pain

RESP: Pulmonary hemorrhage, upper respiratory tract infection

SKIN: Flushing, photosensitivity rash, urticaria

Childbearing Considerations

PREGNANCY

- Trade name, Viagra, is not indicated for use in females.
- It is not known if the trade name, Revatio, can cause fetal harm.
- Use Revatio with caution only if benefit to mother outweighs potential risk to fetus.

LACTATION

- Trade name, Viagra, is not indicated for use in females.
- Trade name, Revatio, appears to be present in breast milk.
- Patient should check with prescriber before breastfeeding if prescribed Revatio.

Nursing Considerations

! **WARNING** Do not administer drug to patients who take nitrates.

- Use sildenafil cautiously in the elderly and patients with hepatic or renal dysfunction,

and men with penile abnormalities that may predispose them to priapism. In addition, use cautiously in patients who have suffered a life-threatening arrhythmia, myocardial infarction, or stroke within the last 6 months or in patients with cardiac failure, coronary artery disease causing unstable angina, hypertension (blood pressure greater than 170/110), related anemias, resting hypotension (blood pressure less than 90/50), retinitis pigmentosa, or sickle cell, as sildenafil therapy has not been studied in these patient groups.

- Also use cautiously in patients with left ventricular outflow obstruction, such as aortic stenosis and idiopathic hypertrophic subaortic stenosis, and those with severely impaired autonomic control of blood pressure, because these conditions increase patient's sensitivity to vasodilators such as sildenafil.
- Monitor patient's blood pressure and heart rate and rhythm before and often during therapy.
- Monitor vision, especially in patients over age 50; who have coronary artery disease, diabetes, hypertension, or hyperlipidemia; or who smoke, because, although rare, sildenafil may cause nonarteritic anterior ischemic optic neuropathy (NAION) that may lead to decreased vision or permanent vision loss. Patients at higher risk for NAION include those who have already experienced it in the past and those who have a low cup to optic disc ratio or retinitis pigmentosa.

! **WARNING** Monitor patient being treated for pulmonary hypertension secondary to sickle cell disease for vaso-occlusive crisis (severe pain and change in color and temperature if extremity is involved). Notify prescriber immediately and prepare to provide supportive care.

PATIENT TEACHING

- Explain that sildenafil used to treat erectile dysfunction may be taken up to 4 hours before sexual activity, but that taking it 1 hour beforehand provides the most effective results.

! **WARNING** Warn patient not to take sildenafil if he also takes any form of organic nitrate, either continuously or intermittently, or other PDE5 inhibitors, including REVATIO (a sildenafil product used to treat another condition), because profound hypotension and death could result. Also caution patient to inform prescriber of all medications taken, as dosage may have to be decreased if a drug such as an alpha blocker has also been prescribed.

- Instruct patient prescribed oral suspension form how to mix it, store it, and discard any remaining suspension after 60 days.
- Tell patient to stop taking drug and contact prescriber if vision decreases suddenly in one or both eyes or if he has a loss of hearing, possibly with dizziness or tinnitus.
- Advise patient taking sildenafil for erectile dysfunction to seek sexual counseling to enhance the drug's effects.
- Urge patient to notify prescriber immediately if erection is painful or lasts longer than 4 hours, to avoid possible penile damage and permanent loss of erectile function.
- Instruct diabetic patient to monitor his blood glucose level frequently because drug may affect glucose control.

silodosin
Rapaflo

Class and Category
Pharmacologic class: Alpha adrenergic blocker
Therapeutic class: Benign prostatic antihyperplasia agent

Indications and Dosages
＊ *To treat symptomatic benign prostatic hyperplasia*
CAPSULES
Adult men. 8 mg once daily. *Maximum:* 8 mg daily.
±**DOSAGE ADJUSTMENT** For patients with moderate renal impairment (creatinine clearance between 30 and 50 ml/min), dosage reduced to 4 mg daily.

Drug Administration
P.O.
- Administer drug with a meal.

- For patient who can't swallow capsules, open capsule and sprinkle contents on a tablespoonful of cool or room-temperature applesauce. Administer within 5 minutes. Patient should not chew mixture. Follow with an 8-ounce glass of cool water. Don't store mixture for future use.

Route	Onset	Peak	Duration
P.O.	2–6 hr	6–7 hr	9–15 hr

Half-life: 13 hr

Mechanism of Action
Binds to postsynaptic alpha$_1$ adreno-receptors located in the bladder base and neck, prostate gland, and prostatic capsule and urethra. Blocking action at these adrenoreceptor sites causes relaxation of smooth muscle in the local area, which improves urine flow and reduces other benign prostatic hyperplasia symptoms.

Contraindications
Hypersensitivity to silodosin and its components, severe hepatic insufficiency (Child-Pugh score 10 or above), severe renal insufficiency (creatinine clearance less than 30 ml/min), use with alpha-blockers (doxazosin, prazosin, terazosin) or strong CYP3A4 inhibitors (clarithromycin, ketoconazole, itraconazole, and ritonavir)

Interactions
DRUGS
alpha-blockers: Possibly increased risk of orthostatic hypotension
antihypertensives: Increased risk of dizziness and orthostatic hypotension
CYP3A4 inhibitors such as clarithromycin, diltiazem, erythromycin, itraconazole, ketoconazole, ritonavir; strong P-glycoprotein inhibitors such as cyclosporine: Increased serum silodosin levels and risk of adverse reactions

Adverse Reactions
CNS: Asthenia, dizziness, headache, insomnia, syncope
CV: Orthostatic hypotension
EENT: Nasal congestion, nasopharyngitis, rhinorrhea, sinusitis
GI: Abdominal pain, diarrhea, elevated liver enzymes, impaired hepatic function, jaundice

GU: Elevated prostate specific antigen level, retrograde ejaculation
SKIN: Pruritus, purpura, rash, **toxic skin eruption**, urticaria
Other: **Angioedema**

Childbearing Considerations

PREGNANCY
- Drug is not indicated for use in women.

LACTATION
- Drug is not indicated for use in women.

REPRODUCTION
- Male infertility is possible and may be reversible, if it occurs.

Nursing Considerations
- Use cautiously in patients with mild renal impairment and mild or moderate hepatic impairment. Patients with moderate renal impairment need dosage adjustment.
- Monitor patient's blood pressure for reduction, especially if he takes an antihypertensive with silodosin.

PATIENT TEACHING
- Instruct patient to take drug with a meal.
- Tell patient who has difficulty swallowing capsules that he may carefully open the capsule and sprinkle the powder on a tablespoonful of applesauce and take within 5 minutes without chewing. He should then drink an 8-oz glass of cool water immediately afterward. Inform him that the applesauce should not be hot and it should be soft enough to be swallowed without chewing.
- Advise patient to avoid hazardous activities until drug's CNS effects are known.
- Advise patient planning cataract surgery or other ocular procedure to tell ophthalmologist that he takes silodosin or has taken it in the past because of potential adverse reactions.

simvastatin
Flolipid, Zocor

Class and Category
Pharmacologic class: HMG-CoA reductase inhibitor (statin)
Therapeutic class: Antilipemic

Indications and Dosages
❋ *As adjunct to treat hyperlipidemia (hypertriglyceridemia, mixed dyslipidemia,* *or primary dysbetalipoproteinemia or hyperlipidemia) to reduce risk of cardiovascular events and coronary heart disease mortality in patients at high risk*

ORAL SUSPENSION, TABLETS
Adults. *Initial:* 10 or 20 mg once daily in the evening. Dosage adjusted at 4-wk intervals, as needed, to achieve target LDL-cholesterol level. *Maintenance:* 5 to 40 mg once daily in the evening. *Maximum:* 40 mg daily (80 mg only for patient who has been taking 80 mg daily chronically for 12 months or more without evidence of muscle toxicity).
❋ *As adjunct to treat homozygous familial hypercholesterolemia*

TABLETS
Adults. *Initial:* 20 to 40 mg once daily in the evening. Dosage adjusted every 4 wk, as needed, to achieve target LDL-cholesterol level. *Maximum:* 40 mg once daily.
❋ *As adjunct to treat adolescent heterozygous familial hypercholesterolemia*

TABLETS (ZOCOR)
Children ages 10 to 17 with girls at least 1 year post-menarche. *Initial:* 10 mg daily in the evening. Adjusted every 4 wk, as needed, to achieve target LDL-cholesterol level. *Maintenance:* 10 to 40 mg once daily in the evening. *Maximum:* 40 mg once daily.

ORAL SUSPENSION (FLOLIPID)
Children ages 10 to 17 with girls at least 1 year post-menarche. 5 to 40 mg once daily in the evening on empty stomach.

±**DOSAGE ADJUSTMENT** For patients with severe renal impairment, initial dosage reduced to 5 mg daily. For patients who are taking diltiazem, dronedarone, or verapamil, daily dosage should not exceed 10 mg; for patients who take amiodarone, amlodipine, or ranolazine, daily dosage should not exceed 20 mg. For patient taking lomitapide, daily dosage reduced by 50% and maximum dosage should not exceed 20 mg (40 mg once daily for patients previously taking 80 mg daily chronically while taking lomitapide). For patients at high risk of coronary artery disease event due to existing CHD, diabetes, peripheral vessel disease, or history of stroke or other cerebrovascular disease and taking oral suspension, initial dosage started and maintained at 40 mg once daily.

Q
R
S

Drug Administration
P.O.

- Administer drug in the evening with or without food for tablet form and on an empty stomach for oral suspension.
- Give drug 1 hour before or 4 hours after giving bile acid sequestrant, cholestyramine, or colestipol.
- Shake oral suspension bottle well for at least 20 seconds before using.
- Use a calibrated device to measure oral suspension dosage.
- Store oral suspension at room temperature and protect from heat. Discard within 30 days after opening.

Route	Onset	Peak	Duration
P.O.	> 3 wk	1.3–2.4 hr	Unknown

Half-life: 1–2 hr

Mechanism of Action

Interferes with the hepatic enzyme hydroxymethylglutaryl-coenzyme A reductase. This action reduces the formation of mevalonic acid, a cholesterol precursor, thus interrupting the pathway necessary for cholesterol synthesis. When the cholesterol level declines in hepatic cells, LDLs are consumed, which in turn reduces the levels of circulating total cholesterol and serum triglycerides.

Contraindications

Active hepatic disease; breastfeeding; concurrent use with concurrent use with strong CYP3A4 inhibitors such as boceprevir, clarithromycin, cobicistat-containing products, erythromycin, HIV protease inhibitors, itraconazole, ketoconazole, nefazodone, posaconazole, telaprevir, or telithromycin; concurrent use with cyclosporine, danazol, or gemfibrozil; hypersensitivity to simvastatin or its components; pregnancy

Interactions
DRUGS

amiodarone, antiretroviral protease inhibitors boceprevir, calcium channel blockers (amlodipine, diltiazem, verapamil), cobicistat-containing products, clarithromycin, colchicine, cyclosporine, danazol, daptomycin, dronedarone, erythromycin, gemfibrozil and other fibrates, itraconazole, ketoconazole, nefazodone, niacin (1 g daily or more), posaconazole, ranolazine, telaprevir, telithromycin, voriconazole: Increased risk of myopathy or rhabdomyolysis
digoxin: Possibly slight elevation in blood digoxin level
oral anticoagulants: Increased bleeding or prolonged PT

FOODS

grapefruit juice (1 or more quarts daily): Increased risk of myopathy or rhabdomyolysis

Adverse Reactions

CNS: Asthenia, cognitive impairment, dizziness, fatigue, headache, insomnia, vertigo
CV: **Atrial fibrillation**, chest pain, edema
EENT: Cataracts, rhinitis, sinusitis
ENDO: Elevated hemoglobin A_{1c} levels, hyperglycemia
GI: Abdominal pain, constipation, diarrhea, elevated liver enzymes, flatulence, gastritis, heartburn, **hepatic failure**, indigestion, nausea, **pancreatitis**, vomiting
GU: Erectile dysfunction, UTI
MS: Immune-mediated necrotizing myopathy, myalgia, myopathy, **rhabdomyolysis**
RESP: Bronchitis, **interstitial lung disease**, upper respiratory tract infection
SKIN: Eczema, pruritus, rash

Childbearing Considerations
PREGNANCY

- Drug may cause fetal harm.
- Drug should not be given during pregnancy.
- Drug should be discontinued immediately when pregnancy becomes known.

LACTATION

- It is not known if drug is present in breast milk.
- Breastfeeding is not recommended during drug therapy.

REPRODUCTION

- Women of childbearing age should be advised to use effective contraception throughout drug therapy.

Nursing Considerations

- Be aware concurrent therapy with niacin (greater than 1 g daily) and simvastatin is not recommended for use with Chinese patients because of increased risk of myopathy.

- Use simvastatin cautiously in elderly patients and those with hepatic or renal impairment.
- Know that 80 mg of simvastatin should be used rarely, since it is associated with a high risk of myopathy. If 40 mg of simvastatin is not sufficiently efficacious, then an alternative agent should be used.
- Monitor serum lipoprotein level, as ordered, to evaluate response to therapy.
- Expect to obtain liver enzymes prior to initiation of simvastatin therapy and then thereafter, as needed.
- Monitor patient for elevated CPK level (as ordered) or for muscle pain, tenderness, or weakness and other symptoms of myopathy; if left unchecked, the more serious form—rhabdomyolysis—may occur, which may lead to renal failure. Risk factors for myopathy include being 65 years or older, of female gender, and having renal impairment or uncontrolled hypothyroidism. If CPK level is significantly elevated or patient has symptoms of myopathy, notify prescriber and expect to withhold drug, as ordered.

PATIENT TEACHING

- Advise patient to take tablet in the evening. Tell patient taking oral suspension form to take drug in the evening on an empty stomach. Instruct patient to shake oral suspension form for at least 20 seconds before measuring dose and to use a calibrated device, not a household spoon, to measure dosage. Inform patient oral suspension may be stored at room temperature but discarded after 30 days.
- Instruct patient to follow low-fat, cholesterol-lowering diet.
- Urge patient to notify prescriber immediately about muscle pain, tenderness, or weakness and other symptoms of myopathy and symptoms of abnormal liver function such as anorexia, dark urine, fatigue, right upper abdominal discomfort, or yellowing of skin.
- Inform female patient of childbearing age of need to use reliable contraceptive method while taking drug. Instruct her to notify prescriber at once if she suspects pregnancy.
- Advise patient to avoid grapefruit juice to decrease risk of drug toxicity.

- Inform patient with diabetes of need to test his blood sugar regularly and to obtain an HbA_{1c} periodically.
- Encourage patient or family to notify prescriber if patient develops or exhibits confusion, forgetfulness, and worsening memory loss.

siponimod
Mayzent

☰ Class and Category
Pharmacologic class: Sphingosine-1-phosphate (S1P) receptor modulator
Therapeutic class: Anti-inflammatory

☰ Indications and Dosages
✳ *To treat relapsing forms of multiple sclerosis, including active secondary progressive disease, clinically isolated syndrome, and relapsing-remitting disease*

TABLETS
Adults with CYP2C9 genotypes *1/*1, *1/*2, or *2/*2. *Initial titration:* 0.25 mg once daily on days 1 and 2; 0.5 mg once daily on day 3; 0.75 mg once daily on day 4; and 1.25 mg once daily on day 5, followed by maintenance dose. *Maintenance:* 2 mg once daily beginning on day 6.
Adults with CYP2C9 genotypes *1/*3 and *2/*3. *Initial titration:* 0.25 mg once daily on days 1 and 2; 0.5 mg once daily on day 3; and 0.75 mg once daily on day 4, followed by maintenance dose. *Maintenance:* 1 mg once daily beginning on day 5.

±**DOSAGE ADJUSTMENT** If one initial titration dose is missed for more than 24 hours, treatment reinitiated with day 1 of the titration regimen. If maintenance treatment is interrupted for 4 or more consecutive daily doses, treatment reinitiated with day 1 of titration regimen.

☰ Drug Administration
P.O.
- Tablets should be swallowed whole and not chewed, crushed, or divided.
- Expect to monitor patient for 6 hours or more after first dose according to manufacturer guidelines.
- Store unopened containers of drug in refrigerator.

- Drug may be stored at room temperature for 3 months. If storage needed for more than 3 months, unopened containers can be stored in refrigerator until needed.

Route	Onset	Peak	Duration
P.O.	Unknown	4 hr	Unknown
Half-life: 30 hr			

Mechanism of Action

Binds with high affinity to S1P receptors 1 and 5. This blocks the capacity of lymphocytes to egress from lymph nodes, reducing the number of lymphocytes in peripheral blood and lymphocyte migration into the central nervous system.

Contraindications

CVA; CYP2C9 *3/*3 genotype; decompensated heart failure requiring hospitalization; history within past 6 months of class III or IV heart failure; hypersensitivity to siponimod or its components; MI, TIA, or unstable angina; presence of Mobitz type II second-degree AV block, third-degree AV block, or sick sinus syndrome, unless a functioning pacemaker is in place

Interactions

DRUGS

class 1a (procainamide, quinidine), class III (amiodarone, sotalol), drugs that decrease heart rate (digoxin, diltiazem, ivabradine, verapamil), QT prolongation drugs: Increased risk of bradycardia or torsades de pointes
antineoplastics, immune-modulating agents, immunosuppressants: Increased risk of additive immune effects
beta-blockers: Additive lowering of heart rate
CYP2C9 inducers, CYP3A4 inducers: Significant decrease in siponimod exposure
CYP2C9 inhibitors, CYP3A4 inhibitors: Significant increase in siponimod exposure, increasing risk of adverse reactions
live attenuated vaccines: Increased risk of infection
nonlive vaccines: Possibly diminished therapeutic effect of vaccine

Adverse Reactions

CNS: Asthenia, CVA (ischemic), dizziness, falling, headache, MI, seizures, tremor
CV: AV block (1st or 2nd degree), bradycardia, hypertension, peripheral edema

EENT: Macular edema
GI: Diarrhea, elevated liver enzymes, nausea
HEME: Lymphopenia
MS: Extremity pain
RESP: Decreased pulmonary function, pulmonary embolism
SKIN: Cutaneous malignancies
Other: Herpes zoster, serious infections

Childbearing Considerations

PREGNANCY

- Drug may cause fetal harm, according to animal studies.
- Use with caution only if benefit to mother outweighs potential risk to fetus.

LACTATION

- It is not known if drug is present in breast milk.
- Patient should check with prescriber before breastfeeding.

REPRODUCTION

- Women of childbearing age should use an effective contraceptive throughout siponimod therapy and for 10 days following drug discontinuation.

Nursing Considerations

- Use siponimod cautiously in patients with a history of significant liver disease because siponimod may affect liver function.
- Ensure that all of the following have been assessed before the initiation of siponimod therapy: complete blood count, CYP2C9 genotype determination, and liver function studies (bilirubin and transaminase levels within past 6 months). Also ensure that patient has had a cardiac examination (ECG, to determine whether preexisting conduction abnormalities are present), ophthalmic evaluation (including an evaluation of the fundus and the macula), current or prior medications (especially drugs that could slow heart rate or affect atrioventricular conduction; antineoplastics, immunosuppressives, or immune-modulating therapies that could cause additive immunosuppressive effects); and vaccinations (patient tested for antibodies to *varicella zoster* virus, with negative test results requiring vaccination prior to starting therapy).
- Know that with the first dose, 6-hour monitoring should be done, especially in patients with sinus bradycardia

(heart rate less than 55 beats/minute) or first- or second-degree AV block and in patients with a history of heart failure or myocardial infarction. First dose should be administered in a setting to manage symptomatic bradycardia. Monitor patient for 6 hours after administering dose, with hourly blood pressure and pulse measurements. Obtain an ECG at the end of day 1. After day 1, determine if patient has any of the following abnormalities (even in the absence of symptoms) and continue monitoring patient until the abnormality resolves: heart rate 6 hours postdose is less than 45 beats per minute, heart rate 6 hours postdose is at the lowest value postdose, or ECG 6 hours postdose shows new-onset second-degree or higher AV block. If postdose symptomatic bradycardia, bradyarrhythmia, or conduction-related symptoms occur, if ECG 6 hours postdose shows new-onset second-degree or higher AV block, or QTc is greater than or equal to 500 msec, expect to initiate appropriate management, as ordered. Begin continuous ECG monitoring and continue monitoring patient until symptoms have resolved. If drug treatment is required, expect patient to be monitored overnight and the 6-hour monitoring period repeated after the second dose. Also, expect a consultation with a cardiologist to be ordered.

- Evaluate patient for signs and symptoms of an infection before siponimod therapy is begun. Review patient's recent CBC results. Know that drug should not be started in patients with a severe active infection until the infection is resolved. Also, be aware that patients should continue to be monitored for infection until at least 3 to 4 weeks after drug is discontinued. Provide treatment for an infection, as prescribed, and expect drug to be temporarily withheld if a serious infection develops. Know that life-threatening infections such as cryptococcal meningitis and disseminated cryptococcal infections have occurred, along with cases of herpes viral infection that may lead to varicella zoster meningitis. Although progressive multifocal leukoencephalopathy has not occurred with siponimod therapy, it has occurred in similar treatment modalities in patients with multiple sclerosis.

- Be aware that patients with a history of uveitis or who have diabetes mellitus are at increased risk of macular edema during siponimod therapy. Monitor patient for any visual changes.
- Monitor patient's liver enzymes, as ordered. Assess patient for signs and symptoms of liver dysfunction such as abdominal pain, anorexia, dark urine, fatigue, jaundice, nausea, rash, and vomiting. Report such findings to prescriber.
- Monitor patient's vital signs throughout siponimod therapy, as bradycardia and hypertension can occur along with conduction defects.
- Be aware of the possibility that posterior reversible encephalopathy syndrome may occur with siponimod therapy. Report any unexpected neurological or psychiatric signs and symptoms to prescriber. If disorder is suspected, expect drug to be discontinued.
- Monitor patient for severe increased disability after siponimod therapy has been discontinued. Although rare, stopping siponimod therapy may exacerbate multiple sclerosis and cause a disease rebound.
- Be aware that it may take up to 4 weeks after siponimod therapy is discontinued for the pharmacodynamic effects on the patient's immune system to end. During this time, caution should be used in prescribing immunosuppressants.
- Assess patient's skin regularly for abnormalities because drug may cause cutaneous malignancies.

PATIENT TEACHING

- Stress importance of taking siponimod exactly as prescribed. If a dose is missed for longer than 24 hours during the titration period, the period will have to be restarted with day 1; if maintenance doses are missed for more than 4 days, a titration period will have to be done again, including a first-dose 6-hour monitoring period. Advise patient not to stop taking drug without first discussing concerns with prescriber.
- Prepare patient for the 6-hour monitoring period required for the first dose.
- Tell patient to swallow tablet whole and not to chew, crush, or divide tablets.
- Tell patient drug may be stored at room temperature for up to 3 months and

should not be refrigerated after container is opened. However, tell patient unopened containers expected to be used after 3 months of obtaining drug should be stored in refrigerator.

- Review infection control measures with patient. Caution patient to avoid anyone with an infection. Tell patient to notify prescriber if infection occurs.
- Warn patient to avoid receiving live attenuated vaccines while taking siponimod and for 4 weeks after drug is discontinued.
- Stress importance of having regular eye examinations during siponimod therapy and tell patient to report any visual changes to prescriber immediately.
- Advise patient to contact prescriber if new-onset or worsening dyspnea occurs.
- Review signs and symptoms of liver dysfunction with patient and tell patient to contact prescriber if present.
- Instruct patient to inspect skin regularly for abnormalities and report any such findings to prescriber.
- Tell patient that upon discontinuation of drug, a rebound effect may occur, exhibited by an exacerbation of the condition.
- Inform women of childbearing age of the possibility of fetal harm with drug therapy; instruct them to use effective contraception throughout therapy and for 10 days after drug is discontinued. Stress importance of reporting suspected or known pregnancy to prescriber at once.
- Advise patient that drug effects last for up to 4 weeks after drug is discontinued.

sirolimus

(rapamycin)

Rapamune

Class and Category

Pharmacologic class: Macrocyclic lactone
Therapeutic class: Immunosuppressant

Indications and Dosages

* *To prevent rejection of kidney transplantation*

ORAL SOLUTION, TABLETS

Adults at high-immunologic risk. *Initial:* Up to 15-mg loading dose on day 1 post-transplantation. *Maintenance:*

5 mg daily beginning on day 2, with dosage adjusted based on trough level taken between days 5 and 7, as needed, with further adjustments made, as needed, every 7 to 14 days. *Maximum:* 40 mg daily.
Adults and adolescents weighing 40 kg (88 lb) or more at low- to moderate-immunologic risk. *Initial:* 6-mg loading dose. *Maintenance:* 2 mg daily, with dosage adjusted according to trough levels, every 7 to 14 days, as needed. *Maximum:* 40 mg daily.
Adolescents weighing less than 40 kg (88 lb) at low- to moderate-immunologic risk. *Initial:* 3-mg/m^2 loading dose. *Maintenance:* 1 mg/m^2 daily.

* *To treat lymphangioleiomyomatosis*

ORAL SOLUTION, TABLETS

Adults. 2 mg daily, dosage adjusted according to trough level 10 to 20 days later, then every 7 to 14 days, as needed, until a stable maintenance dose achieved.

±**DOSAGE ADJUSTMENT** Maintenance dosage adjustment reduced by one-third for patients with mild-to-moderate impaired hepatic function and one-half for patients with severe impaired hepatic function.

Maintenance dosage increased for patients discontinuing concomitant cyclosporine therapy.

Drug Administration

P.O.

- Give initial dose as soon after transplantation as possible, as prescribed and daily dose 4 hours after cyclosporine, as prescribed.
- Administer drug consistently either with or without food to prevent changes in absorption rate.
- Tablets should be swallowed whole and not chewed, crushed, or divided.
- If oral suspension is stored in refrigerator, a slight haze may be present. If so, bring solution to room temperature and then shake gently until haze disappears. Use only the amber oral dose syringe supplied to withdraw prescribed amount of drug from bottle after fitting the oral syringe adapter to the neck of drug bottle. Mix oral solution with at least 2 oz (60 ml) of orange juice or water in a glass or plastic container but not Styrofoam. Don't dilute drug in grapefruit juice or any other liquid. Stir well and have

patient drink solution immediately. Then rinse glass with at least 4 oz (120 ml) of additional liquid, stir vigorously, and have patient drink that liquid to make sure that all of drug is taken.

- Oral solution is usually stored in refrigerator but may be left at room temperature for no more than 15 days; if stored in oral amber syringe, it may be stored at room temperature for 24 hours.
- Discard oral solution after 1 month.
- When storing tablets or oral solution, protect from light.
- Avoid direct contact with skin or mucous membranes; if it occurs, wash area thoroughly with soap and water; rinse eyes with plain water.

Route	Onset	Peak	Duration
P.O.	Unknown	1–6 hr	Unknown

Half-life: 46–78 hr

Mechanism of Action

Inhibits activation and proliferation of T lymphocytes and antibody production. Sirolimus also inhibits cell cycle progression from the G_1 to the S phase, possibly by inhibiting a key regulatory kinase believed to suppress cytokine-driven T-cell proliferation. These actions interfere with body rejecting the transplanted kidney and abnormal growth of muscle-like cells that occur in lymphangioleiomyomatosis.

Contraindications

Hypersensitivity to sirolimus or its components, malignancy

Interactions

DRUGS

cyclosporine; strong CYP3A4 and P-gp inhibitors such as clarithromycin, erythromycin, itraconazole, ketoconazole, telithromycin, voriconazole; weak or moderate CYP3A4 and P-gp inhibitors such as bromocriptine, cimetidine, diapride, clotrimazole, danazol, diltiazem, fluconazole, metoclopramide, nicardipine, protease inhibitors (boceprevir, indinavir, ritonavir, telaprevir),troleandomycin, verapamil: Increased sirolimus concentrations, increasing risk of adverse reactions
strong CYP3A4 and P-gp inducers such as rifabutin, rifampin; weak to moderate

CYP3A4 and P-g[inducers such as carbamazepine, phenobarbital, phenytoin, rifapentine, St. John's wort: Decreased sirolimus concentrations, decreasing effectiveness
live vaccines: Vaccination may be less effective
verapamil: Increased concentrations of verapamil

FOODS

grapefruit juice: Possibly decreased metabolism of sirolimus

Adverse Reactions

CNS: Asthenia, dizziness, fever, headache, insomnia, **posterior reversible encephalopathy syndrome, progressive multifocal leukoencephalopathy (PML),** tremor
CV: Atrial fibrillation, chest pain, **deep vein thrombosis,** hyperlipidemia, hypersensitivity vasculitis, hypertension, hypertriglyceridemia, **pericardial effusion,** peripheral edema, **tachycardia**
EENT: Epistaxis, nasopharyngitis, stomatitis
ENDO: Hyperglycemia
GI: Abdominal pain, ascites, constipation, diarrhea, elevated liver enzymes, **hepatic artery thrombosis** (liver transplant), **hepatotoxicity,** nausea, **pancreatitis,** vomiting
GU: Azoospermia, BK viral nephritis, elevated serum creatinine level, focal segmental glomerulosclerosis, **hemolytic uremic syndrome,** menstrual disorders, **nephrotic syndrome,** ovarian cysts, proteinuria, **pyelonephritis,** UTI
HEME: Anemia, **leukopenia, neutropenia, pancytopenia, thrombocytopenia, thrombocytopenic purpura**
MS: Arthralgia, bone necrosis, low back or flank pain, joint abnormality, myalgia
RESP: Alveolar proteinosis, **bronchial anastomotic dehiscence** (lymphangioleiomyomatosis after lung transplant), dyspnea on exertion, **interstitial lung disease,** pleural effusion, pneumonia, **pulmonary embolism or hemorrhage,** upper respiratory tract infection
SKIN: Acne, **cancer including melanoma and Merkel cell carcinoma, exfoliative dermatitis,** rash
Other: Anaphylaxis; angioedema; cytomegalovirus; delayed wound healing;

Epstein–Barr virus; herpes simplex or zoster; **hypokalemia**; **hypophosphatemia**; increased susceptibility to infection, including opportunistic infections such as tuberculosis and activation of latent viral infections; lymphedema; lymphocele; **lymphoma**; **sepsis**; weight gain or loss

Childbearing Considerations

PREGNANCY

- Drug can cause fetal harm.
- Drug should be discontinued immediately when pregnancy is known.

LACTATION

- It is not known if drug is present in breast milk but due to drug's mechanism of action it may cause serious adverse effects in breastfed infants.
- A decision should be made to discontinue breastfeeding or the drug to avoid potential serious adverse reactions in the breastfed infant.

REPRODUCTION

- Women of childbearing age should be advised to use effective contraception throughout drug therapy and for 12 weeks after drug has been discontinued.
- Both female and male fertility may be affected by drug use; females may develop menstrual disorders (including amenorrhea and menorrhagia) and ovarian cysts and males may develop azoospermia.

Nursing Considerations

- Be aware that sirolimus isn't recommended in liver or lung transplant patients.
- Use sirolimus cautiously in patients who are receiving other drugs known to adversely affect renal function, such as aminoglycosides and amphotericin B; together, they may further decrease renal function.
- Monitor patients with existing or recent (including recent exposure to) chickenpox and patients with herpes zoster for worsening symptoms because they have an increased risk of developing severe generalized disease while taking sirolimus.
- Monitor whole blood sirolimus concentrations, as ordered, in patients receiving concentrated form of drug, patients with hepatic impairment or weighing less than 40 kg (88 lb), and those receiving potent CYP3A4 inducers or inhibitors concurrently.
- Know that when using trough level to determine drug's effectiveness, dosage adjustment should be made only after other factors are taken into account, such as signs, symptoms, and tissue biopsy findings. Keep in mind that interpretation methods vary among laboratories and values aren't interchangeable.
- Monitor serum creatinine level, as ordered, because BK virus-associated nephropathy has occurred with sirolimus therapy. In addition, patients receiving sirolimus and cyclosporine may develop impaired renal function. Notify prescriber of any increases in serum creatinine level because sirolimus or cyclosporine dosage may have to be adjusted or drug discontinued.
- Monitor patient for urinary protein excretion, as ordered. If protein appears in urine, sirolimus may have to be discontinued.
- Monitor patient for signs and symptoms of infection and check CBC results, as ordered, to detect sirolimus-induced blood dyscrasias or changes in neutrophil count, which may indicate infection.
- For patients with hyperlipidemia, keep in mind the potential need to institute dietary changes, an exercise program, or a lipid-lowering drug regimen if blood cholesterol or triglyceride levels increase, because drug may aggravate hyperlipidemia.
- Monitor patients with wounds who are taking sirolimus because drug may impair or delay wound healing, especially in patients with a body mass index greater than 30 kg/m².

PATIENT TEACHING

- Advise patient to take sirolimus consistently either with or without food to prevent changes in absorption rate.
- Advise patient prescribed tablet form not to chew, crush, or split the tablets but to take whole.
- Instruct patient to take daily dose with at least 2 oz (60 ml) of orange juice or water. Caution him not to dilute drug in grapefruit juice or any other liquid. Advise him to stir mixture well and drink immediately, then to add at least another 4 oz (120 ml) of liquid to empty container, stir mixture again,

and drink that liquid to ensure that he has swallowed all of drug.

- Urge patient to avoid people with cold, flu, or other infections because immunosuppression makes him more vulnerable.
- Instruct patient not to take live vaccines during sirolimus therapy.
- Inform patient that sirolimus therapy may increase his risk of skin cancer. Tell him to avoid prolonged sun exposure, sun lamps, and tanning booths. He should use a sunscreen with a high protection factor and wear protective clothing when outdoors.
- Advise patient to keep follow-up appointments for blood tests, as ordered.
- Advise women of childbearing age that sirolimus may be harmful to unborn child. Stress importance of using an effective contraceptive before therapy starts, throughout therapy, and for 12 weeks after therapy is ended. If pregnancy does occur, instruct patient to notify prescriber immediately.

sitagliptin phosphate
Januvia

☰ Class and Category
Pharmacologic class: Dipeptidyl peptidase-4 (DPP-4) inhibitor

☰ Indications and Dosages
* *As adjunct to achieve control of glucose level in type 2 diabetes mellitus*

TABLETS
Adults. 100 mg once daily.
±**DOSAGE ADJUSTMENT** For patients with moderate renal insufficiency (estimated glomerular filtration rate of 30 ml/min to less than 45 ml/min), dosage reduced to 50 mg once daily; for patients with severe renal insufficiency (estimated glomerular filtration rate less than 30 ml/min) or end-stage renal disease requiring hemodialysis or peritoneal dialysis, dosage reduced to 25 mg once daily.

☰ Drug Administration
P.O.
- Administer tablets at about same time daily to maintain consistency.
- Can be given with or without food.

- Tablets should be swallowed whole and not chewed, crushed, or divided.

Route	Onset	Peak	Duration
P.O.	Unknown	1–4 hr	Unknown

Half-life: 12.4 hr

☰ Mechanism of Action
Inhibits the dipeptidyl peptidase-4 enzyme to slow inactivation of incretin hormones. These hormones are released by the intestine throughout the day but increase in response to a meal. When blood glucose level is normal or increased, incretin hormones increase insulin synthesis and release from pancreatic beta cells. One type of incretin hormone, glucagon-like peptide (GLP-1), also lowers glucagon secretion from pancreatic alpha cells, which reduces hepatic glucose production. These combined actions decrease blood glucose level in type 2 diabetes.

☰ Contraindications
Hypersensitivity to sitagliptin or its components

☰ Interactions
DRUGS
digoxin: Slightly increased plasma digoxin level
insulin or insulin secretagogue such as sulfonylureas: Possibly increased hypoglycemic effects

☰ Adverse Reactions
CNS: Headache
CV: **Heart failure**
EENT: Mouth ulceration, nasopharyngitis, stomatitis
GI: Abdominal pain, **acute pancreatitis**, constipation, diarrhea, elevated liver enzymes, nausea, vomiting
GU: **Acute renal failure**, worsening renal function
RESP: Upper respiratory tract infection
MS: Arthralgia (disabling, severe), back or extremity pain, myalgia
SKIN: Bullous pemphigoid, cutaneous vasculitis, rash, **Stevens–Johnson syndrome**, urticaria
Other: **Anaphylaxis, angioedema**

Q
R
S

⬛ Childbearing Considerations

PREGNANCY

- Pregnancy exposure registry: 1-800-986-8999.
- It is not known if drug can cause fetal harm.
- Use with caution only if benefit to mother outweighs potential risk to fetus.

LACTATION

- It is not known if drug is present in breast milk.
- Patient should check with prescriber before breastfeeding.

⬛ Nursing Considerations

- Assess patient's renal function before starting sitagliptin therapy, as ordered, and periodically thereafter. In moderate to severe renal dysfunction, dosage will be reduced and frequency of assessing renal function increased. Also know that renal function should be assessed more frequently in elderly patients because aging can be associated with reduced renal function.

! **WARNING** Monitor patient for hypersensitivity reactions that, although uncommon, may be severe. If present, notify prescriber and expect sitagliptin to be discontinued.

- Monitor patient's blood glucose level, as ordered, to determine effectiveness of sitagliptin therapy.
- Be aware that heart failure has occurred with two other drugs in the same class as sitagliptin. Monitor patient for signs and symptoms of heart failure and if present report immediately to prescriber; provide care according to standard protocols, as ordered; and know that sitagliptin may have to be discontinued.
- Monitor patient for hypoglycemia if drug is used in combination with insulin or insulin secretagogues such as sulfonylureas.

PATIENT TEACHING

- Emphasize the need to follow a diet control program and an exercise program during sitagliptin therapy.
- Warn patient not to chew, crush, or split the tablet before swallowing. Also, tell patient to take drug at about the same time every day with or without food.

! **WARNING** Advise patient to notify prescriber immediately if she has trouble breathing, or has hives, rash, or swelling.

- Inform patient that periodic blood tests will be done to determine effectiveness of drug and to assess kidney function.
- Teach patient how to monitor blood glucose level and when to report changes.
- Alert patient also taking insulin or insulin secretagogues such as a sulfonylurea that hypoglycemia may occur. Instruct patient how to recognize and treat hypoglycemia and to notify prescriber if it occurs.
- Caution patient that taking other drugs in addition to sitagliptin to control his diabetes or taking certain drugs to treat other conditions may lead to hypoglycemia. Review signs, symptoms, and appropriate prescribed treatment for hypoglycemia with him.
- Instruct patient to contact prescriber if he develops other illnesses, such as infection, or experiences surgery or trauma, because his diabetes medication may require adjustment.
- Advise patient to carry identification indicating that she has diabetes.
- Instruct patient to stop taking sitagliptin and report persistent severe abdominal pain, possibly radiating to the back and accompanied by vomiting.
- Review signs and symptoms of heart failure, such as rapid weight increase, shortness of breath, or swelling in feet. Instruct patient to immediately report such to prescriber.
- Tell patient to report development of blisters or erosions while receiving sitagliptin therapy.

sodium bicarbonate

Baking Soda, Sellymin (CAN)

⬛ Class and Category

Pharmacologic class: Electrolyte
Therapeutic class: Antacid, electrolyte replenisher, systemic and urinary alkalizer

⬛ Indications and Dosages

✽ *To treat hyperacidity*

ORAL POWDER

Adults and adolescents. One-half teaspoon every 2 hr, as needed. *Maximum:* 4 teaspoons daily.

TABLETS

Adults and adolescents. 325 mg to 2 g daily to four times a day, as needed. *Maximum:* 16 g daily.

Children ages 6 to 12. 520 mg, repeated once after 30 min, as needed.

✳ *To provide urinary alkalization*

ORAL POWDER

Adults and adolescents. 1 teaspoon every 4 hr. *Maximum:* 4 teaspoons daily.

TABLETS

Adults and adolescents. *Initial:* 4 g, then 1 to 2 g every 4 hr. *Maximum:* 16 g daily.

Children. 23 to 230 mg/kg daily, adjusted as needed.

±**DOSAGE ADJUSTMENT** Dosage reduction possible for elderly patients because of age-related renal impairment.

☰ Drug Administration

P.O.

- Administer 2 hours before or after other oral drugs.
- Mix powder in at least 120 ml of water before administering.
- Use a calibrated device to measure dosage of powder form.

Route	Onset	Peak	Duration
P.O.	Unknown	1–2.5 hr	Unknown

Half-life: Unknown

☰ Mechanism of Action

Buffers excess hydrogen ions, increases plasma bicarbonate level, and raises blood pH, thereby reversing metabolic acidosis. Sodium bicarbonate also increases the excretion of free bicarbonate ions in urine, raising urine pH; increased alkalinity of urine may help to dissolve uric acid calculi. In addition, it relieves symptoms of hyperacidity by neutralizing or buffering existing stomach acid, thereby increasing the pH of stomach contents.

☰ Contraindications

Loss of chloride through vomiting or continuous gastrointestinal suction, use of diuretic therapy known to produce a hypochloremic alkalosis

☰ Interactions

DRUGS

amphetamines, quinidine: Decreased urinary excretion of these drugs, possibly resulting in toxicity

calcium-containing products: Increased risk of milk-alkali syndrome

ciprofloxacin, norfloxacin, ofloxacin: Decreased solubility of these drugs, leading to crystalluria and nephrotoxicity

citrates: Increased risk of systemic alkalosis; increased risk of calcium calculus formation and hypernatremia in patients with history of uric acid calculi

digoxin: Possibly elevated digoxin level

H_2-receptor antagonists, iron preparations or supplements, ketoconazole: Decreased absorption of these drugs

urinary acidifiers (ammonium chloride, ascorbic acid, potassium and sodium phosphates): Counteracted effects of urinary acidifiers

FOODS

dairy products: Increased risk of milk-alkali syndrome with prolonged use of sodium bicarbonate

☰ Adverse Reactions

CNS: Mental or mood changes

CV: Irregular heartbeat, peripheral edema (with large doses), weak pulse

EENT: Dry mouth

GI: Abdominal cramps, thirst

MS: Muscle spasms, myalgia

SKIN: Extravasation of I.V. with necrosis, tissue sloughing, or ulceration

☰ Childbearing Considerations

PREGNANCY

- It is not known if drug can cause fetal harm.
- Use with caution only if benefit to mother outweighs potential risk to fetus.
- Be aware that drug increases risk of metabolic acidosis and edema in pregnant women.

LACTATION

- It is not known if drug is present in breast milk.
- Patient should check with prescriber before breastfeeding.

☰ Nursing Considerations

- Monitor sodium intake of patient taking sodium bicarbonate oral powder because it contains 952 mg of sodium/tsp; and tablets contain 325 mg/3.9-mEq tablet, 520 mg/ 6.2-mEq tablet, and 650 mg/ 7.7-mEq tablet.

- Monitor urine pH, as ordered, to determine drug's effectiveness as urine alkalizer.
- Know that if patient on long-term sodium bicarbonate therapy is consuming calcium or milk, watch for milk-alkali syndrome, characterized by anorexia, confusion, headache, hypercalcemia, metabolic acidosis, nausea, renal insufficiency, and vomiting.

PATIENT TEACHING

- Instruct patient to mix powder with 4 ounces of water before taking drug.
- Advise patient not to take sodium bicarbonate with large amounts of dairy products or for longer than 2 weeks, unless directed by prescriber.
- Caution patient not to take more drug than prescribed, to avoid adverse reactions.
- Direct patient not to take drug within 2 hours of other oral drugs.
- Advise patient to avoid taking other prescribed or OTC drugs without prescriber's approval, because many drugs interact with sodium bicarbonate.

sodium ferric gluconate

(contains 62.5 mg elemental iron per 5 ml)
Ferrlecit

≡ Class and Category

Pharmacologic class: Iron salt, mineral
Therapeutic class: Hematinic

≡ Indications and Dosages

✳ *To treat iron deficiency anemia in patients receiving long-term hemodialysis and supplemental epoetin therapy*

I.V. INFUSION OR INJECTION

Adults. 10 ml (125 mg of elemental iron) per dialysis session. *Maximum:* 125 mg per dose. *Usual:* Minimum cumulative dose of 1 g elemental iron given over eight sequential dialysis treatments. Dosage repeated at lowest dosage needed to maintain target levels of hemoglobin and hematocrit and acceptable limits of blood iron level.

I.V. INFUSION

Children age 6 and over. 0.12 ml/kg (1.5 mg/kg of elemental iron) per dialysis session. *Maximum:* 125 mg per dose.

≡ Drug Administration

I.V.

- For I.V. injection for adults, administer undiluted slowly at a rate of up to 12.5 mg/min per dialysis session.
- For I.V. infusion in adults, dilute in 100 ml of 0.9% Sodium Chloride Injection and infuse immediately over 1 hour per dialysis session.
- For I.V. infusion in children, dilute in 25 ml of 0.9% Sodium Chloride Injection and infuse immediately over 1 hour.
- *Incompatibilities:* Other I.V. drugs or solutions (other than 0.9% Sodium Chloride Injection), parenteral nutrition

Route	Onset	Peak	Duration
I.V.	Unknown	Varies	Unknown

Half-life: 1 hr

≡ Mechanism of Action

Acts to replenish iron stores lost during hemodialysis as a result of increased blood loss or increased iron utilization from epoetin therapy. Iron is an essential component of hemoglobin, myoglobin, and several enzymes, including catalase, cytochromes, and peroxidase, and is needed for catecholamine metabolism and normal neutrophil function. Sodium ferric gluconate also normalizes RBC production by binding with hemoglobin or being stored as ferritin in reticuloendothelial cells of the bone marrow, liver, and spleen.

≡ Contraindications

Hypersensitivity to sodium ferric gluconate or its components

≡ Interactions

DRUGS

oral iron preparations: Possibly reduced absorption of oral iron supplements

≡ Adverse Reactions

CNS: Asthenia, dizziness, fatigue, fever, headache, hypertonia, hypoesthesia, loss of consciousness, nervousness, paresthesia, **seizures,** syncope

CV: Chest pain, generalized edema, hypertension, **hypotension**, phlebitis, tachycardia
EENT: Dry mouth, taste altered
GI: Abdominal pain, diarrhea, nausea, vomiting
HEME: **Hemorrhage**
MS: Back pain, leg cramps
RESP: Cough, dyspnea, upper respiratory tract infection, wheezing
SKIN: Diaphoresis, pallor, pruritus, skin discoloration
Other: **Anaphylaxis**, generalized pain, **hyperkalemia**, **hypersensitivity reactions**, infusion or injection-site reaction including superficial thrombophlebitis, **shock**

⫶ Childbearing Considerations
PREGNANCY
- Drug can cause fetal harm under certain circumstances, especially in the second and third trimesters. For instance, drug may cause circulatory failure in mother, which in turn causes bradycardia in the fetus.
- Be aware that drug also contains benzyl alcohol, which does not appear to have an effect on fetus through maternal drug administration; however, it can cause serious adverse events and death when administered intravenously to neonates and infants.
- Use with caution only if benefit to mother outweighs potential risk to fetus.

LACTATION
- It is not known if drug is present in breast milk. However, benzyl alcohol is possibly present in breast milk and may be transferred to neonate during breastfeeding.
- Patient should check with prescriber before breastfeeding.

⫶ Nursing Considerations
- Be aware that most patients need a minimum cumulative dose of 1 g of elemental iron administered over eight sequential dialysis treatments.

❗ **WARNING** Assess patient for evidence of allergic reaction, including chills, facial flushing, pruritus, and rash, and of a hypersensitivity reaction, including diaphoresis, dyspnea, nausea, severe lower back pain, vomiting, and wheezing. Discontinue drug and notify prescriber immediately if patient develops an allergic or hypersensitivity reaction, and be prepared to provide emergency interventions.

❗ **WARNING** Assess blood pressure often after drug administration because hypotension may occur and may be related to infusion rate or total cumulative dose. Avoid rapid infusion, and be prepared to provide I.V. fluids for volume expansion.

- Expect to monitor blood hemoglobin level, hematocrit, serum ferritin level, and transferrin saturation, as ordered, before, during, and after sodium ferric gluconate therapy. Make sure serum iron level is tested 48 hours after last dose. To prevent iron toxicity, notify prescriber and expect to end therapy if blood iron level is normal or elevated.
- Assess patient for possible iron overload, characterized by bleeding in GI tract and lungs, decreased activity, pale conjunctivae, and sedation.

PATIENT TEACHING
- Warn patient not to take any oral iron preparations during sodium ferric gluconate therapy without first consulting prescriber.
- Inform patient that symptoms of iron deficiency may include decreased stamina, fatigue, learning problems, and shortness of breath.

❗ **WARNING** Stress importance of reporting an allergic reaction that may become serious.

- Tell women of childbearing age to notify prescriber if pregnancy is suspected or occurs.

sodium polystyrene sulfonate
K-Exit (CAN), Kionex, SPS Suspension

⫶ Class and Category
Pharmacologic class: Sulfonated cation-exchange resin
Therapeutic class: Antihyperkalemic

⫶ Indications and Dosages
✳ *To treat hyperkalemia*

ORAL POWDER, SUSPENSION

Adults. 15 g (4 level tsp) once daily to four times a day.

RECTAL POWDER, SUSPENSION

Adults. 30 to 50 g every 6 hr as retention enema, as needed.

Drug Administration

P.O.

- Suspend each dose of oral suspension in a small quantity of water or syrup (about 3 to 4 ml of liquid per gram of resin). Prepare fresh and use within 24 hours.
- Be sure to follow full aspiration precautions (such as keeping patient in an upright position while giving drug), because patients may be at risk of aspiration caused by inhalation of drug particles, especially patients with altered level of consciousness, impaired gag reflex, or who are prone to regurgitation. If needed, administer through gastric feeding tube.
- Administer other oral medication at least 3 hours before or 3 hours after sodium polystyrene sulfonate administration. However, patients with gastroparesis may require a 6-hour separation.

P.R.

- Precede rectal administration with a cleansing enema, as ordered.
- Mix powdered resin in 100 ml of aqueous solution in bag connected to soft, large (French 28) catheter.
- Solution should be at room temperature before administration.
- Have patient lie on his left side with his lower leg straight and upper leg flexed or with his knees to his chest.
- Gently insert the tube into the rectum and well into the sigmoid colon. The solution should flow into the colon by way of gravity and be retained for 30 to 60 minutes or longer, if possible.
- After patient is unable to retain the solution any longer, administer a non-sodium-containing cleansing enema, as prescribed.

Route	Onset	Peak	Duration
P.O.	2–12 hr	2–3 hr	4–6 hr
P.R.	30 min	Unknown	2–3 hr

Half-life: Unknown

Mechanism of Action

Releases sodium ions in exchange for other cations in intestines. Resin enters large intestine and releases sodium ions in exchange for hydrogen ions. As the resin moves through the intestines, hydrogen ions are then exchanged for potassium ions, which are in greater concentration. Bound resin leaves the body in feces, carrying potassium and other ions with it, thereby reducing serum potassium level.

Contraindications

Hypersensitivity to sodium polystyrene sulfonate or its components, hypokalemia, obstructive bowel disease, reduced intestinal motility in neonates

Interactions

DRUGS

nonabsorbable cation-donating antacids and laxatives: Reduced resin's potassium exchange capability, increased risk of systemic alkalosis
sorbitol: May contribute to risk of intestinal necrosis by sorbitol
other orally administered medications: Decreased absorption and reduced effectiveness of these drugs

Adverse Reactions

CV: Peripheral edema
GI: Abdominal cramps, anorexia, **colonic necrosis**, constipation, diarrhea, epigastric pain, fecal impaction, gastric irritation, **GI bleeding**, indigestion, **intestinal necrosis or obstruction**, **ischemic colitis**, nausea, ulcerations, vomiting
GU: Decreased urine output
RESP: Aspiration
Other: **Hypernatremia, hypocalcemia, hypokalemia, hypomagnesemia, metabolic alkalosis**, weight gain

Childbearing Considerations

PREGNANCY

- It is not known if drug can cause fetal harm.
- Use with caution only if benefit to mother outweighs potential risk to fetus.

LACTATION

- It is not known if drug is present in breast milk.
- Patient should check with prescriber before breastfeeding.

Nursing Considerations

- Know that sodium polystyrene sulfonate should not be given to a patient who has not had a bowel movement postsurgery, or in patients who are at risk for developing constipation or impaction (including patients with a history of chronic constipation, inflammatory bowel disease, impaction, ischemic colitis, previous bowel obstruction or resection, or vascular intestinal atherosclerosis) because these factors increase the risk for intestinal necrosis, which may be life-threatening.
- Use sodium polystyrene sulfonate cautiously in patients with heart failure, hypertension, or marked edema.
- Be aware that because the drug doesn't take effect for several hours, it's inappropriate for treating acute, life-threatening hyperkalemia.
- Assess patient for hypokalemia or hypocalcemia. If present, notify prescriber immediately and expect to withhold drug because it reduces calcium and potassium levels. Evidence of hypokalemia includes abdominal cramps, acidic urine, anorexia, drowsiness, ECG changes, hypotension, hypoventilation, muscle weakness, and tachycardia. Evidence of hypocalcemia includes abdominal pain, agitation, anxiety, ECG changes, hypotension, muscle twitching, psychosis, seizures, and tetany.
- Use of sorbitol with sodium polystyrene sulfonate isn't recommended because of increased risk of colonic necrosis and other serious GI effects, such as bleeding, ischemic colitis, and perforation.
- Assess for constipation and fecal impaction after administration. If either occurs, notify prescriber, expect drug to be discontinued, and provide care, as ordered, to relieve constipation or fecal impaction.

PATIENT TEACHING

- Instruct patient not to mix oral form of sodium polystyrene sulfonate with foods and liquids high in potassium content, such as bananas and orange juice.
- Teach patient who will self-administer rectal solution the correct technique and body position. Remind him a cleansing enema may be required before and after drug administration. Tell him to let the solution flow into the colon by gravity and to retain it for at least 30 to 60 minutes, longer if possible.
- Advise patient to notify prescriber immediately about abdominal cramps, nausea, and vomiting.

sodium zirconium cyclosilicate
Lokelma

Class and Category

Pharmacologic class: Potassium binder
Therapeutic class: Potassium reducer

Indications and Dosages

✳ *To treat hyperkalemia in nonlife-threatening situations*

ORAL SUSPENSION

Adults. *Initial:* 10 g three times daily for up to 48 hr. *Maintenance:* 10 g once daily. Dosage increased during maintenance in increments of 5 g at weekly or longer intervals, as needed, based on serum potassium. *Usual maintenance dosage range:* 5 g every other day to 15 g daily.

±**DOSAGE ADJUSTMENT** For patients on chronic hemodialysis, initial dose reduced to 5 mg once daily on nondialysis days. Initial dose of 10 mg may be given if patient's serum potassium level is greater than 6.5 mEq/L. Usual maintenance dose range is 5 to 15 mg once daily, on nondialysis days.

Drug Administration

P.O.

- Empty entire contents of packet into a drinking glass containing about 3 tablespoons of water or more, if patient desires. Stir well and administer immediately. If powder remains in the drinking glass, add more water, stir, and have patient drink immediately. Repeat until no powder remains, to ensure that entire dose has been given.
- Administer other oral drugs at least 2 hours before or after sodium zirconium cyclosilicate.

Route	Onset	Peak	Duration
P.O.	1 hr	1.2 hr	Unknown

Half-life: Unknown

Mechanism of Action

Increases fecal potassium excretion through binding of potassium in the lumen of the gastrointestinal tract. This reduces the concentration of free potassium in the gastrointestinal lumen, thereby lowering serum potassium levels.

Contraindications

Hypersensitivity to sodium zirconium cyclosilicate or its components

Interactions

DRUGS

oral drugs that have pH-dependent solubility: Altered absorption of these drugs, possibly causing altered efficacy or safety

Adverse Reactions

CV: Edema
Other: Hypokalemia

Childbearing Considerations

PREGNANCY

- Drug is not absorbed systemically and is not expected to affect the fetus.

LACTATION

- Drug is not absorbed systemically and is not expected to be present in breast milk.

Nursing Considerations

- Know that sodium zirconium cyclosilicate should not be given to patients with abnormal postoperative bowel motility disorders, bowel obstruction, bowel impaction, or severe constipation, because drug may be ineffective or even worsen these gastrointestinal conditions.
- Be aware that drug has radiopaque properties and may give the appearance of an imaging agent during abdominal X-ray procedures.
- Monitor patient for edema, especially patients who should restrict their sodium intake or are prone to fluid retention, such as those with heart failure or renal disease.
- Monitor patients on hemodialysis for acute illnesses associated with decreased oral intake or diarrhea that can increase the risk of hypokalemia during drug therapy.

PATIENT TEACHING

- Tell patient to empty entire contents of packet into a drinking glass containing about 3 tablespoons of water or more, if patient desires. Tell patient to stir well and drink immediately. If powder remains in the drinking glass, patient should add more water, stir, and drink contents immediately. Repeat until no powder remains, to ensure that entire dose has been given.
- Instruct patient to take other oral drugs at least 2 hours before or after sodium zirconium cyclosilicate administration, to prevent other drugs from not being absorbed properly.
- Advise patient to limit dietary sodium intake, if needed, and to notify prescriber if fluid retention occurs.
- Instruct patient to notify prescriber if an acute illness that restricts intake or causes diarrhea occurs, as dosage of drug may have to be adjusted.
- Tell patient to notify prescriber of sodium zirconium cyclosilicate use prior to an abdominal X-ray.

sofosbuvir
Sovaldi

Class and Category

Pharmacologic class: NS5B polymerase inhibitor
Therapeutic class: Antiviral

Indications and Dosages

⁂ *As adjunct to treat chronic hepatitis C virus (HCV) infection in patients with genotype 1 or 4 who are without cirrhosis or who have compensated cirrhosis and used in combination with pegylated interferon and ribavirin*

TABLETS

Adults who are treatment-naïve. 400 mg once daily for 12 wk.

⁂ *As adjunct to treat chronic hepatitis C virus (HCV) infection in patients with genotype 2 or 3 who are without cirrhosis or who have compensated cirrhosis and used in combination with ribavirin*

ORAL PELLETS, TABLETS

Adults and children age 3 years and over weighing at least 35 kg (77 lb). 400 mg once daily for 12 wk for genotype 2 and 24 wk for genotype 3.
Children age 3 years and over weighing 17 kg (37.4 lb) to less than 35 kg (77 lb).

200 mg once daily for 12 wk for genotype 2 and 24 wk for genotype 3.

Children age 3 years and over weighing less than 17 kg (37.4 lb). 150 mg once daily for genotype 2 and 24 wk for genotype 3.

✳ *As adjunct to treat chronic hepatitis C virus (HCV) infection in patients with hepatocellular carcinoma waiting for a liver transplant in combination with ribavirin*

TABLETS

Adults. 400 mg once daily for 48 wk or until liver transplant becomes available.

☰ Drug Administration

P.O.

- Administer at about the same time daily to maintain consistency. Give with or without food.
- Oral pellet can be administered directly into mouth without chewing or with food. To administer with food at or below room temperature, sprinkle the pellets on one or more spoonfuls of nonacidic foods such as chocolate syrup, ice cream, mashed potato, or pudding and gently mix.
- The mixture should be consumed within 30 minutes and not chewed to avoid a bitter aftertaste.

Route	Onset	Peak	Duration
P.O.	Unknown	0.5–2 hr	Unknown

Half-life: 0.4 hr

☰ Mechanism of Action

Undergoes intracellular metabolism to form an active uridine analogue triphosphate, which is then incorporated into HCV RNA by the NS5B polymerase and acts as a chain terminator.

☰ Contraindications

Hypersensitivity to sofosbuvir or its components

☰ Interactions

DRUGS

amiodarone: Possibly development of serious symptomatic bradycardia

carbamazepine, oxcarbazepine, phenobarbital, phenytoin, rifabutin, rifampin, rifapentine, St. John's wort, tipranavir/ritonavir: Possibly decreased sofosbuvir plasma concentration, leading to reduced effectiveness

☰ Adverse Reactions

CNS: Asthenia, chills, depression (severe), fatigue, fever, headache, insomnia, irritability, **suicidal ideation**

GI: Anorexia, diarrhea, elevated pancreatic enzymes, hyperbilirubinemia, nausea

HEME: Anemia, **neutropenia, pancytopenia, thrombocytopenia**

MS: Elevated creatine kinase, myalgia

SKIN: Pruritus, rash (sometimes with blisters or angioedema-like swelling)

Other: **Angioedema**, flu-like symptoms

☰ Childbearing Considerations

PREGNANCY

- It is not known if drug can cause fetal harm. However, because drug is given in combination with ribavirin or peginterferon alfa and ribavirin, drug combinations can cause fetal harm and are contraindicated in pregnant women and in men whose female partners are pregnant.
- Female patients and female partners of male patients must have a negative pregnancy test prior to drug therapy being initiated.

LACTATION

- It is not known if drug is present in breast milk.
- Drug combinations with ribavirin or peginterferon alfa and ribavirin make breastfeeding contraindicated.

REPRODUCTION

- Be aware that female patients or female partners of male patients must use at least two effective methods of contraception during combination treatment and for at least 6 months after drugs are discontinued.
- Female patients and female partners of male patients must undergo monthly pregnancy tests.

☰ Nursing Considerations

- Know that reducing the dosage of sofosbuvir or interrupting treatment should be avoided to prevent treatment failure. Also be aware that if other drugs used in combination with sofosbuvir are discontinued, sofosbuvir should also be discontinued.

❗ **WARNING** Ensure that all patients have been tested for current or prior HBV infection before sofosbuvir therapy is begun, because in patients coinfected with HBV and HCV, there is risk of hepatitis B virus reactivation

Q
R
S

that may result in fulminant hepatitis, hepatic failure, or even death. If patient tests positive for HBV, monitor patient closely for clinical and laboratory signs, as ordered, of hepatitis flare or HBV reactivation during treatment with sofosbuvir and during posttreatment follow-up. Expect treatment for HBV infection to be given, if needed.

- Monitor patient also receiving amiodarone with sofosbuvir for symptomatic bradycardia that may be severe enough to require pacemaker intervention. Be aware that bradycardia may occur up to 2 weeks after sofosbuvir therapy has begun. Patients at risk include those taking beta-blockers or those with underlying advanced liver disease or cardiac disorders. Expect patient to be hospitalized for cardiac monitoring for the first 48 hours of sofosbuvir therapy. Notify prescriber if bradycardia occurs and expect drug to be discontinued. Known that bradycardia generally disappears after drug is discontinued.

PATIENT TEACHING
- Instruct patient to take sofosbuvir exactly as ordered and not to discontinue it without prescriber knowledge.
- Tell patient to take sofosbuvir every day at a regularly scheduled time.
- Instruct patient taking oral pellet form not to chew the pellets and that pellets can be administered directly into mouth. Alternatively, tell parents pellets can be administered with food that is at or below room temperature by sprinkling the pellets on one or more spoonfuls of nonacidic foods such as chocolate syrup, ice cream, mashed potato, or pudding and gently mixing. The mixture should be consumed within 30 minutes and not chewed to avoid a bitter aftertaste.
- Teach patient how to take his pulse and to report immediately a sudden decrease in pulse rate or signs and symptoms of serious bradycardia, such as chest pain, confusion, dizziness, excessive tiredness, fainting or near-fainting, malaise, memory problems, shortness of breath, or weakness.
- Tell patient to inform all prescribers of sofosbuvir therapy, because drug reacts with many different drugs, which may cause

reduced effectiveness or increased risk of adverse reactions.
- Advise female patients to notify prescriber if pregnancy occurs or is suspected. If patient is also taking ribavirin with sofosbuvir, tell patient to use two reliable contraceptives during treatment and for at least 6 months after stopping ribavirin.
- Tell mothers wishing to breastfeed to discuss breastfeeding with their prescriber.

solifenacin succinate
VESIcare, VESIcare LS

≣ Class and Category
Pharmacologic class: Antimuscarinic
Therapeutic class: Bladder antispasmodic

≣ Indications and Dosages
✳ *To treat overactive urinary bladder with symptoms of frequency, urge incontinence, and urgency*

TABLETS
Adults. 5 mg daily; if tolerated well, increased to 10 mg daily.

✳ *To treat neurogenic detrusor overactivity in pediatric patients*

ORAL SUSPENSION (VESICARE LS)
Children 2 years and older weighing more than 60 kg (132 lb). *Initial:* 5 ml (5 mg) once daily, increased as needed. *Maximum:* 10 ml (10 mg) once daily.

Children 2 years and older weighing more than 45 kg (121 lb) to 60 kg (132 lb). *Initial:* 4 ml (4 mg) once daily, increased as needed. *Maximum:* 8 ml (8 mg) once daily.

Children 2 years and older weighing more than 30 kg (66 lb) to 45 kg (121 lb). *Initial:* 3 ml (3 mg) once daily, increased as needed. *Maximum:* 6 ml (6 mg) once daily.

Children 2 years and older weighing more than 15 kg (33 lb) to 30 kg (66 lb). *Initial:* 3 ml (3 mg) once daily, increased as needed. *Maximum:* 5 ml (5 mg) once daily.

Children 2 years and older weighing 9 kg (19.8 lb) to 15 kg (33 lb). *Initial:* 2 ml (2 mg) once daily, increased as needed. *Maximum:* 4 ml (4 mg) once daily.

±**DOSAGE ADJUSTMENT** For patients with severe renal impairment or moderate hepatic impairment or patients taking ketoconazole or other potent CYP3A4 inhibitors and taking tablet form, dosage limited to 5 mg daily. For children with severe renal impairment or moderate hepatic impairment or patients taking ketoconazole or other potent CYP3A4 inhibitors and taking oral suspension, starting dose maintained with no further titration.

Drug Administration
P.O.
- Tablets should be swallowed whole with a full glass of water and not chewed, crushed, or divided.
- Do not administer oral suspension at same time as with food or other drinks, as this may result in a bitter taste. Shake oral suspension well before using. Use a calibrated device to measure dosage. Follow administration with water or milk. Store at room temperature and discard after 28 days of first opening.

Route	Onset	Peak	Duration
P.O.	Unknown	3–8 hr	Unknown

Half-life: 45–68 hr

Mechanism of Action
Antagonizes the effect of acetylcholine on muscarinic receptors in detrusor muscle, decreasing the muscle spasms that cause inappropriate bladder emptying. This action increases bladder capacity and volume, which relieves the sensation of frequency and urgency and enhances bladder control.

Contraindications
Gastric retention, hypersensitivity to solifenacin or its components, uncontrolled angle-closure glaucoma, urine retention

Interactions
DRUGS
CYP3A4 inducers: Possibly decreased concentration of solifenacin and its effectiveness
ketoconazole, other potent CYP3A4 inhibitors: Increased serum concentrations of solifenacin and increased risk of adverse effects

Adverse Reactions
CNS: Confusion, delirium, depression, dizziness, fatigue, hallucinations, headache, somnolence
CV: **Atrial fibrillation**, hypertension, palpitations, peripheral edema, **prolonged QT interval**, tachycardia, **torsades de pointes**
EENT: Blurred vision, distortion of sense of taste, dry eyes or mouth, glaucoma, nasal dryness, pharyngitis, sialadenitis
GI: Abdominal pain, anorexia, **colonic or intestinal obstruction**, constipation, elevated liver enzymes, fecal impaction, gastroesophageal reflux disease, ileus, indigestion, nausea, vomiting
GU: Renal impairment, UTI, urinary retention
MS: Muscle weakness
RESP: **Airway obstruction from angioedema**, cough, dysphonia
SKIN: Dry skin, **erythema multiforme**, **exfoliative dermatitis**, pruritus, rash, urticaria
Other: **Anaphylaxis**, **angioedema**, flu-like symptoms, **hyperkalemia**

Childbearing Considerations
PREGNANCY
- It is not known if drug can cause fetal harm.
- Use with caution only if benefit to mother outweighs potential risk to fetus.

LACTATION
- It is not known if drug is present in breast milk.
- Patient should check with prescriber before breastfeeding.

Nursing Considerations
- Use cautiously in patients with intestinal atony, myasthenia gravis, or ulcerative colitis because solifenacin may decrease GI motility; in patients with significant bladder outflow obstruction because solifenacin may cause urine retention; in patients with hepatic impairment because solifenacin is metabolized in the liver; and in patients with renal impairment because solifenacin excretion may be impaired.

! **WARNING** Monitor patient closely, even after first dose, for hypersensitivity reactions. Although uncommon, anaphylactic reactions and angioedema have occurred with solifenacin therapy. Be prepared to manage these life-threatening reactions and expect drug to be discontinued if they occur.

- Monitor patient for signs of anticholinergic CNS adverse reactions, especially after treatment is begun or dosage increased.
- Monitor elderly patients, especially those age 75 and over, for adverse reactions because they're at increased risk for solifenacin-induced adverse reactions.

PATIENT TEACHING

- Instruct patient to take solifenacin with a full glass of water and to swallow the tablet whole and not to chew, crush, or divide it.
- Tell parents or caregiver not to administer oral suspension at same time as with food or other drinks, as this may result in a bitter taste. Also instruct to shake oral suspension well before using, use a calibrated device to measure dosage (not a household spoon), and follow administration with water or milk.
- Stress importance of not taking two doses of drug in one day. If a dose is missed, tell patient to take it as soon as possible but if it has been at least 12 hours since last dose, to skip dose and take next dose at usual time.
- Caution patient to avoid exertion in a warm or hot environment because sweating may be delayed, which could increase body temperature and increase risk of heatstroke.
- Advise patient to avoid potentially hazardous activities until drug's CNS effects are known.
- Inform patient that alcohol may cause drowsiness, and urge patient to limit or avoid alcoholic beverages while taking solifenacin.

! WARNING Tell patient to report allergic reaction to prescriber; if serious, instruct patient to seek immediate medical attention and stop taking drug.

solriamfetol hydrochloride
Sunosi

Class and Category

Pharmacologic class: Dopamine and norepinephrine reuptake inhibitor
Therapeutic class: Analeptic
Controlled substance schedule: IV

Indications and Dosages

∗ *To improve wakefulness in patients with excessive daytime sleepiness associated with narcolepsy*

TABLETS

Adults. 75 mg once daily, increased after at least 3 days to 150 mg once daily, if needed. *Maximum:* 150 mg daily.

∗ *To improve wakefulness in patients with excessive daytime sleepiness associated with obstructive sleep apnea*

TABLETS

Adults. 37.5 mg once daily, then doubled at intervals of at least 3 days to maximum dose, as needed. *Maximum:* 150 mg daily.

±**DOSAGE ADJUSTMENT** For patients with moderate renal impairment (an estimated glomerular filtration rate between 30 and 59 ml/min), initial dose reduced or kept at 37.5 mg once daily, with dose increased to a maximum of 75 mg once daily after at least 7 days. For patients with severe renal impairment (an estimated glomerular filtration rate between 15 and 29 ml/min), dosage reduced or kept at 37.5 mg once daily with no titration.

Drug Administration

P.O.

- Split 75-mg tablet in half when dosage calls for 37.5 mg.
- Administer drug when patient wakes in morning. Avoid administering drug within 9 hours of planned sleep because drug may interfere with sleep if taken too late in the day.

Route	Onset	Peak	Duration
P.O.	Unknown	2 hr	9 hr

Half-life: 7.1 hr

Mechanism of Action

Unknown but thought to be related to its activity as a dopamine and norepinephrine reuptake inhibitor.

Contraindications

Hypersensitivity to solriamfetol or its components, use within 14 days of MAO inhibitors

Interactions

DRUGS

dopaminergic drugs: Possibly altered pharmacodynamic effects

drugs that increase blood pressure: Increased risk of hypertension
MAO inhibitors: Increased risk of hypertensive crisis

Adverse Reactions

CNS: Agitation, anxiety, bruxism, disturbances in attention, dizziness, feeling jittery, headache, insomnia, irritability, panic attack, restlessness, thirst, tremor
CV: Chest discomfort or pain, hypertension, palpitations, tachycardia
EENT: Dry mouth
GI: Abdominal pain, anorexia, constipation, diarrhea, nausea, vomiting
RESP: Cough, dyspnea
SKIN: Erythematous rash, excessive diaphoresis, rash, urticaria
Other: **Hypersensitivity reactions,** weight loss

Childbearing Considerations

PREGNANCY

- Pregnancy exposure registry: 1-877-283-6220 or www.Sunosi PregnancyRegistry.com.
- It is not known if drug can cause fetal harm.
- Use with caution only if benefit to mother outweighs potential risk to fetus.

LACTATION

- It is not known if drug is present in breast milk.
- Patient should check with prescriber before breastfeeding.
- If breastfeeding occurs, mother should monitor infant for agitation, anorexia, insomnia, and reduced weight gain.

Nursing Considerations

- Obtain patient's blood pressure prior to beginning solriamfetol therapy; blood pressure must be adequately controlled before drug is given, as hypertension increases risk of adverse cardiovascular events, including cardiovascular death, CVA, or MI.
- Use solriamfetol cautiously in patients with risk factors for major adverse cardiovascular events, especially patients with known cardiovascular and cerebrovascular disease, preexisting hypertension, and patients with advanced age. Also, use caution if patient is taking other drugs that increase blood pressure and heart rate.

- Use solriamfetol cautiously in patients with bipolar disorders or psychosis. Be aware that patients with moderate or severe renal impairment may be at higher risk of psychiatric symptoms because of the prolonged half-life of the drug.

! **WARNING** Monitor patient for hypersensitivity reactions such as erythematous rash, rash, and urticaria.

- Monitor patient's blood pressure and heart rate throughout solriamfetol therapy. Notify prescriber if elevations occur. Expect new-onset hypertension or exacerbations of preexisting hypertension to be treated. Know that if patient experiences increases in blood pressure or heart rate that cannot be managed with a dosage reduction of drug or other appropriate measures, drug will likely be discontinued.
- Monitor patient for psychiatric symptoms such as anxiety, insomnia, and irritability that may occur with solriamfetol therapy.
- Monitor patient for possible emergence or exacerbation of psychiatric symptoms. If they occur, notify prescriber and expect dosage to be reduced or drug discontinued.

PATIENT TEACHING

- Tell patient taking a 37.5-mg dose to split a 75-mg tablet in half.
- Instruct patient to take solriamfetol upon awakening and to avoid taking drug within 9 hours of planned sleep because drug may interfere with sleep if taken too late in the day.

! **WARNING** Alert patient that drug may cause an allergic reaction such as hives or a rash. If present, tell patient to notify prescriber.

- Teach patient how to take a blood pressure and pulse rate. Provide guidelines for when to call prescriber if elevated. Also tell patient to seek emergency care if signs or symptoms of a heart attack or stroke are present.
- Inform patient that anxiety, insomnia, and irritability may occur with drug use. If troublesome, tell patient to discuss with prescriber.

sotalol hydrochloride
Betapace, Betapace AF, Sorine, Sotacor
(CAN), Sotalol I.V., Sotylize

Class and Category
Pharmacologic class: Nonselective beta
blocker
Therapeutic class: Class III antiarrhythmic

Indications and Dosages
⁎ *To treat life-threatening ventricular*
arrhythmias

TABLETS
Adults. *Initial:* 80 mg twice daily, increased,
as needed, in increments of 80 mg every
3 days provided patient's QT interval is less
than 500 msec. *Maintenance:* 160 to 320 mg
daily in divided doses twice daily or three
times a day. *Maximum:* 640 mg daily.
**Children 2 years old and over with normal
renal function:** *Initial:* 1.2 mg/kg three times
daily; may be titrated up to maximum of
2.4 mg/kg three times daily allowing at least
36 hours between dose increments.
**Children under age 2 years with normal
renal function.** Highly individualized.

ORAL SOLUTION (SOTYLIZE)
Adults. *Initial:* 80 mg once or twice daily,
increased, as needed, in increments of 80 mg
every 3 days provided patient's QT interval is
less than 500 msec. Usual: 80 to 160 mg once
or twice daily. *Maximum:* 320 mg once or
twice daily.
**Children 2 years old and over with normal
renal function.** *Initial:* 30 mg/m² three times
daily; may be titrated up to 60 mg/m² three
times daily allowing 36 hr between dosage
adjustments. *Maximum:* 60 mg/m²/dose.
**Children under age 2 years with normal
renal functions.** Highly individualized.

I.V. INFUSION (SOTALOL I.V.)
Adults. *Loading dose:* Highly individualized
and dependent on the creatinine clearance
and target oral dose. *Maintenance:* 75 mg
when substituted for 80-mg oral dose;
112.5 mg when substituted for 120-mg oral
dose; and 150 mg when substituted for
160-mg oral dose. *Maximum:* 150 mg daily.
⁎ *To delay recurrence of atrial fibrillation*
and atrial flutter in patients currently in
sinus rhythm

TABLETS
Adults. *Initial:* 80 mg twice daily, increased
every 3 days in 80-mg increments daily
provided QTc interval is less than 500 msec.
Usual: 120 mg twice daily.

ORAL SOLUTION (SOTYLIZE)
Adults. *Initial:* 80 mg once or twice daily,
increased, as needed, in increments of 80 mg
every 3 days provided patient's QT interval
is less than 500 msec. *Usual:* 120 mg once or
twice daily.

I.V. INFUSION (SOTALOL I.V.)
Adults. *Loading dose:* Highly
individualized and dependent on the
creatinine clearance and target oral dose.
Maintenance: 75 mg when substituted
for 80-mg oral dose; 112.5 mg when
substituted for 120-mg oral dose; and
150 mg when substituted for 160-mg oral
dose. *Maximum:* 150 mg twice daily.
±**DOSAGE ADJUSTMENT** For adult patients
treated for ventricular arrhythmias and with
a creatinine clearance between 30 and
59 ml/min, oral dosage interval reduced
to every 24 hours; if creatinine clearance
is between 10 and 29 ml/min, oral dosage
interval increased to 36 or 48 hours; and if
creatinine clearance is less than 10 ml/min,
dosage individualized. For adult patients with
a creatinine clearance between 40 and
59 ml/min, I.V. dosing interval increased to
every 24 hours.

Drug Administration
P.O.
- Administer consistently at the same time(s)
  daily.
- Give 2 hours before or after antacids
  containing aluminum oxide or magnesium
  hydroxide.
- Oral solution strength is 5 mg/ml. To
  administer an 80-mg dose, 16 ml are required;
  for 120-mg dose, 24 ml are required; for
  160-mg dose, 32 ml are required; for 240-mg
  dose, 48 ml are required; and for a 320-mg
  dose, 64 ml are required.
- Use a calibrated device to measure oral
  solution dosage.
- Store drug at room temperature.

I.V.
- Dilute drug with 120 to 250 ml of 0.9%
  Sodium Chloride Injection, 5% Dextrose in
  Water, or Lactated Ringer's solution.

- Use a volumetric infusion pump for administration.
- Infuse loading dose over 1 hour and maintenance doses over 5 hours each.
- When storing drug at room temperature, protect from light.
- *Incompatibilities:* None listed by manufacturer

Route	Onset	Peak	Duration
P.O.	1–2 hr	2.5–4 hr	Unknown
I.V.	5–10 min	1 hr	Unknown

Half-life: 12 hr

☰ Mechanism of Action

Combines class II and class III antiarrhythmic activity to increase sinus cycle length. This beta blocker decreases AV nodal conduction and increases AV nodal refractoriness. Suppression of SA node automaticity and AV node conductivity decreases atrial and ventricular ectopy.

☰ Contraindications

Acquired or congenital QT syndromes (QT interval greater than 450 ms); bronchial asthma or related bronchospastic conditions; cardiogenic shock; decompensated heart failure; hypersensitivity to sotalol or its components; second- or third-degree AV block, sick sinus syndrome, or sinus bradycardia (less than 50 beats per minute) without functioning pacemaker; serum potassium less than 4 mEq/L

☰ Interactions

DRUGS

antacids: Altered sotalol effectiveness
beta-agonists such as albuterol, isoproterenol, terbutaline: Decreased effects of these drugs
calcium channel blockers: Additive effects on atrioventricular conduction or ventricular function resulting in bradycardia and hypotension
catecholamine-depleting agents such as guanethidine, reserpine; negative chronotropes such as beta-blockers, digitalis glycosides, diltiazem, verapamil: Possibly excessive reduction of resting sympathetic nervous tone resulting in marked bradycardia and/or hypotension causing syncope
class I, II, and III antiarrhythmia; other drugs known to cause QT prolongation: Prolonged refractoriness possibly resulting in prolonged QT interval
clonidine: Increased risk of bradycardia; increased risk of rebound hypertension when clonidine discontinued
insulin, oral antidiabetic drugs: Impaired glucose control, increased risk of hyperglycemia, and masked hypoglycemia

☰ Adverse Reactions

CNS: Anxiety, depression, dizziness, drowsiness, fatigue, insomnia, lethargy, nervousness, weakness
CV: AV conduction disorders, bradycardia, heart failure, hypotension, peripheral vascular insufficiency, prolonged QT interval, sinus arrest or pauses, torsades de pointes, ventricular arrhythmias
EENT: Nasal congestion
ENDO: Hyperglycemia, hypoglycemia
GI: Abdominal pain, constipation, diarrhea, nausea, vomiting
GU: Sexual dysfunction
MS: Muscle weakness
RESP: Bronchospasm, dyspnea, wheezing

☰ Childbearing Considerations

PREGNANCY

- Drug may cause fetal harm such as growth restriction, hyperbilirubinemia, hypoglycemia, increased risk of prolonged QT interval, transient fetal bradycardia, and possible intrauterine death.
- Use with caution only if benefit to mother outweighs potential risk to fetus.
- Breakthrough arrhythmias, including ventricular tachycardia, are increased during pregnancy.

LABOR & DELIVERY

- Risk of arrhythmias increases during labor and delivery.

LACTATION

- Drug is present in breast milk.
- Breastfeeding should not be done during drug therapy.

REPRODUCTION

- Drug may cause erectile dysfunction.

☰ Nursing Considerations

! **WARNING** Expect to obtain baseline QT interval before starting sotalol and periodically throughout therapy, as ordered. This is because drug can cause

Q
R
S

life-threatening ventricular tachycardia associated with QT interval prolongation. Intravenous sotalol should not be initiated if the baseline QTc is longer than 450 ms. If QTc prolongs to 500 ms or greater, notify prescriber at once and expect dose to be reduced or drug discontinued. Be aware that sotalol-induced bradycardia increases the risk of torsades de pointes, especially after cardioversion, and may require emergency pacemaker insertion, especially in children.

- Monitor apical and radial pulses, blood pressure, circulation in limbs, daily weight, fluid intake and output, and respiratory rate, before and during sotalol therapy.
- Monitor patient for heart failure that can occur or worsen during initiation or titration of sotalol because of its beta-blocking effects.
- Know that if prescriber is stopping amiodarone, sotalol shouldn't be started until QT interval has returned to baseline, because of possible adverse cardiac effects.
- Be aware that stopping sotalol abruptly may cause life-threatening reactions such as exacerbations of angina pectoris and myocardial infarction. For this reason, chronic beta blocker therapy such as sotalol is not routinely withheld prior to major surgery. However, be aware that the impaired ability of the heart to respond to reflex adrenergic stimuli may increase the risks of general anesthesia and surgical procedures. Dosage should be gradually reduced over 1 to 2 weeks.
- Monitor serum electrolyte levels because drug can increase risk of torsades de pointes in patients with electrolyte imbalances, especially hypokalemia or hypomagnesemia.
- Assess carefully if patient has diabetes mellitus or thyrotoxicosis because they may mask hypoglycemia and hyperthyroidism.
- Be aware that falsely elevated levels of urinary metanephrine may occur during sotalol therapy when levels are measured by fluorimetric or photometric methods.

! **WARNING** Know that a patient with a history of anaphylactic reaction to a variety of

allergens may have a more severe reaction when taking sotalol and may be unresponsive to the usual doses of epinephrine used to treat the allergic reaction.

PATIENT TEACHING
- Tell patient to take sotalol consistently at the same time(s) daily.
- Advise patient to take drug 2 hours before or after antacids containing aluminum oxide or magnesium hydroxide.
- Tell patient to use a calibrated device to measure oral solution dosage, not a household spoon.

! **WARNING** Advise patient to notify prescriber immediately if he has difficulty breathing or develops a slow or erratic pulse.

- Urge patient to consult prescriber before taking OTC drugs, especially cold remedies, which may decrease sotalol's effectiveness.
- Urge patient to avoid hazardous activities until drug's CNS effects are known.
- Advise mothers that breastfeeding should not be undertaken while taking sotalol.

! **WARNING** Caution patient not to abruptly stop taking sotalol, as life-threatening effects may occur.

spectinomycin hydrochloride
Trobicin

⊫ Class and Category
Pharmacologic class: Aminoglycoside
Therapeutic class: Antibiotic

⊫ Indications and Dosages
✻ *To treat acute cervicitis, proctitis, and urethral gonorrhea caused by susceptible strains of* Neisseria gonorrhoeae

I.M. INJECTION
Adults. 2 g as a single dose.
±**DOSAGE ADJUSTMENT** For patients living in geographic area where antibiotic resistance is known to be prevalent, dosage increased to 4 g as a single dose given as two separate 2-g dose injections.

≡ Drug Administration
I.M.
- Reconstitute drug with 3.2 ml of accompanying diluent (Bacteriostatic Water for Injection with Benzyl Alcohol) to each 2-g vial. Shake vial vigorously before withdrawing dose.
- Inject, using a 20G needle, deep into upper outer quadrant of gluteal muscle.
- A 4-g dose should be divided between two gluteal injection sites.
- Store diluted drug at room temperature and use within 24 hours.

Route	Onset	Peak	Duration
I.M.	Unknown	1–2 hr	Unknown

Half-life: 3 hr

≡ Mechanism of Action
Binds to negatively charged sites on bacterial outer cell membrane, disrupting cell integrity, and binds to bacterial ribosomal subunits, inhibiting protein synthesis. Both actions lead to bacterial cell death.

≡ Contraindications
Hypersensitivity to spectinomycin or its components

≡ Interactions
DRUGS
None reported by manufacturer

≡ Adverse Reactions
CNS: Chills, dizziness, fever, insomnia
GI: Abdominal cramps, nausea, vomiting
SKIN: Urticaria
Other: Anaphylaxis, injection-site pain

≡ Childbearing Considerations
PREGNANCY
- It is not known if drug can cause fetal harm.
- Use with caution only if benefit to mother outweighs potential risk to fetus.

LACTATION
- It is not known if drug is present in breast milk.
- Patient should check with prescriber before breastfeeding.

≡ Nursing Considerations
! **WARNING** Monitor patient for hypersensitivity reactions after administration. Although uncommon, anaphylaxis or anaphylactoid reactions have occurred. If present, notify prescriber and be prepared to provide supportive care with antihistamines, corticosteroids, or epinephrine, as ordered.

- Be aware drug should not be used to treat syphilis.

PATIENT TEACHING
- Tell patient he'll be tested for syphilis at the start of treatment and 3 months later because spectinomycin treatment may delay or mask syphilis symptoms.

! **WARNING** Alert patient that drug may cause an allergic reaction, which could be serious. If present, tell patient to notify prescriber and if serious to seek immediate emergency care.

- Explain risk factors for sexually transmitted diseases, and teach correct condom use.
- Advise patient to encourage sexual partner to be tested for gonorrhea.
- Instruct patient to notify prescriber if signs and symptoms persist after a few days.

spironolactone
Aldactone, CaroSpir

≡ Class and Category
Pharmacologic class: Potassium-sparing diuretic
Therapeutic class: Diuretic

≡ Indications and Dosages
✳ *As adjunct to increase survival and to reduce need for hospitalization for heart failure when used in addition to standard therapy in patients with severe heart failure (NYHA class III–IV) and reduced ejection fraction*

TABLETS (ALDACTONE)
Adults with serum potassium of 5.0 mEq/l or less and an estimated glomerular filtration rate (eGFR) greater than 50 ml/min. *Initial:* 25 mg once daily. Dosage increased to 50 mg once daily, as needed.
Adults with an eGFR between 30 and 50 ml/min. 25 mg every other day.

ORAL SUSPENSION (CAROSPIR)
Adults with a serum potassium of 5.0 mEq/l or less and eGFR greater than

Q
R
S

50 ml/min. *Initial:* 20 mg (4 ml) once daily, increased to 37.5 mg (7.5 ml) once daily, if needed.

Adults with an eGFR between 30 to 50 ml/min. 10 mg (2 ml) once daily.

±**DOSAGE ADJUSTMENT** For heart failure patients who develop hyperkalemia while receiving a dose of 25 mg (tablet) or 20 mg (4 ml) (oral suspension) daily, dosage reduced to 25 mg (tablet) or 20 mg (4 ml) (oral suspension) every other day.

✱ *As adjunct to treat hypertension*

TABLETS (ALDACTONE)

Adults. *Initial:* 25 to 100 mg daily as a single dose or in divided doses for at least 2 wk; gradually adjusted every 2 wk, as needed, if initial dose is less than 100 mg, to control blood pressure. *Maximum:* 100 mg daily.

ORAL SUSPENSION (CAROSPIR)

Adults. *Initial:* 20 mg (4 ml) to 75 mg (15 ml) daily as a single dose or in divided doses for at least 2 wk; gradually adjusted every 2 wk as needed if initial dose less than 75 mg (15 ml). *Maximum:* 75 mg (15 ml) daily.

✱ *To treat edema associated with hepatic cirrhosis*

TABLETS (ALDACTONE)

Hospitalized adults. *Initial:* 100 mg daily as a single dose or in divided doses, for at least 5 days before increasing dosage if given as the only agent for diuresis. *Usual:* 25 to 200 mg daily as a single dose or in divided doses.

ORAL SUSPENSION (CAROSPIR)

Hospitalized adults. *Initial:* 75 mg (15 ml) daily as a single dose or in divided doses, for at least 5 days before increasing dosage if given as the only agent for diuresis. Increased slowly to maximum dose, as needed. *Maximum:* 100 mg (20 ml) daily.

✱ *To treat primary hyperaldosteronism*

TABLETS (ALDACTONE)

Adults waiting for surgery. 100 to 400 mg daily.

Adults unable to have surgery. Highly individualized with lowest effective dosage given to manage condition.

⬚ Drug Administration

P.O.

- Administer drug with or without food but be consistent.
- Shake oral suspension well before use and use a calibrated device to measure dosage. Store at room temperature.

- Do not interchange oral suspension for tablet form, as the two formulations are not interchangeable.

Route	Onset	Peak	Duration
P.O.	2–4 hr	2.5–5 hr	2–3 days

Half-life: 1–2 hr

⬚ Contraindications

Addison's disease, concomitant use of eplerenone, hyperkalemia, hypersensitivity to spironolactone or its components

⬚ Interactions

DRUGS

ACE inhibitors, aldosterone blockers, angiotensin II antagonists, heparin and low-molecular-weight heparin, NSAIDs, other potassium-sparing diuretics, potassium-containing drugs, potassium supplements, trimethoprim: Increased risk of severe hyperkalemia

acetylsalicylic acid: Possibly reduced effectiveness of spironolactone

cholestyramine: Increased risk of hyperkalemic metabolic acidosis

CYP2C8 substrates (repaglinide), CYP3A substrates (midazolam, sirolimus, tacrolimus): Possibly increased exposure of these drugs

digoxin: Possibly increased half-life of digoxin, increasing exposure to digoxin

lithium: Possibly lithium toxicity

NSAIDs: Decreased antihypertensive effect of spironolactone

FOODS

high potassium diet, low-salt milk, salt substitutes: Increased risk of severe hyperkalemia

⬚ Adverse Reactions

CNS: Ataxia, confusion, dizziness, drowsiness, **encephalopathy**, fatigue, fever, headache, lethargy, somnolence

CV: **Hypotension**, vasculitis

EENT: Increased intraocular pressure, nasal congestion, tinnitus, vision changes

ENDO: Breast or nipple pain, gynecomastia, hyperglycemia

GI: Abdominal cramping or pain, anorexia, constipation, diarrhea, flatulence, **gastric bleeding** or ulceration, gastritis, **mixed cholestatic/hepatocellular toxicity**, nausea, vomiting

Mechanism of Action

Normally, aldosterone attaches to receptors on the walls of distal convoluted tubule cells, causing sodium (Na⁺) and water (H₂O) reabsorption in the blood, as shown at left. Spironolactone competes with aldosterone for these receptors, thereby preventing sodium and water reabsorption and causing their excretion through the distal convoluted tubules, as shown below right. Increased urinary excretion of sodium and water reduces blood volume and blood pressure.

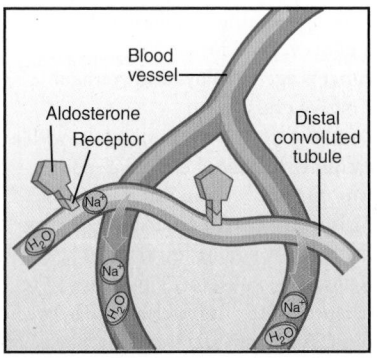
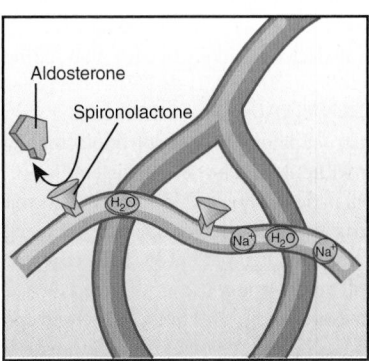

GU: Amenorrhea, decreased libido, impotence, irregular menses, postmenopausal bleeding, **renal failure**, worsening renal function
HEME: Agranulocytosis, aplastic anemia, leukopenia, neutropenia, thrombocytopenia
RESP: Cough, dyspnea
MS: Arthralgia, back and leg pain, leg cramps, muscle weakness, myalgia
SKIN: Alopecia, erythematous or maculopapular cutaneous eruptions, pruritus, **Stevens–Johnson syndrome, toxic epidermal necrolysis,** urticaria
Other: Anaphylaxis, dehydration, **drug reaction with eosinophilia and systemic symptoms (DRESS), hyperkalemia,** hyperuricemia, **hypocalcemia, hypochloremic metabolic alkalosis, hypomagnesemia, hyponatremia**

Childbearing Considerations

PREGNANCY
- Drug may cause fetal harm affecting sex differentiation of the male fetus.
- Drug should be avoided in pregnant women.

LACTATION
- Drug is not present in breast milk but an active metabolite has been found in breast milk.

- Patient should check with prescriber before breastfeeding.

REPRODUCTION
- Women of childbearing age should use effective contraceptive measures throughout drug therapy.

Nursing Considerations

- Expect to evaluate patient's serum potassium level 1 week after spironolactone therapy begins, after each dosage adjustment, monthly for the first 3 months, quarterly for 1 year, and then every 6 months thereafter or as ordered. Notify prescriber if level exceeds 5 mEq/L or patient's renal function deteriorates (serum creatinine level exceeding 4 mg/dl). If patient has severe heart failure, know that potassium supplementation should be discontinued and patient followed closely, because hyperkalemia may be fatal in such patients.
- Evaluate spironolactone's effectiveness by assessing blood pressure and presence and degree of edema.
- Monitor patients with renal impairment closely because risk of adverse reactions is greater in these patients, as well as the elderly, because spironolactone is substantially excreted by the kidneys. Also be aware that patients with impaired renal function are at higher risk for hyperkalemia.

! **WARNING** Monitor patient with hepatic impairment, especially if patient has ascites and cirrhosis, because spironolactone can cause sudden alterations in fluid and electrolyte balance which may cause coma, impaired neurological function, or worsening hepatic encephalopathy. Be aware that patients with hepatic impairment accompanied by ascites and cirrhosis should be given spironolactone initially in a hospital setting.

PATIENT TEACHING

- Instruct patient to take spironolactone with or without food but be consistent.
- Tell patient who can't swallow tablets that drug is available as a suspension. If using suspension, tell patient to shake container well before using, use a calibrated device to measure dosage and not a household spoon, and store suspension at room temperature.
- Teach patient who takes spironolactone for hypertension how to measure his blood pressure. Urge him to monitor it regularly and report pressure greater than 140 mm Hg systolic or 90 mm Hg diastolic to prescriber.
- Caution patient that he may experience dizziness during spironolactone therapy if fluid balance is altered.
- Warn patient to avoid performing hazardous activities, such as driving, until adverse effects of drug are known.
- Instruct patient to inform prescriber of any new condition or new drug therapy, including over-the-counter medications, so that prescriber can evaluate if the patient is at increased risk for hyperkalemia.
- Advise women to report suspected or known pregnancy immediately to prescriber. Alert patient that there is a potential risk to the fetus if it is male because of the drug's anti-androgenic properties. Encourage her to use effective contraceptive measures throughout spironolactone therapy to avoid pregnancy.

stavudine
Zerit

Class and Category
Pharmacologic class: Nucleoside analogue
Therapeutic class: Antiretroviral

Indications and Dosages

✻ *As adjunct to treat human immunodeficiency virus type 1 (HIV-1) infection*

CAPSULES, ORAL SOLUTION
Adults. 40 mg every 12 hr.
Adults weighing less than 60 kg (132 lb). 30 mg every 12 hr.
Neonates at least 14 days old and older and children weighing less than 30 kg (66 lb). 1 mg/kg every 12 hr.
Neonates aged 13 days and younger. 0.5 mg/kg every 12 hr.

±**DOSAGE ADJUSTMENT** For adults with a creatinine clearance between 26 and 50 ml/min and weighing at least 60 kg (132 lb), dosage reduced to 20 mg every 12 hr and if weighing less than 60 kg (132 lb), dosage reduced to 15 mg every 12 hr. For adults with a creatinine clearance between 10 and 25 ml/min and weighing at least 60 kg (132 lb), dosage reduced and interval increased to 20 mg every 24 hr and for adults weighing less than 60 kg (132 lb), dosage reduced and interval increased to 15 mg every 24 hr. For patients on hemodialysis, dosage and interval are the same as for patients with a creatinine clearance of 10 to 25 ml/min, but dosage is administered after the completion of hemodialysis on dialysis days and at the same time of day on nondialysis days. There are no specific recommendations for children with renal insufficiency.

Drug Administration
P.O.
- Administer with or without food but be consistent. Missed doses should be avoided.
- Capsules should be swallowed whole and not chewed, crushed, or opened.
- Pharmacist can prepare an oral solution, if needed. Shake bottle vigorously before using. Use measuring cup provided to measure dose. Store in refrigerator. Discard after 30 days.

Route	Onset	Peak	Duration
P.O.	Unknown	1 hr	Unknown

Half-life: 1–1.6 hr

Mechanism of Action
Inhibits the activity of HIV-1 reverse transcriptase by competing with the natural substrate thymidine triphosphate

to cause DNA chain termination following its incorporation into viral DNA. It also inhibits selective cellular DNA polymerases to markedly reduce the synthesis of mitochondrial DNA.

Contraindications
Concomitant therapy with didanosine, hypersensitivity to stavudine or its components

Interactions
DRUGS
doxorubicin, ribavirin: Possibly interfere with action of stavudine and its effectiveness
hydroxyurea: Increased risk for toxicities such as hepatotoxicity, pancreatitis, and severe peripheral neuropathy
zidovudine: Interferes with action of stavudine, potentially rendering it ineffective

ACTIVITIES
alcohol use: Increased risk of liver damage or pancreatitis

Adverse Reactions
CNS: Chills, fever, headache, insomnia, motor weakness (severe), peripheral neurologic symptoms including neuropathy
ENDO: Cushingoid appearance, fat redistribution, hyperglycemia
GI: Abdominal pain, anorexia, diarrhea, elevated liver and pancreatic enzymes, **hepatic failure or toxicity, hepatomegaly with steatosis** that may become severe, hyperlactatemia (symptomatic), nausea, **pancreatitis**, vomiting
HEME: Anemia, **leukopenia**, macrocytosis, **neutropenia, thrombocytopenia**
MS: Myalgia
SKIN: Rash
Other: Immune reconstitution syndrome, **hypersensitivity reactions, lactic acidosis,** lipoatrophy, lipodystrophy

Childbearing Considerations
PREGNANCY
- Pregnancy exposure registry: 1-800-258-4263.
- It is not known if drug can cause fetal harm.
- Use with caution only if benefit to mother outweighs potential risk to fetus.
- Be aware that the drug in combination with didanosine is contraindicated in pregnant women because of an increased risk of lactic acidosis.

LACTATION
- Drug is present in breast milk.
- The Centers for Disease Control and Prevention recommends that HIV-1 infected mothers not breastfeed to avoid risking postnatal transmission of HIV-1 infection to infants. They also do not recommend breastfeeding because of potential drug-induced adverse reactions in the infant.

Nursing Considerations
- Know that when stavudine is used with other agents with similar toxicities, the incidence of these toxicities may be higher than when stavudine is used alone. For example, use with didanosine may increase risk of hepatotoxicity, pancreatitis, and severe peripheral neuropathy. Know that the combination of didanosine and stavudine should be used with caution during pregnancy and is recommended only if the potential benefit clearly outweighs the potential risk.
- Know that extreme caution is needed when administering stavudine with patients with known risk factors for liver disease, because of increased risk of liver abnormalities that may become severe or even fatal. Be aware that the combination of stavudine along with didanosine and hydroxyurea should be avoided, because of increased risk of hepatotoxicity and hepatic failure that may result in death. Monitor liver enzymes and patient for evidence of worsening liver dysfunction. If present, notify prescriber and expect drug therapy to be interrupted or discontinued.

! **WARNING** Monitor patient closely for signs and symptoms of symptomatic hyperlactatemia or lactic acidosis syndrome which may be severe, such as gastrointestinal (abdominal pain, nausea, vomiting, or unexplained weight loss), generalized fatigue, neurologic symptoms such as motor weakness, and respiratory symptoms (dyspnea, tachypnea). Although being of female gender, having prolonged nucleoside exposure, or obesity increases risk, patients without these risk factors have also developed lactic acidosis and severe hepatomegaly with steatosis. Notify prescriber immediately if patient becomes symptomatic or has laboratory values suggestive of lactic acidosis, pronounced hepatotoxicity, or symptomatic hyperlactatemia. Know that hepatomegaly and steatosis may occur without marked transaminase elevations. If confirmed, expect drug to be discontinued.

- Monitor patient for peripheral neuropathy. Know that motor weakness may mimic Guillain–Barré syndrome, including respiratory failure requiring drug to be discontinued immediately even though symptoms may continue or worsen after drug therapy has been stopped. Be aware that peripheral sensory neuropathy (numbness, pain, or tingling in feet or hands) most often occurs in patients with advanced HIV-1 disease or history of peripheral neuropathy, or in patients receiving other drugs that have been associated with neuropathy, including didanosine.
- Monitor patient for changes in appearance related to fat redistribution, such as the development of breast enlargement, central obesity, cushingoid appearance, dorsocervical fat enlargement (buffalo hump), and facial and peripheral wasting caused by antiretroviral therapy such as stavudine.
- Be aware that immune reconstitution syndrome has occurred in patients treated with combination antiretroviral therapy, including stavudine. The inflammatory response predisposes susceptible patients to opportunistic infections such as cytomegalovirus, *Mycobacterium avium* infection, *Pneumocystis jiroveci* pneumonia, or tuberculosis. Autoimmune disorders such as Graves' disease, Guillain–Barré syndrome, or polymyositis have also occurred. Report sudden or unusual adverse reactions to prescriber.

PATIENT TEACHING

- Tell patient or caregiver that drug may be given with or without food, but should be consistent. Drug should also be taken at about the same time for the two doses and that the doses should be separated by 12 hours.
- Inform patient that capsule must be swallowed whole and not chewed, crushed, or opened.
- Instruct patient or caregiver that oral solution bottle must be shaken vigorously before using. The measuring cup provided should also be used to measure dose. Drug should be stored in refrigerator and discarded after 30 days.
- Advise patient to avoid missing doses of stavudine. If she misses a dose, she should take it as soon as she remembers, but should not double the next dose or take more than prescribed.

! WARNING Inform patient about severe liver disease that may occur with stavudine. Tell her to report signs and symptoms of liver disease, such as acholic stools, anorexia, fatigue, malaise, nausea, tenderness over liver area, or yellowing of skin or whites of the eyes, and to seek immediate medical attention.

! WARNING Instruct patient on early symptoms of lactic acidosis or symptomatic hyperlactatemia, such as abdominal discomfort, dyspnea, fatigue, motor weakness, nausea, unexplained weight loss, or vomiting. If present, tell patient to seek immediate medical attention, as drug may have to be discontinued.

- Warn patient to be alert for signs and symptoms of peripheral neuropathy such as numbness, pain, or tingling in feet or hands. If present, she should notify prescriber.
- Inform patient that stavudine therapy may cause changes in her body appearance because of fat redistribution. Prepare her for the possibility of developing breast enlargement, central obesity, dorsocervical fat enlargement (buffalo hump), facial wasting, and peripheral wasting.
- Instruct patient to report any persistent, severe, or unusual signs and symptoms. Inform patient taking other drugs in combination with stavudine with similar adverse effects that the incidence of adverse reactions may be higher than when stavudine is used alone.
- Alert mothers that breastfeeding is not recommended during stavudine therapy.
- Tell patients with diabetes to monitor their blood glucose closely, as stavudine may increase blood glucose levels. Also tell

patient taking oral solution that it contains 50 mg of sucrose (sugar) per ml.
- Warn patient to avoid alcohol intake while taking drug, because the combination may increase the risk of liver damage or pancreatitis.

streptomycin sulfate

≡ Class and Category
Pharmacologic class: Aminoglycoside
Therapeutic class: Antibiotic

≡ Indications and Dosages
* *To treat gram-negative bacillary bacteremia, chancroid, granuloma inguinale, meningitis, pneumonia, systemic infections, and UTI*

I.M. INJECTION
Adults. 1 to 2 g daily in divided doses every 6 to 12 hr. *Maximum:* 2 g daily.
Children. 20 to 40 mg/kg daily in divided doses every 6 to 12 hr.

* *As adjunct to treat endocarditis caused by* Streptococcus viridans *or* E. faecalis

I.M. INJECTION
Adults. 1 g twice daily for 1 wk (*S. viridans*) or 2 wk (*E. faecalis*) with penicillin. Then, 500 mg twice daily for 1 wk (*S. viridans*) or 4 wk (*E. faecalis*).

±**DOSAGE ADJUSTMENT** For patients over 60 years of age being treated for streptococcal endocarditis, dosage reduced to 500 mg twice daily for entire 2-week period.

* *As adjunct to treat active tuberculosis*

I.M. INJECTION
Adults. 15 mg/kg daily. *Maximum:* 1 g daily. Alternatively, 25 to 30 mg/kg (up to 1.5 g) two or three times weekly. *Maximum:* 1.5 g daily.
Children. 20 to 40 mg/kg daily. *Maximum:* 1 g daily. Alternatively, 25 to 30 mg/kg two or three times weekly. *Maximum:* 1.5 g daily.

* *To treat plague caused by* Yersinia pestis

I.M. INJECTION
Adults. 1 g or 15 mg/kg (up to 1 g) twice daily for at least 10 days.

* *To treat tularemia caused by* Francisella tularensis

I.M. INJECTION
Adults. 1 to 2 g daily in divided doses for 7 to 14 days and until patient is afebrile for 5 to 7 days.

±**DOSAGE ADJUSTMENT** If creatinine clearance is 50 to 80 ml/min, dosage reduced to 7.5 mg/kg I.M. every 24 hr; if 10 to 49 ml/min, 7.5 mg/kg I.M. every 24 to 72 hr; if less than 10 ml/min, 7.5 mg/kg I.M. every 72 to 96 hr.

≡ Drug Administration
I.M.
- Reconstitute drug by adding 4.2 ml of Sterile Water for Injection to each 1-g vial to provide a concentration of 200 mg/ml; 3.2 ml of diluent to provide a 250-mg/ml concentration; and 1.8 ml to provide a concentration of 400 mg/ml.
- Inject deeply into upper outer quadrant of buttocks or mid-lateral thigh in adults and mid-lateral thigh in children.
- Aspirate prior to injecting drug to avoid inadvertent injection into a blood vessel.
- Rotate injection sites to prevent sterile abscess formation.

Route	Onset	Peak	Duration
I.M.	Unknown	1–2 hr	Unknown

Half-life: 2–4.7 hr

≡ Mechanism of Action
Binds to negatively charged sites on the bacteria's outer cell membrane, disrupting cell integrity. Streptomycin also binds to bacterial ribosomal subunits and inhibits protein synthesis. Both actions lead to bacterial cell death.

≡ Contraindications
Hypersensitivity to streptomycin, other aminoglycosides, or their components

≡ Interactions
DRUGS
capreomycin: Possible increased risk of nephrotoxicity or ototoxicity
carbapenems (imipenem): Possible additive or synergistic antibacterial effects against some gram-positive bacteria
cephalosporins: Increased incidence of nephrotoxicity; possible inactivation of streptomycin
colistimethate/colistin, cyclosporine, other aminoglycosides, polymyxin B, vancomycin: Possible increased risk of nephrotoxicity and/or neurotoxicity
diuretics: Increased risk of ototoxicity

Q
R
S

neuromuscular blocking agents including general anesthetics (decamethonium, rocuronium, succinylcholine, tubocurarine): Possible increase in neuromuscular blockade and respiratory paralysis

NSAIDs: Possible increased serum streptomycin concentrations

penicillins: Additive or synergistic antibacterial effects; possible inactivation of streptomycin

Adverse Reactions

CNS: Clumsiness, dizziness, **neurotoxicity**, paresthesia, peripheral neuropathy, **seizures**, unsteadiness, vertigo

EENT: Hearing loss, sensation of fullness in ears, tinnitus, vision loss

GI: Anorexia, nausea, thirst, vomiting

GU: Decreased or increased urine output, **nephrotoxicity**

MS: Muscle twitching

SKIN: Erythema, pruritus, rash, urticaria

Childbearing Considerations

PREGNANCY

- Drug may cause fetal harm by causing congenital deafness.
- Drug should not be used during pregnancy.

LACTATION

- Drug is present in breast milk.
- A decision should be made to discontinue breastfeeding or the drug to avoid potential serious adverse reactions in the breastfed infant.

Nursing Considerations

- Use streptomycin cautiously in patients with renal impairment. In severely uremic patients, single dose can produce high blood level of drug for several days; cumulative effects may produce ototoxicity.
- Expect prescriber to order baseline renal function studies and to assess cranial nerve VIII function (responsible for hearing) at start of streptomycin therapy to allow for later comparisons.
- Monitor serum peak and trough levels, as ordered, to ensure adequate, but not toxic, drug level.

PATIENT TEACHING

- Inform patient that treatment for tuberculosis lasts at least 1 year.
- Urge patient to notify prescriber if he has fullness or ringing in ears, hearing loss, or vertigo.

sucralfate
Carafate

Class and Category

Pharmacologic class: GI protectant
Therapeutic class: Antiulcer

Indications and Dosages

✳ *To treat active duodenal ulcer*

ORAL SUSPENSION, TABLETS

Adults. 1 g four times a day for 4 to 8 wk, possibly less.

✳ *To prevent reoccurrence of duodenal ulcer*

TABLETS

Adults and adolescents. 1 g twice daily.

Drug Administration

P.O.

- Give drug on an empty stomach.
- Administer drug 1 hour before meals and at bedtime.
- Do not give antacids within 30 minutes of sucralfate.

Route	Onset	Peak	Duration
P.O.	1–2 hr	Unknown	6 hr

Half-life: Unknown

Mechanism of Action

May react with hydrochloric acid in the stomach to form a complex that buffers acid. The complex adheres electrostatically to proteins on the ulcer's surface and creates a protective barrier at the ulcer site. Sucralfate also inhibits back-diffusion of hydrogen ions and adsorbs bile acids and pepsin, actions that promote healing of an existing duodenal ulcer and prevent reoccurring ulcer formation.

Interactions

DRUGS

cimetidine, ciprofloxacin, digoxin, fluoroquinolone antibiotics, ketoconazole, l-thyroxine, phenytoin, quinidine, tetracycline, theophylline: Decreased bioavailability of these drugs

Adverse Reactions

CNS: Dizziness, drowsiness, headache, insomnia, light-headedness, vertigo

EENT: Dry mouth

ENDO: Hyperglycemia

GI: Constipation, diarrhea, indigestion, nausea, vomiting
MS: Back pain
RESP: Bronchospasm, dyspnea
SKIN: Pruritus, rash, urticaria
OTHER: Anaphylaxis, angioedema

Childbearing Considerations

PREGNANCY
- It is not known if drug can cause fetal harm.
- Use with caution only if benefit to mother outweighs potential risk to fetus.

LACTATION
- It is not known if drug is present in breast milk.
- Patient should check with prescriber before breastfeeding.

Nursing Considerations
- Use sucralfate cautiously in patients with chronic renal failure because of increased risk of aluminum toxicity.
- Monitor diabetic patient's blood glucose level closely because sucralfate may cause hyperglycemia significant enough to require an adjustment of antidiabetic drug therapy prescribed.

PATIENT TEACHING
- Instruct patient to take sucralfate on an empty stomach at least 1 hour before meals and at bedtime.
- Advise patient not to take antacids within 30 minutes of sucralfate.
- Caution patient to check with prescriber before taking another drug within 2 hours of sucralfate.

sucroferric oxyhydroxide

Velphoro

Class and Category
Pharmacologic class: Polynuclear iron(III) oxyhydroxide
Therapeutic class: Phosphate binder

Indications and Dosages
✱ *To control serum phosphorus levels in patients with chronic kidney disease on dialysis*

CHEWABLE TABLETS
Adults. *Initial:* 500 mg three times daily, increasing or decreasing dosage in 500-mg

increments weekly, as needed. *Maintenance:* 1,500 to 2,000 mg daily. *Maximum:* 3,000 mg daily.

Drug Administration

P.O.
- Give drug with meals and administer all other oral drugs prescribed for patient at a different time, because absorption of the other drugs may be affected.
- Chewable tablets must be chewed and not swallowed whole.
- Chewable tablets do not have to be taken with water or other liquid.

Route	Onset	Peak	Duration
P.O.	Unknown	Unknown	Unknown

Half-life: 6 hr

Mechanism of Action
Phosphate binding takes place by ligand exchange between hydroxyl groups and/or water in sucroferric oxyhydroxide and phosphate in the diet. The bound phosphate is eliminated in feces. Both calcium phosphorus product levels and serum phosphorus levels are reduced as a consequence of the reduced dietary phosphate absorption.

Contraindications
Hypersensitivity to sucroferric oxyhydroxide or its components

Interactions

DRUGS
acetylsalicylic acid, cephalexin, doxycycline, levothyroxine: Absorption of these drugs may be affected

Adverse Reactions
EENT: Abnormal drug distaste, tooth discoloration
GI: Dark-colored feces, diarrhea, nausea
SKIN: Rash

Childbearing Considerations
PREGNANCY
- Drug is not absorbed systemically and not expected to result in fetal exposure.

LACTATION
- Drug is not absorbed systemically and not expected to result in fetal exposure.

Nursing Considerations
- Monitor patient's serum phosphorus levels regularly, as ordered, to determine

drug effectiveness and need for dosage adjustments.

- Monitor patients who have a history of hemochromatosis or other diseases characterized by iron accumulation, patients who develop peritonitis during peritoneal dialysis, and patients with significant gastric or hepatic disorders or following major gastrointestinal surgery, because sucroferric oxyhydroxide effects on these conditions are not known.

Patient Teaching

- Instruct patient to take sucroferric oxyhydroxide with meals.
- Tell patient tablets must be chewed and not swallowed whole. Tell him the tablets may be crushed to aid chewing and swallowing them. Also, tell patient he does not need to drink anything when taking the chewable tablets.
- Inform patient that drug may cause discolored (black) stool but this effect is harmless. Inform patient that drug may also stain teeth.
- Instruct patient to take any concomitant drug therapy at least 2 hours before sucroferric oxyhydroxide.
- Tell patient to report any rash to prescriber.

sufentanil
Dsuvia

Class, Category, and Schedule
Pharmacologic class: Opioid agonist
Therapeutic class: Opioid analgesic
Controlled substance schedule: II

Indications and Dosages
* *To relieve acute pain in a hospital setting, which is severe enough to require an opioid analgesic and for which alternative treatments are inadequate in a medically supervised healthcare setting*

SUBLINGUAL TABLETS
Adults. 30 mcg, as needed with a minimum of 1 hr between doses. *Maximum:* 360 mcg or 12 tablets in 24 hr, and not for use for more than 72 hr.

Drug Administration
P.O.
- Drug is a biohazard drug. Take appropriate precautions.

- Administered only in a hospital setting.
- If patient has a dry mouth, give patient ice chips prior to administering drug.
- Put on gloves and tear open the notched pouch only when ready to administer drug. Be aware that the pouch contains one clear plastic single-dose applicator (SDA) that houses a single blue-colored tablet in the tip.
- Remove the white lock from the green pusher by squeezing the sides together and detaching from pusher. To avoid accidentally ejecting the tablet, avoid touching the green pusher before placing the SDA in patient's mouth for administration.
- To administer, tell patient to open mouth and touch the tongue to the roof of the mouth, if possible. Rest the SDA lightly on patient's lips or lower teeth. Place the SDA tip under the tongue and aim at the floor of patient's mouth or sublingual space. Avoid direct mucosal contact with the SDA tip. Gently depress the green pusher to deliver the tablet to patient's sublingual space.
- Tablet should be allowed to dissolve under the tongue and not chewed or swallowed.
- Visually confirm tablet placement. If tablet is not in patient's mouth, it must be retrieved and disposed of according to institutional CII waste procedures.
- Discard the used SDA in biohazard waste container after administration.
- Patient should not eat or drink, and should minimize talking, for 10 minutes after receiving drug.

Route	Onset	Peak	Duration
P.O.	> 10 min	1 hr	2.3–3.8 hr

Half-life: 164 min

Mechanism of Action
Binds to and activates selective mu-opioid receptors found throughout the central nervous system to produce pain relief.

Contraindications
Acute or severe bronchial asthma in an unmonitored setting or in the absence of resuscitative equipment, gastrointestinal obstruction including paralytic ileus, hypersensitivity to sufentanil or its components, significant respiratory depression

Interactions

DRUGS

5-HT3 inhibitors (used to treat psychiatric disorders), linezolid, methylene blue (intravenous), selective serotonin reuptake inhibitors, serotonin and norepinephrine reuptake inhibitors, tricyclic antidepressants, triptans: Increased risk of serotonin syndrome

anticholinergic drugs: Possibly increased risk of urinary retention and/or severe constipation, which may lead to paralytic ileus

benzodiazepines and other CNS depressants: Increased risk of serious adverse reactions such as coma, hypotension, profound sedation, and severe respiratory depression

CYP3A4 inducers such as carbamazepine, phenytoin, rifampin: Decreased plasma concentration of sufentanil, resulting in decreased efficacy or possible withdrawal symptoms in patients who have developed physical dependence to sufentanil

CYP3A4 inhibitors such as azole-antifungal agents (ketoconazole), macrolide antibiotics (erythromycin), and protease inhibitors (ritonavir): Increased plasma concentration of sufentanil, resulting in increased or prolonged effects

diuretics: Reduced efficacy of diuretics

MAO inhibitors: Increased risk of serotonin syndrome; increased risk of opioid toxicity

mixed agonist/antagonist or partial agonist opioid analgesics such as buprenorphine, butorphanol, nalbuphine, pentazocine: Possibly reduced analgesic effect of sufentanil and possible precipitation of withdrawal symptoms

muscle relaxants: Possibly enhanced neuromuscular blocking action of skeletal muscle relaxants; increased degree of respiratory depression

ACTIVITIES

alcohol use: Increased risk of serious adverse reactions such as coma, hypotension, profound sedation, and severe respiratory depression

Adverse Reactions

CNS: Agitation, anxiety, confusion, disorientation, dizziness, euphoric mood, hallucination, headache, hemiparesis, insomnia, lethargy, memory impairment, mental status changes, **seizures, serotonin syndrome,** somnolence, syncope

CV: **Bradycardia, electrocardiogram abnormalities,** hypertension, **hypotension (severe),** orthostatic hypotension, tachycardia

EENT: Oral hypoesthesia

ENDO: **Adrenal insufficiency**

GI: Abdominal distention or pain, belching, constipation, diarrhea, dyspepsia, elevated liver enzymes, flatulence, gastritis, nausea, postoperative ileus, vomiting

GU: Decreased urine output, oliguria, **renal failure,** urinary hesitation or retention

MS: Muscle spasms

RESP: **Apnea, atelectasis, bradypnea, decreased oxygen saturation and respiratory rate, hypoventilation, hypoxia, life-threatening respiratory depression, respiratory distress or failure**

SKIN: Diaphoresis, flushing, pruritus, rash

Other: **Anaphylaxis,** physiological and physical dependence

Childbearing Considerations

PREGNANCY

- Drug may cause fetal harm.
- Prolonged use of drug during pregnancy can result in neonatal opioid withdrawal syndrome (NOWS), which may be life-threatening if not recognized and treated.
- Use with caution only if benefit to mother outweighs potential risk to fetus.

LABOR & DELIVERY

- Drug is not recommended for use in pregnant women immediately before or during labor. Opioids may alter length of time of labor.
- Opioids cross the placenta and may produce respiratory depression and psycho-physiologic effects in the neonate. Monitor neonate closely for signs of excess sedation and respiratory depression.
- An opioid antagonist, such as naloxone, must be available at the time of delivery in the event it is needed to reverse opioid-induced respiratory depression in the neonate.

LACTATION

- Drug is present in breast milk.
- Patient should check with prescriber before resuming breastfeeding.
- Infants exposed to drug through breast milk should be monitored for excess sedation and respiratory depression.

Q
R
S

REPRODUCTION

- Although drug is given for no more than 72 hours, be aware that chronic use of opioids may reduce fertility in females and males.

Nursing Considerations

- Be aware that excessive use of sufentanil may lead to abuse, addiction, misuse, overdose, and possibly death. Know that sufentanil is available only through a restricted Risk Evaluation and Mitigation Strategy (REMS) program. Monitor patient's intake of drug closely. Alert prescriber if patient has a history of dependence on other opioids.
- Use extreme caution when administering sufentanil to patients with significant chronic obstructive pulmonary disease or cor pulmonale, and to patients having a substantially decreased respiratory reserve, hypercapnia, hypoxia, or preexisting respiratory depression, especially when initiating or titrating therapy. These patients may develop respiratory depression, even with usual therapeutic doses, because sufentanil may decrease patient's respiratory drive to the point of apnea.
- Know that sufentanil may cause sleep-related disorders including central sleep apnea and sleep-related hypoxemia increasing the risk in a dose-dependent fashion. If patient develops central sleep apnea, know that sufentanil dose may have to be decreased.
- Use sufentanil cautiously in cachectic, debilitated, or elderly patients, especially when initiating and titrating therapy, as these patients are at increased risk for adverse effects, especially respiratory depression.

! WARNING Monitor patient for respiratory depression that could become life-threatening quickly, especially when drug is initiated or if patient is accidently exposed to drug. However, know that respiratory depression may occur at any time during sufentanil use and may occur even when used as recommended. If patient develops respiratory depression, expect to give naloxone. Watch for seizures, because naloxone may increase this risk. Take seizure precautions.

- Be aware that sufentanil may increase the frequency of seizures in patients with seizure disorders and may increase risk of seizures in the presence of other conditions associated with seizures. Monitor patient closely.
- Be aware that opioids like sufentanil should not be given to women during pregnancy, while in labor, or when breastfeeding, as newborn or infant may experience neonatal opioid withdrawal syndrome (NOWS). This syndrome may exhibit as excessive or high-pitched crying, poor feeding, rapid breathing, or trembling. If not recognized and treated appropriately, it can become life-threatening.
- Monitor patients closely who may be susceptible to the intracranial effects of carbon dioxide retention from respiratory depression caused by sufentanil therapy, such as patients with head injuries or those who have a preexisting elevation in intracranial pressure.

! WARNING Know that many drugs may interact with opioids like sufentanil to cause serotonin syndrome. Monitor patient closely for signs and symptoms such as agitation, diaphoresis, diarrhea, fever, hallucinations, labile blood pressure, muscle twitching or stiffness, nausea, shakiness, shivering, tachycardia, trouble with coordination, or vomiting. Notify prescriber at once, because serotonin syndrome may be life-threatening. Be prepared to discontinue drug, if possible and ordered, and provide supportive care.

- Monitor effectiveness of sufentanil in relieving pain; consult prescriber as needed.
- Assess patient for constipation and provide a high-fiber diet and adequate fluid intake, if not contraindicated, because constipation can become severe.
- Monitor patient for evidence of physical dependence or abuse. Know that addiction can occur not only in those who obtain drug illicitly but also in patients who are appropriately prescribed drug at recommended doses. Be aware that excessive use of sufentanil may lead to abuse, addiction, misuse, overdose, and possibly death.

- Notify prescriber if serious adverse reactions occur with sufentanil therapy and expect dosage to be reduced.

! **WARNING** Monitor patient's vital signs closely. Know that in addition to respiratory depression, sufentanil may cause severe hypotension, especially in patients whose blood pressure is already compromised by a depleted blood volume or after concurrent administration of drugs that decrease blood pressure. Also be aware that drug may cause bradycardia in some patients.

! **WARNING** Be aware that concomitant use with CYP3A4 inhibitors or discontinuation of CYP3A inducers can result in a fatal overdose of sufentanil.

! **WARNING** Monitor patient for adrenal insufficiency. Although rare, it can be life-threatening. Monitor patient for anorexia, dizziness, fatigue, hypotension, nausea, vomiting, or weakness. Notify prescriber if adrenal insufficiency is suspected and expect diagnostic testing to be done. If diagnosis is confirmed, expect to administer corticosteroids and discontinue sufentanil.

- Monitor patient for decreased bowel motility in postoperative patients receiving sufentanil, as drug may obscure the development of acute abdominal conditions.

! **WARNING** Be aware that sufentanil should only be used concomitantly with benzodiazepine therapy in patients for whom other treatment options are inadequate. If prescribed together, expect dosing and duration of sufentanil to be limited. Monitor patient closely for signs and symptoms of a decrease in consciousness, including coma, profound sedation, and significant respiratory depression. Notify prescriber immediately and provide emergency supportive care, as death may occur.

PATIENT TEACHING
- Instruct patient to allow sufentanil tablet to dissolve under the tongue and not to chew or swallow the tablet. Also advise patient not to drink or eat and to minimize talking for 10 minutes after each dose of the drug.

- Warn patient of possibility of addiction even when taken as prescribed.

! **WARNING** Alert patient that respiratory depression may occur with sufentanil use, especially when drug is first given, and to report any breathing difficulties immediately.

- Caution patient to avoid having alcohol or other drugs brought to him in the healthcare setting because ingesting alcohol, including medications containing alcohol, increases the risk of overdose, respiratory depression, and death, as does taking other types of depressants, including benzodiazepines, together with sufentanil therapy.
- Instruct patient to rise slowly from a lying or sitting position and to lie or sit down if he experiences light-headedness. If effect is frequent or severe, tell him to notify prescriber.
- Urge patient to consume plenty of fluids and high-fiber foods, if not contraindicated, to prevent constipation.
- Alert mother who was breastfeeding before drug given to check with prescriber before breastfeeding is resumed. If breastfeeding occurs, tell mother to monitor infant closely for excess sedation and respiratory depression.

sulfadiazine

Class and Category
Pharmacologic class: Sulfonamide
Therapeutic class: Antibiotic

Indications and Dosages
✶ *As adjunct to treat chloroquine-resistant malaria,* Haemophilus influenzae *acute otitis media (with penicillin) or meningitis (with streptomycin), or toxoplasmosis encephalitis (with pyrimethamine) in patients with or without acquired immunodeficiency syndrome; to prevent or treat meningococcal meningitis; to treat chancroid, inclusive conjunctivitis, nocardiosis, or trachoma; to treat urinary tract infections such as cystitis, pyelitis, or pyelonephritis caused by* Enterobacter *species,* Escherichia coli, Klebsiella *species,* Proteus mirabilis, P. vulgaris, *and* Staphylococcus aureus *after failure with other sulfonamides*

TABLETS

Adults. *Initial:* 2 to 4 g. *Maintenance:* 2 to 4 g daily, divided into 3 to 6 doses.
Infants age 2 months and over and children. *Initial:* 75 mg/kg. *Maintenance:* 150 mg/kg daily divided into 4 to 6 doses. *Maximum:* 6 g daily.

✱ *To prevent rheumatic fever*

TABLETS

Children weighing more than 30 kg (66 lb). 1 g daily.
Children weighing less than 30 kg (66 lb). 500 mg daily.

▤ Drug Administration

P.O.

- Administer consistently at same time daily.
- Give each dose with 8 ounces of water.

Route	Onset	Peak	Duration
P.O.	Unknown	4–6 hr	Unknown
Half-life: 8–17 hr			

▤ Mechanism of Action

Inhibits para-aminobenzoic acid, a bacterial enzyme responsible for synthesizing folic acid, which susceptible bacteria require for growth. By inactivating bacteria, sulfadiazine prevents or alleviates infection.

▤ Contraindications

Breastfeeding; hypersensitivity to sulfadiazine, its components, or other chemically related drugs, such as sulfonamides; infants under the age of 2 months except as adjunctive treatment for congenital toxoplasmosis; pregnancy at term

▤ Interactions

DRUGS

indomethacin, probenecid, salicylates: Increased concentration of sulfadiazine
methotrexate, oral anticoagulants, sulfonylurea hypoglycemic agents, thiazide diuretics, uricosuric agents: Increased effects of these drugs increasing risk of adverse reactions

▤ Adverse Reactions

CNS: Dizziness, fatigue, fever, headache, lethargy, weakness
EENT: Pharyngitis
GI: Anorexia, diarrhea, dysphagia, jaundice, nausea, vomiting
GU: Crystalluria

HEME: Agranulocytosis, aplastic anemia, hemolytic anemia, leukopenia, thrombocytopenia, unusual bleeding or bruising
MS: Arthralgia, myalgia
SKIN: Blisters, erythema, pallor, photosensitivity, pruritus, rash
Other: Drug-induced fever

▤ Childbearing Considerations

PREGNANCY

- It is not known if drug can cause fetal harm.
- Drug is contraindicated in pregnancy at term.
- Use with caution only if benefit to mother not at term outweighs potential risk to fetus.

LACTATION

- Drug is present in breast milk.
- Drug is contraindicated with breastfeeding.

▤ Nursing Considerations

- Use sulfadiazine cautiously in patients with blood dyscrasias or megaloblastic anemia from folate deficiency because drug may cause blood dyscrasias; in those with G6PD deficiency because hemolysis may occur; in those with hepatic or renal impairment because of increased risk of toxicity; and in those with porphyria because drug may precipitate an acute attack.
- Obtain blood sample for CBC and body tissue or fluid specimen for culture and sensitivity tests, as ordered, before giving drug. Expect first dose to be given before results are available.

! **WARNING** Monitor patient for drug-induced fever, which may develop 7 to 10 days after starting sulfadiazine therapy. Signs and symptoms may include abdominal pain, anorexia, ataxia, depression, diarrhea, headache, insomnia, nausea, peripheral neuropathy, tinnitus, and vomiting.

- Monitor fluid intake and output during therapy. Altered fluid balance may increase risk of crystalluria.
- Monitor patient's blood glucose level, and assess for signs and symptoms of hypoglycemia in patients who take an oral antidiabetic drug. Be prepared to respond if hypoglycemia develops.

PATIENT TEACHING

- Instruct patient to take sulfadiazine exactly as prescribed and to complete the full course, even if he feels better.
- Advise patient to take drug with a full glass of water and to drink plenty of fluids during therapy.
- Urge patient to notify prescriber if urine turns reddish brown; this may indicate crystalluria.
- Inform patient about possible dizziness, and urge him to avoid potentially hazardous activities until drug's CNS effects are known.
- Advise patient to avoid prolonged exposure to sunlight and to wear sunscreen and protective clothing when outdoors.
- Urge patient who takes oral contraceptives to use an additional method of birth control during therapy.
- Advise patient who takes an oral antidiabetic drug to check his blood glucose level frequently because of the increased risk of hypoglycemia during therapy.

sulfasalazine

Azulfidine, Azulfidine EN-Tabs, Salazopyrin (CAN), Salazopyrin EN-Tabs (CAN)

▤ Class and Category

Pharmacologic class: Salicylate-sulfonamide
Therapeutic class: Anti-inflammatory

▤ Indications and Dosages

⁎ *To treat mild-to-moderate ulcerative colitis; as adjunct to treat severe ulcerative colitis; to prolong remission period between acute attacks of ulcerative colitis*

DELAYED-RELEASE TABLETS, TABLETS

Adults and adolescents. *Initial:* 1–2 g daily in evenly divided doses every 6 to 8 hr; increased as needed. *Maintenance:* 500 mg every 6 hr.

Children age 6 and over. *Initial:* 40 to 60 mg/kg daily divided into 3 to 6 doses. *Maintenance:* 30 mg/kg daily divided into 4 doses.

⁎ *To treat rheumatoid arthritis in patients who have not responded to salicylates or other NSAIDs*

DELAYED-RELEASE TABLETS

Adults. *Initial:* 500 mg daily during wk 1, increased by 500 mg daily every wk, as needed, up to 2,000 mg daily in divided doses. If no response after 12 wk, increased to 3,000 mg daily. *Maintenance:* 1,000 mg every 12 hr. *Maximum:* 3,000 mg daily.

⁎ *To treat juvenile rheumatoid arthritis in patients who have not responded to salicylates or other NSAIDs*

DELAYED-RELEASE TABLETS

Children ages 6 and over. 30 to 50 mg/kg daily in divided doses twice daily. *Maximum:* 2 g daily.

±**DOSAGE ADJUSTMENT** For patients with ulcerative colitis, initial dosage may be reduced if GI intolerance occurs. For adult patients with rheumatoid arthritis as a means to reduce possible GI intolerance, initial dosage may be reduced to 0.5 to 1 g daily and then increased weekly as needed. For children with juvenile rheumatoid arthritis as a means to reduce possible GI intolerance, initial dosage may be reduced to one-quarter to one-third of expected maintenance dose and then gradually increased weekly to reach maintenance dose.

▤ Drug Administration

P.O.

- Administer drug with meals (immediate-release) or after meals (delayed-release).
- Give drug with a full glass of water.
- Delayed-release tablets should be swallowed whole and not chewed, crushed, or divided.

Route	Onset	Peak	Duration
P.O.	Unknown	3–12 hr	Unknown
P.O./D.R.	Unknown	6 hr	Unknown

Half-life: 6–14 hr

▤ Mechanism of Action

As a prodrug of sulfapyridine and 5-aminosalicylic acid (mesalamine), delivers more sulfapyridine and mesalamine to the colon than either metabolite could provide alone. Sulfapyridine provides antibacterial action along the intestinal wall; mesalamine inhibits cyclooxygenase, thereby decreasing the production of arachidonic acid metabolites and reducing colonic inflammation. It also reduces joint

Q
R
S

inflammation locally caused by rheumatoid arthritis.

Contraindications

Hypersensitivity to salicylates, sulfasalazine or its metabolites, sulfonamides, or their components; intestinal or urinary obstruction; porphyria

Interactions

DRUGS

digoxin: Possibly inhibited absorption and decreased blood level of digoxin
folic acid (vitamin B₉): Decreased folic acid absorption
methotrexate: Increased incidence of gastrointestinal adverse reactions, especially nausea

Adverse Reactions

CNS: Ataxia, chills, depression, fatigue, fever, **Guillain–Barré syndrome**, headache, insomnia, **meningitis**, peripheral neuropathy, **seizures**, vertigo, weakness
CV: Myocarditis, pericarditis, vasculitis
EENT: Hearing loss, orange-yellow tears, oropharyngeal pain, pharyngitis, tinnitus
GI: Abdominal pain, anorexia, **cirrhosis,** diarrhea, elevated liver enzymes, **hepatitis, hepatotoxicity,** indigestion, jaundice, nausea, **pancreatitis,** ulcerative colitis exacerbation, vomiting
GU: Crystalluria, decreased ejaculatory volume, male infertility, **nephritis,** nephrolithiasis, **nephrotic syndrome,** orange-yellow urine, **toxic nephrosis**
HEME: Agranulocytosis, aplastic anemia, hemolytic anemia, hematophagic histiocytosis, leukopenia, neutropenia, thrombocytopenia, unusual bleeding or bruising
MS: Arthralgia, **rhabdomyolysis**
RESP: Cyanosis, eosinophilic infiltration, **idiopathic pulmonary fibrosis, lymphocytic interstitial pneumonitis,** pleuritis pneumonia
SKIN: Acute generalized exanthematous pustulosis (AGEP), alopecia, **erythema multiforme, exfoliative dermatitis,** photosensitivity, pruritus, purpura, rash, **Stevens–Johnson syndrome,** toxic epidermal necrolysis, urticaria
Other: Anaphylaxis, angioedema, drug rash with eosinophilia and systemic symptoms (DRESS), folate deficiency, infections (serious), lupus erythematosus-like syndrome, mononucleosis-like syndrome, **sepsis,** serum sickness syndrome

Childbearing Considerations

PREGNANCY

- It is not known if drug can cause fetal harm. However, drug does pass the placental barrier, increasing risk of kernicterus in the neonate.
- Use with caution only if benefit to mother outweighs potential risk to fetus.

LACTATION

- Drug is present in breast milk.
- Infants less than 2 months of age should not be breastfed, because of risk of kernicterus. Patient should check with prescriber before breastfeeding older infants.
- Be aware that studies are mixed regarding drug causing bloody stools and/or diarrhea in breastfed infants.

REPRODUCTION

- Infertility and oligospermia have been reported in male patients; reversal usually occurs when drug is discontinued.

Nursing Considerations

! WARNING Be aware that patients with hematologic toxicity or hepatic or renal dysfunction may develop serious to life-threatening adverse reactions. Assess patient for fever, jaundice, pallor, purpura, or sore throat prior to drug being given. Monitor BUN and serum creatinine levels, CBC, and liver enzymes, before and periodically during sulfasalazine therapy.

- Expect drug to be withheld while awaiting laboratory results in patients experiencing symptoms of hematologic, hepatic, or renal dysfunction.
- Use sulfasalazine cautiously in patients with a history of recurring or chronic infections because drug may predispose patient to infections. Monitor patients for new infections throughout therapy. If present, notify prescriber.
- Be aware that sulfasalazine doses over 4 g or a blood level over 50 mcg/ml increase the risk of adverse and toxic reactions. Know that serious infections, including fatal sepsis and pneumonia, have occurred in patients taking sulfasalazine.

- Monitor fluid intake and output and urine color, consistency, and pH. Acidic urine may require alkalization to prevent crystalluria.
- Be aware that measurements, by liquid chromatography, of urinary normetanephrine may cause a false-positive test result.

! WARNING Monitor patient, especially during the first month of sulfasalazine therapy, for hypersensitivity or skin reactions that may become life-threatening. At first sign of mucosal lesions, rash, or any other sign of hypersensitivity, stop sulfasalazine therapy and notify prescriber.

PATIENT TEACHING

- Instruct patient to take sulfasalazine with meals (immediate-release) or after meals (delayed-release), to decrease GI distress. Also tell patient to swallow delayed-release tablets whole and not to chew, swallow, or divide them.
- Advise patient to prevent crystalluria by taking drug with a full glass of water and drinking at least 64 oz of fluid per day.
- Instruct patient and family to administer drug around the clock.
- Inform patient that symptom relief may take 2 to 5 days for ulcerative colitis and 4 to 12 weeks for rheumatoid arthritis.
- Alert patient that drug may turn skin and urine orange-yellow.
- Advise contact lens wearer to consider wearing glasses during therapy because drug can permanently stain contact lenses yellow.
- Instruct patient to avoid prolonged sun exposure and to wear protective clothing and sunscreen when outdoors.
- Advise patient to brush with a soft-bristled toothbrush and to use dental floss and toothpicks gently because leukopenic and thrombocytopenic drug effects increase risk of gingival bleeding and infection.
- Urge patient to return for laboratory tests and follow-up visits to monitor drug's effect.

! WARNING Instruct patient to report allergic reactions, fever; jaundice; paleness; skin abnormalities such as skin blistering, discoloration, rash or hives; or sore throat. These may be signs of serious adverse effects. If present, advise patient to notify prescriber immediately and if serious or severe to seek immediate medical attention. Explain that prescriber will order tests to determine the cause and that drug may be withheld until test results are known.

- Instruct mothers who are breastfeeding to stop taking sulfasalazine or stop breastfeeding immediately if their infant develops bloody stools or diarrhea, and to notify prescriber. Also, inform mothers that breastfeeding is not recommended for infants under 2 months of age.

sulindac

Class and Category
Pharmacologic class: NSAID
Therapeutic class: Analgesic, anti-inflammatory

Indications and Dosages
✳ *To decrease pain and inflammation in ankylosing spondylitis, osteoarthritis, and rheumatoid arthritis*

TABLETS
Adults. *Initial:* 150 mg twice daily, adjusted based on patient's response. *Maximum:* 200 mg twice daily.

✳ *To relieve symptoms of acute gouty arthritis, acute subacromial bursitis, and supraspinatus tendinitis*

TABLETS
Adults. 200 mg twice daily for 7 days for acute gouty arthritis and 7 to 14 days for bursitis and tendinitis; decreased to lowest effective dosage after satisfactory response occurs. *Maximum:* 400 mg daily.

Drug Administration
P.O.

- Administer drug with or immediately after meals to decrease GI distress.
- Administer with a full glass of water.
- Have patient remain upright for 20 to 30 minutes after administration to prevent drug from lodging in esophagus and causing esophageal irritation.

Route	Onset	Peak	Duration
P.O.	> 1 wk	3–4 hr	Unknown

Half-life: 7–8 hr

Mechanism of Action

May block the activity of cyclooxygenase, an enzyme needed to synthesize prostaglandins, which mediate the inflammatory response that cause local vasodilation, pain, and swelling. By blocking cyclooxygenase and inhibiting prostaglandins, this NSAID reduces inflammatory symptoms and pain.

Contraindications

Asthma, urticaria, or allergic-type reactions induced by aspirin or other NSAIDs; hypersensitivity to sulindac, other NSAIDs, and their components; in setting of coronary artery bypass graft (CABG) surgery

Interactions

DRUGS

angiotensin-converting enzyme (ACE) inhibitors, angiotensin II antagonists: Decreased antihypertensive effect of these drugs; increased risk of renal impairment in patients with already compromised renal function
cyclosporine: Increased cyclosporine-induced toxicity
diflunisal: Decreased plasma sulindac levels, decreasing effectiveness
dimethyl sulfoxide (DMSO): Decreased sulindac effectiveness, possibly peripheral neuropathy
diuretics: Possibly decreased diuretic effects
lithium: Possibly increased blood level and toxic effects of lithium
methotrexate: Decreased methotrexate excretion, possibly leading to toxicity
other NSAIDs, warfarin: Increased risk of gastrointestinal toxicity including GI bleeding
platelet aggregation inhibitors: Increased risk of bleeding, additive effects of these drugs
probenecid: Increased blood level and adverse and toxic effects of sulindac

ACTIVITIES

alcohol use: Increased risk of adverse GI effects, including GI bleeding

Adverse Reactions

CNS: Aseptic meningitis, chills, CVA, drowsiness, fever, headache, malaise, nervousness, transient ischemic attack
CV: Deep vein thrombosis, edema, heart failure, hypertension, MI, palpitations, peripheral edema, vasculitis
EENT: Tinnitus

ENDO: Hypoglycemia
GI: Abdominal cramps or pain, anorexia, constipation, diarrhea, esophageal irritation, flatulence, gastritis, GI bleeding or ulceration, hepatic failure, hepatitis, hepatotoxicity, indigestion, jaundice, nausea, perforation of intestines or stomach, vomiting
GU: Acute renal failure, decreased urine output, interstitial nephritis, nephrotic syndrome, polyuria, proteinuria
HEME: Agranulocytosis, aplastic anemia, leukopenia, pancytopenia
RESP: Bronchospasm, dyspnea, pulmonary edema, wheezing
SKIN: Diaphoresis, erythema multiforme, exfoliative dermatitis, maculopapular rash, pruritus, purpura, Stevens–Johnson syndrome, toxic epidermal necrolysis, urticaria
Other: Anaphylaxis, angioedema, hypersensitivity reactions

Childbearing Considerations

PREGNANCY

- Drug increases risk of premature closure of the fetal ductus arteriosus if given during the third trimester of pregnancy.
- Drug increases risk of oligohydramnios and neonatal renal impairment if administered at or beyond 20 weeks gestation.
- Drug should be avoided in pregnant women starting at 30 weeks of gestation and onward.
- Drug should only be administered if absolutely necessary to a pregnant woman at 20 weeks up to 30 weeks gestation using the lowest possible dose and shortest duration possible.

LACTATION

- It is not known if drug is present in breast milk.
- A decision should be made to discontinue breastfeeding or the drug to avoid potential serious adverse reactions in the breastfed infant.

REPRODUCTION

- The use of drug may delay or prevent rupture of ovarian follicles, which has caused reversible infertility in some women. Drug should not be used in women who are having difficulty conceiving or are undergoing infertility testing.

≡ Nursing Considerations

- Use sulindac with extreme caution in patients with a history of GI bleeding or ulcer disease because NSAIDs such as sulindac increase risk of GI bleeding and ulceration. Expect to use sulindac for the shortest time possible in these patients.

! WARNING Be aware that serious GI tract bleeding, perforation, and ulceration may occur without warning symptoms. Elderly patients are at greater risk. To minimize risk, give drug with food. If GI distress occurs, withhold drug and notify prescriber at once.

- Use sulindac cautiously in patients with hypertension, and monitor blood pressure closely throughout therapy. Drug may cause hypertension or worsen it.

! WARNING Monitor patient closely for thrombotic events, including MI and stroke, because NSAIDs increase the risk.

- Be aware that if patient has systemic lupus erythematosus and mixed connective tissue disease, monitor him closely because sulindac increases the risk of aseptic meningitis.

! WARNING Know that if patient has bone marrow suppression or is receiving antineoplastic drug therapy, monitor laboratory results (including WBC count), and watch for evidence of infection because anti-inflammatory and antipyretic actions of sulindac may mask signs and symptoms, such as fever and pain.

- Monitor patient closely, especially if patient is elderly or taking sulindac long term; watch for less common but serious adverse GI reactions, including anorexia, constipation, diverticulitis, dysphagia, esophagitis, gastritis, gastroenteritis, gastroesophageal reflux disease, hemorrhoids, hiatal hernia, melena, stomatitis, and vomiting.
- Monitor liver enzymes because, in rare cases, elevated levels may progress to severe hepatic reactions, including fatal hepatitis, hepatic failure, and liver necrosis.
- Watch BUN and serum creatinine levels in elderly patients; those with heart failure, hepatic dysfunction, or impaired renal function; and those taking ACE inhibitors or diuretics, because drug may cause renal failure.
- Monitor CBC for decreased hemoglobin and hematocrit because drug may worsen anemia.

! WARNING Assess patient's skin routinely for rash or other signs of hypersensitivity reaction because sulindac and other NSAIDs may cause serious skin reactions without warning, even in patients with no history of NSAID hypersensitivity. Stop drug at first sign of reaction, and notify prescriber. Know that hypersensitivity syndrome, which could become life-threatening, may develop. Report multiple occurring and multiorgan adverse reactions to prescriber and expect drug to be discontinued. Be prepared to provide emergency supportive care, as ordered.

! WARNING Monitor patient for adventitious breath sounds and dyspnea; sulindac may cause fluid retention, which may precipitate heart failure in susceptible patients.

- Expect patient to undergo audiometric examinations before and periodically during prolonged therapy, as ordered.

PATIENT TEACHING

- Instruct patient to take sulindac exactly as prescribed. Explain that higher doses don't increase effectiveness and may increase risk of adverse reactions.
- Instruct patient to take drug with or immediately after meals to decrease GI distress, to take with a full glass of water, and to remain upright for 20 to 30 minutes after administration to prevent drug from lodging in esophagus and causing esophageal irritation.
- Urge patient to notify prescriber immediately of chills, fever, rash, or sweating, which may indicate hypersensitivity.
- Advise patient to consult prescriber before using acetaminophen, alcohol, aspirin, other NSAIDs, or any OTC drugs during sulindac therapy.
- Caution patient to avoid hazardous activities until drug's CNS effects are known.
- Explain the need for periodic laboratory tests and physical examinations during prolonged therapy to monitor drug effectiveness.

Q.
R
S

- Inform patient that sulindac may increase the risk of serious adverse cardiovascular reactions; urge patient to seek immediate medical attention if signs or symptoms arise, such as chest pain, shortness of breath, slurring of speech, or weakness.
- Tell patient that sulindac also may increase the risk of serious adverse GI reactions; stress the need to seek immediate medical attention for such signs and symptoms as abdominal or epigastric pain, black or tarry stools, indigestion, or vomiting blood or material that looks like coffee grounds.

! **WARNING** Alert patient to the possibility of rare but serious hypersensitivity and skin reactions. Urge him to seek immediate medical attention for blisters, fever, itching, rash, or other indications of hypersensitivity.

sumatriptan
Imitrex Nasal Spray, Tosymra Nasal Spray

sumatriptan succinate
Imitrex, Imitrex STATdose, Onzetra Xsail, Zembrace SymTouch

☰ Class and Category
Pharmacologic class: Serotonin 5-HT$_1$-receptor agonist
Therapeutic class: Antimigraine

☰ Indications and Dosages
∗ *To relieve acute migraine attacks, with or without aura*

TABLETS (IMITREX)
Adults. 25, 50, or 100 mg as a single dose as soon as possible after onset of symptoms, repeated after at least 2 hr, as needed. *Maximum:* 200 mg daily.
±**DOSAGE ADJUSTMENT** For patients with mild-to-moderate hepatic dysfunction, 50 mg is maximum single dose.

SUBCUTANEOUS INJECTION (ZEMBRACE SYMTOUCH)
Adults. *Initial:* 3 mg, repeated after 1 hr, as needed. *Maximum:* 4 (3-mg) injections/24 hr with dosages separated by at least 1 hr.

SUBCUTANEOUS INJECTION (IMITREX)
Adults. *Initial:* 1 to 6 mg (Imitrex) depending on severity of headache, repeated after at least 1 hr, as needed. *Maximum:* 12 mg (two 6-mg injections) in 24 hr with doses separated by at least 1 hr.

NASAL SPRAY (IMITREX)
Adults. 5 mg, 10 mg, or 20 mg given as a single spray in 1 nostril or 10 mg given as a single 5-mg spray in each nostril. One additional dose may be taken if migraine not resolved or another attack occurs after at least 2 hr. *Maximum:* 40 mg daily.

NASAL SPRAY (TOSYMRA)
Adults. 10 mg given as a single spray in 1 nostril. Dose repeated after at least 1 hour if migraine not resolved or another attack occurs. Alternatively, 10 mg given as a single spray in 1 nostril and, if migraine not relieved after 1 hour, another sumatriptan product may be administered. *Maximum:* 30 mg daily with each 10-mg dose separated by at least 1 hour.

NASAL POWDER (ONZETRA XSAIL)
Adults. 22 mg (11 mg in each nostril). One additional dose given after 2 hr if migraine not resolved or another attack occurs. *Maximum:* 44 mg (2 doses) in 24 hours or 22 mg plus one dose of another sumatriptan product, separated by at least 2 hr, in 24 hr.
∗ *To relieve cluster headaches*

SUBCUTANEOUS INJECTION (IMITREX)
Adults. *Initial:* 6 mg, repeated after 1 or 2 hr, as needed. *Maximum:* 2 (6-mg) injections/ 24 hr with dosages separated by at least 1 hr.

☰ Drug Administration
- Administer drug as soon as symptoms of migraine or cluster headaches occur.

P.O.
- Tablets should be swallowed whole and not chewed, crushed, or divided.
- Administer with fluids to help disguise unpleasant taste.

SUBCUTANEOUS
- Needle shield of prefilled syringe contains dry natural rubber, which may cause an allergic reaction if latex sensitive.
- Never administer by any other route.
- Rotate sites.
- Store at room temperature protected from light.

- Inject only in the abdomen or thigh if using an autoinjector.

Imitrex Autoinjector

- Imitrex can be used with an autoinjector device for 4-mg and 6-mg doses only. Use device only if adequate skin and subcutaneous thickness of at least 1/4 inch is present. To use, open lid of the carrying case, tear off tamper-evident seal, and open the lid over the syringe cartridge. Hold pen by the ridges at the top. Take pen out of the carrying case. Check to make sure the white priming rod is not sticking out from the lower end of the pen. If it is, put pen back into the carrying case and press down firmly until a click is felt. Take pen out of the carrying case again. Put pen in the open cartridge pack and turn to the right until it will not turn any more (about a half a turn). Release safety catch by pressing pen firmly against the skin until the gray part of the barrel slides against the blue part and cannot be pressed any further. The gray part of the barrel must stay in contact with the blue part while injecting drug. When injecting, hold pen against the skin for at least 5 seconds. After each use, put pen back into the carrying case to reset the white priming rod before the next use.

Zembrace SymTouch Autoinjector

- Hold device in one hand and pull red cap off with the other hand, being careful not to put or press thumb, fingers, or hand over the yellow needle guard. Place the autoinjector at a 90-degree angle with the yellow needle guard end gently pressed against patient's skin. Press and hold autoinjector down against the skin. A click will be heard as injection starts. Continue to hold the device down until a second click is heard. Wait 5 seconds before removing autoinjector. The yellow needle guard will drop down and lock over the needle. Check that the red plunger rod has filled the drug viewing window, which means the full dose has been given. Do not reuse the autoinjector. Discard.

INTRANASAL POWDER

- Administer by using one 11-mg nosepiece in each nostril.
- To use nosepiece, remove clear device cap from the reusable delivery device, remove a disposable nosepiece from its foil pouch, and click nosepiece into the device body.
- Fully press and promptly release the white piercing button on the device body to pierce the capsule inside the nosepiece. Press piercing button only once and release prior to administration to each nostril.
- Have patient insert nosepiece into the nostril so that it makes a tight seal. Keeping the nosepiece in the nose, have patient rotate device to place mouthpiece into the mouth.
- Have patient blow forcefully through the mouthpiece to deliver the powder into the nasal cavity. Listen for a rattling sound, which indicates patient has blown forcefully.
- After drug is administrated, have patient remove and discard the nosepiece.
- Use same process using a second 11-mg nosepiece in the other nostril to complete the 22-mg dose.

INTRANASAL SPRAY

- Have patient blow nose before administering drug.
- Have patient hold head in an upright position, while gently closing one nostril. Patient should breathe gently out through mouth.
- Hold drug container with thumb supporting container at bottom and index and middle fingers on either side of the nozzle.
- Insert nozzle into open nostril about 1/2 inch. While patient gently takes a breath in through the nose, press the blue plunger firmly to release dose.
- After removing nozzle, have patient gently breathe in through the nose and out through the mouth for 10 to 20 seconds. Patient should not breathe deeply.
- After use, rinse tip of bottle with hot water (don't suction water into bottle) and dry with a clean tissue. Replace cap after cleaning.

Route	Onset	Peak	Duration
P.O.	30 min	2–2.5 hr	Unknown
SubQ	10 min	12 min	9–24 hr
Nasal spray	15–30 min	5–23 min	Unknown
Nasal powder	Unknown	45 min	Unknown

Half-life: 2–2.5 hr

Mechanism of Action

May stimulate 5-HT$_1$ receptors, causing selective vasoconstriction of dilated and inflamed cranial blood vessels in carotid circulation, thus decreasing carotid arterial blood flow and relieving acute migraines and cluster headaches.

Contraindications

History of CVA, basilar or hemiplegic migraine, or transient ischemic attack; hypersensitivity to sumatriptan or its components; ischemic bowel or coronary artery disease; peripheral vascular disease; recent use (within 24 hr) of ergotamine-containing medication, ergot-type medication (such as dihydroergotamine or methysergide), or another 5-hydroxytryptamine 1 (5-HT1) agonist; severe hepatic impairment; uncontrolled hypertension; use of a MAO inhibitor within 14 days; Wolff-Parkinson-White syndrome or arrhythmias associated with other cardiac accessory conduction pathway disorders

Interactions

DRUGS

antidepressants, lithium: Increased risk of serious adverse effects

ergotamine-containing drugs: Possibly additive or prolonged vasoconstrictive effects including serotonin syndrome

fluoxetine, fluvoxamine, paroxetine, sertraline: Possibly hyper-reflexia, incoordination, and weakness

MAO inhibitors: Risk of decreased sumatriptan clearance, increased risk of serious adverse effects

other triptans: Additive vasospastic effects; increased risk of serotonin syndrome

selective serotonin reuptake inhibitors, serotonin–norepinephrine reuptake inhibitors, tricyclic antidepressants: Increased risk of serotonin syndrome

Adverse Reactions

CNS: Anxiety, atypical sensations, dizziness, drowsiness, fatigue, fever, headache, malaise, sedation, **serotonin syndrome, seizures,** vertigo, weakness

CV: Arrhythmias; chest heaviness, pain, pressure, or tightness; **coronary artery vasospasm; ECG changes;** hypertension; **hypotension;** palpitations; peripheral vascular ischemia

EENT: Abnormal vision, blindness or partial vision loss, jaw or mouth discomfort, nasal burning or irritation, nose or throat discomfort, photophobia (P.O., subcutaneous), taste perversion (nasal), tongue numbness or soreness

GI: Abdominal discomfort, **bloody diarrhea, colonic ischemia,** dysphagia

MS: Muscle cramps, myalgia, neck pain or stiffness

SKIN: Diaphoresis, erythema, flushing, pallor, photosensitivity (P.O., subcutaneous), pruritus, rash, urticaria

Other: Anaphylaxis; angioedema; injection-site burning, erythema, hemorrhage, induration, irritation, pain, paresthesia, pruritis, swelling, and urticaria

Childbearing Considerations

PREGNANCY

- It is not known if drug can cause fetal harm.
- Use with caution only if benefit to mother outweighs potential risk to fetus.

LACTATION

- Drug is present in breast milk following subcutaneous administration.
- Patient should check with prescriber before breastfeeding.
- If patient decides to breastfeed, breastfeeding should be avoided for 12 hours after mother takes drug regardless of form used.

Nursing Considerations

- Be aware that sumatriptan shouldn't be given to elderly patients, because they're more likely to have coronary artery disease (CAD) and more pronounced blood pressure increases.
- Assess patient for arrhythmias, chest pain, or other signs of heart disease and monitor blood pressure in patients with CAD before and for at least 1 hour after sumatriptan administration.
- Don't give sumatriptan within 24 hours of another 5-HT$_1$-receptor agonist, such as naratriptan, rizatriptan, or zolmitriptan with the exception of a single dose of another sumatriptan product, provided the doses are separated by at least 1 to 2 hours depending on brand used. Don't give an ergotamine-containing or ergot-type drug within 24 hours of sumatriptan therapy. Doing so increases risk of serious adverse interactions and effects.

! **WARNING** Monitor patient closely for hypersensitivity reactions, including anaphylaxis and angioedema which may be life-threatening. If present, notify prescriber immediately and expect to provide emergency supportive care according to institution emergency protocols.

- Know that for patients with seizure disorder, seizure precautions should be instituted according to facility policy because sumatriptan may lower seizure threshold.

! **WARNING** Monitor patient closely for serotonin syndrome exhibited by agitation, coma, diarrhea, hyperreflexia, hyperthermia, incoordination, labile blood pressure, nausea, tachycardia, or vomiting. Notify prescriber immediately because serotonin syndrome may be life-threatening and provide supportive care.

PATIENT TEACHING
- Advise patient to use sumatriptan as soon as possible after the onset of migraine symptoms.
- Urge patient to contact prescriber and avoid taking sumatriptan if headache symptoms aren't typical.
- Remind patient not to exceed prescribed daily dosage. Inform him that overuse of the drug for 10 or more days per month may lead to exacerbation of headache and may require detoxification. If his use of the drug increases, advise him to notify his prescriber.
- Advise patient to swallow tablets whole and drink fluids to disguise unpleasant taste.
- Show patient suitable sites for subcutaneous injection, and teach him how to load, administer, and discard autoinjector or how to use subcutaneous needle. Tell patient to alert prescriber if he is allergic to latex, as the needle cap of the prefilled syringe is made of a latex derivative.
- Instruct patient not to take a second dose if first dose doesn't provide significant relief.
- Inform patient that he may experience burning, pain, and redness for 10 to 30 minutes after subcutaneous injection.

Suggest that he apply ice to relieve pain and redness.
- Teach patient prescribed the nasal powder or nasal spray forms how to use them correctly.
- Advise patient never to share the medication with another person even if they have the same symptoms, as cross-contamination and severe adverse reactions could occur.
- Encourage patient to lie down in a dark, quiet room after taking drug to help relieve migraine.

! **WARNING** Instruct patient to seek emergency care for chest, jaw, or neck tightness after drug use because drug may cause coronary artery vasospasm; subsequent doses may require ECG monitoring. Also, tell patient to notify prescriber if an allergic reaction occurs and if serious or severe to seek immediate medical attention.

- Urge patient to report palpitations or rash to prescriber.
- Advise patient to avoid potentially hazardous activities until drug's CNS effects are known.
- Alert patient with seizure disorder that drug may lower seizure threshold.
- Encourage yearly ophthalmologic examinations for patients who require prolonged drug therapy.
- Inform woman who is breastfeeding that she should avoid breastfeeding for 12 hours after treatment with sumatriptan to minimize infant exposure to drug.
- Urge patient to inform all prescribers of sumatriptan therapy because of potentially dangerous drug interactions.

suvorexant
Belsomra

☰ Class, Category, and Schedule
Pharmacologic class: Orexin receptor antagonist
Therapeutic class: Hypnotic
Controlled substance schedule: IV

☰ Indications and Dosages
✳ *To treat insomnia characterized by difficulties with sleep onset and/or sleep maintenance*

TABLETS

Adults. 10 mg once nightly within 30 minutes of bedtime, increased, as needed, to 20 mg once daily. *Maximum:* 20 mg once daily at night.

±**DOSAGE ADJUSTMENT** For patients taking moderate CYP3A inhibitors, dosage reduced to 5 mg once per night, with maximum dosage not exceeding 10 mg once per night. For patients taking CNS depressants concurrently, dosage may have to be decreased.

Drug Administration

P.O.

- Administer within 30 minutes of bedtime and when patient has at least 7 hours remaining for sleep.

Route	Onset	Peak	Duration
P.O.	30 min	2 hr	Unknown
Half-life: 12 hr			

Mechanism of Action

Antagonism of orexin receptors blocks the binding of wake-promoting neuropeptides orexin A and orexin B to produce sleep.

Contraindications

Hypersensitivity to suvorexant and its components, narcolepsy

Interactions

DRUGS

CNS depressants: Additive CNS and respiratory depression; increased risk of abnormal behavior and thinking
CYP3A inducers: Decreased effectiveness of suvorexant
CYP3A inhibitors: Increased effect of suvorexant and incidence of adverse reactions
digoxin: Increased serum digoxin levels

ACTIVITIES

alcohol use: Additive CNS depression; increased risk of abnormal behavior and thinking

Adverse Reactions

CNS: Abnormal dreams, amnesia, anxiety, cataplexy-like behaviors (mild), complex sleep behaviors (sleepwalking, engaging in activities while not fully awake), dizziness, hallucinations, headache, impaired daytime wakefulness, leg weakness (temporary), psychomotor hyperactivity, sleep paralysis (temporarily), somnolence, **suicidal ideation**, worsening of depression
CV: Palpitations, tachycardia
EENT: Dry mouth
GI: Diarrhea, nausea, vomiting
RESP: Cough, upper respiratory tract infection
SKIN: Pruritus
Other: Physical and psychological dependence

Childbearing Considerations

PREGNANCY

- It is not known if drug can cause fetal harm.
- Use with caution only if benefit to mother outweighs potential risk to fetus.

LACTATION

- It is not known if drug is present in breast milk.
- Patient should check with prescriber before breastfeeding.
- If breastfeeding takes place, mother should monitor infant for excessive sedation.

Nursing Considerations

- Use suvorexant with extreme caution in patients with a history of alcohol or drug abuse because of risk of addiction.
- Use suvorexant cautiously in debilitated or elderly patients and those with depression or impaired respiratory function.
- Monitor obese patients and women closely for adverse effects because these patients are at increased risk. Be aware that there is a dosage relationship to development of adverse reactions in general.
- Monitor respiratory status, especially in patients with respiratory compromise, who are at increased risk for respiratory depression.
- Institute fall precautions, because drug causes drowsiness.
- Watch patient closely for suicidal tendencies, particularly when therapy starts and dosage changes, because depression may worsen temporarily during these times, possibly leading to suicidal ideation.

PATIENT TEACHING

- Tell patient to take drug 30 minutes before bedtime on an empty stomach with at least 7 hours remaining for sleep time.
- Caution patient to avoid potentially hazardous activities after taking suvorexant;

drug's intended effect is to decrease alertness. Tell patient that CNS depressant effects may persist in some patients for up to several days after drug is discontinued.

- Advise patient that drug may cause abnormal behaviors during sleep that extend into daytime, causing wakefulness impairment. Such behaviors may include driving a car, eating, talking on the phone, or having sex without any recall of the event. If family members notice any such behavior or patient sees evidence of such behavior upon awakening, drug should be withheld and prescriber notified.

- Advise patient to avoid alcohol while taking suvorexant.

- Tell patient to notify prescriber if insomnia worsens or new signs or symptoms occur.

- Urge family or caregiver to watch patient closely for suicidal tendencies, especially when therapy starts or dosage changes.

T

tacrolimus
Astagraf XL, Envarsus XR, Prograf

≡ Class and Category
Pharmacologic class: Calcineurin inhibitor
Therapeutic class: Immunosuppressant

≡ Indications and Dosages
✳ *To prevent organ rejection in patients undergoing allogeneic heart, kidney, or liver transplantation*

CAPSULES (PROGRAF)
Adults having kidney transplantation in combination with azathioprine. 0.2 mg/kg/day given in two equally divided doses every 12 hr beginning with first dose begun between 6 and 24 hr post-transplant but only after renal function has recovered (serum creatinine level of 4 mg/dl or less).

Adults having kidney transplantation in combination with mycophenolate mofetil (MMF)/IL-2 receptor antagonist therapy. 0.1 mg/kg/day given in two equally divided doses every 12 hr beginning with first dose begun between 6 and 24 hr post-transplant but only after renal function has recovered (serum creatinine level of 4 mg/dl or less).

Adults having liver transplantation with corticosteroids only. 0.10 to 0.15 mg/kg/day given in two equally divided doses every 12 hr. Administer first dose 6 hr after transplantation.

Adults having heart or lung transplantation with azathioprine or MMF. 0.075 mg/kg/day given in two equally divided doses every 12 hr. Administer first dose 6 hr after transplantation.

CAPSULES, ORAL SUSPENSION (PROGRAF)
Children having kidney transplantation. 0.3 mg/kg/day given in two equally divided doses every 12 hr.

Children having liver transplantation. 0.15 to 0.20 mg/kg/day (capsules) or 0.2 mg/kg/day (oral suspension) given in two equally divided doses every 12 hr. Administer first dose 6 hr after transplantation.

Children having heart transplantation. 0.3 mg/kg/day (0.1 mg/kg/day if antibody induction treatment is administered) given in two equally divided doses every 12 hr.

I.V. INFUSION (PROGRAF)
Adults having kidney or liver transplantation. 0.03 to 0.05 mg/kg/day beginning no sooner than 6 hr after transplantation.

Adults having heart transplantation. 0.01 mg/kg/day beginning no sooner than 6 hr after transplantation.

Adults having a lung transplantation. 0.01 to 0.03 mg/kg/day beginning no sooner than 6 hr after transplantation,

Children having liver transplantation. 0.03 to 0.05 mg/kg/day beginning no sooner than 6 hr after transplantation.

±**DOSAGE ADJUSTMENT** For patients with hepatic or renal impairment, dosage kept at lower end of range with possible need for further reduction. African-American adults taking capsule form and patients with cystic fibrosis with lung transplantation using either capsules or oral suspension may need higher doses to attain trough concentrations.

✳ *To prevent organ rejection in patients undergoing allogeneic kidney transplantation*

EXTENDED-RELEASE CAPSULES (ASTAGRAF XL)
Adults taking MMF and steroids with basiliximab. *Initial:* 0.15 to 0.2 mg/kg once daily prior to reperfusion or within 48 hr of completion of transplant procedure. Dosage then adjusted to achieve target trough concentration range.

Adults taking MMF and steroids without basiliximab. *Preoperatively:* 0.1 mg/kg as a single dose within 12 hr prior to reperfusion. *Postoperatively:* 0.2 mg/kg as the second dose given at least 4 hr after the preoperative dose and within 12 hr after reperfusion, then adjusted to achieve target trough concentration ranges.

Children with basiliximab MMF and steroids. 0.3 mg/kg once daily administered within 24 hr following reperfusion.

±**DOSAGE ADJUSTMENT FOR ASTAGRAF XL** African-American patients may need higher doses to attain trough concentrations comparable to those of Caucasian patients. For patients with severe hepatic impairment, lower dosage may be required. For patients taking CYP3A inducers or inhibitors, dosage may have to be adjusted.

* *To prevent organ rejection in patients undergoing allogenic kidney transplantation and are converting from a tacrolimus immediate-release product*

XR TABLETS (ENVARSUS XR)

Adults in combination with other immunosuppressants. *Initial:* 80% of total daily dose of immediate-release product given once daily, then adjusted to achieve target whole blood trough concentration range of 4 to 11 ng/ml.

* *To prevent organ rejection in de novo kidney transplant patients*

XR TABLETS (ENVARSUS XR)

Adults in combination with other immunosuppressants. *Initial:* 0.14 mg/kg/day, then titrated, as needed.

± **DOSAGE ADJUSTMENT FOR ENVARSUS XR** African-American patients may need higher doses to attain trough concentrations comparable to those of Caucasian patients. For patients with severe hepatic impairment, lower dosage may be required. For patients receiving CYP3A inducers or inhibitors concomitantly, dosage may have to be adjusted.

⌸ Drug Administration

- Tacrolimus can cause fetal harm. Take special precautions when handling drug.

P.O.

- Do not interchange immediate-release capsules with extended-release capsules or tablets. Also, do not interchange extended-release capsules with extended-release tablets, nor interchange capsules with granules used to make oral suspension.
- Keep in mind when converting patient from parenteral to oral therapy after heart transplantation, expect to give oral form 8 to 12 hours after infusion is discontinued.
- To prepare oral suspension, empty the entire contents of each Prograf granules packet into a glass cup. Add 15 to 30 ml of room-temperature drinking water to the cup. Mix and administer entire contents of cup immediately. Granules will not completely dissolve. For younger patients, the suspension can be drawn up via a non-PVC oral syringe that is dispensed with drug. Refill the cup or syringe with 15 to 30 ml of water and give to patient to

ensure that all of the medication is taken. Do not sprinkle Prograf granules on food.

- Administer Prograf, 12 hours apart, at same time each day with or without food but administer consistently with or without food.
- Administer extended-release form of drug once daily in the morning either 1 hour before a meal or 2 hours after a meal on an empty stomach.
- Capsules and tablets should be swallowed whole and not chewed, crushed, or divided.

I.V.

- Be aware that I.V. tacrolimus therapy should only be given if patient can't tolerate oral tacrolimus. Patient should be switched to oral therapy as soon as possible.
- Dilute drug with 0.9% Sodium Chloride Injection or 5% Dextrose Injection to a concentration of 0.004 to 0.02 mg/ml.
- Once diluted, drug should be stored in glass or polyethylene containers (not PVC containers, because of decreased stability and possible extraction of phthalates).
- Use a PVC-free tubing to administer drug, if situation warrants, such as in pediatric dosing.
- Infuse as a continuous infusion.
- Discard after 24 hours if not used.
- *Incompatibilities:* Solutions of pH 9 or greater such as acyclovir or ganciclovir; PVC containers

Route	Onset	Peak	Duration
P.O.	Unknown	1.5–3 hr	Unknown
P.O./E.R.	Unknown	6 hr	Unknown
I.V.	Rapid	1–2 hr	Unknown
Half-life: 12 hr			

⌸ Mechanism of Action

Inhibits T-lymphocyte activation, possibly by binding to an intracellular protein, FKBP-12. This binding results in formation of a complex of tacrolimus-FKBP-12, calcineurin, calcium, and calmodulin which inhibits phosphatase activity of calcineurin. This inhibition may prevent dephosphorylation and translocation of nuclear factor of activated T-cells, a nuclear component thought to initiate gene transcription for the formation of lymphokines. The result is inhibition of T-lymphocyte activation, which produces immunosuppression.

Contraindications

Hypersensitivity to tacrolimus or its components, hypersensitivity to polyoxyl 60 hydrogenated castor oil (parenteral form)

Interactions

DRUGS

amiodarone, boceprevir, bromocriptine, chloramphenicol, cimetidine, cisapride, clarithromycin, clotrimazole, cyclosporine, danazol, diltiazem, erythromycin, ethinyl estradiol, fluconazole, ganciclovir, itraconazole, ketoconazole, lansoprazole, letermovir, magnesium-aluminum-hydroxide, methylprednisolone, metoclopramide, nefazodone, nelfinavir, nicardipine, nifedipine, omeprazole, protease inhibitors, ritonavir, Schisandra sphenanthera extracts, telaprevir, troleandomycin, verapamil, voriconazole and other CYP3A inhibitors: Possibly increased blood tacrolimus level; increased risk of serious adverse reactions such as neurotoxicity or QT prolongation
carbamazepine, methylprednisolone, phenobarbital, phenytoin, prednisone, rifabutin, rifampin, St. John's wort and other CYP3A4 inducers: Possibly decreased blood tacrolimus level
mycophenolic acid: Possibly increased plasma mycophenolic acid level
vaccines (live or killed): Possibly suppressed immune response and increased adverse effects of vaccine

FOODS

grapefruit, grapefruit juice: Possibly increased blood tacrolimus trough levels in liver transplant patients

ACTIVITIES

alcohol use (Astagraf XL, Envarsus XR): Increased rate of release of tacrolimus; increased risk of serious adverse reactions such as neurotoxicity or QT prolongation

Adverse Reactions

CNS: Asthenia, **coma, CVA,** delirium, dizziness, fever, headache, hemiparesis, insomnia, jittery feeling, **leukoencephalopathy,** mental changes, motor and sensory dysfunction, mutism, **neurotoxicity,** paresthesia, **posterior reversible encephalopathy syndrome, progressive multifocal leukoencephalopathy, seizures,** speech disorder, syncope, tremor

CV: **Atrial and ventricular arrhythmias, cardiac arrest,** chest pain, hypercholesterolemia, hyperlipemia, hypertension, hypertriglyceridemia, myocardial hypertrophy, **MI, myocardial ischemia, pericardial effusion,** peripheral edema, **QT-interval prolongation, torsades de pointes, venous thrombosis**

EENT: Blindness, cortical blindness, deafness, hearing loss, optic atrophy or neuropathy, photophobia

ENDO: Cushingoid features, diabetes mellitus (new onset), hot flashes, hyperglycemia

GI: Abdominal pain, anorexia, ascites, bile duct stenosis, cholangitis, **cirrhosis,** colitis, constipation, diarrhea, dyspepsia, enterocolitis, fatty liver, gastric ulcer, gastroenteritis, gastroesophageal reflux disease, **GI perforation, hepatic cytolysis or failure, hepatic impairment or toxicity, hepatitis,** impaired gastric emptying, jaundice, nausea, **liver necrosis, pancreatitis, veno-occlusive liver disease,** vomiting

GU: BK virus nephropathy, elevated creatinine and BUN levels, hemorrhagic cystitis, **hemolytic uremic syndrome,** micturition abnormality, **nephrotoxicity,** oliguria, **renal failure,** renal impairment, UTI

HEME: **Agranulocytosis,** anemia, **decreased blood fibrinogen, disseminated intravascular coagulation (DIC), febrile neutropenia, hemolytic anemia,** leukocytosis, **leukopenia, neutropenia, pancytopenia, prolonged activated partial thromboplastin time, pure red cell aplasia, thrombocytopenia, thrombocytopenic purpura, thrombotic microangiopathy, thrombotic thrombocytopenic purpura**

MS: Arthralgia, back pain, extremity pain including calcineurin inhibitor–induced pain syndrome

RESP: **Acute respiratory distress syndrome,** atelectasis, **bronchiolitis obliterans syndrome,** bronchitis, cough, dyspnea, **interstitial lung disease, lung infiltration,** pleural effusion, pneumonia, **pulmonary embolism or hypertension, respiratory distress or failure**

SKIN: Flushing, hyperpigmentation, **malignancy,** photosensitivity, pruritus, rash, **Stevens–Johnson syndrome, toxic epidermal necrolysis**

Other: Anaphylaxis, cytomegalovirus infection, **hyperkalemia, hypokalemia, hypomagnesemia, hypophosphatemia,** impaired wound healing, infections, **lymphoproliferative or malignant disorders, multiorgan failure,** opportunistic infections (including activation of latent viral infections), primary graft dysfunction, weight loss

Childbearing Considerations

PREGNANCY

- Pregnancy exposure registry: 1-877-955-6877 or https://www .transplantpregnancyregistry .org/.
- Drug can cause fetal harm such as congenital abnormalities and fetal distress, as well as low birth weight, renal dysfunction, and transient neonatal hyperkalemia at birth.
- Use with caution only if benefit to mother outweighs potential risk to fetus.

LABOR & DELIVERY

- Increased risk for premature delivery (less than 37 weeks) following maternal exposure to drug.

LACTATION

- Drug is present in breast milk.
- Patient should check with prescriber before breastfeeding.

REPRODUCTION

- Advise women of childbearing age to use a reliable method of contraception before drug therapy is begun and throughout drug therapy.
- Female and male fertility may be affected by drug therapy.

Nursing Considerations

- Know that tacrolimus should not be given to patients with congenital long QT syndrome because of increased risk of life-threatening ventricular arrhythmias.
- Know that tacrolimus therapy should not be started within 24 hours of cyclosporine, and vice versa. If tacrolimus or cyclosporine blood levels are elevated beyond 24 hours of either drug being discontinued, know that the other drug should not be started until elevation is resolved.
- Check to be sure patient is up to date on all immunizations according to the standard schedule. If possible, live vaccines should be avoided.

- Expect to give drug with adrenal corticosteroid therapy.
- Know that sirolimus should not be administered with tacrolimus because of the potential for severe adverse reactions.
- Be aware that children usually need higher doses of tacrolimus than adults.

! WARNING Closely monitor patient for anaphylaxis at least during first 30 minutes of I.V. administration. Make sure emergency equipment and drugs, such as aqueous solution of epinephrine and oxygen, are immediately available.

- Monitor patient's blood tacrolimus trough levels regularly, as ordered. Higher trough levels increase risk of toxicity, especially nephrotoxicity and neurotoxicity.
- Monitor blood pressure, especially in patients with history of hypertension, because drug can worsen this condition.
- Monitor results of liver and renal function tests, as ordered, to detect signs of decreased function. Changes in liver function may affect effectiveness of tacrolimus or increase risk of adverse effects.
- Know that tacrolimus may increase serum cholesterol, lipid, and triglyceride levels.
- Monitor patient's blood glucose level closely because tacrolimus may cause post-transplant diabetes mellitus with the need for insulin therapy, especially in African-American and Hispanic patients.
- Monitor patient's serum potassium level, as ordered, because drug can alter it.
- Watch for evidence of neurotoxicity, especially in patients receiving high doses of drug. Evidence of encephalopathy includes headache, impaired consciousness, loss of motor function, psychiatric disturbance, seizures, and tremors.

! WARNING Monitor patient's ECG and electrolytes, as ordered, periodically throughout tacrolimus therapy because drug may prolong the QT interval, especially in patients with bradyarrhythmias, congestive heart failure, electrolyte disturbances, and concomitant use of certain antiarrhythmic drugs.

- Be aware that tacrolimus therapy increases the risk of patient developing serious infections and malignancies. Monitor patient closely, as patient may need to be hospitalized because of life-threatening severity.

PATIENT TEACHING

- Tell patient to inspect her tacrolimus medication when she receives a new prescription and before taking it. If it looks different or dosage instructions have changed, tell patient to alert prescriber, because tacrolimus products are not interchangeable.
- Advise patient to take oral doses of Prograf, 12 hours apart, at same time each day with or without food but be consistent. Advise patient to take oral doses of extended-release form once daily in the morning either 1 hour before a meal or 2 hours after a meal on an empty stomach. Tell patient to swallow capsule or tablet whole and not to chew, crush, or divide capsule or tablet. Instruct patient or caregiver how to mix and administer Prograf oral granules used to make an oral suspension. Warn not to sprinkle granules on food and to take or administer the suspension immediately after preparation.
- Tell patient to avoid consuming alcohol or grapefruit juice or eating grapefruit while taking tacrolimus.
- Advise patient not to stop taking drug without consulting prescriber.
- Instruct patient not to receive virus vaccines during therapy. Urge him to avoid people who have received such vaccines or to wear a protective mask when he's around them.
- Caution patient to avoid having contact with people who have infections during therapy because tacrolimus causes immunosuppression. Stress importance of notifying prescriber if an infection occurs, as it can become severe. Tell patient to report chills; cough; fever; flu-like symptoms; muscle aches; or painful, red, or warm areas on the skin.
- Warn patient that tacrolimus may cause cancer because of its immunosuppressant action. Tell patient to report any unexplained or unusual signs and symptoms to prescriber.
- Emphasize the importance of having repeated laboratory tests while taking tacrolimus, and urge compliance.
- Inform patient that tacrolimus therapy may result in insulin-dependent diabetes.

Tell him to report frequent urination or an increase in fatigue, hunger, or thirst.
- Tell patient to report shortness of breath, swelling anywhere on the body, or tiredness to prescriber.
- Instruct patient to alert all prescribers to tacrolimus therapy and not to take any over-the-counter drugs, including herbal products, without consulting prescriber first.
- Teach patient how to take his blood pressure and provide guidelines for when blood pressure readings should be reported to prescriber.
- Instruct patient to limit exposure to direct sunlight and to wear protective clothing and use broad-spectrum sunscreen when exposure can't be avoided.
- Warn women of childbearing age to use effective contraceptive measures before starting drug and continuing throughout therapy. If pregnancy occurs, tell patient to alert prescriber immediately.
- Tell mothers who wish to breastfeed that breastfeeding is not recommended during tacrolimus therapy.

tadalafil

Adcirca, Alyq, Cialis

≣ Class and Category

Pharmacologic class: Phosphodiesterase-5 (PDE5) inhibitor
Therapeutic class: Erectile dysfunction agent

≣ Indications and Dosages

⚹ *To treat erectile dysfunction*

TABLETS (CIALIS)

Men. *Initial:* 10 mg at least 30 min before sexual activity; dosage decreased to 5 mg or increased to 20 mg, based on clinical response. Alternatively, 2.5 mg once daily without regard to timing of sexual activity, increased to 5 mg once daily, as needed.

±**DOSAGE ADJUSTMENT** For patients who take drug on an as-needed basis and are taking potent CYP3A4 inhibitors such as ketoconazole or ritonavir, dosage shouldn't exceed 10 mg every 72 hr. For patients taking potent CYP3A4 inhibitors and drug once daily, the maximum recommended dose is 2.5 mg daily. For patients with a creatinine clearance of 30 to 50 ml/min, who take drug on an as-needed basis, initial dosage decreased to 5 mg daily and maximum dosage not to exceed 10 mg every 48 hr. For patients with a creatinine clearance of less than 30 ml/min or who are on hemodialysis, who take drug on an as-needed basis, maximum dose should not exceed 5 mg every 72 hr. Once-daily dosing is not recommended for patients with a creatinine clearance less than 30 ml/min. For patients with mild to moderate hepatic dysfunction who take drug on an as-needed basis, dosage should not exceed 10 mg once every day.

✳ *To treat benign prostatic hyperplasia*

TABLETS (CIALIS)

Men. 5 mg once daily.

±**DOSAGE ADJUSTMENT** For patients taking potent CYP3A4 inhibitors such as ketoconazole or ritonavir, dosage reduced to 2.5 mg daily. For patients with a creatinine clearance of 30 to 50 mg/ml, initial dosage reduced to 2.5 mg once daily with possible increase to 5 mg, based upon individual response. Drug is not recommended for patients with a creatinine clearance less than 30 ml/min for this indication.

✳ *To treat benign prostatic hyperplasia and erectile dysfunction*

TABLETS (CIALIS)

Men. 5 mg once daily without regard to timing of sexual activity.

±**DOSAGE ADJUSTMENT** For patients taking potent CYP3A4 inhibitors such as ketoconazole or ritonavir, dosage reduced to 2.5 mg daily. For patients with a creatinine clearance of 30 to 50 mg/ml, initial dosage reduced to 2.5 mg once daily with possible increase to 5 mg, based upon individual response. Drug is not recommended for patients with a creatinine clearance less than 30 ml/min for this indication.

✳ *To treat pulmonary arterial hypertension in order to improve exercise ability in patients classified as group 1 by the World Health Organization*

TABLETS (ADCIRCA, ALYQ)

Adults. 40 mg once daily.

±**DOSAGE ADJUSTMENT** For patients with mild to moderate hepatic or renal impairment or who have already taken ritonavir for at least 1 wk, initial dosage of 20 mg once daily and then increased as tolerated. For patient already taking tadalafil

and being prescribed ritonavir, tadalafil temporarily discontinued for at least 24 hours before ritonavir starts. Then, after at least 1 week of ritonavir, tadalafil restarted at 20 mg once daily and then increased to 40 mg once daily, as tolerated.

☰ Drug Administration

P.O.

- Drug should not be administered concurrently with nitrates.
- Drug used to treat erectile dysfunction on an as-needed basis should be administered at least 30 minutes before sexual activity.
- Drug prescribed daily should be administered at about the same time every day.

Route	Onset	Peak	Duration
P.O.	< 45 min	1.5–6 hr	< 36 hr

Half-life: 17.5 hr

☰ Mechanism of Action

Enhances the effect of nitric oxide released in the penis during sexual stimulation. Nitric oxide activates the enzyme guanylate cyclase, which causes increased levels of cGMP in the corpus cavernosum. This leads to increased blood flow to the penis, thus producing an erection.

By preventing breakdown of cyclic guanosine monophosphate by phosphodiesterase, levels increase leading to smooth muscle relaxation of the pulmonary vasculature and subsequently, vasodilation. Vasodilation causes the pressure within the pulmonary vasculature to decrease, which improves tolerance to exercise and delays worsening of pulmonary arterial hypertension.

☰ Contraindications

Concomitant guanylate cyclase stimulator therapy such as riociguat, continuous or intermittent nitrate therapy, hypersensitivity to tadalafil or its components

☰ Interactions

DRUGS

alpha blockers (alfuzosin, doxazosin, tamsulosin), antihypertensives, nitrates: Increased risk of hypotension, which could become severe

antacids (aluminum hydroxide/magnesium hydroxide): Reduction in rate of absorption of tadalafil

CYP3A4 inducers such as rifampin: Possibly decreased tadalafil exposure
CYP3A4 inhibitors such as ketoconazole, HIV protease inhibitor such as ritonavir: Possible increased tadalafil exposure

FOODS

grapefruit juice: Possibly prolonged tadalafil effects

ACTIVITIES

alcohol use: Potentiated blood pressure–lowering effects

Adverse Reactions

CNS: Asthenia, CVA, dizziness, fatigue, headache, hypesthesia, insomnia, migraine, paresthesia, **seizures**, somnolence, syncope, transient global amnesia, vertigo
CV: Angina pectoris, chest pain, hypertension, **hypotension**, **MI**, postural hypotension, palpitations, peripheral edema, **sudden cardiac death**, tachycardia
EENT: Blurred vision, changes in color vision, conjunctivitis, dry mouth, epistaxis, eyelid swelling, eye pain, hearing or visual loss, increased lacrimation, nasal congestion, nasopharyngitis, nonarteritic anterior ischemic optic neuropathy (NAION), pharyngitis, retinal artery or vein occlusion, tinnitus, visual field defects
GI: Diarrhea, dysphagia, dyspepsia, elevated liver enzymes, esophagitis, gastroesophageal reflux, gastritis, nausea, upper abdominal pain, vomiting
GU: Priapism, spontaneous penile erection, UTI
MS: Arthralgia, back or neck pain, extremity pain, myalgia
RESP: Bronchitis, cough, dyspnea, upper respiratory tract infection
SKIN: Diaphoresis, **exfoliative dermatitis**, flushing, pruritus, rash, **Stevens–Johnson syndrome**, urticaria
Other: Angioedema, flu-like symptoms, **hypersensitivity reactions**

Childbearing Considerations

PREGNANCY

- Cialis is not indicated in female patients.
- Pregnant women with pulmonary arterial hypertension are at risk for heart failure, stroke, preterm delivery, and maternal and fetal death.
- It is not known if Adcirca or Alyq can cause fetal harm.

- Use Adcirca or Alyq with caution only if benefit to mother outweighs potential risk to fetus.

LACTATION

- Cialis is not indicated in female patients.
- It is not known if Adcirca or Alyq is present in breast milk.
- Patient should check with prescriber before breastfeeding when prescribed Adcirca or Alyq.

REPRODUCTION

- Sperm count may be decreased with drug therapy.

Nursing Considerations

- Know that patients with hereditary degenerative retinal disorders, including retinitis pigmentosa, should not receive tadalafil because of the risk of serious ophthalmic adverse reactions.
- Be aware that patients with severe hepatic or renal impairment should not receive tadalafil because its effects in these patients are unknown.
- Use tadalafil cautiously in patients with left ventricular outflow obstruction, such as aortic stenosis and idiopathic hypertrophic subaortic stenosis, and those with severely impaired autonomic control of blood pressure because these conditions increase sensitivity to vasodilators, such as tadalafil.
- Use tadalafil cautiously in patients with conditions that may predispose them to priapism, such as leukemia, multiple myeloma, penile deformities (such as angulation, cavernosal fibrosis, or Peyronie's disease), or sickle cell anemia.
- Monitor blood pressure and heart rate and rhythm before and during therapy.

PATIENT TEACHING

- Explain that, when used as needed to treat erectile dysfunction, tadalafil should be taken at least 30 min before sexual activity to provide the most effective results. If patient is prescribed a daily dose of tadalafil, tell patient to take drug at about the same time every day.

! **WARNING** Tell patient not to take tadalafil if he takes any form of organic nitrate, either continuously or intermittently, because profound hypotension and death could result.

T

- Advise patient taking tadalafil to treat erectile dysfunction to obtain sexual counseling to help enhance the drug's effects.
- Urge patient to notify prescriber immediately if erection is painful or lasts longer than 4 hours, to avoid possible penile damage and permanent loss of erectile function.
- Advise patient to avoid alcohol or grapefruit juice consumption while taking tadalafil.
- Tell male patients taking tadalafil for pulmonary arterial hypertension not to take another form of tadalafil under the brand name of Cialis or any other PDE5 inhibitors to treat erectile dysfunction.

! **WARNING** Tell patient to seek immediate medical attention if he experiences hearing loss that may be accompanied by dizziness or tinnitus or a sudden loss of vision in one or both eyes.

tamoxifen citrate
Nolvadex-D (CAN), Soltamox

Class and Category
Pharmacologic class: Selective estrogen receptor modulator (SERM)
Therapeutic class: Anti-estrogen agent

Indications and Dosages
* *To treat estrogen receptor–positive metastatic breast cancer in men and women*

ORAL SOLUTION, TABLETS
Adults. 20 to 40 mg daily. Dosages greater than 20 mg divided and administered twice daily.

* *As adjuvant treatment of patients with early-stage estrogen receptor–positive breast cancer; to reduce occurrence of contralateral breast cancer when used as adjuvant therapy for the treatment of breast cancer*

ORAL SOLUTION, TABLETS
Adults. 20 mg daily for 5 to 10 years.

* *To reduce the risk of invasive breast cancer in women with ductal carcinoma in situ (DCIS) after radiation and surgery; to reduce the risk of breast cancer in women at high risk*

ORAL SOLUTION, TABLETS
Adults. 20 mg daily for 5 yr.

Drug Administration
P.O.
- Tablets should be swallowed whole and not chewed, crushed, or divided. Tablets should be taken with water.
- Use the dosing cup that comes with drug when measuring dosage of oral solution. Store at room temperature and protect from light. Discard 3 months after opening.

Route	Onset	Peak	Duration
P.O.	Unknown	5 hr	Unknown

Half-life: 5–7 days

Mechanism of Action
May block the effects of estrogen on breast tissue by competing with estrogen for estrogen receptor binding sites. Estrogen may stimulate the growth of cancer cells.

Contraindications
Hypersensitivity to tamoxifen or its components; women at high risk for breast cancer and women with DCIS and a history of deep vein thrombosis or pulmonary embolus or who need coumarin-type anticoagulant therapy

Interactions
DRUGS
bromocriptine: Possibly increased blood tamoxifen level
CYP2D6 inducers: Possibly decreased plasma concentrations of tamoxifen
CYP2D6 inhibitors: Possibly altered tamoxifen efficacy
cytotoxic agents: Increased risk of thromboembolic events
warfarin and other coumarin-type anticoagulants: Increased anticoagulant effect of these drugs

Adverse Reactions
CNS: Confusion, **CVA**, depression, dizziness, fatigue, headache, light-headedness, somnolence, weakness
CV: Edema, hyperlipidemia, **thrombosis**
EENT: Keratopathy, ocular toxicity (including cataracts), optic neuritis, retinopathy
GI: Elevated liver enzymes, **hepatotoxicity**, nausea, vomiting
GU: **Endometrial cancer**, endometrial hyperplasia, endometrial polyps, genital

itching, menstrual irregularities, ovarian cysts, vaginal discharge (females); impotence, decreased libido (males)

HEME: Anemia, **leukopenia, thrombocytopenia**

MS: Transient bone or tumor pain

RESP: **Pulmonary embolism**

SKIN: Bullous pemphigoid, dry skin, **erythema multiforme**, rash, **Stevens–Johnson syndrome**, thinning hair

Other: **Angioedema**, hot flashes, **hypercalcemia**, weight gain

Childbearing Considerations

PREGNANCY

- Drug may cause fetal harm.
- Drug is not recommended during pregnancy.
- A negative pregnancy test must be obtained before drug therapy is begun.

LACTATION

- It is not known if drug is present in breast milk.
- Breastfeeding should not be done during drug therapy and for 3 months following the last dose.

REPRODUCTION

- Women of childbearing age should be advised to use barrier or other nonhormonal contraceptive method if sexually active before starting drug, throughout drug therapy, and for 9 months after drug has been discontinued.
- Male patients with female partners of childbearing age should use effective contraception during drug therapy and for 6 months following the last dose.
- Stress importance of reporting suspected or known pregnancy immediately to prescriber.

Nursing Considerations

! **WARNING** Make sure that patient has been informed about serious or potentially life-threatening adverse effects associated with tamoxifen before therapy begins. Be aware that women with ductal carcinoma in situ and those at high risk for breast cancer are more likely to develop pulmonary emboli, stroke, or uterine cancer than others receiving tamoxifen.

- Know that if patient is premenopausal, drug therapy should begin in the middle of menstruation; if patient's menstrual cycles are irregular, verify that she has had a negative pregnancy test before therapy starts.
- Expect patient to undergo an ophthalmic examination before and periodically during tamoxifen therapy. Also expect to monitor patient for adverse ocular reactions, such as cataracts.
- Assess patient for signs and symptoms of thromboembolic events, such as change in mental status, leg pain, or shortness of breath.
- Periodically monitor patient's cholesterol and triglyceride levels, liver enzymes, and platelet and WBC counts, as ordered.
- Monitor blood calcium level and assess patient for signs and symptoms of hypercalcemia, such as nausea, thirst, and vomiting; tamoxifen may cause hypercalcemia in breast cancer patients with bone metastasis within a few weeks of starting treatment.

PATIENT TEACHING

- Advise patient to swallow tamoxifen tablet whole and not to chew, crush, or divide tablet. Take with water.
- Tell patient prescribed oral solution to use the dosing cup that comes with drug when measuring dosage; store drug at room temperature, protect from light, and discard 3 months after opening.
- Instruct premenopausal patient to use a nonhormonal form of contraception, such as a condom or diaphragm, during tamoxifen therapy. Emphasize that she shouldn't become pregnant while taking drug and for 9 months afterward. Advise her to notify prescriber at once if she becomes pregnant during therapy.
- Instruct male patients with a partner who is of childbearing age to use effective contraception during drug therapy and for 6 months afterward.
- Inform patient of the most common side effects: hot flashes, irregular menses, and vaginal discharge.

! **WARNING** Urge patient to immediately notify prescriber if she notices difficulty breathing, facial swelling, itching, or a rash, because they may signify a hypersensitivity reaction.

T

- Advise patient to notify prescriber if she experiences calf swelling or leg pain during tamoxifen therapy, because they may indicate a blood clot.
- Instruct patient to report signs of hepatotoxicity, such as flu-like symptoms, nausea, tiredness, or yellow skin.
- Advise patient to have regular gynecologic examinations and to notify prescriber about abnormal symptoms, including abdominal or pelvic pain, new breast lumps, and unusual vaginal bleeding or discharge.
- Urge patients who take tamoxifen for prophylaxis to have regular mammograms, because tamoxifen doesn't prevent all breast cancers.
- Emphasize the importance of taking tamoxifen regularly. Urge patient to consult prescriber if adverse reactions, such as nausea and vomiting, are interfering with dosage schedule. These symptoms may be a sign of hypercalcemia.
- Inform women who wish to breastfeed that tamoxifen is not recommended during breastfeeding and for 3 months after drug is discontinued.

tamsulosin hydrochloride

Flomax

Class and Category

Pharmacologic class: Alpha-adrenergic antagonist
Therapeutic class: Benign prostatic hyperplasia (BPH) agent

Indications and Dosages

✳ *To treat BPH*

CAPSULES

Adults. *Initial:* 0.4 mg daily for 2 to 4 wk, increased to 0.8 mg daily if no response to initial dosage. *Maximum:* 0.8 mg daily.

Drug Administration

P.O.

- Administer 30 minutes after same meal each day.
- Capsules should be swallowed whole and not chewed, crushed, or opened.

Route	Onset	Peak	Duration
P.O.	4–8 hr	4–8 hr	9–15 hr

Half-life: 9–13 hr

Mechanism of Action

Blocks alpha$_1$-adrenergic receptors in the prostate. This action inhibits smooth muscle contraction in the bladder neck and prostate, prostatic capsule, and prostatic urethra, which improves the rate of urine flow and reduces symptoms of BPH.

Contraindications

Hypersensitivity to tamsulosin or its components

Interactions

DRUGS

alpha blockers: Additive effects of both drugs
cimetidine: Risk of decreased tamsulosin clearance
CYP2D6 inhibitors (such as paroxetine and terbinafine), CYP3A4 inhibitors (such as erythromycin, ketoconazole): Possibly increased plasma tamsulosin level
phosphodiesterase-5 inhibitors: Increased risk of hypotension

Adverse Reactions

CNS: Asthenia, dizziness, drowsiness, headache, insomnia, syncope, vertigo
CV: Arrhythmia, atrial fibrillation, chest pain, orthostatic hypotension, palpitations, tachycardia
EENT: Amblyopia, diplopia, dry mouth, epistaxis, intraoperative floppy iris syndrome (during cataract and glaucoma surgery), pharyngitis, rhinitis, visual impairment
GI: Constipation, diarrhea, nausea, vomiting
GU: Decreased libido, ejaculation disorders, priapism
MS: Back pain
RESP: Dyspnea, respiratory impairment
SKIN: Desquamation, erythema multiforme, exfoliative dermatitis, pruritus, rash, Stevens–Johnson syndrome, urticaria
Other: Angioedema

Childbearing Considerations

PREGNANCY

- Drug is not indicated for female patients.

LACTATION

- Drug is not indicated for female patients.

Nursing Considerations

- Be aware that prostate cancer should be ruled out before tamsulosin therapy begins.
- Know that if drug is given on an empty stomach, patient's blood pressure should be monitored because of the increased risk of orthostatic hypotension.
- Be aware that if patient doesn't take drug for several days, therapy should be resumed at 0.4 mg/dose, as prescribed.

PATIENT TEACHING

- Instruct patient not to chew, crush, or open tamsulosin capsules and to take drug about 30 minutes after the same meal each day.
- Instruct patient to notify prescriber if he misses several days of therapy, and caution him against restarting drug at previous dosage.
- Advise patient to avoid potentially hazardous activities until drug's CNS effects are known. Mention the need for caution if dosage is increased.
- Advise patient to change position slowly, especially after initial dose and each dosage increase, to minimize effects of orthostatic hypotension.
- Tell patient to inform ophthalmologist of tamsulosin therapy because drug may increase risk for complications with cataract surgery.

tegaserod
Zelnorm

Class and Category

Pharmacologic class: Serotonin-4 (5-HT$_4$) receptor agonist
Therapeutic class: Gastrointestinal agent

Indications and Dosages

✷ *To treat irritable bowel syndrome with constipation*

TABLETS

Adult women under age 65. 6 mg twice daily.

Drug Administration

P.O.

- Administer tablets at least 30 minutes before a meal.

Route	Onset	Peak	Duration
P.O.	Unknown	1 hr	Unknown

Half-life: 4.6–8.1 hr

Mechanism of Action

Enhances basal motor activity, inhibits visceral sensitivity, normalizes impaired motility, and stimulates the peristaltic reflex and intestinal secretion throughout the gastrointestinal tract to relieve the symptoms of irritable bowel syndrome with constipation.

Contraindications

History of angina, MI, stroke, or transient ischemic attack; history of abdominal adhesions, bowel obstruction, suspected sphincter of Oddi dysfunction, or symptomatic gallbladder disease; history of ischemic colitis or other forms of intestinal ischemia; hypersensitivity to tegaserod or its components; severe renal impairment (eGFR less than 15 ml/min)

Interactions

DRUGS

None reported by manufacturer

Adverse Reactions

CNS: Asthenia, dizziness, headache, migraine, **suicidal ideation**, vertigo
CV: Cardiovascular ischemic events, major cardiovascular events
GI: Abdominal pain, diarrhea with volume depletion, dyspepsia, flatulence, increased appetite, ischemic colitis, nausea, **rectal hemorrhage**
HEME: Anemia
MS: Arthropathy, tendinitis
Other: Elevated blood creatine phosphokinase

Childbearing Considerations

PREGNANCY

- It is not known if drug causes fetal harm.
- Use with caution only if benefit to mother outweighs potential risk to fetus.

LACTATION

- It is not known if drug is present in breast milk.
- Breastfeeding is not recommended during drug therapy.

T

Nursing Considerations

- Assess women less than 65 years of age for a history of cardiovascular disease and cardiovascular risk factors before treatment with tegaserod. Know that if patient experiences angina, MI, or stroke during drug therapy, drug should be discontinued.

! **WARNING** Monitor patient for bloody diarrhea, new or worsening abdominal pain, and rectal bleeding during tegaserod therapy, as they may indicate ischemic colitis and hospitalization may be required. Have patient evaluated promptly and know that if ischemic colitis or another form of intestinal ischemia is confirmed, drug should be discontinued and not restarted.

! **WARNING** Monitor patient for volume depletion if diarrhea—one of the most common adverse reactions of tegaserod— occurs. Know that volume depletion may be severe enough to require hospitalization and cause hypotension, hypovolemia, and syncope requiring rehydration.

- Monitor patient for abnormal thoughts, especially worsening of depression and emergence of suicidal thoughts, particularly during initial few months of tegaserod therapy.

PATIENT TEACHING

- Instruct patient to take tegaserod exactly as prescribed and to take drug at least 30 minutes before a meal.

! **WARNING** Tell patient to seek immediate medical attention if she experiences chest pain, or signs and symptoms of a heart attack or stroke, including transient ischemic attack. Also advise patient to inform prescriber if she develops cardiovascular heart disease or other changes in health that could increase cardiovascular risk. Newly diagnosed conditions to report include diabetes mellitus, hyperlipidemia, hypertension, or obesity.

! **WARNING** Review signs and symptoms of ischemic colitis and tell patient that if she develops bloody diarrhea, new or worsening abdominal pain, or rectal bleeding, she should seek medical attention and stop taking tegaserod.

- Encourage patient to increase fluid intake, if not contraindicated, during times of diarrhea. If she experiences fainting, advise her to contact prescriber.
- Urge family or caregiver to watch patient closely for worsening of depression and suicidal tendencies, especially during the initial few months of tegaserod therapy.
- Advise women of childbearing age that breastfeeding is not recommended during tegaserod therapy.

telavancin hydrochloride
Vibativ

Class and Category
Pharmacologic class: Lipoglycopeptide
Therapeutic class: Antibiotic

Indications and Dosages
∗ *To treat complicated skin and skin structure infections caused by gram-positive organisms:* Enterococcus faecalis *(vancomycin-susceptible isolates only),* Staphylococcus aureus, Streptococcus agalactiae, S. anginosus *group (includes* S. anginosus, S. constellatus, *and* S. intermedius), *and* S. pyogenes

I.V. INFUSION
Adults. 10 mg/kg every 24 hr for 7 to 14 days.

∗ *To treat hospital-acquired and ventilator-associated bacterial pneumonia caused by* S. aureus *when alternative treatments are not suitable*

I.V. INFUSION
Adults. 10 mg/kg every 24 hr for 7 to 21 days.

±**DOSAGE ADJUSTMENT** For patients with creatinine clearance of 30 to 50 ml/min, dosage reduced to 7.5 mg/kg every 24 hours. For patient with creatinine clearance of at least 10 but less than 30 ml/min, 10 mg/kg every 48 hours.

Drug Administration
I.V.
- Reconstitute 250-mg vial with 15 ml of a diluent such as 0.9% Sodium Chloride Injection, 5% Dextrose Injection, or Sterile Water for Injection to obtain a concentration of 15 mg/ml. Reconstitute 750-mg vial with

45 ml of a diluent such as 0.9% Sodium Chloride Injection, 5% Dextrose Injection, or Sterile Water for Injection to obtain a concentration of 15 mg/ml. To prevent foaming during reconstitution, allow the vacuum of the vial to pull the diluent from the syringe into the vial. Do not forcefully inject diluent into vial. Do not shake vial or final infusion solution.

- Dilute doses of 150 to 800 mg in 100 to 250 ml of 0.9% Sodium Chloride Injection, 5% Dextrose Injection, or Lactated Ringer's Injection before infusing. Doses less than 150 mg or greater than 800 mg should be further diluted in a volume that yields a final concentration of 0.6 to 0.8 mg/ml.
- Use reconstituted solution within 12 hours if stored at room temperature or 7 days if refrigerated. Use diluted solution within 12 hours if stored at room temperature, 7 days if refrigerated, or 32 days if frozen (includes reconstitution time). The total time in the vial after reconstitution plus time in the infusion bag after dilution must be counted toward these storage times. Discard if time limit exceeds these parameters.
- If same I.V. line is used to infuse other drugs, flush line before and after infusion of telavancin with 0.9% Sodium Chloride Injection, 5% Dextrose Injection, or Lactated Ringer's Injection.
- Infuse over 60 minutes.
- *Incompatibilities:* Other I.V. drugs

Route	Onset	Peak	Duration
I.V.	Unknown	Unknown	Unknown

Half-life: 8 hr

Mechanism of Action

Inhibits cell wall synthesis and alters the permeability of bacterial membranes, causing cell wall lysis and cell death.

Contraindications

Hypersensitivity to telavancin or its components, intravenous unfractionated heparin sodium

Interactions

DRUGS

ACE inhibitors, loop diuretics, NSAIDs: Increased risk of nephrotoxicity
drugs known to prolong the QT interval, such as clarithromycin, disopyramide,
erythromycin, quinidine: Increased risk of prolonged QT interval

Adverse Reactions

CNS: Dizziness, rigors
CV: Prolonged QT interval
EENT: Taste disturbance
GI: Abdominal pain, anorexia, diarrhea, *Clostridium difficile*–associated diarrhea, nausea, vomiting
GU: Elevated creatinine level, foamy urine, nephrotoxicity
HEME: Abnormal coagulation
SKIN: Pruritus, rash
Other: Anaphylaxis, infusion-related reactions such as erythema or pain

Childbearing Considerations

PREGNANCY

- Pregnancy exposure registry: 1-877-484-2700.
- Drug may cause fetal harm such as digital and limb malformations.
- Women of childbearing age should have pregnancy status verified before drug is initiated.
- Drug should not be used in pregnancy unless benefit to mother outweighs potential risk to fetus.

LACTATION

- It is not known if drug is present in breast milk.
- Patient should check with prescriber before breastfeeding.

REPRODUCTION

- Women of childbearing age should use an effective contraceptive during drug therapy and for 2 days after the final dose.
- Drug may impair male fertility.

Nursing Considerations

- Know that telavancin isn't recommended for patients with congenital long QT syndrome, severe left ventricular hypertrophy, uncompensated heart failure or who currently have a prolonged QT interval, because drug may prolong the QT interval, causing life-threatening complications.
- Know that use of intravenous unfractionated heparin sodium is contraindicated with telavancin because the activated partial thromboplastin time (aPTT) test results may be falsely prolonged for up to 18 hours after telavancin administration.

T

- Use cautiously in patients taking drugs known to prolong the QT interval because of increased risk of a prolonged QT interval.
- Obtain baseline serum creatinine level before telavancin therapy starts because preexisting moderate to severe renal impairment may increase mortality in the presence of telavancin therapy and is not recommended in such patients unless the benefit outweighs the potential risk. Expect to monitor patient's serum creatinine level throughout therapy, as ordered, because drug may cause nephrotoxicity, especially in patients with congestive heart failure, diabetes mellitus, hypertension, or preexisting renal disease and in patients taking such nephrotoxic drugs as ACE inhibitors, loop diuretics, and NSAIDs. If renal function declines, notify prescriber and expect to discontinue telavancin.
- Monitor patient for a reaction like red-man syndrome, which causes flushing of upper body, pruritus, rash, or urticaria. If present, stop or slow infusion to resolve.

! WARNING Monitor patient for hypersensitivity reactions during and after infusion of drug. Stop infusion at first sign of skin rash or any other hypersensitivity sign and notify prescriber.

- Monitor patient for diarrhea, which may range from mild to severe and may occur more than 2 months after antibiotic is discontinued. Report diarrhea and, if C. difficile is suspected, expect telavancin to be discontinued. Provide supportive care, such as antibiotic therapy to treat C. difficile, electrolyte and fluid replacement, protein supplementation, and possibly surgical intervention, as needed.
- Be aware that while telavancin doesn't interfere with coagulation, it does interfere with certain tests used to monitor coagulation, such as activated clotting time, APTT, coagulation-based factor Xa tests, INR, and PT. Collect blood samples for coagulation tests as close as possible to administration of next dose of telavancin to minimize interference.

PATIENT TEACHING

- Instruct women of childbearing age to use effective contraception during telavancin therapy and for 2 days after the last dose.

! WARNING Alert patient that drug may cause an allergic reaction. Tell patient to notify medical staff if difficulty breathing or other signs of a hypersensitivity reaction occur.

- Caution patient that diarrhea may occur more than 2 months after antibiotic has been discontinued and to report any persistent or severe episodes to prescriber.
- Warn patient that drug may cause urine to be foamy and taste to be altered.
- Advise patient to alert all prescribers that he takes telavancin because some drugs may interact with it, causing serious adverse effects.

telmisartan
Micardis

Class and Category
Pharmacologic class: Angiotensin II receptor blocker (ARB)
Therapeutic class: Antihypertensive

Indications and Dosages
∗ *To manage hypertension, alone or with other antihypertensives*

TABLETS

Adults. *Initial:* 40 mg daily. *Maintenance:* 20 to 80 mg daily. *Maximum:* 80 mg daily.

∗ *To reduce risk of MI, stroke, or death from cardiovascular causes in patients at high risk who are unable to take ACE inhibitors*

TABLETS

Adults age 55 and over. 80 mg once daily.

Drug Administration
P.O.

- Do not remove tablets from blister until immediately before administration.

Route	Onset	Peak	Duration
P.O.	1–2 hr	30–60 min	24 hr

Half-life: 24 hr

Mechanism of Action
Blocks angiotensin II from binding to receptor sites in many tissues, including adrenal glands and vascular smooth muscle. This action inhibits the aldosterone-secreting and vasoconstrictive effects of angiotensin II, which reduces blood pressure.

Contraindications

Concurrent aliskiren therapy in patients with diabetes, hypersensitivity to telmisartan or its components

Interactions

DRUGS

aliskiren: Increased risk of hyperkalemia, hypotension, and renal dysfunction
digoxin: Increased peak blood digoxin level and risk of digitalis toxicity
lithium: Increased serum lithium levels and toxicity
NSAIDs: Increased risk of renal dysfunction in elderly patients and those with volume depletion and existing renal dysfunction; increased risk of hypotension
potassium-sparing diuretics, potassium supplements: Increased risk of hyperkalemia

FOOD

salt substitutes containing potassium: Increased risk of hyperkalemia

Adverse Reactions

CNS: Asthenia, dizziness, fatigue, headache, syncope, weakness
CV: Atrial fibrillation, bradycardia, chest pain, **congestive heart failure,** hypertension, **hypotension, MI,** orthostatic hypotension, peripheral edema
EENT: Pharyngitis, sinusitis
ENDO: Hypoglycemia (in diabetics)
GI: Abdominal pain, diarrhea, elevated liver enzymes, indigestion, nausea, vomiting
GU: Acute renal failure, erectile dysfunction, renal dysfunction, UTI
HEME: Anemia, eosinophilia, **thrombocytopenia**
MS: Back pain, leg or muscle cramps, myalgia, tendinitis, tendon pain, tenosynovitis
RESP: Cough, upper respiratory tract infection
SKIN: Diaphoresis, erythema, rash, urticaria
Other: Anaphylaxis, angioedema, elevated uric acid level, flu-like symptoms, **hyperkalemia,** hypovolemia

Childbearing Considerations

PREGNANCY

- Drug can cause fetal harm, especially if exposure occurs during the second or third trimester.
- Drug reduces fetal renal function, leading to anuria and renal failure, and increases fetal and neonatal morbidity and death.

It can also cause fetal lung hypoplasia, hypotension, and skeletal deformations such as skull hypoplasia.
- Drug is contraindicated in pregnant women and should be discontinued as soon as possible if pregnancy occurs.

LACTATION

- It is not known if drug is present in breast milk.
- Breastfeeding is not recommended because of potential serious adverse reactions including hyperkalemia, hypotension, and renal impairment in the breastfed infant.

Nursing Considerations

- Give telmisartan cautiously to patients with dehydration or hyponatremia.
- Expect prescriber to add a diuretic to regimen if patient's blood pressure isn't well controlled by telmisartan.
- Check patient's blood pressure regularly. Be prepared to treat symptomatic hypotension by placing patient in supine position and giving normal saline solution, as ordered.
- Monitor BUN and serum creatinine levels and urine output in patients with impaired renal function because they're at increased risk for oliguria, progressive azotemia, and possibly acute renal failure.
- Monitor liver enzymes, as appropriate, and assess for evidence of drug toxicity in patients with severe hepatic disease because they're at increased risk for toxicity from increased drug accumulation.
- Avoid using telmisartan in pregnant women during second and third trimesters because drug can increase the risk of fetal harm.

PATIENT TEACHING

- Advise patient to avoid hazardous activities until telmisartan's CNS effects are known.
- Instruct patient to change position slowly to minimize effects of orthostatic hypotension.
- Urge patient to immediately notify prescriber about diarrhea, dizziness, severe nausea, or vomiting.
- Instruct patient to consult prescriber before taking any new drug.
- Advise patient not to use potassium supplements or salt substitutes that contain potassium without checking with prescriber first.
- Advise patient to drink adequate amounts of fluid during hot weather and when exercising.

T

- Advise female patients of childbearing age to notify prescriber immediately about known or suspected pregnancy.
- Inform mothers not to breastfeed their infant during telmisartan therapy.

temazepam
Restoril

Class, Category, and Schedule
Pharmacologic class: Benzodiazepine
Therapeutic class: Sedative-hypnotic
Controlled substance schedule: IV

Indications and Dosages
✶ *To provide short-term management of insomnia*

CAPSULES
Adults. 7.5 mg, 15 mg, or 30 mg nightly. *Maximum:* 30 mg daily for no longer than 10 consecutive days.

±**DOSAGE ADJUSTMENT** For elderly or debilitated patients, 7.5 mg nightly. *Maximum:* 15 mg daily for no longer than 10 consecutive days.

Drug Administration
P.O.
- Administer drug 30 minutes before bedtime.
- Do not administer more than 10 consecutive days.

Route	Onset	Peak	Duration
P.O.	10–20 min	1.5 hr	Unknown

Half-life: 3.5–18.4 hr

Mechanism of Action
May potentiate the effects of gamma-aminobutyric acid (GABA) and other inhibitory neurotransmitters by binding to specific benzodiazepine receptor sites in cortical and limbic areas of the CNS. By binding to these receptor sites, temazepam increases GABA's inhibitory effects and blocks cortical and limbic arousal.

Contraindications
Hypersensitivity to temazepam, other benzodiazepines, or their components; pregnancy

Interactions
DRUGS
opioids, other benzodiazepines: Increased risk of respiratory depression that could become severe, profound sedation

ACTIVITIES
alcohol use: Increased CNS and respiratory depression that could be severe

Adverse Reactions
CNS: Aggressiveness, anxiety (in daytime), ataxia, complex behaviors (such as sleep driving), confusion, decreased level of consciousness or concentration, depression, dizziness, drowsiness, euphoria, fatigue, headache, insomnia, nightmares, slurred speech, **suicidal ideation**, syncope, talkativeness, tremor, vertigo, wakefulness during last third of night
CV: Palpitations, tachycardia
EENT: Abnormal or blurred vision, increased salivation, **throat tightness**
GI: Abdominal pain, constipation, diarrhea, hepatic dysfunction, jaundice, nausea, thirst, vomiting
GU: Decreased libido
HEME: **Agranulocytosis**, anemia, **leukopenia**, **neutropenia**, **thrombocytopenia**
MS: Muscle spasm or weakness
RESP: Dyspnea, increased bronchial secretions
SKIN: Diaphoresis, flushing, pruritus, rash
Other: **Acute or protracted withdrawal syndrome**, anaphylaxis, **angioedema**, physical and psychological dependence

Childbearing Considerations
PREGNANCY
- Drug may cause fetal harm because of potential for increased risk of congenital malformations as well as neonatal CNS depression when drug is given during last few weeks of pregnancy.
- A pregnancy test should be performed before drug therapy is begun.
- Drug is contraindicated in women who are or may become pregnant.

LACTATION
- It is not known if drug is present in breast milk.
- Patient should check with prescriber before breastfeeding.

REPRODUCTION

- Women of childbearing age should use effective contraception during drug therapy, to prevent pregnancy.

☰ Nursing Considerations

- Use temazepam cautiously in patients with a history of depression or suicidal thoughts.

! **WARNING** Assess patient for history of abuse, misuse, and addiction as well as prior dependence and withdrawal reactions to benzodiazepine use.

! **WARNING** Monitor patient closely for evidence of hypersensitivity reaction, such as dyspnea, nausea, swelling, throat tightness, and vomiting. If present, discontinue temazepam immediately, notify prescriber, and provide supportive care.

- Watch patient closely for suicidal tendencies, particularly when therapy starts and dosage changes, because depression may worsen temporarily during these times and could lead to suicidal ideation.

! **WARNING** Monitor patient for evidence of physical and psychological dependence during therapy.

- Implement safety precautions, according to facility policy, especially in elderly patients, because they're more sensitive to drug's CNS effects and at higher risk for falls.
- Assess patients with respiratory depression, severe COPD, or sleep apnea for signs of ventilatory failure.
- Be aware that temazepam can aggravate acute intermittent porphyria, myasthenia gravis, and severe renal impairment.
- Be aware that temazepam may cause deterioration of cognition or coordination in patients with late-stage Parkinson's disease or worsening psychosis.
- Be aware that drug shouldn't be discontinued abruptly, even after only 1 to 2 weeks of therapy, because doing so may cause an acute withdrawal syndrome that could become life-threatening or a protracted withdrawal syndrome that could last weeks to more than 12 months. Expect to taper dosage slowly for discontinuation purposes.

! **WARNING** Know that opioids should only be used concomitantly with benzodiazepine therapy in patients for whom other treatment options are inadequate. If prescribed together, expect dosing and duration of the opioid to be limited. Monitor patient closely for signs and symptoms of a decrease in consciousness, including coma, profound sedation, and significant respiratory depression. Notify prescriber immediately and provide emergency supportive care, as death may occur.

PATIENT TEACHING

- Instruct patient to take temazepam exactly as prescribed and not to stop or change dosage without consulting prescriber. Warn patient not to take drug for more than 10 consecutive days.
- Explain the risks associated with abrupt cessation, including abdominal cramps, acute sense of hearing, confusion, depression, nausea, numbness, perceptual disturbances, photophobia, sweating, tachycardia, tingling, trembling, and vomiting. Tell patient acute withdrawal syndrome could become life-threatening. Also, warn patient that abrupt cessation may cause protracted withdrawal syndrome that could last weeks to more than 12 months.
- Advise patient to avoid consuming alcohol because it increases drug's sedative effects and the risk of such abnormal behaviors as sleep driving. Also, tell patient that combining alcohol or a benzodiazepine such as temazepam with an opioid could result in severe respiratory depression and even death.
- Caution patient about possible drowsiness. Advise her to avoid potentially hazardous activities until drug's CNS effects are known and to take fall precautions.
- Urge patient to notify prescriber immediately about excessive drowsiness, nausea, and known or suspected pregnancy.

! **WARNING** Instruct patient to stop taking temazepam and seek emergency care if she experiences abnormal swelling, difficulty breathing, nausea, throat tightness, or vomiting.

T

- Advise patient that drug may cause abnormal behaviors during sleep, such as driving a car, eating, talking on the phone, or having sex without any recall of the event. If family notices any such behavior or patient sees evidence of such behavior upon awakening, the prescriber should be notified.
- Urge family or caregiver to watch patient closely for suicidal tendencies, especially when therapy starts or dosage changes.
- Instruct patient to inform all prescribers of temazepam use, especially when pain medication may be prescribed.

tenapanor
Ibsrela

Class and Category
Pharmacologic class: Sodium/hydrogen exchanger 3 (NHE3) inhibitor
Therapeutic class: Gastrointestinal agent

Indications and Dosages
* *To treat irritable bowel syndrome with constipation*

TABLETS
Adults. 50 mg twice daily.

Drug Administration
P.O.
- Administer immediately before breakfast or first meal of the day and immediately before dinner.
- Store tenapanor at room temperature; keep in original container and protect from moisture. Desiccant should not be removed from bottle, nor should drug be subdivided or repackaged.

Route	Onset	Peak	Duration
P.O.	Unknown	Unknown	Unknown

Half-life: Unknown

Mechanism of Action
Reduces absorption of sodium from the small intestine and colon by inhibiting sodium/hydrogen exchanger 3 on the apical surface of the enterocytes, resulting in an increase in water secretion into the intestinal lumen. This accelerates intestinal transit time and results in a softer stool consistency. It also reduces abdominal pain associated with irritable bowel syndrome with constipation by decreasing visceral hypersensitivity and decreasing intestinal permeability.

Contraindications
Children less than 6 years of age, hypersensitivity to tenapanor or its components, known or suspected mechanical gastrointestinal obstruction

Interactions
DRUGS
None reported by manufacturer

Adverse Reactions
CNS: Dizziness
GI: Abdominal pain, abnormal gastrointestinal sounds, diarrhea that could be severe, flatulence, **rectal bleeding**
Other: Hyperkalemia

Childbearing Considerations
PREGNANCY
- Drug is minimally absorbed systemically and not expected to result in fetal exposure.

LACTATION
- It is not known if drug is present in breast milk.
- Drug is minimally absorbed systemically and not expected to result in relevant exposure to breastfed infants.

Nursing Considerations
- Be aware that safety and effectiveness of tenapanor have not been established for children less than 18 years of age.
- Monitor patient for diarrhea. If severe, notify prescriber, suspend dosing, and rehydrate patient, as needed.

PATIENT TEACHING
- Instruct patient to take tenapanor immediately prior to breakfast or first meal of the day and immediately prior to dinner.
- Tell patient if a dose is missed, to skip the missed dose and take next dose at the regular time and not to take two doses at the same time.
- Instruct patient to store tenapanor at room temperature, keep in original container, and protect from moisture. Desiccant should not be removed from the bottle, nor should drug be subdivided or repackaged. Also remind patient to store drug securely and out of the reach of children, as accidental

ingestion, especially by children younger than 6 years of age, may cause severe diarrhea and dehydration.

- Tell patient to stop taking tenapanor and notify prescriber if severe diarrhea occurs.

tenecteplase
TNKase

Class and Category
Pharmacologic class: Tissue plasminogen activator (tPA)
Therapeutic class: Thrombolytic

Indications and Dosages
✳ *To reduce mortality associated with acute MI*

I.V. INJECTION
Adults. Single bolus in individualized dosage based on patient's weight, as follows: 50 mg (10 ml) for patients weighing 90 kg (198 lb) or more; 45 mg (9 ml) for patients weighing 80 to 89 kg (176 to 196 lb); 40 mg (8 ml) for patients weighing 70 to 79 kg (154 to 174 lb); 35 mg (7 ml) for patients weighing 60 to 69 kg (132 to 152 lb); 30 mg (6 ml) for patients weighing less than 60 kg (132 lb). *Maximum:* 50 mg.

Drug Administration
I.V.
- Reconstitute immediately before use because drug contains no antibacterial preservatives. If reconstituted drug isn't used immediately, refrigerate vial at 2° to 8°C (36° to 46°F). Discard solution if not used within 8 hours.
- Use the supplied 10-ml syringe prefilled with Sterile Water for Injection and dual cannula device to reconstitute and administer drug.
- Inject all of the solution into drug vial, directing stream of diluent into powder. Gently swirl—don't shake—vial until contents are completely dissolved. If slight foaming occurs during reconstitution, allow drug to stand undisturbed for a few minutes to allow large bubbles to dissipate. Solution should be colorless to pale yellow and transparent.
- Withdraw prescribed dose from reconstituted drug in vial, using supplied syringe. Once dose is drawn into the

syringe, stand the shield vertically on a flat surface (with green side down) and passively recap the red hub cannula. Remove the entire shield assembly, including the red hub cannula, by twisting counterclockwise. Retain the clear-ended blunt plastic cannula for split septum IV access.

- Although supplied syringe is intended for use with needleless I.V. systems, be aware that it is also compatible with a conventional needle. Follow manufacturer's directions for use with each system.
- Flush any dextrose-containing I.V. lines with 0.9% Sodium Chloride Injection before and after administering drug.
- Administer by first removing green cap and attaching the clear-ended blunt plastic cannula to the syringe. Remove the shield and use the blunt plastic cannula to access the split septum injection port. Because the blunt plastic cannula has two side ports, air or fluid expelled through the cannula will exit in two sideway directions; direct away from face or mucous membranes. Connect syringe directly to I.V. port if using a Luer-lock system. If using conventional needle, attach a large-bore needle (18 G) to the syringe's universal Luer-lock. Administer as a single I.V. bolus rapidly over 5 seconds.
- *Incompatibilities:* Dextrose-containing solutions

Route	Onset	Peak	Duration
I.V.	Immediate	Unknown	20–24 min

Half-life: 90–130 min

Mechanism of Action
Binds to fibrin and converts plasminogen to plasmin. Plasmin breaks down fibrin, fibrinogen, and other clotting factors, resulting in dissolution of a coronary artery thrombus.

Contraindications
Active internal bleeding, aneurysm, arteriovenous malformation, bleeding disorders, brain tumor, history of cerebrovascular accident, hypersensitivity to tenecteplase or its components, intracranial or intraspinal surgery or trauma within past 2 months, severe uncontrolled hypertension

T

≡ Interactions

DRUGS

abciximab, aspirin, clopidogrel, dipyridamole, heparin, oral anticoagulants, ticlopidine: Possibly increased risk of bleeding

≡ Adverse Reactions

CNS: Intracranial hemorrhage
EENT: Epistaxis, gingival bleeding, **laryngeal edema**, pharyngeal bleeding
GI: **GI and retroperitoneal bleeding**
GU: **Genitourinary bleeding**, prolonged or heavy menstrual bleeding
HEME: Hematoma
RESP: Hemoptysis
SKIN: Bleeding at puncture sites, surgical incision sites, or venous cutdown sites; rash; urticaria
OTHER: Anaphylaxis, angioedema

≡ Childbearing Considerations

PREGNANCY

- It is not known if drug can cause fetal harm, although maternal hemorrhage may result in fetal death.
- Use with caution only if benefit to mother outweighs potential risk to fetus.

LACTATION

- It is not known if drug is present in breast milk.
- Patient should check with prescriber before breastfeeding.

≡ Nursing Considerations

! WARNING Monitor patient during and for several hours after tenecteplase has been administered for hypersensitivity reactions, which may include anaphylaxis, angioedema, laryngeal edema, rash, and urticaria. If symptoms occur, notify prescriber, expect drug therapy to be discontinued, and provide supportive care, as prescribed.

! WARNING Monitor patient for evidence of GI bleeding, including bloody or black, tarry stools; bloody or coffee-ground vomitus; and severe stomach pain. Notify prescriber immediately if any of these signs or symptoms develops.

- Assess tenecteplase injection site for signs and symptoms of hematoma, including dark, deep purple bruises under skin and itching, pain, redness, or swelling. Also monitor patient for delayed bleeding at puncture sites, bleeding from surgical incisions, and superficial bleeding.
- Assess for signs and symptoms of genitourinary bleeding (such as hematuria), intracranial bleeding (such as decreased level of consciousness), respiratory tract bleeding (such as hemoptysis), or retroperitoneal bleeding (such as abdominal pain or swelling or back pain). Notify prescriber immediately if patient develops any of these signs or symptoms.
- If serious bleeding (not controllable by local pressure) occurs, expect to discontinue concomitant heparin or oral antiplatelet therapy immediately.
- Avoid I.M. injections and nonessential handling of patient, if possible, for first few hours after drug administration.
- Know that if arterial puncture becomes necessary during first few hours after tenecteplase administration, you should expect to use an upper extremity that's accessible to manual compression. Apply pressure for at least 30 minutes after procedure, use a pressure dressing, and frequently monitor puncture site for signs of bleeding.
- Monitor patients at higher risk for thromboembolism, such as patients with atrial fibrillation or mitral stenosis, while receiving a thrombolytic such as tenecteplase.

PATIENT TEACHING

- Advise patient to immediately report any bleeding, including from gums or nose.
- Instruct patient to limit physical activity during tenecteplase administration to reduce the risk of bleeding or injury.

! WARNING Stress importance of notifying staff immediately if any signs of an allergic reaction occur, including difficulty breathing.

tenofovir alafenamide fumarate

Vemlidy

≡ Class and Category

Pharmacologic class: Nucleoside analog reverse transcriptase inhibitor
Therapeutic class: Antiretroviral

Indications and Dosages

∗ *To treat chronic hepatitis B virus (HBV) infection in patients with compensated liver disease*

TABLETS

Adults. 25 mg once daily.

±**DOSAGE ADJUSTMENT** For patient taking carbamazepine concomitantly, dosage doubled.

Drug Administration

- Administer drug at about the same time daily.
- Give drug with food.
- Administer drug to patients receiving chronic hemodialysis after hemodialysis.

Route	Onset	Peak	Duration
P.O.	Unknown	0.5 hr	Unknown

Half-life: 0.5 hr

Mechanism of Action

Inhibits the activity of HBV reverse transcriptase by competing with the natural substrate, deoxyadenosine 5' triphosphate, and, after incorporation into DNA, by DNA chain termination.

Contraindications

Hypersensitivity to tenofovir alafenamide or its components

Interactions

DRUGS

acyclovir, aminoglycosides, cidofovir, ganciclovir, multiple NSAIDs, valacyclovir, valganciclovir: Increased risk of reduced renal function, increasing tenofovir alafenamide concentrations, which may lead to increased risk of adverse reactions
BCRP and P-gp inhibitors: Possibly increased absorption of tenofovir alafenamide
P-gp inducers such as carbamazepine, oxcarbazepine, phenobarbital, phenytoin, rifabutin, rifampin, rifapentine, St. John's wort: Decreased absorption of tenofovir alafenamide

Adverse Reactions

CNS: Fatigue, headache
CV: Elevated LDL-cholesterol levels
GI: Abdominal pain, diarrhea, dyspepsia, elevated liver or pancreatic enzymes, flatulence, nausea, **pancreatitis, severe acute exacerbation of hepatitis B, severe hepatomegaly with steatosis**, vomiting
GU: **Acute renal failure, acute tubular necrosis,** Fanconi syndrome, glycosuria, renal impairment (new onset or worsening), proximal renal tubulopathy
MS: Back pain, bone density loss, elevated creatine kinase levels
RESP: Arthralgia, cough
SKIN: Rash
Other: **Lactic acidosis**

Childbearing Considerations

PREGNANCY

- Pregnancy exposure registry: 1-800-258-4263.
- It is not known if drug can cause fetal harm.
- Use with caution only if benefit to mother outweighs potential risk to fetus.

LACTATION

- It is not known if drug is present in breast milk.
- Patient should check with prescriber before breastfeeding.

Nursing Considerations

- Know that HIV-1 antibody testing should be done on all HBV-infected patients before initiating therapy with tenofovir, to avoid the development of HIV-1 resistance.
- Obtain an estimated creatinine clearance, serum creatinine, urine glucose, and urine protein in all patients prior to initiating tenofovir therapy and periodically throughout, as ordered, because drug is principally eliminated by the kidneys. Renal impairment may occur, which may become severe in patients with chronic kidney disease. Also, know that patient's serum phosphorus level should be assessed before and during therapy if patient has chronic kidney disease.
- Be aware that tenofovir alafenamide should not be used in combination with any other drug containing tenofovir or adefovir dipivoxil. Also know that tenofovir alafenamide should not be administered with nephrotoxic agents such as high-dose or multiple NSAIDs, because of increased risk of renal dysfunction.

! **WARNING** Monitor patient upon discontinuation of tenofovir for several months, because severe acute exacerbations of hepatitis have occurred when drug has been stopped. Monitoring should include not only an assessment for signs and symptoms of hepatitis, but also laboratory studies such as liver enzymes, as ordered.

T

- Notify prescriber if patient develops a fracture and/or muscle pain or weakness, persistent or worsening bone pain, or pain in extremities, as these symptoms require further evaluation.

> **! WARNING** Monitor patient for signs and symptoms, as well as laboratory findings, of lactic acidosis or pronounced hepatotoxicity that may develop with tenofovir therapy. Know that hepatomegaly and steatosis may occur even in the absence of marked transaminase elevations.

- Be aware that patients who have a history of pathologic bone fracture or other risk factors for bone loss or osteoporosis should be assessed regularly for bone density loss. Patient may benefit from calcium and vitamin D supplementation.

PATIENT TEACHING

- Instruct patient to take tenofovir exactly as prescribed and to avoid missing doses. If a dose is missed, tell patient to take the dose as soon as she remembers it, but not to double the dose. Warn patient not to discontinue drug without consulting prescriber.
- Inform patient that bone density scanning may be ordered during tenofovir therapy.
- Tell patient to avoid high-dose or multiple NSAIDs while taking tenofovir, because of the risk of renal dysfunction.
- Caution patient to report any persistent, severe, or unusual signs and symptoms, including infection, to prescriber.
- Tell patient to inform all prescribers of tenofovir alafenamide therapy, as other drugs containing tenofovir should not be prescribed during therapy.

> **! WARNING** Inform patients who are discontinuing tenofovir to seek medical attention if signs and symptoms of hepatitis reappear. This is because severe acute exacerbations of hepatitis may occur for many months after drug has been discontinued. Encourage patient to comply with regular blood tests performed for several months after drug is discontinued.

- Advise patient to inform all healthcare providers of tenofovir use, because it may interact with other drugs.

tenofovir disoproxil fumarate
Viread

Class and Category
Pharmacologic class: Nucleoside reverse transcriptase inhibitor (NRTI)
Therapeutic class: Antiretroviral

Indications and Dosages
* *As adjunct to treat human immunodeficiency virus type 1 (HIV-1) infection; to treat chronic hepatitis B virus (HBV)*

TABLETS
Adults and children weighing at least 35 kg (77 lb). 300 mg once daily.
Children age 2 and older weighing 28 kg (61.6 lb) to less than 35 kg (77 lb). 250 mg once daily.
Children age 2 and older weighing 22 kg (48.4 lb) to less than 28 kg (61.6 lb). 200 mg once daily.
Children age 2 and older weighing 17 kg (37.4 lb) to less than 22 kg (48.4 lb). 150 mg once daily.

ORAL POWDER
Adults and children age 2 and over weighing less than 35 kg (77 lb) but at least 10 kg (22 lb) who are unable to swallow the tablet. 8 mg/kg once daily. *Maximum:* 300 mg once daily.

±**DOSAGE ADJUSTMENT** For adult patient with a creatinine clearance between 30 and 49 ml/min, dosage interval increased to every 48 hr. For adult patient with a creatinine clearance between 10 and 29 ml/min, dosage interval increased to every 72 to 96 hr. For hemodialysis patient, dosage interval increased to every 7 days or after a total of approximately 12 hours of dialysis. There are no specific recommendations for children with renal dysfunction.

Drug Administration

P.O.
- Weigh patient regularly and obtain dosage adjustment, as needed.
- Measure oral powder using only the supplied dosing scoop. Mix with 2 to 4 ounces of soft food not requiring chewing, such as applesauce, baby food, or yogurt.

Administer mixture immediately to avoid a bitter taste.

- Do not mix powder in a liquid because the powder may float on top of the liquid even after stirring.
- Administer tablets without regard to food intake.

Route	Onset	Peak	Duration
P.O.	Unknown	1–2 hr	Unknown

Half-life: 17 hr

Mechanism of Action

Inhibits the activity of HIV-1 reverse transcriptase and HBV reverse transcriptase by competing with the natural substrate deoxyadenosine 5′ triphosphate and, after incorporation into DNA, by DNA chain termination.

Contraindications

Hypersensitivity to tenofovir disoproxil fumarate or its components

Interactions

DRUGS

atazanavir: Decreased atazanavir concentration decreasing drug effectiveness
atazanavir/ritonavir, darunavir/ritonavir, ledipasvir/sofosbuvir, lopinavir/ritonavir, sofosbuvir/velpatasvir, sofosbuvir/ velpatasvir/voxilaprevir: Increased tenofovir concentration with increased risk of adverse reactions
didanosine: Increased concentration of didanosine with increased risk of adverse reactions
drugs affecting renal function, such as aminoglycosides, acyclovir, cidofovir, ganciclovir, high-dose or multiple NSAIDs use, valacyclovir, valganciclovir: Possibly increased concentration of tenofovir and/or increased concentration of other renally eliminated drugs

Adverse Reactions

CNS: Anxiety, asthenia, depression, dizziness, fatigue, fever, headache, insomnia, peripheral neuropathy
CV: Chest pain, elevated cholesterol and triglycerides
EENT: Nasopharyngitis, sinusitis
ENDO: Hyperglycemia
GI: Abdominal pain, **acute hepatitis (severe)**, anorexia, diarrhea, dyspepsia, elevated liver and pancreatic enzymes, flatulence, **hepatomegaly with steatosis (severe)**, nausea, **pancreatitis**, vomiting
GU: Acute renal failure, acute tubular necrosis, elevated creatinine, **Fanconi syndrome,** hematuria, interstitial nephritis, **renal impairment**
HEME: Anemia, **neutropenia**
MS: Arthralgia, back pain, decreased bone density, elevated bone specific alkaline phosphatase and creatine kinase, muscular weakness, myalgia, myopathy, osteomalacia, **rhabdomyolysis**
RESP: Dyspnea, pneumonia, upper respiratory infections
SKIN: Diaphoresis, maculopapular rash, pruritus, pustular rash, rash, urticaria, vesiculobullous rash
Other: Angioedema, hypokalemia, hypophosphatemia, immune reconstitution syndrome, **lactic acidosis,** lipodystrophy, pain, weight loss

Childbearing Considerations

PREGNANCY

- Pregnancy exposure registry: 1-800-258-4263.
- Studies show no increase in fetal harm when drug is taken during the first and third trimesters.
- Use with caution only if benefit to mother outweighs potential risk to fetus.

LACTATION

- Drug is present in breast milk.
- The Centers for Disease Control and Prevention recommends that HIV-1 infected mothers not breastfeed to avoid risking postnatal transmission of HIV-1 infection to infants. They also do not recommend breastfeeding because of potential drug-induced adverse reactions in the infant.
- Patient taking drug to treat hepatitis B viral infection should check with prescriber before breastfeeding.

Nursing Considerations

- Know that HIV-1 antibody testing should be done on all HBV-infected patients before initiating therapy with tenofovir, to avoid the development of HIV-1 resistance.
- Obtain an estimated creatinine clearance, serum creatinine, urine glucose, and urine

T

protein in all patients prior to initiating tenofovir therapy and periodically throughout, as ordered, because drug is principally eliminated by the kidneys. Renal impairment may occur, which may become severe in patients with chronic kidney disease. Also know that patient's serum phosphorus level should be assessed before and during therapy. Report at any time throughout therapy patient complaints of bone, extremity, or muscle pain or weakness or if patient sustains a fracture, as these may be manifestations of proximal renal tubulopathy and require a prompt evaluation of renal function.

- Be aware that tenofovir should not be used in combination with any other drug containing tenofovir or adefovir dipivoxil. Also know that tenofovir should not be administered with nephrotoxic agents such as high-dose or multiple NSAIDs, because of increased risk of renal dysfunction.

! **WARNING** Monitor patient being treated for hepatitis B upon discontinuation of tenofovir for several months, because severe acute exacerbations of hepatitis have occurred when drug has been stopped. Monitoring should include not only an assessment for signs and symptoms of hepatitis, but also laboratory studies such as liver enzymes, as ordered.

- Notify prescriber if patient develops a fracture and/or muscular pain or weakness, persistent or worsening bone pain, or pain in extremities, as these may be signs and symptoms of proximal renal tubulopathy and require further evaluation.

! **WARNING** Monitor patient for signs and symptoms, as well as laboratory findings, of lactic acidosis or pronounced hepatotoxicity that may develop with tenofovir therapy. Know that hepatomegaly and steatosis may occur even in the absence of marked transaminase elevations.

- Be aware that patients who have a history of pathologic bone fracture or other risk factors for bone loss or osteoporosis should be assessed regularly for bone density loss. Patient may benefit from calcium and vitamin D supplementation.

- Be aware that immune reconstitution syndrome has occurred in patients treated with combination antiretroviral therapy, including tenofovir. The inflammatory response predisposes susceptible patients to opportunistic infections such as cytomegalovirus, *Mycobacterium avium* infection, *Pneumocystis jiroveci* pneumonia, or tuberculosis. Autoimmune disorders such as Graves' disease, Guillain–Barré syndrome, or polymyositis have also occurred. Report sudden or unusual adverse reactions to prescriber.

PATIENT TEACHING

- Instruct patient to take tenofovir exactly as prescribed and to avoid missing doses. If a dose is missed, tell patient to take the dose as soon as she remembers it, but not to double the dose. Warn patient not to discontinue the drug without consulting prescriber.

- Remind patient or caregiver measuring oral powder to use only the supplied dosing scoop, to ensure an accurate dose. Tell him to mix with 2 to 4 ounces of soft food not requiring chewing, such as applesauce, baby food, or yogurt, and to take mixture immediately to avoid a bitter taste. Tell patient not to mix powder in a liquid.

- Inform patient that bone density scanning may be ordered during tenofovir therapy.

- Tell patient to avoid high-dose or multiple NSAIDs while taking tenofovir, because of the risk of renal dysfunction.

- Caution patient to report any persistent, severe, or unusual signs and symptoms, including infection, to prescriber.

- Tell patient to inform all prescribers of tenofovir therapy, as other drugs containing tenofovir should not be prescribed during therapy.

- Inform mothers with HIV not to breastfeed during tenofovir therapy.

! **WARNING** Inform patients who are discontinuing tenofovir after being treated for hepatitis B virus to seek medical attention if signs and symptoms of hepatitis reappear. This is because severe acute exacerbations of hepatitis may occur for many months after drug has been discontinued.

terazosin hydrochloride

Class and Category

Pharmacologic class: Alpha-adrenergic blocker
Therapeutic class: Antihypertensive, benign prostatic hyperplasia (BPH) agent

Indications and Dosages

✱ *To manage hypertension*

CAPSULES

Adults. *Initial:* 1 mg nightly. *Maintenance:* 1 to 5 mg daily as a single dose or in divided doses every 12 hr. *Maximum:* 20 mg daily.

✱ *To treat symptomatic BPH*

CAPSULES

Adults. *Initial:* 1 mg once nightly, increased in increments to 2, 5, and then 10 mg once nightly, as needed, based on symptom improvement and urine flow for a minimum of 4 to 6 wk before dosage increased to 20 mg, if needed. *Maximum:* 20 mg daily.

Drug Administration

P.O.

- Administer once-daily dose at bedtime.
- Dosage will have to be retitrated if consecutive doses are missed for several days.

Route	Onset	Peak	Duration
P.O.	15 min	1 hr	24 hr

Half-life: 12 hr

Mechanism of Action

Blocks postsynaptic alpha$_1$-adrenergic receptors in many tissues, including the bladder neck, the prostate and vascular smooth muscle. This action promotes vasodilation, which reduces blood pressure and improves urine flow.

Contraindications

Hypersensitivity to terazosin or its components

Interactions

DRUGS

phosphodiesterase-5 inhibitors, verapamil: Additive blood pressure–lowering effects and symptomatic hypotension

Adverse Reactions

CNS: Asthenia, dizziness, headache, lethargy, nervousness, paresthesia, somnolence, syncope, vertigo
CV: Chest pain, **hypotension**, orthostatic hypotension, palpitations, peripheral edema, sinus tachycardia
EENT: Blurred vision, dry mouth, intraoperative floppy iris syndrome, nasal congestion, sinusitis
GI: Constipation, diarrhea, nausea, vomiting
MS: Arthralgia, back pain
Other: Flu-like symptoms, weight gain

Childbearing Considerations

PREGNANCY

- It is not known if drug can cause fetal harm.
- Drug is not recommended during pregnancy unless benefit to mother outweighs potential risk to fetus.

LACTATION

- It is not known if drug is present in breast milk.
- Patient should check with prescriber before breastfeeding.

Nursing Considerations

- Be aware that prostate cancer should be ruled out before giving terazosin for BPH.
- Expect prescriber to reduce terazosin dosage if a diuretic or another antihypertensive is added to patient's regimen.
- Monitor blood pressure 2 to 3 hours after initial dose because of possible first-dose hypotension and again after 24 hours to evaluate patient's response.
- Be aware that elderly patients may have exaggerated hypotension and other adverse reactions.

PATIENT TEACHING

- Instruct patient to take terazosin at bedtime.
- Explain possible first-dose hypotension. Advise patient to change position and rise slowly to prevent syncope early in therapy. Suggest lying down or sitting if dizziness or light-headedness occurs.
- Advise patient to avoid hazardous activities until drug's CNS effects are known.
- Instruct patient to notify prescriber if she misses several doses in a row; caution her against resuming therapy at previous dose.
- Advise patient to avoid alcohol use, excessive exercise, exposure to hot

T

weather, or prolonged standing, because these activities can worsen orthostatic hypotension.

- Emphasize the importance of regular follow-up visits with prescriber to evaluate patient's response to drug.

terbinafine hydrochloride

Lamisil

≣ Class and Category

Pharmacologic class: Allylamine derivative
Therapeutic class: Antifungal

≣ Indications and Dosages

* *To treat onychomycosis of fingernails and toenails due to dermatophytes* (tinea unguium)

TABLETS

Adults. 250 mg once daily for 6 wk for fingernail onychomycosis and 12 wk for toenail onychomycosis.

≣ Drug Administration

P.O.

- Administer drug without regard to food.
- Protect tablets from light.

Route	Onset	Peak	Duration
P.O.	Unknown	< 2 hr	Unknown

Half-life: 36 hr

≣ Mechanism of Action

Inhibits the conversion of squalene mono-oxygenase to squalene epoxidase, a key enzyme in fungal biosynthesis. The resulting squalene accumulation weakens cell membranes and creates a deficiency of ergosterol, the fungal membrane component necessary for normal fungal growth.

≣ Contraindications

Active or chronic liver disease, hypersensitivity to terbinafine or its components

≣ Interactions

DRUGS

beta blockers, class 1C antiarrhythmics such as flecainide and propafenone, MAO inhibitors (type B), selective serotonin reuptake inhibitors, tricyclic antidepressants: Possibly increased blood levels of these drugs
cimetidine, other hepatic enzyme inhibitors: Significantly decreased terbinafine clearance, possibly increased adverse reactions
cyclosporine: Increased clearance of cyclosporine and decreased effectiveness of cyclosporine
CYP2C9 and CYP3A4 inhibitors such as amiodarone and ketoconazole: Possibly increased systemic exposure of terbinafine
hepatotoxic drugs: Increased risk of hepatotoxicity
rifampin: Increased clearance and decreased effectiveness of terbinafine
warfarin: Possibly altered prothrombin time

FOODS

caffeine: Decreased caffeine clearance

ACTIVITIES

alcohol use: Increased risk of hepatic dysfunction

≣ Adverse Reactions

CNS: Anxiety, depression, fatigue, fever, headache, hypoesthesia, malaise, paresthesia, vertigo
CV: Myocarditis, pericarditis, thrombotic microangiopathy, vasculitis
EENT: Hearing impairment, loss of smell, reduced visual acuity, taste loss or perversion (possibly severe), tinnitus, visual field defect
GI: Abdominal pain, anorexia, cholestasis, diarrhea, elevated liver enzymes, flatulence, hepatic failure, hepatitis, hepatotoxicity, indigestion, jaundice, nausea, pancreatitis, vomiting
GU: Hemolytic uremic syndrome, nephritis
HEME: Agranulocytosis, anemia, neutropenia (severe), pancytopenia, thrombocytopenia, thrombotic thrombocytopenic purpura
MS: Arthralgia, myalgia, rhabdomyolysis
RESP: Pneumonitis
SKIN: Acute generalized exanthematous pustulosis, alopecia, bullous dermatitis, cutaneous lupus erythematosus, erythema multiforme, exacerbation of psoriasis, exfoliative dermatitis, photosensitivity, psoriasiform eruptions, pruritus, rash, Stevens–Johnson syndrome, toxic epidermal necrolysis, urticaria
Other: Anaphylaxis, angioedema, drug reaction with eosinophilia and systemic

symptoms (DRESS), elevated blood creatine phosphokinase, influenza-like illness, serum sickness-like reaction, systemic lupus erythematosus

Childbearing Considerations

PREGNANCY

- It is not known if drug can cause fetal harm.
- Drug therapy is not recommended to begin during pregnancy because treatment can be postponed until after delivery.

LACTATION

- Drug is present in breast milk.
- Breastfeeding is not recommended during drug therapy.

Nursing Considerations

- Know that because terbinafine has been linked to serious adverse hepatic effects, expect to send nail specimens for laboratory testing to confirm onychomycosis before starting therapy. Also expect to check liver enzymes, as ordered, prior to starting therapy.
- Ensure that patient's liver enzymes have been checked before terbinafine therapy is begun, to rule out preexisting liver disease. Expect to monitor liver enzymes regularly throughout therapy if baseline enzymes are normal.
- Monitor patient for hepatic failure (anorexia, dark urine, fatigue, jaundice, nausea, pale stools, right upper abdominal pain, and vomiting). Know that periodic monitoring of liver enzymes should be done throughout therapy because hepatotoxicity may also occur in patients without preexisting liver disease. Expect to stop drug and obtain liver enzyme tests if these problems develop.

! **WARNING** Monitor patient for serious hypersensitivity or skin reactions such as Stevens–Johnson syndrome or drug reaction with eosinophilia and systemic symptoms (DRESS) syndrome. Know that in addition to skin abnormalities such as rash and urticaria, DRESS may also involve one or more organs. If hypersensitivity reactions persist or progress, notify prescriber and expect drug to be discontinued.

- Monitor patient's complete blood count, as ordered. Know that thrombotic microangiopathy has occurred with

terbinafine use and can be life-threatening. Notify prescriber promptly of any abnormalities, especially unexplained anemia and thrombocytopenia. If thrombotic microangiopathy is confirmed, expect drug to be discontinued.

PATIENT TEACHING

- Emphasize the need to complete the full course of terbinafine therapy to prevent relapse of infection.
- Stress importance of protecting drug from light.
- Discourage consumption of alcohol during therapy.

! **WARNING** Alert patient that drug may cause an allergic or skin reaction. Tell patient to contact prescriber at the first sign of an allergic reaction or rash. If reaction is serious or severe, stress importance of seeking immediate medical attention.

- Tell patient to contact prescriber if onychomycosis doesn't improve in a few weeks.
- Instruct patient to notify prescriber if he develops persistent anorexia, dark urine, fatigue, jaundice, nausea, pale stools, or right upper abdominal pain. Stress importance of stopping terbinafine therapy immediately if any of these symptoms occur.
- Instruct patient to avoid direct sunlight or UV light and to wear sunscreen when outdoors.
- Instruct patient to inform prescriber of any unexplained bleeding or bruising that may occur.
- Advise patient to alert prescriber if loss or perversion of taste occurs and becomes severe enough to cause anxiety, depression, or weight loss.
- Advise women of childbearing age to notify prescriber if pregnancy occurs during drug therapy.

terbutaline sulfate

Class and Category

Pharmacologic class: Beta adrenergic receptor agonist
Therapeutic class: Bronchodilator

Indications and Dosages

* *To prevent or reverse bronchospasm from asthma, bronchitis, or emphysema*

TABLETS

Adults and adolescents age 15 and over. 2.5 to 5 mg three times a day at 6-hr intervals while awake. *Maximum:* 15 mg daily.
Children ages 12 to 15. 2.5 mg three times a day at 6-hr intervals while awake. *Maximum:* 7.5 mg daily.

SUBCUTANEOUS INJECTION

Adults and children age 12 and over. *Initial:* 0.25 mg, repeated in 15 to 30 min, as needed. *Maximum:* 0.5 mg/4-hr period.

Drug Administration

P.O.

- Administer tablets without regard to food.

SUBCUTANEOUS

- Do not use if solution is discolored.
- Inject into the lateral side of the deltoid muscle.
- Protect from light.

Route	Onset	Peak	Duration
P.O.	30–45 min	2–3 hr	4–8 hr
SubQ	6–15 min	30–60 min	1.5–4 hr

Half-life: 6–14 hr

Mechanism of Action

Stimulates beta$_2$-adrenergic receptors in the lungs, which is believed to increase production of cAMP. The increased cAMP level relaxes bronchial smooth muscles, thereby increasing bronchial airflow and relieving bronchospasm.

Contraindications

Hypersensitivity to terbutaline, other sympathomimetic amines, or their components; use to treat tocolysis (oral form)

Interactions

DRUGS

beta blockers: Mutual inhibition of therapeutic effects, increased risk of bronchospasm in asthmatic patients
halogenated anesthetics: Possibly ventricular arrhythmias
MAO inhibitors, tricyclic antidepressants: Possible potentiated action on vascular system causing adverse reactions that could become severe

non-potassium–sparing diuretics (loop or thiazide): Possible ECG changes and/or hypokalemia
sympathomimetics: Increased CNS stimulation and risk of adverse cardiovascular effects, including prolonged QT interval
xanthines (theophylline): Increased CNS stimulation and other additive toxic effects

FOODS

caffeine: Increased CNS stimulation and other additive toxic effects

Adverse Reactions

CNS: Anxiety, dizziness, drowsiness, headache, insomnia, light-headedness, nervousness, restlessness, tremor, weakness
CV: Chest pain, **irregular heartbeat**, palpitations, tachycardia
EENT: Dry mouth, taste perversion
ENDO: Hyperglycemia
GI: Heartburn, nausea, vomiting
MS: Muscle spasms
RESP: Dyspnea
SKIN: Diaphoresis, flushing, rash

Childbearing Considerations

PREGNANCY

- It is not known if drug can cause fetal harm.
- Drug is not recommended during pregnancy unless benefit to mother clearly outweighs potential risk to fetus.

LABOR & DELIVERY

- Drug may interfere with uterine contractility and should be used during labor and delivery only if the benefits clearly outweigh the risk and mother is not in preterm labor.
- Oral form is contraindicated to prevent or treat mother in preterm labor.
- Injectable form is contraindicated for prevention or prolonged treatment (beyond 72 hours) of preterm labor.
- Exposure to drug may increase fetal heart rate and cause neonatal hypoglycemia.

LACTATION

- It is not known if drug is present in breast milk.
- Patient should check with prescriber before breastfeeding.

Nursing Considerations

- Use terbutaline cautiously in patients with cardiovascular disease because drug can adversely affect cardiovascular function. Monitor patient's heart rate and rhythm and blood pressure, and assess for chest pain.

- Assess patient's respiratory rate, depth, and quality; oxygen saturation; and activity tolerance at regular intervals because continuous use of beta$_2$-agonists for 12 months or longer accelerates the decline in pulmonary function.

PATIENT TEACHING

- Teach patient how to give subcutaneous injection, as needed.
- Instruct patient not to increase dose or frequency without consulting prescriber.
- Urge patient to seek immediate medical attention if symptoms worsen.
- Inform patient that she may experience transient nervousness or tremors during terbutaline therapy.

teriflunomide
Aubagio

≣ Class and Category

Pharmacologic class: Pyrimidine synthesis inhibitor
Therapeutic class: Immunomodulator

≣ Indications and Dosages

∗ *To treat relapsing forms of multiple sclerosis, including active secondary progressive disease, clinically isolated syndrome, and relapsing-remitting disease*

TABLETS

Adults. 7 or 14 mg once daily.

≣ Drug Administration

P.O.

- Administer tablets with or without regard to food.

Route	Onset	Peak	Duration
P.O.	Unknown	1–4 hr	Unknown

Half-life: 18–19 days

≣ Mechanism of Action

Inhibits dihydroorotate dehydrogenase, a mitochondrial enzyme involved in de novo pyrimidine synthesis to possibly reduce the number of activated lymphocytes in the central nervous system responsible for the signs and symptoms of multiple sclerosis.

≣ Contraindications

Concurrent therapy with leflunomide; hypersensitivity to teriflunomide, leflunomide, or their components; pregnancy; severe hepatic impairment; women of childbearing age not using reliable contraception

≣ Interactions

DRUGS

BCRP and organic anion transporting polypeptide B1 and B3 (OATP1B1/1B3) substrates such as atorvastatin, nateglinide, pravastatin, repaglinide, rosuvastatin, simvastatin: Increased concentrations of these drugs
CYP1A2 substrates such as alosetron, duloxetine, theophylline, tizanidine: Reduced effectiveness of these drugs
CYP2C8 substrates such as paclitaxel, pioglitazone, repaglinide, rosiglitazone: Possibly increased exposure of these drugs with potential for leading to adverse effects
live vaccines: Increased risk of infection
oral contraceptives containing ethinyl estradiol or levonorgestrel: Increased systemic exposure of these drugs, increasing risk of adverse reactions
organic anion transporter 3 (OAT3) substrates such as cefaclor, cimetidine, ciprofloxacin, furosemide, ketoprofen, methotrexate, penicillin G, zidovudine: Increased exposure of these drugs with possibly increased risk of adverse reactions
warfarin: Decreased peak international normalized ratio

≣ Adverse Reactions

CNS: Anxiety, burning sensation, headache, paresthesia, peripheral neuropathy, sciatica
CV: Hypertension, palpitations
EENT: Blurred vision, conjunctivitis, oral herpes, sinusitis, toothache
GI: Abdominal distention, colitis, diarrhea, elevated liver enzymes, gastroenteritis, **hepatic dysfunction or failure, hepatotoxicity,** nausea, **pancreatitis,** upper abdominal pain
GU: **Acute renal failure,** acute uric acid nephropathy, cystitis, elevated serum creatinine levels
HEME: **Leukopenia, neutropenia, thrombocytopenia**
MS: Manifestation of carpal tunnel syndrome, musculoskeletal pain, myalgia

T

RESP: Acute interstitial pneumonitis, bronchitis, cough, dyspnea, **interstitial lung disease**, upper respiratory infection

SKIN: Acne, alopecia, pruritus, psoriasis or worsening of psoriasis (including pustular psoriasis), **Stevens–Johnson syndrome, toxic epidermal necrolysis**, urticaria

Other: **Anaphylaxis, angioedema, drug reaction with eosinophilia and systemic symptoms (DRESS)**, flu-like symptoms, **hyperkalemia**, infections such as tuberculosis, onset of seasonal allergies, weight loss

Childbearing Considerations

PREGNANCY

- Pregnancy exposure registry: 1-800-745-4447, option 2.
- Drug has the potential to cause fetal harm.
- Drug is contraindicated in pregnant women and in women of childbearing age not using effective contraception.
- A negative pregnancy test must be obtained before drug therapy is begun.
- If pregnancy occurs during drug therapy, drug must be discontinued immediately. Instituting an accelerated drug elimination procedure as soon as pregnancy is detected may decrease the risk to the fetus.

LACTATION

- It is not known if drug is present in breast milk.
- Breastfeeding should not be undertaken during drug therapy.

REPRODUCTION

- Women of childbearing age must use effective contraception during drug therapy, as it is essential that pregnancy be avoided during therapy. Women receiving drug who wish to become pregnant must discontinue drug with prescriber consent and undergo an accelerated drug elimination procedure. Contraceptive measures must continue after drug has been discontinued until plasma concentrations of drug are less than 0.02 mg/L (0.02 mcg/ml).
- Drug is present in semen. Therefore, men or their female partner must use effective contraception as well. If male patient wishes to father a child, drug must be discontinued and an accelerated elimination procedure done or verification that the plasma concentration of drug is less than 0.02 mg/L (0.02 mcg/ml) before attempting to father a child.

Nursing Considerations

- Know that teriflunomide isn't recommended for patients with bone marrow dysplasia, severe immunodeficiency, or severe, uncontrolled infections because of its immunosuppressant effect. It is also not recommended for patients with liver disease or those with a serum alanine aminotransferase level greater than two times the upper level normal prior to initiation of therapy because drug may worsen liver dysfunction.
- Obtain a pregnancy test on all women of childbearing age, as ordered, prior to starting teriflunomide therapy. Know that drug should not be started if pregnancy is suspected or confirmed or in women who refuse to use a reliable contraceptive.
- Know that patients with active acute or chronic infections should not begin drug treatment with teriflunomide until infection is resolved.
- Use cautiously in patients who are over 60 years of age, patients with diabetes, or in patients taking concomitant neurotoxic drugs, because of an increased risk of developing peripheral neuropathy. If peripheral neuropathy occurs during teriflunomide therapy, notify prescriber and expect drug to be discontinued and possibly cholestyramine washout ordered.
- Test patient for latent tuberculosis before starting leflunomide, as ordered. If positive, expect standard medical treatment to be given before teriflunomide therapy starts.
- Obtain baseline blood pressure before starting teriflunomide, and monitor periodically thereafter because drug may cause hypertension.
- Assess liver enzyme (ALT and AST) levels at start of therapy, monthly during first 6 months, and if stable, every 6 to 8 weeks thereafter, as ordered. If levels become elevated greater than threefold upper level normal, notify prescriber and expect teriflunomide therapy to be withheld until underlying cause is determined. If the elevation is thought to be teriflunomide induced, expect to start cholestyramine washout, as ordered, and monitor liver test weekly until normalized. If another cause is found for the elevation, expect to resume teriflunomide therapy.

- Ensure that a complete CBC has been done within the past 6 months prior to starting teriflunomide therapy to use as a baseline. Repeat CBC, as ordered, thereafter if signs and symptoms of bone marrow suppression occur.

! WARNING Monitor patient for hypersensitivity reactions that can become life-threatening, such as anaphylaxis and angioedema. If present, notify prescriber and provide supportive care, as needed and prescribed.

- Notify prescriber if patient develops a serious infection or skin condition because drug may have to be interrupted and charcoal or cholestyramine given to eliminate drug rapidly.

! WARNING Monitor patient's respiratory function closely because drug may cause interstitial lung disease that could become life-threatening. If patient develops a cough and dyspnea, notify prescriber; drug may have to be stopped, and patient may need charcoal or cholestyramine to eliminate drug rapidly.

- Check patient's serum potassium level, as ordered, if symptoms of acute renal failure or hyperkalemia occur.

PATIENT TEACHING

- Tell patient to report signs of respiratory dysfunction, such as cough and dyspnea.

! WARNING Caution woman of childbearing potential not to become pregnant while taking drug because of the high risk of birth defects. Emphasize importance of using reliable forms of birth control and to notify prescriber immediately if pregnancy is suspected. Also advise men and their female partners to use effective contraception to minimize possibility of pregnancy.

- Inform mothers wishing to breastfeed that breastfeeding should not be done during drug therapy.
- Advise patient to avoid live vaccines during teriflunomide therapy.
- Instruct patient to notify prescriber immediately if she develops an infection or skin condition.

! WARNING Instruct patient to stop taking teriflunomide if he develops an allergic reaction, including difficulty breathing; itching or swelling of eyes, face, lips, or throat; fever, rash, or swollen glands; or signs of liver dysfunction such as darkened urine, fatigue, and yellow eyes or skin. In addition, patient should seek immediate medical attention.

teriparatide recombinant human
Bonsity, Forteo

Class and Category
Pharmacologic class: Recombinant human parathyroid hormone (PTH)
Therapeutic class: Antiosteoporotic

Indications and Dosages
* *To treat osteoporosis in postmenopausal women; primary or hypogonadal osteoporosis in men at high risk for fracture; and to treat men and women with glucocorticoid-induced osteoporosis at high risk for fracture*

SUBCUTANEOUS INJECTION
Adults. 20 mcg daily for up to 2 yr.

Drug Administration
SUBCUTANEOUS
- Solution in delivery pen should be colorless and clear.
- Use delivery pen immediately after removal from refrigerator. Return delivery pen to refrigerator as soon as injection is given.
- Inject drug into abdominal wall or thigh while patient is sitting down or lying down because of potential orthostatic hypotension.
- Rotate injection sites.
- Discard delivery pen 28 days after the first injection.
- Protect delivery pen from damage and light while stored.

Route	Onset	Peak	Duration
SubQ	Rapid	30 min	4 hr

Half-life: 1 hr

T

Mechanism of Action

Teriparatide, which contains recombinant PTH, stimulates new bone growth and increases bone density. In a patient with osteoporosis, bone density and mass are diminished by an imbalance between bone destruction and formation. Normally, osteoclasts break down and resorb bone, leaving behind a cavity in a section of bone. Then bone-building cells, called osteoblasts, line the walls of the cavity and stimulate new bone formation. PTH stimulates these actions by attaching to receptors on osteoclasts and osteoblasts, as shown below. Teriparatide binds to cell-surface receptors on osteoblasts and preferentially stimulates osteoblastic over osteoclastic activity. Also, the drug increases the amount of circulating calcium available for bone formation by increasing the intestinal absorption of calcium and phosphate, thus enhancing the rate of calcium resorption from bone, increasing the reabsorption of calcium, and inhibiting the reabsorption of phosphate in the kidneys. These actions stimulate new bone formation and increase bone density to reduce osteoporotic bone changes.

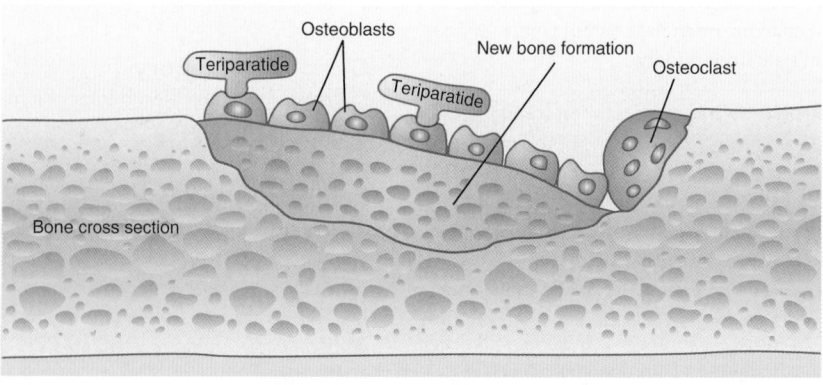

Contraindications

Hypersensitivity to teriparatide or its components

Interactions

DRUGS

digitalis glycosides: Possibly increased risk of digitalis toxicity

Adverse Reactions

CNS: Asthenia, depression, dizziness, headache, insomnia, paresthesia, syncope, vertigo
CV: Angina pectoris, chest pain, hypertension, transient orthostatic hypotension
EENT: Pharyngitis, rhinitis, taste perversion, tooth disorder
ENDO: Hypoparathyroidism
GI: Constipation, diarrhea, indigestion, vomiting
GU: Urolithiasis
MS: Arthralgia, muscle cramps or spasms in back or leg, neck pain
RESP: Cough, dyspnea, pneumonia
SKIN: Cutaneous calcification (including calciphylaxis), diaphoresis, pruritus, rash, urticaria
Other: Anaphylaxis, angioedema, antibody formation against teriparatide, generalized pain, hypercalcemia, hypocalcemia, injection-site reactions (erythema, localized bruising, minor bleeding, pain, pruritus, swelling)

Childbearing Considerations

PREGNANCY

- It is not known if drug can cause fetal harm.
- Drug should be discontinued if pregnancy occurs.

LACTATION

- It is not known if drug is present in breast milk.

- Breastfeeding is not recommended during drug therapy due to risk for osteosarcoma.

⧮ Nursing Considerations

! WARNING Be aware that teriparatide shouldn't be used to treat patients at risk for osteosarcoma (such as those with Paget's disease or a metabolic bone disease other than osteoporosis), unexplained elevations of alkaline phosphatase, open epiphyses, or prior skeletal radiation or malignancy.

! WARNING Be aware that patients with hypercalcemia shouldn't receive teriparatide because drug may worsen hypercalcemia.

- Use drug cautiously in patients with active or recent urolithiasis because drug could worsen this condition.

! WARNING Monitor patient closely for allergic reactions because teriparatide is a peptide agent.

- Monitor patient's blood calcium level, and notify prescriber of any elevation; in persistent hypercalcemia, drug may have to be stopped.
- Monitor patient's blood pressure during the first several doses of drug therapy because of a risk of transient orthostatic hypotension. If this occurs, place patient in a reclining position and alert prescriber.
- Monitor patient for cutaneous calcification, including calciphylaxis, especially in patients with underlying autoimmune disease, concomitant systemic corticosteroid or warfarin use, and kidney failure.

PATIENT TEACHING

- Teach patient how to administer teriparatide by subcutaneous injection and how to properly use the delivery pen device and dispose of needles. Advise her not to share pen device with others.
- Inform patient that each delivery pen can be used for up to 28 days after the first injection but then should be discarded even if it still contains solution.
- Instruct patient to store delivery pen in the refrigerator and to recap it when not in use to protect it from damage and light.
- Tell patient that delivery pen should be used immediately after removal from refrigerator

and should be put back in refrigerator as soon as the injection is given.
- Instruct patient to inject drug into thigh or abdominal wall and to rotate injection sites.
- Caution patient to administer drug in a room where she can immediately sit or lie down if light-headedness or palpitations occur. Advise her to notify prescriber if these symptoms persist or worsen.

! WARNING Alert patient that drug may cause an allergic reaction. Tell patient to notify prescriber, if present, and to seek immediate medical attention if serious.

- Instruct patient to notify prescriber of persistent symptoms of hypercalcemia, such as nausea, vomiting, constipation, lethargy, and muscle weakness.
- Caution patient about potential of developing osteosarcoma.
- Inform mothers wishing to breastfeed that breastfeeding must be avoided while taking drug.

tetracycline hydrochloride

⧮ Class and Category
Pharmacologic class: Tetracycline
Therapeutic class: Antibiotic

⧮ Indications and Dosages
✳ *To treat infections caused by gram-negative and gram-positive organisms*

CAPSULES

Adults. 250 mg four times daily or 500 mg twice daily increased to 500 mg four times daily, as needed for severe infections or those not responding to lower doses.
Children age 9 and over. 25 to 50 mg/kg daily divided into four equal doses every 6 hr.

✳ *To treat moderate to severe acne vulgaris in patients requiring long-term treatment*

CAPSULES

Adults. *Initial:* 1,000 mg daily in divided doses until improvement occurs (usually in 3 wk); then dosage reduced gradually. *Maintenance:* 125 to 500 mg daily, every other day, or intermittently.

✳ *To treat brucellosis caused by susceptible organisms*

CAPSULES

Adults. 500 mg every 6 hr for 3 wk, given with streptomycin.

✱ *To treat gonorrhea caused by* Neisseria gonorrhoeae

CAPSULES

Adults. 500 mg every 6 hr for 7 days.

✱ *To treat syphilis in patients allergic to penicillin*

CAPSULES

Adults. 500 mg every 6 hr for 15 days (for early syphilis of less than 1 yr duration) or 30 days (for late syphilis with more than 1 yr duration except for neurosyphilis).

✱ *To treat uncomplicated endocervical, rectal, or urethral infections caused by* Chlamydia trachomatis

CAPSULES

Adults. 500 mg four times a day for at least 7 days.

±**DOSAGE ADJUSTMENT** For patients with renal impairment, dosage reduced or time intervals extended between doses.

⬚ Drug Administration

P.O.

- Never administer outdated drug because of increased risk of renal toxicity and Fanconi syndrome.
- Administer drug at least 1 hour before meals or 2 hours after meals, because dairy products and some foods may interfere with absorption.
- Administer each dose with a full glass of water while patient is in an upright position and avoid bedtime administration to avoid esophageal or GI irritation.
- Avoid administering other drugs, including antacids, within 3 hours of tetracycline.

Route	Onset	Peak	Duration
P.O.	Unknown	2–4 hr	Unknown

Half-life: 6–12 hr

⬚ Mechanism of Action

Exerts a bacteriostatic effect against a wide variety of gram-negative and gram-positive organisms by passing through the bacterial lipid bilayer, where it binds reversibly to 30S ribosomal subunits. Bound tetracycline blocks the binding of aminoacyl transfer RNA to messenger RNA, thus inhibiting bacterial protein synthesis.

⬚ Contraindications

Hypersensitivity to tetracycline or its components

⬚ Interactions

DRUGS

aluminum-, calcium-, or magnesium-containing antacids; iron supplements (oral); magnesium-containing laxatives; magnesium salicylate; multivitamins (containing manganese or zinc salts); sodium bicarbonate: Possibly impaired absorption of oral tetracycline and formation of nonabsorbable complexes

digoxin: Possibly increased digoxin level

methoxyflurane: Possibly nephrotoxicity

oral anticoagulants: Decreased plasma prothrombin activity

oral contraceptives (containing estrogen): Possibly reduced contraceptive reliability and increased risk of breakthrough bleeding (with long-term tetracycline use)

penicillins: Possibly decreased bactericidal effect of penicillins

FOODS

dairy products and other foods: Possibly impaired absorption of oral tetracycline

⬚ Adverse Reactions

CNS: Dizziness, light-headedness, unsteadiness

EENT: Darkened or discolored tongue, enamel hypoplasia, oral candidiasis, tooth discoloration (in children)

GI: Abdominal pain, diarrhea, **hepatotoxicity**, nausea, rectal candidiasis, vomiting

GU: Vaginal candidiasis

SKIN: Photosensitivity

⬚ Childbearing Considerations

PREGNANCY

- Drug can cause fetal harm such as adverse effects on skeletal and tooth development.
- The use of drug during last half of pregnancy may cause permanent discoloration of the child's teeth.
- Drug should not be used during pregnancy unless there is no alternative and benefit to mother outweighs potential risk to fetus.
- Pregnant women with renal disease may be more prone to develop drug-induced liver failure.

LACTATION

- Drug is present in breast milk.

- A decision should be made to discontinue breastfeeding or the drug to avoid potential serious adverse reactions in the breastfed infant.

REPRODUCTION

- Women who use oral contraceptives containing estrogen need to use another method of contraception while taking tetracycline because estrogen-containing contraceptives may be less effective.

Nursing Considerations

- Avoid giving tetracycline to children age 8 and under because drug may cause permanent brown or yellow tooth discoloration and enamel hypoplasia.
- Be aware that enamel hypoplasia and tooth discoloration may occur in breastfed infants, along with inhibition of linear skeletal growth, oral and vaginal candidiasis, and photosensitivity.
- Assess for photosensitivity, which can develop within a few minutes or up to several hours after exposure to sunlight or other ultraviolet (UV) light. Effects may last for 1 to 2 days after discontinuation of drug.
- Be aware that citric acid in tetracycline preparations may accelerate drug deterioration and that using outdated drug may cause Fanconi's syndrome, characterized by multiple defects in renal tubular function. Symptoms include acidosis, bicarbonate wasting, glycosuria, hypokalemia, osteomalacia, and phosphaturia.

PATIENT TEACHING

- Instruct patient to take oral tetracycline at least 1 hour before meals or 2 hours after meals, because dairy products and some foods may interfere with absorption.
- Advise patient to take each dose with a full glass of water while in an upright position to avoid esophageal or GI irritation.
- Advise patient to avoid taking other drugs, including OTC antacids and other preparations, within 3 hours of oral tetracycline.
- Urge patient to complete entire course of tetracycline therapy even if she feels better.
- Caution her to avoid direct sunlight or UV light and to wear sunscreen when outdoors.
- Advise women who use oral contraceptives containing estrogen to use another method

of contraception while taking tetracycline because contraceptives may be less effective. Tell patient to notify prescriber immediately if pregnancy is known or suspected.
- Emphasize the need to discard outdated tetracycline because of the risk of toxic effects.
- Encourage patient to take safety precautions if she experiences dizziness or other adverse CNS reactions.

tezepelumab-ekko
Tezspire

Class and Category

Pharmacologic class: Human monoclonal antibody
Therapeutic class: Antiasthmatic

Indications and Dosages

✴ **As adjunct for severe asthma maintenance*

SUBCUTANEOUS INJECTION

Adults. 210 mg once every 4 wk.

Drug Administration

SUBCUTANEOUS

- Drug is available in a single-dose glass vial or as a single-dose prefilled syringe.
- Remove drug from refrigerator and allow it to reach room temperature prior to administration, which usually takes about 60 minutes. Do not warm in any other way. Never shake vial or syringe. Do not replace in refrigerator once drug has reached room temperature. Use within 30 days after removal from refrigerator.
- Solution should be clear to opalescent, colorless to light yellow. Solution in prefilled syringe may contain small air bubbles, which should not be removed. Discard if solution is cloudy, discolored, or contains large particulate matters. Avoid use if vial or syringe has been dropped or damaged or if the drug has expired.
- If using the single-dose prefilled syringe, do not remove needle cover until ready to administer drug. Also, avoid touching the activation clips prior to administration, in order to avoid premature activation of the needle safety guard. Remove syringe from tray only by grasping syringe body.

T

- Administer by first gently pinching skin and then inject at a 45-degree angle into abdomen (avoid 2 inches or 5 cm around navel area), thigh, or upper arm. Do not inject where the skin is bruised, hard, red, or tender. When injecting, push the plunger all the way until the plunger head is completely between the needle guard activation clips. After injection, maintain pressure on the plunger head and remove needle from skin. Then release pressure to allow needle guard to cover the needle. Do not recap the syringe.
- Document injection site on patient's record as rotation of sites is advised.

Route	Onset	Peak	Duration
SQ	Unknown	3–10 days	Unknown

Half-life: 26 days

Mechanism of Action

Although the exact mechanism of action has not been identified, the drug binds to human thymic stromal lymphopoietin (TSLP) to block its interaction with the heterodimeric TSLP receptor. Because TSLP occupies a position in the asthma inflammatory cascade, blocking TSLP reduces biomarkers and cytokines associated with airway inflammation present in asthma.

Contraindications

Hypersensitivity to tezepelumab-ekkd or its components

Interactions

DRUGS

None reported by manufacturer

Adverse Reactions

EENT: Allergic conjunctivitis, pharyngitis
MS: Arthralgia, back pain
SKIN: Rash
OTHER: Antidrug antibodies, injection-site reactions (pain, redness, swelling)

Childbearing Considerations

PREGNANCY

- Although it is not known if drug can cause fetal harm, placental transfer of monoclonal antibodies is greatest during the third trimester with potential effects on the fetus greatest during this time.
- Use with caution only if benefit to mother outweighs potential risk to fetus.

LACTATION

- It is not known if drug is present in breast milk.
- Patient should check with prescriber before breastfeeding.

Nursing Considerations

- Know that tezepelumab-ekko should never be used to treat acute asthma symptoms or acute exacerbations such as acute bronchospasm or status asthmaticus.
- Be aware that inhaled or systemic corticosteroid therapy should not be abruptly discontinued when tezepelumab-ekko is initiated but should be done gradually to avoid systemic withdrawal symptoms and/or causing conditions previously suppressed by systemic corticosteroid therapy to worsen.
- Expect patients with a preexisting parasitic (helminth) infection to be treated before drug therapy is begun because it is not known if drug will influence a patient's response to parasitic treatment. Know that if patient develops a parasitic infection during tezepelumab-ekko therapy, the drug should be discontinued until the infection is eradicated.

! **WARNING** Monitor patient for hypersensitivity reactions such as allergic conjunctivitis and rash. Be aware that these reactions usually occur within hours of administering tezepelumab-ekko but may occur as a delayed reaction days later. If a reaction occurs, notify prescriber, as drug may have to be discontinued depending on the severity of the reaction.

! **WARNING** Do not administer live attenuated vaccines to patients receiving tezepelumab-ekko because effects are unknown.

PATIENT TEACHING

- Inform patient not to abruptly discontinue prescribed inhaled or systemic corticosteroid therapy when tezepelumab-ekko therapy is begun. Tell patient that prescriber will gradually reduce corticosteroid dosage, if warranted.

! **WARNING** Warn patient never to treat acute asthma symptoms or acute exacerbations such as acute bronchospasm or status asthmaticus with tezepelumab-ekko. Advise patient to notify prescriber if asthma is uncontrolled or worsens.

! **WARNING** Review allergic reactions to drug with patient such as allergic conjunctivitis and rash. Tell patient that a reaction may occur within hours of receiving the drug or days later. If present, tell patient to notify prescriber, as drug may have to be discontinued depending on the severity of the reaction.

- Advise patient to report signs and symptoms of a parasitic infection to prescriber, as additional treatment will be needed and tezepelumab-ekko therapy may have to be temporarily discontinued.
- Stress importance of patient not receiving any live attenuated vaccines while taking tezepelumab-ekko.

tiagabine hydrochloride
Gabitril

Class and Category
Pharmacologic class: Gamma-aminobutyric acid (GABA) reuptake inhibitor
Therapeutic class: Anticonvulsant

Indications and Dosages
✳ *As adjunct to treat partial seizures*

TABLETS
Adults already taking enzyme-inducing antiepileptic drugs. *Initial:* 4 mg daily; increased by 4 to 8 mg/wk until desired response occurs, given in two to four divided doses daily. *Usual:* 32 to 56 mg daily. *Maximum:* 56 mg daily in two to four divided doses.

Children ages 12 to 18 already taking enzyme-inducing antiepileptic drugs. *Initial:* 4 mg daily for 1 wk, then increased to 8 mg, followed a wk later by increases of 4 to 8 mg/wk until desired response occurs and given in two to four divided doses daily. *Maximum:* 32 mg daily in two to four divided doses.

±**DOSAGE ADJUSTMENT** For patients taking only non-enzyme-inducing antiepileptic drugs, dosage reduced and possibly a slower titration schedule required. For patients with impaired hepatic function, dosage individualized and reduced, or interval extended, if needed.

Drug Administration
P.O.
- Administer drug with food.
- If more than one dose is missed, consult prescriber, as retitration of dose may be required.

Route	Onset	Peak	Duration
P.O.	Rapid	45 min	7–9 hr

Half-life: 7–9 hr

Mechanism of Action
Appears to inhibit neuronal and glial uptake of gamma-aminobutyric acid (GABA), the major inhibitory neurotransmitter in the CNS. Tiagabine makes more GABA available in the CNS to open chloride channels in postsynaptic membranes, thereby leading to membrane hyperpolarization and preventing transmission of nerve impulses.

Contraindications
Hypersensitivity to tiagabine or its components

Interactions
DRUGS
benzodiazepines, CNS depressants: Possibly additive CNS depression
carbamazepine, phenobarbital, phenytoin: Possibly decreased tiagabine effectiveness
St. John's wort: Possibly enhanced metabolism of tiagabine

ACTIVITIES
alcohol use: Possibly additive CNS depression

Adverse Reactions
CNS: Amnesia, anxiety, asthenia, ataxia, confusion, depression, dizziness, drowsiness, EEG abnormalities, hostility, impaired cognition, insomnia, light-headedness, paresthesia, **seizures, status epilepticus, suicidal ideation,** tremor, weakness
EENT: Blurred vision, pharyngitis, stomatitis
GI: Abdominal pain, diarrhea, increased appetite, nausea, vomiting
GU: UTI
MS: Dysarthria
SKIN: Bullous dermatitis, ecchymosis, rash

Childbearing Considerations
PREGNANCY
- Pregnancy exposure registry: 1-888-233-2334 or http://www.aedpregnancyregistry.org/.

T

- Drug may cause fetal harm, based on animal studies.
- Use with caution only if benefit to mother outweighs potential risk to fetus.

LACTATION

- It is not known if drug is present in breast milk.
- Patient should check with prescriber before breastfeeding.

Nursing Considerations

! **WARNING** Expect to taper dosage gradually, as prescribed, because stopping drug abruptly may increase seizure frequency.

- Take seizure precautions because tiagabine has caused seizures and status epilepticus in patients with no history of seizures.
- Watch patient closely for evidence of suicidal tendencies, especially when therapy starts or dosage changes, and report concerns at once.

PATIENT TEACHING

- Instruct patient to take drug with food.
- Advise patient to avoid hazardous activities until drug's CNS effects are known. Also urge her to avoid alcohol use.
- Inform patient who takes a CNS depressant that drug may increase depressant effect.
- Instruct patient not to stop taking tiagabine abruptly. Explain that prescriber usually tapers dosage over 4 weeks to reduce the risk of withdrawal seizures.
- Urge caregivers to watch patient closely for evidence of suicidal tendencies, especially when therapy starts or dosage changes, and to report concerns immediately.

ticagrelor
Brilinta

Class and Category
Pharmacologic class: P2Y$_{12}$ platelet inhibitor
Therapeutic class: Antiplatelet

Indications and Dosages
✷ *To reduce the rate of thrombotic cardiovascular events such as cardiovascular death, myocardial infarction, and stroke in patients with acute coronary syndrome (ACS) or history of myocardial infarction; reduce rate*

of stent thrombosis in patients who have been stented for treatment of ACS

TABLETS

Adults. *Initial:* 180 mg as a loading dose followed by 90 mg twice daily for 1 yr, then 60 mg twice daily.

✷ *To treat coronary artery disease in patients with no history of a prior myocardial infarction or stroke*

TABLETS

Adults. 60 mg twice daily.

✷ *To treat acute ischemic stroke or transient ischemic attack*

TABLETS

Adults. *Initial:* 180 mg as a loading dose followed by 90 mg twice daily for 30 days.

Drug Administration
P.O.

- Expect to administer aspirin with ticagrelor therapy.
- Crush tablets and mix with water for patients who are unable to swallow tablets whole. Know that the mixture can also be administered via a nasogastric tube.

Route	Onset	Peak	Duration
P.O.	30 min	1.5 hr	24 hr

Half-life: 7–9 hr

Mechanism of Action
Reversibly interacts with the platelet P2Y$_{12}$ ADP-receptor to prevent platelet activation.

Contraindications
Active pathological bleeding, history of intracranial hemorrhage, hypersensitivity to ticagrelor or its components

Interactions
DRUGS

aspirin (daily doses above 100 mg): Reduced effectiveness of ticagrelor
CYP3A inducers such as carbamazepine, phenobarbital, phenytoin, rifampin: Reduces ticagrelor exposure, decreasing effectiveness
CYP3A inhibitors such as atazanavir, clarithromycin, indinavir, itraconazole, ketoconazole, nefazodone, nelfinavir, ritonavir, saquinavir, voriconazole: Substantially increases ticagrelor exposure and risk of adverse reactions such as bleeding and dyspnea
digoxin: Altered blood digoxin levels

lovastatin, simvastatin: Increased serum levels of these drugs

opioids: Delayed or reduced absorption of ticagrelor

Adverse Reactions

CNS: Dizziness, fatigue, headache, **intracranial bleeding**

CV: Atrial fibrillation, bradycardia including AV block, chest pain, hypertension, **hypotension (may be severe), intracardiac bleed with cardiac tamponade**

EENT: Epistaxis, intraocular bleeding with permanent vision loss

ENDO: Gynecomastia

GI: Diarrhea, nausea

GU: Elevated serum creatinine level

HEME: Minor or **major bleeding, thrombotic thrombocytopenic purpura**

MS: Back or noncardiac chest pain

RESP: Central sleep apnea, Cheyne-Stokes respirations, cough, dyspnea

SKIN: Bruising, rash

Other: Angioedema, elevated uric acid, **hypovolemic shock**

Childbearing Considerations

PREGNANCY

- It is not known if drug can cause fetal harm.
- Use with caution only if benefit to mother outweighs potential risk to fetus.

LACTATION

- It is not known if drug is present in breast milk.
- Breastfeeding is not recommended during drug therapy.

Nursing Considerations

- Be aware that ticagrelor shouldn't be given to patients with active pathological bleeding or who have a history of intracranial hemorrhage. It should also not be started in patients who are undergoing urgent coronary artery bypass graft (CABG) surgery or who have severe hepatic impairment.
- Know that patients with a history of bradycardia-related syncope not protected by a pacemaker, second- or third-degree AV block, or sick sinus syndrome may be at a higher risk of developing bradyarrhythmias with ticagrelor.
- Be aware that maintenance doses of aspirin above 100 mg may decrease effectiveness of ticagrelor and should be limited to 75 to 100 mg daily.

- Monitor patient closely for bleeding tendencies. Know that risk of bleeding increases with ticagrelor use in older patients as well as patients with a history of bleeding disorders or performance of percutaneous invasive procedures. Risk of bleeding also increases with concomitant use of drugs such as anticoagulant and fibrinolytic therapy, chronic use of nonsteroidal anti-inflammatory drugs, and higher doses of aspirin.
- Be prepared to discontinue ticagrelor therapy, as ordered, 5 days before surgery, if possible. However, drug should be restarted as soon as possible after surgery because of increased risk of myocardial infarction, stroke, and even death.
- Be suspicious of bleeding in a patient who becomes hypotensive and has recently undergone coronary angiography, CABG, PCI, or other surgical procedures, even if the patient does not have any signs of bleeding. Notify prescriber immediately if patient becomes hypotensive, and expect to provide supportive care. Be aware that attempts to manage bleeding should be made without discontinuing drug, if possible, because stopping ticagrelor increases risk of subsequent cardiovascular events.
- Monitor patient for dyspnea that may occur with ticagrelor therapy. If dyspnea is determined to be caused by drug, expect to continue therapy, as no specific treatment is needed and often resolves on its own.
- Avoid abrupt interruption of ticagrelor therapy because doing so increases the risk of myocardial infarction, stent thrombosis, and death.
- Be aware that ticagrelor can give false negative functional tests for heparin-induced thrombocytopenia (HIT) or false negative results in platelet functional tests for patients with HIT.

PATIENT TEACHING

- Warn patient not to discontinue ticagrelor therapy abruptly because of increased risk of life-threatening adverse effects.
- Advise patient unable to swallow the tablet whole to crush it and mix with water immediately before taking drug.
- Caution patient to limit maintenance doses of aspirin to no more than 100 mg daily.

T

! **WARNING** Advise patient to seek immediate emergency care if bleeding occurs and is serious. Also, tell patient to notify prescriber if new or unexpected shortness of breath occurs at night, at rest, or when patient is doing any activity. In addition, patient should report irregular breathing patterns such as breathing that speeds up or slows down or patient experiences short pauses in breathing.

- Instruct patient to take bleeding precautions such as avoiding the use of a razor and brushing teeth with a soft-bristled toothbrush.
- Tell patient to alert all prescribers of ticagrelor therapy.
- Advise women of childbearing age that breastfeeding is not recommended during ticagrelor therapy.

tildrakizumab-asmn
Ilumya

Class and Category
Pharmacologic class: Monoclonal antibody
Therapeutic class: Immunomodulator

Indications and Dosages
* *To treat moderate to severe plaque psoriasis in patients who are candidates for systemic therapy or phototherapy*

SUBCUTANEOUS INJECTION
Adults. 100 mg followed by 100 mg in 4 wk and then 100 mg every 12 wk thereafter.

Drug Administration
SUBCUTANEOUS
- Remove drug from refrigerator and let prefilled syringe sit, in the carton with lid closed, at room temperature for 30 minutes.
- Follow instructions on carton to remove syringe correctly, and remove only when ready to inject. Do not pull off needle cover until ready to inject.
- Inspect syringe contents. Solution should appear clear to slightly opalescent, colorless to slightly yellow. Air bubbles may be present, but there is no need to remove them.
- Pull needle cover straight off (do not twist) and discard.

- Inject drug into abdomen, thighs, or upper arm by pushing down the blue plunger until it can go no further. Remove needle from the skin entirely before letting go of the blue plunger. After the blue plunger is released, the safety lock will draw the needle inside the needle guard.
- If a dose is missed, administer the dose as soon as possible and then resume dosing at the regularly scheduled interval.

Route	Onset	Peak	Duration
SubQ	Unknown	6 days	Unknown

Half-life: 23 days

Mechanism of Action
Selectively binds to the p19 subunit of IL-23 and inhibits its interaction with the IL-23 receptor to inhibit the release of proinflammatory chemokines and cytokines, which reduces inflammation.

Contraindications
Hypersensitivity to tildrakizumab-asmn or its components

Interactions
DRUGS
live vaccines: Increased risk of infection from live vaccine

Adverse Reactions
GI: Diarrhea
RESP: Upper respiratory infections
SKIN: Urticaria
Other: **Angioedema**, antibody formation to tildrakizumab-asmn, injection-site reactions (bruising, edema, erythema, hematoma, hemorrhage, inflammation, pain, pruritus, swelling)

Childbearing Considerations
PREGNANCY
- It is not known if drug can cause fetal harm.
- Use with caution only if benefit to mother outweighs potential risk to fetus.

LACTATION
- It is not known if drug is present in breast milk.
- Patient should check with prescriber before breastfeeding.

Nursing Considerations
- Ensure that patient has been evaluated for tuberculosis prior to start of tildrakizumab-asmn therapy. Know that drug should not

be given to patients with active tuberculosis. Know that patients with a past history of active or latent tuberculosis in whom an adequate course of treatment cannot be confirmed may need antituberculosis treatment before tildrakizumab-asmn is given.

- Know that tildrakizumab-asmn should not be given to patient with a serious infection until the infection resolves or is adequately treated.

- Check patient's immunization history to ensure that patient is current on immunizations before tildrakizumab-asmn therapy is begun. Do not administer a live vaccine while patient is taking tildrakizumab-asmn because of risk of infection.

> **! WARNING** Monitor patient for angioedema and urticaria. If present, notify prescriber, expect drug to be discontinued, and provide supportive care, as ordered.

- Monitor patient for infections, especially respiratory infections. If patient develops a serious infection or is not responding to standard treatment for an infection, alert prescriber, as drug may have to be discontinued.

PATIENT TEACHING

- Inform patient that tildrakizumab-asmn will be given by a health professional. Stress importance of keeping appointments for drug administration.

> **! WARNING** Instruct patient to seek immediate medical attention if she experiences any serious allergic reactions after drug has been administered.

- Review signs and symptoms of infection with patient and tell patient to notify prescriber if present.

tinidazole

☰ Class and Category

Pharmacologic class: Nitroimidazole
Therapeutic class: Antiprotozoal

☰ Indications and Dosages

* *To treat trichomoniasis caused by* Trichomonas vaginalis

TABLETS

Adults. 2 g one time.

* *To treat giardiasis caused by* Giardia duodenalis (G. lamblia)

TABLETS

Adults. 2 g one time.
Children age 3 and over. 50 mg/kg (up to 2 g) one time.

* *To treat intestinal amebiasis caused by* Entamoeba histolytica

TABLETS

Adults. 2 g daily for 3 days.

* *To treat amebic liver abscess caused by* E. histolytica

TABLETS

Adults. 2 g daily for 3 to 5 days.
Children age 3 and over. 50 mg/kg (up to 2 g) daily for 3 to 5 days.

* *To treat bacterial vaginosis in non-pregnant women*

TABLETS

Non-pregnant women. 2 g once daily for 2 days. Alternatively, 1 g once daily for 5 days.

± **DOSAGE ADJUSTMENT** For patients receiving hemodialysis, an additional dose equivalent to one-half the dose prescribed should be given after the dialysis treatment on the days dialysis is performed.

☰ Drug Administration

P.O.

- Administer with food to minimize gastric discomfort.
- If patient is unable to swallow tablets, have pharmacist make an oral suspension. Shake bottle well before use. Use a calibrated device to measure dose. Store at room temperature for up to 7 days.

Route	Onset	Peak	Duration
P.O.	Unknown	1–2 hr	Unknown

Half-life: 12–14 hr

☰ Mechanism of Action

Undergoes intracellular chemical reduction during anaerobic metabolism. After tinidazole is reduced, it damages DNA's helical structure and breaks its strands, which inhibits bacterial nucleic acid synthesis and causes cell death.

☰ Contraindications

Breastfeeding, Cockayne syndrome, hypersensitivity to tinidazole or its components, treatment of trichomoniasis during first trimester of pregnancy

Interactions

DRUGS

cholestyramine: Possibly decreased bioavailability of tinidazole

cyclosporine, tacrolimus: Possibly increased serum cyclosporine and tacrolimus levels

CYP3A4 inducers such as fosphenytoin, phenobarbital, rifampin: Possibly accelerated elimination of tinidazole making it less effective

CYP3A4 inhibitors such as cimetidine, ketoconazole: Possibly prolonged half-life and decreased plasma clearance of tinidazole, increasing plasma tinidazole concentrations

disulfiram: Possibly disulfiram-like effects

fluorouracil: Possibly decreased fluorouracil clearance

lithium: Possibly increased serum lithium levels

oral anticoagulants: Possibly increased anticoagulant effect

oxytetracycline: Possibly diminished effect of tinidazole

phenytoin: Possibly prolongation of the half-life and reduction in the clearance of intravenously administered phenytoin; possibly acceleration of tinidazole elimination, reducing its effectiveness

ACTIVITIES

alcohol use: Possibly disulfiram-like effects

Adverse Reactions

CNS: Ataxia, **coma**, confusion, depression, dizziness, drowsiness, fatigue, fever, headache, insomnia, malaise, peripheral neuropathy, **seizures**, vertigo, weakness

CV: Palpitations

EENT: Bitter or metallic taste, dry mouth, excessive salivation, furry tongue, oral candidiasis, pharyngitis, stomatitis, tongue discoloration

GI: Abdominal cramps, anorexia, constipation, diarrhea, epigastric discomfort, flatulence, hepatic abnormalities, indigestion, nausea, thirst, vomiting

GU: Darkened urine, dysuria, increased vaginal discharge, menorrhagia, UTI, vaginal candidiasis or odor, vulvovaginal discomfort

HEME: Leukopenia, **neutropenia, thrombocytopenia**

MS: Arthralgia, arthritis, myalgia, pelvic pain

RESP: **Bronchospasm**, dyspnea, upper respiratory tract infection

SKIN: Diaphoresis, **erythema multiforme**, flushing, pruritus, rash, **Stevens–Johnson syndrome**, urticaria

Other: **Angioedema**

Childbearing Considerations

PREGNANCY

- It is not known if drug can cause fetal harm, although drug crosses placental barrier.
- Use with caution in the second and third trimester only if benefit to mother outweighs potential risk to fetus.

LACTATION

- Drug is present in breast milk.
- Breastfeeding should be interrupted during drug therapy and for 3 days following drug discontinuation.

REPRODUCTION

- Drug may impair fertility in males, based on animal studies.

Nursing Considerations

- Know that tinidazole has the potential to be carcinogenic. Drug should be used only for approved indications and is not for chronic use.
- Use tinidazole cautiously in patients with blood dyscrasias or CNS disease because tinidazole's adverse effects may worsen these disorders. Also use cautiously in patients with hepatic impairment because a chemically related drug has reduced elimination.

! WARNING Monitor patient for hypersensitivity reactions which could be severe, such as angioedema or severe cutaneous reactions. Alert prescriber, if present, and expect to provide supportive care, as ordered.

- Take seizure precautions. If a seizure or other abnormal neurologic symptoms occur, notify prescriber and expect to stop drug.
- Treat a patient diagnosed with trichomoniasis and her sexual partner with the same dose of tinidazole and at the same time, as ordered, because trichomoniasis is a sexually transmitted disease.
- Monitor patient's total WBC count and differential if retreatment with tinidazole is needed, because adverse hematologic reactions may occur with repeated use.

PATIENT TEACHING

- Tell patient to take tinidazole with food to minimize gastric discomfort.
- Advise patient unable to swallow tablets that drug is available as oral suspension made by the pharmacist.
- Advise patient to avoid alcohol while taking tinidazole and for 3 days afterward because alcohol can cause intense flushing.
- Instruct breastfeeding patient not to breastfeed during therapy and for 3 days after taking last dose.

! **WARNING** Alert patient that drug may cause an allergic reaction, including serious skin reactions. Advise patient to notify prescriber, if present, and if serious to seek immediate medical care.

---

tiotropium bromide

Spiriva HandiHaler, Spiriva Respimat

☰ Class and Category

Pharmacologic class: Anticholinergic
Therapeutic class: Bronchodilator

☰ Indications and Dosages

✳ *To provide long-term maintenance treatment of asthma*

ORAL INHALATION (SPIRIVA RESPIMAT)

Adults and children age 6 and over. 2.5 mcg (2 inhalations) once daily. *Maximum:* 2.5 mcg every 24 hr.

✳ *To provide long-term maintenance treatment of bronchospasm associated with COPD, including chronic bronchitis and emphysema; to reduce COPD exacerbations*

ORAL INHALATION (SPIRIVA HANDIHALER)

Adults. 18 mcg (2 inhalations) once daily. *Maximum:* 18 mcg every 24 hr.

ORAL INHALATION (SPIRIVA RESPIMAT)

Adults. 5 mcg (2 inhalations) once daily. *Maximum:* 5 mcg every 24 hr.

☰ Drug Administration

INHALATION

HandiHaler

- Do not expose capsules to air until ready for use.

- To remove a capsule from the blister pack, open the foil only as far as the stop line, to avoid exposing the rest of the capsules in the blister pack to air. Discard capsules if they are inadvertently exposed to air and won't be used immediately.
- Place capsule into the center chamber of inhalation device and then press and release the button on the side of inhalation device to pierce capsule. Then have patient exhale completely, close her lips around the mouthpiece, inhale slowly and deeply, and then hold her breath for as long as is comfortable.
- Do not use device to give any other drug. The tiotropium capsule must be taken only using the device and never swallowed.
- Have patient rinse mouth after each treatment to help minimize throat dryness and irritation.

Respimat

- Insert the cartridge into the inhaler prior to first use. First, press the safety catch while firmly pulling off the clear base, being careful not to touch the piercing element. Write the date to discard by on label (3 months from the date cartridge is being inserted). Insert narrow end of cartridge into the inhaler. Place inhaler on a firm surface and push down firmly until it clicks in place. Then put the clear base back into place and turn the base in the direction of the arrows on the label until it clicks (half a turn).
- Prime the device by first opening the cap until it snaps fully open and then actuating inhaler (pointed toward the ground) until an aerosol cloud is visible; then repeat the process three more times. If inhaler is not used for more than 3 days, inhaler should be actuated once prior to use; if not used for more than 21 days, inhaler should be activated three times prior to use.
- Have patient breathe out slowly and fully and then hand inhaler to patient asking patient to close lips around the mouthpiece without covering the air vents and pointing inhaler toward back of throat. While having patient take a slow, deep breath through the mouth, have patient press the dose-release button and continue to breathe in. Patient should hold breath for 10 seconds or for as long as it is comfortable. Repeat procedure for second puff. Have patient remove

T

inhaler from mouth and then close cap on inhaler.

- Only clean mouthpiece, including the metal part inside mouthpiece, with a damp cloth or tissue at least 1 time each week.
- The Respimat inhaler should not be used to take any other drug.
- Have patient rinse mouth after each treatment to help minimize throat dryness and irritation.

Route	Onset	Peak	Duration
Inhalation	30 min	1–4 hr	>24 hr

Half-life: 25–44 hr

Mechanism of Action

Prevents acetylcholine from attaching to muscarinic receptors on membranes of smooth muscle cells. By blocking acetylcholine's effects in the bronchi and bronchioles, tiotropium relaxes smooth muscles and causes bronchodilation.

Contraindications

Hypersensitivity to tiotropium or its components

Interactions

DRUGS

anticholinergics: Possibly increased anticholinergic effects

Adverse Reactions

CNS: **CVA**, depression, difficulty speaking, dizziness, insomnia, paresthesia
CV: Angina, **atrial fibrillation**, chest pain, hypercholesterolemia, hypertension, palpitations, peripheral edema, **supraventricular tachycardia**, tachycardia
EENT: Application-site irritation (glossitis, mouth ulceration, pharyngolaryngeal pain), blurred vision, cataract, dry mouth, dysphonia, epistaxis, eye pain, glaucoma, glossitis, hoarseness, increased intraocular pressure, laryngitis, oral candidiasis, pharyngitis, rhinitis, sinusitis, stomatitis, throat irritation, visual halos
ENDO: Hyperglycemia
GI: Abdominal pain, constipation, diarrhea, dysphagia, gastroesophageal reflux, indigestion, **intestinal obstruction**, ileus, vomiting
GU: Difficulty urinating, urine retention, UTI
MS: Arthritis, leg or skeletal pain, myalgia

RESP: Cough, **paradoxical bronchospasm**, upper respiratory tract infection
SKIN: Pruritus, rash, urticaria
Other: **Anaphylaxis**, **angioedema**, candidiasis, dehydration, flu-like symptoms, **hypersensitivity reaction (immediate)**, infection

Childbearing Considerations

PREGNANCY

- It is not known if drug can cause fetal harm.
- Use with caution only if benefit to mother outweighs potential risk to fetus.

LACTATION

- It is not known if drug is present in breast milk.
- Patient should check with prescriber before breastfeeding.

Nursing Considerations

- Use tiotropium cautiously in patients with angle-closure glaucoma, benign prostatic hyperplasia, or bladder neck obstruction.

> **! WARNING** Monitor patient closely after giving first dose of tiotropium for immediate hypersensitivity reactions, including anaphylaxis, angioedema, bronchospasm, and skin reactions. If reaction occurs, notify prescriber and expect to stop tiotropium and provide supportive care. Know that patients with a hypersensitivity to atropine should not receive tiotropium, because tiotropium is a derivative of atropine. Also use tiotropium cautiously in patients who have severe hypersensitivity to milk proteins.

- Know that when tiotropium is used for maintenance therapy in patients with asthma, it may take up to 8 weeks to realize maximum benefits.
- Be aware that tiotropium should never be used to relieve acute bronchospasm.
- Monitor patient's renal function, as ordered, especially in patients with moderate to severe renal impairment, because tiotropium is excreted mainly by the kidneys. Monitor patient with renal dysfunction closely for anticholinergic effects.
- Monitor patient's pulmonary function, as ordered, to evaluate the effectiveness of tiotropium.

PATIENT TEACHING

- Caution patient not to use tiotropium to treat acute bronchospasm and that drug should not be used more often than every 24 hours.

- Instruct patient on the proper use of the HandiHaler or Respimat inhalation device.
- Instruct patient to rinse her mouth after each treatment to help minimize throat dryness and irritation.

! **WARNING** Instruct patient to stop using drug and seek immediate emergency care if an acute allergic reaction occurs.

- Advise patient to tell prescriber about decreased response to tiotropium as well as difficulty urinating, eye pain, palpitations, and vision changes.

tipranavir
Aptivus

Class and Category

Pharmacologic class: Protease inhibitor
Therapeutic class: Antiretroviral

Indications and Dosages

* *As adjunct to treat human immunodeficiency virus type 1 (HIV-1) infection in patients who are treatment-experienced and infected with HIV-1 strains resistant to more than one protease inhibitor*

CAPSULES, ORAL SOLUTION

Adults. 500 mg twice daily coadministered with 200 mg of ritonavir twice daily.
Children ages 2 to 18. 14 mg/kg twice daily with 6 mg/kg of ritonavir twice daily. Alternatively, 375 mg/m^2 twice daily coadministered with ritonavir 150 mg/m^2 twice daily. *Maximum:* 500 mg twice daily coadministered with ritonavir 200 mg twice daily.

±**DOSAGE ADJUSTMENT** For children who develop intolerance or toxicity, dosage reduced to 12 mg/kg with 5 mg/kg ritonavir (or 290 mg/m^2 coadministered with 115 mg/ m^2 ritonavir) twice daily, provided their virus is not resistant to multiple protease inhibitors.

Drug Administration

P.O.

- Administer capsules and oral solution without regard to meals.
- Capsules should be swallowed whole and not chewed, crushed, or opened. Unopened

bottles of capsules should be stored in refrigerator; opened bottle can be stored at room temperature but should be discarded after 60 days of opening bottle.

- Use the provided 5-ml plastic oral dispensing syringe calibrated to measure and deliver oral solution dosage. Store oral solution at room temperature. Discard after 60 days of initially opening bottle.
- When coadministering drug with ritonavir, administer drug with or without food if using ritonavir capsules or solution; administer drug with food if using ritonavir tablets.

Route	Onset	Peak	Duration
P.O.	Unknown	3 hr	Unknown

Half-life: 5–5.6 hr

Mechanism of Action

Selectively inhibits the virus-specific processing of specific polyproteins in HIV-1 infected cells to prevent formation of mature virions.

Contraindications

Coadministration with alfuzosin, amiodarone, bepridil, cisapride, dihydroergotamine, ergonovine, ergotamine, flecainide, lurasidone, lovastatin, methylergonovine, midazolam (oral), pimozide, propafenone, quinidine, rifampin, St. John's wort, sildenafil (for treatment of pulmonary arterial hypertension), simvastatin, triazolam; hypersensitivity to tipranavir or its components; moderate to severe hepatic impairment

Interactions

DRUGS

abacavir, amprenavir, didanosine, dolutegravir, etravirine, fosamprenavir, lopinavir, meperidine, methadone, omeprazole, raltegravir, saquinavir, valproic acid, zidovudine: Decreased concentration of these drugs with possible loss of therapeutic effect
atazanavir: Decreased concentration of atazanavir with possible decreased effectiveness and increased tipranavir concentration with possible increased effect and incidence of adverse reactions
atorvastatin, bosentan, colchicine, desipramine, fluticasone, fluoxetine,

itraconazole, ketoconazole, midazolam (parenteral), paroxetine, quetiapine, rifabutin, rilpivirine, rosuvastatin, salmeterol, sertraline, sildenafil, tadalafil, trazodone, vardenafil: Increased concentration of these drugs, with possible increased effect and incidence of adverse reactions

buprenorphine/naloxone, carbamazepine, phenobarbital, phenytoin: Decreased concentration of tipranavir with possible decreased effectiveness

calcium channel blockers, cyclosporine, pioglitazone, repaglinide, sirolimus, tacrolimus: Possibly decreased concentration of these drugs with possible decreased effectiveness, or increased concentrations of these drugs with possible increased effect and incidence of adverse reactions

clarithromycin: Increased concentration of both drugs, with possible increased effects and incidences of adverse reactions

disulfiram, metronidazole: Possible increased disulfiram effect with tipranavir capsules because of alcohol content

enfuvirtide, fluconazole: Increased tipranavir concentration with possible increased effect and incidence of adverse reactions

ethinyl estradiol-containing drugs: Ethinyl estradiol concentrations decreased by as much as 50%, making oral contraceptive use ineffective; increased risk of estrogen deficiency in women taking drug as hormone replacement; increased risk of nonserious rash

warfarin: Possibly change in international normalized ratio (INR), with possible need for dosage change

Adverse Reactions

CNS: Dizziness, fatigue, fever, headache, insomnia, **intracranial hemorrhage**, malaise, peripheral neuropathy, sleep disorder, somnolence

CV: Elevated cholesterol and triglyceride levels

ENDO: Diabetes mellitus, hyperglycemia

GI: Abdominal distention or pain, anorexia, diarrhea, dyspepsia, elevated liver and pancreatic enzymes, flatulence, gastroesophageal reflux disease, **hepatic failure, hepatic steatosis, hepatitis,** hyperbilirubinemia, nausea, **pancreatitis,** vomiting

GU: Renal insufficiency

HEME: Anemia, **leukopenia, neutropenia, thrombocytopenia**

MS: Myalgia, muscle cramp

RESP: Cough, dyspnea

SKIN: Exanthema, photosensitivity, pruritus, rash

Other: Dehydration, facial wasting, flu-like illness, **hypersensitivity reactions,** lipoatrophy, lipodystrophy (acquired), lipohypertrophy, **mitochondrial toxicity,** weight loss

Childbearing Considerations

PREGNANCY

- Pregnancy exposure registry: 1-800-258-4263.
- It is not known if drug can cause fetal harm, although it does cross the placental barrier.
- Use with caution only if benefit to mother outweighs potential risk to fetus.

LACTATION

- It is not known if drug is present in breast milk.
- The Centers for Disease Control and Prevention recommends that HIV-1 infected mothers not breastfeed, to avoid risking postnatal transmission of HIV-1 infection to infants. They also do not recommend breastfeeding because of potential drug-induced adverse reactions in the infant.

REPRODUCTION

- Drug may reduce the effectiveness of estrogen-based oral contraceptives. Women of childbearing age should use an additional or alternative nonhormonal contraception during drug therapy.

Nursing Considerations

- Know that use of tipranavir and ritonavir in treatment-naïve patients is not recommended.
- Be aware that genotypic or phenotypic testing and/or treatment history should guide tipranavir use.
- Use cautiously in patients with a co-infection with hepatitis B or C or who have elevated transaminase levels or mild hepatic impairment, because these patients are at greater risk of experiencing tipranavir's adverse effect on the liver. Expect to have liver function tests done at initiation of therapy and then monitored frequently throughout course of treatment.

Know that with asymptomatic elevations in ALT or AST greater than 10 times the upper normal limit or elevations between 5 and 10 times the upper normal limit, and patient's total bilirubin greater than 2.5 times the upper normal limit, expect drug to be discontinued. Also monitor patient for clinical signs and symptoms of hepatic dysfunction, such as acholic stools, anorexia, fatigue, jaundice, liver tenderness or enlargement, or nausea. Report findings to prescriber.

- Use cautiously in patients who are at risk for increased bleeding or who are receiving drugs known to increase risk of bleeding, because tipranavir may cause intracranial bleeding.

- Use cautiously in patients with a sulfa allergy, because tipranavir contains a sulfonamide moiety and cross-sensitivity between the two types of drugs is unknown.

- Expect patient's cholesterol and triglyceride levels to be checked before tipranavir therapy is begun and periodically throughout therapy, because drug may cause elevated lipid levels that may require treatment.

- Know that pediatric dosage of tipranavir is based on body weight or body surface area and should not exceed the recommended adult dose.

! **WARNING** Monitor patient for rash, which may become severe, though this is uncommon. If severe, notify prescriber, expect drug to be discontinued, and provide supportive care, as prescribed.

- Monitor patient's blood glucose level. Exacerbation of preexisting diabetes or new-onset diabetes mellitus has occurred in patients receiving protease inhibitor therapy such as tipranavir.

- Be aware that immune reconstitution syndrome has occurred in patients treated with combination antiretroviral therapy, including tipranavir. The inflammatory response predisposes susceptible patients to opportunistic infections such as cytomegalovirus, *Mycobacterium avium* infection, *Pneumocystis jiroveci* pneumonia, or tuberculosis. Autoimmune disorders such as Graves' disease, Guillain–Barré syndrome, or polymyositis have also

occurred. Report sudden or unusual adverse reactions to prescriber.

- Monitor patients with hemophilia, especially type A and B, because hemarthrosis and spontaneous skin hematomas have occurred with protease inhibitors.

PATIENT TEACHING

- Tell patient to take tipranavir exactly as prescribed and not to alter dosage without prescriber knowledge. Also instruct patient to swallow capsule whole and not to chew or open capsules. Advise patient to keep unopened container of capsules in refrigerator but that opened container of capsules may be kept at room temperature.

- Advise patient to use the supplied dosing syringe to measure and give oral solution. Tell patient that bottle may be kept at room temperature but to discard after 60 days of opening bottle.

! **WARNING** Instruct patient to report a skin rash, sensitivity to the sun, or other symptoms such as blister formation, fever, generalized itching, joint pain or stiffness, peeling of skin, redness, or throat tightness and seek immediate medical attention. Also, advise patient to seek medical attention immediately if any unexplained or unusual bleeding or other reaction occurs.

- Tell patient prescribed oral solution form not to take supplemental vitamin E greater than a standard multivitamin, as oral solution of tipranavir contains higher amounts of vitamin E.

- Instruct patient to report any signs and symptoms of liver dysfunction, such as fatigue, loss of appetite, malaise, or yellowing of skin or white areas of her eyes.

- Tell patient to inform all prescribers of tipranavir therapy, because of multiple drug interactions associated with this drug. Stress importance of not taking any over-the-counter preparations, including herbals, without consulting prescriber.

- Inform women receiving estrogen-based hormonal contraceptives to use additional or alternative nonhormonal contraceptives during tipranavir therapy.

- Inform mothers that breastfeeding should not be done during tipranavir therapy.

T

tirofiban hydrochloride

Aggrastat

Class and Category

Pharmacologic class: Glycoprotein IIb/IIIa receptor antagonist
Therapeutic class: Antiplatelet

Indications and Dosages

* *To reduce the rate of thrombotic cardiovascular events (combined endpoint of death, myocardial infarction, or refractory ischemia/repeat cardiac procedure) in patients with non-ST elevation acute coronary syndrome (NSTE-ACS)*

I.V. INFUSION

Adults. *Initial bolus:* 25 mcg/kg within 5 minutes and then maintenance dose of 0.15 mcg/kg/min for up to 18 hr.
±**DOSAGE ADJUSTMENT** For patients with creatinine clearance of 60 ml/min or less, maintenance infusion rate reduced to 0.075 mcg/kg/min, for up to 18 hr.

Drug Administration

I.V.

- Don't dilute premixed 500-ml drug supplied in IntraVia containers. To open container, first tear off its dust cover. Plastic may be somewhat opaque because of moisture absorption but the opacity will diminish gradually. Check for leaks by squeezing the inner bag firmly; if leaks are found, discard. Don't use solution unless it's clear and the seal is intact.
- Withdraw bolus dose from the 15-ml premixed bolus vial into a syringe. Alternatively, bolus dose may be administered from the 100-ml premixed vial or from the 100-ml or 250-ml premixed bag. Do not dilute. Administer bolus dose of 25 mcg/kg within 5 minutes using a syringe or I.V. pump. For patient who weighs 167 kg (367 lb) or more, bolus dose should be administered via syringe from the 15-ml premixed bolus vial, to ensure that delivery time does not exceed 5 minutes.
- Immediately follow bolus dose with maintenance infusion from the 100-ml premixed vial, the 100-ml premixed bag,

or the 250-ml premixed bag via an I.V. pump. Infuse at 0.15 mcg/kg/min up to 18 hours. Discard any leftover portion in vial or bag.
- Drug is compatible with the following drugs administered in the same I.V. line: atropine sulfate, dobutamine, dopamine, epinephrine hydrochloride, famotidine, furosemide, heparin, lidocaine, midazolam, morphine sulfate, nitroglycerin, potassium chloride, propranolol hydrochloride.
- *Incompatibilities:* Diazepam or other drugs except those above

Route	Onset	Peak	Duration
I.V.	Immediate	Unknown	4–8 hr

Half-life: 4–8 hr

Mechanism of Action

Binds to glycoprotein IIb/IIIa receptor sites on the surface of activated platelets. Circulating fibrinogen can bind to these receptor sites and link platelets together, forming a clot that eventually blocks a coronary artery. By binding to receptor sites, tirofiban prevents the normal binding of fibrinogen and other factors and inhibits platelet aggregation.

Contraindications

Active internal bleeding, history of bleeding diathesis or thrombocytopenia following prior exposure to tirofiban, hypersensitivity to tirofiban or its components, major surgical procedure or severe physical trauma within the previous month

Interactions

DRUGS

anticoagulants, antiplatelets, fibrinolytics: Increased risk of bleeding

Adverse Reactions

CNS: Chills, dizziness, fever, headache, **intracranial hemorrhage**
CV: Edema, **hemopericardium**, peripheral edema, sinus bradycardia
GI: **Hematemesis**, nausea, **retroperitoneal bleeding**, vomiting
GU: Hematuria, pelvic pain
HEME: **Severe bleeding, thrombocytopenia**
RESP: **Pulmonary hemorrhage**
SKIN: Diaphoresis, rash, urticaria
Other: **Anaphylaxis, hypersensitivity reactions**, infusion-site bleeding

☰ Childbearing Considerations

PREGNANCY

- It is not known if drug can cause fetal harm, although animal studies suggest it does not.
- Myocardial infarction is a medical emergency in pregnancy, which can be fatal to the pregnant woman and fetus if left untreated.
- Use with caution only if benefit to mother outweighs potential risk to fetus.

LACTATION

- It is not known if drug is present in breast milk.
- Patient should check with prescriber before breastfeeding after receiving drug and condition has stabilized.

☰ Nursing Considerations

> **! WARNING** Keep in mind that if patient is also receiving a heparin infusion, expect to monitor APTT before treatment, 6 hours after heparin infusion starts, and regularly thereafter. Expect to adjust heparin dosage to maintain APTT at about two times the control, as ordered. Notify prescriber immediately if patient develops an abnormally high APTT. Also, assess patient for signs and symptoms of abnormal bleeding and report them to prescriber immediately because potentially life-threatening bleeding may occur.

- Know that after cardiac catheterization or percutaneous transluminal coronary angioplasty, keep patient on bed rest with head of bed elevated. Ensure hemostasis of percutaneous site for at least 4 hours before discharge. Minimize invasive procedures, including epidural procedures, to reduce the risk of bleeding.
- Monitor patient's hemoglobin level, hematocrit, and platelet count, as ordered. Expect to discontinue tirofiban if patient's platelet count is less than 90,000/mm^3. Expect to give a platelet transfusion, as prescribed, if platelet count falls below 50,000/mm^3.

PATIENT TEACHING

- Advise patient to immediately report any bleeding, bruising, headache, pain, or swelling during I.V. infusion of tirofiban.

tizanidine hydrochloride
Zanaflex

☰ Class and Category

Pharmacologic class: Alpha$_2$ adrenergic agonist
Therapeutic class: Antispasmodic

☰ Indications and Dosages

✽ *To manage acute and intermittent increases of muscle tone with spasticity*

CAPSULES, TABLETS

Adults. *Initial:* 2 mg every 6 to 8 hr, as needed, for maximum of 3 doses in 24 hr and then increased gradually by 2 to 4 mg/dose after 1 to 4 days, as needed and as prescribed. *Maximum:* 36 mg daily.

±**DOSAGE ADJUSTMENT** For patients with hepatic dysfunction or renal insufficiency, dosage reduced when drug is being titrated upward.

☰ Drug Administration

P.O.

- Administer capsules or tablets consistently at about the same time of day and do not interchange between formulations.
- Administer consistently either with food or without food.

Route	Onset	Peak	Duration
P.O.	Unknown	1–2 hr	3–6 hr

Half-life: 2.5 hr

☰ Mechanism of Action

Reduces spasticity by decreasing the release of excitatory amino acids. This alpha$_2$-adrenergic agonist's action increases presynaptic inhibition of spinal motor neurons, with the greatest effects on polysynaptic pathways.

☰ Contraindications

Hypersensitivity to tizanidine or its components, use with ciprofloxacin or fluvoxamine

☰ Interactions

DRUGS

alpha$_2$-adrenergic agonists: Possibly significant hypotension

T

ciprofloxacin, fluvoxamine: Significantly decreased blood pressure and increased drowsiness and psychomotor impairment
CNS depressants: Increased additive effects such as excess sedation
CYP1A2 inhibitors (such as acyclovir, amiodarone, cimetidine, famotidine, fluoroquinolones other than strong CYP1A2 inhibitors, mexiletine, oral contraceptives, propafenone, ticlopidine, verapamil, zileuton): Possibly increased plasma tizanidine level; increased risk of bradycardia, hypotension, and sedation

ACTIVITIES

alcohol use: Increased adverse effects of tizanidine, additive CNS depression

⬚ Adverse Reactions

CNS: Anxiety, delusions, drowsiness, dyskinesia, fatigue, fever, hallucinations, slurred speech
CV: Orthostatic hypotension
EENT: Dry mouth, pharyngitis, rhinitis
GI: Abdominal pain, anorexia, constipation, diarrhea, dyspepsia, elevated liver enzymes, **hepatic failure, hepatomegaly,** jaundice, nausea, vomiting
GU: Urinary frequency, UTI
MS: Back pain, muscle weakness, myasthenia
SKIN: Diaphoresis, rash, ulceration

⬚ Childbearing Considerations

PREGNANCY

- It is not known if drug can cause fetal harm.
- Use with caution only if benefit to mother outweighs potential risk to fetus.

LACTATION

- It is not known if drug is present in breast milk.
- Patient should check with prescriber before breastfeeding.

⬚ Nursing Considerations

- Be aware that extreme caution is required if tizanidine is prescribed for a patient with hepatic impairment because drug is extensively metabolized in the liver.
- Monitor hepatic and renal function for first 6 months and periodically thereafter.
- Expect prolonged drug use to inhibit saliva.
- Be aware that tizanidine should be stopped slowly to prevent rebound hypertension, tachycardia, and hypertonia as well as withdrawal.

- Do not switch capsules for tablets and vice versa. While both forms are bioequivalent to each other under fasting conditions (more than 3 hours after a meal), they are not under fed conditions (within 30 minutes of meal). These pharmacokinetic differences may result in delayed or more rapid onset of activity and increased adverse reactions, depending on the nature of the switch. Maintain a consistent schedule of drug administered in a fasting or fed state.

PATIENT TEACHING

- Instruct patient to take tizanidine exactly as prescribed and consistently either with or without food and not to switch between capsules and tablets.
- Caution patient not to stop taking tizanidine suddenly, to prevent adverse effects.
- Advise patient to change positions slowly to minimize effects of orthostatic hypotension.
- Urge patient to avoid alcohol during drug therapy because of its additive CNS effects.
- Tell patient to notify dentist or prescriber if dry mouth lasts longer than 2 weeks.
- Instruct patient to inform all pharmacists and prescribers about any drug he starts or stops taking.

tobramycin

Bethkis, Kitabis Pak, Tobi, Tobi Podhaler, Tobramycin

⬚ Class and Category

Pharmacologic class: Aminoglycoside
Therapeutic class: Antibiotic

⬚ Indications and Dosages

✱ *To treat serious bacterial infections caused by susceptible strains of microorganisms as follows: bone, skin, and skin structure infections caused by* Enterobacter *species,* Escherichia coli, Pseudomonas aeruginosa, Proteus *species, or* Staphylococcus aureus; *central nervous system infections (meningitis) caused by susceptible organisms; complicated and recurrent urinary tract infections caused by* Citrobacter *species,* Enterobacter *species,* E. coli, Klebsiella *species,* Proteus *species,* Providencia, P. aeruginosa, Serratia *species, or* S. aureus; *intra-abdominal infections (including peritonitis) caused by* Enterobacter *species,* E. coli, *or* Klebsiella *species; lower*

respiratory tract infections caused by
Enterobacter *species*, E. coli, Klebsiella
species, P. aeruginosa, Serratia *species, or*
S. aureus; *septicemia caused by* E. coli,
Klebsiella *species, or* P. aeruginosa

I.V. INFUSION, I.M. INJECTION (TOBRAMYCIN)

Adults with serious infection. 1 mg/kg every
8 hr.
Adults with life-threatening infections.
5 mg/kg daily in three to four divided doses,
reduced as soon as clinically appropriate to
3 mg/kg daily divided into 3 equal doses and
given every 8 hr.
Children and neonates over age 7 days.
2 to 2.5 mg/kg every 8 hr or 1.5 mg/kg
every 6 hr.
**Premature or full term neonates age 7 days
or less.** Up to 2 mg/kg every 12 hr.
✳ *To treat pulmonary infection caused by*
P. aeruginosa *in patients with cystic fibrosis*

I.M. INJECTION, I.V. INFUSION (TOBRAMYCIN)

Adults and children. 2.5 mg/kg every 6 hr;
dosage adjusted to achieve peak blood drug
level of 8 to 12 mcg/ml and trough blood
drug level below 2 mcg/ml.

INHALATION (BETHKIS, KITABIS PAK, TOBI)

Adults and children age 6 and older. 1
ampule (300 mg) twice daily 12 hours apart
in alternating periods of 28 days on and
28 days off.

INHALATION (TOBI PODHALER)

Adults and children age 6 years and over.
Four 28-mg capsules inhaled using Podhaler
every 12 hr in alternating periods of 28 days
on and 28 days off.
±**DOSAGE ADJUSTMENT** For patients with
renal impairment, dosage possibly reduced or
dosage interval increased. For obese patients
receiving drug parenterally, dosage calculated
by using the patient's estimated lean body
weight plus 40% of the excess as the basic
weight on which to figure mg/kg.

≡ Drug Administration

I.V.

- Dilute drug by adding 50 to 100 ml of 0.9%
  Sodium Chloride Injection or 5% Dextrose
  Injection for adults and a lesser amount for
  children.

- Infuse over 20 to 60 minutes. Do not infuse
  for less than 20 minutes because peak serum
  concentrations may exceed 12 mcg/ml.
- Flush I.V. line with 0.9% Sodium Chloride
  Injection or 5% Dextrose Injection after
  drug is administered.
- *Incompatibilities:* Other drugs

I.M.

- Withdraw dose directly from drug vial.
- Rotate sites.

INHALATION

- Administer dosages as close to 12 hours
  apart as possible. Do not administer less
  than 6 hours apart.
- Administer last, if other inhaled
  medications are being administered.
- Inhalation capsules should never be
  administered orally.
- Capsules for inhalation should be stored in
  the blister pack and each capsule removed
  immediately before use.
- Always administer capsules with Podhaler
  device. Use a new Tobi Podhaler device
  every 7 days.
- Don't expose ampules for inhalation
  solution to intense light. Refrigerate them or
  store at room temperature for up to 28 days.
- Do not use inhalation solution if it is cloudy.
- Have patient sit up or stand up and breathe
  normally through the mouthpiece of the
  nebulizer to deliver the inhalation solution.
  Nose clips may help patient breathe through
  the mouth.
- Administer nebulizer solution over 15
  minutes or until sputtering from the output
  of the nebulizer has occurred for at least
  one minute using the handheld Pari LC
  Plus reusable nebulizer with Pari Vios air
  compressor.
- Never dilute nebulizer solution or mix it
  with dornase alfa or other medication in the
  nebulizer.

Route	Onset	Peak	Duration
I.V.	Immediate	30 min	8 hr
I.M.	Unknown	30–60 min	8 hr
Inhalation	Unknown	60 min	Unknown

Half-life: 2–4 hr

≡ Mechanism of Action

Inhibits bacterial protein synthesis
by binding irreversibly to one of two

aminoglycoside-binding sites on the 30S ribosomal subunit, resulting in bacteriostatic effects. Bactericidal effects may stem from tobramycin's ability to accumulate within cells so that the intracellular drug level exceeds the extracellular level.

Contraindications

Hypersensitivity to tobramycin, other aminoglycosides, or their components

Interactions

DRUGS

diuretics: Increased risk of aminoglycoside toxicity

general anesthetics, neuromuscular blockers: Possibly increased neuromuscular blockade

other drugs with nephrotoxic, neurotoxic, or ototoxic potential including systemic aminoglycosides: Increased risk of nephrotoxicity, neurotoxicity, and ototoxicity

Adverse Reactions

CNS: Confusion, dizziness, headache, inability to speak, lethargy, malaise, **neurotoxicity**, vertigo

EENT: Hearing loss, laryngitis, oropharyngeal pain, ototoxicity, taste perversion, tinnitus, voice alteration

GI: Anorexia, *Clostridium difficile–associated diarrhea*, diarrhea, elevated liver enzymes, nausea, vomiting

GU: Elevated BUN and serum creatinine levels, **nephrotoxicity**, oliguria, proteinuria, **renal failure**

HEME: Anemia, leukocytosis, **leukopenia**, **neutropenia, thrombocytopenia**

MS: Myalgia

RESP: Bronchospasm, discolored sputum, wheezing

SKIN: Exfoliative dermatitis, pruritus, rash, urticaria

Other: Hypersensitivity reactions, hypocalcemia, hypokalemia, hypomagnesemia, hyponatremia, injection-site pain

Childbearing Considerations

PREGNANCY

- It is not known if drug can cause fetal harm. However, other aminoglycosides have caused fetal harm such as irreversible bilateral congenital deafness.
- Use with caution only if benefit to mother outweighs potential risk to fetus.

LACTATION

- Drug may be present in breast milk.
- A decision should be made to discontinue breastfeeding or the drug to avoid potential serious adverse reactions in the breastfed infant when administering parenteral form of drug.
- Patient should check with prescriber about breastfeeding if inhaled form is taken.
- If breastfeeding occurs with inhaled form, mother should monitor infant for bloody or loose stools and candidiasis (diaper rash, thrush).

Nursing Considerations

- Use cautiously in patients with muscular disorders because tobramycin may aggravate muscle weakness. High-risk patients include those with myasthenia gravis or Parkinson's disease. Also be aware that prolonged respiratory paralysis may occur in patients receiving concomitant neuromuscular blocking agents.
- Obtain fluid and tissue samples for culture and sensitivity testing before and during tobramycin therapy, as ordered. Review results, if available, before therapy starts.
- Expect the serum concentration of tobramycin to be monitored only through venipuncture, as a finger-stick sample may lead to falsely increased measurements of serum levels of the drug, which cannot be completely avoided with handwashing before testing is done.
- Keep in mind that because drug can cause bilateral and irreversible hearing loss, assess for early signs of cochlear and vestibular ototoxicity, including ataxia, dizziness, high-frequency hearing loss, tinnitus, and vertigo. If present, expect an audiogram to be ordered. Drug may have to be discontinued.
- Monitor patient for bronchospasms and wheezing. Notify prescriber immediately if present and be prepared to treat, as prescribed.
- Monitor serum calcium, magnesium, potassium, and sodium levels to detect electrolyte imbalances.

! **WARNING** Be alert for allergic reactions, including anaphylaxis.

- Watch for signs of nephrotoxicity, such as elevated BUN and serum creatinine levels. Be aware that patients with renal dysfunction or who are taking nephrotoxic drugs should have measurements of serum concentrations of tobramycin and renal function done as ordered by prescriber. If nephrotoxicity occurs, drug may have to be discontinued.

- Expect dehydration to increase the risk of nephrotoxicity.
- Monitor patient closely for diarrhea, which may indicate pseudomembranous colitis caused by *C. difficile*. If diarrhea occurs, notify prescriber, expect to withhold tobramycin, and treat with electrolytes, fluids, protein, and an antibiotic effective against *C. difficile*.
- Monitor patients receiving concomitant inhaled and parenteral form of aminoglycoside therapy for toxicities. Obtain regular serum tobramycin levels, as ordered.

PATIENT TEACHING

- Instruct patient on how to administer drug by inhalation. For inhaled tobramycin using ampules, instruct patient to inhale over 15 minutes, using a handheld nebulizer with a compressor. For inhaled tobramycin using capsules, instruct patient always to store capsules in the blister, not to remove capsules until immediately before use, and to use only with the Podhaler.
- Teach patient how to use nebulizer while sitting or standing upright and to breathe normally through its mouthpiece. Nose clips may help patient breathe through her mouth.

! WARNING Alert patient that drug may cause an allergic reaction. If present, tell patient to notify prescriber or if serious to seek immediate emergency care.

- Advise patient to notify prescriber if shortness of breath or wheezing occurs after administration of tobramycin inhalation solution.
- Urge patient to immediately report high-frequency hearing loss and vertigo.
- Instruct female patient to notify prescriber immediately about known or suspected pregnancy.
- Advise mothers who are breastfeeding to monitor their infants for bloody or loose stools and for diaper rash or thrush.

- Urge patient to tell prescriber about diarrhea that's severe or lasts longer than 3 days. Remind patient that watery or bloody stools may occur 2 or more months after antibiotic therapy and may be serious, requiring prompt treatment.
- Remind patient to alert all prescribers about tobramycin therapy, because drug interacts with many other drugs.

tocilizumab
Actemra

Class and Category
Pharmacologic class: Monoclonal antibody (interleukin-6 receptor inhibitor)
Therapeutic class: Antiarthritic (disease-modifying antirheumatic drug [DMARD])

Indications and Dosages
* *To treat moderate to severe active rheumatoid arthritis as monotherapy in patients who have had an inadequate response to one or more disease-modifying antirheumatic drugs (DMARDs) or as adjunct with methotrexate or other nonbiologic DMARDs*

I.V. INFUSION
Adults. 4 mg/kg every 4 wk, increased, as needed, to 8 mg/kg every 4 wk. *Maximum:* 800 mg per infusion.

SUBCUTANEOUS INJECTION
Adults weighing 100 kg (220 lb) or more. 162 mg every wk.
Adults weighing less than 100 kg (220 lb). 162 mg every other wk, followed by increased dosage frequency to every wk, as needed.
* *To treat active systemic juvenile idiopathic arthritis as monotherapy or as adjunct with methotrexate*

I.V. INFUSION
Children age 2 and over weighing 30 kg (66 lb) or more. 8 mg/kg every 2 wk.
Children age 2 and over weighing less than 30 kg (66 lb). 12 mg/kg every 2 wk.

SUBCUTANEOUS INJECTION
Children age 2 and over weighing 30 kg (66 lb) or more. 162 mg once every wk.
Children age 2 and over weighing less than 30 kg (66 lb). 162 mg every 2 wk.
* *To treat active polyarticular juvenile idiopathic arthritis*

I.V. INFUSION

Children age 2 and over weighing 30 kg (66 lb) or more. 8 mg/kg every 4 wk.

Children age 2 and over weighing less than 30 kg (66 lb). 10 mg/kg every 4 wk.

SUBCUTANEOUS INJECTION

Children age 2 and over weighing 30 kg (66 lb) or more. 162 mg once every 2 wk.

Children age 2 and over weighing less than 30 kg (66 lb). 162 mg once every 3 wk.

✳ *To treat giant cell arteritis*

I.V. INFUSION

Adults. 6 mg/kg every 4 wks in combination with a tapering course of glucocorticoids. *Maximum:* 600 mg per infusion.

SUBCUTANEOUS INJECTION

Adults. 162 mg once wk in combination with a tapering course of glucocorticoids. Alternatively, 162 mg once every other wk in combination with a tapering course of glucocorticoids.

✳ *To treat chimeric antigen receptor T-cell-induced severe or life-threatening cytokine release syndrome*

I.V. INFUSION

Adults and children age 2 and over weighing 30 kg (66 lb) or more. 8 mg/kg with up to 3 more doses administered with at least 8 hours between doses, if needed. *Maximum:* 800 mg per infusion.

Adults and children age 2 and over weighing less than 30 kg (66 lb). 12 mg/kg with up to 3 more doses administered at least 8 hr between doses, if needed. *Maximum:* 800 mg per infusion.

✳ **To treat systemic sclerosis–associated interstitial lung disease (SSc-ILD)*

SUBCUTANEOUS INJECTION

Adults. 162 mg once a wk.

± **DOSAGE ADJUSTMENT** Dosage reduction or interruption of dosing may be needed to manage dose-related laboratory abnormalities, including elevated liver enzymes, neutropenia, and thrombocytopenia. See manufacturer guidelines for specific recommendations for dosage adjustments.

▤ Drug Administration

I.V.

- Dilute using either a 100-ml infusion bag or bottle for patients weighing 30 kg or more or a 50-ml infusion bag or bottle for patients weighing less than 30 kg. Diluents to use include 0.45 % or 0.9% Sodium Chloride Injection.
- From the infusion bag, withdraw volume of solution equal to the volume of tocilizumab solution that will be added to infusion bag.
- Slowly add drug from each vial into infusion bag or bottle and gently invert bag to mix while avoiding foaming.
- Discard any unused drug left in vials.
- Once fully diluted with 0.9% Sodium Chloride Injection, solution may be refrigerated or stored at room temperature for up to 24 hours. Once fully diluted with 0.45% Sodium Chloride Injection, solution may be refrigerated for up to 24 hours or stored at room temperature for up to 4 hours. Protect from light.
- If stored in refrigerator, allow solution to reach room temperature prior to infusion.
- Infuse drug with an infusion set, and never give as I.V. push or a bolus.
- Infuse over one hour.
- Drug is compatible with polypropylene, polyethylene, and polyvinyl chloride infusion bags and polypropylene, polyethylene, and glass infusion bottles.
- *Incompatibilities:* Other drugs

SUBCUTANEOUS

- When transitioning from intravenous therapy to subcutaneous therapy, the first subcutaneous dose should be given instead of next scheduled intravenous dose.
- Administer using the prefilled ACTPen autoinjector or prefilled syringe. However, do not use the autoinjector for treatment of SSc-ILD.
- Inspect solution; do not use if cloudy, discolored, or containing particulate matter.
- Inject only in healthy skin areas; do not give into areas where skin is bruised, hard, red, tender or not intact. Also, do not inject into moles or scars.
- Rotate sites.

Route	Onset	Peak	Duration
I.V.	Unknown	Unknown	Unknown
SubQ	Unknown	3–4.5 days	Unknown

Half-life: 5–13 days

▤ Mechanism of Action

Binds to interleukin 6 (IL-6) receptors to interrupt signaling through them. IL-6 is a proinflammatory cytokine produced by various cells, such as B- and T-cells, fibroblasts, lymphocytes, and monocytes. It is also produced by endothelial and synovial cells, leading to local production of IL-6 in joints affected by inflammatory processes such as polyarticular juvenile idiopathic arthritis, rheumatoid arthritis, and systemic juvenile idiopathic arthritis. Binding of IL-6 receptors prevents inflammation-related signals from being relayed, which reduces inflammatory response and relieves signs and symptoms of inflammatory-related arthritis, giant cell arteritis, and cytokine release syndrome.

Contraindications

Absolute neutrophil count below 2,000/mm³, hypersensitivity to tocilizumab or its components, liver enzymes (ALT or AST) above 1.5 times upper limit of normal, platelet count below 100,000/mm³

Interactions

DRUGS

atorvastatin; cytochrome P-450 substrates with a narrow therapeutic index such as cyclosporine, theophylline, warfarin; CYP3A4 substrates such as lovastatin, oral contraceptives, simvastatin; omeprazole: Possibly decreased plasma levels of these drugs with decreased effectiveness
live vaccines: Increased risk of adverse vaccine effects

Adverse Reactions

CNS: Demyelinating disorders, dizziness, headache
CV: Elevated lipid levels, hypertension
EENT: Nasopharyngitis, oral ulceration
GI: Diverticulitis, elevated liver enzymes, gastritis, gastroenteritis, hepatic impairment, **hepatic failure, hepatitis, hepatotoxicity,** jaundice, **pancreatitis, perforation,** upper abdominal pain
GU: UTI
HEME: Neutropenia, thrombocytopenia
MS: Bacterial arthritis
RESP: Bronchitis, pneumonia, upper respiratory tract infection
SKIN: Cellulitis, generalized erythema, pruritus, rash, **Stevens–Johnson syndrome,** urticaria
Other: Anaphylaxis, anti-tocilizumab antibodies, herpes zoster, **immunosuppression,** infections including activation of latent infections, injection-site reactions (erythema, pain, pruritus, swelling), **malignancies, sepsis,** tuberculosis with pulmonary or extrapulmonary disease

Childbearing Considerations

PREGNANCY

- Pregnancy exposure registry: 1-877-311-8972.
- It is not known if drug causes fetal harm. However, drug is increasingly transported across the placental barrier as pregnancy progresses, with the largest amount occurring during the third trimester, which may adversely fetal immune system.
- Use with caution only if benefit to mother outweighs potential risk to fetus, because infants exposed to drug in utero may be at risk for adverse reactions or limited effectiveness when administered live or live attenuated vaccines.

LACTATION

- It is not known if drug is present in breast milk.
- Patient should check with prescriber before breastfeeding.

Nursing Considerations

- Know that tocilizumab isn't recommended for patients with active liver disease or impairment because drug may adversely affect liver function.
- Make sure patient has a tuberculin skin test before therapy starts. If skin test is positive, tuberculosis treatment will have to be started before tocilizumab therapy can begin. Even patients who have tested negative for tuberculosis may develop tuberculosis during therapy. Monitor patient for low-grade fever, persistent cough, and wasting or weight loss; report such findings to prescriber.

! **WARNING** Know that if patient has evidence of an active infection when drug is prescribed, therapy shouldn't start until infection has been treated. Monitor all patients for infections, including invasive fungal infections such as aspergillosis, candidiasis, or pneumocystis; or bacterial, mycobacterial, protozoal, or viral opportunistic infections during and after therapy, especially patients who are taking immunosuppressants. If a serious infection develops, expect prescriber to interrupt drug therapy until infection is controlled.

T

- Obtain a baseline of patient's absolute neutrophil count, liver enzymes, and platelet count before starting tocilizumab therapy, as ordered. Therapy shouldn't begin if patient's absolute neutrophil count is below 2,000/mm^3, ALT or AST level is above 1.5 times the upper limit of normal, or platelet count is below 100,000/mm^3. Monitor these values, as ordered, every 4 to 8 weeks for the first 6 months after drug is initiated and then every 3 months after that, and report abnormalities. Dosage adjustment may be required or drug may have to be discontinued if abnormalities occur. For example, drug should be discontinued if absolute neutrophil count drops below 500 per mm^3.
- Assess patient's lipid parameters about 4 to 8 weeks after drug therapy is begun, because tocilizumab can cause increases in patient's lipid profile. If elevated, expect patient to be managed per clinical guidelines.
- Use tocilizumab cautiously in patients with recurrent infection or increased risk of infection, patients who live in regions where histoplasmosis and tuberculosis are endemic, and patients with a history of CNS demyelinating disorders because they may occur, although rarely, during tocilizumab therapy.

! **WARNING** Stop tocilizumab immediately and notify prescriber if patient has an allergic reaction. Provide supportive care, as needed.

! **WARNING** Know that serious cases of hepatic injury have occurred with tocilizumab therapy, some of which resulted in need for liver transplant or death. Monitor patient's liver enzymes, as ordered, and patient for signs of dysfunction such as abdominal discomfort (upper right), anorexia, dark urine, fatigue, or jaundice. Know that dosage may have to be reduced or drug withheld or discontinued depending on the specific liver enzyme abnormalities present. For example, if liver enzymes are persistently greater than 1 to 3 x upper normal limits, intravenous dosage reduced to 4 mg/kg or drug held until ALT or AST have normalized; subcutaneous dosage frequency increased to every other week or dosage held until ALT or AST have normalized. If values are greater than 3 to 5 x upper normal limits, dosage held until values are less than 3 x the upper normal limits and then recommendations followed until values are less than 1 x the upper normal limits. If values are persistently greater than 3 x the upper normal limits or greater than 5 x upper normal limits, expect drug to be discontinued.

PATIENT TEACHING

- Instruct patient or caregiver on how to administer drug subcutaneously, if prescribed. Tell patient to inspect solution, which should be clear and colorless to pale yellow. If not, prefilled syringe should be discarded. Remind patient or caregiver to rotate sites and never give injection into moles, scars, or areas where the skin is bruised, hard, not intact, red, or tender. Tell how to dispose of syringe properly and to keep syringes, including those discarded, out of reach of children and pets.

! **WARNING** Review the signs and symptoms of an allergic reaction (difficulty breathing, rash, swollen face), and tell patient to seek emergency care immediately if these occur.

- Stress importance of compliance with laboratory tests ordered to monitor for adverse reactions.
- Inform patient that infections, including activation of latent infections such as tuberculosis, may occur during tocilizumab therapy. Instruct him to report persistent, severe, or unusual signs and symptoms to prescriber.

! **WARNING** Instruct patient to contact a healthcare provider immediately about persistent, severe abdominal pain because it could reflect GI perforation. Also, report accompanying loss of appetite, fatigue, dark urine, or yellow skin because this could indicate a liver problem.

- Advise patient to avoid people with infections and to have all prescribed laboratory tests performed.
- Inform patient that risk of developing a malignancy is higher in patients taking tocilizumab, but it is still rare. Emphasize importance of follow-up visits and reporting any sudden or unusual signs or symptoms.

- Caution against receiving live-virus vaccines while taking tocilizumab.
- Advise patient to inform all healthcare providers about tocilizumab use and to inform prescriber about any OTC medications being taken, including herbal remedies and mineral and vitamin supplements.
- Urge woman who becomes pregnant while receiving tocilizumab to contact prescriber.
- Inform women to alert pediatrician of tocilizumab use during pregnancy before live or live attenuated vaccines are given to the infant.
- Stress importance of complying with ordered blood tests during drug therapy.

tofacitinib citrate
Xeljanz, Xeljanz XR

Class and Category
Pharmacologic class: Janus kinase inhibitor
Therapeutic class: Antirheumatic (disease-modifying antirheumatic drug [DMARD])

Indications and Dosages
⁕ *To treat moderate to severe active rheumatoid arthritis as monotherapy in patients who have had an inadequate response or intolerance to methotrexate; or as adjunct to methotrexate or other nonbiologic disease-modifying antirheumatic drugs (DMARDs); to treat psoriatic arthritis in patients who have had an inadequate response or intolerance to methotrexate or other DMARDs; to treat active ankylosing spondylitis in patients who have had an inadequate response or intolerance to one or more tumor necrosis factor (TNF) blockers*

TABLETS
Adults. 5 mg twice daily.

E.R. TABLETS
Adults. 11 mg once daily.

±**DOSAGE ADJUSTMENT** For patients with moderate hepatic impairment or moderate or severe renal insufficiency, or patients taking concomitant CYP3A4 inhibitors such as ketoconazole, or concomitant use with one or more drugs that result in both potent inhibition of CYP2C19 such as fluconazole and moderate inhibition of CYP3A4, dosage of either immediate-release or extended-release tablets reduced to 5 mg once daily.

⁕ *To treat moderate to severe active ulcerative colitis in patients who have had an inadequate response or who are intolerant to TNF blockers*

TABLETS
Adults. *Initial:* 10 mg twice daily for 8 wk followed by 10 mg twice daily for another 8 wk, depending on therapeutic response. *Maintenance:* 5 mg twice daily, increased to 10 mg twice daily, if loss of response occurs, for shortest duration possible before returning to 5 mg twice daily.

E.R. TABLETS
Adults. *Initial:* 22 mg once daily for 8 wk followed by 22 mg once daily for another 8 wk, depending on therapeutic response. *Maintenance:* 11 mg once daily, increased to 22 mg once daily, if needed, for shortest duration possible before returning to 11 mg once daily.

±**DOSAGE ADJUSTMENT** *For immediate-release tablets:* For patients taking a strong CYP3A4 inhibitor such as ketoconazole or a moderate CYP3A4 inhibitor with a strong CYP2C19 inhibitor such as fluconazole and for patients with moderate hepatic impairment or moderate to severe renal impairment, dosage reduced to 5 mg twice daily if patient was taking 10 mg twice daily, and dosage reduced to 5 mg once daily if patient was taking 5 mg twice daily. For patients with an absolute neutrophil count (ANC) between 500 and 1,000 cells/mm^3, dosage reduced to 5 mg twice daily if patient was taking 10 mg twice daily and dosage increased back to 10 mg twice daily when ANC is greater than 1,000. For patients with a hemoglobin less than 8 g/dl or for patient who experiences a decrease of more than 2 g/dl, drug therapy interrupted until hemoglobin values have normalized. For patients who experience an ANC or lymphocyte count less than 500 cells/mm^3, drug discontinued. For patients who are 50 years or older with at least one cardiovascular risk factor, limited to once-daily dosing. *For extended-release tablets:* For patients taking a strong CYP3A4 inhibitor such as ketoconazole or a moderate CYP3A4 inhibitor with a strong CYP2C19 inhibitor such as fluconazole and for patients with moderate hepatic impairment or moderate to severe renal impairment, dosage reduced to 11 mg once daily if patient was taking 22 mg once daily, and dosage reduced to 5 mg

T

once daily if patient was taking 11 mg once daily. For patients with an ANC between 500 and 1,000 cells/mm^3, dosage reduced to 11 mg once daily if patient was taking 22 mg once daily and dosage increased back to 22 mg once daily when ANC is greater than 1,000. For patient taking 11 mg once daily, dosing interrupted and then resumed at 11 mg once daily when ANC is greater than 1,000. For patients with a hemoglobin less than 8 g/dl or for patient who experiences a decrease of more than 2 g/dl, drug therapy interrupted until hemoglobin values have normalized. For patients who experience an ANC or lymphocyte count less than 500 cells/mm^3, drug discontinued. For patients who have at least one cardiovascular risk factor, dosage limited to once daily.

✳ *To treat polyarticular juvenile idiopathic arthritis*

ORAL SOLUTION, TABLETS

Children age 2 and older weighing 40 kg (88 lb) or more. 5 mg twice daily.
Children age 2 and older weighing 20 kg (44 lb) to less than 40 kg (88 lb). 4 mg twice daily.
Children age 2 and older weighing 10 kg (22 lb) to less than 20 kg (44 lb). 3.2 mg (3.2 ml) twice daily.

±**DOSAGE ADJUSTMENT** For patients with moderate to severe renal impairment, moderate hepatic impairment, or who are receiving strong CYPA4 inhibitors such as ketoconazole or a moderate CYP3A4 inhibitor with a strong CYP2C19 inhibitor such as fluconazole, dosage interval reduced to once daily. For patients with a hemoglobin less than 8 g/dl or for patient who experiences a decrease of more than 2 g/dl, drug therapy interrupted until hemoglobin values have normalized. For patients with an ANC between 500 and 1,000 cells/mm^3, dosage interrupted until ANC is greater than 1,000 cells/mm^3 or discontinued if ANC becomes less than 500 cells/mm^3. For patients with confirmed lymphocyte count less than 500 cells/mm^3, dosing discontinued.

▤ Drug Administration

P.O.
- Tablets and oral solution are interchangeable but not with extended-release tablet form.

- For patients undergoing hemodialysis, administer drug after the dialysis session on dialysis days. If drug was taken before dialysis procedure, do not administer a supplemental dose after dialysis.
- Administer oral solution using the included press-in bottle adapter and oral dosing syringe. Push down on cap to remove. Do not shake. Insert press-in bottle adapter for first time use only. After removing air from dosing syringe, insert syringe tip into upright bottle through the opening of the press-in bottle adapter until it is firmly in place. Turn bottle upside down, withdraw dose. If bubbles appear in syringe, fully push plunger in so solution flows back into bottle and withdraw again. Turn bottle upright and place on flat surface. Remove syringe by pulling straight up on the oral dosing syringe barrel. Administer by placing the tip of the syringe into the inside of patient's cheek. Slowly push plunger all the way down. Make sure patient swallows the oral solution. Rinse plunger and barrel after use and allow to air-dry.
- Extended-release tablets should be swallowed whole and not broken, chewed, or crushed.

Route	Onset	Peak	Duration
P.O.	Unknown	0.5–1 hr	Unknown
P.O./E.R.	Unknown	4 hr	Unknown

Half-life: 3–6 hr

▤ Mechanism of Action

Modulates the signaling pathway by inhibiting the enzyme, Janus kinase (JAK). JAK is an intracellular enzyme which transmits signals arising from cytokine or growth factor–receptor interactions on the cellular membrane to influence cellular processes of hematopoiesis and immune cell function. Inhibiting the phosphorylation and activation of Signal Transducers and Activator of Transcription (STATs) needed to influence cellular processes lessens some of the signs and symptoms of conditions being treated.

▤ Contraindications

Hypersensitivity to tofacitinib or its components

Interactions

DRUGS

CYP3A4 potent inducers such as rifampin: Possibly loss or reduced effectiveness of tofacitinib

CYP3A4 potent inhibitors such as ketoconazole, moderate CYP3A4 inhibitors/ potent CYP2C19 inhibitors such as fluconazole: Increased tofacitinib exposure and adverse reactions

immunosuppressive drugs such as azathioprine, cyclosporine, tacrolimus: Potentiated immunosuppression

live vaccines: Increased risk of infection

Adverse Reactions

CNS: CVA, fatigue, fever, headache, insomnia, paresthesia

CV: Elevated lipid levels, hypertension, **MI**, peripheral edema, **thrombosis (arterial or deep vein thrombosis)**

EENT: Esophageal candidiasis, nasopharyngitis, sinus congestion

GI: Abdominal pain, diarrhea, diverticulitis, dyspepsia, elevated liver enzymes, gastritis, hepatic steatosis, liver injury, nausea, vomiting

GU: Elevated serum creatinine levels, UTI

HEME: Anemia, **lymphopenia, neutropenia**

MS: Arthralgia, elevated creatine phosphokinase, joint swelling, musculoskeletal pain, tendinitis

RESP: Cough, dyspnea, **interstitial lung disease**, pneumonia, **pneumocystosis, pulmonary embolism**, upper respiratory infection

SKIN: Cellulitis, erythema, **melanoma**, multidermatomal herpes zoster, **nonmelanoma skin cancers**, rash, pruritus

Other: Bacteria, mycobacterial, invasive fungal, viral or other opportunistic infections such as tuberculosis and other BK viral, cytomegalovirus, cryptococcus, or mycobacterial infections; dehydration; herpes zoster; **lymphoproliferative disorder; malignancies such as breast, colorectal, gastric, lung, lymphoma, malignant melanoma, prostate, and renal cell**

Childbearing Considerations

PREGNANCY

- Pregnancy exposure registry: 1-877-311-8972.
- It is not known if drug causes fetal harm, but animal studies suggest it may.

- Use with caution only if benefit to mother outweighs potential risk to fetus.

LACTATION

- It is not known if drug is present in breast milk.
- Breastfeeding is not recommended during drug therapy and for at least 18 hours after the last dose of immediate-release tablets or 36 hours after the last dose of extended-release tablets.

REPRODUCTION

- Women of childbearing should use effective contraception throughout drug therapy.
- Drug may reduce female fertility.

Nursing Considerations

- Be aware tofacitinib therapy should not be given to a patient who has an active infection, including localized infections.
- Know that tofacitinib should not be given to patients with severe hepatic impairment; tofacitinib should not be initiated in patients with a lymphocyte count less than 500 cells/mm^3, an absolute neutrophil count (ANC) less than 1,000 cells/mm^3, or hemoglobin levels less than 9 g/dl.
- Check with patient to be sure past immunizations received are in line with current immunization guidelines before starting tofacitinib therapy. If the patient needs further immunizations, ensure that it is done before drug therapy begins.
- Screen patient for viral hepatitis, as ordered, prior to starting tofacitinib therapy.
- Check to be sure that the patient has been tested for latent or active tuberculosis before tofacitinib therapy begins. Antituberculosis therapy might be prescribed for patients with a past history of active or latent tuberculosis if completion of treatment cannot be verified. Also, patients who have a negative test for latent tuberculosis may also be prescribed antituberculosis therapy if they have risk factors for tuberculosis.
- Use extreme caution when administering drug to patients with a history of chronic or recurrent infections, exposure to tuberculosis, history of a serious infection or an opportunistic infection, have resided or traveled in areas of endemic mycoses or endemic tuberculosis, or have underlying conditions that may predispose them to infection.

T

! **WARNING** Be aware that tofacitinib therapy increases risk of life-threatening cardiovascular problems and cancer. The prescriber may choose to discontinue drug in patients who develop a malignancy during tofacitinib therapy.

- Use cautiously in patients who may be at increased risk for gastrointestinal perforation, such as a patient with a history of diverticulitis. Monitor patient closely throughout tofacitinib therapy. Notify prescriber if patient experiences new-onset abdominal symptoms suggestive of perforation.
- Use caution when administering nondeformable extended-release form of drug to patients with preexisting severe gastrointestinal narrowing. Rare reports of obstructive symptoms in patients with known strictures have occurred with other drugs utilizing a nondeformable extended-release formula.
- Obtain a CBC to determine patient's baseline, as ordered. Once the baseline is established, expect prescriber to order a lymphocyte level every 3 months; an ANC level after 4 to 8 weeks of therapy and then every 3 months; and a hemoglobin level after 4 to 8 weeks and then every 3 months. These test results will guide the prescriber in making modifications in the patient's treatment plan.
- Be aware that patient taking higher doses for the treatment of rheumatoid arthritis is at increased risk for developing a pulmonary embolism. Also, patients 50 years and older with at least one cardiovascular risk factor treated with 10 mg twice daily have a higher rate of all-cause mortality, including sudden CV death, compared to those treated with 5 mg twice daily or TNF blockers. Dosage limited to once a day in patients 50 years and older who have at least one cardiovascular risk factor.

! **WARNING** Monitor patient for hypersensitivity reactions. If present, notify prescriber and provide supportive care, as ordered.

- Monitor the patient's liver enzymes routinely, as ordered, because drug has been associated with liver damage. Alert prescriber of any abnormalities and expect drug to be withheld during the investigation as to the cause of the elevated liver enzymes. If no other cause can be found, expect prescriber to discontinue drug.
- Know that viral reactivation, including herpes virus reactivation (herpes zoster), has occurred with tofacitinib therapy.
- Expect prescriber to order a lipid profile on the patient 4 to 8 weeks after tofacitinib therapy has begun, because the drug has caused increases in lipid parameters generally within the first 6 weeks of therapy. Expect to manage hyperlipidemia, if present, according to clinical guidelines, as prescribed.
- Monitor patient for signs and symptoms of infection during and after tofacitinib therapy. Know that patients with diabetes mellitus are at increased risk for infection. Notify prescriber if an infection develops and expect to obtain a complete blood count, if ordered. Be aware that drug should be discontinued if the patient has an ANC count or lymphocyte count less than 500. If the patient has an ANC level between 500 and 1,000 or a hemoglobin level greater than a 2 g/dl decrease or less than 8 g/dl, expect drug therapy to be interrupted until the ANC and hemoglobin levels have returned to target range.

! **WARNING** Monitor patient for thrombosis, which may occur with tofacitinib therapy. Patients at increased risk are patients with rheumatoid arthritis taking 10 mg twice daily and are 50 years or older and have at least one cardiovascular risk factor.

PATIENT TEACHING

- Instruct patient to take tofacitinib exactly as prescribed.
- Instruct patient taking extended-release tablets to swallow tablets whole and not to chew, crush, or split tablets. Remind patient taking oral solution to use the press-in bottle adaptor and oral dosing syringe when measuring dose and to store at room temperature.
- Alert patient that an inert tablet shell may be passed in her stool or via colostomy. If present, reassure her that the active medication has already been absorbed by the time patient sees the shell.

! **WARNING** Alert patient that an allergic reaction may occur with drug use. Tell patient to notify prescriber, if present, and to seek immediate medical care if serious.

- Review infection control measures with patient as well as the signs and symptoms of an infection. If an infection occurs, tell patient to notify prescriber immediately.
- Make sure patient understands the serious adverse reactions associated with tofacitinib, such as the development of malignancies and serious infections.
- Stress importance for women of childbearing age to use effective contraception during treatment. Tell female patient to notify prescriber if pregnancy is suspected or known.
- Make women of childbearing age aware that breastfeeding should not be done while taking tofacitinib and for at least 18 hours after the last dose of immediate-release tablets or 36 hours after the last dose of extended-release tablets.
- Inform female patients that tofacitinib therapy may reduce fertility.
- Encourage patient to comply with laboratory blood tests needed to monitor patient's reaction to tofacitinib.
- Advise patient at increased risk for skin cancer to have a periodic skin examination.
- Warn patient to avoid live vaccines while taking tofacitinib.

! **WARNING** Urge patient to seek immediate emergency care if patient experiences chest pain that worsens with breathing, leg pain or tenderness, red or discolored skin in the affected arm or leg, sudden shortness of breath, or swelling of arm or leg.

tolcapone
Tasmar

Class and Category
Pharmacologic class: Catechol-O-methyltransferase (COMT) inhibitor
Therapeutic class: Antiparkinsonian

Indications and Dosages
* As adjunct (with levodopa and carbidopa) to treat idiopathic Parkinson's disease in patients who are experiencing symptom fluctuations and are not responding satisfactorily to or are not appropriate candidates for other adjunctive treatment*

TABLETS
Adults. *Initial:* 100 mg three times a day. *Maximum:* 200 mg three times a day.
± **DOSAGE ADJUSTMENT** For patient with moderate or severe dyskinesia that was present before beginning treatment, dosage may have to be reduced.

Drug Administration
P.O.
- Administer first dose of the day with levodopa/carbidopa and subsequent doses about 6 and 12 hours later.
- Give without regard to food intake.

Route	Onset	Peak	Duration
P.O.	Unknown	2 hr	Unknown

Half-life: 2–3 hr

Mechanism of Action
Prolongs plasma half-life of levodopa by inhibiting catechol-O-methyltransferase (COMT), an enzyme responsible for metabolizing catecholamines—including dopa, dopamine, epinephrine, norepinephrine, and their hydroxylated metabolites. COMT inhibition decreases the metabolizing enzyme for levodopa, which yields a more sustained plasma levodopa level, making it more available for diffusion into the CNS to be converted to dopamine.

Contraindications
Confusion, hyperpyrexia, or rhabdomyolysis with previous use of tolcapone; hepatic dysfunction; hypersensitivity to tolcapone or its components

Interactions
DRUGS
desipramine, levodopa/carbidopa: Possibly increased frequency of adverse effects
warfarin: Possibly altered anticoagulant effects

Adverse Reactions
CNS: Aggression, agitation, compulsive behaviors such as intense urges to perform certain activities excessively (binge eating, gambling, sex, or spending money), confusion, delirium, delusions,

disorientation, dizziness, drowsiness, dyskinesia, fatigue, fever, hallucinations, headache, lethargy, loss of balance, paranoid ideation, psychotic-like behavior, somnolence

CV: Chest pain, orthostatic hypotension
EENT: Dry mouth
GI: Abdominal pain, **acute fulminant liver failure**, anorexia, cholestasis, constipation, diarrhea, elevated liver enzymes, jaundice, vomiting
GU: Bright yellow urine, hematuria
MS: Muscle cramps, **rhabdomyolysis**
RESP: Dyspnea, upper respiratory tract infection
SKIN: Diaphoresis

Childbearing Considerations

PREGNANCY
- It is not known if drug can cause fetal harm.
- Use with caution only if benefit to mother outweighs potential risk to fetus.

LACTATION
- It is not known if drug is present in breast milk.
- Patient should check with prescriber before breastfeeding.

Nursing Considerations
- Ensure that patient has had the risks of tolcapone therapy explained fully to him and has signed the acknowledgment form before starting therapy.
- Know that tolcapone should not be given to patient with a major psychotic disorder because of the increased risk of exacerbating psychosis.
- Use cautiously in patient with severe dyskinesia or dystonia because drug is known to cause rhabdomyolysis.
- Monitor liver enzymes, as ordered, during tolcapone therapy to detect hepatic impairment. Expect to discontinue drug if patient's liver enzymes exceed twice the upper limit of normal or if patient has any signs or symptoms of liver dysfunction, such as persistent anorexia, dark urine, fatigue, jaundice, lethargy, nausea, pruritus, or right upper quadrant tenderness.
- Assess patient for behavioral changes, hallucinations, or new or worsening mental status during tolcapone therapy or after starting or increasing the dose, especially

in patients over age 75. If present, notify prescriber, as dosage may have to be reduced or drug discontinued.
- Anticipate that drug may precipitate or exaggerate preexisting dyskinesia.
- Expect tolcapone to be discontinued if no improvement occurs after 3 weeks of drug therapy.
- Assess patient for skin changes regularly because risk of melanoma is higher in patients with Parkinson's disease. It isn't clear whether risk results from disease or drugs used to treat it.

PATIENT TEACHING
- Instruct patient to take first dose of the day with levodopa/carbidopa and then take remaining doses about 6 and 12 hours later.
- Inform patient that urine may turn bright yellow during tolcapone therapy.
- Advise patient to avoid hazardous activities until drug's CNS effects are known. Inform patient that tolcapone therapy may cause him to fall asleep suddenly during activities of daily living without warning and can occur for the first time even a year after therapy has begun. If this happens, tell patient to notify prescriber and continue to avoid hazardous activities until prescriber has deemed such activities safe. Also warn patient and family that behavioral changes, hallucinations, or new or worsening mental status have occurred with use of tolcapone, especially in patients over the age of 75.
- Urge patient to notify prescriber immediately about darkened urine, decreased appetite, fatigue, jaundice, lethargy, and right-sided abdominal pain.
- Caution patient not to stop taking drug abruptly. Explain that prescriber will supervise tapering of drug dosage.
- Urge patient to have regular follow-up appointments and laboratory tests.
- Urge patient to have regular skin examinations by a dermatologist or other qualified health professional.
- Advise patient to notify prescriber about intense urges that result in performing certain behaviors excessively (such as binge eating, uncontrolled gambling, sex, or spending money) because dosage may have to be reduced or drug discontinued.

tolterodine tartrate
Detrol, Detrol LA

Class and Category
Pharmacologic class: Cholinergic receptor blocker
Therapeutic class: Antispasmodic

Indications and Dosages
☀ *To treat overactive bladder with urinary frequency, urgency, or urge incontinence*

TABLETS
Adults. 2 mg twice daily. Reduced to 1 mg twice daily based on patient response and tolerance.
±**DOSAGE ADJUSTMENT** Dosage reduced to 1 mg twice daily for patients with significant hepatic or renal dysfunction and for patients who are also receiving CYP3A4 inhibitors, such as clarithromycin, ketoconazole, or ritonavir.

E.R. CAPSULES
Adults. 4 mg daily. Reduced to 2 mg daily based on individual response and tolerance.
±**DOSAGE ADJUSTMENT** For patients with mild to moderate hepatic dysfunction, severe renal dysfunction, and for patients receiving CYP3A4 inhibitors, such as clarithromycin, ketoconazole, or ritonavir, dosage reduced to 2 mg once daily.

Drug Administration
P.O.
- Capsules should be swallowed whole and not chewed, crushed, or opened.

Route	Onset	Peak	Duration
P.O.	Unknown	1–2 hr	Unknown
P.O./E.R.	Unknown	2–6 hr	Unknown

Half-life: 2–6.9 hr

Mechanism of Action
Exerts antimuscarinic (atropine-like) and potent direct antispasmodic (papaverine-like) actions on smooth muscle in the bladder, which decreases detrusor muscle contractions. This helps reduce urinary frequency and urgency as well as urge-related incontinence.

Contraindications
Gastric retention; hypersensitivity to tolterodine tartrate, its components, or to fesoterodine fumarate extended-release tablets; uncontrolled angle-closure glaucoma; urine retention

Interactions
DRUGS
fluoxetine: Possibly decreased tolterodine metabolism increasing immediate-release tolterodine blood concentration
other anticholinergics: Increased risk of anticholinergic adverse effects such as blurred vision, constipation, dry mouth, and somnolence
potent CYP3A4 inhibitors such as clarithromycin, itraconazole, ketoconazole, ritonavir: Possibly increased blood tolterodine level

Adverse Reactions
CNS: Confusion, disorientation, dizziness, drowsiness, fatigue, hallucinations, headache, memory impairment, somnolence, worsening of dementia
CV: Chest pain, edema, hypertension, palpitations, **QT prolongation**, tachycardia
EENT: Abnormal vision, blurred vision, dry eyes, dry mouth
GI: Abdominal pain, constipation, diarrhea, flatulence, indigestion, nausea
GU: Dysuria, urine retention, UTI
Other: **Anaphylaxis**, **angioedema**, flu-like symptoms

Childbearing Considerations
PREGNANCY
- It is not known if drug can cause fetal harm.
- Use with caution only if benefit to mother outweighs potential risk to fetus.

LACTATION
- It is not known if drug is present in breast milk.
- A decision should be made to discontinue breastfeeding or drug to avoid potential serious adverse reactions in the breastfed infant.

Nursing Considerations
- Use cautiously in patients with decreased GI motility, myasthenia gravis, or narrow-angle glaucoma because tolterodine could make these conditions worse.

! **WARNING** Monitor patients with a history of bladder outflow obstruction for bladder distention or decreased urine output, because tolterodine poses a risk of urine retention.

- Monitor patients for abdominal bloating or distention or patients with a history of GI obstructive disorders, such as pyloric stenosis, because of increased risk of gastric retention.
- Be aware that drug's antimuscarinic effects may produce blurred vision, dizziness, and drowsiness. If these occur, institute fall precautions according to facility policy.

PATIENT TEACHING

- Tell patient capsules should be swallowed whole and not chewed, crushed, or opened.
- Instruct patient taking tolterodine to report immediately to prescriber any difficulty urinating or infrequent urination, as well as difficulty breathing or swelling that involves the face, lips, throat, or tongue, and to seek emergency medical care.
- Advise patient not to drive or perform activities that require high alertness until drug's CNS and vision effects are known. Instruct her to notify prescriber if blurred vision, dizziness, or drowsiness persists.
- Encourage patient to use sugarless candy, gum, or ice to relieve dry mouth. Advise her to notify prescriber or dentist if dry mouth persists or worsens over 2 weeks.

tolvaptan
Jynarque, Samsca

Class and Category
Pharmacologic class: Vasopressin receptor antagonist
Therapeutic class: Vasopressin antagonist

Indications and Dosages
* *To treat significant hypervolemic and euvolemic hyponatremia (serum sodium level less than 125 mEq/L or symptomatic but less-marked hyponatremia that has resisted correction with fluid restriction), including patients with heart failure or syndrome of inappropriate antidiuretic hormone (SIADH)*

TABLETS
Adults. *Initial:* 15 mg once daily, increased after at least 24 hours to 30 mg once daily. *Maximum:* 60 mg once daily or given for more than 30 days.

* *To slow kidney function decline in patients at risk of rapidly progressing autosomal dominant polycystic kidney disease*

TABLETS (JYNARQUE)
Adults. *Initial:* 45 mg upon waking followed with 15 mg 8 hours later for a total daily dose of 60 mg. Dosage titrated at least a week later to 60 mg upon waking followed with 30 mg 8 hours later for a total daily dose of 90 mg. Dosage further titrated to target dose after another wk with 90 mg upon waking followed with 30 mg 8 hours later for a total daily dose of 120 mg and thereafter.

±**DOSAGE ADJUSTMENT FOR JYNARQUE** For patient taking concomitant moderate CYP3A inhibitors, initial dosage of 45 mg followed by 15 mg reduced to 15 mg and 15 mg 8 hours later; 60 mg followed by 30 mg reduced to 30 mg and 15 mg 8 hours later; and 90 mg followed by 30 mg reduced to 45 mg and 15 mg 8 hours later.

Drug Administration
P.O.
- Administer without regard to food.
- Administer first dose of Jynarque when patient awakes in morning and second dose 8 hours later.
- Avoid administering drug with grapefruit or grapefruit juice.

Route	Onset	Peak	Duration
P.O.	2–4 hr	2–4 hr	Unknown

Half-life: 3–12 hr

Mechanism of Action
Raises serum sodium levels by decreasing urine osmolality and increasing urine output. Tolvaptan does this by preventing attachment of vasopressin to vasopressin V2 receptors on cell membranes in the nephron's collecting duct. Without vasopressin activity, urinary water excretion increases.

Contraindications
Acute need to raise serum sodium urgently; anuria; concomitant use of strong CYP3A inhibitors such as clarithromycin, ketoconazole, indinavir, itraconazole, nefazodone, nelfinavir, ritonavir, saquinavir, telithromycin; hypovolemic hyponatremia; hypersensitivity to tolvaptan or its components; inability of patient to sense or respond appropriately to thirst; significant liver impairment or injury (Jynarque); uncorrected abnormal blood

sodium concentrations or urinary outflow obstruction (Jynarque); use in patients with autosomal dominant polycystic kidney disease outside of FDA-approved REMS (Samsca)

Interactions

DRUGS

ACE inhibitors, angiotensin receptor blockers, potassium-sparing diuretics, potassium supplements: Increased risk of hyperkalemia
CYP3A inducers such as barbiturates, carbamazepine, phenytoin, rifabutin, rifampin, rifapentine, St. John's wort: Decreased serum tolvaptan level and decreased effectiveness
CYP3A inhibitors such as aprepitant, clarithromycin, diltiazem, erythromycin, fluconazole, ketoconazole, indinavir, itraconazole, nefazodone, nelfinavir, ritonavir, saquinavir, telithromycin, verapamil; P-gp inhibitors such as cyclosporine: Increased serum tolvaptan level and risk of adverse reactions
desmopressin: Possibly altered desmopressin activity
digoxin: Increased digoxin level

FOODS

grapefruit juice: Increased serum tolvaptan level

Adverse Reactions

CNS: Asthenia, **CVA**, fever, **osmotic demyelination syndrome**, thirst
CV: Deep vein thrombosis, intracardiac thrombus, ventricular fibrillation
EENT: Dry mouth
ENDO: Diabetic ketoacidosis, hyperglycemia
GI: Anorexia, constipation, **GI bleeding,** hepatic dysfunction, **hepatic injury, ischemic colitis,** nausea
GU: Nocturia, polyuria, **urethral or vaginal hemorrhage**
HEME: Disseminated intravascular coagulation (DIC), prolonged prothrombin time
MS: Rhabdomyolysis
RESP: Pulmonary embolism, respiratory failure
SKIN: Rash
Other: Anaphylaxis, dehydration, **hyperkalemia, hypernatremia, hyponatremia,** hypovolemia

Childbearing Considerations

PREGNANCY

- It is not known if drug can cause fetal harm.
- Use with caution only if benefit to mother outweighs potential risk to fetus.

LACTATION

- It is not known if drug is present in breast milk.
- Breastfeeding is not recommended during drug therapy.

Nursing Considerations

- Know that Jynarque is only available through a restricted program called the Jynarque REMS Program. Ensure that patient has been enrolled and has agreed to comply with ongoing monitoring requirements.
- Expect patients prescribed Jynarque to have bilirubin and liver enzymes evaluated prior to starting Jynarque therapy, again after 2 and 4 weeks of therapy, then monthly for 18 months and every 3 months thereafter because of increased risk of serious liver injury.
- Be aware that tolvaptan should not be given to patients with a creatine clearance of less than 10 ml/min because no benefit can be expected in patients who are anuric.
- Use cautiously in patients with cirrhosis because of increased risk of GI bleeding.

! **WARNING** Give Samsca brand of tolvaptan, initially or if reintroduced, in a hospital setting because too-rapid correction of hyponatremia (more than 12 mEq/L in 24 hour) causes osmotic demyelination (affective changes, coma, dysarthria, dysphagia, lethargy, mutism, spastic quadriparesis, seizures, death). If present, notify prescriber immediately and expect to stop tolvaptan and give hypotonic fluids.

- Monitor fluid and electrolyte balance regularly, especially when starting tolvaptan and adjusting dosage, as ordered. If patient develops hypernatremia, notify prescriber and expect to decrease dose or withhold drug and modify the patient's free-water infusion or intake, as ordered.

- Don't restrict fluids during first 24 hours of therapy because doing so may increase the risk of overly rapid correction of dehydration, hypovolemia, and serum sodium.
- Use of hypertonic saline isn't recommended during tolvaptan therapy because effects are unknown.

! WARNING Monitor patient for signs and symptoms of hepatic dysfunction such as anorexia, dark urine, fatigue, jaundice, and right upper abdominal pain; if present, notify prescriber, and obtain liver enzymes immediately, as ordered. If hepatic dysfunction is confirmed, expect drug to be discontinued. Know that if the cause of hepatic dysfunction is found to be due to something other than tolvaptan therapy, expect drug to be resumed.

PATIENT TEACHING

- Stress to patient receiving Jynarque the need to comply with frequent blood tests to monitor for adverse liver reactions.
- Instruct patient to consume fluids according to thirst during first 24 hours of therapy and not to try to limit fluid intake.
- Tell patient that he'll need to resume fluid restriction and will need continued monitoring of sodium level and fluid status when drug is discontinued.
- Tell patient to notify prescriber if he experiences dark urine or yellowing of eyes and skin, fatigue, loss of appetite, or right upper abdominal pain.
- Inform mothers that breastfeeding is not recommended during drug therapy and to alert prescriber if pregnancy occurs or is suspected.

topiramate

Eprontia, Qudexy XR, Topamax, Topamax Sprinkle, Trokendi XR

Class and Category

Pharmacologic class: Sulfamate-substituted monosaccharide
Therapeutic class: Anticonvulsant

Indications and Dosages

* *To treat partial-onset or primary generalized tonic–clonic seizures*

CAPSULES (TOPAMAX SPRINKLE), ORAL SOLUTION (EPRONTIA), TABLETS (TOPAMAX)

Adults and children age 10 and over. *Initial:* 25 mg twice daily in morning and evening for wk 1; 50 mg twice daily in morning and evening for wk 2; 75 mg twice daily in morning and evening for wk 3; 100 mg twice daily in morning and evening for wk 4; 150 mg twice daily in morning and evening for wk 5; and 200 mg twice daily in morning and evening for wk 6. *Maintenance:* 200 mg twice daily in morning and evening.
Children age 2 to 10 years of age. *Initial:* 25 mg once daily in evening for wk 1. Increased to 25 mg twice daily in morning and evening for wk 2. Increased thereafter by 25 to 50 mg/day each subsequent wk, as tolerated, over the next 5 to 7 wk. *Maintenance:* For children weighing up to 11 kg (up to 24.2 lb), 75 to 125 mg twice daily; for children weighing 12 to 22 kg (26.4 to 48.4 lb), 100 to 150 mg twice daily; for children weighing 23 to 31 kg (50.6 to 68.2 lb), 100 to 175 mg twice daily; for children weighing 32 to 38 kg (70.4 to 83.6 lb), 125 to 175 mg twice daily; and for children weighing more than 38 kg (more than 83.6 lb), 125 to 200 mg twice daily. *Maximum:* Highest maintenance dosage for weight.

EXTENDED-RELEASE CAPSULES (QUDEXY XR, TROKENDI XR)

Adults and children age 10 and over. *Initial:* 50 mg once daily for wk 1; 100 mg once daily for wk 2; 150 mg once daily for wk 3; 200 mg once daily for wk 4; 300 mg once daily for wk 5; and 400 mg once daily for wk 6 and beyond. *Maintenance:* 400 mg once daily.
Children age 2 to less than 10 (Qudexy XR) and children age 6 to less than 10 (Trokendi XR). *Initial:* 25 mg once daily at night for wk 1; 50 mg once daily at night for wk 2; then increased weekly in increments of 25 to 50 mg until minimum maintenance dose reached, usually within 5 to 7 wk. Additional increases in increments of 25 to 50 mg made weekly to maximum maintenance dose, as needed. *Maintenance:* For children weighing up to 11 kg (24.2 lb), 150 to 250 mg once daily at night; for children weighing 12 to 22 kg (26.4 to 48.4 lb), 200 to 300 mg once daily at night; for children weighing 23 to 31 kg (50.6 to 68.2 lb), 200 to 350 mg once

daily at night; for children weighing 32 to 38 kg (70.4 to 83.6 lb), 250 to 350 mg once daily at night; and for children weighing more than 38 kg (83.6 lb), 250 to 400 mg once daily at night. *Maximum:* Highest maximum maintenance dose for weight.

✳ *As adjunct to treat partial seizures, primary generalized tonic–clonic seizures, and seizures associated with Lennox–Gastaut syndrome*

CAPSULES (TOPAMAX SPRINKLE), ORAL SOLUTION (EPRONTIA), TABLETS (TOPAMAX)

Adults and adolescents age 17 and over. *Initial:* 25 to 50 mg daily in divided doses twice daily for 1 wk. Increased by 25 to 50 mg daily every wk thereafter until maintenance dose is reached. *Maintenance:* 200 to 400 mg daily in divided doses twice daily for partial-onset seizures and Lennox–Gastaut syndrome and 400 mg daily in divided doses twice daily for primary generalized tonic-clonic seizures.

Children ages 2 to 17. *Initial:* 1 mg/kg/day to 3 mg/kg daily at night for 1 wk. Increased every 1 to 2 wk by 1 to 3 mg/kg daily in divided doses twice daily until maintenance dose is reached. *Maintenance:* 5 to 9 mg/kg daily in divided doses twice daily.

EXTENDED-RELEASE CAPSULES (QUDEXY XR, TROKENDI XR)

Adults and adolescents age 17 and over. *Initial:* 25 to 50 mg once daily, increased weekly in increments of 25 to 50 mg once daily, as needed. *Maximum:* 400 mg once daily.

Children age 2 to less than 17 years of age (Qudexy XR) and children age 6 to less than 17 (Trokendi XR). *Initial:* 1 to 3 mg/kg/day once daily at night for 1 wk, increased every 1 to 2 wk in increments of 1 to 3 mg/kg/day, as needed. *Maximum:* 9 mg/kg/day or 400 mg daily.

✳ *To prevent migraine headache*

CAPSULES (TOPAMAX SPRINKLE), ORAL SOLUTION (EPRONTIA), TABLETS (TOPAMAX)

Adults and children age 12 and over. *Initial:* 25 mg daily in evening for wk 1; then 25 mg twice daily morning and evening for wk 2; then 25 mg in morning and 50 mg in evening for wk 3, then 50 mg twice daily in morning and evening. *Maintenance:* 50 mg twice daily.

EXTENDED-RELEASE CAPSULES (QUDEXY XR, TROKENDI XR)

Adults and children age 12 and over. *Initial:* 25 mg once daily for wk 1; 50 mg once daily for wk 2; 75 mg once daily for wk 3; and 100 mg once daily for wk 4. *Maintenance:* 100 mg once daily.

±**DOSAGE ADJUSTMENT** For patients with moderate to severe renal impairment, dosage possibly reduced by 50%. For patients undergoing hemodialysis, a supplemental dose may be required during a prolonged period of dialysis.

Drug Administration

P.O.

- Do not break tablets, because of the bitter taste.
- Use a calibrated device to measure dosage of oral solution. Discard unused portion after 60 days.
- Topamax Sprinkle and Qudexy XR capsules may be swallowed whole or opened and sprinkled onto a teaspoon of soft food. Mixture should be swallowed immediately and not chewed or crushed, nor should it be stored.
- Trokendi XR capsules should be swallowed whole and not chewed, crushed, or opened.

Route	Onset	Peak	Duration
P.O.	Unknown	1–4 hr	Unknown
P.O./E.R.	Unknown	20–24 hr	Unknown

Half-life: 21–56 hr

Mechanism of Action

May block the spread of seizures by reducing the length and frequency of excitatory transmission.

Contraindications

Hypersensitivity to topiramate or its components, recent alcohol use defined as within 6 hours prior to and 6 hours after taking topiramate (Trokendi XR)

Interactions

DRUGS

amitriptyline: Possibly high increase in amitriptyline blood concentration increasing risk of adverse reactions

antihistamines, barbiturates, benzodiazepines, CNS depressants, opioid analgesics, skeletal

T

muscle relaxants, tricyclic antidepressants: Additive CNS depression

carbamazepine, phenytoin: Decreased blood topiramate level

hydrochlorothiazide: Possibly increased blood topiramate levels

lithium: Increased risk of lithium toxicity

oral contraceptives: Increased risk of breakthrough bleeding, decreased contraceptive efficacy

other carbonic anhydrase inhibitors such as acetazolamide, zonisamide: Increased risk of kidney stone formation; increased severity of metabolic acidosis

pioglitazone: Possibly decreased exposure of pioglitazone with decreased effectiveness

ACTIVITIES

alcohol use: Additive CNS depression

Adverse Reactions

CNS: Abnormal coordination, aggression, agitation, anxiety, aphasia, apathy, asthenia, ataxia, confusion, decreased concentration, depersonalization, depression, dizziness, dysphasia, emotional lability, encephalopathy, fatigue, fever, gait abnormality, hallucinations, headache, hyperkinesia, hyperthermia, hypoesthesia, hyporeflexia, insomnia, irritability, language problems, memory alterations or loss, mood changes, nervousness, neurosis, paresthesia, personality disorder, psychomotor slowing, psychosis, rigors, seizures, slurred or other abnormalities of speech, somnolence, stupor, suicidal ideation, syncope, thirst, tremor, vertigo

CV: Bradycardia, cardiac arrest, chest pain, edema, hypertension, hypotension, palpitations, vasodilation

EENT: Acute myopia and secondary angle-closure glaucoma syndrome, blurred vision, conjunctivitis, diplopia, dry mouth, edema of the pharynx, epistaxis, gingivitis, glossitis, gum hyperplasia, hearing loss, increased saliva, laryngitis, maculopathy, myopia, nystagmus, otitis media, periorbital pain, pharyngitis, rhinitis, secondary angle-closure glaucoma with acute myopia, sinusitis, taste loss or perversion, tinnitus, tongue edema, vision changes including visual field defects

ENDO: Breast pain, hot flashes, hyperglycemia, hypoglycemia, hypothyroidism

GI: Abdominal pain, anorexia, constipation, diarrhea, dyspepsia, elevated gamma GGT levels, fecal incontinence, flatulence, gastroenteritis, gastroesophageal reflux, hepatic failure, hepatitis, increased appetite, indigestion, nausea, pancreatitis, vomiting

GU: Cystitis, decreased libido, dysmenorrhea, dysuria, frequent urination, hematuria, impotence, kidney stones, leukorrhea, menstrual irregularities, nephrocalcinosis, nocturia, premature ejaculation, prostatic disorder, renal calculi, renal tubular acidosis, urinary frequency or incontinence, UTI, vaginal hemorrhage, vaginitis

HEME: Anemia, bleeding events, increased prothrombin time, leukopenia, purpura, thrombocytopenia

MS: Arthralgia, back pain, decreased bone mineral density (children), dysarthria, involuntary muscle contractions, leg cramps or pain, muscle weakness, myalgia, skeletal pain

RESP: Bronchitis, cough, dyspnea, pneumonia, pulmonary embolism, upper respiratory tract infection

SKIN: Abnormal hair growth, acne, alopecia, bullous skin reactions, decreased or increased sweating, dermatitis, erythema multiforme, eczema, flushing, pallor, pemphigus, pruritus, rash, seborrhea, skin discoloration, Stevens–Johnson syndrome, toxic epidermal necrolysis

Other: Body odor, decreased serum bicarbonate levels, decreased height and weight (children), dehydration, elevated serum alkaline phosphatase, flu-like symptoms, hyperammonemia, hypersensitivity reactions, hyponatremia, hypophosphatemia, increased susceptibility to infection, metabolic acidosis, moniliasis, weight gain or loss

Childbearing Considerations

PREGNANCY

- Pregnancy exposure registry: 1-888-233-2334 or http://www.aedpregnancyregistry.org/.
- Drug can cause fetal harm such as increased risk for cleft lip or palate and being small for gestational age.
- Use with caution only if benefit to mother outweighs potential risk to fetus.

LABOR & DELIVERY

- Drug may cause preterm labor and premature delivery.

- There is a potential for the development of drug-induced metabolic acidosis in the mother and/or in the fetus, which might affect the fetus's ability to tolerate labor.
- Neonates should be monitored for transient metabolic acidosis following birth if mother received drug.

LACTATION

- Drug is present in breast milk.
- Patient should check with prescriber before breastfeeding.
- If breastfeeding occurs, monitor breastfed infant for diarrhea and somnolence.

REPRODUCTION

- Women of childbearing age should use an effective contraceptive throughout drug therapy.

Nursing Considerations

- Obtain baseline serum bicarbonate level before topiramate therapy and monitor periodically throughout therapy, as ordered.
- Obtain baseline height and weight in children, as drug may have negative effects on growth.
- Use topiramate cautiously in patients with impaired hepatic function, or inborn errors of metabolism, or those who are taking valproic acid; these patients may be at higher risk for hyperammonemia, with or without encephalopathy, while taking topiramate. In addition, hypothermia may occur in patients taking valproic acid concomitantly. If present, notify prescriber and expect topiramate or valproic acid therapy to be discontinued.

! **WARNING** Anticipate an increase in seizure activity if topiramate therapy for seizures stops abruptly. Take seizure precautions, as appropriate. Expect drug to be withdrawn gradually if time permits.

- Keep in mind that if patient reports ocular pain or decreased visual acuity, notify prescriber immediately; topiramate may cause increased intraocular pressure and secondary angle-closure glaucoma as well as visual field defects. Expect to stop drug immediately.
- Monitor patient for cognitive-related dysfunction, especially patients who are started on a higher initial dose or have a rapid titration rate.

- Assess for signs of recurrence of renal calculi if patient has a history of this condition.
- Monitor patient for bleeding events, especially patients who have conditions that increase risk of bleeding, who take drugs that cause thrombocytopenia such as other antiepileptic drugs, or who take drugs that affect platelet function or coagulation such as anticoagulants, aspirin, nonsteroidal anti-inflammatory drugs, or selective serotonin reuptake inhibitors.
- Assess patient's skin frequently, as serious skin reactions may occur. If a rash develops, notify prescriber and expect drug to be discontinued.

PATIENT TEACHING

- Instruct patient to swallow tablets and Trokendi XR capsules whole. However, tell patient taking Topamax Sprinkle or Qudexy XR capsules that these capsules may be swallowed whole or opened and sprinkled onto a teaspoon of soft food. Mixture should be swallowed immediately and not chewed or crushed, nor should it be stored. Tell patient receiving oral solution to measure dosage using a calibrated device, not a household spoon. Also, tell patient to discard unused portion of oral solution after 60 days.
- Urge patient to avoid potentially hazardous activities until drug's CNS effects are known.
- Advise patient to watch for decreased sweating and significantly increased body temperature, especially during hot weather, and to notify prescriber immediately if they occur.
- Tell patient to maintain adequate fluid intake to minimize the risk of developing kidney stones.
- Instruct patient to avoid alcohol use completely within 6 hours before and after taking topiramate.
- Advise female patient of possible breakthrough bleeding. If she takes an oral contraceptive, encourage her to use another form of contraception during therapy.
- Caution patient not to stop taking topiramate abruptly, because seizures may occur. Instead, patient should expect drug to be withdrawn gradually if it must be discontinued.

T

- Instruct patient to seek immediate emergency care for blurred vision, other visual disturbances, or periorbital pain.
- Tell patient to notify prescriber if he develops changes in mental status, unexplained lethargy, or vomiting.
- Urge caregivers to watch patient closely for evidence of suicidal tendencies, especially when topiramate therapy starts or dosage changes, and to report concerns at once to prescriber.
- Instruct patient to stop taking drug and notify prescriber if a rash occurs during drug therapy.
- Counsel female patient of childbearing age to use effective birth control.
- Alert parents/caregivers that drug can have a negative effect on growth and decrease bone mineral density. Encourage parents/caregivers to discuss any concerns with prescriber.

torsemide
Demadex, Soaanz

Class and Category
Pharmacologic class: Loop diuretic
Therapeutic class: Antihypertensive, diuretic

Indications and Dosages
✳ *To treat edema in heart failure*

TABLETS
Adults. *Initial:* 10 or 20 mg once daily, adjusted by doubling dose each time to achieve desired effect. *Maximum:* 200 mg daily.

✳ *To treat edema in chronic renal failure*

TABLETS
Adults. *Initial:* 20 mg once daily adjusted by doubling dose each time to achieve desired effect. *Maximum:* 200 mg daily.

✳ *To treat ascites, alone or with an aldosterone antagonist or a potassium-sparing diuretic*

TABLETS (DEMADEX)
Adults. *Initial:* 5 or 10 mg once daily, adjusted by doubling dose each time, as needed, to achieve desired effect. *Maximum:* 40 mg daily.

✳ *To manage hypertension*

TABLETS (DEMADEX)
Adults. *Initial:* 5 mg once daily, increased to 10 mg daily after 4 to 6 wk, if response is inadequate. *Maximum:* 10 mg daily.

Drug Administration
P.O.
- Administer daily dose in morning to prevent nocturia.

Route	Onset	Peak	Duration
P.O.	1 hr	1–2 hr	6–8 hr

Half-life: 3.5 hr

Mechanism of Action
Blocks active chloride and sodium reabsorption in the ascending loop of Henle by promoting rapid excretion of chloride, sodium, and water. Torsemide also increases the production of renal prostaglandins, increasing the plasma renin level and renal vasodilation. As a result, blood pressure falls, reducing preload and afterload.

Contraindications
Anuric patients; hepatic coma; hypersensitivity to torsemide, povidone, or their components

Interactions
DRUGS
ACE inhibitors, angiotensin receptor blockers, antihypertensives: Additive hypotension; increased risk of renal impairment
ACTH, corticosteroids: Possibly increased risk of hypokalemia
aminoglycoside antibiotics, ethacrynic acid: Increased risk of ototoxicity
cholestyramine: Possibly decreased absorption of orally administered torsemide
CYP2C9 inducers such as rifampin: Decreased plasma concentrations of torsemide, possibly decreasing effectiveness
CYP2C9 inhibitors such as amiodarone, fluconazole, miconazole, oxandrolone: Increased plasma concentrations of torsemide and possibly increased risk of adverse reactions
CYP2C9 substrates such as celecoxib or substrates with a narrow therapeutic range, such as phenytoin, warfarin: Possibly decreased effectiveness and safety of these drugs
digoxin: Increased risk of arrhythmias and digitalis toxicity due to hypokalemia or hypomagnesemia
indomethacin: Possibly decreased antihypertensive and diuretic effects of torsemide

lithium: Possibly lithium toxicity
nephrotoxic drugs such as aminoglycosides, cisplatin, NSAIDs: Increased risk of worsening renal function
NSAIDS, salicylates: Increased risk of nephrotoxicity and salicylate toxicity
probenecid, other organic anion drugs: Possibly decreased diuretic effect of torsemide
radiocontrast agents: Increased risk of renal toxicity

Adverse Reactions

CNS: Confusion, dizziness, drowsiness, fatigue, headache, insomnia, lethargy, nervousness, paresthesia, restlessness, thirst, weakness
CV: Chest pain, **ECG abnormalities**, edema, **hypotension**, tachycardia
EENT: Dry mouth, hearing loss, ototoxicity, pharyngitis, rhinitis, tinnitus, visual impairment
ENDO: Hyperglycemia
GI: Abdominal pain, anorexia, constipation, diarrhea, elevated liver enzymes, indigestion, nausea, **pancreatitis**, vomiting
GU: **Azotemia**, elevated blood urea creatinine and nitrogen levels, oliguria, urinary frequency or retention, worsening renal function
HEME: Anemia, **leukopenia, thrombocytopenia**
MS: Muscle spasms, myalgia
RESP: Cough
SKIN: Photosensitivity, pruritus, **Stevens–Johnson syndrome, toxic epidermal necrolysis**
Other: Elevated uric acid levels, **hypocalcemia**, hypochloremic alkalosis, **hypokalemia, hypomagnesemia, hyponatremia**, hypovolemia, thiamine (vitamin B1) deficiency

Childbearing Considerations

PREGNANCY
- It is not known if drug can cause fetal harm.
- Use with caution only if benefit to mother outweighs potential risk to fetus.

LACTATION
- It is not known if drug is present in breast milk.
- Patient should check with prescriber before breastfeeding, as drug may suppress lactation.

Nursing Considerations

- Monitor patient's serum electrolyte levels and fluid intake and output to detect hypovolemia, because dehydration can worsen renal function, causing acute renal failure. Patients at higher risk include patients who are taking renin-angiotensin aldosterone inhibitors or other nephrotoxic drugs or who are salt-depleted. Expect to monitor renal function in patients who experience dehydration.
- Monitor patient with hepatic disease who has ascites or cirrhosis, because a sudden shift in fluid and electrolyte balance may precipitate hepatic coma. Diuretic therapy can also contribute to a variety of disorders such as azotemia, hypokalemia, hyponatremia, hypovolemia, or metabolic alkalosis in these patients, which can cause or worsen hepatic encephalopathy. Know that if this occurs, drug should be withheld or discontinued.

! **WARNING** Expect torsemide-induced electrolyte imbalances, such as hypokalemia and hypomagnesemia, to increase the risk of toxicity and fatal arrhythmias in a patient who takes a digitalis glycoside. Hypokalemia also potentiates the neuromuscular blockade effects of nondepolarizing neuromuscular blockers.

PATIENT TEACHING
- Instruct patient to take daily dose in morning.
- Advise patient to change position slowly to minimize the effects of orthostatic hypotension. Instruct patient to notify prescriber if fainting occurs.
- Tell patient to maintain an adequate fluid intake and to be aware that diarrhea, excessive perspiration, or vomiting can lower blood pressure, possibly causing fainting to occur. Instruct patient to notify prescriber if excessive fluid loss occurs.
- Warn patient not to take any over-the-counter NSAID drug without consulting prescriber first.
- Instruct patient to notify prescriber at once about drowsiness, dry mouth, hearing changes, lethargy, muscle pain, nausea, restlessness, thirst, vomiting, or weakness.
- Advise diabetic patient to monitor her blood glucose level often because drug may raise it.

T

tralokinumab-Idrm
Adbry

Class and Category
Pharmacologic class: Human IgG4 monoclonal antibody
Therapeutic class: Interleukin inhibitor

Indications and Dosages
* *To treat moderate to severe atopic dermatitis in patients whose disease is not adequately controlled with topical prescription therapies or when those therapies are not advised*

SUBCUTANEOUS INJECTION

Adults. *Initial*: 600 mg (four 150-mg injections), followed by 300 mg (two 150-mg injections every other wk). *Maintenance*: After 16 wk of therapy for patients who weigh less than 100 kg (220 lb) and have achieved clear or almost clear skin, 300 mg every 4 wk given, as needed.

Drug Administration
SUBCUTANEOUS

- Remove prefilled syringes from refrigerator by gasping the body of the syringe. Do not shake. Allow syringe to reach room temperature, which usually takes about 30 minutes, before injecting drug. Do not warm any other way and do not remove needle cap during warming. Once syringes have reached room temperature, do not put back into refrigerator. Use within 14 days.
- Solution should appear clear to opalescent, colorless to pale yellow. Discard if solution is cloudy or discolored or there is visible particulate matter present. There may be small air bubbles in the solution. This is normal and not necessary to remove.
- Be aware that drug does not contain preservatives, so any unused drug should be discarded.
- Administer each of the initial four 150-mg injections or the subsequent two 150-mg injections at different injection sites at least 1 inch (3 cm) from other injection sites but within the same body area such as the abdomen (except for 2 inches or 5 cm around navel), thigh, or upper arm. Do not inject into areas that are bruised, scarred, or damaged.
- Document body area used for the injections in patient's record, as the body area used should be rotated with each subsequent set of injections.
- Store unused prefilled syringes in the refrigerator until ready to use. Keep syringes from direct sunlight.

Route	Onset	Peak	Duration
SQ	Unknown	Unknown	Unknown

Half-life: 3 wk

Mechanism of Action
Binds to human interleukin-13 (IL-13), which is a naturally occurring cytokine in the type 2 immune response. This inhibits the action of IL-13 to release proinflammatory cytokines, chemokines, and IgE.

Contraindications
Hypersensitivity to tralokinumab-Idrm or its components

Interactions
DRUGS
None reported by manufacturer

Adverse Reactions
EENT: Conjunctivitis, keratitis
HEME: Eosinophilia
RESP: Upper respiratory infections
OTHER: Anaphylaxis, angioedema, antibody formation against tralokinumab-Idrm, injection-site reactions (pain, redness, swelling)

Childbearing Considerations
PREGNANCY
- It is not known if drug can cause fetal harm.
- Use with caution only if benefit to mother outweighs potential risk to fetus.

LACTATION
- It is not known if drug is present in breast milk.
- Patient should check with prescriber before breastfeeding.

Nursing Considerations
- Ensure that all recommended age-related vaccinations are completed prior to starting tralokinumab-Idrm therapy.
- Know that tralokinumab-Idrm may be used with or without topical corticosteroids. For problem areas, such as those that occur on the face, neck, intertriginous, and genital

areas, topical calcineurin inhibitors may be prescribed but only if problems persist.

- Expect patients with a preexisting parasitic (helminth) infection to be treated before drug therapy is begun because it is not known if drug will influence a patient's response to parasitic treatment. Know that if patient develops a parasitic infection during tralokinumab-Idrm therapy and patient does not respond to antiparasitic therapy, drug should be discontinued until the infection is eradicated.

! **WARNING** Monitor patient for hypersensitivity reactions which could become life-threatening, such as anaphylaxis and angioedema. If a serious reaction occurs, notify prescriber, discontinue drug immediately, and provide supportive care, as ordered.

! **WARNING** Do not administer live attenuated vaccines to patients receiving tralokinumab-Idrm because effects are unknown.

- Question patient often about the presence of eye symptoms because tralokinumab-Idrm may cause conjunctivitis and keratitis.

PATIENT TEACHING

- Inform patient that more than one injection will be needed to receive the dosage of tralokinumab-Idrm prescribed; four injections for the initial dose and two injections for each maintenance dose.
- Instruct patient how to administer a tralokinumab-Idrm subcutaneous injection and sites to use. Stress importance of injecting the drug in the same body area (but at least 1 inch apart from each injection) and to rotate body area sites each time a dose is required.

! **WARNING** Review allergic reactions to drug with patient. Tell patient to notify prescriber or seek immediate emergency care if a serious allergic reaction occurs and to stop drug therapy immediately.

- Advise patient to report signs and symptoms of a parasitic infection to prescriber, as additional treatment will be needed.
- Stress importance of patient not receiving any live attenuated vaccines while taking tralokinumab-Idrm.

- Instruct patient to report eye symptoms to prescriber.

tramadol hydrochloride

ConZip, Qdolo, Ultram, Ultram ER, Zytram XL (CAN)

Class, Category, and Schedule

Pharmacologic class: Opioid agonist
Therapeutic class: Opioid analgesic
Controlled substance schedule: IV

Indications and Dosages

＊ *To relieve pain severe enough to require opioid-like treatment and for which alternative treatment options such as nonopioid analgesics or opioid combination products are inadequate or not tolerated*

ORAL SOLUTION, TABLETS

Adults with chronic pain not requiring rapid onset of analgesic effect. *Initial:* 25 mg daily in morning, then titrated every 3 days in 25-mg increments in separate doses to reach 100 mg daily given as 25 mg four times daily. Then, if further analgesia is needed, total daily dose increased by 50 mg every 3 days to reach 200 mg daily given as 50 mg four times daily. After titration, 50 to 100 mg given, as needed, every 4 to 6 hr. *Maximum:* 400 mg daily.

Adults requiring rapid pain relief. 50 to 100 mg every 4 to 6 hr, as needed. *Maximum:* 400 mg daily.

±**DOSAGE ADJUSTMENT** For patients with creatinine clearance less than 30 ml/min, dosing interval increased to 12 hr with maximum daily dosage not to exceed 200 mg. For patients with severe hepatic dysfunction, dosage reduced to 50 mg every 12 hr. For elderly patients over 75 years of age, total daily dosage reduced to 300 mg/day. For patient already receiving a benzodiazepine or other CNS depressant, initial dose of immediate-release forms may be reduced and then titrated more slowly.

E.R. CAPSULES, E.R. TABLETS

Adults not currently treated with immediate-release form of tramadol. 100 mg once daily, increased in 100-mg increments once daily every 5 days, as needed. *Maximum:* 300 mg once daily.

Adults maintained on tramadol immediate-release form. Dosage calculated using the 24-hr immediate-release dosage rounded down to the next lowest 100-mg increment. Dosage then adjusted as needed. *Maximum:* 300 mg once daily.

Drug Administration

P.O.

- Immediate-release and extended-release capsules and tablets should be swallowed whole and not chewed, crushed, or opened/broken.
- Use a calibrated device to measure oral solution dosage. Store at room temperature.

Route	Onset	Peak	Duration
P.O.	1 hr	2–3 hr	Unknown
P.O./E.R.	Unknown	4–12 hr	Unknown

Half-life: 6–10 hr

Mechanism of Action

Binds with mu receptors and inhibits the reuptake of norepinephrine and serotonin, which may account for tramadol's analgesic effect.

Contraindications

Acute or severe bronchial asthma in the absence of resuscitative equipment or unmonitored setting; children under the age of 12; hypersensitivity to tramadol opioids, or their components; known or suspected gastrointestinal obstruction, including paralytic ileus; postoperative management in children ages 12 to 18 following adenoidectomy and/or tonsillectomy; significant respiratory depression; use within 14 days of MAO inhibitor therapy

Interactions

DRUGS

5-HT3 receptor antagonists, certain muscle relaxants (cyclobenzaprine, metaxalone), drugs that affect the serotonin neurotransmitter system (mirtazapine, trazodone), selective serotonin reuptake inhibitors, serotonin and norepinephrine reuptake inhibitors, tricyclic antidepressants, triptans: Increased risk of serotonin syndrome
anticholinergics: Increased risk of urinary retention and/or severe constipation, which may lead to paralytic ileus

CYP2D6 inhibitors (bupropion, fluoxetine, paroxetine, quinidine): Decreased analgesia or increased tramadol exposure leading to increased risk for serious adverse events including seizures and serotonin syndrome.
antipsychotics, anxiolytics, benzodiazepines, CNS depressants, general anesthetics, muscle relaxants, other opioids, sedatives/hypnotics, tranquilizers: Increased risk of severe respiratory depression and possibly death
CYP3A4 inducers such as carbamazepine, phenytoin, rifampin: Decreased plasma concentration of tramadol and effectiveness with possible onset of withdrawal
CYP3A4 inhibitors such as azole antifungal agents, macrolide antibiotics, protease inhibitors: Increased plasma concentration of tramadol and risk of adverse reactions such as seizures and serotonin syndrome and adverse reactions related to opioid toxicity
digoxin: Possible digoxin toxicity
diuretics: Reduced effectiveness of diuretics
mixed agonist/antagonist, partial agonist opioid analgesics: Possible reduced analgesic effect and/or precipitation of withdrawal symptoms
MAO inhibitors such as linezolid, phenelzine, tranylcypromine: Increased risk of serotonin syndrome, opioid toxicity
muscle relaxants: Enhanced neuromuscular blocking action of skeletal muscle relaxants, increased degree of respiratory depression
warfarin: Possibly altered warfarin effects

ACTIVITIES

alcohol use: Additive CNS depression and respiratory depression that may become severe

Adverse Reactions

CNS: Agitation, anxiety, asthenia, depression, dizziness, emotional lability, euphoria, fatigue, fever, hallucinations, headache, hypertonia, hypoesthesia, insomnia, lethargy, nervousness, paresthesia, restlessness, rigors, **seizures**, **serotonin syndrome**, somnolence, **suicidal ideation**, tremor, vertigo, weakness
CV: Chest pain, orthostatic hypotension, **prolonged QT interval**, **torsades de pointes**, vasodilation
EENT: Blurred vision, dry mouth, nasal or sinus congestion, sore throat, vision changes
ENDO: **Adrenal insufficiency,** **hypoglycemia,** hot flashes

GI: Abdominal pain, anorexia, constipation, diarrhea, indigestion, nausea, vomiting
GU: Androgen deficiency, decreased libido, erectile dysfunction, impotence, infertility, lack of menstruation, urinary frequency, urine retention
MS: Arthralgia; back, limb, or neck pain
RESP: Cough, dyspnea, **respiratory depression (severe)**
SKIN: Diaphoresis, dermatitis, flushing, pruritus, rash
Other: **Anaphylaxis**, flu-like illness, **hyponatremia**, physical and psychological dependence

Childbearing Considerations

PREGNANCY

- Drug may cause fetal harm.
- Prolonged use of drug during pregnancy can result in neonatal opioid withdrawal syndrome (NOWS), which may be life-threatening if not recognized and treated.
- Avoid prolonged use during pregnancy. Use with caution only if benefit to mother outweighs potential risk to fetus.

LABOR & DELIVERY

- Drug is not recommended for use in pregnant women immediately before or during labor. Opioids may alter length of time of labor.
- Opioids cross the placental barrier and may produce respiratory depression and psycho-physiologic effects in the neonate as well as seizure activity. Monitor neonate closely.
- An opioid antagonist, such as naloxone, must be available at the time of delivery in the event it is needed to reverse opioid-induced respiratory depression in the neonate.

LACTATION

- Drug is present in breast milk.
- Breastfeeding should not take place during drug therapy.

REPRODUCTION

- Chronic use of opioids may reduce fertility in females and males.
- Drug may also produce adverse effects on male reproductive hormones and tissues, according to animal studies.

Nursing Considerations

- Be aware that tramadol shouldn't be given to patients with a history of anaphylactoid reactions to codeine or other opioids.
- Avoid giving tramadol to patients with acute abdominal conditions because it may mask evidence and disrupt assessment of the abdomen.
- Be aware that tramadol should not be given to children.
- Be aware that excessive use of tramadol may lead to abuse, addiction, misuse, overdose, and possibly death. Monitor patient's intake of drug closely and for evidence of physical dependence. Alert prescriber if patient has a history of dependence on other opioids. Be aware that a Risk Evaluation and Mitigation Strategy (REMS) is required before tramadol can be prescribed.
- Know that chronic maternal use of tramadol during pregnancy can result in neonatal opioid withdrawal syndrome (NOWS), which may be life-threatening if not recognized and treated appropriately. NOWS occurs when a newborn has been exposed to tramadol for a prolonged period while in utero.
- Use tramadol cautiously in patients who are taking antidepressant drugs or tranquilizers and in patients who use alcohol in excess or who suffer from depression or emotional disturbance.

! **WARNING** Watch for allergic reactions after giving first dose of tramadol, including angioedema, bronchospasm, pruritus, Stevens–Johnson syndrome, toxic epidermal necrolysis, and urticaria. Also watch for signs and symptoms of anaphylaxis, such as dyspnea and hypotension.

! **WARNING** Monitor patient for respiratory depression that could become life-threatening quickly, especially when drug is initiated or dosage is increased. If patient develops respiratory depression, expect to give naloxone. Watch for seizures because naloxone may increase this risk. Take seizure precautions.

- Assess respiratory status often if patient has head injury or increased intracranial pressure because of possible increased carbon dioxide retention and CSF pressure, either of which may cause respiratory depression. Also, be aware that tramadol may constrict pupils, obscuring evidence of intracranial complications.

T

! **WARNING** Monitor patient for hyponatremia (confusion, disorientation), especially in females over the age of 65 and within the first week of therapy. Know that decreased serum sodium levels are often less than 120 mmol/L, which could be life-threatening. Confirm with a serum sodium level and, if present, discontinue drug and initiate appropriate treatment such as fluid restriction, as ordered.

- Monitor patient for hypoglycemia, especially if diabetic, as hospitalization may be required. If suspected, obtain a blood glucose level and, if confirmed, treat appropriately. Notify prescriber as tramadol may have to be discontinued.

! **WARNING** Watch for seizures in patients with epilepsy, a history of seizures, or an increased risk of seizures, such as those with alcohol or drug withdrawal, CNS infection, head injury, or metabolic disorder.

- Expect to taper tramadol rather than stopping it abruptly to avoid acute withdrawal symptoms such as anxiety, diarrhea, insomnia, nausea, pain, panic attacks, paresthesias, piloerection, rigors, sweating, tremor, and upper respiratory symptoms.

! **WARNING** Know that many drugs may interact with tramadol to cause serotonin syndrome. Monitor patient closely for signs and symptoms such as agitation, diaphoresis, diarrhea, fever, hallucinations, labile blood pressure, muscle twitching or stiffness, nausea, shakiness, shivering, tachycardia, trouble with coordination, or vomiting. Notify prescriber at once because serotonin syndrome may be life-threatening. Be prepared to discontinue drug, if possible and ordered, and provide supportive care.

- Monitor patient for adrenal insufficiency. Although rare, it can be life-threatening. Monitor patient for anorexia, dizziness, fatigue, hypotension, nausea, vomiting, or weakness. Notify prescriber if adrenal insufficiency is suspected and expect diagnostic testing to be done. If confirmed, expect to administer corticosteroids and wean patient off tramadol, if possible.

- Monitor patient closely for evidence of suicidal thinking or behavior, especially when therapy starts or dosage changes.

! **WARNING** Be aware that tramadol should only be used concomitantly with benzodiazepine therapy in patients for whom other treatment options are inadequate. If prescribed together, expect dosing and duration of tramadol to be limited. Monitor patient closely for signs and symptoms of a decrease in consciousness, including coma, profound sedation, and significant respiratory depression. Notify prescriber immediately and provide emergency supportive care, as death may occur.

PATIENT TEACHING

- Urge patient to follow prescribed dose limits and dosing intervals to prevent respiratory depression and seizures. Warn patient that excessive or prolonged use can lead to abuse, addiction, misuse, overdose, and possibly death. Encourage patient and family/caretaker to have naloxone on hand in the event of an accidental overdose. Instruct family/caregiver on signs and symptoms of an opioid overdose and how to use naloxone. Stress importance of calling 911 immediately if naloxone is administered.
- Instruct patient prescribed immediate-release tablets or extended-release form to swallow capsule or tablet whole and not to chew, crush, or split tablet/open capsule.
- Tell patient to use a calibrated measuring device and not a household spoon to measure oral solution dosage. Tell patient to store oral solution at room temperature.

! **WARNING** Instruct patient to seek immediate emergency medical care and to stop taking tramadol if a serious allergic reaction occurs.

- Caution patient not to stop tramadol abruptly.
- Instruct patient to avoid hazardous activities until drug's CNS effects are known.
- Warn patient not to consume alcohol or take a benzodiazepine without prescriber knowledge, as severe respiratory depression can occur and may lead to death.
- Inform patient that long-term use of tramadol may decrease sex hormone levels, causing decreased libido, erectile

dysfunction, impotence, infertility, or lack of menstruation. Encourage patient to report any symptoms to prescriber.
- Urge patient to notify prescriber about known, suspected, or intended pregnancy.
- Tell mothers wishing to breastfeed that it is not recommended during drug therapy.
- Urge caregivers to watch patient closely for evidence of suicidal tendencies, especially when therapy starts or dosage changes, and to report concerns at once to prescriber.
- Tell patient to notify prescriber immediately if he develops any persistent, severe, sudden, or unusual adverse reactions.
- Instruct patient to inform all prescribers of tramadol therapy because of potential drug interactions.
- Caution patient to keep tramadol out of the reach of children because even one dose could result in a fatal overdose in a child.
- Warn patient that tramadol may cause severe constipation. Advise patient to maintain adequate hydration, increase fiber in diet, and to seek treatment instructions from prescriber if constipation occurs and is not relieved soon after onset.
- Instruct patient how to dispose of unused tramadol in accordance with local state guidelines and/or regulations.

trazodone hydrochloride

Class and Category
Pharmacologic class: Triazolopyridine derivative
Therapeutic class: Antidepressant

Indications and Dosages
* *To treat major depression*

TABLETS
Adults. 150 mg in divided doses daily, increased by 50 mg/day every 3 to 4 days. *Maximum for outpatients:* 400 mg daily in divided doses. *Maximum for inpatients experiencing more severe depression:* 600 mg daily in divided doses.

Drug Administration
P.O.
- Give drug after a meal or light snack to reduce dizziness.

- Give larger portion of daily dose at bedtime if drowsiness occurs.
- Tablets should be swallowed and not chewed or crushed. Tablet should only be broken along the score lines.

Route	Onset	Peak	Duration
P.O.	Unknown	1–2 hr	Unknown

Half-life: 5–9 hr

Mechanism of Action
Blocks serotonin reuptake along the presynaptic neuronal membrane, causing an antidepressant effect. Trazodone exerts an alpha-adrenergic blocking action and produces modest histamine blockade, causing a sedative effect. It also inhibits the vasopressor response to norepinephrine, which reduces blood pressure.

Contraindications
Hypersensitivity to trazodone or its components, use within 14 days of an MAO inhibitor including intravenous methylene blue and linezolid

Interactions
DRUGS
antibiotics (gatifloxacin), antipsychotics (chlorpromazine, thioridazine, ziprasidone), class IA antiarrhythmics (disopyramide, procainamide, quinidine), class 3 antiarrhythmics (amiodarone, sotalol): Increased risk of prolonged QT interval and cardiac arrhythmia
anticoagulants such as clopidogrel, dabigatran, rivaroxaban, warfarin; antiplatelets such as aspirin: Increased risk of bleeding
barbiturates and other CNS depressants: Enhanced effect of CNS depressants
CYP3A4 inducers (strong) such as carbamazepine, phenytoin, rifampin, St. John's wort: Decreased exposure of trazodone decreasing effectiveness
CYP3A4 inhibitors (strong) such as clarithromycin, indinavir, itraconazole, ketoconazole, and ritonavir: Possibly increased plasma trazodone levels with increased risk of adverse reactions
digoxin, phenytoin: Possibly increased blood levels of these drugs and increased risk of toxicity
MAO inhibitors; other serotonergic drugs such as buspirone, fentanyl, lithium, serotonin

T

uptake inhibitor antidepressants, St. John's wort, tramadol, tricyclic antidepressants, triptans, tryptophan: Increased serotonin effects

ACTIVITIES

alcohol use: Increased CNS depression, risk of hypotension and respiratory depression

Adverse Reactions

CNS: Abnormal coordination or dreams, agitation, anxiety, aphasia, ataxia, balance disorder, chills, confusion, **CVA**, dizziness, drowsiness, extrapyramidal symptoms, fatigue, hallucinations, headache, insomnia, light-headedness, memory impairment, migraine, nervousness, paresthesia, paranoid reaction, psychosis, **seizures, serotonin syndrome**, somnolence, stupor, **suicidal ideation**, syncope, tardive dyskinesia, tremor, vertigo, weakness

CV: Arrhythmias, congestive heart failure, edema, **hypotension**, orthostatic hypotension, palpitations, **prolonged QT interval**, vasodilation

EENT: Angle-closure glaucoma, blurred vision, diplopia, dry mouth

ENDO: Inappropriate ADH syndrome

GI: Abdominal pain, cholestasis, constipation, diarrhea, elevated bilirubin or liver enzymes, indigestion, jaundice, nausea, vomiting

GU: Anorgasmia; ejaculation disorders; decreased libido; priapism; urinary incontinence, retention, or urgency

HEME: Hemolytic anemia, leukocytosis

MS: Back pain, myalgia

RESP: Apnea, dyspnea

SKIN: Alopecia, hirsutism, night sweats, pruritus, psoriasis, rash, urticaria

Other: Hyponatremia

Childbearing Considerations

PREGNANCY

- Pregnancy exposure registry: 1-844-405-6185 or https:/womensmentalhealth.org/clinical-and-research-programs/pregnancyregistry/antidepressants/.
- It is not known if drug can cause fetal harm.
- Use with caution only if benefit to mother outweighs potential risk to fetus.

LACTATION

- Drug may be present in breast milk.
- Patient should check with prescriber before breastfeeding.

Nursing Considerations

- Use trazodone cautiously in patients with cardiac disease, because drug can cause arrhythmias.
- Expect most patients who respond to trazodone to do so by the end of the second week of therapy.
- Closely monitor depressed patients for suicidal thoughts and tendencies. Notify prescriber if they occur, and take suicide precautions according to facility policy.

! WARNING Monitor patient closely for serotonin syndrome exhibited by agitation, coma, diarrhea, hallucinations, hyperreflexia, hyperthermia, incoordination, labile blood pressure, nausea, tachycardia, and vomiting. Notify prescriber immediately, because serotonin syndrome may be life-threatening; provide supportive care.

- Be aware that adverse CNS reactions usually improve after patient completes a few weeks of therapy.

! WARNING Be aware that trazodone therapy may increase the risk of priapism.

PATIENT TEACHING

- Urge patient to avoid taking trazodone on an empty stomach because doing so may increase the risk of dizziness or light-headedness.
- Advise patient that drug may cause mild pupillary dilation, which may lead to an episode of acute angle-closure glaucoma. Encourage patient to have an eye exam before starting therapy to see if he is at risk.
- Caution patient to avoid potentially hazardous activities during therapy until nervous system effects have abated.
- Advise patient not to fast during trazodone therapy because of possible adverse CNS reactions.
- Instruct male patient to notify prescriber immediately about priapism.
- Caution patient not to take aspirin or nonsteroidal anti-inflammatory agents without first discussing use with the prescriber.
- Instruct patient not to stop trazodone therapy abruptly.

- Urge family and caregivers to watch patient closely for abnormal thinking or behavior or increased aggression or hostility. Emphasize importance of notifying prescriber about unusual changes.

triamcinolone

triamcinolone acetonide
Kenalog-10, Kenalog-40, Kenalog-80, Nasacort Allergy 24 Hour, Zilretta

Class and Category
Pharmacologic class: Glucocorticoid
Therapeutic class: Corticosteroid

Indications and Dosages
✳ *To treat a multitude of disorders exhibiting severe inflammation or need for immunosuppression*

I.M. INJECTION (KENALOG-40, KENALOG-80)
Adults. 2.5 to 100 mg daily depending on specific disease entity being treated. *Suggested initial dosage:* 60 mg daily, increased or decreased according to response and duration of relief. *Usual:* 40 to 80 mg, but lower or higher doses may be needed. Dosage adjusted as needed.
Children. *Initial:* 0.11 to 1.6 mg/kg daily in 3 or 4 divided doses. Dosage adjusted as needed.

✳ *To treat hay fever or pollen asthma in patients not responding to pollen administration and other conventional therapy*

I.M. INJECTION (KENALOG-40, KENALOG-80)
Adults. 40 to 100 mg as a single dose for the pollen season.

✳ *To treat acute exacerbations of multiple sclerosis*

I.M. INJECTION (KENALOG-40, KENALOG-80)
Adults. 160 mg for one wk, followed by 64 mg every other day for one month.

✳ *To relieve inflammation caused by acute gouty arthritis, acute nonspecific tenosynovitis, acute or subacute bursitis, epicondylitis, rheumatoid arthritis, and synovitis*

INTRA-ARTICULAR INJECTION (KENALOG-10, KENALOG-40)
Adults. 2.5 to 5 mg for smaller joints and 5 to 15 mg for larger joints, as needed; dosage increased up to 10 mg for smaller joints; up to 40 mg for larger joints, as needed (Kenalog-40).

✳ *To relieve osteoarthritis pain of the knee*

E.R. INTRA-ARTICULAR INJECTION (ZILRETTA)
Adults. 32 mg injected as a single dose in the knee.

✳ *To relieve symptoms of perennial and seasonal allergic rhinitis*

NASAL SPRAY (NASACORT ALLERGY 24 HOUR)
Adults and children age 12 and over. *Initial:* 220 mcg (2 sprays) in each nostril once daily until symptoms improve. *Maintenance:* 110 mcg (1 spray) in each nostril once a day.
Children ages 6 to 12. *Initial:* 110 mcg (1 spray) in each nostril once a day, increased to 220 mcg (2 sprays) in each nostril once a day, as needed, with dosage reduced when symptoms improve. *Maintenance:* 110 mcg (1 spray) in each nostril daily. *Maximum:* 220 mcg or 4 sprays daily.
Children ages 2 to 6. 110 mcg (1 spray) daily in each nostril.

Drug Administration
I.M.
- Shake vial before withdrawing to ensure a uniform suspension.
- Inspect suspension for clumping or granular appearance. If present, do not use.
- Inject immediately after withdrawing from vial and inject deeply into the gluteal muscle.
- A longer needle length may be required in obese patients.
- Rotate sites.

INTRA-ARTICULAR
Kenalog
- Shake vial before withdrawing to ensure a uniform suspension.
- Inspect suspension for clumping or granular appearance. If present, do not use.
- Prescriber should inject immediately after drug is withdrawn from vial.
Zilretta
- Drug is supplied as a single-dose kit.
- Use only diluent supplied in the kit and follow manufacturer guidelines for preparation.

T

- Once diluted, expect prescriber to inject drug immediately to avoid settling of the suspension, or store drug in vial for up to 4 hours at room temperature. Gently swirl vial to resuspend suspension prior to withdrawing drug from vial.
- Do not interchange drug with other formulations of injectable triamcinolone acetonide.

NASAL

- Shake container well before each use.
- Prime container by releasing 5 sprays into the air before first use. If drug not used for 2 weeks or more, reprime by releasing 1 spray before use.
- Have patient gently blow nose before administration.
- Insert nozzle into nostril, pointing away from the septum. Hold other nostril closed and have patient sniff gently while spraying.
- Do not have patient blow nose for at least 15 minutes after administration.

Route	Onset	Peak	Duration
I.M.	24–48 hr	Unknown	30–40 days
Intra-articular	>12 hr	7 hr	28–42 days
Nasal	Unknown	1.5 hr	Unknown

Half-life: 88 min

≡ Mechanism of Action

Triamcinolone:

- decreases peribronchial edema and mucus secretion by inhibiting the binding of allergens to immunoglobulin E antibodies on the surface of mast cells, thereby inactivating the release of chemotactic substances
- decreases inflammation by interfering with leukocyte adhesion to capillary walls
- inhibits the release of leukocytic acid hydrolases, preventing macrophage accumulation at the infection site
- inhibits histamine and kinin release, preventing the formation of scar tissue.

≡ Contraindications

Hypersensitivity to triamcinolone or its components, idiopathic thrombocytopenic purpura (I.M. injection)

≡ Interactions

DRUGS

aminoglutethimide: Possible loss of corticosteroid-induced adrenal suppression

amphotericin B, potassium-depleting agents such as diuretics: Increased risk of hypokalemia
aspirin, NSAIDs: Increased risk of gastrointestinal adverse effects
cholestyramine: Possible increased clearance of corticosteroids
cholinesterase inhibitors: Increased risk of severe muscle weakness in patients with myasthenia gravis
cyclosporine: Possible additive effects of both drugs' activity; increased risk of seizures
CYP3A4 inhibitors such as atazanavir, clarithromycin, cobicistat-containing products, indinavir, itraconazole, ketoconazole, nefazodone, nelfinavir, ritonavir, saquinavir, telithromycin: Decreased triamcinolone clearance, increased risk of adverse effects
digitalis glycosides: Increased risk of arrhythmias and digitalis toxicity
estrogens including oral contraceptives: Increased triamcinolone effects
hepatic enzyme inducers such as barbiturates, carbamazepine, phenytoin, insulin, oral antidiabetic drugs: Increased blood glucose level
isoniazid: Possible decreased concentrations of isoniazid and its effectiveness
macrolide antibiotics: Significant decrease in corticosteroid clearance
toxoids, vaccines: Decreased response to toxoids and vaccines
warfarin: Possible inhibition of response to warfarin

≡ Adverse Reactions

CNS: Depression, dizziness, emotional lability, exacerbated psychosis, fatigue, headache, **increased intracranial pressure with papilledema (pseudotumor cerebri)**, insomnia, malaise, neuritis, neuropathy, paresthesia, personality changes, psychiatric disorders, restlessness, **seizures**, vertigo
CV: Edema, **heart failure**, hypertension
EENT: Altered sense of smell or taste, cataracts, dry mouth, epistaxis (nasal form), glaucoma, hoarseness, nasal congestion, nasal irritation (nasal form), nasal septal perforation (nasal form), oropharyngeal candidiasis, pharyngitis, posterior subcapsular cataracts, rhinorrhea, secondary ocular infection, sinusitis, sneezing
ENDO: Cushing's syndrome, diabetes mellitus, growth retardation (children)

GI: Abdominal pain, constipation, diarrhea, dyspepsia, esophageal ulceration, gastritis, nausea, vomiting

GU: Altered motility and number of spermatozoa, cystitis, postmenopausal **vaginal hemorrhage**, renal disease, UTI, vaginitis

MS: Bone mineral density loss, bursitis, muscle wasting or weakness, myalgia, osteoporosis, tenosynovitis

RESP: **Asthma**, bronchitis, chest congestion, dyspnea, increased cough

SKIN: Ecchymosis, petechiae (parenteral form), photosensitivity, pruritus, rash, striae, urticaria

Other: **Anaphylaxis; angioedema;** decreased resistance to infections; flu-like symptoms; herpes infection; hiccups; impaired wound healing; injection-site atrophy, induration, pain, soreness, and sterile abscess; moon face; weight gain

⊞ Childbearing Considerations

PREGNANCY

- It is not known if drug can cause fetal harm.
- Use with caution only if benefit to mother outweighs potential risk to fetus.
- Infants born to mothers receiving drug during pregnancy should be monitored for hypoadrenalism.

LACTATION

- Drug is present in breast milk.
- Patient should check with prescriber before breastfeeding because drug could interfere with endogenous corticosteroid production, suppress growth, or cause other adverse reactions.

⊞ Nursing Considerations

- Be aware that high doses of corticosteroids such as triamcinolone aren't recommended for patients with cranial trauma who don't require a corticosteroid for another condition, because they increase risk of death.
- Know that triamcinolone should be administered with extreme caution, if at all, in patients who have active or quiescent tuberculosis infection of the respiratory tract, ocular herpes simplex, systemic parasitic or viral infection, or untreated bacterial or fungal infection, because this drug can make these infections worse.
- Use cautiously in patients with active or latent peptic ulcer, diverticulitis, fresh intestinal

anastomoses, and nonspecific ulcerative colitis; there is increased risk of a perforation for these patients. Be aware that signs of peritoneal irritation following gastrointestinal perforation in patients receiving steroid therapy may be minimal or absent.

- Monitor patient with cirrhosis carefully for an enhanced drug effect because increased metabolism of steroids may occur in the presence of cirrhosis.
- Be aware that triamcinolone may reactivate tuberculosis in patients who have a history of it.

! **WARNING** Monitor patient for hypersensitivity. Although rare, triamcinolone has caused anaphylaxis that ended in death. Notify prescriber immediately if hypersensitivity occurs; expect to discontinue triamcinolone therapy and provide emergency supportive care.

- Monitor patients for exposure to high doses, which may result in toxicity evidenced by life-threatening hypotension and metabolic acidosis.

! **WARNING** Know that patients on corticosteroid therapy require an increased dosage of rapidly acting corticosteroids when unusual stress is anticipated, during the stressful event, and for a period after the stressful situation. Assess patient for signs and symptoms of adrenal insufficiency (fatigue, hypotension, lassitude, nausea, vomiting, and weakness) during times of stress, such as infection, surgery, or trauma. Notify prescriber immediately if you detect these signs and symptoms because adrenal insufficiency may be life-threatening. Drug-induced secondary adrenocortical insufficiency may be minimized by gradual reduction of dosage.

- Be aware that, although rare, bone mineral density loss and osteoporosis may occur, which may increase risk of fractures, especially in patients on prolonged triamcinolone therapy.
- Adjust triamcinolone dosage, as prescribed, in patients with changes in thyroid status because metabolic clearance of corticosteroids is decreased in hypothyroid patients and increased in hyperthyroid patients.

T

- Assess patient for signs and symptoms of infection (abnormal symptoms in particular body system, fever, or malaise), because steroid therapy such as triamcinolone increases risk of susceptibility to infections, especially with higher dosages.

PATIENT TEACHING

- Caution patient not to adjust dosage for prescription triamcinolone without consulting prescriber and to follow dosage recommendations when using an over-the-counter preparation.
- Teach patient how to use nasal spray, including how to prime spray pump bottle before use. Caution patient not to get nasal spray in eyes. If this occurs, patient should rinse his eyes well with water.
- Inform patient that maximum benefit of triamcinolone therapy may not occur for up to 2 weeks.

! **WARNING** Alert patient that drug may cause an allergic reaction. Advise patient to notify prescriber if present and if serious to seek immediate medical care.

- Caution patient to avoid exposure to people who have chickenpox or measles, as well as other contagious infections, throughout triamcinolone therapy and for 12 months afterward.
- Advise patient to have periodic eye examinations during long-term therapy because triamcinolone can cause glaucoma or ocular nerve damage.

triamterene
Dyrenium

☰ Class and Category
Pharmacologic class: Potassium-sparing diuretic
Therapeutic class: Diuretic

☰ Indications and Dosages
✽ *To treat edema in cirrhosis, heart failure, and nephrotic syndrome, as well as edema secondary to hyperaldosteronism, idiopathic edema, and steroid-induced edema*

CAPSULES

Adults. *Initial:* 100 mg twice daily and adjusted as needed. *Maximum:* 300 mg daily.

☰ Drug Administration
P.O.
- Administer drug after meals.

Route	Onset	Peak	Duration
P.O.	2–4 hr	1–3 hr	7–9 hr

Half-life: 1.5–2 hr

☰ Mechanism of Action
Inhibits sodium reabsorption in distal convoluted tubules and cortical collecting ducts, causing sodium and water loss and enhancing potassium retention.

☰ Contraindications
Anuria; concurrent therapy with other agents containing triamterene or potassium agents such as potassium-sparing agents (amiloride, spironolactone), potassium salts, potassium substitutes, or potassium supplements; hypersensitivity to triamterene or its components; progressive or severe kidney disease or dysfunction with possible exception of nephrosis; severe hepatic disease

☰ Interactions
DRUGS
ACE inhibitors, potassium-containing drugs such as penicillin G potassium, potassium salts, potassium-sparing diuretics, potassium supplements: Increased risk of hyperkalemia
antihypertensives, anesthetic agents, other diuretics, pre-anesthetic agents, skeletal muscle relaxants (non-depolarizing): Possibly potentiated effects of these drugs
chlorpropamide: Possible increased risk of severe hyponatremia
indomethacin: Increased risk of renal impairment
lithium: Increased risk of lithium toxicity
oral antidiabetic drugs: Altered blood glucose control

☰ Adverse Reactions
CNS: Dizziness, fatigue, headache, weakness
EENT: Dry mouth
ENDO: Hyperglycemia, **hypoglycemia**
GI: Diarrhea, jaundice, nausea, vomiting
GU: **Azotemia**, elevated BUN and serum creatinine levels, renal calculi
SKIN: Photosensitivity, rash

Childbearing Considerations

PREGNANCY

- It is not known if drug can cause fetal harm.
- Use with caution only if benefit to mother outweighs potential risk to fetus.

LACTATION

- It is not known if drug is present in breast milk.
- Breastfeeding is not recommended during drug therapy.

Nursing Considerations

- Be aware that triamterene shouldn't be given to patient with creatinine clearance below 10 ml/min because this condition increases the risk of drug-induced hyperkalemia.
- Monitor serum potassium level during therapy, especially in patient with diabetes mellitus or renal impairment. Also monitor patient's BUN and serum creatinine levels to assess renal function and prevent hyperkalemia.
- Monitor patient for irregular heartbeat, which is usually the first sign of hyperkalemia. If you suspect hyperkalemia, obtain an ECG tracing, as ordered. A widened QRS complex or an arrhythmia requires prompt additional therapy.
- Monitor laboratory test results and watch for signs of metabolic or respiratory acidosis, which may occur suddenly in patient with cardiac disease or uncontrolled diabetes mellitus.
- Monitor patient's serum sodium and uric acid levels, as ordered, because triamterene may worsen preexisting hyponatremia and reduce uric acid clearance, increasing the risk of gout and hyperuricemia.
- Monitor CBC with differential because drug may increase the risk of megaloblastic anemia in patient with folic acid deficiency.

PATIENT TEACHING

- Advise patient to take triamterene after meals.
- Instruct patient to avoid exposure to excessive heat or sunlight to prevent dehydration and, possibly, photosensitivity.
- Explain to patient with a history of gout that drug may increase the risk of attack.
- Advise patient to notify prescriber about ineffective diuresis and unexplained weight gain during therapy.

triazolam
Halcion

Class, Category, and Schedule

Pharmacologic class: Benzodiazepine
Therapeutic class: Sedative-hypnotic
Controlled substance schedule: IV

Indications and Dosages

＊ *To provide short-term management of insomnia*

TABLETS

Adults. 0.25 mg once nightly. *Maximum:* 0.5 mg daily (for patients with inadequate response to usual dose). For patients with low body weight, initial dosage reduced to 0.125 mg.

±**DOSAGE ADJUSTMENT** For elderly or debilitated patients, initial dosage not to exceed 0.125 mg and maximum dosage limited to 0.25 mg daily.

Drug Administration

P.O.

- Administer at bedtime.
- Do not administer with grapefruit juice.

Route	Onset	Peak	Duration
P.O.	15–30 min	0.5–2 hr	6–7 hr

Half-life: 1.5–5.5 hr

Mechanism of Action

Potentiates effects of the inhibitory neurotransmitter gamma-aminobutyric acid, which increases inhibition of the ascending reticular activating system and produces varying levels of CNS depression, including anticonvulsant activity, coma, hypnosis, sedation, and skeletal muscle relaxation.

Contraindications

Concurrent therapy with strong CYP3A inhibitors (itraconazole, ketoconazole, lopinavir, nefazodone, ritonavir); hypersensitivity to triazolam, other benzodiazepines, or their components

Interactions

DRUGS

CNS depressants, other benzodiazepines including anticonvulsants, antihistamines, psychotropic drugs: Additive depressant effects that could become severe, especially respiratory depression and severe sedation

T

CYP3A inducers: Decreased plasma concentration of triazolam significantly decreasing effectiveness

CYP3A inhibitors such as cimetidine, clarithromycin, erythromycin, indinavir, isoniazid, itraconazole, ketoconazole, lopinavir, nefazodone, nelfinavir, oral contraceptives, saquinavir: Increased triazolam concentrations, increased risk of adverse reactions

opioids: Increased risk of respiratory depression or significant worsening of opioid-related respiratory depression

FOODS
grapefruit juice: Increased blood triazolam level and adverse reactions

ACTIVITIES
alcohol use: Increased sedation, respiratory depression that could become severe

Adverse Reactions

CNS: Abnormal behavior, aggression, agitation, anterograde amnesia, altered state of consciousness, anxiety, ataxia, complex behaviors (such as sleep driving), confusion, coordination disorders, delusion, depression, dizziness, drowsiness, dystonia, euphoria, fatigue, grogginess, hallucination, headache, insomnia, irritability, light-headedness, mania, memory impairment, nervousness, nightmares, restlessness, sedation, somnambulism, somnolence, syncope, talkativeness, tremor, vertigo

CV: Chest pain, tachycardia

EENT: Blepharitis, glossitis, stomatitis, taste disturbance, **throat tightness**, tongue discomfort, visual disturbances

GI: Abdominal distress, anorexia, constipation, jaundice, nausea, vomiting

GU: Bladder disorders, libido disorder, menstruation irregularity, urinary incontinence or retention

MS: Aching limbs; backache; dysarthria; muscle cramps, pain, spasticity

RESP: Dyspnea

SKIN: Pruritis

Other: **Anaphylaxis**, **angioedema**, paradoxical drug reaction, physical and psychological dependence, protracted withdrawal syndrome

Childbearing Considerations

PREGNANCY
- Pregnancy exposure registry: 1-866-961-2388 or https://womensmentalhealth.org/clinical-and-research-programs/pregnancyregistry/othermedications/.
- Drug may cause fetal harm if given during the later stages of pregnancy, such as feeding problems, respiratory depression, sedation, and withdrawal at birth.
- Use with caution only if benefit to mother outweighs potential risk to fetus.

LACTATION
- It is not known if drug is present in breast milk.
- Breastfeeding is recommended to be withheld during treatment and for 28 hours after last dose.
- If breastfeeding takes place during drug therapy, monitor infant for feeding problems, respiratory depression, sedation, and withdrawal symptoms (when drug therapy is stopped).

Nursing Considerations
- Evaluate patient's risk for abuse, addiction, and misuse before administering drug for the first time as use of triazolam exposes patient to these risks, which can lead to overdose or death.

! **WARNING** Be aware that triazolam shouldn't be discontinued abruptly, even after only 1 to 2 weeks of therapy. Doing so can cause withdrawal symptoms that could be life-threatening. Monitor patient for abdominal cramps, confusion, depression, diaphoresis, hyperacusis, insomnia, irritability, nausea, nervousness, paresthesia, perceptual disturbances, photophobia, tachycardia, tremor, and vomiting and alert prescriber immediately, if present.

! **WARNING** Assess patient for signs of physical and psychological dependence, and notify prescriber if they occur.

- Monitor patient's ABG results and respiratory depth and rate, as appropriate, because drug may worsen ventilatory failure in patient with pulmonary disease, such as respiratory depression, severe COPD, or sleep apnea. Use drug cautiously in patients with acute intermittent porphyria, myasthenia gravis, and severe renal impairment because it may aggravate these conditions.
- Take safety precautions for elderly patients because triazolam may impair cognitive

and motor function and increase the risk for falls.

- Use drug cautiously in patients with advanced Parkinson's disease because it may worsen cognition, coordination, and psychosis.

! **WARNING** Monitor patient closely for hypersensitivity reactions such as dyspnea, nausea, swelling, throat tightness, and vomiting. If present, stop triazolam immediately, notify prescriber, and provide supportive care.

! **WARNING** Be aware that opioids should only be used concomitantly with benzodiazepine therapy like triazolam in patients for whom other treatment options are inadequate. If prescribed together, expect dosing and duration of the opioid to be limited. Monitor patient closely for signs and symptoms of a decrease in consciousness, including coma, profound sedation, and significant respiratory depression. Notify prescriber immediately and provide emergency supportive care, as death may occur.

PATIENT TEACHING

- Instruct patient to take triazolam exactly as prescribed and not to stop taking it abruptly if taken for more than 2 weeks, because of the risk of having withdrawal symptoms. Alert patient that a protracted withdrawal syndrome lasting weeks to more than 12 months may occur in some patients if drug is abruptly stopped.

! **WARNING** Instruct patient to seek emergency care if she has abnormal swelling, nausea, throat tightness, trouble breathing, or vomiting.

- Advise patient that drug may cause abnormal behaviors during sleep, such as driving a car, eating, having sex, or talking on the phone without any recall of the event. If family notices any such behavior or patient sees evidence of such behavior upon awakening, the prescriber should be notified.
- Caution patient about possible drowsiness during therapy and to avoid performing hazardous activities, if

present. Also, tell patient to take fall precautions.

- Urge patient to avoid alcohol consumption and opioid use because these increase drug's sedative effects, including respiratory depression which can become severe, and risk of abnormal behaviors, such as sleep driving. Also advise patient to avoid grapefruit juice, as it may increase triazolam levels and increase risk of adverse reactions.
- Advise patient to notify prescriber about excessive drowsiness, known or suspected pregnancy, and nausea.
- Instruct patient to inform all prescribers of triazolam use, especially when pain medication may be prescribed.

trospium chloride
Sanctura

≡ Class and Category
Pharmacologic class: Antimuscarinic
Therapeutic class: Bladder antispasmodic

≡ Indications and Dosages
⁎ *To treat overactive bladder with symptoms of urge urinary incontinence, urgency, and urinary frequency*

TABLETS
Adults. 20 mg twice daily.
±**DOSAGE ADJUSTMENT** For patients with severe renal insufficiency (creatinine clearance less than 30 ml/min) and patients age 75 or over, dosage reduced to 20 mg daily.

≡ Drug Administration
P.O.
- Administer with water on an empty stomach 1 hour before meals.
- For patient with severe renal impairment, administer the once-daily dose at bedtime.

Route	Onset	Peak	Duration
P.O.	Unknown	5–6 hr	Unknown

Half-life: 20–35 hr

≡ Mechanism of Action
Antagonizes the effect of acetylcholine on muscarinic receptors in the bladder. Trospium's parasympatholytic action

reduces the tonus of smooth muscle in the bladder. These actions increase maximum cystometric bladder capacity and volume with the first detrusor contraction, which relieves the sensation of frequency and urgency and enhances bladder control.

Contraindications

Gastric retention, hypersensitivity to trospium or its components, uncontrolled angle-closure glaucoma, urine retention

Interactions

DRUGS

anticholinergics: Increased frequency or severity of adverse effects
metformin: Decreased systemic exposure of trospium
morphine, pancuronium, procainamide, tenofovir, vancomycin: Possibly increased plasma concentration of all these drugs as well as trospium
orally administered drugs: Possibly altered absorption of some of these drugs

Adverse Reactions

CNS: Confusion, delirium, dizziness, drowsiness, fatigue, fever, hallucinations, headache, insomnia, light-headedness, syncope
CV: Chest pain, **hypertensive crisis**, palpitations, tachycardia
EENT: Blurred vision; dry eyes, mouth, or throat; visual abnormalities
GI: Abdominal distention or pain, constipation, flatulence, gastritis, indigestion, vomiting
GU: Urine retention
MS: **Rhabdomyolysis**
SKIN: Decreased sweating, dry skin, flushing, rash, **Stevens–Johnson syndrome**
Other: **Anaphylaxis**, **angioedema**

Childbearing Considerations

PREGNANCY

- It is not known if drug can cause fetal harm.
- Use with caution only if benefit to mother outweighs potential risk to fetus.

LACTATION

- It is not known if drug is present in breast milk.
- Patient should check with prescriber before breastfeeding.

Nursing Considerations

- Use trospium cautiously in patients with intestinal atony, myasthenia gravis, or ulcerative colitis because drug may decrease GI motility; patients with significant bladder outflow obstruction because drug may cause urine retention; patients with hepatic impairment because drug's effects on the liver are unknown; and patients with renal impairment because drug excretion may be impaired.

! WARNING Monitor patient for hypersensitivity reactions, which may become severe, such as anaphylaxis and angioedema. Notify prescriber immediately, if present, expect drug to be discontinued, and provide supportive care, as ordered.

- Monitor elderly patients carefully, especially those age 75 or over, for adverse reactions because elderly patients have an increased risk of trospium-induced adverse reactions.
- Monitor patient for anticholinergic central nervous system adverse effects such as confusion, dizziness, hallucinations, and somnolence. If present, notify prescriber and expect a dose reduction or drug to be discontinued.

PATIENT TEACHING

- Instruct patient to take trospium on an empty stomach or at least 1 hour before eating because food delays its absorption. Tell patient with severe renal impairment to take the drug once a day at bedtime.
- Caution patient to avoid performing activities in a warm or hot environment because sweating may be delayed, which could cause a sudden increase in body temperature and heatstroke.
- Advise patient to avoid hazardous activities until drug's CNS effects are known.

! WARNING Emphasize importance of reporting allergic reactions, including swelling of her face, lips, throat, or tongue; stopping trospium therapy; and seeking emergency medical care immediately.

- Advise patient to notify prescriber if he develops confusion, dizziness, hallucinations, or somnolence, as dosage may have to be altered or drug discontinued.

turoctocog alfa pegol
(N8-GP or antihemophilic factor [recombinant], glycopegylated-exei)
Esperoct

Class and Category
Pharmacologic class: Coagulation factor VIII
Therapeutic class: Coagulant

Indications and Dosages
* *To provide on-demand treatment and control of bleeding episodes*

I.V. INFUSION
Adults and children 12 years and older.
For minor bleeding: 40 international units as a single dose. *For moderate bleeding:* 40 international units followed by an additional dose after 24 hr, if needed. *For major bleeding:* 50 international units followed by additional doses, every 24 hr, as needed.
Children less than 12 years of age. *For minor bleeding:* 65 international units as a single dose. *For moderate bleeding:* 65 international units followed by an additional dose after 24 hr, if needed. *For major bleeding:* 65 international units followed by additional doses, every 24 hr, as needed.

* *To provide perioperative management of bleeding*

I.V. INFUSION
Adults and children 12 years and older. *For minor bleeding:* 50 international units, with additional doses given after 24 hr, if needed. *For major bleeding:* 50 international units, with additional doses that may be given every 24 hr for the first week and then every 48 hr until wound healing has occurred.
Children less than 12 years of age. *For minor bleeding:* 65 international units, with additional doses given after 24 hr, if needed. *For major bleeding:* 65 international units with additional doses that may be given every 24 hr for the first week and then every 48 hr until wound healing has occurred.

* *To provide routine prophylaxis to reduce the frequency of bleeding episodes*

I.V. INFUSION
Adults and children 12 years and older.
Initial: 50 international units/kg every 4 days. Regimen then adjusted to less or more frequent dosing based on bleeding episodes.
Children less than 12 years of age. *Initial:* 65 international units/kg twice weekly. Regimen then adjusted to less or more frequent dosing based on bleeding episodes.

±**DOSAGE ADJUSTMENT** Dosing also may be adjusted to achieve a specific target Factor VIII activity level using the following formula:
Dosage (IU) = Body weight (kg) × desired Factor VIII increase (IU/dl or % normal) × 0.5

Drug Administration
I.V.
- Reconstitute drug (if dose requires more than one vial per infusion, reconstitute each vial separately) by first bringing drug vial and prefilled diluent syringe to room temperature. Remove plastic cap from vial. Wipe rubber stopper on vial with a sterile alcohol swab and allow it to dry prior to use. Remove protective paper from vial adapter. Do not remove vial adapter from protective cap. Place vial on a flat and solid surface. While holding the protective cap, place vial adapter over vial and press down firmly on the protective cap until vial adapter spike penetrates the rubber stopper. Carefully remove protective cap from vial adapter. Grasp plunger rod and attach plunger rod to syringe by holding plunger rod by the wide top end. Turn plunger rod clockwise into rubber plunger inside prefilled diluent syringe until resistance is felt. Break off syringe cap from prefilled diluent syringe by snapping at the perforation of cap. Connect prefilled diluent syringe to vial adapter by turning it clockwise until it is secured. Push the plunger rod to slowly inject all the diluent into vial.
- Without removing the syringe, gently swirl vial until all the powder is dissolved. Avoid shaking the vial and foaming the solution.
- Inspect the diluted solution for particulate matter and discoloration. Solution should be clear and have no particles.
- Do not administer drug in the same tubing or container with other drugs.
- Administer the diluted solution immediately or store solution in the vial,

T

with the vial adapter and syringe attached, at room temperature for up to 4 hours, or in refrigerator for up to 24 hours.

- Invert vial and slowly draw solution into syringe. Detach syringe from vial adapter by turning syringe counterclockwise. Attach syringe to the Luer end of an infusion needle set.
- Infuse the reconstituted solution intravenously slowly over about 2 minutes. After infusion, dispose of syringe with the infusion set, vial with the vial adapter, any unused solution, and other waste materials safely.
- Be aware that the prefilled syringe is made of glass with an internal tip diameter of 0.037 inches and is compatible with a standard Luer-lock connector. However, some needleless connectors for intravenous catheters are incompatible with the glass diluent syringes, so their use can damage the connector and affect administration. Consult manufacturer guide for examples. To administer drug through incompatible needleless connectors, withdraw reconstituted drug into a standard 10-ml sterile Luer-lock plastic syringe.
- Store drug vials in refrigerator prior to reconstitution or at room temperature for 3 to 12 months depending on storage temperature. Protect from light.
- *Incompatibilities:* Other drugs

Route	Onset	Peak	Duration
I.V.	Unknown	Unknown	Unknown

Half-life: 14–19 hr

Mechanism of Action

Temporarily replaces the missing coagulation Factor VIII.

Contraindications

Hypersensitivity to turoctocog alfa pegol, or its components, including hamster proteins

Interactions

DRUGS

None reported by manufacturer

Adverse Reactions

SKIN: Pruritus, rash, redness
Other: Antibody formation to turoctocog alfa pegol, **hypersensitivity reactions including anaphylaxis**, injection-site reactions

Childbearing Considerations

PREGNANCY

- It is not known if drug causes fetal harm.
- Use with caution only if benefit to mother outweighs potential risk to fetus.

LACTATION

- It is not known if drug is present in breast milk.
- Patient should check with prescriber before breastfeeding.

Nursing Considerations

! WARNING Monitor patient for hypersensitivity reactions, including anaphylaxis, because drug contains traces of hamster proteins, which may cause allergic reactions in some patients. Early signs of an allergic reaction which can progress to anaphylaxis include angioedema, chest tightness, difficulty breathing, hives, itching, rash, and wheezing. Observe patients closely for any of these signs and symptoms, especially during the early phases of drug administration. If an allergic reaction occurs, stop drug therapy, notify prescriber, and provide supportive care, as indicated and ordered.

- Suspect antibody formation to drug if bleeding is not controlled after drug administration or the expected Factor VIII activity plasma levels are not attained. If this occurs, expect prescriber to order a Bethesda assay to determine if Factor VIII antibodies are present.
- Be aware that Factor VIII activity levels can be affected by the type of activated partial thromboplastin time reagent used in the assay.

PATIENT TEACHING

- Explain to patient how drug is to be administered.

! WARNING Emphasize importance of reporting any unusual effects that might be a sign of an allergic reaction, such as difficulty breathing, hives, itching, rash, swelling of face or tongue, or wheezing. If present, urge patient to seek immediate medical attention and stop drug therapy.

- Instruct patient that if he experiences lack of a clinical response to Factor VIII replacement therapy, he should contact prescriber for further treatment and/or assessment.

U V W

ubrogepant
Ubrelvy

Class and Category
Pharmacologic class: Calcitonin gene-related peptide (CGRP) receptor antagonist
Therapeutic class: Antimigraine

Indications and Dosages
✷ *To treat acute migraine*

TABLETS

Adults. 50 mg or 100 mg followed by a second dose at least 2 hr after initial dose, if needed. *Maximum:* 200 mg/24 hr; treatment of 8 migraines in a 30-day period.

±**DOSAGE ADJUSTMENT** For patient taking concomitant moderate or weak CYP3A4 inducers, all doses kept at 100 mg. For patient taking concomitant moderate or weak CYP3A4 inhibitors or who has severe hepatic or renal impairment, all doses kept at 50 mg and for patient taking a moderate CYP3A4 inhibitor, a second dose should be avoided within 24 hr.

Drug Administration
P.O.
- Do not administer tablets with grapefruit juice.
- Do not administer a second tablet within 24 hours if patient has consumed grapefruit or grapefruit juice.

Route	Onset	Peak	Duration
P.O.	Unknown	1.5 hr	Unknown

Half-life: 5–7 hr

Mechanism of Action
Blocks CGRP, a protein released during a migraine attack, from binding to its receptors, thereby relieving migraine pain.

Contraindications
Concomitant therapy with strong CYP3A4 inhibitors, hypersensitivity to ubrogepant or its components

Interactions
DRUGS

BCRP and/or P-gp inhibitors such as carvedilol, curcumin, eltrombopag, quinidine; CYP3A4 inhibitors (moderate) such as ciprofloxacin, cyclosporine, fluconazole, fluvoxamine; CYP3A4 inhibitors (strong) such as clarithromycin, itraconazole, ketoconazole, verapamil: Significant increase in exposure of ubrogepant and increased risk of adverse reactions
CYP3A4 inducers (strong) such as barbiturates, phenytoin, rifampin, St. John's wort: Significant reduction of ubrogepant exposure and decreased effectiveness

FOODS

grapefruit, grapefruit juice: Increased ubrogepant levels with increase in nausea and sleepiness

Adverse Reactions
CNS: Fatigue, somnolence
EENT: Dry mouth
GI: Nausea

Childbearing Considerations
PREGNANCY
- It is not known if drug can cause fetal harm.
- Use with caution only if benefit to mother outweighs potential risk to fetus.
- Women with migraine may be at increased risk of gestational hypertension and preeclampsia during pregnancy.

LACTATION
- It is not known if drug is present in breast milk.
- Patient should check with prescriber before breastfeeding.

Nursing Considerations
- Be aware that ubrogepant is not indicated for prevention of migraine.
- Use caution when administering drug to elderly patients.

PATIENT TEACHING
- Instruct patient to take ubrogepant exactly as prescribed and not to exceed the maximum dosage.
- Tell patient to inform all prescribers of ubrogepant therapy as well as use of over-the-counter medications or herbal products, because of potential for drug interactions.

U
V
W

- Advise patient to avoid grapefruit or grapefruit juice intake because of increased risk of nausea and sleepiness.
- Instruct patient not to take a second tablet within 24 hours if grapefruit or grapefruit juice was consumed or any of the following medications have been taken: ciprofloxacin, cyclosporine, fluconazole, fluvoxamine, or verapamil.

umeclidinium bromide

Incruse Ellipta

Class and Category

Pharmacologic class: Anticholinergic
Therapeutic class: Bronchodilator

Indications and Dosages

＊ *To provide maintenance treatment for chronic obstructive pulmonary disease (COPD)*

ORAL INHALATION

Adults. 62.5 mcg (1 inhalation) daily.
Maximum: 62.5 mcg in a 24-hr period.

Drug Administration

INHALATION

- Administer drug at the same time of day.
- Open cover of inhaler only when ready to administer drug. If inhaler is opened and closed without drug being inhaled, the dose will be lost. It is not possible to accidentally take a double dose or an extra dose in one inhalation.
- Slide the cover down to expose mouthpiece. A click should be heard. No need to shake inhaler.
- Hand inhaler to patient and have patient breathe out fully while holding inhaler away from mouth. Then have patient put inhaler into mouth and close lips firmly around it, fitting over the curved shape of the mouthpiece. Have patient take one long, steady, deep breath in through the mouth, not the nose.
- Ensure patient does not block the air vent with fingers.
- Have patient remove inhaler and hold breath for about 3 to 4 seconds. Then have patient breathe out slowly and gently.
- Inhaler may be cleaned using a dry tissue before closing the cover, although routine cleaning is not required. Slide the cover up and over the mouthpiece as far as it will go.

Route	Onset	Peak	Duration
Inhalation	Unknown	5–15 min	Unknown

Half-life: 11 hr

Mechanism of Action

Inhibits the muscarinic M_3 receptor in smooth muscle to cause bronchodilation.

Contraindications

Hypersensitivity to umeclidinium or its components, severe hypersensitivity to milk proteins

Interactions

DRUGS

anticholinergics: Possibly additive effects

Adverse Reactions

CNS: Depression, dizziness, headache, vertigo
CV: **Atrial fibrillation, idioventricular rhythm,** supraventricular extrasystole, tachycardia
EENT: Blurred vision, eye pain, nasopharyngitis, pharyngitis, rhinitis, worsening of narrow-angle glaucoma
GI: Abdominal pain (upper), diarrhea, dyspepsia, nausea
GU: Dysuria, urinary retention, UTI, worsening of urinary retention
MS: Arthralgia; back, extremity, or neck pain; myalgia
RESP: Cough, **paradoxical bronchospasm,** respiratory tract infection
SKIN: Pruritus, rash, urticaria
Other: **Anaphylaxis, angioedema**

Childbearing Considerations

PREGNANCY

- It is not known if drug can cause fetal harm.
- Use with caution only if benefit to mother outweighs potential risk to fetus.

LACTATION

- It is not known if drug is present in breast milk.
- Patient should check with prescriber before breastfeeding.

Nursing Considerations

- Know that umeclidinium should not be initiated in patients who are experiencing a rapidly deteriorating or potentially life-threatening episode of COPD.

- Do not administer umeclidinium for relief of acute symptoms. Drug is not a rescue inhaler. Instead, acute symptoms should be treated with an inhaled, short-acting beta$_2$-agonist, as ordered.

! WARNING Monitor patient for hypersensitivity reactions such as anaphylaxis, pruritus, rash, swelling in any area of the body, or urticaria. Expect drug to be discontinued if present. Be prepared to treat according to protocol standards. Know that patients with a severe milk protein allergy should not receive umeclidinium therapy because after inhaling other powder products containing lactose, some patients with a severe milk protein allergy have developed serious hypersensitivity reactions.

- Use with caution in patients with narrow-angle glaucoma or urinary retention because these conditions may worsen with umeclidinium therapy.

! WARNING Monitor patient's respiratory status for paradoxical bronchospasm. Because of its life-threatening nature, notify prescriber immediately, withhold umeclidinium, and prepare to treat patient with an inhaled, short-acting bronchodilator, as ordered. If bronchospasm develops during umeclidinium therapy, expect drug to be permanently discontinued.

PATIENT TEACHING

- Tell patient to take umeclidinium at about the same time every day and not to use more than once in a 24-hour period.
- Remind patient that umeclidinium cannot be used to relieve acute symptoms of COPD. Instead, tell patient to treat acute symptoms with a prescribed inhaled, short-acting beta$_2$ agonist such as albuterol, as prescribed.
- Teach patient how to use the inhaler.
- Urge patient to notify prescriber if her symptoms worsen, if umeclidinium becomes less effective, or if she needs more inhalations of her prescribed short-acting beta$_2$-agonist than usual. This may indicate that patient's condition is worsening.

! WARNING Inform patient that drug may cause paradoxical bronchospasms. If present, tell patient to discontinue drug and notify prescriber. Also, tell patient to notify prescriber immediately if she develops blurred vision; colored images in association with red eyes; eye discomfort, pain, or visual halos.

! WARNING Alert patient that drug may cause an allergic reaction. Tell patient to notify prescriber, if an allergic reaction occurs or, if serious, to seek immediate medical attention. Also, advise patient to notify prescriber immediately if she develops any difficulty passing urine or painful urination, especially if she has a bladder-neck obstruction or if, in a male patient, prostatic hyperplasia is present.

- Instruct patient not to stop taking umeclidinium without prescriber knowledge, because symptoms may recur.

upadacitinib
Rinvoq

Class and Category
Pharmacologic class: Disease-modifying antirheumatic drug (Janus kinase inhibitor)
Therapeutic class: Antirheumatic

Indications and Dosages
✳ *To treat moderate to severe active rheumatoid arthritis in patients who have had an inadequate response or intolerance to one or more tumor necrosis factor (TNF) blockers; to treat psoriatic arthritis*

E.R. TABLETS
Adults. 15 mg once daily.

✳ *To treat refractory, moderate to severe atopic dermatitis in patients who are not adequately controlled with other systemic drugs, including biologics, or when use of those therapies is inadvisable*

E.R. TABLETS
Adults under the age of 65 and children 12 years of age and older weighing at least 40 kg (88 lb). *Initial:* 15 mg once daily, increased to 30 mg once daily, if needed.
Adults 65 years and older. 15 mg once daily.

U
V
W

❋ *To treat moderate to severe active ulcerative colitis in patients who have had an inadequate response or intolerance to one or more TNF blockers.*

Adults: *Induction:* 45 mg once daily for 8 wk. *Maintenance:* 15 mg once daily, increased to 30 mg once daily, if needed, for patient with refractory, severe, or extensive disease

±**DOSAGE ADJUSTMENT** For patients with severe renal impairment (estimated glomerular filtration rate 15 to less than 30 ml/min) who have atopic dermatitis or ulcerative colitis, dosage not to exceed 15 mg once daily for patients with atopic dermatitis and induction dose reduced to 30 mg once daily for 8 wk and maintenance dosage reduced to 15 mg once daily for patients with ulcerative colitis. For patients with mild to moderate hepatic impairment or who are receiving concomitant therapy with strong CYP3A4 and have ulcerative colitis, induction dose reduced to 30 mg once daily for 8 wk and maintenance dose reduced to 15 mg once daily. For patient with atopic dermatitis, psoriatic arthritis, or rheumatoid arthritis who are also receiving concomitant therapy with strong CYP3A4, dosage not to exceed 15 mg once daily. Treatment for all indications interrupted if absolute neutrophil count (ANC) is less than 1,000 cells/mm³ and restarted once ANC is above this value; if absolute lymphocyte count (ALC) is less than 500 cells/mm³ and restarted once ALC is above this value; if hemoglobin (Hb) is less than 8 g/dl and restarted when Hb is above this value; or if drug-induced liver injury is suspected.

Drug Administration

P.O.

- Tablets should be swallowed whole and not chewed, crushed, or split.

Route	Onset	Peak	Duration
P.O./E.R.	Unknown	1.5 hr	Unknown

Half-life: 5–7 hr

Mechanism of Action

Janus kinases are intracellular enzymes, which transmit signals arising from cytokine or growth factor-receptor interactions on the cellular membrane to influence cellular processes of hematopoiesis and immune cell function. Phosphorylation and activation of signal transducers and activators of transcription are inhibited by Janus kinase inhibitors. This action is thought to improve the clinical manifestation of rheumatoid arthritis.

Contraindications

Hypersensitivity to upadacitinib or its components

Interactions

DRUGS

live, attenuated vaccines: Increased risk of infection
strong CYP3A4 inducers such as rifampin: Decreased exposure of upadacitinib with reduced effectiveness
strong CYP3A4 inhibitors such as ketoconazole: Increased upadacitinib exposure with increased risk of adverse reactions

Adverse Reactions

CNS: Fever
CV: Arterial or deep venous thrombosis, elevated cholesterol and triglyceride levels
EENT: Oral candidiasis
GI: Elevated liver enzymes, gastrointestinal perforation, nausea
HEME: Anemia, lymphopenia, neutropenia
RESP: Cough, pneumonia, pulmonary embolism, pulmonary tuberculosis, upper respiratory infection
SKIN: Nonmelanoma skin cancer
Other: Anaphylaxis, angioedema, bacterial, viral (including herpes simplex and herpes zoster), and other opportunistic infections such as extrapulmonary tuberculosis; elevated creatine phosphokinase; invasive fungal infections, including cryptococcosis and pneumocystosis; lymphoma and other malignancies

Childbearing Considerations

PREGNANCY

- Drug has potential to cause fetal harm such as malformations, according to animal studies.
- Pregnancy status should be verified before drug therapy begins.
- Use with caution only if benefit to mother outweighs potential risk to fetus.

LACTATION

- It is not known if drug is present in breast milk.

- Breastfeeding is not recommended during drug therapy and for 6 days after last dose.

REPRODUCTION
- Advise women of childbearing age to use effective contraception during drug therapy and for 4 weeks following last dose.

Nursing Considerations
- Know that upadacitinib is not recommended in patients with an absolute lymphocyte count (ALC) less than 500 cells/mm^3, absolute neutrophil count (ANC) less than 1,000 cells/mm^3, or hemoglobin level less than 8 g/dl. It is also not recommended for patients with severe hepatic impairment.
- Use upadacitinib cautiously in patients at risk for gastrointestinal perforation, such as those with a history of diverticulitis or taking NSAIDs. Notify prescriber immediately if patient develops new-onset abdominal symptoms during drug therapy.

! WARNING Be aware that patients are at increased risk for developing serious infections that may lead to hospitalization or death. Patients at risk include those who were also taking corticosteroids or immunosuppressants such as methotrexate. Know that extreme caution should be used in patients with a history of chronic or recurrent infection. Monitor patient closely for infection during and after treatment, including patients who tested negative for latent tuberculosis prior to initiating therapy. If patient develops an infection, notify prescriber and expect drug therapy to be interrupted until infection is under control.

! WARNING Be aware that patients receiving a similar drug who were 50 years of age or older with at least one cardiovascular risk factor experienced a higher rate of mortality or an increased incidence of thrombosis while taking drug, including sudden cardiovascular death. Monitor patient closely throughout upadacitinib therapy.

- Ensure that patient has been tested for latent tuberculosis before upadacitinib is given. If needed, expect treatment for latent infection to be given prior to upadacitinib therapy being initiated.

! WARNING Monitor patient for hypersensitivity reactions such as anaphylaxis, pruritus, rash, swelling in any area of the body, or urticaria. Expect drug to be discontinued, if present. Be prepared to treat according to protocol standards.

- Know that viral reactivation, including cases of herpes virus reactivation such as herpes zoster and hepatitis B virus reaction, may occur during upadacitinib therapy. Ensure that patient has been screened for viral hepatitis before therapy begins and also during therapy. If hepatitis B virus DNA is detected in a patient receiving upadacitinib, expect a liver specialist to be consulted.
- Check to be sure patient is up to date on immunizations and, if not, is brought up to date, including prophylactic zoster vaccinations, before upadacitinib therapy begins. Live-attenuated vaccines are not recommended during or immediately prior to upadacitinib therapy.
- Expect to monitor patient's ANC, ALC, and hemoglobin levels regularly throughout upadacitinib therapy. Know that treatment should be interrupted if ANC is less than 1,000 cells/mm^3 and then restarted once ANC returns above this value; if ALC is less than 500 cells/mm^3 and then restarted once ALC returns above this value; if hemoglobin is less than 8 g/dl and then restarted once hemoglobin is above this value; or if drug-induced liver injury is suspected.
- Monitor patient's liver enzymes and assess for drug-induced liver injury. If suspected, notify prescriber and expect drug therapy to be interrupted.

! WARNING Monitor patient for any evidence of thrombosis, such as arterial or deep venous thrombosis, or pulmonary embolism that may occur as a result of upadacitinib therapy.

- Expect to monitor patient's lipid parameters 12 weeks after drug therapy is begun, and thereafter according to clinical guidelines for hyperlipidemia, if present. Be aware that statin therapy usually decreases elevations in cholesterol and LDL to pretreatment levels.

PATIENT TEACHING

- Instruct patient to swallow tablets whole and not chew, crush, or split the tablets.

> **! WARNING** Alert patient that drug may cause an allergic reaction. Tell patient to notify prescriber, if present, and to seek immediate emergency attention if serious.

- Teach patient about infection control measures to take while receiving upadacitinib therapy. Tell patient to stay away from anyone who has an infection and to notify prescriber if an infection develops.
- Tell patient to notify prescriber if any prolonged, severe, or unusual signs and symptoms appear.

> **! WARNING** Review signs and symptoms of thrombosis with patient. If present, emphasize importance of stopping drug therapy and seeking emergency medical attention.

- Inform patient that blood tests will be required before and during upadacitinib therapy.
- Advise patients to examine skin regularly, especially if they are at risk for skin cancer. Tell patient to notify prescriber of any abnormal findings.
- Urge women of childbearing age to use effective contraception during drug therapy and for 4 weeks after last dose, as drug may adversely affect fetal development.
- Tell women of childbearing age that breastfeeding is not recommended during upadacitinib therapy and 6 days after last dose.
- Caution patient to avoid receiving live vaccines during or immediately prior to upadacitinib therapy.

ursodiol
(ursodeoxycholic acid)
Actigall, Urso Forte, URSO 250

☰ Class and Category
Pharmacologic class: Bile acid
Therapeutic class: Bile salt replenisher, cholelitholytic

☰ Indications and Dosages

✳ *To prevent gallstone formation in obese patients during rapid weight loss*

CAPSULES (ACTIGALL)
Adults. 300 mg twice daily.

✳ *To dissolve gallstones*

CAPSULES (ACTIGALL)
Adults. 8 to 10 mg/kg daily in divided doses twice daily or three times a day.

✳ *To treat primary biliary cirrhosis*

TABLETS (URSO 250, URSO FORTE)
Adults. 13 to 15 mg/kg daily in two to four divided doses.

☰ Drug Administration
P.O.
- Administer ursodiol with food to increase drug dissolution.
- Give aluminum-containing antacids, cholestyramine, and colestipol at least 1 hour before or 4 hours after ursodiol, because they may decrease drug's effects.

Route	Onset	Peak	Duration
P.O.	Unknown	Unknown	Unknown

Half-life: Unknown

☰ Mechanism of Action
Suppresses biliary secretion, hepatic synthesis, and intestinal reabsorption of cholesterol. Prolonged use prevents or promotes dissolution of gallstones.

☰ Contraindications
For all forms: Hypersensitivity to ursodiol or its components
For Actigall: Additional hypersensitivity to bile salts; presence of calcified cholesterol stones, radiolucent bile pigment stones, or radiopaque stones; when cholecystectomy is not contraindicated
For Urso Forte, URSO 250: Complete biliary obstruction

☰ Interactions
DRUGS
aluminum-containing antacids, cholestyramine, colestipol: Decreased absorption and therapeutic effects of ursodiol
clofibrate, estrogens, oral contraceptives: Interference with ursodiol's therapeutic effects; increased risk of gallstone formation

Adverse Reactions

CNS: Anxiety, asthenia, depression, dizziness, fatigue, fever, headache, malaise, sleep disturbance
CV: Chest pain, hypertension, peripheral edema
ENDO: Hyperglycemia
EENT: **Laryngeal edema**, metallic taste, rhinitis, stomatitis
GI: Abdominal discomfort or pain, cholecystitis, constipation, diarrhea, elevated liver enzymes, esophagitis, flatulence, indigestion, jaundice, nausea, peptic ulcer, vomiting
GU: Elevated creatinine level
HEME: **Leukopenia, thrombocytopenia**
MS: Arthralgia, back pain, myalgia
RESP: Cough
SKIN: Alopecia, diaphoresis, dry skin, pruritus, rash, urticaria
Other: **Angioedema**

Childbearing Considerations

PREGNANCY
- It is not known if drug can cause fetal harm.
- Actigall is not recommended for use during pregnancy.
- URSO 250 and Urso Forte should be used with caution if benefit to mother outweighs potential risk to fetus.

LACTATION
- It is not known if drug is present in breast milk.
- Patient should check with prescriber before breastfeeding.

Nursing Considerations

- Monitor patient's liver enzymes every month for 3 months after ursodiol therapy is begun and then every 6 months thereafter, as ordered. If elevation occurs, notify prescriber, as drug may have to be discontinued.
- Expect drug to be discontinued if gallstones haven't partially dissolved after 12 months of therapy.
- If patient inadvertently takes too much ursodiol, diarrhea will most likely result and may warrant systemic treatment.

PATIENT TEACHING
- Tell patient to take ursodiol with meals.
- Urge patient to take aluminum-containing antacids at least 1 hour before or 4 hours after ursodiol to support absorption.
- Urge patient to notify prescriber immediately if evidence of acute cholecystitis develops, such as acute right-upper-quadrant abdominal pain.
- Inform patient that he may need to take ursodiol for a prolonged period before gallstones dissolve.
- Advise diabetic patient to monitor blood glucose levels during therapy because ursodiol may alter blood glucose control.

ustekinumab
Stelara

Class and Category

Pharmacologic class: Monoclonal antibody
Therapeutic class: Immunomodulator

Indications and Dosages

* *To treat moderate to severe plaque psoriasis in patients who are candidates for phototherapy or systemic therapy*

SUBCUTANEOUS INJECTION

Adults and children ages 6 to 18 weighing more than 100 kg (220 lb). *Initial:* 90 mg followed by 90 mg 4 wk later and then 90 mg every 12 wk.
Adults weighing 100 kg (220 lb) or less and children ages 6 to 18 weighing 60 kg (132 lb) to 100 kg (220 lb). *Initial:* 45 mg followed by 45 mg 4 wk later and then 45 mg every 12 wk.
Children ages 6 to 18 weighing less than 60 kg (132 lb). 0.75 mg/kg, followed by 0.75 mg/kg 4 wk later and then 0.75 mg/kg every 12 wk.

* *To treat active psoriatic arthritis as monotherapy or in combination with methotrexate*

SUBCUTANEOUS INJECTION

Adults. *Initial:* 45 mg, followed by 45 mg 4 wk later, and then 45 mg every 12 wk.
±**DOSAGE ADJUSTMENT** For patients who weigh more than 100 kg (220 lb) and also have coexistent moderate to severe plaque psoriasis in addition to psoriatic arthritis, initial dosage increased to 90 mg followed by 90 mg 4 wk later, and then 90 mg every 12 wk.

* *To treat moderate to severe active Crohn's disease; to treat moderately to severely active ulcerative colitis*

U
V
W

I.V. INFUSION

Adults who weigh more than 85 kg (187 lb). *Initial:* 520 mg as a single infusion.

Adults who weigh more than 55 kg (121 lb) but less than 85 kg (187 lb). *Initial:* 390 mg as a single infusion.

Adults who weigh 55 kg (121 lb) or less. *Initial:* 260 mg as a single infusion.

SUBCUTANEOUS INJECTION

Adults. *Maintenance:* 90 mg 8 wk after initial intravenous dose, then every 8 wk thereafter.

☰ Drug Administration

- Vials should be stored upright in refrigerator and protected from light.
- Do not shake vials before administration.
- Drug should be colorless to light yellow and may contain a few small translucent or white particles. Discard if solution is cloudy or discolored or contains other particulate matter.

I.V.

- Withdraw volume equal to dosage volume from a 250-ml bag of 0.9% Sodium Chloride Injection and discard. Add drug volume to bag and mix gently.
- Diluted solution may be stored for up to 7 hours at room temperature.
- Use only an infusion set with an in-line 0.2 micrometer, non-pyrogenic, low-protein-binding filter for infusion.
- Infuse over at least 60 minutes, with infusion completed within 8 hours after being diluted in the infusion bag.
- Do not infuse in the same I.V. line with other agents.
- *Incompatibilities:* Other drugs

SUBCUTANEOUS

- Needle cover on prefilled syringe contains dry natural rubber and should not be handled if allergic to latex.
- Use a 1-ml syringe with a 27 G, ½-inch needle when using the single-dose vial.
- Inject into any quadrant of abdomen, gluteal region, thighs, or upper arms. Injection of entire prefilled syringe contents is necessary to activate the needle guard.
- Rotate sites, and avoid areas that are bruised, erythematous, indurated, or tender.

Route	Onset	Peak	Duration
SubQ	Unknown	7–13.5 days	Unknown
I.V.	Unknown	Unknown	Unknown

Half-life: 14–45.5 days

☰ Mechanism of Action

Binds to p40 protein subunit used by interleukin (IL)-12 and IL-23 cytokines. These specific cytokines are involved in inflammatory and immune responses, such as natural killer cell activation and CD4⁺ T-cell differentiation and activation. By disrupting signaling mediated by IL-12 and IL-23, signs and symptoms caused by inflammatory and immune responses are diminished or relieved.

☰ Contraindications

Hypersensitivity to ustekinumab or its components

☰ Interactions

DRUGS

live-virus vaccines: Increased risk of adverse vaccine effects

☰ Adverse Reactions

CNS: Depression, dizziness, fatigue, fever, headache, **reversible posterior leukoencephalopathy syndrome**

EENT: Nasopharyngitis, pharyngolaryngeal pain, sinusitis

GI: Abdominal pain, diarrhea, diverticulitis, gastroenteritis, nausea

GU: UTI

MS: Back pain, myalgia, osteomyelitis

RESP: **Cryptogenic organizing pneumonia; eosinophilic pneumonia; interstitial pneumonia;** respiratory tract infections, including opportunistic fungal infections and tuberculosis

SKIN: Cellulitis, erythrodermic psoriasis, pruritus, pustular psoriasis, rash, urticaria

Other: **Anaphylaxis, angioedema,** anti-ustekinumab antibodies, flu-like symptoms, injection-site reactions (bruising, erythema, hemorrhage, induration, irritation, pain, pruritus, swelling), **malignancies (breast, colorectal, head and neck, kidney, melanoma and nonmelanoma disorders of skin, prostate, or thyroid),** serious infection, including bacterial, fungal, and viral infections and reactivation of latent infections

☰ Childbearing Considerations

PREGNANCY

- Pregnancy exposure registry: 1-877-311-8972.
- It is not known if drug can cause fetal harm.
- Use with caution only if benefit to mother outweighs potential risk to fetus.

LACTATION

- It is not known if drug is present in breast milk.
- Patient should check with prescriber before breastfeeding.

☰ Nursing Considerations

- Make sure patient has a tuberculin skin test before therapy starts. If skin test is positive, treatment of latent tuberculosis should start before ustekinumab therapy starts. Also expect antituberculosis therapy to start if patient has a history of latent or active tuberculosis but adequate therapy can't be confirmed or if patient has a negative test for latent tuberculosis but has risk factors for tuberculosis.
- Make sure patient is current with all immunizations before starting ustekinumab therapy because patient shouldn't receive live vaccines during treatment. BCG vaccines shouldn't be given for 1 year before or after ustekinumab therapy.
- Use caution when administering ustekinumab to a patient undergoing allergen immunotherapy because drug may decrease the protective effect of allergen immunotherapy, which in turn may increase the risk of an allergic reaction to a dose of allergen immunotherapy.
- Use ustekinumab cautiously in patients with recurrent infection or increased risk of infection and in patients who live in regions where histoplasmosis and tuberculosis are endemic.

! **WARNING** Know that if patient has evidence of an active infection when drug is prescribed, therapy shouldn't start until infection has been treated. Monitor all patients for infection during therapy, especially those receiving immunosuppressants. Be on the alert for cough, dyspnea, and interstitial infiltrates following one to three doses that may suggest pneumonia has developed. If a

serious infection, an opportunistic infection, or sepsis develops, expect prescriber to stop ustekinumab and start appropriate antimicrobial therapy.

- Be aware that patients with a history of cancer or who have genetic deficiencies in IL-12 or IL-23 should be thoroughly evaluated before ustekinumab therapy starts, because various cancers have occurred in patients being treated with ustekinumab. Monitor patients throughout therapy for persistent, severe, or unusual signs and symptoms.
- Know that comparison of the incidence of antibodies to ustekinumab with the incidence of antibodies to other products may be misleading.

! **WARNING** Monitor patient for hypersensitivity reactions that could become life-threatening. At first sign of hypersensitivity, notify prescriber, expect drug to be discontinued, and provide supportive care.

- Monitor patient for confusion, headache, seizures, and vision disturbances, which may signal reversible posterior leukoencephalopathy syndrome, a rare neurologic disorder that may occur with ustekinumab therapy. If present, notify prescriber, discontinue ustekinumab therapy, and provide appropriate treatment, as ordered.
- Inspect patient's skin regularly for evidence of abnormalities because rapid appearance of multiple cutaneous squamous cell carcinoma has occurred in patients who had preexisting risk factors for nonmelanoma skin cancer. Patients who are over 60 years of age, have a medical history of prolonged immunosuppressant therapy, and those with a history of psoralen plus ultraviolet radiation using UVA bands (PUVA) treatment should be closely monitored.

PATIENT TEACHING

- Inform patient that treatment must be supervised by a healthcare professional.
- Teach patient how to administer drug subcutaneously, if self-administration is ordered by prescriber.
- Inform patient that tuberculosis may occur during ustekinumab therapy. Instruct him

U
V
W

to report low-grade fever, persistent cough, or wasting or weight loss to prescriber.

- Teach patient to recognize and report evidence of infection; drug may have to be stopped. Advise patient to avoid people with infections and to have all prescribed laboratory tests performed.
- Inform patient that the risk of developing certain kinds of cancer is higher in patients taking ustekinumab. Emphasize importance of follow-up visits and reporting any persistent, sudden-onset, or unusual signs or symptoms.
- Caution against receiving live-virus vaccines while taking ustekinumab; doing so may adversely affect the immune system.
- Urge patient to inform all healthcare providers about ustekinumab use and to inform prescriber about all OTC medications being taken, including herbal remedies and mineral and vitamin supplements.

! **WARNING** Alert patient that drug may cause an allergic reaction. Tell patient to notify prescriber immediately if an allergic reaction occurs or if confusion, headaches, seizures, or visual disturbances occur, as drug may have to be discontinued and additional medical attention given.

- Instruct patient to store drug vials standing up straight.

valproate sodium

valproic acid

divalproex sodium

Depakote, Depakote ER, Depakote Sprinkle, Epival (CAN)

Class and Category

Pharmacologic class: Carboxylic acid derivative
Therapeutic class: Anticonvulsant

Indications and Dosages

✴ *To treat as monotherapy or as adjunct complex partial seizures that occur in isolation or associated with other types of seizures*

CAPSULES, DELAYED-RELEASE SPRINKLE CAPSULES, DELAYED-RELEASE TABLETS, EXTENDED-RELEASE CAPSULES, EXTENDED-RELEASE TABLETS, I.V. INFUSION (VALPROIC ACID, VALPROATE SODIUM, DIVALPROEX SODIUM)

Adults and children age 10 and over. *Initial:* 10 to 15 mg/kg/day, increased by 5 to 10 mg/kg daily every wk, as needed. I.V. infusion administered over no less than 60 min. *Maximum:* 60 mg/kg daily.

✴ *To treat as monotherapy or as adjunct simple and complex absence seizures; adjunctive therapy to treat multiple seizure types that include absence seizures*

CAPSULES, DELAYED-RELEASE SPRINKLE CAPSULES, DELAYED-RELEASE TABLETS, EXTENDED-RELEASE CAPSULES, EXTENDED-RELEASE TABLETS, I.V. INFUSION (VALPROIC ACID, VALPROATE SODIUM, DIVALPROEX SODIUM)

Adults. *Initial:* 15 mg/kg/day, increased by 5 to 10 mg/kg daily every wk, as needed. I.V. infusion given over no less than 60 min. *Maximum:* 60 mg/kg/day.

±**DOSAGE ADJUSTMENT** For adults being converted from immediate-release divalproex tablets to delayed-release tablets, dosage increased by 8% to 20% more than total daily dose of immediate-release tablets and given once daily.

✴ *To treat acute manic phase of bipolar disorder*

DELAYED-RELEASE TABLETS (DIVALPROEX SODIUM)

Adults. *Initial:* 750 mg daily in divided doses. *Maximum:* 60 mg/kg daily.

EXTENDED-RELEASE TABLETS (DIVALPROEX SODIUM)

Adults. *Initial:* 25 mg/kg/day once daily, increased as rapidly as possible to achieve therapeutic dose. *Maximum:* 60 mg/kg/day.

✴ *To prevent migraine headache*

DELAYED-RELEASE TABLETS (DIVALPROEX SODIUM)

Adults. *Initial:* 250 mg every 12 hr, increased as needed. *Maximum:* 1 g daily.

EXTENDED-RELEASE TABLETS (DIVALPROEX SODIUM)

Adults. Initial: 500 mg daily for 1 wk, increased, as needed, up to 1 g daily. *Maximum:* 1 g daily.

☰ Drug Administration

P.O.

- Administer with food to minimize GI irritation, if needed.
- Administer drug at least 2 hours before or 6 hours after cholestyramine.
- Delayed-release or extended-release tablets should be swallowed whole and not chewed, crushed, or divided.
- Sprinkle capsules on a small amount of semisolid food just before administration. Administer immediately and ensure that patient does not chew mixture.

I.V.

- Dilute drug with at least 50 ml of 0.9% Sodium Chloride Injection, 5% Dextrose in Water, or Lactated Ringer's solution.
- Diluted solution may be stored for 24 hours.
- Infuse over 60 minutes at a rate not to exceed 20 mg/min. Rapid administration increases risk of adverse reactions and should be avoided.
- Know that patient should be switched from I.V. to P.O. form as soon as possible.
- *Incompatibilities:* None listed by manufacturer

Route	Onset	Peak	Duration
P.O.	Unknown	15–60 min	Unknown
I.V.	Unknown	Unknown	Unknown

Half-life: 4–16 hr

☰ Mechanism of Action

May decrease seizure activity by blocking reuptake of gamma-aminobutyric acid (GABA), the most common inhibitory neurotransmitter in the brain. GABA suppresses the rapid firing of neurons by inhibiting voltage-sensitive sodium channels.

☰ Contraindications

Hepatic impairment; hypersensitivity to valproic acid, valproate sodium, divalproex sodium, or their components; mitochondrial disease caused by POLG mutations; pregnancy or women of childbearing age who are not using effective contraception (for prevention of migraine headaches); suspected POLG-related disorder in children under 2 years of age; urea cycle disorders

☰ Interactions

DRUGS

amitriptyline, nortriptyline: Increased plasma levels of these drugs

aspirin: Increased valproic acid level with possible increased risk of adverse reactions

carbamazepine: Altered concentrations of carbamazepine

carbapenem antibiotics (ertapenem, imipenem, meropenem): Reduced serum valproic acid level, causing loss of seizure control

chlorpromazine: Increased trough plasma levels of valproate

cholestyramine: Decreased bioavailability of valproic acid

clonazepam: Increased risk of absence seizures

CNS depressants: Increased CNS depression

diazepam: Inhibited diazepam metabolism

estrogen-containing hormonal contraceptives: Possibly increased clearance of valproate, which may decrease effectiveness and increase risk of seizures

ethosuximide: Unpredictable blood ethosuximide level

felbamate: Impaired valproic acid metabolism and increased valproate level

lamotrigine: Decreased lamotrigine clearance

phenobarbital, primidone: Possible increased phenobarbital concentrations resulting in CNS depression that could become severe

phenytoin: Increased risk of phenytoin toxicity, loss of seizure control

propofol: Possibly increased blood levels of propofol

rufinamide: Increased rufinamide concentrations

topiramate: Increased risk of hyperammonemia with or without encephalopathy

zidovudine: Clearance decreased for zidovudine resulting in increased concentrations

ACTIVITIES

alcohol use: Additive CNS depression

☰ Adverse Reactions

CNS: Abnormal dreams or thinking, aggression, agitation, amnesia, apathy, asthenia, ataxia, attention disturbance, behavioral deterioration, catatonic reaction, cerebral pseudoatrophy, chills,

U
V
W

cognitive decline, confusion, depression, dizziness, drowsiness, emotional upset, **encephalopathy**, euphoria, fever, gait abnormality, hallucinations, headache, hostility, hyperactivity, hyperesthesia, hypertonia, hypokinesia, **hypothermia**, increased reflexes, insomnia, irritability, lack of coordination, learning disorder, lethargy, **loss of seizure control**, malaise, nervousness, **paradoxical seizures**, paresthesia, parkinsonism, psychomotor hyperactivity, psychosis, sedation, speech disorder, somnolence, **suicidal ideation**, tardive dyskinesia, tremor, twitching, vertigo, weakness

CV: **Bradycardia**, chest pain, edema, hypertension, **hypotension**, orthostatic hypotension, palpitations, peripheral edema, tachycardia, vasodilation

EENT: Amblyopia, conjunctivitis, diplopia, dry eyes, ear or eye pain, glossitis, hearing loss, nystagmus, parotid gland swelling, pharyngitis, rhinitis, sinusitis, spots before eyes, stomatitis, taste perversion, tinnitus

ENDO: Breast enlargement, elevated testosterone level, galactorrhea, hyperandrogenism, hyperglycemia, inappropriate ADH secretion, parotid gland swelling

GI: Abdominal pain, anorexia, constipation, diarrhea, dyspepsia, elevated liver enzymes, fecal incontinence, flatulence, gastroenteritis, **hepatotoxicity**, increased appetite, indigestion, jaundice, nausea, **pancreatitis**, vomiting

GU: Aspermia, azoospermia, cystitis, decreased sperm count or spermatozoa motility, dysuria, enuresis, male infertility, menstrual irregularities, polycystic ovary disease, **tubulointerstitial nephritis**, urinary incontinence, UTI, **vaginal hemorrhage**

HEME: **Agranulocytosis**, anemia, **aplastic anemia**, **bone marrow suppression**, eosinophilia, hematoma, **hypofibrinogenemia**, **leukopenia**, lymphocytosis, macrocytosis, **pancytopenia**, porphyria (acute, intermittent), **prolonged bleeding time**, **thrombocytopenia**

MS: Arthralgia, arthrosis, back pain, bone pain, decreased bone mineral density, dysarthria, fractures, leg cramps, myalgia, neck pain or rigidity, osteopenia, osteoporosis

RESP: Dyspnea, increased cough

SKIN: Alopecia, cutaneous vasculitis, diaphoresis, discoid lupus erythematosus, dry skin, ecchymosis, **erythema multiforme**, furunculosis, hair color or texture changes, hirsutism, maculopapular rash, nail and nail bed disorders, petechiae, photosensitivity, pruritus, rash, seborrhea, **Stevens–Johnson syndrome**, **toxic epidermal necrolysis**

Other: **Anaphylaxis**, decreased carnitine concentration, developmental delay (children), **drug reaction with eosinophilia and systemic symptoms (DRESS)**, **hyperammonemia**, **hyponatremia**, injection-site pain, weight gain or loss

Childbearing Considerations

PREGNANCY

- Pregnancy exposure registry: 1-888-233-2334 or https://www.aedpregnancyregistry.org.
- Drug causes fetal harm such as decreased IQ, major congenital malformations, and neurodevelopmental disorders. Drug may also cause fatal hepatic failure in fetus. In addition, drug may also increase risk of attention deficit/hyperactivity disorder and autism spectrum disorders.
- Drug is contraindicated in pregnant women and in women of childbearing age who are not using effective contraception for treatment of migraines.
- Use with extreme caution only if no alternate is effective in controlling bipolar disorder or epilepsy and the benefit to mother outweighs potential risk to fetus.
- Drug should not be discontinued abruptly if pregnancy occurs during drug therapy for epilepsy, as this can precipitate status epilepticus with resulting maternal and fetal hypoxia and threat to life.

LACTATION

- Drug is present in breast milk.
- Patient should check with prescriber before breastfeeding.
- If breastfeeding occurs, monitor infant for jaundice or unusual bleeding or bruising.

REPRODUCTION

- Women of childbearing age should use effective contraception and be counseled regularly of its importance throughout drug therapy. This is especially important for women planning to become pregnant and girls at the onset of puberty.

- If pregnancy occurs, prescriber should be notified immediately and patient switched to a different drug. However, patient should not discontinue drug abruptly without consulting prescriber and before an alternative drug can be prescribed.
- Drug may cause male infertility.

Nursing Considerations

- Use caution when administering drug to children or patient with history of hepatic disease, patient receiving multiple anticonvulsants, patient with congenital metabolic disorders, severe seizure disorder accompanied by mental retardation, and organic brain disease, because they may be at increased risk for developing hepatotoxicity.
- Ensure that serum liver testing has been done prior to starting therapy and at frequent intervals after that because drug may cause hepatotoxicity that could be fatal.
- Be aware that patient with hypoalbuminemia or another protein-binding deficiency is at increased risk for valproic acid toxicity.

! **WARNING** Watch for evidence of decreased hepatic function, including anorexia, facial edema, jaundice, lethargy, loss of seizure control, malaise, vomiting, and weakness, especially during the first 6 months of treatment. Monitor liver enzymes, as ordered. Notify prescriber immediately if hepatotoxicity is suspected and, if confirmed, expect drug to be discontinued immediately.

- Monitor platelet count, as ordered, for signs of thrombocytopenia, and notify prescriber if they appear.

! **WARNING** Keep in mind hyperammonemia may occur even if liver function test results are normal. Monitor ammonia levels, as ordered. If patient develops unexplained lethargy, vomiting, or changes in mental status with an increase in ammonia level; if asymptomatic ammonia elevations are detected and persist; or if patient develops hypothermia even without hyperammonemia, expect to discontinue valproic acid.

- Watch patient closely for suicidal tendencies, particularly when therapy starts and dosage changes, because depression may worsen temporarily during these times, possibly leading to suicidal ideation.
- Monitor patient's drug level, as ordered, especially early in therapy and if patient takes other drugs, because interactions can alter the blood level.
- Be aware drug may alter urine ketone test and thyroid function tests.

PATIENT TEACHING

- Advise patient to take drug with food and take drug at least 2 hours before or 6 hours after cholestyramine, if prescribed.
- Instruct patient to swallow delayed-release tablets or extended-release capsules whole to prevent irritation to mouth and throat and not to break, chew, crush, or open them. However, immediate-release capsules may be opened and contents mixed with food for easier swallowing. Instruct patient not to chew contents of capsules.
- Tell patient to notify prescriber immediately and withhold further doses of drug, unless advised otherwise by prescriber, if symptoms such as anorexia, facial edema, lethargy, malaise, weakness, and vomiting occur.
- Inform patient to notify prescriber that if medication residue is seen in stools, as plasma valproate levels may have to be checked and possibly an alternative treatment prescribed.
- Advise patient to avoid hazardous activities during therapy because drug may affect mental and motor performance.
- Urge patient to avoid alcohol during therapy.
- Advise patient to notify prescriber if tremor develops during therapy; it may be dose-related.
- Urge family or caregiver to watch patient closely for suicidal tendencies, especially when therapy starts or dosage changes.
- Instruct women of childbearing age to use effective contraception while taking drug and to notify prescriber if pregnancy is suspected or occurs.

valsartan

Diovan

U
V
W

Class and Category

Pharmacologic class: Angiotensin II receptor blocker (ARB)
Therapeutic class: Antihypertensive

⬟ Indications and Dosages

✽ *To manage hypertension, alone or with other antihypertensives*

ORAL SUSPENSION, TABLETS

Adults. *Initial:* 80 or 160 mg once daily, increased as needed and prescribed. *Maximum:* 320 mg/day.

Children ages 1 to 16. 1 mg/kg (up to 40 mg total) once daily, increased as needed and prescribed. *Maximum:* 4 mg/kg (up to 160 mg) daily.

✽ *To treat New York Heart Association (NYHA) class II to IV heart failure*

ORAL SUSPENSION, TABLETS

Adults. *Initial:* 40 mg twice daily, increased to 80 mg twice daily and then 160 mg twice daily, as needed. *Maximum:* 320 mg daily in divided doses.

✽ *To reduce cardiovascular mortality in stable patients with left ventricular failure or dysfunction following an MI*

ORAL SUSPENSION, TABLETS

Adults. *Initial:* 20 mg twice daily starting as early as 12 hr after MI, increased to 40 mg twice daily within 7 days, followed by subsequent adjustments to 160 mg twice daily as tolerated. *Maintenance:* 160 mg twice daily.

⬟ Drug Administration

P.O.

- Tablets and oral suspension are not interchangeable on a milligram-per-milligram basis. Do not combine two dosage forms to achieve a total dose.
- Oral suspension should be used in children ages 1 to 5, in children older than 5 who cannot swallow tablets, and in children for whom the calculated dose does not correspond to the available tablet strengths of the drug.
- Oral suspension form is available in a concentration of 4 mg/ml. Shake suspension well for at least 10 seconds before using. Use a calibrated device to measure dosage. Store suspension up to 30 days at room temperature or up to 75 days in refrigerator.

Route	Onset	Peak	Duration
P.O.	2 hr	2–4 hr	24 hr
Half-life: 6 hr			

⬟ Mechanism of Action

Blocks the hormone angiotensin II from binding to receptor sites in adrenal glands, vascular smooth muscle, and other tissues. This action inhibits aldosterone-secreting and vasoconstrictive effects of angiotensin II, thereby reducing blood pressure. It also reduces renal reabsorption of sodium, which helps to reduce fluid retention that occurs in heart failure.

⬟ Contraindications

Concurrent aliskiren therapy in diabetic patients, hypersensitivity to valsartan or its components

⬟ Interactions

DRUGS

ACE inhibitors, aliskiren, other angiotensin receptor blockers: Increased risk of hypotension, hyperkalemia, and renal dysfunction

antihypertensives, diuretics: Additive hypotensive effect

lithium: Possibly increased serum lithium concentration and toxicity

NSAIDs: Increased risk of renal dysfunction, especially in the elderly and patients with or existing renal dysfunction or volume depletion; decreased hypertensive effect of valsartan

potassium salts, potassium-sparing diuretics, potassium supplements: Possibly hyperkalemia; increased serum creatinine in heart-failure patients

FOODS

high-potassium foods such as bananas or potatoes, potassium-containing salt substitutes: Possibly hyperkalemia

⬟ Adverse Reactions

CNS: Dizziness, fatigue, headache, insomnia, syncope, vertigo

CV: Edema, **hypotension**, orthostatic hypotension, vasculitis

EENT: Blurred vision, pharyngitis, rhinitis, sinusitis

GI: Abdominal pain, diarrhea, elevated liver enzymes, **hepatitis**, indigestion, nausea, vomiting

GU: **Acute renal failure**, increased blood creatinine level

HEME: Thrombocytopenia

MS: Arthralgia, back pain, **rhabdomyolysis**

RESP: Cough, upper respiratory tract infection
SKIN: Alopecia, bullous dermatitis, rash
Other: Angioedema, hyperkalemia, increased incidence of viral infection

Childbearing Considerations
PREGNANCY
- Drug can cause fetal harm. Drug given during the second or third trimester reduces fetal renal function and increases fetal and neonatal morbidity and death. Resulting oligohydramnios can lead to fetal anuria, renal failure, hypotension, lung hypoplasia, and skeletal malformations as well as fetal death.
- Drug is contraindicated in pregnant women. If pregnancy occurs, drug should be discontinued as soon as possible and an alternative drug given instead.

LACTATION
- It is not known if drug is present in breast milk.
- Breastfeeding is not recommended during drug therapy.

REPRODUCTION
- Women of childbearing age need to use an effective contraceptive during drug therapy and to report any suspected or known pregnancy immediately to prescriber.

Nursing Considerations
- Know that valsartan shouldn't be given to patients who are taking a diuretic or have hypovolemia, because there is increased risk of severe hypotension from volume depletion. If severe hypotension occurs, place patient in a supine position, notify prescriber, and expect to give an intravenous infusion of normal saline.
- Check patient's blood pressure often.
- Be aware that maximal blood pressure reduction typically occurs after 4 weeks during therapy.
- Monitor serum potassium level because drug may elevate potassium level by blocking aldosterone secretion. Be aware that hyperkalemia occurs more often in children with underlying chronic kidney disease.
- Obtain a serum creatinine level periodically, as ordered, because changes in renal function can occur during valsartan therapy. Know that patients who are at high risk for renal dysfunction are patients with chronic kidney disease, renal artery stenosis, severe congestive heart failure, or who are volume-depleted. Notify prescriber of an elevated serum creatinine level and changes in voiding patterns because renal dysfunction could lead to acute renal failure.

PATIENT TEACHING
- Instruct patient to take valsartan exactly as prescribed at the same time each day to maintain therapeutic effect.
- Tell patient taking oral suspension form to shake bottle for at least 10 seconds before using and to use a calibrated device to measure dose, not a household spoon. Also tell patient that bottle can be stored up to 30 days if kept at room temperature and up to 75 days if kept in refrigerator.
- Advise patient to avoid hazardous activities until drug's CNS effects are known.
- Advise patient to avoid using potassium-containing salt substitutes without consulting prescriber.
- Instruct female patient of childbearing age to use reliable birth control during therapy and to notify prescriber at once about known or suspected pregnancy, because valsartan will have to be discontinued. Inform mothers that breastfeeding should not be undertaken during drug therapy.
- Urge patient to keep follow-up appointments to monitor progress.
- Tell patients to inform all prescribers of valsartan therapy and any other drug therapy they are taking, including drugs such as ibuprofen and naproxen.
- Tell patient that light-headedness can occur with valsartan therapy, especially during the first days of therapy. If fainting should occur, advise patient to stop taking valsartan and to notify prescriber. Remind patient that diarrhea, excessive perspiration, inadequate fluid intake, or vomiting can lower blood pressure and cause fainting.

vancomycin hydrochloride
Firvanq, Vancocin

U
V
W

Class and Category
Pharmacologic class: Glycopeptide
Therapeutic class: Antibiotic

☰ Indications and Dosages

✻ *To treat pseudomembranous colitis caused by* Clostridium difficile

CAPSULES, ORAL SOLUTION

Adults. 125 mg every 6 hr for 10 days.
Children. 40 mg/kg daily divided into three or four doses for 7 to 10 days. *Maximum:* 2 g daily.

✻ *To treat staphylococcal enterocolitis caused by* Staphylococcus aureus

CAPSULES, ORAL SOLUTION

Adults. 500 mg to 2 g daily divided into three or four doses for 7 to 10 days.
Children. 40 mg/kg daily divided into three or four doses for 7 to 10 days. *Maximum:* 2 g daily.

✻ *To treat serious or severe infections caused by susceptible strains of methicillin-resistant* Staphylococci; *to treat infections that are resistant to other antimicrobial drugs*

I.V. INFUSION

Adults. 500 mg every 6 hr or 1 g every 12 hr infused over no more than 10 mg/min or over at least 60 min, whichever is longer.
Children. 10 mg/kg every 6 hr infused over at least 60 min.
Neonates ages 1 week to 1 month. *Initial:* 15 mg/kg followed by 10 mg/kg every 8 hr infused over at least 60 min.
Neonates under age 1 week. *Initial:* 15 mg/kg followed by 10 mg/kg every 12 hr infused over at least 60 min.

±**DOSAGE ADJUSTMENT** For patients with renal impairment, total daily dose adjusted to equal about 15 times the glomerular filtration rate in ml/min. For elderly patients, dosage reduced depending on renal function. For premature infants, a longer dosing interval may be needed.

☰ Drug Administration

P.O.

- Capsules should be swallowed whole and not chewed, crushed, or opened.
- Shake oral solution well before measuring dose. Use a calibrated device to measure dosage of oral solution. Refrigerate solution when not in use.

I.V.

- Thaw frozen containers at room temperature or under refrigeration. Do not thaw by immersion in water baths or by microwave irradiation. Do not force thaw. Once thawed, check for minute leaks by squeezing the bag firmly. Do not use if leaks are detected. Agitate bag after solution has reached room temperature. If solution remains cloudy or insoluble precipitate is present or any seal is broken, discard. Thawed solution is stable for 72 hours at room temperature or 30 days refrigerated. Do not refreeze.
- Reconstitute 250-mg vial with 5 ml of Sterile Water for Injection, then further dilute with 50 ml of compatible solution; 500-mg vial with 10 ml of Sterile Water for Injection and further dilute with 150 ml of compatible solution; 1.25-mg vial with 25 ml of Sterile Water for Injection and further dilute with 250 ml of compatible solution; and 1.5-g vial with 30 ml of Sterile Water for Injection and further dilute with 300 ml of compatible solution.
- Compatible solutions to use for dilution include 0.9% Sodium Chloride Injection, 5% Dextrose Injection, 5% Dextrose Injection and 0.9% Sodium Chloride Injection, Lactated Ringer's Injection, and Lactated Ringer's and 5% Dextrose Injection.
- After dilution with 0.9% Sodium Chloride Injection or 5% Dextrose Injection, diluted solution may be stored in refrigerator for 14 days; after dilution with other compatible solutions listed above, diluted solution may be stored in refrigerator for 96 hours.
- Infuse each adult dose at no more than 10 mg/min or over at least 60 minutes, whichever is longer. Infuse each dose for children and neonates over at least 60 minutes. Avoid rapid delivery because it may cause hypotension or transient "red man syndrome," characterized by chills; fainting; fever; flushing of face, neck, torso, and upper arms; hypotension; nausea; tachycardia; and vomiting.
- *Incompatibilities:* Beta-lactam antibiotics and other drugs (due to vancomycin's low pH)

Route	Onset	Peak	Duration
P.O.	Unknown	Unknown	Unknown
I.V.	Unknown	End of infusion	Unknown

Half-life: 4–6 hr

☰ Mechanism of Action

Inhibits bacterial RNA and cell wall synthesis; alters permeability of bacterial membranes, causing cell wall lysis and cell death.

Contraindications

Hypersensitivity to corn or corn products when given with dextrose solutions, hypersensitivity to vancomycin or its components

Interactions

DRUGS

aminoglycosides (amikacin, gentamicin, tobramycin), amphotericin B, bacitracin (parenteral), cisplatin, colistin, polymyxin B, viomycin: Additive nephrotoxicity or neurotoxicity

anesthetic agents: Increased risk of erythema and histamine-like flushing

Adverse Reactions

CNS: Chills, depression, dizziness, fatigue, fever, headache, insomnia, vertigo

CV: **Hypotension,** peripheral edema, vasculitis

EENT: Hemorrhagic occlusive retinal vasculitis, ototoxicity

GI: Abdominal pain, constipation, *Clostridioides difficile*–associated diarrhea, diarrhea, flatulence, nausea, vomiting

GU: **Acute kidney injury,** interstitial nephritis, **nephrotoxicity,** UTI

HEME: Anemia, eosinophilia, **neutropenia, thrombocytopenia**

MS: Back pain

RESP: Dyspnea, wheezing

SKIN: **Acute generalized exanthematous pustulosis (AGEP); exfoliative dermatitis;** extravasation with pain, tenderness, thrombophlebitis, and tissue necrosis; linear IgA bullous dermatosis (LABD); pruritus; rash; **Stevens–Johnson syndrome; toxic epidermal necrolysis;** urticaria

Other: **Anaphylaxis, drug reaction with eosinophilia and systemic symptoms (DRESS),** drug-induced fever, **hypokalemia,** injection-site inflammation, superinfection, vancomycin infusion reaction (dyspnea, flushing of upper body, hypotension, urticaria, wheezing) with I.V. administration

Childbearing Considerations

PREGNANCY

- It is not known if oral drug can cause fetal harm.
- Do not use vancomycin injection that contains excipients polyethylene glycol (PEG400) and N-acetyl D-alanine (NADA) during the first or second trimester of pregnancy because of increased risk of fetal spinal malformations. Other formulations of vancomycin should be used instead.
- Use with caution only if benefit to mother outweighs potential risk to fetus.

LACTATION

- Drug is present in breast milk.
- Patient should check with prescriber before breastfeeding.

Nursing Considerations

- Be aware that vancomycin is not indicated for prophylaxis of endophthalmitis, nor should it be administered intracamerally or intravitreally, especially during or after cataract surgery, because it may cause hemorrhagic occlusive retinal vasculitis which may result in permanent vision loss.
- Expect to monitor blood vancomycin concentrations frequently. Higher trough concentrations of 15 to 20 mg/L are commonly targeted now, though they are associated with more nephrotoxicity than the lower trough concentrations previously used.
- Monitor serum vancomycin concentration in patients with colitis or renal impairment because significant increases in blood drug level have occurred in such patients taking multiple oral doses of vancomycin.
- Know that if patient has an inflammatory intestinal disorder, he should be assessed often for adverse reactions because vancomycin absorption may be increased in these conditions.
- Check CBC results and BUN and serum creatinine levels during therapy, especially if patient has renal impairment or takes an aminoglycoside, because systemic vancomycin may cause acute kidney injury.
- Observe I.V. infusion site for evidence of extravasation, including necrosis, pain, tenderness, and thrombophlebitis. If extravasation occurs, discontinue infusion immediately and notify prescriber.
- Assess hearing during therapy. Transient or permanent ototoxicity may occur if patient receives an excessive amount of drug, has an underlying hearing loss, or receives concurrent aminoglycosides.
- Monitor patient closely for diarrhea when receiving intravenous form of vancomycin, because it may indicate pseudomembranous colitis caused by *C. difficile,* a risk with

U
V
W

many antibiotics. If diarrhea occurs during therapy, notify prescriber and expect to withhold drug. If confirmed, treat with fluids, electrolytes, protein, and an antibiotic effective against *C. difficile*.

- Know that oral vancomycin is only used for gastrointestinal *C. difficile* and staphylococcal infections, as it is not absorbed. Patients cannot be converted from I.V. to oral vancomycin for other infections.

! **WARNING** Assess patient's skin regularly because drug can cause severe dermatologic reactions. At the first sign of blisters, mucosal lesions, or a rash, notify prescriber.

PATIENT TEACHING

- Instruct patient to shake oral solution well before each use and to use a calibrated measuring device to measure accurate doses, not a household spoon. Tell patient to store oral solution in refrigerator.
- Advise patient taking capsule form to swallow capsule whole and not to chew, crush, or open capsule.
- Advise patient to notify prescriber if no improvement occurs after a few days.
- Instruct patient to complete full course of vancomycin, as prescribed.
- Instruct patient to notify prescriber if she develops persistent or severe diarrhea.
- Instruct patient to keep follow-up appointments during and after treatment.

! **WARNING** Alert patient that drug may cause severe skin reactions. Tell patient to notify prescriber if blisters, mucosal lesions, or skin rashes occur.

- Tell patient to alert prescriber before drug is given intravenously if she is pregnant or suspects a pregnancy.

vardenafil hydrochloride

Levitra, Staxyn

Class and Category

Pharmacologic class: Phosphodiesterase type 5 (PDE-5) inhibitor
Therapeutic class: Anti-impotence agent

Indications and Dosages

✶ *To treat erectile dysfunction*

TABLETS (LEVITRA)

Adults. 10 mg taken 1 hr before sexual activity; increased to 20 mg or decreased to 5 mg, as needed. *Maximum:* 20 mg and once-daily limit regardless of dosage.

±**DOSAGE ADJUSTMENT** If patient takes ritonavir, vardenafil dosage shouldn't exceed 2.5 mg in 72 hr. If patient takes atazanavir, clarithromycin, indinavir, itraconazole 400 mg daily, ketoconazole 400 mg daily, saquinavir, or another potent CYP3A4 inhibitor, vardenafil dosage shouldn't exceed 2.5 mg in 24 hr. If patient takes erythromycin, itraconazole 200 mg daily, or ketoconazole 200 mg daily, vardenafil dosage shouldn't exceed 5 mg in 24 hr. If patient is 65 or over, initial dosage should be reduced to 5 mg.

ORALLY DISINTEGRATING TABLETS (STAXYN)

Adults. 10 mg taken 1 hr before sexual activity. *Maximum:* 10 mg within 24-hr period.

Drug Administration

P.O.

- Tablets are not interchangeable with oral disintegrating tablets.
- Patient should place orally disintegrating tablet on his tongue immediately after removing it from the blister package and allow it to dissolve. It should not be chewed, crushed, or split and not taken with any liquid.

Route	Onset	Peak	Duration
P.O.	60 min	0.5–2 hr	4 hr

Half-life: 4–6 hr

Mechanism of Action

Enhances effect of nitric oxide (released in the penis by sexual stimulation) and inhibits phosphodiesterase type 5, which increases cGMP level, relaxes smooth muscle, increasing blood flow into the corpus cavernosum to produce an erection.

Contraindications

Concurrent administration of guanylate cyclase stimulators (riociguat), concurrent intermittent or regular nitrate therapy and nitric oxide donors, hypersensitivity to vardenafil or its components

☰ Interactions

DRUGS

alpha blockers, antihypertensives, guanylate cyclase stimulators, nitrates and nitric oxide donors: Profound hypotension
CYP3A4 inhibitors such as erythromycin, indinavir, ketoconazole, ritonavir and other CYP3A4 inhibitors: Increased vardenafil effects
indinavir, ritonavir: Reduced blood levels of indinavir and ritonavir

FOODS

grapefruit juice: Possibly increased vardenafil effect

☰ Adverse Reactions

CNS: Dizziness, headache, **seizures**, transient global amnesia
CV: Hypotension, prolonged QT interval
EENT: Decreased vision, hearing loss, loss of vision in one or both eyes, nasal congestion, nonarteritic anterior ischemic optic neuropathy (NAION), rhinitis, sinusitis, tinnitus
GI: Indigestion, nausea
GU: Priapism
MS: Back pain
SKIN: Flushing
Other: Flu-like symptoms

☰ Childbearing Considerations

PREGNANCY

- Drug is not for use in women.

LACTATION

- Drug is not for use in women.

☰ Nursing Considerations

- Know that vardenafil shouldn't be used by men taking class IA (procainamide, quinidine) or class III (amiodarone, sotalol) antiarrhythmics or by men who have congenital prolonged QT interval. Drug may potentiate prolonged QT interval. It should also not be used in men who have hypotension (resting systolic blood pressure of less than 90 mm Hg), myocardial infarction (within last 6 months), presence of life-threatening arrhythmia, recent history of stroke, severe cardiac failure, uncontrolled hypertension (greater than 170/110 mm Hg), or unstable angina, because drug use could worsen these conditions.
- Use vardenafil cautiously in elderly men, men with penile abnormalities that may predispose them to priapism, or men with mild hepatic impairment (should not be used if patient has moderate to severe hepatic impairment), or renal dysfunction (although it should not be used if patient is on dialysis).
- Also use cautiously in patients with left ventricular outflow obstruction, such as aortic stenosis, and those with severely impaired autonomic control of blood pressure. These conditions increase sensitivity to vasodilators, such as vardenafil.
- Monitor blood pressure and heart rate before and after giving drug, especially if patient takes an alpha blocker, because of increased risk of symptomatic hypotension.
- Monitor patient's vision, especially if he's over age 50; has coronary artery disease, diabetes, hyperlipidemia, or hypertension; or smokes, because vardenafil rarely leads to nonarteritic ischemic optic neuropathy and vision that is decreased, possibly permanently.
- Monitor patient's hearing. Sudden decrease or loss, possibly with dizziness and tinnitus, may occur with vardenafil use. Report such changes immediately, and expect drug to be discontinued.

PATIENT TEACHING

- Alert patient that orally disintegrating tablets contain phenylalanine and should not be taken by patients with phenylketonuria. It also contains sorbitol and should not be taken if he has hereditary problems with fructose intolerance.
- Tell patient to take drug 1 hour before anticipated sexual activity for best results.
- Instruct patient to place a prescribed orally disintegrating tablet on his tongue immediately after removing it from the blister package and allow it to dissolve. He should not crush or split the tablet, and tablet should not be taken with any liquid.

> **! WARNING** Tell patient not to take vardenafil if he takes an organic nitrate, continuously or intermittently, or within 4 hours of taking an alpha blocker, because profound hypotension and death could result.

- Caution patient not to take vardenafil more than once daily or to exceed 20 mg daily for

U
V
W

oral tablet or 10 mg for orally disintegrating tablet. Tell him to call his prescriber or go to the emergency department immediately if he accidentally takes more vardenafil than prescribed.

- Tell patient to stop taking vardenafil and notify prescriber if he has a sudden hearing loss, sudden loss of vision in one or both eyes, or trouble remembering.
- Advise patient to seek sexual counseling to enhance drug's effects.
- Inform patient taking Staxyn that some form of sexual stimulation is needed for an erection to happen.
- Urge patient to notify prescriber at once if erection is painful or lasts longer than 4 hours, to avoid possible penile damage and permanent loss of erectile function.
- Instruct patient to alert all prescribers of vardenafil use.

varenicline tartrate

Champix (CAN), Chantix

☰ Class and Category

Pharmacologic class: Nicotinic receptor partial agonist
Therapeutic class: Nicotinic blocker

☰ Indications and Dosages

✳ *As adjunct to smoking cessation treatment*

TABLETS

Adults. *Initial:* 0.5 mg daily for 3 days; then increased to 0.5 mg twice daily for 4 days, and then increased to 1 mg twice daily for a total of 12 wk of therapy. If effective, an additional 12 wk of therapy may be given.

±**DOSAGE ADJUSTMENT** If patient has severe renal impairment, maximum dosage is 0.5 mg twice daily. If patient is having hemodialysis for end-stage renal disease, maximum dosage is 0.5 mg daily.

☰ Drug Administration

P.O.

- Administer after eating and with a full glass of water.
- Drug may be initiated 1 week before patient's set date to stop smoking. Alternatively, drug may be initiated and then patient quits smoking between day 8 and day 35.

Route	Onset	Peak	Duration
P.O.	Unknown	3–4 hr	24 hr

Half-life: 24 hr

☰ Mechanism of Action

Blocks nicotine from activating $alpha_4beta_2$ receptors by binding to them. This inhibits nicotine stimulation of the central nervous mesolimbic dopamine system, which probably is the area that produces pleasure in and reinforcement of smoking.

☰ Contraindications

Hypersensitivity to varenicline or its components

☰ Interactions

DRUGS

nicotine (transdermal): Increased adverse reactions

ACTIVITIES

alcohol use: May decrease alcohol tolerance, increasing intoxicating effects of alcohol including aggressive behavior and sometimes amnesia of event

☰ Adverse Reactions

CNS: Abnormal dreams, aggression, agitation, anxiety, asthenia, attention difficulties, behavior changes, **CVA**, delusions, depression, dizziness, dysgeusia, fatigue, hallucinations, headache, **homicidal ideation**, hostility, insomnia, irritability, lethargy, loss of consciousness, malaise, mania, mental impairment, panic, paranoia, psychosis, restlessness, **seizures**, sensory disturbances, sleep disorder, sleepwalking, somnambulism, somnolence, **suicidal ideation**, thirst

CV: Angina, chest pain, edema, hypertension, **MI**, peripheral ischemia, **thrombosis, ventricular extrasystole**

EENT: Dry mouth, epistaxis, gingivitis, rhinorrhea

ENDO: Hot flashes, hyperglycemia

GI: Abdominal pain, **acute pancreatitis**, anorexia, constipation, diarrhea, dyspepsia, flatulence, gastroesophageal reflux disease, **GI hemorrhage**, increased appetite, liver enzyme abnormalities, nausea, splenomegaly, vomiting

GU: **Acute renal failure**, polyuria, urine retention

HEME: Leukocytosis, **thrombocytopenia**

MS: Arthralgia, back pain, muscle cramp, musculoskeletal pain, myalgia
RESP: **Asthma**, dyspnea, **pulmonary embolism**
SKIN: Diaphoresis, **erythema multiforme**, pruritus, rash, **Stevens–Johnson syndrome**, urticaria
Other: **Angioedema**, flu-like syndrome, **hyperkalemia, hypersensitivity reactions,** hypokalemia, lymphadenopathy

Childbearing Considerations

PREGNANCY

- It is not known if drug can cause fetal harm.
- Use with caution only if benefit to mother outweighs potential risk to fetus.

LACTATION

- It is not known if drug is present in breast milk.
- Patient should check with prescriber before breastfeeding.
- If breastfeeding occurs, monitor the breastfed infant for excessive vomiting and seizures.

Nursing Considerations

- Know that varenicline is not recommended for use in children 16 years of age and younger.
- Use cautiously in patients with renal disease because varenicline is substantially excreted by the kidneys.
- Review patient's medication history before starting varenicline because dosage adjustments may be needed for drugs such as insulin, theophylline, and warfarin.

! **WARNING** Monitor patient for angioedema, difficult breathing, rash with mucosal lesions, or other signs of hypersensitivity. Report immediately, stop varenicline therapy, and provide supportive emergency care, as prescribed.

- Know that if patient has nausea, the most common adverse reaction to varenicline, notify prescriber. Dosage reduction may help.

! **WARNING** Know that serious neuropsychiatric adverse effects have occurred with varenicline use, even in patients with no prior psychiatric history. Aggressive or unusual behavior directed to self or others may be exhibited. Observe

patient closely. If present, stop drug therapy immediately, notify prescriber, and provide safety measures to protect patient and others.

- Know that even with varenicline therapy, nicotine withdrawal symptoms and worsening of underlying psychiatric illness may occur with smoking cessation. If present, notify prescriber immediately, institute safety measures, and expect drug to be discontinued.
- Watch patient closely for suicidal tendencies, particularly when therapy starts and dosage changes, because depression may worsen temporarily during these times, possibly leading to suicidal ideation.
- Monitor patient for seizures, especially within the first month of therapy, and in patients with a history of seizures or other factors that could lower their seizure threshold.

PATIENT TEACHING

- Tell patient to take drug after eating and with a full glass of water.
- Explain that using nicotine patches while taking varenicline won't increase its effectiveness and may increase adverse reactions such as dizziness, nausea, and vomiting.
- Instruct patient to set a date to quit smoking and then start taking varenicline 1 week before the quit date. Or, patient can begin therapy and then set a date to quit smoking between days 8 and 35 of treatment. Or, if patient is unable or unwilling to quit smoking right away, inform him that he can start taking varenicline and reduce smoking during the first 12 weeks of treatment as follows: during weeks 1–4, reduce number of cigarettes smoked daily by half; during weeks 5–8, reduce number of cigarettes smoked daily to reach one-quarter of the starting daily cigarettes smoked; and during weeks 9–12, keep reducing number of cigarettes smoked until zero is reached by week 12. Know that varenicline can be taken for an additional 12 weeks of therapy after smoking has stopped, if needed.
- Encourage patient to continue trying to stop smoking even if an early relapse occurs during varenicline therapy.

U
V
W

! **WARNING** Tell patient to seek medical attention immediately if he develops difficulty breathing; mucosal lesions; rash or other skin reaction; swelling of his eyes, face, lips, mouth, or neck; or any other signs of hypersensitivity during therapy.

- Inform patient that the most common adverse reactions to varenicline therapy are insomnia and nausea, usually transient. If they persist, patient should notify prescriber; dosage reduction may help.
- Caution patient to avoid hazardous activities until CNS effects of drug are known. Explain that near-miss traffic accidents and other accidental injuries have occurred in patients taking varenicline.
- Explain that strange, unusual, or vivid dreams may occur during therapy. Also inform patient that sleepwalking may occur that can lead to behavior that may be harmful to self, others, or property. If sleepwalking occurs, tell patient to stop taking drug and notify prescriber.

! **WARNING** Tell patient and family or caregiver that nicotine withdrawal can occur even with varenicline use and that aggressive or unusual behavior can occur in patients with or without a history of mental illness. Tell them that if patient has an existing mental illness, varenicline therapy may worsen it. Inform them that sometimes these behaviors may become serious and can be directed to self or others and may be worsened by concomitant use of alcohol. Advise patient to avoid alcohol during varenicline therapy and urge family or caregiver to monitor patient closely for suicidal or homicidal tendencies, especially when therapy starts or dosage changes. Advise patient, family, or caregiver to notify prescriber about abnormal thinking or behavior and to stop taking drug immediately if this occurs.

! **WARNING** Instruct patient to seek emergency medical care if she experiences a seizure or new or worsening symptoms of cardiovascular disease such as calf pain when walking, chest pain, shortness of breath, or sudden onset of difficulty speaking, numbness, or weakness.

- Advise women who are breastfeeding while taking varenicline to monitor infant for excessive vomiting and seizures. If present, tell patient to stop taking varenicline and have infant seen by a pediatrician.

vasopressin
Vasostrict

Class and Category
Pharmacologic class: Posterior pituitary hormone
Therapeutic class: Antidiuretic hormone

Indications and Dosages
✳ *To increase blood pressure in patients in vasodilatory shock (post-cardiotomy or sepsis) who remain hypotensive despite catecholamines and fluids*

I.V. INFUSION
Adults. *Initial:* 0.01 units/min (septic shock) or 0.03 units/min (post-cardiotomy shock), titrated up by 0.005 units/min at 10- to 15-min intervals, as needed. After target blood pressure has been maintained for 8 hr without the use of catecholamines, dosage tapered by 0.005 units/min every hr, as tolerated, to maintain target blood pressure. *Maximum:* 0.07 units/min (septic shock); 0.1 units/min (post-cardiotomy shock).

Drug Administration
I.V.
- Dilute to a concentration of 0.1 units/ml using 0.9% Sodium Chloride Injection or 5% Dextrose in Water by diluting 50 units in 500 ml; if fluid restriction is present, dilute 100 units in 100 ml to yield a concentration of 1 unit/ml..
- Store diluted drug at room temperature for up to 18 hours or refrigerated for up to 24 hours.
- Use an infusion pump to administer drug.
- Infuse continuously starting with 0.03 units/ minute for post-cardiotomy shock or 0.01 units/minute for septic shock. Titrate up by 0.005 units/min at 10- to 15-minute intervals, as needed. Do not exceed 0.1 units/min for post-cardiotomy shock and 0.07 units/min for septic shock.
- After initial entry into the 10-ml multidose vial, vial must be refrigerated. Discard

multidose 10-ml vial after 30 days from first puncture.

- *Incompatibilities:* None listed by manufacturer

Route	Onset	Peak	Duration
I.V.	Rapid	15 min	20 min

Half-life: < 10 min

Mechanism of Action

Vasoconstrictive effects are mediated by vascular V_1 receptors which are directly coupled to phospholipase C, resulting in release of calcium. This leads to vasoconstriction. In addition, vasopressin stimulates antidiuresis via stimulation of V_2 receptors which are coupled to adenyl cyclase. Both of these actions help to raise blood pressure.

Contraindications

Hypersensitivity to vasopressin or its components, hypersensitivity to 8-L-arginine vasopressin, hypersensitivity to chlorobutanol found in the 10-ml multiple-dose vial but not in the 1-ml single-dose vial

Interactions

DRUGS

catecholamines: Additive effect on mean arterial blood pressure and other hemodynamic parameters
drugs suspected of causing diabetes insipidus (clozapine, demeclocycline, foscarnet, lithium): Decreased diuretic and pressor effects of vasopressin
drugs suspected of causing SIADH (chlorpropamide, cyclophosphamide, enalapril, felbamate, haloperidol, ifosfamide, methyldopa, pentamidine, selected serotonin reuptake inhibitors, tricyclic antidepressants): Possibly increased diuretic and pressor effects of vasopressin
furosemide: Increased effect of vasopressin on osmolar clearance and urine flow
ganglionic blocking agents: Increased effect on mean arterial blood pressure
indomethacin: Possibly prolonged effect of vasopressin on cardiac index and systemic vascular resistance

Adverse Reactions

CV: Atrial fibrillation, bradycardia, decreased cardiac index, myocardial ischemia, right heart failure

EENT: Circumoral pallor
ENDO: Reversible diabetes insipidus
GI: Elevated bilirubin levels, mesenteric ischemia
GU: Acute renal insufficiency
HEME: Decreased platelets, hemorrhagic shock, intractable bleeding
MS: Distal limb ischemia
SKIN: Pruritus, rash, urticaria
Other: Hypersensitivity reaction, hyponatremia

Childbearing Considerations

PREGNANCY

- It is not known if drug can cause fetal harm. However, drug can produce tonic uterine contractions, which could threaten pregnancy continuation.
- Use with caution only if benefit to mother outweighs potential risk to fetus. Be aware that dosage increase may be needed in the second or third trimester.

LACTATION

- It is not known if drug is present in breast milk.
- Once condition is stabilized, patient should check with prescriber before breastfeeding.

Nursing Considerations

- Use cautiously in patients with impaired cardiac response, because vasopressin may worsen cardiac output.
- Monitor patient for reversible diabetes insipidus after treatment of vasopressin is completed. Signs to be alert for include dilute urine, hypernatremia, and polyuria. Also monitor patient's serum electrolytes, fluid status, and urine output after vasopressin has been discontinued. Be aware that some patients may require readministration of vasopressin or administration of desmopressin to correct fluid and electrolyte shifts.

! **WARNING** Monitor patient for hypersensitivity reactions, which could be severe. Notify prescriber immediately, if present, and expect to provide supportive care.

- Be aware that a decrease in cardiac index may occur with the use of vasopressin, indicating worsening of cardiac function.

U
V
W

PATIENT TEACHING

! **WARNING** Advise patient to immediately report all adverse reactions, especially allergic reactions such as difficulty breathing or swallowing, hives, or swelling of face or tongue.

- Tell patient to alert staff if discomfort occurs at the infusion site.

venlafaxine hydrochloride
Effexor XR, Venlafaxine E.R.

desvenlafaxine
Khedezla

desvenlafaxine fumarate
Desvenlafaxine ER

desvenlafaxine succinate
Pristiq

Class and Category
Pharmacologic class: Selective serotonin and norepinephrine reuptake inhibitor (SSNRI)
Therapeutic class: Antidepressant

Indications and Dosages
＊ *To treat and prevent relapse of major depression*

E.R. CAPSULES (EFFEXOR XR)
Adults. 75 mg once daily (for some patients, 37.5 mg once daily for 4 to 7 days before increasing to 75 mg daily); then increased by 75 mg daily every 4 days or longer, as needed. *Maximum:* 225 mg daily.

E.R. TABLETS (DESVENLAFAXINE ER, KHEDEZLA, PRISTIQ)
Adults. 50 mg once daily.

E.R. TABLETS (VENLAFAXINE ER)
Adults. *Initial:* 75 mg once daily as single dose (for some patients, 37.5 mg once daily for 4 to 7 days before increasing to 75 mg once daily); then increased by 75 mg once daily every 4 days or longer. *Maximum:* 225 mg daily.

＊ *To treat generalized anxiety disorder*

E.R. CAPSULES (EFFEXOR XR)
Adults. 75 mg once daily (for some patients, 37.5 mg once daily for 4 to 7 days before increasing to 75 mg once daily); then increased by 75 mg once daily every 4 days or longer, as needed. *Maximum:* 225 mg daily.

＊ *To treat social anxiety disorder*

E.R. CAPSULES (EFFEXOR XR), E.R. TABLETS (VENLAFAXINE ER)
Adults. 75 mg once daily.

＊ *To treat panic disorder*

E.R. CAPSULES (EFFEXOR XR)
Adults. *Initial:* 37.5 mg once daily for 7 days, increased to 75 mg once daily, as needed; then increased by 75 mg once daily every 4 days or more, as needed. *Maximum:* 225 mg daily.

± **DOSAGE ADJUSTMENT** *Effexor XR, Venlafaxine ER:* For patients with mild to moderate renal impairment, initial daily dose decreased by 25% to 50%. For patients undergoing dialysis or who have severe renal impairment, daily dose reduced by 50%. For patients with mild to moderate hepatic failure, dose reduced by 50%; for patients with severe hepatic impairment or hepatic cirrhosis, dosage may have to be reduced more than 50%. *Desvenlafaxine ER, Pristiq:* For patient with severe renal impairment and end-stage renal disease, maximum dose is 25 mg daily or 50 mg every other day. *Khedezla:* For patient with severe renal impairment and end-stage renal disease, dosage is 50 mg every other day. *Desvenlafaxine ER, Khedezla, Pristiq:* For patient with hepatic impairment, maximum dosage not to exceed 100 mg daily.

Drug Administration
P.O.
- Administer drug with food and give with a full glass of water.
- Administer drug at the same time each day, morning or evening.
- Capsules and tablets should be swallowed whole and not chewed or crushed.
- If patient has trouble swallowing capsules, open capsule, sprinkle contents on a spoonful of applesauce, and have patient

swallow immediately without chewing, followed by a glass of water.

Route	Onset	Peak	Duration
P.O./E.R.	1–2 wk	5.5–9 hr	Unknown

Half-life: 3–7 hr

Mechanism of Action

Inhibits neuronal reuptake of norepinephrine and serotonin, along with its active metabolite, O-desmethylvenlafaxine. These actions raise norepinephrine and serotonin levels at nerve synapses, elevating mood and reducing anxiety, depression, and panic.

Contraindications

Hypersensitivity to desvenlafaxine, venlafaxine, or their components; use of an MAO inhibitor within 14 days, including intravenous methylene blue and linezolid

Interactions

DRUGS

aspirin, NSAIDs, warfarin and other anticoagulants: Increased risk of bleeding
CYP2D6 substrates such as atomoxetine, desipramine, dextromethorphan, metoprolol, nebivolol, perphenazine, tolterodine: Increased risk of toxicity of these drugs
serotonergic drugs such as amphetamines, buspirone, fentanyl, lithium, MAO inhibitors, other selected serotonin reuptake inhibitors, other serotonin–norepinephrine reuptake inhibitors, St. John's wort, tramadol, tricyclic antidepressants, triptans, tryptophan: Possibly serotonin syndrome

ACTIVITIES

alcohol use: Increased CNS effects

Adverse Reactions

CNS: Abnormal dreams, agitation, amnesia, anxiety, asthenia, attention disturbance, bruxism, **cerebral ischemia**, chills, confusion, delirium, delusions, depersonalization, depression, dizziness, dream disturbances, drowsiness, dyskinesia, extrapyramidal disorder, fatigue, fever, hallucinations, headache, hypesthesia, hypomania, impaired balance and coordination, insomnia, irritability, mania, migraine, mood changes, nervousness, **neuroleptic malignant syndrome**, paresthesia, **seizures, serotonin syndrome**, somnolence, **suicidal ideation**, syncope, tardive dyskinesia, tremor, vertigo

CV: **Arrhythmias, AV block**, chest pain, **congestive heart failure**, elevated cholesterol and triglyceride levels, edema, **extrasystoles**, hypertension, **hypotension, MI**, palpitations, **prolonged QT interval**, sinus tachycardia, **Takotsubo cardiomyopathy**, thrombophlebitis, **torsades de pointes**, vasodilation, **ventricular fibrillation or tachycardia**, worsening of peripheral vascular disease

EENT: Abnormal vision, accommodation abnormality, angle-closure glaucoma, blurred vision, dry mouth, mucous membrane bleeding, mydriasis, pharyngitis, rhinitis, taste alteration, tinnitus

ENDO: Elevated blood prolactin levels, hot flashes, hyperglycemia, syndrome of inappropriate ADH secretion

GI: Abdominal pain, anorexia, colitis, constipation, diarrhea, elevated liver enzymes, flatulence, **GI hemorrhage, hepatitis**, indigestion, nausea, **pancreatitis**, vomiting

GU: Anorgasmia (women), decreased libido, ejaculation disorder, erectile dysfunction, urinary incontinence or urgency, urine hesitancy or retention

HEME: **Abnormal bleeding, agranulocytosis**, anemia, **aplastic anemia**, leukocytosis, **leukopenia, neutropenia, pancytopenia, prolonged bleeding time, thrombocytopenia**

MS: Neck pain, musculoskeletal stiffness, **rhabdomyolysis**

RESP: Cough, **eosinophilic pneumonia**, increased dyspnea, **interstitial lung disease**

SKIN: Diaphoresis, ecchymosis, **erythema multiforme**, pruritus, rash, **Stevens–Johnson syndrome, toxic epidermal necrolysis**

Other: Angioedema, discontinuation syndrome, **hypersensitivity reactions**, hyponatremia, lymphadenopathy, weight gain or loss

Childbearing Considerations

PREGNANCY

- Pregnancy exposure registry: 1-844-405-6185.
- Drug may cause fetal harm, especially if exposure occurs late in third trimester. At birth, neonate may possibly require prolonged hospitalization, respiratory support, and tube feeding.
- Use with caution only if benefit to mother outweighs potential risk to fetus.

U
V
W

LACTATION

- Drug is present in breast milk.
- A decision should be made to discontinue breastfeeding or the drug to avoid potential serious adverse reactions in the breastfed infant.

Nursing Considerations

- Be aware that desvenlafaxine and venlafaxine should not be given to patients with bradycardia, congenital long QT syndrome, hypokalemia or hypomagnesemia, recent acute myocardial infarction, or uncompensated heart failure because of increased risk of prolonged QT interval and torsades de pointes. It should also not be given to patients who are taking other drugs that prolong the QT interval. Expect hypokalemia and hypomagnesemia to be corrected before drug therapy is begun.
- Use cautiously in patients with a history of mania because desvenlafaxine and venlafaxine therapy may worsen condition. Also use cautiously in patients with a history of seizures, and expect to discontinue drug, as ordered, if seizures occur.
- Use cautiously in patients who have medical conditions that might be made worse by an increased heart rate, as in heart failure, hyperthyroidism, or recent MI.

! **WARNING** Be aware that serotonin syndrome in its most severe form may resemble neuroleptic malignant syndrome, which includes autonomic instability with possibly rapid changes in vital signs, hyperthermia, mental status changes, and muscle rigidity. Notify prescriber, withhold drug immediately, and provide supportive care. Expect drug to be discontinued.

- Monitor blood pressure often during therapy because it may cause dose-related sustained increase in supine diastolic pressure. Expect to reduce or stop drug, as prescribed, if increase develops.
- Assess patient's electrolyte balance, as ordered, because drug can cause hyponatremia, especially in elderly patients and in patients who take diuretics or are volume-depleted. If patient has evidence of hyponatremia (confusion, headache, trouble concentrating, unsteadiness, weakness), notify prescriber. If

imbalance is confirmed, expect to stop drug and give appropriate care.

- Watch patient for suicidal tendencies, especially when therapy starts and dosage changes.
- Be aware that false-positive urine immunoassay screening tests for amphetamine and phencyclidine (PCP) have been found in patients taking desvenlafaxine or venlafaxine. Expect different testing to be done to distinguish drug from PCP and amphetamine.

! **WARNING** Know that drug shouldn't be stopped abruptly, because doing so may cause multiple adverse effects, including asthenia, dizziness, flu-like symptoms, headache, insomnia, and nervousness. Notify prescriber if patient experiences aggression, suicidal thoughts, or violent behavior as well as visual changes and increased blood pressure during dosage reduction or discontinuation. Know that discontinuation may have to occur over several months.

- Monitor patient closely for abnormal bleeding that may range from ecchymosis to life-threatening hemorrhage. Know that concomitant use of desvenlafaxine and venlafaxine and drugs known to affect bleeding or coagulation increases the risk of bleeding.

PATIENT TEACHING

- Instruct patient to take drug with food and follow with a full glass of water. Tell her not to chew or crush E.R. capsules or tablets. If she has trouble swallowing capsules, tell her to open capsule, sprinkle contents on a spoonful of applesauce, and swallow immediately without chewing, followed by a glass of water.
- Caution patient not to stop taking drug abruptly, as serious adverse reactions could occur. Tell patient to notify prescriber during a dosage reduction or discontinuation of the drug if aggression, anxiety, irritability, suicidal thoughts, tremor, visual changes, or feelings of violence occur.
- Advise patient that drug may cause mild pupillary dilation, which may lead to an episode of acute angle-closure glaucoma. Encourage patient to have an eye exam before starting therapy to see if he is at risk.

- Advise patient to avoid alcohol during desvenlafaxine or venlafaxine therapy.
- Advise patient not to stop taking desvenlafaxine or venlafaxine abruptly.
- Caution patient to notify prescriber if she becomes pregnant during therapy because she'll need a different antidepressant. Also inform patient that breastfeeding is not recommended during drug therapy.
- Advise patient to tell prescriber about all other prescribed drugs or OTC products she takes because of risk of interactions.
- Urge caregivers to monitor patient closely for suicidal tendencies, especially when therapy starts or dosage changes.
- Caution patient to avoid aspirin and NSAIDs, if possible, while taking desvenlafaxine or venlafaxine.
- Inform patient that urine screening tests for amphetamine and phencyclidine (PCP) may produce a false-positive for several days following discontinuation of desvenlafaxine or venlafaxine therapy, but that other tests may be done to distinguish drug from amphetamine and PCP.

! **WARNING** Tell patient to report immediately sudden-onset, persistent, severe, or unusual symptoms.

- Tell patient to inform all prescribers of desvenlafaxine or venlafaxine therapy and not to take any over-the-counter medications, including herbal preparations, without prescriber knowledge.
- Encourage patient to discuss sexual dysfunction, if present.

verapamil hydrochloride

Calan SR, Verelan, Verelan PM

≣ Class and Category

Pharmacologic class: Calcium channel blocker
Therapeutic class: Antianginal, antiarrhythmic, antihypertensive

≣ Indications and Dosages

✳ *To treat angina at rest, including unstable (crescendo, pre-infarction) angina or vasospastic (Prinzmetal's variant) angina; to treat chronic angina pectoris*

TABLETS

Adults. 80 mg to 160 mg three times daily.

✳ *To manage hypertension*

S.R. CAPSULES (VERELAN)

Adults. *Initial:* 180 mg once daily in the morning and then titrated, as needed, according to the following schedule: 240 mg in the morning; then 360 mg in the morning; and then 480 mg in the morning.

± **DOSAGE ADJUSTMENT** For elderly and low-weight patients, initial dosage reduced to 120 mg once daily and then titrated, as needed, beginning with 180 mg once daily.

S.R. TABLETS (CALAN SR)

Adults. *Initial:* 180 mg once daily in the morning increased, as needed, to 240 mg once daily in the morning. Alternatively, titrated to 180 mg twice daily or 240 mg in the morning and 120 mg in the evening with further increase to 240 mg twice daily, as needed.

± **DOSAGE ADJUSTMENT** For elderly and low-weight patients, initial dosage reduced to 120 mg once daily.

TABLETS

Adults. *Initial:* 120 mg to 360 mg daily given in three divided doses. *Maximum:* 480 mg daily.

E.R. CAPSULES (VERELAN PM)

Adults. *Initial:* 200 mg nightly, increased to 300 mg nightly, then to 400 mg nightly, if needed.

✳ *To treat supraventricular tachyarrhythmias, including atrial fibrillation or flutter*

I.V. INJECTION (VERAPAMIL HYDROCHLORIDE)

Adults and adolescents age 15 and over. *Initial:* 5 to 10 mg; then 10 mg, as needed, if response isn't adequate after 30 min.
Children ages 1 to 15. *Initial:* 0.1 to 0.3 mg/kg (usual single-dose range: 2 to 5 mg); then dosage repeated as needed, if response isn't adequate after 30 min. *Maximum:* 5 mg as the initial dose; 10 mg as a repeat dose.
Infants up to age 1. *Initial:* 0.1 to 0.2 mg/kg (usual single-dose range: 0.75 to 2 mg); then dosage repeated, as needed, if response isn't adequate after 30 min.

≣ Drug Administration

P.O.

- Capsules should be swallowed whole and not chewed or crushed. Capsules may be

U
V
W

opened and sprinkled on a spoonful of applesauce. Mixture should be swallowed immediately without chewing and followed with a glass of cool water. Do not store mixture for later use. Administer Verelan PM capsules at bedtime.

- Tablets should be swallowed whole and not chewed, crushed, or divided.

I.V.

- Maintain continuous ECG monitoring and keep emergency resuscitative equipment and drugs readily available during I.V. therapy.
- Inspect solution before administration; should be clear.
- Administer directly through free-flowing I.V. line with compatible solutions, including 0.9% Sodium Chloride Injection, 5% Dextrose in Water, or Ringer's Injection.
- Inject slowly over at least 2 minutes; at least 3 minutes for elderly patients.
- *Incompatibilities:* Albumin, amphotericin B, hydralazine hydrochloride, Sodium Lactate Injection in polyvinyl chloride bags, solutions with a pH above 6.0, trimethoprim with sulfamethoxazole

Route	Onset	Peak	Duration
P.O.	1–2 hr	1–2 hr	8–10 hr
P.O./E.R.	30 min	5–9 hr	24 hr
I.V.	1–5 min	10–15 min	0.5–1 hr

Half-life: 5–12 hr (P.O.); 2–5 hr (I.V.)

▤ Mechanism of Action

Inhibits calcium movement into coronary and vascular smooth-muscle cells by blocking slow calcium channels in cell membranes. The resulting decrease in intracellular calcium level has the following effects:

- inhibits smooth-muscle cell contractions
- decreases myocardial oxygen demand by relaxing coronary and vascular smooth muscle, reducing peripheral vascular resistance, and decreasing systolic and diastolic pressures
- slows AV conduction time and prolongs AV nodal refractoriness
- interrupts reentry circuit in AV nodal reentrant tachycardias.

▤ Contraindications

Cardiogenic shock, concomitant use of beta blockers (with I.V. verapamil),

hypersensitivity to verapamil (I.V. verapamil) or its components, hypotension, severe heart failure unless secondary to supraventricular tachycardia that responds to verapamil, severe left ventricular dysfunction, sick sinus syndrome or second- or third-degree heart block unless artificial pacemaker is in place, use in atrial fibrillation or flutter and an accessory bypass tract is present such as Lown-Ganong-Levine or Wolff-Parkinson-White syndromes (I.V. verapamil), ventricular tachycardia (with I.V. verapamil)

▤ Interactions

DRUGS

antihypertensives: Hypotensive effects
aspirin: Increased bleeding time
beta blockers: Increased risk of heart failure, hypotension, and severe bradycardia
carbamazepine, cyclosporine, theophylline: Increased risk of toxicity from these drugs
cimetidine: Decreased metabolism and increased blood level of verapamil
clonidine: Increased risk of severe sinus bradycardia
dantrolene: Increased risk of hyperkalemia and myocardial depression
digoxin: Increased blood digoxin level and risk of digitalis toxicity
disopyramide, flecainide: Additive negative inotropic effects
erythromycin, ritonavir: Increased blood verapamil level
HMG-CoA reductase inhibitors such as atorvastatin, lovastatin, and simvastatin: Increased risk of myopathy and rhabdomyolysis
ivabradine: Increased exposure to ivabradine with possible exacerbation of bradycardia and conduction disturbances
lithium: Altered serum lithium levels
mTOR inhibitors such as everolimus, sirolimus, temsirolimus: Increased plasma levels of mTOR inhibitors and verapamil
neuromuscular blockers: Prolonged recovery from neuromuscular blockade
paclitaxel: Decreased paclitaxel clearance
phenobarbital: Increased verapamil clearance
quinidine: Increased risk of quinidine toxicity, increased QT interval, additive negative inotropic effects

rifampin: Decreased bioavailability of oral verapamil

telithromycin: Increased risk of bradyarrhythmias, hypotension

FOODS

grapefruit juice: Increased verapamil level

ACTIVITIES

alcohol use: Increased blood alcohol level and prolonged CNS effects

Adverse Reactions

CNS: Asthenia, confusion, **CVA,** disequilibrium, dizziness, equilibrium disorders, extrapyramidal reactions, fatigue, headache, insomnia, paresthesia, psychosis, shakiness, somnolence, syncope

CV: Abnormal ECG, angina, **AV conduction disorders, bradycardia,** claudication, **heart failure,** hypertension, **hypotension, MI,** palpitations, peripheral edema, tachycardia, vasculitis

EENT: Blurred vision, dry mouth, tinnitus

ENDO: Gynecomastia, hyperprolactinemia

GI: Constipation, diarrhea, elevated liver enzymes, GI distress, nausea

GU: Galactorrhea, impotence, increased urination, menstrual irregularities

MS: Arthralgia, muscle spasms

RESP: Dyspnea, **pulmonary edema**

SKIN: Alopecia, diaphoresis, ecchymosis, **erythema multiforme,** exanthema, flushing, hyperkeratosis, rash, **Stevens–Johnson syndrome,** urticaria

Other: Allergy aggravated

Childbearing Considerations

PREGNANCY

- It is not known if drug causes fetal harm, although it does cross the placental barrier.
- Use with caution only if benefit to mother outweighs potential risk to fetus.

LACTATION

- Drug is present in breast milk.
- Breastfeeding should be discontinued during drug therapy.

Nursing Considerations

- Assess patient with hypertrophic cardiomyopathy or idiopathic hypertrophic subaortic stenosis for early development of hypotension and pulmonary edema, because second-degree AV block and sinus arrest can result.

- Assess for bradycardia and hypotension, and notify prescriber if blood pressure or heart rate declines significantly.
- Know that disopyramide or flecainide shouldn't be given within 48 hours before or 24 hours after verapamil because additive negative inotropic effects can result.
- Institute measures to prevent constipation, including a high-fiber diet and a stool softener, as prescribed.

PATIENT TEACHING

- Direct patient to check her pulse before taking verapamil and to notify prescriber if it's below 50 beats/minute or as instructed by prescriber.
- Inform patient taking capsules to swallow the capsules whole and not chew or crush capsules. Capsules may be opened and sprinkled on a spoonful of applesauce. Mixture should be swallowed immediately without chewing and followed with a glass of cool water. Do not store mixture for later use. Instruct patient that Verelan PM capsules should be taken at bedtime.
- Tell patient tablets should be swallowed whole and not chewed, crushed, or divided.
- Caution patient about possible dizziness and the need to avoid potentially hazardous activities until drug's CNS effects are known.
- Inform patient that adverse skin reactions may subside with continued verapamil use. Advise her to notify prescriber if rash persists.
- Encourage patient to increase dietary fiber intake to help prevent constipation. Advise her to notify prescriber if problem becomes persistent or severe.
- Inform women wishing to breastfeed that breastfeeding is not recommended during drug therapy.

vericiguat
Verquvo

U
V
W

Class and Category

Pharmacologic class: Soluble guanylate cyclase (sGC) stimulator

Therapeutic class: Vasodilator

Indications and Dosages

＊ *To reduce the risk of cardiovascular death and heart failure hospitalization following a hospitalization for heart failure or need for outpatient I.V. diuretics in adults with symptomatic chronic heart failure and ejection fraction less than 45%*

TABLETS

Adults. *Initial:* 2.5 mg once daily. Dose doubled every 2 wk to reach target maintenance dose of 10 mg, as tolerated. *Maintenance:* 10 mg once daily.

Drug Administration

P.O.

- Ensure that a pregnancy test has been done and is negative in women of childbearing age before administering the first dose.
- Administer drug with food.
- Tablet should be swallowed whole. However, for patients unable to swallow the tablet, crush and mix with water immediately before administering drug.

Route	Onset	Peak	Duration
P.O.	Unknown	Unknown	Unknown

Half-life: 30 hr

Mechanism of Action

Stimulates soluble guanylate cyclase (sGC), which is an enzyme in the nitric oxide signaling pathway. When nitric oxide binds to this enzyme, it catalyzes the synthesis of intracellular cyclic guanosine monophosphate (cGMP). cGMP helps to regulate cardiac contractility, cardiac remodeling, and vascular tone. By stimulating sGC, vericiguat increases levels of intracellular cGMP, which causes smooth muscles to relax and vasodilation to occur.

Contraindications

Concomitant therapy with other soluble guanylate cyclase stimulators, hypersensitivity to vericiguat or its components, pregnancy

Interactions

DRUGS

other soluble guanylate cyclase stimulators: Additive effects leading to possibility of serious cardiovascular adverse reactions
PDE-5 inhibitors: Potential for hypotension

Adverse Reactions

CV: Hypotension
HEME: Anemia

Childbearing Considerations

PREGNANCY

- Drug may cause fetal harm such as heart and major blood vessel malformations, according to animal studies.
- Drug is contraindicated during pregnancy.

LACTATION

- It is not known if drug is present in breast milk.
- Mothers should not breastfeed during drug therapy.

REPRODUCTION

- Women of childbearing age should use an effective method of contraception during drug therapy and for 1 month after the final dose.

Nursing Considerations

- Monitor patient's blood pressure for signs of hypotension.
- Assess patient for signs and symptoms of anemia such as fatigue and pallor. Expect to monitor patient's hemoglobin and hematocrit, as well.

PATIENT TEACHING

- Instruct patient to swallow tablet whole. However, if unable to do so, tell patient to crush tablet and mix with water immediately before taking drug.
- Advise women of childbearing age to report suspected or known pregnancy to prescriber immediately.
- Warn mothers not to breastfeed their infant.

vibegron
Gemtesa

Class and Category

Pharmacologic class: Beta-3 adrenergic agonist
Therapeutic class: Bladder muscle relaxant

Indications and Dosages

＊ *To treat overactive bladder with symptoms of urge urinary incontinence, urgency, and urinary frequency*

TABLETS

Adults. 75 mg once daily.

Drug Administration
P.O.
- Administer with a glass of water.
- Tablets may be crushed and mixed with a tablespoon of applesauce and ingested immediately. Follow immediately with a glass of water.

Route	Onset	Peak	Duration
P.O.	Unknown	1–3 hr	Unknown

Half-life: 30.8 hr

Mechanism of Action
Relaxes the detrusor smooth muscle during bladder filling to increase bladder capacity, which reduces overactive bladder symptoms.

Contraindications
Hypersensitivity to vibegron or its components

Interactions
DRUGS
digoxin: Increased serum digoxin concentrations

Adverse Reactions
CNS: Headache
EENT: Dry mouth, nasopharyngitis
GI: Constipation, diarrhea, nausea
GU: Increased residual urine volume, urinary retention, UTI
RESP: Bronchitis, upper respiratory infection
SKIN: Drug eruption, eczema, hot flush, pruritus, rash

Childbearing Considerations
PREGNANCY
- It is not known if drug can cause fetal harm.
- Use with caution only if benefit to mother outweighs potential risk to fetus.

LACTATION
- It is not known if drug is present in breast milk.
- Patient should check with prescriber before breastfeeding.

Nursing Considerations
- Monitor patient for urinary retention, especially if patient has bladder outlet obstruction or is also taking a muscarinic antagonist drug for overactive bladder. If urinary retention develops, notify prescriber and expect drug to be discontinued.
- Monitor effectiveness of drug therapy to ease patient's symptoms.

PATIENT TEACHING
- Instruct patient to swallow tablet whole followed with a glass of water.
- Tell patient unable to swallow tablets that tablet can be crushed and mixed with a tablespoon of applesauce. Patient should immediately follow ingestion of mixture with a glass of water.
- Advise patient to notify prescriber immediately if urinary retention occurs, and expect drug to be discontinued.

vigabatrin
Sabril, Vigadrone

Class and Category
Pharmacologic class: Gamma-aminobutyric acid (GABA) transaminase inhibitor
Therapeutic class: Anticonvulsant

Indications and Dosages
❋ *As adjunct therapy for refractory complex partial seizures in patients with inadequate response to several alternative treatments and for whom potential benefits outweigh the risk of vision loss*

ORAL SOLUTION, TABLETS
Adults, adolescents 17 years and over, and children weighing more than 60 kg (132 lb). *Initial:* 500 mg twice daily, increased weekly in 500-mg increments, as needed. *Maximum:* 1.5 g twice daily.
Children age 2 to 16 years of age weighing more than 25 kg (55 lb) to less than 60 kg (132 lb). *Initial:* 250 mg twice daily, increased weekly, as needed. *Maximum:* 1 g twice daily.
Children age 2 to 16 years of age weighing more than 20 kg (44 lb) to less than 25 kg (55 lb). *Initial:* 250 mg twice daily, increased weekly, as needed. *Maximum:* 750 mg twice daily.
Children age 2 to 16 years of age weighing more than 15 kg (33 lb) to less than 20 kg (44 lb). *Initial:* 225 mg twice daily, increased weekly, as needed. *Maximum:* 650 mg twice daily.
Children age 2 to 16 weighing at least 10 kg (22 lb) to 15 kg (33 lb). *Initial:* 175 mg twice daily, increased weekly, as needed. *Maximum:* 525 mg twice daily.

U
V
W

± DOSAGE ADJUSTMENT For adult patient and children 2 years or older with creatinine clearance 51 to 80 ml/min, dose reduced by 25%; creatinine clearance 31 to 50 ml/min, dose reduced by 50%; creatinine clearance 11 to 30 ml/min, dose reduced by 75%.

* *As monotherapy for pediatric patients with infantile spasms for whom potential benefits outweigh risk of vision loss*

ORAL SOLUTION

Children age 1 month to 2 years. *Initial:* 50 mg/kg/day in two divided doses, increased every 3 days by 25 to 50 mg/kg/day, as needed. *Maximum:* 150 mg/kg/day in two divided doses.

Drug Administration

P.O.

- Mix oral solution by emptying the entire contents of each 500-mg packet needed into a clean cup; dissolve in 10 ml of cold or room-temperature water per packet to a final concentration of 50 mg/ml. Discard if final solution is not clear, colorless, or free of particles. Administer resulting solution immediately using the 3-ml or 10-ml oral syringe supplied by pharmacy.
- Drug may be given with or without food.

Route	Onset	Peak	Duration
P.O.	Unknown	1–2 hr	Unknown
Half-life: 10.5 hr			

Mechanism of Action

Inhibits the action of gamma-aminobutyric acid transaminase (GABA-T), the enzyme responsible for metabolism of the inhibitory neurotransmitter GABA. This increases GABA level in the CNS, which may play a role in suppression of seizure activity. The mechanism of action for infantile spasms is unknown.

Contraindications

Hypersensitivity to vigabatrin and its components

Interactions

DRUGS

clonazepam: Increased risk of clonazepam-associated adverse reactions
phenytoin: Decreased serum phenytoin level

Adverse Reactions

CNS: Abnormal behavior or dreams, abnormal magnetic resonance imaging (MRI) in children age 6 and under, acute psychosis, anxiety, apathy, asthenia, attention disturbance, confusion, coordination abnormality, delirium, depression, dizziness, dystonia, **encephalopathy**, expressive language disorder, fatigue, fever, gait disturbance, headache, hyperreflexia, hypertonia, hypoesthesia, hypomania, hyporeflexia, hypotonia, insomnia, intramyelinic edema (infants), irritability, lethargy, malaise, **malignant hyperthermia**, memory loss, myoclonus, nervousness, paresthesia, peripheral neuropathy, postictal state, **seizures**, sensory disturbance, somnolence, **status epilepticus**, **suicidal ideation**, thirst, tremor, vertigo

CV: Chest pain, edema, peripheral edema

EENT: Asthenopia, blurred vision, deafness, diplopia, eye pain, **laryngeal edema**, nasopharyngitis, nystagmus, optic neuritis, pharyngolaryngeal pain, **stridor**, tinnitus, toothache, tunnel vision, vision loss (permanent and severe), visual field defect

ENDO: Delayed puberty

GI: Abdominal or stomach pain, cholestasis, constipation, decreased liver enzymes, diarrhea, distention, dyspepsia, esophagitis, **GI hemorrhage**, nausea, vomiting

GU: Dysmenorrhea, erectile dysfunction, UTI

HEME: Anemia

MS: Arthralgia; back or limb pain; dysarthria; muscle spasticity, spasms, or twitching

RESP: Bronchitis, cough, **pulmonary edema**, **respiratory failure**, upper respiratory infection

SKIN: Alopecia, maculopapular rash, pruritus, **Stevens–Johnson syndrome**, **toxic epidermal necrolysis**

Other: **Angioedema**, birth defects, developmental delay, flu-like symptoms, **multiorgan failure**, weight gain

Childbearing Considerations

PREGNANCY

- Pregnancy exposure registry: 1-888-233-2334 or https://www.aedpregnancyregistry.org.
- Drug may cause fetal harm, based on animal studies.
- Use with caution only if benefit to mother outweighs potential risk to fetus.

LACTATION

- Drug is present in breast milk.
- Breastfeeding is not recommended during drug therapy.

☰ Nursing Considerations

! WARNING Monitor patient's vision, and make sure patient has been examined by an ophthalmic professional in which visual fields and retinal examination has been performed no later than 4 weeks after vigabatrin therapy has begun and then every 3 months throughout therapy and 3 to 6 months after therapy has been discontinued, because drug can cause progressive and permanent bilateral concentric visual field constriction and severely reduce visual acuity. Be aware that while risk increases with total dose and duration of therapy, all patients are at risk for visual abnormalities even after drug has been stopped. Because of the risk of permanent and possibly severe vision loss, drug can be prescribed and obtained only through the REMS distribution program. Report any visual abnormalities immediately, and expect drug to be discontinued.

- Know that abnormal MRI results have been noted in children 6 years and younger receiving vigabatrin.
- Monitor patient for suicidal ideation throughout therapy but especially when therapy starts or dosage changes.
- Know that when discontinuing vigabatrin therapy, expect to do so gradually by decreasing daily dose by 1 g each week until drug is discontinued, as ordered.
- Know that when discontinuing vigabatrin therapy in children, expect to do so gradually by decreasing dose by 25 to 50 mg/kg/day every 3 to 4 days.
- Monitor patient for evidence of peripheral neuropathy, such as numbness or tingling in feet or toes, progressive loss of reflexes, starting at the ankles, or reduced distal lower limb position sense or vibration. Alert prescriber if abnormalities are present.
- Assess patient routinely for edema, including peripheral edema.

PATIENT TEACHING

! WARNING Explain the risk of possibly permanent vision loss that may occur as blurred vision or tunnel vision before patient starts vigabatrin. Stress the importance of having vision checked every 3 months throughout therapy and 3 to 6 months after drug is discontinued even if patient is an infant. However, inform patient that vision testing may be insensitive and may not detect vision loss before it is severe and has become permanent.

- Warn patient not to stop taking vigabatrin abruptly; she will need to be weaned off drug gradually over several weeks.
- Instruct parents how to mix the oral solution by emptying the entire contents of each 500-mg packet needed into a clean cup and dissolved in 10 ml of cold or room-temperature water per packet. Show parents how to administer the resulting solution using the 3-ml or 10-ml oral syringe supplied by the pharmacist. Remind them that the concentration of the final solution is 50 mg/ml. Stress importance of checking dosage before administering.
- Advise female patient of childbearing age to report suspected or confirmed pregnancy to prescriber because adverse effects are unknown. Also inform that breastfeeding is not recommended during drug therapy.
- Advise patient or caregiver to notify prescriber if patient has unusual behaviors or feelings, especially if related to suicidal ideation and particularly at the beginning of therapy and during dosage adjustments.
- Caution patient not to perform hazardous activities such as operating equipment until CNS effects of drug are known.
- Alert patient to monitor his weight because drug may cause weight gain.

vilazodone hydrochloride
Viibryd

☰ Class and Category
Pharmacologic class: Selective serotonin reuptake inhibitor (SSRI)
Therapeutic class: Antidepressant

☰ Indications and Dosages
✳ *To treat major depressive disorder*

U
V
W

TABLETS

Adults. *Initial:* 10 mg once daily for 7 days, followed by 20 mg once daily for 7 days, then increased to 40 mg once daily as needed.

±**DOSAGE ADJUSTMENT** For patients taking a strong inhibitor of CYP3A4 (clarithromycin, itraconazole, voriconazole), dosage should not exceed 20 mg daily. For patients taking a strong CYP3A4 inducer (carbamazepine, phenytoin, rifampin) for more than 14 days, dosage may be increased up to twofold over 1 to 2 weeks but not exceed 80 mg daily.

Drug Administration

P.O.

- Administer drug with food.

Route	Onset	Peak	Duration
P.O.	Unknown	4–5 hr	Unknown

Half-life: 25 hr

Mechanism of Action

Exerts antidepressant effects by potentiating serotonin activity in CNS and inhibiting serotonin reuptake at the presynaptic neuronal membrane. Blocked serotonin reuptake increases levels and prolongs activity of serotonin at synaptic receptor sites.

Contraindications

Hypersensitivity to vilazodone or its components, use within 14 days of MAO inhibitor therapy

Interactions

DRUGS

amphetamines, buspirone, fentanyl, lithium, MAO inhibitors, serotonin–norepinephrine reuptake inhibitors, serotonin reuptake inhibitors, St. John's wort, tramadol, tricyclic antidepressants, triptans, tryptophan: Increased risk of life-threatening adverse effects such as serotonin syndrome
aspirin, NSAIDs, warfarin, and other anticoagulants: Increased risk of bleeding
CYP3A4 inhibitors such as clarithromycin, itraconazole, voriconazole: Increased blood vilazodone levels with increased risk of adverse effects
digoxin: Possible increased risk of digoxin concentrations

Adverse Reactions

CNS: Abnormal dreams, dizziness, fatigue, feeling jittery, hallucinations, insomnia, irritability, mania, migraine, **neuroleptic malignant syndrome-like reactions,** panic attack, paresthesia, restlessness, **seizures, serotonin syndrome,** sleep paralysis, **suicidal ideation,** tremor
CV: Palpitations, **prolonged QT interval, torsades de pointes, ventricular extrasystoles**
EENT: Angle-closure glaucoma, blurred vision, cataracts, dry eyes or mouth
GI: **Acute pancreatitis,** anorexia, diarrhea, dyspepsia, flatulence, gastroenteritis, **GI bleeding,** increased appetite, nausea, vomiting
GU: Absent or delayed orgasm (females), decreased libido, delayed ejaculation, erectile dysfunction, pollakiuria
HEME: **Bleeding events**
MS: Arthralgia
SKIN: Diaphoresis, drug eruption, night sweats, rash, urticaria

Childbearing Considerations

PREGNANCY

- Pregnancy exposure registry: 1-844 -405-6185 or https://womensmentalhealth. org/clinical-and-research-programs /pregnancyregistry/antidepressants/.
- Drug may cause fetal harm, especially if exposure occurs late in third trimester. Neonate exposed to drug in utero may require prolonged hospitalization, respiratory support, and tube feeding as a result of persistent pulmonary hypertension of the newborn and drug discontinuation syndrome.
- Use with caution only if benefit to mother outweighs potential risk to fetus.

LACTATION

- It is not known if drug is present in breast milk.
- Patient should check with prescriber before breastfeeding.

Nursing Considerations

- Be aware that vilazodone should not be given to patients with bradycardia, congenital long QT syndrome, hypokalemia or hypomagnesemia, recent acute myocardial infarction, or uncompensated heart failure because of increased risk of prolonged QT interval and torsades de pointes. It should also not be given to patients who are taking other drugs that prolong the QT interval. Expect hypokalemia and hypomagnesemia to be corrected before vilazodone therapy is begun.

- Use vilazodone cautiously in a patient with a seizure disorder because drug effect has not been studied in patients with seizures.
- Expect to taper vilazodone therapy gradually when drug is no longer required; abrupt discontinuation can precipitate withdrawal symptoms.

! **WARNING** Monitor patient closely for serotonin syndrome exhibited by agitation, coma, diarrhea, hallucinations, hyperreflexia, hyperthermia, incoordination, labile blood pressure, nausea, tachycardia, or vomiting. Notify prescriber immediately because serotonin syndrome may be life-threatening; provide supportive care.

! **WARNING** Be aware that serotonin syndrome in its most severe form may resemble neuroleptic malignant syndrome, which includes autonomic instability with possibly rapid changes in mental status and vital signs, hyperthermia, and muscle rigidity. Stop drug immediately, and provide supportive care.

- Watch patient closely for suicidal tendencies, particularly when therapy starts and dosage changes, because depression may worsen temporarily during these times, possibly leading to suicidal ideation.
- Watch for mania, which may result from any antidepressant in a susceptible patient.
- Monitor patient closely for evidence of GI bleeding, especially if patient also takes a drug known to cause GI bleeding, such as aspirin, an NSAID, or warfarin.
- Monitor patient's serum sodium level, as ordered, especially in the elderly and patients with volume depletion, because selective serotonin reuptake inhibitors, the class of drugs vilazodone belongs to, have caused hyponatremia. If patient develops a confusion, difficulty concentrating, headache, memory impairment, unsteadiness, and weakness, and sodium level has decreased, notify prescriber and expect drug to be discontinued. Be prepared to provide supportive care.

PATIENT TEACHING

- Instruct patient to take vilazodone with food because drug may not be as effective if taken on an empty stomach.
- Advise patient that drug may cause mild pupillary dilation, which may lead to an episode of acute closure glaucoma. Encourage patient to have an eye exam before starting therapy to see if he is at risk.
- Tell family or caregiver to observe patient closely for suicidal tendencies, especially when therapy starts or dosage changes.
- Tell patient not to take aspirin or NSAIDs during therapy because they increase the risk of bleeding. If patient takes warfarin, tell her to use bleeding precautions and to notify prescriber at once if bleeding occurs.
- Caution patient to alert all prescribers about vilazodone therapy because of potentially serious drug interactions.
- Advise patient to notify prescriber of any persistent, severe, or unusual adverse reactions.
- Encourage patient to address sexual dysfunction with prescriber, if concerned.

vorapaxar
Zontivity

Class and Category
Pharmacologic class: Protease activated receptor-1 (PAR-1) inhibitor
Therapeutic class: Antiplatelet

Indications and Dosages
＊ *As adjunct with aspirin and/or clopidogrel to reduce thrombotic cardiovascular events in patients with a history of myocardial infarction or peripheral arterial disease*

TABLETS
Adults. 2.08 mg once daily.

Drug Administration
P.O.
- No special administration instructions given by manufacturer.

Route	Onset	Peak	Duration
P.O.	1 wk	1–2 hr	Unknown

Half-life: 5–13 days

U V W

Mechanism of Action

Inhibits thrombin-induced and thrombin receptor agonist peptide-induced platelet aggregation.

Contraindications

Active pathologic bleeding; history of intracranial hemorrhage, stroke, or transient ischemic attack; hypersensitivity to vorapaxar or its components

Interactions

DRUGS

strong CYP3A inducers such as carbamazepine, phenytoin, rifampin, St. John's wort: Decreased vorapaxar effectiveness
strong CYP3A inhibitors such as boceprevir, clarithromycin, conivaptan, indinavir, itraconazole, ketoconazole, nefazodone, nelfinavir, posaconazole, ritonavir, saquinavir, telaprevir, telithromycin: Increased vorapaxar exposure and adverse reactions

Adverse Reactions

CNS: Depression, **intracranial hemorrhage**
EENT: Diplopia, oculomotor disturbance, retinal disorder including retinopathy
GI: **GI bleeding**
HEME: Anemia, **bleeding events that may become severe,** iron deficiency
SKIN: Eruptions, exanthema, rash

Childbearing Considerations

PREGNANCY

- It is not known if drug can cause fetal harm.
- Use with caution only if benefit to mother outweighs potential risk to fetus.

LACTATION

- It is not known if drug is present in breast milk.
- Breastfeeding is not recommended during drug therapy.

Nursing Considerations

- Know that vorapaxar should not be given to patients with a history of intracranial hemorrhage, stroke, or transient ischemic attack because of an increased risk for intracranial hemorrhage. Drug should be discontinued in a patient who experiences a stroke while taking vorapaxar.
- Assess patient's bleeding risk before beginning vorapaxar therapy, because vorapaxar increases the risk of bleeding in proportion to the patient's underlying bleeding risk. Factors that may increase the patient's risk of bleeding include the use of certain concomitant drugs such as anticoagulants, chronic nonsteroidal anti-inflammatory drugs, fibrinolytic therapy, selective serotonin reuptake inhibitors, or serotonin–norepinephrine reuptake inhibitors; history of bleeding disorders; low body weight; older age; or reduced hepatic or renal function.
- Know that vorapaxar should not be given to patients with severe hepatic impairment because of increased risk for bleeding.

! **WARNING** Monitor patient for bleeding throughout vorapaxar therapy. Suspect bleeding in patient who is hypotensive and has recently undergone coronary angiography, coronary artery bypass graft surgery, percutaneous coronary intervention, or other surgical procedures. Stop vorapaxar therapy and notify prescriber immediately of suspected or known bleeding. Prepare to support patient according to standard of care, as there is no known treatment to reverse the antiplatelet effect of drug because of its long half-life. Significant inhibition of platelet aggregation has been known to persist for at least 4 weeks after drug has been discontinued.

PATIENT TEACHING

- Tell patient to take vorapaxar exactly as prescribed and not to discontinue drug without discussing it with the prescriber. Inform patient that drug is usually prescribed along with other drugs such as aspirin and/or clopidogrel.
- Inform patient that he may bleed or bruise more easily. Stress importance of promptly reporting any excessive, prolonged, or unanticipated bleeding, or blood in the stool or urine.
- Review safety precautions to avoid bleeding events, such as using an electric razor and soft toothbrush.
- Remind patient to inform all dentists and physicians of vorapaxar use prior to any dental procedure or surgery. Emphasize that the dentist or doctor performing the procedure should talk to the prescriber before stopping drug.
- Tell patient to keep prescriber informed of all dietary supplements, over-the-counter drugs, or prescription drugs he takes.

voriconazole
Vfend

⣿ Class and Category
Pharmacologic class: Triazole
Therapeutic class: Antifungal

⣿ Indications and Dosages
✶ *To treat invasive aspergillosis; to treat serious fungal infections caused by* Scedosporium apiospermum *and* Fusarium *species, including* Fusarium solani, *in patients intolerant of or refractory to other therapy*

I.V. INFUSION
Adults, adolescents age 15 and older regardless of body weight, and adolescents age 12 to 14 weighing 50 kg (110 lb) or more. *Loading dose:* 6 mg/kg at no more than 3 mg/kg/hr every 12 hr for two doses. *Maintenance:* 4 mg/kg at no more than 3 mg/kg/hr every 12 hr for at least 7 days before being switched to an oral form. Maintenance dose reduced to 3 mg/kg every 12 hr for patients unable to tolerate the 4 mg/kg dose.

ORAL SUSPENSION, TABLETS
Adults weighing 40 kg (88 lb) or more, adolescents age 15 and older regardless of body weight, and adolescents age 12 to 14 weighing 50 kg (110 lb) or more. *After 7 days of I.V. therapy:* 200 mg every 12 hr, increased to 300 mg every 12 hr, as needed. **Adults weighing less than 40 kg (88 lb).** *After 7 days of I.V. therapy:* 100 mg every 12 hr, increased to 150 mg every 12 hr, as needed.

I.V. INFUSION
Children age 2 to less than 12 years of age, adolescents age 12 to 14 weighing less than 50 kg (110 lb). *Loading dose:* 9 mg/kg at no more than 3 mg/kg/hr every 12 hr for two doses. *Maintenance:* 8 mg/kg at no more than 3 mg/kg/hr every 12 hr with dosage decreased or increased, as needed in 1 mg/kg steps and given for at least 7 days before being switched to oral form.

ORAL SUSPENSION, TABLETS
Children age 2 to less than 12 years, adolescents 12 to 14 years of age weighing less than 50 kg (110 lb). *After 7 days of I.V. therapy:* 9 mg/kg every 12 hr, with dosage decreased or increased by 1 mg/kg, as needed. *Maximum:* 350 mg every 12 hr.

✶ *To treat candidemia in non-neutropenic patients and other deep-tissue disseminated* Candida *infections involving the abdomen, bladder wall, kidney, skin, or a wound*

I.V. INFUSION
Adults, adolescents age 15 and older regardless of body weight, and adolescents age 12 to 14 weighing 50 kg (110 lb) or more. *Loading dose:* 6 mg/kg at no more than 3 mg/kg/hr every 12 hr for two doses. *Maintenance:* 3 to 4 mg/kg at no more than 3 mg/kg/hr every 12 hr and then switched to oral form when feasible. If it's not possible to switch to oral form, I.V. therapy given for at least 14 days after symptoms resolve or last positive culture, whichever takes longer.
Children age 2 to less than 12 years of age, adolescents age 12 to 14 weighing less than 50 kg (110 lb). *Loading dose:* 9 mg/kg at no more than 3 mg/kg/hr every 12 hr for two doses. *Maintenance:* 8 mg/kg at no more than 3 mg/kg/hr every 12 hr and then switched to oral form when feasible and significant improvement has occurred.

ORAL SUSPENSION, TABLETS
Adults weighing 40 kg (88 lb) or more, adolescents age 15 and older regardless of weight, and adolescents age 12 to 14 weighing 50 kg (110 lb) or more. *After I.V. therapy:* 200 mg every 12 hr for at least 14 days after symptoms resolve or last positive culture, whichever takes longer. **Adults weighing less than 40 kg (88 lb).** *Maintenance:* 100 mg every 12 hr, increased to 150 mg every 12 hr, as needed and given for at least 14 days after symptoms resolve or last positive culture, whichever takes longer. **Children age 2 to less than 12 years, adolescents 12 to 14 years of age weighing less than 50 kg (110 lb).** *After I.V. therapy:* 9 mg/kg every 12 hr with dosage increased or decreased, as needed, in 1 mg/kg steps. *Maximum:* 350 mg every 12 hr.

✶ *To treat esophageal candidiasis*

I.V. INFUSION
Children age 2 to less than 12 years, adolescents age 12 to 14 weighing less than 50 kg (110 lb). *Initial:* 4 mg/kg at no more than 3 mg/kg/hr every 12 hr with dosage increased or decreased, as needed, in 1 mg/kg steps. After at least 5 days of therapy and only after there is significant improvement, therapy switched to oral form.

ORAL SUSPENSION, TABLETS

Adults weighing 40 kg (88 lb) or more, adolescents age 15 and older regardless of weight, and adolescents age 12 to 14 weighing 50 kg (110 lb) or more. 200 mg every 12 hr for at least 14 days and at least 7 days after signs and symptoms resolve.

Adults weighing less than 40 kg (88 lb). 100 mg every 12 hr for at least 14 days and at least 7 days after signs and symptoms resolve.

Children age 2 to less than 12 years, adolescents 12 to 14 years of age weighing less than 50 kg (110 lb). *Maintenance:* 9 mg/kg every 12 hr with dosage increased or decreased, as needed, in 1 mg/kg steps. *Maximum:* 350 mg every 12 hr.

±**DOSAGE ADJUSTMENT** For adult use with efavirenz or phenytoin, maintenance dose increased. For adult patients with mild to moderate hepatic impairment, maintenance dosage reduced. For adult patients with moderate to severe renal impairment (creatinine clearance less than 50 ml/min), only oral drug should be given. No dosage guidelines for children are given by manufacturer.

≣ Drug Administration

P.O.

- Administer at least 1 hour before or 1 hour after a meal.
- Shake oral suspension for about 10 seconds before each use. Use calibrated device to measure dosage. Store at room temperature and discard after 14 days.

I.V.

- Reconstitute powder with 19 ml Sterile Water for Injection to obtain a volume of 20 ml with a concentrate of 10 mg/ml. Solution should be clear. It is recommended to use a standard 20-ml nonautomated syringe to ensure that exact amount of Sterile Water for Injection is dispensed. Discard vial if the vacuum does not pull solution into the vial.
- Shake vial until all powder is dissolved.
- Dilute to final concentration of 5 mg/ml or less using 0.9% Sodium Chloride Injection, 5% Dextrose Injection, or Lactated Ringer's solution (see manufacturer guidelines for other appropriate solutions). This requires withdrawing and discarding at least an equal volume of diluent from infusion bag or bottle before instillation of drug

concentrate. Final concentration should not be less than 0.5 mg/ml nor greater than 5 mg/ml.

- Discard partially used vials after mixing. If infusion isn't administered immediately, store in refrigerator for no longer than 24 hours.
- Administer I.V. infusion over 1 to 3 hours at a concentration of 5 mg/ml or less and no more than 3 mg/kg/hr. Never administer as an I.V. bolus.
- *Incompatibilities:* 4.2% Sodium Bicarbonate infusion, I.V. solutions other than recommended by manufacturer, other I.V. drugs

Route	Onset	Peak	Duration
P.O./I.V.	Unknown	1–2 hr	12 hr

Half-life: Dose-dependent

≣ Mechanism of Action

Prevents fungal ergosterol biosynthesis by inhibiting fungal cytochrome P-450–mediated 14 alpha-lanosterol demethylation. The loss of ergosterol in the fungal cell wall renders the fungal cell inactive.

≣ Contraindications

Coadministration with long-acting barbiturates, carbamazepine, CYP3A4 substrates (astemizole, cisapride, ivabradine, pimozide, or quinidine), efavirenz (doses of 400 mg every 24 hours or higher), ergot alkaloids, lurasidone, naloxegol, rifabutin, rifampin, ritonavir (400 mg every 12 hours), sirolimus, St. John's wort, tolvaptan, venetoclax: hypersensitivity to voriconazole or its components

≣ Interactions

DRUGS

alfentanil: Increased plasma alfentanil level and increased risk of adverse reactions

benzodiazepines: Possibly prolonged sedative effect of benzodiazepines

calcium channel blockers; HMG-CoA reductase inhibitors, such as lovastatin; omeprazole; sirolimus: Possibly increased plasma levels of these drugs, leading to increased risk of adverse reactions and toxicity

carbamazepine, long-acting barbiturates, rifabutin, rifampin, ritonavir, St. John's wort: Decreased plasma voriconazole concentration *cyclosporine, sirolimus, tacrolimus:* Increased serum concentrations of these drugs and risk of toxicity, especially nephrotoxicity

CYP3A4 substrates (astemizole, cisapride, pimozide, quinidine, terfenadine): Increased plasma levels of these drugs, which may lead to prolonged QT interval and, rarely, torsades de pointes

efavirenz: Possibly significant decreased plasma voriconazole levels and increased plasma efavirenz levels

ergot alkaloids (dihydroergotamine, ergotamine): May increase plasma level of ergot alkaloids, leading to ergotism

everolimus, fluconazole, oral contraceptives: Increased plasma voriconazole level and risk of toxicity

fentanyl and other long-acting opiates metabolized by CYP3A4 such as oxycodone: Increased plasma level of fentanyl and other long-acting opiates with increased risk of adverse reactions

HIV protease inhibitors (amprenavir, nelfinavir, ritonavir, saquinavir), non-nucleoside reverse transcriptase inhibitors (delavirdine): Possibly inhibited metabolism of voriconazole leading to increased plasma voriconazole levels and plasma levels of these drugs

methadone: Increased plasma level of methadone, possibly leading to toxicity, including QT-interval prolongation

NSAIDs: Increased plasma NSAID levels leading to possible increased adverse reactions, including toxicity

oral contraceptives: Increased plasma voriconazole level and risk of toxicity; increased plasma levels of oral contraceptives and risk of adverse reactions

phenytoin: Decreased plasma level of voriconazole and increased plasma level of phenytoin

sulfonylureas: Possibly increased plasma level of sulfonylureas and increased risk of hypoglycemia

vinca alkaloids: Possibly increased risk of neurotoxicity

warfarin: Possibly increased PTT

▤ Adverse Reactions

CNS: Affect lability, agitation, anxiety, asthenia, ataxia, chills, depression, dizziness, fever, hallucinations, headache, hypothermia, insomnia, lethargy, paresthesia, **seizures,** syncope, vertigo

CV: Arrhythmias, bradycardia, cardiac arrest, chest pain, hypertension, hypotension, palpitations, peripheral edema, **prolonged QT interval, supraventricular** tachycardia, tachycardia, **torsades de pointes,** vasodilation, **ventricular tachycardia**

EENT: Abnormal or blurred vision, altered or enhanced visual perception, change in color perception, chromatopsia, dry eyes or mouth, eye hemorrhage, keratitis, nasal congestion, nystagmus, optic neuritis, papilledema, photophobia, tinnitus, visual disturbances that could be prolonged

ENDO: Adrenal insufficiency, Cushing's syndrome, hypoglycemia

GI: Abdominal pain or tenderness, cholestasis, cholestatic jaundice, diarrhea, dyspepsia, elevated liver enzymes, **fulminant hepatic failure, hepatitis,** hyperbilirubinemia, jaundice, nausea, **pancreatitis,** vomiting

GU: Abnormal kidney function **or toxicity, acute renal failure,** elevated serum creatinine level

HEME: Anemia, **leukopenia, pancytopenia, thrombocytopenia**

MS: Arthralgia, fluorosis, myalgia, periostitis, skeletal pain

RESP: Respiratory disorders, **respiratory failure,** tachypnea

SKIN: Alopecia, cheilitis, cutaneous lupus erythematosus, dermatitis (allergic or contact), **erythema multiforme, exfoliative dermatitis,** flushing, maculopapular rash, photosensitivity, pruritus, pseudoporphyria, rash, **Stevens–Johnson syndrome, toxic epidermal necrolysis,** urticaria

Other: Anaphylaxis, drug reaction with eosinophilia and systemic symptoms (DRESS), elevated alkaline phosphatase, **hypercalcemia, hypermagnesemia, hyperphosphatemia, hypersensitivity reactions, hypokalemia, hypomagnesemia,** infusion reactions such as phlebitis, **sepsis**

▤ Childbearing Considerations

PREGNANCY

- Drug may cause fetal harm, based on animal studies.
- Use with caution only if benefit to mother outweighs potential risk to fetus.

U
V
W

LACTATION

- It is not known if drug is present in breast milk.
- Patient should check with prescriber before breastfeeding.

REPRODUCTION

- Women of childbearing age should use effective contraception during drug therapy.

Nursing Considerations

- Use voriconazole cautiously in patients hypersensitive to other azoles and in patients at risk for proarrhythmic events (such as those receiving cardiotoxic chemotherapy or concomitant drug therapy known to prolong QT interval, or those who have acquired or congenital QT prolongation, cardiomyopathy, hypokalemia, sinus bradycardia, or symptomatic arrhythmias [existing]), because drug may prolong the QT interval. Know that calcium, magnesium, and potassium imbalances should be corrected before starting voriconazole therapy as well as any time an imbalance occurs during voriconazole therapy. Monitor patient's electrolyte balance closely.
- Determine if patient has any problems with galactose intolerance, glucose–galactose malabsorption, or Lapp lactase deficiency before starting therapy because voriconazole tablets contain lactose and shouldn't be given to patients with these conditions.
- Obtain specimens for fungal culture and other relevant laboratory studies (including histopathology), as ordered, before giving first dose. Expect to begin drug before test results are known.
- Assess patient's liver function, including bilirubin, as ordered, at the start of voriconazole therapy and at least weekly for the first month of treatment then monthly thereafter because, although uncommon, drug has caused serious hepatic reactions, including fatalities. Know that a higher frequency of elevated liver enzymes has been noted in children. Be aware that drug may be discontinued if liver abnormalities occur.
- Monitor renal function, especially serum creatinine level, when giving I.V. form of voriconazole because drug may accumulate in body when creatinine clearance is less than 50 ml/min, increasing the risk of adverse reactions.

! WARNING Observe patient receiving I.V. voriconazole closely for anaphylactoid-type reactions, such as chest tightness, dyspnea, faintness, fever, flushing, nausea, pruritus, rash, sweating, and tachycardia, which may occur immediately after starting infusion. Stop infusion if these reactions occur, and notify prescriber immediately.

- Monitor patient closely throughout therapy for rash, which may indicate a serious cutaneous reaction, such as Stevens–Johnson syndrome. If rash occurs, notify prescriber, and expect that voriconazole may be discontinued. Also, if patient develops pre-malignant skin lesions, drug should be discontinued.
- Monitor diabetic patients also taking sulfonylureas closely for hypoglycemia, and check blood glucose levels regularly.
- Assess patient's visual function, including color perception, visual acuity, and visual field, if voriconazole therapy continues longer than 28 days.
- Monitor patient closely for pancreatitis, especially if patient is a child or has risk factors for acute pancreatitis, such as recent chemotherapy or hematopoietic stem cell transplantation.
- Report skeletal pain to prescriber and expect skeletal x-rays to be done. If fluorosis or periostitis is found, anticipate voriconazole therapy to be discontinued.

PATIENT TEACHING

- Inform patient with galactose intolerance, glucose–galactose malabsorption, or Lapp lactase deficiency that voriconazole tablets contain lactose.
- Instruct patient taking oral voriconazole to take drug at least 1 hour before or 1 hour after a meal.
- Tell patient that frequent blood tests will have to be performed and importance of compliance with schedule.

! WARNING Alert patient that an allergic reaction or skin reaction may occur with drug therapy. Stress importance of alerting prescriber at the first sign (especially of a rash) and to seek immediate emergency care, if serious.

- Instruct patients with diabetes mellitus who are also taking a sulfonylurea to check blood glucose regularly and to monitor self for hypoglycemia, as drug increases risk of hypoglycemia.
- Tell patient to alert all prescribers of voriconazole therapy.
- Caution patient to report any serious, severe, or unusual signs and symptoms to prescriber.
- Instruct women of childbearing age to use effective contraception during therapy and to notify prescriber immediately if pregnancy is suspected.
- Caution patient not to drive at night and to avoid hazardous activities because drug may cause visual disturbances, including blurring or photophobia.
- Advise patient to avoid exposure to direct sunlight or UV light and to wear sunscreen when outdoors.

vortioxetine hydrobromide
Trintellix

Class and Category
Pharmacologic class: Serotonin modulator
Therapeutic class: Antidepressant

Indications and Dosages
✱ *To treat major depressive disorder (MDD)*

TABLETS
Adults. *Initial:* 10 mg once daily, then increased to 20 mg once daily, as tolerated. *Maximum:* 20 mg once daily.

±**DOSAGE ADJUSTMENT** For patients who cannot tolerate higher doses, dosage may be decreased down to 5 mg once daily. For patients taking strong CYP inducers, such as carbamazepine, phenytoin, or rifampin concurrently for longer than 14 days, dosage increased up to three times the original dose and when inducer is discontinued, dosage decreased to original level within 14 days. For patients taking strong CYP2D6 inhibitors such as bupropion, fluoxetine, paroxetine, or quinidine concurrently, dosage reduced by one-half, and when inhibitor is discontinued, dosage increased to original level within 14 days. For patients who are known CYP2D6

poor metabolizers, maximum dosage is 10 mg once daily.

Drug Administration
P.O.
- Administer at about same time daily.

Route	Onset	Peak	Duration
P.O.	1–2 wk	7–11 hr	Unknown

Half-life: 66 hr

Mechanism of Action
Enhances serotonergic activity in the central nervous system through inhibiting the reuptake of serotonin. Enhanced serotonergic activity is thought to relieve symptoms of depression.

Contraindications
Hypersensitivity to vortioxetine or its components; use within 14 days of a MAO inhibitor

Interactions
DRUGS
amphetamines, buspirone, fentanyl, lithium, MAO inhibitors, SNRIs, SSRIs, St. John's wort, tramadol, tricyclic antidepressants, triptans, tryptophans: Increased risk of serotonin toxicity
aspirin, NSAIDs, warfarin, and other anticoagulants and antiplatelets: Increased risk of bleeding
CYP2D6 inducers (strong) such as carbamazepine, phenytoin, rifampin: Decreased plasma vortioxetine levels with possible decreased effectiveness
CYP2D6 inhibitors (strong) such as bupropion, fluoxetine, paroxetine, and quinidine: Increased plasma vortioxetine levels with increased risk of adverse reactions
drugs that are highly protein bound such as warfarin: May increase free concentrations of vortioxetine or other tightly-bound drugs in plasma

Adverse Reactions
CNS: Abnormal dreams, activation of hypomania/mania, aggression, agitation, anger, dizziness, headache, hostility, irritability, **seizures, serotonin syndrome, suicidal ideation,** vertigo
EENT: Altered taste, angle-closure glaucoma, dry mouth
ENDO: Hyperprolactinemia

U
V
W

GI: Acute pancreatitis, constipation, diarrhea, dyspepsia, flatulence, nausea, vomiting

GU: Absent or delayed orgasm (females), decreased libido, ejaculatory delay or failure, erectile dysfunction, sexual performance or sexual satisfaction difficulties

HEME: Abnormal bleeding

RESP: Difficulty breathing

SKIN: Flushing, hyperhidrosis, pruritus, rash, urticaria

Other: Discontinuation disorder, false-positive urine results for methadone, hypersensitivity reactions including anaphylaxis, hyponatremia, weight gain

Childbearing Considerations

PREGNANCY

- Pregnancy exposure registry: 1-844-405-6185 or https://womensmentalhealth.org/clinical-and-research-programs/pregnancyregistry/antidepressants/.
- Drug may cause fetal harm, especially if exposed to drug late in third trimester, which may require prolonged hospitalization, respiratory support, and tube feeding as a result of persistent pulmonary hypertension of the newborn and drug discontinuation syndrome.
- Use with caution only if benefit to mother outweighs potential risk to fetus.

LACTATION

- It is not known if drug is present in breast milk.
- Patient should check with prescriber before breastfeeding.

Nursing Considerations

- Be aware that at least 14 days should elapse between discontinuing a MAO inhibitor used to treat psychiatric disorders and initiation of vortioxetine therapy to avoid risk of patient developing serotonin syndrome. Also, know that at least 21 days should elapse after vortioxetine is discontinued and therapy with a MAO inhibitor used to treat a psychiatric disorder is begun.
- Screen patient for bipolar disorder before vortioxetine therapy is begun. Monitor patient for mania, which may result from use of drug in a susceptible patient, especially patients with bipolar disorder.

- Expect dosage to be decreased to 10 mg once daily for 1 week before vortioxetine is discontinued to avoid patient experiencing dizziness, headaches, mood swings, including muscle tension, runny nose, or sudden outbursts of anger that may occur in the first week of abrupt discontinuation of drug.
- Watch patient closely for suicidal tendencies, particularly when therapy starts and dosage changes, because depression may worsen temporarily during these times, possibly leading to suicidal ideation.
- Monitor patient closely for evidence of increased bleeding such as GI bleeding, especially if patient also takes a drug known to cause GI bleeding, such as aspirin, a NSAID, warfarin, or other anticoagulants.

! **WARNING** Monitor patient closely for serotonin syndrome exhibited by agitation, coma, diarrhea, hallucinations, hyperreflexia, hyperthermia, incoordination, labile blood pressure, nausea, or vomiting. Notify prescriber immediately because serotonin syndrome may be life-threatening, and provide supportive care.

- Monitor patient's serum sodium level because hyponatremia has occurred with use of serotonergic drugs, including vortioxetine. Patients at greater risk include the elderly and patients taking diuretics or who are volume-depleted. Report signs and symptoms of hyponatremia, such as confusion, difficulty concentrating, headache, memory impairment, unsteadiness, or weakness. If left untreated, coma, death, hallucinations, respiratory arrest, seizures, or syncope may occur.

PATIENT TEACHING

- Instruct patient to take drug exactly as prescribed, be consistent with daily administration time, and alert prescriber with concerns.
- Inform patient that nausea is the most common side effect of vortioxetine therapy, and it commonly occurs within the first week of treatment.
- Advise patient that drug may cause mild pupillary dilation, which may lead to an episode of acute angle-closure glaucoma. Encourage patient to have an eye exam before starting therapy to see if he is at risk.

- Tell family or caregiver to observe patient closely for suicidal tendencies, especially when therapy starts or dosage changes and when drug is given to young adults.
- Warn patient not to discontinue drug abruptly, as serious adverse reactions may occur.
- Advise patient to inform all prescribers of vortioxetine therapy.
- Emphasize importance of reporting any persistent, severe, or sudden symptoms to prescriber.
- Alert patients about risk of bleeding when taking drugs known to increase risk of bleeding, such as aspirin, blood thinners, or NSAIDs.
- Tell patient and caregivers to report any signs of abnormal behavior.
- Inform elderly patient or patient who is taking drugs, such as diuretics, that cause him to be dehydrated of the risk of a low sodium level; tell patient to alert prescriber if he experiences new or sudden onset of symptoms.

! **WARNING** Advise patient to seek emergency medical attention if an allergic reaction such as difficulty breathing, hives, rash, or swelling occurs.

- Instruct female patients of childbearing age to notify prescriber if pregnancy occurs or is suspected.
- Tell patient to inform all prescribers of vortioxetine therapy and not to take any over-the-counter medications, including herbal products, without prescriber knowledge.
- Encourage patient to discuss sexual difficulties with prescriber, if present.

warfarin sodium
Coumadin, Jantoven

Class and Category
Pharmacologic class: Coumarin derivative
Therapeutic class: Anticoagulant

Indications and Dosages
* *To prevent and treat venous thrombosis and its extension, pulmonary embolism; to prevent and treat thromboembolic complications associated with atrial fibrillation and/or cardiac valve replacement; to reduce risk of death, recurrent MI, and thromboembolic events such as stroke or systemic embolization after myocardial infarction*

TABLETS
Adults. Highly individualized, based on age, body weight, comorbidities, concomitant medications, race, and sex. *Usual initial:* 2 to 5 mg daily for 2 to 4 days. *Maintenance:* 2 to 10 mg daily based on target INR and PT results.
±**DOSAGE ADJUSTMENT** For Asian, debilitated, or elderly patients and patient with CYP2C9 or VKORC1 genotypes, initial and maintenance dosages reduced and then adjusted based on INR and PT results.

Drug Administration
P.O.
- Administer drug at the same time each evening.
- Drug dosages will be adjusted according to INR values.

Route	Onset	Peak	Duration
P.O.	<24 hr	1.5–3 days	2–5 days

Half-life: 20–60 hr

Mechanism of Action
Interferes with the liver's ability to synthesize vitamin K–dependent clotting factors, depleting clotting factors II (prothrombin), VII, IX, and X. This action, in turn, interferes with the clotting cascade. By depleting vitamin K–dependent clotting factors and interfering with the clotting cascade, warfarin prevents coagulation.

Contraindications
Bacterial endocarditis; bleeding or hemorrhagic tendencies such as active ulceration or overt bleeding of the gastrointestinal, genitourinary, or respiratory tract as well as CNS hemorrhage including cerebral aneurysms and dissecting aorta; blood dyscrasias; cerebral or dissecting aneurysm; cerebrovascular hemorrhage; eclampsia, preeclampsia, or threatened abortion; hypersensitivity to warfarin or its components; major lumbar or regional block anesthesia; malignant hypertension; mental state or condition that leads to lack of patient cooperation, or unsupervised situation; pericardial effusion; pericarditis; pregnancy except in women with mechanical heart valves, who are at

U
V
W

high risk of thromboembolism; recent or planned neurosurgery, ophthalmic surgery, or traumatic surgery resulting in large open surfaces; spinal puncture and other diagnostic or therapeutic procedures with potential for uncontrollable bleeding

Interactions
DRUGS

acyclovir, allopurinol, alprazolam, amiodarone, amlodipine, amprenavir, aprepitant, atorvastatin, atazanavir, bicalutamide, capecitabine, cilostazol, cimetidine, ciprofloxacin, clarithromycin, conivaptan, cotrimoxazole, cyclosporine, darunavir/ ritonavir, diltiazem, disulfiram, erythromycin, enoxacin, etravirine, famotidine, fluconazole, fluoxetine, fluvastatin, fluvoxamine, fosamprenavir, imatinib, indinavir, isoniazid, itraconazole, ketoconazole, lopinavir/ ritonavir, methoxsalen, metronidazole, miconazole, mexiletine, nalidixic acid, nefazodone, nelfinavir, nilotinib, norfloxacin, NSAIDs, oral contraceptives, oxandrolone, phenylpropanolamine, posaconazole, propafenone, propranolol, ranolazine, ritonavir, saquinavir, sulfinpyrazone, terbinafine, telithromycin, thiabendazole, ticlopidine, tigecycline, tipranavir, verapamil, voriconazole, zafirlukast, zileuton: Increased anticoagulant effect of warfarin, increased risk of bleeding
armodafinil, amprenavir, aprepitant, bosentan, carbamazepine, efavirenz, etravirine, modafinil, montelukast, moricizine, nafcillin, phenobarbital, phenytoin, pioglitazone, prednisone, rifampin, rufinamide: Decreased anticoagulant effect of warfarin
herbal remedies (including garlic, ginkgo biloba, and ginseng): Increased anticoagulant effect of warfarin, increased risk of bleeding
other herbal remedies (including co-enzyme Q10, ginseng, St. John's wort): Decreased anticoagulant effect

ACTIVITIES

alcohol use: Increased risk of hypoprothrombinemia
smoking, smoking cessation aids: Altered response to warfarin

Adverse Reactions

CNS: Coma, **intracranial hemorrhage**, loss of consciousness, syncope, weakness
CV: Angina, calcium uremic arteriolopathy (calciphylaxis), chest pain, **hypotension**
EENT: Epistaxis, intraocular hemorrhage
GI: Abdominal cramps and pain, diarrhea, **hepatitis**, jaundice, nausea, vomiting
GU: Hematuria, vaginal bleeding (abnormal)
HEME: Anemia, **potentially fatal hemorrhage**
SKIN: Alopecia, ecchymosis, petechiae, pruritus, purple-toe syndrome, tissue necrosis
Other: Anaphylaxis

Childbearing Considerations
PREGNANCY

- Drug can cause fetal harm such as severe fetal abnormalities as well as fatal hemorrhage.
- Drug is contraindicated in pregnancy (except in pregnant women with mechanical heart valves).
- A pregnancy test should be performed before drug is begun.

LACTATION

- It is not clear if drug is present in breast milk.
- Patient should check with prescriber before breastfeeding.
- If breastfeeding is undertaken, monitor infant for unusual bleeding or bruising.

REPRODUCTION

- Women of childbearing age should use effective contraception during treatment and for 1 month after last dose of drug.

Nursing Considerations

- Ensure that woman of childbearing age has a negative pregnancy test result before warfarin therapy is initiated, because drug may cause fetal harm even in the first trimester.
- Expect to give another parenteral anticoagulant, such as enoxaparin or heparin, with oral warfarin for at least 3 days, or until desired response occurs, before giving warfarin only.
- Avoid I.M. injections during warfarin therapy, if possible, because they can result in bleeding, bruising, and hematoma.
- Monitor INR (daily in acute care setting) and assess for therapeutic effects, as prescribed. Therapeutic INR levels are 2.0 to 3.0 for bioprosthetic heart valve, nonvalvular atrial fibrillation, and venous thromboembolism, and 2.5 to 3.5 after MI and for mechanical heart valve.
- Monitor patient with hepatic impairment closely for bleeding, because hepatic

impairment decreases metabolism of warfarin and impairs synthesis of clotting factors. Expect to monitor patient's INR more frequently.

- Expect treatment to last up to 12 weeks for bioprosthetic heart valve, 1 to 3 months for nonvalvular atrial fibrillation or venous thromboembolism, and for rest of life after MI and for mechanical heart valve replacement.

> **! WARNING** Be aware of the increased risk for intracranial hemorrhage if patient has cerebral ischemia (such as recent transient ischemic attack or minor ischemic stroke) and INR of 3 to 4.5. As prescribed, withhold next warfarin dose and give vitamin K, as ordered, if INR exceeds 4 because of the risk of bleeding.

- Assess for occult bleeding if patient receives I.V. lipid emulsion or other medical product that contains soybean oil. Such products can decrease vitamin K absorption and increase warfarin's anticoagulant effect.
- Monitor patient for persistent, severe, sudden, or unusual signs and symptoms, as warfarin therapy may cause many adverse reactions, including calciphylaxis, a syndrome of blood clots, calcification of blood vessels, and skin necrosis. If diagnosed, expect warfarin therapy to be discontinued and alternative anticoagulation therapy prescribed.

PATIENT TEACHING

- Explain that warfarin therapy aims to prevent thrombosis by decreasing clotting ability while avoiding the risk of spontaneous bleeding.
- Instruct patient to take drug at the same time each evening.
- Advise patient if a dose is missed to take it as soon as it is remembered on the same day, but not to take a double dose the next day to make up for it.
- Urge patient to keep weekly follow-up appointments for blood tests after discharge until PT and INR levels are stabilized.
- Advise patient to avoid alcohol during warfarin therapy.
- Urge patient to take precautions against bleeding, such as using an electric shaver and a soft-bristled toothbrush. Advise him to continue these precautions for 2 to 5 days

after therapy stops, as directed, because anticoagulant effect may persist during this time.

- Caution patient to avoid activities that could cause traumatic injury and bleeding.
- Advise patient to avoid drastic changes in dietary habits, such as eating large amounts of leafy, green vegetables. Explain that dark green, leafy vegetables contain vitamin K that counteracts the effects of warfarin.
- Urge patient to notify prescriber immediately about unusual bleeding and any unexplained symptoms, such as abnormal vaginal bleeding; dizziness; easy bruising; gum bleeding; headache; nosebleeds; prolonged bleeding from cuts; red, black, or tarry stool; red or dark brown urine; swelling; and weakness.
- Advise patient to consult prescriber before taking other drugs—including OTC drugs and herbal remedies—during therapy. Also instruct him to not discontinue any drug, including over-the-counter drugs and herbal products he takes regularly, without consulting the prescriber.
- Instruct female patient of childbearing age to use an effective contraceptive during warfarin therapy and for at least 1 month after warfarin has been discontinued. Also tell patient to notify prescriber immediately if pregnancy occurs or is suspected.
- Tell patient who is breastfeeding to monitor her infant for bleeding or bruising and to notify prescriber immediately if either occurs.

> **! WARNING** Tell patient to contact prescriber immediately if he experiences pain and discoloration of the skin mostly on areas of the body with a high fat content, such as abdomen, breasts, buttocks, hips, and thighs or if he experiences any unusual symptoms. Explain that drug may cause reversible purple-toe syndrome but that this syndrome isn't harmful.

- Urge patient to carry medical identification that reveals he's taking warfarin.
- Tell patient to inform all dentists and healthcare professionals that he is taking warfarin, especially before any procedure or surgery, including dental, is performed.

U
V
W

X Y Z

zafirlukast

Class and Category
Pharmacologic class: Leukotriene receptor antagonist
Therapeutic class: Antiasthmatic

Indications and Dosages
＊ *To prevent or treat chronic asthma*

TABLETS

Adults and children over age 11. 20 mg twice daily.
Children ages 5 to 11. 10 mg twice daily.

Drug Administration
P.O.
- Administer drug at same times daily.
- Give drug on an empty stomach at least 1 hour before or 2 hours after meals.

Route	Onset	Peak	Duration
P.O.	1 wk	3 hr	12 hr

Half-life: 10 hr

Mechanism of Action
Inhibits the selective binding of cysteinyl leukotrienes (arachidonic acid derivatives that usually mediate inflammation in asthma and other inflammatory disorders) by competitively blocking receptor sites. This action causes bronchial relaxation and decreases bronchial hyperresponsiveness, eosinophil movement, mucus secretion, and vascular leakage.

Contraindications
Hepatic impairment including hepatic cirrhosis, hypersensitivity to zafirlukast or its components

Interactions
DRUGS
carbamazepine, tolbutamide: Possibly increased levels of these drugs and, possibly, additive adverse effects
aspirin: Increased blood zafirlukast level
erythromycin: Decreased response to zafirlukast

fluconazole: Increased plasma zafirlukast levels
theophylline: Decreased zafirlukast level; possibly increased theophylline levels
warfarin: Prolonged PT

Adverse Reactions
CNS: Asthenia, depression, dizziness, fever, headache, insomnia, malaise
CV: Edema, vasculitis
GI: Abdominal pain, diarrhea, edema, elevated liver enzymes, **hepatic failure**, **hepatitis**, hyperbilirubinemia, indigestion, nausea, vomiting
HEME: Agranulocytosis, bleeding, eosinophilia
MS: Arthralgia, back pain, myalgia
RESP: Eosinophilic pneumonia
SKIN: Bruising, pruritus, rash, urticaria
Other: Angioedema, generalized pain, **hypersensitivity reactions,** infections

Childbearing Considerations
PREGNANCY
- It is not known if drug can cause fetal harm.
- Use with caution only if benefit to mother outweighs potential risk to fetus.

LACTATION
- Drug is present in breast milk.
- Breastfeeding is not recommended during drug therapy.

Nursing Considerations
- Know that zafirlukast shouldn't be used to treat bronchospasm during an acute asthma attack or status asthmaticus; it can't relieve symptoms quickly enough.
- Assess respiratory depth, quality, and rate, as well as breath sounds, before and during treatment to evaluate response to therapy.

! **WARNING** Monitor patient for hypersensitivity reactions, including angioedema. If present, notify prescriber, withhold drug, and provide supportive care, as prescribed.

- Be aware that if patient is being weaned from corticosteroids while taking zafirlukast, she should be monitored for Churg–Strauss syndrome—a rare allergic reaction characterized by eosinophilia, fever, myalgia, and weight loss—for cardiac complications, neuropathy, and worsening pulmonary symptoms.

PATIENT TEACHING

- Instruct patient to take drug exactly as prescribed, in evenly spaced doses, every day, even during acute exacerbations and symptom-free periods.
- Instruct patient to take drug on an empty stomach at least 1 hour before meals, or 2 hours after.
- Urge patient to continue using prescribed rescue inhalants for acute asthma attacks.
- Teach patient how to use peak-flow meter to monitor pulmonary function.

! **WARNING** Review signs and symptoms of an allergic reaction, including swelling of eyes, face, throat, and tongue. If present, stress importance of seeking emergency medical attention immediately.

- Tell patient to report immediately any evidence of liver dysfunction, such as anorexia, fatigue, flu-like symptoms, jaundice, lethargy, nausea, right upper-quadrant abdominal pain, or pruritus.

zaleplon
Sonata

Class, Category, and Schedule
Pharmacologic class: Pyrazolopyrimidine
Therapeutic class: Hypnotic
Controlled substance schedule: IV

Indications and Dosages
* *Short-term treatment of insomnia*

CAPSULES

Adults up to age 65. 10 mg once nightly as needed, for up to 35 days. *Usual:* 10 mg nightly for 7 to 10 days. *Maximum:* 20 mg nightly.

±**DOSAGE ADJUSTMENT** For patients who are debilitated, elderly, have hepatic impairment or low weight, or take cimetidine, dosage reduced to 5 mg daily.

Drug Administration
P.O.

- Administer immediately before bedtime or after patient has gone to bed and has experienced difficulty falling asleep.
- Avoid giving with or after a heavy, high-fat meal because decreased absorption may reduce drug's effects.

Route	Onset	Peak	Duration
P.O.	30 min	1 hr	3–4 hr

Half-life: 1 hr

Mechanism of Action
Selectively binds with type 1 benzodiazepine (BZ1 or omega$_1$) receptors on the gamma-aminobutyric acid-A receptor complex. This binding produces muscle relaxation and sedation as well as antianxiety and anticonvulsant effects.

Contraindications
Hypersensitivity to zaleplon or its components, past experience of complex sleep behaviors during zaleplon therapy

Interactions
DRUGS

carbamazepine, phenobarbital, phenytoin, rifampin: Reduced zaleplon effects
cimetidine: Increased blood zaleplon level
CNS depressants, diphenhydramine, imipramine, thioridazine: Additive CNS effects
erythromycin, ketoconazole: Increased zaleplon concentration
flumazenil: Reversal of zaleplon's sedation
promethazine: Possibly decreased plasma zaleplon concentration

FOODS

high-fat foods: Prolonged absorption time and reduced effectiveness of zaleplon

ACTIVITIES

alcohol use: Increased CNS depression

Adverse Reactions
CNS: Amnesia, anxiety, complex behaviors (such as sleep driving), depression, dizziness, drowsiness, fever, hallucinations, hypertonia, insomnia, nightmares, paresthesia, **seizures**, **suicidal ideation**, tremor, vertigo
EENT: Dry mouth, gingivitis, glossitis, mouth ulcers, stomatitis, **throat tightness**
GI: Anorexia, colitis, constipation, eructation, esophagitis, flatulence, gastritis, gastroenteritis, increased appetite, indigestion, **melena**, nausea, **rectal bleeding**, vomiting
MS: Back pain
RESP: Dyspnea
SKIN: Photosensitivity, pruritus, rash
Other: **Anaphylaxis**, **angioedema**, physical and psychological dependence

☰ Childbearing Considerations

PREGNANCY

- It is not known if drug can cause fetal harm.
- Drug is not recommended for use in pregnant women because effects are unknown.

LACTATION

- Drug is present in breast milk in small amounts.
- Breastfeeding is not recommended during drug therapy.

☰ Nursing Considerations

- Watch patient closely for suicidal tendencies, particularly when therapy starts and dosage changes, because depression may worsen temporarily during these times, possibly leading to suicidal ideation.
- Monitor patient for signs of drug abuse because zaleplon has an abuse potential similar to that of benzodiazepines and benzodiazepine-like hypnotics.

! WARNING Monitor patient closely for hypersensitivity reactions, such as dyspnea, nausea, swelling, throat tightness, and vomiting. If present, discontinue zaleplon immediately, notify prescriber, and provide supportive care.

PATIENT TEACHING

- Explain that zaleplon is intended for short-term use. Advise against using it for any condition other than insomnia.
- Caution patient against exceeding prescribed dosage.
- Warn patient not to take drug with less than a full night of sleep remaining (7 or 8 hours) because of the risk of next-day psychomotor impairment, including impaired driving.
- Instruct patient to take zaleplon immediately before bedtime or right after having trouble falling asleep, because of drug's rapid onset of action. Also alert patient that a heavy, high-fat meal can interfere with drug's effectiveness.
- Teach patient alternative measures for relaxation and sleep induction.
- Advise patient to consult prescriber before taking other CNS depressants.
- Urge patient to avoid alcohol during zaleplon therapy because it increases risk of abnormal behaviors, such as sleep driving.

! WARNING Warn patient that zaleplon contains FD & C Yellow No. 5 (tartrazine), which can cause an allergic reaction, especially in those with an aspirin sensitivity. Instruct patient to immediately report allergic reactions, such as difficulty breathing or rash, to prescriber.

- Instruct patient to notify prescriber if inability to sleep continues. Dosage may have to be adjusted.
- Caution patient about performing hazardous activities such as driving until the effects of zaleplon are known, because it can cause dizziness and drowsiness. Also warn patient to take fall precautions.
- Instruct patient to stop taking zaleplon and seek emergency care if she has abnormal swelling, nausea, throat tightness, trouble breathing, or vomiting.
- Explain that drug may cause abnormal behaviors during sleep, such as driving a car, eating, having sex, or talking on the phone without any recall of the event. If family notices any such behavior or patient sees evidence of such behavior upon awakening, prescriber should be notified.
- Urge family or caregiver to watch patient closely for suicidal tendencies, especially when therapy starts or dosage changes.

zidovudine
Retrovir

☰ Class and Category

Pharmacologic class: Nucleoside reverse transcriptase inhibitor
Therapeutic class: Antiretroviral

☰ Indications and Dosages

✳ *As adjunct to treat human immunodeficiency viral type (HIV-1) infection*

CAPSULES, SYRUP

Adults. 300 mg twice daily.
Children less than 18 years weighing 30 kg (66 lb) or more. 300 mg twice daily or 200 mg three times daily. Alternatively, 240 mg/m² body surface area (BSA) twice daily or 160 mg/m² BSA three times daily. *Maximum:* 600 mg daily.
Infants at least 4 weeks old and children less than 18 years weighing 9 kg (19.8 lb) to less

than 30 kg (66 lb). 9 mg/kg twice daily or 6 mg/kg three times daily. Alternatively, 240 mg/m² body surface area (BSA) twice daily or 160 mg/m² BSA three times daily. *Maximum:* 18 mg/kg/day divided into two or three doses.

Infants at least 4 weeks old and weighing at least 4 kg (8.8 lb) but less than 9 kg (19.8 lb). 12 mg/kg twice daily or 8 mg/kg three times daily. Alternatively, 240 mg/m² BSA twice daily or 160 mg/m² BSA three times daily. *Maximum:* 24 mg/kg/day in two or three divided doses.

I.V. INFUSION

Adults. 1 mg/kg every 4 hr until oral dosage can be initiated.

✴ *To prevent maternal-fetal HIV-1 transmission*

CAPSULES, SYRUP

Pregnant women at greater than 14 weeks of pregnancy. 100 mg five times daily until start of labor.

I.V. INFUSION

Pregnant women during labor and delivery. *Initial:* 2 mg/kg infused over 1 hr followed by 1 mg/kg/hr until umbilical cord is clamped.

SYRUP

Neonate 12 hr after birth. 2 mg/kg every 6 hr for 6 wk.

I.V. INFUSION

Neonate 12 hr after birth. 1.5 mg/kg infused over 30 min every 6 hr for 6 wk or until oral administration can be initiated.

±**DOSAGE ADJUSTMENT** For adult patients on dialysis or who have a creatinine clearance of less than 15 ml/min, oral dosage reduced to 100 mg every 6 to 8 hr and the intravenous dosage interval increased to every 6 to 8 hr. Patients who develop severe anemia and/or neutropenia may require a dose interruption until marrow recovery occurs.

≡ Drug Administration

P.O.

- Use calibrated device to measure syrup dosage; for neonates, use a syringe with 0.1-ml markings to ensure accurate dosage.
- Store capsules in a cool, dry environment.

I.V.

- Drug vial stopper contains natural rubber latex and should not be handled by someone with a latex allergy.
- Dilute drug with 5% Dextrose Injection to achieve a concentration no greater than 4 mg/ml.

- Use diluted solution within 8 hours if left at room temperature and 24 hours if refrigerated.
- Infuse at a constant rate of 1 mg/kg slowly over 1 hour for adults and 30 minutes for neonates. If given to a pregnant woman during labor, follow initial infusion given over 1 hour by a continuous infusion at a rate of 1 mg/kg/hr until umbilical cord is clamped.
- Drug should never be given as a bolus injection or by rapid infusion, nor should it be administered intramuscularly.
- *Incompatibilities:* None listed by manufacturer

Route	Onset	Peak	Duration
P.O./I.V.	Unknown	30–90 min	Unknown

Half-life: 1–3 hr

≡ Mechanism of Action

After being phosphorylated to its active metabolite, the metabolite inhibits the DNA- and RNA-dependent polymerase activities of HIV-1 reverse transcriptases via DNA chain termination after incorporation of the nucleotide analogue into viral DNA. This destroys activity of the HIV-1 viruses.

≡ Contraindications

Hypersensitivity to zidovudine or its components

≡ Interactions

DRUGS

bone marrow suppressive or cytotoxic agents, such as ganciclovir, interferon alfa, ribavirin: Possibly increased hematologic toxicity of zidovudine

doxorubicin, nucleoside analogues affecting DNA replication such as ribavirin, stavudine: Antagonistic relationship between the two drugs

≡ Adverse Reactions

CNS: Anxiety, asthenia, chills, confusion, decreased reflexes, depression, dizziness, fatigue, headache, insomnia, irritability, loss of mental acuity, malaise, mania, nervousness, neuropathy, paresthesia, **seizures**, somnolence, syncope, tremor, vertigo

CV: **Cardiomyopathy**, chest pain, **congestive heart failure**, **ECG abnormalities**, edema, left ventricular dilation, vasculitis

EENT: Amblyopia; ear discharge, erythema, pain, or swelling; hearing loss; macular edema;

mouth ulcers; nasal congestion or discharge; oral mucosa pigmentation; photophobia; rhinitis; sinusitis; stomatitis; taste perversion

ENDO: Cushingoid appearance, fat redistribution, gynecomastia

GI: Abdominal cramps or pain, anorexia, constipation, diarrhea, dyspepsia, dysphagia, elevated liver or pancreatic enzymes, flatulence, **hepatic decompensation, hepatitis,** hyperbilirubinemia, jaundice, nausea, **pancreatitis, severe hepatomegaly with steatosis,** splenomegaly, vomiting

GU: Hematuria, urinary frequency or hesitancy

HEME: Anemia, **aplastic anemia, granulocytopenia, hemolytic anemia, leukopenia,** macrocytosis, **neutropenia, pancytopenia with marrow hypoplasia, pure red cell aplasia, thrombocytopenia**

MS: Arthralgia, back pain, musculoskeletal pain, muscle spasm, myalgia, myopathy, myositis, **rhabdomyolysis**

RESP: Abnormal breath sounds, cough, dyspnea, wheezing

SKIN: Diaphoresis, pigmentation changes in nails and skin, pruritus, rash, **Stevens–Johnson syndrome, toxic epidermal necrolysis,** urticaria

Other: **Anaphylaxis, angioedema,** elevated CPK and LDH levels, flu-like symptoms, generalized pain, intravenous site irritation or pain, **lactic acidosis,** lymphadenopathy, weight loss

☰ Childbearing Considerations

PREGNANCY

- Pregnancy exposure registry: 1-800-258-4263.
- Drug does not appear to cause fetal harm.
- Use with caution only if benefit to mother outweighs potential risk to fetus, especially in the second and third trimesters.

LACTATION

- Drug is present in breast milk.
- The Centers for Disease Control and Prevention recommend that HIV-1 infected mothers not breastfeed to avoid risking postnatal transmission of HIV-1 infection to infants. They also do not recommend breastfeeding because of potential drug-induced adverse reactions in the infant.

☰ Nursing Considerations

- Use zidovudine cautiously in patients with hepatic dysfunction, including liver cirrhosis, because of potential for hepatic dysfunction during zidovudine therapy.
- Be aware that dosing regimen for the prevention of maternal-fetal HIV-1 transmission includes three phases. First, oral zidovudine is given to the mother beginning after 14 weeks of pregnancy and continued throughout the remainder of pregnancy, stopping at the start of labor. Then drug is given intravenously to the mother during labor until the umbilical cord is cut. Lastly, drug is then given to the newborn beginning 12 hours after birth and continued for 6 weeks.
- Know that pediatric dosage is based upon body weight in kg or alternatively on BSA. In some cases, the dosage calculated by body weight will not be the same as that calculated by BSA.

! WARNING Monitor patient for hypersensitivity reactions during drug therapy. Alert prescriber, if present, and be prepared to provide supportive care.

! WARNING Know that lactic acidosis and severe hepatomegaly with steatosis have occurred with zidovudine therapy, and death has occurred in some patients. Risk factors include presence of obesity, prolonged nucleoside exposure, and being a woman. However, know that lactic acidosis and severe hepatomegaly with steatosis have also occurred in patients with no known risk factors. Expect drug to be discontinued in any patient who develops clinical or laboratory findings suggestive of lactic acidosis or pronounced hepatotoxicity, even in the absence of marked transaminase elevations.

- Monitor patient's hematologic status closely during zidovudine therapy, as ordered. Know that if patient's hemoglobin falls to less than 7.5 g/dl or the reduction is greater than 25% of baseline and/or granulocyte count falls to less than 750 cells/mm^3 or the reduction is greater than 50% of baseline, notify prescriber and expect zidovudine therapy to be withheld until marrow recovery occurs. Even with marrow recovery, adjunctive supportive measures such as epoetin alfa might be required when zidovudine therapy is restarted.

- Know that coadministration of ribavirin and zidovudine is not advised, because ribavirin exacerbates the development of zidovudine-induced anemia.
- Be aware that patients receiving interferon alfa and/or ribavirin in addition to zidovudine should be monitored closely for treatment-associated toxicities, especially anemia, hepatic decompensation, and neutropenia. Dosage reduction or discontinuation of interferon alfa, ribavirin, or both may be required if zidovudine toxicities become serious.
- Be aware that prolonged therapy increases the risk of myopathy and myositis.
- Be aware that immune reconstitution syndrome has occurred in patients treated with combination antiretroviral therapy, including zidovudine. The inflammatory response predisposes susceptible patients to opportunistic infections such as cytomegalovirus, *Mycobacterium avium* infection, *Pneumocystis jiroveci* pneumonia, or tuberculosis. Autoimmune disorders such as Graves' disease, Guillain–Barré syndrome, or polymyositis have also occurred. Report sudden or unusual adverse reactions to prescriber.
- Observe patient for redistribution of body fat, including breast enlargement, central obesity, development of buffalo hump, facial wasting, and peripheral wasting, which may produce a cushingoid-type appearance.

PATIENT TEACHING

- Instruct parents or caregivers to take extra care in measuring dosage when using syrup that will be given to babies and children, to avoid dosage errors. Caution them to use an appropriately sized syringe with 0.1-ml graduation to ensure accurate dosing of the syrup formulation. Do not use the common household teaspoon.
- Tell patient that if she misses a dose of zidovudine, she should take it as soon as she remembers, but should not double the next dose or take more than prescribed.

! **WARNING** Instruct patient to seek immediate medical attention if she experiences a serious allergic reaction, such as having difficulty breathing, hives, or swelling of her face, lips, tongue, or throat.

- Inform patient that periodic laboratory studies will have to be performed and that compliance with these appointments is essential for early detection of adverse reactions. If toxicity develops, inform her that she may need transfusions or zidovudine to be discontinued.
- Alert patient that fat accumulation and redistribution may occur during zidovudine therapy.

! **WARNING** Alert patient that severe conditions may develop while taking zidovudine. Encourage her to stop taking drug and seek medical attention immediately if she experiences any persistent, severe, or unusual symptoms.

- Advise patient to inform all prescribers of zidovudine therapy.

! **WARNING** Inform patient that zidovudine may cause lactic acidosis, which if not treated, could be fatal. Tell patient to seek immediate medical attention if she develops breathing difficulty, cold or numb feeling in her arms and legs, dizziness, fast or uneven heart rate, muscle pain or weakness, nausea, vomiting, or any other unexpected or unusual signs or symptoms.

- Tell mothers that breastfeeding should not be done during zidovudine therapy.

zinc acetate
Galzin

zinc chloride

zinc gluconate
Orazinc

zinc sulfate
Orazinc, Verazinc, Zinc 15, Zinc-220, Zinca-Pak, Zincate

Class and Category
Pharmacologic class: Trace element, mineral
Therapeutic class: Nutritional supplement

☰ Indications and Dosages

* *To prevent zinc deficiency based on recommended daily allowances*

CAPSULES, E.R. TABLETS, LOZENGES, TABLETS

Men and boys age 14 and over. 11 mg daily.
Women. 8 mg daily.
Pregnant women. 11 mg daily.
Breastfeeding women. 12 mg daily.
Adolescent females ages 14 to 18. 9 mg daily.
Pregnant adolescents ages 14 to 18. 12 mg daily.
Breastfeeding adolescents ages 14 to 18. 13 mg daily.
Children ages 9 to 13. 8 mg daily.
Children ages 4 to 8. 5 mg daily.
Children ages 1 to 3. 3 mg daily.
Infants ages 7 to 13 months. 3 mg daily.
Newborns to 6 months. 2 mg daily.

* *To treat zinc deficiency*

CAPSULES, E.R. TABLETS, LOZENGES, TABLETS

Adults and children. Dosage individualized based on severity of deficiency.

I.V. INFUSION

Adults and adolescents. 3 mg daily.
Children weighing 10 kg (22 lb) or more. 50 mcg/kg (up to 3 mg/day) daily.
Children weighing 5 kg (11 lb) to less than 10 kg (22 lb). 100 mcg/kg daily.
Term neonates weighing 3 kg (6.6 lb) to less than 5 kg (11 lb). 250 mcg/kg daily.
Preterm neonates weighing less than 3 kg (6.6 lb). 400 mcg/kg daily.

* *As adjunct maintenance therapy for patients previously treated for Wilson's disease*

CAPSULES

Adults. 50 mg three times a day.
Pregnant women. 25 mg three times a day, increased to 50 mg three times a day if drug effectiveness decreases.
Children age 10 and over. 25 mg three times a day, increased to 50 mg three times a day if drug effectiveness decreases.

☰ Drug Administration

P.O.

- Administer zinc supplements 1 hour before or 2 to 3 hours after meals; at least 2 hours after giving oral iron supplements (to prevent decreased zinc absorption) or copper supplements (to prevent decreased copper absorption); and at least 6 hours before or 2 hours after administering quinolone or tetracycline antibiotics (to prevent decreased absorption of these drugs).
- Have patient let zinc lozenge dissolve in mouth slowly and completely and not to swallow it whole or chew it.
- Capsules and E.R. tablets should be swallowed whole and not chewed, crushed, or divided/opened.

I.V.

- Don't give I.V. zinc preparations that contain benzyl alcohol to neonates or premature infants, because this preservative may cause a fatal toxic syndrome.
- I.V. zinc preparations are not for direct intravenous infusion but must be used as an admixture in parenteral nutrition solutions.
- Prepare final admixture of zinc and parenteral nutrition solution according to manufacturer guidelines.
- Visually inspect solution for precipitates and that the emulsion has not separated, if lipid emulsion has been added. Separation of the emulsion is visible by a yellowish streak or accumulation of yellowish droplets in the admixed emulsion. Discard if any precipitates are noted.
- Penetrate drug vial closure only one time with a suitable sterile transfer device or dispensing set that allows measured dispensing of contents.
- Use drug for admixing promptly once the sterile transfer set has been inserted into the pharmacy bulk package container or not more than 4 hours at room temperature after container closure has been penetrated. Discard any remaining drug. Once zinc is added to parenteral nutrition solution, use promptly after mixing. If not used promptly, store admixture in refrigerator for no longer than 9 days. After removal from refrigerator, use promptly and complete infusion within 24 hr.
- Protect admixture parenteral nutrition solution from light.

Route	Onset	Peak	Duration
P.O.	Unknown	2 hr	Unknown
Half-life: 11 days			

X
Y
Z

Mechanism of Action

Needed for proper function of more than 200 metalloenzymes (those with tightly bound zinc atoms as an integral part of their structure), including alcohol dehydrogenase, alkaline phosphatase, carbonic anhydrase, carboxypeptidase A, and RNA polymerase. Zinc also helps maintain cell membrane, nucleic acid, and protein structure and is essential for certain physiologic functions, including cell growth and division, dark adaptation and night vision, host immunity, sexual maturation and reproduction, taste acuity, and wound healing. This mineral also provides cellular antioxidant protection by scavenging free radicals.

In addition, zinc acetate interferes with intestinal absorption of copper and produces a protein that binds with copper, preventing its transfer to blood. Bound copper is then excreted in stools, thus decreasing copper toxicity in Wilson's disease.

Contraindications

Hypersensitivity to zinc or its components

Interactions

DRUGS

copper supplements: Impaired copper absorption (with large doses of zinc)
oral iron supplements, oral phosphate salts, phosphorus-containing drugs: Decreased zinc absorption
quinolones, tetracyclines: Decreased absorption and possibly decreased effectiveness of these antibiotics
thiazide diuretics: Increased urinary excretion of zinc
zinc-containing preparations: Increased blood zinc level

FOODS

fiber- or phylate-containing foods (such as bran, cereals, whole-grain breads), phosphorus-containing foods (including milk, poultry): Decreased zinc absorption

Adverse Reactions

CNS: Neurologic deterioration
GI: Elevated alkaline phosphate, amylase, and lipase; gastric irritation; nausea; vomiting

Childbearing Considerations

PREGNANCY

- It is not known if drug can cause fetal harm.
- Use with caution only if benefit to mother outweighs potential risk to fetus.
- Be aware that the recommended dosage allowance is increased during pregnancy.

LACTATION

- Drug is present in breast milk.
- Patient should check with prescriber before breastfeeding.

Nursing Considerations

- Monitor patient receiving long-term zinc therapy for sideroblastic anemia, which may result from zinc-induced copper deficiency and is characterized by anemia, bone marrow problems, granulocytopenia, leukopenia, and neutropenia. Be aware that these effects are reversible after zinc is discontinued.
- Monitor patient with preexisting copper deficiency for exacerbation of this condition; zinc can decrease serum copper level.
- Monitor blood alkaline phosphatase level monthly, as ordered; it may increase.
- Be aware that zinc chloride contains aluminum, which may accumulate to the point of toxicity if patient's kidney function is impaired. Assess kidney function regularly.

PATIENT TEACHING

- Explain the need for a zinc supplement.
- Instruct patient to take zinc on an empty stomach, at least 1 hour before or 2 hours after meals. Caution her not to take zinc within 2 hours of iron or copper supplements or phosphorus-containing drugs.
- Instruct patient to let zinc lozenge dissolve in mouth slowly and completely and not to swallow it whole or chew it. Advise her not to take zinc lozenges more often than directed.

ziprasidone hydrochloride

Auro-Ziprasidone, Geodon, Zeldox (CAN)

ziprasidone mesylate

Geodon for Injection

Class and Category

Pharmacologic class: Benzisoxazole
Therapeutic class: Antipsychotic

Indications and Dosages

✳ *To treat schizophrenia*

CAPSULES

Adults. *Initial:* 20 mg twice daily. Dosage increased as indicated every 2 or more days. *Usual:* 20 to 80 mg twice daily. *Maximum:* 80 mg twice daily.

✳ *To treat acute agitation in schizophrenic patients*

I.M. INJECTION

Adults. *Initial:* 10 to 20 mg. 10-mg dose may be given every 2 hr up to maximum dose; 20-mg dose may be given every 4 hr up to maximum dose. *Maximum:* 40 mg daily for no longer than 3 consecutive days.

✳ *To treat acute manic or mixed episodes of bipolar disorder*

CAPSULES

Adults. *Initial:* 40 mg twice daily on day 1; then increased to 60 or 80 mg on day 2 with further adjustments as needed.

✳ *As adjunct to lithium or valproate for maintenance treatment of bipolar I disorder*

CAPSULES

Adults. Same dose patient was initially stabilized on that falls within 40 to 80 mg twice daily.

Drug Administration

P.O.

- Capsules should be swallowed whole and not chewed, crushed, or opened.
- Administer drug with food.

I.M.

- Protect ziprasidone vials from light.
- Reconstitute by adding 1.2 ml Sterile Water for Injection to vial; shake vigorously until drug is dissolved. Each ml of reconstituted solution contains 20 mg ziprasidone. Discard any unused portion.
- Inject only as an I.M. injection.
- Reconstituted drug may be stored for up to 24 hours at room temperature protected from light or up to 7 days if refrigerated and protected from light.

Route	Onset	Peak	Duration
P.O.	Unknown	6–8 hr	12 hr
I.M.	Unknown	1 hr	Unknown

Half-life: 2–7 hr

Mechanism of Action

Selectively blocks dopamine and serotonin receptors in the mesocortical tract of the CNS, thereby suppressing psychotic symptoms.

Contraindications

Concurrent use of other drugs that prolong QT interval, history of arrhythmia or prolonged QT interval, hypersensitivity to ziprasidone or its components, recent acute MI, uncompensated heart failure

Interactions

DRUGS

carbamazepine: Possibly decreased blood ziprasidone level

drugs that prolong QT interval (including dofetilide, pimozide, quinidine, sotalol, sparfloxacin, and thioridazine): Increased risk of prolonged QT interval, torsades de pointes, and sudden death

ketoconazole: Possibly increased blood ziprasidone level

Adverse Reactions

CNS: Agitation, akathisia, amnesia, anxiety, asthenia, **CVA**, depression, dizziness, dystonia, extrapyramidal reactions, headache, hypertonia, hypomania, insomnia, mania, **neuroleptic malignant syndrome**, paresthesia, personality or speech disorder, **serotonin syndrome**, somnolence, **suicidal ideation**, syncope, tardive dyskinesia, tremor

CV: **Bradycardia**, chest pain, hypercholesterolemia, hypertension, orthostatic hypotension, **prolonged QT interval**, tachycardia, thrombophlebitis, vasodilation

EENT: Abnormal vision, dry mouth, increased salivation, rhinitis, **tongue swelling**

ENDO: Dysmenorrhea, hyperglycemia, hyperprolactinemia

GI: Abdominal pain, anorexia, constipation, diarrhea, dysphagia, indigestion, nausea, **rectal bleeding**, vomiting

GU: Priapism, urinary incontinence

HEME: **Agranulocytosis, leukopenia, neutropenia**

MS: Arthralgia, back pain, dysarthria, myalgia

RESP: Cough, **pulmonary embolism**, upper respiratory tract infection

SKIN: Allergic dermatitis, diaphoresis, **exfoliative dermatitis**, furunculosis, rash, **Stevens-Johnson syndrome**, urticaria

Other: Accidental injury, **angioedema, drug reaction with eosinophilia and systemic symptoms (DRESS),** flu-like symptoms, injection-site pain, weight gain

Childbearing Considerations

PREGNANCY

- Pregnancy exposure registry: 1-866-961-2388 or http://womensmentalhealth.org/clinical-and-research-programs/pregnancyregistry/.
- Drug may cause fetal harm, especially during third trimester, as neonates are at increased risk for extrapyramidal and/or withdrawal symptoms following delivery.
- Use with caution only if benefit to mother outweighs potential risk to fetus.

LACTATION

- Drug is present in breast milk.
- Patient should check with prescriber before breastfeeding.
- If breastfeeding occurs, mother should monitor infant for excess sedation, extrapyramidal symptoms, irritability, and poor feedings.

REPRODUCTION

- Drug may increase serum prolactin levels, which may lead to a reversible reduction in fertility in women of childbearing age.

Nursing Considerations

! **WARNING** Know that ziprasidone shouldn't be used to treat elderly patients with dementia-related psychosis because drug increases the risk of death in these patients.

! **WARNING** Assess cardiac rhythm in patients with hypokalemia or hypomagnesemia. Dizziness, palpitations, and syncope may indicate life-threatening torsades de pointes. Be prepared to stop ziprasidone if QT interval is greater than 500 msec.

- Monitor patient, especially elderly women, for involuntary movements, which may become irreversible tardive dyskinesia. If symptoms develop, notify prescriber immediately and be prepared to stop drug.
- Immediately report evidence of neuroleptic malignant syndrome, a rare but potentially fatal adverse reaction including acute renal failure, altered mental status, arrhythmia, blood pressure changes, diaphoresis, hyperpyrexia, irregular pulse, muscle rigidity, myoglobinuria (rhabdomyolysis), and tachycardia.
- Monitor patient's blood glucose and lipid levels routinely, as ordered, because drug increases risk of hypercholesterolemia and hyperglycemia.
- Monitor patient's CBC, as ordered, because serious adverse hematologic reactions may occur, such as agranulocytosis, leukopenia, and neutropenia. Monitor more frequently during first few months of therapy if patient has a history of drug-induced leukopenia, neutropenia, or significantly low WBC count. If abnormalities occur during ziprasidone therapy, watch for fever and other evidence of infection, notify prescriber, and expect to discontinue drug if severe.
- Monitor patient closely for evidence of suicidal thinking or behavior, especially when therapy starts or dosage changes.
- Know that long-standing hyperprolactinemia caused by ziprasidone therapy may cause decreased bone density if associated with hypogonadism.
- Institute fall precautions.

PATIENT TEACHING

- Instruct patient to take ziprasidone with food to increase absorption and to swallow capsule whole, not chewing, crushing, or opening capsule.
- Advise patient to avoid hazardous activities until CNS effects are known. Review fall precautions with patient and family or caregiver.
- Tell family to monitor patient closely for suicidal tendencies; patients with bipolar disorder or psychotic illness are at greater risk.
- Urge patient to rise slowly from lying or seated position to minimize orthostatic hypotension.
- Urge patient to notify prescriber immediately if he develops persistent, severe, sudden-onset, or unusual adverse reactions, especially a fever, rash, or swollen lymph nodes. If present, tell him to stop taking ziprasidone and seek urgent medical care.

zoledronic acid
Reclast, Zometa

Class and Category
Pharmacologic class: Bisphosphonate
Therapeutic class: Antiosteoporotic

Indications and Dosages
✳ *To treat hypercalcemia caused by cancer*

I.V. INFUSION (ZOMETA)
Adults. 4 mg as a single dose. After 7 days, retreatment with 4 mg as a single dose if serum calcium level doesn't remain at or return to normal. *Maximum:* 4 mg/dose.

✳ *As adjunct treatment for patients with multiple myeloma or bony metastasis who are receiving standard antineoplastic therapy and have a creatinine clearance above 60 ml/min*

I.V. INFUSION (ZOMETA)
Adults. 4 mg every 3 to 4 wk.

±**DOSAGE ADJUSTMENT** If patient's creatinine clearance is 50 to 60 ml/min, dosage decreased to 3.5 mg; if it's 40 to 49 ml/min, dosage decreased to 3.3 mg; and if it's 30 to 39 ml/min, dosage decreased to 3 mg.

✳ *To treat postmenopausal osteoporosis in women; to treat osteoporosis in men; to treat and prevent glucocorticoid-induced osteoporosis in patients receiving daily prednisone doses of 7.5 mg or greater for at least 12 months*

I.V. INFUSION (RECLAST)
Adults. 5 mg once yearly.

✳ *To treat Paget's disease of the bone*

I.V. INFUSION (RECLAST)
Adults. 5 mg followed by 1,500 mg elemental calcium daily in divided doses and 800 international units of vitamin D daily for 2 wk.

✳ *To prevent osteoporosis in postmenopausal women*

I.V. INFUSION (RECLAST)
Adults. 5 mg every 2 yr.

Drug Administration
I.V.
- Ensure that patient is hydrated prior to administering drug.
- Expect to administer acetaminophen, if not contraindicated, before zoledronic acid therapy to reduce adverse reactions.
- Reclast comes as a ready-to-infuse solution. Zometa is available as a 4 mg/100 ml single-dose ready-to-use bottle that also doesn't require any further preparation.
- If using 4 mg/5 ml single-dose vial of Zometa for dilution, withdraw dosage and dilute drug in 100 ml of 0.9% Sodium Chloride Injection or 5% Dextrose Injection. Do not store undiluted in a syringe, to avoid inadvertent injection.
- Drug may be refrigerated if not administered immediately. Allow solution to come to room temperature before administration.
- Total time between dilution, storage in the refrigerator, and end of administration for Zometa must not exceed 24 hours and then must be discarded if not used.
- Infuse over no less than 15 minutes. Single dose should not exceed 4 mg.
- Give drug through a separate vented infusion line. Follow infusion by flushing I.V. line with 10 ml of 0.9% Sodium Chloride Injection.
- *Incompatibilities:* Calcium or other divalent cation-containing solutions such as Lactated Ringer's solution

Route	Onset	Peak	Duration
I.V.	4–7 days	Unknown	32 days

Half-life: 146 hr

Mechanism of Action
Inhibits resorption of mineralized bone and cartilage by osteoclasts and induces osteoclast breakdown. In cancer-related hypercalcemia, hyperactive osteoclasts cause bone resorption and release of calcium into blood, which causes polyuria, GI disruption, progressive dehydration, and decreasing GFR. This, in turn, increases renal calcium resorption and worsens hypercalcemia. Zoledronic acid interrupts this process.

Contraindications
Acute renal impairment, creatinine clearance less than 35 ml/min (Reclast); hypersensitivity to zoledronic acid or its components; hypocalcemia (Reclast)

Interactions
DRUGS
aminoglycosides, calcitonin: Possibly additive serum calcium lowering effect

loop diuretics, such as furosemide: Possibly increased risk of hypocalcemia
nephrotoxic drugs, NSAIDs: Increased risk of nephrotoxicity

Adverse Reactions

CNS: Anxiety, asthenia, chills, confusion, depression, dizziness, fatigue, fever, headache, hyperesthesia, hypoesthesia, insomnia, malaise, paresthesia, tremor, vertigo, weakness
CV: **Atrial fibrillation, bradycardia,** chest pain, hypertension, **hypotension,** peripheral edema
EENT: Blurred vision, conjunctivitis, dry mouth, episcleritis, iritis, orbital edema or inflammation, osteonecrosis of external auditory canal, scleritis, sore throat, stomatitis, taste disturbance, uveitis
GI: Abdominal pain, anorexia, constipation, diarrhea, dyspepsia, nausea, vomiting
GU: **Acquired Fanconi syndrome,** elevated serum creatinine level, hematuria, proteinuria, **renal insufficiency or failure,** UTI
HEME: Anemia, **neutropenia, thrombocytopenia**
MS: Arthralgia; atypical subtrochanteric and diaphyseal femoral fractures; incapacitating bone, joint, or muscle pain; muscle cramps or spasms; myalgia; osteonecrosis of the jaw, femur, or hip
RESP: **Bronchospasm,** cough, dyspnea, **exacerbation of asthma, interstitial lung disease,** upper respiratory tract infection
SKIN: Alopecia, dermatitis, diaphoresis, flushing, **Stevens–Johnson syndrome, toxic epidermal necrolysis,** urticaria
Other: **Aggravated malignant neoplasm, anaphylaxis, angioedema,** flu-like illness, **hypersensitivity reactions, hyperkalemia, hypernatremia, hypocalcemia, hypomagnesemia, hypophosphatemia,** infusion-site redness and swelling, weight gain

Childbearing Considerations

PREGNANCY
- Drug can cause fetal harm because there is a theoretical risk, especially skeletal and other abnormalities in fetus, if a woman becomes pregnant after completing a course of bisphosphonate therapy. Time between cessation of drug therapy to conception, the particular bisphosphonate used, and route of administration causing fetal harm are unknown.
- Drug should not be used during pregnancy or in women contemplating a future pregnancy.
- Pregnancy status should be verified before drug is administered.

LACTATION
- It is not known if drug is present in breast milk.
- Drug should not be given during breastfeeding.

REPRODUCTION
- Women of childbearing age should use an effective contraceptive during drug therapy and thereafter.
- Female fertility may be impaired, based on animal studies.

Nursing Considerations

- Be aware that zoledronic acid isn't indicated for hypercalcemia from hyperparathyroidism or other nontumor conditions.
- Verify pregnancy status of women of childbearing age before zoledronic acid therapy is initiated, because drug can cause fetal harm.
- Use cautiously in patients with aspirin sensitivity because bisphosphonates such as zoledronic acid have caused bronchoconstriction in these patients.
- Make sure patient has had a dental checkup before zoledronic acid therapy starts, especially if patient has cancer; is receiving chemotherapy, head or neck radiation, or a corticosteroid; or has poor oral hygiene, because risk of jaw osteonecrosis is increased in these patients, and invasive dental procedures during zoledronic acid therapy may worsen osteonecrosis.
- Expect to aggressively hydrate hypercalcemic patient with I.V. normal saline solution before and during zoledronic acid therapy, as prescribed, to achieve and maintain urine output of about 2 L daily.

! **WARNING** Monitor fluid intake and output often during hydration, and assess patient, especially one with heart failure, for evidence of life-threatening overhydration.

- Monitor patient for adverse reactions, such as fever, flu-like symptoms, headache, and myalgia. Joint swelling may also occur. These reactions usually occur within first 3 days after zoledronic acid administration and resolve within 3 days (although resolution may take up to 14 days for some patients).
- Know that hypocalcemia and mineral metabolism disorders must be treated before zoledronic acid therapy begins.

! **WARNING** Assess patient's renal function, as ordered, before and during zoledronic acid therapy to detect renal deterioration. For patient with a normal serum creatinine level who develops an increase of 0.5 mg/dl within 2 weeks of receiving zoledronic acid, expect to withhold next dose until serum creatinine level is within 10% of patient's baseline value. For patient with an abnormal serum creatinine level who develops an increase of 1.0 mg/dl within 2 weeks of receiving drug, expect to withhold next dose until serum creatinine level is within 10% of baseline value.

- Monitor patient's serum calcium, magnesium, and phosphate levels, as ordered, during zoledronic acid therapy. If hypocalcemia, hypomagnesemia, or hypophosphatemia occurs, expect to give short-term supplemental therapy.
- Assess aspirin-sensitive asthma patients for worsening of respiratory symptoms during zoledronic acid therapy because other bisphosphonates have caused bronchoconstriction in these patients.
- Monitor patient for dehydration. If present, notify prescriber and expect drug to be withheld until dehydration has been corrected.
- Monitor patient for acute phase reaction (APR) that may occur within 3 days following intravenous administration of zoledronic acid. If patient develops flu-like symptoms such as arthralgias, bone pain, chills, fever, flushing, and myalgias, notify prescriber.
- Monitor patient closely for severe and occasionally incapacitating bone, joint, and/or muscle pain. If present, notify prescriber and expect to provide supportive care, as ordered, for pain relief.

PATIENT TEACHING

- Teach patient the importance of eating a nutritious diet, including adequate amounts of calcium and vitamin D. Tell patients with multiple myeloma and bone metastasis of solid tumors to check with prescriber about the need for an oral calcium supplement containing 500 mg of calcium and a multivitamin containing 400 international units of vitamin D.
- Instruct patient to drink at least two glasses of fluid within a few hours before receiving zoledronic acid intravenously.
- Advise patient to alert prescriber about bone, joint, or muscle pain or new or worsening groin, hip, or thigh pain.
- Instruct patient on proper oral hygiene and on need to notify prescriber before undergoing invasive dental procedures.
- Tell patient to notify prescriber if he notices blood or other changes in his urine or a change in amount of urine voided or frequency of voiding pattern. Stress importance of compliance in having regular blood tests that have been ordered to check his kidney function.
- Advise women of childbearing age to use effective contraception during and after zoledronic acid therapy and to notify prescriber immediately if they are or could be pregnant, because drug will have to be stopped. Alert female patients that drug may also impair fertility. Also inform these patients that breastfeeding is also not recommended during zoledronic acid therapy.
- Inform patient not to take other bisphosphonates concurrently, including Reclast if they are prescribed Zometa or Zometa if they are prescribed Reclast.

zolmitriptan
Zomig, Zomig ZMT

☰ Class and Category
Pharmacologic class: Selective 5-hydroxytryptamine agonist
Therapeutic class: Antimigraine

☰ Indications and Dosages
✴ *To treat acute migraine headache with or without aura*

ORAL DISINTEGRATING TABLETS, TABLETS

Adults. *Initial:* 1.25 or 2.5 mg, repeated in 2 hr as needed. *Maximum:* 5 mg as a single dose, 10 mg in 24 hr, or 3 headaches/mo.

NASAL SPRAY

Adults. *Initial:* 2.5 mg (1 spray) repeated in 2 hr as needed. Dosage increased to 5 mg/episode, as needed. *Maximum:* 5 mg as single dose; 10 mg/24 hr; or 4 headaches/mo.

±**DOSAGE ADJUSTMENT** For patient with moderate to severe hepatic impairment, initial oral dosage using tablet form should not be higher than 1.25 mg and maximum dose should not exceed 5 mg in 24 hr. Nasal spray or oral disintegrating tablets are not recommended for these patients. For patient receiving cimetidine concurrently, single dosage should not exceed 2.5 mg and the maximum dosage should not exceed 5 mg in a 24-hr period.

Drug Administration

P.O.

- Do not remove disintegrating tablet from blister pack until just before giving the tablet. Peel foil to open pack; do not push tablet through foil. Have patient put tablet on tongue and let dissolve and then swallow. Do not break orally disintegrating tablet.
- Regular tablet may be broken in half, if needed to achieve correct dose.

NASAL

- Have patient blow nose before use.
- Don't test or prime spray before use, as it is a single-dose device.
- Have patient insert device into nostril and close other nostril with finger.
- Have patient press plunger device while breathing gently in through the nose. Device then removed and patient should then breathe gently through mouth for 5 to 10 seconds.

Route	Onset	Peak	Duration
P.O.	Unknown	1.5–3 hr	Unknown
Nasal	5 min	3 hr	Unknown

Half-life: 2.8–3.7 hr

Mechanism of Action

Constricts dilated and inflamed cranial blood vessels in the carotid circulation and inhibits production of proinflammatory neuropeptides by binding to receptors on intracranial blood vessels and sensory nerves in the trigeminal-vascular system to stimulate negative feedback, which halts the release of serotonin.

Contraindications

History of basilar or hemiplegic migraine, stroke, or transient ischemic attack; hypersensitivity to zolmitriptan or its components; ischemic coronary artery or bowel disease; peripheral vascular disease; recent use (within 24 hours) of another 5-HT$_1$ agonist, ergotamine-containing medication, or ergot-type medication (such as dihydroergotamine or methysergide); uncontrolled hypertension; use of a MAO inhibitor within past 14 days; Wolff-Parkinson-White syndrome or arrhythmias associated with other cardiac accessory conduction pathway disorders

Interactions

DRUGS

5-HT$_{1B/1D}$ agonists: Increased risk of additive vasospastic reactions

cimetidine: Doubled blood zolmitriptan levels; prolonged zolmitriptan half-life

ergot alkaloids: Prolonged vasoconstriction effects

MAO inhibitors: Increased zolmitriptan effects

naratriptan, rizatriptan, sumatriptan: Prolonged zolmitriptan effects

selective serotonin reuptake inhibitors and serotonin norepinephrine reuptake inhibitors: Increased risk of developing serotonin syndrome

Adverse Reactions

CNS: Asthenia, dizziness, hyperesthesia, paresthesia, somnolence, vertigo

CV: Angina, **coronary artery vasospasm**, hypertension, **MI**, palpitations, transient myocardial ischemia, **ventricular fibrillation or tachycardia**

EENT: Dry mouth, vision disturbance

GI: Abdominal pain, **bloody diarrhea**, dysphagia, **GI or splenic infarction**, indigestion, **ischemic colitis**, nausea, vomiting

MS: Myalgia; myasthenia; pain, pressure, or tightness in jaw, neck, or throat

SKIN: Diaphoresis, flushing

Other: **Anaphylaxis, angioedema**

Childbearing Considerations
PREGNANCY
- It is not known if drug can cause fetal harm.
- Use with caution only if benefit to mother outweighs potential risk to fetus.
- Be aware that women with migraine may be at increased risk for preeclampsia during pregnancy.

LACTATION
- It is not known if drug is present in breast milk.
- Patient should check with prescriber before breastfeeding.

Nursing Considerations

! **WARNING** Monitor patient for signs and symptoms of vasoconstriction, which may lead to colonic and vascular ischemia with abdominal pain and bloody diarrhea, especially if patient has ischemic bowel disease or peripheral vascular disease (including Raynaud's phenomenon).

- Monitor elderly patients and those with hepatic impairment for increased blood pressure, and notify prescriber immediately if it occurs.
- Monitor patient closely for signs and symptoms of angina. If patient develops chest pain, notify prescriber.

! **WARNING** Monitor patient closely for signs and symptoms of serotonin syndrome, which may include agitation, coma, diarrhea, hallucinations, hyperreflexia, hyperthermia, incoordination, labile blood pressure, nausea, tachycardia, and vomiting. Notify prescriber immediately because serotonin syndrome may be life-threatening. Be prepared to provide supportive care and discontinue zolmitriptan.

PATIENT TEACHING
- Instruct patient to take zolmitriptan exactly as prescribed. Tell her also not to take more than 10 mg in any 24-hour period, nor should she take drug for more than recommended number of times per month because overuse of drug may lead to exacerbation of headache. Tell her to be alert for migraine-like daily headaches developing or marked increase in frequency of migraine headaches that signals overuse may be occurring. Tell her to notify prescriber, as drug may no longer be as effective and drug withdrawal may be needed.
- Advise patient not to remove disintegrating tablet from blister pack until just before taking the tablet. Instruct her to peel foil back and not to push tablet through the foil. After opening pack, let tablet dissolve on her tongue, and then swallow. Remind her not to break orally disintegrating tablet.
- Teach patient how to administer nasal spray. Caution patient to avoid spraying drug into her eyes.
- Urge patient to notify prescriber about severe or unusual adverse reactions.
- Instruct patient not to take zolmitriptan within 24 hours of other drugs in the same class.
- Tell patient to inform all prescribers of zolmitriptan therapy, because serious drug interactions may occur.

zolpidem tartrate
Ambien, Ambien CR, Edluar, Zolpimist

Class, Category, and Schedule
Pharmacologic class: Imidazopyridine
Therapeutic class: Hypnotic
Controlled substance schedule: IV

Indications and Dosages
* To provide short-term treatment of insomnia
ORAL SPRAY, S.L. TABLETS, TABLETS
Adult men. 5 or 10 mg once nightly for 7 to 10 days. *Maximum:* 10 mg daily.
Adult women. 5 mg once nightly for 7 to 10 days. *Maximum:* 5 mg daily.
±**DOSAGE ADJUSTMENT** For elderly men or debilitated male patients and men with mild to moderate hepatic impairment, dosage possibly reduced to 5 mg at bedtime, with a maximum of 5 mg daily for nursing facility residents.

E.R. TABLETS
Adult men. 6.25 or 12.5 mg once nightly.
Adult women. 6.25 mg once nightly.
±**DOSAGE ADJUSTMENT** For elderly or debilitated patients and those with mild to moderate hepatic impairment, dosage reduced to 6.25 mg once nightly.

X
Y
Z

Drug Administration

P.O.

- Administer on an empty stomach at bedtime for faster sleep onset, but only administer if patient has 7 to 8 hours of sleep time remaining.
- Extended-release tablets should be swallowed whole and not chewed, crushed, or divided.
- Sublingual tablets should be placed under the tongue to dissolve; not swallowed or administered with water.
- Oral spray requires pump to be primed by spraying 5 times before first use or if not used for 14 days. Spray should be directed over tongue while fully pressing down firmly to provide one 5-mg dose.

Route	Onset	Peak	Duration
P.O.	< 30 min	30–120 min	6–8 hr
P.O./E.R.	< 30 min	30–120 min	6–8 hr

Half-life: 1.5–3 hr

Mechanism of Action

May potentiate the effects of gamma-aminobutyric acid (GABA) and other inhibitory neurotransmitters. By binding to specific benzodiazepine receptors in the limbic and cortical areas of the CNS, zolpidem increases GABA's inhibitory effects, blocks cortical and limbic arousal, and preserves deep sleep (stages 3 and 4).

Contraindications

Development of complex sleep behaviors after taking zolpidem, hypersensitivity to zolpidem or its components

Interactions

DRUGS

barbiturates, chlorpromazine, general anesthetics, opioid agonists, other CNS depressants, phenothiazines, tramadol, tricyclic antidepressants: Possibly increased CNS depression and reduced psychomotor function
CYP3A4 inducers such as rifampin, St. John's wort: Decreased effectiveness of zolpidem
CYP3A4 inhibitors such as ketoconazole: Increased risk of zolpidem-induced adverse reactions
sertraline: Increased exposure to zolpidem

Adverse Reactions

CNS: Abnormal thinking, aggressiveness, amnesia, asthenia, ataxia, behavioral changes, complex behaviors (such as sleep driving), confusion, decreased level of consciousness or inhibition, dizziness, drowsiness, euphoria, hallucinations, headache, insomnia, lethargy, paradoxical CNS stimulation (including agitation, euphoria, hallucinations, hyperactivity, and nightmares), **suicidal ideation**, vertigo, worsening of depression
EENT: Application-site reactions from sublingual dose form (blisters, mucosal inflammation, oral ulcers), blurred vision, diplopia, **throat tightness**, visual abnormality
GI: Constipation, diarrhea, elevated liver enzymes, **hepatic injury**, hiccups, indigestion, jaundice, nausea, vomiting
GU: UTI
MS: Arthralgia, myalgia
RESP: Dyspnea, **respiratory depression**, upper or lower respiratory infection
Other: **Anaphylaxis**, **angioedema**, withdrawal symptoms

Childbearing Considerations

PREGNANCY

- Drug can cause fetal harm, as drug used late in third trimester may cause neonates at birth to experience hypotonia, respiratory depression, and sedation.
- Use with caution only if benefit to mother outweighs potential risk to fetus.
- Be aware that women with migraine may be at increased risk for preeclampsia during pregnancy.

LACTATION

- Drug is present in breast milk.
- Patient should check with prescriber before breastfeeding.
- If breastfeeding occurs, infant should be monitored for excess sedation, hypotonia, and respiratory depression. Mother may interrupt breastfeeding by pumping and discarding breast milk during treatment and for 23 hours after last dose.

Nursing Considerations

- Use zolpidem cautiously in patients with additional disorders because it isn't known if zolpidem therapy might aggravate these conditions, especially conditions with respiratory impairment.

- Expect patient to receive no more than a 1-month supply of zolpidem for outpatient therapy, with treatment being as short as possible.

! **WARNING** Keep in mind if zolpidem is withdrawn abruptly (especially after prolonged therapy), monitor patient for withdrawal symptoms, such as abdominal cramps or discomfort, fatigue, flushing, inconsolable crying, light-headedness, nausea, nervousness, panic attack, rebound insomnia, and vomiting.

- Expect that zolpidem will produce anticonvulsant and muscle relaxant effects at high doses.
- Know that if patient takes other CNS depressants, expect to reduce zolpidem dosage, as prescribed.
- Monitor patient closely for suicidal tendencies, particularly when therapy starts or dosage increases, because depression may worsen temporarily during these times, possibly leading to suicide.

! **WARNING** Monitor patient closely for hypersensitivity reactions such as dyspnea, nausea, swelling, throat tightness, or vomiting. If present, discontinue zolpidem immediately, notify prescriber, and provide supportive care.

- Monitor neonates born to mothers using zolpidem late in the third trimester of pregnancy for hypotonia, respiratory depression, and sedation.

PATIENT TEACHING
- Caution patient to take drug exactly as prescribed and not to increase dosage unless directed by prescriber.
- Instruct patient to take drug immediately before bedtime as long as 7 to 8 hours of sleep time remains and to take drug on an empty stomach.
- Advise patient taking extended-release form to swallow tablet whole and not to break, chew, or crush it.
- Instruct patient using sublingual form patient to place tablet under his tongue and allow it to dissolve completely before swallowing. Tell him never to swallow the sublingual tablet whole or take with water.

- Instruct patient how to administer oral spray form, if prescribed.
- Advise patient to notify prescriber immediately about abdominal cramps or discomfort, fatigue, flushing, inconsolable crying, light-headedness, nausea, nervousness, panic attack, and vomiting.

! **WARNING** Instruct patient to stop taking zolpidem and seek emergency care if he has abnormal swelling, nausea, throat tightness, trouble breathing, or vomiting.

- Advise patient that zolpidem may produce abnormal behaviors during sleep, such as driving a car, eating, talking on the phone, or having sex without any recall of the event. If patient's family notices any such behavior or if patient sees evidence of such behavior upon awakening, prescriber should be notified.
- Tell patient that drug may cause drowsiness or decreased level of consciousness and even next-morning impairment from zolpidem use despite feeling fully awake. Advise patient to get a good night's sleep of at least 7 or 8 hours to help minimize this adverse effect. Tell her to take precautions against falling and not to perform any hazardous activity such as driving, especially after taking the drug and during the morning hours.
- Tell family or caregiver to observe patient closely for suicidal tendencies, especially when therapy starts or dosage changes.
- Advise mothers breastfeeding during zolpidem therapy to monitor the infant for excess sedation, hypotonia, and slower-than-normal breathing, because drug passes through into breast milk. Encourage mother instead to interrupt breastfeeding, if possible, and pump and then discard breast milk during zolpidem therapy and for 23 hours after drug administration in order to minimize drug exposure of the breastfed infant.

zonisamide
Zonegran

☰ Class and Category
Pharmacologic class: Sulfonamide
Therapeutic class: Anticonvulsant

Indications and Dosages

* *As adjunct to treat partial seizures in patients with epilepsy*

CAPSULES

Adults and adolescents over age 16. *Initial:* 100 mg once daily or divided and given twice daily. Dosage increased by 100 mg once daily every 2 wk, as needed. *Usual:* 200 to 400 mg once daily or divided and given twice daily. *Maximum:* 400 mg once daily or divided and given twice daily.

±**DOSAGE ADJUSTMENT** For patients with hepatic or renal dysfunction, a slower titration may be required.

Drug Administration

P.O.

- Capsules should be swallowed whole and not chewed, crushed, or opened.

Route	Onset	Peak	Duration
P.O.	Unknown	2–6 hr	Unknown

Half-life: 63–69 hr

Mechanism of Action

May stop seizures and suppress their foci by blocking sodium channels and reducing voltage-dependent, inward currents from calcium channels. This action stabilizes neuronal membranes and suppresses synchronized neuronal hyperactivity.

Contraindications

Hypersensitivity to zonisamide, other sulfonamides, or their components

Interactions

DRUGS

CNS depressants: Additive CNS depressant effects
other carbonic anhydrase inhibitors: Increased risk of hyperammonemia and severity of metabolic acidosis; increased risk of kidney stone formation
topiramate, valproic acid: Increased risk of metabolic acidosis

FOODS

grapefruit juice: Possibly decreased metabolism of zonisamide

ACTIVITIES

alcohol: Additive CNS depressant effects

Adverse Reactions

CNS: Abnormal gait, agitation, anxiety, asthenia, ataxia, confusion, depression, difficulty concentrating, dizziness, **encephalopathy,** fatigue, headache, incoordination, insomnia, irritability, memory loss, nervousness, paresthesia, schizophrenia, **seizures,** somnolence, speech abnormalities, **suicidal ideation,** tremor
CV: Chest pain
EENT: Acute myopia, amblyopia, blurred vision, diplopia, dry mouth, increased intraocular pressure (possibly leading to permanent vision loss), nystagmus, periorbital pain, pharyngitis, rhinitis, secondary closure angle glaucoma, taste alteration, tinnitus, visual disturbances
GI: Abdominal pain, **acute pancreatitis,** anorexia, constipation, diarrhea, dyspepsia, nausea, vomiting
GU: Renal calculi
HEME: Anemia, **leukopenia, thrombocytopenia**
MS: Elevated creatine phosphokinase levels, **rhabdomyolysis**
RESP: Increased cough
SKIN: Ecchymosis, pruritus, rash
Other: Angioedema, **drug reaction with eosinophilia and systemic symptoms (DRESS),** flu-like symptoms, **hyperammonemia (with or without encephalopathy), metabolic acidosis,** weight loss

Childbearing Considerations

PREGNANCY

- Pregnancy exposure registry: 1-888-233-2334 or https://www.aedpregnancyregistry.org/.
- Drug may cause serious fetal harm.
- Use with caution only if benefit to mother outweighs potential risk to fetus.
- Neonates of mothers treated with drug should be monitored for metabolic acidosis.

LACTATION

- Drug is present in breast milk.
- A decision should be made to discontinue breastfeeding or the drug to avoid potential serious adverse reactions in the breastfed infant.

REPRODUCTION

- Women of childbearing age should use effective contraception during drug therapy.

Nursing Considerations

- Obtain a serum bicarbonate level before starting zonisamide and then periodically during therapy, as prescribed, because drug may cause metabolic acidosis, especially in patients with predisposing conditions or therapies or who are younger in age.

> **! WARNING** Monitor results of patient's CBC and other laboratory tests for signs of blood dyscrasias because zonisamide is a sulfonamide and can be absorbed systemically. Systemic absorption may result in life-threatening reactions, including agranulocytosis, aplastic anemia, and other blood dyscrasias; fulminant hepatic necrosis; Stevens–Johnson syndrome; and toxic epidermal necrolysis.

- Be aware that patients receiving doses of 300 mg daily or more are at increased risk for adverse CNS reactions, including decreased concentration, drowsiness, fatigue, and impaired speech.
- Monitor patient for symptoms of hyperammonemia such as lethargy, unexplained change in mental status, or vomiting. If suspected, obtain serum ammonia levels, as ordered. Know that drug-induced hyperammonemia may resolve or decrease in severity with a decrease of the daily dose.
- Monitor BUN and serum creatinine levels for signs of abnormally decreased glomerular filtration rate (GFR). Expect some decrease in GFR during first 4 weeks of treatment and return to baseline within 2 to 3 weeks after drug is discontinued.
- Monitor patient for signs and symptoms of renal calculi.
- Be aware that zonisamide shouldn't be discontinued abruptly because doing so may increase frequency of seizures.
- Monitor patient closely for evidence of suicidal thinking or behavior, especially when therapy starts or dosage changes.

PATIENT TEACHING

- Inform patient that zonisamide is usually prescribed with other anticonvulsants and that she should continue to take all drugs as prescribed.
- Instruct patient to swallow zonisamide capsules whole and not to break them open or chew them.
- Inform patient that prescriber may have to adjust zonisamide dosage over several weeks or months before stable dose is achieved.
- Advise patient to use caution when driving or performing other activities that are hazardous or require mental alertness because zonisamide commonly causes decreased concentration, dizziness, and somnolence, particularly during first month of therapy.
- Advise patient to wear a medical identification bracelet or necklace or carry medical identification with information about her seizure disorder.
- Encourage patient to drink six to eight glasses of water each day to prevent kidney stones, unless contraindicated.
- Advise patient to rise slowly from a lying or seated position to reduce the risk of dizziness.
- Urge caregivers to watch closely for evidence of suicidal tendencies, especially when therapy starts or dosage changes, and to report concerns immediately to prescriber.
- Instruct women of childbearing age to notify prescriber immediately if pregnancy is suspected or known, as drug will have to be replaced. Also alert patient that breastfeeding is not recommended.

> **! WARNING** Instruct patient to notify prescriber immediately if an allergic reaction occurs, seizures worsen, signs of blood abnormalities (easy bruising, fever, oral ulcers, sore throat) are present, signs of kidney stones occur (abdominal pain, blood in urine, sudden back pain), signs of hyperammonemia (change in level of consciousness and/or cognitive function with lethargy and/or vomiting) occur, or a skin rash develops. She should also report signs and symptoms such as fast breathing, fatigue, irregular heartbeat, loss of appetite, or palpitations as well as blurred vision, visual disturbances, or periorbital pain.

- Tell patient to seek emergency care if sweating decreases significantly from normal with or without a fever.

Appendices

Emergency Use Authorization

With the recent COVID-19 pandemic, a number of Emergency Use Authorizations (EUAs) have been issued in an effort to curtail the severity of the infection and rising death rates. But what is an EUA? Not understanding what an EUA is has caused many people to question the safety of the tests, drugs, and vaccines used in the fight against COVID-19. This, in turn, has caused some to avoid using any product with an EUA status.

The Food and Drug Administration's (FDA) use of an EUA is not something new that came about because of the COVID-19 pandemic. The EUA program was established in 2004 when bioterrorist attacks, including the use of anthrax, were a major concern. Since then EUAs have been issued for the H1N1 virus, Ebola, Avian Flu, and Middle Eastern Respiratory Syndrome (MERS), to name a few prior to the COVID-19 pandemic.

For an EUA to be issued, the secretary of Health and Human Services (HHS) must first determine that a disease or other health condition poses an emergency threat to the general public. A declared public health emergency can be caused by an infectious disease or biological, chemical, nuclear, and radiological threats. Once such a threat is recognized and declared, the FDA then looks at products that are in development but not yet fully approved but are showing promising results to diagnose, treat, or prevent the health problem. They also look at products that may be able to be modified to help combat the life-threatening threat to public health safety.

The FDA then works with manufacturers to help them decide whether to and when to submit an EUA request for their product. Once submitted, the FDA reviews the information including the totality of the scientific evidence known thus far. After a thorough review, the FDA may authorize medical products that have not yet received full FDA approval or authorize unapproved uses of approved medical products to diagnose, treat, or prevent severe or life-threatening disease or conditions. This is because an EUA can only be issued for a product when there are no adequate, approved, and available alternatives that can be used for the emergency being declared and when the known and potential benefits outweigh the potential risks.

Under normal circumstances, a product seeking FDA "full approval" must meet rigorous safety and efficacy standards, which could take years. In an emergency situation, the time line is condensed but the product must still meet FDA standards before it can be issued under an EUA. Once an EUA is given, the product still continues to be monitored and evaluated by the FDA. For example, the Pfizer and Moderna vaccines used to prevent or lessen the effects of COVID-19 were granted EUA status in 2021 but have now gone on to receive full FDA approval.

When a product is issued an EUA, it does not mean that the authorization cannot be revised or revoked. An example of this was when the FDA issued an EUA for the drug hydroxychloroquine in the initial fight against COVID-19. As it continued to evaluate the drug, it became clear that the drug did not provide a significant benefit and in fact posed risks that outweighed any benefit derived from the use of the drug in the battle against COVID-19. Thus, the FDA retracted the EUA for this drug.

Finally, it is important to understand that when a health emergency is declared, there is usually an outpouring of resources and energy geared to one goal: developing products to use to diagnose, prevent, or treat the situation at hand. To that end, manufacturers can elect to prioritize their work centered on that product adding countless hours of manpower required to achieve FDA approval under the safety guidelines required by the FDA. For example, the various COVID-19 vaccines were already in clinical development months before the manufacturers submitted applications for EUAs.

In summary, the issuing of an EUA still requires the product to undergo a thorough investigation. Clinical trials are still needed but are shortened because time is of the essence to treat the emergency. Once released for use to diagnose, treat, or prevent the emergency, the product continues to be under the scrutiny of the FDA, making the product as safe as possible for use in the emergency.

Safety Guidelines for Opioid Use

Pain relief has been a long-standing goal in health care for patients with pain. Patients may experience short-term pain as a result of an illness, injury, or medical or surgical procedure. Others experience chronic or persistent pain, defined as pain that lasts longer than 3 months or beyond normal tissue healing, which can drastically alter quality of life.

Opioids are powerful pain-reducing drugs, and their efficacy has made them increasingly popular for both short- and long-term pain management. However, opioids are also addictive, especially when used inappropriately. This has led to their abuse and misuse in society, along with a sharp increase in recent years of opioid-related overdoses and deaths.

In an effort to address the opioid crisis in the United States, the Food and Drug Administration (FDA) has formulated and implemented a plan called the *FDA Opioids Action Plan*. This plan details seven measures the FDA is using to combat this problem and includes:

- Expanding the use of advisory committees to approve any new drug application for an opioid that does not have abuse-deterrent properties, as well as seeking expert advice on opioid labeling regarding use by children.
- Providing clearer information to prescribers of opioids by making certain changes to immediate-release opioid labeling similar to those issued in 2013 for extended-release or long-acting opioid analgesics.
- Requiring drug companies to address issues of abuse and misuse associated with long-term use of their opioid drug products, provide predictors of opioid addiction, and explore other important issues related to opioid addiction through adherence to postmarketing requirements.
- Increasing training for prescribers on pain management and safe prescription use of opioid drugs.
- Encouraging the development of abuse-deterrent formulations, especially generic opioid formulations.
- Making naloxone more accessible to treat opioid overdose while at the same time encouraging drug companies to develop new classes of analgesics that would be as effective as opioids but not carry the same risks.
- Increasing the patient's understanding of the risks associated with opioids, and the risks of misuse by other persons who obtain them.

As a result of the FDA Opioids Action Plan, drug companies are now required to address several safety issues in their opioid drug labels (package inserts). Changes to individual sections of the drug label reflective of these safety issues are summarized here:

- **Boxed Warning**—Now includes warnings about addiction, abuse, and misuse; life-threatening respiratory depression; accidental ingestion; neonatal opioid withdrawal syndrome (NOWS); and any significant drug product-specific interactions that could raise the risk of adverse reactions associated with opioid use.
- **Indications and Usage**—Modified to emphasize that opioids are to be reserved for the management of pain only if alternative treatment options such as nonopioid analgesics cannot be used or are ineffective and the pain is severe enough to require an opioid analgesic.
- **Contraindications**—Includes patients with significant respiratory depression and patients with acute or severe bronchial asthma in an unmonitored setting or in the absence of resuscitative equipment.
- **Warning and Precautions**—Addresses each of the components found in the boxed warning as well as risks associated with concurrently administered central nervous system depressants; life-threatening respiratory depression in patients with chronic pulmonary disease, in the elderly or patients who are cachectic or debilitated; and the potential development of adrenal insufficiency with opioid use.
- **Adverse Reactions**—Lists all the serious adverse reactions addressed in the "Warnings and Precautions" section of the drug label as well as adding adrenal insufficiency and serotonin syndrome to the postmarketing section.
- **Drug Interactions**—Includes any significant drug-specific interactions that would increase the opioid effect as well as interactions between opioids and central nervous system depressants, including alcohol and between opioids and serotonergic drugs.
- **Specific Populations**—Additional information included regarding NOWS and potential for neonatal respiratory depression during delivery or with breastfeeding; potential risk for infertility with chronic use; and increased risk for respiratory depression in the elderly.
- **Drug Abuse and Dependence**—Details information about opioid abuse and dependence.
- **Overdosage**—Adds or modifies information to address seriousness and current treatment of opioid overdose.
- **Patient Counseling**—Includes information to be given to the patient on addiction, abuse, and misuse of opioids; risk of life-threatening respiratory depression or accidental ingestion; interactions with alcohol and other CNS depressants; potential for adrenal insufficiency and serotonin syndrome and what to report; potential for development of NOWS and embryo-fetal toxicity during pregnancy, respiratory depression in infants during delivery and with breastfeeding; how to dispose of the unused opioid; and the addition of a medication guide.

In addition, the Centers for Disease Control (CDC) has also released recommendations for use of opioids in treating chronic pain. These recommendations exclude patients who are in active cancer treatment, palliative care, or end-of-life care.

The CDC recommends that opioids not be used as first-line therapy in the treatment of chronic pain. Instead, nonpharmacologic therapies such as cognitive behavioral therapy or exercise, or nonopioid pharmacologic therapies such as NSAIDs, should be tried first. If opioids are prescribed, the CDC recommends that they be combined with nonpharmacologic or nonopioid pharmacologic therapy to provide greater benefits and lower opioid dosage requirements.

When opioids are used, the lowest possible effective dosage should be prescribed and therapy should start with immediate-release opioids rather than extended-release or long-acting opioids. In addition, the quantity prescribed should not go beyond the expected need for pain relief.

Closer follow-up is also recommended, with regular monitoring of patients to determine effectiveness of the prescribed pain measures. It is especially important to ascertain that the opioid is not causing harm. If benefits do not outweigh harm, it is recommended that the opioid dosage be reduced and then discontinued, if needed.

It is very important that the patient's response to pain relief measures be accurately measured and assessed. Only then can the goal to provide effective pain relief without causing the patient harm be achieved. Although opioid therapy has its place in pain management, it is important to understand that opioids are not always necessary and, if used inappropriately, can cause much harm, not only to the patient but to society in general.

Data from Food and Drug Administration. (2016). Fact sheet—FDA opioids action plan. Retrieved from https://www.fda.gov/newsevents/newsroom/factsheets/ucm484714.htm

Parenteral Insulin Preparations

For each category of insulin, the following table lists the species; common trade names; onset, peak, and duration; and key nursing considerations.

CATEGORY, SPECIES, AND TRADE NAMES	KEY NURSING CONSIDERATIONS
Rapid-acting insulin	

Onset: 10–20 min   **Peak**: 30–90 min   **Duration**: 2–5 hr

Human • Admelog (insulin lispro) • Apidra (insulin glulisine) • Fiasp (insulin aspart) • Humalog (insulin lispro) • Lyumjev (insulin lispro-aabc) • NovoLog (insulin aspart) • NovoRapid (insulin aspart) (CAN) **Concentrated** • Humalog U-200	• Only mix with NPH (intermediate-type) insulin, if needed, except for Humalog U-200, which should not be mixed with any other insulin. Administer immediately after mixing. • When mixing rapid-acting insulin with a longer-acting insulin, always draw the rapid-acting insulin into the syringe first to avoid dosage errors. • Be aware that Lyumjev comes in two strengths: U-100 and U-200. The U-200 prefilled pen contains 2 times as much insulin per 1 milliliter as standard U-100 insulin. • When giving SubQ, given Admelog within 15 minutes before or meal or immediately after a meal; give Humalog up to 15 minutes before a meal or immediately after a meal; give Lyumjev at the start of a meal or up to within 20 minutes after starting a meal; give NovoLog and NovoRapid 5 to 10 minutes before a meal; give Apidra up to 15 to 20 minutes before a meal, and give Fiasp up to 2 minutes before a meal or up to 20 minutes after starting a meal. When giving rapid-acting insulin (except for Fiasp) via an insulin pump, do not dilute or mix with any other insulin, change the insulin in the reservoir at least every 48 hours (Apidra), 6 days (NovoLog, NovoRapid), and 7 days (Humalog). Change the infusion sets and insertion site at least every 3 days. • Be aware that 1 unit of rapid-acting insulin has the same glucose-lowering ability as 1 unit of short-acting insulin. • Rapid-acting insulin is available as a cartridge. Make sure to use the correct device for the brand of insulin prescribed, and don't add any other insulin to the cartridge. • Assess patient taking insulin concurrently with a thiazolidinedione for signs and symptoms of heart failure. If heart failure develops, provide supportive care, as ordered, and expect the thiazolidinedione to be discontinued or dosage reduced. • Know that Fiasp's onset is 5 to 10 minutes; Lyumjev duration is 6 hours. • Admelog and Lyumjev (U-100 only) may also be given as a continuous subcutaneous infusion without being diluted and not mixed with other insulins when given in the pump. Either may also be given as an intravenous infusion but only after dilution. Fiasp can also be used in insulin infusion pumps and to treat pediatric patients. • Do not repeatedly inject insulin into areas of lipodystrophy or localized cutaneous amyloidosis because hyperglycemia may occur; and a sudden change in the injection site to an unaffected area may cause hypoglycemia.

(continues)

Parenteral Insulin Preparations *(continued)*

CATEGORY, SPECIES, AND TRADE NAMES	KEY NURSING CONSIDERATIONS

Short-acting insulin

Onset: 30–60 min   **Peak:** 1.5–4 hr   **Duration:** 5–8 hr

Human
- Humulin-R
- Novolin ge Toronto (CAN)
- Novolin R
- ReliOn Novolin R

Concentrated
- Humulin-R U-500

- Don't use short-acting insulin if it's cloudy, discolored, or unusually viscous.
- Use the U-500 strength to treat insulin resistance, as prescribed. Be very careful to use conversion chart if U-500 strength is being administered using U-100 syringes. Also, make sure the right strength of the short-acting insulin is being administered, as severe hypoglycemia and death have occurred because of dispensing, prescribing, and administration errors.
- Mix short-acting insulin with other insulin types, if needed.
- Do not repeatedly inject insulin into areas of lipodystrophy or localized cutaneous amyloidosis because hyperglycemia may occur; and a sudden change in the injection site to an unaffected area may cause hypoglycemia.
- Administer SubQ, I.M., or I.V., as prescribed. Use a continuous SubQ infusion pump, if ordered. The catheter tubing and reservoir insulin should be changed every 48 hours or as specified by the pump manufacturer.
- When giving SubQ or I.M. injections, give the short-acting insulin 15 to 30 minutes before a meal or bedtime snack.
- Assess patient taking insulin concurrently with a thiazolidinedione for signs and symptoms of heart failure. If heart failure develops, provide supportive care, as ordered, and expect the thiazolidinedione to be discontinued or dosage reduced.

Intermediate-acting insulin

Onset: 1–3 hr   **Peak:** 4–12 hr   **Duration:** 12–24 hr

Human
- Humulin N
- Novolin ge NPH (CAN)
- Novolin N
- ReliOn Novolin N

- Don't use intermediate-acting insulin if it contains precipitate that is clumped or granular or that clings to the sides of the vial.
- Roll the vial gently between your palms to mix; don't shake it. Also gently turn the prefilled syringe up and down several times before using to achieve a uniform mixture.
- Administer by SubQ injection only, 30 minutes before a meal or bedtime snack.
- Be aware that intermediate-acting insulin rarely produces a blood glucose level that's as close to normal as possible. So expect to mix it with a rapid-acting or short-acting insulin, as prescribed, for optimum blood glucose control.
- Assess patient taking insulin concurrently with a thiazolidinedione for signs and symptoms of heart failure. If heart failure develops, provide supportive care, as ordered, and expect the thiazolidinedione to be discontinued or dosage reduced.
- Do not repeatedly inject insulin into areas of lipodystrophy or localized cutaneous amyloidosis because hyperglycemia may occur; and a sudden change in the injection site to an unaffected area may cause hypoglycemia.

CATEGORY, SPECIES, AND TRADE NAMES	KEY NURSING CONSIDERATIONS

Long-acting insulin

Onset: 1–1.5 hr   **Peak:** None   **Duration:** 24–28 hr

Human
- Basaglar (insulin glargine)
- Detemir (insulin detemir) (CAN)
- Glargine (insulin glargine) (CAN)
- Lantus (insulin glargine)
- Levemir (insulin detemir)
- Semglee (insulin glargine-yfgn)

- Don't use long-acting insulin if it contains precipitate that is clumped or granular or that clings to the sides of the vial.
- Do not mix insulin detemir or insulin glargine with another insulin or solution.
- Know that insulin degludec is now approved for use in children age 1 year and over.
- Roll the vial gently between your palms to obtain a uniform mixture; don't shake it.
- Administer by the SubQ route only. Inject insulin glargine once daily at any time, keeping the daily injection time consistent. Inject insulin detemir prescribed once daily with the evening meal or at bedtime; inject insulin detemir prescribed twice daily with the morning meal and with the evening meal, at bedtime, or 12 hours after the morning dose.
- Give insulin glargine at bedtime, if possible, so that additional insulin can be given while patient is awake if effects decline before 24 hours pass. If insulin glargine is given in the morning and its effects don't last 24 hours, hyperglycemia may occur while patient sleeps.
- Assess patient taking insulin concurrently with a thiazolidinedione for signs and symptoms of heart failure. If heart failure develops, provide supportive care, as ordered, and expect the thiazolidinedione to be discontinued or dosage reduced.
- Do not repeatedly inject insulin into areas of lipodystrophy or localized cutaneous amyloidosis because hyperglycemia may occur; and a sudden change in the injection site to an unaffected area may cause hypoglycemia.

Ultra-long-acting insulins

Onset: 1–6 hr   **Peak:** None   **Duration:** 36–42 hr

- Toujeo (insulin glargine)
- Tresiba (insulin degludec)
Concentrated
- Tresiba U-200

- Don't use ultra-long-acting insulin if it contains precipitate that is clumped or granular or that clings to the sides of the vial.
- Roll the vial gently between your palms to obtain a uniform mixture; don't shake it.
- Be aware that Toujeo contains 3 times as much insulin (300 units/ml) in 1 ml as standard insulin (100 units/ml) and is not for use in children. Toujeo Max SoloStar holds 900 units of insulin glargine—more than any other long-acting insulin pen in the United States—and provides up to 160 units/ml in a single injection and allows for 2-unit increment adjustment. In comparison, Toujeo Solo Star pen contains 450 units of insulin glargine with a maximum dose of 80 units per injection, and dosage must be adjusted in 1-unit increments.
- Administer by the SubQ route only. Inject once daily at any time of day but keep time consistent.
- Assess patient taking insulin concurrently with a thiazolidinedione for signs and symptoms of heart failure. If heart failure develops, provide supportive care, as ordered, and expect the thiazolidinedione to be discontinued or dosage reduced.
- Do not repeatedly inject insulin into areas of lipodystrophy or localized cutaneous amyloidosis because hyperglycemia may occur; and a sudden change in the injection site to an unaffected area may cause hypoglycemia.

(continues)

Parenteral Insulin Preparations *(continued)*

CATEGORY, SPECIES, AND TRADE NAMES	KEY NURSING CONSIDERATIONS

Combination insulins

Onset: 30 min   **Peak:** 1–12 hr   **Duration:** 18–24 hr

Human
Intermediate-acting/rapid acting
- Humalog Mix 25 (CAN)
- Humalog Mix 50 (CAN)
- Humalog Mix 75/25
- Humalog Mix 50/50
- NovoLog Mix 50/50
- NovoLog Mix 70/30

Intermediate-acting/ short-acting
- Humulin 30/70 (CAN)
- Humulin 70/30
- Novolin 70/30
- Novolin ge 30/70 (CAN)
- Novolin ge 40/60 (CAN)
- Novolin ge 50/50 (CAN)
- NovoMix 30 (CAN)
- ReliOn Novolin 70/30

Ultra-long-acting/rapid-acting
- Ryzodeg 70/30

- Don't use combination insulin if it contains precipitate that is clumped or granular.
- Know that Ryzodeg 70/30 is now approved for use in children age 1 year and over.
- Roll the vial gently between your palms to mix; don't shake it. Also gently turn the prefilled syringe up and down several times before using to achieve a uniform mixture.
- Administer combination insulin by the SubQ route only, 30 minutes before a meal.
- Be aware that Canadian and American products contain the same insulin ratio but express it differently. For example, the Canadian Humulin 30/70 and the American Humulin 70/30 both contain 30 units of a short-acting insulin and 70 units of an intermediate-acting insulin. Canadian products list the short-acting insulin first; American products list it second.
- Know that Ryzodeg 70/30 is composed of 70% long-acting insulin and 30% rapid-acting insulin.
- Assess patient taking insulin concurrently with a thiazolidinedione for signs and symptoms of heart failure. If heart failure develops, provide supportive care, as ordered, and expect the thiazolidinedione to be discontinued or dosage reduced.
- Do not repeatedly inject insulin into areas of lipodystrophy or localized cutaneous amyloidosis because hyperglycemia may occur; and a sudden change in the injection site to an unaffected area may cause hypoglycemia.

Combination insulins and glucagon-like peptide-1 receptor agonists

Onset: 4–6 hr   **Peak:** 8–20 hr   **Duration:** 24–28 hr

Long-acting insulin/GLP-1 receptor agonist
- Xultophy 100/3.6 (insulin degludec/liraglutide)
- Soliqua 100/33 (insulin glargine/ lixisenatide)

- Know that onset, peak, and duration are determined by the insulin contained in the combination.
- Expect the same adverse reactions that occur with the individual drugs making up the combination product.
- Monitor for hypoglycemia that may become life- threatening, especially with lifestyle or medication changes.
- Monitor renal function in patients with renal impairment or severe GI adverse reactions, as acute kidney injury can occur.
- Evaluate patient's serum potassium level as ordered, because severe hypokalemia has occurred.
- Assess patient concurrently taking a thiazolidinedione for signs and symptoms of heart failure. If heart failure develops, provide supportive care, as ordered, and expect dosage to be reduced or drug discontinued.
- Monitor patient for signs and symptoms of pancreatitis.
- Do not repeatedly inject insulin into areas of lipodystrophy or localized cutaneous amyloidosis because hyperglycemia may occur; and a sudden change in the injection site to an unaffected area may cause hypoglycemia.

Oral Allergen Extracts

Prevention of allergy symptoms in patients diagnosed with an allergy has historically required an extended period of desensitization through the administration of injections given in a healthcare setting. Many patients do not have the time or resources required to undergo such a rigorous desensitization process. A new form of treatment using a sublingual route that the patient can self-administer (after the first dose) is now available for certain types of allergens as summarized in the following chart.

GENERIC AND TRADE NAMES	INDICATIONS	USUAL ADULT DOSAGES	NURSING CONSIDERATIONS FOR ALLERGEN EXTRACTS
grass pollen Grastek	To treat grass pollen–induced allergic rhinitis	2800 Bioequivalent Allergy Unit (1 tablet) sublingual once daily	▪ Know that allergen extracts are contraindicated in patients with severe, unstable asthma; in patients with a history of any severe systemic allergic reaction, severe local reaction after taking any sublingual allergen immunotherapy, or eosinophilic esophagitis; or in patients with a hypersensitivity to any of the inactive ingredients (gelatin, mannitol, or sodium hydroxide).
mixed pollens allergen extract Oralair	To treat grass pollen–induced allergic rhinitis	300 Index of Reactivity (1 tablet) sublingual once daily	▪ Monitor patient closely for allergic reactions that could become severe and life-threatening, such as anaphylaxis and severe laryngopharyngeal constriction.
ragweed extract Ragwitek	To treat short-term ragweed pollen–induced allergic rhinitis with or without conjunctivitis	12 AMB a 1-Unit (1 tablet) sublingual once daily	▪ First dose must be administered in a healthcare setting and patient observed for at least 30 minutes after administration for signs and symptoms of an allergic reaction.

Less Commonly Used Drugs

A
acarbose   Glucobay (CAN), Precose

Indications and Dosages
* As adjunct to diet and exercise to control blood glucose level in type 2 diabetes mellitus

TABLETS

Adults. *Initial:* 25 mg three times daily with first bite of each meal, increased at 4- to 8-wk intervals, as needed. *Maintenance:* 50 mg to 100 mg three times daily. *Maximum:* 50 mg three times daily for patients weighing 60 kg (132 lb) or less; 100 mg three times daily for patients weighing more than 60 kg.

±DOSAGE ADJUSTMENT For patients at increased risk for gastrointestinal adverse effects, initial dosage started at 25 mg once daily with frequency increased gradually until 25 mg three times daily is reached.

aclidinium bromide   Tudorza Pressair

Indications and Dosages
* To provide long-term maintenance treatment of bronchospasm associated with chronic obstructive pulmonary disease (COPD), including chronic bronchitis and emphysema

INHALATION AEROSOL

Adults. 1 inhalation (400 mcg) twice daily.

alfuzosin hydrochloride   Uroxatral, Xatral (CAN)

Indications and Dosages
* To treat signs and symptoms of benign prostatic hyperplasia

E.R. TABLETS

Adults. 10 mg daily taken with same meal each day.

alirocumab   Praluent

Indications and Dosages
* To reduce risk of myocardial infarction, stroke, and unstable angina requiring hospitalization in patients with established cardiovascular disease; as adjunct to diet alone or in combination with other lipid-lowering therapies to treat primary hyperlipidemia (including heterozygous familial hypercholesterolemia) in patients who require additional lowering of LDL-C

SUBCUTANEOUS INJECTION

Adults. *Initial:* 75 mg once every 2 wk, increased to 150 mg once every 2 wk, as needed. Alternatively, 300 mg once every 4 wk. *Maximum:* 150 mg once every 2 wk or 300 mg once every 4 wk

* As adjunct to other LDL-C lowering therapies to treat homozygous familial hypercholesterolemia to reduce LDL-C; to treat heterozygous familial hypercholesterolemia in patients undergoing apheresis

SUBCUTANEOUS INJECTION

Adults. 150 mg every 2 wk.

±DOSAGE ADJUSTMENT For patient receiving 300 mg every 4 weeks whose LDL-C reduction is inadequate, dosage split with 150 mg given once every 2 wk.

alosetron hydrochloride   Lotronex

Indications and Dosages
* To treat women with severe diarrhea-predominant irritable bowel syndrome (IBS) who have chronic IBS symptoms (usually lasting 6 months or longer) with no gastrointestinal tract anatomic or biochemical abnormalities present and who haven't responded to conventional therapy

TABLETS

Adults. *Initial:* 0.5 mg twice a day for 4 wk, then increased up to 1 mg twice daily, if needed.

±DOSAGE ADJUSTMENT For patient who develops constipation with initial dosage, drug discontinued until constipation is resolved and then restarted at 0.5 mg once a day.

alvimopan   Entereg

Indications and Dosages
* To accelerate GI recovery in hospitalized patients after partial large- or small-bowel resection with primary anastomosis

CAPSULES

Adults. *Initial:* 12 mg 30 min to 5 hr before surgery, followed by 12 mg twice daily, starting the day after surgery for up to 7 days or until discharge. *Maximum:* 24 mg/day with a maximum of 15 doses total.

anakinra   Kineret

Indications and Dosages
* To reduce signs and symptoms and slow structural damage in moderate to severe active rheumatoid arthritis in patients who have not responded to disease-modifying antirheumatics

SUBCUTANEOUS INJECTION

Adults. 100 mg daily.

* *To treat neonatal-onset multisystem inflammatory disease (NOMID) in patients with cryopyrin-associated periodic syndrome (CAPS)*

SUBCUTANEOUS INJECTION

Children. *Initial:* 1 to 2 mg/kg daily or dosage split into twice-daily administration followed by dosage adjustments in 0.5 to 1.0 mg/kg increments, as needed. *Maximum:* 8 mg/kg daily

±DOSAGE ADJUSTMENT Interval reduced to every other day in severe renal insufficiency or end-stage renal disease (creatinine clearance less than 30 ml/min).

apomorphine hydrochloride   Apokyn

≣ **Indications and Dosages**

* *To treat hypomobility "off" episodes (end-of-dose wearing-off and unpredictable on/off episodes) in advanced Parkinson's disease as acute, intermittent treatment*

SUBCUTANEOUS INJECTION

Adults. *Initial when patient is in an "off" state:* 0.2 ml (2 mg) as a test dose. If tolerated, a second 0.2-ml (2-mg) dose given at least 2 hr after test dose and adjusted as needed in 0.1-ml (1-mg) increments every few days. *Maximum:* 0.6 ml (6 mg) as a single dose, 2 ml (20 mg) total daily dose, and no more than 5 doses per day.

±DOSAGE ADJUSTMENT For patients who tolerate 0.2 ml (2 mg) but who do not respond adequately, a 0.4-ml (4-mg) dose may be given under medical supervision, with standing and supine blood pressure checked every 20 min for 1 hr at the next observed "off" period, as long as it is at least 2 hr after the initial 0.2-ml (2-mg) test dose. If tolerated, a dose 0.1 ml (1 mg) lower may be given as needed and increased in 0.1-ml (1-mg) increments every few days as needed to a maximum dose of 0.6 ml (6 mg). If patient doesn't tolerate a 0.4-ml (4-mg) test dose, a 0.3-ml (3-mg) test dose may be given under medical supervision, with standing and supine blood pressure checked every 20 min for 1 hr at the next observed "off" period, as long as it is at least 2 hr after the initial 0.4-ml (4-mg) test dose. If tolerated, a 0.2-ml (2-mg) dose can be started as needed and increased to no more than 0.3 ml (3 mg)

if needed after a few days. For patients with mild to moderate renal impairment, the initial dose should be reduced to 0.1 ml (1 mg).

arformoterol   Brovana

≣ **Indications and Dosages**

* *To provide maintenance treatment of bronchoconstriction in patients with COPD, including chronic bronchitis and emphysema*

INHALATION SOLUTION

Adults. 15 mcg (contents of one 2-ml vial) twice daily (morning and evening) via nebulization. *Maximum:* 30 mcg daily.

auranofin   Ridaura

≣ **Indications and Dosages**

* *To treat active rheumatoid arthritis in patients who are intolerant to or unresponsive to nonsteroidal anti-inflammatory drugs (NSAIDs)*

Adults. *Initial:* 6 mg daily or 3 mg twice daily, increased after 6 mo to 3 mg three times daily, if needed and tolerated.

azilsartan medoxomil   Edarbi

≣ **Indications and Dosages**

* *To manage hypertension, alone or with other antihypertensives*

TABLETS

Adults. 80 mg once daily.

±DOSAGE ADJUSTMENT For patients who are receiving high doses of diuretics, initial dosage is decreased to 40 mg once daily.

B

bromocriptine mesylate   Alti-Bromocriptine (CAN), Cycloset, Parlodel, Parlodel Snap Tabs

≣ **Indications and Dosages**

* *To treat amenorrhea, galactorrhea, hypogonadism, and infertility from hyperprolactinemia*

CAPSULES, TABLETS (PARLODEL)

Adults and adolescents age 15 and over. *Initial:* 1.25 to 2.5 mg daily. Increased by 2.5 mg every 2 to 7 days as needed. *Maintenance:* 2.5 to 15 mg daily.

Children ages 11 to 15 years with a prolactin-secreting pituitary adenoma. 1.25 to 2.5 mg daily. Increased as needed and tolerated. *Maintenance:* 2.5 to 10 mg daily.

* *To treat Parkinson's disease*

CAPSULES, TABLETS (PARLODEL)

Adults. *Initial:* 1.25 mg twice daily. Increased by 2.5 mg every 14 to 28 days, as needed. *Maximum:* 100 mg daily.

＊ *To treat acromegaly*

CAPSULES, TABLETS (PARLODEL)

Adults and children age 15 and over. *Initial:* 1.25 to 2.5 mg for 3 days. Then increased by 1.25 to 2.5 mg every 3 to 7 days, if needed. *Maintenance:* Usually 20 to 30 mg daily. *Maximum:* 100 mg daily.

＊ *To control blood glucose level in type 2 diabetes mellitus, with diet and exercise*

TABLETS (CYCLOSET)

Adults. *Initial:* 0.8 mg once daily. Increased weekly in increments of 0.8 mg, as needed. *Maximum:* 4.8 mg daily.

±DOSAGE ADJUSTMENT For patients taking Cycloset and a moderate CYP3A4 inhibitor such as erythromycin, dosage not to exceed 1.6 mg once daily.

C

cefadroxil

☰ Indications and Dosages

＊ *To treat UTI caused by* Escherichia coli, Klebsiella *species, or* Proteus mirabilis

CAPSULES, TABLETS

Adults. For uncomplicated lower UTI, 1 to 2 g once daily or in divided doses every 12 hr. For all other UTIs, 2 g daily in divided doses every 12 hr.

ORAL SUSPENSION

Adults. For uncomplicated lower UTI, 1 to 2 g once daily or in divided doses every 12 hr. For all other UTIs, 2 g daily in divided doses every 12 hr.

Children. 30 mg/kg daily in divided doses every 12 hr. *Maximum:* Adult dosage.

＊ *To treat skin and soft-tissue infections caused by staphylococci or streptococci*

CAPSULES, TABLETS

Adults. 1 g daily or 500 mg every 12 hr.

ORAL SUSPENSION

Adults. 1 g daily or 500 mg every 12 hr.

Children. 30 mg/kg daily in divided doses every 12 hr. *Maximum:* Adult dosage.

＊ *To treat pharyngitis and tonsillitis caused by group A beta-hemolytic streptococci*

CAPSULES, TABLETS

Adults. 1 g daily or 500 mg twice daily for 10 days.

ORAL SUSPENSION

Adults. 1 g daily or 500 mg twice daily for 10 days.

Children. 30 mg/kg daily as a single dose or in equally divided doses every 12 hr for 10 days. *Maximum:* 1 g daily or 500 mg twice daily for 10 days.

±DOSAGE ADJUSTMENT For adult patients with renal impairment, initial dose of 1 g; then maintenance of 0.5 g every 12 hr if creatinine clearance is 25 to 50 ml/min; 0.5 g every 24 hr if creatinine clearance is 10 to 25 ml/min; and every 36 hr if creatinine clearance is 0 to 10 ml/min.

cevimeline hydrochloride   Evoxac

☰ Indications and Dosages

＊ *To treat dry mouth associated with Sjögren's syndrome*

CAPSULES

Adults. 30 mg three times daily. *Maximum:* 90 mg daily.

D

dantrolene sodium   Dantrium, Dantrium Intravenous, Revonto, Ryanodex

☰ Indications and Dosages

＊ *To treat chronic spastic conditions caused by severe chronic disorders, such as cerebral palsy, multiple sclerosis, spinal cord injury, and stroke*

CAPSULES

Adults. *Initial:* 25 mg once daily for 7 days. Then dosage increased to 25 mg three times a day for 7 days followed by 50 mg three times a day for 7 days, followed by 100 mg three times a day, if needed. *Maximum:* 400 mg daily.

Children. *Initial:* 0.5 mg/kg once daily for 7 days. Then dosage increased to 0.5 mg/kg three times daily for 7 days followed by 1 mg/kg three times a day for 7 days, followed by 2 mg/kg three times a day, if needed. *Maximum:* 100 mg four times daily.

＊ *To manage preoperatively malignant hyperthermia-susceptible surgical patients*

CAPSULES

Adults and children. 4 to 8 mg/kg daily in divided doses three times daily or four times daily 1 or 2 days before surgery, with last dose given 3 to 4 hr before surgery.

I.V. INFUSION (DANTRIUM INTRAVENOUS, REVONTO)

Adults and children. *Initial:* 2.5 mg/kg 60 to 75 min before anesthesia and infused over

1 hr. Additional individualized doses given as needed during surgery.

I.V. INJECTION (RYANODEX)

Adults and children. 2.5 mg/kg about 75 min before anesthesia and injected over 1 min. Additional individualized doses given as needed during surgery.

* *To treat malignant hyperthermic crisis*

I.V. INJECTION (DANTRIUM INTRAVENOUS, REVONTO, RYANODEX)

Adults and children. *Initial:* 1 mg/kg by rapid bolus; repeated, as needed, until symptoms subside or cumulative dose of 10 mg/kg has been reached and if symptoms reappear.

* *To treat postmalignant hyperthermic crisis*

CAPSULES

Adults and children. 4 to 8 mg/kg daily in divided doses four times daily for 1 to 3 days.

I.V. INFUSION (REVONTO)

Adults and children. *Initial:* Individualized dosage beginning with 1 mg/kg or more as needed if oral therapy can't be used.

---

darunavir ethanolate   Prezista

≣ Indications and Dosages

* *As adjunct to treat human immunodeficiency virus (HIV) infection*

ORAL SUSPENSION, TABLETS

Adults who are treatment-naïve or who are treatment-experienced with no darunavir-resistance-associated substitutions. 800 mg once daily with ritonavir 100 mg once daily with food.

Adults who are treatment-experienced with at least one darunavir-resistance-associated substitution, adults with no baseline resistance information, and pregnant women. 600 mg twice daily with ritonavir 100 mg twice daily with food.

Children ages 3 to 17 weighing 40 kg (88 lb) or more who are treatment-naïve or who are treatment-experienced with no darunavir-resistance-associated substitutions. 800 mg once daily with ritonavir 100 mg once daily with food.

Children ages 3 to 17 weighing 40 kg (88 lb) or more who are treatment-experienced with at least one darunavir resistance-associated substitution. 600 mg twice daily with ritonavir 100 mg twice daily with food.

Children ages 3 to 17 weighing 30 kg (66 lb) to less than 40 kg (88 lb) who are treatment-naïve or who are treatment-experienced with no darunavir-resistance-associated substitutions. 675 mg once daily with ritonavir 100 mg once daily with food.

Children ages 3 to 17 weighing 30 kg (66 lb) to less than 40 kg (88 lb) who are treatment-experienced with at least one darunavir-resistance-associated substitution. 450 mg twice daily with ritonavir 60 mg twice daily with food.

Children ages 3 to 17 weighing 15 kg (33 lb) to less than 30 kg (66 lb) who are treatment-naïve or who are treatment-experienced with no darunavir-resistance-associated substitutions. 600 mg once daily with ritonavir 100 mg once daily with food.

Children ages 3 to 17 weighing 15 kg (33 lb) to less than 30 kg (66 lb) who are treatment-experienced with at least one darunavir-resistance-associated substitution. 375 mg twice daily with ritonavir 48 mg twice daily with food.

Children age 3 and over weighing at least 10 kg (22 lb) but less than 15 kg (33 lb) who are treatment-naïve or who are treatment-experienced with no darunavir resistance-associated substitutions. 35 mg/kg once daily with ritonavir 7 mg/kg once daily with food.

Children age 3 and over weighing at least 10 kg (22 lb) but less than 15 kg (33 lb) who are treatment-experienced with at least one darunavir-resistance-associated substitution. 20 mg/kg twice daily with ritonavir 3 mg/kg twice daily with food.

---

diflunisal

≣ Indications and Dosages

* *To relieve mild to moderate pain*

TABLETS

Adults. 1 g followed by 0.5 g every 8 to 12 hr. Alternatively, 500 mg followed by 250 mg every 8 to 12 hr. *Maximum:* 1.5 g daily.

* *To reduce inflammation in osteoarthritis or rheumatoid arthritis*

TABLETS

Adults. 0.5 to 1 g daily in divided doses twice daily. *Maximum:* 1.5 g daily.

± **DOSAGE ADJUSTMENT** Dosage reduced for elderly patients.

dimethyl fumarate   Tecfidera

☰ Indications and Dosages

* *To treat relapsing forms of multiple sclerosis, including active secondary progressive disease, clinically isolated syndrome, and relapsing-remitting disease*

DELAYED-RELEASE CAPSULES

Adults. *Initial:* 120 mg twice daily for 7 days; then increased to 240 mg twice daily. *Maintenance:* 240 mg twice daily.

±**DOSAGE ADJUSTMENT** Dosage decreased to 120 mg twice daily for up to 4 weeks for patients who cannot initially tolerate maintenance dose.

dolutegravir sodium   Tivicay, Tivicay PD

☰ Indications and Dosages

* As adjunct to treat human immunodeficiency virus type 1 (HIV-1) in combination with other antiretroviral agents; as adjunct with rilpivirine as a complete regimen for the treatment of HIV-1 infection in adults to replace the current antiretroviral regimen in those who are virologically suppressed (HIV-RNA less than 50 copies/ml) on a stable antiretroviral regimen for at least 6 months with no history of treatment failure or known substitutions associated with resistance to either antiretroviral agent

TABLETS (TIVICAY)

Adults who are treatment-naïve, treatment-experienced INSTI-naïve, or virologically suppressed and switching to dolutegravir plus rilpivirine. 50 mg once daily.

Adults who are treatment-naïve or treatment-experienced INSTI-naïve who are currently receiving certain CYP3A or UGTIA inducers such as carbamazepine, efavirenz, fosamprenavir/ritonavir, rifampin, or tipranavir/ritonavir; adults who are INSTI-experienced who have certain INSTI-associated resistance substitutions or clinically suspected INSTI resistance. 50 mg twice daily.

ORAL SUSPENSION (TIVICAY PD)

Children who are treatment-naïve or treatment-experienced INSTI-naïve and weigh at least 20 kg (44 lb) or more. 50 mg once daily.

Children who are treatment-naïve or treatment-experienced INSTI-naïve and weigh at least 14 kg (30.8 lb) but less than 20 kg (44 lb). 40 mg once daily.

Children 4 weeks and older who are treatment-naïve or treatment-experienced INSTI-naïve and weigh 20 kg (44 lb) or greater. 30 mg once daily.

Children 4 weeks and older who are treatment-naïve or treatment-experienced INSTI-naïve and weigh 14 kg (30.8 lb) to less than 20 kg (44 lb). 25 mg once daily.

Children 4 weeks and older who are treatment-naïve or treatment-experienced INSTI-naïve and weigh 10 kg (22 lb) to less than 14 kg (30.8 lb). 20 mg once daily.

Children 4 weeks and older who are treatment-naïve or treatment-experienced INSTI-naïve and weigh 6 kg (13.2 lb) to less than 10 kg (22 lb). 15 mg once daily.

Children 4 weeks and older who are treatment-naïve or treatment-experienced INSTI-naïve and weigh 3 kg (6.6 lb) to less than 6 kg (13.2 lb). 5 mg once daily.

±**DOSAGE ADJUSTMENT** For children: Concurrent therapy with certain CYP3A or UGTIA inducers such as carbamazepine, efavirenz, fosamprenavir/ritonavir, rifampin, or tipranavir/ritonavir, dosage frequency increased to twice daily regardless of weight.

dupilumab   Dupixent

☰ Indications and Dosages

* *To treat moderate to severe atopic dermatitis when disease is not adequately controlled with topical prescription therapies or when those therapies are not advisable*

SUBCUTANEOUS INJECTION

Adults and children age 6 to 17 years of age weighing 60 kg (132 lb) or more. *Initial:* 600 mg (given as two 300-mg injections), followed by 300 mg every other wk.

Children age 6 to 17 years of age weighing 30 kg (66 lb) to less than 60 kg (132 lb). *Initial:* 400 mg (given as two 200-mg injections), followed by 200 mg every other wk.

Children age 6 to 17 years weighing 15 kg (33 lb) to less than 30 kg (66 lb). *Initial:* 600 mg (given as two 300-mg injections), followed by 300 mg every 4 wks.

* *As add-on maintenance treatment of moderate to severe asthma*

SUBCUTANEOUS INJECTION

Adults and children age 12 and over with an eosinophilic phenotype. 400 mg (two 200-mg injections) followed by 200 mg every

2 wk. Alternatively, 600 mg (two 300-mg injections) followed by 300 mg every 2 wk. **Adults and children age 12 and over who are oral corticosteroids-dependent or also have co-morbid moderate to severe atopic dermatitis.** 600 mg (two 300-mg injections) followed by 300 mg every 2 wk. **Children age 6 to 11 years weighing 30 kg (66 lb) or more.** 200 mg every 2 wk. **Children age 6 to 11 years weighing 15 kg (33 lb) to less than 30 kg (66 lb).** 100 mg every 2 wk or 300 mg every 4 wk.

* *As add-on maintenance treatment in patients with inadequately controlled chronic rhinosinusitis with nasal polyposis*

SUBCUTANEOUS INJECTION
Adults. 300 mg every other week.

E

entacapone   Comtan

▤ Indications and Dosages

* *As adjunct to carbidopa and levodopa to treat end-of-dose "wearing-off" in patients with Parkinson's disease*

TABLETS
Adults. 200 mg with each dose of carbidopa and levodopa. *Maximum:* 1,600 mg daily.

eprosartan mesylate   Teveten

▤ Indications and Dosages

* *To control blood pressure in patients with essential hypertension*

TABLETS
Adults. *Initial:* 600 mg daily. *Usual:* 400 mg to 600 mg once daily or in 2 divided doses. *Maximum:* 800 mg once daily or in divided doses twice daily.

± **DOSAGE ADJUSTMENT** For patients with moderate to severe renal impairment, dosage reduced to 600 mg once daily or in divided doses twice daily.

etelcalcetide   Parsabiv

▤ Indications and Dosages

* *To treat secondary hyperparathyroidism in patients with chronic kidney disease on hemodialysis*

I.V. INJECTION
Adults. *Initial:* 5 mg three times a wk at the end of hemodialysis treatment, followed by titration in 2.5- or 5-mg increments no more frequently than every 4 wk, as indicated by an elevation of PTH levels above the recommended target range. *Maintenance:* Highly individualized, ranging from 2.5 mg to 15 mg three times a wk.

± **DOSAGE ADJUSTMENT** For patients with a corrected serum calcium below the lower limit of normal but at or above 7.5 mg/dl and who do not have symptoms of hypocalcemia, dose possibly decreased or temporarily withheld. If drug temporarily withheld, dose restarted at a lower dose when the PTH is within target range and hypocalcemia has been corrected. For patients with a corrected serum calcium below 7.5 mg/dl or patients who have symptoms of hypocalcemia, dose withheld until corrected serum calcium is within normal limits, symptoms of hypocalcemia have been resolved, and predisposing factors for hypocalcemia have been addressed. Dose restarted at a dose 5 mg lower than the last administered dose. If last administered dose was 2.5 mg or 5 mg, dose restarted at 2.5 mg.

etodolac

▤ Indications and Dosages

* *To manage osteoarthritis and rheumatoid arthritis*

CAPSULES, TABLETS
Adults. 300 mg twice daily or three times daily. Alternatively, 400 mg twice daily or 500 mg twice daily. *Maximum:* 1,000 mg daily.

E.R. TABLETS
Adults. 400 to 1,000 mg daily.

* *To manage juvenile rheumatoid arthritis*

E.R. TABLETS
Children ages 6 to 16 weighing greater than 60 kg (132 lb). 1,000 mg once daily.
Children ages 6 to 16 weighing 46 kg (101 lb) to 60 kg (132 lb). 800 mg once daily.
Children ages 6 to 16 weighing 31 kg (68 lb) to 45 kg (99 lb). 600 mg once daily.
Children ages 6 to 16 weighing 20 kg (44 lb) to 30 kg (66 lb). 400 mg once daily.

* *To relieve mild to moderate pain*

CAPSULES, TABLETS
Adults. *Initial:* 400 mg and then 200 to 400 mg every 6 to 8 hr. *Maximum:* 1,000 mg daily.

evolocumab   Repatha

▤ Indications and Dosages

* *Adjunct to diet as monotherapy or in combination with other lipid-lowering therapies to treat primary hyperlipidemia*

including heterozygous familial hypercholesterolemia to reduce low-density lipoprotein cholesterol (LDL-C); to reduce the risk of coronary revascularization, myocardial infarction, or stroke in patients with established cardiovascular disease

SUBCUTANEOUS INJECTION
Adults. 140 mg every 2 wk or 420 mg once a month.

* *As adjunct to diet and other LDL-lowering therapies to treat heterogeneous familial hypercholesterolemia to reduce LDL-C*

SUBCUTANEOUS INJECTION
Children 10 years and older. 140 mg every 2 wk or 420 mg once a month.

* *Adjunct to diet and other LDL-lowering thera-pies to treat homozygous familial hypercholes-terolemia in patients to reduce LDL-C*

SUBCUTANEOUS INJECTION
Adults and children age 10 years and older. 420 mg once a month increased to 420 mg every 2 wk if effectiveness is not achieved in 12 weeks.

F
fenoprofen calcium   Nalfon

≡ Indications and Dosages
* *To manage mild to moderate pain*

CAPSULES
Adults. 200 mg every 4 to 6 hr, as needed.

* *To relieve pain, stiffness, and swelling from osteoarthritis or rheumatoid arthritis*

CAPSULES
Adults. 400 to 600 mg 3 times daily or 4 times daily. *Maximum:* 3,200 mg daily.

ferumoxytol   Feraheme

≡ Indications and Dosages
* *To treat iron deficiency anemia in patients with chronic kidney disease or who are intolerant to oral iron or who have had an unsatisfactory response to oral iron*

I.V. INFUSION
Adults. 510 mg administered over at least 15 min followed by another 510 mg in 3 to 8 days administered over at least 15 min. Dose repeated after 1 or more months, as needed.

G
guanfacine hydrochloride   Intuniv

≡ Indications and Dosages
* *To manage hypertension, alone or with other antihypertensives*

TABLETS
Adults. 1 mg daily at bedtime, increased as needed to 2 mg after 3 to 4 wk. Increased to 3 mg if needed after another 3 to 4 wk. *Maintenance:* 2 or 3 mg daily.

* *To treat attention deficit hyperactivity disorder (ADHD); adjunct therapy with stimulant medications*

E.R. TABLETS (INTUNIV)
Adults and children age 6 and over. *Initial:* 1 mg once daily, increased, as needed, by 1 mg/wk. *Maintenance:* 1 to 4 mg once daily. *Maximum:* 4 mg once daily.

±**DOSAGE ADJUSTMENT** For patients starting guanfacine therapy while currently on a moderate or strong CYP3A4 inhibitor or a moderate or strong CYP3A4 inhibitor is added after starting guanfacine therapy, dosage reduced by half. When a moderate or strong CYP3A4 inhibitor is stopped but guanfacine therapy is not, dosage increased back to recommended level. For patient taking a moderate or strong CYP3A4 inducer when starting guanfacine therapy or a moderate or strong CYP3A4 inducer is added, dosage doubled gradually over 1 to 2 weeks. When a moderate or strong CYP3A4 inducer is stopped but guanfacine therapy is not, dosage decreased to recommended level over 1 to 2 weeks.

I
isoproterenol hydrochloride   Isuprel

≡ Indications and Dosages
* *To manage bronchospasm during anesthesia*

I.V. INJECTION
Adults. 0.01 to 0.02 mg as a diluted solution, repeated as needed.

* *As adjunct to treat cardiogenic shock, congestive heart failure, hypoperfusion states, low cardiac output, and septic shock*

I.V. INFUSION
Adults. 0.5 mcg to 5 mcg/min with infusion rate determined by central venous pressure, heart rate, systemic blood pressure, and urine output.

* *To treat Adams–Stokes attacks, cardiac arrest, or heart block*

I.V. INFUSION
Adults. *Initial:* 0.02 to 0.06 mg followed by 0.01 to 0.02 mg infused at 5 mcg/min.

±**DOSAGE ADJUSTMENT** If time is not of the upmost importance, initial therapy may be given as an I.M. or subcutaneous injection with an adjusted dose.

K
ketoprofen

☰ Indications and Dosages

＊ *To treat symptoms of osteoarthritis or rheumatoid arthritis*

CAPSULES

Adults. *Initial:* 75 mg three times daily or 50 mg four times daily. *Maximum:* 300 mg daily.

E.R. CAPSULES

Adults. *Maintenance:* 200 mg daily.

＊ *To relieve mild to moderate pain; pain associated with dysmenorrhea*

CAPSULES

Adults. *Initial:* 25 to 50 mg every 6 to 8 hr, as needed. May be increased to 75 mg every 6 to 8 hr, as needed. *Maximum:* 300 mg daily.

±**DOSAGE ADJUSTMENT** For debilitated, elderly, and small patients, dosage reduced. For patients with mild renal dysfunction, maximum daily dose reduced to 150 mg daily; for patients with more severe renal impairment (glomerular filtration rate less than 25 ml/min), end-stage renal disease, or liver dysfunction, maximum daily dose reduced to 100 mg.

L
letermovir   Prevymis

☰ Indications and Dosages

＊ *To prevent cytomegalovirus (CMV) infection and disease in CMV seropositive recipients of an allogenic hematopoietic stem cell transplant*

I.V. INFUSION, TABLETS

Adults. 480 mg once daily initiated between day 0 and day 28 posttransplantation and continued through day 100 posttransplantation. Infusion should be administered at a constant rate over 1 hr.

±**DOSAGE ADJUSTMENT** For patients taking concurrent therapy with cyclosporine, dosage deceased to 240 mg once daily. If cyclosporine is discontinued, dosage resumed at 480 mg once daily. If cyclosporine dosing is interrupted due to high cyclosporine levels, no dose adjustment is needed.

liothyronine sodium (L-triiodothyronine, sodium L-triiodothyronine, T₃, thyronine sodium)   Cytomel, Triostat

☰ Indications and Dosages

＊ *To treat primary, secondary, and tertiary hypothyroidism*

TABLETS (CYTOMEL)

Adults. *Initial:* 25 mcg daily and increased by 25 mcg every 1 to 2 wk until response occurs. *Maintenance:* 25 to 75 mcg daily

±**DOSAGE ADJUSTMENT** For elderly patients and patients with underlying cardiac disease, initial dose reduced to 5 mcg once daily and increased in 5-mcg increments every 1 to 2 weeks, as needed.

＊ *To treat acquired or congenital hypothyroidism*

TABLETS (CYTOMEL)

Adults and children. *Initial:* 5 mcg daily. Increased by 5 mcg every 3 to 4 days until desired response occurs. *Maintenance:* Highly individualized.

±**DOSAGE ADJUSTMENT** For pediatric patients at risk for cardiac failure, initial dose may have to be reduced. For pediatric patients at risk for hyperactivity, initial dosage reduced by 75% with increases done in 25% increments of the full replacement dose on a weekly basis until the full recommended replacement dose is reached. For pregnant women, dosage may have to be increased.

＊ *As adjunct to radioiodine therapy and surgery in the management of well-differentiated thyroid cancer*

TABLETS (CYTOMEL)

Adults. Highly individualized but usually higher doses required.

＊ *As a diagnostic test in suppression tests to differentiate suspected mild hyperthyroidism or thyroid gland autonomy*

TABLETS (CYTOMEL)

Adults. 75 to 100 mcg daily for 7 days with radioactive iodine uptake being determined before and after the 7-day administration period.

＊ *To treat myxedema coma or premyxedema coma (severe hypothyroidism)*

I.V. INJECTION (TRIOSTAT)I

Adults. *Initial:* 25 to 50 mcg. Repeated according to patient's response, as needed. Then P.O. therapy is resumed as soon as possible.

±**DOSAGE ADJUSTMENT** When treating myxedema coma in patients with known or suspected cardiovascular disease, initial dose decreased to 10 to 20 mcg.

M

meclofenamate sodium

▤ Indications and Dosages

* *To relieve pain and inflammation in rheumatoid arthritis and osteoarthritis*

CAPSULES

Adults and adolescents over age 14. 200 to 400 mg in divided doses every 6 to 8 hr, as needed.

* *To relieve mild to moderate pain*

CAPSULES

Adults and adolescents over age 14. 50 mg every 4 to 6 hr, as needed. Increased to 100 mg every 4 to 6 hr, as needed.

* *To treat hypermenorrhea and primary dysmenorrhea*

CAPSULES

Adults and adolescents over age 14. 100 mg three times daily for up to 6 days starting with the onset of menstrual flow.

mepolizumab   Nucala

▤ Indications and Dosages

* *Adjunct to maintenance treatment of patients with severe asthma who have an eosinophilic phenotype*

SUBCUTANEOUS INJECTION

Adults and children age 12 and older. 100 mg once every 4 wk.

Children age 6 to 11. 40 mg once every 4 wk.

* *To treat eosinophilic granulomatosis with polyangiitis (EGPA)*

SUBCUTANEOUS INJECTION

Adults. 300 mg once every 4 wk given as 3 separate 100-mg injections.

metaxalone

▤ Indications and Dosages

* *As adjunct to relieve discomfort caused by acute, painful musculoskeletal conditions*

TABLETS

Adults and children over age 12. 800 mg three times daily or four times daily.

misoprostol   Cytotec

▤ Indications and Dosages

* *To reduce the risk of NSAID-induced gastric ulcers*

TABLETS

Adults. 200 mcg four times daily given with food with last dose at bedtime every day.

±**DOSAGE ADJUSTMENT** Dosage reduced to 100 mcg four times daily if patient can't tolerate 200-mcg dose.

moexipril hydrochloride

▤ Indication and Dosages

* *To manage hypertension without diuretic therapy*

TABLETS

Adults. *Initial:* 7.5 mg daily 1 hr before a meal and increased, as needed. *Maintenance:* 7.5 to 30 mg as a single dose or in divided doses twice daily. 1 hr before meals. *Maximum:* 60 mg/day.

* *To manage hypertension with thiazide diuretic therapy*

TABLETS

Adults. *Initial:* 3.75 mg daily 1 hr before a meal. Increased gradually, as ordered, until blood pressure is controlled. *Maintenance:* 7.5 to 30 mg as a single dose or in divided doses twice daily, 1 hr before meals. *Maximum:* 60 mg/day.

±**DOSAGE ADJUSTMENT** For patients with creatinine clearance of 40 ml/min or less, initial dosage reduced to 3.75 mg daily and increased, as ordered, to maximum of 15 mg daily.

N

neostigmine methylsulfate   Bloxiverz, Neostigmine Methylsulfate

▤ Indications and Dosages

* *To reverse nondepolarizing neuromuscular blockade after surgery*

I.V. INJECTION

Adults and children. 0.03 mg/kg (drugs with shorter half-lives) or 0.07 mg/kg (drugs with longer half-lives or need for more rapid recovery) given over at least 1 min with atropine or glycopyrrolate administered prior to or concomitantly. *Maximum:* 0.07 mg/kg or 5 mg, whichever is less.

O

orlistat   Alli, Xenical

* *As adjunct to manage obesity, including weight loss and weight maintenance along with a reduced-calorie diet; to reduce the risk of weight gain*

CAPSULES

Adults and adolescents. 120 mg three times a day with fat-containing meals.

oxacillin sodium

⬛ Indications and Dosages

✳ *To treat mild to moderate infections caused by penicillinase-producing strains of Staphylococcus*

I.V. INFUSION, I.M. OR I.V. INJECTION

Adults. 250 to 500 mg every 4 to 6 hr for mild or moderate infections and 1 g every 4 to 6 hr for severe infections. I.V. infusion rate depends on solution used for dilution and adjusted so that the total dose is administered before the drug loses its stability in the solution used (see manufacturer instructions). I.V. injection given over 10 min.

P
paricalcitol   Zemplar

⬛ Indications and Dosages

✳ *To prevent and treat secondary hyperparathyroidism in patients with chronic stage 3 or 4 renal failure*

CAPSULES

Adults and adolescents age 16 and over whose baseline iPTH level is 500 pg/ml or less. *Initial:* 1 mcg daily or 2 mcg three times weekly with doses separated by at least 1 day. *Maintenance:* Dosage adjusted at 2- to 4-wk intervals based on the intact parathyroid hormone (iPTH) level relative to baseline and serum calcium and phosphorus levels to maintain an iPTH level within target range.

Adults and adolescents age 16 and over whose baseline iPTH level exceeds 500 pg/ml. *Initial:* 2 mcg daily or 4 mcg three times weekly with doses separated by at least 1 day. *Maintenance:* Dosage adjusted at 2- to 4-wk intervals based on the iPTH level relative to baseline and serum calcium and phosphorus levels to maintain an iPTH level within target range.

Children ages 10 to 16. *Initial:* 1 mcg three times weekly with doses separated by at least 1 day. *Maintenance:* Dosage adjusted every 4 wk based on the iPTH level relative to baseline and serum calcium and phosphorus levels to maintain an iPTH level within target range.

✳ *To prevent and treat secondary hyperparathyroidism associated with chronic stage 5 renal failure in patients on hemodialysis or peritoneal dialysis*

CAPSULES

Adults and adolescents age 16 and over. *Initial:* Baseline iPTH (pg/ml) divided by 80 three times weekly with doses separated by at least 1 day. *Maintenance:* Individualized based on most recent iPTH level (pg/ml) divided by 80 and current serum calcium and phosphorus levels to maintain iPTH level within target range.

Children ages 10 to 16. *Initial:* Baseline iPTH (pg/ml) divided by 120 rounding down to nearest whole number. *Maintenance:* Individualized and titrated based on most recent iPTH level and serum calcium and phosphorus levels to maintain an iPTH level within target range.

I.V. INJECTION

Adults. *Initial:* 0.04 to 0.1 mcg/kg (2.8–7 mcg) administered as a bolus no more frequently than every other day at any time during dialysis, with dosage increased by 2 to 4 mcg at 2- to 4-wk intervals, as needed. *Maintenance:* Individualized and titrated based on most recent iPTH level and serum calcium and phosphorus levels to maintain an iPTH level within target range.

Children age 5 years and older with a baseline intact PTH less than 500 pg/ml. *Initial:* 0.04 mcg/kg administered as a bolus three times weekly, no more frequently than every other day, and given at any time during dialysis. *Maintenance:* Individualized and titrated based on most recent iPTH level and serum calcium and phosphorus levels to maintain an iPTH level within target range.

Children age 5 and older with a baseline intact PTH of 500 pg/ml or greater. *Initial:* 0.08 mcg/kg three times a weekly, no more frequently than every other day, and given at any time during dialysis. *Maintenance:* Individualized and titrated based on most recent iPTH level and serum calcium and phosphorus levels to maintain an iPTH level within target range.

patiromer sorbitex calcium   Veltassa

⬛ Indications and Dosages

✳ *To treat hyperkalemia*

ORAL SUSPENSION

Adults. *Initial:* 8.4 g once daily, increased once a week or longer or decreased, as needed, in increments of 8.4 g to reach desired serum potassium concentration. *Maximum:* 25.2 g once daily.

peginesatide   Omontys

≡ Indications and Dosages

* *To treat anemia due to chronic kidney disease in patients on dialysis*

I.V. OR SUBCUTANEOUS INJECTION

Adults not currently treated with another erythropoiesis-stimulating agent (ESA). 0.04 mg/kg once monthly.

Adults converting from epoetin alfa. Based on the weekly dose of epoetin alfa at the time of substitution, first dose given 1 wk after the last epoetin alfa dose was administered and then continued monthly.

Adults converting from darbepoetin alfa. Based on the weekly dose of darbepoetin alfa at the time of substitution, first dose given at the next scheduled dose of darbepoetin alfa in place of it.

±**DOSAGE ADJUSTMENT** For patient experiencing a rapid rise in hemoglobin (more than 1 g/dl in the 2 wk prior to the next dose or more than 2 g/dl in 4 wk), dosage reduced by 25% or more. For the patient whose hemoglobin level is approaching or exceeding 11 g/dl, dosage reduced or drug withheld until hemoglobin levels begin to decrease. If drug was withheld, dosage restarted at a dosage that is 25% less than the previously administered dose. For patient who does not exhibit at least an increase in hemoglobin of more than 1 g/dl after 4 wk of therapy, dosage increased by 25%.

pentazocine lactate   Talwin

≡ Indications and Dosages

* *To relieve pain severe enough to require opioid treatment and for which alternative treatment options such as nonopioid analgesics or opioid combination products are inadequate or not tolerated; to use as preanesthetic or preoperative sedation as a supplement to surgical anesthesia*

I.M., I.V., OR SUBCUTANEOUS INJECTION

Adults. *Initial:* 30 mg every 3 to 4 hr, as needed. *Maximum:* 30 mg/single dose I.V., 60 mg/single dose I.M. or subcutaneously, or 360 mg/24 hr for all parenteral forms. I.V. injection given slowly.

* *To relieve obstetric pain*

I.V. INJECTION

Adults. 20 mg given slowly when contractions become regular; repeated two or three times every 2 to 3 hr, as needed.

I.M. INJECTION

Adults. 30 mg as a single dose.

* *To provide premedication for sedation*

I.M. INJECTION

Children age 1 and older. 0.5 mg/kg as a single dose.

pentosan polysulfate sodium   Elmiron

≡ Indications and Dosages

* *To relieve bladder discomfort or pain caused by interstitial cystitis*

CAPSULES

Adults. 100 mg three times a day for up to 3 mo, possibly followed by another 3 mo if no improvement and no adverse reactions.

pentoxifylline

≡ Indications and Dosages

* *To treat intermittent claudication in patients with peripheral vascular disease*

E.R. TABLETS

Adults. 400 mg three times a day with meals for 8 weeks.

±**DOSAGE ADJUSTMENT** For patients who have severe renal impairment (creatinine clearance below 30 ml/min), dosage reduced to 400 mg once a day. For patients who experience adverse GI or CNS reactions, dosage may be reduced to 400 mg twice daily.

peramivir   Rapivab

≡ Indications and Dosages

* *To treat acute uncomplicated influenza in patients who have been symptomatic for no more than 2 days*

I.V. INFUSION

Adults and adolescents. 600 mg as a single dose given over 15 to 30 min.

Children ages 2 to 13 years. 12 mg/kg as a single dose given over 15 to 30 min. *Maximum:* 600 mg as a single dose.

±**DOSAGE ADJUSTMENT** For adult patients with a creatinine clearance between 30 and 49 ml/min, dosage reduced to 200 mg. For adult patients with a creatinine clearance between 10 and 29 ml/min, dosage reduced to 100 mg. For children with a creatinine clearance between 30 and 49 mg/kg, dosage reduced to 4 mg/kg. For children with a creatinine clearance between 10 and 29 ml/min, dosage reduced to 2 mg/kg.

perampanel Fycompa

≣ Indications and Dosages

* *Adjunct therapy for treatment of primary generalized tonic–clonic seizures in patients with epilepsy*

ORAL SUSPENSION, TABLETS

Adults and children age 12 and over.
Initial: 2 mg once daily at bedtime, then increased in 2-mg increments weekly, as needed. *Maintenance:* 8 to 12 mg once daily at bedtime. *Maximum:* 12 mg daily at bedtime.

* *To treat partial-onset seizures as adjunctive or monotherapy*

ORAL SUSPENSION, TABLETS

Adults and children age 4 and over. *Initial:* 2 mg once daily at bedtime, then increased in increments of 2 mg weekly, as needed. *Maintenance:* 8 to 12 mg.

±**DOSAGE ADJUSTMENT** For elderly patients, dosage titration done every 2 wk. For patients with mild to moderate hepatic impairment, dosage increased every 2 wk in 2-mg increments until target dose is achieved. For patients with mild hepatic impairment, maximum daily dosage is 6 mg daily at bedtime; for patients with moderate hepatic impairment, maximum daily dosage is 4 mg daily at bedtime. For patients with moderate renal impairment, a slower titration may be considered. For patients taking moderate or strong CYP3A4 enzyme inducers, including enzyme-inducing AEDs such as carbamazepine, oxcarbazepine, or phenytoin, initial dosage increased to 4 mg once daily.

perindopril erbumine Coversyl (CAN), Coversyl Plus (CAN)

≣ Indications and Dosages

* *To manage hypertension*

TABLETS

Adults. *Initial:* 4 mg once daily or in divided doses twice daily, increased as prescribed until blood pressure is controlled or maximum dosage is reached. *Usual:* 4 to 8 mg daily. *Maximum:* 16 mg daily.

* *To reduce risk of cardiovascular death or nonfatal MI in patients with stable coronary artery disease*

TABLETS

Adults. *Initial:* 4 mg once daily for 2 wk; then increased as tolerated to 8 mg once daily. *Maintenance:* 8 mg daily.

±**DOSAGE ADJUSTMENT** For patient with renal impairment with a creatinine clearance greater than 30 ml/min, initial dosage reduced to 2 mg daily and dosage should not exceed 8 mg daily.

perphenazine

≣ Indications and Dosages

* *To treat psychotic disorders, such as schizophrenia*

TABLETS

Hospitalized adults and adolescents.
8 to 16 mg twice daily to four times a day, adjusted as needed and tolerated. *Maximum:* 64 mg daily.

Nonhospitalized adults and adolescents.
4 to 8 mg three times daily, adjusted as needed and tolerated.

* *To treat severe nausea and vomiting*

TABLETS

Adults and adolescents. 8 to 16 mg daily in divided doses, decreased as appropriate. *Maximum:* 24 mg daily.

±**DOSAGE ADJUSTMENT** Initial dose possibly reduced and gradually increased for debilitated, elderly, or emaciated patients.

phentolamine mesylate

≣ Indications and Dosages

* *To diagnose pheochromocytoma*

I.V. INJECTION

Adults. 5 mg as a single dose injected rapidly.
Children. 1 mg as a single dose injected rapidly.

I.M. INJECTION

Adults. 5 mg as a single injection.
Children. 3 mg as a single injection.

* *To manage hypertension before or during pheochromocytoma surgery*

I.V. OR I.M. INJECTION

Adults. 5 mg 1 to 2 hr before surgery, repeated as needed. During surgery, 5 mg I.V., as needed.
Children. 1 mg 1 to 2 hr before surgery, repeated as needed. During surgery, 1 mg I.V., as needed.

* *To prevent dermal necrosis or sloughing after extravasation of I.V. norepinephrine*

I.V. INJECTION

Adults. 10 mg/L of I.V. fluid that contains norepinephrine at rate determined by patient response.

✳ *To treat dermal necrosis or sloughing after extravasation of I.V. norepinephrine*

INTRADERMAL INJECTION

Adults. 5 to 10 mg in 10 ml of normal saline solution infiltrated in affected area within 12 hr of extravasation.

pindolol   SynPindol (CAN)

▤ Indications and Dosages

✳ *To manage hypertension*

TABLETS

Adults. *Initial:* 5 mg twice daily, increased by 10 mg daily every 3 to 4 wk, as prescribed. *Maximum:* 60 mg daily (U.S.), 45 mg daily (Canada).

potassium iodide (KI, SSKI)   ThyroSafe, ThyroShield

▤ Indications and Dosages

✳ *To prevent radioactive iodine from getting into the thyroid gland during a nuclear radiation emergency*

ORAL SOLUTION, TABLETS

Adults and children over age 12 to 18 weighing at least 68 kg (150 lb). 130 mg once daily for as long as directed by public health officials.

Children over age 12 to 18 weighing at least 68 kg (150 lb). 130 mg once daily for as long as directed by public health officials.

Children age 3 to 12 and children over age 12 to 18 weighing less than 68 kg (150 lb). 65 mg once daily for as long as directed by public health officials.

Children over age 1 month to 3 years. 32.5 mg once daily for as long as directed by public health officials.

Infants at birth to 1 month. 16.25 mg for as long as directed by public health officials.

pralidoxime chloride (2-PAM chloride, 2-pyridine   Protopam Chloride)

▤ Indications and Dosages

✳ *As adjunct to reverse organophosphate pesticide toxicity*

I.V. INFUSION

Adults. *Initial:* 1 to 2 g in 100-ml 0.9% Sodium Chloride Injection infused over 15 to 30 min until muscarinic signs and symptoms disappear; may be repeated in 1 hr and then every 10 to 12 hr if muscle weakness persists.

Children. *Initial:* 20 to 50 mg/kg (not to exceed 2,000 mg/dose) in 100-ml 0.9% Sodium Chloride Injection infused over 15 to 30 min followed by a continuous infusion of 10 to 20 mg/kg/hr. Alternatively, an initial intermittent infusion of 20 to 50 mg/kg (not to exceed 2,000 mg/dose) given over 15 to 30 min. Dosage may be repeated in 1 hr and then every 10 to 12 hr if muscle weakness persists.

±**DOSAGE ADJUSTMENT** For patient with pulmonary edema, dosage given slowly (over not less than 5 min) as a 50 mg/ml solution in water.

I.M. INJECTION

Adults and children weighing 40 kg or more. *For mild symptoms:* 600 mg (2 ml). May repeat dose after 15 min and again after an additional 15 min, as needed. If at any time after the first dose patient develops severe symptoms, two additional 600-mg doses may be given in rapid succession for a total cumulative dose of 1,800 mg. *For severe symptoms:* 600 mg (2 ml) administered three times in rapid succession for a total dose of 1,800 mg. *For persistent symptoms:* After three injections of 600 mg each have been given, series may be repeated beginning about 1 hr after administration of the last injection.

Children weighing less than 40 kg. *For mild symptoms:* 15 mg/kg. May repeat dose after 15 min and again after an additional 15 min, as needed. If at any time after the first dose patient develops severe symptoms, two additional 15-mg/kg doses may be given in rapid succession for a total cumulative dose of 45 mg/kg. *For severe symptoms:* 15 mg/kg administered three times in rapid succession for a total dose of 45 mg/kg. *For persistent symptoms:* After three injections of 15 mg/kg each have been given, series may be repeated beginning about 1 hr after administration of the last injection.

✳ *To treat anticholinesterase overdose secondary to myasthenic drugs (including ambenonium, neostigmine, and pyridostigmine)*

I.V. INJECTION

Adults. *Initial:* 1 to 2 g, followed by 250 mg every 5 min, as indicated.

✳ *To treat exposure to nerve agents*

I.V. INJECTION

Adults. *Initial:* 1 atropine-containing autoinjector followed by 1 pralidoxime-containing autoinjector as soon as atropine's effects are evident; both injections repeated every 15 min for two additional doses if nerve agent symptoms persist.

±**DOSAGE ADJUSTMENT** Dosage reduced for patients with renal insufficiency.

primidone   Sertan (CAN)

prasterone   Intrarosa

≡ **Indications and Dosages**

٭ *To treat moderate to severe dyspareunia, a symptom of vaginal and vulvar atrophy, due to menopause*

VAGINAL INSERTS

Adult postmenopausal women. 6.5 mg (1 insert) daily at bedtime.

primidone   Sertan (CAN)

≡ **Indications and Dosages**

٭ *To control focal, grand mal, or psychomotor epileptic seizures, as monotherapy or as adjunctive therapy*

CHEWABLE TABLETS, ORAL SUSPENSION, TABLETS

Adults and children age 8 and over who have received no previous treatment. *Initial:* 100 or 125 mg at bedtime for first 3 days; then increased to 100 or 125 mg twice daily for next 3 days, followed by 100 or 125 mg three times a day for next 3 days. On 10th day, begin maintenance dosage as prescribed. *Maintenance:* 250 mg three times a day or four times a day, adjusted as needed. *Maximum:* 2 g daily.

Adults and children age 8 and over who already receive other anticonvulsants. *Initial:* 100 or 125 mg at bedtime and gradually increased to maintenance level as the other drug is gradually decreased. The transition period should be longer than 2 wk.

Children up to age 8. *Initial:* 50 mg at bedtime for first 3 days; then increased to 50 mg twice daily for next 3 days, followed by increase to 100 mg twice daily for next 3 days. On 10th day, begin maintenance dosage. *Maintenance:* 125 to 250 mg three times a day or 10 to 25 mg/kg/day in divided doses.

propantheline bromide

≡ **Indications and Dosages**

٭ *As adjunct to treat peptic ulcer disease*

TABLETS

Adults. 15 mg three times a day before meals and 30 mg at bedtime, adjusted as needed and tolerated.

±**DOSAGE ADJUSTMENT** For elderly patients with mild symptoms or patients of below-average weight, dosage possibly reduced to 7.5 mg three times a day or four times a day.

pyrazinamide

≡ **Indications and Dosages**

٭ *As adjunct to treat tuberculosis, along with other antitubercular drugs*

TABLETS

Adults and children. 15 to 30 mg/kg daily; or, 50 to 70 mg/kg 2 times/wk for the initial 2 months of a 6-month or longer treatment regimen with other antituberculous drugs. *Maximum:* 3 g daily.

±**DOSAGE ADJUSTMENT** For patients with HIV infection, longer course of therapy may be needed.

R

reteplase   Retavase

≡ **Indications and Dosages**

٭ *To treat acute ST-elevation myocardial infarction (STEMI) to reduce the risk of death and heart failure*

I.V. INJECTION

Adults. 10 units over 2 min; repeated once after 30 min.

riluzole   Exservan, Rilutek, Tiglutik

≡ **Indications and Dosages**

٭ *To treat amyotrophic lateral sclerosis*

ORAL FILM ORAL SUSPENSION, TABLETS

Adults. 50 mg every 12 hr taken 1 hr before or 2 hr after a meal.

rotigotine   Neupro

≡ **Indications and Dosages**

٭ *To treat Parkinson's disease*

TRANSDERMAL

Adults in early stage. *Initial:* Apply 2 mg every 24 hr once daily, increased weekly in increments of 2 mg every 24 hr, as needed. *Maximum:* 6 mg every 24 hr.

Adults in advanced stage. *Initial:* Apply 4 mg every 24 hr once daily, increased weekly in increments of 2 mg every 24 hr, as needed. *Maximum:* 8 mg every 24 hr.

٭ *To treat moderate to severe primary restless leg syndrome*

TRANSDERMAL

Adults. *Initial:* Apply 1 mg every 24 hr once daily, increased weekly in increments of 1 mg every 24 hr, as needed. *Maximum:* 3 mg every 24 hr.

rufinamide   Banzel

≣ Indications and Dosages

✳ *As adjunct treatment of seizures associated with Lennox–Gastaut syndrome*

TABLETS

Adults and adolescents age 17 and over. *Initial:* 200 to 400 mg twice daily, increased in daily increments of 200 to 400 mg twice daily, every 2 days until reaching 1,600 mg twice daily. *Maximum:* 1,600 mg twice daily.

Children age 1 to less than 17. *Initial:* 5 mg/kg twice daily, increased in daily increments of 5 mg/kg twice daily, every 2 days until reaching 22.5 mg/kg twice daily or 1,600 mg twice daily, whichever is less.

±**DOSAGE ADJUSTMENT** For patients undergoing dialysis, dosage may have to be increased. For patients also receiving valproate, initial dosage reduced to less than 400 mg daily in adults and less than 10 mg/kg daily in children.

S

secnidazole   Solosec

≣ Indications and Dosages

✳ *To treat bacterial vaginosis*

ORAL GRANULES

Adult women. 2 g as a single dose.

✳ *To treat trichomoniasis*

ORAL GRANULES

Adult women and female sexual partners. 2 g as a single dose.

secukinumab   Cosentyx

≣ Indications and Dosages

✳ *To treat moderate to severe plaque psoriasis in patients who are candidates for phototherapy or systemic therapy*

SUBCUTANEOUS INJECTION

Adults. 150 or 300 mg (given as 2 150-mg injections) once a wk for 5 doses, then 150 or 300 mg (given as 2 150-mg injections) every 4 wk.

Children age 6 years and older weighing 50 kg (110 lb) or more. 150 mg once a wk for 5 doses, then 150 mg every 4 wk.

Children age 6 years and older weighing less than 50 kg (110 lb). 75 mg once a wk for 5 doses, then 75 mg every 4 wk.

✳ *To treat psoriatic arthritis in patients with coexistent moderate to severe plaque psoriasis*

SUBCUTANEOUS INJECTION

Adults. 150 or 300 mg (given as two 150-mg injections) once a wk for 5 doses, then 150 or 300 mg (given as two 150-mg injections) every 4 wk.

✳ *To treat active psoriatic arthritis*

SUBCUTANEOUS INJECTION

Adults. *Initial:* 150 mg weekly for 5 doses, followed by 150 mg every 4 wk. Alternatively, 150 mg every 4 wk. Dosage may be increased to 300 mg (given as 2 150-mg injections) every 4 wk, if needed. *Maximum:* 300 mg every 4 wk.

Children age 2 years and older weighing 50 kg (110 lb) or more. 150 mg weekly for 5 doses, followed by 150 mg every 4 wk.

Children age 2 years and weighing 15 kg (33 lb) to less than 50 kg (110 lb). 75 mg weekly for 5 doses, followed by 75 mg every 4 wk.

✳ *To treat ankylosing spondylitis*

SUBCUTANEOUS INJECTION

Adults. *Initial:* 150 mg weekly for 5 doses, followed by 150 mg every 4 wk. Alternatively, 150 mg every 4 wk. Dosage may be increased to 300 mg (given as two 150-mg injections) every 4 wk, if needed. *Maximum:* 300 mg every 4 wk.

✳ *To treat non-radiographic axial spondyloarthritis*

SUBCUTANEOUS INJECTION

Adults. *Initial:* 150 mg weekly for 5 doses, followed by 150 mg every 4 wk. Alternatively, 150 mg every 4 wk.

✳ *To treat active enthesitis-related arthritis*

SUBCUTANEOUS INJECTION

Adults and children age 4 years and older weighing 50 kg (110 lb) or more. *Initial:* 150 mg weekly for 5 doses, followed by 150 mg every 4 wk.

Adults and children age 4 years and older weighing 15 kg (33 lb) to less than 50 kg (110 lb). *Initial:* 75 mg weekly for 5 doses, followed by 75 mg every 4 wk.

T

tapentadol hydrochloride   Nucynta, Nucynta ER, Nucynta Oral Solution

Controlled substance schedule: II

Indications and Dosages

* To relieve pain severe enough to require opioid treatment and for which alternative treatment options such as nonopioid analgesics or opioid combination products are inadequate or not tolerated

ORAL SOLUTION, TABLETS

Adults. *Initial:* 50, 75, or 100 mg repeated every 4 to 6 hr, as needed. *Maximum:* 700 mg on first day; 600 mg daily thereafter

± **DOSAGE ADJUSTMENT** On first day of therapy, second dose may be given as soon as 1 hr after first dose, if needed. For patients with moderate hepatic impairment (Child–Pugh Class B), dosage should not exceed 50 mg for each episode, intervals between doses should be at least 8 hours, and no more than 3 doses should be given in a 24-hour period.

E.R. TABLETS

Adults. *Initial:* 50 mg every 12 hours, increased by 50 mg no more than twice daily every 3 days, as needed. *Maximum:* 250 mg twice daily.

± **DOSAGE ADJUSTMENT** For patients with moderate hepatic impairment taking ER tablets, initial dosage reduced to 50 mg once daily and increased as needed to maximum dosage of 100 mg once daily.

* To relieve neuropathic pain associated with diabetic peripheral neuropathy and for which alternative treatment options are inadequate when a continuous, around-the-clock opioid analgesic is needed for an extended period of time

E.R. TABLETS

Adults. *Initial:* 50 mg twice daily, increased by 50 mg twice daily, as needed, no sooner than every 3 days. *Maximum:* 250 mg twice daily.

± **DOSAGE ADJUSTMENT** For patients with moderate hepatic impairment, initial dosage reduced to 50 mg once daily and increased as needed to maximum dosage of 100 mg once daily.

tedizolid   Sivextro

Indications and Dosages

* To treat acute bacterial skin and skin structure infections caused by the following gram-positive microorganisms: Enterococcus faecalis, Staphylococcus aureus (including methicillin-resistant and methicillin-susceptible isolates),

Streptococcus agalactiae, S. anginosus group (including S. anginosus, S. constellatus, and S. intermedius), and S. pyogenes

TABLETS

Adults. 200 mg once daily for 6 days.

I.V. INFUSION

Adults. 200 mg infused over 1 hr once daily for 6 days.

theophylline   Elixophyllin, Theo-24

Indications and Dosages

* As adjunct to inhaled beta-2 selective agonists and systemically administered corticosteroids to treat acute exacerbations of symptoms and reversible airflow obstruction associated with asthma and other chronic lung diseases such as chronic bronchitis and emphysema

ELIXIR, TABLETS

Adults, children, and infants. Loading and maintenance doses highly individualized based upon the following factors: age and weight of patient; currently using or not using a theophylline drug; nonsmoker or smoker; presence or absence of sepsis with multi-organ failure, or shock; and presence of underlying heart, liver, or lung conditions.

* To treat symptoms and reversible airflow obstruction associated with chronic asthma and other chronic lung diseases such as chronic bronchitis and emphysema

ELIXIR, E.R. CAPSULES, E.R. TABLETS, TABLETS

Adults, children, and infants. Highly individualized based upon age and weight of patient, serum theophylline concentrations, and underlying heart, liver, or lung conditions.

tigecycline   Tygacil

Indications and Dosages

* To treat community-acquired bacterial pneumonia caused by Haemophilus influenzae (beta-lactamase negative isolates), Legionella pneumophila, and Streptococcus pneumoniae (penicillin-susceptible isolates), including cases with concurrent bacteremia; to treat complicated intra-abdominal infections caused by Bacteroides fragilis, B. thetaiotaomicron, B. uniformis, B. vulgatus, Citrobacter freundii, Clostridium perfringens, Enterobacter cloacae, Enterococcus faecalis (vancomycin-susceptible isolates only), Escherichia coli, Klebsiella oxytoca, K. pneumoniae,

Peptostreptococcus micros, Staphylococcus aureus *(methicillin-susceptible isolates only), and* Streptococcus anginosus *(group only); to treat complicated skin and skin structure infections caused by* B. fragilis, E. coli, E. faecalis *(vancomycin-susceptible isolates only),* S. aureus *(methicillin-susceptible and resistant isolates),* S. agalactiae, S. anginosus *group (includes* S. anginosus, S. constellatus, *and* S. intermedius*), and* S. pyogenes

I.V. INFUSION

Adults. *Initial:* 100 mg infused over 30 to 60 min followed by 50 mg infused over 30 to 60 min every 12 hr for 5 to 14 days for complicated skin and skin structure infections and intra-abdominal infections; 7 to 14 days for community-acquired bacterial pneumonia.

±**DOSAGE ADJUSTMENT** For patients with severe hepatic impairment, initial dosage of 100 mg should be followed by a reduced maintenance dosage of 25 mg every 12 hr.

trandolapril

☰ Indications and Dosages

✳ *To manage hypertension*

TABLETS

Adults. *Initial:* 1 mg (2 mg for African Americans daily), increased every wk based on clinical response. Dosage may be given in two daily doses if antihypertensive effect diminishes before 24 hr. *Usual:* 2 to 4 mg daily. *Maximum:* 8 mg daily.

✳ *To treat heart failure or left-ventricular dysfunction after MI*

TABLETS

Adults. *Initial:* 1 mg daily, increased, as needed, toward target dose of 4 mg once daily.

±**DOSAGE ADJUSTMENT** Initial dosage reduced to 0.5 mg for patients also receiving a diuretic, those with cirrhosis, or those with a creatinine clearance of less than 30 ml/min.

tranexamic acid

☰ Indications and Dosages

✳ *To treat cyclic heavy menstrual bleeding*

TABLETS

Adults. 1,300 mg three times daily for a maximum of 5 days during monthly menstruation

±**DOSAGE ADJUSTMENT** For patient with a serum creatinine level above 1.4 mg/dl but

equal to or less than 2.8 mg/dl, 1,300 mg two times a day for a maximum of 5 days during menstruation; for patient with a serum creatinine level above 2.8 mg/dl but equal to or less than 5.7 mg/dl, 1,300 mg once daily for a maximum of 5 days during menstruation; for patient with a serum creatinine level above 5.7 mg/dl, 650 mg once daily for a maximum of 5 days during menstruation.

✳ *To treat patients with hemophilia to reduce or prevent hemorrhage and reduce need for replacement therapy during and following tooth extraction*

I.V. INFUSION

Adults. *Initial:* 10 mg/kg infused at 50 mg/min immediately before tooth extraction together with replacement therapy, followed by 10 mg/kg three times a day or four times a day, as needed, for up to 8 days.

±**DOSAGE ADJUSTMENT** For patients with moderate to severe renal impairment with a serum creatinine of 1.36 to 2.83 mg/dl, dosage reduced to 10 mg/kg twice daily; for a serum creatinine of 2.83 to 5.66 mg/dl, dosage reduced to 10 mg/kg daily; and for a serum creatinine greater than 5.66 mg/dl, dosage reduced to 5 mg/kg every 24 hours or 10 mg/kg every 48 hours.

V

valacyclovir hydrochloride   Valtrex

☰ Indications and Dosages

✳ *To treat herpes labialis*

CAPLETS, ORAL SUSPENSION

Adults and children age 12 and over. 2 g twice daily for 1 day given 12 hr apart with therapy begun at the earliest symptom (burning, itching, tingling).

✳ *To treat initial episode of genital herpes in immunocompetent patients*

CAPLETS, ORAL SUSPENSION

Adults. 1 g twice daily for 10 days.

✳ *To treat recurrent episodes of genital herpes in immunocompetent patients*

CAPLETS, ORAL SUSPENSION

Adults. 500 mg twice daily for 3 days, with therapy begun at the first sign of recurrence.

✳ *To suppress chronic recurrent episodes of genital herpes in immunocompetent patients*

CAPLETS, ORAL SUSPENSION
Adults. 1 g once daily. Alternatively, for patient with history of 9 or fewer episodes per year, 500 mg once daily.

* *To suppress chronic recurrent episodes of genital herpes in patients with HIV-1 viral infection who have a CD4+ cell count equal to or greater than 100 cells/mm[3]*

CAPLETS, ORAL SUSPENSION
Adults. 500 mg twice daily.

* *To reduce transmission of genital herpes for immunocompetent source partner in patient with history of 9 or fewer episodes per year*

CAPLETS, ORAL SUSPENSION
Adults. 500 mg once daily for source partner.

* *To treat herpes zoster in patients who are immunocompetent*

CAPLETS, ORAL SUSPENSION
Adults. 1 g three times daily for 7 days begun at the earliest sign or symptom of herpes zoster.

Children ages 2 to 18. 20 mg/kg three times daily for 5 days. *Maximum:* 1 g three times daily.

±**DOSAGE ADJUSTMENT** For adult patients with renal impairment being treated for herpes labialis, dosage reduced to 1 g twice daily for 1 day if creatinine clearance is between 30 and 49 ml/min; dosage reduced to 500 mg twice daily for 1 day if creatinine clearance is between 10 and 29 ml/min; and dosage reduced to a 500-mg single dose if creatinine clearance is less than 10 ml/min. For patients with renal impairment being treated for initial episode of genital herpes, dosage reduced to 1 g every 24 hr if creatinine clearance is between 10 and 29 ml/min, and dosage reduced to 500 mg every 24 hr if creatinine clearance is less than 10 ml/min. For immunocompetent patients with renal impairment being treated for recurrent episode of genital herpes, or for suppressive therapy, dosage reduced to 500 mg every 24 hr if creatinine clearance is 29 ml/min or less, and for alternate therapy if renal-impaired patient has had 9 or fewer recurrences per year, dosage reduced to 500 mg every 48 hr. For HIV-1–infected patients with renal impairment using drug to suppress chronic recurrent episodes of genital herpes, dosage reduced to 500 mg every 24 hr if creatinine clearance is 29 ml/min or less. For adult patients with renal

impairment being treated for herpes zoster, dosage reduced to 1 g every 12 hr if creatinine clearance is between 30 and 49 ml/min; dosage reduced to 1 g every 24 hr if creatinine clearance is between 10 and 29 ml/min, and reduced to 500 mg every 24 hr if creatinine clearance is less than 10 ml/min.

valbenazine   Ingrezza

☰ Indications and Dosages
* *To treat tardive dyskinesia*

CAPSULES
Adults. Initial: 40 mg once daily, increased after 1 wk to 80 mg once daily.

±**DOSAGE ADJUSTMENT** For patients with moderate or severe hepatic impairment or for patients taking a strong CYP3A4 inhibitor concomitantly, dosage kept at 40 mg once daily. For patients who are known CYP2D6 poor metabolizers or who are taking strong CYP2D6 inhibitors concomitantly, dosage reduction may be considered.

valganciclovir hydrochloride   Valcyte

☰ Indications and Dosages
* *To treat cytomegalovirus (CMV) retinitis*

ORAL SOLUTION, TABLETS
Adults. *Induction:* 900 mg twice daily for 21 days with food. *Maintenance:* 900 mg once daily.

* *To prevent CMA disease in heart, kidney, and kidney-pancreas transplant adults at high risk*

ORAL SOLUTION, TABLETS
Adults who have received a heart or kidney-pancreas transplant. 900 mg once daily with food starting within 10 days of transplantation until 100 days posttransplantation.

Adults who have received a kidney transplant. 900 mg once daily with food starting within 10 days of transplantation until 200 days posttransplantation.

* *To prevent CMA disease in children with a heart or kidney transplant*

ORAL SOLUTION, TABLETS
Infants 1 month of age and over, children up to 16 years who have received a heart transplant. Dosage calculated individually and given once daily with food and started within 10 days of transplantation until

100 days posttransplantation. *Maximum:* 900 mg once daily.

Infants 4 months of age and over, children up to 16 years who have received a kidney transplant. Dosage calculated individually and given once daily with food and started within 10 days of transplantation until 200 days posttransplantation. *Maximum:* 900 mg once daily.

±**DOSAGE ADJUSTMENT** For pediatric patients, the dosage is calculated based on the formula: $7 \times BSA \times CrCl$ with maximum calculated creatinine clearance used in the formula to be no more than 150 mg/min. For adult patients with a creatinine clearance between 40 and 59 ml/min, induction dosage reduced to 450 mg twice daily and maintenance dosage reduced to 450 mg once daily. For adult patients with a creatinine clearance between 25 and 39 ml/min, induction dosage reduced to 450 mg once daily and maintenance dosage reduced to 450 mg every 2 days. For adult patients with a creatinine clearance between 10 and 24 ml/min, induction dosage reduced to 450 mg every 2 days and maintenance dosage reduced to 450 mg twice weekly.

vedolizumab   Entyvio

▤ Indications and Dosages

∗ *To treat moderate to severe Crohn's disease or ulcerative colitis*

I.V. INFUSION

Adults. 300 mg infused over 30 min, followed by 300 mg 2 and 6 wk later, and then every 8 wk thereafter.

Z

zanamivir   Relenza

▤ Indications and Dosages

∗ *To treat acute uncomplicated illness due to influenza A and B viral infection in patients who have been symptomatic for no more than 2 days*

ORAL INHALATION

Adults and children ages 7 years and over. 10 mg twice daily about 12 hr apart for 5 days. The first two doses should be taken on the first day with at least 2 hr separating the doses if 12-hr stretch is not feasible.

∗ *To prevent influenza*

ORAL INHALATION

Adults and children ages 5 years and over in a household setting. 10 mg once daily for 10 days.

Adults and adolescents in a community setting. 10 mg once daily for 28 days.

Selected Antihistamines

Antihistamines are usually used to relieve immediate hypersensitivity reactions. They're also used as antiemetics (especially in motion sickness), antidyskinetics, antitussives, sedatives, and adjuncts to preoperative or postoperative analgesia.

Antihistamines are contraindicated in patients taking drugs that prolong the QT interval (including itraconazole, ketoconazole, mibefradil, some macrolide antibiotics, quinidine, and zileuton). They're also contraindicated in patients hypersensitive to antihistamines or their components.

The table below includes trade names; usual dosages; and onset, peak, and duration for antihistamines that your patient is most likely to use daily or intermittently to control symptoms of allergic rhinitis. When caring for a patient who takes an antihistamine, individualize your plan of care but be sure to include these general interventions:

- Use antihistamines cautiously in patients with a history of glaucoma, peptic ulcer, or urine retention because anticholinergic effects may worsen these conditions.
- Assess patient for hypokalemia and correct the imbalance, as prescribed, before antihistamine therapy to reduce the risk of arrhythmias.
- Obtain a detailed medication history before antihistamine therapy to help prevent drug interactions.
- Give antihistamines with food if GI distress occurs.
- Urge patient to avoid alcohol and other CNS depressants during antihistamine use because the combination can cause additive CNS depression.
- Monitor blood pressure because these drugs' anticholinergic effects may cause hypertension.
- Be aware that short- and long-acting antihistamines may be combined and H_2 blockers added to increase antihistamine effects.
- Be aware that products containing pseudoephedrine should be used for less than 7 days.

GENERIC AND TRADE NAMES	USUAL ADULT DOSAGE	ONSET, PEAK, AND DURATION
acrivastine Semprex-D (also include pseudoephedrine)	8 mg/60 mg P.O. every 4 to 6 hr. *Maximum:* Four times a day	**Onset:** 30 min **Peak:** Unknown **Duration:** 6 to 8 hr
azatadine Optimine	1 to 2 mg P.O. every 8 to 12 hr. *Maximum:* 2 mg in 24 hr	**Onset:** 15 to 60 min **Peak:** 4 hr **Duration:** 12 hr
azelastine Astelin	1 to 2 sprays (137 mcg/spray) in each nostril twice daily	**Onset:** In 3 hr **Peak:** Unknown **Duration:** 12 hr
Astepro 0.1%	1 to 2 sprays (137 mcg/spray) in each nostril twice daily	
Astepro 0.15%	2 sprays (205.5 mcg/spray) in each nostril once daily	
carbinoxamine maleate Arbinoxa, Palgic	4 to 8 mg P.O. three times a day or four times a day. *Maximum:* 24 mg in 24 hr (Immediate Release)	**Onset:** 30 min **Peak:** Unknown **Duration:** 4 hr (Arbinoxa, Palgic), 17 hr (Karbinal ER)
Karbinal ER	6 to 16 mg P.O. every 12 hr (Extended Release)	
cetirizine hydrochloride Zyrtec Zyrtec D (also includes pseudoephedrine)	5 to 10 mg P.O. daily 5 mg/120 mg every 12 hr	**Onset:** 30 to 60 min **Peak:** 1 hr **Duration:** Up to 24 hr

(continues)

Selected Antihistamines *(continued)*

GENERIC AND TRADE NAMES	USUAL ADULT DOSAGE	ONSET, PEAK, AND DURATION
desloratadine Clarinex, Clarinex Reditabs	5 mg P.O. daily	**Onset:** Unknown **Peak:** 3 hr (Clarinex Reditabs); unknown for other types **Duration:** Unknown
Clarinex-D 12 hr (also contains pseudoephedrine)	2.5 mg/120 mg P.O. twice daily	
Clarinex-D 24 hr (also contains pseudoephedrine)	2.5 mg/240 mg P.O. once daily	
fexofenadine hydrochloride Allegra	60 mg P.O. twice daily or 180 mg P.O. daily	**Onset:** 1 hr **Peak:** 2 to 3 hr **Duration:** 12 hr
Allegra-D-12 hr (also includes pseudoephedrine)	60 mg/120 mg P.O. every 12 hr	
Allegra-D-24 hr (also includes pseudoephedrine)	180 mg/240 mg P.O. once daily	
levocetirizine dihydrochloride Xyzal	2.5 to 5 mg P.O. daily in evening	**Onset:** Less than 1 hr **Peak:** 0.9 hr **Duration:** 24 hr
loratadine Claritin	10 mg P.O. daily	**Onset:** 1 to 3 hr **Peak:** 8 to 12 hr **Duration:** At least 24 hr
Claritin-D12 (also includes pseudoephedrine)	5 mg/120 mg P.O. every 12 hr	
Claritin-D24 (also includes pseudoephedrine)	10 mg/240 mg P.O. every 24 hr	
olopatadine hydrochloride Patanase	2 sprays (665 mcg/spray) in each nostril twice daily	**Onset:** Unknown **Peak:** 15 to 120 min **Duration:** Unknown

Selected Ophthalmic Drugs

Although less commonly prescribed than oral drugs, drugs instilled into the eyes are frequently brought into the clinical setting by patients with chronic conditions. In most cases, the patient or a family member has administered these preparations at home. Your patient teaching should include a review of proper administration and storage of these drugs. Have the patient or a family member demonstrate proper use of the drug to make sure it will be administered correctly at home. Use this time to reassess the patient's ability to continue self-medication. Also, instruct him to report any changes in the condition being treated, either negative or positive. A properly educated patient not only ensures safe drug administration, but also is more likely to detect adverse reactions that require a dosage reduction or drug discontinuation, thus preventing the development of more serious health problems.

The following chart lists the generic and trade names, FDA-approved indications, and usual adult dosages for those ophthalmic preparations you're most likely to see in your practice setting. The drugs are divided according to therapeutic use.

GENERIC AND TRADE NAMES	INDICATIONS	USUAL ADULT DOSAGES
Ophthalmic antibiotics		
bacitracin AK-Tracin	To treat surface bacterial infections affecting the conjunctiva and cornea	1/4-in to 1/2-in strip of ointment applied to conjunctival sac, 1 to 3 times daily or as needed
besifloxacin 0.6% Besivance	To treat bacterial conjunctivitis due to susceptible organisms	1 gtt in affected eye(s) three times a day 4 to 14 hr apart for 7 days
chloramphenicol 1% Diochloram, Pentamycetin/HC, Sopamycetin (CAN)	To treat severe surface bacterial infections affecting the conjunctiva and cornea	Apply small amount of ointment to lower conjunctival sac every 3 to 6 hr and as needed for at least 48 hr after eye resumes normal appearance
ciprofloxacin hydrochloride 0.3% Ciloxan	To treat corneal ulcers due to *Pseudomonas aeruginosa, Staphylococcus aureus, S. epidermidis, Streptococcus pneumoniae,* and possibly *Serratia marcescens* and *S. viridans*	2 gtt in affected eye every 15 min for first 6 hr, then 2 gtt every 30 min for rest of first day; on day 2, 2 gtt in affected eye every hr; on days 3 to 14, 2 gtt in affected eye every 4 hr
	To treat bacterial conjunctivitis due to *Haemophilus influenzae, S. aureus, S. epidermidis, S. pneumoniae* and *S. viridans*	1 or 2 gtt in conjunctival sac of affected eye every 2 hr while awake for first 2 days and then 1 or 2 gtt every 4 hr while awake for next 5 days; or 1/2-in strip of ointment in affected eye three times a day for 2 days, then twice daily for next 5 days
erythromycin Ilotycin	To treat superficial eye infections involving conjunctiva and/or cornea	1 cm (0.39 in) of ointment applied in infected eye up to 6 times/day, depending on severity of infection
	As adjunct to prevent ophthalmia neonatorum due to *Neisseria gonorrhoeae* or *Chlamydia trachomatis*	1 cm (0.39 in) of ointment applied in each eye
gatifloxacin 0.5% Zymaxid	To treat bacterial conjunctivitis due to *Staphylococcus aureus, S. epidermidis, Streptococcus mitis, S. pneumoniae,* and *Haemophilus influenzae*	1 gtt in affected eye every 2 hr while awake, up to eight times daily on day 1; then 1 gtt twice daily to four times a day while awake on days 2 to 7

(continues)

Selected Ophthalmic Drugs (continued)

GENERIC AND TRADE NAMES	INDICATIONS	USUAL ADULT DOSAGES
Ophthalmic antibiotics (continued)		
gentamicin sulfate Garamycin, Genoptic, Gentacidin, Gentak	To treat bacterial infections such as blepharitis, blepharo-conjunctivitis, conjunctivitis, corneal ulcers, dacryocystitis, keratoconjunctivitis, or meibomianitis due to susceptible organisms	1 or 2 gtt every 4 hr or, for severe infection, up to 2 gtt/hr; alternatively, 1/2-in strip of ointment applied to lower conjunctival sac twice daily or three times daily
levofloxacin 0.5% Quixin	To treat bacterial conjunctivitis due to susceptible organisms	On days 1 and 2: 1 or 2 gtt every 2 hr while awake, up to 8 times/day; on days 3 to 7: 1 or 2 gtt every 4 hr while awake, up to 4 times/day
moxifloxacin 0.5% Vigamox Moxeza 0.5%	To treat bacterial conjunctivitis due to *Staphylococcus aureus, S. epidermidis, S. haemolyticus, S. hominis, Streptococcus pneumoniae, S. viridans* group, *Haemophilus influenzae,* and *Chlamydia trachomatis*	1 gtt three times a day for 7 days
ofloxacin 0.3% Ocuflox	To treat conjunctivitis due to *Staphylococcus aureus, S. epidermidis, Streptococcus pneumoniae, Enterobacter cloacae, Haemophilus influenzae, Proteus mirabilis,* and *Pseudomonas aeruginosa* To treat bacterial corneal ulcers due to *S. aureus, S. epidermidis, S. pneumoniae, E. cloacae, H. influenzae, Propionibacterium mirabilis, Propionibacterium aeruginosa, Serratia marcescens,* and *Propionibacterium acnes*	1 or 2 gtt in conjunctival sac every 2 to 4 hr for first 2 days; then 1 to 2 gtt four times a day for up to 5 more days 1 or 2 gtt every 30 min while awake and 1 or 2 gtt every 4 to 6 hr after retiring for 2 days; then 1 or 2 gtt/hr while awake for up to 7 more days; then 1 to 2 gtt four times a day until end of treatment
sulfacetamide sodium 10% Bleph-10, Ocu-Sol 10, Ocu-Sol 15, Ocu-Sol 30, Sodium Sulamyd, Sulf-10, Sulfac 10%	To treat conjunctivitis and other superficial eye infections due to susceptible organisms	1 or 2 gtt solution in lower conjunctival sac every 2 to 3 hr initially, with dosage tapered by increasing time interval between doses as condition improves for up to 10 days; or 1/4-in to 1/2-in strip of ointment in conjunctival sac four times a day and bedtime
sulfacetamide sodium ointment 10%, solution 15% Isopto Cetamide	As adjunct to treat trachoma	2 gtt in lower conjunctival sac every 2 hr

GENERIC AND TRADE NAMES	INDICATIONS	USUAL ADULT DOSAGES
Ophthalmic antibiotics *(continued)*		
tobramycin Tobrasol 0.3%, Tobrex, To-mycine (CAN)	To treat external superficial ocular infections and its adnexa due to susceptible organisms	1 to 2 gtt every 1 to 4 hr, depending on severity of infection; or 1/2-in strip of ointment applied to lower conjunctival sac every 8 to 12 hr for mild to moderate infections or every 3 to 4 hr for severe infections
tobramycin 0.3% (3 mg) and dexamethasone 0.1% (1 mg) TobraDex	To treat steroid-responsive inflammatory ocular conditions for which a corticosteroid is indicated and where superficial bacterial ocular infection or a risk of bacterial ocular infection exists	1 to 2 gtt every 4 to 6 hr; during first 24 to 48 hr, dosage may be increased to 1 to 2 gtt every 2 hr; or apply 1/2-in strip of ointment into the conjunctival sac up to four times a day
Ophthalmic antiviral drugs		
acyclovir 3% Avaclyr	To treat acute herpetic keratitis (dendritic ulcers) in patients with herpes simplex virus	1 cm ribbon of ointment into the lower cul-de-sac of the affected eye 5 times a day (about 3 hours apart while awake) until corneal ulcer heals and then 1 cm ribbon 3 times a day for 7 days
ganciclovir gel 0.15% Zirgan	To treat acute herpes keratitis (dendritic ulcers)	1 gtt five times daily (about every 3 hr while awake) until corneal ulcer heals; then 1 gtt three times a day for 7 days
Ophthalmic anti-inflammatory drugs		
bromfenac 0.09% Xibrom (0.09%)	To treat postoperative inflammation and reduce ocular pain after cataract extraction	1 gtt in operative eye twice daily starting 24 hr after cataract surgery and continuing through first 2 wk of postoperative period
Bromday (0.09%) Prolensa (0.07%)	To treat postoperative inflammation and reduce ocular pain after cataract extraction	1 gtt in operative eye once daily, starting 24 hr before cataract surgery and continuing through first 2 wk of postoperative period
BromSite	To treat postoperative inflammation and prevent ocular pain associated with cataract extraction	1 gtt in operative eye twice daily (morning and evening) 1 day before surgery, day of surgery, and 14 days postoperatively
cetirizine hydrochloride 0.24% Zerviate	To treat ocular itching associated with allergic conjunctivitis	1 gtt in affected eye(s) twice daily.

(continues)

Selected Ophthalmic Drugs *(continued)*

GENERIC AND TRADE NAMES	INDICATIONS	USUAL ADULT DOSAGES
Ophthalmic anti-inflammatory drugs *(continued)*		
dexamethasone Maxidex **dexamethasone sodium phosphate 0.1%** AK-Dex	To treat allergic conjunctivitis; corneal injury from chemical or thermal burns or from penetration of foreign bodies; inflammatory conditions of the anterior segment of globe, conjunctiva, cornea, or eyelids; iridocyclitis; suppression of graft rejection after keratoplasty; and uveitis	1 or 2 gtt of suspension or solution every hr during day and every 2 hr at night initially. When response occurs, 1 gtt every 4 hr; or apply 1/2-in to 1-in strip of ointment up to four times daily, then tapered to once daily
diclofenac sodium 0.1% Voltaren, Voltaren Ophtha (CAN)	To treat postoperative inflammation after removal of cataract	1 gtt in conjunctival sac four times a day, starting 24 hr after surgery through first 2 postoperative wk
	To provide temporary relief of pain and photophobia in corneal refractive surgery	1 or 2 gtt in operative eye 1 hr before surgery. Then 1 or 2 gtt 15 min after surgery. Then 1 gtt four times a day, starting 4 to 6 hr after surgery for up to 3 days, as needed
difluprednate 0.05% Durezol	To treat inflammation and pain associated with ocular surgery	1 gtt in conjunctival sac of affected eye(s) four times a day for 2 wk starting 24 hr after surgery. Then 1 gtt twice daily for 1 wk
	To treat endogenous anterior uveitis	1 gtt into conjunctival sac of affected eye four times a day for 14 days, then tapered as needed
fluorometholone 0.1% Fluor-Op, FML Forte, FML Liquifilm, FML S.O.P. **fluorometholone acetate** Eflone, Flarex	To treat corticosteroid-responsive inflammation of the anterior segment of the globe, bulbar and palpebral conjunctiva, and cornea	1 gtt in conjunctival sac twice daily to four times a day or, in severe conditions, up to every 4 hr during first 1 to 2 days, as needed; or 1.5-in strip of ointment in conjunctival sac once daily to three times a day
		1 or 2 gtt in conjunctival sac four times daily or, in severe conditions, up to every 2 hr during first 1 or 2 days, as needed
ketorolac tromethamine Acular 0.5%	To relieve ocular itching due to seasonal allergic conjunctivitis	1 gtt in conjunctival sac of each eye four times a day
	To treat postoperative inflammation in patients who have undergone cataract extraction	1 gtt in operative eye four times a day, starting 24 hr after surgery through first 2 postoperative wk
Acuvail 0.45%	To relieve pain and treat postoperative inflammation in patients who have undergone cataract extraction	1 gtt in affected eye twice daily, starting 1 day before surgery, continuing through day of surgery and first 2 wk of postoperative period
Acular LS 0.4%	To reduce ocular burning/stinging and pain following corneal refractive surgery	1 gtt in affected eye four times daily for up to 4 days following procedure

GENERIC AND TRADE NAMES	INDICATIONS	USUAL ADULT DOSAGES

Ophthalmic anti-inflammatory drugs (continued)

loteprednol etabonate Alrex 0.2%	To relieve seasonal allergic conjunctivitis	1 gtt of 0.2% suspension in affected eyes four times a day
Lotemax 0.5% Inveltys 1%	To treat postoperative inflammation following ocular surgery	1 or 2 gtt in conjunctival sac of operated eye four times a day, beginning 24 hr after surgery and continuing through first 2 wk of postoperative period
	To treat steroid-responsive inflammatory conditions of the anterior segment of the globe, bulbar and palpebral conjunctiva, and cornea	1 or 2 gtt in conjunctival sac of affected eye four times a day. Initially, dosage may be increased during first week to 1 gtt every hour, as needed
medrysone 1.0% HMS Liquifilm	To treat allergic conjunctivitis, episcleritis, epinephrine sensitivity, and vernal conjunctivitis	1 gtt into conjunctival sac up to every 4 hr
olopatadine hydrochloride 0.1% Patanol	To treat signs and symptoms of allergic conjunctivitis	1 gtt twice daily at 6- to 8-hr intervals
olopatadine hydrochloride 0.7% Pazeo	To treat ocular itching associated with allergic conjunctivitis	1 gtt into conjunctival sac in each affected eye once daily
prednisolone acetate suspension 1% Econopred Plus, Omnipred, Pred Forte, Pred Mild **prednisolone sodium phosphate solution 1%** AK-Pred, Prednisol	To treat steroid-responsive inflammation of the anterior segment of globe, cornea, and bulbar and palpebral conjunctiva; to treat corneal injury from chemical, radiation, or thermal burns, or penetration of foreign bodies	1 or 2 gtt in conjunctival sac twice daily to four times a day (suspension) or 1 gtt in conjunctival sac every 4 hr (solution) unless severe, then initially every hr during day and every 2 hr at night until response noted, then decreased to 1 gtt every 4 hr
rimexolone 1% Vexol	To treat anterior uveitis	1 or 2 gtt in conjunctival sac every hr while awake in first wk; 1 gtt every 2 hr while awake in second wk; then tapered until uveitis resolves
	To treat postoperative inflammation after ocular surgery	1 or 2 gtt in conjunctival sac of affected eye four times a day, starting 24 hr after surgery and continuing through first 2 postoperative wk

Ophthalmic cycloplegic mydriatics

atropine sulfate 1% Isopto Atropine, Minims Atropine (CAN)	To treat acute iritis or uveitis	Small strip of ointment applied to conjunctival sac up to twice daily
	To produce dilation for cycloplegic refraction	1 gtt 40 min before refraction. *Maximum:* 2 gtt

(continues)

Selected Ophthalmic Drugs *(continued)*

GENERIC AND TRADE NAMES	INDICATIONS	USUAL ADULT DOSAGES
Ophthalmic cycloplegic mydriatics *(continued)*		
cyclopentolate hydrochloride 0.5%, 1%, 2% AK-Pentolate, Cyclogyl, Minims Cyclopentolate (CAN), Pentolair	To produce mydriasis and cycloplegia required in specific diagnostic procedures	1 or 2 gtt of 0.5%, 1%, or 2% solution in each eye; then 1 or 2 gtt in 5 to 10 min, as needed
homatropine hydrobromide 2%, 5% Isopto Homatropine, Minims Homatropine (CAN)	To dilate pupils for cycloplegic refraction To treat uveitis	1 or 2 gtt in each eye, repeated in 5 to 10 min as needed 1 or 2 gtt in affected eye(s) every 3 to 4 hr
phenylephrine 2.5%, 10%	To dilate pupil	1 gtt per eye at 3- to 5-minute intervals up to maximum of 3 drops per eye.
tropicamide 0.5%, 1% Mydriacyl, Opticyl, Tropicacyl	To produce mydriasis To dilate pupils for cycloplegic funduscopic exam	1 to 2 gtt of 1% solution, repeated in 5 min, as needed 1 to 2 gtt of 0.5% solution in eyes 15 to 20 min before exam, repeated every 30 min as needed
Ophthalmic miotics		
acetylcholine chloride Miochol-E	To produce papillary miosis in cataract surgery, penetrating keratoplasty, iridectomy, and other anterior segment surgery	0.5 to 2 ml gently into anterior chamber before or after sutures secured or after lens placement in cataract surgery
carbachol 0.01% Carbastat, Miostat	To produce papillary miosis in ocular surgery; to reduce intensity of intraocular pressure elevation in first 24 hr after cataract surgery	0.5 ml (solution) into anterior chamber before or after sutures secured or after lens placement in cataract surgery
carbachol 0.75%, 1.5%, 2.25%, 3% Carboptic, Isopto Carbachol	To treat open-angle glaucoma	1 or 2 gtt up to three times a day
flurbiprofen sodium 0.03% Ocufen	To inhibit intraoperative miosis	1 gtt in affected eye every 30 min, beginning 2 hr before surgery, up to total of 4 gtt

GENERIC AND TRADE NAMES	INDICATIONS	USUAL ADULT DOSAGES
Ophthalmic miotics *(continued)*		
pilocarpine 1%, 2%, 4% Akarpine, Isopto Carpine, Miocarpine (CAN), Pilocar, Pilopine HS, Pilostat	To treat primary open-angle glaucoma	1 gtt up to four times a day; or 1-cm (0.39-in) ribbon of 4% gel at bedtime
pilocarpine hydrochloride Akarpine, Isopto Carpine, Minocarpine (CAN), Pilocar, Pilopine HS, Pilostat	To treat acute angle-closure glaucoma as emergency therapy	1 gtt of 2% solution every 15 to 60 min for up to four doses
pilocarpine hydrochloride 1.25% Vuity	To treat presbyopia	1 gtt of 1% solution
pilocarpine nitrate 1% Minims Pilocarpine (CAN)	To treat mydriasis due to mydriatic or cycloplegic drug therapy	1 gtt in each eye once daily
proparacaine hydrochloride 0.5% AK-Taine, Alcaine, Ophthetic, Parcaine	To provide deep anesthesia during cataract extraction	1 gtt every 5 to 10 min for 5 to 7 doses
	To provide anesthesia during removal of eye sutures	1 or 2 gtt 2 to 3 min before procedure
	To provide anesthesia during removal of foreign bodies	1 or 2 gtt in affected eye before surgery
	To provide anesthesia during tonometry	1 or 2 gtt immediately before measurement
tetracaine 0.5% Pontocaine	To provide eye anesthesia (short term)	1 or 2 gtt, as needed
travoprost 0.004% Travatan Z	To reduce elevated intraocular pressure caused by ocular hypertension or open-angle glaucoma	1 gtt in affected eye (s) once daily in evening
Miscellaneous ophthalmic drugs		
alcaftadine 0.25% Lastacaft	To prevent itching associated with allergic conjunctivitis	1 gtt in each eye once daily
apraclonidine hydrochloride 0.5% Iopidine	As adjunct in patients on maximally tolerated medical therapy who require additional intraocular pressure (IOP) reduction	1 or 2 gtt in affected eye(s) three times daily
azelastine hydrochloride 0.05% Optivar	To treat itching of the eye associated with allergic conjunctivitis	1 gtt in affected eye twice daily

(continues)

Selected Ophthalmic Drugs *(continued)*

GENERIC AND TRADE NAMES	INDICATIONS	USUAL ADULT DOSAGES
Miscellaneous ophthalmic drugs *(continued)*		
bepotastine besilate 1.5% Bepreve	To treat itching of the eye associated with allergic conjunctivitis	1 gtt in affected eye twice daily
betaxolol hydrochloride Betoptic 0.5%, Betoptic S 0.25%	To treat chronic open-angle glaucoma or ocular hypertension	1 or 2 gtt of 0.5% solution twice daily or 1 gtt of 0.25% solution twice daily
bimatoprost 0.01%, 0.03% Lumigan	To reduce elevated IOP in patients with open-angle glaucoma or ocular hypertension	1 gtt in affected eye daily in evening
brimonidine tartrate Alphagan 0.2%, Alphagan P 0.1%, 0.15%	To reduce IOP in open-angle glaucoma or ocular hypertension	1 gtt in affected eye three times daily, about 8 hr apart
brimonidine tartrate 0.025% Lumify	To remove eye redness	1 gtt in affected eye(s) every 6 to 8 hr
brinzolamide 1% Azopt	To reduce IOP in ocular hypertension or open-angle glaucoma	1 gtt three times a day
brinzolamide 1% and brimonidine tartrate 0.2% Simbrinza	To reduce IOP in open-angle glaucoma or ocular hypertension	1 gtt in affected eye three times a day
carteolol hydrochloride 1% Ocupress	To treat chronic open-angle glaucoma or intraocular hypertension	1 gtt in conjunctival sac of affected eye twice daily
cyclosporine 0.09% cyclosporine emulsion 0.05% Restasis	To increase tear production in keratoconjunctivitis sicca	1 gtt every 12 hr
cysteamine 0.44% Cystaran	To treat corneal cystine crystal accumulation in patients with cystinosis	1 gtt in each eye, every waking hr
cysteamine 0.37% Cystadrops	To treat corneal cystine crystal accumulation in patients with cystinosis	1 gtt in each eye four times a day during waking hours
dipivefrin hydrochloride 0.1% Ophtho-Dipivefrin (CAN), Propine	To reduce IOP in chronic open-angle glaucoma	1 gtt every 12 hr
dorzolamide hydrochloride 2 % Trusopt	To treat increased IOP in ocular hypertension or open-angle glaucoma	1 gtt in conjunctival sac of affected eye three times a day

Miscellaneous ophthalmic drugs *(continued)*

GENERIC AND TRADE NAMES	INDICATIONS	USUAL ADULT DOSAGES
echothiophate iodide Phospholine Iodide	To reduce elevated IOP	1 gtt twice daily (morning and at bedtime). Alternatively, 1 gtt once daily or once every other day (at bedtime)
	To diagnose pediatric accommodative esotropia	1 gtt in both eyes once daily at bedtime for 2 or 3 weeks
	To treat pediatric accommodative esotropia	1 gtt in both eyes every other day. *Maximum:* 1 gtt in both eyes every day
emedastine difumarate Emadine	To treat allergic conjunctivitis	1 gtt in affected eye up to four times a day
ketotifen fumarate 0.025%, 0.035% Alaway, Zaditor	To treat allergic conjunctivitis	1 gtt in affected eye twice daily every 8 to 12 hr, but no more than twice daily
latanoprost 0.005% Xalatan, Xelpros	To reduce IOP in ocular hypertension or open-angle glaucoma	1 gtt in conjunctival sac of affected eye daily in evening
latanoprostene bunod 0.024% Vyzulta	To reduce IOP in ocular hypertension or open-angle glaucoma	1 gtt in affected eye(s) once daily in evening
levobunolol hydrochloride AKBeta, Betagan, Novo-Levobunolol (CAN)	To treat chronic open-angle glaucoma or ocular hypertension	1 or 2 gtt of 0.5% solution once daily or 0.25% solution twice daily
levocabastine hydrochloride 0.05% Livostin	To treat signs and symptoms of seasonal allergic conjunctivitis	1 gtt four times a day
lifitegrast 5% Xiidra	To treat dry eye disease	1 gtt twice daily (about 12 hr apart) in each eye
metipranolol 0.3% OptiPranolol	To reduce IOP in ocular hypertension or open-angle glaucoma	1 gtt in affected eye twice daily
naphazoline hydrochloride Ak-Con 0.1%, Albalon 0.1%, Clear Eyes 0.012%, Naphcon A 0.025%, Vasocon 0.05%	To treat ocular congestion, irritation, or itching	1 gtt of 0.1% solution every 3 to 4 hr; or 1 gtt of 0.012% to 0.03% solution up to four times a day for no more than 72 hr
nedocromil sodium 2% Alocril	To treat itching associated with both seasonal and perennial allergic conjunctivitis	1 or 2 gtt twice daily
netarsudil 0.02% Rhopressa	To reduce IOP in ocular hypertension or open-angle glaucoma	1 gtt in affected eye(s) once daily in evening
netarsudil 0.02% and latanoprost 0.005% Rocklatan	To reduce IOP in open-angle glaucoma or ocular hypertension	1 gtt in affected eye(s) once daily in evening

(continues)

Selected Ophthalmic Drugs *(continued)*

GENERIC AND TRADE NAMES	INDICATIONS	USUAL ADULT DOSAGES
Miscellaneous ophthalmic drugs *(continued)*		
oxymetazoline hydrochloride	To provide relief from eye redness due to minor eye irritations	1 or 2 gtt in conjunctival sac four times a day (at least 6 hr apart) for no more than 72 hr
oxymetazoline hydrochloride 0.1% Uplifted	To treat acquired blepharoptosis	1 gtt in ptotic eye(s) once daily
proparacaine hydrochloride 0.5% AK-Taine, Alcaine, Ophthetic, Parcaine	To provide deep anesthesia during cataract extraction	1 gtt every 5 to 10 min for 5 to 7 doses
	To provide anesthesia during removal of eye sutures	1 or 2 gtt 2 to 3 min before procedure
	To provide anesthesia during removal of foreign bodies	1 or 2 gtt in affected eye before surgery
	To provide anesthesia during tonometry	1 or 2 gtt immediately before measurement
sodium chloride, hypertonic Altachlore, Muro-128 2%, Muro-128 5%, Muroptic-5	To provide temporary relief from corneal edema	1 or 2 gtt every 3 to 4 hr; or 1/4-in of ointment applied every 3 to 4 hr
tafluprost 0.0015% Zioptan	To reduce IOP in ocular hypertension or open-angle glaucoma	1 gtt in conjunctival sac in affected eye(s) once daily in evening
tetracaine 0.5% Pontocaine	To provide eye anesthesia (short term)	1 or 2 gtt, as needed
tetrahydrozoline hydrochloride 0.05% Eye-Sine, Murine Plus, Optigene 3, Tetrasine, Visine	To treat allergic conditions, conjunctival congestion, and irritation	1 gtt up to four times a day or as directed
timolol hemihydrate 0.25%, 0.5% Betimol **timolol maleate 0.25%, 0.5%** Apo-Timop (CAN), Timoptic **timolol maleate extended-release gel solution 0.25%, 0.5%** Timoptic-XE	To reduce IOP in ocular hypertension or open-angle glaucoma	1 gtt of 0.25% solution in affected eye twice daily, increased to 1 gtt of 0.5% solution, as needed; then 1 gtt daily; or 1 gtt extended-release gel solution in affected eye daily
travoprost 0.003% Izba **travoprost 0.004%** Travatan	To reduce elevated IOP in patients with open-angle glaucoma or ocular hypertension	1 gtt in affected eye daily in evening
unoprostone isopropyl 0.15% Rescula	To reduce elevated IOP in patients with open-angle glaucoma or ocular hypertension	1 gtt in affected eye twice daily

Selected Topical Drugs

Topical drugs consist of an active drug prepared in a specified medium that promotes absorption through the skin. Media commonly are chosen based on drug solubility; rate of drug release; ability to hydrate the outer skin layer; ability to enhance penetration; drug stability; and interactions between the chosen medium, skin, and active ingredient.

Topical media include aerosols, creams, gels, lotions, ointments, powders, tinctures, and wet dressings. Aerosols, gels, lotions, and tinctures are convenient for application to the scalp and other hairy areas. Acutely inflamed areas are best treated with drying preparations, such as lotions, tinctures, and wet dressings. Chronic inflammation does well with applications of lubricating preparations, including creams and ointments.

Because of its physical properties, the skin can act as a holding area for many drugs, allowing slow penetration and prolonged duration of action. (This characteristic makes it important to understand the patient's allergies.) However, when administering topical or transdermal drugs that aren't prescribed for a specific location, keep in mind that penetration properties may vary in different areas of the body. For example, the axillae, face, scalp, and scrotum are more permeable than the limbs, and ventral surfaces typically are more permeable than dorsal surfaces.

Topical Drug Types

Topical drugs are classified as antibacterials, antifungals, antivirals, corticosteroids, retinoids, and other miscellaneous preparations.

- Antibacterials may be useful in the early treatment of minor skin infections and wounds. Minor skin infections may respond well to topical drugs applied at the infection site. Minor wounds should be treated at the site and in the immediately surrounding area to prevent other pathogens from colonizing the area.
- Antifungals usually are used to treat mucocutaneous infections, such as tineas, primarily ringworm and athlete's foot. Systemic use of antifungals is limited by their potentially toxic adverse effects, most commonly hepatic or renal damage. All fungi are completely resistant to conventional antibacterial drugs.
- Antivirals are used to inhibit viral replication. They work by targeting any one of the steps involved in viral replication: penetration into

susceptible host cells; uncoating of the viral nucleic acid; synthesis of regulatory proteins, RNA and DNA, and structural proteins; assembly of viral particles; and release of the virus from the cell. Topical antivirals such as penciclovir can shorten the duration of herpetic lesions, lessen lesion pain, and minimize viral shedding.

- Corticosteroids reduce the signs and symptoms of inflammation. Topical corticosteroids cause vasoconstriction, probably by suppressing cell degranulation. They also cause decreased cell permeability by reducing histamine release from basal and mast cells.
- Retinoids, typically derivatives of vitamin A, are very effective in treating acne vulgaris, although the acne may appear to worsen before it improves. Retinoids are also useful for reducing wrinkles. When applied to the skin, retinoids remain primarily in the dermis; less than 10% of the drug is absorbed into the circulation. Prolonged use of retinoids promotes new dermal growth, new blood vessel formation, and thickening of the epidermis. Because these drugs are absorbed systemically and may have teratogenic effects, they shouldn't be used by pregnant women.
- Miscellaneous topical drugs are used to treat a variety of topical skin conditions, including dry skin, ichthyosis, parasitic infestations, psoriasis, and unwanted hair growth.

Administration Tips

Before you apply a topical drug, clean the site and let it dry. Use gloves or a finger cot during application to prevent the drug from being absorbed through your own skin. Inform your patient of any expected discomfort, such as temporary burning or stinging. After application, cover the site only if required; some topical drugs shouldn't be covered with an occlusive dressing.

Be sure to teach the patient and a family member correct administration technique. Also, review possible adverse reactions, highlighting those that should be reported to the prescriber. Stress the importance of complying with the drug regimen because some topical drugs require weeks or months of therapy to eradicate the underlying condition.

The following table includes the generic and trade names of many commonly prescribed topical drugs as well as their FDA-approved indications and usual adult dosages.

Selected Topical Drugs *(continued)*

GENERIC AND TRADE NAMES	INDICATIONS	USUAL ADULT DOSAGES
Antibacterials		
azelaic acid cream 20% Azelex	To treat mild to moderate inflammatory acne vulgaris	Gently massage thin film into affected area twice daily, morning and evening.
azelaic acid foam 15% Finacea Foam **azelaic acid gel 15%** Finacea Gel	To treat inflammatory papules and pustules of mild to moderate rosacea	Apply thin layer to entire facial area twice daily, morning and evening.
bacitracin zinc	To treat topical infections; to prevent infection in minor skin wounds such as abrasions, minor burns, and cuts	Apply light dusting of powder or thin film of ointment to affected area once daily to three times a day up to 1 wk.
benzoyl peroxide Benzac, Brevoxyl, Clearasil, Desquam, Fostex, Triaz, ZoDerm	To treat mild to moderate inflammatory acne vulgaris	Apply to affected area once daily, gradually increasing to twice daily or three times a day.
clindamycin and benzoyl peroxide Acanya 1.2%/2.5%, Benzaclin 1%/5%, Duac 1.2%/5%, Nevac 1.2%/5%	To treat acne vulgaris	Apply once or twice daily (morning and/or evening) to affected areas.
clindamycin 1.2% and tretinoin 0.025% Veltin Gel, Ziana Gel	To treat acne vulgaris	Apply pea-sized amount to affected areas once daily in evening.
clindamycin phosphate Cleocin 1%, Clinda-Derm 1%, Clindagel 1%, Clindesse 2%, Clindets 1%, Dalacin T Topical Solution 1% (CAN), Evoclin 1%	To treat inflammatory acne vulgaris To treat bacterial vaginosis	Apply to affected area once or twice daily (morning and evening). 1 applicatorful (100 mg) intravaginally at bedtime for 7 days.
dapsone gel 7.5% Aczone	To treat acne vulgaris	Apply pea-sized amount in thin layer to entire face or other affected areas once daily.
dapsone gel 5% Aczone	To treat acne vulgaris	Apply pea-sized amount in thin layer to entire face or other affected areas twice daily.
erythromycin 1.5%, 2% Akne-Mycin, A/T/S, Ery-Derm, Erygel, Erythrogel, ETS (CAN), Sans-Acne (CAN), Staticin	To treat inflammatory acne vulgaris	Apply to affected areas once or twice daily (morning and evening).
erythromycin 3% and benzoyl peroxide 5% Benzamycin	To treat moderate inflammatory acne vulgaris	Apply to affected areas twice daily, morning and evening.
gentamicin sulfate Garamycin, G-myticin	To prevent or treat superficial skin infections due to susceptible bacteria; to treat superficial burns	Apply small amount to skin in affected area three or four times a day.

GENERIC AND TRADE NAMES	INDICATIONS	USUAL ADULT DOSAGES
Antibacterials *(continued)*		
mafenide acetate Sulfamylon	As adjunct to treat second- and third-degree burns	Apply 1/16-in layer aseptically to affected areas once or twice daily.
metronidazole 0.75%, 1% MetroCream, MetroGel, MetroGel-Vaginal, MetroLotion, Noritate	To treat inflammatory papules and pustules of acne rosacea	Apply thin film to affected area once or twice daily (morning and evening).
	To treat bacterial vaginosis	1 applicatorful (37.5 mg) intravaginally at bedtime or twice daily for 5 days.
minocycline 1.5% Zilxi	To treat inflammatory lesions of rosacea	Apply topical foam over all areas of the face once daily, gently rub into skin
mupirocin 2% Bactroban, Bactroban Cream, Bactroban Nasal, Bactroban Ointment, Centany Nasal	To treat impetigo due to *Staphylococcus aureus* and *Streptococcus pyogenes*	Apply to affected areas three times a day up to 10 days.
	To treat secondary infections of traumatic skin lesions due to *S. aureus* and *S. pyogenes*	Apply thin film and cover with a gauze dressing three times a day for 10 days.
	To eradicate nasal colonization of methicillin-resistant *S. aureus*	Apply half of the contents of a unit-dose tube to each nostril twice daily for 5 days.
neomycin sulfate Myciguent	To prevent or treat superficial bacterial infections	Rub fingertip-size dose into affected area once daily to three times a day for no more than 1 week.
ozenoxacin Xepi	To treat impetigo due to *Staphylococcus aureus* or *Streptococcus pyogenes*	Apply thin layer to affected area (not exceeding 100 cm^2) twice daily for 5 days.
povidone-iodine 0.75%, 10% Betadine, Betadine Cream, Betadine Spray	To disinfect wounds and burns	Apply or spray to affected area, as needed.
	To prepare skin for surgical incision	Wet skin with water, then apply 1 cc/20–30 sq inches using 7.5% solution. Lather and scrub site for 5 minutes, then rinse. Follow with 10% solution painted on skin and allowed to dry.
silver sulfadiazine 1% Flamazine (CAN), Silvadene, Thermazine	To prevent and treat wound sepsis in second- and third-degree burns	Apply 1/16-in layer aseptically once to twice daily to clean debrided burns; reapply promptly if removed.
sulfacetamide sodium 10% Klaron	To treat acne vulgaris	Apply thin film twice daily.

(continues)

Selected Topical Drugs *(continued)*

GENERIC AND TRADE NAMES	INDICATIONS	USUAL ADULT DOSAGES
Antifungals		
butenafine hydrochloride 1% Lotrimin Ultra, Mentax	To treat tinea corporis, tinea cruris, or tinea versicolor	Apply to affected surrounding area once daily for 2 wk.
Lotrimin Ultra, Mentax	To treat interdigital tinea pedis due to *Epidermophyton floccosum, Trichophyton mentagrophytes,* or *T. rubrum*	Apply to affected and immediately surrounding area once daily for 4 wk or twice daily for 1 wk.
butoconazole nitrate 2% Femstat 3	To treat vulvovaginal mycotic infections caused by *Candida* species	1 applicatorful (100 mg) intravaginally at bedtime for 3 days.
Gynazole-1	To treat vulvovaginal infections caused by *Candida albicans*	1 applicatorful (100 mg) intravaginally once anytime day or night; may repeat course for total of 6 days in pregnant women (second and third trimester only).
ciclopirox olamine Loprox Cream 0.77%	To treat candidiasis, tinea corporis, tinea cruris, tinea pedis, and tinea versicolor	Massage gently into affected and surrounding area twice daily, morning and evening.
Loprox Shampoo 1%	To treat seborrheic dermatitis	Apply 5 ml to scalp (10 ml for long hair), lather and leave on scalp for 3 minutes, then rinse. Repeat twice weekly for 4 weeks with minimum of 3 days between applications.
ciclopirox olamine 8% Penlac	To treat onychomycosis of the fingernails and toenails	Apply evenly to entire nail surface and surrounding 5 mm of skin at bedtime for up to 48 wk.
clotrimazole Canesten (CAN), Desenex, Femcare, FungiCURE, Fungoid, Gyne-Lotrimin, Lotrimin, Mycelex, Trivagizole	To treat superficial fungal infections (tinea corporis, tinea cruris, tinea pedis, tinea versicolor, candidiasis)	Apply thin film and massage into affected and surrounding area twice daily, morning and evening, for 2 to 8 wk.
	To treat vulvovaginal candidiasis	Insert 100-mg vaginal tablet at bedtime for 7 days; or 500-mg vaginal tablet at bedtime for 1 day; or 1 applicatorful intravaginally at bedtime for 7 days (or 3 days if using Trivagizole).
	To treat oropharyngeal candidiasis	Dissolve oral troche over 15 to 30 min 5 times/day for 14 days.
	To prevent oropharyngeal candidiasis	Dissolve oral troche over 15 to 30 min three times a day for duration of chemotherapy or until corticosteroid dosage is reduced to maintenance levels.

GENERIC AND TRADE NAMES	INDICATIONS	USUAL ADULT DOSAGES
Antifungals *(continued)*		
econazole nitrate 1% Ecostatin (CAN)	To treat tinea corporis, tinea cruris, tinea pedis, tinea versicolor	Rub into affected area once or twice daily for at least 2 wk (4 wk for tinea pedis).
	To treat cutaneous candidiasis	Rub into affected area twice daily (morning and evening) for 2 wk.
Ecoza	To treat interdigital tinea pedis	Apply to affected areas once daily for 4 wk.
efinaconazole 10% Jublia	To treat onychomycosis of the toenail(s) due to *Trichophyton rubrum* and *Trichophyton mentagrophytes*	Apply solution to affected toenail(s) once daily for 48 wk using the integrated flow-through brush applicator.
gentian violet 1%, 2%	To treat candidiasis	Apply 1% solution to affected area two or three times daily for 3 days.
	To help protect against skin infection in minor burns, cuts, or scrapes	Apply small amount of 2% solution to affected area once to three times daily.
ketoconazole 1%, 2% Ketozole, Nizoral	To treat tinea corporis, tinea cruris, tinea pedis, and tinea versicolor due to susceptible organisms; to treat cutaneous candidiasis	Apply thin film to affected and immediately surrounding area daily for at least 2 wk (6 wk for tinea pedis).
Ketozole Shampoo 2%, Nizoral AD Shampoo 1% Extina 2%, Xolegel 2%	To treat tinea versicolor	Apply Nizoral AD Shampoo 1% to wet hair, lather, massage for 1 min, leave drug on scalp for 3 min, then rinse and repeat 2 times/wk for 4 up to 8 wk (with at least 3 days between shampoos), then intermittently, as needed. Alternatively, apply Ketozole Shampoo 2% one time only to wet hair, lather, massage for 1 min, leave drug on scalp for 5 min, then rinse.
	To treat seborrheic dermatitis	Apply to affected and immediately surrounding area twice daily for 4 wk.
luliconazole 1% Luzu	To treat interdigital tinea pedis	Apply to affected area and about 1 in of the immediate surrounding area(s) once daily for 2 wk.
	To treat tinea cruris and tinea corporis	Apply to affected area and about 1 in of the immediate surrounding area(s) once daily for 1 wk.

(continues)

Selected Topical Drugs *(continued)*

GENERIC AND TRADE NAMES	INDICATIONS	USUAL ADULT DOSAGES
Antifungals *(continued)*		
miconazole nitrate 2% Fungoid, Micatin, Monistat 1, Monistat 3, Monistat 7, Zeasorb-AF	To treat tinea corporis, tinea cruris, tinea pedis; cutaneous candidiasis; and common dermatophyte infections	Apply cream sparingly (or powder or spray liberally) over affected area twice daily for 2 wk (4 wk for tinea corporis and tinea pedis).
	To treat tinea versicolor	Apply sparingly to affected area daily for 2 wk.
	To treat vulvovaginal candidiasis	Insert into vaginal canal at bedtime for 7 days (100 mg), repeated, as needed; insert 200-mg strength into vaginal canal at bedtime for 3 days; or insert 1,200-mg strength into vaginal canal as a single treatment.
	To treat onychomycosis	Brush tincture on affected areas of nail surface, beds, and edges and under nail surface once or twice daily for up to several months; or spray on clean, dry, affected nails, holding actuator down for 1 or 2 sec once or twice daily.
naftifine hydrochloride 2% Naftin	To treat tinea corporis, tinea cruris, and interdigital tinea pedis	Apply to affected area and 1/2-in margin surrounding area once daily for 2 wk.
nystatin Nadostine (CAN), Nilstat, Nystop	To treat cutaneous and muco-cutaneous infections due to *Candida albicans*	Apply cream to affected area twice daily or as indicated; or apply powder twice daily or three times a day.
oxiconazole nitrate Oxistat, Oxizold (CAN)	To treat tinea corporis, tinea cruris, and tinea pedis	Apply to affected and surrounding area once or twice daily for 2 wk (4 wk for tinea pedis).
	To treat tinea versicolor	Apply cream to affected and surrounding area daily for 2 wk.
selenium sulfide 1%, 2.5% Selsun, Versel (CAN)	To treat tinea versicolor	Apply to scalp, lather with small amount of water, wait 10 min, then rinse, once daily for 7 days.
	To treat dandruff and seborrheic scalp dermatitis	Massage into wet scalp, wait 2 to 3 min, rinse, and repeat 2 times/wk for 2 wk, then once daily for 2, 3, or 4 wk.
sertaconazole nitrate 2% Ertaczo	To treat interdigital tinea pedis caused by *Epidermophyton floccosum, Trichophyton mentagrophytes,* and *Trichophyton rubrum*	Apply to affected areas both between the toes and the immediately surrounding healthy skin twice daily for 4 wk.
sulconazole nitrate 1% Exelderm	To treat tinea corporis, tinea cruris, and tinea versicolor	Massage small amount gently into affected and surrounding areas once or twice daily (tinea pedis) for 3 wk.

GENERIC AND TRADE NAMES	INDICATIONS	USUAL ADULT DOSAGES
Antifungals (continued)		
tavaborole Kerydin	To treat onychomycosis of the toenails due to *Trichophyton mentagrophytes* or *Trichophyton rubrum*	Apply to affected toenails, including under the tip of each toenail, once daily for 48 wk.
terbinafine hydrochloride 1% Lamisil	To treat tinea versicolor	Apply to affected area twice daily for 1 or 2 wk.
	To treat tinea corporis and tinea cruris	Apply thin film to affected area once or twice daily for 1 wk.
	To treat interdigital tinea pedis	Apply between the toes twice daily for 1 wk (interdigital tinea pedis) or to affected area daily for 1 wk.
	To treat tinea pedis involving bottom or sides of feet	Apply to affected area twice daily (morning and evening) for 2 wk.
terconazole 0.4%, 0.8% Terazol 3, Terazol 7	To treat vulvovaginal candidiasis	1 applicatorful (20 mg) intravaginally at bedtime for 3 days (0.4%) or 1 applicatorful (40 mg) for 7 days (0.8%); or insert 80-mg vaginal suppository at bedtime for 3 consecutive days.
tioconazole GyneCure Ovules (CAN), Vagistat-1	To treat vulvovaginal candidiasis	Insert 1 applicatorful (300 mg) or 1 suppository (300 mg) intravaginally at bedtime as a single dose.
tolnaftate 1% Absorbine Footcare, Aftate for Athlete's Foot, Aftate for Jock Itch, Dr. Scholl's Athlete's Foot, Genaspore, NP-27, Pitrex, Quinsana Plus, Tinactin, Ting, Zeasorb-AF	To treat tinea corporis, tinea cruris, tinea manuum, tinea pedis, and tinea versicolor	Apply to affected and surrounding areas twice daily, morning and evening, for 4 wk (2 wk for tinea cruris); continue for 2 wk after symptoms subside or up to 6 wk.
Antivirals		
acyclovir 5% Zovirax	To treat initial genital herpes and selectively for non-life-threatening mucocutaneous herpes simplex in immunocompromised patients	Apply ointment every 3 hr (6 times/day) for 7 days. Use finger cot, rubber glove, or applicator stick for both forms to prevent herpetic whitlow.
	To treat herpes labialis in immunocompetent patients	Apply cream to affected area 5 times a day for 4 days.
docosanol 10% Abreva	To treat recurrent herpes labialis of lips and face	Apply cream gently and completely to affected area five times daily, starting with first visible sign of lesion and continuing until lesion is healed.
penciclovir 1% Denavir	To treat recurrent herpes labialis of lips and face	Apply every 2 hr while awake for 4 days.

(continues)

Selected Topical Drugs *(continued)*

GENERIC AND TRADE NAMES	INDICATIONS	USUAL ADULT DOSAGES
Corticosteroids		
alclometasone dipropionate 0.05% Aclovate	To relieve inflammatory and pruritic manifestations of corticosteroid-responsive dermatoses	Apply thin film to affected area and massage twice daily to three times a day.
amcinonide 0.01% Cyclocort	To relieve inflammatory and pruritic manifestations of corticosteroid-responsive dermatoses	Apply thin film to affected area and massage twice daily (lotion) or twice daily to three times a day (cream, ointment).
betamethasone benzoate 0.05% Beben (CAN), Uticort	To relieve inflammatory and pruritic manifestations of corticosteroid-responsive dermatoses	Apply thin film or a few drops to affected area once or twice daily up to 45 g/wk (ointment, cream), 50 g/wk (gel), or 50 ml (lotion).
betamethasone dipropionate 0.05% Diprolene, Diprolene AF, Diprosone, Topilene (CAN)	To relieve inflammatory and pruritic manifestations of corticosteroid-responsive dermatoses	Apply thin film or a few drops to affected area once or twice daily.
betamethasone valerate 0.1% Betatrex, Beta-Val, Luxiq, Valisone	To relieve inflammatory and pruritic manifestations of corticosteroid-responsive dermatoses	Apply foam to scalp, and massage until foam disappears, twice daily (morning and evening). Apply thin film of cream or ointment 1 to 3 times daily. Apply a few drops of lotion twice daily (morning and evening).
clobetasol propionate 0.025% Impoyz	To treat moderate to severe plaque psoriasis	Apply thin layer to affected skin and rub in gently twice daily, up to 50 g/wk for 2 wk.
clobetasol propionate 0.05% Dermovate (CAN), Embeline, Temovate	To relieve inflammatory and pruritic manifestations of corticosteroid-responsive dermatoses	Apply thin film to affected area and rub in gently twice daily (morning and evening), up to 50 g/wk, for 2 wk.
Olux	To relieve moderate to severe inflammatory and pruritic manifestations of corticosteroid-responsive dermatoses of scalp	Apply to affected area of scalp twice daily, once in morning and once at night, up to 50 g/wk, for 2 wk.
desonide 0.05% DesOwen, Tridesilon, Verdeso	To relieve inflammatory and pruritic manifestations of corticosteroid-responsive dermatoses	Apply thin film to affected area twice daily to four times a day.
desoximetasone 0.05% Topicort	To relieve inflammatory and pruritic manifestations of corticosteroid-responsive dermatoses	Apply thin film to affected skin areas twice daily.
desoximetasone 0.25% Topicort spray	To treat plaque psoriasis	Spray a thin film on to affected skin areas twice daily (rub in gently) for no more than 4 weeks.

GENERIC AND TRADE NAMES	INDICATIONS	USUAL ADULT DOSAGES
Corticosteroids *(continued)*		
diflorasone diacetate 0.05% Florone, Psorcon	To relieve inflammatory and pruritic manifestations of corticosteroid-responsive dermatoses	Apply thin film to affected area once daily to four times a day.
fluocinolone acetonide 0.01% Derma Smooth FS, Fluoderm (CAN), Fluolar (CAN), Fluonid (CAN), Synalar, Synamol (CAN)	To relieve inflammatory and pruritic manifestations of corticosteroid-responsive dermatoses	Apply thin film to affected area twice daily to four times a day.
	To treat seborrheic dermatoses	Use shampoo on scalp daily.
	To treat scalp psoriasis	Apply oil to affected areas on scalp and leave overnight.
fluocinonide 0.05% Lidemol (CAN), Lidex	To relieve inflammatory and pruritic manifestations of corticosteroid-responsive dermatoses	Apply thin film to affected area twice daily to four times a day.
flurandrenolide Cordran 0.05%, Cordran Tape, Drenison 0.05% (CAN)	To relieve inflammatory and pruritic manifestations of corticosteroid-responsive dermatoses	Apply thin film to affected area and massage twice daily to three times a day; or apply tape every 12 to 24 hr.
fluticasone propionate 0.05% Cutivate	To treat atopic dermatitis; to relieve inflammatory and pruritic manifestations of corticosteroid-responsive dermatoses	Apply thin film once or twice daily (atopic dermatitis) or twice daily (dermatoses).
halcinonide 0.1% Halog	To relieve inflammatory and pruritic manifestations of corticosteroid-responsive dermatoses	Apply sparingly and massage two to three times a day.
halobetasol propionate 0.05% Lexette, Ultravate	To treat plaque psoriasis	Apply thin film to affected area and rub in gently twice daily, up to 50 g/wk, for 2 wk.
halobetasol propionate 0.01% Bryhali		Apply thin layer to affected area and rub in gently once daily, up to 50 g/wk and for no longer than 8 wk.
halobetasol propionate 0.01% and tazarotene 0.045% Duobrii	To treat plaque psoriasis	Apply thin layer once daily to cover only affected areas and rub in gently.

(continues)

Selected Topical Drugs *(continued)*

GENERIC AND TRADE NAMES	INDICATIONS	USUAL ADULT DOSAGES
Corticosteroids *(continued)*		
hydrocortisone 0.25% Cetacort	To relieve inflammatory and pruritic manifestations of corticosteroid-responsive dermatoses	Apply thin film (aerosol foam, cream, lotion, ointment, solution) to affected area once daily to four times a day.
hydrocortisone 0.5% Cetacort, Cortate (CAN), Delacort, Dermtex HC, Emo-Cort (CAN), Hydro-Tex		
hydrocortisone 1% Ala-Cort, Cort-Dome, Cortizone 10, Emo-Cort (CAN), Nutracort, Synacort		
hydrocortisone 2% Ala-Scalp HP, Dermasorb HC		
hydrocortisone 2.5% Anusol-HC, Emo-Cort (CAN), Hytone, Nutracort, Stie-Cort, Synacort, Texacort		
hydrocortisone acetate 0.1% Corticreme (CAN)		
hydrocortisone acetate 0.5% Corticaine, Cortacet (CAN), Cortoderm (CAN), Hyderm, Lanacort, Novo-Hydrocort (CAN)		
hydrocortisone acetate 1%, 2%, 2.5% Cortaid, Corticreme (CAN), Cortoderm (CAN), Hyderm (CAN), Maximum Strength Cortaid, Micort HC-Lipocream, Novo-Hydrocort (CAN)	To relieve inflammatory and pruritic manifestations of corticosteroid-responsive dermatoses	Apply thin film (aerosol foam, cream, lotion, ointment, solution) to affected area once daily to four times a day.
hydrocortisone acetate 1% and pramoxine hydrochloride 1% topical aerosol foam Epifoam		
hydrocortisone butyrate 0.1% Locoid	To relieve inflammatory and pruritic manifestations of corticosteroid-responsive dermatoses	Apply to affected area twice daily to three times a day.
hydrocortisone probutate 0.1% Pandel		Apply to affected area once or twice daily.
hydrocortisone valerate 0.2% Westcort		Apply to affected area two to three times daily.

GENERIC AND TRADE NAMES	INDICATIONS	USUAL ADULT DOSAGES
Corticosteroids (continued)		
hydrocortisone acetate, polymyxin B sulfate, and neomycin sulfate Cortisporin	To treat corticosteroid-responsive dermatoses (short term) with mild bacterial infection	Apply sparingly and massage twice daily to four times a day.
mometasone furoate 0.1% Elocom (CAN), Elocon	To relieve inflammatory and pruritic manifestations of corticosteroid-responsive dermatoses	Apply thin film or a few drops to affected area daily.
prednicarbate 0.1% Dermatop	To relieve inflammatory and pruritic manifestations of corticosteroid-responsive dermatoses	Apply thin film to affected area twice daily.
triamcinolone acetonide 0.025%, 0.5% Aristocort, Aristocort A, Aristocort D (CAN), Kenalog, Triacet, Triaderm (CAN), Trianide Mild (CAN)	To relieve inflammatory and pruritic manifestations of corticosteroid-responsive dermatoses	Apply thin film of 0.025% to affected area twice daily to four times a day; apply 0.1% or 0.5% two to three times daily.
triamcinolone acetonide 0.1% Aristocort, Aristocort A, Aristocort R (CAN), Delta-Tritex, Flutex, Kenac, Kenalog, Kenalog-H, Triacet, Triaderm (CAN), Trianide Regular (CAN) **triamcinolone acetonide 0.5%** Aristocort, Aristocort A, Aristocort C (CAN), Flutex, Kenalog, Triacet	To relieve inflammatory and pruritic manifestations of corticosteroid-responsive dermatoses	Apply thin film (cream) to affected area twice daily to four times a day; 0.025% lotion or ointment once or twice daily; 0.1% lotion or ointment once daily; or 0.5% ointment once daily.
triamcinolone acetonide topical aerosol 0.2% Kenalog	To relieve inflammatory and pruritic manifestations of corticosteroid-responsive dermatoses	Spray affected area three times a day to four times a day.
Retinoids		
adapalene 0.1% Differin	To treat acne vulgaris	Apply thin film to affected area at bedtime.
tazarotene 0.1% Avage	As adjunct to treat mitigation of facial fine wrinkling, facial mottled hyper- and hypopigmentation, and benign facial lentigines	Apply pea-size amount to affected area at bedtime.

(continues)

Selected Topical Drugs *(continued)*

GENERIC AND TRADE NAMES	INDICATIONS	USUAL ADULT DOSAGES
Retinoids *(continued)*		
tazarotene 0.05%, 0.1% Avage, Tazorac	To treat acne; to treat mild to moderately severe facial acne vulgaris	Apply thin film to affected area at bedtime.
tazarotene 0.1% Fabior	To treat acne vulgaris	Apply thin layer to affected areas of the face and upper trunk once daily in the evening.
tazarotene 0.045% Arazlo	To treat moderate to severe acne vulgaris	Apply a thin layer to affected areas once daily.
tretinoin 0.025% Avita, Renova, Retin-A, Retin-A Micro, Stieva-A (CAN), Tretin-X **tretinoin 0.05%** Altreno	To treat acne vulgaris	Apply pea-size amount to clean, dry affected area at bedtime.
tretinoin and benzoyl peroxide 0.1%, 3% Twyneo	To treat acne vulgaris	Apply a thin layer to affected areas once daily.
trifarotene 0.005% Aklief	To treat acne vulgaris	Apply thin layer to affected areas of the face and/or trunk once daily in the evening.
Miscellaneous topical drugs		
abametapir 0.74% Xeglyze	To treat head lice	Apply to dry hair in amount sufficient to coat the hair and scalp thoroughly; leave on for 10 minutes, then rinse off with water.
adapalene 0.1% and benzoyl peroxide 2.5% gel Epiduo **adapalene 0.3% and benzoyl peroxide 2.5% gel** Epiduo Forte	To treat acne vulgaris	Apply pea-size amount to each clean, dry affected area once daily.
ammonium lactate 12% Lac-Hydrin	To treat dry, scaly skin and ichthyosis vulgaris	Apply to affected area, and rub in twice daily.
anthralin Anthranol 1 (CAN), Anthranol 2 (CAN), Anthranol 3 (CAN), Anthrascalp (CAN), Drithocreme, Dritho-Scalp, Psoriatec, Zithranol, Zithranol-RR	To treat chronic psoriasis To treat chronic scalp psoriasis	Apply sparingly and massage into affected lesions daily. Apply to lesions daily for 1 wk.
becaplermin Regranex	To treat lower-extremity diabetic neuropathic ulcers that extend into the subcutaneous tissue or beyond and that have an adequate blood supply	Amount applied to ulcers daily calculated based on size of ulcer.

GENERIC AND TRADE NAMES	INDICATIONS	USUAL ADULT DOSAGES
Miscellaneous topical drugs *(continued)*		
brimonidine 0.33% Mirvaso	To treat rosacea	Apply pea-sized amount onto each of the five areas of the face once daily. Do not apply to eyes or lips.
calcipotriene 0.005% Dovonex, Sorilux	To treat plaque psoriasis	Apply cream or scalp lotion in a thin layer twice daily up to 8 wk. Apply thin layer of ointment once or twice daily up to 8 wk.
calcipotriene hydrate 0.005% and betamethasone dipropionate 0.064% Taclonex	To treat plaque psoriasis	Apply suspension to affected areas and rub in gently once daily for up to 8 wk.
Taclonex Scalp	To treat moderate to severe plaque psoriasis of the scalp	Apply suspension to affected scalp areas and rub in gently once daily for 2 to 8 wk or until skin clears.
	To treat psoriasis vulgaris	Apply ointment to affected skin; rub in gently and completely once daily for up to 4 wk.
capsaicin 0.025%, 0.075%, 0.1% Capsin, Zostrix	To provide temporary pain relief from rheumatoid arthritis and osteoarthritis; to relieve neuralgias from pain following shingles (herpes zoster) infection	Apply to affected area no more than four times a day.
chlorhexidine gluconate 4% Betasept, Hibiclens	To clean skin wounds	Rinse area, apply minimal amount to cover, then wash and rinse thoroughly.
	To prepare skin for surgical incision	Apply liberally to surgical site and swab for at least 2 minutes. Dry with sterile towel and repeat once.
clascoterone 1% Winlevi	To treat acne vulgaris	Apply thin uniform layer of cream twice daily, in morning and evening, to affected areas
clotrimazole and betamethasone dipropionate 0.05%/1% Lotrisone	To treat symptomatic inflammatory tinea corporis, tinea cruris, and tinea pedis	Apply thin layer and massage cream gently into affected and surrounding skin areas twice daily for 2 wk (tinea corporis, tinea cruris) or for 4 wk (tinea pedis).
coal tar Denorex, Pentrax, Zetar, Zetar Shampoo	To treat psoriasis	Add 15 to 20 ml to lukewarm bath, immerse affected area for 15 to 20 min, and rinse thoroughly 3 to 7 times/wk.
	To treat dandruff or scalp seborrhea	Massage into wet scalp, rinse, repeat application and wait 5 min, then rinse again.

(continues)

Selected Topical Drugs *(continued)*

Miscellaneous topical drugs *(continued)*

GENERIC AND TRADE NAMES	INDICATIONS	USUAL ADULT DOSAGES
crisaborole 2% Eucrisa	To treat mild to moderate atopic dermatitis	Apply thin layer of ointment twice daily to affected areas
crotamiton 10% Eurax	To treat scabies	Massage into cleansed body from chin to soles of feet, and reapply after 24 hr; change bed linens next day, and bathe 48 hr after second dose; repeat in 7 to 10 days if new lesions appear.
	To treat symptomatic pruritic skin	Massage gently into affected areas until absorbed. Repeat as needed.
desoximetasone 0.05% Topicort	To relieve inflammatory and pruritic manifestations of corticosteroid-responsive dermatoses	Apply thin film twice daily to affected areas.
diclofenac sodium 1% Voltaren	To treat osteoarthritis pain	Apply 2.25 inches (2 grams) for upper body areas and 4.5 inches (4 grams) for lower body area of gel to affected area four times daily, every day.
diclofenac sodium 3% Solaraze	To treat actinic keratoses	Massage gel gently onto affected lesion areas twice daily for 60 to 90 days.
doxepin hydrochloride 5% Zonalon	To treat moderate pruritus associated with atopic dermatitis and chronic lichen simplex	Apply thin film to affected area four times a day (every 3 to 4 hr) for up to 8 days.
eflornithine hydrochloride 13.9% Vaniqa	To retard unwanted hair growth	Apply thin film to affected area of face and chin twice daily (at least 8 hr apart); don't wash treated area for at least 4 hr.
fluocinolone acetonide 0.01%, hydroquinone 4%, tretinoin 0.05% TRI-LUMA Cream	To treat severe facial melasma	Apply a thin film lightly and uniformly to hyperpigmented areas of melasma including about 1/2 in of skin surrounding each lesion daily at least 30 min before bedtime.
fluorouracil cream Carac 0.5% Efudex 2%, 5%	To treat actinic and solar keratoses of face and anterior scalp	Apply to lesions twice daily for 4 wk.
	To treat actinic or solar keratosis	Apply to lesions twice daily for 2 to 4 wk.
	To treat superficial basal cell carcinoma	Apply 5% preparation twice daily in sufficient amounts to cover lesions for up to 12 wks.
Fluoroplex 1%	To treat actinic or solar keratosis	Apply to lesions twice daily for 2 to 6 wk.

GENERIC AND TRADE NAMES	INDICATIONS	USUAL ADULT DOSAGES
Miscellaneous topical drugs *(continued)*		
glycopyrronium 2.4% Qbrexza	To treat primary axillary hyperhidrosis	Apply once daily to both axillae using a single cloth.
hexachlorophene 3% Phisohex	To use as a surgical scrub	Wet hands and forearms with water, apply 5 ml of solution and rub into a copious lather for 3 min, then rinse; repeat once.
	To use for bacteriostatic cleansing	Wet hands with water, pour 5 ml into palm and work up a lather, then apply to area to be cleaned. Rinse thoroughly.
hydrocortisone acetate 1%, polymyxin B sulfate, bacitracin zinc, and neomycin sulfate Cortisporin	To treat corticosteroid-responsive dermatoses associated with secondary bacterial infection	Apply small amount to affected areas twice daily to four times a day for up to 7 days.
hydroquinone Claripel 4%, Eldopaque 2%, Eldoquin 2% and 4%, Melanex 3%	To treat hyperpigmentation and melanin	Apply twice daily to the affected areas for no longer than 2 mo.
imiquimod 2.5%, 3.75% Zyclara	To treat facial or scalp actinic keratoses	Apply 2.5% or 3.75% to affected area daily for two 2-wk treatment cycles separated by a 2-wk no-treatment period.
	To treat external genital and perianal warts	Apply 3.75% cream to the external genital and perianal warts until total clearance or up to 8 wk.
imiquimod 5% Aldara	To treat external genital and perianal warts	Apply thin layer to affected area and rub in 3 times/wk at bedtime for up to 16 wk; remove with soap and water after 6 to 10 hr.
	To treat actinic keratosis on face and scalp	Apply to affected area on face or scalp (but not both concurrently) for 16 wk.
	To treat superficial basal cell carcinoma	Apply to affected area 5 times per wk for 6 wk prior to bedtime and leave on skin for about 8 hrs, then wash area with mild soap and water.
ingenol mebutate 0.015%, 0.05% Picato	To treat actinic keratosis	Apply 0.015% gel to face and scalp once daily for 3 consecutive days; apply 0.05% gel to trunk and extremities once daily for 2 consecutive days.

(continues)

Selected Topical Drugs (continued)

GENERIC AND TRADE NAMES	INDICATIONS	USUAL ADULT DOSAGES
Miscellaneous topical drugs (continued)		
ivermectin 0.5% Sklice	To treat head lice	Apply to dry hair in amount sufficient to coat the hair and scalp thoroughly; leave on for 10 minutes, then rinse off with water.
ivermectin 1% Soolantra	To treat inflammatory lesions of rosacea	Apply pea-sized amount for each affected area of the face (chin, each cheek, forehead) once daily.
lidocaine 2.5% and prilocaine 2.5% EMLA	For local anesthesia	Apply 1 disk or thick layer of 2- to 2.5-g cream occlusively for at least 1 hr before the start of routine procedure or 2 hr before the start of painful procedure.
malathion 0.5% Ovide	To treat pediculus humanus capitis (head lice and their ova) of scalp hair	Apply to dry hair in amount just sufficient to wet the hair and scalp thoroughly; then let hair dry naturally. After 8 to 12 hr, shampoo and rinse hair and use a fine-toothed comb to remove dead lice and eggs. If lice are still present after 7 to 9 days, repeat application.
mequinol 2%, tretinoin 0.01% Solage	To treat solar lentigines	Apply solution twice daily, morning and evening, at least 8 hr apart. Avoid application to surrounding skin, and do not bathe for 6 hr after application.
nitroglycerin 0.4% Rectiv	To treat moderate to severe pain associated with chronic anal fissure	Apply 1 in of ointment intra-anally every 12 hr for up to 3 wk.
oxybutynin chloride 10% Gelnique	To treat overactive bladder with symptoms of urge urinary incontinence, urgency, and frequency	Apply 1 sachet of gel or 1 activation of metered-dose pump once daily to clean, dry, intact skin on abdomen, upper arms/shoulders, or thighs.
permethrin 1% Nix	To prevent or treat head lice	Wash and dry hair, saturate scalp, leave on hair for 10 min, then rinse; remove nits with provided comb; repeat in 7 days if living mites are still present.
permethrin 5% Acticin, Elimite	To treat scabies	Massage into skin from head to soles of feet, and remove after 8 to 10 hr; repeat in 14 days if living mites are still present.

GENERIC AND TRADE NAMES	INDICATIONS	USUAL ADULT DOSAGES
Miscellaneous topical drugs *(continued)*		
pimecrolimus 1% Elidel	To treat mild to moderate atopic dermatitis as a second-line therapy	Apply to affected areas twice daily for up to 6 wk.
podofilox 0.5% Condylox	To treat anogenital warts (gel)	Apply gel to anogenital warts for 3 days, then withhold for 4 days; repeat cycle up to four times.
	To treat external genital warts (gel or solution)	Apply gel or solution to external genital warts every 12 hr in the morning and evening for 3 days, then withhold for 4 days; repeat cycle up to four times.
pyrethrin and piperonyl butoxide Licide, Pronto, RID	To treat body, head, and pubic lice	Apply to dry hair or affected body area. Massage through all hairy areas until hair is wet. Leave on hair for 10 min; then wash with warm water and rinse thoroughly. Repeat in 7 to 10 days.
ruxolitinib 1.5% Opzelura	To treat mild to moderate atopic dermatitis in non-immunocompromised patients	Apply thin layer to affected areas of up to 20% body surface area. *Maximum:* 60 g/wk
spinosad 0.9% Natroba	To treat head lice	Apply to dry scalp and hair using only the amount needed to cover the scalp and hair. Rinse off with warm water after 10 min. Repeat in 7 days if live lice are still seen.
tacrolimus 0.03% and 0.1% Protopic	To treat moderate to severe atopic dermatitis in patients unresponsive to other therapies	Apply thin layer to affected areas twice daily, rubbing in gently and completely.
tirbanibulin 1% Klisyri	To treat actinic keratosis of face or scalp	Apply to affected area(s) once daily for 5 consecutive days.
urea 41%, 45% Utopic	To treat hyperkeratotic conditions	Apply to affected area twice daily and rub in.

Selected Combination Antiviral Drugs

Combination antiviral drugs are used to treat viral infections, such as human immunodeficiency virus (HIV) and hepatitis C infections.

The following table lists the generic and trade names, indications, and usual adult dosages for some commonly used combination antivirals. Although you must individualize your care for a patient who receives an antiviral, be sure to include these general interventions in your plan of care:

- Avoid administering HIV drugs all at once.
- If patient takes an antacid, administer it 1 hour before or 2 hours after an antiviral because antacids may reduce antiviral absorption.
- Monitor hepatic enzyme levels to detect elevations and help prevent hepatotoxicity.
- Monitor BUN and serum creatinine levels to detect signs of impaired renal function.
- Monitor I.V. injection site for pain or phlebitis, which may result from the high pH of reconstituted solutions.
- Assess the immunosuppressed patient for opportunistic infections during antiviral therapy.
- Inform female patient that oral contraceptives may be ineffective when taken with HIV drugs. Suggest alternate contraceptive methods.

GENERIC AND TRADE NAMES	INDICATIONS	USUAL ADULT DOSAGES
Antivirals used for HIV infection		
abacavir sulfate, dolutegravir, and lamivudine Triumeq	To treat HIV-1 infection	600 mg abacavir, 50 mg dolutegravir, and 300 mg lamivudine (1 tablet) P.O. once daily
abacavir sulfate and lamivudine Epzicom	As adjunct to treat HIV-1 infection	600 mg abacavir and 300 mg lamivudine (1 tablet) P.O. daily
abacavir sulfate, lamivudine, and zidovudine Trizivir	As adjunct or as monotherapy to treat HIV-1 infection	300 mg abacavir, 150 mg lamivudine, and 300 mg zidovudine (1 tablet) P.O. twice daily
atazanavir sulfate and cobicistat Evotaz	As adjunct to treat HIV-1 infection	300 mg atazanavir and 150 mg cobicistat (1 tablet) P.O. once daily
bictegravir sodium, emtricitabine, and tenofovir alafenamide Biktarvy	To treat HIV-1 infection	50 mg bictegravir, 200 mg emtricitabine, and 25 mg tenofovir alafenamide (1 tablet) P.O. once daily.
cabotegravir and rilpivirine Cabenuva	To treat HIV-1 infection in adults and adolescents weighing at least 35 kg (77 lb)	*Initial:* 600 mg of cabotegravir and 900 mg of rilpivirine I.M. given on last day of current antiretroviral therapy or oral lead-in, if used. *Maintenance:* 400 mg of cabotegravir and 600 mg of rilpivirine I.M. monthly. Alternatively, 600 mg cabotegravir and 900 mg rilpivirine I.M. given 1 month apart for 2 consecutive months followed by same dosage every 2 months.
darunavir and cobicistat Prezcobix	As adjunct to treat HIV-1 infection	800 mg darunavir and 150 mg cobicistat (1 tablet) P.O. once daily

GENERIC AND TRADE NAMES	INDICATIONS	USUAL ADULT DOSAGES
Antivirals used for HIV infection *(continued)*		
darunavir, cobicistat, emtricitabine, and tenofovir alafenamide Symtuza	To treat HIV-1 infection	800 mg darunavir, 150 mg cobicistat, 200 mg emtricitabine, and 10 mg tenofovir alafenamide (1 tablet) P.O. once daily.
dolutegravir sodium and lamivudine Dovato	To treat HIV-1 infection	50 mg dolutegravir and 300 mg lamivudine (1 tablet) P.O. once daily
dolutegravir and rilpivirine Juluca	To treat HIV-1 infection	50 mg dolutegravir and 25 mg rilpivirine (1 tablet) P.O. once daily with a meal
doravirine, lamivudine, and tenofovir disoproxil fumarate Delstrigo	To treat HIV-1 infection	100 mg doravirine, 300 mg lamivudine, and 300 mg tenofovir disoproxil fumarate (1 tablet) P.O. once daily
efavirenz, emtricitabine, and tenofovir disoproxil fumarate Atripla	As adjunct or monotherapy to treat HIV-1 infection in adults weighing at least 40 kg (88 lb) or more	600 mg efavirenz, 200 mg emtricitabine, and 300 mg tenofovir disoproxil fumarate (1 tablet) P.O. once daily, at bedtime
efavirenz, lamivudine, and tenofovir disoproxil fumarate Symfi Symfi Lo	To treat HIV-1 infection in patients weighing at least 40 kg (88 lb) or more To treat HIV-1 infection in adults and children weighing at least 35 kg (77 lb)	600 mg efavirenz, 300 mg lamivudine, and 300 mg tenofovir disoproxil fumarate (1 tablet) P.O. once daily 400 mg efavirenz, 300 mg lamivudine, and 300 mg tenofovir disoproxil fumarate (1 tablet) P.O. once daily
elbasvir and grazoprevir Zepatier	To treat chronic hepatitis C virus (HCV), genotype 1 or 4 infection in adults and children 12 years of age and older weighing at least 30 kg (66 lb)	50 mg elbasvir and 100 mg grazoprevir (1 tablet) P.O. once daily
elvitegravir, cobicistat, emtricitabine, tenofovir alafenamide Genvoya	To treat HIV-1 infection	150 mg elvitegravir, 150 mg cobicistat, 200 mg emtricitabine, and 10 mg tenofovir alafenamide (1 tablet) once daily
elvitegravir, cobicistat, emtricitabine, tenofovir disoproxil fumarate Stribild	To treat HIV-1 infection	150 mg elvitegravir, 150 mg cobicistat, 200 mg emtricitabine, 300 mg tenofovir (1 tablet) P.O. once daily with food
emtricitabine, rilpivirine, tenofovir disoproxil fumarate Complera	To treat HIV-1 infection	200 mg emtricitabine, 25 mg rilpivirine, 300 mg tenofovir (1 tablet) P.O. daily with meal

(continues)

Selected Combination Antiviral Drugs *(continued)*

GENERIC AND TRADE NAMES	INDICATIONS	USUAL ADULT DOSAGES
Antivirals used for HIV infection *(continued)*		
emtricitabine, rilpivirine, tenofovir alafenamide fumarate Odefsey	To treat HIV-1 infection	200 mg emtricitabine, 25 mg rilpivirine, and 25 mg tenofovir alafenamide (1 tablet) P.O. once daily
emtricitabine and tenofovir alafenamide Descovy	To treat HIV-1 infection	200 mg emtricitabine and 25 mg tenofovir alafenamide (1 tablet) P.O. once daily in combination with other antiretrovirals
emtricitabine and tenofovir disoproxil fumarate Truvada	As adjunct to treat HIV-1 infection in patients weighing at least 17 kg (37.4 lb)	*Weighing at least 35 kg (77 lb):* 200 mg emtricitabine and 300 mg tenofovir disoproxil fumarate (1 tablet) P.O. once daily *Weighing 28 kg (61.6 lb) to less than 35 kg (77 lb):* 167 mg emtricitabine and 250 mg tenofovir disoproxil fumarate (1 tablet) P.O. once daily *Weighing 22 kg (48.4 lb) to less than 28 kg (61.6 lb):* 133 mg emtricitabine, 200 mg tenofovir disoproxil fumarate (1 tablet) P.O. once daily *Weighing 17 kg (37.4 lb) to less than 22 (48.4 lb):* 100 mg emtricitabine and 150 mg tenofovir disoproxil fumarate (1 tablet) P.O. once daily
lamivudine and raltegravir Dutrebis	As adjunct to treat HIV-1 infection	150 mg lamivudine and 300 mg raltegravir (1 tablet) P.O. twice daily
lamivudine and tenofovir disoproxil fumarate Cimduo	As adjunct to treat HIV-1 infection in patients weighing 35 kg (77 lb) or more	300 mg lamivudine and 300 mg tenofovir disoproxil fumarate (1 tablet) P.O. once daily
lamivudine and zidovudine (3TC/AZT, 3TC/ZDV) Combivir	As adjunct to treat HIV-1 infection in patients who weigh 50 kg (110 lb) or more	150 mg of lamivudine and 300 mg of zidovudine P.O. twice daily
lopinavir and ritonavir Kaletra	As adjunct to treat HIV-1 infection	800 mg lopinavir and 200 mg ritonavir once daily or 400 mg lopinavir and 100 mg ritonavir P.O. twice daily
Antivirals used for hepatitis C infection		
dasabuvir, ombitasvir, paritaprevir, and ritonavir Viekira XR	To treat chronic hepatitis C virus genotype 1b infection without cirrhosis or with compensated cirrhosis	600 mg dasabuvir, 24.99 mg ombitasvir, 150 mg paritaprevir, and 99.99 mg ritonavir (3 ER tablets) P.O. once daily.
elbasvir and grazoprevir Zepatier	To treat chronic hepatitis C with genotype 1 or 4	50 mg elbasvir and 100 mg grazoprevir (1 tablet) P.O. once daily

GENERIC AND TRADE NAMES	INDICATIONS	USUAL ADULT DOSAGES
Antivirals used for hepatitis C infection *(continued)*		
glecaprevir and pibrentasvir Mavyret	To treat chronic HCV genotype 1, 2, 3, 4, 5, or 6 without cirrhosis or with compensated cirrhosis; to treat HCV genotype 1 infection in patients previously treated with a regimen containing an HCV NS5A inhibitor or an NS3/4A protease inhibitor, but not both	300 mg glecaprevir and 120 mg pibrentasvir (3 tablets) P.O. once daily for 8 weeks (HCV genotype 1, 2, 3, 4, 5, or 6 with no cirrhosis or compensated cirrhosis); 12 weeks (HCV genotype 1 with previous treatment with an NS3/4/4A protease inhibitor without prior treatment with an NS5A inhibitor); 16 weeks (HCV genotype 1 with an NS5A inhibitor without prior treatment with an NS3/4A protease inhibitor)
ledipasvir and sofosbuvir Harvoni	To treat chronic hepatitis C genotype 1, 4, 5, or 6 in patients without cirrhosis or with compensated cirrhosis; as adjunct to treat chronic hepatitis C genotype 1 in patients with decompensated cirrhosis or genotype 1 or 4 in liver transplant recipients without cirrhosis or compensated cirrhosis	90 mg ledipasvir and 400 mg sofosbuvir (1 tablet) P.O. once daily
ombitasvir, paritaprevir, and ritonavir Technivie	As adjunct to treat chronic hepatitis C genotype 4 in patients without cirrhosis	25 mg ombitasvir, 150 mg paritaprevir, and 100 mg ritonavir (2 tablets) P.O. once daily in morning
sofosbuvir and velpatasvir Epclusa	To treat chronic hepatitis C genotype 1, 2, 3, 4, 5, or 6 in patients with compensated cirrhosis or without cirrhosis, or with decompensated cirrhosis when used in combination with ribavirin	400 mg sofosbuvir and 100 mg velpatasvir (1 tablet) P.O. once daily for 12 wk (adults); dosage based on weight and given once daily for 12 wk (children age 3 years and older)
sofosbuvir, velpatasvir, and voxilaprevir Vosevi	To treat chronic hepatitis C genotype 1, 2, 3, 4, 5, or 6 in patients with compensated cirrhosis or without cirrhosis in patients previously treated with an HCV regimen containing an NS5A inhibitor or genotype 1a or 3 infection previously treated with an HCV regimen containing sofosbuvir without an NS5A inhibitor	400 mg sofosbuvir, 100 mg velpatasvir, and 100 mg voxilaprevir (1 tablet) P.O. once daily

Common Cancers and Antineoplastic Drug Therapy

Antineoplastic drugs are commonly used in the treatment of many types of cancer today. Most of these drugs work by inhibiting cell proliferation, which leads to cell death. They're most effective at killing actively dividing cells.

Cell-specific antineoplastics exert their actions during one or more phases of the cell cycle. S-phase antineoplastics interfere with deoxyribonucleic acid (DNA) synthesis; M-phase drugs interfere with the formation of microtubules and disrupt mitosis.

Most antineoplastics impair DNA in one of the following four ways:
- preventing separation of DNA strands
- inhibiting DNA repair
- mimicking DNA bases
- disrupting the triplicate codons or producing oxygen-free radicals that damage the DNA.

Antineoplastic drugs are cytotoxic, which means that they affect both neoplastic cells and normal cells. As a result, they may cause serious and sometimes life-threatening adverse reactions.

Antineoplastics are most harmful to normal cells that exhibit rapid activity and growth, such as bone marrow tissue, the epithelium of the GI mucosa, and hair follicles. When these drugs suppress bone marrow activity, the patient may develop leukopenia, thrombocytopenia, or anemia. When they affect the GI mucosa, the patient may experience nausea, vomiting, anorexia, bowel dysfunction, and mucosal ulcerations. When antineoplastic drugs affect the hair follicles, the result is hair loss (alopecia), one of the most common adverse reactions.

Although not life-threatening, hair loss can be emotionally traumatic for patients, especially women. However, the recent FDA approval of scalp-cooling caps to spare hair loss as a result of chemotherapy can help to prevent baldness in many patients.

The following chart lists the most common cancers (excluding nonmelanoma skin cancers) in the order of prevalence according to the American Cancer Society. The most common type of cancer for women is breast cancer and the most common type of cancer for men is prostate cancer.

The antineoplastic drugs that may be used initially to treat these common cancers are listed under each cancer type. Adult dosages for these cancers are usually based on body weight in kilograms and subsequent dosages are adjusted according to the type and severity of adverse reactions that have occurred during the last cycle. Antineoplastic therapy is given in cycles of a certain number of days or weeks based on protocol for that type of cancer and the patient's reaction to the drugs given during the previous cycle. For example, if the patient experiences bone marrow suppression from the previous cycle, the degree of suppression will determine if the antineoplastic drug regimen is withheld until the blood counts improve or the dosages of the drugs used are decreased.

It is imperative that the nurse monitor patients receiving antineoplastic therapy closely for adverse reactions, because reactions can occur suddenly and can often become serious or life-threatening quickly.

CANCER TYPE	COMMON ANTINEOPLASTIC DRUG THERAPY
Breast cancer	▪ Anthracyclines: Examples include doxorubicin (Adriamycin) and epirubicin (Ellence) ▪ Taxanes: Examples include paclitaxel (Taxol) and docetaxel (Taxotere) ▪ 5-fluorouracil (5-FU) ▪ carboplatin (Paraplatin) ▪ cyclophosphamide (Cytoxan) Combinations of 2 or 3 of these drugs are most often administered. Advanced breast cancer ▪ Anthracyclines: Examples include doxorubicin (Adriamycin), epirubicin (Ellence), and pegylated liposomal doxorubicin (Doxil) ▪ Platinum agents: Examples include carboplatin (Paraplatin) and cisplatin (Platinol, Platinol-AQ) ▪ Taxanes: Examples include albumin-bound paclitaxel (Abraxane), docetaxel (Taxotere), and paclitaxel (Taxol) ▪ capecitabine (Xeloda) ▪ eribulin (Halaven) ▪ gemcitabine (Gemzar) ▪ ixabepilone (Ixempra) ▪ nab-paclitaxel (Abraxane) ▪ vinorelbine (Navelbine) Most often, advanced breast cancer is treated with a single antineoplastic agent, although a combination such as carboplatin plus paclitaxel may be administered depending on the clinical status of the patient.
Prostate cancer	▪ cabazitaxel (Jevtana) ▪ docetaxel (Taxotere) ▪ estramustine (Emcyt) ▪ mitoxantrone (Novantrone)
Lung cancer	▪ carboplatin (Paraplatin) ▪ cisplatin (Platinol, Platinol-AQ) ▪ docetaxel (Taxotere) ▪ doxorubicin (Adriamycin) ▪ etoposide (VePesid, VP-16) ▪ gemcitabine (Gemzar) ▪ paclitaxel (Taxol) ▪ pemetrexed (Alimta) ▪ vinorelbine (Navelbine) Various combinations of these drugs are often administered.
Colorectal cancer	▪ 5-fluorouracil (5-FU) ▪ capecitabine (Xeloda) ▪ irinotecan (Camptosar) ▪ oxaliplatin (Eloxatin) ▪ trifluridine and tipiracil (Lonsurf) Combinations of 2 or more of these drugs are often administered.

(continues)

Common Cancers and Antineoplastic Drug Therapy (continued)

CANCER TYPE	COMMON ANTINEOPLASTIC DRUG THERAPY
Melanoma	<ul><li>carboplatin (Paraplatin)</li><li>cisplatin (Platinol, Platinol-AQ)</li><li>dacarbazine (DTIC)</li><li>nab-paclitaxel (Abraxane)</li><li>paclitaxel (Taxol)</li><li>temozolomide (Temodar)</li><li>vinblastine (Alkaban-AQ, Velban)</li></ul>
Bladder cancer	Used with radiation:<ul><li>5-fluorouracil (5-FU)</li><li>cisplatin (Platinol, Platinol-AQ)</li><li>mitomycin (Mitomycin-C, MTC)</li></ul>Used without radiation:<ul><li>carboplatin (Paraplatin)</li><li>cisplatin (Platinol, Platinol-AQ)</li><li>docetaxel (Taxotere)</li><li>doxorubicin (Adriamycin)</li><li>gemcitabine (Gemzar)</li><li>methotrexate (MTX, Otrexup, Trexall)</li><li>paclitaxel (Taxol)</li><li>vinblastine (Alkaban-AQ, Velban)</li></ul>Combinations such as carboplatin and either paclitaxel or docetaxel (for patients with poor kidney function); cisplatin and gemcitabine; methotrexate, vinblastine, doxorubicin, and cisplatin (called MVAC); or cisplatin, methotrexate, and vinblastine (called CMV) may be used. However, if adverse reactions are severe, single drugs as listed earlier may have to be administered instead.
Lymphoma (Non-Hodgkin)	<ul><li>cyclophosphamide (Cytoxan, Neosar)</li><li>doxorubicin (Adriamycin)</li><li>vincristine (Oncovin, Vincasar)</li></ul>
Kidney (renal cell) cancer	Antineoplastic drugs are usually not effective in treating kidney cancer and are not standard treatment. However, the following drugs may be used after targeted drugs and/or immunotherapy have already been tried.<ul><li>5-fluorouracil (5-FU)</li><li>capecitabine (Xeloda)</li><li>floxuridine (FUDR)</li><li>gemcitabine (Gemzar)</li><li>vinblastine (Alkaban-AQ, Velban)</li></ul>

CANCER TYPE	COMMON ANTINEOPLASTIC DRUG THERAPY
Acute myeloid leukemia	<ul><li>cytarabine (Cytosar-U)</li><li>daunorubicin (Cerubidine)</li><li>idarubicin (Idamycin)</li><li>mitoxantrone (Novantrone, OTN Mitoxantrone)</li></ul> Additional antineoplastic drugs that may be used include: <ul><li>6-mercaptopurine (6-MP, Purinethol)</li><li>6-thioguanine (6-TG, Tabloid)</li><li>azacitidine (Vidaza)</li><li>cladribine (Leustatin, 2-CdA)</li><li>decitabine (Dacogen)</li><li>etoposide (VePesid, VP-16)</li><li>fludarabine (Fludara)</li><li>hydroxyurea (Hydrea)</li><li>methotrexate (MTX, Otrexup, Trexall)</li><li>topotecan (Hycamtin)</li></ul>
Endometrial cancer	<ul><li>carboplatin (Paraplatin)</li><li>doxorubicin (Adriamycin)</li><li>liposomal doxorubicin (Doxil)</li><li>paclitaxel (Taxol)</li></ul>

Selected Antihypertensive Combinations

Antihypertensive drugs are used along with lifestyle changes to manage hypertension. Antihypertensive combinations, which commonly include one or two antihypertensives and a diuretic, are used to simplify patients' drug regimens and, in some cases, to enhance drug actions.

The table below lists the generic and trade names; functional classes; usual adult dosages;

ANTIHYPERTENSIVE COMBINATION TRADE NAMES	ANTIHYPERTENSIVE GENERIC NAMES	DIURETIC GENERIC NAMES
Aldoril-15	methyldopa 250 mg	hydrochlorothiazide (HCTZ) 15 mg
Aldoril-25	methyldopa 250 mg	HCTZ 25 mg
Aldoril D30	methyldopa 500 mg	HCTZ 30 mg
Aldoril D50	methyldopa 500 mg	HCTZ 50 mg
Amturnide 150/5/12.5	aliskiren 150 mg, amlodipine 5 mg	HCTZ 12.5 mg
Amturnide 300/5/12.5	aliskiren 300 mg, amlodipine 5 mg	HCTZ 12.5 mg
Amturnide 300/5/25	aliskiren 300 mg, amlodipine 5 mg	HCTZ 25 mg
Amturnide 300/10/12.5	aliskiren 300 mg, amlodipine 10 mg	HCTZ 12.5 mg
Amturnide 300/10/25	aliskiren 300 mg, amlodipine 10 mg	HCTZ 25 mg
Apresazide 25/25	hydralazine hydrochloride (HCL) 25 mg	HCTZ 25 mg
Apresazide 50/50	hydralazine HCl 50 mg	HCTZ 50 mg
Apresazide 100/50	hydralazine HCl 100 mg	HCTZ 50 mg
Atacand HCT 16/12.5	candesartan cilexetil 16 mg	HCTZ 12.5 mg
Atacand HCT 32/12.5	candesartan cilexetil 32 mg	HCTZ 12.5 mg
Atacand HCT 32/25	candesartan cilexetil 32 mg	HCTZ 25 mg
Avalide-150	irbesartan 150 mg	HCTZ 12.5 mg
Avalide-300	irbesartan 300 mg	HCTZ 12.5 mg
Azor 5/20	amlodipine 5 mg, olmesartan 20 mg	None
Azor 5/40	amlodipine 5 mg, olmesartan 40 mg	
Azor 10/20	amlodipine 10 mg, olmesartan 20 mg	
Azor 10/40	amlodipine 10 mg, olmesartan 40 mg	
Benicar HCT 20/12.5	olmesartan medoxomil 20 mg	HCTZ 12.5 mg
Benicar HCT 40/12.5	olmesartan medoxomil 40 mg	HCTZ 12.5 mg
Benicar HCT 40/25	olmesartan medoxomil 40 mg	HCTZ 25 mg
Capozide 25/15	captopril 25 mg	HCTZ 15 mg
Capozide 25/25	captopril 25 mg	HCTZ 25 mg
Capozide 50/15	captopril 50 mg	HCTZ 15 mg
Capozide 50/25	captopril 50 mg	HCTZ 25 mg
Diovan HCT 80/12.5	valsartan 80 mg	HCTZ 12.5 mg
Diovan HCT 160/12.5	valsartan 160 mg	HCTZ 12.5 mg
Diovan HCT 160/25	valsartan 160 mg	HCTZ 25 mg
Diovan HCT 320/12.5	valsartan 320 mg	HCTZ 12.5 mg
Diovan HCT 320/25	valsartan 320 mg	HCTZ 25 mg
Dyazide 37.5/25	triamterene 37.5 mg	HCTZ 25 mg

and onset, peak, and duration for commonly used antihypertensive combinations. For information about the mechanisms of action, interactions, adverse reactions, and nursing considerations related to antihypertensive combinations, review the entries for the specific antihypertensives and diuretics that they contain.

FUNCTIONAL CLASSES	USUAL ADULT DOSAGES	ONSET, PEAK, AND DURATION
Centrally acting anti-adrenergic and thiazide diuretic	1 tab twice daily or three times daily 1 tab twice daily 1 tab daily 1 tab daily	**Onset:** Unknown **Peak:** 4 to 6 hr **Duration:** 12 to 24 hr
Direct renin inhibitor, calcium channel blocker, and thiazide diuretic	1 tab once daily 1 tab once daily 1 tab once daily 1 tab once daily 1 tab once daily	**Onset:** Unknown **Peak:** 3 to 8 hr **Duration:** Unknown
Peripherally acting arterial dilator and thiazide diuretic	1 cap once or twice daily 1 cap once or twice daily 1 cap once or twice daily	**Onset:** 20 to 30 min **Peak:** 1 to 2 hr **Duration:** 2 to 4 hr
Angiotensin II receptor antagonist and thiazide diuretic	1 tab once or twice daily 1 tab daily 1 tab daily	**Onset:** 1 to 2 wk **Peak:** Within 4 wk **Duration:** Unknown
ACE inhibitor and thiazide diuretic	1 tab daily 1 tab daily	**Onset:** Unknown **Peak:** Unknown **Duration:** Unknown
Calcium channel blocker and angiotensin II receptor antagonist	1 tab daily 1 tab daily 1 tab daily 1 tab daily	**Onset:** Unknown **Peak:** 1 to 6 hr **Duration:** 24 hr
Angiotensin II receptor antagonist and thiazide diuretic	1 tab daily 1 tab daily 1 tab daily	**Onset:** Unknown **Peak:** Unknown **Duration:** Unknown
ACE inhibitor and thiazide diuretic	1 tab daily to three times a day 1 tab once or twice daily 1 tab once daily to three times a day 1 tab once or twice daily	**Onset:** 15 to 60 min **Peak:** 60 to 90 min **Duration:** 6 to 12 hr
Angiotensin II receptor blocker and thiazide diuretic	1 or 2 tabs daily 1 tab daily 1 tab daily 1 tab daily 1 tab daily	**Onset:** 2 hr **Peak:** 6 hr **Duration:** 24 hr
Potassium-sparing diuretic and thiazide diuretic	1 or 2 caps or tabs daily	**Onset:** 2 to 4 hr **Peak:** 1 day **Duration:** 7 to 9 hr

(continues)

Selected Antihypertensive Combinations *(continued)*

ANTIHYPERTENSIVE COMBINATION TRADE NAMES	ANTIHYPERTENSIVE GENERIC NAMES	DIURETIC GENERIC NAMES
Edarbyclor 40/12.5 Edarbyclor 40/25	azilsartan 40 mg azilsartan 40 mg	chlorthalidone 12.5 mg chlorthalidone 25 mg
Exforge 5/160 Exforge 10/160 Exforge 5/320 Exforge 10/320	amlodipine 5 mg, valsartan 160 mg amlodipine 10 mg, valsartan 160 mg amlodipine 5 mg, valsartan 320 mg amlodipine 10 mg, valsartan 320 mg	None
Exforge HCT 5/160/12.5 Exforge HCT 10/160/12.5 Exforge HCT 5/160/25 Exforge HCT 10/160/25 Exforge HCT 10/320/25	amlodipine 5 mg, valsartan 160 mg amlodipine 10 mg, valsartan 160 mg amlodipine 5 mg, valsartan 160 mg amlodipine 10 mg, valsartan 160 mg amlodipine 10 mg, valsartan 320 mg	HCTZ 12.5 mg HCTZ 12.5 mg HCTZ 25 mg HCTZ 25 mg HCTZ 25 mg
Hyzaar 50/12.5 Hyzaar 100/12.5 Hyzaar 100/25	losartan potassium 50 mg losartan potassium 100 mg losartan potassium 100 mg	HCTZ 12.5 mg HCTZ 12.5 mg HCTZ 25 mg
Inderide 40/25 Inderide 80/25 Inderide LA 80/50 Inderide LA 120/50 Inderide LA 160/50	propranolol HCL 40 mg propranolol HCl 80 mg propranolol HCl 80 mg propranolol HCl 120 mg propranolol HCl 160 mg	HCTZ 25 mg HCTZ 25 mg HCTZ 50 mg HCTZ 50 mg HCTZ 50 mg
Lopressor HCT 50/25 Lopressor HCT 100/25 Lopressor HCT 100/50	metoprolol tartrate 50 mg metoprolol tartrate 100 mg metoprolol tartrate 100 mg	HCTZ 25 mg HCTZ 25 mg HCTZ 50 mg
Lotensin HCT 5/6.25 Lotensin HCT 10/12.5 Lotensin HCT 20/12.5 Lotensin HCT 20/25	benazepril HCl 5 mg benazepril HCl 10 mg benazepril HCl 20 mg benazepril HCl 20 mg	HCTZ 6.25 mg HCTZ 12.5 mg HCTZ 12.5 mg HCTZ 25 mg
Lotrel 2.5/10 Lotrel 5/10 Lotrel 5/20 Lotrel 5/40 Lotrel 10/20 Lotrel 10/40	amlodipine 2.5 mg, benazepril HCl 10 mg amlodipine 5 mg, benazepril HCl 10 mg amlodipine 5 mg, benazepril HCl 20 mg amlodipine 5 mg, benazepril 40 mg amlodipine 10 mg, benazepril HCl 20 mg amlodipine 10 mg, benazepril 40 mg	None None None None None None
Maxzide-25 37.5/25 Maxzide 75/50	triamterene 37.5 mg triamterene 75 mg	HCTZ 25 mg HCTZ 50 mg
Micardis HCT 40/12.5 Micardis HCT 80/12.5 Micardis HCT 80/25	telmisartan 40 mg telmisartan 80 mg telmisartan 80 mg	HCTZ 12.5 mg HCTZ 12.5 mg HCTZ 25 mg

FUNCTIONAL CLASSES	USUAL ADULT DOSAGES	ONSET, PEAK, AND DURATION
ACE inhibitor and thiazide-like diuretic	1 tab daily 1 tab daily	**Onset:** Unknown **Peak:** 6 hr **Duration:** 24 hr
Calcium channel blocker and angiotensin II receptor blocker	1 or 2 tabs daily 1 tab daily 1 tab daily 1 tab daily	**Onset:** Unknown **Peak:** 6 to 12 hr **Duration:** 24 hr
Calcium channel blocker, angiotensin II receptor blocker, and thiazide diuretic	1 tab daily 1 tab daily 1 tab daily 1 tab daily 1 tab daily	**Onset:** Unknown **Peak:** 2 to 6 hr **Duration:** Unknown
Angiotensin II receptor blocker and thiazide diuretic	1 or 2 tabs daily 1 tab daily 1 tab daily	**Onset:** Unknown **Peak:** 6 hr **Duration:** 24 hr or more
Beta blocker and thiazide diuretic	1 or 2 tabs twice daily 1 or 2 tabs twice daily 1 cap daily 1 cap daily 1 cap daily	**Onset:** Unknown **Peak:** 1 to 1.5 hr **Duration:** Unknown
Beta blocker and thiazide diuretic	2 tabs daily or 1 tab twice daily 1 or 2 tabs daily or 1 tab twice daily 2 tabs daily or 1 tab twice daily	**Onset:** 1 hr **Peak:** 1 to 2 hr **Duration:** Unknown
ACE inhibitor and thiazide diuretic	1 tab daily 1 tab daily 1 tab daily 1 tab daily	**Onset:** 1 hr **Peak:** 2 to 4 hr **Duration:** 24 hr
Calcium channel blocker and ACE inhibitor	1 or 2 caps daily 1 cap daily 1 cap daily 1 cap daily 1 cap daily 1 cap daily	**Onset:** Unknown **Peak:** Unknown **Duration:** 24 hr
Potassium-sparing diuretic and thiazide diuretic	1 tab daily 1 tab daily	**Onset:** 2 to 4 hr **Peak:** 1 day **Duration:** 7 to 9 hr
Angiotensin II receptor antagonist and thiazide diuretic	1 tab once or twice daily 1 tab once or twice daily 1 tab once daily	**Onset:** Within 3 hr **Peak:** In 4 wk **Duration:** Several days to 1 wk

(continues)

Selected Antihypertensive Combinations *(continued)*

ANTIHYPERTENSIVE COMBINATION TRADE NAMES	ANTIHYPERTENSIVE GENERIC NAMES	DIURETIC GENERIC NAMES
Moduretic	amiloride 5 mg	HCTZ 50 mg
Prinzide 10/12.5 Prinzide 20/12.5	lisinopril 10 mg lisinopril 20 mg	HCTZ 12.5 mg HCTZ 12.5 mg
Tekamlo 150/5 Tekamlo 150/10 Tekamlo 300/5 Tekamlo 300/10	aliskiren 150 mg, amlodipine 5 mg aliskiren 150 mg, amlodipine 10 mg aliskiren 300 mg, amlodipine 5 mg aliskiren 300 mg, amlodipine 10 mg	None None None None
Tekturna HCT 150/12.5 Tekturna HCT 150/25 Tekturna HCT 300/12.5 Tekturna HCT 300/25	aliskiren 150 mg aliskiren 150 mg aliskiren 300 mg aliskiren 300 mg	HCTZ 12.5 mg HCTZ 25 mg HCTZ 12.5 mg HCTZ 25 mg
Timolide 10/25	timolol maleate 10 mg	HCTZ 25 mg
Tribenzor 20/5/12.5 Tribenzor 40/5/12.5 Tribenzor 40/5/25 Tribenzor 40/10/12.5 Tribenzor 40/10/25	amlodipine 5 mg, olmesartan 20 mg amlodipine 5 mg, olmesartan 40 mg amlodipine 5 mg, olmesartan 40 mg amlodipine 10 mg, olmesartan 40 mg amlodipine 10 mg, olmesartan 40 mg	HCTZ 12.5 mg HCTZ 12.5 mg HCTZ 25 mg HCTZ 12.5 mg HCTZ 25 mg
Twynsta 40/5 Twynsta 40/10 Twynsta 80/5 Twynsta 80/10	telmisartan 40 mg, amlodipine 5 mg telmisartan 40 mg, amlodipine 10 mg telmisartan 80 mg, amlodipine 5 mg telmisartan 80 mg, amlodipine 10 mg	None None None None
Uniretic 7.5/12.5 Uniretic 15/12.5 Uniretic 15/25	moexipril HCL 7.5 mg moexipril 15 mg moexipril HCl 15 mg	HCTZ 12.5 mg HCTZ 12.5 mg HCTZ 25 mg
Valturna 150/160 Valturna 300/320	aliskiren 150 mg, valsartan 160 mg aliskiren 300 mg, valsartan 320 mg	None None
Vaseretic 10/25	enalapril maleate 10 mg	HCTZ 25 mg
Zestoretic 10/12.5 Zestoretic 20/12.5 Zestoretic 20/25	lisinopril 10 mg lisinopril 20 mg lisinopril 20 mg	HCTZ 12.5 mg HCTZ 12.5 mg HCTZ 25 mg
Ziac 2.5/6.25 Ziac 5/6.25 Ziac 10/6.25	bisoprolol fumarate 2.5 mg bisoprolol fumarate 5 mg bisoprolol fumarate 10 mg	HCTZ 6.25 mg HCTZ 6.25 mg HCTZ 6.25 mg

FUNCTIONAL CLASSES	USUAL ADULT DOSAGES	ONSET, PEAK, AND DURATION
Potassium-sparing diuretic and thiazide diuretic	1 or 2 tabs daily	**Onset:** 2 hr **Peak:** 6 to 10 hr **Duration:** 24 hr
ACE inhibitor and thiazide diuretic	1 or 2 tabs daily 1 or 2 tabs daily	**Onset:** 1 hr **Peak:** 6 hr **Duration:** 24 hr
Direct renin inhibitor and calcium channel blocker	1 or 2 tabs daily 1 tab daily 1 tab daily 1 tab daily	**Onset:** Unknown **Peak:** 3 to 8 hr **Duration:** 24 hr
Direct renin inhibitor and thiazide diuretic	1 tab daily 1 tab daily 1 tab daily 1 tab daily	**Onset:** Unknown **Peak:** 1 to 2.5 hr **Duration:** Unknown
Beta blocker and thiazide diuretic	2 tabs daily or 1 tab twice daily	**Onset:** Unknown **Peak:** 1 to 2 hr **Duration:** Unknown
Angiotensin II receptor antagonist, calcium channel blocker, and thiazide diuretic	1 tab daily 1 tab daily 1 tab daily 1 tab daily 1 tab daily	**Onset:** Unknown **Peak:** 1 to 6 hr **Duration:** 24 hr
Angiotensin II receptor antagonist and calcium channel blocker	1 tab daily 1 tab daily 1 tab daily 1 tab daily	**Onset:** Unknown **Peak:** 1 to 6 hr **Duration:** Unknown
Potassium-sparing diuretic and thiazide diuretic	1 tab daily 1 tab daily 1 tab daily	**Onset:** 1 hr **Peak:** 3 to 6 hr **Duration:** 24 hr
Direct renin inhibitor and angiotensin II antagonist	1 tab daily 1 tab daily	**Onset:** Unknown **Peak:** 1 to 3 hr **Duration:** Unknown
ACE inhibitor and thiazide diuretic	1 tab once or twice daily	**Onset:** 1 hr **Peak:** 4 to 6 hr **Duration:** 24 hr
ACE inhibitor and thiazide diuretic	1 or 2 tabs daily 1 or 2 tabs daily 1 or 2 tabs daily	**Onset:** 1 hr **Peak:** 6 hr **Duration:** 24 hr
Beta blocker and thiazide diuretic	1 or 2 tabs daily 1 or 2 tabs daily 1 or 2 tabs daily	**Onset:** Unknown **Peak:** Unknown **Duration:** Unknown

Selected Obstetrical Drugs

Obstetrical drugs are used during pregnancy for a variety of reasons, such as control of nausea and vomiting, pain relief, and assistance in the labor and delivery process. Drugs used to control nausea and vomiting throughout pregnancy and analgesics used to provide pain relief, especially during the labor and delivery process, are covered in the main section of the *Nurse's Drug Handbook*. While other drugs may be used during pregnancy, not all have FDA approval for such use. For example, misoprostol, a synthetic prostaglandin, is used to treat ulcers. However, it may also be used for indications not approved by the FDA, such as assisting in the termination of a pregnancy, evacuation of the uterine contents in a missed abortion, and dilating the cervix prior to labor. These uses are considered "off-label" uses because they have not been FDA approved. In adherence with the standard of only including FDA-approved indications in the *Nurse's Drug Handbook*, following are selected obstetrical drugs that are FDA approved for use with pregnancy issues.

GENERIC NAME AND TRADE NAME	INDICATIONS	ADULT DOSAGES
dinoprostone Cervidil, Prepidil, Prostin E$_2$	Initiation and/or continuation of cervical ripening in patients at or near term in whom there is a medical or obstetrical indication for the induction of labor	10 mg intravaginally designed to release 0.3 mg/hr of the drug over a 12-hr period; removed upon onset of active labor or 12 hr after insertion
hydroxyprogesterone caproate Makena	To reduce risk of preterm birth in women who are carrying only one fetus and who have a history of singleton spontaneous preterm birth	250 mg (1 ml) I.M. once weekly begun between 16 wk, 0 days and 20 wk, 6 days of gestation and continued weekly until wk 37 or delivery, whichever comes first
oxytocin Pitocin	To initiate or improve uterine contractions in situations where there are fetal or maternal concerns, so as to achieve a vaginal delivery	*Initial:* 0.5 mU (milliunits)/min to 1 mU/min I.V., increased in increments of 1 to 2 mU/min every 30 to 60 min, as needed; once desired frequency of contractions has been reached and labor has progressed to 5 to 6 cm dilation, dosage may be decreased by 1 to 2 mU/min every 30 to 60 min

GENERIC NAME AND TRADE NAME	INDICATIONS	ADULT DOSAGES
	To produce uterine contractions during the third stage of labor and to control postpartum bleeding or hemorrhage	10 to 40 units added to existing intravenous solution being infused (maximum 40 units to 1,000 ml of solution) and infused at a rate to sustain uterine contraction and control atony
		Alternatively, 10 units (1 ml) I.M. after delivery of placenta
	To treat incomplete, inevitable, or elective abortion	*Initial:* I.V. infusion rate highly individualized (10 units mixed in 500 ml of saline or 5% dextrose-in-water solution)
		Maximum: 30 units in a 12-hr period
ulipristal acetate ELLA	To prevent pregnancy following unprotected intercourse or contraceptive failure	30 mg (1 tablet) as soon as possible within 120 hours (5 days) after unprotected intercourse or contraceptive failure

Vitamins

As you know, an adequate daily intake of vitamins is essential to vital bodily functions, such as embryonic development (vitamin A), regulation of serum calcium and phosphate (vitamin D), and blood clotting (vitamin K).

Vitamins are classified as one of two types: fat soluble (vitamins A, D, E, and K) and water soluble (vitamin C and all forms of vitamin B). Fat-soluble vitamins can accumulate in body tissue over time; when excessive amounts are ingested through diet or supplementation, severe and life-threatening toxicity can develop. Water-soluble vitamins don't accumulate in the body; they are excreted daily so that

GENERIC AND TRADE NAMES	RECOMMENDED DAILY INTAKE
vitamin A (retinol) Aquasol A	*Adult men and boys over age 10.* 1,000 mcg/day. *Adult women and girls over age 10.* 800 mcg/day. *Pregnant women.* 800 mcg/day. (900 mcg/day [CAN].) *Breastfeeding women.* 1,200 to 1,300 mcg/day. (1,200 mcg/day [CAN].) *Children ages 7 to 10.* 700 mcg/day. (700 to 800 mcg/day [CAN].) *Children ages 4 to 7.* 500 mcg/day. *Neonates and children to age 4.* 375 to 400 mcg/day. (400 mcg/day [CAN].)
vitamin B₁ (thiamine hydrochloride) Betaxin (CAN), Bewon (CAN), Biamine	*Adult men and boys over age 10.* 1.2 to 1.5 mg/day. (0.8 to 1.3 mg/day [CAN].) *Adult women and girls over age 10.* 1 to 1.1 mg/day. (0.8 to 0.9 mg/day [CAN].) *Pregnant women.* 1.5 mg/day. (0.9 to 1 mg/day [CAN].) *Breastfeeding women.* 1.6 mg/day. (1 to 1.2 mg/ day [CAN].)

toxicity is not usually a concern with excessive intake.

The following chart lists the generic and trade names of fat-soluble and water-soluble vitamins, the recommended daily intake to prevent vitamin deficiency, dosages when deficiency occurs, other indications and dosages for vitamin therapy, and guidelines for parenteral administration of vitamins.

OTHER INDICATIONS AND DOSAGES	PARENTERAL ADMINISTRATION GUIDELINES
TO TREAT VITAMIN A DEFICIENCY CAPSULES, ORAL SOLUTION, TABLETS **_Adults and adolescents._** Dosage individualized based on severity of deficiency, as prescribed. I.M. INJECTION **_Adults and children age 8 and over._** 15,000 to 30,000 retinol equivalent (RE)/day (50,000 to 100,000 IU/day) for 3 days, followed by 15,000 RE/day (50,000 IU/day) for 2 wk. **_Children ages 1 to 8._** 1,500 to 4,500 RE/day (5,000 to 15,000 IU/day) for 10 days; for severe deficiency, 5,250 to 10,500 RE/day (17,500 to 35,000 IU/day) for 10 days. **_Infants to age 1 year._** 1,500 to 3,000 RE/day (5,000 to 10,000 IU/day) for 10 days; for severe deficiency, 2,250 to 4,500 RE/day (7,500 to 15,000 IU/day) for 10 days. I.V. INFUSION **_Adults and children._** Dosage individualized as part of total parenteral nutrition solution, as prescribed. **_TO TREAT XEROPHTHALMIA_** CAPSULES, ORAL SOLUTION, TABLETS **_Children age 1 and over._** 60,000 RE (200,000 IU) as a single dose. Dose repeated on day 2 and again in 4 wk. **_Children ages 6 months to 1 year._** 30,000 RE (100,000 IU) as a single dose. Dose repeated on day 2 and again in 4 wk. **_AS AN ADJUNCT TO TREAT MEASLES_** CAPSULES, ORAL SOLUTION, TABLETS **_Children age 1 and over._** 60,000 RE (200,000 IU) as a single dose when measles are diagnosed. **_Children ages 6 months to 1 year._** 30,000 RE (100,000 IU) as a single dose when measles are diagnosed.	▪ Be aware that anaphylaxis and death have occurred after I.V. administration of vitamin A; I.V. administration is restricted to special solutions, such as in total parenteral nutrition solution. Typically, parenteral administration of vitamin A is by I.M. injection. ▪ Take precautions to protect vitamin A solution from exposure to light because it's light sensitive.
TO TREAT VITAMIN B$_1$ DEFICIENCY (BERIBERI) ELIXIR, TABLETS **_Adults._** 5 to 10 mg t.i.d. **_Children and infants._** 10 mg/day. I.V. or I.M. injection **_Adults._** _Initial:_ 5 to 100 mg every 8 hr, switched to P.O. vitamin B$_1$ therapy as soon as possible and continued for total of 1 mo.	▪ Be aware that I.V. administration of vitamin B$_1$ has caused severe and life-threatening reactions, especially with repeat administration. Monitor patient closely for angioedema, GI bleeding, respiratory distress, throat tightness, urticaria, vascular collapse, and weakness during and after administration.

(continues)

Vitamins *(continued)*

GENERIC AND TRADE NAMES	RECOMMENDED DAILY INTAKE
vitamin B$_1$ *(continued)*	***Children ages 7 to 10.*** 1 mg/day. (0.8 to 1 mg/day [CAN].) ***Children ages 4 to 7.*** 0.9 mg/day. (0.7 mg/day [CAN].) ***Children ages 1 to 4.*** 0.3 to 0.7 mg/day. (0.3 to 0.6 mg/day [CAN].)
vitamin B$_3$ (niacin) Endur-Acin, Nia-Bid, Niac, Niacels, Niacor, Nico-400, Nicobid Tempules, Nicolar, Nicotinex Elixir, Novo-Niacin (CAN), Slo-Niacin	***Adult men and boys age 11 and over.*** 15 to 20 mg/day. (14 to 23 mg/day [CAN].) ***Adult women and girls age 11 and over.*** 13 to 15 mg/day. (14 to 16 mg/day [CAN].) ***Pregnant women.*** 17 mg/day. (14 to 16 mg/day [CAN].) ***Breastfeeding women.*** 20 mg/day. (14 to 16 mg/day [CAN].) ***Children ages 7 to 11.*** 13 mg/day. (14 to 18 mg/day [CAN].) ***Children ages 4 to 7.*** 12 mg/day. (13 mg/day [CAN].) ***Neonates and children to age 4.*** 5 to 9 mg/day. (4 to 9 mg/day [CAN].)
vitamin B$_6$ (pyridoxine hydrochloride) Beesix, Doxine, Nestrex, Pyri, Ro- dex, Vita-bee 6	***Adult men and boys age 11 and over.*** 1.7 to 2 mg/day. ***Adult women and girls age 11 and over.*** 1.4 to 1.6 mg/day. ***Pregnant women.*** 2.2 mg/day. ***Breastfeeding women.*** 2.1 mg/day. ***Children ages 7 to 10.*** 1.4 mg/day. ***Children ages 4 to 6.*** 1.1 mg/day. ***Neonates and children to age 3.*** 0.3 to 1 mg/day.

OTHER INDICATIONS AND DOSAGES

PARENTERAL ADMINISTRATION GUIDELINES

TO TREAT WERNICKE'S ENCEPHALOPATHY
I.V. OR I.M. INJECTION
Adults. Initial: 100 mg I.V. *Maintenance:* 50 to 100 mg I.V. or I.M. daily until normal recommended daily intake is achieved.

- Rotate sites for I.M. administration of vitamin B_1 to help prevent induration and tenderness that may occur following administration.
- Be aware that I.M. administration may be painful; use the Z-track method of administration.
- Know that because of incompatibilities, parenteral vitamin B_1 shouldn't be added to alkaline or neutral solutions; also, don't mix it with oxidizing and reducing agents, including barbiturates, carbonates, citrates, and copper.
- Take precautions to protect vitamin B_1 solution from exposure to light because it's light sensitive.

TO TREAT VITAMIN B_3 DEFICIENCY
E.R. CAPSULES, E.R. TABLETS, ORAL SOLUTION, TABLETS
Adults and children age 11 and over. Dosage individualized based on severity of deficiency, as prescribed. *Maximum:* 6 g/day.
I.V. INJECTION
Adults and children age 11 and over. 25 to 100 mg at least twice daily.
Children to age 11. Up to 300 mg daily I.M. injection
Adults and children age 11 and over. 50 to 100 mg at least 5 times/day.
Children to age 11. Dosage individualized based on severity of deficiency.

TO TREAT HYPERLIPIDEMIA (NIACIN ONLY)
E.R. CAPSULES, E.R. TABLETS, ORAL SOLUTION, TABLETS
Adults. Initial: 1,000 mg t.i.d. Dosage increased by 500 mg/day every 2 to 4 wk, as needed. *Maintenance:* 1 to 2 g t.i.d. *Maximum:* 6 g/day.
DOSAGE ADJUSTMENT To reduce or prevent facial flushing, initial dosage reduced to 100 mg/day (tab) or 500 mg/day (E.R. tab), and then gradually increased to 3 to 4 g/day.

- Be aware that I.V. administration of vitamin B_3 may cause CNS or CV adverse reactions, such as arrhythmias, dizziness, headache, peripheral vasodilation, and syncope. Rate of I.V. administration shouldn't exceed 2 mg/min, regardless of method of I.V. administration.
- Know that vitamin B_3 must be diluted for I.V. use. For direct injection, dilute to 2 mg/ml; for intermittent or continuous infusion, dilute dose in 500 ml of normal saline or other compatible solution.
- Give I.M. injection following routine I.M. administration guidelines. Vitamin B_3 doesn't need to be diluted for I.M. injection.
- Be aware that parenteral administration shouldn't be used to treat hyperlipidemia.

TO TREAT VITAMIN B_6 DEFICIENCY
E.R. CAPSULES, TABLETS
Adults and children. Dosage individualized based on severity of deficiency, as prescribed.
E.R. TABLETS
Adults. Dosage individualized based on severity of deficiency, as prescribed.
I.V. INFUSION
Adults and children. Dosage individualized as part of total parenteral nutrition.

- Be aware that I.M. or SubQ administration of vitamin B_6 may cause injection-site burning or stinging. Before giving injection, alert patient that this adverse effect may occur.
- Know that I.V. administration is given as part of a multivitamin solution; follow the guidelines for administering an I.V. multivitamin solution as recommended for the product being used.

(continues)

Vitamins *(continued)*

GENERIC AND TRADE NAMES	RECOMMENDED DAILY INTAKE
vitamin B$_6$ *(continued)*	**Children ages 7 to 10.** 1.4 mg/day. **Children ages 4 to 6.** 1.1 mg/day. **Neonates and children to age 3.** 0.3 to 1 mg/day. **Adult men and boys age 11 and over.** 1.7 to 2 mg/day. **Adult women and girls age 11 and over.** 1.4 to 1.6 mg/day. **Pregnant women.** 2.2 mg/day. **Breastfeeding women.** 2.1 mg/day.
vitamin B$_9$ (folic acid) Apo-Folic (CAN), Folvite, Novo-Folacid (CAN)	**Adult men and boys age 11 and over.** 150 to 400 mcg/day. (150 to 220 mcg/day [CAN].) **Adult women and girls age 11 and over.** 150 to 400 mcg/day. (145 to 190 mcg/day [CAN].) **Pregnant women.** 400 to 800 mcg/day. (445 to 475 mcg/day [CAN].) **Breastfeeding women.** 260 to 800 mcg/day. (245 to 275 mcg/day [CAN].) **Children ages 7 to 11.** 100 to 400 mcg/day. (125 to 180 mcg/day [CAN].) **Children ages 4 to 7.** 75 to 400 mcg/day. (90 mcg/day [CAN].) **Neonates and children to age 4.** 25 mcg/day. (50 to 80 mcg/day [CAN].)
vitamin B$_{12}$ (cyanocobalamin, hydroxocobalamin)	**Adults age 19 and over.** 2.4 mcg/day. **Pregnant women.** 2.6 mcg/day. **Breastfeeding women.** 2.8 mcg/day. **Adolescents ages 14 to 19.** 2.4 mcg/day. **Children ages 9 to 14.** 1.8 mcg/day. **Children ages 4 to 9.** 1.2 mcg/day. **Children ages 1 to 4.** 0.9 mcg/day. **Infants ages 6 to 12 months.** 0.4 mcg/day. **Neonates and infants to 6 months.** 0.5 mcg/day.

OTHER INDICATIONS AND DOSAGES

PARENTERAL ADMINISTRATION GUIDELINES

TO TREAT PYRIDOXINE DEPENDENCY SYNDROME
I.V. OR I.M. INJECTION
Adults and children age 11 and over. 30 to 600 mg daily.
Infants with seizures. *Initial:* 10 to 100 mg, then individualized based on severity of deficiency, as prescribed.

TO TREAT DRUG-INDUCED PYRIDOXINE DEFICIENCY
I.V. OR I.M. INJECTION
Adults and children age 11 and over. 50 to 200 mg/day for 3 wk, then 25 to 100 mg/day, as needed.

- Know that vitamin B_6 may increase AST (SGOT) levels. Be aware that at least one manufacturer warns against I.V. administration of vitamin B_6 to patients with heart disease.
- Take precautions to protect vitamin B_6 solution from exposure to light because it's light sensitive.

TO TREAT VITAMIN B9 DEFICIENCY
TABLETS
Adults and children. Dosage individualized based on severity of deficiency, as prescribed.
I.V. INFUSION, I.M. OR SUBCUTANEOUS INJECTION
Adults and children. 0.25 to 1 mg daily until hematologic response occurs.

- Be aware that some vitamin B_9 solutions contain benzyl alcohol. Don't administer these solutions to neonates or immature infants because of a risk of fatal toxic syndrome, which may include circulatory, CNS, renal, and respiratory impairment and metabolic acidosis.
- Know that unless ordered otherwise, you should dilute 5 mg/ml of vitamin B_9 with 49 ml of sterile water for injection to provide a solution containing 0.1 mg of vitamin/ml.
- Know that parenteral administration may cause anaphylaxis. Parenteral administration should be used only in patients with severe vitamin deficiency or in those with severely impaired GI absorption.
- Be aware that SubQ administration should be injected deep.
- Take precautions to protect vitamin B_9 solution from exposure to light because it's light sensitive.

TO TREAT VITAMIN B12 DEFICIENCY
Caused by nutritional intake imbalance (not for use to treat pernicious anemia)
LOZENGES, TABLETS
Adults and children. Dosage individualized based on severity of deficiency, as prescribed.
Caused by pernicious anemia; malabsorption disorders (tropical or nontropical sprue, partial or total gastrectomy, regional enteritis, gastroenterostomy, ileal resection); or malignancies, granulomas, strictures, or anastomoses involving the ileum.
SUBCUTANEOUS INJECTION
(CYANOCOBALAMIN)
Adults. *Initial:* 30 mcg daily for 5 to 10 days, then switched to I.M. administration for maintenance therapy.

- Be aware that parenteral vitamin B_{12} solution is incompatible with many drugs, including ascorbic acid, chlorpromazine hydrochloride, dextrose, heavy metals, phytonadione, prochlorperazine edisylate, and warfarin sodium. Also know that alkaline or strongly acidic solutions and oxidizing or reducing agents are also incompatible with vitamin B_{12} solution. Do not administer vitamin with other drugs.
- Know that both cyanocobalamin and hydroxocobalamin may be administered by I.M. injection, but only cyanocobalamin may be administered as a SubQ injection. Be alert to which form is being administered to ensure correct route of administration.

(continues)

Vitamins *(continued)*

GENERIC AND TRADE NAMES	RECOMMENDED DAILY INTAKE
vitamin B₁₂ *(continued)*	**Children ages 7 to 10.** 1 mg/day. (0.8 to 1 mg/day [CAN].) **Children ages 4 to 7.** 0.9 mg/day. (0.7 mg/day [CAN].) **Children ages 1 to 4.** 0.3 to 0.7 mg/day. (0.3 to 0.6 mg/day [CAN].)
vitamin C (ascorbic acid) Ascorbic Acid, Cecon Drops, Cenolate, Cevi-Bid, Vicks Vitamin C Drops	**Adult men.** 90 mg/day. **Adult women.** 75 mg/day. **Pregnant women age 19 and over.** 85 mg/day. **Breastfeeding women age 19 and over.** 120 mg/day. **Adolescent boys ages 14 to 19.** 75 mg/day. **Adolescent girls ages 14 to 19.** 65 mg/day. **Pregnant girls ages 14 to 19.** 80 mg/day. **Breastfeeding girls ages 14 to 19.** 115 mg/day. **Children ages 9 to 14.** 45 mg/day. **Children ages 4 to 9.** 25 mg/day. **Children ages 1 to 4.** 15 mg/day. **Infants ages 7 to 12 months.** 50 mg/day. **Neonates and infants to age 7 months.** 40 mg/day. *DOSAGE ADJUSTMENT* Recommended daily intake for people who smoke is 100 mg/day because of an increased utilization of vitamin C. Recommended daily intake should be increased to promote wound healing and for those with a chronic illness, fever, hemovascular disorder, or infection; the amount of vitamin C increase depends on the severity of the underlying condition.

OTHER INDICATIONS AND DOSAGES	PARENTERAL ADMINISTRATION GUIDELINES

Children. *Initial:* 1,000 to 5,000 mcg given in single daily doses of 100 mcg over 2 or more wk. *Maintenance:* 60 or more mcg/mo.

I.M. INJECTION (CYANOCOBALAMIN OR HYDROXOCOBALAMIN)

Adults. *Initial:* 30 mcg daily for 5 to 10 days. *Maintenance:* 100 to 200 mcg every mo.

Children. *Initial:* 1,000 to 5,000 mcg, given in single daily doses of 100 mcg over 2 or more wk. *Maintenance:* 60 or more mcg/mo.

DOSAGE ADJUSTMENT Dosage adjusted, as needed, to maintain normal hematologic morphology and an erythrocyte count greater than 4.5 million/mm.

Adults. *Initial.* 1 mg/wk for 3 wk. *Maintenance:* 250 mcg/mo.

TO TREAT FAMILIAL SELECTIVE B$_{12}$ MALABSORPTION
I.M. INJECTION (CYANOCOBALAMIN)

TO TREAT HEREDITARY DEFICIENCY OF TRANSCOBALAMIN II
I.M. INJECTION (CYANOCOBALAMIN)
Adults. 1 to 2 mg/wk.

- Be aware that SubQ administration of cyanocobalamin should be injected deeply.
- Know that vitamin B$_{12}$ is excreted more rapidly after I.V. injection; I.V. administration isn't recommended.
- Take precautions to protect vitamin B$_{12}$ solution from exposure to light because it's light sensitive.

TO TREAT VITAMIN C DEFICIENCY (SCURVY)

E.R. CAPSULES; LOZENGES; ORAL SOLUTION; E.R. TABLETS; TABLETS; SUBCUTANEOUS, I.M. OR I.V. INJECTION

Adults. 100 to 250 mg once or twice daily until skeletal changes and signs and symptoms of hemorrhagic disorder are reversed (usually within 2 to 21 days).

ORAL SOLUTION; TABLETS; SUBCUTANEOUS, I.M., OR I.V. INJECTION

Infants and Children. 100 to 300 mg/day in divided doses until skeletal changes and signs and symptoms of hemorrhagic disorder are reversed (usually within days).

- Be aware that I.M. injection is the preferred parenteral route for administering vitamin C, although it may be administered I.V. or SubQ when necessary.
- Rotate sites for I.M. and SubQ administration to help prevent transient mild soreness that may occur following administration. Inform patient that this adverse effect may occur.
- Avoid rapid administration, if giving I.V. vitamin C, to prevent dizziness or faintness.
- Administer vitamin C solution by itself because it's incompatible with many drugs.
- Be aware that vitamin C solution rapidly oxidizes in air and in alkaline solutions. Take precautions to protect vitamin solution from exposure to air and light.
- Open vitamin C ampules carefully because increased pressure may develop after prolonged storage.

(continues)

Vitamins *(continued)*

GENERIC AND TRADE NAMES	RECOMMENDED DAILY INTAKE
vitamin D2 (ergocalciferol) Calciferol, Calciferol Drops, Drisdol, Drisdol Drops, Ostoforte (CAN), Radiostol Forte (CAN)	*Adults and children ages 11 and over.* 200 to 400 IU/day. (100 to 200 IU/day [CAN].) *Pregnant and breastfeeding women.* 400 IU/day. (200 to 300 IU/day [CAN].) *Children ages 7 to 11.* 400 IU/day. (100 to 200 IU/day [CAN].) *Children ages 4 to 7.* 400 IU/day. (200 IU/day [CAN].) *Neonates and children to age 4.* 300 to 400 IU/day. (200 to 400 IU/day [CAN].)
vitamin E (alpha tocopherol) Amino-Opti-E, Aquasol E, E-Complex 600, E-Vitamin succinate, Liqui-E, Pheryl E, Vita-Plus E, Webber Vitamin E (CAN)	*Adult men and adolescent boys.* 16.7 IU/day. (10 to 16.7 IU/day [CAN].) *Adult women and adolescent girls.* 13 IU/day. (8.3 to 11.7 IU/day [CAN].) *Pregnant women.* 16.7 IU/day. (13 to 15 IU/day [CAN].) *Breastfeeding women.* 18 to 20 IU/day. (15 to 16.7 IU/day [CAN].) *Children ages 7 to 10.* 11.7 IU/day. (10 to 13 IU/day [CAN].) *Children ages 4 to 7.* 11.7 IU/day. (8.3 IU/day [CAN].) *Infants and children to age 4.* 5 to 10 IU/day. (5 to 6.7 IU/day [CAN].)

OTHER INDICATIONS AND DOSAGES

PARENTERAL ADMINISTRATION GUIDELINES

TO TREAT VITAMIN D₂ DEFICIENCY
CAPSULES, ORAL SOLUTION, TABLETS
Adults and children. Dosage individualized based on severity of deficiency, as prescribed.

TO TREAT VITAMIN D-RESISTANT RICKETS
CAPSULES, ORAL SOLUTION, TABLETS
Adults. 12,000 to 150,000 IU units daily.

TO TREAT VITAMIN D-DEPENDENT RICKETS
CAPSULES, ORAL SOLUTION, TABLETS
Adults. 10,000 to 60,000 IU daily. *Maximum:* 150,000 IU daily.
Children. 3,000 to 10,000 IU daily. *Maximum:* 50,000 IU daily.

TO TREAT OSTEOMALACIA CAUSED BY LONG-TERM ANTICONVULSANT USE
CAPSULES, ORAL SOLUTION, TABLETS
Adults. 1,000 to 4,000 IU daily.
Children. 1,000 IU daily.

TO TREAT FAMILIAL HYPOPHOSPHATEMIA
CAPSULES
Adults. 50,000 to 100,000 IU daily.

TO TREAT HYPOPARATHYROIDISM
CAPSULES
Adults. 50,000 to 150,000 IU daily.
Children. 50,000 to 200,000 IU daily.

TO TREAT INTESTINAL MALABSORPTION
I.M. INJECTION
Adults and children. 10,000 IU daily.

- Be aware that vitamin D₂ is usually given orally. However, I.M. injection may be required for patients with biliary, GI, or liver disease associated with malabsorption of vitamin D analogues.
- Take precautions to protect parenteral vitamin D₂ solution from exposure to light because light causes it to decompose.

TO TREAT VITAMIN E DEFICIENCY
CAPSULES (ADULTS ONLY), ORAL SOLUTION, TABLETS
Adults and children. Dosage individualized based on severity of deficiency, as prescribed.

Know that vitamin E isn't administered parenterally.

Interferons

Interferons are classified as biological response modifiers or antineoplastics. They fall into three major categories—alpha, beta, and gamma—which are described below.

The table on the following pages lists the trade names, indications, usual adult dosages, adverse reactions, and nursing considerations for these interferons.

Interferon alpha

Highly purified proteins produced by a recombinant DNA process, drugs in this category exhibit antiviral and antitumor activity. Antiviral activity depends on their inhibition of viral protein synthesis. Antitumor activity results from their ability to exert a cytostatic effect, reducing the rate of cell proliferation by delaying RNA and protein production. This delay induces cells to enter a resting stage. These drugs also increase the activity of human natural killer (NK) cells, which have the ability to lyse certain tumor cells and normal targets. They also selectively increase the number of cytotoxic T cells, thereby affecting tumor growth. Phagocytic activity of macrophages also is increased.

Interferon alfacon

This specific form of interferon is produced by fermentation of genetically engineered *Escherichia coli*. It's structurally and functionally related to interferon beta and has greater biological activity than other interferon alfas.

Interferon beta

Produced by fibroblasts and epithelial cells, drugs in this category neutralize the activity

GENERIC AND TRADE NAMES	INDICATIONS AND USUAL ADULT DOSAGES
Interferon alpha drugs	
interferon alfa-n3 Alferon N	*To treat condyloma acuminatum:* 250,000 international units intralesionally at base of wart 2 times/wk for up to 8 wk.
peginterferon alfa-2a PEGASYS	*As monotherapy to treat patients with chronic hepatitis C who have compensated liver disease and contraindications or significant intolerance to other hepatitis C virus antiviral drugs; as adjunct to treat patients with chronic hepatitis C and compensated liver disease in combination with other antiviral drugs; to treat patients with chronic hepatitis B who have compensated liver disease and evidence of viral replication and liver inflammation:* 180 mcg/wk SubQ for individualized length of time for chronic hepatitis C and 48 wk for chronic hepatitis B.
peginterferon alfa-2b PEG-Intron Sylatron	*As adjunct to treat patients with chronic hepatitis C who have compensated liver disease and have never received an interferon alpha:* 180 mcg/wk SubQ for 48 wk. *To treat patients with chronic hepatitis C:* 1 mcg/kg/wk (PEG-Intron) SubQ every wk on the same day of the wk for 1 yr. *As adjunct to treat patients with chronic hepatitis C in combination with ribavirin:* 1.5 mcg/kg (PEG-Intron) SubQ every wk on the same day of the wk for 48 wk for genotype 1 and 24 wk for genotype 2 or 3. *As adjunct treatment of melanoma with microscopic or gross nodal involvement within 84 days of definitive surgical resection:* 6 mcg/kg/wk (Sylatron) SubQ for 8 doses followed by 3 mcg/kg/wk (Sylatron) SubQ for up to 5 yr.
recombinant interferon alfa-2b Intron A	*To treat hairy cell leukemia:* 2 million international units/m² I.M. or SubQ 3 times/wk for up to 6 mo. *To treat condyloma acuminatum:* 1 million international units (using only the 10-million units/ml strength) intralesionally at base of wart (up to 5 warts/course) 3 times/wk on alternate days for 3 wk. If response is inadequate 12 to 16 wk after initial treatment, repeat course, as prescribed.

of endogenous interferon gamma (IFNG), the substance believed to be responsible for triggering the autoimmune process that leads to multiple sclerosis. In multiple sclerosis, an initial viral infection may stimulate IFNG production by T cells. Then IFNG induces macrophages to produce proteinases that degrade the myelin sheath around the nerves and spinal cord. Cytotoxic T cells then move to the site of inflammation, recognizing antigens as receptor sites, where they attack the tissue affected by IFNG, resulting in progressive neurologic dysfunction. Interferon beta drugs interfere with IFNG production by lymphocytes and the mRNA transcription caused by IFNG. As a result, cytotoxic T cells can't locate receptor sites and cause further damage in the CNS.

Interferon gamma

Produced from genetically engineered *E. coli*, this type of interferon is chemically and therapeutically distinct from interferon alpha. Drugs in this category have potent phagocyte-activating properties. By enhancing oxidative metabolism, they produce toxic oxygen metabolites in phagocytes, which permits more efficient killing of certain fungi, bacteria, and protozoal microbes. Enhanced antibody-dependent cellular cytotoxicity and NK-cell activity reduce the risk of developing a serious infection in patients with chronic disease. These drugs also stimulate production of cytokines, such as interleukin-1-beta, and regulate the immune system by suppressing the IgE level and inhibiting collagen production.

ADVERSE REACTIONS

CNS: Depression, dizziness, fatigue, headache, **homicidal or suicidal ideation**, peripheral neuropathy, psychosis, **seizures**, vertigo
CV: Hypertriglyceridemia, hypertension, **hypotension**, palpitations, **pericarditis**
EENT: Dry mouth, hearing loss
ENDO: Diabetic ketoacidosis, hyperglycemia
GI: Anorexia, diarrhea, **hepatotoxicity**, nausea, vomiting
GU: Renal failure
HEME: Anemia, **leukopenia, pure red cell aplasia, thrombocytopenia, thrombotic thrombocytopenic purpura**
MS: Myositis, **rhabdomyolysis**
RESP: Pulmonary fibrosis or hypertension
SKIN: Alopecia, rash, **Stevens–Johnson syndrome, toxic epidermal necrolysis**, urticaria
Other: Anaphylaxis, angioedema, bacterial infections, flu-like symptoms, liver or renal graft rejection, **sepsis**, systemic lupus erythematosus

NURSING CONSIDERATIONS

- Use interferon alpha drugs cautiously in patients with renal impairment and in elderly patients.
- Be aware that cross-sensitivity may occur among interferon alpha drugs.
- Be aware that interferon alpha drugs aren't interchangeable.
- Be aware that patients who are sensitive to mouse immunoglobulin also may be sensitive to recombinant interferon alfa-2a.
- Ensure that patient is well hydrated, if not contraindicated, at the start of and throughout therapy, to reduce the risk of hypotension.
- Reconstitute by adding 3 ml of diluent provided by manufacturer and swirling gently to dissolve.
- Be aware that reconstitution of peginterferon alfa-2a, interferon alfa-n3, and ropeginterferon alfa-2b-njft is not necessary.
- Don't shake vial. Discard vial if left at room temperature for more than 12 hours.
- Be aware that cross-sensitivity with interferon alfa-n3 to egg protein, mouse immunoglobulin, or neomycin may occur.
- Be aware that cross-sensitivity may occur with *Escherichia coli*–derived products.
WARNING Know that because interferon alpha drugs may cause or aggravate fatal or life-threatening autoimmune, ischemic, infectious, or neuropsychiatric disorders, patient should be monitored periodically with clinical and laboratory evaluations; expect drug to be discontinued if he develops severe or worsening signs and symptoms of these conditions.

(continues)

Interferons *(continued)*

GENERIC AND TRADE NAMES	INDICATIONS AND USUAL ADULT DOSAGES

Interferon alpha drugs *(continued)*

To treat AIDS-related Kaposi's sarcoma: 30 million international units/m^2 (using 50 million international units/ml) I.M. or SubQ 3 times/wk.

To treat chronic hepatitis B: 5 million international units/day or 10 million international units 3 times/wk I.M. or SubQ for 16 wk.

To treat chronic hepatitis C: 3 million international units I.M. or SubQ 3 times/wk.

To treat malignant melanoma: 20 million international units/m^2 as I.V. infusion over 20 min for 5 consecutive days/wk for 4 wk, followed by 10 million international units/m^2 SubQ 3 times/wk for 48 wk.

As adjunct to treat follicular lymphoma: 5 million international units/m^2 3 times/wk SubQ for up to 18 months.

ropeginterferon alfa-2b-njft
Besremi

To treat polycythemia vera: Initial: 100 mcg SubQ (50 mcg if receiving hydroxyurea) every 2 weeks, with dosage increased by 50 mcg every 2 weeks, as needed. *Maximum:* 500 mcg/dose.

Interferon alfacon-1 drugs

interferon alfacon-1
Infergen

To treat chronic hepatitis C in patients with compensated liver disease: 9 mcg SubQ 3 times/wk, at intervals of at least 48 hr, for 24 wk. If inadequate response or relapse occurs, 15 mcg SubQ 3 times/wk, for up to 48 wk.

As adjunct with ribavirin to treat chronic hepatitis C: 15 mcg daily for up to 48 wk.

Interferon beta drugs

interferon beta-1a
Avonex

To treat relapsing forms of multiple sclerosis: 30 mcg I.M. once/wk.

Rebif

To treat relapsing forms of multiple sclerosis: Initial: 20% of maintenance dose 3 times/wk SubQ, and increased over 4-wk period to the targeted maintenance dose. *Maintenance:* 22 mcg or 44 mcg SubQ 3 times/wk.

interferon beta-1b
Betaseron, Extavia

To treat relapsing forms of multiple sclerosis: 0.0625 mg SubQ every other day for wk 1 and 2, increased to 0.125 mg SubQ every other day for wk 3 and 4, increased to 0.1875 mg SubQ every other day for wk 5 and 6, and increased to 0.25 mg SubQ every other day on wk 7 and thereafter.

peginterferon beta-1a
Plegridy

To treat relapsing forms of multiple sclerosis: 63 mcg SubQ or I.M. on day 1, 94 mcg SubQ or I.M. on day 15, and 125 mcg SubQ or I.M. on day 29 and every 14 days thereafter.

ADVERSE REACTIONS	NURSING CONSIDERATIONS
	▪ Obtain CBC before and regularly during treatment, as ordered, because interferon alpha drugs may cause bone marrow suppression. Expect drug to be discontinued if patient develops severe decreases in neutrophil or platelet count. ▪ Implement bleeding and infection control measures, according to facility policy. ▪ Administer acetaminophen, as prescribed, to prevent or treat fever or headache. ▪ Expect patient taking ropeginterferon alfa-2b-njft and hydroxyurea to be weaned off of hydroxyurea by reducing the total biweekly dose by 20 to 40% every 2 wks during wks 3–12 with hydroxyurea discontinued by week 13.
CNS: Anxiety, confusion, decreased concentration, depression, insomnia, nervousness **EENT:** Abnormal vision **HEME: Leukopenia, thrombocytopenia**	▪ Be aware that use of interferon alfacon-1 isn't recommended for patients with autoimmune hepatitis or psychiatric disorders. ▪ Be aware that cross-sensitivity may occur with other interferon alfa drugs or E. coli–derived products. ▪ Don't shake vial. ▪ Implement bleeding and infection control measures, according to facility policy. ▪ Monitor patient for signs and symptoms of vision abnormalities.
CNS: Anxiety, confusion, depression, dizziness, emotional lability, fatigue, headache, **seizures, suicidal ideation,** weakness **CV: Cardiomyopathy,** palpitations, tachycardia, **thrombotic microangiopathy,** vasodilation **EENT:** Retinal vascular disorders **ENDO:** Thyroid dysfunction **GI: Autoimmune hepatitis,** diarrhea, elevated liver enzyme levels, nausea, **pancreatitis,** vomiting **GU: Hemolytic-uremic syndrome** **HEME:** Anemia, including **hemolytic, leukopenia, pancytopenia, thrombocytopenia** **RESP: Bronchospasm** **SKIN:** Alopecia, pruritus, skin discoloration, urticaria **Other: Anaphylaxis, angioedema,** flu-like symptoms, immunogenicity, infection, injection-site reactions (including necrosis), systemic lupus erythematosus, weight changes	▪ Use beta interferons with extreme caution in patients with depression or seizure disorder. ▪ Be aware that cross-sensitivity may occur with human albumin or natural or recombinant interferon beta. ▪ Reconstitute following manufacturer's directions and refrigerate. Use interferon beta-1a within 6 hours of reconstitution. Use interferon beta-1b within 3 hours of reconstitution. ▪ Implement bleeding and infection control measures, according to facility policy. ▪ Be aware the rubber cover of Plegridy prefilled syringe for I.M. injection contains natural rubber latex. ▪ Pregnancy exposure registry for peginterferon beta-1a: 1-866-810-1462 or https://www.plegridypregnancyregistry.com/

(continues)

Interferons *(continued)*

GENERIC AND TRADE NAMES	INDICATIONS AND USUAL ADULT DOSAGES

Interferon gamma drugs

interferon gamma-1b
Actimmune

To reduce frequency and severity of serious infections associated with chronic granulomatous disease or to delay progression of severe, malignant osteopetrosis in patients with body surface area greater than 0.5 m²: 50 mcg/m² (1 million international units/m²) SubQ 3 times/wk.

To reduce frequency and severity of serious infections associated with chronic granulomatous disease or to delay progression of severe, malignant osteopetrosis in patients with body surface area of 0.5 m² or less: 1.5 mcg/kg/dose SubQ 3 times/wk.

ADVERSE REACTIONS	NURSING CONSIDERATIONS
CNS: Fatigue, headache **GI:** Diarrhea, nausea, vomiting **HEME:** Leukopenia **SKIN:** Rash **Other:** Flu-like symptoms	• Use gamma interferon cautiously in patients previously exposed to cytotoxic drugs or radiation therapy. • Be aware that cross-sensitivity may occur with *Escherichia coli*–derived products. • Know that stopper on vial is a derivative of latex, which may cause allergic reactions to those sensitive to latex. • Discard vial if left at room temperature for more than 12 hours. • Implement bleeding and infection-control measures, according to facility policy. • Administer acetaminophen, as prescribed, to prevent or treat fever and headache.

Compatible Drugs in a Syringe

The table below lets you know at a glance whether particular drugs are compatible for at least 15 minutes when mixed together in a syringe for immediate administration. However, keep in mind that drugs listed as compatible when mixed in a syringe may not be compatible when prepared for other routes of administration. Drug combinations prepared for immediate administration usually require a more concentrated solution than those prepared for infusion.

Key: C = Compatible; I = Incompatible; n/a = Compatibility information not available, no recommendations can be given.

	ATROPINE	CHLORPROMAZINE	DEXAMETHASONE	DIAZEPAM	DIPHENHYDRAMINE	DROPERIDOL	FUROSEMIDE	GLYCOPYRROLATE	HALOPERIDOL
atropine		C	n/a	n/a	C	C	n/a	C	I
chlorpromazine	C		n/a	n/a	C	C	n/a	C	n/a
dexamethasone	n/a	n/a		n/a	I	n/a	n/a	n/a	n/a
diazepam	n/a	n/a	n/a		n/a	n/a	n/a	I	n/a
diphenhydramine	C	C	I	n/a		C	n/a	C	I
droperidol	C	C	n/a	n/a	C		I	C	n/a
furosemide	n/a	n/a	n/a	n/a	n/a	I		n/a	n/a
glycopyrrolate	C	C	I	C	C	C	n/a		C
haloperidol	n/a	n/a	n/a	n/a	C	n/a	n/a	n/a	
heparin	C	I	n/a	I	n/a	I	C	n/a	I
hydromorphone	C	C	n/a	n/a	C	n/a	n/a	C	C
hydroxyzine	C	C	n/a	n/a	C	C	n/a	C	I
ketorolac	n/a	n/a	n/a	I	n/a	n/a	n/a	n/a	I
lidocaine	n/a	n/a	n/a	n/a	n/a	n/a	n/a	C	n/a
lorazepam	n/a	n/a	n/a	n/a	n/a	n/a	n/a	n/a	n/a
meperidine	C	C	n/a	C	C	C	n/a	C	n/a
metoclopramide	C	C	n/a	n/a	C	C	I	n/a	n/a
midazolam	C	C	n/a	n/a	C	n/a	n/a	C	C
morphine	C	C	n/a	n/a	C	C	n/a	C	I
pentobarbital	C	I	n/a	n/a	I	I	n/a	I	n/a
prochlorperazine	C	n/a	n/a	n/a	C	C	n/a	C	n/a
scopolamine	C	C	n/a	n/a	C	C	n/a	C	n/a

HEPARIN	HYDROMORPHONE	HYDROXYZINE	KETOROLAC	LIDOCAINE	LORAZEPAM	MEPERIDINE	METOCLOPRAMIDE	MIDAZOLAM	MORPHINE	PENTOBARBITAL	PROCHLORPERAZINE	SCOPOLAMINE
n/a	C	C	n/a	n/a	n/a	C	C	C	C	C	C	C
I	C	C	n/a	n/a	n/a	C	C	C	I	I	C	C
n/a	C	n/a	n/a	n/a	n/a	n/a	C	n/a	n/a	n/a	n/a	n/a
I	n/a	n/a	I	n/a	n/a	n/a	n/a	n/a	n/a	n/a	n/a	n/a
n/a	C	C	n/a	n/a	n/a	C	C	C	C	I	C	C
I	n/a	C	n/a	n/a	n/a	C	C	C	C	I	C	C
C	n/a	n/a	n/a	n/a	n/a	n/a	I	n/a	n/a	n/a	n/a	n/a
n/a	C	C	n/a	C	n/a	C	n/a	C	C	I	C	C
I	C	I	I	n/a	n/a	n/a	n/a	n/a	I	n/a	n/a	n/a
	n/a	n/a	n/a	C	n/a	I	C	n/a	C	n/a	n/a	n/a
n/a		C	I	n/a	C	n/a	n/a	C	n/a	C	I	C
n/a	C		I	C	n/a	C	C	C	C	I	C	C
n/a	I	I		n/a	n/a	n/a	n/a	n/a	n/a	n/a	I	n/a
C	n/a	C	n/a		n/a	n/a	C	n/a	n/a	n/a	n/a	n/a
n/a	C	n/a	n/a	n/a		n/a	n/a	n/a	n/a	n/a	n/a	n/a
I	n/a	C	n/a	n/a	n/a		C	I	I	C	C	C
C	C	n/a	n/a	C	n/a	C		C	C	n/a	C	C
n/a	C	C	n/a	n/a	n/a	C	C		C	I	I	C
C*	n/a	C	n/a	n/a	n/a	n/a	C	C		I	C	C
n/a	C	I	n/a	n/a	n/a	I	I	I	I		I	C
n/a	I	C	I	n/a	n/a	C	C	I	C	I		C
n/a	C	C	n/a	n/a	n/a	C	C	C	C	C	C	

* Compatible only with morphine doses of 1, 2, and 5 mg.

Drug Formulas and Calculations

When giving drugs, you must be familiar with drug formulas and calculation methods to make sure your patient receives the prescribed drug in the correct dosage, strength, or flow rate. This appendix offers a quick review of ways to calculate the strength of a solution, drug dosages, and I.V. flow rates.

Calculating the Strength of a Solution

Most solutions are prepared in the required strength by the pharmacy or medical supply source.

But sometimes only a concentrated form is available, and you'll need to dilute the solution or solid to administer the prescribed strength.

When a solid form of a drug is used to prepare a solution, the drug must be completely dissolved. Solid drug forms, such as tablets, crystals, and powders, are considered 100% strength. (An exception to this is boric acid, which is only 5% at full strength.) The final diluted solution is stated in terms of liquid measurement. To prepare a solution, you'll need to add the prescribed solid or liquid form of the drug (the solute) to the prescribed amount of diluent (the solvent). Two of the most common clinical diluents are normal saline solution and sterile water.

You can use two formulas to calculate the strength of a solution, as shown in the examples below.

Method 1: Calculating percentage and volume
Use the following formula:

$$\frac{\text{Weaker solution}}{\text{Stronger solution}} = \frac{\text{Solute}}{\text{Solvent}}$$

Example: You need to dilute a stock solution of 100% strength to a 5% solution. How much solute will you need to add to obtain 500 ml of the 5% solution?

Calculate as follows:

$$\frac{5\ (\%)\ (\text{Weaker solution})}{100\ (\%)\ (\text{Stronger solution})} = \frac{X\ (g)\ (\text{solute})}{500\ ml\ (\text{solvent})}$$

$$100\ X = (500)(5)\ \text{or}\ 2{,}500$$

$$X = 25\ g$$

Answer: You'll need to add 25 g of solute to each 500 ml of solvent to prepare a 5% solution.

Method 2: Calculating percentage and volume
Use the following formula:

$$\frac{(\text{Desired strength})}{(\text{Available strength})} \times \frac{\text{Total amount of}}{\text{desired solution}} = X \frac{(\text{amount of undiluted drug}}{\text{needed to make solution})}$$

Example: You need to make 100 ml of a 20% solution, using an 80% solution. How much of the 80% solution must you add to the sterile water to yield a final volume of 100 ml of a 20% solution?

Calculate as follows:

$$\frac{20\ (\%)(\text{Desired strength})}{80\ (\%)(\text{Available strength})} \times \frac{100\ ml\ (\text{Total amount}}{\text{of desired solution})} = X\frac{0.20}{0.80} = 0.25$$

$$0.25 \times 100\ (ml) = X$$

$$X = 25\ ml\ \text{of 80% solution}$$

Answer: You'll need to add 25 ml of the 80% solution to the water to make a final volume of 100 ml of a 20% solution.

Calculating Drug Dosages

You may be required to calculate drug dosages when you need to administer a drug that's available only in one measure, but prescribed in another. You should also be prepared to convert various units of measure, such as milligrams (mg) to grains (gr), and dry measurements to liquid. You can use three common methods of ratio and proportion to calculate drug dosages, as shown in the examples below.

CALCULATING ORAL DRUG DOSAGES

Example: You need to give a patient 0.25 mg of digoxin, which comes only in 0.125-mg tablets. How many tablets will you need to give him to attain the proper dosage?

Method 1: Using labeled amount of drug

In this method, true proportions between the drug label and the prescribed dose are used to determine ratio and proportion. The drug label, which states the amount of drug in one unit of measurement—in this case, 0.125 mg in each tablet of digoxin—is the first ratio, expressed as follows:

$$\text{milligrams : tablets} = \text{milligrams : tablets}$$

$$0.125 \text{ mg (amount of drug) : 1 tablet (unit of measure)}$$

The prescribed dose—in this case, 0.25 mg—is the second ratio; it must be stated in the same order and units of measure as the first, as follows:

$$0.125 \text{ mg : 1 tablet} = 0.25 \text{ mg : X (tablets)}$$

Calculate as follows:

$$0.125 \text{ X} = 0.25 \text{ mg}$$
$$X = \frac{0.25}{0.125}$$
$$X = 2$$

Answer: You'll need to give the patient 2 tablets of digoxin 0.125 mg.

Be sure to use critical thinking to assess whether your answer is correct. Because the amount of drug prescribed is greater than the amount of drug in one tablet, it's reasonable to expect the required number of tablets to be greater than one.

Method 2: Using an established formula

To determine the correct number of digoxin tablets to give using this method, use the following formula:

$$\frac{\text{Prescribed dose}}{\text{Dose available}} \times \text{Quantity (unit of measure)} = \text{X (unknown quantity to be given)}$$

Calculate as follows:

$$\frac{0.25 \text{ mg}}{0.125 \text{ mg}} \times 1 \text{ tablet} = \text{X (number of 0.125-mg tablets)}$$

$$\frac{0.25}{0.125} = \text{X}$$

$$2 = \text{X}$$

Answer: You'll need to give the patient 2 tablets of digoxin 0.125 mg.

Method 3: Calculating according to proportion size

This method uses the same components as method #1, but the ratio is based on proportions according to size. To determine the correct number of digoxin tablets to give using this method, use the following formula:

$$\frac{\text{Smaller}}{\text{Larger}} = \frac{\text{Larger}}{\text{Smaller}}$$

Substitute 0.125 into the smaller part and 0.25 into the greater part of the first ratio. Critical thinking leads us to believe that you'll need more than 1 tablet of the weaker 0.125-mg strength to equal the stronger 0.25 mg. Set up the proportion as follows:

Calculate as follows:

$$\frac{0.125 \text{ mg}}{0.25 \text{ mg}} = \frac{1 \text{ (tablet)}}{X \text{ (tablets)}}$$

$$0.125 \text{ X} = 0.25$$

$$X = \frac{0.25}{0.125}$$

$$X = 2 \text{ tablets}$$

Answer: You'll need to give the patient 2 tablets of digoxin 0.125 mg.

CALCULATING PARENTERAL DRUG DOSAGES

The same methods used for calculating oral drugs and solutions can be used for preparing parenteral injections.

Example: You need to administer a prescribed dose of 1 mg morphine sulfate from a unit-dose cartridge containing 4 mg/2 ml. How many milliliters will you need to give to equal the prescribed dose of 1 mg?

Method 1: Using labeled amount of drug

Using the same ratio as for oral drugs, the drug label—in this case, 4 mg—is the first ratio, and the prescribed dose—in this case, 1 mg—is the second ratio, expressed as follows:

4 mg (the amount of drug) : 2 ml (the unit of measure)

Calculate as follows:

$$4 \text{ mg} : 2 \text{ ml} = 1 \text{ mg} : X \text{ ml}$$

$$4X = 2$$

$$X = \frac{2}{4}$$

$$X = 0.5 \text{ ml}$$

Answer: You'll need to give 0.5 ml of morphine sulfate to equal the prescribed dose of 1 mg.

Method 2: Using an established formula

Use this formula:

$$\frac{\text{Prescribed dose}}{\text{Dose available}} \times \text{Quantity (unit of measure)} = X \text{ (unknown quantity to be given)}$$

Calculate as follows:

$$\frac{1 \text{ mg}}{4 \text{ mg}} \times 2 \text{ ml} = X \text{ (number of ml)}$$

$$\frac{2}{4} = X$$

$$X = 0.5 \text{ ml}$$

Answer: You'll need to give 0.5 ml of morphine sulfate to equal the prescribed dose of 1 mg.

Method 3: Calculating according to proportion size

To determine the correct amount of morphine sulfate to give using this method, use the following formula:

smaller : greater = smaller : greater
milligrams : milligrams = milliliters : milliliters

Critical thinking leads us to believe that 1 mg is less than 4 mg and that you'll need less than 2 ml to give 1 mg of the drug; therefore, 1 mg goes into the smaller part of the first ratio, and X goes into the smaller part of the second ratio. Set up the proportion as follows:

$$1 \text{ mg} : 4 \text{ mg} = X \text{ (ml)} : 2 \text{ ml}$$

$$4X = 2$$

$$X = \frac{2}{4}$$

$$X = 0.5 \text{ ml}$$

Answer: You'll need to give 0.5 ml of morphine sulfate to equal the prescribed dose of 1 mg.

Calculating I.V. Flow Rates

When an I.V. solution is delivered by gravity, you must calculate the number of drops needed per minute for proper infusion. To calculate I.V. flow rates, you need to know three things:

- The drip factor—or the number of drops contained in 1 ml for the type of I.V. set you'll be using. This information is provided on the individual package label.
- The amount and type of fluid that you'll infuse as prescribed on the physician's order sheet
- The infusion duration time in minutes.

Once you've gathered this information, you can calculate the I.V. flow rate using the following equation:

$$\frac{\text{Total number of ml}}{\text{Total number of minutes}} \times \text{drip factor (gtt/ml)} = \text{flow rate (gtt/min)}$$

Example 1: If the physician prescribes 1,000 ml of D_5W to infuse over 10 hours, and the drip rate for your administration set is 15 drops (gtt)/ml, calculate as follows:

$$\frac{1,000 \text{ ml}}{10 \text{ hours} \times 60 \text{ minutes}} \times 15 \text{ gtt/m} = X \text{ gtt/minute}$$

$$\frac{1,000 \text{ ml}}{600 \text{ minutes}} \times 15 \text{ gtt/m} = X \text{ gtt/minute}$$

$$1.67 \text{ ml/minute} \times 15 \text{ gtt/m} = X \text{ gtt/minute}$$

$$25.05 \text{ gtt/minute} = X$$

Answer: To infuse, round off 25.05 to 25 gtt/minute or according to your institution's policy.

Example 2: If the physician prescribes 500 ml of half-normal (0.45%) saline solution to infuse over 2 hours, and the drip rate for your administration set delivers 10 gtt/ml, calculate as follows:

$$\frac{500 \text{ ml}}{2 \text{ hours} \times 60 \text{ minutes}} \times 15 \text{ gtt/m} = X \text{ gtt/minute}$$

$$\frac{1,000 \text{ ml}}{120 \text{ minutes}} \times 15 \text{ gtt/m} = X \text{ gtt/minute}$$

$$4.67 \text{ ml/minute} \times 15 \text{ gtt/m} = X \text{ gtt/minute}$$

$$41.7 \text{ gtt/minute} = X$$

Answer: To infuse, round off 41.7 to 42 gtt/minute or according to your institution's policy.

Note: When preparing for I.V. administration using a controlled infusion device, the electronic flow-regulator will either count drops using an electronic eye or use a controlled pumping action to deliver the fluid in milliliters. Your final calculation will be based on the unit of measure used by the device: drops per minute or ml per hour.

Weights and Equivalents

The following three tables show approximate equivalents among systems of measurement.

Table 1 Liquid Equivalents Among Household, Apothecaries', and Metric Systems

HOUSEHOLD	APOTHECARIES'	METRIC
1 teaspoon (tsp)	1 fluid dram	5 milliliters (ml)
1 tablespoon (tbs)	0.5 fluid oz	15 ml
2 tbs (1 ounce [oz])	1 fluid oz	30 ml
1 cupful	8 fluid oz	240 ml
1 pint	16 fluid oz	473 ml
1 quart (qt)	32 fluid oz	946 ml (1 liter)

**Table 2 Solid Equivalents Among
Apothecaries' and Metric Systems**

APOTHECARIES'	METRIC
15 grains (gr)	1 gram (g) (1,000 milligrams [mg])
10 gr	0.6 g (600 mg)
7.5 gr	0.5 g (500 mg)
5 gr	0.3 g (300 mg)
3 gr	0.2 g (200 mg)
1.5 gr	0.1 g (100 mg)
1 gr	0.06 g (60 mg) or 0.065 g (65 mg)
0.75 gr	0.05 g (50 mg)
0.5 gr	0.03 g (30 mg)
0.25 gr	0.015 g (15 mg)
1/60 gr	0.001 g (1 mg)
1/100 gr	0.6 mg
1/120 gr	0.5 mg
1/150 gr	0.4 mg

Table 3 Solid Equivalents Among Avoirdupois, Apothecaries', and Metric Systems

AVOIRDUPOIS	APOTHECARIES'	METRIC
1 gr	1 gr	0.065 g
15.4 gr	15 gr	1 g
1 ounce (oz)	480 gr	28.35 g
437.5 gr	1 oz	31 g
1 pound (lb)	1.33 lb	454 g
0.75 lb	1 lb	373 g
2.2 lb	2.7 lb	1 kg

Equianalgesic Doses for Opioid Agents

An equianalgesic dose of a synthetic opioid agonist is the dose that produces the same level of analgesia as 10 mg of I.M. or subQ morphine, the principal opioid obtained from opium poppies. If your patient is switched from one opioid to another, expect to use the equianalgesic dose to decrease the risk of adverse reactions while increasing the likelihood of adequate pain relief. The chart below compares equianalgesic doses (oral and parenteral) for adults and children who weigh 50 kg (110 lb) or more.

OPIOID	ORAL DOSE	PARENTERAL DOSE
codeine	200 mg (not recommended)	120 to 130 mg
hydrocodone	30 mg	Not applicable
hydromorphone	7.5 mg	1.5 mg
levorphanol	4 mg	2 mg
meperidine	300 mg	75 to 100 mg
morphine (around-the-clock dosing)	30 mg	10 mg
morphine (single or intermittent dosing)	60 mg	10 mg
oxycodone	30 mg	Not applicable

Abbreviations

The following abbreviations, which are common to nursing practice, may be used throughout the text.

ABG	arterial blood gas	H_2	histamine$_2$
ACE	angiotensin-converting enzyme	HDL	high-density lipoprotein
ADH	antidiuretic hormone	HEME	hematologic
AIDS	acquired immunodeficiency syndrome	HIV	human immunodeficiency virus
		HMG-CoA	hydroxymethylglutaryl-coenzyme A
ALT	alanine aminotransferase	HPV	human papilloma virus
ANA	antinuclear antibodies	hr	hour
APTT	activated partial thromboplastin time	HSV	herpes simplex virus
		HZV	herpes zoster virus
AST	aspartate aminotransferase	ICP	intracranial pressure
ATP	adenosine triphosphate	I.D.	intradermal
AV	atrioventricular	IgA	immunoglobulin A
BUN	blood urea nitrogen	IgE	immunoglobulin E
°C	degrees Celsius	I.M.	intramuscular
cAMP	cyclic adenosine monophosphate	INR	international normalized ratio
(CAN)	Canadian drug trade name	I.V.	intravenous
cap	capsule	IVPB	intravenous piggyback
CBC	complete blood count	kg	kilogram
cGMP	cyclic guanosine monophosphate	KIU	kallikrein inactivator units
CK	creatine kinase	L	liter
Cl	chloride	LA	long-acting
cm	centimeter	lb	pound
CMV	cytomegalovirus	LD	lactate dehydrogenase
CNS	central nervous system	LDL	low-density lipoprotein
COPD	chronic obstructive pulmonary disease	LOC	level of consciousness
		LR	lactated Ringer's solution
CSF	cerebrospinal fluid	M	molar
CV	cardiovascular	m^2	square meter
CVA	cerebrovascular accident	MAO	monoamine oxidase
D$_5$LR	dextrose 5% in lactated Ringer's solution	mcg	microgram
		mEq	milliequivalent
D$_5$NS	dextrose 5% in normal saline solution	mg	milligram
		MI	myocardial infarction
D$_5$/0.2NS	dextrose 5% in quarter-normal saline solution	min	minute
		ml	milliliter
D$_5$/0.45NS	dextrose 5% in half-normal saline solution	mm	millimeter
		mm^3	cubic millimeter
D$_5$W	dextrose 5% in water	mmol	millimole
D$_{10}$W	dextrose 10% in water	mo	month
D$_{50}$W	dextrose 50% in water	MS	musculoskeletal
dl	deciliter	msec	millisecond
DNA	deoxyribonucleic acid	Na	sodium
DS	double-strength	NaCl	sodium chloride
EC	enteric-coated	NG	nasogastric
ECG	electrocardiogram	ng	nanogram
EEG	electroencephalogram	NPH	human isophane insulin
EENT	eyes, ears, nose, and throat	NPO	nothing by mouth
ENDO	endocrine	NS	normal saline solution
E.R.	extended release	0.225NS	quarter-normal saline (0.225%) solution
°F	degrees Fahrenheit		
FDA	Food and Drug Administration	0.45NS	half-normal saline (0.45%) solution
g	gram	NSAID	nonsteroidal anti-inflammatory drug
GABA	gamma aminobutyric acid		
GFR	glomerular filtration rate	NYHA	New York Heart Association
GI	gastrointestinal	OTC	over the counter
gtt	drop	oz	ounce
GU	genitourinary	PCA	patient-controlled analgesia
H$_1$	histamine$_1$	P.O.	by mouth

P.R.	by rectum		S.L.	sublingual
PSVT	paroxysmal supraventricular tachycardia		S.R.	sustained-release
			stat	immediately
PT	prothrombin time		SubQ	subcutaneous
PTCA	percutaneous transluminal coronary angioplasty		supp	suppository
			tab	tablet
PTT	partial thromboplastin time		T_3	triiodothyronine
PVC	premature ventricular contraction		T_4	thyroxine
RBC	red blood cell		USP	United States Pharmacopeia
REM	rapid eye movement		UTI	urinary tract infection
RESP	respiratory		VLDL	very-low-density lipoprotein
RNA	ribonucleic acid		WBC	white blood cell
RSV	respiratory syncytial virus		WK, wk	week
SA	sinoatrial			
sec	second			

- Generic and alternate names: lowercase initial letter
- Trade names: uppercase initial letter
- Tables: *t* after page number

E

K

L

M

U

V

W

X

Y

Z